ABNORMAL LABORATORY FINDINGS (continued)
Robert M. DuFort

Malassimilation
  Malabsorption
  Maldigestion
Lymphangiectasia
Starvation
Liver Failure
Hypoadrenocorticism

Cholinesterase
  Decreased
Organophosphates
Carbamates

Cobalamin (B₁₂)
  Decreased
Bacterial Overgrowth

Creatinine
  Increased
Azotemia
  Prerenal
  Renal
  Postrenal
  Decreased
Decreased Muscle Mass

Creatine Kinase (CK)
  Increased
Muscle Inflammation
  Immune Mediated
  Eosinophilic Myositis
  Masticatory Muscle Myositis
  Endocarditis
  Infectious
    Toxoplasmosis
    Neosporum caninum
Nutritional
  Hypokalemia
    (Polymyopathy)
  Taurine Deficiency
Trauma
Exertional Myositis
Surgical
Intramuscular Injections
Hypothermia
Pyrexia
Prolonged Recumbency
Postinfarct Ischemia
  Cardiomyopathy
  Disseminated Intravascular
    Coagulation

Fibrinogen
  Increased
Inflammation
Pregnancy
  Decreased
Liver Failure
Coagulopathies
Primary Hypofibrinogenemia

Folate
  Increased
Bacterial Overgrowth

Fructosamine
  Increased
Diabetes Mellitus
  Decreased
Spurious
Hypoproteinemia
Anemia (False)

**Gamma Glutamyltransferase
(GGT)**
  Increased
Cholestasis
  Intrahepatic
  Extrahepatic
Drugs (Canine)
  Glucocorticoids
Anticonvulsants
  Primadone
  Phenobarbital
  Decreased
Spurious
Hemolysis

Globulin
  Increased
Dehydration (Albumin and Total
  Protein)

Inflammation
Gammopathy
  Monoclonal
    Plasma Cell Myeloma
    Ehrlichia
    Dirofilariasis
  Polyclonal
    Chronic Inflammatory
      Disease
    Feline Infectious Peritonitis
    Dental Disease
    Dermatitis
    Inflammatory Bowel Disease
    Parasitic Diseases
    Immune-Mediated Diseases
    Neoplasia
  Decreased
Neonatal
Immunodeficiency
  Congenital
  Acquired
Blood Loss
Protein-Losing Enteropathy

Glucose
  Increased
Endocrine
  Acromegaly
  Diabetes Mellitus
  Hyperadrenocorticism
Stress (Cats)
Drugs
  Intravenous Glucose
    Administration
  Glucocorticoids
  Xylazine
  Progestagens (Ovaban and
    Others)
  Decreased
Liver Failure
Endocrine
  Hypoadrenocorticism
  Hypopituitarism
Starvation
Neoplasia
Hyperinsulinism
  Iatrogenic
  Insulinoma
  Idiopathic
    Puppies
    Toy Breed Dogs
Septicemia
Polycythemia
Leukemia
Glycogen Storage Disease
Artifact
  Delayed Serum Separation

Iron
  Increased
Hemolysis
  Decreased
Chronic Blood Loss
Dietary Deficiency

Lactate Dehydrogenase (LDH)
  Increased
Organ/Tissue Damage
Hemolysis
  In Vivo
  In Vitro
Hepatocytes
Muscle
Kidney
Spurious
  Failure to Separate Serum from
    RBCs

Lipase
  Increased
Pancreatic Disease
  Pancreatitis
  Necrosis
  Neoplasia
Enteritis
Renal Disease
Glucocorticoids

Magnesium
  Decreased
Dietary
Diabetic Ketacidosis

Potential Causes:
  Gastrointestinal
    Malabsorption
    Chronic Diarrhea
  Renal
    Glomerular Disease
    Tubular Disease
  Drugs
    Diuretics
    Amphotericin B
  Others

Phosphorus
  Increased
Reduced GFR
  Renal
    Acute
    Chronic
  Postrenal
Hemolysis
Hyperthyroidism
Neonates
Intoxication
  Hypervitaminosis D
  Jasmine Ingestion
Dietary Excess
Iatrogenic
  Phosphate Enemas
  Intravenous Phosphate
    Administration
Osteolysis
Hypoparathyroidism
Spurious
  Delayed Serum Separation
  Decreased
Hyperparathyroidism
  Primary
  Nutritional Secondary
Neoplasia
  PTH-Like Hormone
  C-Cell Thyroid Tumors
Insulin Therapy
Diabetic Ketoacidosis
Dietary Deficiency
Eclampsia
Hyperadrenocorticism

Potassium
  Increased
Renal Failure
  Distal RTA
  Oliguric/Anuric
Postrenal
  Obstruction
  Ruptured Bladder
Spurious
  Breed Idiosyncrasy (Akitas)
  Leukemias
  Thrombocytosis
  Collection in Potassium
    Heparin
  Collection in Potassium EDTA
Hypoadrenocorticism
Acidosis
  Diabetic Ketoacidosis
Diffuse Tissue Damage
  Massive Muscle Trauma
  Postischemic Reperfusion
Dehydration
Hypoaldosterone
Drugs
  Propranolol
  Potassium-Sparing
    Diuretics
  ACE Inhibitors
  Decreased
Alkalosis
Dietary Deficiency (Feline)
Potassium-Free Fluids
Bicarbonate Administration
Drugs
  Penicillins
  Amphotericin B
  Loop Diuretics
GI Fluid Loss (K⁺-Rich)
Hyperadrenocorticism
Hyperaldosterone
Insulin Therapy
Renal
  Postobstructive Diuresis
  Renal Tubular Acidosis
  Dialysis

Hypokalemic Periodic
  Paralysis
  Burmese
  Pit Bull
Renal Failure
  Chronic Polyuria

Protein, Total
  Increased
Dehydration (Albumin and
  Globulin)
Hyperglobulinemia
Spurious
  Hemolysis
  Lipemia
  Decreased
Hemorrhage
External Plasma Loss
GI Loss
Overhydration
Liver Failure
Glomerular Loss

Sodium
  Increased
Hyperaldosterone
GI Fluid Loss (Na⁺-Poor)
  Vomiting
  Diarrhea
Diabetes Insipidus
Renal Failure
Dehydration
Insensible Fluid Loss
  Fever
  Panting
  High Ambient Temperature
Decreased Water Intake
  Limited Water Access
  Primary Adipsia
Increased Salt Intake
  Intravenous
  Oral
Spurious
  Serum Evaporation
  Decreased
Hypoadrenocorticism
Diabetes Mellitus
GI Fluid Loss (Na⁺-Rich)
  Vomiting
  Diarrhea
Hookworms
Burns
Chronic Effusions
Excess ADH
Diuretics
Hypotonic Fluids
Diet (Severe Sodium Restriction)
Psychogenic Polydipsia
Renal Failure (Polyuric)
Spurious
  Hyperlipidemia

Thyroxine (T₄)
  Increased
Hyperthyroidism
Anti-T₄ Autoantibodies
  Decreased
Hypothyroidism
Nonthyroid Illness
Drugs
  Corticosteroids
  Phenobarbital

Triiodothyronine (T₃)
  Increased
Hyperthyroidism
Anti-T₃ Autoantibodies
  Decreased
Hypothyroidism

**Trypsinogen-Like Immunoreactivity
(TLI)**
  Increased
Pancreatitis
Postprandial
  Decreased
Pancreatic Exocrine Insufficiency

Expert CONSULT

Activate your access at expertconsult.com

① REGISTER

- Visit **expertconsult.com**.
- Click **"Register Now."**
- Fill in your **user information.**
- Click **"Create Account."**

② ACTIVATE YOUR BOOK

- Scratch off your **Activation Code** below and enter it into the **"Add a title"** box.
- **You're done!** Click on the book's title under **"My Titles."**

For technical assistance, email **online.help@elsevier.com** or call **800-401-9962** (inside the US) or **+1-314-995-3200** (outside the US).

Scratch off Below
Ettinger / Feldman

ZNGEEWZ

Activation Code

TEXTBOOK OF
VETERINARY INTERNAL MEDICINE
DISEASES OF THE DOG AND THE CAT
SEVENTH EDITION

VOLUME 1

STEPHEN J. ETTINGER, DVM

Pet DRx Corporation
California Animal Hospital Veterinary Specialty Group
Los Angeles, California

EDWARD C. FELDMAN, DVM

School of Veterinary Medicine
University of California
Davis, California

SAUNDERS

ELSEVIER

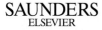

3251 Riverport Lane
St. Louis, Missouri 63043

TEXTBOOK OF VETERINARY INTERNAL MEDICINE, Two-volume set: 978-1-4160-6593-7
SEVENTH EDITION   Volume 1: 9996062775
                                                       Volume 2: 999606283X

Copyright © 2010, 2005, 2000, 1995, 1989, 1983, 1975 by Saunders, an imprint of Elsevier Inc.

"Biomarkers and Omics" by N. Emenaker and J. Kagan is in the Public Domain.

All rights reserved. No part of this publication may be reproduced or transmitted in any form or by any means, electronic or mechanical, including photocopying, recording, or any information storage and retrieval system, without permission in writing from the publisher. Permissions may be sought directly from Elsevier's Rights Department: phone: (+1) 215 239 3804 (US) or (+44) 1865 843830 (UK); fax: (+44) 1865 853333; e-mail: healthpermissions@elsevier.com. You may also complete your request on-line via the Elsevier website at http://www.elsevier.com/permissions.

Notice

Knowledge and best practice in this field are constantly changing. As new research and experience broaden our knowledge, changes in practice, treatment and drug therapy may become necessary or appropriate. Readers are advised to check the most current information provided (i) on procedures featured or (ii) by the manufacturer of each product to be administered, to verify the recommended dose or formula, the method and duration of administration, and contraindications. It is the responsibility of the practitioner, relying on their own experience and knowledge of the patient, to make diagnoses, to determine dosages and the best treatment for each individual patient, and to take all appropriate safety precautions. To the fullest extent of the law, neither the Publisher nor the Editors assume any liability for any injury and/or damage to persons or property arising out of or related to any use of the material contained in this book.

The Publisher

Library of Congress Cataloging-in-Publication Data

Textbook of veterinary internal medicine : diseases of the dog and the cat / [edited by] Stephen J. Ettinger, Edward C. Feldman. – 7th ed.
    p. ; cm.
    Includes bibliographical references and index.
    ISBN-13: 978-1-4160-6593-7 (set, hardcover : alk. paper)
    ISBN-13: 978-9996062773 (v. 1)
    ISBN-10: 9996062775 (v. 1)
    ISBN-13: 978-9996962837 (v. 2)
    [etc.]
1. Dogs–Diseases. 2. Cats–Diseases. 3. Veterinary internal medicine. I. Ettinger, Stephen J.
II. Feldman, Edward C. III. Title:
Diseases of the dog and cat.
    [DNLM: 1. Dog Diseases–diagnosis. 2. Dog Diseases–therapy. 3. Cat Diseases–diagnosis.
4. Cat Diseases–therapy. SF 991 T355 2010]
    SF991.T48 2010
    636.7'0896–dc22
                                                            2009030709

Vice President and Publisher: Linda Duncan
Publisher: Penny Rudolph
Associate Developmental Editor: Lauren Harms
Publishing Services Manager: Patricia Tannian
Senior Project Manager: Kristine Feeherty
Design Direction: Charlie Seibel
Cover Art: Tate Museum of London
Back Cover Art: Tyne & Wear Museums, Laing Art Gallery, Newcastle

Printed in Canada

Last digit is the print number: 9 8 7 6 5 4 3 2 1

Working together to grow
libraries in developing countries

www.elsevier.com | www.bookaid.org | www.sabre.org

ELSEVIER   BOOK AID International   Sabre Foundation

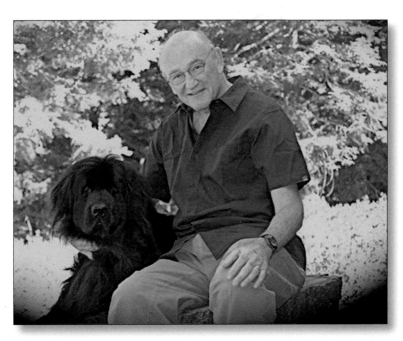

**Stephen J. Ettinger, DVM, DACVIM
(Internal Medicine and Cardiology)**

California Animal Hospital Veterinary Specialty Group
Los Angeles, California

*The Physical Examination of the Dog and Cat
Clinical Problem Solving: The Steps That Follow the History
and Physical Examination
Euthanasia
Diseases of the Trachea and Upper Airways
Biomarkers of Cardiovascular Disease
Guidelines for the Diagnosis and Treatment of Canine Chronic
Valvular Heart Disease
Therapy of Arrhythmias*

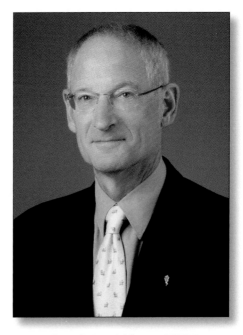

**Edward C. Feldman, DVM,
DACVIM
(Internal Medicine)**

Professor of Small Animal Internal
Medicine
Chairman, VM: Medicine & Epidemiology
School of Veterinary Medicine
University of California
Davis, California

*Polyuria and Polydipsia
Electrolyte Disorders: Potassium (Hyper/
Hypokalemia)
Disorders of the Parathyroid Glands
Ovarian and Estrous Cycle Abnormalities*

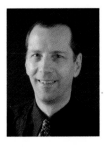

Anthony Abrams-Ogg, DVM, DACVIM (SAIM)
Associate Professor
Department of Clinical Studies
Ontario Veterinary College
University of Guelph
Guelph, Ontario, Canada
Nonregenerative Anemia

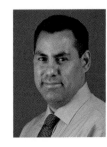

Ale Aguirre, DVM, DACVIM
Chief of Internal Medicine
VETMED Consultants
Phoenix, Arizona
*Diseases of the Gallbladder and
Extrahepatic Biliary System*

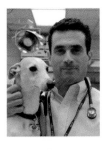

Mark J. Acierno, MBA, DVM, DACVIM
Associate Professor
Department of Veterinary Clinical
Science
Louisiana State University
Baton Rouge, Louisiana
*Micturition Disorders and Urinary
Incontinence*
Rhinoscopy, Nasal Flushing, and Biopsy
Continuous Renal Replacement Therapy

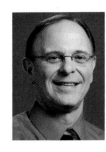

A. Rick Alleman, DVM, PhD, DABVP, DACVP
Professor
Department of Physiological Sciences
College of Veterinary Medicine
University of Florida
Gainesville, Florida
Cytology of Internal Organs

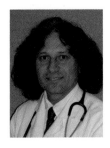

P. Filippo Adamo, DVM, DECVN
Section Chief, Neurology/
Neurosurgery
Bay Area Veterinary Specialists
San Leandro, California
*Cerebrospinal Fluid Collection,
Myelography, Epidurography, and
Discography*

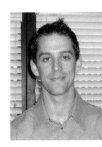

Justin Allen, DVM
Cardiology Resident
California Animal Hospital Veterinary
Specialty Group
Los Angeles, California
Cyanosis

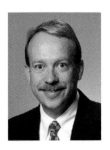

Larry G. Adams, DVM
Professor, Small Animal Internal
Medicine
Purdue University
West Lafayette, Indiana
*Canine Ureteral and Lower Urinary
Tract Diseases*

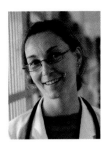

Karin Allenspach, DVM, FVH, PhD, DECVIM-CA, FHEA, MRCVS
Senior Lecturer in Small Animal
Internal Medicine
The Royal Veterinary College
Department of Veterinary Clinical
Sciences
University of London
North Mymms, Hatfield, United
Kingdom
Diseases of the Large Intestine

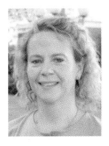

Verena K. Affolter, DVM, PhD, DECVP
Associate Professor of Clinical
Dermatopathology
Department of Pathology,
Microbiology, Immunology
University of California
Davis, California
Canine and Feline Histiocytic Diseases

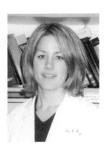

Kelly Anderson-Wessberg, DVM, DACVIM (Cardiology)
Veterinary Specialty Center
Buffalo Grove, Illinois
Coughing

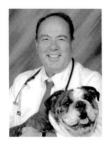

James M.G. Anthony, BSc (Agr.), DVM, MRCVS, FAUD, DAVDC, DEVDC, PAg
Associate Professor, Veterinary Dentistry and Oral Surgery
Department of Small Animal Clinical Sciences
Western College of Veterinary Medicine
University of Saskatchewan
Saskatoon, Saskatchewan
Head, Dentistry and Oral Surgery
Department of Dentistry
VCA All-Care Animal Referral Center
Fountain Valley, California
Tumors of the Mouth, Head, and Neck

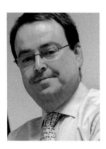

David J. Argyle, BVMS, PhD, DECVIM-CA (Oncology), MRCVS
William Dick Professor of Clinical Studies
Royal (Dick) School of Veterinary Studies
The University of Edinburgh Hospital for Small Animals
Edinburgh, Scotland, United Kingdom
Gene Therapy
Diseases of the Spleen

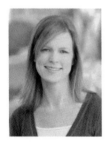

Katharine Arnell, DVM
Internal Medicine Resident
Department of Internal Medicine
Veterinary Specialty Hospital of San Diego
San Diego, California
Hepatic Biopsy Techniques

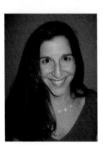

Lillian R. Aronson, DVM, DACVS
Associate Professor of Surgery
School of Veterinary Medicine
University of Pennsylvania
Philadelphia, Pennsylvania
Renal Transplantation

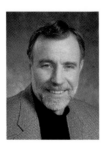

Clarke Atkins, DVM, DACVIM (Internal Medicine & Cardiology)
Jane Lewis Seaks Distinguished Professor of Companion Animal Medicine
College of Veterinary Medicine
North Caroline State University
Raleigh, North Carolina
Heartworm Disease

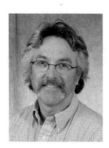

Rodney S. Bagley, DVM
Professor, Neurology and Neurosurgery
Department of Clinical Sciences
College of Veterinary Medicine
Washington State University
Pullman, Washington
Neurophysiology

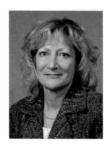

Claudia J. Baldwin, DVM, MS, DACVIM
Associate Professor
Department of Veterinary Clinical Sciences
College of Veterinary Medicine
Iowa State University
Ames, Iowa
Vaginal-Vulvar and Preputial Discharge

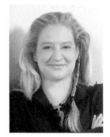

Kirstie A. Barrett, DVM, DACVIM (Cardiology)
Cardiology Department
California Animal Hospital Veterinary Specialty Group
Los Angeles, California
Cardiac Emergencies
Bronchodilators

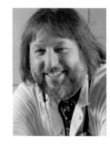

Joseph W. Bartges, DVM, PhD, DACVIM, DACVN
Professor of Medicine and Nutrition
Acree Endowed Chair of Small Animal Research
Department of Small Animal Clinical Sciences
College of Veterinary Medicine
The University of Tennessee
Knoxville, Tennessee
Hematuria and Other Conditions Causing Discolored Urine
Nutritional Management of Renal Conditions
Urinary Tract Infections

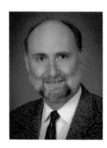

John E. Bauer, DVM, PhD, DACVN
Professor and Mark L. Morris Professor of Clinical Nutrition
College of Veterinary Medicine and Biomedical Sciences
Texas A&M University
College Station, Texas
Antioxidants, Nutraceuticals, and Dietary Supplements

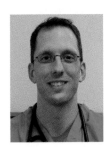

Matthew W. Beal, DVM, DACVECC
Associate Professor
Emergency & Critical Care Medicine
Department of Small Animal Clinical
  Sciences
College of Veterinary Medicine
Michigan State University
East Lansing, Michigan
Thoracic Trauma

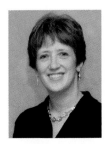

**Ellen N. Behrend, VMD, PhD,
  DACVIM**
Professor
Department of Clinical Sciences
Auburn University
Auburn, Alabama
Polyphagia

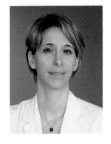

**Marie-Claude Bélanger, DMV, MS,
  DACVIM**
Associate Professor
Department of Clinical Sciences
University of Montreal
Montreal, Quebec, Canada
Innocent Heart Murmurs
Echocardiography

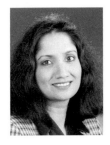

Neeli Bendapudi, PhD
Associate Professor, Marketing
Fisher College of Business
The Ohio State University
Columbus, Ohio
Clueing in Customers

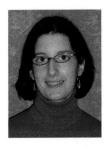

**Noemi Benitah, DVM, DACVIM
  (SAIM)**
Staff Internist
Department of Small Animal Internal
  Medicine
Red Bank Veterinary Hospital
Tinton Falls, New Jersey
*Electrolyte Disorders: Sodium (Hyper/
  Hyponatremia)*

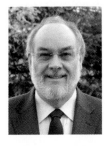

**David Bennett, BSc, BVetMed, PhD,
  DVM, DSAO, FHEA, MRCVS**
Professor
University of Glasgow
Glasgow, Scotland, United Kingdom
Immune-Mediated and Infective Arthritis
Canine and Feline Osteoarthritis

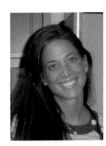

Allyson C. Berent, DVM, DACVIM
Staff Veterinarian: Interventional
  Radiology/Medicine
Director of Interventional Endoscopy
The Animal Medical Center
New York, New York
Tracheal Stenting in Collapsed Trachea
Hepatic Vascular Anomalies

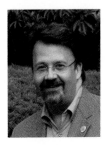

**Philip J. Bergman, DVM, DACVIM
  (Oncology)**
Chief Medical Officer
BrightHeart Veterinary Centers
Armonk, New York
Cancer Vaccines and Immunotherapy
Hemangiosarcoma

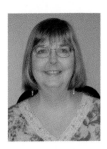

Deborah C. Bernreuter, DVM, MS
Veterinary Clinical Pathologist
IDEXX Laboratories, Inc.
Irvine, California
*Cytology of the Skin and Subcutaneous
  Tissues*

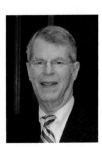

Leonard L. Berry, PhD
Presidential Professor for Teaching
  Excellence
Distinguished Professor of Marketing
M.B. Zale Chair in Retailing and
  Marketing Leadership
Mays Business School
Professor of Humanities in Medicine
College of Medicine Health Science
  Center
Texas A&M University
College Station, Texas
Clueing in Customers

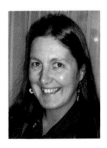

**Sonya V. Bettenay, BVSc (Hons),
  DEd, FACVSc, DECVD**
Dermatologie Department
Fachklinik Haas & Link
Industrie Str. 6
Germering, Germany
Skin Scrapings and Skin Biopsies

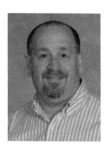

David S. Biller, DVM, DACVR
Professor
Department of Clinical Sciences
College of Veterinary Medicine
Kansas State University
Manhattan, Kansas
Mediastinal Disease

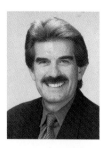

Byron L. Blagburn, MS, PhD
Distinguished University Professor
Department of Pathobiology
College of Veterinary Medicine
Auburn University
Auburn, Alabama
Fecal Examination

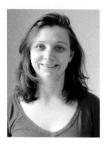

Amanda K. Boag, MA, VetMB, DACVIM, DACVECC, FHEA, MRCVS
Lecturer in Emergency and Critical Care
Department of Veterinary Clinical Science
The Royal Veterinary College
North Mymms
Hatfield, Hertfordshire, United Kingdom
Nosocomial Infection and Resistant Bacteria

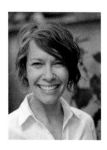

Elise Mittleman Boller, DVM, DACVECC
Matthew J. Ryan Veterinary Hospital
University of Pennsylvania
Philadelphia, Pennsylvania
Shock

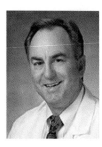

John D. Bonagura, DVM, MS, DACVIM
Professor and Head of Clinical Cardiology Services
Department of Veterinary Clinical Sciences
College of Veterinary Medicine
The Ohio State University
Columbus, Ohio
Congenital Heart Disease

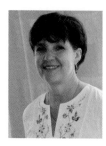

Dawn M. Boothe, DVM, PhD, DACVIM (Internal Medicine), ACVCP
Professor
Department of Anatomy, Physiology & Pharmacology
Department of Clinical Sciences
Director, Clinical Pharmacology
College of Veterinary Medicine
Auburn University
Auburn, Alabama
Antifungal Drug Therapy

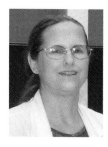

Mary H. Bowles, DVM, DACVIM
Associate Professor
Veterinary Clinical Sciences
Oklahoma State University
Stillwater, Oklahoma
Unblocking the Urethra of the Male Cat
Probiotics

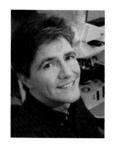

Mathew Breen, DVM, PhD
Professor
College of Veterinary Medicine
North Carolina State University
Raleigh, North Carolina
Clinical Genomics

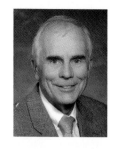

Edward B. Breitschwerdt, DVM, DACVIM
Professor of Medicine and Infectious Disease
Department of Clinical Sciences
North Carolina State University
Raleigh, North Carolina
Canine Bartonella

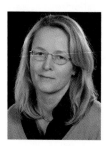

Catharina Brömel, DVM, DACVIM (SAIM)
School of Veterinary Medicine
University of California
Davis, California
Buccal Mucosal Bleeding Time

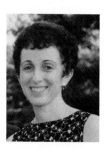

Marjory B. Brooks, DVM, DACVIM
Department of Population Medicine & Diagnostic Sciences
Associate Director, Comparative Coagulation Section
Animal Health Diagnostic Center
Ithaca, New York
Immune-Mediated Thrombocytopenia, von Willebrand Disease, and Platelet Disorders

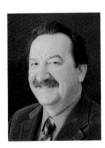

Claudio Brovida, DVM
ANUBI Ospedale per Animali da
  Compagnia
Moncalieri, Italy
*World Small Animal Veterinary
  Association (WSAVA) Guidelines*

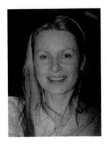

**Narelle Lila Brown, BVSc (Hons),
  BSc, MACVS, MVS**
Animal Referral Hospital
Department of Small Animal Medicine
South Strathfield
New South Wales
Australia
Sneezing and Nasal Discharge

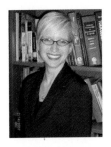

Ahna G. Brutlag, DVM
Assistant Director of Veterinary
  Services
SafetyCall International and Pet Poison
  Helpline
Bloomington, Minnesota
*Topical Toxins
Chemical Toxicities*

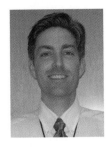

C.A. Tony Buffington, DVM
Professor of Veterinary Clinical
  Sciences
Adjunct Professor of Urology
The Ohio State University Veterinary
  Hospital
Columbus, Ohio
Lower Urinary Tract Disorders in Cats

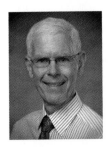

**Barret J. Bulmer, DVM, MS,
  DACVIM (Cardiology)**
Associate Professor
Department of Clinical Sciences
Oregon State University
Corvallis, Oregon
*Angiotensin Converting Enzyme
  Inhibitors and Vasodilators*

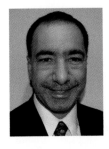

**William Burkholder, DVM, PhD,
  DACVN**
Center for Veterinary Medicine
Division of Animal Feeds
Food and Drug Administration/Center
  for Veterinary Medicine
Rockville, Maryland
Food Safety and Toxicities

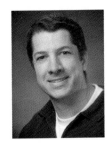

**Patrick M. Burns, BVSc, MACVSc,
  DACVA**
Clinical Instructor
Veterinary Clinical Sciences
The Ohio State University
Columbus, Ohio
Post Professional Researcher
College of Medicine
Dorothy M. Davis Heart and Lung
  Research Institute
Columbus, Ohio
Venomous Bites and Stings

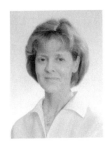

Mary Beth Callan, VMD, DACVIM
Associate Professor of Medicine
Department of Clinical Studies
School of Veterinary Medicine
University of Pennsylvania
Philadelphia, Pennsylvania
Petechiae and Ecchymoses

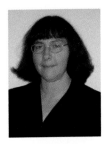

**Karen L. Campbell, DVM, MS,
  DACVIM, DACVD**
Professor and Section Head, Specialty
  Medicine
Department of Veterinary Clinical
  Medicine
University of Illinois
Urbana, Illinois
*Changes in Pigmentation
Other External Parasites*

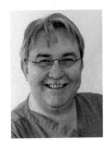

**Didier-Noël Carlotti, Doct-Vét, Dip
  ECVDAquivet**
Clinique Vétérinaire, Parc d'Activités
Mermoz Eysines
Bordeaux, France
*Cutaneous and Subcutaneous Lumps,
  Bumps, and Masses
Genital Dermatoses
Management of Canine Atopy*

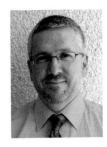

Anthony P. Carr, VMD
Professor
Department of Small Animal Clinical
  Sciences
Western College of Veterinary
  Medicine
Saskatoon, Saskatchewan, Canada
Treatment of Hypertension

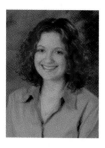

Valerie L. Case, DVM
Resident
Department of Internal Medicine
California Animal Hospital Veterinary
  Specialty Group
Los Angeles, California
Melena and Hematochezia

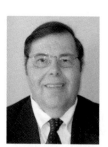

James L. Catalfamo, MS, PhD
Department of Population Medicine
  and Diagnostic Sciences
College of Veterinary Medicine
Cornell University
Ithaca, New York
*Immune-Mediated Thrombocytopenia,
  von Willebrand Disease, and Platelet
  Disorders*

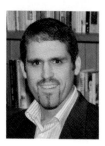

**Nick Cave, BVSc, MVSc, MACVSc,
  DipACVN**
Senior Lecturer in Small Animal
  Medicine and Nutrition
Institute of Veterinary, Animal and
  Biomedical Sciences
Te Kunenga Ki Pūrehuroa
Massey University
Private Bag
Palmerston North, New Zealand
Immunology and Nutrition

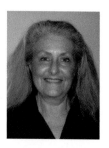

Sharon A. Center, DVM, DACVIM
College of Veterinary Medicine
Cornell University
Ithaca, New York
*Toxic, Metabolic, Infectious, and
  Neoplastic Liver Diseases*

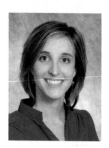

**Sofia Cerda-Gonzalez, DVM,
  DACVIM (Neurology)**
Assistant Professor
Department of Clinical Sciences
College of Veterinary Medicine
Cornell University
Ithaca, New York
Disorders of Skeletal Muscles

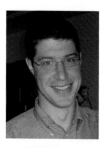

Greg Chambers, DVM
Akron Veterinary Internal Medicine
  Practice
Metropolitan Veterinary Hospital
Akron, Ohio
*Abdominal Distension, Ascites, and
  Peritonitis*

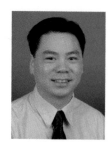

**Daniel L. Chan, DVM, DACVECC,
  DACVN, MRCVS**
Lecturer in Emergency and Critical
  Care
Department of Veterinary Clinical
  Sciences
The Royal Veterinary College
North Mymms
Hatfield, Hertfordshire, United
  Kingdom
Parenteral Nutritional Support

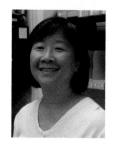

**Ruthanne Chun, DVM, DACVIM
  (Oncology)**
Clinical Associate Professor
Medical Sciences
School of Veterinary Medicine
University of Wisconsin
Madison, Wisconsin
*Urogenital and Mammary Gland
  Tumors*

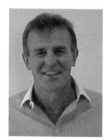

**David Buchanan Church, BVSc, PhD,
  MACVSC, MRCVS**
Professor of Small Animal Studies
Department of Veterinary Clinical
  Sciences
The Royal Veterinary College
North Mymms
Hatfield, Hertfordshire, United
  Kingdom
*Electrolyte Disorders: Potassium (Hyper/
  Hypokalemia)*

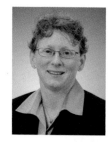

**Joan R. Coates, BS, DVM, MS,
  DACVIM (Neurology)**
Associate Professor, Department of
  Veterinary Medicine and Surgery
Neurology & Neurosurgery Service
  Leader, Department of Neurology &
  Neurosurgery
Veterinary Medical Teaching Hospital
University of Missouri
Columbia, Missouri
Brain Disease

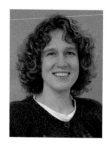

**Leah A. Cohn, DVM, PhD, DACVIM
  (SAIM)**
Professor of Veterinary Medicine
Department of Veterinary Medicine
  and Surgery
Veterinary Medical Teaching Hospital
University of Missouri
Columbia, Missouri
*Glucocorticoid Therapy
Pulmonary Parenchymal Disease*

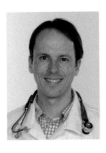

Etienne Côté, DVM, DACVIM (Cardiology, SAIM)
Assistant Professor
Department of Companion Animals
Atlantic Veterinary College
University of Prince Edward Island
Charlottetown, Prince Edward Island,
 Canada
Innocent Heart Murmurs
Electrocardiography and Cardiac
 Arrhythmias

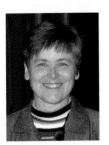

Melanie Craven, DVM
College of Veterinary Medicine
Cornell University
Ithaca, New York
Rectoanal Disease

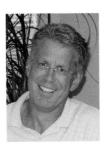

P. Cynda Crawford, DVM, PhD
Maddie's Shelter Medicine Program
Department of Small Animal Clinical
 Sciences
College of Veterinary Medicine
University of Florida
Gainesville, Florida
Feline Immunodeficiency Virus
Feline Leukemia Virus
Canine Viral Diseases

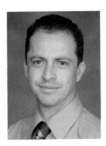

Paul A. Cuddon, BVSc (Hons), DACVIM (Neurology)
Associate Professor
Department of Clinical Sciences
Colorado State University
Fort Collins, Colorado
Electromyography and Nerve Conduction
 Velocity Studies

Ronaldo Casimiro da Costa, DMV, MSc, PhD, DACVIM (Neurology)
Assistant Professor and Service Head,
 Neurology and Neurosurgery
Department of Veterinary Clinical
 Sciences
College of Veterinary Medicine
The Ohio State University
Columbus, Ohio
Ataxia, Paresis, and Paralysis

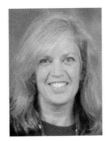

Autumn P. Davidson, DVM, MS, DACVIM (Internal Medicine)
Clinical Professor
Department of Medicine and
 Epidemiology
School of Veterinary Medicine
University of California
Davis, California
Staff Internist
Department of Medicine
VCA Animal Care Center of Sonoma
Rohnert Park, California
Transcervical Catheterization in the
 Bitch
Coccidioidomycosis
Aspergillosis
Ovarian and Estrous Cycle
 Abnormalities

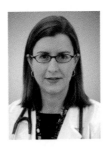

Harold Davis, BA, RVT, VTS (Emergency and Critical Care)
Manager, Emergency and Critical Care
 Service
Veterinary Medical Teaching Hospital
University of California
Davis, California
Venous and Arterial Puncture

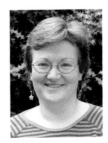

Susan Dawson, DVM, PhD, BVMS
Faculty of Veterinary Science
University of Liverpool
Leahurst, Neston Wirral Cheshire,
 United Kingdom
Other Feline Viral Diseases

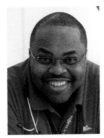

Amy DeClue, DVM, MS, DACVIM
Assistant Professor
College of Veterinary Medicine
University of Missouri
Columbia, Missouri
Sepsis and the Systemic Inflammatory
 Response Syndrome

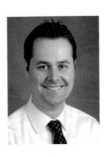

Sean J. Delaney, DVM, MS, DACVN
Sr. Executive Vice President, Chief
 Nutrition Officer
Natura Pet Products, Inc.
Davis, California
Nutritional Management of Endocrine
 Disease
Home-Prepared and Raw Diets

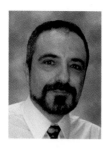

Helio Autran de Morais, DVM, MS, PhD, DACVIM (SAIM and Cardiology)
Associate Professor
Department of Clinical Sciences
Oregon State University College of Veterinary Medicine
Corvallis, Oregon
Diseases of the Spleen

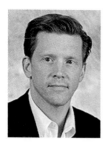

Jennifer J. Devey, DVM, DACVECC
Fox Valley Animal Referral Center
Appleton, Wisconsin
Hyperbaric Medicine
Gastric Lavage
Acute Abdomen
Crystalloid and Colloid Fluid Therapy

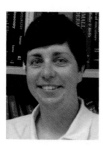

Curtis W. Dewey, DVM, MS, DACVIM (Neurology), DACVS
Associate Professor and Section Chief, Neurology/ Neurosurgery
Department of Clinical Sciences
Cornell University
Ithaca, New York
Inflammatory, Infectious, and Other Multifocal Brain Diseases

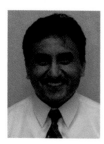

Ravinder S. Dhaliwal, DVM, MS, DACVIM, DABVP
Department of Oncology
PetCare Veterinary Hospital
Santa Rosa, California
Department of Oncology
VCA All Care Animal Referral Center
Fountain Valley, California
Consultant
Antech Diagnostics
Irvine, California
Tumors of the Mouth, Head, and Neck

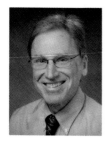

Stephen P. DiBartola, DVM, DACVIM
Professor of Medicine
Department of Veterinary Clinical Sciences
College of Veterinary Medicine
The Ohio State University
Columbus, Ohio
Clinical Approach and Laboratory Evaluation of Renal Disease

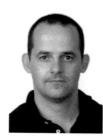

Peter J. Dickinson, DVM
Associate Professor, Chief Neurology/ Neurosurgery
Department of Surgical and Radiological Sciences
School of Veterinary Medicine
University of California
Davis, California
Muscle and Nerve Biopsy
Brain Biopsy

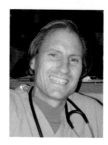

Marianne Diez, DVM, PhD, DECVCN
Associate Professor
Nutrition Unit
Faculty of Veterinary Medicine
University of Liège
Liège, Belgium
Obesity

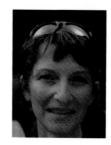

Kenneth J. Drobatz, DVM, MSCE
Professor and Chief Section, Critical Care
Associate Chair, Department of Clinical Studies
School of Veterinary Medicine
Director, Emergency Services
Mathew J. Ryan Veterinary Hospital
University of Pennsylvania
Philadelphia, Pennsylvania
Global Approach to the Trauma Patient
Clinical Evaluation of the Respiratory Tract

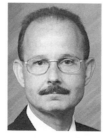

Robert M. DuFort, DVM, DACVIM
IDEXX Laboratories, Inc.
Davis, California
Abnormal Laboratory Findings

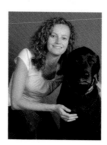

Marilyn E. Dunn, DMV, MVSc, DACVIM
Associate Professor
Department of Clinical Sciences
University of Montreal
St. Hyacinthe, Quebec, Canada
Acquired Coagulopathies

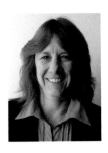

Karen Ehnert, DVM, MPVM, DACVPM
Associate Professor (Adjunct)
Veterinary Medicine
Western University of Health Sciences
Pomona, California
Senior Veterinarian
County of Los Angeles
Department of Public Health
Veterinary Public Health and Rabies
  Control
Los Angeles, California
Zoonotic Disease Problems

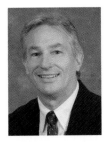

Bruce E. Eilts, DVM, MS, DACT
Professor of Theriogenology
Department of Veterinary Clinical
  Sciences
Louisiana State University
Baton Rouge, Louisiana
*Contraception and Pregnancy
  Termination in the Dog and Cat
Cystic Endometrial Hyperplasia and
  Pyometra*

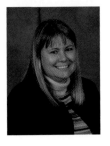

Denise A. Elliott, BVSc (Hons), PhD, DACVIM, DACVN
Health and Nutritional Sciences
  Director
The Americas Royal Canin, SAS
Aimargues, France
*Body Composition of the Dog and Cat
Nutritional Management of the Lower
  Urinary Tract Conditions
Dietary and Medical Considerations in
  Hyperlipidemia*

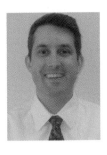

Joshua Elliott, DVM, MA
Columbia River Veterinary Specialists
Vancouver, Washington
Jaundice

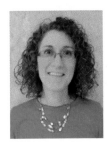

Nancy Emenaker, PhD
Program Director
National Institutes of Health, National
  Cancer Institute
Bethesda, Maryland
Biomarkers and "Omics"

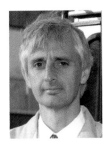

Gary C.W. England, BVetMed, PhD, DVM, DVR, DipVRep, DECAR, DACT, FHEA, FRCVS
Foundation Dean & Professor of
  Comparative Veterinary
  Reproduction
School of Veterinary Medicine &
  Science
University of Nottingham
Loughborough, Leicestershire, United
  Kingdom
*Canine Female Infertility
Care of the Neonate and Fading Pups*

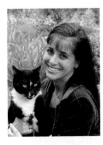

Amara H. Estrada, DVM, DACVIM (Cardiology)
Associate Professor of Cardiology
Department of Small Animal Clinical
  Sciences
University of Florida
Gainesville, Florida
Artificial Pacing of the Heart

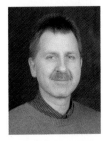

Dominik Faissler, DVM, DECVN
Department of Clinical Sciences
Cummings School of Veterinary
  Medicine at Tufts University
North Grafton, Massachusetts
Tremor Syndromes

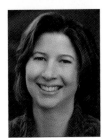

Andrea J. Fascetti, VMD, PhD, DACVIM, ACVN
Professor, Nutrition
Department of Veterinary Medicine
University of California
Davis, California
*Nutrition of Healthy Dogs and Cats in
  Various Adult Stages*

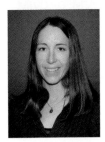

Wendy D. Fife, DVM, MS, DACVR
Veterinary Radiologist
Diagnostic Imaging PC
Boulder, Colorado
*Abdominal Ultrasound: Aspirations and
  Biopsies*

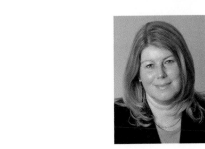

Andrea Fischer, DVM (Habil.), DACVIM (Neurology), DECVN
Center of Clinical Veterinary Medicine
Clinic of Small Animal Medicine
Ludwig Maximilian University of
  Munich
Munich, Germany
*Tetanus
Botulism*

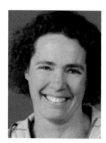

Janet E. Foley, DVM, PhD
Professor
School of Veterinary Medicine
University of California
Davis, California
*Veterinary Diagnosis of Bacterial,
Fungal, and Viral Disease*

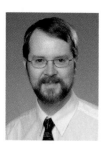

Peter Foley, MSc, DVM, DACVIM
Assistant Professor
Department of Companion Animals
Atlantic Veterinary College
University of Prince Edward Island
Charlottetown, Prince Edward Island,
Canada
*Constipation, Tenesmus, Dyschezia, and
Fecal Incontinence*

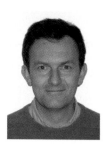

Jacques Fontaine, DVM, DECVD
Consultant in Dermatology
University of Liège
Liège, Belgium
Clinique Vétérinaire
Brussels, Belgium
Papules and Pustules

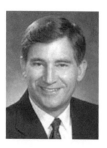

Richard B. Ford, DVM, DACVIM
Professor Emeritus
College of Veterinary Medicine
North Carolina State University
Raleigh, North Carolina
*Companion Animal Vaccines and
Vaccination*

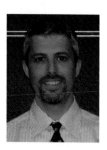

Marnin A. Forman, DVM, DACVIM
Staff Internist
Med Vet, Medical and Cancer Center
for Pets
Worthington, Ohio
Anorexia

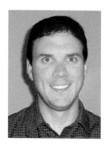

**Scott Forney, DVM, DACVIM
(Cardiology)**
California Animal Hospital Veterinary
Specialty Group
Los Angeles, California
Dyspnea and Tachypnea

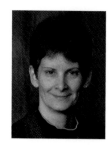

**S. Dru Forrester, DVM, MS,
DACVIM**
Scientific Affairs
Hill's Pet Nutrition, Inc.
Topeka, Kansas
Adjunct Faculty
Department of Clinical Sciences
College of Veterinary Medicine
Kansas State University
Manhattan, Kansas
*Cystocentesis and Urinary Bladder
Catheterization*

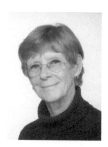

**Catharina Linde Forsberg, DVM,
PhD, DECAR**
Professor
Division of Reproduction
Swedish University of Agricultural
Sciences
Uppsala, Sweden
*Artificial Insemination in the Dog
Abnormalities in Canine Pregnancy,
Parturition, and Periparturient Period*

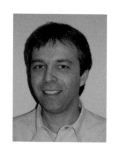

Thierry Francey, DVM, DACVIM
Department of Clinical Veterinary
Medicine
University of Bern
Bern, Switzlerand
Prostatic Diseases

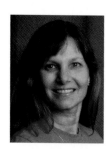

Linda Frank, MS, DVM, DACVD
Professor of Dermatology
Department of Small Animal Clinical
Sciences
University of Tennessee
Knoxville, Tennessee
Alopecia

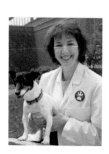

**Lisa M. Freeman, DVM, PhD,
DACVN**
Professor
Department of Clinical Sciences
Tufts Cummings School of Veterinary
Medicine
North Grafton, Massachusetts
Nutritional Modulation of Heart Disease

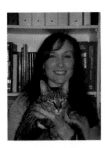

Angela E. Frimberger, BS, VMD
Director
Veterinary Oncology Consultants
Wauchope, Australia
Principles of Chemotherapy

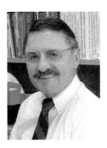

William Gengler, DVM, DAVDC
Associate Dean of Clinical Affairs
Department of Surgical Sciences
School of Veterinary Medicine
University of Wisconsin
Madison, Wisconsin
Gagging

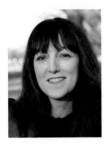

Virginia Luis Fuentes, VetMB, PhD, DVC, MRCVS, DipACVIM, DipECVIM (Cardiology)
Senior Lecturer
Department of Veterinary Clinical Sciences
The Royal Veterinary College
Hatfield, Hertfordshire, United Kingdom
Inotropes: Inodilators

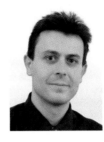

Alexander James German, BVSc, PhD, CertSAM, DECVIM-CA, MRCVS
Senior Lecturer in Small Animal Medicine
Department of Veterinary Clinical Sciences
University of Liverpool
Liverpool, Merseyside, United Kingdom
Obesity Biology and Management
Diseases of the Small Intestine

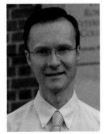

Oliver A. Garden, BSc, BVetMed, PhD, FHEA, MSB, MRCVS, DACVIM, DECVIM-CA
Senior Lecturer in Internal Medicine and Immunology
Department of Veterinary Clinical Sciences
The Royal Veterinary College
Royal College Street
London, United Kingdom
The Queen Mother Hospital for Animals
The Royal Veterinary College
North Mymms
Hatfield, Hertfordshire, United Kingdom
Immune-Mediated Diseases and Therapies

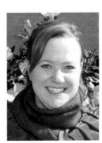

Roger Gfeller,[†] DVM, DACVECC
Chief of Emergency and Critical Care
Animal Emergency Referral Center
Torrance, California
Gastric Lavage

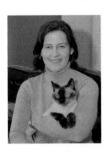

Laura D. Garrett, DVM, DACVIM (Oncology)
Clinical Assistant Professor
Veterinary Clinical Medicine
University of Illinois
Urbana, Illinois
Urogenital and Mammary Gland Tumors

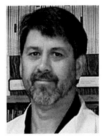

Tracy Gieger, DVM, DACVIM, DACVR
Assistant Professor
Department of Veterinary Clinical Sciences
Louisiana State University
Baton Rouge, Louisiana
Bleeding Disorders: Epistaxis and Hemoptysis

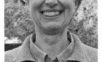

Rosalind M. Gaskell, BVSc, PhD, MRCVS
Professor
Faculty of Veterinary Science
University of Liverpool
Leahurst, Neston Wirral Cheshire, United Kingdom
Other Feline Viral Diseases

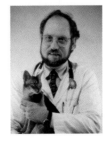

Urs Giger, DVM, MS, FVH
Charlotte Newton Sheppard Professor
Department of Clinical Studies
School of Veterinary Medicine
University of Pennsylvania
Philadelphia, Pennsylvania
Professor
Department of Small Animal Medicine
Vetsuisse Faculty University of Zurich
Zurich, Switzerland
Polycythemia and Erythrocytosis

[†]Deceased.

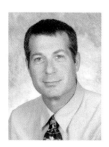

Richard E. Goldstein, DVM, DACVIM, DECVIM-CA
Associate Professor of Medicine
Department of Clinical Sciences
Cornell University
Ithaca, New York
Swollen Joints and Lameness
Leptospirosis
Lyme Disease

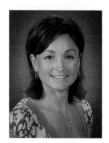

Rebecca E. Gompf, DVM, MS, DACVIM
Associate Professor of Cardiology
Department of Small Animal Clinical
Sciences
College of Veterinary Medicine
University of Tennessee
Knoxville, Tennessee
Cough Suppressants and Sedation of the Cardiac Patient

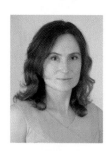

Sonya G. Gordon, DVM, DVSc, DACVIM (Cardiology)
Associate Professor
Department of Small Animal Clinical
Sciences
College of Veterinary Medicine and
Biomedical Science
Texas A&M University
College Station, Texas
Beta Blocking Agents

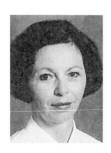

Kinga Gortel, DVM, MS, DACVD
Veterinary Dermatologist
C.A.R.E. Centre Animal Hospital
Calgary, Alberta
Canada
Scaling and Crusting Dermatoses
Ear Flushing

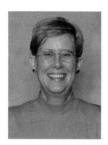

Jacqueline L. Grandy, DVM†
Former Research Associate
Department of Surgical and
Radiological Sciences
School of Veterinary Medicine
University of California
Davis, California
Diseases of the Spinal Cord

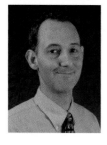

David C. Grant, DVM, MS, DACVIM
Department of Small Animal Clinical
Sciences
Virginia-Maryland Institute
Regional College of Veterinary
Medicine
Blacksburg, Virginia
Cystocentesis and Urinary Bladder Catheterization

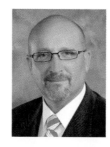

Thomas K. Graves, DVM, PhD, DACVIM
Associate Professor of Small Animal
Medicine
College of Veterinary Medicine
University of Illinois
Urbana, Illinois
Hypercortisolism in Cats (Feline Cushing's Syndrome)

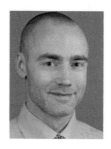

Leigh G. Griffiths, VetMB, MRCVS, DSAS (Soft Tissue), DACVIM (Cardiology), PhD
Assistant Professor of Cardiology
University of California
Davis, California
Anesthesia for the Cardiac Patient

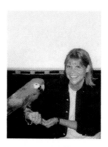

Amy M. Grooters, DVM
Professor
Companion Animal Medicine
Louisiana State University
Baton Rouge, Louisiana
Histoplasmosis, Blastomycosis, Sporotrichosis, Candidiasis, Pythiosis, and Lagenidiosis
Cryptococcosis

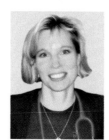

Timothy J. Gruffydd-Jones, DVM
The Feline Centre
University of Bristol
Langford, Bristol
United Kingdom
Feline Inflammatory Liver Disease

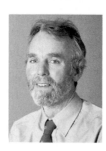

Danièlle A. Gunn-Moore, BSc, BVM&S, PhD, FHEA, MACVSc, RCVS, Specialist in Feline Medicine, MRCVS
Professor of Feline Medicine and Head
of Companion Animal Sciences
Royal (Dick) School of Veterinary
Studies, Division of Clinical
Veterinary Sciences
University of Edinburgh
Edinburgh, Scotland
United Kingdom
Mycobacterial Infections in Cats and Dogs

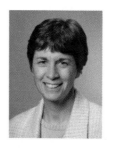

Lynn F. Guptill, DVM, PhD, DACVIM
Associate Professor
Department of Veterinary Clinical
Services
Purdue University
West Lafayette, Indiana
Feline Bartonella

---

†Deceased.

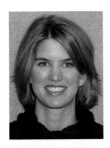

Eileen Sullivan Hackett, DVM, MS, DACVS, DACVECC
Assistant Professor
Department of Clinical Sciences
Colorado State University Sciences
Fort Collins, Colorado
Constant Rate Infusions

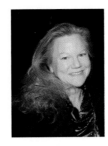

Cathleen A. Hanlon, VMD, PhD, DACVPM
Director and Professor, Rabies
Laboratory
College of Veterinary Medicine
Kansas State University
Manhattan, Kansas
Rabies

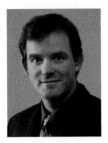

Tim Hackett, DVM, MS
Associate Professor of Emergency and
Critical Care Medicine
Department of Clinical Sciences
Colorado State University
Fort Collins, Colorado
Constant Rate Infusions

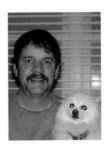

Steven S. Hannah, PhD
Director of Molecular Nutrition
Nestlé Purina Pet Care Company
St. Louis, Missouri
Nutritional Genomics

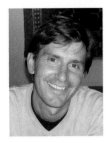

Jens Häggström, DVM, PhD, DECVIM-CA (Cardiology)
Professor
Department of Clinical Sciences
Faculty of Veterinary Medicine and
Animal Science
The Swedish University of Agricultural
Sciences
Uppsala, Sweden
Acquired Valvular Heart Disease

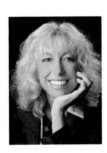

Katrin Hartmann, DVM (Habil.), DECVIM-CA
Center of Clinical Veterinary Medicine
Clinic of Small Animal Medicine
Ludwig Maximilian University of
Munich
Munich, Germany
Tetanus
*Feline Infectious Peritonitis and Feline
Coronavirus Infection*

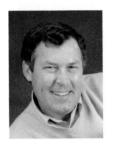

Kevin A. Hahn, DVM, PhD, DACVIM (Oncology)
Director of Research and Chief
Medical Officer
Pet Nutrition Center
Hill's Pet Nutrition, Inc.
Topeka, Kansas
Rational Use of Diagnostic Tests

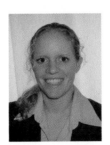

Andrea M. Harvey, BVSc, DSAM (Feline), DipECVIM-CA
FAB Clinical Fellow in Feline Medicine
Department of Clinical Veterinary
Science
University of Bristol Veterinary School
Langford House
Langford, Bristol, United Kingdom
Feline Inflammatory Liver Disease

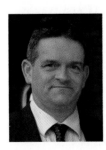

Edward J. Hall, MA, VetMB, PhD
Professor
Department of Clinical Veterinary
Science
University of Bristol
Langford, Bristol, United Kingdom
Diseases of the Small Intestine

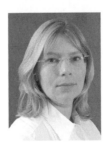

Elizabeth Head, BSc, MA, PhD
Assistant Professor in Residence
Department of Neurology
Institute for Brain Aging & Dementia
University of California
Irvine, California
Cognitive Dysfunction in Aged Dogs

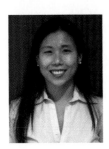

Eveline Han, VMD, DACVIM
Veterinary Internal Medicine and
Allergy Specialists
New York, New York
Pleural and Extrapleural Diseases

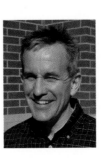

Peter W. Hellyer, DVM
Department of Clinical Sciences
College of Veterinary Medicine and
Biomedical Sciences
Fort Collins, Colorado
*Clinical Pain Identification, Assessment,
and Management*

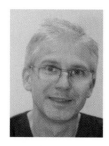

Philippe Hennet, DVM, DAVDC, DEVDC
Clinique Vétérinaire Advetia
Paris, France
Dental Nutrition

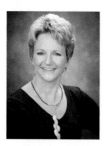

Rebecka S. Hess, DVM, DACVIM
Associate Professor
Department of Clinical Studies
School of Veterinary Medicine
University of Pennsylvania
Philadelphia, Pennsylvania
Insulin-Secreting Islet Cell Neoplasia

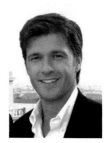

Carolyn J. Henry, DVM, MS, DACVIM (Oncology)
Professor of Oncology
Department of Veterinary Medicine
 and Surgery
College of Veterinary Medicine
Veterinary Medical Teaching Hospital
University of Missouri
Columbia, Missouri
Paraneoplastic Syndromes

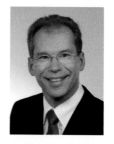

Johannes Hirschberger, DVM (Habil.), DECVIM-CA (Oncology), DECVIM-CA (Internal Medicine)
Clinic of Small Animal Medicine
Center of Clinical Veterinary Medicine
Ludwig Maximilian University of
 Munich
Munich, Germany
Feline Injection-Site Sarcoma

William E. Herndon, DVM, DACVIM (Cardiology)
Staff Cardiologist
California Veterinary Specialists
Carlsbad, California
Edema

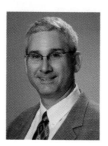

Daniel F. Hogan, DVM, DACVIM (Cardiology)
Associate Professor—Cardiology
School of Veterinary Medicine
Purdue University
West Lafayette, Indiana
Arterial Thromboembolic Disease

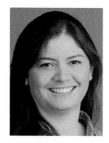

Melissa Herrera, DVM, DACVIM
Assistant Professor of Clinical Small
 Animal Internal Medicine
School of Veterinary Medicine
University of California
Davis, California
Pheochromocytoma

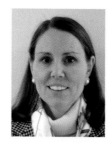

Ann E. Hohenhaus, DVM, DACVIM (Oncology & Internal Medicine)
Head, Jaqua Transfusion Medicine
 Service
The Animal Medical Center
New York, New York
*Blood Transfusions, Component
 Therapy, and Oxygen-Carrying
 Solutions*

Eric J. Herrgesell, DVM, DACVR
Veterinary Medical Imaging
Abdominal Ultrasonography

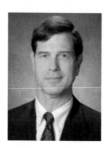

R. Bruce Hollett, DVM, MS, DACT
Associate Professor and Director
Department of Large Animal Medicine
 and Dean's Office
College of Veterinary Medicine
The University of Georgia
Athens, Georgia
Brucellosis

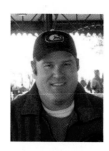

Michael E. Herrtage, MA, BVSc, DVSc, DVR, DVD, DSAM, DECVIM-CA, DECVDI, MRCVS
Professor of Small Animal Medicine
Department of Veterinary Medicine
University of Cambridge
Cambridge, Cambridgeshire, United
 Kingdom
Diseases of the Nose and Nasal Sinuses

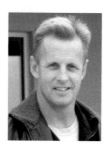

David Holt, BVSc, DACVS
Professor of Surgery
Department of Clinical Studies
School of Veterinary Medicine
University of Pennsylvania
Philadelphia, Pennsylvania
Hepatic and Splenic Emergencies

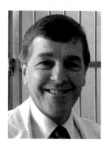

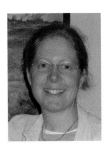

Kate Hopper, BVSc, PhD, DACVECC
Assistant Professor
Small Animal Emergency and Critical
  Care
Department of Veterinary Surgery and
  Radiological Sciences
University of California
Davis, California
Oxygen Therapy

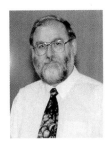

**Johnny D. Hoskins, DVM, PhD,
  DACVIM**
Professor Emeritus
Veterinary Clinical Medicine
Louisiana State University
Baton Rouge, Louisiana
Neonatal and Pediatric Nutrition

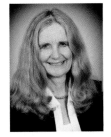

**Lynn Rolland Hovda, RPH, DVM,
  MS, DACVIM**
SafetyCall International and Pet Poison
  Helpline
Bloomington, Minnesota
Plant Toxicities
Human Prescription and Street Drugs

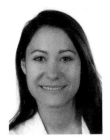

Cornelia Huttinger, DVM
Medizinische Kleintierklinik
Clinic of Small Animal Medicine
University of Munich
Munich, Germany
Feline Injection-Site Sarcoma

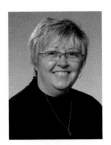

Sherri L. Ihle, DVM, MS, DACVIM
Associate Professor
Department of Companion Animals
Atlantic Veterinary College
University of Prince Edward Island
Charlottetown, Prince Edward Island,
  Canada
Failure to Grow

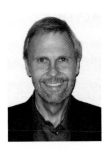

Peter J. Ihrke, VMD, DACVD
Professor of Dermatology
School of Veterinary Medicine
University of California
Davis, California
Pruritus

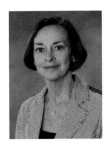

**Marion L. Jackson, DVM, MVetSc,
  PhD, DACVP**
Professor of Veterinary Pathology
Western College of Veterinary
  Medicine
University of Saskatchewan
Saskatoon, Saskatchewan, Canada
Leukocytes in Health and Disease

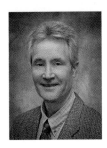

**Albert E. Jergens, DVM, PhD,
  DACVIM**
Professor
Department of Veterinary Clinical
  Sciences
College of Veterinary Medicine
Iowa State University
Ames, Iowa
*Interventional Endoscopy/Interventional
  Imaging*
Diseases of the Esophagus
*Host-Microbial Interactions in
  Gastrointestinal Health*

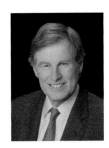

**Kenneth A. Johnson, MVSc, PhD,
  FACVSc, DACVS, DECVS**
Clinical Professor of Orthopaedics
University of Sydney
Sydney, Australia
Skeletal Diseases

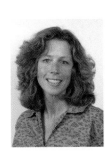

**Lynelle R. Johnson, DVM, MS, PhD,
  DACVIM**
Associate Professor
Department of Veterinary Medicine:
  Medicine & Epidemiology
University of California
Davis, California
Fine Needle Aspiration and Lung Biopsy

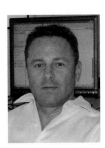

Ron Johnson, DVM, PhD, DACVCP
Associate Professor
Biomedical Sciences
University of Guelph
Guelph, Ontario, Canada
Compounding Drugs

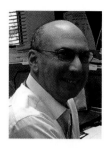

Jacob Kagan, PhD, MS
National Cancer Institute
Bethesda, Maryland
Biomarkers and "Omics"

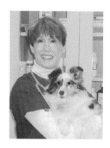

Rebecca Kirby, DVM, DAVCIM, DACVECC
Animal Emergency Center
Glendale, Wisconsin
Gastrointestinal Emergencies

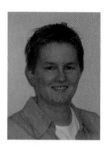

Heidi B. Kellihan, DVM, DACVIM (Cardiology)
Clinical Assistant Professor of Cardiology
Department of Medicine
University of Wisconsin
Madison, Wisconsin
Pulmonary Hypertension and Pulmonary Thromboembolism

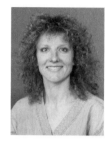

Karen L. Kline, DVM, MS, DACVIM (Neurology)
Staff Neurologist
Department of Neurology
VCA Veterinary Specialty Center of Seattle
Lynnwood, Washington
Altered States of Consciousness: Stupor and Coma

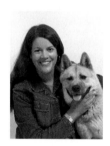

Karen M. Kelly, DVM, DABVP (Canine & Feline)
Associate Veterinarian
Southern California Veterinary Hospital
Woodland Hills, California
Home Euthanasia

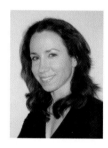

Marguerite F. Knipe, DVM
Department of Surgical & Radiological Sciences
School of Veterinary Medicine
University of California
Davis, California
Sleep Disorders

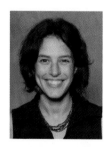

Efrat Kelmer, DVM, MS, DACVECC
Clinical Assistant Professor
Department of Small Animal Clinical Sciences
College of Veterinary Medicine
University of Tennessee
Knoxville, Tennessee
Cardiopulmonary Arrest and Resuscitation

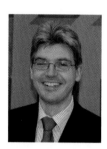

Hans S. Kooistra, DVM, PhD, DECVIM
Associate Professor
Department of Clinical Sciences of Companion Animals
University of Utrecht
Utrecht, Netherlands
Growth Hormone Disorders: Acromegaly and Pituitary Dwarfism

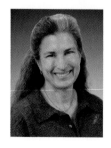

Marie E. Kerl, DVM, DACVIM (SAIM), DACVECC
Associate Teaching Professor
Department of Veterinary Medicine & Surgery
University of Missouri
Columbia, Missouri
Acid-Base, Oximetry, and Blood Gas Emergencies
Renal Tubular Diseases

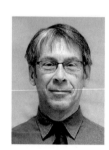

Stephen Kruth, BA, DVM
Professor
Department of Clinical Studies
University of Guelph
Guelph, Ontario, Canada
Immune-Mediated Hemolytic Anemia and Other Regenerative Anemias

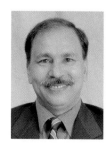

Safdar A. Khan, DVM, MS, PhD, DABVT
Senior Director of Toxicology Research
ASPCA Animal Poison Control Center
Adjunct Toxicology Instructor
College of Veterinary Medicine
University of Illinois
Urbana, Illinois
Intoxication versus Acute, Nontoxicologic Illness: Differentiating the Two

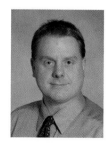

Butch KuKanich, DVM, PhD, DACVCP
Assistant Professor
Department of Anatomy and Physiology
Kansas State University
Manhattan, Kansas
Over-the-Counter Human Medications

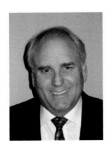

W. Douglas Kunz, MS, DVM
Medical Director
Animal Medical Hospital
Palm Springs, California
Euthanasia

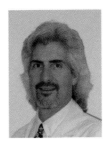

Michael R. Lappin, DVM, DACVIM
Professor
Department of Clinical Science
College of Veterinary Medicine and
  Biomedical Sciences
Colorado State University
Fort Collins, Colorado
*Laboratory Diagnosis of Infectious
  Disease*
Protozoal Infections

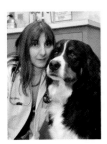

Mary Anna Labato, DVM, DACVIM
Clinical Professor
Section Head Small Animal Medicine
Department of Clinical Sciences
Staff Veterinarian
Foster Hospital
Cummings School of Veterinary
  Medicine
Tufts University
North Grafton, Massachusetts
*Micturition Disorders and Urinary
  Incontinence*
Rhinoscopy, Nasal Flushing, and Biopsy
Continuous Renal Replacement Therapy

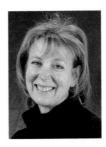

**Martha Moon Larson, DVM, MS,
  DACVR**
Professor
Department of Small Animal Clinical
  Sciences
Virginia-Maryland Regional College of
  Veterinary Medicine
Virginia Polytechnic Institute and State
  University
Blacksburg, Virginia
Mediastinal Disease

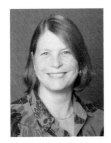

**Dottie P. Laflamme, MS, DVM, PhD,
  DACVN**
Senior Research Scientist
Nestlé Purina Pet Care Research
  Center
St. Louis, Missouri
Nutritional Genomics

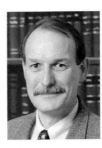

**Richard A. LeCouteur, BVSc, PhD,
  DACVIM (Neurology)**
Professor
Department of Surgical & Radiological
  Sciences
University of California
Davis, California
Muscle and Nerve Biopsy
Brain Biopsy
Diseases of the Spinal Cord

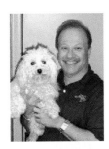

**Gary Landsberg, BSc, DVM, DACVB,
  dip ECVBM-CA**
North Toronto Animal Clinic
Thornhill, Ontario, Canada
Cognitive Dysfunction in Aged Dogs

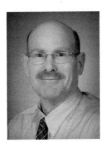

George E. Lees, DVM, MS, DACVIM
Professor of Internal Medicine
Department of Small Animal Clinical
  Sciences
Texas A&M University
College Station, Texas
Familial Renal Disease in Dogs

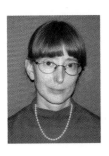

Cathy Langston, DVM, DACVIM
Head of Nephrology, Urology, and
  Hemodialysis
Animal Medical Center
New York, New York
Peritoneal Dialysis
Renal Emergencies
Acute Uremia
Renal Transplantation

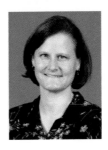

Julie K. Levy, DVM, PhD, DACVIM
Professor
Maddie's Shelter Medicine Program
College of Veterinary Medicine
University of Florida
Gainesville, Florida
Feline Immunodeficiency Virus
Feline Leukemia Virus

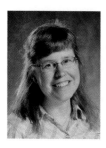

Kerstin Lindblad-Toh, PhD
Broad Institute of MIT and Harvard
Cambridge, Massachusetts
Uppsala University
Uppsala, Sweden
The Genome

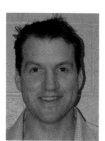

Julius M. Liptak, BVSc, MVCS, FACVSc, DACVS, DECVS
Small Animal Surgeon and Surgical Oncologist
Alta Vista Animal Hospital
Ottawa, Ontario, Canada
Bone and Joint Tumors

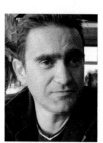

Remo Lobetti, BVSc, MMedVet (Med), PhD, DECVIM-CA (Internal Medicine)
Bryanston Veterinary Hospital
Bryanston, Gauteng
Johannesburg, South Africa
Tropical Diseases

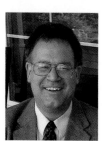

Randall Lovell, BS, DVM
Division of Animal Feeds Feed Safety Team
Food and Drug Administration/Center for Veterinary Medicine
Rockville, Maryland
Food Safety and Toxicities

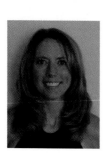

Lori L. Ludwig, VMD, MS, DACVS
Associate
Department of Surgery
Veterinary Surgical Care
Mount Pleasant, South Carolina
Pleural and Extrapleural Diseases

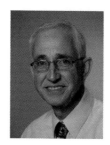

Andrew Urs Luescher, Dr Med Vet, PhD, DACVB, ECVBM-CA
Associate Professor
Department of Veterinary Clinical Sciences
Director, Animal Behavior Clinic
Department of Veterinary Teaching Hospital
Purdue University
West Lafayette, Indiana
Behavioral Disorders
Preventive Behavior Care

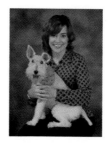

Kristin MacDonald, DVM, PhD, DACVIM (Cardiology)
Veterinary Cardiologist
VCA Animal Care Center of Sonoma
Rohnert Park, California
Myocardial Disease: Feline

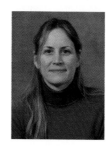

Amy L. MacNeill, DVM, PhD, DACVP
Assistant Professor
Department of Pathobiology
University of Illinois
Urbana, Illinois
Cytology of Internal Organs

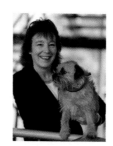

Jill E. Maddison, BVSc, PhD, FACVSc, MRCVS
Director of Professional Development
The Royal Veterinary College
North Mymms
Hatfield, Hertfordshire, United Kingdom
Adverse Drug Reactions

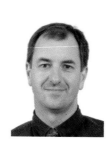

David J. Maggs, BVSc (Hons), DACVO
Associate Professor
Department of Surgical & Radiological Sciences
University of California
Davis, California
Ocular Manifestations of Systemic Disease

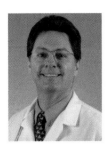

F.A. (Tony) Mann, DVM, MS, DACVS, DACVECC
Professor
Department of Veterinary Medicine and Surgery
Director of Small Animal Emergency and Critical Care Services
Veterinary Medical Teaching Hospital
University of Missouri
Columbia, Missouri
Cardiopulmonary Arrest and Resuscitation
Initial Evaluation of Respiratory Emergencies

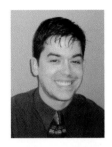

Christopher L. Mariani, DVM, PhD, DACVIM (Neurology)
Assistant Professor of Neurology
North Carolina State University
Raleigh, North Carolina
Peripheral Nerve Disorders
Neuromuscular Junctional Disease

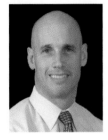

Stanley L. Marks, BVSc, PhD, DACVIM (Internal Medicine, Oncology), DACVN
Professor
Department of Medicine and Epidemiology
School of Veterinary Medicine
University of California
Davis, California
Nasoesophageal, Esophagostomy, Gastrostomy, and Jejunal Tube Placement Techniques
The Principles and Implementation of Enteral Nutrition
Enteric Bacterial Disease

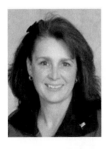

Diane E. Mason, DVM, PhD
Kansas State University
Veterinary Medical Teaching Hospital
Manhattan, Kansas
Diseases of the Ear

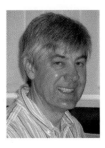

Ian S. Mason, BVetMed, PhD, CertSAD, DECVD, MRCVS
Purton Stoke, Wiltshire, United Kingdom
Erosions and Ulcerations

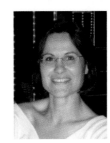

Luisa Mateus, DVM
Associate Professor
Division of Reproduction and Obstetrics
Faculty of Veterinary Medicine
Technical University of Lisbon
Lisbon, Portugal
Cystic Endometrial Hyperplasia and Pyometra

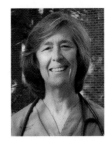

Karol A. Mathews, DVM, DVSc, DACVECC
Professor
Emergency & Critical Care Medicine
Department of Clinical Studies
Ontario Veterinary College
University of Guelph
Guelph, Ontario, Canada
Nonsteroidal Anti-Inflammatory Analgesics

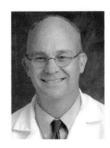

Michael E. Matz, DVM, DACVIM
Staff Internist
Veterinary Specialty
Center of Tucson
Tucson, Arizona
Flatulence
Endoscopic Procedures for Evaluation of the Gastrointestinal Tract

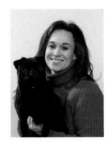

Elisa M. Mazzaferro, MS, DVM, PhD, DACVECC
Director of Emergency Services
Department of Emergency and Critical Care
Wheat Ridge Veterinary Specialists
Wheat Ridge, Colorado
Heatstroke

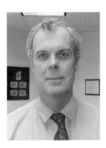

Daniel G. McChesney, BS, MS, PhD
Director, Office of Surveillance and Compliance
Food and Drug Administration/Center for Veterinary Medicine
Rockville, Maryland
Food Safety and Toxicities

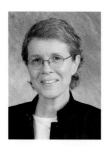

Margaret C. McEntee, DVM, DACVIM, DACVR
Professor
Department of Clinical Sciences
College of Veterinary Medicine
Cornell University
Ithaca, New York
Soft-Tissue Sarcomas

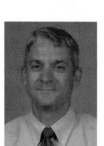

Andrew Lee McGraw, DVM
Resident, Small Animal Internal
   Medicine
Department of Clinical Sciences
College of Veterinary Medicine
Auburn University
Auburn, Alabama
Reproductive Emergencies

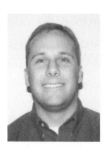

Leo J. "Ty" McSherry, DVM, DACVP
Clinical Pathologist
Antech Diagnostics
Lake Success, New York
*Techniques for Bone Marrow Aspiration
   and Biopsy*

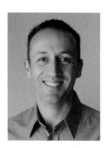

Carlos Melian, DVM, PhD
Director
Department of Veterinary Teaching
   Hospital
Universidad de Las Palmas de Gran
   Canaria
Clinica Veterinaria Atlantico
Las Palmas de Gran Canaria, Spain
Hyperadrenocorticism in Dogs

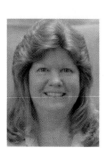

Sandra R. Merchant, DVM, DACVD
Professor of Dermatology
Department of Veterinary Clinical
   Sciences
Louisiana State University
Baton Rouge, Louisiana
*The Skin as a Sensor of Internal
   Medicine Disorders*

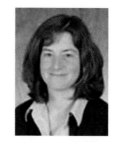

**Kathryn M. Meurs, DVM, DACVIM
(Cardiology)**
Department of Veterinary Clinical
   Sciences
College of Veterinary Medicine
Washington State University
Pullman, Washington
Myocardial Disease: Canine

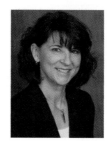

**Patrice M. Mich, DVM, MS, DABVP
(Canine/Feline), DACVA**
Post Doctoral Fellow in Integrative
   Pain Medicine
Department of Clinical Sciences
Colorado State University
Fort Collins, Colorado
Medical Director
OrthoPets United and OrthoPets
   Center for Animal Pain Management
Denver, Colorado
*Clinical Pain Identification, Assessment,
   and Management*

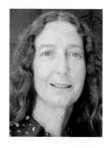

**Kathryn E. Michel, DVM, MS,
DACVN**
Associate Professor of Nutrition
Department of Clinical Studies
School of Veterinary Medicine
University of Pennsylvania
Philadelphia, Pennsylvania
Nutritional Assessment

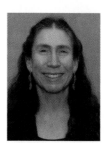

Kristina G. Miles, DVM, MS, DACVR
Associate Professor
Department of Veterinary Clinical
   Sciences
College of Veterinary Medicine
Iowa State University
Ames, Iowa
*Interventional Endoscopy/Interventional
   Imaging*

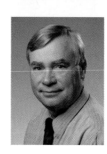

**James B. Miller, DVM, MS, DACVIM
(SAIM)**
Professor
Department of Companion Animals
Atlantic Veterinary College
University of Prince Edward Island
Charlottetown, Prince Edward Island,
   Canada
*Hyperthermia and Fever of Unknown
   Origin*

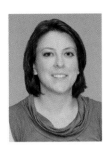

Kelly Mitchell, DVM
Ontario Veterinary College
University of Guelph
Guelph, Ontario, Canada
*Immune-Mediated Hemolytic Anemia
and Other Regenerative Anemias*

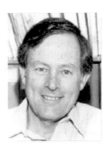

James G. Morris, M. Agr. Sc., PhD
Professor Emeritus
Department of Molecular Biosciences
University of California
Davis, California
*Nutrition of Healthy Dogs and Cats in
Various Adult Stages*

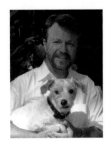

**Carmel T. Mooney, MVB, MPhil,
PhD, DECVIM-CA, MRCVS**
Senior Lecturer
University Veterinary Hospital
University College Dublin
Belfield
Dublin, Ireland
Hyperthyroidism

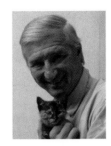

**Ralf S. Mueller, Dr.med.vet., Dr.
habil., DACVD, FACVSc, DECVD**
Professor
Center of Clinical Veterinary Medicine
Clinic of Small Animal Medicine
Ludwig Maximilian University of
Munich
Munich, Germany
Skin Scrapings and Skin Biopsies

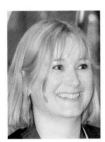

**Antony S. Moore, BVSc, MVSc,
DACVIM (Oncology)**
Veterinary Oncology Consultants
Wauchope, New South Wales,
Australia
Practical Chemotherapy

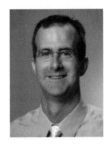

**James F. Naughton, DVM, MS,
DACVR**
Clinical Assistant Professor, Radiology
Department of Veterinary Clinical
Sciences
School of Veterinary Medicine
Purdue University
West Lafayette, Indiana
Cytology of Internal Organs

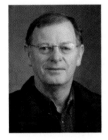

Peter F. Moore, BVSc, PhD
Professor
Department of VM Pathology,
Microbiology and Immunology
University of California
Davis, California
Canine and Feline Histiocytic Diseases

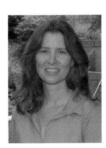

**O. Lynne Nelson, DVM, DACVIM
(Cardiology)**
Associate Professor of Cardiology
Washington State University
Pullman, Washington
Pleural Effusion

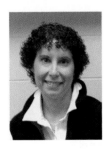

Karen A. Moriello, DVM, DACVD
Clinical Professor of Dermatology
School of Veterinary Medicine
Department of Medical Sciences
University of Wisconsin
Madison, Wisconsin
Body Odors
*Problem-Oriented Differential Diagnosis
of Autoimmune Skin Diseases*

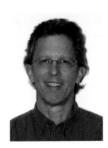

Richard W. Nelson, DVM, DACVIM
Professor, Internal Medicine
Department of Medicine and
Epidemiology
School of Veterinary Medicine
University of California
Davis, California
Canine Diabetes Mellitus
Pheochromocytoma

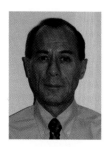

Patrick Nguyen, DVM, PhD, DECVCN
Professor
Nutrition & Endocrinology Unit
National Veterinary School of Nantes
Nantes, France
Obesity

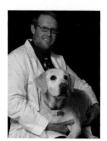

Brook A. Niemiec, DVM, DAVDC, Fellow AVD
Chief of Staff
Southern California Veterinary Dental Specialties
San Diego, California
President
San Diego Veterinary Training Center
San Diego, California
Founding Consultant
VETDentalRad.com
Monument, Colorado
Ptyalism

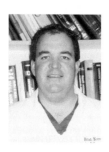

Brian C. Norman, DVM, DACVIM (Internal Medicine)
Medical Director
California Animal Hospital Veterinary Specialty Group
Los Angeles, California
Transtracheal Wash and Bronchoscopy

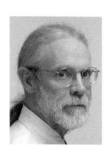

Dennis P. O'Brien, DVM, PhD, DACVIM (Neurology)
Chancellor's Chair in Comparative Neurology
Department of Veterinary Medicine & Surgery
Neurologist, Neurology & Neurosurgery Service
Veterinary Medical Teaching Hospital
University of Missouri
Columbia, Missouri
Brain Disease

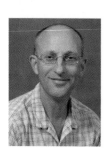

Robert T. O'Brien, DVM, MS, DACVR
Department of Veterinary Clinical Medicine
University of Illinois
Urbana, Illinois
Diseases of the Spleen

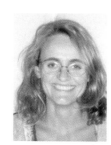

Lisbeth Høier Olsen, DVM, DrVetSci
Associate Professor
Department of Basic Animal and Veterinary Sciences
University of Copenhagen
Copenhagen, Denmark
Acquired Valvular Heart Disease

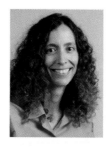

Theresa Ortega-Simpson, BS, DVM, DACVIM
Internist
Small Animal Internal Medicine
Veterinary Medical and Surgical Group
Ventura, California
Pallor

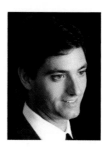

João S. Orvalho, DVM, DACVIM (Cardiology)
Specialist in Clinical Cardiology
Veterinary Medical Center
University of California
San Diego, California
Electrocardiographic Techniques

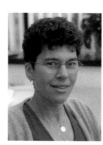

Cynthia M. Otto, DVM, PhD, DACVECC
Associate Professor of Critical Care
Department of Clinical Studies
University of Pennsylvania
Philadelphia, Pennsylvania
Shock

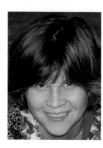

Catherine A. Outerbridge, DVM, MVSc, DACVIM, DACVD
Department of Medicine and Epidemiology
School of Veterinary Medicine
University of California
Davis, California
Hepatocutaneous Syndrome

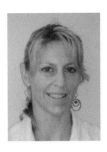

**Beth Overley, DVM, DACVIM
(Oncology)**
Center for Animal Referral and
    Emergency Services
Langhorne, Pennsylvania
Rational Use of Diagnostic Tests

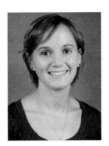

Sally C. Perea, DVM, MS, DACVN
Senior Nutritionist
Natura Pet Products, Inc.
Davis, California
*Nutritional Management of Endocrine
    Disease*
Home-Prepared and Raw Diets

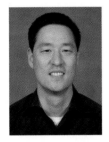

**Mark A. Oyama, DVM, DACVIM
(Cardiology)**
Associate Professor
Department of Clinical Studies
University of Pennsylvania
Philadelphia, Pennsylvania
Congenital Heart Disease

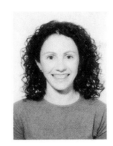

**M. Dolores Pérez-Alenza, DVM,
PhD**
Professor
School of Veterinary Medicine
Complutense University of Madrid
Madrid, Spain
Hyperadrenocorticism in Dogs

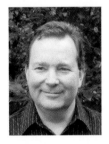

**Stephen W. Page, BSc(Vet), BVSc,
DVCS, MVCS, MAppSc(Env Tox),
MACVSc (Pharmacology)**
Director
Advanced Veterinary Therapeutics
Berry, New South Wales, Australia
Adverse Drug Reactions

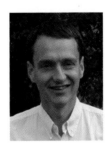

**Henrik Duelund Petersen, DVM,
DrVetSci**
Zealand Pharma A/S
Glostrup, Denmark
Acquired Valvular Heart Disease

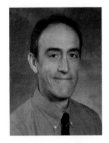

Mark G. Papich, DVM, DACVCP
Professor of Clinical Pharmacology
College of Veterinary Medicine
North Carolina State University
Raleigh, North Carolina
Antibacterial Drug Therapy

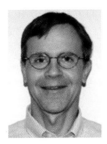

Mark E. Peterson, DVM, DACVIM
The Caspary Institute and Bobst
    Animal Hospital of the Animal
    Medical Center
New York, New York
Hyperadrenocorticism in Dogs

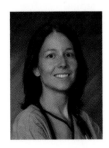

Dominique Paquette, DVM
Department of Neurology
California Animal Hospital
Los Angeles, California
Peripheral Cranial Neuropathies

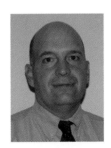

**Jean-Paul Petrie, DVM, DACVIM
(Cardiology)**
Clinical Cardiologist
Hudson Valley Veterinary Cardiology,
    LLC
Sloatsburg, New York
*Thoracic and Pericardial Taps and
    Drains*
Venous and Lymphatic Disorders

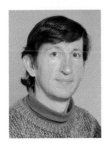

**Peter J. Pascoe, BVSc, DACVA,
DiplECVAA**
Professor of Anesthesiology
Department of Surgical and
    Radiological Sciences
School of Veterinary Medicine
University of California
Davis, California
Pulse Oximetry

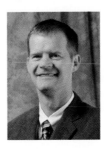

Jonathan D. Plant, DVM, DACVD
Medical Advisor for Dermatology
Banfield, The Pet Hospital
Portland, Oregon
Scaling and Crusting Dermatoses

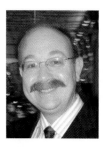

Michael Podell, MSc, DVM, DACVIM (Neurology)
Adjunct Professor
College of Veterinary Medicine
University of Illinois
Urbana, Illinois
Neurology and Neurosurgery
Animal Emergency and Referral Center
Northbrook, Illinois
Seizures

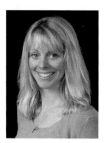

Rachel E. Pollard, DVM, PhD, DACVR
Department of Surgical and
 Radiological Sciences
University of California
School of Veterinary Medicine
Davis, California
Abdominal Ultrasonography

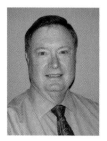

David J. Polzin, DVM, DACVIM
Professor and Chief of Internal
 Medicine
Department of Veterinary Clinical
 Sciences
College of Veterinary Medicine
University of Minnesota
St. Paul, Minnesota
Chronic Kidney Disease

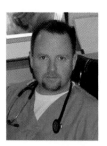

Brian A. Poteet, MS, DVM, DACVR, DABSNM
Director
Department of Gulf Coast Veterinary
 Diagnostic Imaging
Gulf Coast Veterinary Specialists
Houston, Texas
Veterinary Nuclear Medicine
Digital Radiology: DICOM, PACS

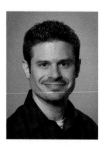

Barrak Pressler, DVM, PhD, DACVIM
Assistant Professor of Internal
 Medicine
Department of Veterinary Clinical
 Sciences
Purdue University
West Lafayette, Indiana
Urinary Tract Infections

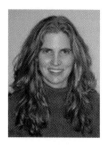

Jennifer Prittie, DVM, ACVIM, ACVECC
Staff Criticalist
Animal Medical Center
New York, New York
Renal Emergencies

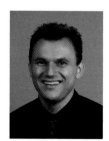

Robert Prošek, DVM, MS, DACVIM, DECVIM-CA
Clinical Assistant Professor
University of Florida
Gainesville, Florida
Adjunct Professor of Cardiology
University of Florida
Director
Animal Heart Centers
Veterinary Specialists Inc.
Veterinary Institute for Interventional
 Therapy
Florida
Abnormal Heart Sounds and Heart
 Murmurs
Biomarkers of Cardiovascular Disease

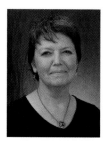

Beverly J. Purswell, DVM, PhD, DACT
Professor
Department of Large Animal Clinical
 Sciences
Virginia Maryland Regional College of
 Veterinary Medicine
Virginia Polytechnic Institute and State
 University
Blacksburg, Virginia
Vaginal Disorders

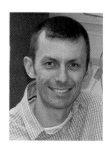

Alan Radford, DVM, BSc, BVSc, PhD
Faculty of Veterinary Science
University of Liverpool
Leahurst, Neston Wirral Cheshire,
 United Kingdom
Other Feline Viral Diseases

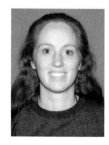

MaryAnn G. Radlinsky, DVM, DACVS
College of Veterinary Medicine
University of Georgia
Veterinary Teaching Hospital
Athens, Georgia
Diseases of the Ear

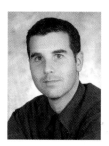

Kenneth M. Rassnick, DVM, DACVIM (Oncology)
Assistant Professor
Department of Clinical Sciences
College of Veterinary Medicine
Cornell University
Ithaca, New York
Tumors of the Skin

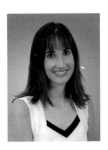

Carol R. Reinero, DVM, DACVIM, PhD
Assistant Professor
University of Missouri
Columbia, Missouri
Initial Evaluation of Respiratory Emergencies

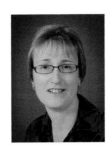

Kenita S. Rogers, BS, DVM, MS
Associate Dean for Professional Programs
Staff Oncologist
College of Veterinary Medicine and Biomedical Sciences
Texas A&M University
College Station, Texas
Mast Cell Disease

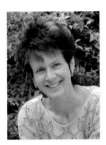

Claudia Reusch, DVM, DECVIM-CA
Professor
Clinic for Small Animal Internal Medicine
Vetsuisse Faculty
University of Zurich
Zurich, Switzerland
Feline Diabetes Mellitus

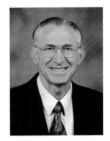

Quinton R. Rogers, PhD
Distinguished Professor of Physiological Chemistry
Department of Molecular Biosciences
School of Veterinary Medicine
University of California
Davis, California
Nutrition of Healthy Dogs and Cats in Various Adult Stages

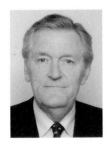

Keith Richter, DVM, DACVIM
Hospital Director and Staff Internist
Veterinary Specialty Hospital of San Diego
San Diego, California
Laparoscopy
Hepatic Biopsy Techniques

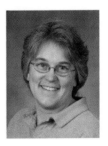

Margaret V. Root Kustritz, DVM, PhD, DACT
Associate Professor
Department of Veterinary Clinical Sciences
University of Minnesota
St. Paul, Minnesota
Effect of Age at the Time of Spay or Castration on Long-Term Health of Dogs and Cats

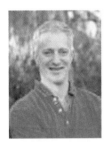

Darlene L. Riel, RVT, VTS (SAIM)
Manager, Gourley Clinical Teaching Center
University of California
Davis, California
Jugular Catheterization and Central Venous Pressure

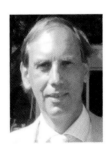

Jan Rothuizen, DVM
Professor
Clinical Sciences of Companion Animals
Faculty of Veterinary Medicine
University of Utrecht
Utrecht, Netherlands
World Small Animal Association (WSAVA) Guidelines
General Principles in the Treatment of Liver Disease

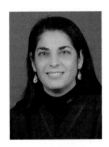

Ad Rijnberk, DVM
University of Utrecht
Utrecht, Netherlands
Diabetes Insipidus

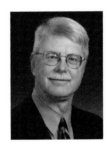

Philip Roudebush, DVM, DACVIM
Adjunct Professor
Department of Clinical Sciences
Kansas State University
Manhattan, Kansas
Director
Department of Scientific Affairs
Hill's Pet Nutrition, Inc.
Topeka, Kansas
Adverse Reactions to Foods: Allergies versus Intolerance

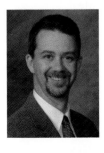

Mark C. Rochat, DVM, MS, DACVS
Professor
Department of Veterinary Clinical Sciences
Oklahoma State University Center for Veterinary Health Sciences
Stillwater, Oklahoma
Arthrocentesis and Arthroscopy

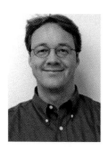

Craig G. Ruaux, BVSc, PhD, MACVSc, DACVIM
Assistant Professor, Small Animal Medicine
Department of Clinical Sciences
Oregon State University
Corvallis, Oregon
Nutritional Management of Hepatic Conditions

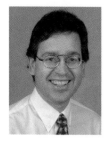

Elke Rudloff, DVM, DACVEC
Director of Education
Animal Emergency Center and Specialty Services
Glendale, Wisconsin
Abdominocentesis and Diagnostic Peritoneal Lavage
Gastrointestinal Emergencies

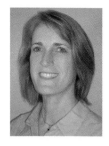

John E. Rush, DVM, MS, DACVIM (Cardiology), DACVECC
Tufts Cummings School of Veterinary Medicine
North Grafton, Massachusetts
Nutritional Modulation of Heart Disease

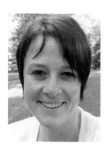

Helena Rylander, DVM, DACVIM (Neurology)
Clinical Assistant Professor
Department of Medical Sciences
School of Veterinary Medicine
University of Wisconsin
Madison, Wisconsin
Neurologic Manifestations of Systemic Disease

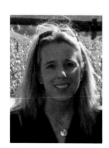

Veronique Sammut, DVM, MS, DACVIM (Neurology)
VetSurg & Neurology
Los Angeles, California
Vestibular Disease

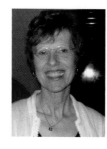

Auke C. Schaefers-Okkens, DVM, PhD, Founding Diplomate ECAR
Department of Clinical Sciences of Companion Animals
Faculty of Veterinary Medicine
University of Utrecht
Utrecht, Netherlands
Estrous Cycle and Breeding Management of the Healthy Bitch

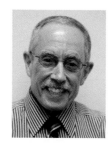

Michael Schaer, DVM, DACVIM, DCVECC
Professor and Special Assistant to the Dean
Department of Small Animal Clinical Sciences
University of Florida
College of Veterinary Medicine
Gainesville, Florida
Diabetic Ketoacidosis and Hyperglycemic Hyperosmolar Syndrome

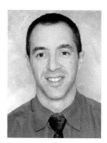

Scott J. Schatzberg, DVM, PhD, DACVIM (Neurology)
Assistant Professor of Neurology
Department of Small Animal Medicine and Surgery
College of Veterinary Medicine
University of Georgia
Athens, Georgia
Neurologic Examination and Neuroanatomic Diagnosis

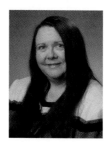

Patricia A. Schenck, DVM, PhD
Diagnostic Center for Population and Animal Health
Section Chief, Endocrine Diagnostic Section
College of Veterinary Medicine
Michigan State University
Lansing, Michigan
Electrolyte Disorders: Ca-P and Mg
Dietary and Medical Considerations in Hyperlipidemia

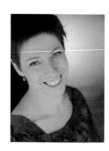

Margie A. Scherk, DVM, DABVP (Feline)
Editor, *Journal of Feline Medicine and Surgery*
Catslnk
Vancouver, British Columbia, Canada
Toxic, Metabolic, Infectious, and Neoplastic Liver Diseases

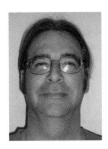

Thomas Schermerhorn, VMD, DACVIM
Associate Professor
Department of Clinical Sciences
Kansas State University
Manhattan, Kansas
Cachexia

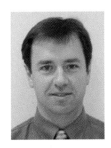

Rance K. Sellon, DVM, PhD, DACVIM
Associate Professor
Department of Veterinary Clinical
 Sciences
College of Veterinary Medicine
Washington State University
Pullman, Washington
Canine Viral Diseases

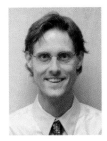

Nick A. Schroeder, DVM, DACVIM (Cardiology)
Veterinary Specialists of South Florida,
 Florida Diuretics
Cooper City, Florida
Diuretics

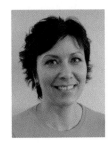

Cecile T. Siedlecki, DVM, ACVIM (Oncology)
Bay Area Veterinary Specialists
San Leandro, California
Lymph Node Aspiration and Biopsy

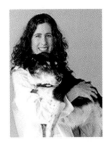

Rhonda L. Schulman, DVM, DACVIM
Internist
Animal Specialty Group
Los Angeles, California
Weakness

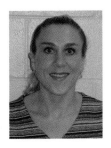

Deborah C. Silverstein, DVM, DACVECC
Assistant Professor of Critical Care
University of Pennsylvania
Philadelphia, Pennsylvania
*Clinical Evaluation of the Respiratory
 Tract*

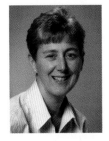

J. Catharine R. Scott-Moncrieff, MA Vet. MB, MS
Professor
Department of Veterinary Clinical
 Sciences
School of Veterinary Medicine
Purdue University
West Lafayette, Indiana
Hypothyroidism
Hypoadrenocorticism

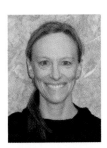

Amelia M. Simpson, DVM, DACVS
Veterinary Surgical Center of Portland
Portland, Oregon
Pleural and Extrapleural Diseases

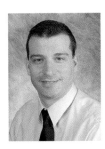

Peter V. Scrivani, DVM, DACVR
Assistant Professor
Department of Clinical Services
Cornell University
Ithaca, New York
Imaging Neurologic Patients

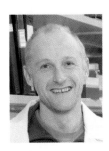

Kenneth W. Simpson, BVM&S, PhD, DACVIM, DECVIM-CA
College of Veterinary Medicine
Cornell University
Ithaca, New York
Diseases of the Stomach

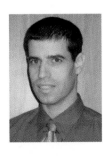

Gilad Segev, DVM, DECVIM-CA
Lecturer
Koret School of Veterinary Medicine
Hebrew University, Jerusalem
Rehovot, Israel
Proteinuria

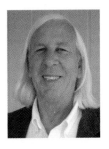

D. David Sisson, DVM, DACVIM (Cardiology)
Professor
Director, Small Animal Services
Department of Clinical Sciences
Oregon State University
Corvallis, Oregon
Pathophysiology of Heart Failure
Congenital Heart Disease

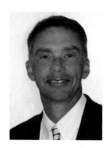

Mark M. Smith, DVM, DACVS, AVDC
Center for Veterinary Dentistry and Oral Surgery
Gaithersburg, Maryland
Oral and Salivary Gland Disorders

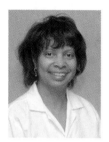

Saralyn Smith-Carr, DVM, PhD, DACVIM
Associate Professor
Small Animal Internal Medicine
Department of Clinical Sciences
College of Veterinary Medicine
Auburn University
Auburn, Alabama
Reproductive Emergencies

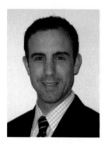

Jason W. Soukup, BS, DVM, DACVD
Veterinary Dentistry and Oral Surgery
School of Veterinary Medicine
University of Wisconsin–Madison
Madison, Wisconsin
Periodontitis

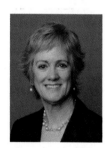

Candace A. Sousa, DVM, DABVP, DACVD
Senior Veterinary Specialist
Pfizer Animal Health
Sacramento, California
Fleas, Flea Allergy, and Flea Control

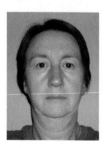

Jennifer A. Spencer, MSc, PhD
Instructor
Department of Pathobiology
College of Veterinary Medicine
Auburn University
Auburn, Alabama
Fecal Examination

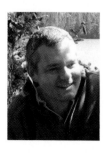

Jörg M. Steiner, DVM, PhD, DACVIM, DECVIM-CA
Associate Professor and Director of the GI Laboratory
Texas A&M University
College Station, Texas
Canine Pancreatic Disease

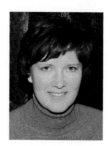

Rebecca L. Stepien, DVM, MS, DACVIM (Cardiology)
Clinical Professor of Cardiology
Department of Medical Sciences
School of Veterinary Medicine
University of Wisconsin–Madison
Madison, Wisconsin
Diagnostic Blood Pressure Measurement
Pathophysiology of Systemic Hypertension and Blood Pressure Assessment

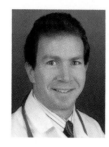

Michael Stone, DVM, DACVIM (SAIM)
Clinical Assistant Professor
Department of Clinical Studies
Cummings School of Veterinary Medicine at Tufts University
North Grafton, Massachusetts
Associate Veterinarian
Veterinary Internal Medicine Mobile Specialists
North Woodstock, Connecticut
Systemic Lupus Erythematosus

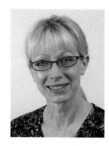

Beverly K. Sturges, DVM, MS, DACVIM
Assistant Clinical Professor
Neurology and Neurosurgery
Department of Surgical & Radiological Sciences
University of California
Davis, California
Sleep Disorders

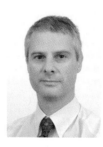

Simon Swift, MA, Vet MB, CertSAC, MRCVS
Rutland House Referrals
St. Helens, United Kingdom
Aldosterone Inhibitors

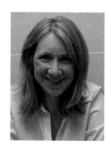

Jane E. Sykes, BVSc (Hons), PhD
Medicine & Epidemiology
University of California
Davis, California
Ehrlichia, Anaplasmosis, Rocky Mountain Spotted Fever, and Neorickettsial Infection
Hemoplasmosis

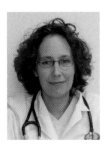

Harriet M. Syme, BVetMed, PhD, FHEA, DACVIM, DECVIM-ca, MRCVS
Senior Lecturer, Small Animal Internal Medicine
The Royal Veterinary College
North Mymms
Hatfield, Hertfordshire, United Kingdom
Canine Ureteral and Lower Urinary Tract Diseases

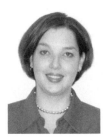

Rebecca S. Syring, DVM, DACVECC
Staff Veterinarian
Department of Clinical Studies
University of Pennsylvania
Philadelphia, Pennsylvania
Traumatic Brain Injury

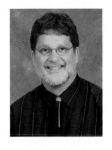

Joseph Taboada, DVM, DACVIM
Professor of Small Animal Internal Medicine
School of Veterinary Medicine
Louisiana State University
Baton Rouge, Louisiana
Histoplasmosis, Blastomycosis, Sporotrichosis, Candidiasis, Pythiosis, and Lagenidiosis
Cryptococcosis

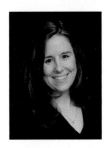

Kendall Taney, DVM, DAVDC
Partner
Center for Veterinary Dentistry and Oral Surgery
Gaithersburg, Maryland
Oral and Salivary Gland Disorders

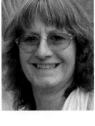

Polly M. Taylor, MA, VetMB, PhD, DECVAA, MRCA, MRCVS
Honorary Senior Lecturer
Department of Clinical Veterinary Science
University of Bristol
Langford, Bristol, United Kingdom
Hypothermia

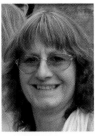

Alain P. Théon, DVM, MS, PhD, DACVR-RO1
Professor
School of Veterinary Medicine
University of California
Davis, California
Practical Radiation Therapy

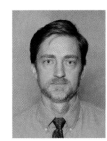

William B. Thomas, DVM, MS
Associate Professor, Neurology and Neurosurgery
College of Veterinary Medicine
University of Tennessee
Knoxville, Tennessee
Movement Disorders

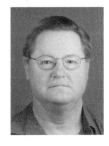

William P. Thomas, DVM, DACVIM (Cardiology)
Professor
Department of Medicine and Epidemiology
University of California
Davis, California
Congenital Heart Disease

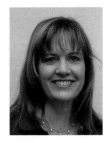

Melanie D. Thompson, DVM, MVSc, DACVIM
Internist
Small Animal Internal Medicine
Veterinary Medical and Surgical Group
Ventura, California
Ear Vein Blood Glucose Monitoring

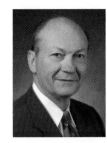

Walter R. Threlfall, DVM, MS, PhD, ACT
Director of Veterinary Continuing Education
College of Veterinary Medicine
The Ohio State University
Columbus, Ohio
Breeding Soundness Examination of the Stud Dog

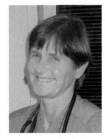

Anna Tidholm, DVM, PhD, DECVIM
Associate Professor
Albano Animal Hospital
Danderyd, Sweden
Pulse Alterations
Calcium Channel Blockers

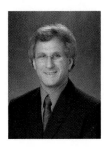

Anthony H. Tobias, BVSc, PhD, DACVIM (Cardiology)
Associate Professor
Veterinary Clinical Sciences Department
College of Veterinary Medicine
University of Minnesota
St. Paul, Minnesota
Pericardial Diseases

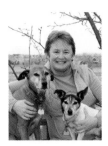

Todd L. Towell, DVM, MS, DACVIM
Manager, Scientific Communication
Department of Scientific Affairs
Hill's Pet Nutrition, Inc.
Topeka, Kansas
Nutrition-Related Skeletal Disorders

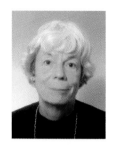

Anjop J. Venker-van Haagen, DVM, PhD, DECVS
Former Associate Professor of
  Veterinary Ear Nose & Throat
  Diseases
Faculty of Veterinary Medicine
University of Utrecht
Utrecht, Netherlands
Diseases of the Nose and Nasal Sinuses

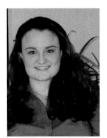

Anne M. Traas, DVM, DACT (Small Animal Reproduction)
Scientist IV, Pharmaceutical Clinical
  Development (R&D)
Boehringer Ingelheim Vetmedica, Inc.
St. Joseph, Missouri
Feline Reproduction

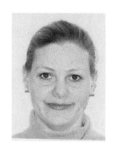

Susan W. Volk, VMD, PhD, DACVS
Assistant Professor of Surgery
School of Veterinary Medicine
University of Pennsylvania
Philadelphia, Pennsylvania
Hepatic and Splenic Emergencies

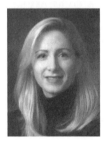

Teresa R. Tucci, DVM, DACVO
Ophthalmologist
Veterinary Specialists, Inc.
Homestead, Florida
Ophthalmologist
Department of Ophthalmology
All Animal Clinic
Key West, Florida
Acute Vision Loss in Small Animals

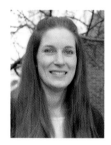

Lori S. Waddell, DVM, DACVECC
Adjunct Assistant Professor
Section of Critical Care, Department
  of Clinical Studies
School of Veterinary Medicine
University of Pennsylvania
Philadelphia, Pennsylvania
Systemic Anaphylaxis
Hypotension

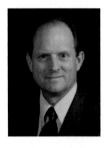

David C. Twedt, DVM, DACVIM
Professor
Department of Clinical Sciences
Colorado State University
Fort Collins, Colorado
Vomiting
*Endoscopic Procedures for Evaluation of
  the Gastrointestinal Tract*

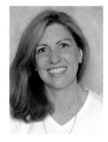

Cynthia R. Ward, VMD, PhD, DACVIM
Associate Professor of Medicine
Department of Small Animal Medicine
  and Surgery
University of Georgia
Athens, Georgia
Gastrointestinal Endocrine Disease

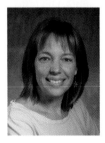

Shelly L. Vaden, DVM, PhD, DACVIM
Professor, Internal Medicine
College of Veterinary Medicine
North Carolina State University
Raleigh, North Carolina
Glomerular Diseases

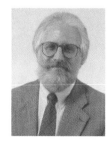

Robert J. Washabau, VMD, PhD, DACVIM (SAIM)
Professor of Medicine and Department
  Chair
Department of Veterinary Clinical
  Sciences
College of Veterinary Medicine
University of Minnesota
St. Paul, Minnesota
Feline Pancreatic Disease

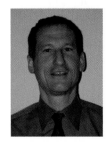

David M. Vail, DVM, MS, DACVIM (Oncology)
Professor of Oncology
University of Wisconsin
Madison, Wisconsin
Hematopoietic Tumors

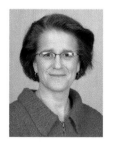

Cynthia R.L. Webster, DVM
Professor
Department of Clinical Science
Tufts Cummings School of Veterinary
  Medicine
Grafton, Massachusetts
*History, Clinical Signs, and Physical
  Findings in Hepatobiliary Disease*

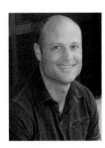

Chick Weisse, VMD, DACVS
Staff Veterinarian: Interventional
  Radiology/Surgery
Director of Interventional Radiology
The Animal Medical Center
New York, New York
Tracheal Stenting in Collapsed Trachea
Hepatic Vascular Anomalies

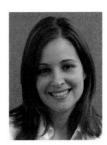

Carmenn Schaefer Woolley, DVM,
  DACVIM (SAIM)
Staff Internist
Department of Small Animal Internal
  Medicine
Bay Area Veterinary Specialists
San Leandro, California
Dysphagia and Regurgitation

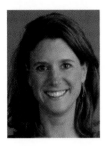

Jodi L. Westropp, DVM, PhD,
  DACVIM
Associate Professor
School of Veterinary Medicine
University of California
Davis, California
Lower Urinary Tract Disorders in Cats

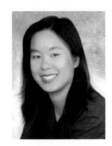

Kristine Yee, DVM, DACVIM
  (Cardiology)
Resident
Department of Cardiology
California Animal Hospital Veterinary
  Specialty Group
Los Angeles, California
Syncope

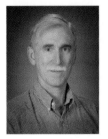

Michael D. Willard, DVM, MS,
  DACVIM
Professor
Department of Small Animal Clinical
  Services
Texas A&M University
College Station, Texas
Diarrhea
Inflammatory Canine Hepatic Disease

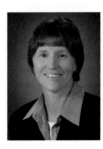

Debra L. Zoran, DVM, PhD,
  DACVIM-SAIM
Associate Professor and Chief of
  Medicine
Texas A&M University
College Station, Texas
The Unique Nutritional Needs of the
  Cat
Nutritional Management of
  Gastrointestinal Conditions

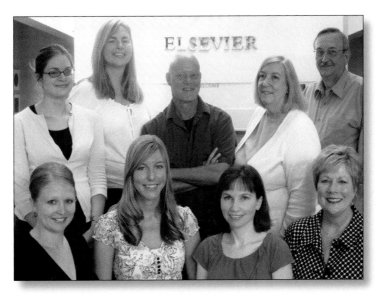

Bottom row, left to right: Shelly Stringer, Senior Developmental Editor; Lauren Harms; Associate Developmental Editor; Kristine Feeherty, Senior Project Manager; Penny Rudolph, Publisher. *Top row, left to right:* Leah Guerrero, Editorial Assistant; Lynn Hoops, Marketing Manager; Bruce Siebert, Producer; Patricia Tannian, Publishing Services Manager; Charlie Seibel, Book Designer.

As we complete the seventh edition of this textbook, we already are gathering information and ideas for the eighth! What started out years ago as an enjoyable way to collect information and write our own thoughts down on paper has been transformed into a greater effort, that of collecting the knowledge of our colleagues and collating it into a thorough, up to date, and scientifically fascinating resource. How this all happens is still somewhat of an enigma to us. Traditionally, many books the size and scope of this one have section editors to help with the preparation. We chose not to take advantage of section editors because the two of us understand the need to publish as quickly as possible after authors have completed their work. Consequently, we take the sole responsibility for putting this textbook together. This means finding authors, some experienced after participating in previous editions of this textbook, some who are well recognized but first-time contributors, and some who have just begun to establish their areas of expertise. All have been willing to devote time and energy to making their efforts coincide and coordinate with that of their peers and co-contributors.

Making the volumes flow together with cross-referencing and minimizing repetition has been a goal. However, there are subjects seen from different perspectives by individuals with differing areas of expertise. Certain subjects presented more than once may create the illusion of repetition, but we see each interpretation as adding value to the book. These different points of view have been purposefully presented.

This edition presents many changes and additions as compared with the first six editions. To avoid adding weight and length, some older subject matter was removed, as was some material no longer considered requisite to an internal medicine textbook. Contributors were asked to consolidate what they could. We altered the format in keeping with changing times. This edition has become quite "electronic." The entire book is online, and this electronic version will truly be a "living volume" where important changes, corrections, and additions may be found. We have added significant amounts of digitized material. Digital loops, videos, pictures, and charts can be found in the online textbook.

The videos alone are educational and exciting. Videos that could not be included in the written version because of length or simply an inability to put so much data in text are the most important new feature, unique to this edition. The use of color, for the first time throughout both written and electronic versions, also makes this seventh edition far superior to any of our previous efforts. Practitioners and students can find pictures and digitized videos of an astounding number of medical techniques and procedures. These can be seen (in several senses of the word) as supporting the notion that the seventh edition stands alone as an incredible teaching resource. Maneuvering through the book is exciting and fun! It is the intent of the editors to keep this material flowing, to increase and add more material throughout the life of the edition, and to update the literature continuously so that the reader may continue to use the Web site version as an up-to-the-minute resource of small animal internal medicine. References have been omitted from the written version in an attempt to be "green" (i.e., to save trees)! Instead, they are available on the Web site's living edition. Where possible, the references are linked to PubMed and should be easily resourced by the reader looking to explore the referenced works.

Other new aspects in this edition start at the beginning of the book. Here, the reader is taken to the heart of today's veterinary small animal internal medical practice. Pedagogy of learning and understanding diagnostic techniques is followed by a practical yet detailed discussion of genomics, both theoretical and practical. While recognizing the importance of the canine and feline genome, we also wish to emphasize the human-animal bond and the reality of euthanasia as part of our responsibility as veterinarians.

The introductory chapters are followed by chapters that lead readers through a guide to disease by clinical signs. Virtually every chapter here has been rewritten, renewed, or updated. Almost all chapters have at least one algorithm. High quality and thorough algorithms are extremely difficult to create but offer readers an opportunity to learn how to proceed from a potentially vague or nonspecific owner concern to a diagnosis. Further, algorithms are often employed when reviewing a patient's record to be certain that a question, physical examination finding, test, or differential diagnosis has not been overlooked. Here, and throughout the textbook, diagnostic techniques used in small animal internal medical practice demonstrate the "normal" as well as typical deviations from normal. These are available as videos, clips, pictures, and data on the Web site that make the chapters more valuable than ever before.

The importance of nutrition in medicine and the contribution of exciting new knowledge in understanding and diagnosing infectious diseases are presented. The traditional approach to understanding abnormalities in each of the organ systems follows. Each section has been expanded. Newer areas are emphasized with the inclusion of distinctly separate chapters. This is particularly true for nutrition, oncology, and infectious diseases. In most sections, information presented has been parsed into smaller subject areas to allow participation of more contributors with defined excellence. As a result, there are more than 300 primary authors for this edition and a much larger overall total number of participants. The textbook contributors include colleagues/specialists from around the world. We anticipate that this edition will be internationally accepted to a degree not previously achieved.

We welcome and thank all contributors for their time, effort, and willingness to share their knowledge. We commend them for adhering to strict timelines and wish to acknowledge them formally here. Without their cooperation, the content could never have been presented in such a brief time span that begins with chapter submission and culminates with publication. Readers have access to material that is incredibly "fresh." In many cases, chapters have been published within a few months of the time that data contained therein were published in peer-reviewed scientific journals!

We cannot thank the staff at Elsevier enough for their help, encouragement, and reliability. Penny Rudolph, our editor, has guided us tirelessly in this effort. Shelly Stringer, Lauren Harms, and Kristine Feeherty have been collegial, tireless, effective, and on time, and have provided the editors a partnership beyond our expectations when we began to "reinvent the wheel" for the seventh time! The electronic EMSS system has provided us with an advanced editorial and collection system that also exceeded our expectations. Kudos to our colleagues and partners in St. Louis.

Steve (Ettinger) and Ed (Feldman) have their own families and colleagues to individually acknowledge as this effort draws to a close. Steve's wife Pat never seems to tire of his being away from the family and in his study working on "the book." Steve is grateful that his younger children Michael, Robbie, and Ricky, even at their age, seem to understand the importance of this effort. His older children, Nicole and Andrew, already know the value of the textbook to their lives and their dad's professional life. To his nearly lifelong professional working partners, Ed Feldman and Etienne Côté, nothing short of "I love you" is due. Ed's wife Shawn has accepted this book as an anchor that sometimes limits their time together, but it also provides mutual understanding with regard to the love and respect they both have for animals and, specifically, the importance of pets in today's impersonal world. Ed's daughters Shaina and Rhonda, together with his son-in-law Steve, understand the importance of this work. Rowan Harper Feldman will learn, too, how her dad spent hours on the book in Guatemala while awaiting release of her visa so that she could join her new mom and dad on their trip back home. Heartfelt love is sent to Steve and Pat, Jimmy and Mary, Orin and Pat, the Monday night crew, and to all our relatives for their support. Tears flow and our hearts soar like eagles when we think of Shaina, Jennifer, Marilyn, Marie, Carol, Scott, Nan, and Tom joining us in Guatemala to help care for our beautiful and youngest little daughter.

We wish to acknowledge the pets that represent the core of the profession we serve. Katie (our Newf), Eliza (our Lab), Billy Gatito, Tooshie, and the lily-eating Jose (our DSHs), Jet (our noisy bird), and the fish and gecko, Spot, that live with our families, all speak to the importance we place on the human animal bond.

We offer our appreciation to our colleagues who consistently give us their feedback for each edition. We appreciate the compliments and continue to welcome your suggestions. No book of this size is without error. Now, we can add information and make corrections regularly on the Web version for you. Our medicine has changed enormously since 1975 when we began this effort. "One medicine" incorporates human and animal science, and the human-animal bond is what makes this book what it is. Thank you for allowing us to enjoy a space at your practice, home, and now on your computer!

Stephen Ettinger, Los Angeles, California
Edward Feldman, Berkeley, California
August 2009

Nothing in the world can take the place of persistence. Talent will not; nothing is more common than unsuccessful men with talent.
Genius will not; unrewarded genius is almost a proverb.
Education will not; the world is full of educated derelicts.
Persistence and determination alone are omnipotent.

—Calvin Coolidge (1872-1933)

CONTENTS

SECTION IV
Critical Care

SECTION V
Toxicology

SECTION I
The Real Basics of Veterinary Medicine

CHAPTER 1

The Physical Examination of the Dog and Cat

Stephen J. Ettinger

To Be a Great Physician, You Must Understand the Whole Story*

We physicians all have heroes during our training. We all remember the great physicians. I contend that the great physicians differ from the good physicians because they understand the entire story. Only when we understand the complete story do we make consistent diagnoses.

Each patient represents a story. That story includes their diseases, their new problem, their social situation, and their beliefs.

How do we understand the story? We must develop excellent communication skills and gather the history in appropriate depth. We must perform a targeted physical examination based on the historical clues. We must order the correct diagnostic tests, and interpret them in the context of the history and physical exam. Once we collect the appropriate data, we then should construct that patient's story.

The story includes making the correct diagnosis or diagnoses. The story must describe the patient's context. Who is this patient? What are the patient's goals? How might the patient's personal situation impact our treatment options?

Sir William Osler said, "The good physician treats the disease; the great physician treats the patient who has the disease." The great physician understands the patient and the context of that patient's illness.

Dr. Robert Centor, Professor of Medicine at the University of Alabama, Birmingham

The physical examination begins long before the veterinarian ever touches the animal. The traditional teachings of look, smell, and listen are as important as ever. Excellent veterinarians avoid making diagnostic decisions driven by laboratory-derived data that bypass the physical examination. Correlation of all data is relevant to the determination of an appropriate diagnosis. This chapter is dedicated to the concept that veterinarians must bring together data from the history, physical examination, and diagnostic tests to care for an animal in the context of its life—including the life the owner envisions for the pet. The second chapter that follows helps the reader to utilize this book and instructs on the benefits of the algorithm as part of the decision-making process. Note that the algorithm by itself has extremely limited value without an excellent physical examination and the historical aspects being considered. I encourage the young and inexperienced clinician to carefully peruse both this and the next chapter to help identify the necessary parts of the decision-making system that ultimately results in a sustainable diagnosis.

When possible, the animal's temperature and weight should be recorded before the veterinarian enters the examination room. This provides the nursing staff the chance to communicate with the animal's caretaker, gather pertinent information, note changes in weight, and identify the owner's concerns or requests.

This also is a good time for the staff to record any drugs currently administered, the prophylactic agents used (e.g., for heartworms, ectoparasites, internal parasites and other endemic processes that affect the living region of that area), the animal's vaccination status, and its reproductive status (i.e., spayed, neutered, or last heat cycle). Receiving information on the current medications and diet being administered can save valuable doctor time and should be noted in the record. Notation of medication administration should always be accompanied by the owner's perception of its efficacy, since this information may influence future treatment and prognosis. Nursing and technical staff may also utilize this time to provide valuable information to the client on subjects that the veterinarian often speeds through. Such examples include new vaccine programs, wellness programs, microchipping information, behavioral hints, and products to aid in training and health.

The process should be as expeditious as possible, and every effort should be made to provide the client with an on-time, efficient examination. Reading material (magazines of interest to a wide variety of clients and their children) should be available if there is a likelihood of the pet's caretaker having to wait. Pet owners should be given an indication as to the doctor's schedule and the length of any delay. Providing the client

*Medscape General Medicine, 9(1):59, 2007. © 2007 Medscape.

with this information can offset frustration, anger, or anxiety. If the hospital has new client brochures about its methods and services, this is a good time to deliver these and to allow the client to browse through the material.

OBSERVING THE PET AND MEETING THE CARETAKER: THE HISTORY

Every veterinarian approaches a pet in his or her own way. With time, it becomes second nature. It is important to develop proper animal handling skills. Furthermore, clients observe a great deal during this process and may determine long before any recommendations are made just how trusting they will be. Gentle care, compassion, concern, and attention cannot be emphasized enough.

The process begins as the veterinarian enters the area where the owner and pet are waiting. A friendly greeting and a small but appropriate amount of banter are usually appreciated. An occasional client makes it clear that the veterinarian should get down to business immediately, and in such situations, it is wise to do so. People appreciate being greeted and particularly like being acknowledged. Asking owners about something specific to them assures them that the veterinarian knows who they are. If the case is a referral, noting the distance traveled or offering a kind word about the trip acknowledges the client in an important way. It is not a technique easily taught, and it is not difficult to see whether the veterinarian "gets it" quickly and learns to communicate or simply turns away from such contact.

The importance of letting each client know that the veterinarian cares about him or her and the pet cannot be overemphasized. This must be done in a genuine way, reflected in dialog, attention, body language, and actions, and not in a lip service way, such as just having "We care" or some other logo stamped on hospital leashes or stationery. Every successful veterinarian can relate tales about brilliant doctors whom clients dislike! The smartest veterinarian may never have the opportunity to demonstrate his or her skills if concern and caring are not expressed in a way that is meaningful to the client. In fact, clients are likely to be antagonistic toward veterinarians who fail to express compassion. Complaints are likely to be made much more frequently about an arrogant veterinarian than about one who is poorly trained or medically inadequate but friendly and compassionate. Professionals with a disproportionately higher number of malpractice claims may be readily separated from those with fewer claims by evaluation of their examination room attitude.

A skilled veterinarian or physician understands that no part of the entire examination is as important as carefully listening to the client. Therefore, adequate time must be allowed for this interaction in an environment that enhances the process. Examination rooms should be comfortable and inviting. Privacy for clients is necessary, because the situation may be a difficult one for them. Decisions that may seem routine and perhaps even minor to the veterinarian may not be perceived as such by the owner.

If there has been a delay, it is paramount that the doctor acknowledges this upon entering the room. The veterinarian should show clients the courtesy of recognizing that they have been waiting. Unnecessary interruptions should be minimized, and every hospital should have a policy in this regard. In a large critical care office, delays and interruptions do occur, but these must be limited. Phone calls should be restricted to those that are professionally relevant or urgent. When such calls interrupt me while with new clients, I explain that I need to speak with other owners about their hospitalized pet, yet I do try to make it clear that I am focusing on their own pet's problems.

It is important to get the owners' version of the history and not one that has been "dictated" to them. For example, when questioned, the owners may acknowledge that a friend or family member told them about the supposed problem. Further questioning may determine that the owners themselves have not noted any clinical signs that warrant concern.

Computers today are commonly used to make notations during the history and examination process. It is important to physically place these in such a way that eye contact with the owner is not lost. If the owner feels that the computer takes precedence to the history, an important part of the examination and history taking may be lost; or worse, the owner may feel disregarded and dissatisfied. Benefits of computer tablets include their being portable and easily managed in front of the client.

There is no single technique for the examination process. Because this chapter is intended to explain my method of examination, I will delineate the regimen I follow, a process learned over decades of experience. When possible, I try to immediately make eye and physical contact with the pet. Even before beginning the process of taking a history, I try to welcome the pet. First, I make a brief attempt at greeting the animal by extending the back of my hand to its face. For this, cats and smaller dogs can be placed on the examination room table. Usually, with medium to large dogs, I kneel down on the examination room floor to greet the animal (I use a gardener's pad to protect my knees). Of course, some dogs and cats (those in cages, particularly) let me know beforehand that they are not ready for such a greeting. Then, I bypass the greeting and make a light comment to the owners about the pet not wishing me well (after all, I say, "Who likes going to the doctor?"). This begins a conversation with the owners that acknowledges the possibility of the pet being fearful and allows the owners to let me know how they feel about the process.

Clients are likely to want to tell the veterinarian what they know, think, or understand about the pet's problems. Regardless of how clearly and confidently clients relate their interpretation of their companion's difficulties, it is essential for the examiner to "go back to square one" and self-interpret the pet's problem. Thus, the client's opinion and the veterinarian's analysis run in parallel: Enough confidence must be placed in the client's story to solidify the trust being developed during this important part of the examination, but the veterinarian must also think independently enough to avoid being led down the wrong path of deduction. I like to give clients a few minutes to express themselves, regardless of the relevance, because what they have to say is likely to be important to the ultimate outcome of the process. For example, clients may refuse to acknowledge how sick the pet is, or they may be worried about "cancer" or may focus on something that may not be pertinent. Clients' comments provide valuable insight into their concern and desire to care for the pet. There are different levels of owner commitment, and pets thus receive varied levels of medical attention.

Clients may offer information obtained from friends, breeders, or sources such as the Internet and may wish to have the veterinarian go over this material. A reasonable technique the veterinarian can use that precludes taking time away from the office call is to acknowledge the request and inform the caretaker that the material will be reviewed once the examination and early decision-making processes have been completed.

An owner's expectations may seem to convey that, "OK, you are the doctor, so you tell me what is wrong." A different tack then becomes necessary, and the approach changes from "Tell me what you have observed" to "It appears that your dog (or cat) has been losing weight; tell me, has this been a recent occurrence?" This may be all that is necessary to get the owners to begin talking about their pet.

Not every owner-veterinarian experience is informative. Valuable information is noted in the record. If the client refuses to provide a history or begins to attack another veterinarian, these comments should be noted in the record. The record provides not only a future legal defense but also a guide to further owner communication for myself and my colleagues. Clients who have been dissatisfied with the results of prior care reasonably object when the same medications are prescribed for their pet. It suggests that the current veterinarian has not been listening. Inquiring in an unobtrusive manner about the owners' needs and desires helps define their wishes and permits the veterinarian to provide options from which the owners can choose.

Specifics about drugs currently being administered should be reviewed. The drug's name, dosage, and frequency of administration are significant. The veterinarian should also ask about prior drugs that may have been prescribed, including over-the-counter (OTC) products, prescriptions from other veterinarians, and holistic products. This is the time to inquire about the foods the animal is currently fed, prior diets provided, canned or kibbled formulations, supplements added, and treats given. The specifics of oral, topical, and injectable prophylactic products administered at home should be identified.

Information should be gathered regarding out-of-area travel and areas where the pet (or other pets in the family) previously may have lived. Clients should be questioned about the welfare of other pets currently living in the household. The vaccination history is needed for each pet in the household, particularly when laboratory tests for infectious diseases affected by prior exposure or vaccines are under consideration.

The history and the owner's story are equally important. These convey to the examiner the owner's perceptions, needs, and desires during this initial period of acquaintance or contact. I find that this can be the most useful time of the examination process. I can touch the pet, gently stroke it, feel the quality of the haircoat and skin, determine the hydration status, and generally get a good idea of the animal's physical well-being (e.g., debilitated or well conditioned, obese or thin, and so on) (Figures 1-1 and 1-2).

This is also a convenient time to gently examine the pet without the animal being fearful, because a pet may be more aware of its owner's voice than of the veterinarian going over its body. This also allows me to determine the animal's behavior and gives the client a feeling of assurance that I am getting to know or am reacquainting myself with the pet. Pets generally seem less fearful while I am at their eye level and when I refer to them by name. Thus the physical examination begins while the history is still being taken.

It is not always possible to begin the examination process during this period, and I do not make a distinct effort to perform every examination this way. If the dog or cat is sitting anxiously (i.e., protectively or in a frightened manner) in the client's lap, I avoid this contact and dwell on the pet and the owner's story. Pets relax during this period and are less fearful of me as time goes by. A truly frightened or fractious animal presents a different situation, which may require use of a muzzle or, even better, an examination away from the owner in an environment that no longer requires the pet to feel it is protecting the owner. It is important to remember that owners should not be allowed to hold their pets during any examination process that entails a likelihood of injury to anyone in contact with a frightened or injured pet. This remains a chronically differing point of view amongst veterinarians. Many clients wish to hold their own pet, yet the veterinarian is responsible for any injuries that may occur. Too, the pet is often more likely to be irritable and protective while being held by the owner. On the other hand, many owners feel uncomfortable not holding their pet. Thus, the examining doctor must use caution, experience, and the cues provided by the owner and the animal to determine what is the best approach under these circumstances. Most importantly, remember to be very careful and to avoid situations that are likely to result in a bite wound injury to the owner, the veterinarian, or anyone else in close proximity to the pet. When a dog or cat reacts adversely to the veterinarian, it is important to back off slowly, reassess the process, and move forward in a manner that is safe for all involved. Usually the client recognizes the need for this. When the client insists on holding a fractious animal, the veterinarian needs to step up and identify the need for a safe process to continue, often with the client out of direct sight.

INITIATING THE PHYSICAL EXAMINATION

The physical examination commences when the veterinarian enters the examination room. The clinician should look at the general appearance of the pet, note odors, and observe irregularities. A severely sick or crisis presentation requires a different approach from that used for a dog or cat with a mild or chronic problem. Clients must also be observed and evaluated. They are prone to be particularly anxious in severe or acute life-threatening situations, although such anxiety may manifest in a spectrum of ways (ranging from a quiet, stunned composure to near-hysteria) that the skilled veterinarian will consider when beginning the discussion with the owner. In these and less emotionally charged situations, the veterinarian should assess the owner's state when first approaching the pet. Intense questioning may be inappropriate if the owner feels that the pet needs immediate medical attention.

When observing the patient, the veterinarian should listen for abnormal breathing sounds or grunting. The animal's body size and posture also should be observed: a plantigrade stance could suggest a neuropathy; neck ventroflexion in cats may indicate hypokalemia; fat pets may be overfed, hypothyroid, or inactive; thin pets may be systemically ill or underfed. It is true that owners may point out these irregularities, but they may misinterpret such changes or may simply not be cognizant of their significance. In a desire to "wish well" for the pet, the owner also may fail to provide information for fear of its significance. The veterinarian has the responsibility to seek out this information.

Examples of signs and symptoms the veterinarian may observe upon entering the examination area are presented in this textbook under the section "Clinical Manifestations of Disease." The chapters in this section are not "complete," because the variety of maladies and the manifestations of disease are infinite. Suffice it to say that the examination process must not be so quick or superficial that an obvious underlying problem is overlooked.

If the animal is ambulatory and has a history of lameness, neurologic deficit, or weakness, it is essential that the veterinarian watch the animal move. This may be done before or after the hands-on physical examination process. At some point during this initial phase of the examination, the veterinarian must observe the pet's gait. This may require having the pet walk on a surface with adequate traction and preferably with the owner as the handler. Lameness, signs of neurologic deficits, or irregularity in gait and appearance is noted. The physical examination is continued, and the clinician attempts to mechanically evaluate any specific lameness or suggestion of a localized abnormality (e.g., patella luxation, stifle cruciate drawer sign, elbow pain or mass).

Nestlé PURINA

BODY CONDITION SYSTEM

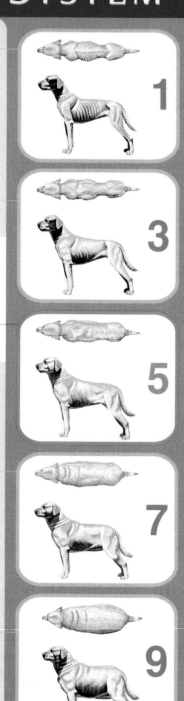

TOO THIN

1 Ribs, lumbar vertebrae, pelvic bones and all bony prominences evident from a distance. No discernible body fat. Obvious loss of muscle mass.

2 Ribs, lumbar vertebrae and pelvic bones easily visible. No palpable fat. Some evidence of other bony prominence. Minimal loss of muscle mass.

3 Ribs easily palpated and may be visible with no palpable fat. Tops of lumbar vertebrae visible. Pelvic bones becoming prominent. Obvious waist and abdominal tuck.

IDEAL

4 Ribs easily palpable, with minimal fat covering. Waist easily noted, viewed from above. Abdominal tuck evident.

5 Ribs palpable without excess fat covering. Waist observed behind ribs when viewed from above. Abdomen tucked up when viewed from side.

TOO HEAVY

6 Ribs palpable with slight excess fat covering. Waist is discernible viewed from above but is not prominent. Abdominal tuck apparent.

7 Ribs palpable with difficulty; heavy fat cover. Noticeable fat deposits over lumbar area and base of tail. Waist absent or barely visible. Abdominal tuck may be present.

8 Ribs not palpable under very heavy fat cover, or palpable only with significant pressure. Heavy fat deposits over lumbar area and base of tail. Waist absent. No abdominal tuck. Obvious abdominal distention may be present.

9 Massive fat deposits over thorax, spine and base of tail. Waist and abdominal tuck absent. Fat deposits on neck and limbs. Obvious abdominal distention.

The BODY CONDITION SYSTEM was developed at the Nestlé Purina PetCare Center and has been validated as documented in the following publications:

Mawby D, Bartges JW, Moyers T, et. al. *Comparison of body fat estimates by dual-energy x-ray absorptiometry and deuterium oxide dilution in client owned dogs.* Compendium 2001; 23 (9A): 70

Laflamme DP. *Development and Validation of a Body Condition Score System for Dogs.* Canine Practice July/August 1997; 22:10-15

Kealy, et. al. *Effects of Diet Restriction on Life Span and Age-Related Changes in Dogs.* JAVMA 2002; 220:1315-1320

Call 1-800-222-VETS (8387), weekdays, 8:00 a.m. to 4:30 p.m. CT

Nestlé PURINA

Figure 1-1 Body condition chart for the dog. (Used by permission from Nestlé Purina Petcare.)

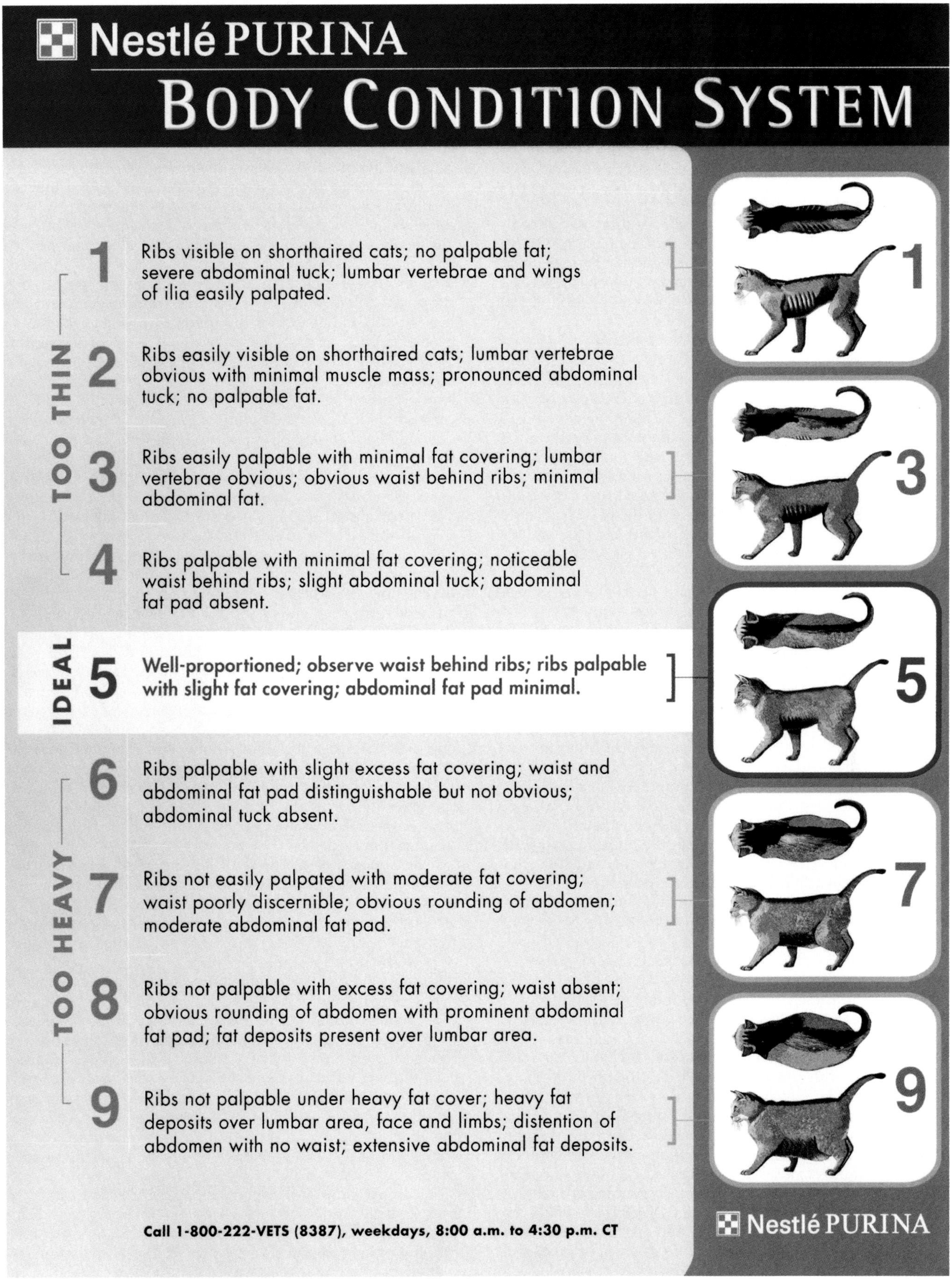

▦ Nestlé PURINA

BODY CONDITION SYSTEM

TOO THIN

1 Ribs visible on shorthaired cats; no palpable fat; severe abdominal tuck; lumbar vertebrae and wings of ilia easily palpated.

2 Ribs easily visible on shorthaired cats; lumbar vertebrae obvious with minimal muscle mass; pronounced abdominal tuck; no palpable fat.

3 Ribs easily palpable with minimal fat covering; lumbar vertebrae obvious; obvious waist behind ribs; minimal abdominal fat.

4 Ribs palpable with minimal fat covering; noticeable waist behind ribs; slight abdominal tuck; abdominal fat pad absent.

IDEAL

5 Well-proportioned; observe waist behind ribs; ribs palpable with slight fat covering; abdominal fat pad minimal.

TOO HEAVY

6 Ribs palpable with slight excess fat covering; waist and abdominal fat pad distinguishable but not obvious; abdominal tuck absent.

7 Ribs not easily palpated with moderate fat covering; waist poorly discernible; obvious rounding of abdomen; moderate abdominal fat pad.

8 Ribs not palpable with excess fat covering; waist absent; obvious rounding of abdomen with prominent abdominal fat pad; fat deposits present over lumbar area.

9 Ribs not palpable under heavy fat cover; heavy fat deposits over lumbar area, face and limbs; distention of abdomen with no waist; extensive abdominal fat deposits.

Call 1-800-222-VETS (8387), weekdays, 8:00 a.m. to 4:30 p.m. CT

▦ Nestlé PURINA

Figure 1-2 Body condition chart for the cat. (Used by permission from Nestlé Purina Petcare.)

A review of previous examination notes for prior irregularities can aid the clinical assessment. For example, comparing the size of a mass with previous findings is something clients appreciate, particularly if the records clearly identify prior dimensions, appearance, and location. Measurement of lesions with calipers or a ruler is good for review and trend purposes. Current availability of digital photography make this a useful technique to consider, particularly if these digitized images can be attached to the record.

Neurologic changes, such as diminished conscious proprioception, diminished muscle tone, limb dragging, or unusual pain during compression of the muscles or lumbosacral compression, are noted and may require further investigation to point to a diagnosis. Something can be said for performing at this time the "stand back" examination, which allows the veterinarian to observe breathing patterns or abdominal changes.

Every seasoned veterinarian has developed his or her own method of performing the physical examination, derived from a wealth of experience. For example, animals are frightened by a large figure looming overhead and are less anxious when approached at eye level. Therefore, as mentioned before, I prefer to kneel on the examination room floor to perform the physical examination (except for cats and small dogs). I find I am better able to perform auscultation completely and thoroughly in this way, and I also am able to palpate more thoroughly while having a good presence with the pet. Particularly with the neophyte examiner, there is something to be said for having most animals in the same position each time for the examination.

After the initial greeting, I prefer to stroke the pet to gain a more generalized knowledge of the overall body status. The body composition score is assessed (see Figures 1-1 and 1-2), as is hydration status, weight change, physical appearance, and the condition of the haircoat. Masses (size, shape, and appearance) are noted. I then examine the entire torso by touch, attempting to define the patient's status. Findings may include abdominal enlargement (fluid, fat, distention, pain), discomfort, and skin or musculoskeletal abnormalities (masses, changes in the haircoat, open wounds, fleas, dirt, ticks, or other abnormalities). Looking for bumps, lumps, or irregularities, I am able to distinguish lymph node changes, pain or swelling in the joints or limbs, physical deformities, and the nature of the femoral pulse. I evaluate the pulse, including its rate, quality, and character (see Chapter 67), and listen for any irregularities while auscultating the heart.

Swelling in the form of edema or fluid collections is correlated with other changes. Edema is identified as being generalized, localized to one limb or region, or associated with abdominal fluid and is noted to be pitting, cold, warm, or oozing in nature.

Specific lameness associated with trauma is identified and may provide an obvious cause; however, the veterinarian should not make that assumption without giving reasonable consideration to other possible causes (e.g., a pathologic fracture in a dog with osteosarcoma). I like to run both hands down the animal's body to check for asymmetry in body form.

Skin and coat changes must be evaluated in light of the animal's living arrangements, as established in conversation with the caretaker. Indoor pets should not have foreign body material in the coat; fleas, flea dirt, ticks, and other ectoparasites should not be present. Hair loss or thinning is a clue to clinical disease and should be noted. Hair loss should be assessed as unilateral or bilateral, and its full significance should be identified in the records. Coat changes must also be correlated with other body changes that may indicate a systemic illness, such as Cushing's disease. Areas of skin change should be evaluated and comments made with respect to the potential benefit of skin or hair culture, skin scraping,

skin biopsy or allergy testing. Pets that live outdoors are more likely to have ectoparasites, weather-related haircoat changes, or bite wounds. As with the indoor pet, these skin conditions must be correlated with the clinical signs and recommendations made accordingly. Coats with a strong odor of perfume or smoke may indicate to the examiner possible problems with regard to allergic lung disease, highly reactive lungs, or an animal that has been in or around a fire.

My preference is to progress the physical examination from the head toward the tail. First, hydration status and mucous membrane color and moisture should be identified. Pain on dorsiflexion or ventroflexion or lateral movement of the head and neck is significant and may be noted when the head is first moved. Pain noted on movement of the head and neck may also be an indication of lower back disease and the pet is reacting to any movement that may induce such pain. The head first should be examined superficially for any changes or problems, such as hair loss or swelling. Areas of discomfort or irregularity are observed. The appearance of the mucous membranes (e.g., pallor gives reason to suspect anemia, hypoperfusion, or hypoxemia), oral cavity, pharynx, and teeth are recorded. Signs of drooling, discharge, or malodor from the oral region should be apparent at this time. It is important for the veterinarian to speak to the owner about the condition of the pet's teeth and gums; it also is important for the owner to see, if possible, any unexpected finding in the oral cavity.

A brief cranial nerve examination can be included during this portion of the examination process. The way the pet holds its mouth closed, the functions both of sensation and of motor ability of the maxillary muscles, and the appearance of the eyes may be relevant. Monitoring for superficial and deep changes within the globes and the periorbital region extends this process. Ophthalmic sensitivity, squinting, or photophobia is recorded. Any discharge is noted and described as to color, composition, and volume and whether the discharge is unilateral or bilateral. Tear production is recorded (Schirmer tear testing), as is nasolacrimal duct patency (e.g., dry, cracked nasal tissue). If nystagmus, strabismus, or other deviations of one or both globes are noted, the veterinarian continues the examination while looking for signs of conjunctival color changes or inflammation. Pupillary size, symmetry, and integrity are noted, as is the pupillary light response, both direct and consensual. Sensation in the eyelids and the surrounding tissue is observed.

The appearance of the skull, the muscles of mastication, and the muscles around the head are noted. Clients frequently suggest that a mass has developed in the occipital region associated with weight loss as the temporal muscles atrophy (external occipital protuberance). Enophthalmos can be a sign of periorbital fat loss and may relate to myositis, weight loss, cachexia, or a primary ophthalmic process. Pain, swelling, or heat in any region is observed. More detailed examination of the eyes, including direct and/or indirect ophthalmoscopy, may be completed at this time; or, if there are suggestions of change, the examiner first may complete the rest of the physical and then perform this part of the eye examination.

Airflow through the nostrils can be quickly assessed using a stethoscope and contralateral compression of the nares or by allowing the pet to breathe onto a metal surface (e.g., a countertop in the examination room) or glass microscope slide.

Examination of the ears, pinnae, and ear canals is expected by the client and is an important part of **every** veterinary physical examination. This is particularly relevant in the new puppy or kitten examination as a check for ear mites, inflammation, or odor. An owner may report that a pet has difficulty eating or chewing, but the problem may in fact be caused by pain from one or both ear canals. Discharge, unusual odor, or discoloration of the canal tissue may be noted. Owners are more likely to notice abnormal conditions of the pinnae (e.g., aural hematoma), but even without such information, the pinnae must be examined. Superficial examination of the ear canal can usually be accomplished in the examination room without difficulty, allowing the veterinarian to discuss chronic ear disease with the owners while showing them the abnormality. Videootoscopy is a preferred technique by some veterinarians to show the caregiver changes in the ear canal.

The integrity of the jaw bite must be determined, as well as the loss of teeth, or the presence of extra teeth. The color of the mucous membranes, capillary refill time, ulcers, color of the tongue, discolorations, and neurologic integrity are identified. The teeth are examined for calculus, caries, fractures, displacement, or discoloration. Abnormalities are recorded and mentioned to the owner. Signs of dental wear due to fence biting or rock chewing should be noted, as well as any resulting sensitivity. Gingival hyperplasia, masses, gingivitis, or ulcers may correlate with clinical signs. In first-time puppy or kitten examinations, evaluation for cleft palate or other congenital defects is required. With an uncooperative or fractious animal, examination of the oral cavity can be a daunting procedure. When the pet resists such an examination, removal to a treatment area away from the owner often allows further examination without difficulty. Special attention is always required in dogs that are aggressive, drooling, or have a behavioral change. Concern for a rabid patient is always paramount.

Evaluation of the pharyngeal region is limited to external palpation during the physical examination. In some dogs, depressing the caudal tongue with the index finger allows visualization of the tonsils and oropharynx. However, comprehensive visualization is rarely possible, and if an indication of an abnormality exists in the pharyngeal or laryngeal region, a more thorough examination under sedation should be encouraged. The tongue should be elevated (using dorsally directed pressure with the thumb externally, between the mandibles) to assess the sublingual region, such as for linear foreign bodies in cats. The laryngeal region should be checked for sensitivity, pain, or masses or institution of the gag reflex. Detection of visible or palpable deformities and monitoring of the laryngeal apparatus may yet be possible without sedation.

Moving to the ventral cervical region, the veterinarian evaluates for masses, tracheal sensitivity, and enlargement of the lymph nodes or thyroid gland. At the thoracic inlet, the clinician examines for lymph node enlargement, crepitus (subcutaneous air leakage), or other masses. Asymmetry of the thorax (scapula, muscles, rib cage, masses, or fat accumulation) should be correlated with signs, as should kyphosis or sternal deformities. Breathing difficulty can be associated with changes in the appearance of the rib cage. Fluid accumulation in the thoracic cavity, significant pleural or pulmonary disease, and some muscle disturbances cause the rib cage to feel or appear abnormal. Congenital thoracic deformities may cause respiratory signs. Peritoneal-pericardial diaphragmatic hernia (PPDH) may be associated with deformities of the xiphoid region of the sternum, such that the examiner can insert a finger into the thoracic cavity and sometimes actually touch the heart.

My preference is to complete the entire physical examination before auscultating lung and heart sounds. These portions of the physical examination are described in Chapters 64 and 66. When palpating the thorax, the examiner should notice the location of the palpable apex beat of the heart. Normally this is over the left fourth to sixth intercostal space at the level of the costochondral junction. Deviations imply cardiac or thoracic cavity diseases. Similarly, palpation of a cardiac thrill is indicative of an extremely loud heart murmur (greater than grade 4/6). Cardiac thrills are usually found at the apex beat

but may be displaced; they should be identified and correlated with the heart sounds and clinical signs.

Progressing caudally to the abdomen, the examiner first should note whether the abdominal wall is pumping rapidly, a possible sign of anxiety, tachypnea, or dyspnea. Tachypnea and dyspnea are observed; they are not recognized through auscultation.

The general appearance of the abdomen is the first thing the clinician should assess. Distended, tucked up, muscular and firm, painful, tense, soft and doughy are all terms used to describe the abdomen. Abdominal pain should be characterized as coming from the abdomen, and distinguished from impostors such as pain caused by musculoskeletal dysfunction (e.g., disk disease) or just plain annoyance with being examined. Not all pets are happy to be in the veterinarian's office, and many display their displeasure this way; it should not be mistaken for a pathologic process.

Examination of the abdomen, as with all other parts of the body, should be performed systematically. Examining the outside of the abdomen and spinal column first and then moving deeper with systematic palpation allows the clinician to review body systems in an organized manner.

During either the initial portion of the abdominal examination or at this time, the veterinarian has the opportunity to examine the mammary glands and surrounding tissue. Large lumps in the mammary tissue are usually easily recognized; however smaller, nondiscrete lesions may require more intensive evaluation and palpation. Carefully moving the finger tips up or down the chain on both sides permits the examiner to note discrepancies in the tissue. Likewise, enlargement of the sublumbar lymph nodes may be noted. In the male, changes in and around the prepuce are identified. Preputial discharge, a small amount of a thin, yellowish color, which is normal, may not be readily seen unless the pet is placed in lateral recumbency. Extruding the penis to appreciate changes in the mucosa or sheath of the penis helps explain abnormal findings or a history of licking. In the male cat, evaluation of the penis and its surrounding area is important, particularly in cases of suspected feline urinary tract disease. Neutered tomcats have small to no spines present on the penis, in contrast to intact tomcats.

Palpation of the abdomen is an individually determined technique. I like to examine animals both from behind and from the side. When examining the abdomen from behind, I am able to palpate for bilateral changes, to assess the kidneys more accurately, and to identify midabdominal masses. Lateral palpation provides a clearer indication of hepatomegaly, splenomegaly, bladder stones, or an enlarged bladder. Occasionally it is helpful to pick up the pet and allow it to stand on the hind legs so that the abdominal viscera falls caudally, permitting a more comprehensive examination.

Distention of the abdominal cavity requires differentiation. In general, there are four major causes of abdominal enlargement: fluid or fat accumulation, muscle laxity, and abdominal organ enlargement. The examination begins with gentle ballottement to determine whether the cause is obesity, pregnancy, fluid accumulation, one or more masses, internal obstruction, muscle weakness, or simply poor muscle condition. Correlating the findings of this examination with the weight and temperature allows the veterinarian to consider abnormal results.

It is generally easier to perform a complete abdominal palpation examination on the cat and many smaller dogs than it is on larger dogs. In cats, it is frequently possible to palpate the intestines, spleen, kidneys, and bladder carefully. In larger companion animals this may not be possible, but there is still much that can be appreciated, such as enlargement of abdominal organs, masses, and fluid collections. In cats, palpation of an enlarged spleen often is a sign suggesting mast cell disease, lymphoma, or another neoplastic process. In dogs, a large, irregular splenic margin strongly suggests hemangiosarcoma or hematoma, although other causes of splenomegaly must be considered (see Chapters 194 and 327). Differentiation from other abdominal masses may be done initially through the physical examination and later by radiographic and/or ultrasonographic monitoring.

Pain upon palpation of the abdomen is a significant sign. Pain requires distinction between referred spinal pain, abdominal pain, generalized pain, and discomfort. The acute abdomen needs correlation with laboratory tests and clinical signs. Pain should be localized, if possible, as cranial, midabdominal, caudal, or generalized. Palpation for masses and the detection of enlarged viscera comprise an art that is not replaced by more sophisticated, expensive, and complicated tests. Pain in the abdomen is a clear indicator for further testing, including radiography, ultrasonography, and laboratory analyses. It also must be correlated with the clinical history. Malaise, failure to move or change position, fever, and nausea may be explained by abdominal pain, whereas a fractious cat, ears back and pupils dilated, that has a tense abdomen may simply be displeased with being examined.

Distention of the abdomen must be correlated with clinical signs (e.g., hair loss, polyuria/polydipsia, paper-thin, scaly skin), fluid collection, pregnancy, neurologic changes, and disease, most notably liver and splenic neoplasia. Urinary bladder distention should be palpable and defined. The kidneys often can be palpated bilaterally if enlarged in the dog and are usually palpable normally in the cat. In most dogs and cats, the left kidney normally can be palpated under all circumstances except when the animal is obese. The right kidney of the dog usually can be palpated only when it is enlarged or displaced. The presence of a large or painful prostate should be noted and correlated with clinical signs. Symmetric enlargement of the fat pads and muscles of the lumbar region (love handles) are commonly seen in an older pet, particularly if it is gaining weight.

Palpation of the abdomen is best completed with the dog or cat standing and with the examiner's fingers kept close together. If the thumb is allowed to rest on the spinal tissue and extreme pressure is exerted, the examiner may misinterpret pain as abdominal rather than spinal (induced by the thumb pressure).

The examination of the caudal abdomen is completed by rectal palpation, which is performed in older male dogs or when signs suggest lower bowel dysfunction, possible lower urinary tract problems, or hind end disorders of an orthopedic or neurologic nature. Rectal palpation has increased in importance with the increased prevalence of abdominal sonography, because lesions within the pelvic canal usually cannot be imaged well sonographically. Prostatic abnormalities are likely to be palpated per rectum in all but the largest male dogs. Correct palpation of the prostate is done with the index finger of one hand and simultaneous cupping with the other hand (via external, dorsocaudal pressure on the caudal abdomen to elevate the prostate gland toward the palpating finger). This is especially useful for larger dogs and/or shorter index fingers. A normal rectal examination identifies a symmetric, bilobed, nonpainful, rubbery-textured prostate gland with a median raphe that clearly separates the two lobes. The peripheral tissue should evoke no pain or irregularity along the canal wall or the bony pelvic structure surrounding the gland. A thin, flat tube is usually palpable on either side of the pelvic symphysis, and this is the urethra. A thickened, ropy urethra may be felt in cases of urethritis or transitional cell carcinoma. Rotation of the hand so the palm points dorsally then allows the examiner to palpate the aortic trifurcation and aortic pulse, and may allow the palpation of sacral (sublumbar) lymph nodes if enlarged. A complete rotation of the wrist

(180° in each direction) is warranted, to identify masses or other abnormalities of the pelvic canal.

Upon entering the rectum, the examiner palpates the anal sacs at the 4 and 8 o'clock positions to determine whether they are enlarged and if they can be readily expressed. The ease with which these glands can be expressed and the type of fluid released aids the evaluation for anal sac disease. Many clients worry considerably about "full" anal sacs, and it is important to identify problems if they exist. It also is necessary to establish adequate dietary measures in dogs with problems so that the anal sacs can be expressed spontaneously when the animal has a bowel movement. Serious anal sac disease does occur in the feline species, albeit uncommonly. The rectal tissue should be neither rough nor painful.

While examining the rectal region and tissue, the clinician should check the animal for evidence of constipation, obstipation, or generally dry, hard stools. Such problems lead to difficulty defecating. The perianal region should be examined for masses and, particularly when straining to defecate occurs, for perineal hernia, either unilateral or bilateral. Perineal hernias are detected by lateral deflection of the index finger immediately after entering the rectum (i.e., no farther than the first or second joint of the inserted finger). If the examiner probes too deeply past that point, this important lesion will be missed. Rectal prolapse must be differentiated from ilealcolic intussusception because of different etiologies and treatments for each. Prolapse is associated with the inability to pass a blunt instrument only to the level of the pelvic inlet. Perianal fistulas are readily identified on the physical examination; however, they are often so painful that examination of this area is made difficult without sedation. During this portion of the examination, the tail is checked for skin lesions and for pain on motion. Animals experiencing tail pain, and occasionally urinary and/or anal sphincter problems, should be examined with injury to the tail region in mind. Tails that have been caught in doors or pulled aggressively (more common in the cat) may develop neurologic problems involving the urinary bladder, anal sphincter, and/or the ability to move the tail.

The testicles and scrotum should be examined in the intact male for pain, skin lesions, and variability in the size and shape of one or both testicles. The presence of one or no testicles in the intact male is an important diagnostic clue. Retention or neoplasia of one or both testicles may correlate with the presenting clinical signs. In the puppy examination, the presence or absence of testicles may indicate a congenital defect and must be identified to the pet owner because the purchase agreement may need to be reviewed. It is important to note the presence of an inguinal (flanker) testis because showing and breeding would be inappropriate, and the pet may be infertile. Explanation of these changes to the new puppy owner is relevant particularly if the pet was purchased for breeding purposes.

In females, examination of the vulvar region is important in determining the presence of discharges, the state of estrus, or the presence of skin conditions that may be responsible for licking or irritability of the hind region. Asking questions that relate to the timing of the last or latest heat cycle may elicit insightful information relevant to pseudopregnancy or pyometra in the intact bitch. Vaginal swabs taken to evaluate the state of the vaginal mucosa are a quick, easy way to determine the presence of pus or red cells in the canal and the current hormonal status of the bitch. Females not in estrus usually do not tolerate internal vaginal palpation, so it is not routinely part of the physical examination. If there is a further requirement for such an examination, it may require additional restraint or sedation.

Prior to examining the limbs, particularly in cases of lameness, the examining veterinarian must evaluate the mobility and flexibility of the head and neck. Particularly in larger breeds of dogs, cervical conditions cause neck guarding and failure to thrive, with nondescript signs of pain, lameness, and malaise. Intermittent or recurrent problems may not be immediately obvious on the physical examination. Dogs that are difficult to examine or animals with acutely painful conditions may be better evaluated under conscious sedation.

Rear leg pain, weakness, and wobbliness may be signs of a neurologic disorder, such as cervical disease, thoracolumbar disease, and/or lumbosacral disease. The physical examination should include compression of the tissues along the spinal canal and the lumbosacral region. Sensitivity alone may be inadequate grounds for making a diagnosis and may only point to one of several conditions that must be considered in the differential diagnosis. Neurologic changes, including postural tone, conscious proprioception, or muscle atrophy, assist the process of evaluating disease states (see Chapter 258).

Evaluation and examination of the limbs, including bilateral femoral pulses, lymph nodes, joints, foot pads, and interdigital regions, can reveal important clues to the presence of internal medical problems. Joint disease, often silent or less than immediately obvious, is easily overlooked unless specific attention is paid to joint swelling or discomfort. The examiner should flex each of the patient's carpi with moderate pressure to assess for signs of joint pain that would otherwise not be recognized; animals with nonspecific signs, especially suggesting intermittent neck or back pain, may in fact be found to have polyarthritis thanks to this physical clue. It is important to observe symptomatic cats out of the carrier, on the floor in a safe, escape-proof room. Swelling, heat, and pain in one or more joints can explain many signs, including lameness, malaise, and fever. Swelling of the peripheral subcutaneous tissues provides reason for further evaluation. Claudication or painful or non–weight-bearing lameness directs the examiner to the affected limb. Thorough examination of the limbs for differentiation of warmth, pulses, or swellings may yield a direct clue to the cause of lameness.

Deep palpation of the bony tissue provides information relevant to both medical and orthopedic problems. Taking into account the age and health of the animal is relevant, because some diseases are specific to young, growing dogs (panosteitis), whereas others would be expected in older, overweight dogs (cruciate rupture, osteoarthritis, bone cancer). Although a general evaluation of the joints is required whenever lameness is present, it is always performed with the realization that only with the animal under conscious sedation or general anesthesia can it be determined with certainty whether a joint problem exists. Cats are usually easier to palpate than dogs, and larger-breed dogs are often difficult to examine without sedation. With that as a given, it is often advantageous to discuss with the client the benefits of radiographs and a joint tap (arthrocentesis) under sedation so that a more complete examination can be done. Palpation of the hips and evaluation for coxofemoral disease must be distinguished from examination for lumbosacral problems and stifle disorders. The opportunity to evaluate these findings in greater detail may be left to a sedated state accomplished at another time. When radiographs of a limb are to be taken, the examiner should remember the benefit of evaluating both limbs to evaluate the significance of the changes noted by comparing symmetry. Other orthopedic problems, including patellar disease in small to midsize dogs, may be more easily identified without sedation.

No lameness examination is complete without evaluation of the footpads and interdigital regions. It is of paramount importance to examine these tissues carefully for infiltrating problems, particularly where foreign bodies are a possibility, and to distinguish interdigital cysts, digital tumors, and pad burns.

COMPLETING THE PHYSICAL EXAMINATION

Every hospital has its own set of paperwork. Smaller veterinary clinics may not require much in the way of formal documentation, but this is the time to complete a well-written medical record. The traditional "SOAP" method provides the entire hospital and others with a record of the physical examination and history findings and of the plan for moving forward with the pet's care.

No physical examination is complete until the results are listed in the examination report and an assessment is made of the findings. This is the time for the veterinarian to identify in the records his or her recommendations for proceeding with the case. It is here that the client or caregiver can once again participate in the caregiving process. The veterinarian needs to summarize the findings, note the pertinent points, and identify how the case should proceed. Noting the findings alone without recommending a course of action does not complete the process. The owner must be informed of the possible courses of action, the advantages and drawbacks of each, and the estimated cost of such work. It is recommended that the veterinarian also note in the record, in addition to the subjective and objective findings, the likely rule-outs and tentative clinical assessment. A definitive diagnosis need not be made at this time, but identifying the rule-outs helps to portray a thought process in progress. If the prognosis is potentially poor or guarded, the examining veterinarian should discuss this with the owner at this point. Clients who fail to "hear" bad news may be very surprised to see that the veterinarian had written such news in the record one or more times in the course of record keeping. From a medical-legal point of view, keeping the client informed and up-to-date is very necessary. From the outset, discussing serious findings with the client ensures better practitioner-client communication.

CHAPTER 2

Clinical Problem Solving: The Steps That Follow the History and Physical Examination—*The Pedagogy of Clinical Medicine*

Stephen J. Ettinger

While modern medicine is aided by a dazzling array of technologies, like MRI scans and DNA analyses, language is still the bedrock of clinical practice. It is also essential that even the most astute doctors doubt their thinking, repeatedly considering the possibility that they may be wrong.[1]

In his 2007 book, *How Doctors Think*, Jerome Groopman makes a case for the point that there is a common and powerful temptation felt by patients and doctors alike to have a simple answer to complicated problems.[2] This is true not only for physicians but for all in the healing arts professions. We often speak unintentionally, not objectively but from faith, resulting in confirmational bias. The doctor reaches the diagnosis he or she wishes the outcome to be. This happens when the doctor selectively accepts or ignores information thus leading to decisions based on a desired outcome. Such skewing of decisions on the doctor's part ultimately of course leads to poor care. When there is a psychological commitment to the animal patient, the owner, or the diagnosis, distorted conclusions are likely to occur (thus the axiom that a smart physician does not have him[her] self for a doctor!!).

It has been demonstrated in medicine that the majority of medical errors are due to flaws in physician thinking and not to technical mistakes.[2] Groopman goes on to suggest that 80% of errors could be accounted for by a cascade of cognitive errors and that based on autopsies (of which far more are completed in people than pets) 10% to 15% of all diagnoses are wrong! Further, the average diagnostic error in interpreting medical images is between 20% and 30%.

How then can we avoid such errors and learn from those who have preceded us? We have divided this textbook into sections for the express purpose of easing the process of teaching and learning. Medical information is presented in a variety of ways that allow the reader to view the subject matter from different points of view. Some of the information overlaps; this is necessary because medical subjects are understood from the viewpoint of clinical signs as well as by organ system review. Many clinical signs overlap organ systems so that the process of understanding the "sign" bridges different fields. The initial chapters of the book deliberately deal with medical perspectives that do not conveniently fit into a single subject area and are too broad in scope to belong to one specific discipline or field. A subject such as pain control, while rather specific to a patient, is general in terms of the material it covers. Pain is a significant clinical problem, but is not related to an organ system or disease process and therefore the general principles of treating pain are presented. This is true as well for the other chapters in the beginning of the text such as genetics and euthanasia.

Problems and chief complaints are described first in the book because in fact this is what is first recognized by the pet's owner. This means that the reader will view common problems before specific organ systems are identified. An example is the clinical sign of polyuria or polydipsia. Caused by many different conditions, this sign is not specific to a single system; it is far more generalized. The reader must approach the process not on the basis of evaluating a single disease but rather knowing how to dissect the simple sign in an orderly manner to appropriately reach a conclusion.

Why do we need specific learning aids? Due to the variance of the readership level, facts must be made readily available and distinguishable for the reader. The beginning reader/student must have the opportunity to learn in the best way possible. There are limitations of human performance and ability, especially prominent in the early periods of introduction to a topic. This book is a clinical text, and many readers have yet to be exposed to clinical approaches to disease, instead having learned the structural basis of science without having been introduced to the vagaries of clinical medicine. For these readers, the ability to memorize has finite limitations and decision-making trees or algorithms may be helpful early on in deciphering clinical facts. Combining algorithms with the clinical factual materials and digital recordings on the website allows the brain to more comprehensively assimilate the problems at hand.

A textbook must be more than a compilation of facts. One does not learn how to write good prose just by reading the dictionary. The facts in a veterinary textbook must be placed in a context that favors their application, and that structure may be initiated through algorithms. Much like a symphony, there are many notes but the musical score helps turn the notes into a melody. The musician (clinician) infuses his/her own style into the music while a good algorithm helps to turn an otherwise chaotic collection of information into something that flows logically.

The raw information is the vocabulary of disease, and the decision-making process transforms this vocabulary into a functional language. It is not enough to have bricks and mortar; these must be placed together in a logical sequence in order to build something that can, like a well-built building, stand firmly on its own.

ALGORITHMS

An interesting phenomenon happens virtually every year, when a new staff of interns and residents begin work. I have been surprised to see very intelligent young veterinarians become almost speechless when asked to list the differential diagnoses for a common disorder, such as vomiting, fever, or polyuria-polydipsia. These bright individuals seem to "freeze" because the combination of recall (just how many facts can be remembered right away?) and application (analyzing the relevance of those facts for a given case) is overwhelming to them, even when the question is fairly simple. This grows even further when a client (or mentor) with high expectations is added to the equation. This may be what the young clinician first experiences. We know that the material is there, but the building blocks and mortar have yet to be set firmly in place.

This important and common stumbling block can be overcome by navigating carefully using a "road" map. These maps that are developed and refined in the minds of skilled clinicians over entire careers are first presented to the neophyte as algorithms. Diagnostic and therapeutic processes are best served when algorithms are used in conjunction with guidelines or standards of care, with the evolving protocols that enhance evidence-based medical decisions. Algorithms are diagnostic trees built much the same way that engineers or architects build structures with a broad base designed to include all possible considerations. Algorithms present information sequentially, with segments of information joined by decision points. They mimic the process of clinical problem solving that veterinarians should use daily in practice.

The algorithm serves as a powerful tool for case management—diagnosing, treating, and reviewing decisions. This process is no better represented than in the integration of algorithms, standards of care, evidence-based decision making, and record management. The astute and trained clinician does not require a written algorithm to review because the process is already natural and built in. It is important to remember that this book is intended for the student at every level. Diagnostic and treatment decisions are exceptionally complex processes. Algorithms "parse" the process into individual steps, and each step requires a minimal number of data bits for the student to review to make the decision process more likely to be successful. Small subsets of data bits are easier for the clinician to appreciate and utilize. *If the system is overloaded, the brain fails to account for all of the subsets within. This alone supports the analytical process of algorithms for the neophyte.*

HOW DO WE DEAL WITH INFORMATION AND WHEN?

In medicine there is always risk of too much information. This causes a problem for the uninitiated student. Test results and other data arrive in increasing quantities. The clinician must determine how to manage this information in a meaningful way. Some information may be critically important while other information is trivial (irrelevant, incorrect, laboratory error, or simply misinterpreted) and deserves to be discarded. Often the student or clinician becomes lost or feels as if he or she is drowning in the data base. Overall there is too much information, and this may ultimately impair decision making. There may be a tendency to jump to conclusions or to choose only a few facts with which to make decisions. The student or clinician then is at risk for missing the diagnosis (or just overlooking the most important facts). This is not unlike triangulation of a GPS position—usually three points are required to specifically identify the present position, and if only two are used the result may be incorrect. Too, there is a level of uncertainty that can paralyze the decision-making process, and without a "road map" to direct the student, he/she can be paralyzed to inaction based on the overwhelming amount of data presented.

The experienced clinician has frequently seen a particular pattern over and over throughout the career and will quickly recognize a condition and knows what it is and what to do. The inexperienced doctor may need to rely on evaluation of data (or at least that which is recognized, perceived, or identified). The inexperienced individual gains from the use of diagnostic trees because instead of grasping at a wrong diagnosis based on a misdirected "gut feeling," he/she may consciously work through the process (properly excluding those points that are irrelevant to the case) to correctly identify the problem and be able to accurately begin an assessment. In *How Doctors Think*,[2] the author describes physician mistakes based on attitudes or feelings about the patient or simply a certainty of the diagnosis before fully evaluating the case and thus missing the diagnosis. "The doctor becomes increasingly convinced of the truth of his misjudgment, developing a psychological commitment to it. He becomes wedded to his distorted conclusion" (Groopman, p. 25).[2]

Diagnosis and treatment decisions are exceptionally complex processes except in glaringly simple medical situations (a laceration or a bite wound). Clinical algorithms can be helpful and direct, especially for run of the mill or routine diagnoses or treatments. The diagnostic tree or algorithm allows the uninitiated to "parse" the process into individual steps. Since the mind works far better with smaller amounts of data at a time, each step in this process requires only a minimal number of data bits to analyze and thus to ultimately support the analytical process.

One of the negative factors when using algorithms is that students often "do as they see," and they rarely if ever see a skilled clinician using a hardcopy of an actual algorithm. This occurs because that clinician has already learned and firmly imprinted in his/her mind the logical and most important steps in dealing with conditions seen every day. For that clinician, the algorithm exists, but has become second nature through repeated use and refinement. The daily chore of examining a patient is far more complex than what one sees an experienced veterinarian doing superficially (the familiar placement of the stethoscope on the thorax but in fact recognizing an unusual arrhythmia, a murmur, the palpation of enlarged lymph nodes or identifying a thoracic wall abnormality). A good clinician thinks the algorithm through in his/her own mind during the process of working the patient up, possibly without even realizing he/she has done so. Thus, algorithms do not replace good clinicians, but they may help the uninitiated to become good clinicians by helping them to organize the thought process and avoid mistakes.

WHAT MAKES A GOOD DECISION TREE OR ALGORITHM?

A decision tree is based on factual evidence that leads to a set of appropriate conclusions. The process is one that clearly and concisely displays logic tied to action and findings. These actions and findings must be simple and not convoluted, so that the reader does not become lost following the logic. *Ultimately diagnostic trees guide a veterinarian through the inevitable act of distilling a large amount of information into a commitment.*

Algorithms are used most effectively during the transition phase when students are moving from basic science knowledge, where things are more often definitely yes or no than they are in the clinics. During his preclinical years in training, this author remembers clearly not being able to understand why the diagnosis of cancer was not always a simple black and white process. That concept became abundantly obvious shortly thereafter and 45 years later it looms as even more complex! Before the student has much experience, pathways of thought are often not yet formed. This is a good time for the learning tree or algorithm to be used. Once the pathways are formed there may be less of a need for them. Everyone learns differently. While algorithms belong in a curriculum to catch the people who learn well from them, this should not be at the undue expense of others who do not learn well this way. Such people will hopefully find other, equally logical and methodical, ways of learning.

Some believe that students need to learn their skills first and that methods to simplify this, using what they see as a "cookbook approach," cause the brain to be lazy. Others believe that in medicine the human brain should have the "stuff down cold" and the person using this information should then have the skills to decide what to use and when to use it. While these arguments are cogent, they fail to provide uniformly good medicine that deals with every case and every interpreter of the facts. Medicine is not a "fight" between the smart and not so smart but rather an attempt to heal, to provide relief of suffering and discomfort. Any method to improve on diagnosis and treatment should be utilized to quickly and efficiently obtain the maximum effect for the benefit of the patient and owner. Evidence-based medicine, rapidly becoming a canon of our profession, demands the use of facts in reaching our decisions and more often than not this approach does provide better answers. Prepared algorithms and practice guidelines in the form of decision-making trees can result in better medicine being offered.

POINTS TO PONDER BEFORE CHOOSING TO USE DECISION TREE ANALYSES

- Use easy to apply, clear, and clinically relevant methods of approaching a problem. Complex, out of reach algorithms do not help the student reach a logical conclusion and should be avoided.
- Avoiding "cookbook" medicine is something that only the user can make happen. If the reader follows the decision-making tree without an active thought process, there is a likelihood of error; this separates the professional from the neophyte. When symptoms are vague, confusing, multiple, or the laboratory tests are inexact, algorithms are not going to be as useful as they are in more straightforward conditions.
- No algorithm is complete without recognizing that the tree itself is never complete and that the assumptions used to reach a specific point may be incomplete. The benefits of the decision-making tree require a thorough knowledge base first. Being able to add to or alter the algorithm when deviation occurs is part of the process.
- Be able to "step out" of the algorithm as required or if it is advantageous to do so. Every case is different, and it is hard to find one size to fit all. Empower the user of the decision-making tree to think independently and to challenge decisions that do not offer appropriate answers.
- Shades of gray lend themselves less well to binary thought processing than black and white. The more complex the process, the greater the likelihood of shades of gray. Vague or confusing signs lead to incorrect decisions if they are seen as not being absolute.
- Complicated medical processes may not be as amenable to the "algorithmic process," in part because we have already fallen off the edge and into the realm of the "gray" or more complex processes that interfere with simple decision-making steps. This is the time to encourage thinking outside the box instead of following inappropriate pathways.

How to Use Decision-Making Trees

Help the user to understand the general order and hierarchy of decisions. Help students understand what algorithms or decision-making trees can and cannot do. Appreciate that algorithms are complementary to, and not substitutes for, independent thinking and decision making. Teach that we cannot put a set of standard decisions into place that will obviate the need for critical analysis.

Continuously remind the clinician to look at the patient with the disease process and not just the disease. Never fail to look at the patient. Be certain that the decisions coming from an algorithm are appropriate and reasonable for the patient being examined. Inappropriate evaluation of laboratory data will take the unsuspecting evaluator down the wrong pathway.

How to Use the Algorithms in This Textbook

Ultimately it is up to the student to utilize the algorithm properly. First, the history and physical examination (see Chapter 1) must be thorough and correct. Knowing the history of the patient is an integral part of utilizing the decision tree (algorithm). Ask questions of the caregiver in order to more fully explore the options from the tree. Unanswered questions need to be explored, not ignored. Follow through in a logical sequence. An incorrect or incomplete history leads one down the wrong decision-making road—e.g., polyuria and stranguria differ, but if only "urinary accidents" are described by the owner and the veterinarian fails to inquire further. The final decision is also likely to be incorrect and the diagnosis and treatment wrong. If the majority of errors are due to flaws in thinking and not technical mistakes, then not considering multiple possibilities leads to choices that are also incorrect.

I recommend that the student make a copy of the algorithm and work through the decision-making process. Write down the findings on the page. DO NOT GUESS at the result because the correct decision depends on choosing the right pathway. Once gone down the wrong pathway, the information and approach continues to be wrong. A dog straining to urinate, who lifting his leg and frequently squirting small amounts of urine because of a calculus obstruction, is not polyuric; vomiting and regurgitation differ; a productive cough or retching of mucus relate not to the GI system but to respiratory or cardiac dysfunction. Good history taking and careful observation go a long way towards making the correct diagnosis.

Produce a clinical picture that fits with the history and the physical examination. Judicious use of laboratory analyses is important, but if a laboratory test is not consistent with the history and physical examination, repeat the test or rethink the information provided. False positives and negatives do occur and interfere with reaching the diagnosis. A free catch urine sample with bacteria but without white cells, polyuria, or straining is not likely to equate to a urinary tract infection despite the bacteria. Breed predispositions do not automatically mean that a specific disease is present. A Wheaten Terrier with polydipsia does not automatically equate to a glomerulonephropathy; a Boxer dog with a murmur does not automatically identify a congenital subaortic stenosis.

BEYOND ALGORITHMS—THE SOAP

The algorithms in this textbook represent the basic framework for handling a general category of problems. They reliably identify as effective a process as is feasible considering the availability of relevant facts. Regardless, they also quickly fall apart when symptoms are vague, multiple, or confusing, and they should not be considered as the absolute final answer to handling a patient's signs and symptoms. Be willing to think outside the box.

As a veterinarian gains experience, he or she gradually adds information and gains confidence in the mental algorithm. Uncommon outcomes and unusual variants allow the decision tree to sprout additional branches. The process of learning and thinking has really begun. Decision trees do however prevent what Groopman[2] claims often influences the clinical choice, which is "the last bad choice."

The methodical approach begins by identifying and noting the subjective (S) and objective (O) information. This remains true whether one has been in practice a day or a decade. Enthusiasm, optimism, and a desire to help, while vital to success, may cause the clinician to jump to conclusions or deviate from a logical approach. When a client refuses diagnostic tests that are recommended, that is not grounds for ignoring the whole process of methodical reasoning. Rather, it represents a pause in the reasoning process—a temporary halt that can be restarted if the patient experiences a recurrence of the problem, if deterioration is noted, or if further analysis is necessary after what may have been a "shotgun approach" to the problem. By using and noting the SOAP in the record and relating to the client the plans for future investigation and incorporating these suggestions into the medical record, the client understands that the process may continue and gains confidence in the doctor's ability and desire to continue to investigate and care for the problem. This then is the invitation to the remainder of the book and to continuing to care for the patient. In 1925, Francis Weld Peabody said about human medicine what remains equally true today in all medicine, "For the secret of the care of the patient is in caring for the patient."[3]

REFERENCES

The reference list can be found on the companion Expert Consult Web site at *www.expertconsult.com*.

CHAPTER 3

Clueing in Customers*

Leonard L. Berry
Neeli Bendapudi

Nobody likes going to the hospital. The experience is at best unnerving, often frightening, and, for most of us, a potent symbol of mortality. What's more, it's very hard for the average patient to judge the quality of the "product" based on direct evidence. You can't try it on, you can't return it if you don't like it, and you need an advanced degree to understand it—yet it's vitally important. Therefore when we're considering a doctor or a medical facility, most of us unconsciously turn detective, looking for evidence of competence, caring, and integrity—processing what we can see and understand to decipher what we cannot.

The Mayo Clinic doesn't leave the nature of that evidence to chance. By carefully managing a set of visual and experiential clues, Mayo tells a consistent and compelling story about its service to customers: At Mayo Clinic, the patient comes first. From the way it hires and trains employees, to the way it designs its facilities, to the way it approaches care, Mayo offers patients and their families concrete and convincing evidence of its strengths and values. The results are exceptionally positive word of mouth and abiding customer loyalty, which have allowed Mayo Clinic to build what is arguably the most powerful brand in health care—with very little advertising—in an industry where few institutions have any brand recognition beyond their local markets.

It's called "evidence management": an organized, explicit approach to presenting customers with coherent, honest evidence of your abilities. Evidence management is a lot like advertising, except that it turns a company into a living, breathing advertisement for itself. Other organizations manage evidence well, too. Ritz Carlton, for example, very effectively communicates outstanding personal service: Employees at all levels take note of customer preferences and are empowered to solve problems on the spot, continually tailoring the experience to each person. Mayo Clinic does not have all the answers; health care is a highly inventive industry, and many institutions could serve as fine examples to business. However, during our extensive study of the Mayo organization over a 5-month period, we saw evidence-management practices that rival or surpass anything we've seen in the corporate sector, practices that are applicable outside of health care. As part of our research design, we interviewed approximately 1000 Mayo employees and patients, observed hundreds of doctor-patient visits at two of Mayo's three major campuses (Scottsdale, Arizona, and Rochester, Minnesota; the third is in Jacksonville, Florida), and stayed in the hospitals overnight as patients. In almost every experience and interaction, in subtle and not-so-subtle ways, we got the message that at Mayo Clinic, the patient comes first (Box 3-1).

Many businesses sell products that are intangible or technically complex—financial and legal services, software, and auto repair are just a few—and their customers naturally look for clues that can help explain what they don't understand or see. In fact, in just about any organization, the clues emitted by people and things (humanics and mechanics, respectively, as introduced to the management literature by Lewis Carbone and Stephan Haeckel) tell a story to customers or potential customers. The question for managers is whether the clues tell the intended story. Mayo Clinic's effectiveness at designing and managing evidence offers a lesson other service organizations would do well to heed: Understand the story you want

---

*Used by permission from Harvard Business Review, February 2003.

Box • 3-1

The Research

Mayo Clinic has three major campuses (Rochester, MN; Scottsdale, AZ; and Jacksonville, FL); primary care clinics in more than 60 communities; 21 owned or managed hospitals; more than 2800 staff physicians; medical technology, medical publishing, laboratory, and health care benefits-administration businesses; and revenue in excess of $4 billion. It serves more than 500,000 individual patients annually.

For this article, we conducted the largest service study ever done at Mayo Clinic. During a 5-month period, we interviewed approximately 1000 Mayo patients, physicians, nurses, allied health staff, and managers at the original Rochester campus and the Scottsdale campus. We also collected data as participant observers, checking into the hospitals as patients, observing surgeries in the operating room and more than 250 doctor-patient interactions in the examination room, making hospital rounds, and flying on the Mayo One emergency rescue helicopter service. We formally studied service delivery in 14 medical specialties selected to provide a cross-section of the practice: cardiac surgery, cardiology, dermatology, emergency medicine, endocrinology, family medicine, gastroenterology, medical and radiation oncology, neurology, orthopedic surgery, preventive medicine, thoracic surgery, transplant surgery, and urology. Mayo Clinic gave us complete access to study its service culture and processes, and the Mayo Clinic Institutional Review Board approved our study.

to tell, and then make sure your people and your facilities provide evidence of that story to customers, day in and day out.

CLUES IN PEOPLE

When we interviewed Mayo patients, we were struck by how consistently they described their care as being organized around their needs rather than the doctors' schedules, the hospital's processes, or any other factor related to Mayo's internal operations. The actions of Mayo staff members, according to what we were told, clearly signal the patient-first focus. Here are representative remarks: "My doctor calls me at home to check on how I am doing. She wants to work with what is best for my schedule." "When I had a colonoscopy, [my doctor] waited to tell me personally that I had a polyp because he remembered that my husband died from small bowel cancer, and he knew that I would be worried I may have the same thing." "My oncologist is…the kindest man I have ever met. He related some of his personal life to me. I was more than my problem to him. He related to me as a person."

Such glowing praise isn't limited just to the doctors and nurses. One patient, for example, was "amazed" at how well the people at the registration desk handle requests: "People who come up to the desk are nervous, or angry, or abusive. These ladies at the registration desk just keep their cool. I wish they could train the customer service reps in department stores."

It's no accident that employees communicate a strong, consistent message to patients. Mayo explicitly and systematically hires people who genuinely embrace the organization's values. The clinic emphasizes the importance of those values through training and ongoing reinforcement in the workplace, a practice that began in the very early part of the twentieth century, when Drs. William and Charles Mayo started the organization. Indeed, William Mayo's credo—"The best interest of the patient is the only interest to be considered"—guides hiring decisions to this day.

It's difficult to get a job at Mayo Clinic because of intellect or technical skill alone. Demonstrated task competence is essential, of course, but the hiring managers are also trained in behavioral interview techniques, and they are expected to use them to elicit an applicant's values. A candidate may be asked, for instance, to discuss a time when he set a development goal for himself and how he met that goal or to describe the proudest moment in his career or even the moment he found most frustrating. Interviewers avoid discussing hypothetical situations that allow candidates to figure out the "right" answer and instead probe for specific details that reflect true experiences and perspectives. For example, a candidate who identifies making a difference in a patient's life as his or her proudest moment may be more attuned to Mayo's values than one who mentions achieving a career milestone.

The people who make the cut—indeed, the people who are drawn to Mayo in the first place—are those who take pride in having the freedom to put patients first. We heard many doctors and nurses say that they appreciate being allowed to practice medicine as they feel it should be practiced. Those feelings of pride and the alignment of employees' attitudes with Mayo's values contribute to lower staff turnover across the board. Annual turnover among hospital nurses is only 4% at Mayo versus 20% for the industry as a whole—continuity that, in turn, helps boost the quality of care.

Once hired, all new employees go through an orientation process specifically designed to reinforce the patient-first mentality. The program for nonphysician employees—whether janitors, accountants, or nurses—is designed to help all staff people understand how their jobs affect patients' care and well-being. If housekeeping fails to maintain sanitary conditions, for instance, a patient's health may be compromised no matter how excellent the medical care received. Storytelling figures heavily in these programs, with the emphasis on how employees have used Mayo values to make difficult decisions on patients' behalf.

Storytelling continues in the workplace because, once people are away from the classroom, the idea of putting the patient first can seem distant and sometimes even unrealistic, given the stress and unpredictability of day-to-day work. Consider, for instance, one story featured at several orientation sessions and widely disseminated throughout the organization. A critically ill patient was admitted to the Scottsdale hospital shortly before her daughter was to be married, and she was unlikely to live to see the wedding. The bride told the hospital chaplain how much she wanted her mother to participate in the ceremony, and he conveyed this to the critical care manager. Within hours, the hospital atrium was transformed for the wedding service, complete with flowers, balloons, and confetti. Staff members provided a cake, and nurses arranged the patient's hair and makeup, dressed her, and wheeled her bed to the atrium. A volunteer played the piano and the chaplain performed the service. On every floor, hospital staff and visiting family and friends ringed the atrium balconies, "like angels from above," to quote the bride. The wedding scene provided not only evidence of caring to the patient and her family but also a strong reminder to the staff that the patient's needs come first. They got the message: We heard the story multiple times in our interviews with employees.

Another story was initially told at a leadership development program for rising Mayo administrators. In one session,

Mayo staff members shared experiences that showed how the service philosophy affects care. An emergency room physician told of a patient who walked into the ER with severe shortness of breath. When told she had a bacterial infection requiring immediate surgery, the woman expressed concern about her sick dog, which was in her illegally parked truck. The attending nurse assured her that he would move the truck and take care of the dog, but when he walked outside, what he saw was not a pickup but a semi, which he wasn't licensed to drive. He was about to have it towed—for $700—when he stopped to consider ways he might save the patient the expense. In the end, the nurse took it upon himself to obtain permission to park the truck at a nearby shopping center for a few days and find a fellow nurse—a former trucker—to drive the truck there. He took the dog to a veterinarian and then cared for it in his own home while the patient recovered. When asked what prompted him to do this, the nurse replied, "At Mayo Clinic, the patient's needs come first."

Various events celebrating exceptional service on behalf of patients further reinforce employees' commitments. The Rochester campus hosts an annual Heritage Week, celebrating the clinic's history and values and reinforcing their relevance to Mayo's work today through historical presentations and displays, lectures, ecumenical and liturgical services, concerts, and social events. Employees, retirees, volunteers, patients, visitors, and members of the community are invited. Mayo Rochester also recognizes exceptional service with its quarterly campus-wide Karis Award (*Karis* is Greek for caring). All staff members are eligible and can be nominated by a coworker, patient, or family member; the identity of the nominator is not disclosed, which removes political considerations from the process. One 1999 winner, a world-renowned colorectal surgeon with numerous scientific recognitions told his tablemates at the award luncheon that he cherished the Karis more than any other award he's received, calling it, "The only award I have for just being a really good doctor."

CLUES IN COLLABORATION

In 1910, William Mayo said, "In order that the sick may have the benefit of advancing knowledge, union of forces is necessary… It has become necessary to develop medicine as a cooperative science." Dr. Mayo's vision profoundly influences the organization's approach to care. Patients experience the Mayo Clinic as a team of experts who are focused on patients' needs above all else. They perceive an integrated, coordinated response to their medical conditions and, often, to related psychological, social, spiritual, and financial needs. Elsewhere, doctors may be reluctant to admit to any gaps in their knowledge. Not so at Mayo. Mayo Clinic assembles the expertise and resources needed to solve the patient's problem. If a Mayo doctor can't answer a question and needs to bring someone else onto a team, she freely admits it to the patient. The doctors meet with one another and with the patient—visible evidence that they are collaborating to solve the patient's problem rather than passing it from one doctor to another. One patient we interviewed expressed a common sentiment when he said, "I have a lot of problems, and I like that I can go to Mayo and be seen by a team of specialists who work together to see the big picture." Collaboration is particularly important because the institution's reputation has become so well known that patients often come in looking for a miracle. Many have consulted several other doctors and consider Mayo the last resort, so the physicians there regularly see patients with complex problems and high expectations, a situation that puts the doctors under extra pressure to make the right diagnoses and treatment decisions and not miss often subtle medical distinctions.

Mayo Clinic encourages this type of collaboration through various organizational incentives. All physicians are salaried, so they don't lose income by referring patients to colleagues, and the organization explicitly shuns the star system, downplaying individual accomplishments in favor of organizational achievements. In the words of one cardiovascular surgeon, "By not having our economics tied to our cases, we are free to do what comes naturally… to help one another." Doctors who are focused on maximizing their incomes or who want to be the star of the show don't work for Mayo Clinic. A surgeon specializing in the liver explained, "The kind of people who are attracted to work for Mayo Clinic have a value system that places the care of those in need over personal issues such as salary, prestige, and power. There is little room for turf battles. It is never a problem to add [a new case] on to the workload of the day. It's simply the best thing to do for the patient."

Mayo also supports teamwork with its use of technology. Staff members partner via a combination of face-to-face and remote collaboration using a sophisticated internal paging, telephone, and videoconferencing system that connects people quickly and easily. Remote teamwork through voice or virtual interaction is just as common as in-person teamwork at hallway or bedside consults. One physician told us, "I never feel I am in a room by myself, even when I am." Recently, for example, a Mayo ENT specialist in Scottsdale called together 20 doctors from all three campuses to discuss a difficult case-a patient with skin cancer at risk for metastasis and, owing to the necessary surgery, nerve injury and disfigurement. The team, assembled in a day, met by videoconference for an hour and a half and reached a consensus for a course of treatment, including specific recommendations on how aggressively to sample the patient's lymph nodes and how best to reconstruct the surgical wound.

Mayo's electronic medical record (EMR) improves the clinic's ability to present a seamless, collaborative organization and manage the evidence that patients see. The EMR provides an up-to-date narrative of the patient's symptoms, diagnoses, test results, treatment plans, procedures, and other related data, connecting in- and outpatient information and communicating across disciplines in outpatient practices. This connection is critical to patient-first decisions in ways that patients don't necessarily see. One emergency room physician said it had prevented her from intubating a patient who had asked not to be resuscitated, for instance, and others told of the importance of the EMR in managing patient medications to avoid allergic reactions or dangerous drug interactions. However, patients also notice and appreciate the single source of information, as we heard repeatedly in our research. One patient told us, "On my last visit, the doctor pulled up all my test scores from the past five years on a computer and showed me the trends, and we discussed what to do. I thought that was excellent." In short, patients told us in numerous interviews that Mayo's team service gave them a sense that the organization was coordinating its resources to provide the best possible care, with the patients' needs foremost in employees' minds.

CLUES IN TANGIBLES

In health care, the visual clues about an institution's core values and the quality of care are particularly difficult to separate from the actual service because people spend significant time in the facility—some stay for days or even weeks. The physical environment is also connected to medical outcomes: The potential of design to promote healing through stress reduction has been documented in dozens of studies. For these reasons, more medical institutions are making an effort to create open, welcoming spaces with soft, natural light. Mayo Clinic goes further with its design philosophy, which is perhaps as well honed and articulated as that of any major service provider in America, and pays strict attention to how every detail affects the patient's experience.

From public spaces to exam rooms to laboratories, Mayo facilities have been designed explicitly to relieve stress, offer a place of refuge, create positive distractions, convey caring and respect, symbolize competence, minimize the impression of crowding, facilitate way finding, and accommodate families. In the words of the architect who designed Mayo Rochester's new 20-story Gonda Building, "I would like the patients to feel a little better before they see their doctors." A well-designed physical environment has a positive impact on employees as well, reducing physical and emotional stress—which is of value not only to employees but also to patients because visible employee stress sends negative signals. In our interviews, patients commented on the lack of apparent stress; one said, "It did not seem like a doctor's office when we went to Mayo. There was no tension."

The Gonda Building has spectacular wide-open spaces, a marble stairwell and floor, glasswork sculpture suspended above, and a multistory wall of windows looking onto a garden. The building's soaring lobby houses a cancer education center because, as one administrator put it, "The more visible the center, the more you remove the stigma of having cancer." The lobby of Mayo Clinic Hospital in Scottsdale is also visually stunning, with its atrium, indoor waterfall, stonework, and wall of windows overlooking a mountain range.

Mayo doesn't limit its facilities' clue management to public spaces. After all, the scary stuff in a medical facility happens elsewhere—in the catheterization lab, in diagnostic imaging, in the hospital room. At Mayo hospitals, staff members write the names of attending doctors and nurses on a white board in every patient's room, which helps stressed-out patients and families keep track of multiple caregivers and serves as a visible clue that there's a real person they can talk with about any concerns. In-hospital showers, microwave ovens, and chairs that convert to beds are available for family members because, as one staff member explained, "People don't come to the hospital alone." The pediatric section of Mayo's St. Mary's Hospital in Rochester transformed artwork by local schoolchildren into a colorful array of wall and ceiling tiles. The resuscitation equipment in pediatric examination rooms is hidden behind a large picture (which slides out of the way when the equipment is needed). While the hospital was under construction at the Scottsdale campus, officials arranged to have an automobile lifted into the building so physical rehabilitation patients would be able to practice getting in and out of a car in the privacy of a hospital.

Environmental clues in the outpatient setting are orchestrated just as carefully. Mayo Clinic buildings include quiet, darkened private areas where patients can rest between appointments. Public spaces are purposely made softer with natural light, color, artwork, piano music, and the sights and sounds of fountains. In examination rooms, the physician's desk is adjacent to a sofa large enough for the patient and family members, a design that removes the desk as a barrier between doctors and their patients.

Mayo also understands that the way employees present themselves sends a signal to patients. Patients don't encounter doctors in casual attire or white coats. Instead, the more than 2800 staff physicians wear business attire, unless they are in surgical scrubs, to convey professionalism and expertise. It's a dress code that some outside Mayo have called "pretentious"; yet we'd argue that it's no more pretentious than, say, the dress code for airline pilots. Airline passengers don't want to see their pilot in a polo shirt, and patients feel the same way about doctors. In effect, Mayo Clinic doctors—just like service workers in many other industries—work in a uniform; it is a visible clue that communicates respect to patients and their families.

Such attention to visual clues extends to the minutest detail. Mayo Rochester employee Mary Ann Morris, the administrator of General Service and the Office of Patient Affairs, often tells a story about her early days with the organization. She was working in a laboratory—a job that required her to wear a white uniform and white shoes—and after a hectic morning getting her two small children to school, she arrived at work to find her supervisor staring at her shoes. The supervisor had noticed that the laces were dirty where they threaded through the eyelets of Morris's shoes and asked Morris to clean them. Offended, Morris said that she worked in a laboratory, not with patients, so why should it matter? Her boss replied that Morris had contact with patients in ways she didn't realize—going out on the street wearing her Mayo name tag, for instance, or passing patients and their families as she walked through the halls—and that she couldn't represent Mayo Clinic with dirty shoelaces. "Though I was initially offended, I realized over time [that] everything I do, down to my shoelaces, represents my commitment to our patients and visitors," Morris told us. "Twenty-eight years later, I still use the dirty shoelace story to set the standard for the service level I aspire to for myself and my coworkers."

A dirty shoelace might seem minor, given the important work of caring for the ill, but a shoelace is something a customer can see, whereas medical expertise and technical ability are not. It's a piece of evidence—a small but integral part of the story Mayo tells to its customers. We aren't arguing that "patients first" is the only story a medical institution might choose to tell patients. A hospital might instead choose to signal, "We hire the smartest doctors," and manage the evidence with prominent displays of academic credentials and awards, a lecture series, and heavy publicity about new research. What Mayo Clinic has done better than just about any organization we can think of, however, is clearly identify a simple, consistent message and then manage the evidence—the buildings, the approach to care, and yes, even the shoelaces—to support that message, day in and day out.

CHAPTER 4

The Genome

Kerstin Lindblad-Toh

Mammalian genomes comprise approximately 3 billion letters that encode ~20,000 protein coding genes and a large number of noncoding RNAs and other signals that ensure that genes are turned on and off at the correct time and place in the body. These genomic blueprints support both development and physiological processes in all mammals. To date, roughly 30 mammalian genomes have been sequenced, among these notably that of the human, mouse, dog, and cat. Together with the actual genome sequence, a number of other resources are typically generated such as maps of variation, tools to measure gene expression, and tools to map disease genes. Here we describe the canine and feline genomes and the associated tools for gene mapping and comment on how genetic information is becoming more and more applicable to veterinary care.

INTRODUCTION

There are typically two reasons why mammalian genomes are sequenced. First, all mammalian species help us understand the human genome through comparative analysis, where we look for genes and other functional elements. These elements are conserved (similar) across species, whereas unimportant portions of the genome change randomly with time. Second, some species are important based on their genetics. These include two types of model organisms; biomedical models such as dog, cat, and mouse that will help us unravel genetic disease and livestock animals such as cattle, sheep, and pig where performance-enhancing traits are more commonly studied.

Based on the complexity of a mammalian genome—each containing 2.5 to 3 billion A, C, G, or Ts—it is often not easy to identify the small fraction of the genome that contains important information. For this purpose, comparative genomics has been used to find the important features in the human and other mammalian genomes. When the mouse and human genomes were first compared, it became clear that the number of genes was lower than previously estimated and that although protein-coding genes make up only ~1.5% of the human genome, a total of 5% of the human genome showed the signal of being more conserved than what could be expected by random chance.[1] Thus a quest began to find all the functional elements (both genes and noncoding elements) in the human genome by sequencing many mammals.[2]

The dog and cat came early in the line of sequenced genomes based on their biomedical and veterinary relevance.[3] Genetic diseases in dogs and cats have long been clinically characterized and tools for trait mapping developed, with the first genetic variant, a point mutation causing hemophilia B, described in 1989.[4] It is therefore not surprising that the dog was the fourth mammal to be sequenced (Figure 4-1).

In 2005, a high-quality genome sequence of the dog genome was first described together with other resources to aid trait mapping in the dog.[5] Shortly thereafter the cat genome was sequenced to a lower quality.[6] However, a complete sequence is underway and is expected to have the same high quality and associated tools as for the dog.

THE CANINE GENOME

The dog, *Canis familiaris*, was sequenced based on its important position in the mammalian tree and its potential for disease gene mapping. Since dogs share many common diseases and most of their genes with their human owners, disease genes discovered in either genome should have relevance for both man and his best friend. In addition, the unique breeding history of the domestic dog makes this species ideally suited for genetic studies.

The assembled dog sequence covers ~99% of the 2.4 billion base pair genome comprised of 38 chromosomes from a single female Boxer. The remarkably high quality of the genome sequence, and the speed at which it was produced (Box 4-1, Figure 4-2), reflected continuing improvements in sequencing and assembly technology since the initiation of the human genome sequence project, which took approximately 10 years to complete.[7,8]

In conjunction with the sequencing, approximately 2.5 million single nucleotide polymorphisms (SNPs) were identified in the Boxer, 10 additional breeds, and 5 other canids, forming the dense, genome-wide marker set necessary for disease gene mapping and phylogenetic analyses.

Both the genome and the extensive SNP set complement existing genetic resources in the dog community to facilitate comprehensive studies of gene expression, genome rearrangements, the proteome, RNAi, and the generation of tools for disease gene mapping and comparative as well as population genetic studies.

Genome Features

Regions of the dog and human genomes that share a common ancestry are called *segments of conserved synteny* and are identified by assessing sequence similarity. The common ancestry reveal similarities and changes in the genomes since their evolutionary split, and are especially useful for pairing orthologous genes (genes derived from a common ancestral gene) (Figure 4-3).

When pair-wise maps of conserved synteny are made from high-quality genomic alignments of dog, human,[7] mouse,[1] rat,[9] and chicken. The human[8] and rodent maps each cover ~94% of the dog genome, whereas a nonmammalian species, such as the chicken genome, covers only ~76% of the dog genome due to a dearth of regions with clear common ancestry between the two species.[1,7,8,9] Given that dog is an outgroup to the primate and rodent lineages in the evolutionary tree (see Figure 4-1), we see clearly that rodents have undergone the highest number of genomic rearrangements relative to humans. While dogs have fewer chromosomal rearrangements than rodents, they still have significantly more than humans (230 dog-human conserved segments at 500 kb resolution, 310 dog-mouse segments).

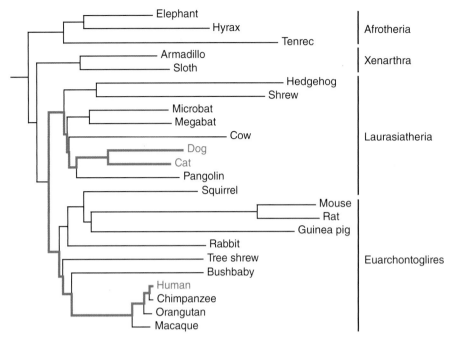

Figure 4-1 Dog is the first sequenced organism from the Laurasiatheria clade. Human, mouse, and rat were first fully sequenced. After dog many additional mammals are being sequenced, including cat. Note that dog and cat are closely related to each other and more closely related to human than mouse, based on the number of base changes.

Box • 4-1

How to Sequence a Genome

It is important to choose the right individual when sequencing a genome. The highest-quality genome sequence is usually generated by sequencing a single female individual with as little variation in her genome as possible. This ensures that the two chromosomes (one from mother one from father) are as alike as possible and therefore as easily decoded and assembled as possible. A female also yields good sequence from the X chromosome, but no Y chromosome sequence.

In whole genome shotgun (WGS) sequencing, the genome is randomly fragmented and ~700 bp reads are generated from each of the fragment's ends. Typically each letter in the genome is sequenced 7 times. Using sequence overlap, the reads are then rejoined into continuous segments *(contigs)*, much like how one would assemble a jigsaw puzzle. Contigs are linked together by paired end reads into larger units called *supercontigs*. Supercontigs are typically anchored to the chromosomes using fluorescent in situ hybridization (FISH).[15] Often a mammalian genome will consist of a few hundred supercontigs, each up to a hundred million bases in size. Usually more than 95% of the sequence is determined, excluding centromers and telomers.

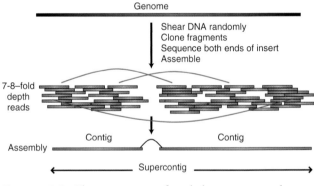

Figure 4-2 The strategy of whole genome shotgun sequencing.

genome relative to both human and mouse (note that most of the "junk" DNA in mammalian genomes are repeats), and b) rates of ancestral base deletion that are approximately equal in the dog and human lineages, but higher in mouse.[5] Consequently, and despite our more recent common ancestry with mouse, the human genome shares approximately 650 Mb more ancestral sequence with dog than with mouse. Due to the low rate of both large-scale deletions and new repeat insertions, the dog genome content is hence likely closer to the ancestral eutherian mammalian genome, in terms of the proportion of the present day sequence, than either human or mouse is.

DOGS HAVE ROUGHLY 20,000 GENES

Defining and examining the protein-coding portion of the dog genome is essential for understanding both the genome itself and its evolutionary relationship to other mammals. For

The total size of the sequenced dog genome is ~2.4 gigabases. Thus, the euchromatic portion of the dog genome is approximately 450 Mb (19%) smaller than the human genome and 150 Mb (6%) smaller than the mouse genome. This size difference is noticeable within the average segment of conserved synteny (see Figure 4-3) and can be attributed to two different factors: a) a lower rate of repeat insertions in the dog

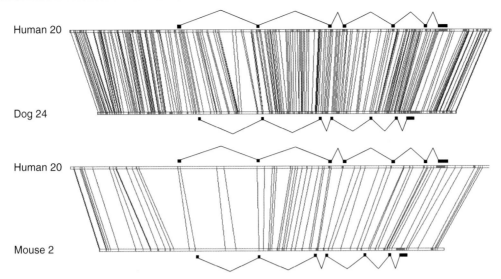

Figure 4-3 The human and dog genomes are more similar to each other than either one is to mouse. The segments of genomes of dog, human, and mouse that have evolved from the same segment in the common ancestor line up well, as can be seen from a 300-kb region on human 20, dog 24, and mouse 2. Note that more uniquely alignable sequences exist between dog and human (more closely spaced anchors) and that both the dog and mouse genomes are smaller than the human genome. These types of alignments are used to generate maps of conserved synteny between species (covering ~94% of the dog genome) and are very useful for translating information about genes *(black lines at top and bottom of drawing)* between species.

example, the evolution of the species is reflected in both the changes within protein-coding genes, which can reveal species-specific positive selection, and gene expansions leading to the development of more specialized gene functions.

By using conserved synteny and the paired relationships of genes between species, we were able to refine the gene sets. This yielded a gene count of ~19,500 dog genes, while human and mouse have closer to 20,500 genes. Most of these genes have 1:1 orthologs (a single corresponding gene) in all three species.

While in general dogs have few gene family expansions, a few notable exceptions have been discovered. The two families with the largest numbers of dog-specific genes are the histone H2Bs and the alpha interferons.[5,10] A third well-known case of dog gene expansion, compared to human, is the set of olfactory receptor genes.[11]

Genes under particularly strong selection in a species may show a higher relative rate of evolution, as measured by Ka/Ks (mutations that cause amino acid changes vs. those that do not). Comparison of the relative evolutionary constraints on the human, dog, and mouse orthologs for ~14,000 genes grouped according to function showed that the relative rate of evolution (strength of selection) between the functional groups was highly correlated in the three species. For example immune genes evolve quickly, whereas genes defining developmental processes evolve slowly. In contrast, the absolute rate of evolution (total number of amino acid substitutions) was significantly higher in the dog lineage than in human, but lower than in mouse. This reflects the pattern for the noncoding portions of the genome, where a rate of ~0.35 substitutions/site is seen between human and dog (compared to ~0.45 between human and mouse).[5]

There was evidence for dog-specific accelerated evolution in some gene families. These were primarily related to metabolism, and may contain promising candidates for studies of

molecular adaptation in carnivores. Some nervous system–related genes appear to have diverged faster in dog and human relative to mouse, but not relative to each other, suggesting similar selection pressures and possible convergence.

Other Features in the Genome

While 1.5% of mammalian genomes encode proteins, an additional 3.5% is highly conserved noncoding sequence, suggesting that these features have other important functions including many types of noncoding RNAs. Comparative analyses of multiple mammals have identified novel transcription factor binding sites, miRNA binding sites,[12] enhancers,[13] and insulators.[12] All of these elements are necessary for regulating the expression of the protein-coding genes.

Population Genetics and its Effect on the Genome

The unique breed structure of the domestic dog population may make disease gene mapping studies especially powerful.[14] To fully utilize this potential, researchers need both a large, uniformly spaced marker set and a good understanding of the extent of linkage disequilibrium in their study population. While many excellent maps and mapping reagents have been produced by the community over the past 15 years, the full genome sequence for the first time made it possible to develop an extensive SNP map.[15-18] To capture the diversity of the dog population, the Boxer sequence was compared to small amounts of sequence from each of nine diverse dog breeds and four gray wolves, and a single coyote. In addition, the Boxer was compared to the 1.5× Poodle assembly.[19] Finally, the Boxer's two chromosomes were themselves compared. Altogether 2.5 million SNPs were discovered. On average ~72% of SNPs were polymorphic in any third random breed. Thus, these SNPs will be useful for genome scans and chromosome marker panels, in addition to localizing the position of a mutation within and across breeds.[5]

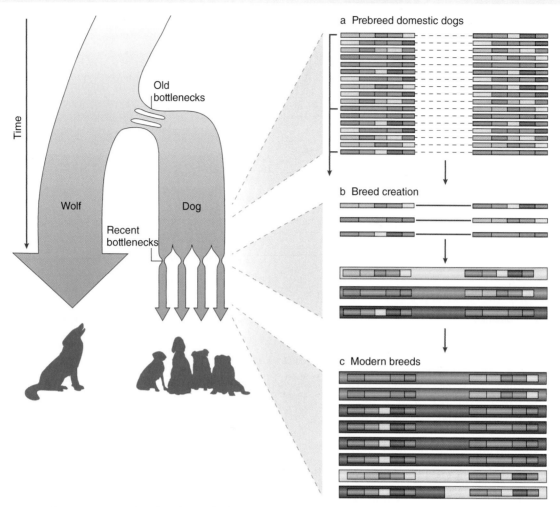

Figure 4-4 Two bottlenecks in the history of dog breeds shape the genome. Two population bottlenecks in dog population history, one old and one recent, shaped haplotype structure (pieces of chromosome inherited together without recombination) in modern dog breeds. First, the domestic dog diverged from wolves ~15,000 years ago.[21] Within the past few hundred years, modern dog breeds were created. Both bottlenecks influenced the haplotype pattern of current breeds. *a*, Before the creation of modern breeds, the dog population had the short-range haplotypes expected given its large size and long time since the domestication bottleneck. *b*, In the creation of modern breeds, a small subset of chromosomes was selected from the pool of domestic dogs. The long-range patterns carried on these chromosomes became common within the breed. *c*, In the short time since breed creation, these long-range patterns have not yet been substantially broken down by recombination. Long breed haplotypes, however, still retain the underlying short ancestral haplotype blocks from the domestic dog population, and these are revealed when one examines chromosomes across many breeds. (From Karlsson EK, Lindblad-Toh K: Leader of the pack: gene mapping in dogs and other model organisms. Nat Rev Genet 9[9]:713-725, 2008.)

History Suggests Long Haplotypes within Breeds and Short Haplotypes across Breeds

Canine population history includes two population bottlenecks, the more recent of which occurred in just the last few hundred years when humans created genetically isolated dog breeds (Figure 4-4).[20,21]

It is well established that recent bottlenecks create long linkage disequilibrium (LD) in populations, facilitating trait mapping, whereas for ancient bottleneck events, the LD has broken down into shorter blocks. In dogs one would expect two effects; short LD in the domestic dog population as a whole and long LD within breeds. This would suggest a two-stage mapping strategy, where the disease locus is first identified within a single breed and then narrowed using multiple breeds (Figure 4-5).[5]

To assess the feasibility of a two-stage approach, the genome project completed a detailed analysis of the haplotype structure in breeds and in the dog population. In breeds, each haplotype block is 500 kb to 1 Mb long (a reflection of the long LD) and has 3 to 6 haplotypes specific to each breed.[5,22] In the whole dog population, haplotype blocks and LD are much shorter, about 10 kb.[5,22] Only three to five common ancestral haplotypes are observed for each haplotype block, and haplotypes are shared between distantly related breeds.

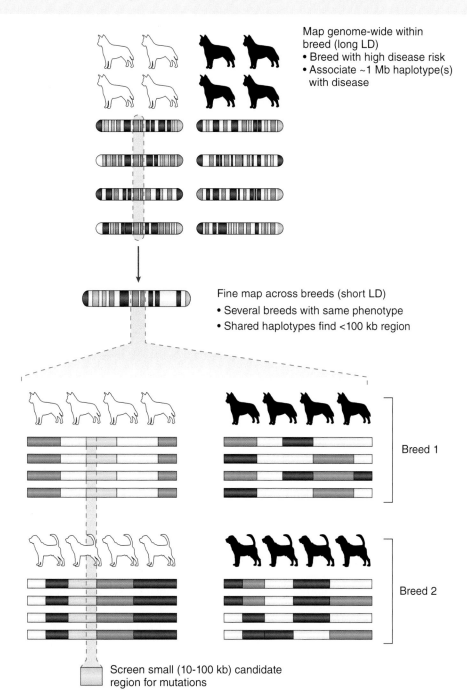

Map genome-wide within
breed (long LD)
• Breed with high disease risk
• Associate ~1 Mb haplotype(s)
  with disease

Fine map across breeds (short LD)
• Several breeds with same phenotype
• Shared haplotypes find <100 kb region

Breed 1

Breed 2

Screen small (10-100 kb) candidate
region for mutations

Figure 4-5 Two-stage mapping strategy. A two-stage approach takes full advantage of the long linkage disequilibrium *(LD)* within breeds and the short ancestral haplotypes shared across breeds, allowing traits to be mapped with relatively few samples.[5] Based on this genome structure, a two-stage mapping strategy is advantageous. In the first step, genome-wide association mapping using >15,000 single nucleotide polymorphisms is employed in a breed with a high disease risk. Secondly, fine mapping of the disease-associated region will be performed in the initial breed together with several related breeds. This permits rapid narrowing of the region to enable mutation screening of part of a gene or a few genes at most. (From Karlsson EK, Lindblad-Toh K: Leader of the pack: gene mapping in dogs and other model organisms. Nat Rev Genet 9[9]:713-725, 2008.)

This sharing of ancestral haplotypes across breeds has important implications for the design of trait-mapping studies. Most disease mutations are likely to predate breed creation, as dog breeds are young and have had little time to accumulate novel mutations. Thus, when several breeds suffer from high prevalence of the same disease, they may share the same causative mutation, carried into each breed on the same ancestral haplotype. However, detecting these shared ancestral blocks in a cross-breed study requires a marker density sufficient to detect 5- to 10-kb ancestral haplotypes, probably a SNP every 1 to 2 kb. Thus, a genome-wide scan is most efficiently done in a single breed, with more breeds added in the fine-mapping stage (see Figure 4-5). To increase the likelihood that different breeds share the same mutation, several studies have focused on identifying the relationship between breeds.[23]

Arrays for Genome-Wide Association Mapping

As part of the dog genome project, the number of SNPs and the number of dogs needed for genome-wide association (GWA) in a breed were estimated.[5] To search the entire genome for the location of a trait locus, 15,000 SNPs proved sufficient. The number of dogs needed in a study using 15,000 SNPs varies depending on the inheritance pattern. For a simple Mendelian recessive trait mapping, the disease allele requires just 20 cases and 20 controls; for a dominant trait, 50 cases and 50 controls suffice. Complex traits are more difficult to model accurately, as the power to detect disease-predisposing alleles varies depending on the relative risk conferred by the allele, the allele frequency, and any interaction with other alleles and the environment. Using a simple model, 100 cases and 100 controls detect a fivefold risk allele in 98% of datasets. While alleles conferring a fivefold increased risk may be uncommon in human populations, the reduced genetic diversity of breed populations, and remarkable high disease prevalence, suggests it is a fair estimate in purebred dogs.

To enable GWA mapping using ~15,000 SNPs, the Broad Institute of Harvard and MIT collaborated with Affymetrix to generate a genome-wide SNP genotyping array.[24] Today, three different genome-wide arrays are available with sufficient SNP coverage for GWA in a breed. These arrays are now being used to map both simple and complex traits, with several studies already published including the white spotting locus, the hair ridge and dermoid sinus in Rhodesian Ridgebacks,[25] cone-rod dystrophy in Dachshunds,[26] and canine epiphyseal dysplyasia in Chinese Crested dogs.[27]

THE FELINE GENOME

The feline genome is relatively closely related to the canine genome but sufficiently different that an independent genome sequence is required. An approximately twofold coverage sequence was generated in 2005 as part of an effort to understand the human genome. The complete genome sequence is expected in 2009. The rational for sequencing the feline genome is similar as for the canine genome. There are specific diseases enriched in certain breeds and a breed structure that makes gene mapping easier than in humans. There is also an active research community that has been developing genetic tools.

The 2× genome of an Abyssinian female cat covers roughly 80% of the genome sequence, as expected when each base is sampled only twice. A preliminary analysis suggests the cat has an average mammalian genome with ~20,000 genes and good similarity to other mammals.[6] A more detailed gene analysis will be possible when the complete genome sequence becomes available, where gene family expansions are more accurately captured. To assist trait mapping, the two chromosomes of the sequenced cat were compared, several types of markers that can be used for mapping was identified including ~300,000 SNPs and ~200,000 short tandem repeats (STRs).

By using ~300 SNPs from the genome project as well as a panel of STRs, the relationship of 120 cat breeds was determined.[28] In addition, the number of SNP markers required for genome-wide association was estimated to >50,000 SNPs. This is at least threefold more than for the dog, but an order of magnitude fewer than in humans.

The generation of a complete genome sequence and many SNPs from multiple breeds will allow the development of better tools for mapping and should lead to the identification of many more disease genes in the coming years.

APPLICATIONS TO VETERINARY CARE

Already prior to the sequencing of the canine and feline genomes, many studies had identified genes and mutations for inherited diseases in cats and dogs. However, with the availability of a genome sequence, knowledge of all genes and their relationship to other mammals, as well as the availability of good tools for disease gene identification, the number of identified genes will snowball over the next few years!

The primary benefit of finding disease genes will be a better understanding of the different diseases and hence the ability to develop better drugs. However, breeders will also want to use genetic tests for guidance in breeding. In some cases, this may be complicated, if most individuals within a breed are predisposed to one or another disease. In addition, for common diseases such as cancers, multiple genetic risk factors as well as environmental factors may govern an individual's risk for the disease. One way may simply be to avoid the worst risk factor combinations, perhaps by taking treatment outcomes for different genetic risk factors into account. Thus, veterinarians may be called upon to interpret and help guide owners based on test results, much like a genetic councilor. This may at times generate conflicts, if one balances the positive effect for a single individual of breeding away from a common risk factor versus the detrimental effects of loss of diversity for the breed as a whole. One such example is the SOD1 mutation present as a major risk factor for degenerative myelopathy.[29] This is a late-onset disease with a high allele frequency in multiple breeds. Because of the frequency, breeding away from this mutation will have to be done very carefully. Perhaps it might even be more productive to find the modifier genes leading to a relatively early onset and breed away from those instead. Knowledge from genetic tests could also potentially lead owners to put dogs down unnecessarily, so it will be important for veterinarians to read up on the specific breed frequencies, onset age, and treatment options and outcomes for certain mutations to know how to best handle such situations.

Still, one clear benefit of genetic testing could be if the choice of drug can be guided by the genetic risk factors of the affected individual. Such long-term benefits, however, will require the cooperation of clinicians, geneticists, and drug companies to develop more targeted drugs and to determine genotype/drug response correlations.

REFERENCES

The reference list can be found on the companion Expert Consult Web site at *www.expertconsult.com*.

CHAPTER 5

Gene Therapy

David J. Argyle

Gene therapy is the introduction of nucleic acids (DNA or RNA) into cells in vivo to treat a disease.[1] The concept of transferring genes into tissues to treat or cure diseases is not a new idea, having been discussed since the early 1960s. However, it is the advances in recombinant DNA technology that have improved our ability to manipulate genetic material and allowed the field of gene therapy to become a clinical reality.[2] While originally conceived as a way of treating life-threatening single-gene defects (e.g., inborn errors of metabolism, severe combined immunodeficiency), gene therapy has become widely applied to a number of other diseases that may involve multiple genetic abnormalities (e.g., cancer) but are refractory to conventional therapies.[3] Since the first human clinical gene therapy trial in 1990, the development of efficient delivery systems and appropriate model systems has been vigorously explored.[2] In this chapter we will discuss the elements for successful gene therapy and how this may be applied to diseases of small animals.

THE ELEMENTS OF GENE THERAPY

Gene therapy typically involves the insertion of a functioning gene into cells to correct a cellular dysfunction or to provide a new cellular function.[2] For example, diseases such as cystic fibrosis, combined immunodeficiency syndromes, muscular dystrophy, hemophilia, and many cancers result from the presence of defective genes. Gene therapy can be used to correct or replace the defective genes responsible. However, for effective gene therapy there is a requirement for the following[4]:

- The disorder has a known genetic defect.
- The therapeutic gene has to be delivered to sufficient number of target cells in the body, thus requiring a vehicle or vector for delivery.
- The therapeutic gene has to be expressed at a sufficient level and for a length of time appropriate for the disease.
- The treatment must be safe.

It has long been regarded that the development of an efficient and safe mechanism for gene delivery has been the major hurdle to gene therapy becoming accepted clinical practice.

VECTOR SYSTEMS

The ideal vector would deliver the gene of interest (transgene) specifically to the cell where the gene would be expressed efficiently. The vector would be easy and cheap to manufacture and would be nonimmunogenic. Unfortunately, the ideal vector does not exist, but currently there are two broad approaches for introducing genetic material into cells: viral and nonviral (Table 5-1).

Viral Vectors: Early studies on the viral etiology of cancer suggested their potential as vectors for gene therapy, by virtue of their ability to transduce cells and give up their genetic material to the host. However, it was not until molecular methods were developed to allow us to manipulate the viral genome that this potential could be realized. At the time of

Table • 5-1

Gene Therapy Vectors and Their Properties

FEATURE	RETROVIRUS	LENTIVIRUS	ADENOVIRUS	AAV	NONVIRAL
Entry into Target Cell	Receptor binding: Transduction	Receptor binding: Transduction	Receptor binding: Transduction	Receptor binding: Transduction	Transfection
Chromosomal Integration	Yes	Yes	No	No (unless *rep* gene included)	No
Transgene Expression	From integrated DNA in host genome	From integrated DNA in host genome	Episomal	Episomal	Episomal
Length of Transgene Expression	Long-term due to integration	Long-term due to integration	Medium term, expression >1 year reported	Medium term, expression >1 year reported	Short-term
Emergence of Replication Competent Vector	Possible	Possible	Possible but very low risk	Possible but very low risk	N/A
Infects Quiescent Cells	No	Yes	Yes	Yes	Yes
Risk of Oncogene Activation	Yes	Yes	No	No	No
Manufacture	Complex	Complex	Complex	Complex	Easy

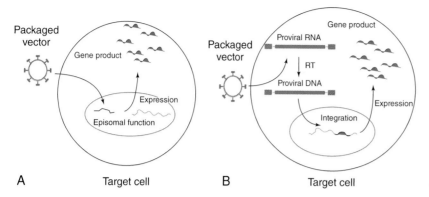

Figure 5-1 Viral gene delivery. **A,** Adenoviral vectors are produced in "producer cell lines." They enter the cell by transduction and their genetic material is transported to the nucleus. In contrast to retroviruses, the DNA is not integrated into the host genome, but gene expression is achieved episomally. **B,** Retroviral vectors are also produced in specialized producer cell lines. They enter the cell by transduction, but their RNA genome is reverse transcribed (by a reverse transcriptase *[RT]*) into proviral DNA. This integrates into the host genome, where expression of the transgene takes place.

writing, over 70% of gene therapy trials to date have utilized viral vectors.[2]

The most common viral vectors and their properties are outlined in Table 5-1. The great advantage to viral vectors for gene delivery is their ability to infect cells and our ability to exploit their replicative machinery (Figure 5-1).

The majority of systems utilize replicative defective viruses to overcome concerns that recombination within the host may lead to the production of wild-type virus with pathogenic potential. The common systems rely on oncogenic retroviruses (e.g., murine leukemia virus [MuLV]) or adenoviruses (e.g., human AD5), but great strides are also being made with lentiviral vectors (particularly human immunodeficiency virus-1 [HIV-1]) and adeno-associated viral vectors (AAV).[5-10]

Nonviral Gene Delivery: Concerns relating to virus safety and an inability to produce high enough viral titers have led to the development of nonviral delivery systems for gene therapy.[11-15] Of the developed nonviral gene-transfer approaches, two methods have been used fairly often in human clinical trials. One involves the simple direct injection of DNA plasmids containing the transgene (naked DNA) into a tissue. This has been used in approximately 14% of human clinical trials, most often in muscle (e.g., in models of Duchenne muscular dystrophy, as DNA vaccines, or directly into tumors for the treatment of cancer). The second method uses cationic liposomes to coat the plasmid DNA and has been used in around 9% of human clinical trials.[2] This lipid coating is considered to facilitate plasmid entry into the cell. The expression of genes from plasmids within cells does usually not result in integration of the DNA into the host-cell genome, and expression is typically short lived.[1]

VECTOR DELIVERY

A further barrier to the clinical development of gene therapy has been the inability to develop efficient vector delivery systems. Using viral vectors, systemic delivery is hindered by rapid clearance of viruses from the body by the immune and complement systems. To overcome this, a number of strategies have been employed:

• Removal of target cells from the body (e.g., hematopoietic stem cells), ex vivo delivery of the transgene using the viral vector, and the return of the target cells to the patient[16] (Figure 5-2)
• Direct injection of virus into target tissue (e.g., for tumor therapy)[3]
• Studies have been performed that describe cellular delivery of viruses by the systemic route. In this, viral producer cells are delivered to the patient and virus production is triggered when the cells reach the target

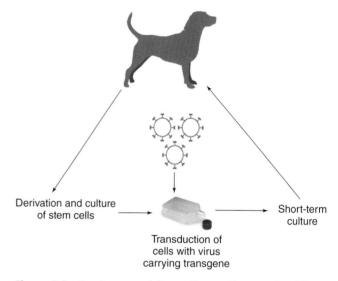

Figure 5-2 Ex vivo gene delivery. Stem cells are isolated from the patient and cultured. The cells are transduced by viral vectors carrying the gene of interest and then returned to the patient.

tissue. T cells, macrophages, and dendritic cells have been explored as potential cell delivery systems with varying success. However, this is technically challenging and cumbersome.[17-21]

For plasmid DNA, systemic delivery is also very limited. Intravenous injection usually leads to accumulation of the vector in the liver. If this is not the target tissue, then it becomes difficult to achieve high levels of gene expression in the appropriate organ. Consequently, the majority of studies have involved direct injection into target tissues using either naked DNA, liposome-encapsulated DNA, or "biolistic" technology. In the latter, naked DNA is adsorbed onto gold particles and fired into tissues at high pressure. The pressure comes from a "gene gun" that utilizes helium to provide the motive force for gene delivery. Limited veterinary studies have been performed using this technology[22] (Figure 5-3).

For intravenous delivery there are some exciting developments utilizing nanomedicine technology. Lower-generation polypropylenimine dendrimers are small molecules that form nanoparticle complexes with DNA and allow the efficient transport of DNA into cells. This system has been used to efficiently transport transgenes systemically in a mouse model to allow high-level gene expression in the target tissue.[23]

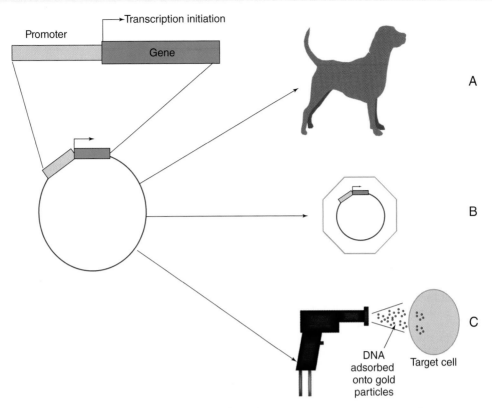

Figure 5-3 Nonviral gene delivery. DNA plasmid vectors contain a gene cassette that incorporates the therapeutic transgene under the control of a promoter. The plasmid can be delivered by direct injection as naked or liposome encapsulated DNA (**A**), by direct injection or systemically wrapped in nanomedicine particles (**B**), or by direct injection utilizing a helium driven "biolistic" gene gun (**C**).

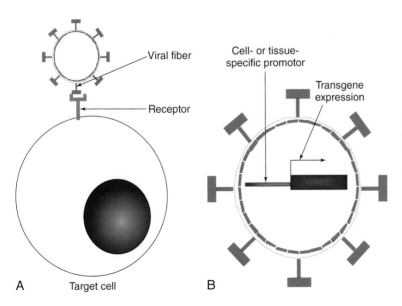

Figure 5-4 Vector targeting. The specificity of viral vectors can be improved utilizing either transductional targeting (**A**) where the viral surface protein are modified so they will only enter the cell of interest; or transcriptional targeting (**B**) where the expression of the therapeutic transgene is under the control of a tissue or cell-specific promoter. Transcriptional targeting can also be employed in nonviral vectors.

VECTOR TARGETING

Another key element of gene therapy is to provide levels of targeting to ensure the transgene is only expressed in the target tissue and normal tissue is spared. In viral vector systems, targeting strategies have been adopted that utilize modification of the viral coat (transductional targeting) and/or regulation of the expression of the transgene (transcriptional targeting)[4] (Figure 5-4).

An example of transductional targeting is the use of modified fibers on the surface of adenoviruses that only allow the virus to enter cells with specific receptors. Transcriptional targeting has been utilized in both viral and nonviral systems and capitalizes on tissue-specific expression of certain genes.[23-30] Although every gene is represented in every cell of the body, expression of any one gene requires specific transcription factors that may be unique to a particular cell or tissue type. Certain genes have been identified that are expressed in target cells but are not expressed in normal cells (e.g., telomerase in cancer cells) or are only expressed in a specific tissue type (e.g., prostate-specific antigen). By using the promoter sequences for these genes to drive transgene expression, targeted expression in specific tissue types can be achieved.

TARGET DISEASES

Monogenic Deficiency Diseases

This group of diseases have been described in both man and domestic animals (e.g., various immunodeficiency syndromes, metabolic storage diseases, hemophilia) and the first human gene therapy trial was in the treatment of adenosine deaminase (ADA) deficiency, a single-gene defect that causes severe immunodeficiency.[1,31] Monogenic deficiency diseases (MDDs) lend themselves to a gene therapy approach, the defective gene being replaced by an exogenous correct version of the same gene. The major hurdle to this therapy, however, is to maintain gene expression for the life of the patient, a goal that is rarely achieved. To this end, most attempts at treatment have involved using a patient's stem cells (i.e., long-lived, self-renewing cells) to express the transgene. In this, cells are removed from the patient, the transgene is introduced to the cells ex vivo, and the cells are returned to the patient. The major problem with this approach has been the ability to achieve long-term gene expression.[16]

While this is very important in human medicine, the treatment of MDD in veterinary patients has been limited. In veterinary medicine, we have the advantage of being able to adopt breeding programs to allow recognized single-gene abnormalities to be removed from particular breeding lines. However, the dog has proved a useful and valuable tool as a model for developing MDD therapies in people, and it is noteworthy that the only really successful gene therapy trials have been accomplished in canine patients.[31-33] For example, gene therapy approaches have been used to correct canine X-linked severe combined immunodeficiency syndromes, canine hemophilia, and retinal dystrophy (RPE65 mutation) associated with the Briard breed. In the hemophilia and retinopathy studies, an AAV vector was used to deliver the correct version of the appropriate gene by direct injection. In the retinopathy model an AAV vector (carrying RPE65 gene) was injected subretinally and helped restore vision in young dogs, but not older dogs (older than 30 months).

Cancer

Despite advances in surgical techniques and the use of radiotherapy and chemotherapy, cancer still remains a disease of high mortality in both human and veterinary medicine, warranting the investigation of alternative treatments. Gene therapy has the potential to play a major role in the development of new cancer therapeutic agents, the following being examples of how this is being developed.

Corrective Gene Therapy The increased understanding of the molecular events in cancer has made possible the identification of defective genes involved in the cancer phenotype. The "cancer genes" are either oncogenes or tumor suppressor genes and are in fact normal genes involved in the tight regulation of the cell cycle. Oncogenes have a positive effect on cellular proliferation (the gas pedal), and tumor suppressor genes have a negative effect (the brakes). Defects in either oncogenes or tumor suppressor genes can promote the cancer phenotype.
- *Correcting mutated tumor suppressor genes:* One of the most studied genes in cancer development has been the tumor suppressor gene *p53*. *p53* acts as a genomic

guardian for the cell, being switched on when a cell's DNA is damaged. The product of this gene causes the cell to either stop dividing or become apoptotic (programmed cell death) depending on the degree of damage. In many cancers this gene is defective, and so damaged cells fail to stop dividing and can accumulate further damaging events, which can allow selection for a malignant phenotype. There have been a number of studies that have addressed this by attempting to replace the defective *p53* gene with its normal counterpart.[3,34] However, there are problems associated with this approach including (1) the inability of our current technology to be able to efficiently deliver a normal *p53* gene to every cancer cell in a tumor mass and (2) cancer is a multigenetic abnormality, and the delivery of one correct gene to a tumor cell may still not have the desired phenotypic effect.[1]
- *Targeting mutated oncogenes:* In comparison to tumor suppressor genes, this situation in cancer requires the expression of the oncogene to be blocked rather than increased. One way of achieving this utilizes the recently described method of RNA interference. In this, short 21bp oligonucleotide fragments (specific for the oncogene mRNA in question) are introduced into the cell. These oligonucleotides cause specific degradation of the target mRNA and provide an efficient mechanism for blocking expression of mutated oncogenes[3,35]

Destruction of Cancer Cells through Delivery of "Suicide Genes" Typically this approach involves the delivery of a gene (usually an enzyme) to cancer cells that has the ability to convert a relatively nontoxic prodrug to an active compound within the cancer cell (gene-directed enzyme prodrug therapy [GDEPT]) (Figure 5-5).

At the clinical level, the gene would be delivered to the patient's tumor and the enzyme activity would be confined to the cancer cells.[1,36] The patient would then be given a prodrug systemically. In the cancer cells, this novel enzyme can convert the prodrug to a more active compound that has the ability to kill the cancer cell. However, due to the low

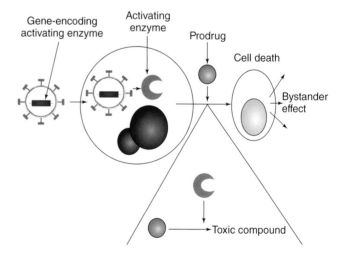

Figure 5-5 Gene-directed enzyme prodrug therapy. In gene-directed enzyme prodrug therapy (GDEPT), an activating gene is delivered to the cancer cells. A relatively inactive prodrug is then given to the patient systemically. In cells processing the activating gene, the prodrug is converted to a highly toxic drug, which can kill the cancer cell. The advantage of this system is the evidence of bystander effect. In this, only a small proportion of cancer cells need to receive the activating gene, as toxic metabolites leak across gap junctions and kill surrounding cancer cells.

efficiency of existing vectors, the success of this therapy will be largely dependent on the extent of the bystander effect. In this, the activation of the prodrug in the cell causes cell death and also leakage of toxic metabolites to neighboring cells. Consequently, it is estimated that only a small fraction of the cells need receive the gene for there to be a dramatic effect on tumor volume. Further, in mouse models, a distant bystander effect on tumor metastases has been demonstrated that is mediated through the patient's immune system.[37] These systems have been combined with transcriptionally targeted vectors (described above) to improve the eventual therapeutic index.

Gene-Directed Immunotherapy It has been demonstrated that cell-mediated immune responses are important components of the antitumor immune response. Cytokines are small glycoprotein molecules that orchestrate immune response, tissue repair, and hematopoiesis, and it has been demonstrated that the relative amounts of individual cytokines can direct the immune system towards either a mainly humoral or mainly a cell-mediated response. In particular, cytokines such as IL-2, interferon-gamma, IL-12, and IL-18 have the ability to promote cell-mediated responses and have allowed the development of a number of clinical gene therapy approaches to cancer using these cytokines genes.[38-43] This approach has also been adopted in a number of small-scale veterinary studies including canine malignant melanoma. In both human and veterinary studies, encouraging antitumor responses have been reported. However, often the response to therapy is highly variable among patients. Up until recently it was considered that this local cytokine response was required to reverse T cell anergy and to allow the immune system to attack the malignant cells. More recently it has become clear that a large part of immune tolerance of cancer cells is mediated through the presence of T regulatory cells within the tumor mass. It is highly probable that future gene therapy cytokine studies will have to be designed with this in mind, where there is a requirement for both promotion of cell-mediated responses and inhibition of T regulatory cells.[44]

Delivery of Chemoprotective Genes In an alternative approach to gene therapy for cancer, this method involves the delivery of genes to normal cells of the bone marrow to protect them against the cytotoxic effects of conventional chemotherapeutic drugs. In particular, the multidrug resistance gene (MDR) has been cloned and delivered to normal bone marrow cells in attempt to protect bone marrow cells from the toxic effects of conventional chemotherapy.[45-47]

The Use of Replication-Competent Viral Vectors Progress has been made in the development of replication-competent viruses that conditionally replicate in cancer cells. As an example, the Onyx 015 vector is an E1b-deleted adenovirus that conditionally replicates in cells with a nonfunctional *p53* gene.[48] p53 protein has the potential to shut down cell cycling when infected with wild-type adenovirus but is prevented from doing so through the actions of the product of viral E1b. E1b-deficient viruses cannot replicate in normal cells with *p53* intact. However, in cells that have no functional p53 protein, viral replication can proceed and cause cell lysis (Figure 5-6).

Many other conditionally replicating viruses are being developed that rely on specific cancer cell defects (e.g., reoviruses that conditionally replicate in cells with intact *Ras* signaling pathways) or are transcriptionally targeted.[49-54] *p53* mutations in domestic species such as the dog and cat have also been well characterized, and this may provide targets for therapy particularly for diseases such as canine osteosarcoma and feline vaccine-associated sarcomas.

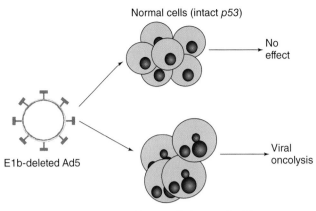

Figure 5-6 Conditionally replicating adenovirus. The Onyx 015 vector is an E1b-deleted adenovirus that conditionally replicates in cells with a nonfunctional *p53* gene. p53 protein has the potential to shut down cell cycling when infected with wild-type adenovirus but is prevented from doing so through the actions of the product of viral E1b. E1b-deficient viruses cannot replicate in normal cells with *p53* intact. However, in cells that have no functional p53 protein, viral replication can proceed and cause cell lysis.

Miscellaneous Approaches to Cancer Gene Therapy The multigenetic abnormalities of cancer lend themselves to multiple gene therapy approaches. In addition to those described above there is vigorous exploration of:
- Gene delivery of sodium iodide symporter genes to tumors to allow them to concentrate radioactive iodine.[3]
- Delivering proapoptotic genes to cancer cells.[3]
- Delivering antiangiogenesis genes to cancers to inhibit growth of their blood supply.[3]

It is highly likely that one individual approach to cancer will be insufficient to cure or control particular cancers. However, it is possible that a combination of treatments, with or without conventional therapies, will prove to provide the best therapeutic solution.

Other Disease Targets
Cancer and MDDs have dominated the gene therapy arena. However, the previous decade has demonstrated that gene therapy technologies can be applied to a broad range of acquired diseases. For further information, the reader is advised to read the associated references:

Infectious Diseases An obvious target for gene therapy in human medicine has been HIV.[55,56] Since HIV predominantly infects cells of the hematopoietic system, pluripotent stem cells constitute potential targets for the introduction of foreign anti-HIV genes. Reimplantation of the genetically modified stem cells into AIDS patients should theoretically allow the repopulation of the host with mature CD4+ cell populations expressing novel molecules that might interfere with viral replication and slow the progression of the disease. This is just one of many strategies being adopted for this disease, others include:
- ***Introduction of suicide genes:*** E.g., cells modified with suicide genes (see cancer section above) for negative selection of HIV-infected cells.
- ***RNA interference (RNAi):*** As with the cancer therapies described above, these are short 21bp oligonucleotides that cause inhibition of gene expression in a sequence-specific fashion. To date, small interfering RNAs have

been used in vitro to target viral genes like *tat* and *rev* and cellular genes like CCR5 with great success.

A direct consequence of this may be the development of appropriate therapies for diseases such as feline immunodeficiency virus (FIV) in cats.

Inflammatory Disease   As the veterinary profession has become adept at controlling the major life-threatening infectious diseases of companion animals, we are now faced with an aging population of patients. Osteoarthritis (OA) in both dogs and cats has become a major and significant problem with few therapeutic solutions. Currently the use of nonsteroidal antiinflammatory drugs (NSAIDs) enables the control of pain but is not disease modifying. There are several studies underway currently developing gene therapy strategies for OA. One of these approaches has been to develop delivery systems to target joint tissue with genes that will inhibit the inflammatory environment (e.g., TNF [tumor necrosis factor] receptor, IL-1RAP [interleukin 1 receptor antagonist protein]). The aim is to produce a therapy that is truly disease modifying and improve the welfare in this chronically painful condition.[57]

Cardiac Disease   With increasing knowledge of basic molecular mechanisms governing the development of heart failure (HF), the possibility of specifically targeting key pathologic players is evolving. Technology allowing for efficient in vivo transduction of myocardial tissue with long-term expression of a transgene enables translation of basic mechanistic knowledge into potential gene therapy approaches. Gene therapy in HF is in its infancy clinically with the predominant amount of experience being from animal models. Nevertheless, this challenging and promising field is gaining momentum as recent preclinical studies in larger animals such as dogs have been carried out with encouraging results.[58]

SAFETY CONSIDERATIONS IN GENE THERAPY

In 1999, gene therapy suffered a major setback with the death of a patient as a direct result of adenovirus gene therapy. One of the major considerations in gene therapy revolves around issues of safety, in particular:

- Inappropriate inflammatory responses caused by vector delivery (e.g., adenoviruses)
- The generation of replication-competent viruses, although this is unlikely with new-generation vectors
- Insertional mutagenesis caused by integrating viruses (e.g., retroviruses)

Many of these issues are resolving with the development of new-generation vectors.[1] As an example, above we discussed the use of a patient's stem cells to harbor an integrated retrovirus expressing a correct version of a gene. Because it is difficult to control where the retrovirus will insert, there is always a risk of insertional mutagenesis, putting the patient at increased risk of cancer. However, one group has recently described the use of zinc finger nucleases (engineered DNA-editing enzymes) that allow the insertion of DNA to a site of choice within the genome.[59] This adds a further level of safety in a high-risk procedure.

CONCLUSION

Gene therapy promises a completely new approach to the treatment of diseases such as cancer and osteoarthritis and represents the newest area of pharmacology. There are a number of technical issues that need to be resolved before gene therapy becomes established clinical practice, such as safety issues surrounding the delivery and efficiency of the vectors. Despite gene therapy being very much in its infancy, the field is advancing at a rapid rate and is highly likely to become an established clinical tool.

REFERENCES

The reference list can be found on the companion Expert Consult Web site at *www.expertconsult.com.*

CHAPTER **6**

Clinical Genomics

Matthew Breen

WHAT IS CLINICAL GENOMICS?

As a rapidly expanding field, the term *clinical genomics* is being used as an umbrella to encompass an increasing number of activities. In general terms, clinical genomics can be grossly described as the use of information obtained from genomics activities for medical purposes. Genomics activities in this context include, but are certainly not limited to, areas of research based on DNA sequencing, gene discovery, DNA copy number, gene expression, and haplotype association. It is perhaps the ability to be able to most appropriately associate relevant clinical/medical information to the emerging

molecular information that provides us with the single largest challenge over the coming decades. As such, sophisticated bioinformatics tools are being developed simultaneously to support the need to combine genomics data with molecular medicine and to allow appropriate delivery of this information to medical decision makers.

With the human genome sequence completed and available in the public domain, and either complete or ongoing genome sequences becoming available for a variety of species of veterinary significance, including animals and their pathogens, it is evident that what is being developed for application to human clinical genomics today will become available to veterinary medicine soon after. With such a growth rate it is not feasible to represent all areas in this introductory chapter, and so we will skim the surface and select examples that serve to illustrate how this field is progressing.

CLINICAL GENOMICS IN VETERINARY MEDICINE

Cost of Veterinary Health Care

As is the case with human health, the care of animals comes at a price, be they companion animals that live in and around our homes, livestock that provide us with food, or captive and free-ranging wildlife. According to a recent market analysis, the estimated global sales of veterinary medicines is currently in the region of $11 billion, of which around two thirds represents sales for the noncompanion animal, primarily food animal, sector and one third for the companion animal sector (http://www.marketreports.com). There is, however, a major difference between the health care of companion versus food animals in so far as food animals rarely reach old age and generally end their lives at a time selected by the industry and with consideration of their economic value. As a consequence, health care costs associated with food animals are generally for younger individuals. Companion animals, however, share a close bond with humans and so are generally allowed to live out the natural course of their lives. As with improvements to human health, advances in veterinary health care translates to prolonged lifespan of companion animals and a consequential increase in age-related diseases/illnesses. Overall there is huge investment in the health and welfare of our pets, raging from routine vaccinations and the numerous preventive medications for flea, tick, and heartworm controls, to the development of sophisticated treatments for chronic illnesses, such as nonsteroidal antiinflammatory drugs for canine arthritis.

A report of the global veterinary pharmaceutical market noted recently that the growth of the pharmaceutical market for companion animals is now at a rate comparable to that of human health care (http://www.bioportfolio.com). Establishing the actual overall cost of veterinary health are in the USA is not easy, though the American Pet Products Manufacturers Association (APPMA) estimates that in 2008 Americans will spend almost $10.5 billion on the overall health care for their pets. The APPMA estimate that the average lifetime cost of a medium-size dog is $10,400, with small dogs costing slightly less and a large one slightly more. Caring for a cat is comparable, with lifetime cost averaging $10,600.

The cost of providing health care for our pets is increasing to a level that prohibits many owners from being able to pay for the treatment required. For example, a 2008 report by Sainsbury's Finance in the UK revealed that veterinary health care costs are now rising at three times the level of inflation and that between 2003 and 2008 in the UK 1,600,000 cats and dogs were euthanized because their owners could not afford the medical costs associated with caring for their pet. During the same period an additional 2,500,000 were not treated due to cost, potentially exposing these animals to pain and suffering (http://www.money.co.uk).

Diagnostic Screening for Genetic Disease and Cancer in Animals

In considering the role and subsequent potential impact of clinical genomics in veterinary medicine, it is important to appreciate that the technological advancements and progress have stemmed largely from the application of genomics sciences information to human disease management. Genetic differences in drug metabolism and drug responses have been described for almost half a century, and the emergence of genome sequence data along with methods to amplify DNA and assays to determine gene sequences have revolutionized our ability to perform large-association studies with huge cohorts. To mention just one example, cardiovascular disease in humans is the leading cause of death the USA, with an age-adjusted death rate in the population of 241/100,000.[1] Approximately 71% of all deaths associated with heart disease in the USA are as a result of coronary heart disease.[2] Almost half of all deaths associated with cardiac arrest occur before medical treatment can be initiated following the arrest, and so identifying disease status early and implementing appropriate health management are key to reducing mortality.[3] As such, human cardiovascular disease has received a lot of attention towards identifying genetic risk factors associated with genetic predisposition. Studies conducted almost a decade ago revealed that the risk for myocardial infarction was higher for people who have an affected first-degree female relative than for those with an affected first-degree male relative.[4] Similarly, around the same time data indicated the presence of protective genotypes, for example in regards to sequence variation in the gene coding for lipoprotein.[5] Gene association studies are ongoing to determine the effect of genetic variations on the etiology, progression, and response to therapy for patients diagnosed with cardiovascular disease. Knowledge of such genetic risk factors for a plethora of diseases will facilitate discoveries of disease prevention as well as improve disease management. While lagging behind human medicine, the same approach applies to veterinary medicine.

With the recent availability of genome sequences for a variety of veterinary species, including dog (canFam2), horse (equiCab1), cat (felCat3), cow (bosTau4), and chicken (galGal3) (http://genome.ucsc.edu), the development of clinical genomics applications to veterinary species is inevitable.

Numerous traits, inherited disorders, and genes have been characterized in a wide range of animals, many of which are appropriately summarized as part of the Online Mendelian Inheritance in Animals (OMIA) database (http://omia.angis. org.au). This database contains useful information as well as references and appropriate links to relevant *PubMed* and gene records at the National Center for Biotechnology Information (NCBI). One could dedicated an entire volume to discuss the impact that clinical genomics has, or will have, on many of these diseases. For the present brief discussion we will concentrate of just a few relatively well-known examples that span the breadth of the species concerned.

Genetic/Diagnostic Testing

HYPP in horses Equine hyperkalemic periodic paralysis (HYPP) is a disease caused by spikes in serum potassium levels that can cause episodes of variable-intensity chronic muscle twitching (fasciculations) and delayed muscle relaxation (myotonia).[6] It appears that this disease arose in a single male American Quarter Horse, born in 1968, who developed a magnificent physique and was aptly named "Impressive." Such was his performance and conformation that Impressive went on to sire over 2000 offspring and is believed to have over 55,000 descendents. Many of these descendents shared his dramatic physical stature and became outstanding and prolific stallions and broodmares. However, the Impressive line is plagued with HYPP, which was shown to be an autosomal dominant disorder caused by just a single-point mutation/ single-base substitution* in the equine adult skeletal muscle sodium channel alpha subunit gene.[6-8] Only horses descended from Impressive have been shown to have this mutation. Of great interest is that the same gene is known also to cause HYPP in humans. With the polymerase chain reaction (PCR) already established, identifying the mutation at the level of DNA sequence allowed the development of a diagnostic PCR test for the presence of this mutant allele. In addition, knowledge of the mutation allowed for the development of an oligo-specific hybridization assay. With the ability to accurately and reliably detect the mutation, the American Quarter Horse Association (AQHA) determined that, as of 2007, all foals descended from Impressive are required to be parentage verified and HYPP genotyped. Any AQH foal that is shown to be homozygous for the mutant allele will not be eligible for AQHA registration (http://www.aqha.com/association/registration/hypp.html). By adopting this policy, the AQHA is hoping to minimize the transmission of the disease allele in subsequent generations through a process of controlled breeding.

Freemartinism in cattle Freemartinism is a condition that has been known for decades. The condition is the most frequent form of intersexuality in cattle and among the most severe forms of sexual abnormality seen in cattle. Mixed-sex twins cogestating in the same uterus frequently exchange placental fluids as a consequence of placental anastomosis, resulting in the fetuses developing XX/XY chimerism. The masculinization effect on the female reproductive tract is variable, but generally results in the female calf presenting with an underdeveloped reproductive tract and small ovaries, leading to infertility. In dairy farming, the economic impact of this condition, when undetected, is in the cost of raising a female calf to adulthood before becoming aware of her infertility and thus her inability to produce milk. Early detection is therefore a key factor. For many years, freemartinism in cattle was detected by assessment of metaphase chromosome preparation generated from a short-term (48 to 72 hours) mitogenically stimulated peripheral lymphocyte culture of a fresh blood sample. The ease of identifying the metacentric sex chromosomes among the acrocentric autosomal complement of cattle allows for rapid screening of individual metaphase spreads. However, cytogenetic screening in livestock is used less widely now than it was 20 years ago, being replaced by faster, more sensitive molecular-based approaches that also have no requirement for transport and processing of viable cells.[9] For example, PCR-based testing was developed for detecting Y-specific cattle chromosome material in heifer DNA samples and is still used widely to identify freemartin cattle.[10-12] The molecular approach offers a considerably faster throughput and thus provides significant cost saving. In addition, direct comparison of molecular versus cytogenetic screening for freemartinism has demonstrated the increased sensitivity of the PCR approach.[13]

Genetic testing for canine diseases Of all companion and livestock species, the domestic dog has perhaps received the most attention with regards to the prevalence of genetic diseases and the need to develop diagnostic tests to effectively identify individuals affected by or susceptible to such diseases. Inherited disorders in the domestic dog have been recognized for over a century, starting with those associated with very visible, striking phenotypes, such as skeletal malformations, to the "hidden" but well-established biomedical disorders, and now to a series of "new" diseases that have defined DNA mutations. There are numerous resources that provide detailed information and links to describe the vast range of inherited disease in dogs, one such being the IDID (inherited disease in dogs) based at the University of Cambridge, UK (http://www.vet.cam.ac.uk/idid) as well as components of the OMIA database (http://omia.angis.org.au) mentioned earlier.[14] Within the IDID database there are data for over 1000 canine genetic

diseases, the majority of which are reported to be autosomal recessive monogenic disorders. Of great interest is the fact that many genetic diseases in purebred dogs are generally reported to affect one or just a few closely related breeds, reflecting their shared ancestry in breed development and subsequent restricted gene pool. In the genomics era of the early 21st century, combining accurate phenotype with tools for rapid genotyping means that discovering the underlying genetic basis for single-gene inherited diseases is becoming a considerably less daunting task. The genetic lesions associated with over 50 single-gene defects in the canine genome have now been characterized, allowing the development of molecular-based, rapid screening tests to determine the genotype of individuals. Many of the earlier genetic tests for dogs were based on detection of a "marker locus," the genotype of which is tightly "linked" to, and thus used to represent, the actual disease gene. However, with such association testing there is always the chance that some genetically "normal" individuals may present with an "affected" haplotype. As more of these tests are based on detection of the actual mutation, rather than a closely linked marker locus, the risk of false positives is eliminated and certainty of genetic diagnosis becomes absolute. It is therefore important for owners/breeder/veterinarians seeking to use a genetic test to be fully aware of the nature of the test being offered and to consider this when reviewing the results. The aim of this molecular screen is to identify those dogs, even at birth, that will develop a particular disease later in life. As important, genetic testing is also aimed at identifying asymptomatic carriers of disease, dogs who will not be affected by the particular disease during their lifespan, but whose genome is hiding a copy of the mutant allele, and who may therefore propagate the disease in subsequent generations. Knowledge of the genotype of a disease locus allows for informed breeding programs to aid in reducing the frequency of the mutant allele in the population, ultimately reducing incidence of the clinical manifestation of the associated disease.

The study of dog diseases that are likely associated with a complex inheritance pattern (e.g., hip dysplasia, cancers) is increasing as our abilities improve to design, implement, and analyze the huge volume of genomics data now able to be produced.

Inherited genetic diseases in the dog affect almost every system of the body, and since many of the phenotypes closely resemble acquired disorders, the ability to accurately diagnose the genetic basis is key if we wish to see any impact on the health of future generations.

Cancer Cytogenetics

Clinical genomics has resulted in the development of sophisticated tests of increasing importance in the detection, prevention, and management of cancer. The presence of chromosome aberrations have been described in over 25,000 human neoplasms representing 75 different types of cancer (http://cgap.nci.nih.gov/Chromosomes/Mitelman). In human medicine, the identity of cytogenetic aberrations has been shown also to assist in the localization of cancer-associated genes and even selection of the most appropriate therapeutic approach. The application of molecular cytogenetics to the analysis of human neoplasia has revolutionized the way in which we interrogate tumor cells for cytogenetic changes, whether they are numerical or structural in origin. The first cytogenetic aberration observed in human cancer that was associated with a pathogenic event also provides a classic example of the impact of clinical genomics. The Philadelphia chromosome (Ph[1]) is a cytogenetic aberration observed in over 80% of adults diagnosed with chronic myelogenous leukemia (CML).[15] Using classical cytogenetics, this rearrangement was shown to

---

*The HYPP mutation is a missense transversion, changing a C to a G and resulting in the generation of the amino acid leucine in place of the normal phenylalanine.

involve an exchange of chromosomal material between the distal ends of human chromosomes (HSA) 9 and 22, generating a derivative chromosome 22 described as t(9;22) (q34;q11).[16] Using locus-specific fluorescence in situ hybridization (FISH), the Philadelphia chromosome may be observed in affected cells in which the gene ABL (usually located at HSA 9q34) is adjacent to the gene BCR (usually located at HSA 22q11). The chimeric activity of the BCR-ABL fusion gene results in elevated tyrosine kinase activity, and it is this that is crucial to the oncogenic potential. In simple terms, the BCR-ABL protein tells the bone marrow to keep making abnormal white blood cells. To halt progression of the disease thus requires this inappropriate signal to be blocked, an effect of the BCR-ABL kinase antagonist, imatinib mesylate (Gleevec®).[15] In blocking the signal given by the BCR-ABL protein, Gleevec acts to stop the formation of new abnormal cells. While this effect does not apply to all patients with CML, it is sufficiently effective that Gleevec therapy is now considered standard of care for patients shown to present with the Philadelphia chromosome. The presence of the Philadelphia chromosome is generally determined with molecular cytogenetics, though PCR-based tests are also available. Since Imatinib mesylate actually inhibits several protein tyrosine kinases including platelet-derived growth factor receptor (PDGFR) and c-kit, which are preferentially expressed in tumor cells, this therapy is in ongoing studies to evaluate its effects in other cancers.[17-20]

From a veterinary perspective, CML is rare and those cases reported in the dog face a poor prognosis.[21-24] A recent study aimed at demonstrating the evolutionarily conserved cytogenetic changes in corresponding human and dog cancers showed that some dogs diagnosed with CML also present with a BCR-ABL translocation (the "Raleigh" chromosome)[24] (Figure 6-1).

These data suggest that, cost aside, treatment with Gleevec (using careful monitoring for liver toxicity) could be an option for therapy of these canine CML cases.

EMERGING APPROACHES TO CLINICAL GENOMICS

The development of DNA sequence-based microarrays allow the genotype of an individual to be surveyed at ever-increasing resolution. In addition, gene expression microarrays (gene chips) are available to allow one to determine simultaneously the level of activity for several thousand genes within a cell population. Currently, gene expression microarrays are commercially available for numerous veterinary species, including dog, horse, cattle, pig, and chicken. Similarly, microarrays are being developed for veterinary species that genotype simultaneously tens of thousands of discrete regions within a signal genome, evaluating the genome of an individual for variation at the level of single nucleotides. These single nucleotide polymorphisms (SNPs) may be grouped together to develop specific haplotypes that are associated with a particular complex disease. Using these approaches, it is now possible to study several hundred individuals, grouped according to a shared "phenotype" in a relatively short timeframe. Through the use of complex statistical algorithms and bioinformatics, significant phenotype-genotype associations may be revealed, involving small regions of the genome. Subsequent study of these regions will then reveal the underlying genes involved and hence provide the means to develop appropriate diagnostic processes.

Currently the application of advanced genomic technologies for routine health is cost prohibitive, even for human medicine. The most recent animal genome to be sequenced and assembled was the horse, costing in the region of $15

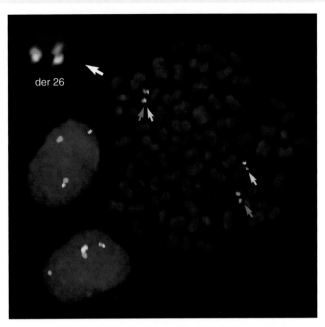

Figure 6-1 Detection of the "Raleigh" chromosome in dogs by molecular cytogenetics. Two canine BAC clones, representing BCR on dog chromosome 9 and ABL on dog chromosome 26, were labeled with an orange or green reporter, respectively. When hybridized to cells from a canine patient with chronic myelogenous leukemia, it is evident in the metaphase spread that in addition to a copy of dog chromosomes 9 (*yellow arrow*) and 26 (*green arrow*) the BCR-ABL probes are adjacent on one chromosome indicating the presence of a 9/26 translocation (*inset*). This translocation is also evident in the two interphase nuclei, where one orange and green locus are juxtaposed. (From Breen M, Modiano JF: Evolutionarily conserved cytogenetic changes in hematological malignancies of dogs and humans—man and his best friend share more than companionship. Chromosome Res 16[1]:145-154, 2008.)

million. However, with the race for the $1000 genome sequence now ongoing, it is conceivable that, as with human health, within the next decade having an animal's genome sequenced for the purposes of health management could become a central component of routine veterinary care.[25,26] The ultimate in clinical veterinary genomics would be individualized medicine based on the genetic health status of our animals.

SUMMARY

In human medicine it is clear that the development of genomics-based diagnostics will continue to precede development of new therapeutics. Without doubt, clinical genomics will begin also to play a more active role in advancing veterinary medicine. How this is approached could, and should, have a major impact on decisions taken regarding diagnosis, prognosis, and treatment strategies for our pets, livestock, and managed wildlife populations. The only certainty as we enter this new era of personalized medicine is that it will happen, and do so at an increasing rate. The veterinary community needs to be prepared to meet the expectations of their clients as well as the needs of their patients.

REFERENCES

The reference list can be found on the companion Expert Consult Web site at *www.expertconsult.com*.

CHAPTER 7

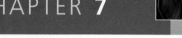

Rational Use of Diagnostic Tests

Kevin A. Hahn
Beth Overley

After obtaining a medical history, veterinarians next proceed with the physical examination of the pet. While physical examination can provide some of the most useful information a veterinarian can obtain, conclusions are subjective and dependent on many variables, including the experience of the veterinarian. Information about the accuracy, precision, sensitivity, and specificity of physical examination findings is also lacking. Thus, these examination findings serve as guideposts to suggest the need for further diagnostic tests that can rule out, confirm, or diagnose states of health and disease. The benefits of performing additional tests, however, are dependent upon judicious and rational test selection, the accurate performance of the tests, and appropriate interpretation and application of results.

SCREENING TESTS

Diagnostic tests are often used to screen asymptomatic patients and identify risk factors for occult disease. Screening tests should be generally noninvasive, inexpensive, and of minimal risk to the patient. Screening tests should have high diagnostic *sensitivity*, which means few false negative results would be expected, as the goal of testing is to rule out the presence of disease. Screening tests should be used to screen for diseases that (1) have serious consequences if left undetected, (2) are reasonably prevalent within the population, and (3) have treatment options readily available. Should a positive result be obtained, a more accurate, confirmatory test should then be performed.

One example of a screening test would be the urine cortisol-to-creatinine ratio $(Cort:Crt)_u$, which is used to screen symptomatic patients for canine hyperadrenocorticism.[1,2] The $(Cort:Crt)_u$ ratio tests for the presence or absence of urinary cortisol excretion and is noninvasive and inexpensive. It also has a high diagnostic sensitivity, which means that a negative result strongly indicates that the patient most likely does not have the disease.[1,2] Urinary cortisol excretion can be caused by both pathologic and physiologic processes, however, and the test cannot distinguish between the two. Therefore, the $(Crt:Crt)_u$ test is not a confirmatory test as it has poor *specificity*, which means there are many false positives. If a patient tests positive, additional tests are required to definitively diagnose hyperadrenocorticism.

DIAGNOSTIC TESTS

Diagnostic tests are often performed to establish a diagnosis or differentiate between two diagnoses in symptomatic patients. Since the goal is to definitively identify a specific disease state, these tests should have good *specificity*, which means there should be few false positive results. Tests with high diagnostic specificity are often used after screening tests to confirm diagnoses. In addition to confirming a disease state, diagnostic tests may also reveal additional information as well

about the severity of disease. They can yield useful prognostic information and establish a baseline for treatment monitoring and disease progression.

Often, several diagnostic modalities can be used to seek a diagnosis in a symptomatic patient. Each test has unique characteristics of which a clinician should be aware. For example, both thoracic radiographs and computed tomography (CT) scan can be used to evaluate pulmonary metastases. CT scan is the more sensitive modality due to superior contrast resolution and diminished anatomic superimposition.[3,4] CT may be less specific though, since it detects more lesions, many of which may be nonneoplastic. It would make sense to use CT scan as a screening test. However, it is less readily available, more expensive, and requires general anesthesia, which increases risk to the patient and cost to the owner. Therefore, radiographs are still more commonly used. However, situations exist where CT scan should be strongly considered. For example, prior to thoracotomy for pulmonary mass excision, CT scan should be recommended to better characterize lymph node size and determine the presence of smaller lesions, since both findings strongly affect prognosis.[5]

In general, less expensive, less invasive, and less risky tests are offered first, although owners should be made aware that more expensive, more invasive tests may follow if diagnosis is not achieved. For example, fine needle aspiration and cytologic evaluation are often recommended prior to surgical removal and biopsy of a mass. For many tumor types, such as lymphoma and mast cell tumors, diagnosis is usually easily achieved with cytology, and knowledge of the diagnosis prior to surgery augments treatment planning. For spindle cell tumors, such as fibrosarcoma or hemangiopericytoma, diagnostic cytologic samples are not always obtained, and a biopsy may need to be performed to achieve a definitive diagnosis.[6]

USEFUL CHARACTERISTICS OF DIAGNOSTIC TESTS

Accuracy and Precision

Accuracy is the measure of a test result's accordance with results determined by a gold standard. It is the frequency with which a given test correctly identifies a patient as having a disease, or put another way, how closely the mean of test data points accords to the mean of the reference standard. A test with high diagnostic accuracy has relatively few false results in comparison to true results.

Precision is the measure of a test result's reproducibility. If repeated testing is performed on an individual patient's sample, the results from each testing should be similar to each other if the test is, in fact, precise. For instance, if a white blood cell count from an individual patient is run 2 to 3 times on a particular hematology analyzer, the results would be considered precise if the results from each testing were in concordance with each other. Results from a hematology analyzer would be expected to be more precise than results from manual differentials.[7] However, it must be confirmed that this is the case, particularly when results from a particular test do not accord with expectations or with a patient's clinical presentation. Put a different way, precision can be thought of as the standard deviation, or how tightly data points cluster around a mean. To achieve valid results, tests must be both accurate and precise.

Gold Standards

To determine the diagnostic accuracy of any given test, there must be a valid and accurate *gold standard* to which test results can be compared. A *gold standard*, ideally, is a reference standard for a particular disease that perfectly distinguishes diseased from nondiseased patients. For some diseases, gold standards are well established. One example would be the use of the adrenocorticotropic hormone (ACTH) stimulation test to determine the presence of hypoadrenocorticism in dogs.[8] Unfortunately, in many other disease states (e.g., pancreatitis), a gold standard either does not exist or is difficult, expensive, or risky to perform. When gold standards are invasive, risky, or expensive, other tests are often developed to confirm and/or support the diagnosis of a given disease. Results from a less invasive, less expensive test are then compared with results from the gold standard to determine the test's clinical utility. This is how a test's diagnostic sensitivity and specificity are determined. If no gold standard exists, sensitivity and specificity are wholly unreliable.

Sensitivity and Specificity

Sensitivity and specificity are characteristics used to define tests. *Sensitivity* characterizes the probability that test results are positive in patients afflicted with a given disease. For test x, if all patients actually afflicted with the disease of interest test positive (no diseased patients have negative tests), then test sensitivity is 100%. Tests with high diagnostic sensitivity make good screenings tests. A negative test result would indicate the patient does not have the disease. A common mnemonic used to remember this is Sn-N-out (high SeNsitivity + Negative result = rule OUT disease).[9]

Specificity characterizes the probability that test results are negative in patients *not afflicted* with a given disease. For test x, if all patients not afflicted with the disease of interest test negative, test specificity is 100%. A positive test result would indicate the patient has the disease. The mnemonic for specificity is Sp-P-in (high Specificity + Positive result = rule IN disease).[9]

Sensitivity and specificity are static characteristics of a diagnostic test, but they are only valid if the test is used to evaluate patients with similar demographics to those evaluated when these test characteristics were determined. If the demographics of patients in a clinical practice differ, the reported sensitivity and specificity of a given test may not be valid in that situation. For example, specificity and sensitivity for a given test would most likely be different in dogs and cats. They may also differ in older versus younger, symptomatic versus asymptomatic, or even in larger versus smaller patients. It is important to note that many diagnostic tests are evaluated first using patients who have severe disease and in control groups who are young and well. Compared with the general population, these groups may have more results that are truly positive (for patients with more advanced disease) and more results that are truly negative (since control groups are young and healthy). Thus, reported test sensitivity and specificity are often higher than would be expected in the general population, where a broader spectrum of health and disease is found. Clinicians should be aware of this when generalizing test results to their own practice.

Sensitivity and specificity also depend on cut-off values used to distinguish diseased states from nondiseased states. If the cut-off values are modified, sensitivity may be enhanced at the expense of specificity, or vice versa. For example, a recent paper used the ACTH stimulation test as a valid gold standard for diagnosing canine hypoadrenocorticism, and the authors used it to determine the sensitivity and specificity of the Na:K ratio at different cutoff points. Diagnostic sensitivity at cut-off values of 28 and 24 were 96% and 79%, respectively. Diagnostic specificity at cutoff values of 28 and 24 were 97% and 100%, respectively.[10] *Receiving operator curve analysis* can help identify cut-off values that optimize both sensitivity and specificity.

Positive and Negative Predictive Values

Predictive values differ from sensitivity and specificity in that they take into account the *prevalence* of disease in the test population. They help answer the clinically relevant question that, given a positive test result, what is the probability that a patient actually has a given disease?

First, *prevalence* is defined as the number of patients within a population that have a particular disease at a specific time, or the probability that a patient in a given population is afflicted with a specific disease. Predictive values are predicated upon prevalence and are therefore often called "post-test" probabilities, since they modify the probability of disease in a given patient using result information obtained from a particular test.

Positive predictive value is the probability that given a positive test result, a patient is afflicted with the disease in question. A high positive predictive value means a positive test result reliably indicates the presence of disease in a patient.

Negative predictive value is the probability that given a negative test result, a patient is not afflicted with the disease in question. A high negative predictive value means that a negative test result reliably indicates the absence of disease in a patient.

Predictive values are predicated both on prevalence and on the specificity and sensitivity characteristics of the test in question. If test specificity is low, the positive predictive value will be poor and the likelihood of a false positive result will be high. This is important, because costs associated with false positives may be considerable in terms of owner stress, inappropriate treatment, and unnecessary testing.

In general, for understanding and applying predictive values, it is important to remember that

1. Decreased prevalence improves the predictive value of a negative test.
2. Increased prevalence improves the predictive value of a positive test.
3. Increased sensitivity improves the predictive value of a negative test.
4. Increased specificity improves the predictive value of a positive test.

Studies in human medicine indicate that a majority of general practitioners tend to overestimate the value of a positive test result and are unable to interpret numerical information about the diagnostic accuracy of screening tests.[11] Thus, it makes sense to provide an example to further elucidate these concepts. Table 7-1 shows a graphical depiction of the concepts discussed. The results of testing with a gold standard are those listed under the columns titled *Disease State*. The results of the hypothetical test being used are listed in the rows titled *Test Result*.

Using this chart, let's try a few hypothetical examples. Table 7-2 can be copied and then used to mathematically work through situations to better understand how different factors relate to each other.

In this example of disease X, 100 people have been tested using a gold standard. In this population, the prevalence of

Table • 7-1

		DISEASE STATE			
		POSITIVE (+)	**NEGATIVE (−)**		
Test result	Positive (+)	True positive (TP)	False positive (FP)	Test positive = TP + FP	**Positive predictive value (PPV)** = TP/(TP + FP)
	Negative (−)	False negative (FN)	True negative (TN)	Test negative = TN + FN	**Negative predictive value** = TN/(FN + TN)
		Disease positive = TP + FN **Sensitivity** = TP/(TP + FN)	Disease negative = TN + FP **Specificity** = TN/(FP + TN)	The entire population = TP + FP + FN + TN **Prevalence (pretest probability)** = (TP + FN)/ (TP + FP + FN + TN)	

Table • 7-2

		DISEASE STATE			
		POSITIVE (+)	**NEGATIVE (−)**		
Test result	Positive (+)	A	B		**PPV** = C
	Negative (−)	D	E		**NPV** = F
		Disease positive = G **Sensitivity** = I	Disease negative = H **Specificity** = J	**Prevalence** = K	

disease was found to be 10%. Thus, 10 patients in the population have the disease; 90 do not. Using this data, we can fill in the information in boxes G (10), H (90), and K (0.1 or 10%). We are looking to evaluate the accuracy of a new, noninvasive test called Y. We test the same 100 patients with new test Y. Of the 10 patients known to be positive for disease X, 8 out of the 10 test positive with the new test. We can now fill in boxes A (8) and D (2) and determine test sensitivity in box I (0.8 or 80%). Note that so far we have only evaluated patients who have the disease. *Sensitivity only looks at the proportion of true and false results in diseased patients.* In this case, there are two falsely positive. If only 1 of the 10 diseased patients were falsely positive, sensitivity would be higher at 90% and there would be *fewer false positives.*

In another example, consider 90 patients whom we know for certain are not afflicted with disease X. We test all 90 using new test Y. Five test positive; 85 test negative. Using this information, we can now fill in boxes B (5) and E (85) and determine the specificity of test Y in box J (94%). *Specificity only looks at the proportion of true and false results in patients who do not have the disease.* If the test were 100% specific, all patients who tested negatively would not have the disease. Thus, a positive test would rule in disease.

In clinical practice, patients do not present with an already known disease state. They more often present with clinical signs and findings suggestive of a given disease. If we accurately know the prevalence of the disease in the population and the sensitivity and specificity of the test being used, we can determine what the probability is that a patient actually has the disease in question given a positive test result. Using the example above for test Y and disease X, we know the disease prevalence of the population is 10%, test specificity is

94%, and test sensitivity is 80%. We are assuming disease prevalence is representative of the population from which the patient being tested comes from. If not, results may not be accurate. Given the provided information, we can determine predictive values in box C (62%) and F (98%). We can conclude that given the information provided, if a patient tests positive with new test Y, there is a 62% chance the patient actually has disease X. If a patient has a negative test result, there is a 98% chance that the patient does not have the disease. Or, if a patient tests negatively, there is only a 2% chance the patient actually has disease X.

This exercise should be repeated keeping sensitivity and specificity unchanged but altering the prevalence of disease to 30% (box G = 30 and box H = 70). Keeping sensitivity at 80%, box A = 24 and box D = 6. Keeping specificity at 94%, box B = 4 and box E = 66. Though the numbers in each column have changed, the proportions have not. *Sensitivity and specificity do not change with prevalence.* However, the predictive values do. Positive predictive value has improved (86%) and negative predictive value has decreased (92%). The same exercise can next be repeated keeping prevalence unchanged and altering specificity and sensitivity. Doing these exercises will again reconfirm the four numbered principles listed previously in this chapter.

OTHER CONSIDERATIONS

A test is only as good as the data that support and validate it. The following are considerations that should be used to understand and evaluate the diagnostic accuracy of a given test result in a given patient.

Reference Standards

Ideally, reference standards for a test should be determined by testing a sizeable population (>60) of animals representative of the patient being tested. Accuracy may differ according to age of patient, species, sex, diet, weight, time of day, and activity status.

For example, reference ranges for hemoglobin concentration are age- and sex-dependent.[12,13] As another example, an antigen-based heartworm test is the gold standard, antemortem diagnostic test for dogs; however, cats often have low worm burden, unisex worm infestations, or immature worm infestations that are not readily detected by these tests.[14,15] Thus, sensitivity is much lower in cats, and this test would not be appropriate as a gold standard for testing cats.

Established reference ranges and interpretation of results are only valid for the methods and the laboratory described. Reference ranges generally represent the range of test results from a subpopulation of healthy patients, and values that apply to 95% of the subjects evaluated are included within the range. Thus, patients who consistently fall slightly outside of the range but do not have progressive changes in their results may be, in fact, normal. Test results should always be interpreted in light of other clinical findings. Additionally, the more tests performed, the greater the chance that a falsely abnormal result may ensue. For example, if a healthy patient were subjected to 20 independent tests, there would be a 64% probability of finding at least one abnormal result.[16]

Interfering Factors

External factors such as feeding schedule, sample processing, or medications can interfere with test results. A high-fat meal prior to evaluation of a serum chemistry analysis will alter values associated with lipid metabolism and cholesterol. Diuretics may affect sodium and potassium values. Cephalosporins may cause spurious serum creatinine levels. Corticosteroids and most all chemotherapy drugs severely decrease lymphocyte levels. Lipemia may decrease sodium levels, depending on the testing method used. Corticosteroids may increase alkaline phosphatase levels. If blood samples are not processed quickly after being drawn, glucose levels will often be artificially lowered. In general, if test results do not correlate with clinical findings or expected results, the veterinarian should view the results with suspicion and consider repeating them for confirmation.

PATIENT PREPARATION

The preparation of the patient is important for certain tests. For example, a fasting state is needed for optimal glucose and triglyceride measurements. Controlled conditions are frequently needed for endocrinology testing. Careful attention must be paid to patient identification and specimen labeling. Knowing when the specimen was collected may be important. For instance, phenobarbital levels cannot be interpreted appropriately without knowing whether the specimen was drawn just before ("trough" level) or after ("peak level") drug administration. Drug levels cannot be interpreted if they are drawn during the drug's distribution phase (e.g., digoxin levels drawn during the first 6 hours after an oral dose). Substances that have a circadian variation (e.g., cortisol) can be properly interpreted only with knowledge of the time of day the sample was drawn.

During specimen collection, other principles should be remembered. Specimens should not be drawn above an intravenous line, as this may contaminate the sample with intravenous fluid. Lysis of cells during collection of a blood specimen will result in spuriously increased serum levels of substances concentrated in cells (e.g., lactate dehydrogenase and potassium). Certain test specimens may require special handling or storage (e.g., blood gas specimens). Delay in delivery of specimens to the laboratory can result in ongoing cellular metabolism and therefore spurious results for some studies (e.g., low blood glucose).

CONCLUSION

Obtaining a proper medical history, performing a complete physical examination, and having a thorough understanding of the accuracy, precision, sensitivity, specificity, and indications of the diagnostic test will result in optimum patient management.

REFERENCES

The reference list can be found on the companion Expert Consult Web site at *www.expertconsult.com*.

CHAPTER 8

Euthanasia

W. Douglas Kunz
Stephen J. Ettinger

As veterinarians, we are very fortunate to be advocates for the wellbeing of our patients from their first visit to the end of life considerations. When we recommend a diagnostic procedure, a surgery, or medication, we are acting for the well-being of the animal under our care. At times, we also must be advocates for the humane demise of our patients. This is a unique position for practitioners of the healing arts. It provides us with certain rights and obligations that no other health care professional has. In turn, it usually engenders a very special bond that exists between veterinarian and client.

Most other health care professionals are very envious of the relationship that exists and between the veterinary doctor and client. This is something we as veterinarians deal with daily. We are often loved by our clients for our humaneness, but the toll it takes on us and our staff associates should also not be ignored. Nor should the responsibility of making appropriate decisions regarding euthanasia be dealt with lightly.

We are presented with the request to euthanize a beloved pet for a variety of reasons. These reasons can vary from deterioration of the quality of life to the point that euthanasia is a kind relief from suffering to the cast off pet whose owner is unwilling or unable to find another home for it. Whereas the former is a much easier process for the practice team as all know that a compassionate service is being performed, the latter can be very difficult because we are in fact being asked to kill a healthy pet. Of course, there are numerous other reasons for euthanasia such as a severely injured or ill pet whose owner does not have the financial resources for treatment, the pet that has severe, irresolvable behavioral problems, or a puppy born with birth defects that the owner is unwilling to treat or which may not be amenable to intervention. Some veterinarians are asked to provide euthanasia services to a local animal shelter,[1] resulting in a situation that poses other unique considerations.

We also do not know all of the circumstances leading up to the decision on the part of the owner to ask that their pet be put to sleep. Occasionally, the difficult task of euthanasia is requested because the pet is a burden to the owner, affecting the mental and/or physical health of that person or because the owner may have passed away and there is no one to care for the pet that may have some very special needs. The number of excuses, reasons, and simply requests made of the veterinarian for such services seems to grow exponentially daily and each day brings on a new request that the DVM had never experienced or thought about previously.

In the course of treating pets it sometimes becomes necessary to gently suggest to an owner that the time has come for them to consider releasing their beloved pet from a circumstance that no longer provides significant quality of life. Not infrequently the client will acknowledge this suggestion and indicate that he/she too was thinking this might be appropriate but was afraid the veterinarian would not agree. This has important repercussions upon the ongoing doctor-client relationship. Before such a step is undertaken, however, it is important to consider the situation. We must be certain that the care the DVM is providing is in fact all that is available or requested for this pet. Under such circumstances a second opinion consultation or a referral to a specialist may be in order. It is clearly important to recognize this in advance because the decision to euthanize is not one easily taken and one that is often not forgotten by the client, but rather dwelled upon in some detail. If the client feels that the DVM did not judiciously use all of the available resources in his/her community to help this pet, very negative feelings may develop. This could affect the client and the client's decision to return at a later date with another pet. Further, making such a recommendation without consideration of other options also leaves the DVM open to question by the client. Should the client decide that this is not the right course and then seek independent review of the case, there can be more serious problems if the animal is subsequently successfully treated after the first DVM recommends euthanasia.

The discussion of euthanasia involves four key factors[2]:
1. Clear communication of the pet's conditions.
2. Assessing the client's feelings and desires, and empathizing with them.
3. Explanation of the process and options associated with euthanasia.
4. Giving grief support and providing outside support resources.

If a pet's condition has deteriorated to the point where the quality of life is poor, how can we best communicate this to the owner? Honest communication describing the professional assessment helps provide the basis for client decision making. Such a conversation may go as follows: "Robert, Fluffy's heart failure has progressed to a point that medication is no longer effective in maintaining his quality of life. His lungs are being compressed by fluid so that he can't obtain sufficient oxygen for the body to function properly. This is why he is reluctant to lie down." A similar discussion could take place with any medical condition that has impaired the quality of life to the point of suggesting euthanasia. There are schemes[2] to assess the quality of life, but it always is a judgment call based on our knowledge and experience as practitioners of veterinary medicine. Some clients respond immediately and clearly that such an option is not something to be considered. If so, note this directly in the record and proceed with caring for the patient as the owner requests. Decision making, especially when the DVM differs in opinion from the owner, is very difficult. However, it is the choice of the owner and not the DVM. Assuming all professional efforts are made to help the pet, then the DVM has the responsibility to provide humane care and comfort as best as possible for the pet and the owner.

To assess what the pet owner is thinking and feeling, ask questions about the pet's behavior at home. This helps the client to acknowledge the diminished quality of life. Such general questions may be, "Robert, how is Fluffy's day? Is it an effort for him or is there still pleasure in his day?" "Robert, what do you think would be best for Fluffy at this point? I understand that you are very sad about this but tell me how you are feeling?" Reassurance to the client at this point is helpful. "Robert, I know this is difficult. I know how much you love Fluffy and that you do not want him to suffer." Another phrase could be, "Sometimes the ultimate act of kindness and selflessness is to let Fluffy go. By making this decision, you are willing to feel the loss and sadness, so that Fluffy will find relief." Often, agreeing with the client will also help. Many clients suggest that the pet is going to heaven, to be with another past pet, to go where things are better. This is not the time or place to differ with the hopes and desires of the owner. It is their pet, their belief system, and their decision. The DVM should not be the decision maker. Often, even suggesting a time period for treatment, say "another day or two to see if this medication will help before we make this difficult choice" may be enough. At times the client will then ask if it really will make any difference and this can be a time for the DVM to offer his/her opinion.

Another process that may occur in the office or on the telephone is the client who is requesting that euthanasia services be provided at their home or at another special place. Each DVM has a distinct policy regarding such situations. Even if this is not something the DVM does, often there is another DVM in the region who does provide such a service. Emotions tend to run very high in such circumstances and separating the client from others, giving them privacy, and being alone with their pet are all very beneficial to the owner's sense of loss and need for privacy. It is far easier if the client chooses an alternative route to euthanasia in the hospital than it is to have a distraught and disgruntled client at the hospital office.

The process of euthanasia in the clinic should be explained along with the option to be present or not. The discussion should include how the client wishes the pet's remains to be handled. Private cremation or burial are options. In many larger cities, when disposal is requested, it may mean rendering of the body. While this is not something pleasant to discuss, the owner should not be told a lie but rather the facts must be presented. Fees for euthanasia (which can be substantial) and for the disposal of the body should be discussed. Client complaints in this area are not unusual, in part because this occurs during the grieving process and at this stage of the process the client may be angry at what is perceived to be high fees for something that is so unpleasant for the pet's owner. It is here that one hears complaints about inappropriate fees, price gouging, or simply, "You are supposed to love pets, but you charged me so much more money than it should have been."

One area for discussion prior to euthanasia is whether children should participate or be in the room when this is taking place. Of course, ultimately it is the owner's choice, however often they will request the opinion of the veterinarian. Generally our belief is that anyone who cares for the pet and wishes to view the procedure should be there. Occasionally one of the adults will stay and one will leave, again a personal option. Sometimes the client will ask only to see the pet momentarily after the euthanasia is completed. With respect to the children, we recommend that children too young to really understand the process not be permitted to view the procedure because it may frighten them or make them leery of anything given to them by injection at some later date. On the other hand, young children who love and know their pet, who understand what is happening, and who wish to be with their pet and their parents should be acknowledged and given the privilege of viewing the process and being with their pet. Lying to children about this process is not recommended, and we as veterinarians should not participate in extending an untruth told to them. We want them to understand suffering, humane care, and the role the veterinarian plays in the important human-animal bond process.

If the pet is to be euthanized during the office visit, dealing with the charges and payment should be handled with sensitivity. A possible scenario might be, "While we take Fluffy away for a few minutes to place a catheter in his vein, my nurse has a form for you to sign and she will take care of your bill with you so that you won't have to stop at the desk after we put Fluffy to sleep." If euthanasia will take place at a future visit, fees should be collected prior to entering the exam room on the day of euthanasia. Some[2] have suggested that a dedicated room with soft lighting, candles, and flowers be used for euthanasia. The reality is that in many clinics cramped for space this is not possible. In one small multidoctor clinic, when euthanasia is to take place, an announcement is made over the intercom asking, "Dr. Green to come to the office." This alerts the staff that it is a sensitive time and to act accordingly. A solemn and sensitive environment is created toward not only the pet's owner and family, but also toward other clients who may be aware of what is to take place. Try to have the staff prepared for the euthanasia and avoid loud noises or laughter on the part of the other hospital personnel when such a serious problem is being attended to. Often, this simple process is not recognized and causes discontent on the part of the pet's owner. More often, the soft, compassionate staff expressing their true feelings to the client helps to assuage guilt and sadness and allows the process to move along smoothly. If at all possible, set aside a more quiet time of the day for the client to come for this service. It provides the client with a quieter atmosphere and one that is less hectic. If this is anticipated to be a difficult and long, drawn-out process, do not schedule it for the end of the day, when closing the clinic interferes with the client remaining with the patient. Some clients will stay for significant periods of time causing havoc with the hospital's staff.

The process of the euthanasia itself can be very moving and comforting to the owner if properly prepared. In virtually every case where the client wishes to see and be with the pet, an intravenous catheter should be placed first. Always have saline filled syringes to check on the patency of the catheter even if it was just placed. Explain to the owner the actual process that you choose to use. Some veterinarians prefer only to use euthanasia solution, others administer the solution after a short acting anesthetic such as Propofol is given, and others prefer to give diazepam or another tranquilizer first to lessen any impact that the pentobarbital solution will have on the central nervous system. The important thing is to explain in detail what will happen, to have an assistant in the room to help hold the pet, and, if the owner wishes to hold the pet as well, to allow them to do so without hampering the process of injecting the euthanasia solution. Infusions, given slowly and efficiently, help the process. Often the pet relaxes quickly, but the veterinarian should continue to administer all of the drugs and should not withhold medication assuming that the pet has died. Not at all unusual is for the pet to continue to breathe for another few moments or for the heart to continue beating. These bodily processes disturb the client and can make them feel distrustful. Some clients believe that veterinarians want to experiment on their pets, and they must be assuaged by assuring them that the pet is really dead, that the heart has stopped beating, and that the respirations have ceased. Some clients (rarely) ask to listen with the stethoscope to assure themselves that the pet is dead, and if they do, it certainly behooves the DVM to allow that to happen without comment. We prefer at this time is to speak softly to those in the room, offer them the opportunity for alone time with their pet, and to quietly leave the room.

After the procedure is completed it is appropriate to express support and sympathy to the client. Ask if they would like a few moments alone with their deceased pet and, if so, withdraw. Explain once again that there may be some muscle twitching which is normal, a deep breath or final expiratory effort may be made, and as the muscles begin to relax the pet might even urinate. Explain that these are normal signs. Also, many owners expect the DVM to listen for heart sounds with a stethoscope—they see it daily on TV and in the movies and such a step may be comforting despite the fact that you know the pet died moments ago during the injection process. Some clients express concern that the eyes are not closed; they should be told that this usually does not occur in people either (again the TV and movie expectation). Everything should be done with respect for the client. A phone call a few days later to ask how the client is doing is appropriate, as is a sympathy card or a donation to any of the several foundations that accept donations on behalf of a deceased pet. One of our clinics (SE) has sent personalized letters to clients for years, always with a hand-written note on the letter. Clients return with another pet years later, often expressing the importance of the written note that was personalized.

If on the follow-up phone call the client is struggling to cope with the loss, it would be appropriate to refer the client to a grief counselor. Be prepared by consulting with a local mental health care professional to know what resources are available in your community. If you have mental health care professionals whom you work with, be prepared to offer names to the client. We like to have both psychologists and psychiatrists on our lists and also both men and women so that the client, if he or she so chooses, may also find comfort in choosing a health care professional who is acceptable. Lengthy discussions regarding the final days, health condition, or laboratory tests often occur with the client who remains unwilling to accept the loss of the pet. While it is more than appropriate to discuss these with the client, to record such discussions in the record, and to be prepared to assist the client in understanding the process, it is also important to recognize when the process goes beyond normal grief and requires professional help. Remember too that anger is part of this process. Offering to discuss the situation with the client in the majority of cases is all that is required, along with the usual points discussed above. If more is needed, be prepared to offer some help but do not allow lengthy discussions to occur if they remain unfruitful and offensive. Offering to continue discussions at a later date, providing written material on the disease process, or even allowing the client to come and review the x-rays and discuss the problem in the office can be helpful. One good method of helping the client is to offer to see them in the office on a no-charge appointment. Be certain that you are prepared with the records, lab tests, and radiographs to show them. Also be certain that the client understands the time limit set for the appointment, so that it does not become a long, nonstop period for rehashing the anger and anxiety. Often a good ending can be made by explaining that your time has elapsed and that you do have another client waiting. Advise the client that if he/she feels that another appointment is necessary, your staff would assist them in making the appointment. At this time the staff and client should be advised that there will be a consultation fee for further visits.

Euthanasia can be a difficult time for the pet owner. If the veterinarian and staff are sensitive and caring throughout the process, long-term relationships through multiple pets' lives are often the result. It is of particular importance to help the client not feel guilty over their decision.[3] By implementing and practicing dialogs such as those described above and establishing procedures to empathetically deal with euthanasia, the client and the staff benefit. Role playing at staff development meetings can be an aid to teach the skill needed for this difficult task. If the staff has been prepared and trained to provide this important service, the process will flow with compassion and professionalism.

One critical component of euthanasia is the method by which the office handles the disposition of the body. More clients are lost to other hospitals here than at any point in the process, other than the lack of professionalism and sensitivity on the part of the DVM and staff to the client. It is essential for the hospital to have a well-organized system for determining how the body is to be disposed of. Carefully identifying the body, the pet's name spelled properly, the owner's name spelled properly, and the choices of the owner are incredibly important. Methods for holding the body must also be considered. A hospital should have a time limit for which bodies can be held and the client must be informed of this. Without doing so, a client may not realize the difficulty in holding a body and may think it perfectly acceptable to call back after a month to advise on their desires for disposition

of the body. Of course by then the body is gone and the client may be very unhappy. Have a limited number of options available to the client, carefully and repeatedly make certain that this is understood, and have the staff do the same with the owner. Then be certain that there is a hospital policy for who handles the body, how it is handled, and what is to become of it. Lost bodies that were intended for private burial and/or cremation cause untold havoc, anxiety, displeasure, and the loss of a client. Such problems simply should not occur in a well-organized facility. Every aspect of this process should also be clearly noted in the medical record and signed by the person acknowledging the decisions being made by the owner.

The process of euthanasia also impacts the veterinary staff. Patients that we have cared for over the years become special to us as well, and we may suffer their loss. It has been suggested[4] that staff have regular opportunities to discuss their feelings and express themselves. This can ward off burnout or compassion fatigue and build the regard for each other as well as team relationships.[4] Staff who have been especially close to the client, the pet, or the medical process may express personal feelings about being present at the time of euthanasia and if possible these feelings should be acknowledged.

Similarly, allowing the staff to express their feelings to clients is a wonderful way to let the client know how much everyone cares. While we usually only write and sign letters to the client from the DVM, there is every reason to have the staff participate in this process as well when the pet has been especially close to the staff or cared for by them over a very long period of time.

Euthanasia represents the end of what may have been a long relationship with a client and his or her pet. During this period much has been shared in the lives of the family and the veterinary hospital. A good closure is really important to the client and the veterinarian. We were fortunate to have taken care of the important member of the family and to have shared in many experiences. Closure is helpful to all involved and often represents not only closure but a new beginning. This may be veterinary medicine at its very best!

Selected Web site links for those seeking additional sources of information on euthanasia or pet loss:

http://www.avma.org/animal_health/brochures/euthanasia/ pet/pet_euth_brochure.asp
http://www.deltasociety.org/
http://www.vetmed.wsu.edu/PLHL/
http://www.pethospice.org/NHFP%20FRAME.htm

REFERENCES

The reference list can be found on the companion Expert Consult Web site at *www.expertconsult.com*.

CHAPTER 9

Home Euthanasia

Karen M. Kelly

Historically, euthanasia has been viewed in veterinary medicine as an uncomfortable medical procedure. In the past, family members were often discouraged from being with their pet and the pet was often euthanized away from the owner. Today, the human-animal bond has changed how veterinarians respond to the human emotional needs created by this significant relationship. Owners view their pets as family members, and this deep connection leads pet owners to have certain expectations in regards to euthanasia. An at-home euthanasia provides pet owners with a peaceful, quiet environment outside of the clinical setting to say goodbye to their companion. Most owners want their pet to be at home to alleviate the stress associated with transporting their pet to the hospital and do not want to feel that their pet's last memory was of the hospital or an unpleasant experience.[1,2]

CONSIDERATIONS WHEN PERFORMING HOME EUTHANASIA

Performing a home euthanasia is obviously very different than euthanasia in a clinical setting. There are special considerations when performing this service. When euthanasia is performed well, it eases and comforts people at a time of great emotional grief. When performed without skill, it can cause great distress and prolonged grief to the pet owner. It is essential to have a special protocol for home euthanasia. Equally important is communicating this process in detail to the pet owner prior to the home visit. This will prepare them for what they will witness and go a long way in helping the owner feel comforted and reassured. Owners will often have questions concerning the presence of other animals and children at the euthanasia as well as how their pet will react to the procedure. Aftercare options and fees along with payment options should also be addressed prior to visiting the home. It is unpleasant and awkward to do this when first entering the home or after the euthanasia has been performed.

PROCESS OF HOME EUTHANASIA

Skilled facilitation of the home euthanasia is most important. The veterinarian must have good technique and express sensitivity and compassion. All paperwork should be first addressed when entering the home. Take the time to relax for a moment with the family and address any questions or concerns. Explain to the family that this is a two- to three-step process. First and most important is the initial sedative injection that will be given to relax the pet, which takes 5 to 10 minutes to take effect (Table 9-1). This allows the family to cuddle with their pet and the veterinarian to comfort and express compassion to the family and pet while the sedative takes effect. Once the pet has settled down and is more relaxed, a stronger anesthetic agent such as Telazol (tiletamine HCL/zolazepam HCL) is given to achieve complete anesthesia and unconsciousness (see Table 9-1). Telazol (tiletamine HCL/zolazepam HCL) is chosen because of its quick, profound, and predictable anesthetic qualities. Advise the owner that after the Telazol (tiletamine HCL/zolazepam HCL) is given their pet will be in a deep unconscious sleep within 5 to 10 minutes and will not feel anything beyond this point.

Once the pet is unconscious and immobilized the final injection of euthanasia solution should be given (see Table

Table • 9-1

Euthanasia Drugs and Effects

DRUGS AND ROUTES OF ADMINISTRATION	DOGS	CATS	TIME TO EFFECT AND SIDE EFFECTS
Butorphanol tartrate	0.5-1 mg/kg	0.5-1 mg/kg	First sedative, takes 5-10 minutes for heavy
Xylazine HCl	0.1-0.5 mg/kg	0.1-0.5 mg/kg	sedation. Xylazine HCL can cause drooling and
Subcutaneous			emesis in cats.
Telazol (tiletamine HCL/zolazepam)	3-5 mg/kg	3-5 mg/kg	Fast, rapid predictable effect. Unconsciousness in
Intramuscular			5-10 minutes. Tongue may come out of mouth.
Subcutaneous			IM injection can sting.
Pentobarbitol sodium with phenytoin			Predictable quick death in 2-3 minutes after
Intravenous	1 mL for each 4-5 kg of body weight	1 mL for each 4-5 kg of body weight	intravenous injection and 10-15 minutes after intraperitoneal and intrathoracic injection.
Intraperitoneal (cats)		3 mL for each 4-5 kg of body weight	
Intrathoracic (cats)			

9-1). Assure the owners once again that the pet will not feel anything and their friend is unconscious and peaceful. The advantage of inducing unconsciousness in the home prior to giving the euthanasia injection is twofold. Firstly, the pet is immobilized so no restraint is needed to administer the final intravenous injection, and secondly, when owners witness their pet struggling against restraint, they become very upset. Some house call veterinarians do not bring an assistant, so it is not possible to do an intravenous injection without unconsciousness. The pet is now in lateral recumbancy and the lateral saphenous is most accessible. A proper tourniquet is most important.[3] Veterinary brand tourniquets have not proven to be effective. They are often difficult to release and manipulate, therefore making it hard to hold the syringe and needle in place. A human elastic CBC tourniquet with a quick release button allows the veterinarian to effortlessly release the tourniquet with one hand while holding the syringe and needle in place with the other hand. The elastic band can be tightened down around the leg very firmly, causing the vein to become very visible and allowing easy access. In most cases, an intravenous catheter is not practical in a home environment. The leg should always be shaved to assist with visualization of the vein. Once the pet has died, advise the owner the heart has stopped and their pet has died.

HOME EUTHANASIA OF CATS

Special consideration with cats is worth mentioning. If the veterinarian is in the home without technical assistance, he or she should always hold the cat for the first and second sedative injections to prevent a bite from the cat to the owner. From experience, some cats can be fractious and bite their owners. Always explain to the owner they will be able to hold and cuddle with their cat after the initial injections are administered.

Administration of the euthanasia solution to cats requires special consideration. It is often very difficult to access a cat's vein, especially in chronically ill geriatric cats. Therefore the euthanasia solution is administered intrathoracically or intraperitoneally after the cat has become unconscious from the Telazol. It then typically takes 5 to 10 minutes for cardiac arrest to occur.

References

The reference list can be found on the companion Expert Consult Web site at *www.expertconsult.com*.

SECTION II
Clinical Veterinary Medicine

CHAPTER 10

Hyperthermia and Fever of Unknown Origin

James B. Miller

Obtaining a body temperature measurement is important in the evaluation of all dogs and cats, especially those thought to be critically ill. A rectal temperature higher than 102.5° F is considered elevated in the unstressed dog or cat. The method of measurement must also be taken into account, because ear, axillary, or toe web measurements will be lower than a simultaneously obtained rectal temperature.

Too frequently, a veterinarian may associate any elevation in body temperature with true fever. The assumption often is made that the fever is caused by an infectious agent, even if there is no obvious cause. If the patient's fever resolves after antibiotics are given, the assumption is made that it was caused by a bacterial infection. A normal body temperature often is assumed to mean the absence of disease. This approach to fever, hyperthermia, or normothermia can be misleading and result in improper diagnoses and therapy (or the lack thereof).

THERMOREGULATION

The thermoregulatory center for the body is located in the central nervous system (CNS) in the region of the anterior hypothalamus (AH). Changes in ambient and core body temperatures are sensed by the peripheral and central thermoreceptors, and the information is conveyed to the AH via the nervous system. Thermoreceptors sensing that the body is below or above its normal temperature (normal "set point") will stimulate the AH to cause the body to increase heat production and reduce heat loss through conservation if the body is too cold or dissipate heat if the body is too warm (Figure 10-1).

Through these mechanisms, dogs and cats can maintain a narrow core body temperature range in a wide variety of environmental conditions. With normal ambient temperatures, most body heat is produced by muscular activity, even while at rest. Cachectic, anesthetized, or animals with severe neurologic impairment may not be able to maintain a normal set point or generate a normal febrile response.

HYPERTHERMIA

Hyperthermia is the term used to describe any elevation in core body temperature above accepted reference values for that species. Hyperthermia is a result of the loss of equilibrium in the heat balance equation such that heat is produced or stored in the body at a rate in excess of heat lost through radiation, convection, or evaporation. The term *fever* is reserved for those hyperthermic animals where the set point in the AH has been "reset" to a higher temperature. In hyperthermic states other than fever, the hyperthermia is not a result of the body attempting to raise its temperature but is due to the physiologic, pathologic, or pharmacologic intervention where heat gain exceeds heat loss. Box 10-1 outlines the various forms of hyperthermia.

True Fever

True fever is a normal response of the body to invasion by a pathogen or injury and is part of the *acute-phase response*. Other parts of the acute-phase response include increased neutrophil numbers and phagocytic ability, enhanced T and B lymphocyte activity, increased acute phase protein production by the liver, increased fibroblast activity, and increased sleep. Fever and the other parts of the acute-phase response are initiated by exogenous pyrogens that lead to the release of endogenous pyrogens.

Exogenous Pyrogens True fever may be initiated by a variety of substances, including infectious agents or their products, immune complexes, tissue inflammation or necrosis, and several pharmacologic agents, including many antibiotics. Collectively, these substances are called *exogenous pyrogens*. Their ability to directly affect the thermoregulatory center is probably minimal and they act by causing host release of endogenous pyrogens. Box 10-2 lists some of the more important known exogenous pyrogens.

Endogenous Pyrogens In response to stimuli by an exogenous pyrogen, proteins (cytokines) released from cells of the immune system trigger the febrile response. Macro-

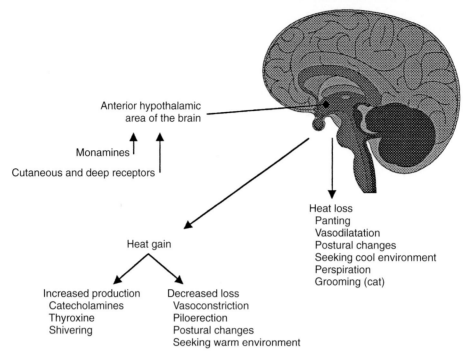

Figure 10-1 Schematic representation of normal thermal regulation.

Box • 10-1

Classification of Hyperthermia

True Fever
Production of endogenous pyrogens

Inadequate Heat Dissipation
Heat stroke
Hyperpyrexic syndromes

Exercise Hyperthermia
Normal exercise
Hypocalcemic tetany (eclampsia)
Seizure disorders

Pathologic or Pharmacologic Origin
Lesions in or around the anterior hypothalamus (AH)
Malignant hyperthermia
Hypermetabolic disorders
Monoamine metabolism disturbances

Box • 10-2

Exogenous Pyrogens

Infectious Agents
Bacteria (Live and Killed)
Gram-positive
Gram-negative
Bacterial Products
Lipopolysaccharides
Streptococcal exotoxin
Staphylococcal enterotoxin
Staphylococcal proteins
Fungi (Live and Killed)
Fungal products
Cryptococcal polysaccharide
Cryptococcal proteins
Virus
Rickettsia
Protozoa
Nonmicrobial Agents
Soluble antigen-antibody complexes
Bile acids
Pharmacologic agents
    Bleomycin
    Colchicine
    Tetracycline (cats)
    Levamisole (cats)
Tissue inflammation/necrosis

phages are the primary immune cell involved, although T and B lymphocytes and other leukocytes may play significant roles. The proteins produced are called *endogenous pyrogens* or *fever-producing cytokines*. Although interleukin-1 (IL-1) is considered the most important cytokine, at least 11 cytokines capable of initiating a febrile response have been identified (Table 10-1).

Some neoplastic cells are also capable of producing cytokines that lead to a febrile response. The cytokines travel via the blood stream to the AH, where they bind to the vas-cular endothelial cells within the AH and stimulate release of prostaglandins (PGs), primarily prostaglandin E_2 (PGE$_2$) and possibly prostaglandin E_{2a} (PGE$_{2a}$). The set point is raised, and the core body temperature rises through increased heat production and conservation (Figure 10-2).

Inadequate Heat Dissipation

Heat Stroke   Heat stroke is a common form of inadequate heat dissipation. Exposure to high ambient temperatures may increase heat load at a faster rate than the body can dissipate the heat. This is especially true in larger breeds of dogs and brachycephalic breeds. Heat stroke may occur rapidly in the dog, especially in closed environments with poor ventilation (e.g., inside a car with windows closed), even on moderately hot days. Environmental temperatures inside a closed car exposed to the direct sun may exceed 120° F (48° C) in less than 20 minutes, even when the outside temperature is only 75° F (24° C). Death may occur in less than an hour, especially in the breed types mentioned. Heat stroke will not respond to antipyretics used in true fever. The animal must be treated with total body cooling immediately if a fatal outcome is to be avoided. Water baths and rinses using cool (but not cold) water best accomplish total body cooling. If the water is too cold, a tendency exists for peripheral vasoconstriction, which will inhibit heat loss and slow the cooling process. Cool water, gastric lavage, or enemas have also been suggested. Cooling should be discontinued when body temperature approaches normal to avoid potential hypothermia. In addition to total body cooling, treatment for vascular collapse and shock should be instituted with severe hyperthermia (greater than 107° F [41.6° C]) or when clinical judgment warrants its use. Intravenous crystalloid solutions given at shock doses and glucocorticoids are indicated in an attempt to prevent permanent organ damage and disseminated intravascular coagulopathy (DIC).

Hyperpyrexic Syndrome   Hyperpyrexic syndrome is associated with moderate-to-severe exercise in hot and humid climates. This syndrome may be more common in hunting dogs or dogs that "jog" with their owners. In humid environments, a tendency exists toward a zero thermal gradient for dry heat loss leading to a net heat gain. In addition, severe exercise may cause the cardiovascular system to supply skeletal muscles with adequate blood flow while compromising peripheral heat loss by not allowing proper vasodilation in the skin. Many hunting dogs and dogs that run with their owners will continue to work or run until they become weak, begin to stagger, and then collapse. In suspected cases, owners should obtain a rectal thermometer. If increased, the owner or the veterinarian should evaluate the dog's rectal temperature at the first sign of weakness or not wanting to continue to exercise. Owners should be instructed that rectal temperatures above 106° F (41° C) require immediate total body cooling, and temperatures above 107° F (41.6° C) are an immediate threat of permanent organ damage or death.

Exercise Hyperthermia

The body temperature will slowly rise with sustained exercise because of increased heat production associated with muscular activity. Even when extreme heat and humidity are not factors, dogs will occasionally reach temperatures that would require total body cooling. This is especially true in dogs not accustomed to exercise, those that are overweight, or those with respiratory disease. Puppies seen for vaccinations are often excited and have been active since being placed in a car, for example. Activity and probable release of catecholamines results in the increased body temperatures obtained on physical examination. These dogs will display features suggestive of attempting to dissipate excess body heat and are neither febrile nor ill.

Table • 10-1

Proteins with Pyrogenic Activity

ENDOGENOUS PYROGEN	PRINCIPAL SOURCE
Cachectin/tumor necrosis factor-α (TNF-α)	Macrophages
Lymphotoxin/tumor necrosis factor-β (TNF-β; LT)	Lymphocytes (T and B)
Interleukin-1α (IL-1α)	Macrophages and many other cell types
Interleukin-1β (IL-β)	
Interferon-α	Leukocytes (esp. monocyte-macrophages)
Interferon-β	Fibroblasts
Interferon-γ	T lymphocytes
Interleukin-6 (IL-6)	Many cell types
Macrophage inflammatory protein 1α	Macrophages
Macrophage inflammatory protein 1β	
Interleukin-8 (IL-8)	

Adapted from Beutler B, Beutler SM: The pathogenesis of fever. In Bennett JC, Plum F, editors: Cecil textbook of medicine, ed 20, Philadelphia, 1996, Saunders, p 1535.

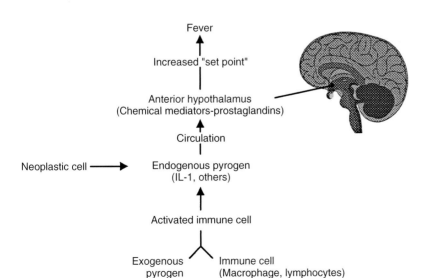

Figure 10-2 Schematic representation of the pathophysiology of fever. *IL-1*, Interleukin-1.

Eclampsia (hypocalcemia) results in extreme muscular activity that can lead to significant heat production resulting in severe hyperthermia. Total body cooling should be initiated in conjunction with specific eclampsia therapy if the dog or cat is hyperthermic. Be cautious of lowering body temperature too quickly and of decreases to subnormal levels.

Seizure disorders as a result of organic, metabolic, or idiopathic causes are encountered frequently. Hyperthermia associated with severe muscular activity can be a feature, especially if the seizures are prolonged or occur in clusters. The initial concern of the clinician should be to stop the seizures; however, when significant hyperthermia is present, total body cooling is recommended.

Pathologic and Pharmacologic Hyperthermia

These types of hyperthermia encompass several disorders that lead to impairment of the heat balance equation. Lesions in the hypothalamus may obliterate the thermoregulatory center leading to impaired response to both hot and cold environments. Malignant hyperthermia, as reported in the dog and cat, can lead to a myopathy initiated by pharmacologic agents, including inhalation anesthetics (especially Halothane) and muscle relaxants such as succinylcholine. Extreme muscle rigidity causes production of excess body heat. Removal of the offending causative agent and total body cooling may prevent death. Hypermetabolic disorders may lead to hyperthermic states. Endocrine disorders such as hyperthyroidism and pheochromocytoma can lead to an increased metabolic rate, vasoconstriction, or both, resulting in excess heat production and decreased ability to dissipate heat. These conditions rarely lead to severe hyperthermia requiring total body cooling.

BENEFITS AND DETRIMENTS OF HYPERTHERMIA

Benefits

Fever is part of the acute-phase response and is a normal response of the body. Even poikilotherms such as fish and reptiles will respond to a pyrogen by seeking higher environmental temperatures to raise their body temperatures. It would be logical to think that a true fever is beneficial to the host. Most studies have shown that a fever will reduce the duration of and mortality from many infectious diseases. A fever decreases the ability of many bacteria to use iron, which is necessary for them to live and replicate. Blocking the fever with nonsteroidal antiinflammatory agents in rabbits with *Pasteurella* infections significantly increases mortality rates. Many viruses are heat sensitive and cannot replicate in high temperatures. Raising the body temperature in neonatal dogs with herpes infections significantly reduces the mortality rate.

Detriments

Hyperthermia leads to an increased metabolic state and oxygen consumption that raise both caloric and water requirements by approximately 7% for each degree Fahrenheit (0.6° C) above accepted normal values. In addition, hyperthermia leads to suppression of the appetite center in the hypothalamus, but usually not the thirst center. Animals that have sustained head trauma or a cerebrovascular accident may suffer more severe brain damage if coexisting hyperthermia is present.

Body temperatures above 107° F (41.6° C) often lead to increases in cellular oxygen consumption that exceed oxygen delivery, resulting in deterioration of cellular function and integrity. This may lead to disseminated intravascular coagulation with thrombosis and bleeding, or serious damage to organ systems including the brain (cerebral edema and subsequent confusion, delirium, obtundation, seizures, coma), heart (arrhythmias), liver (hypoglycemia, hyperbilirubinemia), gastrointestinal tract (epithelial desquamation, endotoxin absorption, bleeding), and kidneys. Additional abnormalities might include hypoxemia, hyperkalemia, skeletal muscle cytolysis, tachypnea, metabolic acidosis, tachycardia, tachypnea, and hyperventilation.

Exertional heat stroke and malignant hyperthermia may lead to severe rhabdomyolysis, hyperkalemia, hypocalcemia, myoglobinemia and myoglobinuria, and elevated levels of creatine phosphokinase. Fortunately, true fevers rarely lead to body temperatures of this magnitude and are usually a result of other causes of hyperthermia that should be managed as medical emergencies.

Clinical Approach

When a dog or cat has an increased body temperature, an effort should be made to approach the problem in a logical manner to avoid erroneous conclusions (Figure 10-3).

A complete history and physical examination should be performed unless the problem is of extreme nature (temperature greater than 106° F [41° C]) and the animal is obviously attempting to dissipate heat (panting, postural changes) or comatose. In such cases, immediate total body cooling and supportive care should be initiated. In other cases, specific questions concerning previous injuries or infections, exposure to other animals, disease in other household pets, previous geographic environment, and previous or current drug therapy may be beneficial. Through this type of questioning and a complete physical examination, the clinician can frequently decide if the increased body temperature is true fever. Temperatures less than 106° F (41° C), unless prolonged, are usually not life threatening, and caution should be taken on using antipyretics before a proper clinical evaluation.

Fever of Unknown Origin

Fever of unknown origin (FUO) is defined in human medicine as a fever that has lasted 3 weeks and has a cause that has not been determined through laboratory evaluation and radiographs. In veterinary medicine, most clinicians consider any animal with an increased body temperature that does not have any historical or physical finding that would explain this abnormality to be an FUO. Although research involving a large number of patients with FUO has been completed in humans, there is relatively little in the veterinary literature to help explain the most common causes of apparent FUO in dogs or cats. The information given in this chapter is based primarily on clinical experience. Most dogs and cats with FUO probably have an infection or suffer from the byproducts derived from those agents.

The prevalence of the causative infectious agent varies depending on the area where the clinician practices and the previous travel history of the pet. Although bacterial infections are probably the most common cause of FUO in the dog, in some geographic locations, systemic fungal diseases or rickettsial infections might be more common. Endocarditis, pyelonephritis, prostatitis, closed pyometra, pyothorax, and other deep abscesses should be considered in a dog with FUO. In the cat, viral diseases such as feline leukemia virus (FeLV), feline infectious peritonitis (FIP) virus, and feline immunodeficiency virus (FIV) are common infectious causes of FUO and may exceed bacterial infections as the leading cause.

Another common cause of FUO in the dog and cat are immune-mediated diseases. Most immune-mediated diseases occur in young adult dogs. Immune complexes are a potent stimulator for the release of fever-producing cytokines and frequently lead to temperatures of 105° F (40.5° C) or 106° F (41° C). Neoplasia is not as common as immune-mediated disease in causing fevers but should always be considered,

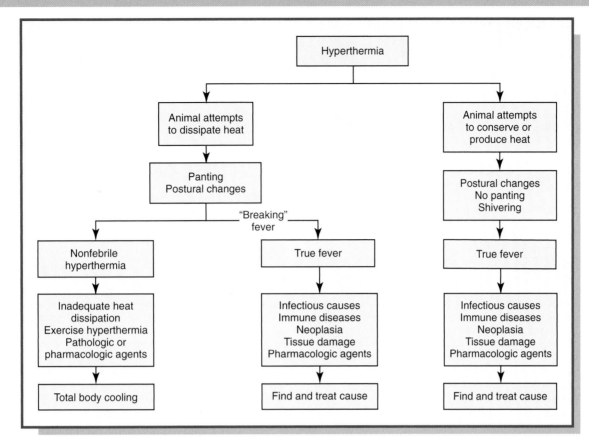

Figure 10-3 Algorithm for treatment of hyperthermia.

especially in older animals. Another, often overlooked, cause of fever is tissue trauma. Trauma often causes mild fever (103° F to 104° F [39.6° C to 40° C]) 1 or 2 days postsurgery when there has been significant muscle involvement. Most of these animals do not have infections and probably should not be treated with antibiotics without additional evidence of infection. Evaluating for infectious disease, immune-mediated disease, neoplasia, and causes of tissue trauma will usually lead to a final diagnosis, even when no obvious cause for the fever exists.

NONSPECIFIC THERAPY FOR FEBRILE PATIENTS

Mild to moderate elevations in body temperature are rarely fatal and may be beneficial to the body. As stated before, hyperthermia may inhibit viral replication, increase leukocyte function, and decrease the uptake of iron by microbes (which is often necessary for growth and replication). If a fever exceeds 107° F, a significant risk of permanent organ damage and disseminated intravascular coagulation exists. The benefits of nonspecific therapy versus its potential negative effects should be considered before initiating such management.

Nonspecific therapy for true fever usually involves inhibitors of prostaglandin synthesis. The compounds most commonly used are the nonsteroidal antiinflammatory drugs. These products inhibit the chemical mediators of fever production and allow normal thermoregulation. They do not block the production of endogenous pyrogens. These products

are relatively safe, although acetylsalicylic acid is potentially quite toxic to cats and cyclooxygenase-2 (COX-2) inhibitors are relatively safer. Dipyrone, an injectable nonsteroidal antiinflammatory drug sometimes used in cats, may lead to bone marrow suppression, especially when given over a prolonged period.

Total body cooling with water or fans, or both, in a febrile patient will reduce body temperature; however, the thermoregulatory center in the hypothalamus will still be directing the body to increase the body temperature. This may result in a further increase in metabolic rate, oxygen consumption, and subsequent water and caloric requirements. Unless a fever is life threatening, this type of nonspecific therapy is counterproductive.

Glucocorticoids block the acute-phase response, fever, and most other parts of this (adaptive) response. In general, their use should be reserved for those patients in whom the cause of the fever is known to be noninfectious and blocking the rest of the acute-phase response will not be detrimental (and may prove beneficial). The most common indications include some immune-mediated diseases in which the fever plays a significant role and glucocorticoid therapy is often part of the chemotherapeutic protocol (e.g., immune-mediated hemolytic anemia, immune-mediated polyarthritis).

Phenothiazines can be effective in alleviating a true fever by depressing normal thermoregulation and causing peripheral vasodilation. The sedative qualities and potential for hypotension caused by the phenothiazines should be considered before administration to the febrile patient.

CHAPTER 11

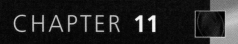

Hypothermia

Polly M. Taylor

MAINTANENCE OF NORMAL BODY TEMPERATURE

Mammalian body temperature is maintained closely around a constant set point at which cellular function is optimal. There are a number of complex mechanisms that maintain body temperature within tight control. The anterior hypothalamus maintains overall control of body temperature. It responds to local increases or decreases in temperature and also to neural input from warm and cold receptors in the skin, the abdominal viscera, and the spinal cord.

To maintain constant temperature, heat generated by muscular activity and metabolism is matched to heat loss. Temperature is regulated largely by control of heat loss from the body surface via the classic routes of heat exchange: conduction, convection, evaporation, and radiation (Web Figure 11-1). Heat is also lost from the respiratory tract through evaporation and in urine and feces. If the body becomes too cold, heat is retained in the body core through peripheral vasoconstriction, which prevents warm blood reaching the body surface. Piloerection insulates the skin by trapping a layer of stationary air. Some additional heat is generated through muscle activity, such as shivering and voluntary movement. Adrenergic chemical thermogenesis may also have a role in maintaining body temperature. Behavioral responses to cold are important in preventing heat loss; for example, moving into shelter and warmth, curling up, and dams protecting the young. Heat is lost by reversal of these processes, such that vasodilation of superficial blood vessels allows warm central blood to reach the skin. Panting increases evaporation from the respiratory tract. In some species, sweating is stimulated to provide the most effective heat loss through evaporation. Dogs and cats do not sweat from the skin, and loss via the respiratory tract through panting is the most significant form of active heat loss.

DEVELOPMENT OF HYPOTHERMIA

Hypothermia develops when either the methods of heat production and conservation are overwhelmed by a cold environment or when the mechanisms of heat retention are impaired. Smaller animals, in which the ratio of body surface area to volume is high, are more likely to develop hypothermia. Old, sick, or otherwise debilitated animals are also more likely to become hypothermic as heat generation and temperature control may be impaired. Neonates, with underdeveloped temperature-regulating mechanisms, are particularly susceptible. Hypothermia leads to a progressive failure of bodily functions, ultimately leading to cardiac standstill and death. In man, a core body temperature of 35° C is regarded as hypothermia. Although animal temperatures are slightly higher than human temperatures, the definitions of degrees of hypothermia applied in human medicine serve well in other species as a guide to the expected degree of malfunction (Figure 11-1). Initially, as core body temperature decreases below 36° C, respiratory rate, pulse rate and arterial blood pressure fall. As temperature decreases below 34° C, muscular control and neural function begin to fail, consciousness is depressed, and metabolism is slowed. As temperature falls further, more life-threatening abnormalities develop.[1] Acidosis and electrolyte imbalance may occur and, below 30° C, even in the absence of any drugs, cardiac dysrhythmias are likely to develop and temperature regulatory mechanisms fail. Hence, animals with a body temperature below 30° C are unlikely to regain normal temperature without treatment. Progressive metabolic and respiratory failure takes place when body temperature is below 28° C, with a high risk of ventricular fibrillation; cardiac standstill occurs at around 20° C.

Normal cats and, particularly, dogs withstand cold environments well. For instance, dogs immersed in water at 20° C

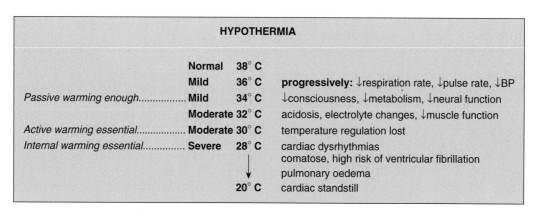

	HYPOTHERMIA	
	Normal	38° C	
	Mild	36° C	progressively: ↓respiration rate, ↓pulse rate, ↓BP
Passive warming enough................	Mild	34° C	↓consciousness, ↓metabolism, ↓neural function
	Moderate	32° C	acidosis, electrolyte changes, ↓muscle function
Active warming essential................	Moderate	30° C	temperature regulation lost
Internal warming essential..............	Severe	28° C	cardiac dysrhythmias
			comatose, high risk of ventricular fibrillation
			pulmonary oedema
		20° C	cardiac standstill

Figure 11-1 The effects of hypothermia. *BP*, Blood pressure.

can maintain heat regulation for 5 hours with less than a 1° C fall in body temperature. By far the most common cause of hypothermia in small animals is the disruption of normal control mechanisms by sedation and anesthesia,[2] which impair hypothalamic function and behavioral responses. Many anesthetics and sedatives cause some degree of peripheral vasodilation, which itself allows more heat loss. As a consequence, most small animals are likely to lose body heat during anesthesia. Exposure to a cold environment or near drowning is a much less common cause of hypothermia in animals. In these circumstances, normal heat retention mechanisms are simply overwhelmed by the environmental conditions. The consequences of cold-exposure hypothermia and its treatment are essentially the same as for anesthesia-induced hypothermia. Hypothermia is likely to be more severe after cold exposure, but there is the advantage of being uncomplicated by the effects of surgery or drugs.

Anesthetic-associated heat loss and the resultant decrease in body temperature slow drug metabolism and lead to prolonged recovery from anesthesia.[3] If severe, it is possible that cardiac function may be affected sufficiently to cause death. More commonly, postoperative hypothermia causes morbidity or death through the consequences of a slow recovery. A long period of unconsciousness increases the likelihood of unresolved obstructed airways and prolonged hypoxia. Shivering will worsen this effect through increased oxygen and energy demands. Lack of movement in an animal still under the influence of vasodilating anesthetics and sedatives leads to a vicious circle of further heat loss and reduced drug metabolism, prolonging recovery and further increasing the chance of airway obstruction and hypoxia.

PREVENTION AND TREATMENT

It is a great deal easier to prevent heat loss during anesthesia than to try to restore the temperature of a cold, unconscious dog or cat at the end of a long surgical procedure. Effort should be made from the start of anesthesia to maintain body temperature between 36° and 38° C. Body temperature needs to be monitored in order to prompt appropriate treatment; this is easily achieved by measuring rectal temperature, which has been shown to correlate well with core temperature.[4] Much can be done to prevent hypothermia by passive methods, largely insulation, although active methods using external heat are usually required where body cavities are exposed. Warming the limbs rather than the trunk has been shown to be particularly effective.[5]

Passive Warming Most heat is lost through conduction to colder surfaces in contact with the animal, such as the operating table, and through evaporation of body fluids and liquids used for surgical preparation. The animal should be insulated from colder surfaces and from the surrounding air, and it should be kept as dry as possible. A warm operating theatre may reduce heat loss into the surroundings, but working in an environment at body temperature is unpleasant; some heat loss by conduction into air circuits flowing around the animal will still occur unless it is insulated. Insulation between the operating table and the animal is easy to achieve with foam padding and other positioning aids. It is also easy to insulate the whole animal by wrapping any exposed parts with bubble wrapping or aluminium foil (Web Figure 11-2). A compromise between the ultimate asepsis and the best heat retention must be made by clipping the minimal amount of hair and wetting the smallest area compatible with the proposed surgery. At all costs, excess scrub water must be dried up. No animal should lie in a pool of scrub liquid during surgery.

It is impossible to prevent evaporation from the exposed surgical site. Intestinal surgery is the worst in this regard because large surface areas of serous membrane may be exposed. Regular flushing with warm (38° to 40° C) saline helps to reduce the amount of evaporation of body fluid and may help to prevent heat loss. Heat is also lost through the respiratory tract. Use of low-flow rebreathing circuits that retain both heat and moisture are advantageous in this respect. Heat and moisture exchangers placed between the endotracheal tube and the breathing circuit help to retain moisture and hence heat, as evaporation is reduced. However, these exchangers increase dead space and may be inappropriate for the cats and small dogs that most need heat retention.

Active Warming Active methods to prevent heat loss are usually required during surgery of the body cavities. Abdominal lavage with saline warmed to around 43° C has been shown to increase body temperature in dogs undergoing celiotomy.[6] External warming can usually be provided by using heated pads, infrared lights, heated gels, and hot-air circulators. Circulating water-heated pads are the safest because they do not become too hot; electrically heated pads or any non–thermostatically controlled system may burn an unconscious dog or cat unable to move away from the heat source.[7] Gel pads that are catalyzed into an exothermic reaction when changing state to a stiff form are useful in cats and small dogs (Web Figure 11-3). The heat generated is not excessive, lasts for 1 to 2 hours, and the stiffened gel bag can be used to position the animal. They are "regenerated" after use by placing in boiling water until the gel state returns. By far the most effective of the active-heating systems are the hot-air blankets, in which hot air is blown into a perforated blanket that is placed about the animal under the surgical drapes (Web Figure 11-4). An extremely wet animal will initially be cooled as the result of evaporation, but in all other circumstances this method has proved extremely effective.

Treatment of hypothermia depends on its severity and cause. After anesthesia, active warming is required as homeostatic mechanisms are impaired. Where the environment has caused hypothermia, normal heat-generating mechanisms will be more effective, and passive methods such as insulation with warm, dry blankets may be sufficient (see Figure 11-1). Extreme hypothermia (core temperature 30° C) requires internal active warming with intravenous fluids at 40° C and gastric, colonic, or peritoneal lavage with fluids at 40° to 42° C. This is to prevent further core cooling, which occurs when surface warming causes vasodilation, thereby allowing cold, peripheral blood to circulate into the body core.

References

The reference list can be found on the companion Expert Consult Web site at *www.expertconsult.com*.

CHAPTER 12

Clinical Pain Identification, Assessment, and Management

Patrice M. Mich
Peter W. Hellyer

In recent years, greater understanding of the biology of pain is complemented by a profound paradigm shift in our recognition of pain as a significant health threat in nonhuman patients and in our commitment to aggressively treat it. This chapter is an overview of current pain science concepts including terminology, physiology, pathophysiology, pain recognition and assessment in veterinary patients, and therapeutics. An exhaustive treatise of the rapidly growing field of pain medicine is beyond its scope. This chapter provides a basic understanding of the practice of veterinary pain medicine with guidelines for clinical pain assessment and management.

NEUROPHYSIOLOGY AND PATHOPHYSIOLOGY OF PAIN

Terminology and Definitions

Pain is an unpleasant sensory and emotional experience associated with actual or potential tissue damage or is described in terms of such damage. The inability to communicate in no way negates the possibility that an individual is experiencing pain and is in need of appropriate pain relieving treatment.[1]

Animal pain is an aversive sensory and emotional experience representing an awareness by the animal of damage or threat to the integrity of tissues.[2]

The activation of specially modified receptors and neural pathways by noxious stimuli results in the peripheral process referred to generically as *nociception*. In contrast, the experience of pain is the final product of a complex information-processing network that results in perception; perception takes place only at higher levels of the central nervous system (CNS) as a direct result of nociception. Pain is the conscious recognition of discomfort resulting from injury, disease, or emotional distress as evidenced by biologic or behavioral changes or both. It is a subjective and emotional experience that may be accompanied by feelings of fear, anxiety, and panic. Pain elicits protective motor actions, results in learned avoidance, and may modify species-specific traits of behavior including social behavior.[3] *Acute pain* is the result of a traumatic, surgical, or infectious event that is abrupt in onset, does not persist much beyond the inciting insult, and is generally alleviated by commonly administered analgesic drugs. *Chronic pain* persists beyond the normal duration of acute disease or injury despite resolution of disease or healing of injury; chronic pain may also result from a persistent pathologic process or nerve injury (neuropathic pain). Chronic pain is seldom sufficiently alleviated by routinely used analgesics and often requires a multimodal approach including, but not limited to, pharmacologic analgesics, tranquilizers or psychotropic drugs, physical therapy, environmental manipulation, acupuncture, and behavioral conditioning.

Simply put, acute pain is a symptom of disease or injury with the protective function of warning the organism of impending or actual tissue damage. Clearly then, acute pain is important; indeed congenital or acquired insensitivity to pain leads to heightened risk of injury and premature death.[4,5] In contrast, chronic pain is a disease itself.[6] Chronic pain does not serve a biologic function and is associated with significant morbidity.

There is an extensive nomenclature associated with the science of pain. Below we include a list of commonly used terms.

Afferent: toward the CNS.

Algology: the science and study of pain phenomena.

Allodynia: pain caused by a stimulus that does not normally provoke pain. However there is no increased response to a stimulus that normally evokes pain.

Analgesia: the absence of pain in the presence of stimuli that would normally be painful.

Anesthesia: the absence of all sensory modalities in the body or in a body part.

Breakthrough pain: intermittent flare of more severe pain in an otherwise adequately controlled acute or chronic pain setting.

Cancer pain: pain resulting from primary tumor growth, metastatic disease, or the toxic effects of chemotherapy and radiation.

Causalgia: a syndrome of prolonged burning pain, allodynia, and hyperpathia after a traumatic nerve lesion, often combined with vasomotor and sudomotor (sweating) dysfunction and later trophic changes.

Central sensitization: a state in which second- and third-order neurons in the CNS respond excessively to normal input from the periphery. An amplified signal from the periphery (peripheral sensitization) can be further amplified centrally. The mechanism involves molecular, cellular, and circuit changes within the CNS including N-methyl-D-aspartic acid receptor (NMDA)–mediated potentiation in the dorsal horn. Central sensitization is typically transient; however, if the driving input from the periphery is sustained it can persist indefinitely (e.g., osteoarthritic pain).

Deafferentation pain: pain caused by loss of sensory input into the CNS, as occurs with avulsion of the brachial plexus or other types of peripheral nerve lesions, or caused by pathology of the CNS.

Dermatome: segmental region of skin and subcutaneous tissue supplied by a specific sensory nerve.

Dysesthesia: an unpleasant abnormal sensation whether spontaneous or evoked. Hyperalgesia and allodynia are examples.

Efferent: away from the CNS.

Hyperalgesia: an increased response to a stimulation that is normally painful. Stimulated nociceptors respond at a lower threshold and more vigorously.

Hyperesthesia: an increased sensitivity to stimulation, excluding the special senses.

Hyperpathia: a pain syndrome in which there is increased response to a stimulus that is normally painful. This may include symptoms of hyperalgesia, hyperesthesia, dysthesia, and allodynia. Pain may be explosive and localization may be inaccurate. Radiating and delayed responses are possible.

Hypoalgesia: a diminished response to stimulation that is normally painful.

Hypoesthesia: a diminished sensitivity to stimulation, excluding special senses.

Inflammatory pain: spontaneous pain and hypersensitivity to pain in response to tissue damage and inflammation.

Interventional pain management: minimally invasive procedures in which analgesic drugs are injected or pain-relieving devices are implanted in order to provide longer-term relief of chronic pain.

Local anesthesia: the temporary loss of sensory function, with or without loss of motor function, in a restricted region of the body.

Myofascial pain: focal pain within a muscle or associated connective tissue resulting in decreased and painful range of motion, stiffness, and muscle spasm.

Neuralgia: pain along the distribution pathway of a nerve or nerves.

Neuritis: an inflammation of a nerve or nerves.

Neuropathic pain: spontaneous pain and hypersensitivity to pain in association with damage to or a lesion of the nervous system (peripheral nervous system [PNS] or CNS). Neuropathic pain is often burning, stabbing, or buzzing and may be paroxysmal.

Neuroplasticity: a characteristic of the nervous system such that it can reorganize itself at both the receptor and neuronal levels in response to injury, disease, or environmental processes.

Nociception: the reception, conduction, and central nervous processing of nerve signals generated by the stimulation of primary afferent nerves.

Nociceptor: a free ending on primary afferent neurons preferentially responsive to a noxious stimulus or to a stimulus that would become noxious if prolonged. This term may be used to indicate the entire primary afferent neuron.

Nociceptor threshold: the minimum strength of stimulus that will cause a nociceptor to generate a nerve impulse.

Noxious stimulus: a stimulus (e.g., mechanical, thermal, chemical) of intensity and quality adequate to trigger nociceptive reactions.

Pain (detection) threshold: the least experience of pain that a subject can recognize. The point at which a subject just begins to feel pain when a noxious stimulus is being applied in an ascending trial or the point at which pain disappears in a descending trial. The pain detection threshold is relatively constant among individuals and species. In most cases it is higher than the nociceptor threshold.

Pain tolerance: the greatest level of pain that a subject will tolerate. Pain tolerance varies considerably among individuals, both human and animal. It is influenced greatly by pharmacologic and nonpharmacologic analgesic intervention as well as an individual's prior experience, environment, and stress level.

Pain tolerance range: the arithmetic difference between the pain detection threshold and the pain tolerance threshold.

Paresthesia: an abnormal sensation, whether spontaneous or evoked. Paresthesias are not painful (as opposed to dysesthesias).

Peripheral sensitization: a state in which tissue injury and inflammation lower the threshold for firing of nociceptive afferents. The mechanism involves synthesis of prostaglandins and release of inflammatory cytokines, chemokines, peptide neurotransmitters, growth factors, nitric oxide, and reactive oxygen species. The result is hyperalgesia and allodynia.

Radiculopathy: a pathologic disturbance of function in one or more nerve roots.

Reflex: an involuntary, purposeful, and orderly response to a stimulus not necessarily associated with pain perception. The anatomic basis for the reflex arc consists of a receptor, a primary afferent nerve fiber associated with the receptor, a region of integration in the spinal cord or brain stem (synapses), and a lower motor neuron leading to an effector organ such as skeletal muscles (somatic reflexes), smooth muscles, or glands (visceral reflexes).

Regional analgesia: the loss of sensation to a part of the body supplied by a specific nerve or nerves as a result of disrupting conduction of sensory impulses.

Sedation: CNS depression mediated by the cerebral cortex whereby the patient is drowsy but arousable.

Somatic pain: well-localized pain arising from any body tissue other than viscera.

Suffering: an unpleasant emotional state or an undesirable mental state that people or animals would normally prefer to avoid. Suffering can refer to a wide range of intense and objectionable subjective states such as fear and frustration. It can be of either physical or psychologic origin.

Tolerance: a shortened duration and/or decreased response to analgesics often associated with a significant increase in the average dose required to achieve desired effect. Most commonly attributed to opiate use.

Tranquilization: a state of calmness mediated through the reticular activating system in which the patient is relaxed and, though awake, relatively unaware of surroundings.

Trigger point: a focal hypersensitive site in muscle or connective tissue, usually associated with myofascial pain syndromes.

Visceral pain: a type of pain arising from stretching, distention, or inflammation of visceral organs. Distinct from somatic pain, it is described as deep, cramping, aching, and poorly localized. It may result in referred pain to somatic regions.

Wind-up: a form of neuroplasticity in which repeated high-intensity stimulation of nociceptors leads to long-lasting increases in excitability of central neurons through structural modifications at presynaptic and postsynaptic sites, particularly in the dorsal horn of the spinal cord. The more correct term is *central sensitization*.

Neuroanatomy and Physiology of Pain Pathways

A simplified model of pain pathways describes progression from periphery to the CNS via transduction, transmission, modulation, projection, and finally, perception (Figure 12-1).

Transduction occurs in the periphery at the terminal ends of sensory primary afferent nerve fibers. Nociceptors are the specialized termini of these fibers, which respond to noxious stimuli. A so-called minimal or adequate stimulus is required to activate nociceptors above their threshold; this results in transduction of noxious stimuli into nerve impulse signals. Known activating stimuli for nociceptors include mechanical, thermal, or chemical stimuli. Nociceptors may be monomodal or polymodal (responding to more than one stimulus type). Distinct from mono- and polymodal nociceptors are the silent nociceptors.[7,8] Under normal stimulating circumstances these nociceptors are insensitive due to a relatively high threshold. An adequate stimulus is only achieved following the release of tissue inflammatory mediators at the site of injury that reduce the threshold for response. As a result, these previously silent nociceptors can be activated by a variety of thermal and mechanical stimuli. This is an example of peripheral sensitization and hypersensitivity.

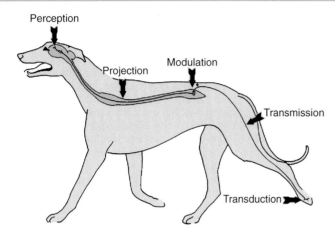

Figure 12-1 Schematic pathways in the neuroanatomic description of pain. Noxious stimuli are transduced into electrical stimuli, transmitted to the spinal cord (where peripheral ascending and descending modulation occurs), and finally are relayed to the brainstem and brain for perception. Descending pathways from higher centers also modulate pain signals.

Transduced signals are propagated along the primary afferent neuron as action potentials in a process called **transmission**. Primary afferent neurons transmitting noxious signals are of two classes: (1) fast-conducting (5 to 30 m/sec), lightly myelinated Aδ fibers ,which are associated with sharp or superficial pain; and (2) slow-conducting (0.5 to 2 m/sec), unmyelinated C fibers, which are associated with a dull, burning type of pain, so-called second pain or deep pain.[9] A third class of primary afferent neuron, Aβ, constitutes myelinated, fast-conducting fibers transmitting nonnoxious sensory information such as touch, pressure, and proprioception. Primary afferent neurons synapse in the dorsal horn of the spinal cord on a number of different neurons, including nociceptive-specific second-order neurons, nonnociceptive-specific so-called wide-dynamic range (WDR) neurons, and interneurons. WDR neurons receive information from Aβ, Aδ, and C fibers. **Modulation** occurs in the dorsal horn of the spinal cord and suprasegmentally resulting in increased or decreased nerve impulse propagation. Further description of modulation is included below.

Second-order projection neurons constitute ascending, projection pathways, the most important of which, outside the head in nonhuman animals, are the spinocervicothalamic and spinoreticular tracts (Figure 12-2).

The former is chiefly concerned with superficial pain and is the primary conscious pain pathway in carnivores.[10,11] The latter is primarily associated with transmission of deep and visceral pain.[12] Second-order neurons **project** to cortical (primary somatosensory cortex, anterior cingulate cortex, insular cortex, and forebrain) as well as several subcortical sites including the reticular formation, nucleus raphe magnus of the medulla, periaqueductal grey matter (PAG) of the midbrain, the hypothalamus, the thalamus, and the limbic system. These projections result in physiologic responses to pain beyond conscious perception, including arousal; altered sympathetic tone; ascending and descending modulation of pain due to release of norepinephrine, serotonin, enkephalin, endorphin, and dynorphin; emotional distress; and memory consolidation. Anatomic data show a high degree of connectivity among these areas. Plasticity, redundancy, and resilience among pain pathways exist such that functions usually performed by one region can be taken over by another.

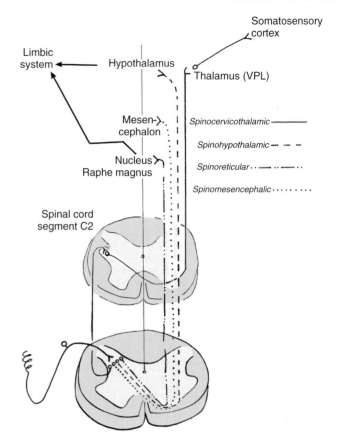

Figure 12-2 Sensory pathways associated with pain signals. *VPL,* Ventral lateral nucleus.

Once the pain signal has reached the brain cortex, conscious perception is possible. Perception is recognition, integration, and processing of sensory information. The ability of a given stimulus to result in the conscious perception of pain and in physiologic response to pain is dependent on modification in the periphery, within the spinal cord, the brainstem, and in cortical regions of the brain. Perception of pain requires consciousness; thus an anesthetized patient cannot perceive a painful stimulus. Importantly, such a patient is capable of all nociceptive responses short of perception and upon recovery from anesthesia is subject to all adverse effects of the unmitigated pain process.

Neuromodulation and Response to Pain
The Cartesian model of pain imagines the somatosensory system like a simple line of communication directly linking and not altering pain signals as they are transmitted from the body (periphery) to the brain (cortex) for conscious perception. Further, this model suggests that the stimulus in the periphery is predictably and proportionately transmitted. Modern pain science has revealed that pain pathways are in fact highly labile, and modulation in the periphery, the spinal cord, brainstem, and higher centers is the rule not the exception. Peripheral nociception is altered by changes in nociceptive threshold chiefly as a result of nociceptive sensitizers and activators. These are inflammatory mediators and neuropeptides (e.g., substance P, bradykinin, serotonin, histamine, prostaglandin, interleukin-1, tumor necrosis factor-α) released from damaged tissue that directly stimulate nociceptors, increase their sensitivity, and recruit silent nociceptors. The direct result is **peripheral sensitization** that leads to **primary hyperalgesia,** a state of increased responsiveness to noxious stimuli, and **allodynia,** a state in which normally nonnoxious

stimuli are capable of activating nociceptors. Modulation of peripheral sensitization is an important target in pain control.

Central nociception is also capricious. Changes in excitability of neurons and glial cells in the spinal cord result in **central sensitization,** a process whereby nerve fibers are "trained" to respond more vigorously to further stimulation. This occurs due to bombardment of second-order neurons with high-intensity, high-frequency stimuli from the periphery (primarily C-fibers). The result is presynaptic membrane modulation and increased release of excitatory neurotransmitter, glutamate, along with substance P, BDNF (brain-derived neurotrophic factor), and calcitonin gene–related peptide (CGRP).[13] Substance P and BDNF are neuromodulatory neurotransmitters that bind to G protein–coupled receptors. Neurotransmitters act on excitatory (α-amino-3-hydroxyl-5-methyl-4-isoxazole-propionate [AMPA], kainite, NMDA) and inhibitory (γ-aminobutyric acid [GABA] and glycine) receptors. NMDA receptors on the postsynaptic membrane, normally silent, are activated by increased glutamate. The consequence is increased calcium influx and subsequent upregulation of receptors resulting in increased membrane sensitivity, so-called spinal facilitation of pain or wind-up. In addition to subcellular modification, neuronal change occurs. WDR neurons are among those cells chiefly associated with wind-up. WDR neurons are capable of receiving information from somatic and visceral structures, noxious and non-noxious stimuli. As a result of high-frequency stimulation, previously nonnoxious stimuli are capable of causing pain, individual peripheral sensory neuron receptive fields expand, and stimulation of one tissue can be perceived as originating in a distant tissue (i.e., referred pain). Additionally, tactile, nonnoxious impulses reaching the WDR neurons via $A\beta$ neurons can inhibit transmission of noxious impulse; this is sometimes called the *gate control theory*, first introduced by Melzack and Wall.[14]

And yet it is more complicated than this. Recent data implicate the role of immune and glial cells in the development of pain disorders. It is clear that neurons alone are not responsible for pain in its many manifestations. So-called neuronal support structures such as microglia, astrocytes, oligodendrocytes, fibroblasts, endothelial cells, Schwann cells, and satellite cells compose 80% to 90% of neurologic tissue and are likely involved in a complex network of intercellular communication for pain signaling and processing.[15] It appears that this communication is multidirectional from support cells to neurons and from neurons to support cells, using gap junctions and chemical modulation (e.g., chemokines, cytokines, nitric oxide, neurotransmitters, excitatory amino acids, prostaglandins).

Specifically, work with microglia and astrocytes in the CNS has redefined our image of the synapse into a tripartite model involving the classical presynaptic and postsynaptic cells accompanied by intimately associated astrocytes.[16,17] Astrocytes comprise 40% to 50% of all glial cells and outnumber neurons. In the basal state astrocytes provide energy and neurotransmitter precursors for neurons. They also provide trophic support. Astrocytes become activated in response to CNS trauma, ischemia, neurodegeneration, and inflammation. Activation is characterized by increased production of proinflammatory substances such as interleukin-1 (IL-1), tumor necrosis factor (TNF), and nitric oxide (NO). For example, NO, produced by activated glia and neurons, potentiates IL-1–induced cyclooxygenase 2 (COX 2), an important enzyme in the synthesis of inflammatory prostaglandins and a target for nonsteroidal antiinflammatory drugs.[18]

Microglia serve in immune surveillance and host defense. In the basal state they act as sentinels with a stellate morphology designed to sample extracellular fluid for endogenous danger signals via toll-like receptors (TLR). Activation signals come from neuromodulators, neurotransmitters, and glial excitatory chemokines released from injured sensory neurons. Activation of these receptors leads to activation of microglia resulting in release of chemical modulators and increased gap junction protein connexin. The overall result is coordinated intercellular response to injury leading to hypersensitivity extending beyond the site and magnitude of the original insult. Indeed a number of investigators have documented upregulation of microglia in models of opioid tolerance, neuropathic pain, and opioid-induced hypersensitivity.[19] Current research suggests that microglia are activated first (initiation of pain facilitation), and this leads to astrocytes activation and resultant persistence of the pain state.[20] Glial cells are not involved in normal pain processing. As such glial dysregulation has become an active area of research for drug discovery in the treatment of chronic pain states, the most promising of which includes gene therapy for the upregulation of spinal antiinflammatory IL-10 and intrathecal glial activation inhibitors.[21]

Finally, activity in the spinal cord is further modulated by descending antinociceptive systems originating in suprasegmental structures. Midline nuclei of the midbrain and medulla, such as the periaqueductal grey and the nucleus raphe magnus, respond to input both from ascending spinoreticular and spinocervicothalamic tracts and from descending pathways from higher cerebral centers (e.g., limbic and cortical regions). These nuclei release neurotransmitters for antinociceptive systems including serotonin, norepinephrine, epinephrine, and endogenous opiates. Cortical and noncortical structures include forebrain; cingulate, insular, and somatosensory cortices; thalamic nuclei; amygdala; hypothalamus; and basal ganglia structures such as the globus pallidus.

It is important to note that the above is a highly simplified, albeit useful, overview of the enormously complex peripheral, dorsal horn, and central sensitization and modification processes.

PAIN IDENTIFICATION AND ASSESSMENT

The prevention and management of pain is fundamental to the practice of medicine; as practitioners we pledge an oath to alleviate patient suffering. The Joint Commission mandated in the year 2000 that human hospitals in the United States must measure and manage pain defining it as the fifth vital sign. Further, the Joint Commission view of pain is that of a condition existing concurrent with many other conditions, but one that warrants specific attention in its own right such that processes must be developed to support improvements in its management. Similarly, the American Animal Hospital Association along with the American Association of Feline Practitioners established pain management guidelines for dogs and cats in 2007.[22] In veterinary medicine, pain may be considered as a vital sign, along with temperature, pulse rate, and respiratory rate. In establishing pain as a vital sign and in establishing guidelines, these organizations acknowledged that pain relief is good medical practice.

In the not-so-distant past pain in nonhuman species was considered either not present, not clinically relevant, or clinically important only insofar as it protected an animal from self-injury. Today the existence, let alone coexistence, of these historical, Cartesian dogmas is untenable. Pain science has shown that human and animal neural pathways are similar with regard to the transduction, transmission, modulation, and projection of pain. However, the presence of these pathways does not, itself, mean that animals experience pain. Traditionally, the awareness or perception of pain as a brain function is considered the highest step in the pain pathway. Pain is defined by the International Association for the Study of Pain as an unpleasant sensory and emotional experience associated with actual or potential tissue damage. The key here is the term *emotional experience* and herein lies the debate over animal pain. Because we do not as yet have the scientific tools to investigate emotional states in our nonhuman species, we are obliged to infer from behavioral change. Consequently, pain in nonhuman animals has been alternatively defined as an aversive sensory experience that elicits protective motor actions, results in learned avoidance, and may modify species-specific traits of behavior, including social behavior.[23]

Veterinary pain science has led the way in acknowledging the existence of animal pain and the importance of alleviating it. The continuing challenge is how best to recognize such pain in order to effectively prevent and treat it. Unlike the other vital signs, pain is difficult to measure and quantify. The tools to measure pain in veterinary patients will undoubtedly change as more clinical and research information becomes available.

Pain Assessment by Proxy

Despite more than a decade of increased interest in pain assessment in veterinary species, the science of accurately measuring pain in animals in general, and dogs and cats in particular, is still in its infancy. Rightly or wrongly, much of this work has focused on the development of pain scales as a means of clinically quantifying pain experienced by individuals. As stated previously, pain has been described as a personal sensory and emotional experience; thus objectifying such experiences for another is inherently difficult. Additionally, efforts to do so in veterinary medicine are hampered by the nature of the patient population, which is nonverbal and tremendously diverse including such differences as species, breed, environment, and age as well as differences in clinical pathology. At this time, no "gold standard" exists to assess pain in animals.

In contrast, human pain science has yielded a number of potentially useful clinical assessment tools that may offer guidance in veterinary pain science. Perhaps the closest comparisons in the human patient population are neonates, infants, people with severe learning disabilities, and those who are mentally and/or verbally disabled. These patients require pain assessment by proxy (i.e., physician, nurse, parent). These populations, particularly neonates and infants, have been extensively studied in the last 25 years. The result has been a proliferation of scales used to assess pain in patients of different developmental levels, in different settings, and in different clinical conditions. Scale refinement continues to create tools that are sensitive and specific for pain. In the absence of direct verbal communication with the patient, the foundation of these scales has been behavior change, both the loss of normal behavior and the development of new, abnormal behavior. A similar process is occurring in veterinary medicine, albeit with the additional challenge of creating scales that are species (and possibly breed?) specific. Similar to nonverbal humans, veterinary patient pain must be assessed by proxy (i.e., veterinarian, technician or nurse, or owner), and this assessment is based largely on behavioral change. Although it is difficult to assess pain in general and in animals particularly, the inability of the patient, human or animal, to accurately communicate pain and suffering does not obviate our responsibility. Both medical and veterinary practitioners are obligated to produce clinically relevant, reliable, and validated pain assessment tools for patients incapable of verbally self-reporting.

With this in mind criteria for an ideal pain scale are presented in Box 12-1.

Because ideal pain scales do not exist for every species and every medical condition, some basic recommendations should be kept in mind. When evaluating a patient for pain, it is

---

Box • 12-1

Characteristics of an Ideal Pain Scale

Patient characteristics:
1. Species specific
2. Breed specific (there may be differences in genetic sensitivities to pain and the demonstration of behaviors indicating pain)
3. Environmental and rearing specific (e.g., individual animal versus group, home versus clinic)
4. Developmental/age specific (e.g., neonates versus pediatrics versus adult versus geriatric)
5. Gender specific (the role of gender in pain perception is still unclear)
6. Cause of pain specific (e.g., pathology-induced pain, procedural pain, surgical pain)
7. Body-region specific (e.g., facial pain, ocular pain, abdominal pain)
8. Character of pain state–specific (i.e., adaptive, maladaptive)
9. Pain intensity–specific (spectrum from none to severe)
10. Recognize individual variations

Pain scale indices and criteria should be:
1. Clearly defined
2. Consistently useable by different individuals
3. Have clearly understood strengths and weaknesses
4. Be able to differentiate differences in the intensity and degree of pain
5. Be straightforward and practical to use
6. Be validated according to carefully considered standards
7. Be a useful tool to guide clinical decision making

---

essential to be aware of the *normal behavior* for that species, age, and individual. Deviations from normal behavior suggest pain, anxiety, disease or treatment effect, or some combination of these. The *purpose* of a given scale is of paramount importance because pain varies depending upon origin and duration. Therefore, a pain scale developed to evaluate acute postoperative pain after orthopedic surgery may be of little help in assessing, for example, abdominal pain or chronic back pain. Pain scales should be used as a *guide* to identify behavioral changes that may indicate insufficiently controlled pain and as a way to track response to therapy. Accordingly, numerically based pain scales should not be used to deny or dispense analgesia based on an arbitrary number.

Current State of Assessing Pain in Animals

Assessing *extreme* pain in animals is relatively simple provided the veterinarian and staff are aware of normal behavior for that species and individual. However, many of the most challenging cases involve patients that experience pain between none and severe. In fact, the absence of pain can be an exceedingly difficult clinical assessment. Lack of outward expression of pain does not rule out the existence of uncontrolled pain. Beyond the seemingly simple determination of pain or no pain is the equally difficult assessments of the degree of pain and the ability of that animal to cope with its pain. In a 1996 survey of Canadian veterinarians, Dohoo and Dohoo found that one of the main factors that determined if veterinarians routinely administered analgesic drugs postoperatively was the veterinarian's perception of the degree of pain felt by animals.[24] The fact that 51.5% of those veterinarians surveyed never used analgesics highlights the clinical importance of being able to recognize pain in the species under a veterinarian's care. Even among veterinary personnel committed to treating pain, weighing the benefits of an analgesic protocol (i.e., decreased pain intensity) with its side effects (e.g., sedation, nausea) can be challenging. As recently as 2005 Williams et al reported that among New Zealand veterinary professionals 42% of respondents felt their knowledge in the area of assessment and treatment of pain was inadequate.[25] A similar survey of French veterinarians in 2004 revealed 58.8% considered their methods of pain quantification and control to be inadequate.[26] Until recently many veterinarians and their staff never received formal training in the recognition of pain. This may explain these survey results. Fortunately, pain medicine is now more frequently incorporated into the core curriculum in veterinary schools, and continuing education programs often feature basic and state-of-the-art lectures on topics relevant to pain in animals.

As more studies focus on species-specific pain behaviors, the ability to recognize and treat pain in animals will improve; however, the assessment of pain in animals will remain a subjective and inaccurate undertaking for the near future. The question may be posed then, is it appropriate to assume that a painful procedure in people will also be painful in an animal? Indeed, the vast majority of pain studies are carried out in animals with results extrapolated to people, leading to the development of new drugs, new techniques, and ultimately to clinical trials for human therapy. Recognizing that marked differences exist in species pain tolerance, in demonstration of overt signs of pain, and in responses to therapeutic interventions, it nevertheless defies logic and ethics for the scientific community to use animals to understand pain in people while simultaneously denying that pain exists or is important in animals. Thus, it is appropriate at this time to assume if a condition causes pain in people, it will also cause some degree of pain in animals. For animals, pain may be more or less than that experienced by a person; therefore, the veterinarian must determine how well the patient is coping with its pain.

Modern veterinary pain medicine is now moving beyond this relatively crude though nonetheless ethically appropriate method of assessing pain. The evaluation methods described in this chapter have been extrapolated from human medicine (e.g., visual analogue scale) or specifically designed to assess acute postoperative pain in dogs and cats. These methods can be adapted to other species provided the veterinarian recognizes that pain behaviors are likely to be different among species. Importantly, all of the methods described are subjective and prone to the error of either underestimating or overestimating degree of pain. Although some pain scales include physiologic parameters, all of the pain scales used in animals rely on the recognition or interpretation (or both) of behavior to some extent. The most useful scales determine the presence or absence of specific behaviors while minimizing the interpretation of those behaviors. Even if the amount of pain is correctly estimated, determining how well the individual animal is coping with pain may be difficult. All of the current pain scales are subject to some degree of interobserver variability. Regardless of the pain assessment tool used, it is important that all pain assessors within the practice receive training on its use. One should not assume that untrained individuals can provide the same level of accuracy in assessing animal pain as compared with trained individuals familiar with the species being observed. Finally, it should be recognized that all of these methods are used to assess the effects of physical pain and that none have been designed to evaluate mental or psychologic dimensions of pain experienced by animals.

Physiologic (Objective) Assessment of Acute Pain

In general, pain assessments can be categorized as primarily objective or subjective. Physiologic data (e.g., heart rate, respiratory rate, arterial blood pressure, pupil dilation) may be useful in objectively assessing response to a noxious (painful) stimulus in a lightly anesthetized animal. Physiologic responses also occur in conscious patients as a result of acute pain or other stressors, but not with the same degree of reliability as in anesthetized patients. CNS and cardiopulmonary reflexes control cardiovascular and respiratory function to maintain a state of homeostasis; therefore, reflex control mechanisms may dampen physiologic responses to pain. In addition, physiologic parameters are not specific enough to differentiate pain from other stressors such as anxiety, fear, or concurrent metabolic conditions (e.g., anemia). Holton et al found that heart rate and respiratory rate were not useful indicators of pain in hospitalized dogs following surgery.[27] However, pupil dilation was significantly correlated with the pain score (numeric rating scale) in dogs following surgery. Nevertheless, the authors indicated that pupil size is unlikely to be a useful parameter to assess pain in hospitalized dogs. Likewise, physiologic measurements, including heart rate, respiratory rate, rectal temperature, plasma cortisol and β-endorphin concentrations, did not differentiate between cats that underwent surgery (tenectomy, onychectomy) and control cats that were anesthetized and bandaged, but had no surgery.[28]

The reader should note that some pain scales use physiologic data and some do not. In the authors' opinion, physiologic parameters are useful in assessing responses to noxious stimuli in patients under general anesthesia or for transient periods in conscious patients. The longer a conscious patient experiences pain, the less useful are physiologic parameters in assessing the degree of pain. When physiologic responses are used to assess pain, it is important to be aware of their limitations and to assess the selected parameter in light of baseline physiologic data. As such, changes in heart rate, respiratory rate, and other physiologic responses together may be more useful in assessing the patient than any absolute value for each criterion.

Behavioral (Subjective) Assessment of Acute Pain

Subjective evaluation of pain in animals relies on observation and interpretation of animal behavior. Pain may be indicated by loss of normal behaviors or appearance of abnormal behavior. In general, pain behaviors are easier to recognize in dogs as compared to cats. For example, dogs in pain may appear restless, agitated, or even delirious. This is particularly true during recovery from anesthesia after surgery. At the other end of the spectrum, dogs may be lethargic, withdrawn, dull, or obtunded. These dogs may not pay attention to environmental stimuli. The normal sleep-wake cycle may be disrupted, resulting in less sleep than normal. Normal activity such as grooming or eating may decrease or stop. Dogs may bite, lick, chew, or shake painful areas. Painful dogs may adopt abnormal body postures in an attempt to relieve or cope with pain in a given area. For example, dogs with abdominal pain (e.g., pancreatitis) may assume a posture with a rigid torso and arched back. Dogs with abdominal or thoracic pain may be reluctant to lie down in spite of obvious exhaustion. Although dogs do not have the same degree of motor control over their facial muscles as do primates, changes in facial expression can be used in some dogs to detect pain. Some examples include ears held back or in a down position, eyes wide open with dilated pupils or partially closed with a dull appearance, and a "fixed stare" with no acknowledgement of surroundings. Some dogs may display a type of grimace uncharacteristic of the dog when not painful. Disuse or guarding of a painful area is a fairly reliable indicator of pain. The dog's gait may be abnormal or the dog may appear stiff. Vocalization may indicate pain in the dog; however, it is an insensitive and nonspecific indicator of pain. Vocalization may occur as a whimper, whine, yelp, groan, grunt, yowl, or any combination. Finally, interactive behaviors are frequently changed in the painful animal. Dogs may become more aggressive and resist handling or palpation. In contrast, they may become more timid than usual and seek increased contact with caregivers.

By way of comparison, behavioral changes indicating pain in the cat may be quite different. Painful cats may simply hide in the back of their cage and demonstrate what appears to be fear or anxiety to the casual observer. A cat sitting quietly in the back of the cage after surgery may be in pain; however, pain would not be recognized if the caregiver expects to see more active signs of pain such as pacing, agitation, or vocalizing. Cats may continue to purr even when painful. Alternatively, a painful cat may growl fiercely with ears flattened striking at approaching objects or may attempt escape. On the other hand, extremely frightened cats will behave much the same. Excessive grooming or lack of grooming can both indicate pain in the cat. Some possible indicators of pain in cats include hunched posture, statuelike appearance, reduced or absent appetite, hiding, and tail flicking; these are also indicators of apprehension and anxiety in the cat. Whether assessing a dog or cat, a lack of familiarity with normal behaviors makes recognition of pain-induced behaviors difficult or impossible.[29]

In both dogs and cats behavioral changes indicative of pain may be too subtle or take too long to recognize under routine clinical situations. Sporadic observation of animal behavior may not reveal signs of pain. Except in the most severe circumstances, the signs of pain may be "masked" by more obvious behavior that is stereotypic of the species being observed. For instance, dogs may wag their tail and greet an observer at the cage door in spite of being in pain.[30] Cats may hiss or purr when approached, but when observed further may return to licking obsessively at a wound. It is incumbent on the observer to take sufficient time for thorough assessment and frequent reassessment keeping in mind normal behavior for the species, breed, and individual character of the patient.

Types of Acute Pain Scales

Preemptive Scoring System The preemptive scoring system (Box 12-2) is a subjective tool based on estimating the amount of pain an animal is likely to experience after a given procedure.

Preemptive scoring systems assign a level of pain (none, mild, moderate, severe) based on the procedure performed and the amount of tissue trauma involved. The guiding principle is if a procedure is likely to cause pain in a human, then it is likely to cause a similar degree of pain in animals. In general, the greater the amount of tissue trauma induced by a procedure, the greater the assigned level of pain. Preemptive scoring systems are useful in *planning* perioperative analgesic strategies. Procedures inducing moderate to severe pain often require the use of multiple analgesic drugs and techniques to adequately manage pain. Preemptive scoring systems are not useful in actually determining the degree of pain felt by an individual patient or in assessing response to therapy. Therefore, the reader is urged to keep in mind that individual patients may experience more or less pain than predicted by the preemptive pain scale.

Semiobjective Scales

Visual analog scale The visual analog scale (VAS) is a semiobjective pain intensity assessment tool consisting of a straight, horizontal line, 100 mm in length, bracketed with

---

Box • 12-2
Preemptive Scoring System

Preemptive Scoring System used to anticipate the amount of pain induced by surgical procedures.

1. Minor Procedures: No Pain
   Physical examination, restraint
   Radiography
   Suture removal, cast application, bandage change*
   Grooming
   Nail trim
2. Minor Surgeries: Minor Pain
   Suturing, debridement
   Urinary catheterization
   Dental cleaning
   Ear examination and cleaning
   Abscess lancing
   Removing cutaneous foreign bodies
3. Moderate Surgeries: Moderate Pain
   Ovariohysterectomy, castration, cesarean section
   Feline onychectomy
   Cystotomy
   Anal sacculectomy
   Dental extraction
   Cutaneous mass removal
   Severe laceration repair
4. Major Surgeries: Severe Pain
   Fracture repair, cruciate ligament repair
   Thoracotomy, laminectomy, exploratory laparotomy
   Limb amputation
   Ear canal ablation

Printed with permission from A roundtable discussion: rethinking your approach to sedation, anesthesia, and analgesia. Veterinary Medicine Publishing, 1997.
The pain categories are only a "best guess" of the amount of pain a certain procedure induces. In general, the more tissue trauma, the greater the pain. Individual animals may be more or less painful than the category suggests.
*Setting of fractures and some bandage changes can be quite painful.

---

descriptors of pain intensity (e.g., no pain, worst pain possible) on either end of the line (Figure 12-3).

The human patient draws a vertical line across the scale in a position that best represents his or her degree of pain. The length is then measured from 0 to the patient's mark to quantify pain. The patient may be asked to assess pain at the current time or the worst pain that occurred since the last assessment. The VAS has been used extensively in people and is generally considered useful in assessing pain and the response to therapy. The scale avoids the use of imprecise descriptive terms and provides many points from which to choose (100). The chief advantages of the VAS are ease of use and that it provides a general appraisal of worsening or improving pain. A disadvantage of the standard VAS used to rate pain intensity is that pain is a multidimensional experience and pain intensity is only one aspect of that experience. Also, the use of the VAS may result in greater variability of pain scores than the simple descriptive scale (SDS) described below. The VAS may erroneously appear more sensitive compared with other scales resulting in overinterpretation or excessive confidence

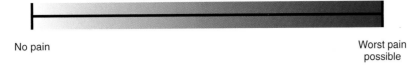

No pain   Worst pain
                                                    possible

Figure 12-3 Visual analogue scale (VAS) used to estimate an animal's current pain status. The scale is a 100-mm line representing the entire spectrum of pain, from no pain to the worst pain possible. The observer draws a line that best represents the animal's estimated pain.

in the results. Disadvantages of the VAS as applied in veterinary medicine occur primarily because the scale relies on an observer to identify and interpret pain behaviors. Thus observer bias may play a key role in assessing pain, leading to the possibility of overdiagnosing or underdiagnosing pain. Variability in visual acuity among observers may affect the accuracy of the VAS. Interobserver variability, when more than one observer evaluates an animal, affects the accuracy of the VAS. The sensitivity of the VAS has not been determined in animals; therefore, changes in VAS score should be interpreted in light of overall patient appearance.

Simple descriptive scale The SDS is a semiobjective scoring system that typically consists of four or five categories or descriptions of pain intensity (Box 12-3).

Each description is assigned a whole number, which becomes the patient's pain score. This differs from the preemptive scoring system in that the SDS assigns a score based on observation of the animal and not the nature of the procedure performed. Advantages of the SDS are that it is simple to use and the results are not affected by visual acuity (no drawing of a line required). A disadvantage of the SDS is that it is not sensitive, consisting of only four or five categories. Therefore, it may overestimate or underestimate the degree of pain and the efficacy of analgesic therapy. As with other assessment tools, observer bias may play a key role in determining pain score.

Numerical rating scale The numerical rating scale (NRS) is a semiobjective scoring system that comprises multiple categories from which to evaluate the patient, including descriptive definitions of pain for each category. The NRS generally uses categories that are assigned whole numbers and the importance of each category is not weighted (Web Box 12-1).

The NRS prompts the observer to evaluate certain aspects of the patient that might be overlooked (e.g., appearance of the eyes, interactive behaviors, physiologic parameters). Advantages of the NRS include a more thorough patient evaluation than what is compelled by the VAS or SDS, an easy method to tabulate pain score, and numerous categories on which to base an assessment of patient comfort. Disadvantages of the NRS include lack of condition and species specificity in descriptions, lack of accuracy and little improvement over the SDS. Categories are generally scored by whole numbers, suggesting that equal differences exist between categories although this may not be true. In spite of numerous categories, painful animals may go undiagnosed. For example, a dog with severe abdominal pain may not receive a high enough number to be considered painful when using a scale designed to assess surgical pain. In the postsurgical patient, NRS may be too insensitive to detect differences in some animals that receive analgesics. Thus NRS may only be able to identify those animals with extreme pain that overtly demonstrate pain behaviors and would have been identified otherwise.

While some studies support the use of these semisubjective scales in veterinary patients,[28] other studies report the VAS,

> ## Box • 12-3
>
> ### *Simple Descriptive Scale*
>
> Simple descriptive scale (SDS) used to estimate an animal's current pain status.
> 0 No Pain
> 1 Mild Pain
> 2 Moderate Pain
> 3 Severe Pain
> 4 Most Severe (Extreme) Pain

SDS, and the NRS are unreliable in veterinary medicine and, because they are purely ordinal, may not provide the necessary discriminatory properties required for assessment of modern analgesia.[31] For example, Quinn et al found that the VAS and NRS do not replace force plate analysis, which most accurately reflects subtle lameness.[32] Clearly, more consistent, quantitative measures of pain are needed, and this has lead to the development of scales that variably rely on specific behavior assessment.

Behavior-Based Scales
Combined behavioral and physiologic response scale The University of Melbourne Pain Scale (UMPS) is based on specific behavioral and physiologic responses in dogs. The UMPS includes multiple descriptors in six categories of behaviors related to pain (Web Box 12-2).

Advantages of the UMPS may include increased accuracy over the Preemptive Scoring System, VAS, SDS, or NRS and an ability to weigh the importance of certain behaviors or parameters. The evaluation of multiple factors increases the sensitivity and specificity of the UMPS. Most importantly the UMPS relies on detailed behavioral observations and evaluates changes in behavior or demeanor, thereby limiting interpretation and observer bias. Disadvantages of the UMPS are limited validation to date and specific patient types, procedures, and conditions in which the UMPS would be expected to be accurate are ill-defined. The UMPS was designed to evaluate dogs after surgery; therefore the accuracy of the scale for other uses or for use in cats has not been established. The UMPS may not be sensitive enough to detect small changes in pain behaviors, particularly if patient evaluations are performed only periodically. The UMPS requires some knowledge of the demeanor of the patient before anesthesia and surgery. Although the veterinary staff may have some knowledge of this, actual temperament when truly comfortable at home is likely not known. This is true of all behavior-based scales.

Behavioral response scale The Glasgow Composite Pain Tool (Web Box 12-3) is based on specific behavioral signs believed to represent pain in the dog.

The behaviors incorporated into the scale were derived from a questionnaire posed to veterinarians. The terms used to represent pain behaviors were distilled from an extensive descriptor list using a variety of statistical methods. The advantages of this scale include limited interpretation and bias by the observer, which provides increased accuracy over the Preemptive Scoring System, VAS, SDS, and NRS. In using this tool, the observer is asked to identify whether a behavior is present, rather than to interpret the meaning of the behavior. Most importantly, the terms used to describe individual behaviors are specifically defined, thereby decreasing uncertainty in using the scale. Physiologic data are not included,

making the scale easier to use than the UMPS and perhaps more accurate. Nevertheless, an evaluation of physiologic parameters can be added when evaluating any patient. Disadvantages of the scale are limited validation in animal studies and a lack of a numeric scoring system that would allow for comparison of scores over time. Furthermore, this scale is limited in application and is perhaps most effective in dogs postsurgically. In 2005 a short form of the Glasgow Composite Pain Tool (Box 12-4) was introduced that includes a numeric rating scale.

The shorter format allows for easier and potentially increased use.

Box • 12-4

Short Form of the Glasgow Composite Pain Scale

Dog's Name _____
Hospital Number _____Date / /   Time
Surgery: Yes / No (delete as appropriate)
Procedure or Condition _____

In the sections below, please circle the appropriate score in each list and sum these to give the total score.

A. Look at dog in kennel.
  Is the dog?

(i)		(ii)	
Quiet	0	Ignoring any wound or painful area	0
Crying or whimpering	1	Looking at wound or painful area	1
Groaning	2	Licking wound or painful area	2
Screaming	3	Rubbing wound or painful area	3
		Chewing wound or painful area	4

> In the case of spinal, pelvic, or multiple limb fractures, or where assistance is required to aid locomotion, do not carry out section B and proceed to C.
> *Please tick if this is the case* ☐ *then proceed to C.*

B. Put lead on dog and lead out of the kennel.

  When the dog rises/walks is it?

C. If it has a wound or painful area, including abdomen, apply gentle pressure 2 inches around the site.

  Does it?

(iii)		(iv)	
Normal	0	Do nothing	0
Lame	1	Look around	1
Slow or reluctant	2	Flinch	2
Stiff	3	Growl or guard area	3
It refuses to move	4	Snap	4
		Cry	5

D. Overall.
  Is the dog?   *Is the dog?*

(v)		(vi)	
Happy and content or happy and bouncy	0	Comfortable	0
Quiet	1	Unsettled	1
Indifferent or nonresponsive to surroundings	2	Restless	2
Nervous or anxious or fearful	3	Hunched or tense	3
Depressed or nonresponsive to stimulation	4	Rigid	4

Total Score (i + ii + iii + iv + v + vi) = _____

Copyright University of Glasgow, Pain and Welfare Group: Short form pain questionnaire. Available at: http://www.gla.ac.uk/vet/research/cascience/painandwelfare/cmps.htm. Accessed May 13, 2009.

Composite behavioral pain scale A modified pain scale is presented in Web Figures 12-1 and 12-2.

This scale is a composite scale derived from the UMPS, Glasgow Composite Pain Tool and its short form, and the SDS. The format is intended to incorporate the most practical features of other scales in a single-page, user-friendly design. Physiologic data is not included although changes in heart rate, respiratory rate, and arterial blood pressure can be added. Use of the scale employs both an observational period and a hands-on evaluation of the patient. In general, the assessment begins with quiet observation of the patient in its cage at a relatively unobtrusive distance. Afterwards, the patient as a whole (wound as well as the entire body) is approached to assess reaction to gentle palpation, indicators of muscle tension and heat, response to interaction, etc. Some specific features include:

1. The scale utilizes a generic 0-4 scale with quarter marks along with a color scale as a visual cue for progression along the 5-point scale.
2. Realistic artist's renderings of animals at various levels of pain add further visual cues. Additional drawings provide space for recording sites of pain, warmth, and muscle tension; this allows documentation of specific areas of concern in the medical record. A further advantage of these drawings is that the observer is encouraged to assess the overall pain state of the patient in addition to focusing on the primary lesion.
3. The scale includes psychologic and behavioral signs of pain as well as palpation responses. The scale uses body tension as an evaluation tool, a parameter not addressed in other scales.
4. There is a provision for nonassessment in the resting patient. To the authors' knowledge this is the only scale that emphasizes the importance of delaying assessment in a sleeping patient while prompting the observer to recognize patients that may be inappropriately obtunded by medication or a more serious health concern.

Advantages of this scale include ease of use with minimal interpretation required. Specific descriptors for individual behaviors are provided, which decreases interobserver variability. Additionally, a scale is provided for both the dog and the cat. This is the only comprehensive feline pain scale as of this writing. A disadvantage of this scale is a lack of validation by clinical studies comparing it to other scales. Further, its use is largely limited to and is intended for use in acute pain. These scales have been in use at Colorado State University Veterinary Medical Center for the past 2 years.

Assessment of Chronic Pain

Assessment tools described to this point are most appropriately applied to acute pain. However, a number of pathologic states, such as osteoarthritis, cancer, otitis, and dental disease, cause both significant and chronic pain. The clinical signs of this type of pain will depend on the underlying cause and may range from subtle to obvious. Additionally, chronically painful animals may experience acute flare-ups of pain that require a different medical approach. For example, a dog with osteoarthritis may experience an episode of acute pain after excessive strenuous activity.

In general, the clinical signs of chronic pain may be relatively subtle and difficult to recognize during a brief examination in the veterinary clinic. A separate examination is recommended in order to fully evaluate chronic pain syndromes. Clinical signs suggestive of pain include decreased activity, reluctance to get up or play, changes in sleeping patterns, changes in appetite, changes in social interactions and grooming habits, and other behavioral changes (e.g., withdrawal, aggression). Obviously, these clinical signs are also suggestive of numerous other medical conditions that may or may not be associated with pain. Careful history taking, a thorough physical examination, appropriate laboratory tests, diagnostic imaging and, occasionally, response to test dose analgesic therapy are all used to diagnose the underlying cause of pain.

A key aspect of assessing and treating the veterinary patient with chronic pain is the absolute requirement for a close working relationship with the patient's caregiver (owner). The working party of the Association of Veterinary Teachers and Research Workers (AVTRW) recommends an overall pain assessment based on observation by a person able to distinguish subtle changes in demeanor, behavior, and locomotion.[23] In a clinical situation, this is often the owner. The findings should then be interpreted by a person with knowledge and experience in pain assessment (a veterinarian). Hielm-Bjorkman et al, in studying canine chronic hip dysplasia, agreed with this recommendation, indicating that owners' observations of changes in both behavior and demeanor of their dogs may be more useful than behavioral evaluations made by veterinarians, as the latter are unlikely to know how the dog usually reacts in different situations.[33] Promising work using psychometric methods by Hielm-Bjorkman, Wiseman-Orr, and others has focused on the development of owner questionnaires as instruments of discriminative and evaluative chronic pain assessment.[33,34] In validating the Glasgow University Veterinary questionnaire (GUVQuest), Wiseman-Orr et al found 84.9% of questionnaire results correctly identified chronic pain in dogs, while 93.8% correctly identified control (not chronically painful). However, of the chronic pain cases, 50% of these owners answered no to the question: Do you think your dog is in pain? These results suggest (1) this tool can be used to screen for chronic pain in dogs, but not to rule it out, and (2) many owners are not able to correctly identify chronic pain in their dogs although their observations are critically important in helping the clinician to make the diagnosis. A short form of the GUVQuest is undergoing field testing and validation (Wiseman-Orr, personal communication, 2008).

Like acute pain, no gold standard exists for measuring chronic pain states in veterinary patients. Validated, sensitive, and reliable species- and condition-specific chronic pain scales are needed. As more research is done in the field of veterinary chronic pain science, owner questionnaires and various health-related quality of life assessment tools (HRQL) may prove to be valuable in standardizing pain assessment and quantifying response to therapy. Prototypical HRQL tools address three primary factors: physical, behavioral (psychologic), and social in terms of both quantitative and qualitative assessment.[35,36] A sample HRQL assessment tool is included in Web Figure 12-3. This scale has not been validated; it has been used as a teaching tool and in a veterinary hospice program at Colorado State University.

Other assessment tools are being evaluated in the laboratory including objective video analysis (e.g., Ethovision and the Observer, www.Noldus.com), pressure-sensitive walkways (e.g., I-scan Pressure Measurement System, Tekscan, Inc., South Boston, Mass.), activity monitors (omni directional accelerometer, e.g., ActiCal Mini Mitter, Respironics, Inc., Bend, Ore.), temporospatial analysis of gait (e.g., GAITRite, www.gaitrite.com), pressure mats (e.g., Footscan gait system, RSscan International, Olen, Belgium), and kinematic motion capture (e.g., Qualisys Motion Capture System, Qualisys AB, Gothenburg, Sweden). As yet these techniques have not been refined and are not directly applicable to the clinical patient.

Chronic pain is an individual, dynamic, and poorly understood clinical condition. Undoubtedly the ultimate method for evaluating the chronic pain patient may be a combination of validated HRQL tools and objective movement-assessment techniques. Despite the challenges, pain assessment and treatment must be individualized and persistently evolving. Paramount to the delivery of appropriate care in the patient suffering chronic pain is periodic reevaluation with a discriminative eye toward therapy adjustment.

CLINICAL PAIN MANAGEMENT CONCEPTS

Pain States

Clinically relevant, pathologic, painful states can be somewhat arbitrarily divided into three main categories. Acute pain is defined as pain that follows bodily injury, disappears with healing, and tends to be self-limiting. The current foundation of acute pain therapy is the opiate drug class and recently, the nonsteroidal antiinflammatory drug (NSAID) class as well. Adjunctive therapies include alpha-2 agonists, local anesthetic techniques, NMDA receptor antagonists, acupuncture, low-level laser therapy, and physiotherapy, among others. Increasingly, it is clear that untreated acute pain results in chronic and neuropathic pain, both of which are notoriously unresponsive to opiates. Chronic pain lasts several weeks or more and persists beyond the expected healing time. Neuropathic pain is pain that originates from injury or involvement of the PNS or CNS with motor, sensory, or autonomic deficits. Chronic and neuropathic pain treatment involves pharmacologic, nonpharmacologic, surgical, interventional, manual, physical, and rehabilitation therapy. Management of the chronic pain patient requires tailoring treatment to the individual as well as frequent reassessment. Other painful states maybe classified within these three general categories and include cancer pain, inflammatory pain, visceral pain, somatic pain, myofascial pain, and breakthrough pain.

Therapeutic Modalities

Pharmacologic In this section we will describe current therapies for the management of painful states starting with a summary of pharmacologic agents. Attention will be focused primarily on the most recent developments in algologic pharmacology since much has been written elsewhere regarding administration and dosing of commonly used agents. Table 12-1 includes a list of selected analgesic drugs and dosing schemes.

Opioids Opiates are powerful, broad-spectrum analgesics and remain the cornerstone of acute pain management. Exogenously administered opioids (opiates) such as morphine, hydromorphone, fentanyl, and buprenorphine achieve their analgesic action through mimicking the effect of endogenous opioids. These compounds bind to μ-, κ-, and δ-opioid receptors found in the periphery, spinal cord, and supraspinal centers. These receptors are G protein–coupled and ultimately decrease release of neurotransmitter through their interaction with voltage-gated calcium channels. Much has been published on the central effects of opiates as well as recommended dosing schemes (doses, routes, and frequency). A list of frequently used opioids and common dosing schemes is found in Table 12-1. This is by no means a complete list. Note that oral bioavailability in dogs and cats is limited. However, recent studies have demonstrated acceptable bioavailability for transbuccal administration of buprenorphine in cats.[37] In a research setting transbuccal buprenorphine provide sedation and mechanical analgesia in dogs (KR Mama et al, unpublished data). The results of these studies suggest a useful and effective method for outpatient treatment.

In the past decade research has focused on peripheral opioid mechanisms in an attempt to curtail undesirable effects of exogenously administered systemic opiates and to improve efficacy in chronic and neuropathic pain states. Undesirable systemic side effects include CNS depression, bradycardia, respiratory depression, excitement, decreased gastrointestinal motility, emesis, increased bladder tone with spasm of ureteral smooth muscle, paradoxical pain, and opiate antinociceptive tolerance. Species variability in response has been noted; in particular, cats may be more sensitive to excitatory effects and dogs appear to be prone to emesis. Capitalizing on the peripheral endogenous opioid system (PEOS) is a promising future strategy for achieving effective analgesia while minimizing these side effects.[38,39]

The PEOS includes peripheral opioid receptors (POR) and peripheral leukocyte-derived opioids (PLDO): endomorphins, endorphins, enkephalins, and dynorphins. In order to activate the PEOS, tissue must have sufficient numbers of leukocytes able to secrete PLDO and functional PORs in sufficient numbers. Inflammation due to tissue damage results in accumulation of PLDO-secreting leukocytes at the site of injury. Perhaps the predominant contributors promoting leukocyte accumulation and PLDO secretion are the chemokines, small proteins important in the trafficking of immune cells and in coordinating the immune response.[40,41] Inflammation also increases the number and efficiency of PORs expressed on primary sensory neurons.[42] PORs are synthesized in the dorsal root ganglion and transported distally to peripheral sensory nerve endings.[43,44] PORs are inactive under normal conditions; however, with tissue injury and inflammation the action of bradykinin improves opioid receptor coupling to G protein–signaling systems.[45] Mousa et al found that during localized inflammatory pain, endogenous peripheral nerve growth factor (NGF) enhances susceptibility to locally applied opioids by upregulating the number and efficacy of morphine opioid receptors in primary afferent neurons. NGF, known to be increased in peripheral inflammation and to increase enkephalin binding sites, may be the major contributor to upregulation in POR number and efficacy.[46]

Clinically, attempts to mimic or augment the PEOS represent a unique opportunity to utilize the powerful analgesic effect of opiates while minimizing untoward systemic effects. Experimental trials and clinical studies show peripheral opiates are effective, particularly in the presence of inflammation. Houghton et al have shown that the local application of a low dose of morphine can effectively reduce nociception in a rat model of bone damage. This analgesic effect was mediated through μ-opioid receptor action in bone.[47,48] Reuben et al found a positive effect with local morphine administration after iliac bone graft harvest in humans undergoing spinal fusion surgery. Since donor site pain has been reported to persist up to 2 years, these results are significant.[49,50] Kalso et al reviewed 36 randomized controlled studies examining the effect of intraarticular opiates and pain following knee surgery in humans. In this study a small amount of morphine administered into a sequestered site of known inflammation produced more analgesia than a similar amount administered systemically.[51] Although morphine has been shown to provide peripheral effects in addition to its central effects, newer opiates (DAMGO {[D-Ala2, N-MePhe4, Gly-ol]-enkephalin}, endomorphin-1 and 2, 14-O-methyloxymorphone) with peripheral specific action may possess improved safety and side-effect profiles over opiates currently in clinical use.[52-54]

In summary, much is known about the central effects of opiates and they are likely to remain a critical and effective tool in the management of acute pain; however, their side effects, loss of efficacy with prolonged use, and relative ineffectiveness in chronic pain states are undesirable. Recent information on the PEOS may obviate these limitations and may be the harbinger of a new generation of analgesics and analgesic modalities.

Table • 12-1

Selected Analgesic Agents

DRUG	CANINE DOSE (MG/KG)	FELINE DOSE (MG/KG)
Opioids		
Buprenorphine	0.005-0.02 SC, IM, IV, buccal q4-8h	0.005-0.02 SC, IM, IV, buccal q4-8h
Butorphanol	0.2-1.0 SC, IM q2-4h	0.1-0.5 SC, IM q2-4h
	0.1-0.5 IV q0.5-2h	0.1-0.2 IV q1-2h
Fentanyl	0.01-0.04 SC, IM q30-60min	0.005-0.02 SC, IM q30-60min
	0.002-0.005 IV q30-60min	0.001-0.003 IV q30-60min
	0.005-0.02 mg/kg/h CRI intra op	0.005-0.01 mg/kg/h CRI intra op
	0.001-0.005 mg/kg/h CRI post op	0.001-0.003 mg/kg/h CRI post op
Hydromorphone	0.05-0.2 SC, IM, IV q4-6h	0.03-0.1 SC, IM q4-6h
	0.05-0.1 IV q4-6h	0.01-0.05 IV q4-6h
	0.05-0.1 mg/kg/h CRI	0.01-0.05 mg/kg/h CRI
Methadone	0.5-1.0 SC, IM q2-4h	0.2-0.5 SC, IM, IV q2-4h
	0.2-0.5 IV	0.1-0.3 IV
	0.025-0.2 mg/kg/h CRI	0.025-0.1 mg/kg/h CRI
Morphine	0.25-1.0 SQ, IM q4-6h	0.05-0.2 SQ, IM q4-6h
	Caution histamine release with IV bolus	Caution histamine release with IV bolus
	0.05-0.1 mg/kg/h CRI	
	0.1 preservative free epidural q12-24h	0.1 preservative free epidural q12-24h
Nalbuphine	0.5-1.0 SC, IM q1-4h	0.2-0.5 SC, IM q1-4h
	0.03-0.5 IV q1-4h	0.03-0.3 IV q1-4h
Naloxone	0.001-0.02 SQ, IM, IV as needed for opiate reversal	0.001-0.02 SQ, IM, IV as needed for opiate reversal
Oxymorphone	0.025-0.2 SC, IM, IV q2-4h	0.025-0.1 SC, IM, IV q2-4h
Remifentanil	0.02-0.06 mg/kg/h CRI intra op	0.02-0.06 mg/kg/h CRI intra op
	0.004-0.01 mg/kg/h CRI post op	0.004-0.01 mg/kg/h CRI post op
NSAIDs		
Carprofen	2.2 PO, SC q12h	1-4 SC single dose
	4.4 PO, SC q24h	Not recommended for oral use
Deracoxib	1-2 q24h	
Firocoxib	5 PO q24h	
Meloxicam	0.1 PO, SC q24h	0.05 PO, SC q1-4 days
Tepoxalin	10 PO q24h	
Local Anesthetics		
Bupivacaine	1-2 SC, intrapleural	1-2 SC, intrapleural
	0.3-1 epidural	0.3-1 epidural
EMLA	Topical application under occlusive dressing for 30-60 min	Topical application under occlusive dressing for 30-60 min
Lidocaine	1-2 SC, IV, epidural	1-2 SC, IV, epidural
	0.025-0.05 mg/kg/min	0.025-0.05 mg/kg/min
Alpha-2 Agonists		
Atipamezole	0.05-0.1 SC, IM to reverse medetomidine or dexmedetomidine	0.05-0.1 SC, IM to reverse medetomidine or dexmedetomidine
Dexmedetomidine	0.0005-0.003 IV bolus	
	0.0005-0.001 mg/kg/h CRI	
Medetomidine	0.005-0.01 IM	0.005-0.01 IM
	0.001-0.005 IV	0.001-0.005 IV
	0.001-0.003 mg/kg/h CRI	0.001-0.003 mg/kg/h CRI
NMDA Receptor Antagonists		
Amantadine	3-5 PO q24h	3-5 PO q24h
Ketamine	0.010-0.020 mg/kg/h CRI intra op	0.010-0.020 mg/kg/h CRI intra op
	0.002-0.005 mg/kg/h CRI post op	0.002-0.005 mg/kg/h CRI post op
Methadone	0.1-0.5 SC, IM, IV q2-4h	0.1-0.3 SC, IM, IV q2-4h
	0.025-0.2 mg/kg/h CRI	0.025-0.1 mg/kg/h CRI
Other		
Acetaminophen	10-15 PO q8-12h	Contraindicated
Gabapentin	5-40 PO q8-12h	5-20 PO q8-12h
Tramadol	1-5 mg/kg q6-8h	0.25-1 mg/kg q6-8h

NSAIDs NSAIDs are a diverse group of agents that possess analgesic, antiinflammatory, antipyretic, and opioid-sparing effects. These drugs are typically classified according to their mechanism of action, inhibition of cyclooxygenase (COX) enzymes. COX enzymes are important in the synthesis of prostaglandins from arachidonic acid.[55] Prostaglandins are ubiquitous and in turn mediate a variety of critical physiologic functions throughout the body including maintenance of renal function, platelet aggregation, secretion of the protective gastric layer (bicarbonate and mucus), as well as inflammation and pain. The existence of at least two isoforms, COX1 and COX2, is well established, and now a splice variant of COX1, so-called COX3, is under scrutiny.[56,57] The specific roles of these isoforms and their relative degree of inducibility continue to be debated. However, COX1 is widely viewed as primarily constitutive and COX2 is thought to be inducible. COX1 generates prostaglandins responsible for mucosal defense, platelet aggregation, and renal function. Inasmuch as COX2 can increase up to twentyfold in the presence of tissue injury and is a known mediator of nociception, COX2 selective agents have been considered more desirable and safer than COX1 specific or nonspecific agents in the treatment of pain.[58,59] The hypothesis that COX1 mediates homeostatic physiologic functions and COX2 important pathophysiologic functions has driven the development of COX2-specific NSAIDs such as the veterinary products carprofen, meloxicam, deracoxib, and tolfenamic acid.[60] Most NSAIDs that inhibit COX result in the diversion of arachidonic acid to the lipoxygenase pathway (5-LOX) resulting in increased synthesis of leukotrienes, potent mediators of inflammation. This suggests that a dual inhibitor of the COX2 and 5-LOX pathways might be an ideal analgesic agent with an improved safety profile. Currently tepoxalin is the only veterinary-approved drug with dual action.[61-64]

NSAIDs are powerful analgesics and are currently one of the most prescribed classes of drugs in both human and veterinary medicine; however, common side effects of NSAIDs should not be underestimated. These include: gastrointestinal toxicity (vomiting, diarrhea, ulceration),[65-68] idiosyncratic hepatotoxicosis,[69] and renal dysfunction especially in the face of hypovolemia.[70] Consequently, the use of NSAIDs requires clinical judgment because the constitutive functions of these enzymes must be considered. These agents should not be administered to patients with acute renal insufficiency, hepatic insufficiency, gastrointestinal ulceration, coagulopathy, hypotension, hypovolemia, or dehydration. NSAIDs should not be used concurrently with corticosteroids or other NSAIDs. There appears to be no consistent recommendation for washout period between corticosteroid use or use of other NSAIDs prior to administration of a new NSAID. Practitioners should bear in mind that response to NSAIDs, both analgesic and adverse, varies greatly among NSAIDs, between and within individuals. Patients may respond favorably to one NSAID product and not another. Cats are exquisitely sensitive to the adverse effects of NSAIDs presumably by virtue of limited glucuronidation pathways.[71-73] As such, toxic plasma levels are easily attained with doses considered safe for an equivalently sized dog. Meloxicam is currently the only NSAID approved for use in cats in the United States. These authors urge caution and careful monitoring of gastrointestinal and renal function when using this product chronically in cats. Currently approved NSAIDs in dogs include: carprofen, deracoxib, etodolac, firocoxib, ketoprofen, meloxicam, tepoxalin, and tolfenamic acid. Off-label compounds include aspirin, piroxicam, and, in dogs only, acetaminophen. For a review of commonly used NSAIDs see Table 12-1.

Local anesthetic agents Local anesthetics prevent nerve transmission by inhibiting the generation and propagation of nerve impulses via reversible blockade of sodium channels within the neuronal membrane. The result is the prevention of neuronal depolarization and nerve conduction. With progressive increase in concentration of local anesthetic, autonomic, somatic sensory, and somatic motor blockade is achieved. The interruption of transmission of nociceptive information from the periphery to the spinal cord has the added advantage of decreasing central sensitization and wind-up by preventing the bombardment of WDR neurons in the dorsal horn.

Cocaine was the first local anesthetic used by Kollar in 1884. The first synthetic local anesthetic, procaine, was introduced by Einhorn in 1905. Since then more rapid and longer-acting agents have been developed. Local anesthetic techniques such as local tissue infiltration (so-called line block), intrapleural block, intravenous local, regional nerve blockade, and epidural or intrathecal administration are well described in small animal medicine.[74-77] Recently, the use of local anesthetics in regional anesthesia has enjoyed an upsurge in use in small animal veterinary practice and is now considered a key component in multimodal analgesia and balanced anesthesia. Regional anesthesia is an alternative to or an adjunct of intravenous and inhalational anesthesia both of which are associated with increased potential risk to the patient as compared to local anesthetics. Additionally, the use of nerve stimulator/locator devices and ultrasound guidance has improved accuracy and thus effectiveness of regional nerve blockade. In one author's practice (PMM), the use of femoral and sciatic blockade has virtually replaced the use of epidural analgesia for stifle procedures in the dog and cat.

Commonly used local anesthetics in small animal practice include lidocaine, mepivacaine, ropivacaine, and bupivacaine. These agents differ most importantly in their time to onset and duration of action as well as in their relative toxicity. Toxicity occurs as a consequence of systemic absorption resulting in cardiovascular system (CVS) and CNS signs. CNS toxicity can be recognized as tremoring and/or seizures. All local anesthetics have the potential to cause peripheral nerve fiber damage when used in high enough concentration and if injected directly into a nerve fascicle. Careful attention to dose and increased resistance to injection will minimize this risk. CVS toxicity is less likely with lidocaine, but may cause bradycardia and hypotension, whereas intravenous injection of bupivacaine can lead to sudden, CPR-resistant cardiovascular collapse. CVS toxicities have been treated with bretylium, magnesium, and, more recently, 20% intravenous lipid.[78] Ropivacaine and levobupivacaine have been advocated as newer, longer-acting agents equipotent to bupivacaine with less cardiotoxicity.

Rate of absorption depends on site, dose, physicochemical properties of the agent, and the addition of epinephrine. Rate of absorption from least to greatest systemic absorption by site is caudal epidural → epidural → brachial plexus → sciatic → femoral. Greater lipid solubility and protein binding of local anesthetics lead to longer duration of action and less systemic absorption, which may alter site-specific absorption characteristics. Importantly, inadvertent IV administration results in severe toxicity regardless of lipid solubility and protein binding (e.g., bupivacaine). Lidocaine and mepivacaine are associated with rapid onset (3 to 5 minutes) and relatively short duration (60 to 120 minutes), while bupivacaine and ropivacaine have a longer time to onset (20 minutes) and longer duration (hours) depending on dose and location.[75,79] Ropivacaine is reported to be less toxic with a shorter motor blockade than bupivacaine.[80,81]

Local analgesic effects may be augmented with the addition of other agents. For example, coadministration of local anesthetics with opioids, especially intraarticularly, has shown synergistic effect in human beings.[82-85] This has not been beneficial for regional nerve blocks because opioid receptors are primarily located at nerve terminals, not midnerve, and there is presumably little inflammation at these more proximal nerve sites. As stated previously, inflammation appears to be critical in the PEOS. Thus far no randomized controlled studies have been published on the coadministration of intraarticular opioid and local anesthetic in veterinary patients. Epinephrine can prolong the duration of block, increase the intensity of the block, and decrease systemic absorption 10% to 30%.[86] This effect is likely due to vasoconstriction mediated by alpha-1 adrenergic receptor agonism since most local anesthetics except ropivacaine cause vasodilation. Typical dose recommendation is 1:200,000 for peripheral nerve block.[79] The rationale for the addition of sodium bicarbonate for alkalinization of local anesthetics is to increase the percentage of local anesthetic existing in the lipid-soluble, neutral, active form. The pH of commercial preparations is 3.9 to 6.4 and may be even lower if packaged with epinephrine. Since the pKa of most local anesthetics is 7.6 to 8.9, only about 3% of anesthetic is in the active form. Alkalinization increases this value to about 10% if the pH is raised to 6.0 to 8.0; above this level precipitation occurs.[87] Alpha-2 agonists such as clonidine have a long history in human local anesthesia dating back to at least the 1980s.[88] More recently dexmedetomidine has been favorably studied in intravenous regional anesthesia.[89,90] The mechanism of action of alpha-2 agonists is not clear although there is some evidence to suggest that coadministration results in central neuraxial and peripheral nerve analgesic synergy.[91] Recently, Lamont and Lemke reported promising effects of medetomidine on mepivacaine-induced radial nerve blockade in the dog.[92]

Finally, the eutectic mixture of lidocaine and prilocaine (EMLA) can be used for transcutaneous local anesthesia. It has been evaluated as a percutaneous analgesic before venipuncture in dogs, cats, rabbits, and rats.[93] Efficacy is reported after 60-minutes application with an occlusive dressing.

Alpha-2 agonists Alpha-2 adrenoreceptor antagonists have been used extensively to provide sedation and analgesia in small animal patients. The first commonly used drug in this class was xylazine, a relatively nonspecific agent with an alpha-2 to alpha-1 ratio of 160:1. In the late 1980s more specific alpha-2 adrenoreceptor agonists were introduced. These included medetomidine 1620:1, detomidine 260:1, romifidine (340:1). The analgesic effect of these drugs is mediated by CNS-localized noradrenergic and nonnoradrenergic neurons. Alpha-2 receptors are located both presynaptically and postsynaptically and analgesia appears to be mediated at both sites. CNS sites of action include the dorsal horn of the spinal cord, the brainstem, and the locus ceruleus (LC) of the pons. Noradrenergic neurons of the LC extend to all segments of the spinal cord and modulate noradrenergic input from higher structures such as the PAG of the midbrain. Activation of alpha-2 receptors in the LC ultimately results in decreased release of norepinephrine; this decrease disinhibits activity in adjacent nuclei, which subsequently results in increased release of norepinephrine at their axonal termini in the dorsal horn. The final result is activation of spinal (dorsal horn) presynaptic and postsynaptic alpha-2 receptors to produce analgesia.[94]

Medetomidine is the most commonly used alpha-2 adrenoreceptor agonist since its release in the United States along with its antagonist atipamezole in 1996. In early 2008 dexmedetomidine, the pure S-enantiomer of the racemic medetomidine, was introduced into the veterinary market and likely will surpass medetomidine. Although twice as potent as medetomidine, the two are essentially the same drug; similar effects and side effects can be anticipated.[95-98]

Alpha-2 agonists are used as a component of total intravenous anesthesia; as a preanesthetic sedative-analgesic agent; as a constant-rate infusion supplement to inhalant anesthesia and in the postoperative period; in epidural and intrathecal injections; intraarticularly; and as a synergistic supplement to local anesthetics in regional nerve blockade. Table 1 includes a list of selected alpha-2 agonists.

Although powerful analgesics, the alpha-2 agonists have equally impressive clinical side effects. Of these the most significant are the cardiovascular effects. Alpha-2 agonists bind to postsynaptic alpha-2 receptors to mediate smooth muscle contraction of blood vessels. The resultant vasoconstriction produces hypertension accompanied by a reflexive, baroreceptor-mediated decrease in heart rate. Cardiac output is diminished by as much as 40% to 50%. After the initial phase of hypertension, central alpha-2 adrenoreceptor effects result in decreased sympathetic tone with concomitant reduced blood pressure, heart rate, and cardiac output.[99,100] Because of these profound CVS effects, careful patient selection is indicated in using this class of drugs for adjunctive analgesia.

NMDA receptor antagonists (methadone, ketamine, dextromethorphan, amantadine) The NMDA receptor is an excitatory amino acid receptor expressed on the central terminals of primary afferent fibers. Activation of these receptors by glutamate results in sensitization of spinal neurons and has been implicated in the development and modulation of prolonged pain states in animal models.[101,102] NMDA antagonists may reduce pain, opiate consumption, or both by two non–mutually exclusive mechanisms. First is the more widely recognized reduction in central hypersensitivity, and second is the fact that NMDA antagonists have also been shown to reduce opiate tolerance in many animal and human studies.[103,104] Opiate tolerance is defined as the decrease in analgesic activity after previous exposure to the same or similar drug; this can occur over a period of hours to weeks.[105,106] Additionally, NMDA receptor–mediated central sensitization/wind-up is associated with opiate-induced abnormal pain (i.e., prolonged opiate administration produces paradoxical pain).[107-109] Laulin et al have reported that a single dose of opiate can induce a lasting increase in basal pain sensitivity leading to hyperalgesia.[110] A number of studies suggest that NMDA receptor antagonists may prevent opiate-induced tolerance and antinociception and may act synergistically with opiates to provide superior analgesia.[111-114] Clinically, combined treatment with an NMDA antagonist and an opiate may decrease opiate-induced side effects because heightened analgesia may allow a lower overall opiate dose. Such combinations have been shown to be well tolerated and safe in human clinical trials.[115,116]

Clinically relevant NMDA receptor antagonists in veterinary medicine include methadone, ketamine, amantadine, and dextromethorphan. Methadone is structurally unrelated to other opium-derived analgesics and exists as a racemic mixture. Each enantiomer has a separate mode of action; the D-isomer noncompetitively antagonizes the NMDA receptor and inhibits norepinephrine reuptake; the l-isomer is a weak μ-opioid agonist.[117] This may explain reduced opioid-related side effects when using methadone. Additionally methadone is a δ-opioid receptor agonist that may desensitize morphine-induced tolerance mechanisms.[118] Methadone may be of use in mitigating opioid-induced tolerance and help in the treatment of neuropathic pain.[119] Methadone has a short half-life in the dog (1.75 to 4.3 hours) and has poor bioavailablity.[120] In these authors' practice methadone is used as an adjunct analgesic, as bolus (0.1 to 0.6 mg/kg q2-6 hours), or constant-rate infusion (0.02 to 0.2 mg/kg/hr), particularly in breakthrough pain and in combating central sensitization in the acute setting.

Ketamine is a noncompetitive NMDA antagonist and has been used in the intraoperative and acute postoperative setting to reduce central sensitization/wind up.[112] The results of a systematic review of human clinical studies showed that ketamine and dextromethorphan produced a significant preventive analgesic benefit in 58% and 67% of studies, respectively.[103] In recent studies ketamine reduces postoperative opiate consumption while maintaining better analgesia than opiates alone.[121,122] Although a number of laboratory studies have reported the role of ketamine in the management of opiate-induced hyperalgesia,[111,123,124,125] thus far only three veterinary clinical trials have shown an advantage in the use of ketamine perioperatively. Slingsby et al evaluated the use of ketamine administered either pre- or post-ovariohysterectomy in dogs.[126] Dogs in the preoperative ketamine administration group required less rescue analgesia, and administration of ketamine postoperatively delayed the onset of postoperative wound hyperalgesia. Wagner et al showed that a constant-rate infusion (CRI) of ketamine improved pain control in forelimb amputations in dogs.[127] Sarrau et al showed that a ketamine CRI postoperatively in dogs undergoing mastectomy improved patient feeding behavior.[128] None of these studies showed an opiate-sparing effect; however, in veterinary patients it is more difficult to elucidate this effect since pain assessment and analgesic delivery are by proxy. More studies are required to further assess the use of ketamine as an opiate-sparing analgesic, particularly studies involving prolonged use of opiates.

Ketamine is not recommended for use as a single agent but as an adjunct in a multimodal analgesic plan. Intravenous doses are considerably smaller than those used for anesthesia (0.5 mg/kg bolus followed by 10 to 20 µg/kg/min intraoperatively and 1 to 3 µg/kg/min postoperatively). Ketamine has been used intrathecally, but caution is warranted due to a report of spinal pathology associated with chronic intrathecal ketamine administration in dogs.[129]

Dextromethorphan is the d-isomer of levomethorphan, lacks opioid activity, and has NMDA antagonist effects. Although best known for its antitussive effects, it has been shown to prevent the development of tolerance to morphine in rats[130] and potentiate the antinociceptive effects of morphine, methadone, and meperidine.[114,131,132] Interestingly this effect appears to be limited to µ-opioid agonists; there appears to be no advantage to combining dextromethorphan (or ketamine) with δ- or κ-opioid agonists.[133] Kukanich showed that oral bioavailability in the dog is 11% while plasma half-life after IV administration is approximately 2 hours.[134] These results suggest that if there is a role for dextromethorphan in multimodal analgesia, it is as a constant-rate infusion.

Since methadone, ketamine, and dextromethorphan are not recommended for oral NMDA-receptor antagonism, their use in chronic, at-home therapy is limited. Amantadine is a possible solution to this problem. Amantadine was synthesized in 1964 as an antiviral drug, but has since gained notoriety in the treatment of Parkinson's disease in humans. Kornhuber and others have shown amantadine to be a noncompetitive low-affinity NMDA-receptor antagonist.[135,136] Amantadine used perioperatively has been shown to decrease morphine consumption by 32% in humans[137] and has been used to treat neuropathic pain in humans.[138,139] Snijdelaar et al reported that the NMDA receptor contributes to synergism between amantadine and morphine in a second-phase formalin response test in rats.[113] In dogs with osteoarthritic pain refractory to NSAID, physical activity was improved by the addition of amantadine 3 to 5 mg/kg q24 hour for 21 days.[140] To our knowledge no reports have been published on the pharmacokinetics of amantadine in dogs and cats.

Other analgesic agents (tramadol, gabapentin, acetaminophen) Tramadol is a centrally acting agent with multimodal analgesic effects. First, it has modest affinity for the µ-opioid receptor (tramadol: 2500-fold to 4000-fold less than morphine; O-desmethyltramadol, the M1 metabolite: 9-fold to 450-fold less than morphine) and no κ or δ affinity.[141] The M1 metabolite appears to be responsible for µ-opioid agonist effect.[142] A second nonopioid mechanism is suggested by the characteristic of only partial naloxone reversibility.[143] Tramadol inhibits neuronal uptake of the monoamine neurotransmitters, norepinephrine and serotonin, involved in descending inhibitory pathways in the CNS; this action prolongs antinociceptive effects.[143] Oral dosing of tramadol in dogs results in rapid absorption with 65% to 75% bioavailability.[144,145] Approximately 99% of the parent compound is metabolized to the active M1 metabolite and the drug is excreted unchanged by the kidneys. Pypendop reported oral bioavailability in cats as 93%.[146] In comparison to morphine, advantages of tramadol include less sedation, less respiratory depression, improved oral bioavailability, and tramadol is not currently a controlled substance. Side effects include decreased seizure thresholds, serotonin syndrome, nausea/vomiting, and in some animals altered behavior.

Clinical trials in humans have shown mixed effects with some reporting analgesic effects of other opiates are superior to tramadol, similar to tramadol, or synergistic with tramadol. These disparate results may be due to suboptimal dosing, type of pain studied, preoperative versus postoperative treatment, and the use of adjunctive analgesics. In one clinical trial in humans the use of tramadol decreased morphine use by 30%.[147] Some have advocated concurrent use of tramadol with other opiate analgesics in light of tramadol's multimodal mechanism. One concern is that because both agents possess µ-agonist effects, an infra-additive effect may result. Several studies refutes this,[147-149] while another supports it.[150] The latter however used a low dose and only tested once at 20 minutes. As of this writing, current practice appears to support concurrent use of tramadol and other µ-agonists. There are few veterinary studies on the clinical use of tramadol. Ko et al found a 40% sevoflurane MAC reduction in cats, which was reversible with administration of naloxone.[151] Steagal et al found little effect on nociceptive thresholds when tramadol (1 mg/kg) was used alone, but an increase in threshold when tramadol was used in conjunction with acepromazine in cats.[152] Interestingly, in the latter study 2 of 8 cats became dysphoric on this dose of tramadol. One study reported similar effects on postovariohysterectomy analgesia for morphine and tramadol in dogs.[153]

Nausea and vomiting are commonly reported in people and often an antiemetic is recommended. Caution is advised with the use of ondansetron as the analgesic effect of tramadol is impaired by this 5-HT3 (serotonin)–receptor antagonist.[154,155] This drug is contraindicated in patients receiving monoamine oxidase inhibitors (MAOIs) or selective serotonin (5-hydroxytryptamine; 5-HT) reuptake inhibitors (SSRIs) due to the increased risk of serotonin syndrome. This is of particular concern in the older patient in which multiple drugs may be prescribed for a variety of chronic conditions.

Although it is appealing to consider tramadol as a sole agent in treating pain by virtue of its side effect profile, oral bioavailability, and lack of DEA control, lack of strong analgesic efficacy limits the use of tramadol as a sole agent in the treatment of severe pain.[156] In the authors' practice tramadol is used alone to treat mild pain and adjunctively in a multimodal plan for treating moderate to severe pain. Dogs are treated at 2 to 5 mg/kg BID-QID.[144] Cats appear to be more sensitive to tramadol and may exhibit altered behavior; therefore 0.5 to 1.0 mg/kg is recommended as a starting dose.

Gabapentin, l-aminoethyl cyclohexane acetic acid, was originally developed and licensed as an antiepileptic agent in the early 1990s. Additionally, gabapentin is well established as an effective treatment for neuropathic pain.[157,158] There is increasing evidence for its use in the perioperative setting as well.[159] Gabapentin's mechanism of action remains an area of intense research and has been attributed to effects on several receptors and ion channels. These include activation of $GABA_B$ receptors and K_{ATP} channels, and inhibition of AMPA receptors and voltage-gated Ca^{2+} channels.[160] Recent data suggests effects are mediated through altered trafficking of calcium channels to the neuronal cell membrane, ultimately resulting in decreased neurotransmitter release.[161,162]

Oral bioavailability in the dog is reported as 80% with a serum half-life of 2.9 hours.[163] Side effects include somnolence, fatigue, and weight gain; however, in general gabapentin appears to be well tolerated at a wide range of doses. Although specific dosing has not been established in dogs and cats, extrapolation from human data and anecdotal veterinary evidence suggest a starting dose range of 5 to 10 mg/kg PO BID to TID, which is commonly increased up to 50 mg/kg PO BID to TID.[4] Despite increasing use of gabapentin in the treatment of pain in dogs and cats, we are aware of only one blinded, controlled clinical trial in dogs (Wagner AE et al, unpublished). These authors have used gabapentin extensively in the treatment of chronic pain in dogs and cats. Pregabalin is a structural analogue to gabapentin and is indicated for the treatment of neuropathic pain in humans. Use in veterinary species is limited; safety, efficacy, and dosing have not been established.

Acetaminophen (paracetamol) possesses low antiinflammatory activity and as such is not considered a classic NSAID. Furthermore, its exact mechanism of action is unclear although recent evidence suggests indirect activation of the cannabinoid CB(1) receptor.[164,165] The so-called COX3, splice variant of COX1, has been suggested as an additional mechanism for acetaminophen. Canine COX3 protein was expressed in transfected insect cells and was selectively inhibited by acetaminophen.[166] However, in humans and rodents an acetaminophen-sensitive COX3 protein is not expressed; this is considered evidence that, at least in these species, acetaminophen does not inhibit COX3.[166]

Acetaminophen is not approved for use in veterinary species, but has been used effectively for the treatment of breakthrough pain in dogs at a dose of 10 to 15 mg/kg BID for up to 5 consecutive days.[167] Additional benefits of acetaminophen include minimal risk of thrombocytopenia, bleeding, and gastrointestinal side effects. Hepatopathy is of concern and routine serum chemistry evaluation is warranted. Acetaminophen should not be used in cats due to inadequate cytochrome P_{450}-dependent hydroxylation (glucuronidation) and subsequent fatal methemoglobinemia.

Nonpharmacologic Analgesic Modalities In addition to the rapidly growing list of pharmaceutical options, the pain management armamentarium for the veterinary practitioner includes a wide variety of nonpharmacologic techniques. Among these are acupuncture, rehabilitation, nutraceutical supplements, low-level laser, massage, transcutaneous electric nerve stimulation (TENS), and herbal supplements. The body of literature critically examining these is relatively small as of

this writing, although a great deal of interest in developing evidence-based support is evident. A complete examination of these topics is beyond the scope of this chapter.

Perhaps the most studied and most recognized of these nonpharmacologic modalities is acupuncture. Traditional Chinese Medicine (TCM) used metaphor-based medical descriptions to explain acupuncture's mechanism of action. Modern acupuncture research has uncovered the neuroanatomic basis for these actions. In the 1970s, articles began appearing in the veterinary medical literature indicating recognition of the link between acupuncture and the autonomic nervous system.[168] In the mid-1980s, anatomist and acupuncturist Houchi Dung published a number of studies on the nerve-acupuncture point relationship throughout the body.[169-174] In 2004, Kothbauer further delineated the relationships between acupuncture points and nerves in his anatomical review of acupuncture point locations in cattle.[175] In general, we now recognize that acupuncture works by modulating activity in the central, peripheral, and autonomic nervous systems.[176,177] Furthermore, acupuncture point stimulation has clear local and spinal effects, but also affects supraspinal processing of neurologic information. Therefore, the use of acupuncture in pain management likely alters the transmission, modulation, and projection of pain stimuli in addition to its effects on pain perception.

In 2006 Habacher et al published a systematic review of veterinary acupuncture literature. They found there is no compelling evidence to recommend or reject acupuncture for any condition in domestic animals and concluded that some encouraging data exist that warrant further investigation in independent rigorous trials.[178] Since that time only a few veterinary studies have been published, only two of which are relevant to analgesia. Hayashi et al found that electroacupuncture combined with standard Western medical treatment was effective and resulted in shorter time to return of ambulation and deep pain perception than did use of Western treatment alone in dogs with signs of thoracolumbar intervertebral disk disease.[179] Cassu et al found an improved effect of bilateral versus unilateral electroacupuncture in dogs using a thermal pain model.[180] For further information regarding clinical veterinary acupuncture, the reader is referred to *Xie's Veterinary Acupuncture* (H. Xie and V. Preast, Blackwell); *Veterinary Acupuncture: Ancient Art to Modern Medicine*, ed 2 (A.M. Schoen, Mosby); and *Essentials of Western Veterinary Acupuncture* (S. Lindley and M. Cummings, Wiley Blackwell).

For information regarding rehabilitation therapy please refer to the veterinary rehabilitation and therapy edition of *Veterinary Clinics of North America: Small Animal*, November 2005. For introductory information regarding massage; low-level laser, cryo, and heat therapy; and TENS see Millis' chapter in the *Handbook of Veterinary Pain Management*, ed 2 (J.S. Gaynor and W.W. Muir, Mosby). For basic information regarding complementary and alternative medicine (CAM), including herbal, manual, magnet and homeopathic therapy, consult Robinson's chapter in the same text.

REFERENCES

The reference list can be found on the companion Expert Consult Web site at *www.expertconsult.com*.

SKIN AND SUBCUTANEOUS

CHAPTER 13

The Skin as a Sensor of Internal Medicine Disorders

Sandra R. Merchant

Cutaneous manifestations of internal disease are common but may be fairly subtle. As our expertise is strengthened in the field of veterinary dermatology, clinicians continue to discover these subtle clues within the skin that alert them to further investigate internal organ systems. In certain diseases, skin change may be the first clinical sign noted. In some conditions, cutaneous and systemic signs occur together. Lastly, the skin may reflect a general catabolic and cachectic stage brought about by the primary disease process.

FUNGAL DISEASES

Deep mycoses are fungal infections of internal organs that can spread hematogenously to the skin. Primary inoculation of the skin is rare. Infections that can cause nodules, plaques, and draining tracts include *Blastomyces dermatitidis*, *Histoplasma capsulatum*, *Cryptococcus neoformans*, and *Coccidioides immitis*. Because of the accessibility of the skin, nodules and draining tracts can be easily aspirated for culture or biopsied for histology to aid in diagnosis and choice of therapy.

Pythiosis is a cutaneous, gastrointestinal, or systemic infection caused by *Pythium insidiosum*, an aquatic oomycete. It affects the gastrointestinal tract but can also cause skin disease. Cutaneous lesions include boggy, ulcerated, poorly circumscribed nodules with proliferative foci that resemble infected granulation tissue and may involve deeper tissue.[1]

Lagenidium spp. is another oomycete pathogen that can cause skin disease. Most dogs with lagenidiosis have lesions in sites other than the gastrointestinal tract. Two species of *Lagenidium* have been isolated from dogs with cutaneous lesions. *Lagenidium caninum* causes uniformly fatal dermatologic and disseminated disease in dogs. Lesions are firm dermal or subcutaneous nodules or ulcerated, indurated, and edematous deep cellulitis with necrosis and draining tracts that are locally invasive.[1] *Lagenidium karlingii* causes a chronic ulcerative nodular dermatitis and does not appear to extend past local tissues.[1]

PROTOZOAL DISEASES

Neosporosis is caused by the protozoal organism *Neospora caninum*. Older dogs most likely become ill from reactivation of a chronic subclinical infection. These dogs can display widespread draining nodules or, less commonly, a rapidly spreading pruritic ulcerative dermatitis of the eyelids, neck, thorax, and perineum.[2] Leishmaniasis is a protozoal infection caused by a variety of *Leishmania* spp. The most common sign is progressive, symmetric alopecia with exfoliative dermatitis primarily on the head, pinnae, and extremities. Nasodigital hyperkeratosis and periocular alopecia is also common. An ulcerative dermatitis, onychogryposis, paronychia, sterile pustular dermatitis, nasal depigmentation with erosion and ulceration, and nodular dermatitis may be seen. Feline leishmaniasis with cutaneous ulcerative or nodular lesions is rare.

ALGAL DISEASES

Prototorecosis is caused by *Prototheca* a saprophytic achlorophyllous alga. Skin lesions are rare and are characterized by nodules, draining ulcers and crusty exudates on the trunk, extremities, and mucosal surfaces. Only cutaneous protothecosis has been reported in the cat. Lesions consist of large, firm, cutaneous nodules found on the limbs or feet.[3] Lesions have also been seen on the nose, forehead, pinna, and base of the tail.

VIRAL DISEASES

Canine distemper can cause hyperkeratosis of the nasal planum and foot pad (hard pad disease). Young puppies may develop a widespread impetigo.[4]

Canine herpes virus can have an erythematous rash consisting of papules or vesicles and subcutaneous edema of the ventral abdominal and inguinal regions.[5]

Feline herpes virus 1 infection can cause a pruritic ulcerative facial dermatitis concentrating around the nasal planum, bridge of nose, and periocular region of adult cats.[6]

Feline rhinotracheitis is an infection with an alpha herpes virus. Occasionally, cats have oral and cutaneous ulcers that are usually multiple and can occur anywhere on the body.[7]

Canine rabies virus infection may cause an animal to constantly lick at the site of viral inoculation and cause a self-inflicted ulceration.[8]

The most characteristic clinical sign of *pseudorabies virus* infection is an intense pruritus, usually around the head region resulting in self-inflicted ulceration of the skin and underlying tissues.[9]

Clinical signs of *feline leukemia virus* (FeLV) include chronic or recurrent gingivitis or pyoderma, seborrhea, exfoliative dermatitis, pruritus, and cutaneous horns. A facially distributed, pruritic crusting dermatosis has been seen secondary to FeLV infection.

Feline immunodeficiency virus (FIV)–infected cats may have chronic or recurrent abscesses, chronic bacterial infection of the skin and ears, and increased incidence of fungal, ringworm, and *Demodex* infections. Generalized papules with crusts, alopecia, and scaling of the head and limbs have been noted in cats that are FIV positive.

BACTERIAL DISEASES

Male dogs infected with *Brucella canis* may have scrotal dermatitis due to licking.[10]

Dogs infected with *Rickettsia rickettsii* may have erythema, petechia, edema, and occasional necrosis of the oral, ocular, and genital mucous membranes. These problems may also affect the pinna, nose, ventrum, and scrotum.[11] English Springer Spaniels with suspected phosphofructokinase deficiency are more likely to develop dermal necrosis than are animals in which treatment is delayed.

Dogs infected with *Ehrlichia* spp. may have skin disease consisting of crusting of the bridge of the nose, pustular and purpuric lesions secondary to vasculitis, as well as an intensely pruritic papular and crusting dermatitis.

IMMUNE MEDIATED DISEASES

Erythema multiforme, a disease of immunologic dysregulation, usually causes acute erythematous macules and papules that spread peripherally and clear centrally. The lesions are most commonly seen at the mucocutaneous junctions, nasal mucosa, pinnae, axilla, and inguinal regions. Erythema multiforme can be associated with infectious diseases and neoplasia and less likely as a manifestation of a drug eruption.

Toxic epidermal necrolysis (TEN) is acute in onset. It is believed to be caused by a lymphocyte and macrophage–mediated mechanism of immunologic injury. Drugs are the most common known inciting cause but neoplasia and infection have also been documented. Widespread painful erythema rapidly proceeds to full-thickness necrosis of the epidermis. The most common areas affected are oral mucosa, footpad, face, and skin of the trunk.

Skin lesions associated with *systemic lupus erythematosus* (SLE) may be nonspecific or take the form of cutaneous lupus erythematosus lesions that are specific skin syndromes characterized by certain clinical and histopathologic findings. Cutaneous manifestations of SLE include seborrheic disease, alopecia, diffuse or regional erythema, cutaneous or mucocutaneous vesicles and bullae, footpad ulcers and hyperkeratosis, panniculitis, refractory secondary bacterial infection, and nasal dermatitis.

Vasculitis is most commonly believed to be immunologically mediated and may be initiated by a hypersensitivity reaction, food allergy, insect sting/arthropod bite reaction, canine mast cell tumor, feline collagenolytic granuloma, rabies vaccine reaction, coexisting disease (infections, malignancies, lupus), precipitating factors (e.g., drugs, vaccines), or idiopathic. Systemic signs may be present including anorexia, depression, and pyrexia.

Cutaneous lesions include poorly healing ulcers typically located in the center of the footpads. In addition, erosions, ulcerations, and crusting that either affect the pinnal margin or form an oval lesion on the concave aspect of the pinna have been noted (Web Figures 13-1 and 13-2).

Vasculitis reactions do not necessarily remain cutaneous. Systemic vasculitis is a much more serious and possibly life-threatening entity.

Sweet's syndrome (acute neutrophilic dermatitis) is also called *superficial suppurative necrolytic dermatitis of Miniature Schnauzers*. Dogs are febrile and depressed, then develop acute erythema of the ventral chest, abdomen, medial thighs, head, and all four extremities, followed shortly by erosions with suppuration, patchy hair loss and apparent deep pyoderma with lymphadenopathy. It has been described in dogs following topical therapy with D-limonene–containing shampoos, as well as other types of shampoos, Rimadyl administration, snake bite, and as an idiopathic condition.

Well's syndrome (acute eosinophilic dermatitis) is an eosinophilic dermatitis with edema. In many cases, skin disease in the dog develops within a week after being treated for severe vomiting and or diarrhea. In some cases, gastrointestinal signs occur simultaneously with skin lesions. Skin lesions can develop without gastrointestinal signs. Typically, dogs develop diffuse erythroderma with large hemorrhagic coalescing or targetoid macules or papules that are most severe on the abdomen.[12] Dermal edema and pruritus are variable. This may be a unique syndrome with a causal drug association.

Hemolytic uremia syndrome, a cutaneous and renal glomerular vasculopathy, has been described in Greyhounds. Dogs with this condition may have skin disease alone, systemic signs coincident with typical skin lesions, cutaneous disease prior to systemic signs, or manifestations of azotemia before cutaneous ulcerations. Systemic signs include pyrexia, polyuria, polydipsia, vomiting, dark stools, lethargy, and acute renal failure. Cutaneous signs include multiple palpable purpura primarily on the limbs varying from pinpoint to 10 cm in diameter that subsequently ulcerate and discharge a serosanguineous fluid. The ulceration may extend into the subcutaneous tissues. Pitting edema of the extremities may occur. This syndrome is presumed to be a vasculopathy secondary to a verotoxin elaborated by *E. coli* obtained from eating raw beef products. A genetic predisposition or a propensity for feeding raw beef products to Greyhounds may explain the breed susceptibility.

Dermatomyositis is a familial, idiopathic (vascular?) condition of the skin and muscle of Collies, Shetland Sheepdogs, and other breeds. The disease is usually seen in dogs between 6 weeks and 6 months of age. The most common clinical sign of myositis is asymptomatic atrophy of the muscles of mastication and distal limbs. Skin lesions occur in areas of mechanical trauma and are commonly seen on the face, especially around the eyes, on the tips of the ears, on carpal and tarsal regions, on the digits, and on the tip of the tail. Early lesions include pustules vesicles, papules, or small nodules progressing to crusting or alopecia. Ulceration can be seen in severely affected dogs.

NEOPLASIA

Nodular dermatofibrosis is a disease seen primarily in German Shepherd Dogs but has been reported in other breeds. Clinical signs include numerous firm dermal-to-subcutaneous nodules. Systemic conditions seen in association with these multiple skin tumors include polycystic kidneys, renal cystadenomas or cystadenocarcinomas, and uterine leiomyomas. Most kidney involvement is bilateral. Asymptomatic small intestinal polyps may be seen.

Dermatologic manifestations of canine *testicular tumors* are uncommon. Dermatologic manifestations in the male feminization syndrome seen most often with Sertoli cell tumors include bilaterally symmetric nonpruritic alopecia. Other dermatologic manifestations of testicular tumors include seborrhea, ceruminous otitis externa, macular melanosis of the inguinal and perianal skin, and a linear erythematous or melanotic macular change that is present along the ventral aspect of the prepuce extending to the scrotum. Occasionally, a dog will have a papular, pruritic eruption.

Lymphomatoid granulomatosis is an angiocentric and angiodestructive lymphoreticular proliferative and granulomatous disease that predominately involves hundreds of nodules within the lungs and lung consolidation. The condition may involve other organs, including the skin. It is thought to represent a variety of angiocentric peripheral T-cell lymphoma. Skin lesions consist of multiple cutaneous plaques and nodules, some of which progress to become punctate to crateriform ulcers. The lesions involve the face, eyelids, mucocutaneous junctions, and trunk (Web Figure 13-3).

Noncutaneous signs include lameness, weakness, weight loss, and respiratory signs such as dyspnea and coughing.

Pheochromocytomas are endocrine tumors arising from the adrenal medulla. Episodic panting or dyspnea and increased bronchovesicular sounds, weight loss, anorexia, depression, weakness, and collapse are some of the systemic abnormalities noted. The dermatologic manifestation is intermittent flushing, especially of the pinna.

Paraneoplastic syndromes consist of clinical signs that are associated with malignancies but not directly related to tumor invasion. In the dog, these paraneoplastic syndromes include the crusting/fissuring dermatosis associated with necrolytic migratory erythema, nodular skin disease seen with nodular dermatofibrosis, paraneoplastic pemphigus vulgaris associated with a thymic lymphoma, suspect paraneoplastic pemphigus foliaceous from a Sertoli cell tumor, and necrotizing panniculitis associated with pancreatic carcinoma or severe pancreatitis. In the cat, these paraneoplastic dermatoses include the skin fragility syndrome seen with feline adrenal neoplasia, exfoliative dermatosis associated with feline thymoma, and a unique bilaterally symmetrical, ventral glistening, paraneoplastic alopecia associated with pancreatic carcinoma, bile duct carcinoma, and thymoma.

Paraneoplastic pruritus has been seen associated with lymphosarcoma in the dog, squamous cell carcinoma in a cat, and liver disease or cholangiohepatitis in the cat.

ENDOCRINOPATHIES

Dermatologic manifestations of *hypothyroidism* consist of a dry, scaly coat, bilaterally symmetrical nonpruritic trunkal alopecia, rat tail, and variable degrees of hyperpigmentation diffusely affecting the trunk, ventral neck, or abdomen. In addition, lichenification, myxedema, vesicular mucinosis, haircoat color change, comedones, hypertrichosis, seborrhea oleosa, seborrhea sicca, seborrheic dermatitis, and *Malassezia* dermatitis have been reported.

Cushing's syndrome or signs of excess exposure to glucocorticoids include hair loss, comedones, and thin, inelastic skin. Other changes include hyperpigmentation, seborrhea sicca, telangiectasia, increased prominence of surgical scars, lack of hair regrowth after shaving, and adult onset generalized demodicosis. Calcinosis cutis is seen in 5% of dogs.

Approximately one half of cats with *hyperthyroidism* have an unkempt haircoat, with excessive shedding and matting of the hair. Changes in hair texture, partial hair loss, and increased nail growth also are features of feline hyperthyroidism. In cats with areas of complete alopecia, behavioral changes associated with excessive grooming have been documented.

Diabetes mellitus, an endocrinopathy, is not usually associated with any cutaneous abnormality. However, otitis externa, pyoderma, seborrheic skin disease, demodicosis, thin skin, alopecia, and xanthomatosis have been reported in diabetic animals.

Necrolytic migratory erythema (diabetic dermatopathy, hepatocutaneous syndrome, superficial necrolytic dermatitis, metabolic necrolytic dermatopathy, or metabolic epidermal necrosis) has been seen in older dogs with a glucagon-producing pancreatic endocrine tumor, Cushing's disease, hyperglucagonemia, glucagon-secreting liver metastasis, hepatopathy secondary to ingestion of mycotoxins, phenobarbital/phenytoin administration, and hepatopathy of unknown origin. The disease has been reported in a cat with pancreatic carcinoma.

Presenting clinical complaints in the dog range from none to depression, lethargy, polydipsia, diabetes mellitus, liver disease, and skin disease. Cutaneous lesions consist of erythematous crusting plaques, crusting erosions, ulcerations, and alopecia primarily of the face, mucocutaneous junctions, ears, feet, footpads, genitalia, and ventrum (axilla and groin). Pressure points can also be similarly affected. Footpads are most commonly affected with marked hyperkeratosis and fissuring. Vesicular lesions can be seen but are not commonly found.

Demodicosis of the dog is most often caused by *Demodex canis*. Of the two demodectic mites in the cat, *Demodex cati* is most often linked to immunosuppression.

Adult-onset canine generalized demodicosis consisting of generalized patchy or diffuse alopecia with erythema, scaling, crusting, and follicular plugging is most likely caused by suppression of the immune system including administration of immunosuppressive drugs and serious systemic disease (e.g., hyperadrenocorticism, hypothyroidism, diabetes mellitus, blastomycosis and other deep mycoses, lymphosarcoma, hemangiosarcoma, and mammary adenocarcinoma). Estrus, whelping, heartworm disease, and intestinal parasite infestation have been associated with canine generalized demodicosis.

Immunosuppression to include diabetes mellitus, respiratory infection, FeLV infection, SLE, toxoplasmosis, feline endocrine alopecia, FIV infection, hyperadrenocorticism, feline infections peritonitis (FIP), neoplasia, and immunosuppressive drugs (glucocorticoids and progestagens) should be considered potential initiating factors for feline generalized demodicosis. Clinical signs include multifocal to generalized patches of alopecia with variable scaling, macules, papules, erythema, hyperpigmentation, crusting, and symmetrical alopecia of the head, neck, legs, and trunk.

REFERENCES

The reference list can be found on the companion Expert Consult Web site at *www.expertconsult.com*.

CHAPTER 14

Alopecia

Linda Frank

Alopecia is a common reason for presentation of a dog or cat to the veterinarian. The alopecia may be focal or diffuse, patchy or generalized. There are many different causes of alopecia and virtually every dermatosis can have an alopecic component. When evaluating the dog or cat for alopecia, a thorough history and physical examination are in order. Knowing the signalment, history, presence or absence of pruritus, and determining the distribution of the alopecia as well as its association with an inflammatory component may be key to helping determine the ultimate cause of the alopecia.

The causes of alopecia can be divided into two basic categories: pruritus-induced alopecia and nonpruritic alopecia (Figure 14-1).

If the hair is not traumatically being removed, then it could be falling out on its own. Nonpruritic alopecias can be further subdivided into inflammatory and noninflammatory causes (see Figure 14-1).

ALOPECIA SECONDARY TO PRURITUS

Alopecia commonly occurs secondary to pruritus because the pet is scratching, licking, or chewing off the hair. This may not be as obvious in the cat because excessive grooming may not be observed by the owner but may be the cause of the alopecia. Common causes of alopecia secondary to pruritus include allergies, ectoparasites, bacterial skin infections, and

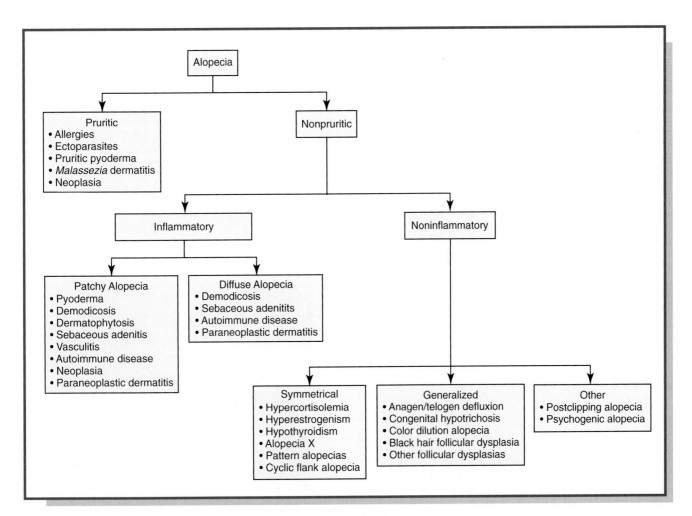

Figure 14-1 Algorithm for alopecia.

Malassezia dermatitis. In older animals, neoplastic diseases such as epitheliotrophic lymphoma or mast cell tumor and paraneoplastic syndromes can also be associated with pruritus-induced alopecia. Clinically, pruritus-induced alopecias are usually characterized by broken hairs where the animal has been scratching. This can be observed by performing a trichogram and examining the tips of the hairs microscopically. Normal, noncut hair should have a tapered tip while a hair scratched at or chewed off will have a blunted tip (Web Figure 14-1).

This technique will not work for dogs that are groomed and clipped regularly, as all of their hairs will be blunted. Evidence of excoriations supporting pruritus may also be observed in the alopecic areas; however, in cats the skin may have no evidence of trauma.

NONPRURITIC ALOPECIA

Inflammatory Alopecias

Inflammation causes hair to fall out multifocally at the inflammatory sites. This is typified in short-coated dogs with bacterial folliculitis, dermatophytosis, demodicosis, or sebaceous adenitis in which the hair loss presents as a patchy or "moth-eaten" appearance to the coat (Figure 14-2).

The lesions might not overtly appear inflammatory; however, the multifocal pattern of the alopecia should make you suspicious of an inflammatory cause. Even if the dog is pruritic, it would be hard to imagine a dog scratching hair out in these focal locations. Hairs may epilate easily from the periphery of these inflammatory alopecic sites. In addition, autoimmune diseases such as pemphigus foliaceus or alopecia areata and neoplastic conditions such as epitheliotrophic lymphoma could result in areas of inflammatory alopecia (Web Figure 14-2}.

Vasculitis from immune-complex deposition secondary to infectious or immune-mediated diseases may cause multifocal alopecia due to local ischemia. Clinically the lesions resemble dermatophytosis in that they are circular and alopecic; however, they often look noninflammatory (thin skin, no erythema or crusting) unless cutaneous necrosis and ulceration occur. A common example of focal ischemic alopecia is rabies vaccine–induced vasculitis (Figure 14-3).

Internal neoplasia may also be associated with alopecia. This is a presumed inflammatory alopecia although the pathomechanism of the alopecia is unknown. Paraneoplastic alopecia has been described in cats associated with pancreatic

and biliary carcinoma.[1] The alopecia is acute and progressive with easy epilation of hair and smooth thin skin (Web Figure 14-3).

Noninflammatory Alopecias

Alopecia may also develop when there is no associated dermal inflammation. This is grouped under a broad category of noninflammatory causes of alopecia, which would include endocrine diseases but also many nonendocrine causes (see Figure 14-1). Noninflammatory alopecias are usually diffuse and symmetrical (Figure 14-4) and may be associated with either abnormal hair growth, in which the defect occurs during the active anagen phase of the hair cycle, or hair cycle abnormalities, in which a new anagen phase of the hair cycle is not initiated.

In general, hairs do not epilate easily from the majority of these noninflammatory alopecic conditions.

Hair Cycle Review   The hair cycle consists of the resting telogen phase, the active anagen growth phase, and the catagen phase, which is the involution from anagen to telogen. Shedding, or exogen, is separate from the hair cycle and is independent of whether a new hair cycle is starting. The hair cycle of most dogs and likely all cats is a telogen-predominant cycle in which the anagen phase is short and hairs regain in the resting or telogen phase for the majority of the hair cycle.[2] The short anagen phase genetically determines the length of the coat and may be of different durations for different regions of the body. The telogen hairs are well anchored and do not epilate easily. Therefore, the presence of telogen hairs is not necessarily pathologic. In contrast to a telogen-predominant cycle, people, poodles, and likely dogs that need regular clipping have an anagen-predominant cycle in which the anagen phase of the hair cycle is prolonged. Animals with anagen-predominant hair cycles are more likely to develop alopecia from chemotherapeutic agents.

Abnormal Hair Growth   In pets with noninflammatory alopecia associated with abnormal hair growth, the defect occurs during the anagen phase of the cycle. There are only a few conditions that fall into this category; they include follicular dysplasias, congenital hypotrichosis, color dilution alopecia, and black hair follicular dysplasia. Follicular dysplasias are most recognized in certain breeds such as the Chinese Crested dog, Mexican Hairless dog, and the Sphinx cat in which the alopecia is a breed characteristic. Congenital hypotrichosis is not well described in small animals, but the alopecia occurs either at birth or within the first 6 months of life and

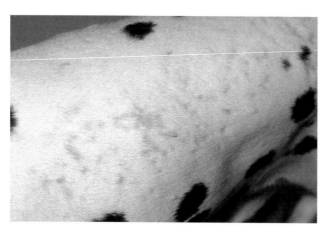

Figure 14-2   A Dalmatian with patchy alopecia secondary to pyoderma.

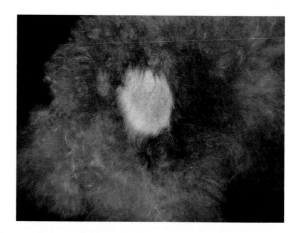

Figure 14-3   A Miniature Poodle with focal alopecia of the right hip secondary to rabies vaccine-induced vasculitis.

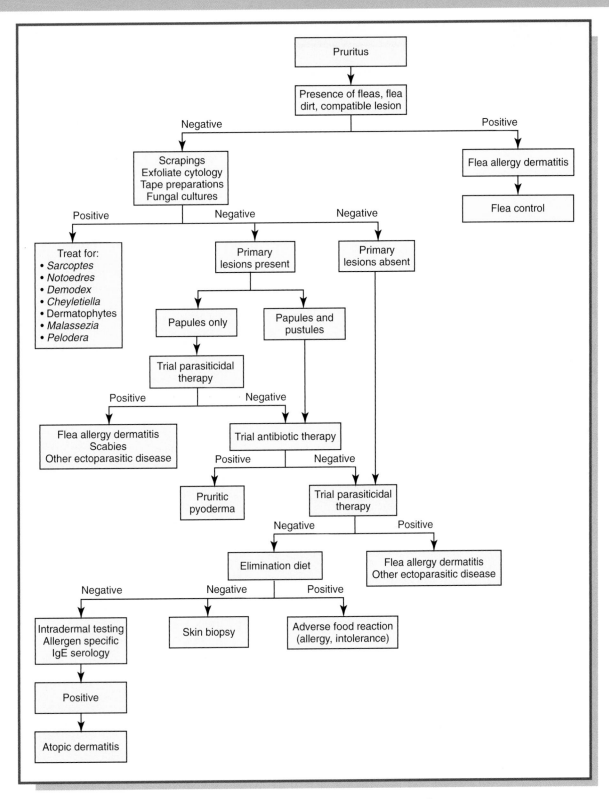

Figure 15-1 Algorithm for diagnosis and management of pruritus.

Table • 15-1

Pruritic Canine Dermatoses

DISEASE	SITE	LESIONS
Flea allergy dermatitis A, E, F	Bilaterally symmetric, dorsal lumbosacral, caudal thighs, groin, axilla, caudal half of body	Papules, plaques, alopecia, erythema, lichenification, hyperpigmentation, excoriations, fibropruritic nodules
Canine scabies A	Ventrum, pinnae margins, face, elbows, partially bilaterally symmetric	Papules, plaques, erythema, alopecia, crusts, excoriations, alopecia
Demodicosis A	Periorbital, commisures of mouth, forelegs, generalized	Alopecia, erythema, crusts, follicular plugging, hyperpigmentation, comedones, secondary pyoderma
Pyoderma A	Groin, axilla, ventrum, interdigital webs, generalized, pressure points	Pustules, crusted papules, erythema, alopecia, target lesions, coalescing collarettes, hyperpigmentation
Atopic dermatitis A, F	Face, periorbital, ears, caudal carpi and tarsi, feet, (dorsum), otitis externa, axilla, pinna, generalized	Erythema, alopecia, excoriations, lack of primary lesions, lichenification, hyperpigmentation
Malassezia dermatitis A, E, F	Ventral neck, groin, skinfolds, face, feet, ventrum	Erythema, exudative or dry, alopecia, hyperpigmentation, lichenification
Cornification defects B	Generalized, ears, preen body	Scales, crusts, alopecia, erythematous plaques
Acral lick dermatitis A	Anterior carpal, metacarpal, radial, metatarsal, tibial regions	Firm, alopecic plaque, central irregular ulcer, hyperpigmented halo
Food allergy A	Face, feet, ears, generalized	Erythema, alopecia, excoriations, lack of primary lesions
Contact dermatitis C	Hairless areas, feet (ventrum), genitals, groin, axilla, generalized	Erythema, exudation, lichenification, hyperpigmentation, papules
Drug eruptions C	Anywhere, localized or generalized, face, ears, scrotum	Pleomorphic, erythema, papules, coalescing target lesions
Endoparasitic migration in puppies C	Face, feet, generalized	Erythema, alopecia, excoriations, lack of primary lesions
Cheyletiellosis B, E	Dorsum of thorax, generalized	Large scales, crusts, alopecia, erythema
Chiggers B, E, F	Ventrum, legs, anywhere	Erythema, scales, crusts, papules, alopecia
Superficial necrolytic dermatitis C	Footpads, face, mucocutaneous junctions, genitals, groin	Adherent crusts, ulcers, excoriations, erythema, fissured pads
Psychogenic pruritus C	Carpi, tarsi, feet (especially forelegs), perianal, generalized	Erythema, alopecia, excoriations, lack of primary lesions
Pediculosis C, E, F	Dorsum, generalized	Scales, crusts, alopecia, papules
Tail-dock neuroma C	Previously docked tail	Erythema, excoriations, alopecia
Rhabditic dermatitis D, E, F	Ventrum, legs, groin	Erythema, papules, alopecia, crusts, scale

A, Common; *B*, less common; *C*, uncommon; *D*, rare or controversial; *E*, regional; *F*, seasonal.

and feline pruritus despite effective modern products. Because lesions seen with canine superficial pyoderma may be pleomorphic, trial use of antibiotics may be indicated in undiagnosed pruritic crusted papular dermatoses. Although response to corticosteroids is suggestive of underlying allergic disease, superficial pyoderma commonly respond partially to corticosteroid therapy.

COST CONTAINMENT

Skin scrapings, surface cytology, trial therapy for ectoparasites, and, surprisingly, skin biopsy, are the most cost-effective diagnostic procedures for the pruritic animal.

Table • 15-2

Pruritic Feline Dermatoses

DISEASE	SITE	LESION
Flea allergy dermatitis A, E, F	Neck, dorsum, lumbosacral, caudal and medial thighs, groin, ears	"Miliary dermatitis," erythema, alopecia, eosinophilic plaques
Eosinophilic plaque A, E, F	Ventral abdomen, medial thighs, anywhere	Raised, ulcerated, erythematous alopecic plaques, secondary to allergy (primarily flea allergy dermatitis)
Otodectic acariasis A	Ears, head, neck, rarely generalized	Otitis externa, excoriations, "miliary dermatitis"
Food allergy A	Head, neck, ears, generalized	Erythema, excoriations, alopecia, lack of primary lesions, "miliary dermatitis"
Atopic dermatitis A, F	Head, neck, ears, generalized	"Miliary dermatitis," erythema, excoriations, alopecia
Self-induced pruritic hair loss (atopic dermatitis, food allergy, flea allergy) B	Bilaterally symmetric, caudal and lateral thighs, ventral abdomen, perineum	Alopecia, hair stubble, erythema, papules, underlying skin may be normal
Self-induced psychogenic hair loss C	Bilaterally symmetric, stripe(s) on dorsal thorax, caudal and lateral thighs, ventral abdomen, perineum, forelegs	Alopecia, hair stubble, normal underlying skin
Cheyletiellosis B, E	Dorsum of thorax, generalized	Large scales, crusts, seborrhea, "miliary dermatitis"
Demodicosis B, E	Trunk, ventral, generalized	Alopecia, scaling
Mosquito-bite hypersensitivity C, E, F	Bilaterally symmetric, dorsal muzzle, planum nasale, periorbital, pinnae, paw pad margins	Papules, crusts, alopecia, erosion, exudation, fistulation
Pediculosis C, E, F	Dorsum, generalized	Scales, crusts, alopecia
Feline scabies C, E	Head, ears, neck, generalized, partially bilaterally symmetric	Erythema, papules, crusts, excoriations, alopecia
Pruritic dermatophytosis C	Head, neck, ears, generalized	Erythema, alopecia, hair stubble, "miliary dermatitis," hyperpigmentation
Drug eruptions C	Anywhere, localized or generalized, pinnae, face	Pleomorphic, erythema, papules, coalescing target lesions
Pemphigus foliaceus D, F?	Bilaterally symmetric, face, planum nasale, ears, interdigital webs, nipples, generalized	Crusts, vesicopustules, alopecia

A, Common; *B*, less common; *C*, uncommon; *D*, rare or controversial; *E*, regional; *F*, seasonal.

GOALS OF THERAPY

Successful long-term management of a pruritic dog or cat requires definitive diagnosis. Repetitive parasiticidal therapy on a weekly basis for 3 or 4 weeks will rule out most contagious ectoparasitic diseases such as canine or feline scabies. However, management of flea allergy dermatitis is a lifelong endeavor requiring control of fleas on the affected animal and all in-contact dogs and cats. Atopic dermatitis responds best to allergen-specific immunotherapy. Secondary pyoderma and *Malassezia* dermatitis are common sequelae to most pruritic skin diseases and must be assessed for and managed long-term. If corticosteroids are used adjunctively for the long-term management of allergic skin disease, short-acting oral corticosteroids such as prednisolone or methylprednisolone are recommended on an alternate-day basis. Data suggests that prednisolone is more predictably absorbed in the cat than prednisone. Corticosteroids are contraindicated in the treatment of canine demodicosis and pyoderma. Many pruritic animals require long-term adjunctive topical management with shampoos and emollients or antipruritic rinses.

CHAPTER 16

Cutaneous and Subcutaneous Lumps, Bumps, and Masses

Didier-Noël Carlotti

Cutaneous and subcutaneous lumps, bumps, and masses include hematomas, abscesses, urticaria and angioedema, neoplasms, and pseudoneoplasms.

CLINICAL AND HISTOPATHOLOGIC DEFINITIONS

A hematoma is a focal extravasation of blood with purpura (bruising) and pain, whereas an abscess is a localized collection of pus with pain, heat, and sometimes purpura. Urticaria is referred to as a group of wheals (sharply circumscribed, raised, edematous lesions) that appear and disappear rapidly. Angioedema is a large swelling in a distensible region such as the face and limbs.

Clinically, pseudoneoplasms and neoplasms appear as nodules, plaques, and masses. Ulceration always indicates a severe pathologic process. Pseudoneoplasms include cysts, nevi, keratoses, granulomas, and pyogranulomas and other lesions. *Pseudoneoplasm* is a better term than *pseudotumor* because the term *tumor* is clinical and should refer to a localized hypertrophy of a tissue or an organ, neoplastic or not. Cysts are epithelial lesions containing grayish keratinous material (Web Figure 16-1) or serous material, such as apocrine cysts, which appear fluctuant, bluish, and well circumscribed (Web Figures 16-2 and 16-3).

A hamartoma is a malformation formed by components of a normal organ arranged erroneously. A nevus is a cutaneous hamartoma that may arise from any skin component. Collagenous nevi are single or multiple nodules characterized histologically by large areas of collagen hyperplasia. In German Shepherd Dogs, multiple collagenous nevi may appear, particularly on the limbs, in association with renal adenocarcinomas and uterine leiomyomas (nodular dermatofibrosis syndrome) (Web Figure 16-4).

Organoid (i.e., pilosebaceous) and epidermal nevi are variable in shape and may be linear (Web Figure 16-5).

Vascular nevi are seen often (but not only) on the scrotum in dogs (Web Figure 16-6).

Keratoses are solid, elevated, and circumscribed lesions characterized by a hyperproduction of keratin. They show up as greasy nodules and plaques (seborrheic keratoses) (Web Figure 16-7), squamocrustous plaques (actinic keratoses, lichenoid keratoses) (Web Figure 16-8), or cutaneous horns (Web Figure 16-9).

A granuloma is a circumscribed tissue reaction characterized by an organized infiltration of mononucleated phagocytes (histiocytes and macrophages) that may occur when foreign bodies, bacteria (Web Figures 16-10 through 16-13), fungi (Figure 16-1) (Web Figures 16-14 through 16-15), parasites (Web Figure 16-16), or any material penetrates or deposits into the skin. If an acute inflammatory process does not destroy the "invader," macrophages become epithelioid. A granuloma may persist until the cause has been eliminated.

"Pyogranuloma" means granulomatous reaction with many neutrophils.

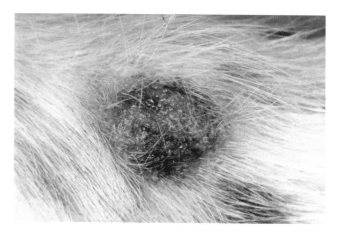

Figure 16-1   Kerion in a dog *(Microsporum gypseum)*.

Lesions of calcinosis circumscripta are pink-colored plaques located on pressure points or in the tongue that contain chalky material (Web Figures 16-17 and 16-18).

Hard erythematous plaques containing whitish material characterize calcinosis cutis, as seen in canine Cushing's syndrome (Web Figure 16-19).

Eosinophilic lesions in the cat are indolent ulcer (Web Figure 16-20), eosinophilic plaque (Web Figure 16-21), and eosinophilic granuloma (the latter often appearing linear) (Web Figure 16-22).

Nodular sterile panniculitis is characterized by deep nodules that fistulize, expressing an oily material (Web Figure 16-23).

Canine juvenile cellulitis is characterized by facial swelling (Web Figure 16-24).

Nodular lesions can be seen in canine sterile granuloma and pyogranuloma syndrome (Web Figure 16-25), as well as in canine histiocytosis, particularly on the face in the latter, with a "clown nose" appearance (Web Figure 16-26).

Other various pseudoneoplasms include acral lick dermatitis (Web Figure 16-27), idiopathic lichenoid dermatitis (coalescent plaques) (Web Figure 16-28), feline plasma cell pododermatitis or stomatitis (Web Figure 16-29 and 16-30), and idiopathic focal mucinosis seen in Doberman Pinschers.

CAUSE AND PATHOPHYSIOLOGY

Hematomas are the result of trauma causing the rupture of blood vessels. They appear frequently after minor trauma in dogs with coagulopathies. Abscesses are the result of the collection of degenerated neutrophils and necrotic tissue cells when an infectious agent has penetrated into and under the skin. Usually a peripheral membrane forms from necrotic tissue and fibrin. Urticaria and angioedema are caused by immediate hypersensitivity reactions generated by insect bites (e.g., Hymenoptera), food, drugs, airborne allergens (atopy), and nonimmunologic stimuli such as contact with irritant material (e.g., weeds such as *Urtica dioica;* insects such as *Thaumetopoea pityocampa* [caterpillar]; physical stimuli such as cold, heat, and sunlight; and even psychogenic factors). Cysts may be traumatic (epidermoid), hereditary (dermoid), follicular, or pilar (i.e., trichilemmal) caused by retention of material (i.e., keratin, glandular products) as a result of congenital or acquired loss of follicular orifices. Apocrine cysts are idiopathic. Nevi may be congenital, and the mechanism of their formation is unknown. However, nodular dermatofibrosis is due to an autosomal dominant gene. Keratoses are idiopathic except actinic keratoses and some cutaneous horns, which are associated with various skin neoplasms or feline leukemia virus (FeLV) infection in the cat.

Bacterial granulomas and pyogranulomas include canine furunculosis caused by cocci such as *Staphylococcus intermedius,* botryomycosis (bacterial pseudomycetoma) caused by various bacteria that may cause a granulomatous reaction (Web Figure 16-31), and nocardiosis and mycobacterioses (atypical mycobacterial infection, feline leprosy, and tuberculosis, which is rare) (Web Figure 16-32).

Fungal granulomas and pyogranulomas include kerions (inflammatory reaction to a dermatophyte) and pseudomycetomas caused by the subcutaneous development of a dermatophyte (*Microsporum canis* in cats, mainly) (Web Figure 16-33), subcutaneous (intermediate) mycoses (sporotrichosis, pythiosis, mycetomas, phaeohyphomycosis, zygomycosis), and deep (systemic) mycoses (blastomycosis, coccidioidomycosis, histoplasmosis, aspergillosis, cryptococcosis [Web Figure 16-34], prototheocosis, paecilomycosis, trichosporonosis).

Endogenous or exogenous foreign bodies can cause granulomas. Endogenous foreign bodies are usually hair and keratin (leading to bacterial furunculosis), calcium (calcinosis circumscripta, idiopathic, Cushing's syndrome), and lipids (xanthomas in case of hyperlipidemia in cats, associated with diabetes mellitus or hereditary). Exogenous foreign bodies include sutures and weed material. Parasitic granulomas include tick bites, canine dracunculosis, canine filariasis, canine leishmaniasis (the nodular form is seen more frequently in short-haired dogs such as the Boxer) (Web Figure 16-35), feline toxoplasmosis, and canine cysticercosis.

Arthropod bites (e.g., mosquitoes, spiders) lead to eosinophilic furunculosis (particularly on the face in dogs and cats) with a granulomatous reaction. Some granulomas are idiopathic: lesions of the feline eosinophilic granuloma complex (although most of the cases are caused by flea allergy dermatitis, feline atopic dermatitis, or food hypersensitivity), canine eosinophilic granuloma, sterile granuloma and pyogranuloma syndrome (due to a proliferation of macrophages), canine cutaneous reactive histiocytosis (caused by a proliferation of normal histiocytes that are dendritic cells), canine sarcoidosis, canine juvenile cellulitis (perhaps viral), nodular sterile panniculitis (the result of an inflammatory process of subcutaneous fat), and amyloidosis. Acral lick dermatitis is often a deep bacterial folliculitis and furunculosis caused by constant licking attributed to an allergic pruritus or behavioral disorder. Lichenoid dermatitis may be idiopathic or an immune-mediated disease as well as feline plasma cell pododermatitis and stomatitis sometimes associated with FeLV, feline immunodeficiency virus (FIV)-infection, or both.

Cutaneous and subcutaneous neoplasms include epithelial (epidermal and follicular), glandular (sebaceous, sweat, and hepatoid gland), mesenchymal (fibrocytic, histiocytic, vascu-

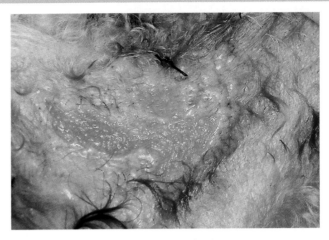

Figure 16-2 Carcinomatosis in a dog: cutaneous metastatic mammary adenocarcinoma.

lar), melanocytic and round cell tumors (mast cell, histiocytic, lymphoma), and metastatic (secondary) (Figure 16-2) (Web Figure 16-36).

Mammary neoplasms can be considered as subcutaneous. Most of the neoplasms have an unknown cause. Viruses can cause specific tumors such as papillomas in dogs and fibrosarcomas and carcinomas in situ (Bowen's disease) in cats. Other causes include irritation, trauma, and actinic exposure. The latter is likely to be the cause of squamous cell carcinoma of the face and ears in the cat (particularly of white color). It is not clear whether repeated vaccinations can lead to fibrosarcomas in cats. Benign neoplasms can be harmful if they reach a large size, are located in particular areas (face, eyelids, external ear canal, mouth, feet, genitals, anus), or both. Malignant neoplasms are invasive and will cause the necrosis of surrounding cells, leading to ulceration.

DIAGNOSIS

Diagnosis of cutaneous and subcutaneous lumps, bumps, and masses is based upon history, physical examination, and complementary aids (Figure 16-3).

Signalment of the animal may be of some importance. Neoplastic lesions occur mostly in adults and old dogs. However, viral papilloma and histiocytoma (Langerhans' cell tumor) will be seen mainly in young animals. Intact male cats are prone to develop abscesses as the result of fighting. Mammary tumors and their cutaneous metastases occur in female dogs, whereas perianal gland tumors occur most frequently in intact males. Most neoplasms, however, have no sex predilection. Breed predispositions are recognized for many superficial neoplasms. The Boxer is known to be predisposed to many, as they are for nodular leishmaniasis. The German Shepherd Dog is predisposed to keratinous cysts and nodular dermatofibrosis. Persian cats are predisposed to dermatophytic pseudomycetoma.

History of the lesions should be taken into account. Important points are the existence of previous similar lesions, association to general disease, known trauma, and rapidity of onset. Obviously, hematomas, abscesses, urticaria, and angioedema appear rapidly. Some lymphomas can develop rapidly. Feline eosinophilic plaques, urticaria and angioedema, some cases of calcinosis cutis, and mast cell tumors are pruritic. Hematomas, abscesses, and some tumors may be painful.

Physical examination should include evaluation of the lesions, local lymph nodes, and distant sites such as lungs. This

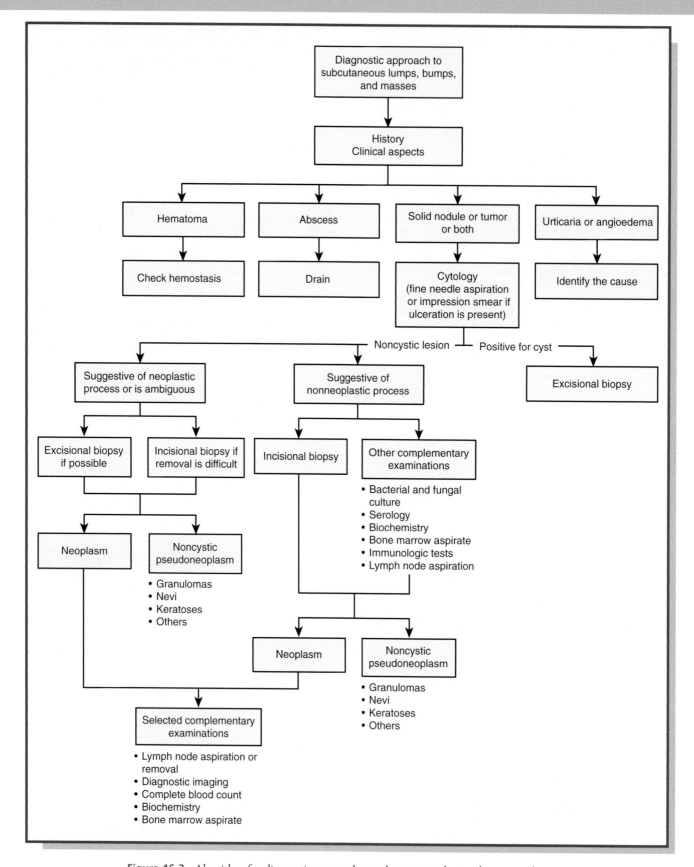

Figure 16-3 Algorithm for diagnostic approach to subcutaneous lumps, bumps, and masses.

strategy applies to most lumps, bumps, and masses, using the TNM approach (tumor, node, metastasis). The lesions should be characterized by localization, size, shape, pedunculated appearance, consistency, depth, and whether or not they are freely movable, ulcerated, or both. For instance, feline eosinophilic granuloma and canine epidermal nevus can be linear; hematomas and most benign neoplasms are not attached to underlying tissues, whereas most of abscesses and malignant neoplasms are attached. Abscesses evolve from firm to fluctuant stages, whereas most pseudoneoplasms and neoplasms are firm (except apocrine cysts and some angiomas and angiosarcomas). Benign neoplasms can be pedunculated. Feline indolent ulcer, eosinophilic plaques, some malignant neoplasms, and canine acral lick dermatitis ulcerate. Enlargement of local lymph nodes can be caused by inflammation (even in case of a neoplastic process) or metastasis. General lymph node enlargement can result from severe infections and lymphosarcoma. Metastasis can rarely be suspected clinically, except for cutaneous metastasis of mammary neoplasms (see Figure 16-2 and Web Figure 16-36) and when an abnormal abdominal mass is palpated.

Cytologic techniques usable for lumps, bumps, and masses are impression, scrape, swab, and fine needle aspiration smears. No contraindications exist. Cytology allows rapid identification of cell types. High cellularity and a homogeneous cell population characterize neoplasms. Cytologic criteria of malignancy include pleomorphism, high nucleocytoplasmic ratios, large nucleoli, and atypical mitoses. In many nonneoplastic lesions, the cytologic examination is highly suggestive of the diagnosis (e.g., pyoderma, fungal diseases, eosinophilic plaques). Fine needle aspiration cytology of a local lymph node can help to differentiate an inflammatory reaction from malignancy.

Histology has a fundamental role in establishing specimens' diagnoses. Incisional biopsy specimens can be obtained with a scalpel or a punch, particularly when cytology is ambiguous. Results aid in selecting appropriate medical therapy, surgery, or both. The sample should be biopsied at the margin of the lesion to incorporate some normal-looking tissue, should not be larger than 1 cm, and should be put in 10 times its volume of 10% formalin. No contraindication exists for incisional biopsy because it does not increase risk of metastasis. The wound should be repaired, and the biopsy site should be removed by further surgery. General anesthesia may be required, and wound repair can be difficult. Excisional biopsy can also be performed, particularly when cytology is ambiguous, when the surgical removal of the lesion is easy, and when physical examination suggests a nonneoplastic or benign neoplastic lesion. If lesions are multiple, excisional biopsy of a typical mass should be considered. Immunohistochemistry and polymerase chain reaction (PCR) can be useful in diagnosing certain pseudoneoplasms.[1] The removal of a lymph node for histopathologic analysis can be helpful and has no harmful consequence. Radiology, ultrasonography, or both are useful in many instances (e.g., a lesion appearing to be attached to an underlying bone or suspicion of lung or abdominal metastasis). In particular instances other complementary examinations can be useful for the diagnosis of pseudoneoplasms: bacterial and fungal cultures, serologic tests, biochemistry, bone marrow and lymph node cytology and immunologic and allergic tests.

PROGNOSIS

The prognosis of cutaneous or subcutaneous (or both) lumps, bumps, and masses is obviously linked to diagnosis, location of the lesion or lesions, and continuing evaluation (TNM). Establishing a prognosis based on physical examination only and clinical neglect (waiting for a possible enlargement of the lesion or lesions) are unacceptable errors.

TREATMENT

Treatment should be based upon diagnosis and prognosis. Medical treatment of urticaria and angioedema, hematomas, and abscesses is almost always successful. The result of treatment of granulomatous pseudoneoplasms can lead to complete cure, particularly when a bacterial or superficial fungal agent has been identified. Surgical excision of cysts, nevi, keratoses, feline plasma cell podal lesions, and benign neoplasms is usually successful. Treatment for malignancies is rarely curative, but long remissions can be obtained, particularly if the owners wish to cooperate.

REFERENCES

The reference list can be found on the companion Expert Consult Web site at *www.expertconsult.com*.

CHAPTER 17

Erosions and Ulcerations

Ian S. Mason

Erosions and ulcers are skin defects with a wide range of causes. Erosions are superficial breaks in the continuity of epithelia that fail to breach the intact basement membrane and usually heal without scarring. Ulcers are deeper and extend through the basement membrane into the underlying dermis. They heal slowly and residual scarring is common. It may be impossible to distinguish between ulcers and erosions without histology. In some diseases, ulcers and erosions occur concurrently, whereas in other conditions only one type of lesion may be present.

Ulcers and erosions may result from a variety of conditions (Box 17-1).

Trauma, including self-trauma associated with pruritus, may lead to eroded and ulcerated lesions. Infectious diseases can lead to defects in the epithelial surface. In canine skin, bullae and vesicles are thin walled and rupture promptly after formation, leading to erosions and ulcers. Chemical and physical factors such as urine scalding, irritant contact dermatitis, and thermal injury may also be responsible for defects in cutaneous continuity.

Erosive and ulcerative diseases in dogs and cats may affect the mucous membranes with or without concurrent cutaneous involvement. Animals with oral lesions usually have halitosis, dysphagia, or both. Clinicians often suspect autoimmune and immune-mediated diseases in animals with erosions and lacerations. However, these diseases are uncommon or rare.

APPROACH TO THE DIAGNOSIS

Diagnosis may be difficult. Ulcers and erosions have many possible causes. Therefore the diagnostic approach must be carefully planned and thorough (Figure 17-1).

History may yield important clues. Obese or short-legged breeds of dogs are predisposed to intertriginous (or body fold) pyoderma and urine scalding. Older animals are more susceptible to metabolic and neoplastic disorders. Concurrent systemic signs may indicate that lesions are the result of metabolic disease or a drug eruption (assuming the animal has received therapy). Determining whether pruritus is present and at which stage it developed is helpful. If early pruritus is present, it is possible that this is a primary pruritic disease, such as that caused by hypersensitivity or ectoparasitism, and that the lesions are the result of self-trauma. Late onset of pruritus may be more difficult to assess and may arise in a large number

---

Box • 17-1

Differential Diagnosis of Ulcers and Erosions Affecting Skin and Mucous Membranes

Canine Diseases
Infectious
Bacterial pyoderma
    Surface:
        Acute moist dermatitis (pyotraumatic dermatitis)
        Intertrigo
    Deep:
        Folliculitis/furunculosis (including pyotraumatic
            folliculitis)
        Oral bacterial infections (aerobic/anaerobic)
Fungal
Yeast infections (*Malassezia pachydermatis, Candida* spp.)
Systemic/subcutaneous
Parasitic
Demodicosis
Metabolic
Calcinosis cutis (hyperadrenocorticism)
Uremia/renal failure
Necrolytic migratory erythema/metabolic epidermal necrosis
Neoplastic
Epitheliotropic lymphoma
Squamous cell carcinoma
Physical, Chemical
Drug reactions
Solar injury
Thermal injury (freeze or burn)
Urine scald
Immune-Mediated/Autoimmune
Discoid lupus erythematosus
Pemphigus group
Uveodermatologic syndrome
Miscellaneous autoimmune subepidermal vesiculobullous
    diseases:
    Bullous pemphigoid
    Epidermolysis bullosa acquisita
    Linear IgA bullous disease
    Mucocutaneous pemphigoid
    Bullous systemic lupus–type 1

Miscellaneous
Arthropod bites
Dermatomyositis
Dystrophic epidermolysis bullosa
Idiopathic ulceration of Collies
Junctional epidermolysis bullosa
Toxic epidermal necrolysis/erythema multiforme

Feline Diseases
Infectious
Viral:
    Calicivirus and herpesvirus
Bacterial:
    Atypical mycobacteriosis
Fungal:
    Subcutaneous and systemic mycoses
    Cryptococcosis
    Sporotrichosis
Metabolic
Uremia/renal disease
Neoplastic
Fibrosarcoma
Lymphoma
Squamous cell carcinoma
Physical/Chemical
Drug reactions
Thermal
Immune-Mediated/Autoimmune
Bullous pemphigoid
Pemphigus foliaceus
Toxic epidermal necrolysis/erythema multiforme
Miscellaneous/Idiopathic
Arthropod bites
Dystrophic epidermolysis bullosa
Eosinophilic plaque
Idiopathic ulceration of dorsal neck
Indolent ulcer
Junctional epidermolysis bullosa

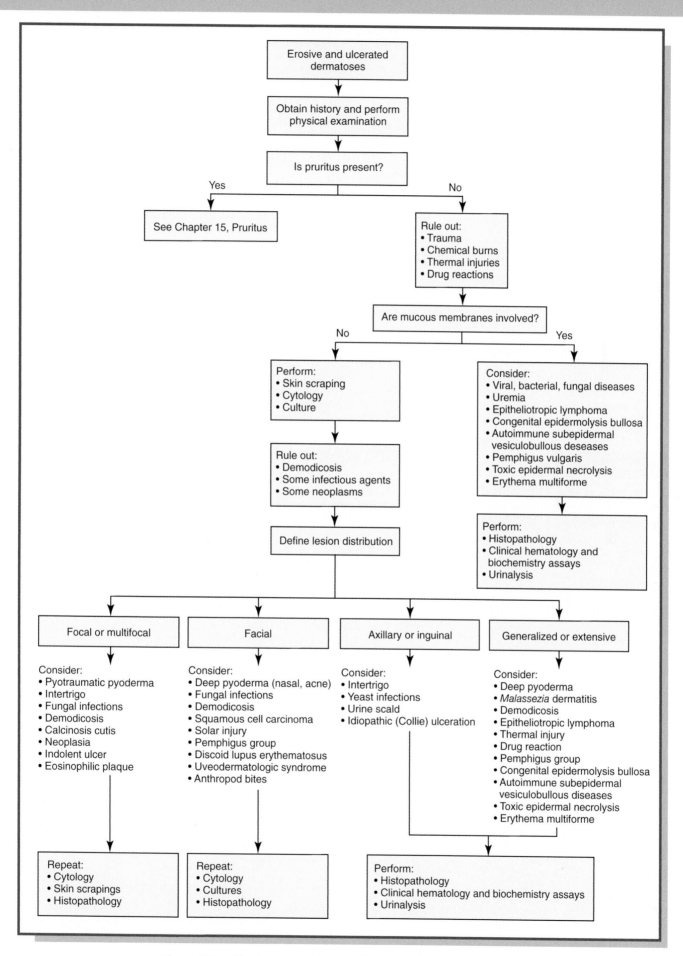

Figure 17-1 Algorithm for evaluation of erosive and ulcerated dermatoses.

of diseases. Chronic sun exposure, especially of poorly pigmented skin, may lead to actinic lesions including neoplasia.

General and dermatologic examination will greatly aid the establishment of a differential diagnosis and enable the clinician to identify any concurrent systemic disease. The distribution of lesions may be extremely helpful (Box 17-2).

Involvement of mucous membranes indicates the presence of uremia, renal failure, or both; viral, bacterial, or yeast infection; certain immune-mediated disorders (bullous pemphigoid, pemphigus vulgaris), or epitheliotropic lymphoma,

Initial diagnostic tests such as cytologic examination of impression smears and microscopy of skin scrapings are useful. However, the majority of causes will be identified by histopathology, and biopsy specimens should be taken early in the development of this group of diseases.

INFECTIOUS CAUSES OF EROSIONS AND ULCERS

Viral Diseases

Feline calicivirus and feline herpesvirus (FHV) infections usually cause upper respiratory tract disease and conjunctivitis. Rarely, they may lead to cutaneous ulceration, typically on the feet. A tentative clinical diagnosis of feline calicivirus and FHV can usually be based on results of the history and physical examination.

Bacterial Disease

Pyoderma and other bacterial diseases may be difficult to recognize because these infections are pleomorphic. If doubt exists as to whether the lesions are the result of bacterial infection, histopathology should be performed. Concurrent systemic antimicrobial therapy is indicated while awaiting the pathologist's findings. If histopathology results indicate that the lesions are bacterial in origin but little improvement has been seen after antimicrobial therapy, it is likely that the infection is secondary. A second biopsy sampling is indicated after antibacterial therapy to allow examination of tissue without secondary infection.

Surface bacterial infections in dogs are characterized by erosion. Intertrigo (skin fold pyoderma) affecting lip, vulvar, facial, tail, or body folds is readily recognized clinically. Impression cytology and culture of the folds may reveal evidence of bacterial infection, usually *Staphylococcus pseudintermedius*, but the yeast *Malassezia pachydermatis* may also be involved. Pyotraumatic dermatitis ("hot spots" or acute moist dermatitis) is another form of canine surface pyoderma that is readily recognized clinically. However, in some cases, the infection is deeper than it would appear on clinical examination (this is termed *pyotraumatic folliculitis*). The distinction between these two forms is made by histopathology and is important because glucocorticoid therapy is contraindicated in the deeper form.

Deep pyoderma in dogs may be characterized by erosion and ulceration; examples include nasal pyoderma and German Shepherd Dog pyoderma. These may be confused with immune-mediated disorders. As previously discussed, histopathology and antimicrobial therapy may be of value. Aerobic and anaerobic bacterial infection may affect the mucous membranes. Such infections are often secondary

---

Box • 17-2

Distribution of Ulcers and Erosions as a Diagnostic Clue

Axillary/Inguinal
Fungal (*Malassezia pachydermatis*, *Candida* spp.) (D)
Idiopathic ulceration of Collies (D)
Intertrigo (D)
Urine scald (D)

Focal/Multifocal
Calcinosis cutis (D)
Demodicosis (D)
Eosinophilic plaque (C)
Indolent ulcer (C)
Intertrigo (D)
Neoplasia (D, C)
Pyoderma (principally pyotraumatic dermatitis or folliculitis) (D)
Systemic/subcutaneous mycosis (D, C)

Facial
Arthropod bites (D, C)
Bullous pemphigoid (D, C)
Deep pyoderma (D)
Demodicosis (D)
Dermatomyositis (D)
Discoid lupus erythematosus (D)
Linear IgA bullous disease (D)
Pemphigus foliaceus/erythematosus (D, C)
Solar injury (D, C)
Squamous cell carcinoma (C)

Systemic/subcutaneous mycosis (D, C)
Uveodermatologic syndrome (D)

Mucocutaneous
Bacteria (aerobic/anaerobic) (D, C)
Bullous pemphigoid (D, C)
Bullous systemic lupus-type 1 (D)
Epidermolysis bullosa aquisita (D)
Epitheliotropic lymphoma (D)
Fungal (*M. pachydermatis*, *Candida* spp.) (D)
Mucocutaneous pemphigoid (D)
Pemphigus vulgaris (D)
Toxic epidermal necrosis/erythema multiforme (D, C)
Uremia (D, C)
Viral infection (calicivirus/herpesvirus) (C)

Generalized/Extensive
Bullous pemphigoid (D)
Deep pyoderma (D)
Demodicosis (D)
Drug reaction (D, C)
Epitheliotropic lymphoma (D)
Malassezia dermatitis (D)
Pemphigus group (D, C)
Thermal injury (D, C)
Toxic epidermal necrolysis/erythema multiforme (D, C)

D, Dog; *C*, cat.

to dental disease, immunosuppression, and systemic diseases.

Opportunist or atypical mycobacterial infections may occur when feline skin is inoculated with soil or water harboring the organism via traumatic injury. Affected cats exhibit chronic nonhealing wounds and ulcers with draining tracts. Systemic signs are usually absent.

Fungal Disease

In recent years, infection of the skin surface associated with the yeast *M. pachydermatis* has been recognized in dogs. Ulceration is not a feature, but the affected skin may be eroded. Lesions usually occur in intertriginous regions, particularly in predisposed breeds (Basset Hounds, West Highland Terriers, and English Cocker Spaniels). The lesions are characterized by intense erythema, a yellow waxy crust, and malodor. Dermatophytosis may lead to eroded and ulcerated lesions in dogs and cats. Diagnosis is based on cytology, culture, and response to antifungal therapy.

Subcutaneous and systemic fungal infections are far less common. Impression smears and histopathology are indicated. Therapy is dependant on the organism involved.

OTHER CAUSES OF EROSIONS AND ULCERS

Parasitic Infections

Infestation with mites such as *Sarcoptes scabiei* or *Cheyletiella* spp. may lead to self-induced erosions and ulcers. Severe cases of demodicosis may, less commonly, lead to ulceration. Skin scrapings are diagnostic and mandatory.

Metabolic Disease

Calcinosis cutis is caused by accumulation of calcium in the skin, usually as a result of hyperadrenocorticism (naturally occurring or iatrogenic). Ulcers may develop over these mineral plaques. Histopathology is diagnostic. Treatment of the underlying systemic disease is usually curative.

Hepatic cirrhosis or pancreatic adenocarcinomata may lead to cutaneous ulceration that particularly affects the feet and perineum of older dogs. This disease has a range of synonyms, including hepatocutaneous syndrome, necrolytic migratory erythema, and metabolic epidermal necrosis.

Uremia as the result of renal failure may lead to oral ulceration. In cats, diabetes mellitus and hyperadrenocorticism may also lead to this phenomenon. Signs of systemic disease are usually present (e.g., anorexia, depression, dehydration). Halitosis is a feature. Urinalysis along with clinical biochemistry and hematology are usually diagnostic.

Neoplasia

Squamous cell carcinoma is a common feline neoplasm particularly affecting the extremities of white or lightly pigmented cats (e.g., ear tips, planum nasale). White English Bull Terriers are also predisposed. The prevalence of squamous cell carcinoma is greater in warmer climates. Waterproof, high sun–protection factor cream should be applied to animals at risk. Ideally, access to sunshine should be restricted.

Epitheliotropic lymphoma leads to nodular, scaling, eroded, and erythematous skin lesions in older dogs. Oral lesions (erythema, erosion) occur in the majority of cases. The prognosis is grave, with therapy having little influence on survival time.

Diagnosis of cutaneous neoplasia is by histopathology, although cytology of fine needle aspirates and impression smears may be helpful.

Physical and Chemical Diseases

Such diseases can usually be diagnosed with history: exposure to extreme cold or scalding, recent treatment with medicaments, or (in the case of urine scalding) clinical examination. Solar-induced disease may be more difficult to diagnose because the onset is chronic and some manifestations of solar dermatoses may resemble other diseases.

Immune-Mediated and Autoimmune Diseases

Although this group is ascribed much significance by clinicians, these diseases are uncommon or rare. Lesions arise when tissue is damaged as a result of an inappropriate immunologic response. In autoimmune diseases, antibodies directed against a tissue component elicit an inflammatory response that may lead to cleavage of the epidermis from the underlying dermis (e.g., bullous pemphigoid, epidermolysis bullosa acquisita) or splitting within the epidermis itself (e.g., the pemphigus group). In some diseases, the precise pathologic mechanism is unknown (e.g., discoid lupus erythematosus).

The differentiation of the different immune-mediated diseases is important and made by histopathology. The different diseases respond to different forms of therapy, and the prognosis varies between them. If a definitive diagnosis is not obtained, there is a risk of treating a benign disease too aggressively with immune-suppressive agents.

Miscellaneous Diseases

Dermatomyositis is a hereditary disorder primarily affecting the face and distal limbs of Rough and Shetland Collie (Shelties) pups, leading to alopecia, erosions, ulceration, and scarring. It probably arises from immune-mediated vasculitis. Idiopathic ulceration is also seen in these breeds; previously it was thought that it may share its cause and pathogenesis with dermatomyositis. However, recent evidence suggests that it may be a form of lupoid dermatitis.

Idiopathic ulceration principally affects the ventral abdomen and groin and usually occurs in middle-aged Rough and Shetland Collie dogs. The prognosis is guarded because it is refractory to treatment in most cases.

Congenital diseases may affect the basement membrane and lead to ulceration and erosion. Examples include junctional epidermolysis bullosa and dystrophic epidermolysis bullosa.

CHAPTER 18

Papules and Pustules

Jacques Fontaine

Papules and pustules are important primary lesions observed in dogs, giving the practitioner an opportunity to potentially discriminate the cause of a dermatitis (Table 18-1 and Figure 18-1).

Papules and pustules are rarely observed in cats. A papule is a small (up to 1 cm), well–circumscribed, solid elevation of the skin. Papules are usually erythematous but can have any color (Web Figure 18-1).

Papules can affect the epthithelium or the dermis. A pustule is a small, focal collection of yellow-green fluid, containing polymorphonuclear leukocytes, localized in the epithelium (Web Figure 18-2).

Pustules may appear following neutrophil-mediated inflammation, as observed in bacterial folliculitis, or they may be caused by gradual polymorphonuclear leukocyte accumulation in a preexisting clear vesicle, as occurs in pemphigus foliaceous.

Papules may develop into pustules and crusts. Pustules naturally will form crusts and epidermal collarettes. Some diseases do not develop into pustules (hypersensitivity reaction).

The most important point in approaching the differential diagnosis regarding papules/pustules is to clarify if the lesions are follicular or nonfollicular. Follicular lesions indicate a pathologic process centered on the hair unit. The main causes are bacterial folliculitis, demodicosis, or dermatophytosis.

Nonfollicular lesions indicate a pathologic process affecting the epidermis, the dermis, or the dermo-epidermal junction.

FOLLICULAR LESIONS

Bacterial Pyoderma

Bacterial pyoderma is probably the most common dermatitis in dogs. In cats, pyoderma is quite rare (Web Figure 18-3). The exception in cats would be deep pyodermas and abscesses derived from fighting bites. If papules/pustules are the most characteristic lesions observed in bacterial pyoderma, other cutaneous signs that may be observed include erythema, scaling, focal alopecia, and crusting. Pruritus is often observed that induces excoriations.

Bacteria are normal residents of the canine skin (staphylocci spp., mainly *Staphylococcus intermedius*; *Micrococcus* spp.; *Clostridium* spp.; *Acinetobacter* spp.; *Propionibacterium acnes*; and *Streptococcus* alpha-hemolytic). In some conditions, the bacterial populations can change in quantity (overgrowth) and quality (usually *S. intermedius* but sometimes *Pseudomonas*, *Escherichia coli*, *Proteus mirabilis*, *Corynebacterium* spp., and *Staphylococcus aureus*) inducing a dermatitis. Pyoderma must be then considered as a secondary disease where the adherence of bacteria at the surface of the skin is modified and bacterial overgrowth occurs. The classical disease associ-

Table • 18-1

Differential Diagnoses in Dogs with Papules and Pustules

DISEASES	PAPULES	PUSTULES	PRURITUS	CLUES	DIAGNOSTIC TEST
Bacterial pyoderma	Yes	Yes	Variable (often)	The most frequent cause	Cytology: neutrophils, phagocytized bacteria
Demodicosis	Yes	Yes	Rare (except if pyoderma)	Furuncles Alopecia Comedons	Skin scraping, hair plucks, cytology showing parasites
Dermatophytosis	Rare	Very unusual	Variable	Alopecia	Wood lamp, trichogram, fungal cultures
Sarcoptic mange	Yes	No	Yes	Crusts	Skin scrapings, therapeutic trial
Cheyletiellosis	Rare	No	Variable (often)	Scales	Skin scrapings, therapeutic trial
Otacariosis	Rare	No	Yes	Otitis	Otoscopy, skin scrapings
Trombiculosis	Yes	Very unusual	Yes	Red bugs seen	Red bugs seen (feet)
Hypersensitivity	Yes	Very unusual	Yes	Rule out all other dermatitis	Rule out all other dermatitis. No specific test available.
Pemphigus	Yes	Yes (fugacious)	Variable	Acanthocytes Crusts	Pustule cytology, biopsy
Early stage neoplasia	Yes	No	Variable	Nodules	Cytopuncture, biopsy

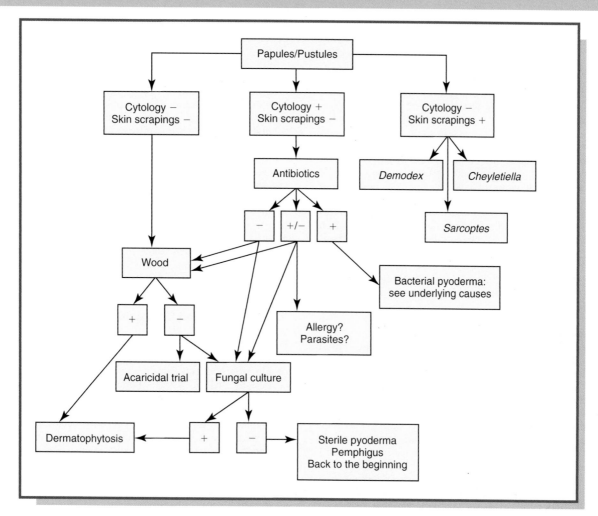

Figure 18-1 Algorithm: papules/pustules diagnosis. (Modified from Mueller RS: The dog with papules, pustules and crusts. In Mueller RS, editor: Dermatology for small animal practitioner, Jackson, Wyo, 2000, Teton NewMedia.)

ated with recurrent pyoderma is canine atopic dermatitis. Other causes to be ruled out include parasitic dermatitis (demodicosis), immunodeficiency secondary to hypothyroidism or hyperadrenocorticism, and keratinization dysfunctions. Depending on the level of the bacterial infection, pyodermas are classified as surface pyoderma, superficial pyoderma, or deep pyoderma. The most "classic" pustules are observed in superficial pyoderma.

Demodicosis

Canine demodicosis is one of the more common skin diseases encountered in veterinary practice. *Demodex canis* is considered as a normal component of canine cutaneous ecology. This parasite can, in some circumstances, overpopulate an area and cause dermatitis. Two forms of demodicosis are recognized: a localized form and a generalized form.

Localized demodicosis occurs most commonly in dogs less than 1 year of age. The typical lesions are patches of erythema and alopecia. Spontaneous remissions occur in most. Generalized demodicosis (involvement of a body region; more than four focal areas; or more than one paw) can induce formation of follicular papules (often associated with erythema, comedones, and follicular casts). Secondary bacterial complications that include pustules and furunculosis are often observed. Demodicosis can typically be diagnosed with deep skin scrapings, hair plucks, or via cytology of an intact pustule (Web Figure 18-4).

Demodex is often observed in pus without staining the slide.

Dermatophytosis

Dermatophytoses are infections of the skin and its appendages caused by a group of closely related species of fungi, dermatophytes (*Microsporum* spp., *Trichophyton* spp., or *Epidermophyton* spp.). Dermatophytes are filamentous fungi having a important tropism for keratin-containing structures (epidermis and follicular units). Dermatophytes produce enzymes that can digest the complex proteins of keratin and then induce skin lesions: papules, pustules, alopecia. While papules and pustules are classically observed in people who have dermatophytosis, such lesions are rarely observed in dogs and cats because they are hidden by fur (they can be observed in nude pets) (Web Figure 18-5).

In rare cases, pustules with acantholytic cells can be observed in *Trichophyton mentagrophytes* infection. This condition must be differentiated from the pemphigus foliaceus.

NONFOLLICULAR LESIONS

Impetigo

Impetigo is a variant of a bacterial superficial pyoderma where the lesions are not centered on the hair follicle. Papules and pustules are classically observed on the ventrum in young dogs. When the condition is observed in older animals, it is usually associated with immunodeficiency. Treatment is similar for all bacterial superficial pyodermas (antibiotics).

Sarcoptic Mange

Sarcoptic mange is a highly contagious, nonseasonal, pruritic skin condition caused by infestation with *Sarcoptes scabiei var. canis*. Sarcoptic mange occurs commonly in dogs but has occasionally been reported in cats. In dogs, the disease typically presents as an intensely pruritic, papulocrustous dermatosis classically affecting the pinnal margins, the elbows, and the hocks. Periumbilical papules and crusts can sometimes be observed. In a late stage of the disease, papules and crusts can be observed in all parts of the body (Web Figure 18-6).

Definitive diagnosis is based on the demonstration of mites and/or eggs by skin scrapings. Microscopic diagnosis is often difficult. Determination by enzyme-linked immunosorbent assay may be useful but is not available everywhere in the world. An alternative and commonly used diagnostic "test" is response to a therapeutic trial (a favorable response to therapy is only a proof of a parasitic problem, not a confirmation of sarcoptic mange infestation).

Cheyletiellosis

Cheyletiellosis is an extremely contagious dermatitis caused by mites living on the skin surface. *Cheyletiella* spp. are not specific to the host and may readily transfer between dogs, cats, and rabbits. Humans in contact with pets carrying *Cheyletiella* spp. may also be transiently infested. Young animals are particularly susceptible. The lesions typically occur on the dorsum and are mainly characterized by excessive scaling (sometimes associated to a mild erythema). In rare cases, a papular eruption can be observed (hypersensitivity reaction) (Web Figure 18-7).

Cheyletiella can be the cause of pyotraumatic dermatitis or recurrent pyoderma. In cats, papulocrustous lesions (miliary dermatitis) may also develop. Pruritus is variable from one case to another and an asymptomatic carrier status can exist (treat all the pets in contact). As recommended for sarcoptic mange, a therapeutic trial is indicated in suspected cases.

Otoacariosis

Otodectes cynotis is a well known parasite of the ear canals of dogs and cats. Rarely, the parasites can move from the ear canal to the skin surface. A papulocrustous dermatitis (miliary dermatitis) may be then observed.

Neotrombiculosis (Harvest Mite)

The harvest mites (*Neotrombicula automnalis*, also known as red bugs) during their larval stage can attach the skin to various animals, including dogs, cats or humans. *Neotrombicula* can induce a papular reaction that can cause intense pruritus. The skin areas most frequently affected are the folds in the feet but also the ventral thorax and abdomen (the zone in contact with the grass where the larvae live) (Web Figure 18-8).

Hypersensitivity (Fleas, Contact Hypersensitivity, Atopic Dermatitis)

It is commonly accepted that there is no typical primary lesion for hypersensitivity reactions. Some pets have primary erythematous macular, papular eruptions or pustules. It is obviously quite difficult to discriminate a primary reaction from a secondary response to infection.

Microscopic examinations of lesional skin biopsies after challenging with allergens in the surface of the epidermis in sensitized dogs show the recruitment of inflammatory cells (neutrophils and eosinophils) in the epidermis and the formation of intraepidermal microabcesses. In cats, miliary dermatitis is a classical form of papulocrustous dermatitis evoking a response to a hypersensitivity process (atopic dermatitis, food allergy, flea bite hypersensitivity). The differential diagnosis must nevertheless consider: dermatophytosis, cheyletiellosis, staphylococcal folliculitis.

Immune-Mediated Dermatitis: Pemphigus Foliaceus (PF)

Pemphigus is a rare immune-mediated vesicobullous to pustular skin disease that is characterized by acantholysis or loss of adhesion between keratinocytes.

Lesions include papulo-pustules, crusts, erosions, ulcers, and alopecia (Web Figure 18-9).

Pustules are sometimes difficult to observe because they are fragile and quickly evolve to become a crust. Acantholytic cells characteristic of the PF can be observed in intact pustules or under a recently formed crust. Some cases may remain localized to the head, face, and pinnae (especially in cats), while others may generalize. In some cases lesions (crusts) can be limited to the footpads. Pruritus is quite common in the generalized form.

Neoplasia

Early in development, some round-cell neoplasias (mast cell tumor, lymphoma, histiocytoma) can be misinterpreted as a benign papule (Web Figure 18-10).

This is rarely observed because usually these papular lesions are hidden by the hair or are not considered important at the beginning. When the lesions become more severe (stage with multiple tumors), it is often possible to observe some beginning lesions evocating a papule.

References

The reference list can be found on the companion Expert Consult Web site at *www.expertconsult.com*.

CHAPTER 19

Scaling and Crusting Dermatoses

Kinga Gortel
Jonathan D. Plant

PATHOPHYSIOLOGY

Scaling and crusting are common findings in many cutaneous diseases (Figure 19-1, Table 19-1).

Scaling refers to the accumulation of loose fragments of cornified cells on the skin surface (Figure 19-2, Web Figure 19-1).

Normal desquamation of cornified cells is not visible to the naked eye, so scales are only seen when loss occurs in larger flakes. Scales are usually secondary lesions in chronically inflamed skin but may also be primary lesions in conditions such as primary seborrhea and ichthyosis.

Crusting occurs when dried exudates or secretions adhere to the surface of the skin (Figure 19-3).

Crusts may be composed of thick scales, pus, blood, serum, or other exudates. They are also usually secondary, occurring on skin traumatized due to pruritus or in any pustular dermatosis. Crusts may be primary in some conditions such as miliary dermatitis and zinc-responsive dermatosis.

SIGNALMENT

Species

Skin diseases differ greatly in incidence between dogs and cats. Pyoderma should be one of the first considerations when scaling or crusting is seen in dogs. In contrast, cats are uncommonly affected by pyoderma, but dermatophytosis is a prime cause of lesions in this species.

Age

The age of onset of the skin lesions can be helpful in narrowing down the differential diagnoses, particularly in very young or geriatric dogs and cats. Puppies and kittens that develop scaling within the first several months of life should be evaluated for infections (such as demodicosis in dogs and dermatophytosis in cats) and congenital dermatoses. In geriatric dogs, in addition to the more common causes of scaling, consideration should be given to cutaneous lymphoma, demodicosis, superficial necrolytic dermatitis, and other metabolic or endocrine disorders.

Breed

Breeds with an inherited predisposition to the development of primary scaling and crusting disorders include American Cocker Spaniels, English Springer Spaniels, West Highland White Terriers, Basset Hounds, Irish Setters, Doberman Pinschers, and Labrador Retrievers. Breed predispositions are also noted in many other dermatoses that lead to scaling and crusting, including canine atopic dermatitis, hypothyroidism, and sebaceous adenitis.

HISTORICAL FINDINGS

The history can be helpful in narrowing the list of differential diagnoses in an animal with scaling or crusting. The age and site of onset should be established. A most important consideration is the degree of accompanying pruritus. Diseases that are often severely pruritic include sarcoptic acariasis, atopic dermatitis, flea bite hypersensitivity, food hypersensitivity, *Malassezia* dermatitis, and cutaneous lymphoma. The owner should also be questioned as to seasonality of the scaling and crusting. If other in-contact animals or humans are affected, this should be taken into consideration. The response of the lesions and pruritus, if present, to previous treatments such as antibiotics, steroids, or antifungal medications is helpful.

PHYSICAL EXAMINATION

Lesions

Scaling and crusting are often found concurrently. The skin should be examined for pustules, papules, excoriation, erythema, and ulceration. The shape and pattern of crusted or scaly areas should be noted (e.g., circular, epidermal collarettes, discrete, multifocal).

Distribution

Scaling and crusting dermatoses may be generalized or have site predilections. Site predilections include but are not limited to the nasal planum (e.g., pemphigus foliaceus, discoid lupus erythematosus, idiopathic hyperkeratosis, squamous cell carcinoma), footpads (e.g., pemphigus foliaceus, zinc-responsive dermatosis, superficial necrolytic dermatitis, plasma cell pododermatitis), and ear pinnae (e.g., sarcoptic acariasis, ear margin seborrhea).

DIAGNOSTIC PLAN

Skin scrapings and cytologic examination are simple and often useful for evaluating dogs or cats with scaling and crusting.

Skin scrapings are most useful for finding *Demodex canis* in dogs and *Notoedres cati* in cats. They are far less sensitive for canine *Sarcoptes scabei*. Other parasites including *Cheyletiella*, *Demodex gatoi*, and lice are found with varying success on skin scrapings. Some ectoparasites are groomed and licked off the coat and may be found using fecal floatation technique. In addition to skin scrapings, clear tape may be pressed on the skin and examined microscopically to look for surface-dwelling ectoparasites.

Text continued on p. 93

 To view a video on this topic, go to **www.expertconsult.com.**

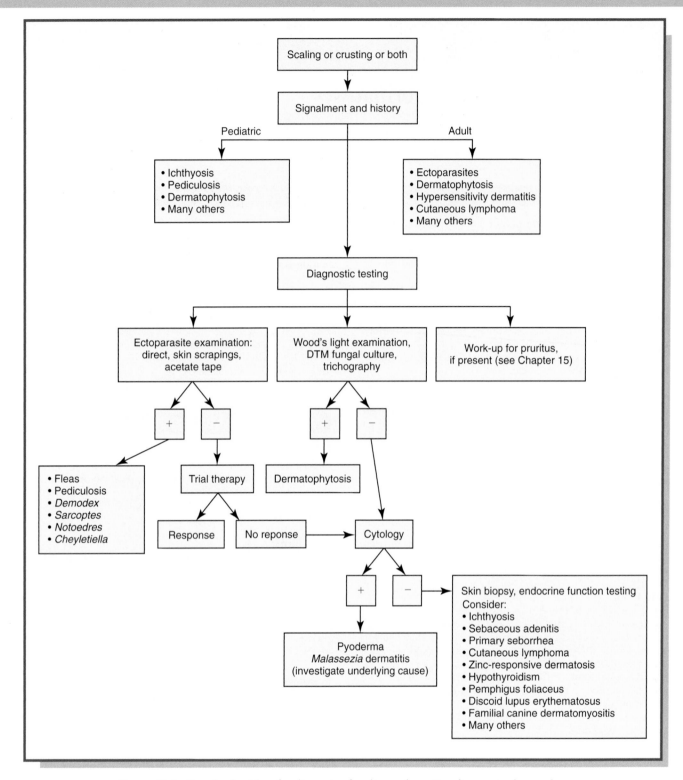

Figure 19-1 Sample algorithm for diagnosis of scaling and crusting diseases in dogs and cats. Prioritizing the differential diagnoses alters the order and choice of diagnostic tests (e.g., cytology may be more appropriate as the first step in certain conditions). *DTM,* Dermatophyte test medium.

Table • 19-1

Scaling and Crusting Diseases of Dogs and Cats

DISEASE	SPECIES	LESION	SIGNALMENT	LESION DISTRIBUTION	FREQUENCY	PRURITUS	DIAGNOSIS
Bacterial							
Superficial folliculitis	Dog, (Cat)	Crusts, scales, collarettes, pustules	Varies—most common cause of crusting in dog	Trunk	VC	– to ++	CS, Cyt, BC, Bx
Deep pyoderma	Dog, Cat	Crusts, ulcers	Varies	Trunk, feet, chin	C	+	CS, Cyt, BC, Bx
Mucocutaneous pyoderma	Dog	Crusts, ulcers	German Shepherd Dog or other	Lips, peribuccal	U	+ (painful)	CS, Bx, Cyt
Pyotraumatic dermatitis	Dog	Moist crust, exudation, erythema	Any (often flea-related)	Face, neck, caudal trunk	VC	++	CS
Fungal							
Dermatophytosis	Cat, Dog	Crusts, scales, alopecia, erythema	Young most frequently Should always be considered in cats	Head, extremities, trunk	C	– to ++	DTM, Wood's light, trichogram
Malassezia dermatitis	Dog, Cat	Crusts, scales, erythema, lichenification	Adult most frequently	Axillary, groin, interdigital, facial	C	+++	Cyt
Deep fungal infection (blastomycosis, cryptococcosis, other)	Dog, Cat	Nodules with possible crusting; systemic signs may be seen	Any	Depends on species of fungus and host	U	Variable	Bx, Cyt, confirmatory blood tests
Parasitic							
Ctenocephalides felis (flea)	Dog, Cat	Scales, erythema	Any	Lumbosacral, neck	C	+	CS, parasite exam
Sarcoptes scabei	Dog	Crusts, scales, excoriations, alopecia, erythema	Any	Pinnal margins, lateral elbows, ventrum	C	+++	SS, response to therapy
Demodex canis	Dog	Crusts, scales, exudation, alopecia, erythema	Young or immunocompromised adults	From single lesions on the head to generalized	C	– to +	SS
Cheyletiella spp.	Dog, Cat	Scales—may be very excessive	Young most frequently	Dorsal trunk to generalized	U	– to ++	SS, tape impression
Notoedres cati	Cat	Crusts, scales	Any	Head, feet, generalized	U	– to +++	SS
Pediculosis	Dog, Cat	Pruritus, nits may resemble scales attached to hair	Any	Variable	U	+ to +++	CS, SS, trichogram

BC, Bacterial culture; Bx, skin biopsy; C, common; CS, clinical signs; Cyt, cytology; DTM, dermatophyte test medium fungal culture; Hx, history; IgE, allergen-specific serum IgE assay; IDAT, allergen-specific intradermal allergy test; MDB, minimum data base (complete blood count, serum biochemistry, urinalysis); NSF, no significant findings; R, rare; SS, skin scraping; U, uncommon; VC, very common; +, positive; –, negative.

Continued

Table • 19-1

Scaling and Crusting Diseases of Dogs and Cats—cont'd

DISEASE	LESION	SPECIES	SIGNALMENT	LESION DISTRIBUTION	FREQUENCY	PRURITUS	DIAGNOSIS
Protozoal							
Leishmaniasis	Scales, alopecia, onychogryphosis	Dog, (Cat)	Any, Foxhounds	Muzzle, periocular, pinnae	Regionally variable	–	Bx, Cyt, serology, other
Viral							
Feline leukemia virus	Crusts, scales, erosions	Cat	Any	Face, pinnae, perioral, feet, trunk	U	++	Serology, Bx
Allergic							
Atopic dermatitis	Erythema, alopecia, crusts (excoriation), scales, others	Dog, Cat	All, dogs often 1-5 years old	Face, ears, feet, ventrum	C	+ to +++	CS, IDAT, IgE
Food hypersensitivity	Erythema, crusts (excoriation), others	Dog, Cat	All, any age	Any	C	+ to +++	Food trial
Flea bite hypersensitivity	Erythema, crusts (excoriation), others	Dog, Cat	All	Caudal dorsum, ventrum, thighs	C	++ to +++	Response to flea control
Miliary dermatitis	Small hemorrhagic crusts	Cat	All (often associated with fleas)	Dorsum	C	++	CS
Endocrine and Metabolic							
Hyperadrenocorticism	Alopecia, cutaneous atrophy, calcinosis cutis, crusts (pyoderma)	Dog, (Cat)	Middle aged, older	Trunk	C	– (calcinois cutis ++)	MDB, hormone assays, imaging, Bx
Hypothyroidism	Scaling, dry skin, pyoderma, +/– alopecia	Dog	Middle aged, often large breed	Generalized	C	–	MDB, thyroid assay
Necrolytic migratory erythema	Severe adherent crusting	Dog, (Cat)	Old	Muzzle, footpads, pressure points	R	+ to ++ (painful)	Bx, MDB, imaging, liver assays, plasma amino acids
Immune-Mediated							
Pemphigus foliaceus	Crusts, pustules	Dog, Cat	Any age and sex; Akita, Chow Chow, others	Nasal planum, muzzle, pinnae, foot pads, trunk	U	– to +	Bx

Disease	Lesions	Species	Breed/Age	Location	Incidence	Pruritus	Tests
Discoid lupus erythematosus	Crusts, depigmentation erosions, ulcers	Dog, (Cat)	Collies, Shetland Sheepdog, and other breeds	Nasal planum, muzzle	U	–	Bx
Erythema multiforme	Crusts, vesicles erythema, target lesions, erosions, ulcers	Dog, Cat	Any	Axillae, groin, mucocutaneous junctions	U	–	Bx
Congenital and Hereditary							
Primary seborrhea	Excessive scaling, or greasy skin	Dog, (Cat)	Onset before 6 months, American Cocker Spaniel and others	Generalized	U	– to ++, esp. with secondary infections	Bx
Ichthyosis	Excessive generalized scaling, mild to very severe	Dog, (Cat)	Present from birth, Golden Retriever, West Highland White Terrier, other	Generalized	R	–	Bx
Schnauzer comedo syndrome	Comedones that may become crusted	Dog	Miniature Schnauzer	Dorsum	C	–	CS, Bx
Familial canine dermatomyositis	Alopecia, scaling, depigmentation	Dog	Onset before 6 months, Collie, Shetland Sheepdog, other	Face, pressure points	U	–	Cs, Bx
Keratinization Defects							
Secondary seborrhea	Excessive scaling, or greasy skin	Dog, Cat	Any age	Depends on primary cause	C	– to +++ depending on cause	CS, any appropriate tests for primary disease
Vitamin A-responsive dermatosis	Marked follicular plugging, hyperkeratotic plaques	Dog	Cocker Spaniel, other, adult onset	Generalized, more pronounced on ventrum	U	– to ++	CS, Bx
Ear margin dermatosis	Follicular casts and scaling	Dog	Dachshund, others	Ear margins, lateral and medial	U	–, may become painful	CS, Bx

BC, Bacterial culture; *Bx*, skin biopsy; *C*, common; *CS*, clinical signs; *Cyt*, cytology; *DTM*, dermatophyte test medium fungal culture; *Hx*, history; *IgE*, allergen-specific serum IgE assay; *IDAT*, allergen-specific intradermal allergy test; *MDB*, minimum data base (complete blood count, serum biochemistry, urinalysis); *NSF*, no significant findings; *R*, rare; *SS*, skin scraping; *U*, uncommon; *VC*, very common; +, positive; –, negative.

Continued

Table • 19-1

Scaling and Crusting Diseases of Dogs and Cats—cont'd

DISEASE	LESION	SPECIES	SIGNALMENT	LESION DISTRIBUTION	FREQUENCY	PRURITUS	DIAGNOSIS
Environmental							
Solar dermatitis	Erythema, scaling, may progress to exudation and crusting	Dog, Cat	Light-haired animals, outdoor exposure	Nasal planum and bridge of nose, pinnae (Cat), ventrum (Dog)	C in sunny areas	− to +	CS, Bx
Nutritional							
Zinc-responsive dermatosis	Crusts, scales, erythema, alopecia	Dog	Siberian Husky, Alaskan Malamute; young adults	Periocular, perioral, mucocutaneous junctions, pressure points	U	− to +	Bx
Fatty acid deficiency	Scales	Dog, Cat	Any	Generalized	R	− to ++	Dietary Hx
Other							
Cutaneous lymphoma	Lesions highly variable but may include severe scaling	Dog , Cat	Older animals	Generalized or localized	U	− to +++	Bx
Granulomatous sebaceous adenitis	Hyperkeratosis, alopecia, follicular casts, may be erythematous	Dog, (Cat)	Young to middle aged, Standard Poodle, Akita, and others	Face, trunk, pinnae, become generalized	C	− to ++	CS, Bx
Otitis externa	Scale, erythema, otic exudate If scale on outer pinnal margins, consider *Sarcoptes*	Dog, (Cat)	Any	Pinnae, ear canal	C	++	Otoscopic examination, Cyt, BC

BC, Bacterial culture; *Bx,* skin biopsy; *C,* common; *CS,* clinical signs; *Cyt,* cytology; *DTM,* dermatophyte test medium fungal culture; *Hx,* history; *IgE,* allergen-specific serum IgE assay; *IDAT,* allergen-specific intradermal allergy test; *MDB,* minimum data base (complete blood count, serum biochemistry, urinalysis); *NSF,* no significant findings; *R,* rare; *SS,* skin scraping; *U,* uncommon; *VC,* very common; *+,* positive; *−,* negative.

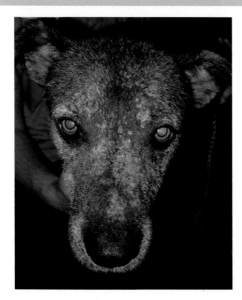

Figure 19-2 Scaling in a dog with juvenile generalized demodicosis.

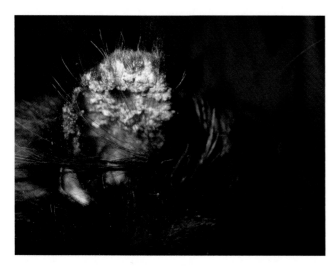

Figure 19-3 Thick crusting on the pinna of a cat with pemphigus foliaceus.

Samples for cytologic examination of the skin may be collected directly from the surface of greasy or moist skin by impression smears, or after the removal of crusts or adherent scales (Web Figure 19-2).

If pustules are present their contents can be smeared on a slide. Waxy or dry samples benefit from gentle heat fixing. A modified Wright's stain (e.g., Diff-Quik) is recommended for examining slides. Cytology is most useful for confirming and quantitating bacteria and yeast. Inflammatory responses of skin can also be evaluated, as neutrophils, eosinophils, and mononuclear cells are easily differentiated. The presence of numerous acantholytic cells among neutrophils suggests pemphigus but is occasionally encountered in other inflammatory conditions. An additional technique particularly well-suited to detecting *Malassezia* is the tape impression preparation. Using this method, the tape is stained and examined under oil immersion to reveal the yeast.

Examination for fungi should be attempted when dermatophytosis is suspected. Cats with scaling and crusting should always be cultured for dermatophytes unless another cause is readily identified. A Wood's light examination is an adequate preliminary test, but a DTM (dermatophyte test medium) fungal culture should always be inoculated if dermatophytosis is suspected. Trichograms, the direct examination of plucked hair, are far less sensitive for dermatophytes. Trichograms can, however, reveal parasites such as *Demodex*, louse eggs (nits), as well as excessive "plugs" of keratin around the hair shafts suggestive of sebaceous adenitis or keratinization disorders.

Skin biopsies are needed to make a definitive diagnosis in some scaling and crusting disorders, including immune-mediated diseases, neoplastic conditions, and primary keratinization disorders. Any unusual, severe, or poorly responsive lesions are good candidates for histopathologic examination. Crust and scale must be included in the sample, so the biopsy sites should never be cleaned or scrubbed, and extra crusts may even be submitted. Hair may be gently cut with scissors without disrupting any surface material. If secondary infection with *Malassezia* or bacteria is present, it is advantageous to treat before the biopsy samples collected. Biopsy samples should be selected so as to represent early lesions such as papules, pustules, depigmentation, or erythematosus skin as well as the more mature lesions of scales and crusts.

A minimum data base (complete blood count, serum chemistry, urinalysis) is most useful in middle-aged and older animals when endocrine or metabolic causes are suspected. Thyroid hormone and adrenal function testing should be considered if history and physical examination indicate that such conditions are likely. Bacterial culture should be performed when bacteria are still found on cytology despite adequate treatment for pyoderma, or if rod-shaped bacteria are noted rather than the typical cocci of *Staphylococcus*.

TREATMENT

Whenever possible, the specific cause of scaling and crusting dermatoses should be identified and addressed. Even more than other cutaneous conditions, diseases with excessive scaling and crusting can benefit greatly from appropriate topical therapy. Active ingredients should be selected based on the underlying condition and are most frequently applied as shampoos and conditioners. Active ingredients may be keratolytic, keratoplastic, degreasing, antimicrobial, antiparasitic, antiinflammatory, antipruritic, or moisturizing. Many dogs with generalized scaling and crusting disorders will benefit from frequent bathing (twice a week or more).

CHAPTER 20

Changes in Pigmentation

Karen L. Campbell

The most important factor in the coloration of skin and hair is its content of melanin. Melanin is produced by melanocytes located in the basal layer of the epidermis and in the outer root sheath and hair matrix of hair follicles. Melanocytes originate in the neural crest and migrate to the skin during early embryogenesis. The production of melanin is affected by genetics, hormones, heat, injury, solar or ionizing radiation, heavy metals, and other factors.[1,2] Changes in any of these factors can increase or decrease pigment production.

Hypopigmentation is the general term for a decrease in pigment. *Leukoderma* is the term for a lack of pigment in the skin; *leukotrichia* is a lack of pigment in the hair. A decrease in pigment in the hair is called *graying* or *poliosis*. *Hyperpigmentation* is the general term for an increase in pigment. *Melanoderma* is the term for increased pigment in the skin; *melanotrichia* is increased pigment in the hair. *Aurotrichia* is the term for hair that is gold colored.

Pigmentary changes are frequently seen in veterinary medicine; some are only of cosmetic concern while others are associated with systemic disease. Figure 20-1 provides an algorithm for evaluation of changes in pigmentation.

HYPOPIGMENTATION

Decreased pigmentation may be due to melanocyte destruction, dysfunction, or an abnormal distribution of melanosomes. Hypopigmentation may be hereditary or acquired.

Hereditary Hypopigmentation

Albinism Albinism is a hereditary absence of pigment, usually due to a deficiency in tyrosinase, an enzyme required for melanin production. Pigment is absent from both skin and hair, the eyes are usually blue. Albinism in cats and dogs is an autosomal recessive trait.

Piebaldism Piebaldism refers to the presence of white spots where melanocytes are absent. This is inherited as a dominant trait in dogs.

Waardenburg-Klein Syndrome Waardenburg-Klein syndrome has been reported in cats, Bull Terriers, Sealyham Terriers, Collies, and Dalmatians. Affected animals have an absence of melanocytes in areas of their skin and hair, have blue or heterochromic eyes, and are also deaf. It is inherited as an autosomal dominant trait with variable penetrance.

Canine Cyclic Hematopoiesis Canine cyclic hematopoiesis is a lethal autosomal recessive disease of Collies characterized by a gray haircoat (Figure 20-2), light-colored nose, and cyclic episodes of neutropenia every 12 to 14 days resulting in recurrent episodes of sepsis and amyloidosis. This is an autosomal recessive disease in which the dilute coat color is linked to a dysfunction of the pluripotential stem cells in the bone marrow.[3,4]

Chédiak-Higashi Syndrome Chédiak-Higashi syndrome is a rare, autosomal recessive disease in blue smoke Persian cats. It is characterized by partial oculocutaneous albinism with abnormal function of granulocytes and platelets resulting in bleeding problems, recurrent infections, and death at a young age.

Graying Age-associated graying results from a reduction of melanocyte replication and is most commonly seen in German Shepherd Dogs, Irish Setters, Labrador Retrievers, and Golden Retrievers.

Vitiligo Certain breeds of dogs and Siamese cats develop macular leukoderma and leukotrichia involving the nose, lips, ears, buccal mucosa, and facial skin (Figure 20-3).

Other areas of the haircoat and the footpads and claws may also be affected. Breeds of dogs most commonly affected include Belgian Tervuren dogs, German Shepherd Dogs, Collies, Rottweilers, Doberman Pinschers, and Giant Schnauzers. Antimelanocyte antibodies have been identified in the serum of some affected dogs. Biopsies typically reveal a complete absence of melanocytes in depigmented areas of skin.

Nasal Hypopigmentation (Dudley Nose, Snow Nose) Season-associated lightening in color of the planum nasale during winter months is common in Siberian Huskies, Golden Retrievers, Labrador Retrievers, and Bernese Mountain Dogs and is referred to as "snow nose." The nose darkens in the spring and summer. Many other breeds of dogs (including Afghan Hounds, Samoyeds, Siberian Huskies, Yellow Labrador Retrievers, German Shepherd Dogs, Golden Retrievers, Poodles, Doberman Pinschers, Irish Setters, and Pointers) have a gradual fading of their nose from black at birth to a chocolate brown or paler color. The color change may be permanent or may wax and wane. A nose that undergoes this form of depigmentation is commonly referred to as a "Dudley nose."

Acquired Hypopigmentation

Postinflammatory Inflammation affecting the epidermis or basement membrane zone may result in destruction or "drop-out" of melanocytes and a loss of pigment. Discoid lupus erythematosus is a common cause of nasal depigmentation (Figure 20-4).

Pemphigus erythematosus, systemic lupus erythematosus, pemphigus foliaceus, uveodermatologic syndrome, bullous pemphigoid, mucocutaneus pyoderma, and drug eruptions may also result in depigmentation of the nose and other areas. Infectious causes of nasal or skin depigmentation include leishmaniasis, blastomycosis, sporotrichosis, and bacterial folliculitis. Contact dermatitis may result in depigmentation of the skin of the nose, lips, and foot pads. Rubber may contain chemicals such as dihydroquinone and monobenzyl ethers, which interfere with melanin production. This

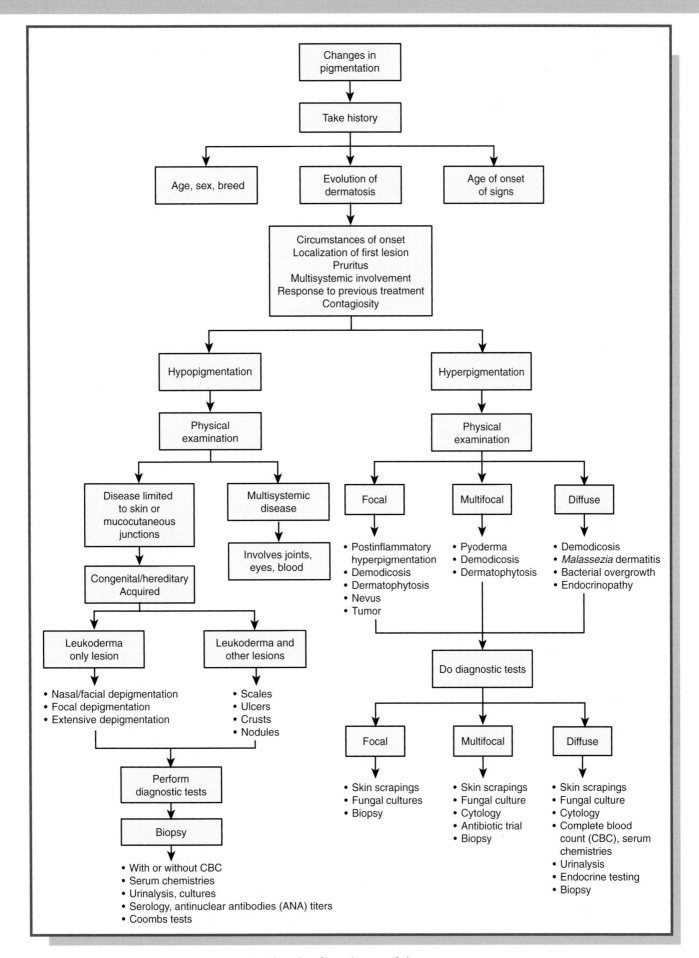

Figure 20-1 Algorithm for evaluation of changes in pigmentation.

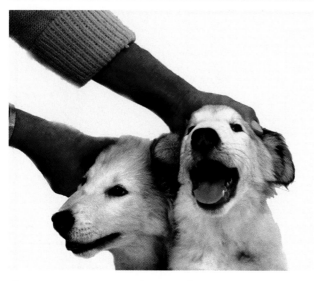

Figure 20-2 Gray coat color in Collies serves as a phenotypic marker for cyclic neutropenia; affected dogs have a cyclic maturation arrest in the bone marrow at the level of differentiation from the stem cell.

can result in depigmentation of areas in contact with the rubber.

Drug-Related Hypopigmentation Ketoconazole, procainamide, and vitamin E have been reported to cause diffuse lightening of coat color in some dogs. Subcutaneous injections of glucocorticoids and progestational compounds may result in localized areas of hypopigmentation. Chemicals such as monobenzyl ethers and hydroquinone interfere with pigment production; these chemicals are used in human medicine to depigment areas of skin.[5]

Nutritional/Metabolic Deficiencies in zinc, pyridoxine, pantothenic acid, and lysine have been associated with graying of the hair. Copper is another cofactor required for pigment production, and a copper deficiency has been reported to cause black hairs to develop a reddish-brown color. Recent studies in black cats have shown that diets low in tyrosine and/or phenylalanine cause such animals to develop reddish-brown haircoats that return to normal when the diet contains more than 18 g/kg of tyrosine + phenylalanine.[6-8] Other conditions that have been associated with hair becoming reddish in color include copper deficiency, hypothyroidism, hyperadrenocorticism, hyperestrogenism, hyperprogesteronism, chlorine exposure, and chronic exposure to ultraviolet light.

Neoplasia Associated Nasal depigmentation, leukoderma and leukotrichia are sometimes associated with epitheliotropic T cell lymphoma, basal cell tumors, mammary adenocarcinoma, and gastric carcinomas.

Idiopathic Leukotrichia and patchy hypopigmentation have been reported as idiopathic conditions in black Newfoundlands and also in black and chocolate Labrador Retrievers. Siamese cats may be affected with unilateral or bilateral periocular leukotrichia, which is sometimes associated with upper respiratory infections, pregnancy, dietary deficiencies, or systemic illnesses while in other cases there is no apparent precipitating cause.

HYPERPIGMENTATION

Hyperpigmentation or melanoderma is associated with increased melanin in the epidermis. Hyperpigmentation may be hereditary, acquired, or associated with pigmented tumors.

Hereditary Hyperpigmentation

Lentigenes Lentigenes are darkly pigmented macules that most often develop in the ventral abdomen. These may develop over a period of several months in healthy adult dogs. These are sometimes referred to as "tar spots." The skin in affected areas is heavily pigmented but otherwise normal. If the skin is thickened and scaly, the lesion is probably due to a papillomavirus infection (discussed under acquired hyperpigmentation). Orange cats commonly develop hyperpigmented macules involving their lips, nose, gingiva, and eyelids (Figure 20-5).

This condition is termed *lentigo simplex* and has no adverse health effects.

Canine Acanthosis Nigricans Acanthosis nigricans is a cutaneous reaction pattern characterized by bilateral hyperpigmentation and lichenification of axillary skin. Dachshunds are thought to have a primary, hereditary form of acanthosis nigricans that develops in dogs under 1 year old. Lesions start with hyperpigmentation of axillary skin and progress to alopecia, lichenification, and seborrheic changes that are often associated with bacterial and yeast infections. The lesions may spread to involve the forelimbs, ventral neck, chest, abdomen, and others sites. Acanthosis nigricans developing in other breeds or in older Dachshunds is usually a postinflammatory form associated with friction, intertrigo, allergies, or endocrine disease with secondary bacterial and *Malassezia* dermatitis.

Acromelanism Dark areas seen on the points (feet, tail, ears) of Siamese, Himalayan-Persian, Balinese, and Burmese cats are the result of a temperature-dependent enzyme controlling melanin production in hair bulbs. Temperatures above approximately 95° F (35° C) inhibit the enzyme resulting in production of lighter-colored hairs. Kittens of these breeds are born white with pigmented hairs replacing white ones on the cooler extremities during hair cycles following birth.

Acquired Hyperpigmentation

Postinflammatory Leukotrienes, thromboxanes, and other mediators of inflammation stimulate melanocytes to increase melanin production, which down-regulates inflammation by scavenging free radicals. Allergies, *Malassezia* dermatitis, bacterial pyoderma, dermatophytosis, demodecosis, scabies, and actinic and intertrigo dermatitis are examples of inflammatory skin diseases commonly associated with cutaneous hyperpigmentation (Figure 20-6).

Melanotrichia may develop as a response to inflammation affecting hair follicles, dermis, or panniculus (e.g., sebaceous adenitis, panniculitis, vaccine reactions).

Endocrine Related Hyperadrenocorticism, hypoadrenocorticism, hypothyroidism, hyperestrogenism, and other sex hormone imbalances may result in diffuse hyperpigmentation. adrenocorticotropic hormone (ACTH) and other pituitary hormones may stimulate melanogenesis. When hair loss precedes hyperpigmentation, ultraviolet light may be the factor, leading to increased melanin production. Dogs with hyperadrenocorticism treated with o,p'-DDD may develop a darker haircoat, perhaps due to increasing concentrations of ACTH or to direct affects of mitotane on the G (graying) locus.

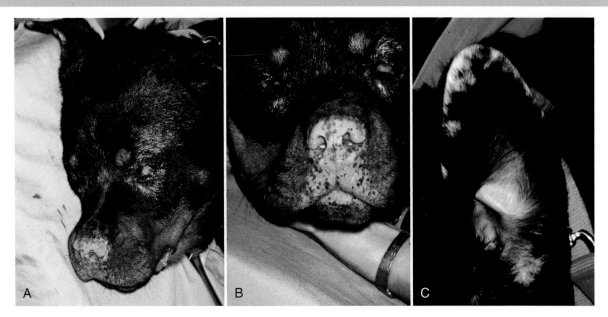

Figure 20-3 Vitiligo is characterized by a loss of pigment in the skin and hairs; this condition may be familial in Rottweilers and other breeds of dogs. **A,** Side view of head of Rottweiler with vitiligo. **B,** Front view showing nasal depigmentation and poliosis in periocular regions. **C,** Close up showing white hairs replacing black ones on the margins of the ear pinnae.

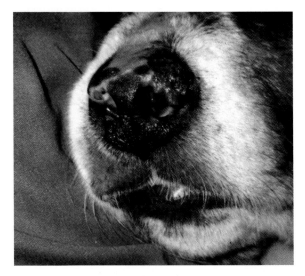

Figure 20-4 Discoid lupus erythematosus is the most common cause of planum nasale depigmentation in dogs.

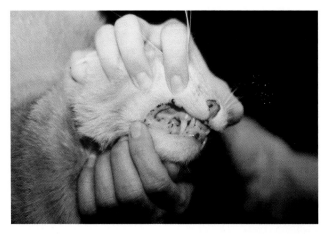

Figure 20-5 Lentigo simplex is characterized by the development of asymptomatic, pigmented macules that develop on the lips, eyelids, planum nasale and gingivae of young-adult, orange cats.

Papillomavirus Associated Canine papillomaviruses can result in several different cutaneous lesions. Pugs appear to be at risk for the development of papillomavirus-associated, slightly raised, scaly, hyperpigmented macules and plaques[9] involving their groin, abdomen, ventral thorax, and neck. Similar lesions have also been described in Miniature Schnauzers, an American Staffordshire Terrier, and a Pomeranian (Figure 20-7).[2,10]

The lesions may transform into squamous cell carcinomas in some patients. Canine papillomavirus is also associated with exophytic papillomas that appear as cauliflower-like nodules or keratinous plaques which may be pink or flesh colored, or brown or black.

Pigmented Tumors and Tumorlike Lesions Many tumors and tumorlike lesions are pigmented, with the color varying with the type of cells involved in the lesions. Apocrine cysts are generally bluish (Figure 20-8).

Cutaneous hemagiomas and hemangiosarcomas may appear red, dark purple, or bluish-black in color. Histiocytic, lymphocytic and plasmacytic tumors may appear pink, red, or purple. Tumors that frequently appear black in color

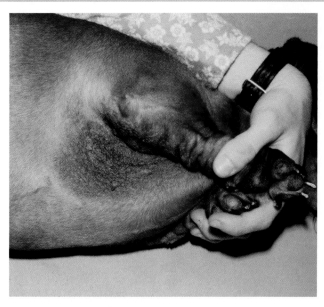

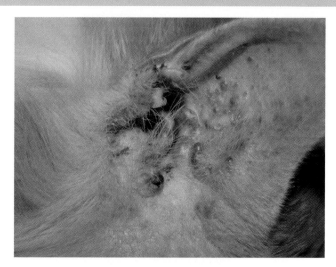

Figure 20-8 Apocrine cysts appear bluish in color; these are located in the external ear canal of an adult cat.

Figure 20-6 Postinflammatory hyperpigmentation of the axillae is commonly associated with underlying atopic dermatitis and chronic *Malassezia* infections in dogs.

include melanomas, melanocytomas, and basal cell tumors. Other tumors that may appear dark brown or black include squamous cell carcinomas, trichoblastomas, and fibromas.

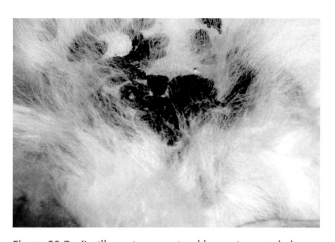

DIAGNOSTIC TESTS

Signalment, history, and physical examination findings are helpful in formulating differential diagnosis for pigmentary disorders. Cutaneous cytology, skin scrapings, and fungal cultures are helpful in the diagnosis of underlying causes for postinflammatory hyperpigmentation. Skin biopsies for histopathologic evaluation are fundamental for the diagnosis of hypopigmentation and for tumor-associated hyperpigmentation.

REFERENCES

The reference list can be found on the companion Expert Consult Web site at *www.expertconsult.com*.

Figure 20-7 Papillomavirus-associated hyperpigmented plaques on the ventral abdomen of a Pomeranian.

Fleas, Flea Allergy, and Flea Control

Candace A. Sousa

Flea infestations of pets and the home environment are a common occurrence. Fleas are responsible for the production and transmission of several diseases of humans and their pets. The flea that causes most of the problems is *Ctenocephalides felis felis*, the common cat flea. In one study it accounted for 92% to 99% of the fleas found on dogs and cats, respectively.[1]

LIFE CYCLE OF THE FLEA

The flea passes through four stages in its life cycle. It undergoes a complete metamorphosis at each stage.[2] At any time approximately 57% of the fleas are eggs, 34% are larva, 8% are pupa, and only about 1% are present as adults. The life cycle can be completed in as little as 12 days or take as long as 174 days and is dependent on the ambient temperature and humidity.[3]

Flea eggs are oval, pearly white, nonsticky, and about 0.5 mm in length.[4] The egg hatches between 1 and 10 days of being deposited on the host and falling off into the environment, depending on the ambient temperature and humidity (ideal conditions are 70% relative humidity and 35° C [95° F]).[2-4]

Flea larvae emerge from the egg after hatching. The larva of *C. felis felis* has three stages or larval "instars." The larvae are about 2 mm long, slender, white, and covered with short hairs. They feed on organic debris and blood-containing feces from adult fleas. The larvae are negatively phototactic (move away from light) and positively geotactic (move toward the ground).[2,4] Therefore when indoors the larvae avoid direct sunlight and move under furniture, appliances, and into carpet fibers. Outdoors, they move into shaded areas under bushes, trees, and leaves. Five to 11 days are required for the larvae to molt twice, during which they grow to about 5 mm in length. The larvae are extremely susceptible to heat and desiccation. They can survive only if the relative humidity is greater than 50% or when soil moisture is between 1% and 20%.[3]

Temperatures greater than 35° C (95° F) and less than 3° C (35° F) for more than 40 hours per month are also deleterious to survival. The mature larvae produce a sticky cocoon in which to pupate. Environmental debris may adhere to the cocoon, which helps it go undetected and provides excellent protection against insecticides. Pupation lasts from 5 to 9 days. Environmental locations suitable for a high rate of larval survival are termed *hot spots* or *source points*.

The preemerged adult flea is the stage that can extend the longevity of the flea life cycle. They can survive for up to 140 days in the cocoon if protected from desiccation. In the cocoon they are also protected from most insecticides. Physical pressure and changes in light, temperature, and carbon dioxide are thought to be stimuli for emergence of the adult flea.

Newly emerged fleas can survive in the environment from 10 to 62 days, again depending on the temperature and humidity.[5] Once on the host, the flea begins feeding within seconds and becomes an obligate parasite. The animal's grooming activity is the primary cause of mortality of ectoparasites. The flea feeds by piercing the skin of the host and inserting the tip of the labrum epipharynx to extract capillary blood.[6] Saliva is introduced by way of the salivary pump and used as an anticoagulant.[4] The female flea consumes an average of 14 µL of blood per day (equivalent to 15% of her body weight).[7] About 72 female fleas will remove 1 mL of blood daily. Male fleas consume less blood than females but feed more frequently.[2] Once fleas feed and initiate reproduction, they become dependent on a constant source of blood or they will die within a couple of days. During feeding, female fleas excrete large quantities of incompletely digested blood ("flea dirt") in long, tubular coils or fine pellets.[2]

The first of multiple matings occurs on the host within 8 to 24 hours. Egg production begins within 36 to 48 hours of the first blood meal, reaches maximum production between 4 and 9 days, and may continue for more than 100 days. Egg production peaks at 40 to 50 per day and averages 27 eggs per day for the first 50 days. A single female flea may deposit over 2000 eggs during her lifetime.[4,8]

FLEA ALLERGY

Flea allergy dermatitis (FAD) is the most common veterinary dermatologic condition in the world. It begins with the bite of a flea; 89% of fleas feed within 5 minutes.[9] The saliva of the flea contains amino acids, aromatic compounds, fluorescent materials, polypeptides, and phosphorus.[10] In the dog the antigenic substances carry a molecular weight of 18,000 to 45,000 Da with the major allergen weighing 30,000 to 32,000 Da.[11]

Dog owners notice scratching, chewing, licking, biting, and other signs of pruritus. Sixty-one percent of flea-allergic dogs develop clinical signs between 1 and 3 years of age.[12] As animals age, with continued exposure to fleas, the degree of hypersensitivity may wane. FAD is uncommon in dogs less than 6 months of age. Dogs with FAD usually have papules, crusts, salivary stains, excoriations, and erythema in a wedge-shaped pattern over the lumbosacral region, caudal thighs, proximal tail, ventral abdomen, and around the umbilicus (Figures 21-1 and 21-2). After chronic itching, the areas become alopecic, lichenified, hyperpigmented, and the dog develops an odor related to secondary infections with *Staphylococcus intermedius* and *Malassezia pachydermatis*.

Cats with flea allergy dermatitis are also pruritic. Cats can be quite efficient at removing fleas with their barbed tongues. As with dogs, the most common locations for flea allergy dermatitis in cats are the dorsal lumbosacral region, caudal thighs, and ventral abdomen (Figure 21-3). Clinical lesions can include alopecia and excoriations. In addition, they commonly develop miliary crusts in these areas as well as around the neck. Some cats will manifest their pruritus as "fur mowing" while others may create eosinophilic plaques from intense licking.

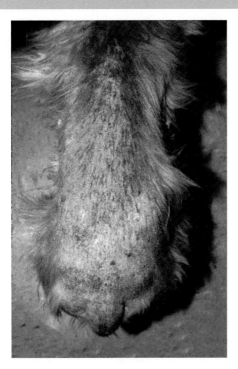

Figure 21-1 Dorsal lumbosacral region of an Afghan Hound with flea allergy dermatitis. Note the distribution of the alopecia. Skin is erythematous and crusted.

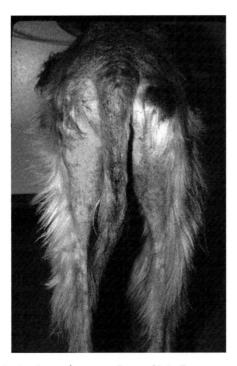

Figure 21-2 Same dog as in Figure 21-1. Dermatitis extends onto the caudal thighs.

A diagnosis of FAD is based on the age of onset of the pruritus, the distribution of the pruritus and clinical signs, and the observation of fleas, flea feces, or both. Many dogs and cats that are allergic to the bite of a flea have very few fleas on them at any time because their excessive grooming activity removes the fleas. Some of those dogs and cats have recurrent tapeworm *(Dipylidium caninum)* infestations from

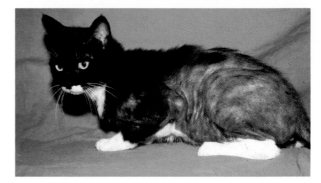

Figure 21-3 Cat with flea allergy dermatitis. Pruritus has resulted in partial alopecia of the entire caudal half of the trunk.

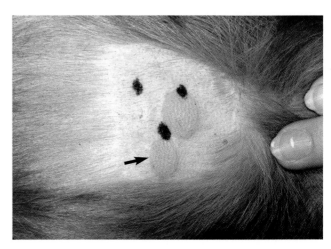

Figure 21-4 Positive immediate reaction (*arrow*) to an intradermal test for flea allergy in a dog (compared with a negative and positive control).

ingestion of the fleas. The diagnosis of FAD in dogs can be confirmed with an intradermal skin test with flea antigen (Figure 21-4).

Treatment of FAD is a 3-step process. Most important is the elimination of the fleas from the animal and prevention of reinfestation with the use of both on-animal and on-premise flea control. The second step involves providing the animal with relief from the allergic reaction and pruritus. Moderate doses of short-acting oral corticosteroids used for 5 to 10 days will usually be sufficient. Lastly, any secondary infections need to be treated with the appropriate oral and/or topical medications.

FLEA CONTROL

The goals of flea control are to eliminate the adult fleas on all the animals in the household and immature fleas in the environment. The best approach incorporates mechanical, physical, and chemical measures. Source points should be identified and treated aggressively. Carpets, pet bedding, and resting areas in the home should be well-vacuumed using a vacuum with a power head. Pet bedding should be washed. Dead vegetation should be cleaned away from animal resting areas outside. A wide variety of chemicals can be used on pets and in the environment; however, no single, "miracle" flea product exists that can be used on both animals and their surroundings.

Many formulations exist for delivering the insecticides to the pet. Shampoos act to mechanically remove the fleas, but because the active ingredients are rinsed off, they have minimal residual action. This problem can be overcome by using a final rinse (dip) that contains an insecticidal product. Many flea sprays are alcohol based and quickly kill adult fleas. Unfortunately, most contain pyrethrins, and unless the chemical is microencapsulated, their duration of action is less than 1 day. Powders, foams, concentrated solutions (spot treatments), and collars are all available and are formulated with a variety of chemicals. Several of the chemicals are also sold in oral formulations (Table 21-1).

None of the current flea products on the market prevent flea blood feeding before the flea is killed. Flea allergy dermatitis may be related to the degree of hypersensitivity of an individual animal, the number of fleas, and the amount of salivary antigen injected through feeding. A reduced flea burden and reduction in flea feeding, rather than complete elimination of all fleas, leads to clinical improvement.

It is not known how much of the flea salivary antigen is needed to induce the symptoms of flea allergy dermatitis. Research done on cats demonstrated that, even with superior flea control, fleas may feed and consume large amounts of blood before they are killed. Compared to untreated controls, imidacloprid was shown to reduce flea blood consumption by 43% 14 days after application. By day 14, fipronil had no effect on decreasing the amount of blood that fleas ingested before they were killed. Selamectin was shown to reduce flea feeding by greater than 95% through day 21 after application and still by close to 90% by day 28. Weekly administration of oral nitenpyram reduced blood feeding by greater than 98%. It is possible that systemically absorbed flea preventatives such as selamectin, nitenpyram, and spinosad may be more effective "antifeedants" than topically applied products as they may paralyze the feeding mechanism (pharyngeal pump) of the flea and thus may be more effective at preventing flea allergy dermatitis.[9,13]

In the indoor environment, hand spraying either by a professional or the owner is the preferred method of delivering the chemicals. This allows the product to be applied directly on the areas most frequented by the pets ("source points"). Large pieces of furniture must be moved to ensure that the spray reaches the areas of larval migration.

Outdoors, sprays are very useful and their application should be concentrated in the areas frequented by the animals, especially those that are shaded, have a mild temperature, and contain organic matter.

REFERENCES

The reference list can be found on the companion Expert Consult Web site at *www.expertconsult.com*.

Table • 21-1

Commercial Products to Control Parasites

PRODUCT	ACTIVE INGREDIENT	MANUFACTURER	REGISTRY	YEAR	SPECIES	FLEA ADULTS	EGGS/ LARVAE	TICKS	HW
Revolution	selamectin	Pfizer AH	FDA	1999	D > 6 wks C > 8 wks	X	X	X (dogs)	X
Program	lufenuron	Novartis	FDA	1994	D > 4 wks C > 4 wks		X (eggs)		
Sentinel	lufenuron milbemycin	Novartis	FDA	1998	D > 4 wks		X (eggs)		X
Capstar	nitenpyram	Novartis	FDA	2003	D > 4 wks C > 4 wks	X			
Prac-Tic	pyriprole	Novartis	EU	2007	D > 8 wks	X		X	
Advantage	imidacloprid	Bayer	EPA	1996	D > 7 wks C > 8 wks	X			
Advantix	imidacloprid permethrin	Bayer	EPA	2002	D > 7 wks	X		X	
Advantage-Multi	imidacloprid 10% moxidectin 2.5% (D) 1% (C)	Bayer	FDA	2007	D > 7 wks C > 9 wks	X			X
Frontline Topspot	fipronil	Merial	EPA	1997	D > 8 wks C > 8 wks	X		X	
Frontline Plus	fipronil methoprene	Merial	EPA	2000	D > 8 wks C > 8 wks	X	X	X	
ProMeris for Cats	metaflumizone	Fort Dodge	EPA	2007	C > 8 wks	X			
ProMeris for Dogs	metaflumizone amitraz	Fort Dodge	EPA	2007	D > 8 wks	X		X	
Vectra	dinotefuran pyriproxfen	Summit Vet	EPA	2008	C > 8 wks	X		X	
Vetra 3D	dinotefuran permethrin pyriproxfen	Summit Vet	EPA	2007	D > 7 wks	X	X	X	
Comfortis	spinosad	Eli Lilly	FDA	2007	D > 14 wks	X			

Organo(thio)phosphates: acephate, azamethiphos, azinphos-methyl, chlorpyrifos, chlorpyrifos-methyl, chlorfenvinphos, diazinon, dichlorvos, dicrotophos, dimethoate, disulfoton, ethion, fenitrothion, fenthion, isoxathion, malathion, methamidophos, methidathion, methyl-parathion, mevinphos, monocrotophos, oxydemeton-methyl, paraoxon, parathion, phenthoate, phosalone, phosmet, phosphamidon, phorate, phoxim, pirimiphos-methyl, profenofos, prothiofos, sulprophos, tetrachlorvinphos, terbufos, triazophos, trichlorfon

Carbamates: alanycarb, aldicarb, bendiocarb, benfuracarb, carbaryl, carbofuran, carbosulfan, fenoxycarb, furathiocarb, methiocarb, methomyl, oxamyl, pirimicarb, propoxur, thiodicarb, triazamate

Pyrethroids: allethrin, bifenthrin, cyfluthrin, cyhalothrin, cyphenothrin, cypermethrin, alpha-cypermethrin, beta-cypermethrin, zeta-cypermethrin, deltamethrin, esfenvalerate, etofenprox, fenpropathrin, fenvalerate, imiprothrin, lambda-cyhalothrin, permethrin, prallethrin, pyrethrin I and II, resmethrin, silafluofen, tau-fluvalinate, tefluthrin, tetramethrin, tralomethrin, transfluthrin, profluthrin, dimefluthrin

X, On-label claim; *AIC*, aids in control; *C*, cat; *D*, dog; *EPA*, Environmental Protection Agency; *EU*, European Union; *FDA*, Food and Drug Administration; *HW*, heartworm; *MAO*, monoamine oxidase; *MOA*, mode of action.

OTODECTES	SARCOPTES	INTERNAL	DEMODEX	BITING LICE	MOSQUITOES	MOA
X	X	X (cats; dogs in EU)		X (EU)		Selamectin binds to glutamate-gated chloride channels in the parasites' nervous system, increasing their permeability and allowing for the rapid and continued influx of chloride ions into the nerve cell. This inhibits nerve activity and causes paralysis.
						Lufenuron, a benzoylphenyl urea, inhibits the formation of chitin (a polymer of *N*-acetyl glucosamine), which is a major component of insect exoskeletons. During each larval molt, chitin is reformed by polymerization. Lufenuron interferes with polymerization and deposition of chitin, killing developing larvae either within the egg or after hatching.
		X				
						Imidacloprid works by binding to postsynaptic nicotinic acetylcholine receptors in insects. This inhibits cholinergic transmission, resulting in paralysis and death.
					Repels	
X (cats)		X				
	AIC				X	Fipronil binds to γ-aminobutyric acid (GABA) receptors of insects, inhibiting the flux of Cl⁻ ions into nerve cells, which results in hyperexcitability.
	AIC				X	
			X (EU)			Metaflumizone attacks the flea nervous system by targeting voltage dependent sodium channels along the presynaptic and postsynaptic nerves and blocking the influx of sodium resulting in disruptions of neuronal impulses that results in reductions in feeding, loss of coordination, paralysis and death of fleas (an axonal insecticide as compared with a synaptic insecticide). Amitraz is an alpha-2 agonist and an MAO inhibitor.
					X	Dinotefuran is a third-generation neonicotinoid with an MOA similar to imidacloprid.
						The spinosyns have a novel mode of action, primarily targeting binding sites on nicotinic acetylcholine receptors (nAChRs) that are distinct from those at which other insecticides exert their activity, leading to disruption of acetylcholine neurotransmission. Spinosad also has secondary effects on GABA neurotransmission that may potentiate its flea killing activity.

Growth regulators: a) chitin synthesis inhibitors: benzoylureas: chlorfluazuron, diflubenzuron, flucycloxuron, flufenoxuron, hexaflumuron, lufenuron, novaluron, teflubenzuron, triflumuron; buprofezin, diofenolan, hexythiazox, etoxazole, clofentazine; b) ecdysone antagonists: halofenozide, methoxyfenozide, tebufenozide, azadirachtin; c) juvenoids: fenoxycarb, methoprene, pyriproxyfen; d) lipid biosynthesis inhibitors: spirodiclofen, spiromesifen, spirotetramat

Nicotinic receptor agonists/antagonists compounds: clothianidin, dinotefuran, imidacloprid, thiamethoxam, nitenpyram, acetamiprid, thiacloprid; the thiazol compound of formula r¹

GABA antagonist compounds: acetoprole, endosulfan, ethiprole, fipronil, pyrafluprole, vaniliprole, pyriprole, the phenylpyrazole compound of formula r²

Macrocyclic lactone insecticides: abamectin, emamectin, milbemectin, milbemycin, moxidectin, lepimectin, spinosad

Avermectins: doramectin, ivermectin, selamectin (all are FDA not EPA)

CHAPTER 22

Genital Dermatoses

Didier-Noël Carlotti

There are specific diseases with lesions potentially or usually restricted to the external genital organs. In addition there are also those conditions with extensive lesions that consequently affect the genital area. Dermatoses of the first category are uncommon in dogs; they are extremely rare in cats.

MAIN GENITAL DERMATOSES IN THE HUMAN BEING

In man, lesions of the penis include psoriasis of the glans, lichen planus, Queyrat's erythroplasia (Bowen's disease), syphilis, genital herpes, warts of the penis (vegetations or condylomas), genital molluscum contagiosum, candidiasis of the glans (balanitis), scabies, vesico-bullous erythema multiforme, genital pemphigus, balanitis xerotica obliterans (scleroatrophic lichen). Lesions of the scrotum include lichen planus, angiokeratomas, epidermoid cysts, sebocystomatosis, syphilis, scabies, Behçet's disease, and neurodermatitis of the scrotum. These lesions do not exist in dogs and cats except for superficial pemphigus in the dog.

In woman, vulvar lesions include perivulvar seborrheic dermatitis, lichen planus, Bowen's disease and Bowenoid papulosis, leukoplasia, syphilis, genital herpes, warts, genital molluscum contagiosum, candidiasis, bullous pemphigoid of the infant, Behçet's disease, acanthosis nigricans, scleroatrophic lichen, and localized neurodermatitis. Again, none of these diseases has been reported in dogs and cats except acanthosis nigricans in the dog and neoplasia. In addition, neoplasia can develop in men and women (e.g., squamous cell carcinoma, basocellular epithelioma).

GENITAL DERMATOSES IN THE DOG

In the male, lesions of the prepuce/sheath include:
- Bacterial folliculitis/furunculosis (Figure 22-1)

- Localized demodicosis (Figure 22-2)
- Vasculitis (Web Figure 22-1)
- Autoimmune skin diseases (cutaneous lupus, bullous diseases) (Web Figures 22-2, 22-3 and 22-4)
- Linear dermatosis of the prepuce (estrogen-secreting testicular tumor) (Figure 22-3)
- Linear epidermal nevus (see Web Figure 16-5)
- Vascular nevus (see Web Figure 16-6)
- Various neoplasms (e.g., Sticker's sarcoma, hemangiosarcoma, and mast cell tumor)
  Lesions of the scrotum include:
- *Contact dermatitis,* the most common disease of this area (Figure 22-4 and Web Figure 22-5)
- Frostbite, solar erythema, traumas
- Intertrigo
- *Malassezia* dermatitis

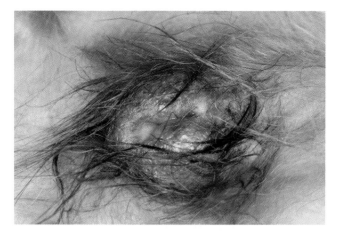

Figure 22-2   Localized demodicosis of the prepuce in a dog (the patient had no lesions elsewhere).

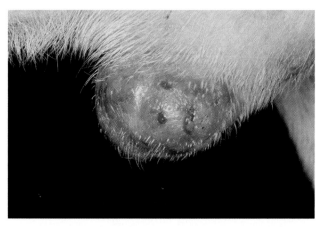

Figure 22-1   Localized bacterial folliculitis/furunculosis of the prepuce in a dog (the patient had no lesions elsewhere).

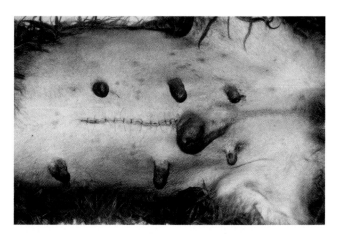

Figure 22-3   Linear dermatosis of the prepuce in a dog with estrogen-secreting testicular tumor (note the gynecomastia). The intraabdominal tumor has been surgically removed.

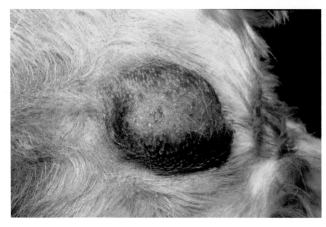

Figure 22-4 Chronic contact dermatitis due to floor detergents on the scrotum in a dog.

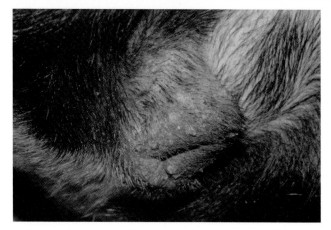

Figure 22-6 Localized demodicosis of the vulva in a dog (the patient had a few lesions elsewhere).

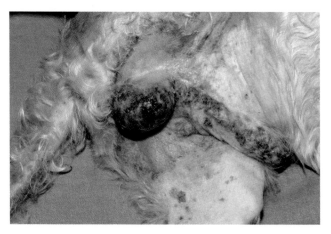

Figure 22-5 Lesions of superficial necrolytic dermatitis (hepato-cutaneous syndrome) on the scrotum and sheath in a dog.

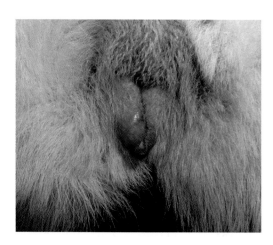

Figure 22-7 Bacterial furuncle on the vulva in a dog.

- Protothecosis
- Babesiosis (Web Figure 22-6)
- Cuterebrosis
- Brucellosis
- Infection with *Erysipelothrix rhusiopathiae*
- Rocky Mountain spotted fever
- Superficial necrolytic dermatitis (Figure 22-5)
- Autoimmune diseases (lupus, bullous diseases)
- Erythema multiforme
- Fixed pigmented erythema
- Cutaneous histiocytosis (Web Figure 22-7)
- Vascular hamartoma
- Neoplasms: squamous cell carcinoma (sometimes exophytic), apocrine adenocarcinoma, myxoma and fibrosarcoma, hemangioma, recurrent cystic hemangioma and hemangiosarcoma, plasmocytoma, lymphoma (epitheliotropic or not), histiocytoma and benign fibrous histiocytoma, mast cell tumor (frequent with sometimes confusing clinical aspects: poorly circumscribed edema) (Web Figure 22-8), melanoma
  In the female:
- Intertrigo (Web Figure 22-9)
- *Malassezia* dermatitis
- Demodicosis (Figure 22-6)

- Bacterial furunculosis (Figure 22-7)
- Contact dermatitis (Web Figure 22-10)
- Autoimmune diseases (lupus, bullous diseases) (Web Figure 22-11)
- Endocrine disorders, particularly hyperestrogenism (Web Figure 22-12)
- Neoplasms (poorly documented)
  It is possible to add to this list, more so in the female than in the male, all allergic dermatitis involving the abdomen with hypertrophy/lichenification/hyperpigmentation of the vulva or the sheath (even the scrotum) (Figure 22-8).

DIAGNOSIS

The diagnosis of genital lesions is based on history, physical examination, and a particular differential diagnostic approach, preceding diagnostic tests. Hubert has proposed to classify these diseases in four categories[1]:
- Erythematosquamous
- Purpuric
- Nodular
- Alopecic

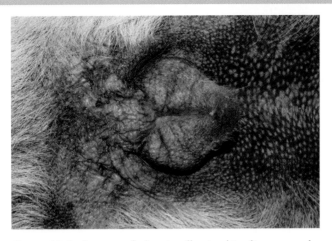

Figure 22-8 Lesions of chronic allergic skin disease on the vulva in a dog. Lichnification and hyperpigmentation were generalized.

He underlines the value of a history of pruritus or pain.

Cerundolo classifies scrotal lesions as multifocal or diffuse, but also in four types[2]:
- Erythema, macules, papules, crusts, and scales
- Crusts and ulceration
- Hyperpigmentation
- Edema and sloughing

TREATMENT

Treatment is specific to the disease condition present and usually follows the standard dermatologic therapies for such conditions elsewhere on the body. See other chapters and diagnoses for specific therapies (Web Figures 22-13, 22-14, and 22-15).

CONCLUSION

This chapter of canine dermatology has perhaps been neglected, perhaps because of the assumed minor importance. However, a systematic approach is beneficial. Contact dermatitis of the scrotum in the male dog is too often ignored.

REFERENCES

The reference list can be found on the companion Expert Consult Web site at *www.expertconsult.com*.

CHAPTER 23

Other External Parasites

Karen L. Campbell

External parasites are major causes of distress and disease in dogs and cats. Some parasites cause only mild irritation, whereas others are associated with severe inflammation and secondary infections. Many ectoparasites serve as vectors or intermediate hosts of other diseases.

Table 23-1 provides a scheme for the identification of major ectoparasites of dogs and cats.

FAMILY DEMODICIDEA

Demodex spp. live as commensals in the skin of most mammals. Most species (including *D. canis* (Web Figure 23-1), *D. injai* (Web Figure 23-2) and *D. cati*) spend their entire life cycle in the hair follicles and sebaceous glands of their host.

A few species (including *D. gatoi* (Web Figure 23-3) and the short-tailed demodectic mite of dogs, *D. cornei*) are found within the epidermis.

It is thought that most follicular infections develop during the early weeks of life, with the commensal population in bitches and queens being transferred to in-contact areas of puppies and kittens. However, the short-tailed forms of the mites may be transferred between adult animals of the same species.

Localized demodicosis in dogs is most common in puppies between 3 to 6 months of age. Skin lesions develop secondary to localized overgrowth of mites on the face (Web Figure 23-4) or forelimbs and consist of one or more localized areas of alopecia, erythema, and scaling.

Clinicians make the diagnosis by doing deep skin scrapings and finding the characteristic "cigar-shaped" mites with short, stubby legs. Factors that may predispose dogs to *Demodex* overgrowth include other parasites, poor nutrition, immunosuppressive drug therapy, and stress—these factors should be identified and corrected. Specific antimite therapy is rarely warranted because the majority of localized cases resolve in 1 to 3 months without treatment. Topical benzoyl peroxide gel or lotion may be applied once daily to help prevent secondary bacterial infections and aid in mite removal from the follicles. Skin scrapings should be repeated in 4 weeks. If lesions are still present and the mite count is still high with a large proportion of immature forms, the condition may be progressing to generalized demodicosis.

Generalized demodicosis in dogs is classified as juvenile onset (affecting dogs 3 to 18 months of age) or adult onset

Table • 23-1

Scheme for Identification of Arthropod Ectoparasites of Dogs and Cats

ADULTS WITH EIGHT LEGS, TWO BODY DIVISIONS (CEPHALOTHORAX, ABDOMEN), NO ANTENNAE, SIMPLE EYES, AND NO WINGS	CLASS ARACHNIDA	ADULTS WITH SIX LEGS, THREE BODY PARTS (HEAD, THORAX, AND ABDOMEN)	CLASS INSECTA
Flattened dorsoventrally, mouthparts of chelicera, hypostome, palp	Suborder Metastigmata (ticks)	Adults wingless, laterally flattened	Order Siphonaptera (fleas)
Dorsal shield (scutum)	Family Ixodidae	Head with genal and pronotal combs	Genus *Ctenocephalides*
Inornate scutum, anal groove forming an arch, lack festoons	Genus *Ixodes*	Flat head (length of head = twice height of head)	*Ctenocephalides felis*
Inornate scutum, has festoons, basis capituli is hexagonal	Genus *Rhipicephalus*	Round head (length of head < twice height of head)	*Ctenocephalides canis*
Ornate scutum, has festoons, basis capituli is rectangular	Genus *Dermacentor*	No combs on head, angular forehead	Genus *Echidnophaga*
Ornate scutum, has festoons, mouthparts are longer than basis capituli, the second palpal segment is twice as long as the third	Class Amblyomma	No combs on head, rounded forehead	Genus *Pulex*
Soft bodied	Family Argasidae	Adults wingless, flattened dorsoventrally, stout legs with claws	Order Phthiraptera (lice)
Mite with respiratory pore in middle of body	Suborder Mesostigmata	Long nose, sucking mouthparts	Suborder Anoplura (sucking lice)
Chelicerae long and stylelike, 750-1000 μm body, long legs, red color after feeding, found near bird roosts or nests	Genus *Dermanyssus*	On dog	*Linognathus setosus*
Mite without a respiratory pore	Suborder Astigmata	Wide head, biting mouthparts	Suborder Mallophaga (biting lice)
Round body 400-430 μm, terminal anus, short stubby legs with long unsegmented pedicels	Genus *Sarcoptes*	On cat	*Felicola subrostrata*
Round body 200-500 μm, dorsal anus, legs with medium-length, unsegmented pedicels	Genus *Notoedres*	On dog in United States (broad body)	*Trichodectes canis*
Oval body 300-400 μm, terminal anus, anterior legs are long with short, unsegmented pedicels and large suckers, rear legs have suckers in males and are rudimentary with whiplike setae in females	Genus *Otodectes*	On dog in tropics (slender body)	*Heterodoxus spiniger*
430-520 μm elongated body, flaplike sternal extensions, terminal suckers on all legs, found "clasping" hairs on cats	Genus *Lynxacarus*	Adults with one pair of wings	Order Diptera (flies)
Mite with stigmata opening on the gnathosoma	Suborder Prostigmata		
100-400 μm slender "cigar-shaped" body	Family Demodicidae		
Found in hair follicles of dogs	*Demodex canis, D. injai*		
Found in subcorneal location in dogs, stubby body	*Demodex cornei*		
Found in hair follicles of cats	*Demodex cati*		
Found in subcorneal location in cats, stubby body	*Demodex gatoi*		
400 μm oval body with large palpal claws, M-shaped gnathosomal mouthpart	Family Cheyletiellidae		
Found on cats, cone-shaped sensory organ on genu I	*Cheyletiella blakei*		
Found on dogs, heart-shaped sensory organ on genu I	*Cheyletiella yasguri*		
Found on rabbits, globose-shaped sensory organ on genu I	*Cheyletiella parasitovorax*		

(affecting middle-aged to older dogs that often are immunocompromised by hyperadrenocorticism, hypothyroidism, diabetes mellitus, immunosuppressive drug therapy, or neoplasia). Clinical signs are variable. Patchy to multifocal alopecia, erythema, and silvery-gray scales are common. The affected skin (Web Figures 23-5 and 23-6) may become lichenified, hyperpigmented, pustular, and crusted or ulcerated. Secondary bacterial infections may progress to life-threatening sepsis.

Peripheral lymphadenopathy is common. Deep skin scrapings usually reveal numerous demodectic adults, nymphs, and larvae or ova (or both). Mixed infections with *D. canis* plus short-tailed and long-bodied forms of *Demodex* mites are sometimes found. An assessment of the general health of the dog should be made, and any underlying diseases or concurrent infections should be treated.

The first product approved for the treatment of canine demodicosis in the United States is Mitaban (amitraz, Pfizer). It is licensed to be used at a concentration of 0.025% applied as a dip every 2 weeks. Amitraz is monoamine oxidase (MAO) inhibitor and an alpha-2 adrenergic agonist. There are many safety concerns with the use of this product: Side effects may include lethargy, depression, ataxia, anorexia, vomiting, diarrhea, bradycardia, hypothermia, pruritus, and hyperglycemia. Amitraz should not be used concurrently with other MAO inhibitors or if the patient or owner is diabetic. Small dogs have a higher incidence of side effects and fatalities have been reported in Chihuahuas.[1] Effective alternatives to amitraz, although not FDA-approved for treating demodicosis, include ivermectin and milbemycin.[2] Collies and other dogs with mutations in MDR1 genes are highly susceptible to ivermectin toxicosis.[3] Dogs can be tested for their MDR1 genotype by submitting cheek swabs for DNA analysis to the College of Veterinary Medicine at Washington State University (www.vetmed.wsu.edu/vpl). It is recommended that ivermectin be initiated with 0.05 mg/kg PO on days 1 to 2, with an increase to 0.1 mg/kg PO on days 3 to 4, and continuing to increase by increments of 0.05 mg/kg until 0.4 mg/kg/day is reached. Ivermectin should be discontinued immediately in any dog showing depression, ataxia, mydriasis, or other signs of toxicity. Collies and other breeds that cannot tolerate high doses of ivermectin can usually be treated with milbemycin oxime. A recommended protocol for milbemycin is 0.5 mg/kg PO days 1 to 2, with increases of 0.5 mg/kg increments until 2.0 mg/kg/day is reached. Signs of milbemycin toxicosis include mydriasis, ataxia, lethargy, and stupor. Two new products that have shown efficacy in the treatment of demodicosis are imidacloprid 10% + moxidectin 2.5% spot-on (Advantage Multi, Bayer) and metaflumizone + amitraz spot-on (Promeris, Fort Dodge).[4,5] Both of these spot-on products are labeled for use once monthly; however, preliminary studies have shown improved efficacy when applied every 2 weeks. Promeris is labeled for use in the treatment of canine demodicosis. Therapy for demodicosis should be continued until two negative skin scrapings have been obtained at monthly intervals and rechecks should be scheduled for 2, 6, and 12 months after cessation of therapy to monitor for relapses.

Localized demodicosis is rare in cats and usually affects the eyelids, periocular region, ear canal, or head and neck. Lesions include patchy alopecia with scaling and crusting or a ceruminous otitis externa (pruritus is variable). Clinicians make the diagnosis by finding mites on superficial and deep skin scrapings, ear swabs, or both. Treatment may include topical rotenone or lime sulfur solution.

Generalized demodicosis is rare and generally less severe in cats than in dogs. It may be associated with an underlying immunosuppressive or metabolic disease such as feline immunodeficiency virus (FIV), feline leukemia virus (FeLV), toxoplasmosis, systemic lupus erythematosus, or diabetes mellitus. Clinical signs include variable pruritus; multifocal, patchy, or symmetrical alopecia with or without erythema; scaling; crusting; macules; and hyperpigmentation. Mites may be found on superficial (*D. gatoi*) or deep (*D. cati*) skin scrapings. Most cats will respond favorably to weekly dips with 2% lime sulfur solution. *D. gatoi* may be contagious; thus in-contact cats should be evaluated and treated if infected. Cats that are not cured by lime sulfur dips may respond to oral ivermectin at 0.3 mg/kg once weekly.[1]

FAMILY SARCOPTIDAE

Sarcoptes scabiei var. canis primarily affects dogs but can also cause disease in cats, foxes, and humans. Dogs can be infested with mites from foxes and humans. The life cycle is approximately 24 days and completed on the host. Off-host survival time depends upon the relative humidity and temperature. Adult mites are small (200 to 400 μm), oval, and white with two pairs of short legs (Web Figure 23-7).

The anus is at the posterior edge of the body. The mites initially affect relatively hairless areas of skin such as the ear pinnae (Web Figure 23-8) and elbows.

Female mites burrow through the epidermis at a rate of 2 to 3 mm/day. They lay their eggs in the resulting tunnel. Eggs hatch into larvae that burrow to the surface of the skin, where they feed. Many dogs develop a hypersensitivity reaction to mite antigens. As few as 10 to 15 mites may produce severe clinical signs in a hypersensitive individual. Clinical signs include an intensely pruritic, nonseasonal dermatitis with papules, excoriations, and hair loss. Affected areas typically develop a thick, yellowish crust. Diagnosis is based on history of a contagious, nonseasonal, intensely pruritic dermatitis involving the pinnal margins, elbows, hocks and ventral abdomen, and chest plus finding mites or mite eggs or feces in superficial skin scrapings. An ELISA test available in Europe is reported to have a sensitivity of 84.2% and a specificity of 89.5%.[6] A presumptive diagnosis may be made based on response to treatment trials. Effective licensed treatments include weekly applications of 2% lime sulfur solution or monthly applications of 6 to 12 mg/kg selamectin.[7] Effective off-label treatments include ivermectin 0.2 to 0.3 mg/kg PO every 7 days for four to six treatments or milbemycin oxime at 2 mg/kg PO every 7 days for four to six treatments. As in the treatment of demodicosis, it is advisable to initiate treatment with either ivermectin or milbemycin at much lower doses with daily increases until the target dose is reached while monitoring for side effects. The target dose is then given once weekly for at least 3 weeks past resolution of clinical signs. In-contact dogs should be treated to eliminate possible asymptomatic carriage of the mites. Imidacloprid 10% + moxidectin 2.5% and metaflumizone + amitraz spot-ons have also been reported as being effective.[8-10]

Notoedres cati primarily parasitizes cats but may also affect foxes, dogs, rabbits, and humans. Notoedric mange is highly contagious and frequently occurs in epizootics in endemic areas. The mites are smaller than *S. scabiei*, have medium-length unjointed sucker-bearing stalks on their legs, more body striations, and a dorsal anus. Clinical signs include intense pruritus and dry, crusted lesions (Web Figure 23-9) that first appear on the medial edges of ear pinnae and spread over ears, head, face, and neck.

Some cases also involve the feet and perineal regions. Diagnosis is confirmed by finding the mites, nymphs, larvae, and ova in superficial skin scrapings. Traditional therapy is 2% lime sulfur solution applied weekly for 4 to 8 weeks. Other effective treatments include selamectin (6 to 12 mg/kg topically every 30 days), ivermectin (0.3 mg/kg PO or SQ every

14 days for two treatments), or doramectin (0.3 mg/kg SQ once).

FAMILY PSORPTIDAE

Otodectes cynotis infests the external ear canal and adjacent skin of dogs, cats, foxes, and ferrets. The prevalence in feral cats in the United States has been reported at 25% to 37%. Although ear pruritus and copious production of a dark "coffee grounds–like" cerumen are common, 10% of infested animals may exhibit no clinical signs. Diagnosis is made by finding mites on otoscopic examination or on microscopic examination of material from ear swabs or ear flushes. Adult mites are 300 to 400 µm, white, with a terminal anus and 4 pairs of legs (Web Figure 23-10).

All legs of the male have short, unjointed stalks with suckers. Only the front two pairs of legs of female mites have suckers; the fourth pair of legs are rudimentary and do not extend beyond the body margin. Topical ceruminolytics should be used to remove cerumen and debris from the external ear canal. Topical otic acaricidal products are effective as is topical selamectin. Systemic ivermectin has been used with variable results. Fipronil spray or spot-on may also be effective; however, fipronil should not be used in the ear itself. In-contact animals should be evaluated and treated as appropriate for the species.

GENUS *Lynxacarus*

Lynxacarus radovski is a hair-clasping fur mite of domestic cats. These mites (Web Figure 23-11) have elongated bodies, 430 to 520 µm long, with a flaplike sternal extension containing the first two legs and used to grasp the hair of the host.

Some cats develop widespread papular crusts, whereas others show no clinical signs from the infestation. Techniques for collecting the mites include acetate tape impressions, hair plucks, and superficial skin scrapings. Effective treatments include topical pyrethrin sprays, 2% lime sulfur dips, and systemic ivermectin. The mite is contagious to other cats and may cause a papular rash in humans; it is not considered contagious to dogs.

FAMILY CHEYLETIELLA

Cheyletiella spp. mites (Web Figure 23-12) are easily recognized by their big palpal claws, M-shaped gnathosomal mouthparts, and comblike tarsal appendages. The sensory organs on genu I may be used to identify different species.

The sensory organ of *C. yasguri* (primary host is dog) is heart shaped, of *C. blakei* (primary host is cat) is cone shaped, and of *C. parasitovorax* (primary host is rabbits) is globe shaped. These three mite species are freely contagious from one host species to another and can transiently affect humans. The mites do not burrow but move rapidly in pseudotunnels in epidermal debris. The entire life cycle is completed on the host. The ova are smaller than louse nits and are attached to host hairs by fine fibrillar strands. Adult female mites may live up to 10 days in the environment. Clinical signs associated with infestation include a dorsally oriented dry scaling and variable pruritus. Some cats develop miliary dermatitis. Diag-nosis is made by finding mites or ova on acetate tape impressions, on superficial skin scrapings, or in fecal flotations. Affected and in-contact dogs, cats, and rabbits should be treated with topical parasiticides (e.g., 2% lime sulfur dip, fipronil, pyrethrin, selamectin). Systemic ivermectin is also effective. Treatment should be continued for 4 to 8 weeks, and the environment should be also be treated with an acaricidal spray approved for use in homes.

FAMILY IXODIDAE

Ixodid (hard) ticks possess a sclerotized dorsal shield plate on the idiosoma known as a *scutum*. These ticks are intermittent feeders, remaining attached for several days. The number of hosts upon which they feed varies from one to three among the different species of ticks. Ticks are important as vectors of protozoan, viral, and rickettsial diseases. Some are also involved in producing tick paralysis. When animals are infested with a small number of ticks, manual removal can be accomplished by soaking the tick in alcohol, grasping the head with a forceps, and applying firm traction. With heavier infestations the animal may be treated with fipronil or a pyrethrin or pyrethroid (dogs only). Amitraz collars may be used to prevent tick attachment. A spot-on formulation of metaflumizone + amitraz provides >90% control of ticks for at least 35 days after application.[11] Environmental control includes mowing and cutting of brush and grass, plus use of environmental pesticides approved for control of ticks.

FAMILY ARGASIDAE

Argasid ticks are soft bodied and lack a scutum. The only argasid tick of importance in small animals is the spinose ear tick, *Otobius megnini*. Adult ticks are not parasitic; however, larvae and nymphs infest the external ear canals of dogs and rarely cats. Clinical signs include an acute onset of otitis externa with severe inflammation and waxy exudate. Diagnosis is made by visualizing the ticks and removing them.

ORDER PHTHIRAPTERA

Lice are highly host specific, with their life cycles completed on the host. Most can only survive a day or two off a host. Sucking lice have mouthparts adapted for sucking the blood of the host. *Linognathus setosus*, the "long-nosed" louse, is the only sucking louse found on dogs. Biting lice have relatively larger heads and ventrally located mouthparts. The claws are smaller than those of sucking lice. The most common biting louse on dogs is *Trichodectes canis* (Web Figure 23-13, *A* and *B*); *Felicola subrostrata* is a biting louse found on cats.

Lice are easily killed by 2% lime sulfur dips, pyrethrin or carbaryl powders or sprays, and most other parasiticides used for fleas. Grooming equipment should be thoroughly cleaned.

REFERENCES

The reference list can be found on the companion Expert Consult Web site at *www.expertconsult.com*.

CHAPTER 24

Edema

William E. Herndon

Abnormal collection of interstitial fluid is called *edema*. The collection of cavity fluid (pericardial, pleural, and peritoneal) should be included in the category of edema, given the importance of serosal transudation (removal of fluid from the interstitial space of suspended organs, such as the heart, lung, liver, and intestine, via the serosal surface and lymphatic drainage). Edema (American English), oedema (British English), previously known as hydropsy, interferes with the normal delivery of nutrients and removal of byproducts of cellular metabolism. The clinical manifestation of edema depends on the organ(s) affected. In veterinary medicine, edema is commonly recognized in the central nervous system (altered mentation, neurologic dysfunction), lung (cough, tachypnea, dyspnea), intestines (anorexia, vomiting, diarrhea, weight loss), and skin/subcutaneous (visually recognizable). The purpose of this chapter is to review normal fluid compartments, fluid movement dynamics, mechanisms of edema formation, and to provide a general schematic for recognizing disease processes causing edema. For specific information regarding central nervous system edema, please refer to Chapter 259.

PHYSIOLOGY AND PATHOPHYSIOLOGY

Body fluids are distributed among the intracellular and extracellular compartments, the latter containing intravascular and interstitial components. The dynamics of fluid flow from the intravascular space to the interstitial space is determined by the Starling equation[1]:

$$J_V = K_f([P_c - P_i] - \sigma[\pi_c - \pi_i])$$

J_v is the net fluid movement between compartments; K_f is the filtration coefficient, which is the product of water permeability (L_p) and microvascular surface area (A); P_c and P_i are the hydrostatic pressures within the vascular and interstitial space, respectively; σ is the osmotic reflection coefficient; and π_c and π_i are the colloid osmotic pressures exerted by the plasma and interstitial space, respectively. Under physiologic circumstances, the cardiovascular system delivers nutrients necessary for cellular function and removes waste products of metabolism. To do this effectively requires net filtration of fluid across capillaries and venules from the intravascular space into the interstitial space that bathes cells. Normally, the net hydrostatic pressure difference (P_c minus P_i) is greater than the net colloid osmotic pressure difference (π_c minus π_i), favoring net filtration from the intravascular into the interstitial space. This plasma filtrate is then removed via the lymphatic system and returned to the systemic venous circulation, usually entering in the cranial thoracic cavity via the lymphatic duct.

Physiologic factors are present to help limit the collection of excessive interstitial fluid. The interstitial matrix has a principle role in regulating hydrostatic pressure via changes in compliance ($\Delta V/\Delta P$). Interstitial collagen and fibroblasts provide tension, compressing an interstitial matrix composed mainly of glycosaminoglycan and hyaluronate.[2] Increases in filtration rates and subsequent interstitial volume result,

initially, in large relative increases in interstitial pressure, helping to limit further edema. Further increases in interstitial volume tend to have a diminishing effect on increasing interstitial pressure, particularly in organs such as the lung. Increased interstitial volume decreases interstitial colloid osmotic pressure, helping to limit further increases in edema. Also, increased interstitial fluid augments lymphatic flow.

Pathophysiologic conditions from a variety of causes may result in the accumulation of interstitial fluid (edema). The most common abnormalities that result in edema formation are increased microvascular surface area and improper vascular dilation (A), decreased plasma colloid osmotic pressure (π_c), increased microvascular permeability to water (L_p) and protein (σ), and increased venous hydrostatic pressure (P_c). Impaired lymphatic flow, mechanical or functional, can result in edema secondary to decreased removal of interstitial fluid (Figure 24-1).

Also, some inflammatory and anaphylactic conditions may increase interstitial compliance ($\Delta V/\Delta P$) by decreasing the tension generated from collagen and fibroblasts; consequently, increasing interstitial fluid volume does not result in increasing pressure (P_i) as it normally would to help limit edema formation.[3] Common causes of edema in small animal veterinary medicine are listed in Box 24-1.

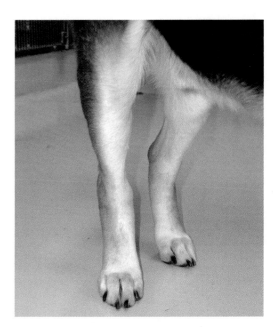

Figure 24-1 Hind leg edema from lymphatic obstruction secondary to lymphoma in a German Shepherd Dog. (Courtesy Dr. Louis-Philippe de Lorimier.)

Box • 24-1

Common Causes of Edema in Small Animal Veterinary Medicine

Increased microvascular surface area and permeability to water and protein
- Sepsis
- Acute respiratory distress syndrome
- Infection
  - Fungal
  - Bacterial
  - Viral
- Pancreatitis

Decreased colloid osmotic pressure
- Hypoproteinemia (peritoneal → pleural → lung)
  - Hepatic disease
  - Glomerular disease
  - Intestinal malabsorption/protein loss
  - Lymphangiectasia
  - Malnutrition

Decreased lymphatic drainage
- Neoplasia
- Radiation therapy
- Postsurgical

Mixed mechanisms
- Noncardiogenic pulmonary edema
  - Head trauma
  - Seizures
  - Electrocution
  - Upper airway obstruction
- Heartworms (lung)
- Anaphylaxis (lung, cats; gastrointestinal, dogs)
- Cirrhosis (peritoneal)
- Organ torsion

Increased venous hydrostatic pressure
- Budd-Chiari–like syndrome
- Pericardial disease (peritoneal → pleural)
- Primary structural heart disease
  - Left-sided heart disease
    - Dog (lung → pleural → peritoneal)
    - Cat (lung → pleural)
  - Right-sided heart disease
    - Dog (peritoneal → pleural → pericardial)
    - Cat (peritoneal, pericardial, pleural)
- Thrombosis
- Iatrogenic fluid overload
- Heartworm (peritoneal → pleural)

Modified from Ettinger ST, Barrett KA: Ascites, peritonitis, and other causes of abdominal distention. In Ettinger ST, Feldman EC, editors: Textbook of veterinary internal medicine, ed 4, Philadelphia, 1995, Saunders, p 64.

THERAPY

Therapy for edema varies depending on the underlying etiology and mechanism(s) of edema formation. In many circumstances, a mixed mechanism of edema formation may be present with a given disease process. For example, in patients with noncardiogenic pulmonary edema secondary to seizure (Figure 24-2), edema may be present secondary to transient increased P_c, decreased lymphatic drainage, and/or increased L_p and σ.

Also, a given disorder may result in edema formation via a secondary mechanism. For example, a patient may present with protein-losing nephropathy, hypoalbuminemia, and peritoneal effusion. This disease often causes peritoneal effusion secondary to decreased π_c. Instead, the peritoneal effusion may be caused by portal vein thrombosis from a hypercoagulable state secondary to loss of antithrombin III. In patients with pulmonary edema from increased pulmonary venous hydrostatic pressure (P_c) secondary to degenerative mitral valve disease (Figure 24-3), initial therapy to reduce vascular hydrostatic pressures using diuretics are the core of short- and long-term therapy (see Chapter 241), although additional medications may be indicated (see Chapters 238, 239, 243, and 244).

Diseases causing edema secondary to decreased plasma π_c may benefit from specific fluid therapies and nutritional

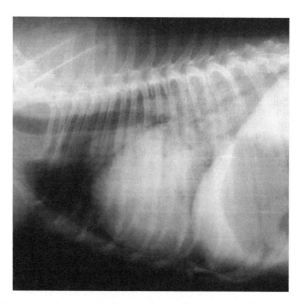

Figure 24-2 Lateral chest radiograph in a dog following a seizure. Noncardiogenic pulmonary edema is present. The caudodorsal distribution of the edema is common in dogs with noncardiogenic pulmonary edema. In clinical practice, two orthogonal radiographic views are recommended.

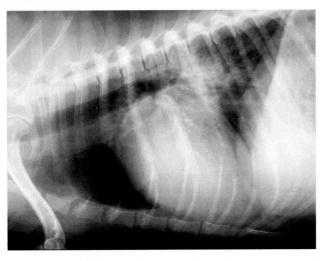

Figure 24-3 Pulmonary edema secondary to degenerative mitral valve disease in a dog. The perihilar distribution of the edema is common in dogs with congestive heart failure. In clinical practice, two orthogonal radiographic views are recommended.

support (see Chapters 129 and 174-176). In general, the underlying cause of edema formation should be treated specifically, while additional therapies should be directed toward maximizing patient comfort while attempting to return tissue function to physiologic states.

REFERENCES

The reference list can be found on the companion Expert Consult Web site at *www.expertconsult.com.*

CHAPTER 25

Hepatocutaneous Syndrome

Catherine A. Outerbridge

Hepatocutaneous syndrome (HS) is an uncommon skin disease associated with systemic metabolic disease. It has also been called *superficial necrolytic dermatitis (SND), metabolic epidermal necrosis, diabetic dermatopathy,* and *necrolytic migratory erythema (NME).* This disease was first described in a dog in 1968.[1] The first English-language reference comparing the disease to the human disease NME was in 1986, when the disease was described in four dogs with diabetes mellitus and was thus first called diabetic dermatopathy.[2] The disease has been most commonly described in older dogs, although a histologically equivalent disease occurring in cats and the black rhinoceros has been reported.[3,4] The etiopathogenesis of this disease is unclear, but it is likely multifactorial. Because different disease processes appear to cause similar histologic skin lesions, it might be more correct to refer to the skin disease as either SND or metabolic epidermal necrosis.

COMPARATIVE ASPECTS WITH NECROLYTIC MIGRATORY ERYTHEMA AND THEORIES OF PATHOGENESIS

NME is a histologically similar disease that is seen in humans. Most often NME occurs in association with a glucagon-

secreting tumor. Glucagonoma syndrome in humans is characterized by the skin lesions of NME, hyperglycemia resulting from carbohydrate intolerance or diabetes mellitus, weight loss, hypoaminoacidemia, and anemia. Humans with NME usually have a profound hypoaminoacidemia, presumed to result from the catabolic gluconeogenic effects of glucagon. However, NME has been diagnosed in some humans with normal plasma amino acid concentrations, and these have often been patients with non–glucagonoma-associated disease. Non–glucagonoma-associated NME has been reported in humans with celiac disease, chronic malabsorption, cirrhosis, non–alpha islet cell tumors, pancreatitis, hepatitis, inflammatory bowel disease, and heroin abuse.

Unlike people with NME, association with glucagonoma has not been consistently demonstrated in the majority of dogs with the skin lesions of SND. Afflicted dogs commonly have a characteristic concurrent hepatopathy, thus the use of the term HS. The hepatic pathology seen in dogs with HS has not been reported to occur in those dogs with confirmed glucagonoma-associated SND. In addition to the association with hepatic pathology, some dogs with the skin lesions of SND have a history of phenobarbital or primidone administration,[5,6] or gastrointestinal signs and malabsorption.[7] The severe vacuolar liver disease seen in the majority of dogs with the skin lesions of SND and the association in some

ETIOLOGY AND PATHOGENESIS

The etiology and pathogenesis of CAD are complex and combine intrinsic and extrinsic factors. Intrinsic factors include genetic and/or breed predisposition, the production of IgE, the role of many cells (antigen-presenting cells, Th2 cells, IgE-producing B cells, mast cells, eosinophils, and neutrophils), numerous mediators of inflammation (histamine, serotonin, leukotrienes, and cytokines), and an alteration of stratum corneum intercellular lipids. The paradigm Th2/Th1 (cells that counterregulate) exists in CAD. Extrinsic factors include numerous environmental allergens: seasonal allergens (grass, weed, or tree pollens) and nonseasonal allergens (house dust mites, storage mites, danders, molds, and even fabrics or insects other than flea). House dust mites and epidermal antigens seem to be important in both North America and Europe whereas pollen and mold antigens appear to be of major importance in North America but of minor importance in Europe.

Among house dust mites, *Dermatophagoides farinae* is much more important than *Dermatophagoides pteronyssinus*. Atopic dogs, in general, do not recognize allergens that are important for man (Der f 1, Der f 2 and Der p 1, Der p 2, respectively), but a 98/109 kDa polypeptide, a chitinase, Der f 15. Recently a new major allergen has been identified: Der f 18. Studies on pollen major allergens for dogs have been done only with the Japanese cedar, *Cryptomeria japonica*. Dogs recognize EP-5 of Cry j 1, whereas man recognizes EP-1. The allergens penetrate the organism percutaneously as well as via the respiratory and digestive routes. The percutaneous route predominates. House dust mites and their allergens can be found around dogs and on their skin and hair as well.

In dogs and people, atopic dermatitis promotes the development of staphylococcal or *Malassezia* infections. Infection leads to staphylococcal folliculitis and microbial overgrowth (particularly *Staphylococcus intermedius* and *Malassezia pachydermatis*), which contribute to inflammation and pruritus. Furthermore, microbial infections can initiate and perpetuate clinical signs of CAD and also promote immunologic reactions triggering the allergic process. Several studies demonstrate clearly that CAD predispose to flea allergy dermatitis (FAD), a common disease in developed countries.

At the present time, there is insufficient evidence to support or refute any association between CAD and cutaneous adverse food reactions. There is obviously a clinical overlap: some cases of clinically defined CAD will respond to an elimination diet whereas there are pruritic dermatoses other than CAD that will do the same. It has been suggested that food allergy can mimic CAD *sensu stricto* (linked to aeroallergens) while others will include food allergy as a cause of CAD. Regardless, all dogs suspected of having CAD should be treated, at least in part, with an elimination diet.

THRESHOLD PHENOMENON AND SUMMATION OF EFFECTS

1. Threshold phenomenon: A certain allergic load may be tolerated by an individual without any disease manifestations, but slight increases may exceed the threshold and initiate clinical signs.[2]
2. Summation of effects: Concomitant diseases fostering pruritus may raise an animal above its pruritic threshold. Therefore *all* factors contributing to pruritus must be investigated: e.g., a subclinical allergy in combination with a flea infestation or a mild pyoderma may produce marked discomfort while one condition might be asymptomatic.[2]

CLINICAL SIGNS AND DIAGNOSIS

The criteria set out by T. Willemse (1986) have been unanimously accepted to establish the diagnosis of canine atopic dermatitis. The demonstration of in vivo or in vitro sensitization is, for many dermatologists, an important criterion for the diagnosis and treatment of CAD, even if the diagnosis is clinical. Among all criteria, pruritus (notably facial, auricular, and pedal), young age of onset, breed or familial predilection, and chronicity are important.

TREATMENT OF DERMATOSES THAT ARE RELATED OR SECONDARY TO ATOPIC DERMATITIS

Treatment of Microbial Infections
An adequate antibacterial treatment regimen for secondary pyoderma, based upon systemic antibiotics and appropriate antibacterial topicals, may return the animal to a quasi-normal state. Such dogs may only be treated when clinical reoccurrences of pyoderma are noted and/or if the clinical signs of CAD become a concern. Also, some atopic dogs will respond to a well–carried out antibiotic treatment, even without visible signs of secondary pyoderma. A true bacterial overgrowth (BOG) syndrome is plausible. One may utilize antibiotics in any dog with abundant cocoid surface flora after cytological tests, as an empiric therapeutic test.[3] The same reasoning is undoubtedly applicable as well to cases of *Malassezia* dermatitis. Systemic (ketoconazole) and topical antifungal therapy are required with a careful follow-up.

Treatment of FAD
A well-conducted flea control regimen can eliminate the FAD and, therefore, in certain cases can enable the animal to fall under its pruritic threshold. In such a case, atopic dermatitis treatment is not necessary if clinical signs are not obvious. If this not the case, the atopic dermatitis should be treated while maintaining absolute antiparasitic treatment.

Management of Food Reactions
As discussed above, food intolerance may resemble CAD and a food elimination diet is always reasonable.

Treatment of Keratoseborrhoeic Skin Disease
A keratoseborrhoeic disorder can occur in CAD particularly with chronic disease. Treatment is mainly topical although systemic essential fatty acids used in the treatment of CAD may have an effect on seborrhoea. Shampoos and moisturizing agents are valuable in keratoseborrhoeic skin disorders.

Treatment of Otitis Externa
Otitis externa is a major feature of canine atopic dermatitis that causes inflammation of the external ear canal and ear pinnae. Secondary infections occur (bacterial and fungal) and perpetuating factors such as hyperplasia of epidermis and both sebaceous and apocrine glands lead to chronicity. It is typically erythematoceruminous at the beginning of the disease, eventually becoming suppurative. The associated lesions of the ear pinnae (lichenification, alopecia, crusting) require therapy. Ear cleansing must be repeated regularly (e.g., twice or three times a week). Numerous easy-to-use and effective commercial otic preparations are available. They contain active substances such as antibiotic, antifungal, and corticosteroid agents. Selection must be made after performing a smear and bacterial culture, and sensitivity testing if the smear shows

rods and/or if the otitis is suppurative. Corticosteroids included in otic preparations reduce pruritus, pain, and proliferative reactions. They also decrease cerumen secretion. Systemic antibiotic therapy is often useful in otitis externa due to CAD, particularly if it is suppurative, because of associated otitis media. Surgical therapy can be avoided in many circumstances with appropriate medical therapy. Surgical failure is often due to failure to recognize and control CAD.

Treatment of Pyotraumatic Dermatitis

Lesions of pyotraumatic dermatitis are common in CAD. They are poorly understood. They should be differentiated from pyotraumatic folliculitis. Although there may be a spontaneous healing in a few days, treatment is beneficial. Clipping and cleansing with antiseptic shampoos can be followed by the application of creams containing antibiotics and corticosteroids. If pruritus or pain is a concern, a short course of systemic glucocorticoid treatment may be useful.

SPECIFIC TREATMENT

Allergenic Eviction

Totally avoiding an offending allergen may enable an animal to fall beneath its pruritic threshold, identical in this instance to the allergic threshold. This avoidance can be illusive in the case of pollens. It may be possible to eliminate environmental feathers, fabrics, and molds. However, the role of these allergens in dogs' atopic dermatitis is minimal and, moreover, feathers and fabrics are mostly sources of house dust mite allergen. Various methods exist to exterminate house dust mites. Their elimination may be effective in human atopic dermatitis: One study on CAD had the same conclusion.[4]

Allergen Specific Immunotherapy (ASIT)

Specific immunotherapy (hyposensitization, desensitization) has been used in humans, since the beginning of the twentieth century, to treat asthma and allergic rhinitis but never in dermatology (it is also used in cases of hypersensitivity to Hymenoptera bites). It first was reported in dogs in the 1940s, expanded in North America in the 1960s, and in Europe in the 1980s. Many mechanisms are proposed, including the production of IgG-blocking antibodies, which combine with allergens before they combine with the IgE, and action on Th2-Th1 substitution, which leads to a reduction in the interleukin-4 production and an increase in the IFN-γ production. The interleukin-4 offers potential for the IgE synthesis and increases the number of weak-affinity IgE receptors or their CD23 soluble form. The IFN-γ inhibits IgE synthesis. The choice of allergens depends on in vivo or in vitro test results. Selection of allergens is essential and should include house dust mites, storage mites, molds, danders, and tree, weed and grass pollens. There could be a cross reactivity between storage mite extracts and *Dermatophagoides farinae* and *D. pteronyssinus* extracts. As grasses have a strong antigenic relationship, the use of a mixture of grass pollen extracts is acceptable.

Skin tests represent the reference to identify the responsible allergens if they are correctly carried out. The ELISA (enzyme-linked immunosorbent assay) serologic diagnosis is attractive due to its simplicity. It is used to assay the allergen-specific IgE in a patient's serum, using anti-IgE antibodies. Correlation with skin testing, arbitrarily considered the gold standard, has been evaluated in several studies. Specificity (rare false positives) and sensitivity (rare false negatives) are variable depending on arbitrary thresholds of positivity. Therefore, the reliability of many tests is doubtful. There is also controversy about testing being reproducible. Recently an innovative technique using human-specific IgE receptors (FcR1), instead of anti-IgE serum, has been proposed. Contrary to skin testing, conventional and FcR1-based ELISA testing can be performed in animals with severe cutaneous lesions and in animals previously treated with antihistamines or even glucocorticoids.

It is important to realize that a positive intradermal skin test or in vitro test is only an indication that an animal has developed specific IgE toward allergens and does not necessarily imply that the dermatologic problem is due to atopic disease. *Tests should always be interpreted in the light of the animal's history and clinical signs.* No standardization exists for the ASIT methods used. Only aqueous extracts are used in North America, whereas in Europe, long-acting extracts are available. It seems that the combination of molds and pollen extracts alters their quality (due to the presence of protease in the mold extracts) and that different types of vials are necessary. Immunotherapy is efficient in man as testified in the results obtained in allergic rhinitis. The results are more or less difficult to evaluate in dogs. They depend on the animal's age and diagnostic criteria, evaluation criteria (telephone follow-up, clinical score), follow-up duration, and recognition of "loss of follow-up" as setbacks. Presently, it is considered that 50% to 80% of animals respond to immunotherapy in open studies.

T. Willemse demonstrated in 1984 the method's efficacy through a double blind placebo controlled study. The 9-month evaluation seems important: it is usual that improvement at this stage is followed by success. Factors that influence results (apart from the diagnostic value and the clinical criteria of each one) include the allergen identification method, specificity, allergen's nature (*Dermatophagoides* spp.), number of allergens, breed, age, and patients' follow-up. The use of highly purified allergens (Der f 15 and Der f 18?) could improve results. No study has yet proven that the use of corticosteroids during desensitization would have a harmful effect on efficacy. Rare cases of secondary effects have been mentioned in an anecdotal manner (urticaria, angioedema, anaphylaxis). An exacerbation of clinical signs is often noticed in the hours following injections. Limited local reactions that are spontaneously reversible often appear with alum precipitated extracts. A majority of veterinary dermatologists believe that the efficacy and absence of secondary effects justifies *ad vitam eternam* hyposensitization. Empirically, it is common for clinical signs to reappear in a period of months to years after treatment has been stopped.

SYMPTOMATIC TREATMENT

This is useful at the beginning of immunotherapy (within the first year in successful cases) or on a long-term basis in failed cases (total or partial), or even in cases where immunotherapy is not required (aged animal, owner's hesitation, or even clinically slightly worrisome cases apart from a few signs). Symptomatic therapy is also indicated for canine atopic–like dermatitis.

Glucocorticoids

Corticosteroids are the most effective medications for the symptomatic treatment of allergic dermatitis. However there is no consistency in response from individual to individual. Further, the effect wanes over time and, therefore, the required dose increases. Topical glucocorticoid ointments, creams, and gels are useful in veterinary dermatology for localized lesions and perhaps have been neglected. Many traditional veterinary formulations are combinations of antimicrobials and glucocorticoids. Tachyphylaxis, atrophy, and microbial infections can occur in case of overuse. Several

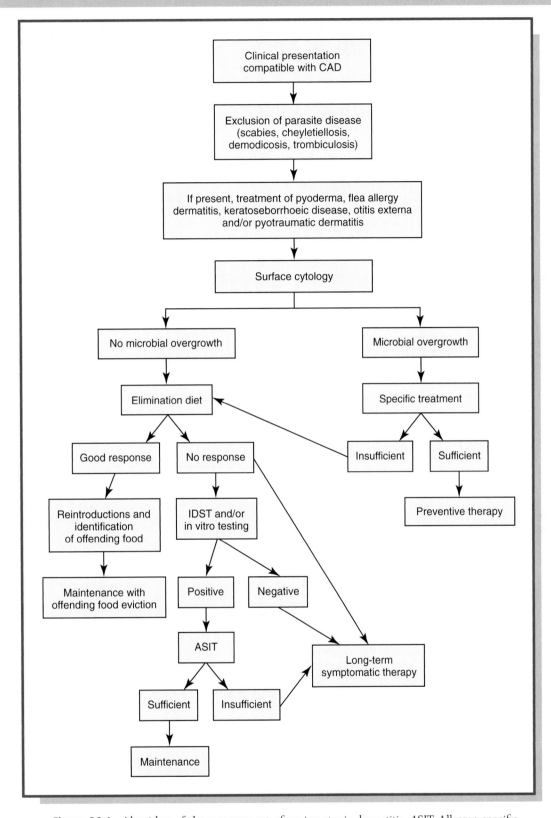

Figure 26-1 Algorithm of the management of canine atopic dermatitis. *ASIT,* Allergen specific immunotherapy; *CAD,* canine atopic dermatitis; *IDST,* intradermal skin testing.

glucocorticoids are also available in lotions, rinses, sprays, and shampoos. A new class of glucocorticoids, the diesters, is used in human dermatology because of reduced systemic effects. Hydrocortisone aceponate, for example, is now available as a medium-sized spray for use in dogs.

Systemic glucocorticoid therapy should be limited to oral administration of prednisolone or methylprednisolone (0.5 to 1 mg/kg/day for 5 to 7 days followed by 1 mg/kg every other day, for as little time as possible). Systemic corticosteroids have significant side effects including polyuria-polydipsia, polyphagia, hepatomegaly, inhibition of the hypothalamo-hypophyso-adrenal axis, dryness of the skin and the haircoat, and even iatrogenic Cushing's syndrome with alopecia. Secondary infections (pyoderma, demodicosis, dermatophytosis) can occur. Regarding steroid use: use them infrequently and at the lowest possible dose, preferably every other day, and only if alternative antipruritic medications have been deemed inefficient.

Nonsteroidal Topicals

These include antipruritic sprays, rinses, or lotions including microemulsions developed to complement shampoos specifically designed for canine atopic dermatitis. Tacrolimus, a calcineurin inhibitor with immunomodulatory properties, has been shown to be effective in the treatment of localized lesions of canine atopic dermatitis. All shampoos are likely to remove allergens and rehydrate the skin, effects that are believed helpful in CAD. Antiseborrhoeic shampoos and humectant sprays may be used to treat xerosis. Shampoos containing fatty acids may help in allergic skin disorders. Shampoos with an antipruritic effect and microemulsion shampoos specifically designed for canine atopic dermatitis have been shown to be useful.

Antihistamines

Anti-H1 antihistamines, which block H1 receptors, may be useful (anti-H2 are inefficient), but many have little or no efficacy. A few have been shown to have medium efficacy: clemastine, chlorpheniramine-hydroxyzine combination (first generation), oxatomide (second generation). Trimeprazine, which alone is inefficient, has proven to reduce the need for prednisone. There is a synergic effect between the essential fatty acids and antihistamines.

Essential Fatty Acids

Essential fatty acids (EFA) have been the subject of many clinical studies in dogs, although not used in human atopic dermatitis. The fatty acids that have been studied are polyunsaturated and administered by oral route, especially omega-3 series eicosapentaenoic acid (EPA) and omega-6 series gamma linolenic acid (GLA). They could have an antiinflammatory activity and could also reinforce the defective cutaneous barrier of atopic dogs. There are still doubts on the real efficacy of EFA in CAD, especially since various elements have not yet been made clear: the dosage (varying from 2 to 10 times the advised doses), minimal duration of the therapeutic test to predict efficacy (1 to 12 weeks), optimal ratio between omega-3 and omega-6 (between 5 and 10), the function of cofactors, criteria to select responder dogs, responder breeds, and synergy with other antiinflammatory agents. They are to be principally used with other antipruritic treatments. A dietary approach, based on a high quantity of omega-3 and the ratio of omega-3/omega-6, may also be helpful. They have few side effects.

Cyclosporine

Cyclosporine, an orally administered calcineurin inhibitor, is an effective drug for the treatment of CAD, as shown in several controlled studies. After a few weeks of daily administration it is possible to administer the drug only every other day or twice a week. A long-term treatment (several months) is justified and in some instances the treatment can be stopped. This molecule has become, despite its high cost, an effective symptomatic treatment of CAD, particularly in severe forms. Its efficacy is dose dependent but the assay of its blood level has no value since it cannot predict the clinical response. Secondary effects are limited and are mainly gastrointestinal, with more rarely gingival hyperplasia, verrucous lesions, or hypertrichosis. The long-term secondary effects known in man (renal insufficiency, hypertension) have not been reported in dogs. Last but not least cyclosporine does not enhance the risk of secondary infections.[5]

Other Nonsteroidal Systemic Antiinflammatory/Antipruritic Agents

Antidepressor and psychotropic drugs, leukotriene inhibitors, misoprostol, phosphodiesterase inhibitors have shown a low to moderate efficacy. IFN-γ and IFN-ω have shown promising effects. Various agents, including an injectable formulation of fatty acid copolymers, a phytotherapy preparation of Chinese herbs, MS-antigen (a peptide extracted from urine of allergic humans), and aminopterin (an antifolate), have given interesting results.

CONCLUSION: COMBINATION THERAPY CASE MANAGEMENT

A complete dermatology and allergy workup is necessary to establish the diagnosis of CAD, mainly based on clinical signs (Figure 26-1).

Long-term management of CAD is difficult. Each case is different and deserves a "combination therapy," which associates treatment of complications, eventual allergen-eviction measures and allergen-specific immunotherapy (both acting on the pruritic threshold), and symptomatic therapy (Web Figures 26-1 and 26-2).

It is the key to success.

References

The reference list can be found on the companion Expert Consult Web site at *www.expertconsult.com*.

CHAPTER 27

Obesity Biology and Management

Alexander James German

DEFINITION

Obesity is defined as an accumulation of excessive amounts of adipose tissue in the body. In humans, strict definitions exist on degree of adiposity, all based upon epidemiologic data that indicate that overweight subjects have reduced longevity.[1] Companion animals are currently classified as overweight when their body weight is more than 15% above their "optimal body weight," and classified as "obese" when their body weight exceeds 30% of optimal.[2] These data suggest, as in humans, adverse consequences develop when dogs and cats are not in optimal body condition.[3-5]

PREVALENCE

Obesity is an escalating global problem in humans, and current estimates suggest that almost two thirds of adults in the United States are overweight or obese.[6,7] Recent studies have estimated the prevalence of overweight/obesity in the pet population to be between 34% and 41%.[4,5,8,9] Although most investigators would agree that the incidence of obesity in pets is increasing, there are limited data to support this concern.

RISK FACTORS

Control of body weight requires the accurate matching of caloric intake to caloric expenditure over time. Despite dramatic fluctuations in caloric intake, normal animals are able to maintain a stable body weight.[10] Obesity arises when energy intake exceeds expenditure for a significant period of time. Dietary factors, coupled with exercise, are undoubtedly important. The number of meals and snacks fed, the feeding of table scraps, and being present when owners prepared or ate their own meal have all been implicated in canine obesity.[11] Interestingly, the type of diet (prepared pet food versus homemade) does not appear to predispose to obesity.[11] Type of commercial diet is important, with obese dogs being more likely to have been fed grocery rather than premium brand foods. In cats, feeding premium foods,[3] feeding food free choice, and feeding fresh meat or table scraps have all been implicated in contributing to obesity.[12-15]

Some diseases (e.g., hypothyroidism and hyperadrenocorticism) can predispose to the development of obesity, but account for less than 1% of cases. Factors of importance include gender and neuter status, age, and breed. Recent work has suggested that genetics play a key role in development of human obesity.[16] Given the breed predispositions that are reported in dogs (e.g., Labrador Retriever, Cavalier King Charles Spaniel, Cocker Spaniel, Beagle) and cats (e.g., Domestic Shorthair),[4,5] genetic influences are likely. Nonetheless, although rare single-gene defects are an occasional cause

of obesity in humans, they have not yet been recognized in companion animals.

Middle age is a particular risk factor for being overweight in both cats and dogs.[4,5] Neutering predisposes to obesity in both species and most recent studies suggest that the effect is due to an alteration in behavior, leading to increased food intake and decreased activity.[17-22] Gender itself is also a predisposing factor in some studies on dogs, with females overrepresented. Other recognized associations in dogs include indoor lifestyle, inactivity, and middle age.[4,5,8] In cats, middle age and apartment dwelling are possible risk factors.[3] Certain pharmaceuticals (e.g., glucocorticoids, anticonvulsant drugs, progestagens) can stimulate polyphagia and could predispose to weight gain if extra food is offered. Other studies have implicated owner factors (human obesity, female gender, close owner-pet relationship), and feeding behavior as risk factors for overweight and obesity in both dogs and cats.[11,15]

PATHOLOGIC CONSEQUENCES

In humans, the medical importance of obesity lies in the effect on mortality and predisposition to other diseases.[6] Obese humans have a reduced lifespan and are more likely to suffer from diseases such as type II diabetes mellitus, hypertension, coronary heart disease, certain cancers (e.g., breast, ovarian, prostate), osteoarthritis, respiratory disease, and reproductive disorders. Similarly, obesity has detrimental effects on health and longevity of dogs and cats.

PATHOGENESIS OF OBESITY-ASSOCIATED DISEASES

Secondary disease associations result either from "mechanical" or "endocrine" effects of excessive white adipose tissue (WAT) deposition. "Mechanical" effects of excess adipose tissue deposition include excessive weight bearing on joints and bones (exacerbating orthopedic diseases), constriction of collapsible structures (exacerbation of upper respiratory tract disorders and urinary incontinence), inability to groom, and reduced heat dissipation due to the insulating effect of fat (exacerbating heat stroke). Disturbance of normal endocrine function of WAT is also recognized as a major pathogenetic mechanism in obesity. WAT is now known to secrete a range of "chemical" factors that can have a regulatory effect on many body systems.[23-25] Of particular note is the range of cytokines, chemokines, and other inflammation-related proteins (collectively termed *adipokines*) secreted by WAT as tissue mass rises. Indeed, obesity is characterized by a state of chronic mild inflammation.[25] Increases in the production certain "inflammatory" adipokines (e.g., leptin, tumor necrosis factor-α, interleukin-6, plasminogen activator inhibitor-1, and haptoglobin) have been causally linked to the development of the metabolic syndrome and other disorders linked to the obese state.[23-25] Inflammatory adipokine gene expression has recently been documented in canine WAT samples.[26,27] Further, plasma leptin concentrations have been shown to be independently associated with insulin sensitivity in lean and overweight cats,[28] suggesting that similar pathogenetic mechanisms may exist in companion animals.

EFFECTS ON LONGEVITY

A long-term colony-based research study, comparing lifelong *ad libitum* feeding with energy restriction (~75% of *ad libitum*), has demonstrated *ad-libitum*–fed dogs tend to be overweight, have a shorter lifespan, and have increased risk of associated disease.[29-34]

DISEASE ASSOCIATIONS

Obesity is reported to be a major risk factor for a variety of disorders (Table 27-1).[3-5,29-49]

The most important associations include orthopedic disease in dogs, and diabetes mellitus in both species. In humans, tissues become "insulin resistant" with excessive caloric intake, and plasma concentrations of insulin increase in direct proportion to increasing body mass index (BMI) in both men and women. Thus, obesity, particularly abdominal obesity, is a major determinant of insulin resistance and hyperinsulinemia. A percentage of cats with diabetes mellitus have a form of the disease resembling non–insulin dependent type 2 diabetes of humans. Obesity is a major risk factor for diabetes in cats. Further, weight loss can resolve insulin resistance and clinical signs of diabetes in some cats. An association between obesity and canine diabetes mellitus has been reported. In one study, diabetic dogs were ~2.5 times more likely to be overweight (at the time of diagnosis) than controls, and almost 4 times as likely to have been overweight throughout life. The exact pathogenetic mechanisms underlying this association are unclear but, given that the most common type of canine diabetes resembles human type 1 (insulin dependent), mechanisms are likely to differ from those in humans and cats. Nonetheless, research does suggest that insulin resistance can develop in overweight dogs. However, given that cases of

Table • 27-1

Reported Disease Associations in Canine and Feline Obesity

| DISEASE CATEGORY | SPECIES | |
	CAT	DOG
Orthopedic	Increased lameness	Cruciate ligament disease
		Osteoarthritis
		Humeral condylar fractures
		Intervertebral disk disease
		Hip dysplasia
Endocrine	Diabetes mellitus	Hypothyroidism
		Hyperadrenocorticism
		Diabetes mellitus
		Metabolic syndrome (experimental)
Lipid disorders	Hepatic lipidosis	Mild hypercholesterolemia, hypertriglyceridemia, increased plasma NEFA and triglyceride concentrations (experimental) associated with insulin resistance
Alimentary	Oral cavity disease	Oral cavity disease
	Increased gastrointestinal disease risk	Pancreatitis
	Predisposition to diarrhea	
Urogenital	Urinary tract disease	Urinary tract disease
		USMI
		Calcium oxalate urolithiasis
		Transitional cell carcinoma
		Glomerular disease (experimental)
		Dystocia
Cardiorespiratory		Tracheal collapse
		Affect on cardiac function
		Expiratory airway dysfunction
		Hypertension
		Portal vein thrombosis
		Myocardial hypoxia
Integument	Increased risk of dermatoses	—
Oncologic	Increased neoplasia risk	Variable neoplasia risk (increased in some but not all studies)
		Transitional cell carcinoma
Other		Increased anesthetic risk
		Decreased heat tolerance

NEFA, Nonesterified fatty acids; *USMI,* urethral sphincter mechanism incompetence.

canine diabetes mellitus usually require lifelong insulin therapy, weight management strategies do not lead to resolution of diabetes mellitus. In humans, metabolic syndrome is a group of risk factors associated with both insulin resistance and cardiovascular disease and thrombosis. Some of these criteria have been applied to dogs, and this species is often used as a model of metabolic syndrome.

MEASUREMENT OF OBESITY IN COMPANION ANIMALS

All measures of adiposity involve defining body composition, or the "relative amounts of the various biologic components of the body." Dual-energy x-ray absorptiometry (DEXA) has recently been shown to be a precise and reliable method for repeated analysis,[50] and can be used to monitor weight loss in a referral setting.[51,52]

However, for first-opinion practice, there is a need for quick, cheap, and noninvasive methods of body composition measurement. A number of body condition scoring schemes combine visual assessment and palpation to assess adipose tissue mass.[8,53,54] When used by trained individuals, scores are relatively repeatable among observers and correlate well with body fat mass determined by DEXA.[53-55] Regular body condition assessment is a simple method for monitoring the state of health of companion animals. Increases in condition score can readily be identified and suggest that the animal is becoming overweight, while decreases signal the possibility of underfeeding or a developing disease process. Further, the current body condition score of an obese individual can be used as a guide to setting target weight for weight loss, by estimating that each point (on a 9-integer condition score) or half point (on a 5-integer condition score) correlates with ~10% to 15% increase in body weight.[53-55] Despite the simplicity and usefulness of such systems, veterinarians appear to use them infrequently.[56]

TREATMENT

In humans, the most successful approach for treatment of severe obesity is bariatric surgery, but this is not considered to be ethically justifiable in companion animals. Dietary therapy remains a common approach to obesity management, and microsomal membrane transfer protein (MTP) inhibitor drugs have recently received approval for the treatment of canine (but not feline) weight loss.[57] Whichever strategy is adopted, long-term success can only come from altering lifestyle long-term (i.e., by increasing activity and altering feeding behavior [implementing calorie control]).

Dietary Management

It is preferable to use purpose-formulated diets to achieve weight loss. Such diets are restricted in fat and calories while supplemented with protein and micronutrients. The mean energy requirement for weight loss in dogs is 60% of required calories at target weight.[51] Cats should be fed an average of 32 kcal/kg of target body weight during weight loss.[52] With these restrictions, the mean rate of weight loss is 0.8% body weight/week for both species.[51,52] Close monitoring is required and energy intake must progressively be reduced to ensure continued weight loss.[51,52] Using a high-protein diet is important since such diets minimize loss of lean tissue, although weight loss is not more rapid.[51,52,58,59] Supplementation of micronutrients ensures that deficiency states do not arise.

Dietary supplementation of L-carnitine, in weight-reduction diets, has been shown to maintain lean tissue during weight loss.[60,61] Possible mechanisms for this protective effect on lean tissue include enhancing fatty acid oxidation and energy availability for protein synthesis during times of need. Recent studies have highlighted the benefit of combining high protein and high fiber for improving satiety.[62] Such formulations appear to be optimal for weight loss diets (Figure 27-1).

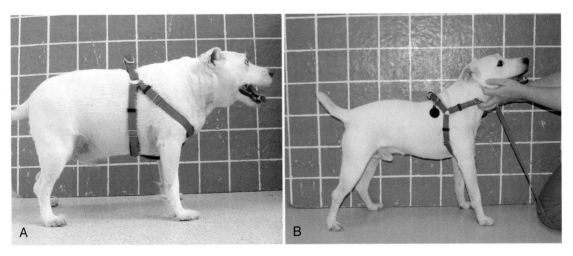

Figure 27-1 **A,** Photograph of an obese 7-year-old neutered male Jack Russell Terrier, presenting with collapse and exercise intolerance. On physical examination, the dog weighed 15.6 kg (34 lb), and condition score was 9/9. **B,** Photograph of the same dog, 181 days later, after successful weight loss on a high-protein high-fiber diet. Body weight had decreased to 9.15 kg (20 lb), and condition score was 5/9. No clinical signs were evident. Total weight lost was 41% of starting body weight, at a rate of 1.6%/week.

Pharmaceutical Therapy and Weight Loss

Two pharmaceutical products have recently been licensed for use in dogs, but NOT in cats.[57,63] Both are MTP inhibitors, which have a local effect at the level of the intestinal epithelial cell, blocking the assembly and release of lipoprotein particles into the bloodstream. Dietary caloric intake is decreased partly by decreasing lipid absorption, but predominantly by decreasing appetite. Both drugs are less potent when administered in conjunction with a low-fat balanced diet. This seems counterintuitive but is explained by understanding that the drugs only work when given orally (so it is a local effect in the intestine), not by injection. Unpublished experimental work suggests that these drugs lead to release of a gut neuropeptide, which acts on the satiety center in the hypothalamus. The exact neuropeptide involved is not known but is suspected to be peptide YY. Although speculative, it would appear that the more fat that builds up in the enterocytes, the stronger the satiety signal. Therefore, on a low-fat diet, more drug would be required to achieve the same effect. While elegant, it does lead to a major dilemma if using drugs for weight loss: that the drugs are most effective in pets fed the wrong diets (high fat), and continuing with that diet after drug discontinuation leads to more rapid weight rebound. Fat content comprising at least 10% of dry matter is recommended.

Dirlotapide is licensed in the United States and Europe, and can be used continuously for up to 12 months. Weight loss occurs at a steady rate (0.75%/week on average), but periodic increases in dose are required to maintain weight loss. Significant amounts of weight loss have been demonstrated in clinical trials.[63] Mitratapide is licensed in Europe only, and has a similar mechanism of action to dirlotapide. Rather than long-term continuous dosing, this drug is used short term and in conjunction with dietary management and behavioral modification.

Side effects, usually gastrointestinal (e.g., vomiting and diarrhea), can occur with either drug in as many as 20% of dogs. Owners should be forewarned that gastrointestinal problems may occur. While these drugs provide an easy avenue for weight loss, appetite returns rapidly after discontinuation of therapy. Unless other strategies (feeding and behavioral) are implemented after stopping either medication, a rapid and predictable rebound in body weight will occur.

Lifestyle Management

Increasing physical activity is a useful adjunct in a weight-management regimen, since it promotes fat loss and may help to preserve lean tissue during weight loss. The exact program must be tailored to the individual, and take account of any concurrent medical concerns. Suitable exercise strategies in dogs include walking, swimming, hydrotherapy, and treadmills. Exercise in cats can be encouraged by increasing play activity, using cat toys (e.g., fishing rod toys), motorized units, and feeding toys. Cats can also be encouraged to "work" for their food by moving the food bowl between rooms prior to feeding, or by the use of feeding toys.

Monitoring of Weight Loss

In addition to the above strategies, it is essential that an entire weight reduction regimen be supervised. This is labor intensive, requires some degree of expertise and training in owner counseling, and often requires a dedicated staff member. It is essential to continue to monitor body weight after ideal weight has been achieved to ensure that weight that was lost is not regained. As previously discussed, a rebound effect has been demonstrated after weight loss in dogs.[64]

PREVENTION

As with most medical diseases, prevention is better than cure. The health and welfare of all dogs and cats can be improved dramatically by preventing obesity, rather than by instituting treatment once the problem has developed. Advice on correct nutrition and exercise should be included in all puppy consultations and continued for all pets whenever they are seen. Discussion of body weight and body condition should be incorporated into every routine checkup (e.g., annual vaccination). By monitoring body weight and body condition score throughout life, increasing adiposity can rapidly be identified and rectified. Finally, veterinarians should be alert to the weight gain that can occur as a consequence of neutering. It is advisable to schedule two to three weight checks in the first 6 to 12 months after neutering to identify those animals at risk of weight gain and correct it before it becomes a problem.

REFERENCES

The reference list can be found on the companion Expert Consult Web site at *www.expertconsult.com.*

CHAPTER 28

Cachexia

Thomas Schermerhorn

A standard definition for cachexia is difficult to provide. In clinical practice, cachexia is the term used to describe the weight loss, loss of muscle, and anorexia that accompany many chronic disease conditions. However, it is important to recognize that cachexia is not simply caused by inadequate nutrient intake and that cachexia and starvation are not equivalent physiologic processes. Two biochemical features distinguish malnutrition caused by cachexia from that caused by starvation. First, unlike starvation, inflammation is a consistent feature of cachexia. Cachexia causes marked activation of the inflammatory cascade, which is characterized by a pronounced acute phase inflammatory response and excessive production of proinflammatory cytokines such as interleukins (IL-1 and IL-6, among others) and tumor necrosis factor-alpha (TNF-α). Cytokines stimulate the ubiquitin pathway, which is a central pathway in protein turnover. Ubiquitin complexes with target cellular proteins and stimulates their metabolism via the proteasome system. Second, cachexia is associated with a rise in resting energy expenditure, which increases as a consequence of altered protein, fat, and carbohydrate metabolism. Loss of body muscle and adipose tissues is marked and an insulin-resistant state may develop. Despite the similar clinical appearance, activation of the ubiquitin-proteasome system and increased energy expenditure are not features of starvation.

A diagnosis of cachexia should be considered for any dog or cat with marked weight loss, severe muscle loss, and decreased appetite in the setting of a chronic inflammatory response or cancer. By this definition, cachexia is not a specific diagnosis but a state of disordered metabolism that can be caused by a variety of diseases.

When evaluating an emaciated dog or cat, it is important to determine, from diagnostic and therapeutic standpoints, whether the condition has developed as a result of inadequate nutrient intake (maldigestion, malabsorption, or underfeeding, for example) or represents true cachexia.

HISTORY

Dogs and cats with cachexia may be brought to veterinarians principally for weight loss or for signs associated with an underlying condition. The carefully obtained history should include questions about appetite, caloric intake, daily exercise, and environment. Some animals with cachexia have weight loss with preservation of appetite; the loss of body condition may be noted before the onset of anorexia in some cases. Dogs and cats with malnutrition as a result of starvation, malabsorption, or maldigestion typically have a good appetite. However, the level of appetite is variable in animals with cachexia, ranging from normal to complete anorexia. Lethargy, weakness, and exercise intolerance may be marked and in some cases are worse than would be expected if simply the result of poor physical condition. The dietary history should be carefully reviewed and include the type and quantity of food offered (including any dietary supplements provided), the possibility that other pets at home might be competing for food, and the pet's level of appetite. It is important to distinguish those animals that have an appetite but cannot prehend or swallow food from those who have no appetite but can chew and swallow normally. Diagnostic considerations suggested by various patient history findings are presented in Box 28-1.

PHYSICAL AND LABORATORY FINDINGS

Cachexia has few specific indicators other than the marked loss of body condition that is a characteristic finding; muscle may be lost disproportionately to fat in some animals with cachexia. Similarly, laboratory findings are not specific for cachexia. Serum protein levels are variable even in the presence of a systemic inflammatory response. For example, elevated fibrinogen levels (as a component of the acute phase response) in humans with neoplasia may be offset by reduced albumin synthesis. Increases in hormone concentrations, such as cortisol and insulin, may be observed in animals with cachexia; these changes may result from or be the cause of cachexia-induced alterations in metabolism. In general, an

individual patient's physical and laboratory findings will be representative of the underlying disease rather than specific indicators of cachexia. No compelling reasons exist to perform specific laboratory tests to make a diagnosis of cachexia. Instead, cachexia is largely a clinical diagnosis that is made when appropriate physical findings are present in a dog or cat with a disease associated with a chronic inflammatory response.

DIAGNOSTIC PLAN

A general algorithm for making a diagnosis of cachexia is shown in Figure 28-1.

It is important to recognize cachexia because animals with this condition may not respond as expected to therapeutic interventions and nutritional support.

THERAPY

Successful therapy of the primary disorder is the most efficacious means of reversing the metabolic abnormalities that underlie the development of cachexia. Nutritional support is the cornerstone of specific therapy for cachexia. Hypercaloric feeding is intended to supply the dog or cat with sufficient

---

Box • 28-1

Diagnostic Considerations for Patients with Marked Weight Loss

Dietary History—Inadequate
Starvation
Underfeeding
Poor-quality food

Dietary History—Adequate
Environmental/housing factors
    Competition for food from other pets
    Limited access to food
Oral and dental disease
Impaired use of nutrients
    Specific nutrient deficiency
    Maldigestion of any cause
    Malabsorption of any cause
    Diabetes mellitus
    Protein-losing disease
        Nephropathy
        Gastroenteropathy
    Cardiac disease*
Elevated metabolism
    Hyperthyroidism
    Chronic fever of any cause*
End-stage renal disease*
Neoplasia*
Chronic infection*
Chronic inflammation of any cause (e.g., immunologic disease*)

Note: Patients may present with or without a loss of appetite.
*Diseases typically associated with cachexia in humans and animals.

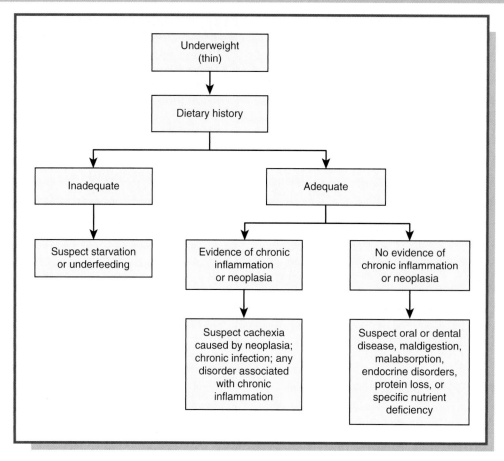

Figure 28-1   Algorithm for making a diagnosis of cachexia.

calories to meet increased maintenance caloric needs (because of hypermetabolism), prevent additional weight loss, and promote weight gain. Unfortunately, hypercaloric feeding alone may not be sufficient therapy for animals with true cachexia. People with cachexia who receive hypercaloric feeding gain weight, but the increase in body weight is almost exclusively the result of an increase in adipose tissue without change in lean body mass. Thus it appears that simple feeding therapy may not be sufficient in all situations to reverse the abnormal protein catabolism that accompanies cachexia.

Pharmacologic therapies that have been used for cachexia in humans that may prove useful for the treatment of animals include nutritional supplements (including fish oils), appetite stimulants, anabolic agents, antiinflammatory drugs, and cytokine inhibitors. Although some of these drugs have been extensively used for other indications in small animals, information is limited about their efficacy when used for cachexia. Specific inhibitors of the ubiquitin system, which inhibit the effects of cachexia at the molecular level, may eventually be developed.

CHAPTER 29

Failure to Grow

Sherri L. Ihle

Growth is a complex process that results in an increase in size of an individual. In dogs and cats, growth primarily occurs during the first 6 to 24 months of life. When an animal does not increase in size at the normal rate or to a normal extent, a "failure to grow" is identified. The owner of the affected pet may notice the problem and bring the animal to the veterinarian, or the animal's small size may be first noticed during a routine physical examination. In veterinary medicine, determination of normal growth is sometimes difficult because breed sizes vary and mixed breed pets predominate. Comparing littermates, when possible, can be helpful in making and assessing the individual's growth rate and pattern.

PATHOPHYSIOLOGY

Genetic, hormonal, metabolic, and nutritional factors influence growth. To meet its full genetic potential, an animal must have growth hormone (somatotropin) to stimulate insulin-like growth factor-I (IGF-I) production, which in turn stimulates skeletal growth, protein synthesis, and cell proliferation. Full IGF-I activity requires the presence of thyroid hormone. The animal must also consume sufficient calories and nutrients; digest, absorb and retain the nutrients; transport the nutrients to the necessary tissues; and be able to use the nutrients for metabolic maintenance and growth. A defect in any of the previously mentioned processes can disrupt, delay, or stop normal growth (Box 29-1; Figure 29-1).

Box • 29-1

Causes of Growth Failure in Dogs and Cats

Small Stature and Poor Body Condition
Dietary problem
Underfeeding
Poor-quality diet
Cardiac disorder
    Congenital anomaly
    Endocarditis
Hepatic dysfunction
    Portosystemic vascular anomaly
    Hepatitis
    Glycogen storage disease
Esophageal disease
    Megaesophagus
    Vascular ring anomaly (e.g., persistent right aortic arch)
Gastrointestinal disease
    Parasites
    Inflammatory bowel disease
    Obstruction (e.g., foreign body, intussusception)
    Histoplasmosis
Exocrine pancreatic insufficiency
Renal disease
    Renal failure (congenital or acquired)
    Glomerular disease
    Pyelonephritis
Inflammatory disease
Hormonal disease
    Diabetes mellitus
    Hypoadrenocorticism
    Diabetes insipidus
    Juvenile hyperparathyroidism (dogs)

Small Stature and Good Body Condition
Chondrodystrophy
Hormonal disease
    Congenital hypothyroidism
    Congenital hyposomatotropism (pituitary dwarfism)
    Hyperadrenocorticism

Genetic Abnormalities of Bone Growth

An inherited endochondral ossification defect in chondrodystrophic animals results in angular limb deformities and subnormal height.

Deficient Nutrient Intake

Gastrointestinal parasitism, resulting in a "relative" deficiency in nutrition, is the most common cause of retarded growth in puppies and kittens. Growth retardation due to parasitism is potentially reversible with proper therapy. If an insufficient amount of food or food of poor quality is consumed, nutrients will not be available to provide substrates and energy for tissue growth. Oral disease may cause pseudoanorexia. Regurgitation or vomiting because of esophageal or gastric disorders could cause insufficient food to reach the intestines for digestion and absorption. Maldigestion or malabsorption can result in decreased uptake of nutrients. Renal, hepatic, cardiac, inflammatory, and hypoadrenal disease can suppress the appetite. Absorption and transport of nutrients from the intestines to other tissues can also be inadequate with cardiac disease.

Caloric or Nutrient Loss

Fever can result in excess caloric loss as body heat. In diabetes mellitus, glucose is lost in the urine. However, in diabetes mellitus, it is the inability to utilize calories that leads to failure to grow or weight loss, rather than the loss of calories into the urine. Proteins and salts can also be lost in the urine in animals with glomerular and renal tubular disease, respectively. Several intestinal disorders can result in protein-losing enteropathy. As previously noted, parasitism is the most common cause of "lost" nutrients.

Abnormal Metabolism

Carbohydrate metabolism can be altered in inflammatory disease, renal disease, and hepatic disease. Protein production can also be decreased with hepatic disease. Hypothalamic or pituitary aplasia or neoplasia (e.g., craniopharyngioma) can result in low growth hormone and IGF-I concentrations. Hypothyroidism can decrease the activity of growth hormone. Because insulin has a positive effect on IGF-I production, insulin deficiency caused by diabetes mellitus or malnutrition can slow growth. Cortisol excess, whether endogenous or exogenous in origin, can inhibit the secretion of growth hormone, which in turn causes failure to grow. An extremely rare form of juvenile hyperparathyroidism in German Shepherd Dogs has also been reported to cause stunted growth.

HISTORICAL FINDINGS

The animal with subnormal growth may be brought to the veterinarian for that problem or the small body size may be noted during routine physical examination. In either case, the owner of the dog or cat should be questioned as to the size of the pet's parents and littermates, if known. If the parents and littermates are also at the lower end of the range of breed size, the small stature of the pet may not be worrisome. However, if the pet is noticeably smaller than its littermates, the problem should be investigated. When the family history is unknown, the pet's size should be compared with that of others in the breed. For the mixed breed dog, the predominant breed should be determined based on physical characteristics, and that breed's average size should be the standard for comparison.

Duration of the Problem

Determining whether the animal's growth has been slow since birth or whether it was normal and then suddenly seemed to stop can be helpful. In the former case, congenital defects

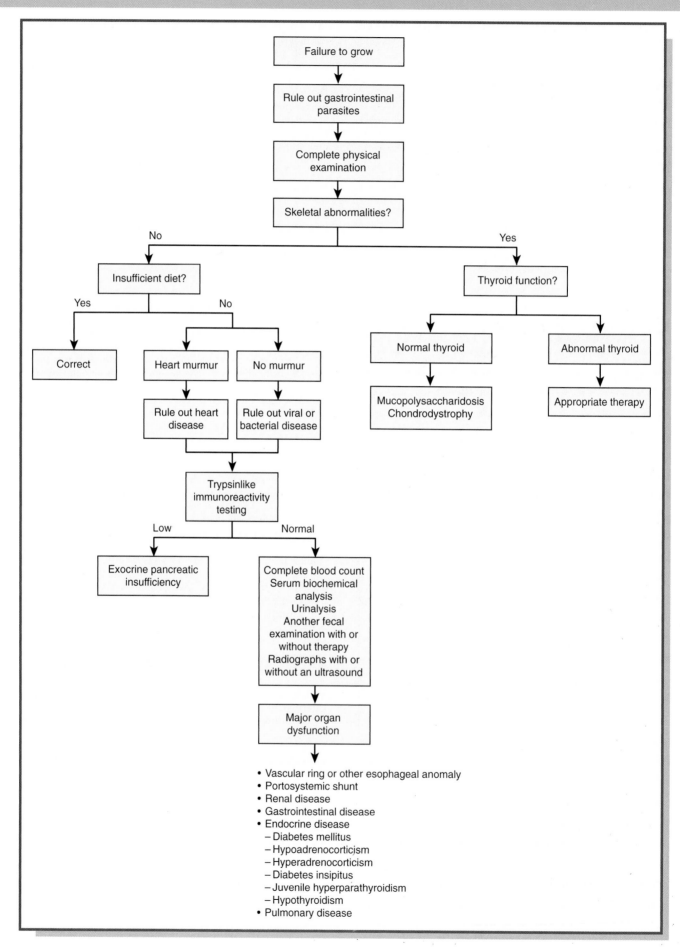

Figure 29-1 Algorithm for diagnostic evaluation of the dog or cat with failure to grow.

should be strongly considered, whereas in the latter case, acquired disorders must also be considered.

Diet

A detailed nutritional history should be obtained as to type of food, amount of food consumed, appetite, and feeding schedule. A less palatable or nonpalatable diet may not be consumed in adequate quantities to support growth while a diet of poor quality may fail to supply adequate nutrients for normal growth and development. A poor appetite, despite the feeding of a palatable, high-quality food, suggests the presence of a systemic illness causing inappetence or anorexia. Conversely, if the animal is always hungry and internal parasites have been ruled out or treated, underfeeding (because of inadequate owner knowledge of the pet's nutritional needs), a disorder causing a "relative" lack of calories (e.g., exocrine pancreatic insufficiency), or an increased nutrient loss (e.g., diabetes mellitus, renal disease, intestinal disease) should be considered.

Concurrent Clinical Signs

The owner should also be questioned about the presence or absence of other clinical signs, which may help define the cause of the problem. Regurgitation usually indicates a pharyngeal or esophageal problem. Vomiting suggests a gastrointestinal problem or systemic illness (e.g., renal disease, hepatic disease, hypoadrenocorticism). Diarrhea or voluminous stools may be seen with disorders causing maldigestion (e.g., exocrine pancreatic insufficiency) or malabsorption (e.g., severe parasitism, inflammatory bowel disease, histoplasmosis). If polyuria is present, diabetes mellitus, renal disease, hepatic dysfunction, or hypercalcemia (juvenile hyperparathyroidism) should be considered. Seizures, episodic abnormal behavior, vomiting, and diarrhea may be signs of hepatic dysfunction. Exercise intolerance or syncope can suggest a congenital cardiac abnormality. Poor response to housebreaking measures or to obedience training, or a lack of normal puppy play activities, can suggest the mental dullness of congenital hypothyroidism, or the encephalopathy of hepatic failure. Poor response to housebreaking measures may also be seen with ectopic ureters or the polyuria of kidney abnormality. Glucocorticoid therapy for an unrelated problem may have slowed the pet's growth. Although the absence of these historical findings does not eliminate these disorders as possible problems, their presence can guide the diagnostic plan.

PHYSICAL EXAMINATION FINDINGS

Although some animals examined as a result of poor growth will have no other clinical abnormalities, in many animals a thorough physical examination can provide valuable clues as to the organ system or systems responsible for the problem. The animal's general appearance and body condition should be assessed. A short animal with a poor body condition is more likely to have a nutritional, metabolic, or cardiac abnormality, whereas a short animal with a good body condition is likely to have a hormonal problem or be chondrodysplastic (see Box 29-1). Chondrodysplastic animals and many animals with congenital hypothyroidism will also have an abnormal skeletal conformation (e.g., angular limb deformities). Symmetrical truncal alopecia, the prolonged presence of a soft puppy haircoat, or thin, scaly skin suggests thyroid hormone deficiency, growth hormone deficiency, or cortisol excess. Mental dullness can be seen with hypothyroidism or hepatic encephalopathy. Hepatic failure can also result in cortical blindness.

The head and neck should be examined for pale mucous membranes (anemia of chronic disease), icterus (hepatic disease), oral pain (dysphagia), and lymphadenopathy (inflammatory disease or neoplasia). The thorax should be carefully ausculted for a murmur (congenital cardiac disease, other cardiac dysfunction), bradycardia (hypoadrenocorticism), or abnormal lung sounds (pulmonary disease). On abdominal palpation, enlarged or shrunken kidneys can indicate a renal problem, and hepatomegaly can suggest hepatic disease or dysfunction. Thickened bowel walls may be felt in the presence of inflammatory bowel disease, or a mass lesion may be palpated in the pet with a foreign body or intussusception.

DIAGNOSTIC PLAN

Decisions concerning the initial diagnostic plan should be based on the animal's body condition and any abnormalities identified from the history and physical examination (see Figure 29-1). Food consumption should always be evaluated (see Historical Findings). If food intake is in question, a brief feeding trial can provide information on appetite and caloric consumption in relation to change in body weight. Multiple fecal examinations and possible deworming should be performed to eliminate severe parasitism as the cause of malnutrition. If the animal has been given a medication that may have slowed growth, the medication should be discontinued, if possible, and subsequent growth monitored. A complete blood count (CBC) should be evaluated for anemia, inflammation, or eosinophilia. Eosinophilia, when documented, most often indicates parasitism, but cortisol deficiency, neoplasia, and other differentials should be considered. Results of a serum biochemical profile can suggest renal, hepatic, or gastrointestinal disease; diabetes mellitus; hypoadrenocorticism; hyperadrenocorticism; hypothyroidism; or hyperparathyroidism. A urinalysis may show proteinuria, isosthenuria, hyposthenuria, glucosuria, or inflammatory sediment. Radiographs can be used to detect a cardiopulmonary abnormality, organomegaly, a small liver or kidneys, intestinal foreign body, or skeletal abnormalities. Ultrasonography may help to further characterize radiographic abnormalities and detect structural abnormalities within an organ. An electrocardiogram may be helpful in assessing potential hyperkalemia (in an emergency) and congenital cardiac abnormalities. Radiographic contrast studies can be used to characterize congenital cardiac abnormalities, to identify portosystemic vascular anomalies, and to detect partial gastrointestinal obstructions. Hepatic function tests can identify the need for further investigation of the liver. Gastrointestinal function tests (e.g., serum trypsin–like immunoreactivity, serum cobalamin and folate) can be used to identify occult gastrointestinal disease causing maldigestion or malabsorption. Biopsy may be needed if gastrointestinal, hepatic, or renal disease is identified. Hormonal tests can be used to detect hypothyroidism, hyperadrenocorticism, hypoadrenocorticism, and hyperparathyroidism; an assay for growth hormone is not currently available on a commercial basis, but an IGF-I assay is available for the dog.

TREATMENT

Treatment of the animal that exhibits growth failure varies widely based on the underlying pathology. Some disorders can be well managed medically, and others require surgical correction.

CHAPTER 30

Swollen Joints and Lameness

Richard E. Goldstein

Although lameness has numerous causes, this chapter focuses on lameness associated with nontraumatic inflammatory joint disease. Assessment for swelling or pain of accessible joints should be a routine component of the physical examination of dogs and cats. Arthritis can be categorized based on cause.

Degenerative joint disease is caused by chronic changes to the joint capsule, cartilage, and synovium associated with minimal to no active inflammation. Degenerative joint disease, although painful, is not typically associated with systemic inflammatory signs. Inflammatory joint diseases can be classified as septic or nonseptic (immune mediated). Inflammatory joint disease is typically associated with one or more of the signs consistent with those of systemic disease. These usually include fever, leukocytosis, inappetence, or lethargy. Arthritis can also be classified based on the number of joints involved. Monoarthritis implies involvement of a single joint, whereas polyarthritis involves multiple joints.

SEPTIC ARTHRITIS

Septic arthritis is defined by presence of bacteria in the synovial or joint fluid, observed on cytologic evaluation or with bacterial culture. Septic arthritis occurs as a result of hematogenous (more common in neonates) spread or external penetrating wounds. It is not always possible to distinguish septic arthritis from immune-mediated arthritis, especially when multiple joints are involved or no obvious penetrating wound is seen. Joint fluid cultures, although worthwhile, are frequently negative even when bacteria are evident on cytologic examination. Neutrophils predominate in the joint fluid of infectious and immune-mediated arthritis. Degenerative changes in neutrophils, however, are more indicative of a septic process. The number and type of joints involved may help the clinician differentiate septic from nonseptic arthritis. Single joint involvement and involvement of proximal joints (hip, shoulder, stifle, and elbow) are usually septic. Multiple, distal joint (carpi, tarsi) involvement is most commonly seen immune-mediated disease. When a septic process is possible, a period of antimicrobial therapy can be recommended, even if no bacteria are observed on joint fluid cytology and joint fluid cultures are pending or negative.

IMMUNE-MEDIATED POLYARTHRITIS

Immune-mediated polyarthritis is the most common polyarthritis in companion dogs and cats. The cause of this condition is likely a type III hypersensitivity reaction, in which immune complexes are deposited in the synovial membrane and an inflammatory cascade is initiated. The immune stimulus is frequently unknown, hence the commonly used term *idiopathic polyarthritis*. Immune-mediated polyarthritis can be categorized both radiographically and histologically into the common nonerosive form and the uncommon erosive condition.

EROSIVE POLYARTHRITIS

Erosive polyarthritis in dogs is similar to human rheumatoid arthritis. These similarities include the progressive, severe, deforming course of the disease and the erosive radiographic appearance of affected joints. In humans, specific antibodies, collectively known as rheumatoid factor (RF), are commonly identified. An IgM antibody, considered the canine RF, has been identified in some dogs with erosive arthritis. Although the term *rheumatoid arthritis* has been used in veterinary medicine, it is preferable to use the descriptive term *erosive arthritis* in dogs.

RF is a nonsensitive and nonspecific marker of erosive or immune-mediated arthritis in dogs, making the assay's clinical utility highly questionable. Radiographic findings commonly seen in dogs with this form of arthritis include erosions involving the articular surface or the loss of trabecular bone density in the epiphyses. The destructive process is progressive. Radiographically, this process appears in the subchondral or juxtaarticular bone as poorly demarcated radiolucent foci. Erosive arthritis has been reported in many breeds but is thought to occur more frequently in small-breed dogs, 2 to 6 years of age. A specific form of erosive arthritis has been reported in Greyhounds.

Erosive polyarthritis has been reported in cats and has been termed *progressive feline polyarthritis*. This is a disease that occurs more commonly in male cats between 1.5 and 5 years of age. It may be an immune-mediated hypersensitivity type III reaction to chronic viral immune stimulation, secondary to chronic feline syncytium-forming virus infection. Two forms of the disease exist: (1) the deforming type, a severely erosive condition that is similar to canine erosive arthritis, and (2) the more common proliferative form. Both forms can be associated with severe systemic signs of disease, including lymphadenopathy, swollen joints, and muscle wasting.

NONEROSIVE POLYARTHRITIS

This is the most common form of immune-mediated polyarthritis in dogs and cats. The source of the antigenic stimulation is usually not known. Nonerosive polyarthritis has been reported to occur secondary to chronic infectious disease, systemic lupus erythematosus (SLE), lymphocytic plasmacytic synovitis, use of certain drugs, and malignancies. It may also be a component of immune-mediated diseases, such as inflammatory bowel disease or chronic hepatitis.

Clinical signs typically include cyclic fever, lethargy, anorexia, and varying degrees of pain, lameness, and swollen joints. A stiff gait characterized as "walking on egg shells" is frequently observed, but some affected dogs have a normal gait. The distal joints (carpi and tarsi) are most commonly affected. Pain, redness, and swelling range from severe to absent. Some dogs exhibit pain that is difficult to localize. Others have signs of back or neck pain. This could be a result of inflammation of the vertebral articulations or concurrent meningitis. Lymphadenopathy and muscle wasting can be profound. Nonerosive polyarthritis can be seen in any breed at any age but most commonly occurs in young dogs (between 1 and 6 years of age). The condition appears to be overrepresented in German Shepherd Dogs, Doberman Pinschers, Collies, Spaniels, Retrievers, Terriers, and Poodles. Specific syndromes involving immune-mediated polyarthritis have been identified in certain breeds of dogs, such as swollen hock syndrome in Shar-Peis and arthritis in Akitas.

Infectious disease can cause a secondary immune-mediated polyarthritis as a result of chronic immune stimulation inducing immune complex deposition in the synovial tissue. Diseases frequently associated with secondary immune-mediated polyarthritis include heartworm disease, canine ehrlichiosis, anaplasmosis (caused by *Anaplasma phagocytophilum*, previously known as *Ehrlichia equi*) Rocky Mountain spotted fever, Lyme disease, and others. Chronic bacterial infections such as discospondylitis, pyelonephritis, prostatitis, and endocarditis can also cause a secondary immune-mediated polyarthritis.

Systemic lupus erythematosus is suspected when polyarthritis is accompanied by immune-mediated hemolytic anemia, thrombocytopenia, glomerulonephritis, or immune-mediated dermatopathies. The value of antinuclear antibody (ANAs) testing is controversial. This syndrome is thought to occur more commonly in females and in German Shepherd Dogs, Collies, Shetland Sheepdogs, Beagles, and Poodles.

Lymphocytic-plasmacytic synovitis has been reported most commonly in German Shepherd Dogs and other large-breed dogs. This condition is thought to be associated with degenerative joint disease, such as arthritis in the stifle joint after rupture of the cranial cruciate ligament. The diagnosis can be confirmed with histologic evaluation of the synovium.

Drug-induced immune-mediated polyarthritis appears to be rare. It has been reported to occur as a result of trimethoprim-sulfadiazine therapy in a group of Doberman Pinschers. Immune-mediated polyarthritis has been suspected in some cases after vaccinations (e.g., vaccinations for Lyme disease).

Inflammatory joint disease (septic or immune mediated) should be suspected in the following instances (Figure 30-1):
- The dog or cat with joint pain, joint swelling, generalized pain, or reluctance to rise.
- Joint pain or swelling that is apparent during the physical examination.

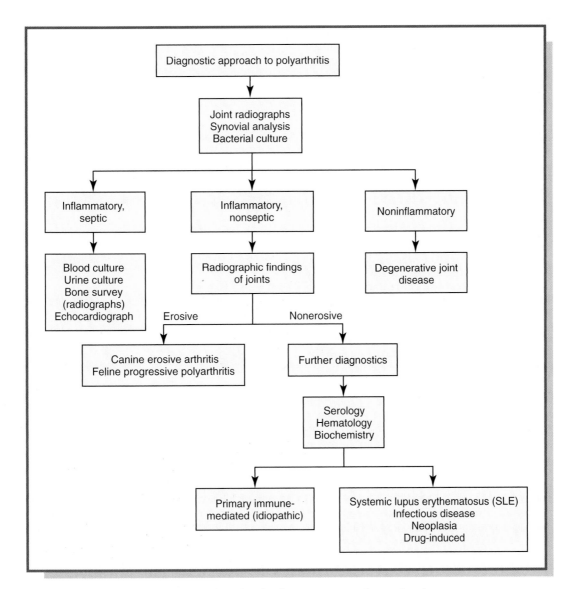

Figure 30-1 Algorithm for diagnostic approach to polyarthritis.

- The dog or cat that has abnormalities that could result from a systemic inflammatory condition: fever or leukocytosis.
- When immune-mediated disease is suspected in other organ systems (i.e., immune-mediated hemolytic anemia, thrombocytopenia, steroid responsive sterile meningitis, glomerulonephritis).

ARTHROCENTESIS AND JOINT FLUID ANALYSIS

Joint fluid analysis is the single most important test performed in the diagnosis of inflammatory arthritis. Joint taps are usually simple to perform and are associated with minimal morbidity or complications (see Chapter 101). Aspiration of synovial fluid (joint taps) and cytologic analysis are necessary to define the involvement of a joint (Figure 30-2).

Affected joints, even severely affected, may not appear swollen or painful. Joint taps should also be performed as part of the diagnostic investigation of a fever or leukocytosis of unknown origin or when other immune-mediated disease is suspected. In a recent study, 20% of dogs with a fever of unknown origin had immune-mediated polyarthritis. Unfortunately, the information clinicians can obtain from joint fluid analysis is limited. Increased numbers of neutrophils appear in joint fluid of both septic and immune-mediated arthritis, making the differentiation between the two difficult, and joint fluid cultures are frequently negative even in the obvious presence of bacteria.

Multiple joints should always be sampled, including those that do not appear to be clinically involved in the disease process. It is recommended that both carpi and both tarsi joints be sampled along with at least one elbow and stifle. Hip and shoulder joints are not commonly tapped unless they appear to be diseased.

GROSS EXAMINATION

Fluid from a normal joint is clear, light straw–colored, and has a sticky, viscous feel, forming a strand when a drop is paced between a fingertip and the thumb, which are then slowly pulled apart, or between a glass slide and a fingertip, which is slowly moved away from the slide (Figure 30-3).

More than a few drops should not be easily obtained from a normal joint. If the fluid is discolored, turbid, lacks viscosity, or is aspirated in excessive amounts, then joint disease is likely. Blood contamination, only partially mixed in with the joint fluid, may occur.

CYTOLOGIC EVALUATION

Normal joint fluid contains less than 2500 to 3000 white blood cells (WBCs) per milliliter and few red blood cells (RBCs). At least 90% of white cells in normal joints are mononuclear. Inflamed joints (septic or immune mediated) will typically have over 5000 WBCs and over 10% neutrophils. The WBC or neutrophil count can be estimated by multiplying the average number of cells seen in each high-power field by 1000. The presence of bacteria or degenerate changes in the neutrophils is suggestive of septic and not immune-mediated arthritis, as is a positive bacterial culture. WBC counts can be markedly increased

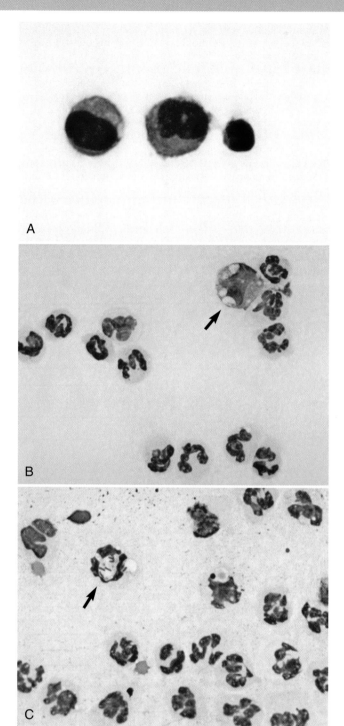

Figure 30-2 A, Normal: Two quiescent mononuclear phagocytes (larger) and a small mature lymphocyte are seen in this low-cellularity direct smear of normal canine synovial fluid. These are the predominant cell types in health in all species. **B,** Nonseptic arthritis: Numerous well-preserved neutrophils and a macrophage *(arrow)* are seen in this highly cellular direct smear of synovial fluid from a cat with immune-mediated polyarthritis. Neutrophils typically are less than 10% in healthy cats. **C,** Septic arthritis: Numerous neutrophils and a few red blood cells (RBCs) are seen in this highly cellular direct smear of synovial fluid from a dog with septic arthritis. The reader should note cellular debris in the background and several degenerate neutrophils, including one that contains several bacterial rods *(arrow)*. (Courtesy Dr. Tracy W. French, Dip. ACVP, Cornell University.)

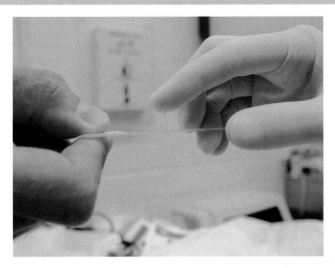

Figure 30-3 A demonstration of the method to grossly assess joint fluid viscosity. A drop is placed on a glass slide. It is gently touched with a fingertip that is then slowly moved away. The reader should note the strand of viscous fluid typical for normal joint fluid viscosity.

with septic or immune-mediated disease processes, approaching 100,000 WBC/mL of joint fluid including over 90% neutrophils.

If sufficient joint fluid is obtained, then additional testing of the fluid is possible, including protein content, glucose concentrations, and a mucin clot test. Clinically these tests are not often performed and are thought to have little additional value if cytology and culture have been performed.

ADDITIONAL TESTING

A minimum data base, including a complete blood count (CBC), a serum biochemistry profile, and a urinalysis, is recommended in any dog or cat with suspected inflammatory arthritis. Radiographs of the joint are indicated if septic or erosive arthritis is suspected. A search for possible sources of bacterial infection should be undertaken if septic arthritis is suspected and no obvious penetrating wound or source of infection is evident. This search could include blood and urine cultures, thoracic and abdominal radiographs, and spinal radiographs to identify discospondylitis, abdominal ultrasound, and possibly cardiac echocardiogram for bacterial endocarditis.

If immune-mediated polyarthritis is suspected, then a search for the source of chronic immune stimulation and additional manifestations of immune-mediated disease should be undertaken. The chronic immune stimulation could be a primary immune disorder (idiopathic) or a result of chronic infection, inflammation, or neoplasia. Additional diagnostics in this case could include the previously mentioned testing listed for septic arthritis, a Coombs' test, and serology for ANAs and RF. Serology for exposure to rickettsial agents such as *Ehrlichia* species, *Borrelia burgdorferi*, *Anaplasma phocytophilum*, systemic fungal infections, and for occult heartworm infestation may be indicated, depending on the prevalence in the region and a possible travel history. Positive results of any of these tests must be taken as part of the entire clinical, hematological and biochemical picture. Positive Coombs' test, RF, and ANA are all nonspecific findings perhaps strengthening the possibility of more general immune-mediated disease or SLE. Positive titers to some of the previously mentioned infectious agents (i.e., *Ehrlichia canis* and *Anaplasma phagocytophilum*) may be indicative of previous exposure and not necessarily active disease.

CHAPTER 31

Body Odors

Karen A. Moriello

Webster's Dictionary defines odor as "That characteristic of a substance which makes it perceptible to the sense of smell whether it be pleasant or unpleasant." From a clinical perspective, the definition of odor would have to be expanded to include whether the odor is normal or abnormal. Whether clinicians realize it or not, the use of smell is an intricate part of the physical examination process. Depending upon the disease process, it can also be involved in the diagnostic, therapeutic, and monitoring process.

PEOPLE, PETS, VETERINARIANS, AND THE BODY ODOR ISSUE

Body odor has a biologic purpose. In general, smell and body odor for all species are important in species recognition, social interactions, and mate selection. In the animal phylum, changes in body odor and pheromones are driven by genetics and evolutionary trends. In the human species, one other major driving force exists—changing social trends. For example, body odor in one era may be considered normal or even desirable but in another deemed socially unacceptable. The issue of environmental odors (i.e., room odors) is almost equally important to people. Manipulation of personal and environmental odors (out of the "unpleasant" and into the "neutral or pleasant" spectrum) is an important social trend (and a commercial industry). Further complicating this issue is the increased recognition that body odor may be an early warning sign of health issues (e.g., fruity apple odor of ketoacidosis as the result of diabetes mellitus or starvation) or a human health hazard (e.g., mold). Veterinarians increasingly have to navigate the issue of "the pet's body odor" with clients.

This is difficult at times because the current norm is "pleasant odor" or "no odor." The clinician's task is to determine whether the body odor in question is a sign of disease or whether it is within the realm of normal for the pet in question. If the latter is true, then clinicians must find a way to make the pet's odor more acceptable to the owner.

PATHOPHYSIOLOGY

Body odor in animals varies with species, breed, sex, age, and overall health. For example, dog breeds with naturally oily coats (e.g., Retrievers, Cocker Spaniels) often have a stronger dog odor than dogs that do not (e.g., Boston Terriers). The conformation of some breeds may predispose them to odor problems. The most notable example includes any breed with redundant skin or lip folds. In the healthy dog or cat, skin secretions contain insignificant amounts of odorous substances. Skin odor is the result of bacterial decomposition of secretions from sebaceous glands, epidermal lipids, and epitrichial and atrichial sweat glands. Epitrichial glands are present on haired skin just below sebaceous glands and open onto the surface via the piliary canal. These glands are largest and most numerous in mucocutaneous junctions, interdigital spaces, and over the dorsal back and lumbosacral areas. Not surprisingly this is often where odor concentrates in pets. Atrichial glands are located only on footpads. Sweat contains unsaturated fatty acids, ammonia constituents, and their volatile salts. Sebum and epidermal lipids on the skin surface are degraded by lipases of gram-positive bacteria to glycerol and unsaturated fatty acids, which are further metabolized to odorous compounds. It is these byproducts that give sebum its antibacterial and antifungal properties. Some of the acids produced by the degradation of these lipids, butyric and caproic acids, are quite volatile and emit a cheesy, rancid odor. Oral odor may be associated with systemic illnesses, such as uremia, diabetes mellitus, or periodontal disease. Malodor associated with periodontal disease is due to the production of volatile sulfur components. Oral odors are most often the result of byproducts of bacterial metabolism resulting from bacteria colonization of plaque, gingival sulci, and the dorsal surface of the posterior tongue. Oral odors may also be the result of something the pet has ingested (e.g., fecal material).

CLINICAL APPROACH

The starting point of any medical visit is the owner's complaint. In general, pets with the problem of body odor fall into one of four broad categories (see the following) as determined by the history and physical examination. In the case of body odor, what the clinician simply sees and smells may accomplish the initial sorting. After this, the clinician can then determine how best to proceed (Figure 31-1 and Box 31-1).

In most cases the veterinarian needs to determine if the underlying cause is due to a systemic disease, pure dermatologic disease, external factors, or lack of client education.

"Normal pets" are considered to be malodorous by the client but not by the clinician. In general, the clinician's initial assessment is that the pet's body odor is within the normal range for the species (e.g., cat owners first acquiring a dog may not be aware of species differences), age (e.g., puppies have a unique odor), sex (e.g., intact tomcats are more odorous than neutered male cats), breed (e.g., Hound Dogs'

odor versus Poodles'), hair length, etc. Furthermore, a thorough, literal "sniff exam" (nose to tail, dorsum to ventrum, feet, and ears) of the patient reveals no unusual odors. Finally, no evidence of a dermatologic or medical disease exists. The key sorting aspect of this group is that the veterinarian considers the animal to smell normal, and no history or physical evidence of illness or skin disease exists. In these situations, client education and suggestions for bathing routines that are tolerable and safe for the pet are indicated.

The clinician should be aware of two subsets in the normal pet group. The first is a subset of normal pets with owners who complain of odors that "come and go." In these situations the cause may be anal sac expression, something the dog ate (e.g., onions, garlic), flatulence, "wet dog" smell, a change in the dog's regular dog food (some specialty diets, especially fish based, cause the dog to "smell fishy"). In warm weather, many dogs will drool excessively, and this will mat the haircoat around the face, chest, and forelegs, leading to an offensive odor. Warm weather often results in increased moisture on the skin, and this can lead to bacterial degradation and odor. In addition, many owners of dogs with allergic skin disease report acute episodes where the skin becomes warm, the dog "literally sweats," and then is very odorous.

The second subset includes those pets that smell normal to the clinician, but the owner reports that there has been a change in how the dog smells. It is critical to carefully examine these patients for evidence of subtle signs of skin disease because these owners may be reporting a valid finding. A recent study found that 86% of owners that were blindfolded and only allowed to use their sense of smell were consistently able to differentiate their dog's body odor from that of another simply by sniffing a blanket. This finding amazed both owners and investigators. What is pertinent to veterinarians is that owners may very well "know" what their dog smells like when it is normal and when it is not.

Malodorous Pet with an Obvious Cause
These are patients with unmistakable odor from urine, feces, skunk, flatulence, and "I rolled in the compost heap" odors. This group could also include the pets with obvious skin or medical problems, where the source of the odor (infected fracture, ears, seborrheic skin, pyotraumatic dermatitis, and so on) is easily found. Animals with severe halitosis are also included here (Box 31-2).

The key sorting aspect of this group is that the clinician immediately knows where the odor is coming from, what is causing it, what needs to be done to eliminate it, and whether or not further medical or dermatologic diagnostics are needed. In these situations, client education may be as simple as recommendations on how to remove the odor (e.g., skunk) or more complicated discussions on the need to treat existing infections and perform appropriate diagnostic tests to investigate the underlying cause.

Malodorous Pets with Obvious Systemic Illnesses
These are patients that are malodorous, but more importantly are systemically ill. This might be determined by historical or physical examination findings (or both); changes in body odor might have been what prompted the client to finally bring the animal for examination. The key sorting aspect of this group is an obvious state of ill health associated with the body odor. In general, cats rarely are presented for the problem of body odor. When they are, it is usually for one of three reasons. First, a strong odor emanates from an ear, mouth, or body region. This should prompt the clinician to look for infections, injuries, neoplasia, myiasis, etc. Second, the cat is soiling itself with urine, feces, or both or not removing it from the haircoat. This could be for any number of reasons, such as physical inability to groom (e.g., obesity, arthritis) or neuromuscular

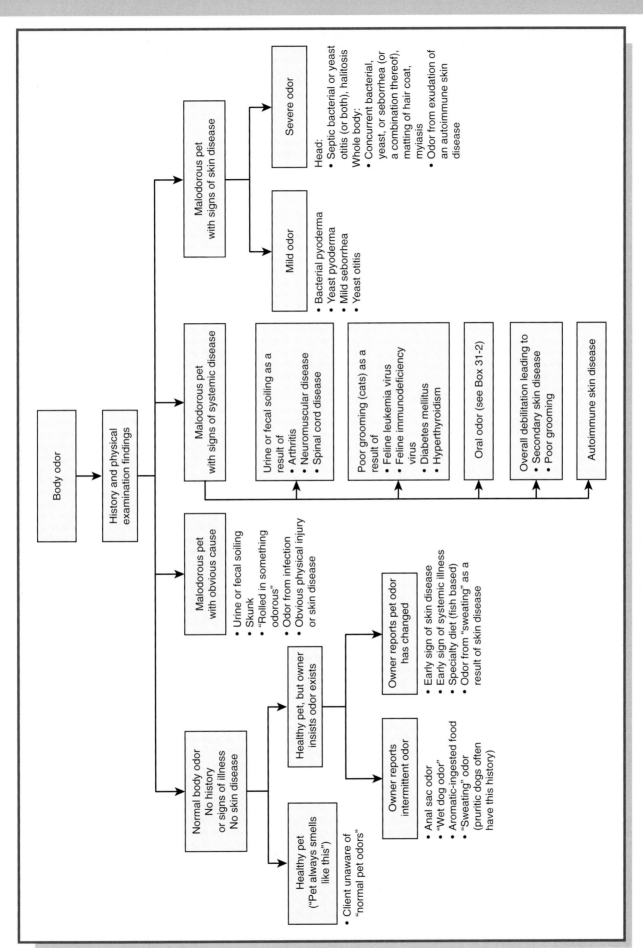

Figure 31-1 Algorithm for presenting complaint of body odor.

Box • 31-1

General Recommendations for Control of Odor

Normal Pets without Skin Disease
- Client education for the owner
- Keep the haircoat short; no feathering haircuts.
- Clip hair from inner pinnae.
- Avoid cloth dog collars that can become impregnated with the pet's body odor.
- Bathe pet in a veterinary hypoallergenic shampoo only as often as to keep odor free.
- Dry pet after exposure to rain or after swimming to avoid wet-dog smell.
- Use veterinary coat deodorizers only.

Skunk Odor
- Liberal application of "Skunk Off"
- Keep pet dry to prevent reemergence of skunk odor (it may take several weeks for the odor to dissipate completely).

Urine, Fecal Matter, and Odors Associated with "Rolled in Something Dead"
- Clip any mats from haircoat.
- Bathe pet in grooming or flea shampoo first to remove gross debris, and rinse well.
- Bathe a second time in a degreasing shampoo such as benzoyl peroxide; odors are often held in skin and hair lipids.

Pets with Odor and Skin Disease
- Complete appropriate diagnostics, and begin appropriate systemic therapy.
- Administer appropriate sedation, analgesia, or anesthesia, if needed.
- Clean or flush ears as needed.
- Grooming recommendations:

- Clip haircoat from inner ear pinnae and around ears, if necessary.
- Clip hair mats and areas of lip fold pyoderma.
- Clip haircoat of medium- or long-haired dogs.
- Bathing recommendations:
  - Always prebathe pet with grooming or flea shampoo to remove gross debris before using a medicated shampoo; rinse well (this step facilitates efficacy of medicated shampoo product).
  - Bathe pet in antimicrobials or antiseborrheic shampoo (it may work best if the client alternates between two shampoos).
  - Severely odorous pets should be bathed daily until client deems pet acceptable.
  - Most pets require two to three baths per week during medical treatment.
- Warnings:
  - Some shampoos are irritating; do not use if pet seems uncomfortable after use.
  - If haircoat becomes excessively dry, decrease frequency of bathing.
  - Dogs with primary seborrhea will require aggressive bathing for life to control disease and odor.
- *Consumer Warning:*
  - *Clients searching for ways to control their pet's body odor will encounter many over-the-counter food supplements with claims to "naturally" deodorize the pet. Some of these products are additives to water and some are additives to diets. To date there are no scientific studies that substantiate these claims. The safety of these products is unknown and clients should be encouraged to consult with their veterinarian before using any of these products.*

---

injury. Third, the cat could just be generally odorous to the client. These cats usually have stopped grooming themselves, and their haircoat is matted or greasy. This situation should prompt the clinician to look for a systemic illness (e.g., hyperthyroidism, diabetes mellitus, neoplasia). Dogs with systemic illness may be mildly or severely malodorous. Mild odors are usually caused by concurrent skin infections triggered by debilitation. The skin odor in these patients usually is not noticeable to the clinician until the dog is physically examined. Severely odorous dogs almost always have the odor localized to one area (e.g., mouth odor caused by uremia), a site of injury and infection (open fracture with secondary infection), or excrement on their haircoat because of some cause of immobility. In these situations, client education must focus on a need to aggressively pursue the cause of the illness, whereas the odor issue is addressed as part of the therapy for the health and wellbeing of the patient (e.g., treatment of urine or fecal soiling).

Malodorous Pets with Skin Disease
Without a doubt, most obviously odorous animals will fall into this group. For the vast majority of patients, the key sorting aspect of this group is an otherwise healthy pet with a history of skin disease, blatantly obvious skin disease, skin disease found during the examination, or a combination of these factors. When working with these patients, the clinician should remember several key points:
- The most common cause of body or ear odor is almost always some combination of bacterial pyoderma, *Malassezia* pyoderma, and seborrhea (usually oily).
- Many of these patients are severely pruritic. The pruritus is most likely caused by a combination of the microbial infections, inflammatory degradation products of oily seborrhea, the presence of an underlying pruritic disease (e.g., atopy), or a combination of these factors.
- The duration of the skin problem, presence or absence of underlying primary seborrhea, and severity of the skin infections (superficial or deep) mostly determine the severity of the odor. Other factors such as length of the haircoat, presence or absence of hair mats, and exposure to moisture can also affect the severity of the odor.
- The odor will most likely resolve with appropriate systemic and topical treatment of the superficial microbial infections and seborrhea; it may or may not return.

Box • 31-2

Common Causes of Halitosis in Dogs and Cats

Oral Diseases
Periodontal disease (gingivitis, periodontitis, abscessation)
Neoplasia (melanoma, fibrosarcoma, squamous cell carcinoma)
Foreign body or trauma (fractures, electrical cord injury)
Pharyngitis
Stomatitis, lymphocytic-plasmacytic feline stomatitis

Respiratory Diseases
Rhinitis and/or sinusitis
Neoplasia
Pneumonia or pulmonary abscess

Dermatologic Diseases
Lip fold pyoderma
Ulcerative mucocutaneous pyoderma
Feline or canine eosinophilic granulomas
Pemphigus complex, bullous pemphigoid, lupus erythematosus
Drug eruptions
Cutaneous lymphoma
Exposure to dimethyl sulfoxide (DMSO)

Metabolic Diseases
Renal failure/uremia
Diabetic ketoacidosis

Gastrointestinal Diseases
Megaesophagus
Inflammatory bowel disease
Exocrine pancreatic insufficiency

Neoplasia
Constipation (cats)

Dietary
Aromatic foods (onions, garlic)
Fetid foodstuffs (e.g., ingestion of carrion)
Coprophagy

Grooming Behavior
Anal sacculitis
Vaginitis/balanoposthitis
Lower urinary tract infections

Adapted from Veterinary guide to odor and disease: the oral cavity and dermatology, Yardley, Pa, 1997, Veterinary Learning Systems.

This depends on whether the underlying trigger of microbial infections is still present, whether the patient has a previously undiagnosed primary disorder of keratinization, and whether the pruritus has resolved. If not, the return of the body odor is almost guaranteed because it will trigger secondary microbial infections and seborrhea.

• Recurrent otic or skin odor always means an underlying skin disease is present. Whether diagnostics beyond skin scrapings, flea combing, skin and ear cytology, and possibly a fungal culture are indicated in malodorous pets with skin disease depends on the patient's history and physical examination.

Note: A subgroup of malodorous pets exists with skin disease and signs of systemic illness (e.g., anorexia, persistent or waxing and waning fevers, depression, reluctance to walk, weight loss, dehydration). This triad (odor, skin disease, illness) should alert the clinician to the possibility that the patient has a severe, life-threatening condition such as deep pyoderma with or without demodicosis, drug reactions, immune-mediated diseases, deep fungal infections with cutaneous manifestations, or toxic epidermal necrolysis. An immediate aggressive dermatologic evaluation is needed: skin scrapings, bacterial cultures, impression smears of exudate, and skin biopsy, in addition to appropriate medical diagnostics and supportive care pending diagnosis.

CHAPTER 32

Ocular Manifestations of Systemic Disease

David J. Maggs

Clinicians tend to consider the eye and adnexa as unique structures that are dissimilar to nonocular tissues. This can lead to omission of the ophthalmic examination in patients with systemic disease or omission of the general physical examination in patients presented with ophthalmic disease. In fact, the eye is a complex aggregate of tissues with marked anatomic and functional similarities to tissues found in most other organ systems. Viewed in this manner, the eyes provide a unique opportunity for direct observation of tissue types that are otherwise not visible without invasive techniques or special instrumentation.

Table • 32-1

Correlations between Ocular and Nonocular Tissues

TISSUE TYPE	VISIBLE OCULAR CORRELATES
Mucous membrane	Conjunctiva
Vascular tissue	Conjunctiva, uvea, retina
Neural tissue	Retina, optic nerve
Lymphoid tissue	Uvea, conjunctiva, third eyelid
Glandular tissue	Meibomian glands, conjunctival goblet cells, third eyelid gland
Connective	Sclera, cornea
Smooth muscle tissue	Iris, upper eyelid (Muller's muscle), third eyelid
Interstitial space	Anterior chamber, subretinal space, vitreous
Hematologic	Conjunctiva, uvea, retina

The major correlations between ocular and nonocular tissues are summarized in Table 32-1.

This table identifies ocular tissues that should be examined carefully in animals with systemic disease and nonocular tissues that should be examined in those with ocular disease. For example, in a dog or cat with generalized lymphadenopathy, the conjunctiva, third eyelid gland, and uveal tract should be closely examined because they also contain lymphoid tissue or cells. Likewise, a thorough general physical examination of the pet with retinal disease may reveal more widespread vascular, neurologic, or hematologic disease.

The following is a description of specific ocular conditions, arranged by affected ocular tissue, that are often associated with systemic disease. This chapter highlights the correlation between ocular and systemic tissues. It does not provide an exhaustive description of the diagnostic approach or therapies.

SURFACE OCULAR DISEASE

The eyelids, conjunctiva, cornea, and sclera are intimately related, physiologically and anatomically. They provide a protective surface for the eye, and all three tissues are susceptible to the same insults that cause surface (dermatologic) disease elsewhere. Therefore a thorough dermatologic history and a complete dermatologic examination may be helpful in animals with surface ocular disease. The diagnostic approach to lesions involving eyelids, conjunctiva, or cornea is identical to that used for skin. It includes incisional or excisional biopsy, scrapings, and viral, fungal, chlamydial, and mycoplasmal or bacterial culture.

Ocular surface tissues may also be affected as "innocent bystanders" in more serious orbital disease or intraocular conditions such as uveitis or glaucoma. Retropulsion of the globe and thorough intraocular exam with measurement of intraocular pressure (IOP) will identify such animals.

Eyelids

Although blepharitis may represent more widespread dermatitis, special consideration should be given to unique palpebral anatomy. Meibomian glands are specialized sebaceous glands that can be primarily infected; particularly with *Staphylococcus* and *Demodex* spp. Altered immune responses can exacerbate clinical signs at this site. Immunodeficiency may encourage colonization by organisms such as dermatophytes or *Demodex* spp., whereas an exuberant immunologic response such as hypersensitivity to *Staphylococcus* spp. may cause more severe inflammation. Eyelid margins represent a clearly visible mucocutaneous junction that could be involved in primary immune-mediated dermatitis such as the pemphigoid diseases or *systemic lupus erythematosus (SLE)*. Other immune-mediated diseases such as vasculitis or uveodermatologic syndrome (also known as Vogt-Koyanagi-Harada [VKH] or VKH-like syndrome) may also be more obvious or more severe in periocular skin.

Altered lid position, with or without altered pupil size or globe deviation, can also represent central, peripheral, or disseminated neurologic disease, specifically dysfunction of cranial nerve (CN) III or VII or decreased sympathetic tone (Horner's syndrome). Clinical localization of the lesion or lesions is important, particularly for Horner's syndrome—the triad of enophthalmos (with protrusion of the third eyelid), ptosis, and miosis. Because of the circuitous, three-neuron route by which sympathetic neurons course from the hypothalamus to the eye, Horner's syndrome can result from disease involving the brain, spinal cord, brachial plexus, thorax and mediastinum, neck, temporal bone and tympanic bulla, or orbit. Diagnostic procedures should be directed at each specific area to eliminate definitive causes. However, even with intensive diagnostic testing, approximately 50% of cases of Horner's syndrome are idiopathic and usually resolve within 2 months.

Conjunctiva

Conjunctival disease is seen alone, with blepharitis or keratitis, or may reflect inflammation of deeper structures such as the sclera, meibomian glands, orbital contents, third eyelid gland, or intraocular tissues. The rich vascularity of conjunctiva and its almost transparent epithelium also make it an excellent site for detection of hematologic (cyanosis, anemia, icterus) or vascular disease.

Feline herpesvirus (FHV-1) and *Chlamydophila felis* (formerly *Chlamydia psittaci*) are primary conjunctival pathogens of cats. Although cats undergoing primary FHV-1 exposure generally demonstrate concurrent signs of upper-respiratory infection, cats infected with *C. felis* and those undergoing a recrudescent FHV-1 episode may demonstrate few or mild nonocular clinical signs. Despite an apparent lack of systemic signs, recent evidence confirms that cats harbor and shed *C. felis* from nonocular sites. Studies also suggest that systemic therapy is more effective than topical therapy at decreasing clinical signs and shedding of *C. felis*.

Conjunctivitis in dogs is usually not associated with systemic disease. Ligneous conjunctivitis is an uncommon but important exception. This is a chronic, membranous conjunctivitis in which gross thickening of conjunctiva occurs bilaterally. Younger, female Doberman Pinschers may be predisposed. Other mucous membranes may also be involved, and the majority of affected dogs also have evidence of upper-respiratory or urinary tract disease. Histology reveals a characteristic amorphous, eosinophilic hyaline material throughout the subconjunctiva.

Cornea and Sclera

Corneal clarity is important for normal vision. Attentive owners may often note early or subtle corneal pathologic changes. Although altered corneal appearance may represent primary keratitis or intraocular disease (particularly uveitis or glaucoma), corneal opacification that begins at or is most notable at the limbus is often an indicator of systemic disease. For example, lymphosarcoma (LSA) tends to cause a homogenous, creamy-pink discoloration of the peripheral corneal stroma. Corneal lipidosis is an important differential diagnosis in these cases and may occur secondary to any disease causing systemic hyperlipidemia. Hypothyroidism is one of the most common causes; however, hyperadrenocorticism, diabetes mellitus, and familial hypertriglyceridemia should also be considered. Serum triglycerides and cholesterol should both be assessed in animals with corneal lipidosis. Rarely, corneal opacification in dogs or cats will be caused by mucopolysaccharidosis.

Although hyperadrenocorticism and diabetes mellitus are associated with prolonged corneal wound healing, dogs with diabetes mellitus have also recently been shown to have significantly decreased corneal sensitivity relative to normal dogs. This may represent a manifestation of diabetic neuropathy, making dogs less likely to blink and produce reflex tears to protect their corneas. In addition, multiple growth factors are transferred to the cornea by sensory nerves, and these are likely to be reduced in such dogs. This likely contributes to the poor wound healing observed in these pets. Therefore therapy and monitoring of corneal disease, especially ulceration, should be more intense in diabetic dogs.

Keratoconjunctivitis Sicca

Decreased aqueous tear production with subsequent keratoconjunctivitis sicca (KCS) is common in dogs but uncommon in cats. In dogs it is usually caused by idiopathic lymphocytic-plasmacytic dacryoadenitis. Rarely, cats or dogs with KCS have immune-mediated destruction of the salivary glands and associated xerostomia (Sjögren's-like syndrome), sometimes clinically apparent as dysphagia. KCS in association with xeromycteria (dry nose) should prompt investigation of neurogenic KCS caused by damage to afferent or efferent pathways of lacrimal innervation. Lacrimal stimuli are transmitted by CN V, and efferent (parasympathetic) fibers are carried first by CN VII and peripherally by CN V. Because these same neural pathways are involved in the production of moisture for the nasal mucosa, ipsilateral xeromycteria evidenced by a dry, crusty nostril may be seen. Diagnostic efforts should be directed at disease processes along the paths of CN V and VII, particularly in the region of the tympanic bullae.

KCS may also occur as a result of drug therapy. Drugs incriminated in decreased tear production include systemically or topically administered atropine, systemically administered sulfa drugs, etodolac, and general anesthesia within the preceding 2 days. Dogs with marginal tear production before administration of these drugs, and those weighing less than 12 kg (in the case of trimethoprim sulfa), appear to be at increased risk of developing KCS. Dose and duration of therapy are less relevant. Restoration of tear production and corneoconjunctival health does not always occur upon discontinuation of the offending drug; therefore Schirmer tear test (STT) results should be monitored before and during therapy.

Finally, KCS may occur as a component of systemic disease but may be overlooked unless a STT test is performed. Systemic infection with canine distemper virus (CDV) is associated with usually transient KCS, while cats undergoing primary infection with FHV-1 may experience transient KCS followed by a period of decreased tear mucin production and associated tear film instability for over 1 month following infection. Dysautonomia (Key-Gaskell syndrome) can cause bilateral reduced aqueous tear secretion, nonresponsive dilated pupils, and protrusion of the third eyelids. Associated systemic signs of autonomic dysfunction, including urinary and fecal incontinence, bradycardia, hypotension, dysphagia, and dry nose are usually more noticeable than the ocular signs; however, ocular signs may help to confirm the diagnosis. Although an association between low STT values and hyperadrenocorticism, diabetes mellitus, or hypothyroidism has been shown in dogs, no association between endocrinopathies and KCS has been proven.

UVEAL TRACT

Uveal pathology is commonly seen with systemic disease. The uveal tract includes the iris, ciliary body, and choroid and is the major vascular supply for the avascular components of the eye (cornea, lens, outer retina). It is composed of a large network of arterioles, venules, and fine capillaries and therefore is a sensitive indicator of vascular or hematologic conditions such as vasculitis, hypertension, anemia, and hyperviscosity (see Fundus). Loss of vascular integrity may be apparent in the anterior chamber as breakdown of the blood-aqueous barrier. This appears differently, based on the extent of breakdown and the presence or absence of inflammatory mediators within the anterior chamber and surrounding tissues. With minimal breakdown, albumin and other small serum proteins are detectable in the anterior chamber as aqueous flare. The aqueous humor may be thought of as a directly visible area of interstitial space, and if serum contents are seen within this space, the possibility of similar plasma "leakage" in other, less visible nonocular interstices should also be considered.

Detection of aqueous flare requires that a beam of light emanating from a bright and focal source be viewed transversely, preferably with some magnification, as it traverses the anterior chamber. This examination should be done with dim ambient light. A slit lamp biomicroscope provides the optimal combination of these conditions; however, a direct ophthalmoscope turned to the smallest spot of light and held within 1 cm of the corneal surface provides a focal light source and can be used in general practice to detect flare. By definition, albumin, and therefore aqueous flare, will be approximately evenly distributed throughout the anterior chamber. Cellular debris (hyphema, dispersed white blood cells [WBCs], or hypopyon) or larger proteins, particularly fibrin in the anterior chamber, suggests more major vascular compromise or potent, cytokine-mediated extravasation of cells. These blood constituents are more likely to settle into the ventral anterior chamber. Depressing the pet's nose so that the eyes are elevated within the orbits will often assist in seeing this region.

Fine uveal capillary beds can act as a biologic "filter" that traps organisms, particularly fungi, or metastatic neoplastic cells. It is frequently involved in systemic infectious disease or as a site of metastatic neoplasia. The uvea also contains the major aggregations of lymphoid cells and is therefore a common site for LSA. It is also frequently involved in specific or nonspecific ocular inflammatory responses (uveitis) that may reflect broader immunopathology such as infectious or neoplastic disease. The list of organisms that have been associated with uveitis is expanding and is somewhat species specific. In cats, feline infectious peritonitis (FIP), feline immunodeficiency virus (FIV) (principally a retinochoroiditis), feline leukemia virus (FeLV) (principally via LSA), *Toxoplasma gondii*, mycobacteria, and the systemic mycoses (principally a chorioretinitis) have traditionally been associated with uveitis. More recently, intraocular detection of other organisms such as FHV-1, *Bartonella* spp., and some *Ehrlichia* spp. has led to suggestions that these organisms also warrant consideration as causative agents in feline uveitis. Despite this expanding list of differential diagnoses and thorough diagnostic testing (sometimes including enucleation and histopathology), a definitive cause of uveitis is not identified in 50% to 70% of affected cats.

The list of infectious organisms causing uveitis in dogs includes fungal organisms, *Leishmania donovani*, *Ehrlichia platys* or *canis*, *Rickettsia rickettsii*, *Brucella canis*, *Toxoplasma gondii*, canine adenovirus, and *Leptospira* spp. In addition, dogs appear to be more susceptible to immune-mediated uveitis than cats. One example is lens-induced uveitis, in which lens proteins leak from a cataractous or ruptured lens and overwhelm normal immune tolerance of these proteins. Another example is uveodermatologic (VKH-like) syndrome in which the immunopathology is directed at melanocytes throughout the body. Because of the preponderance and visibility of melanin-containing cells in the uveal tract and skin, clinical manifestations of disease in these two tissues are most dramatic.

It is incorrect to suggest that the clinical appearance of uveitis can be used to determine a definitive cause. However, noting whether the uveal inflammation appears more cellular or granulomatous, blood tinged, or proteinaceous may help prioritize diagnostic efforts (Figure 32-1).

Finally, the iris (anterior uvea) forms the pupil and therefore often provides clinical evidence of neurologic disease. Pupillary abnormalities suggestive of systemic disease include feline "spastic pupil syndrome" in which intermittent periods of anisocoria are seen without obvious iridal or afferent neurologic defects. Most cats are FeLV-positive or become so soon after diagnosis but may not have other systemic signs of infection when pupil abnormalities are noted. Virally induced pathology of CN III is suspected. Pupilomotor abnormalities with normal vision and without ocular inflammation are also seen with dysautonomia (mydriasis) and Horner's syndrome (miosis).

LENS

The two most common conditions affecting the lens are cataract and lens dislocation (subluxation or luxation). Lens dislocation usually occurs secondary to severe intraocular disease, particularly uveitis, which may be a sign of systemic disease. Although lens dislocation may also occur as a primary event in predisposed dog breeds such as Terriers, these pets do not have evidence of the generalized connective tissue disorders seen in some humans.

Although the majority of canine cataracts are hereditary in origin, almost all dogs with diabetes mellitus will develop cataracts within 12 months of diagnosis. By contrast, the most common cause of feline cataracts is uveitis. Cats with diabetes rarely develop cataracts. Other systemic causes of cataracts include altered nutrition (especially orphan animals raised on milk replacement products), hypocalcemia with or without hyperphosphatemia (as seen with hypoparathyroidism), electric shock, lightning strike, and senility.

FUNDUS

The ocular fundus is not a single structure. Rather, it is a collective term describing all structures in the posterior portion of the globe that can be viewed with the ophthalmoscope. Visible structures will vary but may include retinal pigment epithelium (if pigmented), neurosensory retina, optic nerve head, retinal vasculature, sclera, tapetum, or choroid. The fundic examination therefore provides a unique opportunity to directly visualize a large cranial nerve (optic nerve), sensitive neural tissue (retina), large venules and arterioles (retinal vessels), and a massive capillary bed (choroid). For this reason, a fundic examination should be performed in all animals with systemic disease.

The choroid is perhaps the fundic tissue most commonly affected in animals with systemic disease. Because of its position immediately subjacent to the retina and its critical role in retinal nutrition and function, signs of choroidal disease are frequently first noted once they affect the retina. The classic example is retinal detachment, which may be caused by primary retinal disease but frequently reflects choroidal effu-

sion. As a result of these close anatomic and physiologic relationships, the terms *chorioretinitis* and *retinochoroiditis* are used to reflect inflammation of these two tissues. The difference between these two terms is subtle, with the intent that the first-mentioned tissue is the one believed to be primarily involved. For example, the systemic mycoses have a predilection for the choroid and so cause a marked chorioretinitis. By contrast, CDV targets neurologic tissue in general and, within the eye, retinal tissue specifically. Insults to the subjacent choroid usually also occur, and the disease is typically referred to as a retinochoroiditis.

Optic Nerve and Retina

Although primary dysfunction of the optic nerve or retina occurs, altered appearance of these tissues often represents disease of the adjacent central nervous system (CNS) or subjacent choroid (see Uveal Tract). Optic neuritis and retinitis may therefore reflect more widespread meningoencephalitis or uveitis. Causes include infectious agents (CDV, systemic mycoses, or *Toxoplasma gondii*), immune-mediated diseases such as granulomatous meningoencephalitis, or neoplasia involving the CNS, meninges, orbit, or choroid. Diagnosis frequently involves cerebrospinal fluid (CSF) analysis and cross-sectional imaging. Optic nerve edema without hemorrhage, exudates, or blindness is termed *papilledema* and is seen in association with increased intracranial pressure. Therefore fundic examination is recommended in all animals suspected of having CNS disease, especially when a CSF tap is planned.

Taurine deficiency in cats has been associated with retinal degeneration that begins as a focal rhomboid area of subtle increased granularity of the area centralis (lateral to the optic disc), progresses to involve retina on both sides of the optic papilla, and ultimately affects the whole retina. Affected cats should also be screened for dilated cardiomyopathy. This syndrome is sometimes called *feline central retinal degeneration (FCRD)* because abnormal dietary or tissue taurine concentration is not always established.

Sudden acquired retinal degeneration (SARD) describes a rapid onset of complete blindness in middle-aged to older dogs with initially normal fundic examination findings. Generalized retinal degeneration becomes clinically evident within 4 to 6 weeks of blindness. Complete and irreversible loss of photoreceptor function takes place without any clinically or histologically detectable inflammation. Female dogs appear overrepresented and many are moderately overweight. Many have a history suggestive of hyperadrenocorticism and some may have clinical signs, blood work, or both that support the diagnosis. The cause of the apparent hyperadrenocorticism is unknown, but unlike the vision loss, systemic signs typically resolve without treatment. This disease must be differentiated from blindness as the result of optic nerve or CNS disease (particularly a functional pituitary tumor with blindness secondary to pressure effects at the optic chiasm). This can be accomplished with advanced imaging under general anesthesia; however, it is completed more simply, safely, and inexpensively by demonstrating an extinguished electroretinogram in the dog with SARD. Sight is never regained; however, owners should be reassured that this is a nonpainful disease that does not involve other ocular tissues.

Vascular and Hematologic Disease

Direct visualization of retinal (and sometimes choroidal) blood vessels permits assessment of many hematologic abnormalities, including anemia (where obvious attenuation or paleness of vessels exists), hyperlipidemia (where retinal vessels take on a creamy orange hue), and hyperviscosity (where increased vessel tortuosity sometimes is noted).

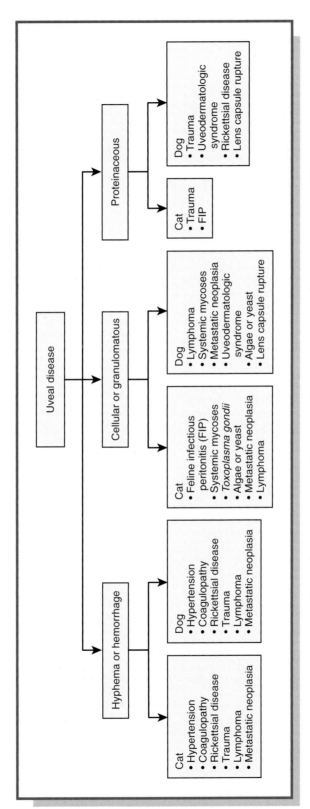

Figure 32-1 The nature of the exudates in patients with uveitis can be used to prioritize but not to eliminate differential diagnoses.

Anemia, hyperviscosity, and systemic hypertension also alter tissue perfusion and vessel wall viability and can be associated with segmental vascular constriction and sacculations of retinal vessels (so-called box-carring), "sludging," and extravasation of blood or plasma into the choroid, retina, and subretinal space. This is clinically apparent as intraretinal or subretinal edema or hemorrhage or as retinal detachment.

Some hypertensive cats also have iridal aneurysms and hyphema. A recent retrospective study of hypertensive cats established that concurrent chronic renal failure, hyperthyroidism, diabetes mellitus, hyperaldosteronism, and cardiac or neurologic abnormalities were common; however, the majority of cats with systemic hypertension are brought to veterinarians after owners observe apparent vision loss.

CHAPTER **33**

Acute Vision Loss in Small Animals

Teresa R. Tucci

Vision loss is seldom truly acute; more commonly it is a sudden recognition of blindness in the patient as perceived by the owner. Multiple lesions in the visual system and central nervous system (CNS) can result in bilateral blindness. Acute vision loss is more apparent to the owner compared with progressive vision loss. Gradual vision loss enables the pet to acclimate and memorize its surroundings. Many times the owner may not realize their pet is blind until an abrupt environmental change occurs, such as rearranging the furniture or moving the pet to another location. The goal of this chapter is to provide the proper guidelines for a comprehensive ophthalmologic examination, which enables the veterinarian to accurately assess acute vision loss in a dog or cat (Box 33-1).

ABNORMALITIES RESULTING IN BLINDNESS

Blindness is a bilateral functional complete loss of vision to which attributing causes are numerous. Three categories are listed in the initial approach to locate a lesion that has caused blindness:
1. Lesions interfering with formation of an image onto the retina
2. Lesions preventing the transmission of an image (peripheral → central)
3. Lesions inhibiting image interpretation (CNS)
   Lesions limiting the formation of the image onto the retina are caused by the absence of a normally clear ocular media (cornea, aqueous humor, lens, and vitreal humor). Disruption of this media results in varying degrees of blindness (see Box 33-1).
   Lesions affecting the retina and its ability to transmit images to the brain or visual pathway (optic nerve, optic chiasm, optic tracts, lateral geniculate nuclei, and optic radiations) are listed (Boxes 33-2 and 33-3).
   Central blindness, also referred to as *cortical blindness*, results when interpretation of an image is absent (Box 33-4).

VISUAL ASSESSMENT

A complete historical timeline is essential for obtaining a thorough ophthalmic examination. Discerning information,

---

BOX • 33-1

Ocular Media Abnormalities Causing Blindness

Cornea
- Edema (glaucoma, endothelial degeneration, immune-mediated keratitis such as keratouveitis caused by canine adenovirus-1, neurotropic keratitis, trauma
- Cellular infiltrate (bacterial, fungal, viral, neoplastic)
- Vascular invasion (chronic corneal exposure such as nonhealing corneal ulcer "Boxer ulcer")
- Fibrosis (scar formation)
- Degenerations (lipid, genetic)

Aqueous Humor
- Fibrin (immune-mediated anterior uveitis, bacterial, fungal, rickettsial, foreign body, postsurgical, FCoV/FeLV/FIV in cats, neoplasia, trauma)
- Hyphema (trauma, foreign body, neoplasia, thrombocytopenia, clotting deficiencies)
- Hypopyon (penetrating foreign body, postoperative, septicemia, bacterial/fungal keratitis or uveitis, endophthalmitis)
- Lipid aqueous (postprandial)

Lens
- Cataracts (genetic, nutritional, metabolic/diabetic, toxic, traumatic, chronic uveitis, postradiation therapy, lighting/electrocution, lens luxation)

Vitreal Humor
- Hemorrhage (systemic hypertension, retinal detachment, traumatic, clotting deficiency, rat toxicity, foreign body, neoplasia)
- Hyalitis (vitreal humor inflammation, numerous infectious diseases especially in cats [FeLV, FIV, FCoV], penetrating foreign body causing cellular infiltrate)

FCoV, Feline coronavirus; *FeLV,* feline leukemia virus; *FIV,* feline immunodeficiency virus.

Box • 33-2

Retinal Lesions Causing Blindness

Retinopathies
- Glaucoma (acute/chronic)
- Sudden acquired retinal degeneration syndromes (SARD)
- Progressive retinal atrophy (rod-cone dysplasia, rod dysplasia, progressive rod-cone degeneration [PRA])
- Central progressive retinal atrophy
- Feline central retinal degeneration (taurine deficiency)
- Toxicity (fluoroquinolone overdose in cats, ivermectin toxicity)
- Postinflammatory atrophy

Retinal Detachment Syndromes
- Exudative/transudative retinal detachments (systemic hypertension, mycoses, viral, bacterial, rickettsial, immune-mediated choroiditis, prototothecosis, toxoplasmosis, IV fluid overload)
- Neoplasia
- Retinal dysplasia
- Hereditary/congenital (Collie eye anomaly, Australian Shepherd anomaly, retinal dysplasia syndrome)

Chorioretinitis
- Canine distemper virus, systemic mycoses, brucellosis, feline coronavirus, immune-mediated disease, toxoplasmosis, uveodermatologic syndrome in Akitas, granulomatous meningoencephalitis, bacterial septicemia

Box • 33-3

Abnormalities Resulting in Failure to Transmit the Visual Message

- Viral diseases (canine distemper encephalitis, feline coronavirus)
- Systemic and ocular mycoses
- Neoplasia
- Traumatic avulsion of optic nerves (proptosis)
- Granulomatous meningoencephalitis
- Hydrocephalus
- Optic nerve hypoplasia
- Immune-mediated optic neuritis
- Vitamin A deficiency

Box • 33-4

Abnormalities Resulting in Failure to Interpret the Visual Message

- Viral (canine distemper virus and feline coronavirus)
- Granulomatous meningoencephalitis
- Systemic mycoses
- Trauma
- Heatstroke
- Hypoxia
- Hydrocephalus
- Hepatoencephalopathy
- Neoplasia
- Storage disease
- Posticata
- Meningitis
- Cerebral malfunctions
- Vascular infarcts
- Ivermectin toxicity
- Seizures, traumatic cerebrovascular accidents

terization of blindness will assist in lesion localization. For example, a patient with night blindness (nyctalopia) but good day vision would indicate retinal atrophy, or a patient with poor day vision (hemeralopia) but good night vision may indicate that the patient has cataracts. Amaurosis defines blindness with no cause. Mechanical blindness (exophthalmia, facial nerve paralysis, elevated third eyelid [Horner's syndrome]) will give the examiner an area of focus when deciphering the clinical findings.

Motion Detection
Evaluation of motion detection in animals is done by tossing an object (cotton balls) across the animal's field of view and monitoring the response, such as a head or eye movement tracking the object. The sensitivity of tactile hairs/cilia, especially in cats, makes it important not to touch or create air currents or sound, which stimulate these hairs creating a similar response.

Obstacle Course
Creating an obstacle course in an exam room allows the examiner to determine if the patient can navigate an unknown environment. Any large solid object can be used (chairs, wastebaskets or cones). It is important to perform this test in both bright and dim light and to perform several trials. Animals with neurologic deficits or those unwilling or unable to walk through the course are not good candidates for this test. The animal avoids the obstacles to pass this test. If the patient is unable to visualize objects and hesitates or bumps into the objects, that animal is likely blind.

Menace Response
The normal response to a menace response test is avoidance such as moving the head away from the object or blinking the eyes. This response is a learned behavior and is therefore typically absent in puppies and kittens under 12 weeks of age. A palpebral reflex (intact facial nerve CN VII) and eyelid function should be elicited and present prior to evaluating a menace response. Severe buphthalmia, exophthalmia, or blepharospasm will prevent blinking and obtaining a menace

such as previous developmental, hereditary, traumatic, or systemic disease problems, is essential for accurate diagnosis of the dog or cat's acute blindness. A history of prior neurologic disturbances or drug usage may confuse lesion localization of visual deficits. Direct observation of the structure within the eye is unique and may lead directly to the diagnosis without clinical pathology or invasive tests.

An orderly sequence during an ophthalmic examination is essential in obtaining a detailed analysis of the eye. Typically, ocular structures are examined beginning with the superficial structures and then proceeding to deeper structures. Charac-

response. An intact menace response requires an intact visual cortex, whereas a dazzle reflex and corneal reflex are strictly subcortical responses. Dazzle reflex is mediated by reflex centers in the rostral colliculi and can evaluate optic nerve function while not stimulating the trigeminal nerve.

Visual Placing and Postural Reactions

This test is performed by holding the animal cradled in a horizontal position with its front legs free to move and then moving the patient toward the edge of the tabletop. A visual patient will respond by lifting the legs before touching the table. A blind patient will move the legs after the legs touch the tabletop. Stairs can be used to perform this test on dogs too large to hold.

Pupillary Light Reflexes

Pupillary light reflexes (PLR) do not provide a test of vision but rather offer a starting point in lesion localization. No special equipment is needed for this test. Using a focal light source in a dimly lit room, the examiner can adequately assess the PLR in a small animal. Brachycephalic breeds such as Boston Terriers and Chinese Pugs can sometimes be more difficult to examine because of their lateral globe position. Nervous patients may require a few minutes for the sympathetic nervous system response to lessen. Stimulation of the sympathetic nervous system causes mydriasis (pupil dilation), giving the examiner the illusion of absent or diminished PLR. Prior to PLR testing always ensure the pupils are of equal size in both bright and dim light. Unequal pupil size (anisocoria) is commonly pathologic in small animal.

The PLR pathway requires normal optic nerve function, optic chiasm, optic tracts, pretectal and accessory oculomotor nuclei (Edinger-Westphal), oculomotor nerves (parasympathetic portion), and functional iridal muscles. The retinas too are required for the PLR pathway. Marked retinal pathology may be present while still maintaining a diminished to normal PLR. Iris atrophy and opacification of the cornea, anterior chamber, or lens are additional complications that can diminish the PLR or prevent observation of the pupil. In this situation the lesion may or may not be localized to the globe.

SPECIAL DIAGNOSITIC TESTS

Electroretinography (ERG) is a highly sensitive test interpreted by specialists to evaluate the function of the photoreceptors (rods and cones) using light stimulation. Because of its ability to differentiate between photoreceptor disease and optic nerve or CNS lesions, the ERG is beneficial in dogs and cats with acute vision loss when ophthalmoscopic examination proves normal.

Ocular ultrasonography is a useful tool in diagnosis of intraocular or retrobulbar lesions when opacification of the ocular media, such as corneal edema, cataracts, or severe enophthalmos, is present.

Computed tomography (CT) and magnetic resonance imaging (MRI) scans are excellent diagnostic tools used to localize lesions that may otherwise go undetected or undiagnosed.

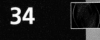

CHAPTER 34

Abdominal Distension, Ascites, and Peritonitis

Greg Chambers

ABDOMINAL DISTENSION

Abdominal distension can be an emergency situation and should be evaluated quickly, especially if accompanied by abdominal pain or discomfort, weakness, profound lethargy, trouble breathing, fever, tachycardia, poor pulses, pale mucous membranes, or if the capillary refill time is greater than 2 seconds. For further instruction on the acute abdomen, please see Chapter 125. Causes for abdominal distension can be separated into five main categories: tissue, fluid, gas, feces, or abdominal musculature weakness (Table 34-1 and Figure 34-1).[1]

Increased amounts of tissue can be due to enlargement of organs (hepatomegaly, splenomegaly, renomegaly, prostatomegaly), pregnancy, fat (obesity, lipoma), neoplasia (cancers of the liver, spleen, kidneys, intestinal tract, prostate, adrenal glands, pancreas, bladder, ovaries, uterus, lipomas, or more generalized neoplasia such as carcinomatosis or lymphosarcoma). Some granulomatous diseases have also been described (pythiosis, aspergillosis).

Fluid accumulation can cause abdominal enlargement by collecting free in the abdomen, inside organs, or in cysts (Web Figures 34-1 and 34-2).

See ascites and peritonitis sections for causes of peritoneal effusions. Fluid can also collect in the gastrointestinal tract (ileus, obstruction, or food bloat), uterus (pyometra and cystic endometrial hyperplasia), urinary bladder (upper or lower motor urinary bladder, obstruction of the urethra), or the kidney (hydronephrosis). Cyst formation can cause abdominal distension. Cysts include those identified as perinephric or paraprostatic and those associated with polycystic kidney or liver disease.

Gas accumulation can occur in the intestinal tract as a result of gastric dilation or volvulus, ileus, torsion, or obstruction. Gas can be present in an emphysematous gallbladder, urinary bladder, or in certain liver diseases. Free gas in the abdomen is typically caused by perforation of a gas-containing organ like the intestines, gas formation by bacteria as in septic peritonitis, trauma, or iatrogenic such as with surgery or laparoscopy.

Table • 34-1

Common Causes of Abdominal Distension

FLUID	WEAK ABDOMINAL MUSCLES	TISSUE	FECES	GAS
Peritoneal effusion	Hyperadrenocorticism	Pregnancy	Obstipation	Gastric dilation or volvulus
Congestion		Organ enlargement	Megacolon	Obstruction or ileus of GI tract
Cyst formation		Neoplasia		Postsurgery
Hydronephrosis		Granuloma		GI tract rupture
Obstruction or ileus of GI tract		Fat		Bacterial peritonitis
Pyometra				

GI, Gastrointestinal.

The last two categories include abdominal musculature weakness (predominantly from hyperadrenocorticism) and feces accumulation (obstipation).

PERITONEAL EFFUSIONS INCLUDING ASCITES AND PERITONITIS

Ascites is defined as an accumulation of serous fluid in the peritoneal cavity and is usually reserved for a transudate that is associated with liver or right heart failure. Unfortunately it is also used by some to refer to any fluid in the peritoneal cavity. In this chapter, the term *peritoneal effusion* is utilized and further classification of the effusion is determined after the fluid has been analyzed. Peritoneal effusions can be divided into 10 different categories: pure transudates, modified transudates, nonseptic exudate, septic exudate, hemorrhagic effusion, bilious effusion, chylous effusion, pseudochylous effusion, malignant effusions, and eosinophilic effusions (Table 34-2; see Figure 34-1).[2,3]

Pure transudates are defined as having <1000 cells, <2.5 total solids, and a specific gravity of <1.017. They occur secondary to decreases in oncotic pressure such as in hypoalbuminemia (from protein-losing nephropathy, protein-losing enteropathy, liver failure, burn wounds, or from repeated removal of peritoneal or pleural fluid), increased hydrostatic pressure (portal hypertension, Budd-Chiari syndrome, or right heart failure) an in rare cases from increased permeability of the vasculature (vasculitis).

Modified transudates are defined as having >1000 but <10,000 cells, between 2.5 and 5.0 total solids, and a specific gravity of >1.017 and <1.025. This group is a catchall between pure transudates and exudates and therefore has a multitude of different cells that can be present as well as a large number of causes such as: increases in hydrostatic pressure and vasculitis as previously described with pure transudates, neoplasia, granulomas, postsurgery or postlaparoscopy, splenic or intestinal torsions, and infarctions.

Exudates are defined as having >5000 cells, >3.0 total solids and >1.025 specific gravity. The cellular component is chiefly made up of neutrophils and macrophages. Causes for exudates include perforation of bowel, neoplasia, pancreatitis, recent surgery, bile duct or gallbladder rupture, urinary tract rupture (bladder, urethral or ureteral), and feline infectious peritonitis. For further information please see the peritonitis section of this chapter.

Hemorrhagic effusions are defined as having >1000 cells, >3.0 total solids and >1.025 specific gravity. The effusion should closely resemble the peripheral blood with red blood cells and some white blood cells such as neutrophils and lymphocytes. The only exception is platelets, which are usually not present unless the bleed occurred in the hour previous to diagnosis. The samples rarely are able to coagulate due to the lack of platelets. Differentials for hemorrhagic effusions include coagulopathies, fracture of the liver or spleen, neoplasia, avulsion of renal arteries, and iatrogenic such as in postoperative patients.

Chylous abdominal effusions have variable cell counts, >2.5 total solids, and >1.018 specific gravity. The predominant cell early on is the lymphocyte but can become the neutrophil secondary to inflammation as the effusion becomes more chronic. The effusion triglyceride level is usually 2 to 3 times greater than the serum triglyceride with the effusion cholesterol being less than the serum cholesterol. Differentials include lymphangiectasia, strangulation or rupture of the lymph vessels by neoplasia, right heart failure, or lymphoproliferative diseases including the mesenteric lymph nodes. Pseudochylous effusion is rare and usually has high cholesterol and low triglyceride concentrations as compared with serum.

Bilious effusions are similar to exudates but contain bilirubin crystals. Bilirubin concentrations in the effusion are higher than in serum. The principle cell involved is the neutrophil, which may contain some bile pigments. Bile effusions occur secondary to rupture of the bile duct or gallbladder. This happens secondary to trauma, cholelithiasis, pancreatitis, or necrotizing cholecystitis.

Malignant effusions are often a subtype of modified transudates or exudates that contain neoplastic cells. Care should be taken in interpreting malignancy on cytology due to normal mesothelial cells displaying criteria that could be mistaken for neoplasia. Review by pathologist is essential.

Eosinophilic effusions present as modified transudates or exudates with greater than 10% eosinophils. These effusions are often caused by lymphoma, systemic mast cell tumors, aberrant larval migrans, fungal disease, or disseminated eosinophilic granulomatosis.

DIAGNOSIS

A complete blood count can be helpful in diagnosis of peritoneal effusions. Increases or decreases in white blood cell count may increase the suspicion of sepsis. Decrease in platelet count could help diagnose coagulopathies such as immune-mediated thrombocytopenia or disseminated intravascular coagulation (DIC) that may be causing hemoabdomen. An increased eosinophil count could be associated with disseminated eosinophilic granulomatosis or mast cell tumors. Low red blood cell counts could be associated with hemoabdomen.

A biochemistry panel and urinalysis should be completed on all patients with abdominal distension and can help in the

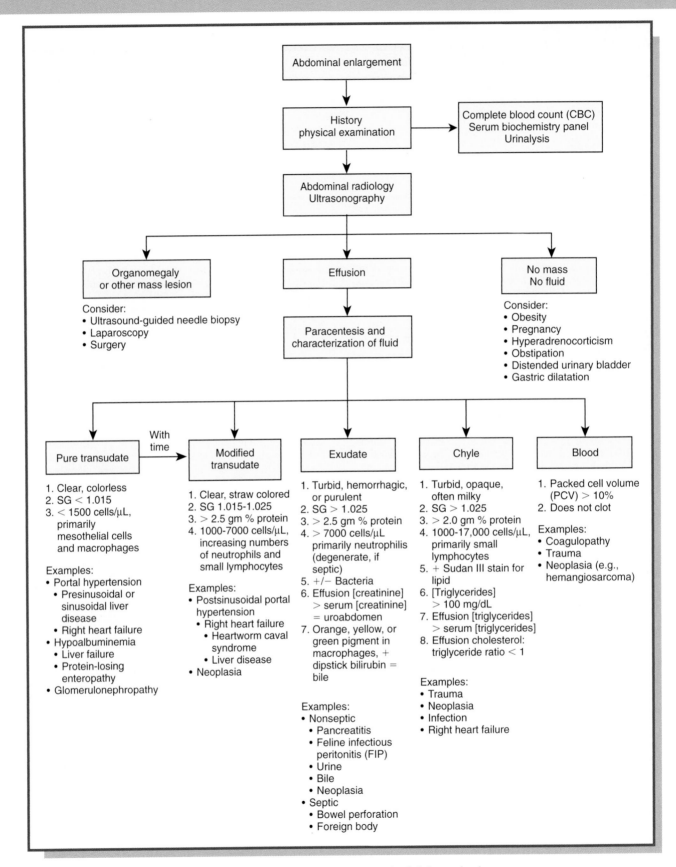

Figure 34-1 Algorithm for diagnostic approach of abdominal enlargement.

Table • 34-2

Common Effusions

	NUCLEATED CELLS/μL	TOTAL SOLIDS (G/dL)	SPECIFIC GRAVITY	SPECIFIC CHARACTERISTICS
Transudates				
Pure transudate	< 1000	<2.5	<1.017	Usually few cells present
Modified transudate	>500	>2.5	>1.017	Some mesothelial cells, neutrophils, red
	<10,000	<5.0	<1.025	blood cells, macrophages and mature lymphocytes can be present in low numbers
Hemorrhagic effusion	>1000	>3.0	>1.025	Appears similar to peripheral blood with a large proportion of red blood cells and usually without platelets being present
Exudates				
Nonseptic exudate	>5000	>3.0	>1.025	Mostly neutrophils and macrophages are present with or without neoplastic cells (no bacteria are usually seen although a culture should be submitted to make sure bacteria were not missed on cytology)
Septic exudate	>5000	>3.0	>1.025	Same as above with bacteria present within cells (although culture is needed for definitive diagnosis)
Bilious effusion	>5000	>3.0	>1.025	Neutrophils and macrophages predominate often with bilirubin crystals seen inside of the macrophages (again culture should be submitted)
Chylous effusion	Variable	>2.5	>1.025	Mature lymphocytes predominate often with neutrophils and macrophages being present in chronic effusions

diagnosis of sepsis, chronic liver disease, urinary obstruction, hyperadrenocorticism, hypoalbuminemia, and protein-losing nephropathy.

Radiographs of the abdomen should be taken and may help in the diagnosis of pregnancy, peritoneal effusion, organomegaly, mass lesions, carcinomatosis, free air, large deposits of adipose tissue, obstipation, gastric dilation, and volvulus.

With the exceptions of pregnancy, obstipation, and large deposits of adipose being present on abdominal radiographs, thoracic radiographs should also be performed. Bicavitary effusions, interstitial nodular patterns, pericardial disease, right heart enlargement, and caudal vena cava size are just some of the essential information acquired with radiography.

Abdominal ultrasound is indicated in animals with abdominal mass lesions or organomegaly, or if peritoneal effusion is present. Abdominal ultrasound is invaluable in the diagnosis and acquisition of small amounts of peritoneal effusion, the presence of cystic disease, mass lesions, organ enlargement, early pregnancy, pyometra, and pancreatitis. Echocardiology should be completed if there is any question of right heart abnormalities or pericardial effusion.

Any peritoneal effusate obtained via aspiration should be evaluated in-house and sent to a pathologist for thorough analysis and cytology. See above section on peritoneal effusions for more detail. Individual situations may require further diagnostics. In cases of hemoabdomen a prothrombin time and partial thrombin time should be completed and possibly even a buccal mucosal bleeding time. In uroabdomen, the creatinine and potassium concentrations of the effusion will be higher than that of serum. Bilirubin levels should be higher in the effusion than the blood in cases of bilious effusion. A straw-colored, translucent, viscous fluid with a total protein greater than 3.5 in a feline is highly suspicious of feline infectious peritonitis. Please see the peritonitis section of this chapter for methods of differentiating septic from nonseptic exudates.

PERITONITIS

Peritonitis is defined as inflammation of the peritoneum. Primary peritonitis is inflammation of the peritoneum without any preexisting abdominal pathology (e.g., feline infectious peritonitis). Secondary peritonitis is the predominant form and occurs in conjunction with abdominal pathology (e.g., perforation of gastrointestinal tract). Secondary peritonitis can be further divided into septic and nonseptic. This determination is most easily made by culture of the peritoneal effusion (most often an exudate). In early cases of peritonitis peritoneal effusion may not be present. In these cases a diagnostic peritoneal lavage may be needed. This is rarely the case: within 2 to 3 hours after contamination of the abdomen with gastrointestinal, chylous, bilious, hemorrhagic, pancreatic, or urinary leakage, there is a significant amount of fluid and leukocytes present.

A positive culture is the definitive diagnosis for septic exudate and should be performed in all cases of exudates. Unfortunately cultures can take many days before they can be considered positive or negative and a more timely determination of a septic exudate is needed to give the patient a better chance of a positive outcome. In-house cytology of the exudate should be performed. If any intracellular bacteria, plant fibers, or intestinal flora are present, the exudate should be considered septic. Unfortunately these cytologic changes are not always present and further testing may be needed. A glucose level can be taken of the effusion by way of a handheld glucometer and compared to blood glucose. If the blood glucose is 20 mg/dL higher than the peritoneal effusion, sepsis is highly likely.[4] This is because the bacteria metabolize glucose present in the effusion. Some malignant effusions can also have a similar decrease in glucose because malignant cells utilize the glucose. Another method for determination of septic effusions is to compare the blood/effusion levels of lactate. If peritoneal effusion is >2.5 mmol/L and higher than the blood lactate, a septic effusion is likely in the dog.[5] This measurement of the lactate is not useful in cats.

TREATMENT

Specific treatment should be directed at the underlying cause of abdominal distension or peritoneal effusion (e.g., a diet for obese patients, medications for hyperadrenocorticism, etc.). Surgery should be included in the treatment of uroabdomen, hemoabdomen, septic exudates, and bilious effusions after initial stabilization.

General treatment may also be utilized for dogs or cats with chronic peritoneal effusions, such as those with right heart failure. Abdominocentesis may be used when the patient has a decreased appetite, becomes lethargic, has difficulty breathing, or finds it difficult to get comfortable while lying down. Care should be taken to not drain the abdomen too often or without cause as electrolyte disturbances, hypoalbuminemia, infection and bleeding are just some of the complications that can ensue.

Critical patients are not able to display signs of discomfort with abdominal distension and need to be monitored closely to prevent abdominal compartment syndrome. *Abdominal compartment syndrome* is defined as impaired organ function secondary to increased intraabdominal pressure.[6] Intraabdominal pressure should be monitored by way of a urinary Foley catheter and monometer centered at the umbilicus of the recumbent patient. The bladder should be drained and 0.5 to 1 mL/kg of 0.9% sodium chloride should be infused prior to application of the manometer. Pressures should be monitored in the case of progressive abdominal distension, azotemia, elevated central venous pressures, evidence of increased intracranial pressure, tachypnea, and tachycardia in patients with recent abdominal surgery or peritoneal effusions. Normal pressures in the dog are 0 to 5 cm water. Pressures after surgery are <15 cm water. If the intraabdominal pressure is 10 to 20 cm water, the patient should be closely monitored; if the pressure is 20 to 35 cm water, active decompression should be considered. If the pressure is >35, decompression of the abdomen is required.

REFERENCES

The reference list can be found on the companion Expert Consult Web site at *www.expertconsult.com.*

CHAPTER 35

Weakness

Rhonda L. Schulman

Weakness is a common owner concern. In veterinary medicine, the terms *fatigue* and *lethargy* are often used synonymously with weakness. Fatigue is the inability to continue performing a task after multiple repetitions, whereas *weakness* means an inability to *initially* perform the task. Lethargy refers to a lower level of consciousness, drowsiness, stupor, or inactivity. The term *asthenia* defines a state of exhaustion in the absence of muscle weakness that can accompany many disease conditions including cardiovascular and metabolic disorders. In dogs and cats, it is usually impossible to distinguish between these states. For the purposes of this chapter the term weakness will be used interchangeably to include fatigue, lethargy, and asthenia. Since many diseases can result in similar, nonspecific signs of weakness, this presentation can be a diagnostic challenge (Figure 35-1). While few diseases can be eliminated or definitively diagnosed during initial evaluation, the dog or cat's signal-

ment, history, and physical examination are used to prioritize differential diagnoses and narrow the focus of specific diagnostic testing.

Signalment will assist in ordering the list of potential differential diagnoses. Be aware of breed-associated conditions that can result in weakness, for example, cardiovascular disease in Cavalier King Charles Spaniels, hypoadrenocorticism in Standard Poodles, portosystemic shunt in Yorkshire Terriers, or hydrocephalus in Chihuahua. All these conditions occur in other breeds and in mixed breed dogs and cats. The age of the pet may be more in accordance with some differentials. Puppies and kittens will be more likely to suffer from intestinal parasitism, dietary indiscretion, congenital disease, portosystemic shunt, hypoglycemia, toxin exposure, or an infectious disease. Old age may not be a cause of weakness; however, geriatric pets may have chronic progressive weakness secondary to endocrine disorders, musculoskeletal pain,

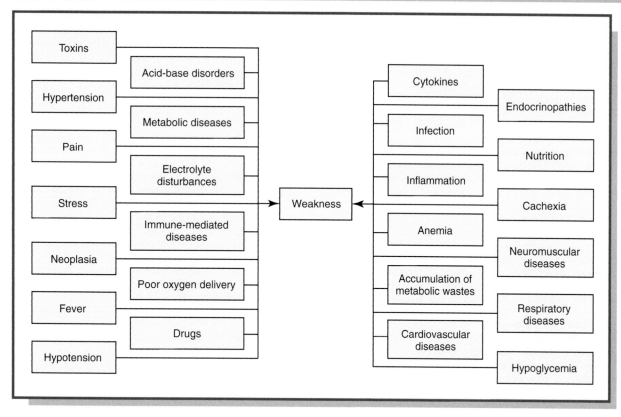

Figure 35-1 Causes of weakness. For a more detailed description of weakness, see Web Figure 35-1 on www.expertconsult.com.

cardiovascular disease, neoplastic conditions, or major organ dysfunction. Immune-mediated diseases are more prevalent in young to middle-aged female dogs.

The pet's history can provide many important clues as to the cause of the weakness. In addition to routine questions regarding time course, concurrent illnesses, medications, and familial history, the owners should be asked about any associations with either exercise or time of day. For example, pets with disorders of glucose homeostasis may typically display symptoms either after eating or fasting. Classically, myasthenic dogs exhibit profound weakness after short bursts of normal activity. Travel history to areas with endemic infectious diseases should raise suspicions for conditions not routinely diagnosed locally.

A thorough physical examination is mandatory. Pain on manipulation of joints or long bones may suggest an underlying orthopedic problem or polyarthritis, manifesting as weakness. Dermatologic signs such as symmetrical alopecia and recurrent pyoderma might indicate an endocrine disorder. Primary cardiovascular disease may be apparent during examination of mucous membranes, capillary refill time, cardiac auscultation, and peripheral pulses. Because neurologic disorders can cause weakness, a complete neurologic examination may be indicated.

In some dogs and cats, a specific finding during the initial physical examination and laboratory analysis results in a definitive diagnosis; unfortunately, many of the conditions resulting in weakness have nonspecific clinical signs and laboratory findings. As a result the initial diagnostic evaluation is used to prioritize differential diagnoses and identify diagnostic tests. This chapter discusses the different mechanisms and diseases that result in weakness.

SPECIFIC MECHANISMS AND DISEASES

Metabolic Diseases

Metabolic diseases are among the most common causes of weakness. Major organ dysfunction can result in weakness through many pathways, such as accumulation of metabolic products, cytokine production, electrolyte imbalances, acid-base disorders, anemia of chronic disease, and nutritional disturbances. Renal and hepatic failure are two examples of metabolic diseases that cause weakness by multiple mechanisms. Biochemical evaluation is essential in the diagnosis of metabolic disorders.

Electrolyte Disorders

Electrolyte imbalances accompany a multitude of conditions and are often the disease component that leads to weakness. Mild changes in serum electrolyte concentrations rarely cause weakness. Thus, if only mild changes are noted in a serum electrolyte concentration, further causes of weakness should be sought. Severe changes in potassium, either increases or decreases, are associated with weakness. Significant hypokalemia may result from excessive loss (gastrointestinal, urinary) or be iatrogenic in nature (fluid diuresis, diuretics). Hyperkalemia, as is seen with hypoadrenocorticism and urinary tract obstruction or rupture, also results in weakness. Sodium imbalances, both increases and decreases, can result in weakness. Hyponatremia is seen in hypoadrenocorticism, congestive heart failure, liver diseases, and losses through the gastrointestinal system and third space. Hypernatremia may be seen with hyperaldosteronism, salt poisoning, and free-water loss.

Perturbations in calcium homeostasis are important potential causes of weakness. Hypocalcemia produces excessive excitability of the nervous system, manifested as tetany and possibly seizures. Between bouts of tetany, dogs and cats typically appear weak. Common causes of hypocalcemia include hypoparathyroidism, renal disease, ethylene glycol toxicity, and eclampsia. Hypercalcemia may also result in weakness and lethargy. Significant hypercalcemia may arise from neoplasia, especially lymphoma, and primary hyperparathyroidism and less commonly from renal failure or toxicities. Hypomagnesemia, prevalent in critically ill pets because of renal and gastrointestinal losses coupled with decreased intake, may also result in weakness. Hypomagnesemia may be seen in conjunction with hypokalemia and/or hypocalcemia.

Acid-Base Disorders

Disturbances in blood pH can accompany many metabolic conditions and can be seen with pulmonary disease. Drugs and toxins may also lead to acidosis or alkalosis. Weakness can be seen with either disorder. Significant alterations in bicarbonate on serum chemistry should raise suspicion for an acid-base disorder and may indicate additional diagnostic testing.

Inflammatory Conditions

Inflammation accompanies many disease processes such as pancreatitis, hepatitis, neoplasia, infectious disease, and immune-mediated conditions. Systemic inflammation can result in pyrexia, negative energy balance, cytokine production, anemia, and acid-base disorders, all exacerbating signs of weakness. Many of these changes are mediated by increased cytokine production in response to the inflammatory stimuli. Certain cytokines, such as interleukin (IL)-1, IL-6, and interferon (IFN)-α, directly cause fatigue via central pathways. Cachexins, such as IL-1, IL-6, IFN-α, and tumor necrosis factor (TNF)-α suppress hunger, promote muscle wasting, and contributes to weakness. At high concentrations, TNF-α decreases myocardial contractility and vascular smooth muscle tone, resulting in systemic hypotension. Cytokine inhibition of erythropoiesis, resulting in anemia, indirectly contributes to weakness.

Infectious Diseases

Bacterial, viral, fungal, rickettsial, protozoal, or parasitic agents can infect any organ or body system. The clinical signs may point to the involved organ, such as coughing with respiratory disease or dysuria with prostatitis, as well as nonspecific signs of infection, such as weakness, inappetence, lymphadenopathy, and pyrexia. The infecting agent may produce toxins that cause weakness.

Immune-Mediated Diseases

Generalized weakness or exercise intolerance is a common component of many immune-mediated disorders. Immune-mediated diseases may lead to anemia, joint or muscle disease with resultant pain, hepatic or renal dysfunction, inflammation, and chronic wasting. Through any or all of these mechanisms, dogs and cats suffering from a variety of immune-mediated diseases may appear weak. Dogs with immune-mediated polyarthritis often have weakness as their only presenting sign, although pain may result in a reluctance to move and apparent weakness.

Anemia

Anemia, with the resultant decrease in oxygen delivery to the tissues, can cause weakness. The presence of weakness or exercise intolerance does not specify the pathophysiologic mechanism resulting in the anemic state. Often more severe signs will be seen with acute blood loss than will be noted with more chronic cases, even if the magnitude of the anemia is greater in the chronic case. With chronic disease, the pet has time to adapt to the anemia, and clinical signs may be subtle.

Endocrine Diseases

Weakness can be seen with almost every endocrine disease including diabetes mellitus, hypothyroidism, hypoadrenocorticism, hyperadrenocorticism, hyperparathyroidism, hypoglycemia, hypoparathyroidism, and pheochromocytoma. Hyperthyroidism uncommonly manifests as weakness. Until a severe crisis occurs, owners and veterinarians may not observe early, nonspecific, episodes of weakness caused by hypoadrenocorticism. Relative adrenal insufficiency may exacerbate the weakness seen in critically ill animals. Endocrine disturbances can result in weakness via various mechanisms. Many endocrinopathies, such as hypoadrenocorticism, hypoparathyroidism, and hyperparathyroidism, and diabetes mellitus can produce weakness as the result of electrolyte abnormalities. Endocrinopathies may cause muscle atrophy, which develops secondary to alterations in protein and carbohydrate metabolism. Neuropathies and myopathies resulting in weakness may be seen with diabetes mellitus and hypoglycemia, as well as hyperadrenocorticism and hypothyroidism. Endocrinopathies can also cause pertubations in blood pressure.

Cardiovascular Disease

Cardiovascular disease may be detected or suspected during physical examination; however, unless the dysfunction is of sufficient severity to induce exercise intolerance, the clinician must continue evaluation for concurrent conditions that may be the actual cause of weakness. Heart murmurs will frequently be ausculted. Crackles may be heard if the pet is suffering from left heart failure. Right heart failure can produce a variety of abnormalities that may be detected on physical exam, including jugular pulses, ascites, and decreased heart and lung sounds secondary to pleural effusion. Often, the biggest diagnostic challenge is establishing that a heart murmur does not signify heart disease of a nature sufficient to induce exercise intolerance. Cardiovascular disease results in the clinical sign of weakness caused by poor cardiac output leading to diminished oxygen delivery to the tissues or by cardiac cachexia. Valvular disease tends to cause exercise intolerance only when it has progressed to congestive failure. Because of the associated septicemia, bacterial endocarditis usually results in extreme lethargy. Arrhythmias may manifest as intermittent weakness. Diseases resulting in pericardial effusion often produce profound weakness and potentially sudden collapse.

Blood Pressure

Alterations in blood pressure can produce weakness, often episodically. Hypotension can result from cardiac dysfunction, hypovolemia, or decreased vascular tone. Hypotension creates poor perfusion and oxygen delivery. Systemic hypertension damages many organs, including the heart, brain, kidneys, and eyes. Systemic hypertension is usually a secondary problem in dogs and cats with underlying diseases including heart disease, renal disease, hyperthyroidism, hyperadrenocorticism, and diabetes mellitus. Caution must be exercised when treating hypertension to not create hypotension.

Respiratory Diseases

Similar to heart disease, respiratory disease may be obvious during the initial physical examination. Owner concerns frequently include coughing, alterations in respiration, or nasal discharge. Changes in lung sounds and respiratory rate or effort are often detected during physical examination. Respiratory diseases that result in exercise intolerance are commonly infectious or inflammatory in nature. Thoracic radiographs, arterial blood gas analysis, and bronchoalveolar lavage or tracheal wash are often necessary diagnostics. Pulmonary hypertension can also lead to weakness. Pulmonary hypertension may occur secondary to heartworm disease or chronic pulmonary disease and carries a guarded prognosis.

Neuromuscular Diseases

Brain Any disorder affecting the brain can cause weakness. The neurologic exam will localize the problem as being central in origin. Encephalitis caused by infectious agents, inflammatory conditions, or immune-mediated disease; cerebral vascular accidents (embolism or hemorrhage); space-occupying lesions (neoplasia, granulomas, or hydrocephalus); vestibular disease (central or peripheral); and idiopathic epilepsy can cause chronic or intermittent weakness. Additionally, many medications that act on the central nervous system (CNS) result in lethargy or exercise intolerance. The minimum data base may help further define the cause. Often more advanced diagnostics such as imaging of the brain or analysis of the cerebrospinal fluid (CSF) will be necessary to fully diagnose the underlying condition.

Spinal Cord Disease Lesions affecting the spinal cord between C1 to T2 can result in quadriparesis. More caudal lesions may cause paraparesis. Causes of spinal cord disease include trauma, degenerative disk disease, vascular accidents, neoplasia, infectious diseases, and inflammatory conditions. Chronic, progressive conditions are more likely to result in the vague signs of weakness compared with the more recognizable problem of acute paraparesis. In addition to the minimum data base, imaging and CSF analysis may be required to determine the underlying cause of spinal cord disease.

Neuropathies Disorders affecting peripheral nerves can result in generalized weakness. The neurologic examination of affected dogs and cats typically reflect lower motor neuron dysfunction with reduced or absent reflexes. Causes of polyneuropathy include polyradiculoneuritis; paraneoplastic disorders; endocrine diseases including diabetes mellitus, hyperadrenocorticism, and hypothyroidism; drugs and toxins (vincristine, lead); infectious agents *(Toxoplasma, Neospora)*; and developmental disorders. Weakness may also result from disruption of neuromuscular transmission. Myasthenia gravis can be either acquired or congenital. Severe exercise intolerance is often a hallmark of this disorder. Other neuromuscular disorders include tick paralysis and botulism. Specialized testing such as electromyography, nerve and muscle biopsy, and serology for antibodies to the acetylcholine receptor are often necessary to establish the diagnosis.

Myopathies Disorders of muscle may cause weakness. Generalized myopathies may result from infectious, inflammatory, congenital, paraneoplastic, or immune-mediated diseases. In humans, significant age-related muscle weakening is seen. This weakening is seen due to a loss in muscle mass as well as changes in muscle fiber type. It is likely the same changes occur in animals and may explain some weakness seen in geriatric patients.

Neoplasia Neoplasia can lead to weakness through many different pathways. Associated inflammation may result in the release of a variety of cytokines that can cause fatigue, cachexia, and anemia. Tumors may specifically release substances such as insulin, steroids, thyroid and parathyroid hormones, catecholamines, and estrogen that cause or exacerbate weakness. Some tumors such as hemangiosarcoma can cause severe, acute blood loss. Cancers can also result in anemia via disseminated intravascular coagulopathy (DIC). Neoplastic invasion or embolization can instigate organ failure. Finally, cancer can produce weakness from pain. In humans, weakness associated with cancer is so common that cancer-related fatigue (CRF) has been accepted as an independent diagnosis. It is considered distinct from the tiredness experienced by healthy individuals in that it is not relieved by rest or sleep. In addition to being present at the time of diagnosis, CRF will be experienced by virtually all patients undergoing either chemotherapy or radiation therapy. Cancer-related fatigue can persist for months to years following therapy in humans.

Physical and Psychologic Stress

Stress is the major cause of fatigue in humans. Psychologic causes of lethargy are much harder to evaluate in animals, but should not be completely discounted. Events that can cause clinically significant anxiety (thunderstorms, fireworks, boarding) or chronic stress (social status, deprivation, illness, pain) may result in generalized weakness. Stress of any nature can activate the hypothalamic-pituitary-adrenal axis, with resultant increased levels of corticotropin-releasing hormone (CRH) and cortisol. Hyperactivity of this axis can lead to depression and weakness. CRH may play a specific role in the development of fatigue. It has also been suggested that primary hypothalamic dysfunction may be important in the cause of generalized weakness.

Exercise intolerance may be seen in an animal pushed beyond its physical capabilities. This can occur both in animals that are not used to exercise and in fit animals that overexert themselves during activities such as hunting and racing.

Pain

Animals may appear exercise intolerant if they are in pain. Animals with spinal, bone, or joint pain are often quite reluctant to move. Physical examination may elucidate musculoskeletal or neurologic pain. Abdominal pain can result from distention, inflammation, or ischemia of organs. These pets may display a hunched appearance and resent abdominal palpation. Visceral pain is less localized and may be harder to pinpoint. Chronic progressive pain may result in slower onset of nonspecific decreased activity level, decreased appetite, or weakness attributed to age-related change rather than pain; examples include glaucoma, oral pain, and end-stage otitis externa.

Nutritional Derangements

Nutritional derangements may be the patient's primary problem or may be a reflection of chronic disease. Changes or reduction in protein synthesis, altered glucose homeostasis, or dyslipoproteinemias may all result in weakness. Specific vitamin and mineral deficiencies may also cause weakness. Nutritional disorders may arise from an inadequate diet, either in content or calories. The patient may not be able to use or synthesize nutrients appropriately or may lose them excessively. Liver, pancreatic, kidney, and gastrointestinal disease may all cause weakness via nutritional deficits. Lipid disorders can arise from endocrinopathies such as diabetes mellitus, hypothyroidism, and hyperadrenocorticism; renal disease; liver disease; pancreatitis; diet; or familial causes. Any chronic condition can lead to cachexia. The clinical signs of cachexia are anorexia, weight loss, and muscle wasting. Cachectic patients suffer from a negative energy balance and metabolic derangements. These changes are often mediated by the same cytokines that cause fatigue.

Drugs

A complete history is essential for the patient with lethargy or weakness. Many medications including anticonvulsants, antihistamines, glucocorticoids, tranquilizers, narcotics, antibiotics, chemotherapeutics, diuretics, and cardiovascular agents can result in side effects, including weakness. If the onset of exercise intolerance coincides with the administration of a new medication, it may be prudent to discontinue that medication or lower the dose.

UROGENITAL

CHAPTER 36

Vaginal-Vulvar and Preputial Discharge

Claudia J. Baldwin

VAGINAL-VULVAR DISCHARGE

When veterinarians examine a female dog or cat that has a genital discharge, it is usually a vulvar discharge, composed of fluid, cells, and/or tissue, that originates from the uterus, vagina, urinary tract, vestibule, or vulva. Such discharges may occur in both intact and neutered females. Other causes of a vaginal-vulvar discharge that need to be considered are sex hormone–producing ovarian disorders (neoplasia or remnant), generalized mucosal disease, exudative perivulvar dermatitis, and bleeding diathesis arising from disorders of blood coagulation.

Normal physiologic vaginal-vulvar discharges, which originate from the uterus, are expected in the intact bitch and queen during the reproductive cycle. During proestrus, the bitch produces a serosanguineous discharge of varying volume. During estrus, the discharge becomes less bloody and usually is straw colored. During early diestrus, the discharge is scant and, if present, is mucoid to dark red. The queen does not normally exhibit appreciable discharge. During late gestation, either the queen or bitch may display a mucoid discharge. At parturition, both produce a clear to green-black discharge that signifies amniotic fluid and separation of placentas, respectively. Normal lochia is red/green/brown; it usually diminishes to undetectable levels by 3 weeks postgestation in the bitch but may not be appreciable in the queen (vaginal discharge postwhelping may persist normally for a longer period in some dogs).

The etiology of a pathologic vaginal-vulvar discharge (Table 36-1) can be considered using the "DAMNIT" diagnostic scheme.

This broad scheme provides clinicians with a logical, inclusive list for the origin and potential causes of discharge in both intact and ovariohysterectomized (OHE) females. (*D* stands for degenerative or developmental, *A* for allergic or autoimmune, *M* for metabolic, *N* for neoplastic or nutritional, *I* for iatrogenic, idiopathic, or inflammatory [infectious or immune related], *T* for toxic or traumatic.)

HISTORY

The history, inclusive of the age and breed, is important in determining the reproductive status of the female. Information on the date of OHE or the last estrus, pregnancy, or parturition may assist the clinician in choosing diagnostics. When there is a question as to whether an OHE has been performed, the clinician should inspect the skin along the caudal abdominal midline for a surgical incision line.

The history may include a continuous or intermittent discharge, licking, and/or "scooting." Developmental or inherited conditions likely would manifest in a younger female, whereas neoplastic disease would be more common in an older female. Clinical signs of systemic illness (e.g., fever, anorexia) would be expected with inflammatory, infectious, disseminated neoplastic, traumatic, or toxic disorders. A drug administration history is important as some drugs used for treatment of other conditions (e.g., diethylstilbestrol for hormonal responsive urinary incontinence) may produce discharge.

PHYSICAL EXAMINATION

A complete physical examination should be performed, including abdominal palpation to detect organomegaly (ovarian, uterine, or bladder) or discomfort. Inspection of the vulva and perineal region may reveal edema, often associated with estradiol influence, inflammation, or trauma; primary or secondary dermatitis; or anatomic abnormalities (e.g., enlarged clitoris, infantile vulva, or ventral vulvar displacement) (Web Figure 36-1).

A rectal examination in bitches allows palpation of the cranial vestibule, the urethra, and a variable portion of the vagina.

CYTOLOGY

Whenever there is a vaginal discharge in a dog, the reproductive evaluation should include collection of discharge from the vestibule with a cotton swab (or in a container, if copious) or, of greater value, a sample should be obtained from the vaginal vault cranial to the urethral opening using a cotton swab. Cytologic evaluation is important to characterize the discharge further. A bloody vaginal discharge in a dog with "intermediate" cells and, certainly, with "superficial" vaginal epithelial cells would be indicative of a dog in proestrus or

Table • 36-1

Source and Etiology of Pathologic Vaginal-Vulvar Discharges

	SOURCE		ETIOLOGY	
ORGAN OR DISORDER	DEVELOPMENTAL/ DEGENERATIVE ORIGIN	NEOPLASTIC	INFLAMMATORY/INFECTIOUS/ IATROGENIC	TRAUMATIC/TOXIC
Uterus/stump	Healing failure post-OHE, SIPS	Various	CEH/pyometra, metritis	Parturient
Vagina	Vaginal bands/septa	Various	Primary and secondary	Breeding, postpartum, FB
Urinary tract	Ectopic ureter, sphincter laxity Vaginal abnormality	TCC	Cystitis/urethritis Iatrogenic	Calculi
Vestibule	Vulvovestibular stricture	Various	Primary or secondary	Breeding, postpartum, FB
Vulva	Ventral displacement/agenesis Infantile/intersex	Various	Clitoral enlargement	FB
Generalized mucosal disease			Immune mediated Infectious	Irritant
Ovarian disorders	Cystic disease/remnant	E2-secreting tumor	Ovarian remnant	
Perivulvar dermatitis			Pyoderma	Irritant
Bleeding diathesis	Inherited deficiency		Iatrogenic platelet dysfunction	Vit K antagonism

CEH, Cystic endometrial hyperplasia; *E2,* estradiol; *FB,* foreign body; *OHE,* ovariohysterectomy; *SIPS,* subinvolution of placental sites (etiology is nondegeneration of trophoblastic cells); *TCC,* transitional cell carcinoma; *Vit,* vitamin.

estrus (see Chapter 297). Cats in proestrus do not have a bloody vaginal discharge. In addition, changes in vaginal cytology are neither as useful nor as obvious in cats.

Large amounts of clear discharge are relatively acellular and most often of urinary bladder origin. Analysis of fluid to determine compatibility with urine (chemical and microscopic) is indicated, as is comparison of results with those from a voided sample or one obtained by cystocentesis. A mucoid discharge displays few cells cytologically, usually healthy appearing neutrophils. With mucopurulent to purulent discharges, neutrophil numbers are increased, often with a large number of degenerate cells. Serosanguineous to sanguinous discharges contain red blood cells with either healthy appearing neutrophils or degenerate neutrophils, indicating inflammation, unless the dog is in late proestrus or estrus. In these latter two stages, white blood cells are virtually always absent. Discharges that are greenish black or a mixture of red, green, and brown derive this coloration from red blood cell breakdown pigment and tissue particles when associated with abortion (Web Figures 36-2, 36-3, and 36-4).

Vaginal-Vulvar Examination

Once fluid has been collected, a digital vaginal examination is indicated. Examination may not be possible without sedation in juvenile small breed dogs, cats, or if pain/discomfort is present. The digital examination should be performed before vaginoscopy, because structural abnormalities can easily be "passed by" if the clinician is relying only on what is seen.

Digital examination allows evaluation of the vulva, vestibule, urethral papilla, vaginovestibular region, and possibly the caudal vagina. Normal anestrous or OHE females have narrowing at the vulvovestibular junction and also at the vaginovestibular junction (the cingulum). Abnormal findings such as circumferential strictures or vaginal septa or bands (commonly at the cingulum) or narrowing of the lumen and altered mucosal texture should be noted, as should straining

or discomfort. Digital examination may elucidate the cause of the discharge.

Vaginoscopy can be performed in many dogs without sedation. A rigid pediatric proctoscope can be used in medium to large dogs. Other instruments (e.g., a flexible or rigid endoscope) allow visualization in cats and smaller dogs. Insufflation and adequate lighting are essential. Shorter instruments with a light source can be used to examine the vestibule, clitoris, and fossa.

With the information gained from these examinations, the clinician may approach the problem with more clarity (Figure 36-1) (see Chapter 304).

Other diagnostic testing may be indicated. If the dog or cat has signs of systemic illness, a complete blood count (CBC), serum biochemistry, and complete urinalysis should be performed. If the abdomen is painful, the uterus enlarged, and/or the discharge is characterized as purulent, a pyometra should be considered and cystocentesis should be avoided to prevent entrance into or damage to the uterus and contamination of the abdomen. Bacterial culture of the discharge, preferably from the vagina and collected with a guarded or sheathed culturette to avoid contamination, is indicated for a systemically ill animal or if an infectious process is suspected. Susceptibility testing of the cultured organisms is indicated to determine the appropriate therapy. Imaging of the abdomen and urogenital system by means of plain and contrast radiology (i.e., vaginogram, vagino-urethrogram), as well as ultrasound and possibly computerized tomography, may be indicated.

Assessment of reproductive hormonal status is important when evaluating both intact and OHE females. Increased estradiol concentrations and vaginal cytology suggestive of estradiol influence (finding "superficial" vaginal epithelial cells) is consistent with normal proestrus or estrus, follicular cysts, ovarian secreting neoplasia, or ovarian remnant, although estradiol concentrations may fluctuate. Stimulation tests using human chorionic gonadotropin or gonadotropin-releasing hormone, which induce ovulation with resultant increases in

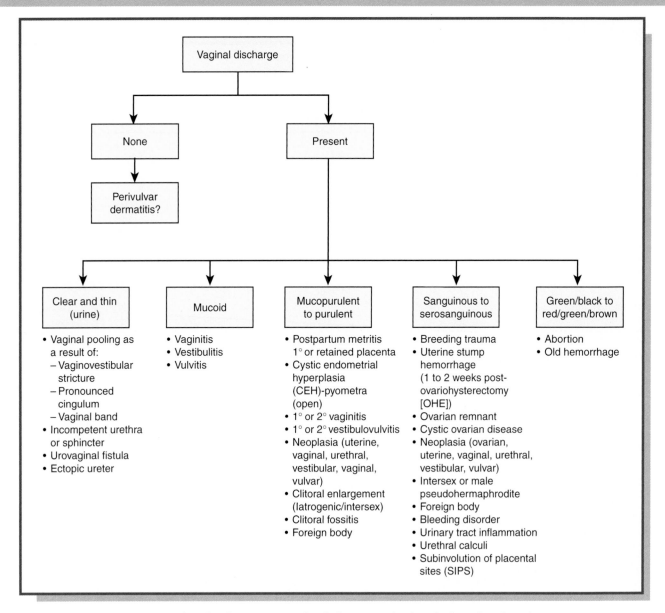

Figure 36-1 Algorithm for assessment of pathologic vaginal-vulvar discharge based on character of discharge and digital examination.

the progesterone concentration, may be diagnostic for follicular cysts or ovarian remnant (see Chapter 298). Measurement of serum progesterone for evidence of the luteal phase of the reproductive cycle may also be helpful with suspected cystic endometrial hyperplasia (CEH)/pyometra in both intact and OHE females, because the majority of females with this disorder have an elevated progesterone concentration or have received exogenous progestational therapy (see Chapter 302).

Biopsy and histology of masses found in the reproductive tract can further characterize their significance and allow prognostication. Coagulation system testing should be considered in a female with a serosanguineous to sanguineous discharge. Mucosal hemorrhage is characteristic of a primary system (platelet and vascular) defect but may also be associated with a coagulation factor abnormality. Iatrogenic, inherited, and acquired disorders should be considered.

At times no cause may be apparent for a vaginal-vulvar discharge. Common causes of chronic vaginitis include mor-

phologic abnormalities of the reproductive or urinary tract, resulting in urinary incontinence or pooling. Juvenile vaginitis, seen in the prepubertal bitch, is almost always self-limiting. Vaginitis in the queen is unusual (see Chapter 304).

PREPUTIAL DISCHARGE

Preputial discharges are composed of fluid and cells that originate from the urinary bladder, prostate gland, testes and epididymis, urethra, and mucosa of the penis and penile sheath. Discharges may be present in both intact and neutered males, and they are much more common in the dog than in the cat. Other causes that should be considered are sex hormone–induced conditions (e.g., hermaphroditism), generalized mucosal disease, or bleeding diathesis caused by disorders of blood coagulation.

Normal discharge in the male is typified as a small amount of grayish-white to yellow material that may be seen at the

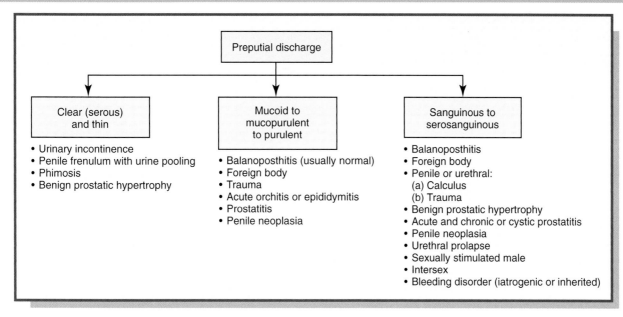

Figure 36-2 Algorithm for assessment of pathologic preputial discharge based on character of discharge and examination.

preputial orifice as moist or dried exudate. It may be difficult to determine, upon inspection of the preputial orifice and surrounding skin and haircoat, whether the volume present is normal. Careful examination of the genitalia is indicated. Abnormal discharge in the male may be investigated by means of the source of origin and the gross appearance of the discharge. Abnormal discharge may be characterized grossly as clear or serous, mucoid to mucopurulent to purulent, and sanguinous or serosanguineous (see the section Cytology, above, for the cytologic characteristics).

HISTORY

It is important to determine the age, breed, and reproductive status of the animal. It also should be ascertained whether the male has been castrated and if so, whether one or both testes were removed. Reproductive activity is of importance. The duration and historical character of the discharge should also be noted. The presence of systemic signs that precede or are associated with discharge would be expected with inflammatory or infectious disease, neoplasia, and traumatic or toxic causes.

PHYSICAL EXAMINATION

A complete physical examination should be performed, with particular attention given to the scrotum, testes (if present), and prepuce. Edema of the scrotum or enlargement or asymmetry of testicular or epididymal tissues is important. In the dog, the prostate gland can be evaluated by simultaneous abdominal and rectal palpation for size, symmetry, and pain. The size of the urinary bladder can also be evaluated by abdominal palpation. The prepuce and penis should be palpated, and the prepuce then should be retracted, caudal to

the bulbus glandis in the dog, to allow visual inspection of the entire penis. Digital and visual inspection of the preputial space (using a blunt instrument) may be indicated (Web Figures 36-5 and 36-6).

Although prepubertal neutering is not associated with preputial discharge, visual inspection of the penis may yield results that differ from intact or postpuberally neutered males. In dogs castrated prior to puberty, the penile tissue may appear less developed. In cats castrated prior to puberty, it may be more difficult to completely extrude the penis for visualization (see Chapter 300).

OTHER DIAGNOSTIC TESTING

Based on the appearance of the discharge, historical information, and physical examination findings, a list of differential diagnoses can be generated (Figure 36-2).

Further evaluation might include a CBC, serum biochemical profile, and urinalysis, as well as imaging of the testicles, prostate, or urinary bladder by means of ultrasound or radiology. Evaluation of testicular or prostatic secretions may be possible through semen collection or prostatic massage. Additional diagnostics may include bacterial culture with susceptibility determination, fine needle aspiration, or biopsy (see Chapter 314). Coagulation system testing should be considered for a male with a serosanguineous to sanguinous discharge. Mucosal hemorrhage is characteristic of a primary system defect but may also be associated with a coagulation factor abnormality; iatrogenic, inherited, and acquired disorders should be considered.

The above evaluation may well lead to a definitive diagnosis. In the absence of definite findings, the male should be reevaluated at a later date. Comparison of subsequent findings with the original data may lead to a definitive diagnosis or management plan.

CHAPTER **37**

Polyuria and Polydipsia

Edward C. Feldman

Concerns about a pet's atypical or unusual urination habits are a common reason for owners to seek veterinary assistance. For example, a dog or cat may urinate excessive volumes, urinate more frequently than "normal," appear to be incontinent, urinate for an unusually long time, no longer seem house-broken, or urinate in atypical or unacceptable locations. Some owners seek veterinary care because they think their pet is drinking too much water, but this is a less common concern than those previously mentioned.

PHYSIOLOGY OF WATER METABOLISM

Water consumption and urine production are controlled by complex interactions between plasma osmolality, fluid volume in the vascular compartment, the thirst center, the kidneys, the pituitary gland, and the hypothalamus. Dysfunction in any of these can result in apparent incontinence or polyuria (PU). Polyuria typically results in polydipsia (PD). Vasopressin (antidiuretic hormone [ADH]) plays a key role in the control of renal water resorption, urine production, urine concentration, and water balance. In the presence of ADH and dehydration, the average healthy dog or cat has the capacity to produce urine with an osmolality well above 2000 mOsm/kg. If a dog or cat is chronically deficient in ADH or is chronically unable to respond to ADH at the renal tubular level, the urine may be as dilute as 20 mOsm/kg.

Plasma osmolality and its principal determinant, the plasma sodium concentration, normally are maintained within remarkably narrow ranges. Stability is achieved through adjustment of total body water concentrations to maintain balance with the plasma sodium concentration. Water balance is controlled by an integrated system that involves precise regulation of water intake via thirst mechanisms and control of renal water loss via ADH secretion and action. Water is continuously lost through the urine, respiratory tract, and feces. Lost water is replaced by that consumed. The urine-concentrating capacity can reduce but not eliminate water loss.

ADH, a nonapeptide, is synthesized in the hypothalamus and secreted from the posterior pituitary gland. The primary sites of ADH activity are epithelial cells in the renal distal tubules and collecting ducts. Here, ADH acts to increase the hydro-osmotic permeability of these cells. The fluid in the tubular lumen normally is dilute, and the fluid in the interstitial space, through which the tubules traverse, is concentrated. Therefore, if water is allowed to diffuse passively along concentration gradients, it flows from the lumen of the nephron, in which the fluid is dilute, into the hypertonic milieu that normally exists in the interstitial space of the renal medulla. If ADH is present, the volume of fluid in the nephron decreases, the osmolality of that fluid increases, and water is conserved. Thus the "normal" animal has the capacity to secrete ADH in response to appropriate stimuli such as increasing plasma osmolality or decreasing plasma volume, both of which follow dehydration. Secretion of ADH and the ability to respond to ADH at the level of the renal tubules and collecting ducts allow the body to conserve water. In the absence of ADH (central diabetes insipidus) or if renal tubular cells are resistant to the action of ADH (nephrogenic diabetes insipidus), the cells lining this portion of the nephron are resistant to diffusion of both water and solutes. Hence, the hypotonic filtrate formed in the more proximal portion of the nephron passes unmodified through the distal tubule and collecting duct. This water diuresis is associated with large volumes of urine that has a low osmolality.

It should be noted that 85% to 90% of the fluid filtered by the glomerulus is reabsorbed isosmotically with sodium and glucose in the proximal portion of the nephron. Sodium then is selectively reabsorbed from the remaining fluid, making the fluid in the distal nephron hypotonic. However, if a poorly reabsorbed solute, such as urea or glucose, is present in excess in the glomerular filtrate, fluid resorption from the proximal tubule is impaired. Because of this physiologic process, an abnormally increased volume of fluid reaches the distal nephron and can overwhelm its capacity to reabsorb water. Consequently, urine volume increases despite the presence of ADH. This type of polyuria is called *solute diuresis*.

DIAGNOSTIC APPROACH TO POLYURIA, POLYDIPSIA, AND OTHER ABNORMALITIES IN URINATION

The First Step: Collecting the Urine

It may be difficult to distinguish "inappropriate" urination (frequency with or without straining or hematuria) from polyuria at the time an owner phones the hospital to make an appointment. Therefore, it is strongly recommended that all cat and dog owners with any "chief complaint" that could be associated with polyuria be encouraged to catch a urine sample from their pet (Figure 37-1).

That urine (even if only a few drops) should be collected in a clean container with a lid and brought with the pet at the time of initial evaluation. Owners of medium- to large-breed male dogs rarely have difficulty collecting urine. Owners of female dogs rarely have difficulty if they utilize a relatively flat container. In both situations, they should approach their pet slowly and discreetly. Owners of small dogs, especially female dogs, may find success in collecting urine if the container lid is used for collection. Owners of cats can try placing plastic wrap on top of their cats' litter and collecting urine after the cat uses the litter box. Alternatively, owners can replace absorbable litter with nonabsorbable litter (using any type of gravel, such as that used in an aquarium). In this situation, the urine can simply be poured into a container. The easiest method for cat owners to collect urine is simply to remove almost all litter from a litter box. Most cats will still use the box, but since there is insufficient litter to absorb the urine it can be poured into a container.

The Next Step: Evaluating the Urine

When the owner arrives at the veterinary hospital, the urine they collected can be evaluated prior to the pet being exam-

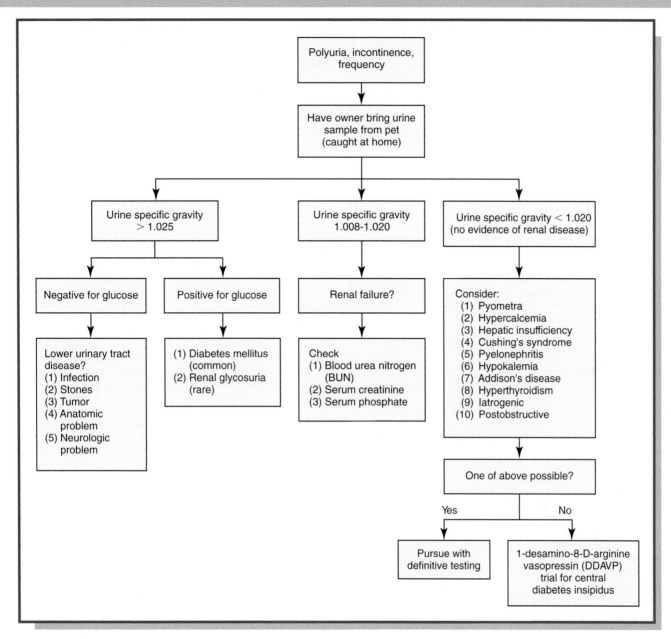

Figure 37-1 Algorithm for polyuria, incontinence, and frequency.

ined. The urine specific gravity should be noted and a "dip stick" test completed. Urine is usually considered normally "concentrated" if the specific gravity is >1.025. Since the owner has collected the urine sample from the pet while that animal was in its home environment, problems in interpretation associated with water being withheld prior to an automobile trip or a pet not consuming typical amounts of water due to nervousness or fear are not encountered. The truly polyuric dog or cat will almost always have dilute urine (specific gravity <1.012), "relatively" dilute urine (specific gravity >1.012 but <1.022), or it will have glucose in the urine.

Concentrated Urine without Glucose

If the urine bought to the hospital by the owners is concentrated (specific gravity >1.025) and it has no glucose, it is likely that the animal has a lower urinary tract condition. In this situation the veterinarian must consider the possibility of urinary tract infection, bladder calculi, bladder mass, anatomic abnormality, neurologic problems, or behavior issues that may explain the owner's observations. Appropriate testing for these conditions (culture, abdominal imaging, etc.) can be recommended if the history and physical examination support such an approach.

Concentrated Urine with Glucose

Most dogs and cats with diabetes mellitus are first examined after an owner has observed polyuria. These animals frequently also have polydipsia, polyphagia, and weight loss. Less commonly, a diabetic dog is brought in for veterinary examination after an owner notes that it has become acutely blind due to cataract formation. A dog or cat also may be brought in for treatment of vomiting, diarrhea, anorexia, listlessness, or other systemic signs secondary to developing diabetic ketoacidosis. Regardless, almost all diabetic dogs and cats have a urine specific gravity of 1.025 to 1.045 and glycosuria. The diagnosis of diabetes mellitus should be strongly suspected simply by noting a positive reaction in the glucose reagent portion of the urine test strip within seconds of removing the strip from the urine. Thus diabetes mellitus can be tentatively diagnosed in dogs and cats before the pet is ever examined by the veterinarian. A diagnosis of diabetes mellitus should always be confirmed by assessing the blood glucose for hyperglycemia (see Chapters 290 and 291).

Rarely, a dog or cat with glycosuria has a blood glucose concentration within reference limits. In this situation, the veterinarian should consider the possibility of renal glycosuria. Renal glycosuria is rare and is the result of a renal tubular defect. Renal glycosuria can be congenital in Basenji and Norwegian Elkhound breeds, but it can occur in any dog or cat (see Chapter 316). In cats, stress may cause glycosuria secondary to stress-induced hyperglycemia, although most cats with stress-induced hyperglycemia do not have glycosuria because the blood glucose never exceeds renal threshold. This concern should be minimized by collecting the urine at home.

Isosthenuric Urine (Urine Specific Gravity of 1.008 to 1.012): Chronic Renal Failure

The term *isosthenuria* usually implies that the urine specific gravity or osmolality is the same as that of serum or plasma. Using this criterion, urine with a specific gravity of 1.008 to 1.012 is isosthenuric. However, for clinical purposes, it is important to remember that a dehydrated animal has a plasma osmolality greater than normal due to loss of water and abnormal retention of solutes (e.g., urea). In this setting, a urine specific gravity as high as 1.020 may be "isosthenuric" despite being greater than the classic 1.008 to 1.012. In other words, what happens if a cat or dog is examined and is thought to be 3% to 10% dehydrated? If the animal has a normal hypothalamus, pituitary, and kidneys, it should have responded to this degree of water loss by secreting maximum amounts of ADH (it has been demonstrated repeatedly that a 3% to 5% decrease in body weight due to water loss is associated with this response). The urine of such an animal, therefore, should reflect maximum release of ADH, and the specific gravity should be well in excess of 1.035. If the dog or cat has a urine specific gravity of 1.018, for example, it should not be considered to have responded appropriately to dehydration.

The primary concern a veterinarian should have when an animal has polyuria and a urine specific gravity within the isosthenuric range is renal insufficiency or failure. In chronic renal failure, a compensatory increase in glomerular filtration rate by surviving nephrons occurs, and a commensurate increase in fluid volume is presented to the distal renal tubules. The increase in the tubular flow rate causes less urea and sodium to be reabsorbed. The result is an osmotic diuresis, which may be exaggerated by a reduction in the renal medullary concentration gradient. A serum chemistry evaluation (BUN and creatinine) should be the first step in determining the presence or absence of renal disease as a cause of polyuria (see Chapter 311).

Urine Specific Gravity <1.020: Pyometra

Any ill female dog or cat should be considered a candidate for having pyometra until proven otherwise. This is appropriate because dogs or cats with a uterine infection can quickly deteriorate secondary to overwhelming sepsis. Dogs and cats that may have pyometra typically have a history of being in estrus 2 to 10 weeks previously, and most have a purulent vaginal discharge. For any animal in which pyometra is suspected, a complete blood count (CBC) should be assessed for evidence of systemic infection and abdominal imaging (radiographs or ultrasound scans) should be obtained and examined for uterine enlargement. Dogs and cats with pyometra may develop polyuria and dilute urine because of the effects of endotoxin from *Escherichia coli*, the bacteria most commonly associated with pyometra. Because this endotoxin interferes with the action of ADH at the level of the renal tubules, these animals have a reversible form of nephrogenic diabetes insipidus (see Chapter 285).

Urine Specific Gravity <1.020: Hypercalcemia

Hypercalcemia has several common causes. Some, but not all, of the conditions associated with hypercalcemia are lymphosarcoma, chronic renal failure, hypoadrenocorticism, primary hyperparathyroidism, vitamin D toxicosis, granulomatous disease (histoplasmosis, blastomycosis), multiple myeloma, apocrine gland carcinomas of the anal sac and other cancers. Therefore, if a dog or cat has a urine specific gravity of less than 1.020, one should assess the serum calcium concentration. If the serum calcium concentration is abnormally increased, tests needed to rule in or rule out the various causes of hypercalcemia can be considered. An increased serum calcium concentration may interfere with the action of ADH at the renal tubular level, causing a reversible form of acquired nephrogenic diabetes insipidus. Other explanations for polyuria in hypercalcemic animals include damage to ADH receptors in the renal tubules, inactivation of adenyl cyclase, or decreased transport of sodium and chloride into the renal medullary interstitium (see Chapter 286).

Urine Specific Gravity <1.020: Hepatic Insufficiency

Although not common, some dogs with significant hepatic insufficiency have an inability to concentrate urine. Clues to the presence of liver insufficiency include a decrease in one or more of the following "liver function" test results on a routine serum biochemical profile: albumin, BUN, cholesterol, or glucose. In addition, an afflicted dog may have microhepatica or a liver that appears otherwise abnormal on radiography or ultrasonography. Dogs with some or many of these abnormalities could be further assessed with preprandial and postprandial bile acids, a radio-labeled liver scan, or hepatic biopsy. Although not well understood, one plausible explanation for dilute urine in animals with liver insufficiency is loss of renal medullary hypertonicity secondary to impaired BUN production. BUN is an important component of the renal medullary concentration gradient. Decreases in this gradient result in polyuria with compensatory polydipsia (see Chapter 274). Another potential contributor to dilute urine is impaired metabolism of cortisol and subsequent cortisol excess (Cushing's syndrome: see below).

Urine Specific Gravity <1.020: Canine Cushing's Syndrome

Polyuria is an extremely common clinical sign in dogs with Cushing's syndrome (CCS) (excess cortisol concentrations do not commonly cause polyuria in cats). The urine specific gravity in at least 85% of dogs with iatrogenic or naturally occurring CCS is less than 1.020 and can be as low as 1.001. The cause of this polyuria remains obscure, although most of these dogs appear to have secondary and reversible ADH deficiency (central diabetes insipidus). Dogs with CCS typically have additional clinical signs, such as polydipsia, polyphagia, panting, muscle weakness, alopecia, pot belly, and thin skin. Routine laboratory abnormalities commonly include increases in serum alkaline phosphatase and alanine aminotransferase activities, increased serum cholesterol concentration, and a decreased or low-normal BUN. Confirmation requires appropriate pituitary-adrenocortical function tests (see Chapters 292 and 293).

Urine Specific Gravity <1.020: Pyelonephritis

Infection and inflammation of the renal pelvis can adversely affect the countercurrent mechanism in the renal medulla. This results in isosthenuria, polyuria, secondary polydipsia and, eventually, renal failure. A dog or cat with bacterial pyelonephritis may have nonspecific signs of lethargy, anorexia, and fever. Neutrophilic leukocytosis may be noted on the CBC. Urinalysis may reveal white blood cells, casts, bacteria, and red cells. Recurrent urinary tract infection may increase suspicion of pyelonephritis. Urine cultures should be performed on cystocentesis samples, but these may or may not be positive for bacteria. Confirmation of this diagnosis usually requires imaging of the kidneys (see Chapter 313).

Urine Specific Gravity <1.020: Hypokalemia

Hypokalemia is thought to interfere with the action of ADH in the renal tubules, creating a reversible form of nephrogenic diabetes insipidus. This electrolyte disturbance is more common in cats than in dogs, more commonly causes muscle weakness than polyuria, and usually occurs secondary to other disorders (see Chapter 311).

Urine Specific Gravity <1.020: Hypoadrenocorticism (Addison's Disease)

Most dogs with Addison's disease are young to middle-aged females. Despite normal kidney function and severe hypovolemia, animals in an Addisonian crisis frequently have a urine specific gravity of less than 1.030 due to the hyponatremia caused by mineralocorticoid deficiency. Hyponatremia reduces the renal medullary concentration gradient, impairing the ability to produce concentrated urine. Although "relatively" dilute urine is typical of a dog or cat with hypoadrenocorticism, related signs are overshadowed by the more worrisome and obvious signs of weakness, listlessness, vomiting, diarrhea, anorexia, and weight loss. The combination of signalment and findings of hyperkalemia and hyponatremia should raise suspicion of Addison's disease (see Chapter 294).

Urine Specific Gravity <1.020: Hyperthyroidism

Polyuria and polydipsia are common in hyperthyroid cats and dogs. Although the exact mechanism of the polyuria is unclear, it is likely that increases in renal blood flow cause a decrease in renal medullary concentration. This impairs water resorption from the distal nephron. Concurrent renal insufficiency may also contribute to these signs. The tentative diagnosis of hyperthyroidism is based on palpation of a thyroid nodule or mass, and confirmation requires a finding of abnormally increased serum total or free thyroxine concentration (see Chapter 288).

Urine Specific Gravity <1.020: Iatrogenic

Several drugs may cause polydipsia and polyuria, including some that are commonly used, such as glucocorticoids, diuretics, and anticonvulsants.

Urine Specific Gravity <1.020: Postobstructive Diuresis

Postobstructive diuresis is most often encountered after a urethral obstruction has been relieved in cats, but it may occur in dogs. These animals often show dramatic increases in BUN secondary to the obstruction, which accounts for a marked osmotic diuresis after the obstruction has been relieved.

CENTRAL DIABETES INSIPIDUS (CDI), NEPHROGENIC DIABETES INSIPIDUS (NDI), AND PSYCHOGENIC (PRIMARY) POLYDIPSIA (PP)

It should be emphasized that CDI, NDI, and PP are quite uncommon. Most causes of polydipsia and polyuria can be identified from the signalment, history, physical examination, urinalysis (especially if the urine is caught by the owner before leaving the home environment), CBC, and serum biochemistry profile. Primary nephrogenic diabetes insipidus (NDI) is an extremely rare condition. However, *secondary* and often reversible NDI accounts for the polyuria in many of the conditions previously discussed. If an animal has dilute urine and does not appear to have any of the previously discussed conditions, it would be fair to assume that the animal does not have primary or secondary NDI. The dog or cat is more likely to have CDI or PP.

The veterinarian then can ask the following question: Does this animal drink a lot because it urinates a lot (CDI), or does it urinate a lot because it drinks a lot (PP)? If CDI is present, the serum osmolality should be high-normal or increased. If PP is present, the serum osmolality should be low-normal or decreased. Thus the serum osmolality becomes a reasonable, cost-effective, and simple test to run. Because the veterinarian has reached a point where it is likely that one of these two conditions may exist and because CDI is much more common than PP, trial therapy at home is recommended using oral DDAVP (synthetic ADH, which is commercially available as 0.1- or 0.2-mg tablets). The dose is empirical. It is recommended that a 20-kg dog be given 0.1 mg three times a day for about 7 days and that a 40-kg dog be given 0.2 mg three times a day for about 7 days. The dosage for dogs and cats weighing more or less than this can be so adjusted. The response in dogs or cats with CDI is quick and obvious (certainly less than 7 days). Owners can collect urine on a daily basis during the trial to substantiate their clinical impressions regarding response. If the pet responds, CDI is likely while Cushing's syndrome remains a possibility. The dose of DDAVP can be slowly tapered to determine the minimum required for long-term treatment. The use of synthetic ADH in the form of nasal drops placed in the eyes is more cumbersome than tablet administration. However, some dogs and cats demonstrate a better response to the eye drops than to oral medication.

The author considers a water deprivation test to be far more dangerous than warranted for the information derived. Remember, the first goal in a water deprivation test is to dehydrate a dog or cat to the point of 3% to 5% loss in body weight. If the test is carried out too long, the dehydration can quickly become life threatening. Additionally, since there are no consistent or reliable treatments for NDI or for PP, benign trial therapy can also serve as a diagnostic tool. Animals that do respond to ADH therapy most likely have hyperadrenocorticism or CDI. Those that don't are more likely to have hyperadrenocorticism (some dogs with Cushing's syndrome respond to ADH therapy and some do not), secondary NDI, or PP. At no point is a water deprivation test warranted.

CHAPTER 38

Micturition Disorders and Urinary Incontinence

Mary Anna Labato
Mark J. Acierno

Micturition is a two-stage process involving the passive storage and the active voiding of urine. Conditions that interfere with these stages are termed *micturition disorders* and are often divided into neurogenic and nonneurogenic based on their underlying causes. Neurogenic disorders are further categorized as lower motor neuron disorders (atonic bladder with overflow incontinence), upper motor neuron disorders (automatic bladder), detrusor-urethral dyssynergia, and dysautonomia. Nonneurogenic disorders, typically mechanical obstructions, include such processes as infection, inflammation, calculi, and neoplasia.

Incontinence is defined as an involuntary escape of urine during the storage phase of the urinary cycle. This can appear clinically in a variety of ways; however, the most common presentation is intermittent or continuous dribbling of urine combined with episodes of normal voiding. Causes of incontinence include urethral sphincter incompetence, an anatomic abnormality in the termination of the urethra, inability of the bladder to expand in capacity, spasms of the bladder, and nerve damage.[1-3]

ANATOMY AND PHYSIOLOGY OF THE URINARY BLADDER

The body of the bladder is composed of the detrusor smooth muscle. The outlet conduit consists of the trigone and proximal urethra. The smooth muscle fibers of the detrusor continue into the proximal urethra, forming a functional internal urethral sphincter. The distal urethra is composed of skeletal muscle functioning as an external sphincter. During the storage phase of micturition, the bladder functions as a low-resistance, high-capacity vessel and the urethra as a high-resistance barrier. During the voiding phase, the bladder acts as a muscular pump and the urethra as a low-resistance vessel.

CONTROL OF MICTURITION

Functional control of the bladder and urethra is attained through a combination of autonomic and somatic interactions (Web Figure 38-1).

Sympathetic innervation regulates the filling phase of micturition and is supplied via the hypogastric nerve, composed of preganglionic fibers exiting the lumbar spinal cord (L1 to L4 in dogs and L2 to L5 in cats) and synapsing in the caudal mesenteric ganglion. Alpha-adrenergic fibers synapse in smooth muscles in both the trigone and proximal urethra and stimulation results in contraction of these muscles forming a functional internal urethral sphincter. Beta-adrenergic fibers synapse in the detrusor muscle; stimulation results in bladder relaxation. Sensory receptors embedded in the bladder wall relay stretch information via the pelvic nerve to the spinal cord. The information is relayed to the brainstem, where it is

integrated with information from the forebrain. Assuming that it is an appropriate time to void, the impulse to empty the bladder is carried down the spinal cord. Parasympathetic innervation dominates the emptying phase of micturition and is derived from the pelvic nerve (sacral spinal cord segments S1 to S3). Stimulation results in bladder contraction. Somatic innervation, supplied via the pudendal nerve, arises from sacral spinal cord segments S1 to S3 and provides stimulation to the striated urethral musculature.

MICTURITION DISORDERS (Figure 38-1)

Neurogenic Causes

Lower Motor Neuron Disorder (Detrusor Areflexia with Sphincter Areflexia)   Lower motor neuron disorders result from lesions involving the sacral spinal cord segments or pelvic nerve, including intervertebral disk disease, cauda equina syndrome, sacroiliac luxations, sacrococcygeal fracture/separation, and tumors (e.g., spinal lymphoma). The bladder typically is large, distended, easily expressed. The incontinence is continuous (overflow incontinence), and a loss of perineal, bulbospongiosus, and detrusor reflexes is noted.

Upper Motor Neuron Disorder (Detrusor Areflexia with Sphincter Hypertonus)   Upper motor neuron disorders result from a lesion involving the spinal cord above the sacral spinal cord segments, such as intervertebral disk disease, tumor, or trauma. This disorder causes incomplete reflex detrusor contraction and spasticity of the urethral sphincter, resulting in incomplete bladder emptying. The bladder is large, turgid, and initially extremely difficult to express. The animal has a history of inability to urinate, and concomitant hindquarter paresis or paralysis frequently is seen.

Detrusor-Urethral Dyssynergia   In detrusor-urethral dyssynergia, initiation of the detrusor reflex is followed by involuntary contraction of the urethral sphincter. The term *detrusor-urethral dyssynergia* refers to involuntary contraction of the external urethral sphincter in the distal urethra (detrusor-striated sphincter dyssynergia) or contraction of smooth muscle in the bladder neck and proximal urethra (detrusor-smooth sphincter dyssynergia) during detrusor contraction. The condition is caused by lesions (masses, degeneration) in the reticulospinal tract. Increased sympathetic activity of both the smooth and striated urethral musculatures may arise from a lesion cranial to or involving the caudal mesenteric ganglion.

Dysautonomia   Dysautonomia is a result of dysfunction of the autonomous nervous system. The cause is unknown. It is a rare disease seen mostly in cats in Great Britain, but it has been recognized in dogs and cats worldwide. Clinical signs are acute and involve many autonomic abnormalities (mydriasis,

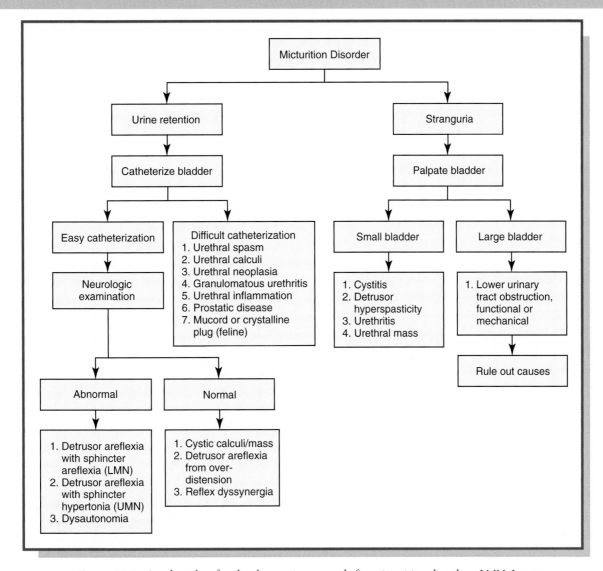

Figure 38-1 An algorithm for the diagnostic approach for micturition disorders. *LMN,* Lower motor neuron; *UMN,* upper motor neuron.

Table • 38-1

Differential Diagnoses for Urinary Incontinence

LARGE BLADDER	SMALL BLADDER
Overflow incontinence	Urethral sphincter mechanism incontinence
Lower motor neuron bladder (detrusor atony)	Detrusor hyperspasticity
Upper motor neuron bladder (automatic bladder)	Ectopic ureter(s)

prolapsed third eyelids, constipation). Urine dribbling and dysuria often are presenting clinical signs due to an atonic bladder.

Nonneurogenic Causes of Micturition Disorders

Nonneurogenic disorders typically involve mechanical obstructions and include such processes as infection, inflammation, calculi, and neoplasia.

Detrusor Atony from Overdistention or Overflow Incontinence This condition results from a mechanical or functional outflow obstruction that causes the tight junctions of the detrusor muscle to separate. Subsequent contractions of the detrusor muscle are weak and ineffectual. Functional outflow obstruction may have a neurogenic component that is usually the result of excessive sympathetic stimulation to the urethra. Common examples of mechanical obstruction are urethral obstruction (especially in cats from mucoid or crystalline plugs), urethral calculi, neoplasia of the trigone or urethra, severe urethritis, urethral stricture, and prostatic disease. As a result of a functional or mechanical obstruction, urine volume increases until the intravesicular pressure overcomes urethral resistance resulting in urine dribbling. Typically, the animal has a history of urine outflow obstruction followed by urinary incontinence. Abdominal palpation reveals a large, flaccid bladder. Neurologic examination reveals intact perineal and bulbospongiosus reflexes, yet the detrusor reflex is weak or absent. There is a large residual urine volume. Urodynamic studies such as the cystometrogram and urethral pressure profile may aid in diagnosis.

Urinary Incontinence (Table 38-1)
Neurogenic causes (Figure 38-2) In dogs incontinence is rarely the sole neurologic abnormality (see above, under

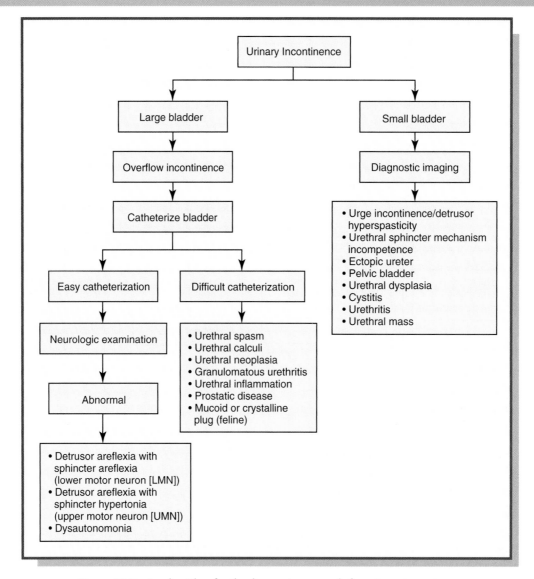

Figure 38-2 An algorithm for the diagnostic approach for urinary incontinence.

neurogenic micturition disorders) detected on physical examination. Treatment of the incontinence and prognosis for resolution or clinical control depend primarily on the underlying cause.[4]

Nonneurogenic Causes

Urethral sphincter mechanism incompetence (USMI) USMI is the most common nonneurogenic cause of incontinence in dogs. This is most often seen in medium to large breed middle-aged neutered female dogs and is often referred to as "spay incontinence." It has also been diagnosed in relatively young pets and may even present as a congenital abnormality. Incontinence is typically intermittent, especially when the dog is at rest or asleep. The volume of urine lost may be small drops or large puddles. There are several structural and physiologic factors that may play a role in the development of this condition. These include aging and relative lack of estrogen, which may affect the collagenous support structures of the urogenital region as well as decrease the availability and/or responsiveness of alpha receptors. Abnormal positioning or morphology of the bladder or urethra can contribute to functional failure (pelvic bladder, urethral dysplasia, overriding urethra). Obesity or vaginal structural abnormalities can contribute to development of clinical signs. Breed predispositions suggest underlying genetic factors.

Hormone-responsive incontinence is one of the most frequently diagnosed disorders. It is a disorder of older spayed female dogs (mean age of occurrence is 8 years); however, it has been documented in animals as young as 8 to 9 months. It is seen primarily in spayed female dogs, predisposed because of decreased sex hormones believed to contribute to normal urethral muscle tone. Hormone-responsive incontinence has been reported infrequently in neutered male dogs and female cats. Urethral incompetence is the most common nonhormonal cause of urinary incontinence in small animals. The cause is thought to be urethral smooth muscle incompetence or urethral malposition (Web Figure 38-2).[5]

Incontinence is typically intermittent especially when the dog is at rest or asleep. The volume of urine lost may be small drops or large puddles.

Detrusor hyperspasticity (instability, urge incontinence) Detrusor hyperspasticity is characterized by involuntary bladder contractions resulting in the frequent voiding of small volumes of urine. Hyperspasticity secondary to infection, neoplasia, or uroliths is called *urge incontinence* while cases in which no underlying cause is determined are referred to as *idiopathic detrusor instability*.[5] The syndrome is commonly seen in cats with cystitis or "idiopathic feline lower urinary tract disorders."

Ectopic ureter(s)   Ectopic ureter (EU) and other congenital urethral malformations are a common cause of urinary incontinence. The abnormal entry of the ureter(s) into the distal urethra or vagina from a congenital malformation results in continuous or intermittent dribbling of urine

HISTORY AND DIAGNOSIS

When an animal is examined for a urine retention or urinary incontinence problem, it is of utmost importance to obtain a complete history, including reproductive status; age at neutering; age at the onset of the problem; previous medical problems, especially those involving the urogenital system; previous history of trauma; medications being given; and an accurate description of the abnormality (see Figure 38-2).

If the animal is having difficulty urinating, two other questions are important: How frequent is urination? Is there stranguria, and if so, is any urine being passed? If there is incontinence, is it continuous or intermittent? Is the animal aware of the incontinence? Does it occur only at rest/asleep or while the animal is awake and moving?

A complete physical and neurologic examination should be performed, with particular attention paid to the urogenital system. The bladder should be palpated carefully before and immediately after voiding to evaluate the extent of distension, tone, and the ease with which the bladder may be expressed manually. Lower motor neuron lesions generally are associated with easy manual expression and reduced sphincter tone. Upper motor neuron lesions generally are associated with difficult manual expression and increased sphincter tone. In the neurologic examination, the innervation of the urogenital system should be evaluated. The perineal reflex evaluates the pudendal nerve. The bulbospongiosus reflex evaluates the integrity of both the pudendal nerve and the sacral spinal segments

A rectal examination should be done to evaluate the prostate gland, pelvic diaphragm, and anal tone. Observe the animal urinating to verify the micturition abnormality. The residual urine volume should be measured. The animal is allowed to void until urine is no longer passed, the bladder is catheterized, and the volume of any remaining urine is measured. In a normal animal, the residual volume should not exceed 0.4 mL/kg. Catheterization of the bladder also assesses the patency of the urethra.

A minimum data base should include a complete blood count (CBC), serum biochemical profile, and urinalysis with culture. In most cases the CBC and chemistry profile are within normal limits, unless a postrenal azotemia has developed from an obstructive process. The urinalysis may reflect evidence of infection, inflammation, and/or neoplasia. Survey and specialized radiographic studies may be useful. Survey radiographs should be checked for any obvious abnormalities in the bladder, urethra, pelvis, or spine. Contrast radiographic studies (intravenous urography, urethrocystography, vaginourethrography) should be evaluated for bladder wall thickening, calculi, prostatic enlargement, urethral strictures, and skeletal abnormalities in the pelvis. An abdominal ultrasound examination may be useful for evaluating bladder wall thickness, examining the prostate, evaluating sublumbar lymph nodes, and ruling out calculi or tumors. A myelogram or magnetic resonance imaging may be indicated to evaluate for spinal cord compression, as with cauda equina syndrome, or intervertebral disk disease.

In patients with a compatible history, the diagnosis of EU has traditionally been confirmed by performing specialized radiographic examinations. Studies now suggest that these methods can correctly identify only 70% to 78.2% of ectopic ureters. Use of rigid cystoscopy has been shown to correctly identify 100% of ectopic ureters while helical computed tomography (CT) is capable of identifying 91% of cases. These newer modalities are the preferred method of diagnosis.

Urodynamic studies used to evaluate micturition disorders routinely consist of a cystometrogram and urethral pressure profile; electromyography also may be a part of the study. The cystometrogram is a pressure-volume recording that measures bladder volume, threshold volume and pressure, maximum contraction pressure, and the detrusor reflex. The urethral pressure profile measures intraurethral tone and identifies and localizes areas of increased or decreased resistance. Electromyography can evaluate coordination of muscular activity between the detrusor and the urethral sphincter.

TREATMENT (Web Table 38-1)

Lower Motor Neuron Bladder
Treatment involves manual expression of the bladder three or four times daily. In the absence of a correctable lesion, long-term therapy is often unrewarding. Complications include urine scalding and recurrent urinary tract infections. Bethanechol, a parasympathomimetic, may be administered in an attempt to increase detrusor contractions.

Upper Motor Neuron Bladder
Voluntary control is lost, and manual expression is difficult if not impossible. In the absence of a correctable lesion, the spinal reflexes resume in days to weeks and involuntary micturition is initiated when the threshold capacity of the bladder is reached (automatic bladder). Initially it is difficult to express the bladder manually. Baclofen, a skeletal muscle relaxant, decreases muscle tone by exerting a depressive effect on the central nervous system. It inhibits medullary interneurons and spinal reflexes, and it decreases spasticity by reducing the activity of gamma efferent neurons. Because of the risk of bladder rupture, the patient should be catheterized aseptically at least three times daily to empty the bladder completely. An indwelling catheter should not be used because of the risk of urinary tract infection. Frequent urinalyses with culture and sensitivity should be performed. Concurrent administration of antibacterial agents may be indicated, especially with long-term intermittent catheterization.

Detrusor-Urethral Dyssynergia
Treatment involves decreasing sympathetic tone or the use of muscle relaxants (see Web Table 38-1). Alpha-adrenergic blocking agents (e.g., phenoxybenzamine, prazosin, and terazosin) can be used to decrease internal sphincter resistance. In addition to its alpha-1 antagonism in urethral smooth muscle, prazosin can cause a centrally mediated decrease in somatic input to the external urethral sphincter. Skeletal muscle relaxants (e.g., baclofen, diazepam, and dantrolene) can be used to decrease external sphincter resistance.

Dysautonomia
Treatment options include administration of bethanechol and frequent bladder emptying by means of catheterization or manual expression.

Urinary Incontinence/Urethral Incompetence
Alpha-adrenergic agonists are the preferred treatment for USMI. Phenylpropanolamine, a nonselective adrenergic agonist, is commonly used to treat this condition. Total reso-

lution of incontinence can be expected in more than 85% of cases. Side effects include hypertension, restlessness, irritability, tachycardia, increased intraocular pressure, and hepatic glycogenolysis. Use of this drug is contraindicated in pets with hypertension, diabetes mellitus, or glaucoma. Diethylstilbestrol (DES) is a synthetic estrogen that has been successfully used to treat USMI. Potential side effects include bone marrow suspension, alopecia, behavior change, and signs consistent with estrus; however, most dogs tolerate the medication well. Testosterone cypionate or methytestosterone may be used in male dogs. Minimal side effects have been noted except for prostatic enlargement. In some instances, animals develop a tolerance for hormonal replacement. Additional therapy with a sympathetic alpha agonist that increases urethral tone is then indicated.[6] The most successful drugs are the sympathomimetic alpha-adrenergic agonists, which directly increase urethral smooth muscle tone. The drug of choice is phenylpropanolamine; an alternate drug is ephedrine or pseudoephrine.[7] Imipramine is a tricyclic antidepressant agent that causes inhibition of norepinephrine reuptake at the synaptic level and results in increased urethral tone. Historically, cases of USMI that were nonresponsive to pharmacologic management have been treated with a variety of surgical approaches such as a colposuspension and urethral imbrication.[8] Recently, studies have shown that endoscopic injection of glutaraldehyde cross-linked collagen or extracellular matrix (ACell Vet, Columbia, Md.) into the urethral submucosa can provide significant relief from incontinence.[9] Sixty-eight percent of dogs treated with this method attained full urinary continence after the procedure while an additional 25% experienced a significant improvement. The primary limitation of this procedure seems to be its temporary nature as many dogs return to incontinence over time.

Urge Incontinence (Detrusor Hyperreflexia)

Direct-acting smooth muscle relaxants such as flavoxate are promising in the treatment of this syndrome. These drugs also have a mild anticholinergic effect. Start with the lowest possible dosage and slowly increase until signs are alleviated or side effects are encountered.[10] Other recommended drugs include oxybutynin, dicyclomine, and propantheline bromide.[11-14]

Ectopic Ureter(s)

The surgical transposition of the ureter(s) to the trigonal area has historically been the treatment of choice. For reasons that are not entirely clear, pets with ectopic ureter often have postsurgical urethral incompetence. The urethral pressure profile can be helpful in predicting which dogs will be continent, continent with medication (alpha-adrenergic agonists), and incontinent following surgery. Hydronephrosis is also a relatively common presurgical finding in EU pets. Therefore, presurgical abdominal ultrasound should be used to evaluate the architecture of the kidney.

Recently, endoscopic guided laser ablation has been utilized to treat ectopic ureters. Dogs with ectopic ureters that transverse intramurally (95% of all cases) are candidates for this minimally invasive procedure. The procedure may be performed on an outpatient basis at the time of cystoscopic ectopic ureter diagnosis, avoiding the need for more than one anesthetic procedure for fixation.[15]

OUTCOME

The prognosis for return to normal function depends on the underlying cause of the micturition disorder. The prognosis is good for acute mechanical obstruction associated with resolving obstructive or irritative disease, acute reversible neurologic lesions, and detrusor atony from overdistention. The prognosis is less favorable for chronic detrusor atony or idiopathic functional obstructive disorders. A complete return to normal voiding may not occur, and long-term treatment may be necessary.

REFERENCES

The reference list can be found on the companion Expert Consult Web site at *www.expertconsult.com*.

CHAPTER 39

Hematuria and Other Conditions Causing Discolored Urine

Joseph W. Bartges

NORMAL URINE

Normal urine is typically transparent and yellow or amber upon visual inspection. Two pigments are primarily responsible for the yellow coloration: urochrome and urobilin. Urochrome is a sulfur-containing oxidation product of the colorless urochromogen. Urobilin is a degradation product of hemoglobin. Because the 24-hour urinary excretion of urochrome is relatively constant, highly concentrated urine will be amber in color, whereas dilute urine may be transparent or light yellow in color. The intensity of the color is in part related to the volume of urine collected and in part related to the concentration of urine produced; therefore, it should be interpreted in the context of the urine specific gravity. Caution must be used not to overinterpret the significance of urine color as part of a complete urinalysis. Significant disease may exist when urine is normal in color. Abnormal urine color may be caused by presence of several endogenous or exogenous pigments. Although abnormal urine color usually indicates a problem, it provides relatively nonspecific information. Causes of abnormal urine color should initially be investigated by examining urine sediment and then with appropriate laboratory tests. Detection of abnormal urine color should prompt questions related to diet, medications being given to the pet, environment, and collection technique. Knowledge of urine color may also be important in interpreting colorimetric test results because it may induce interference with the test.

DISCOLORED URINE

Urine color that is anything other than yellow or amber is abnormal. There are many potential causes of discolored urine (Table 39-1).

The most common abnormal urine color in dogs and cats is red, brown, or black, which may be caused by hematuria,

hemoglobinuria, myoglobinuria, and bilirubinuria (Figure 39-1).

Pale Yellow Urine

Urine that is pale yellow or clear in appearance may be normal or may be indicative of a polyuric state. Urine may be appropriately dilute if it is associated with recent consumption or administration of fluids, consumption of a diet containing low quantities of protein or high quantities of sodium chloride, glucocorticoid excess, or administration of diuretics. Urine would be considered to be inappropriately concentrated if it were dilute in the presence of dehydration. Diseases that may be associated with persistently dilute urine include diabetes insipidus, hyperadrenocorticism, hypoadrenocorticism,

Table • 39-1

Potential Causes of Discolored Urine

URINE COLOR	CAUSES	URINE COLOR	CAUSES
Yellow or amber	Urochromes Urobilin	Yellow-brown or green-brown	Bile pigments
Deep yellow	Highly concentrated urine Quinacrine* Nitrofurantoin* Phenacetin* Riboflavin (large quantities)* Phenolsulfonphthalein (acidic urine)*	Brown to black (brown or red-brown when viewed in bright light in thin layer)	Melanin Methemoglobin Myoglobin Bile pigments Thymol* Phenolic compounds* Nitrofurantoin* Nitrites* Naphthalene* Chlorinated hydrocarbons* Aniline dyes* Homogentisic acid*
Blue	Methylene blue Indigo carmine and indigo blue dye* Indicans* Pseudomonas infection* Water-soluble chlorophyll* Rhubarb* Toluidine blue* Triamterene* Amitriptyline* Anthraquinone* Blue food dye*	Colorless	Very dilute urine (diuretics, diabetes mellitus, diabetes insipidus, glucocorticoid excess, fluid therapy, overhydration)
Green	Methylene blue Dithiazanine Urate crystalluria Indigo blue* Evan's blue* Bilirubin Biliverdin Riboflavin* Thymol* Phenol* Triamterene* Amitriptyline* Anthraquinone* Green food dye*	Milky white	Lipid Pyuria Crystals

Continued

Table • 39-1

Potential Causes of Discolored Urine—cont'd

URINE COLOR	CAUSES	URINE COLOR	CAUSES
Red, pink, red-brown, red-orange, or orange	Hematuria	Brown	Methemoglobin
	Hemoglobinuria		Melanin
	Myoglobinuria		Sulfasalazine*
	Porphyrinuria		Nitrofurantoin*
	Congo red		Phenacetin*
	Phenolsulfonphthalein (following alkalinization)		Naphthalene*
			Sulfonamides*
	Neoprontosil		Bismuth*
	Warfarin (orange)*		Mercury*
	Food pigments (rhubarb, beets, blackberries)*		Feces (rectal-urinary fistula)
			Fava beans*
	Carbon tetrachloride*		Rhubarb*
	Phenazopyridine		Sorbitol*
	Phenothiazine*		Metronidazole*
	Diphenylhydantoin*		Methocarbamol*
	Bromsulphalein (following alkalinization)		Anthracin cathartics*
	Chronic heavy metal poisoning (lead, mercury)*		Clofazimine*
			Primaquine*
	Rifampin*		Chloroquine*
	Emodin*		Furazolidone*
	Phenindione*		Copper toxicity
	Eosin*		
	Rifabutin*		
	Acetazolamide*		
	Red food dye*		
Orange-yellow	Highly concentrated urine		
	Excess urobilin		
	Bilirubin		
	Phenazopyridine		
	Sulfasalazine*		
	Fluorescein sodium*		
	Flutamide*		
	Quinacrine*		
	Phenacetin*		
	2,4-d*		
	Acetazolamide*		
	Orange food dye*		

*Observed only in human beings.

hypercalcemia, hyperthyroidism, and renal failure. The reader is reminded that dogs and cats with uncomplicated diabetes mellitus, while typically extremely polyuric, usually have urine specific gravities of 1.025 to 1.045. If urine is pale yellow or clear, the urine specific gravity is often less than 1.015. A simple test to determine whether polyuria is persistent is to determine the urine specific gravity of an owner-collected morning sample. Other tests should include serum biochemical analysis and a complete urinalysis. Additional testing may include measurement of serum thyroxine concentration, adrenal function testing, or monitoring urine specific gravity after several days of vasopressin administration.

Red, Brown, or Black Urine

Presence of red, brown, or black urine suggests blood, hemoglobin, myoglobin, or bilirubin (see Figure 39-1). A positive occult blood reaction is obtained when urine contains any of these substances. Discoloration of urine may also result in false-positive reactions on other urine dipstick test pads. Analysis of urine sediment will reveal the presence of red blood cells if the discoloration is due to hematuria. If no red blood cells are present on microscopic examination of urine sediment, hemoglobin, myoglobin, or bilirubin should be suspected. Examination of plasma color may aid in differentiating these potential explanations. If the discolored urine is due to myoglobin, the plasma will be clear because myoglobin in plasma is not bound significantly to a carrying protein, which results in filtration and excretion of myoglobin. If the plasma is pink, it is suggestive of hemoglobin. If the plasma is yellow, it is suggestive of bilirubin; serum bilirubin concentration should also be increased. Myoglobinuria is indicative of muscle damage; serum creatine kinase activity is often increased in this setting. Hemoglobinemia is indicative of intravascular hemolysis resulting from immune-mediated, parasite-mediated, or drug-mediated destruction of red blood cells. Hyperbilirubinemia may result from liver disease, posthepatic obstruction, or hemolysis.

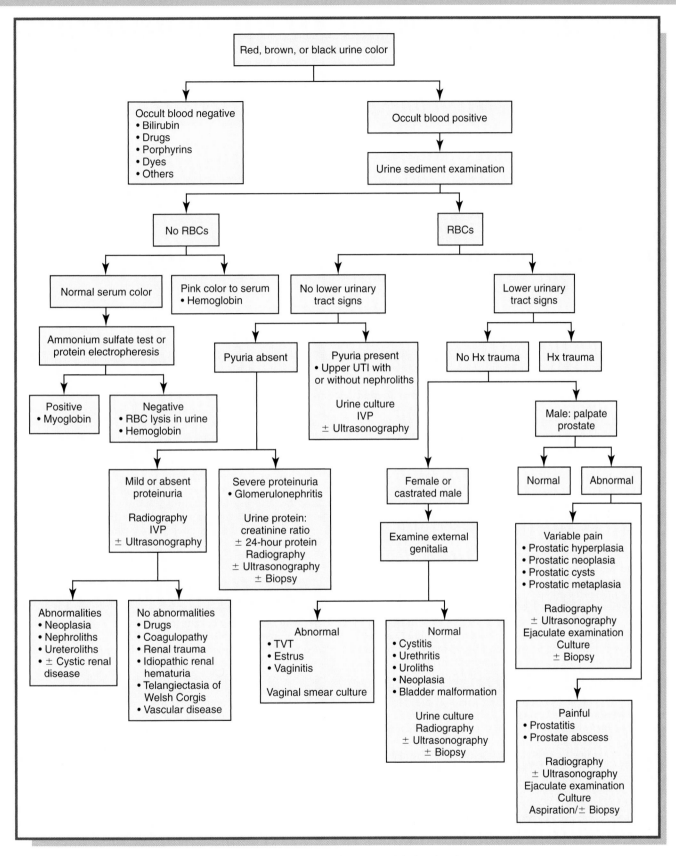

Figure 39-1 Algorithm for diagnosis of red-, brown-, or black-colored urine. *Hx,* History; *IVP,* intravenous pyelogram; *RBC,* red blood cell; *TVT,* transmissible venereal tumor; *UTI,* urinary tract infection.

Milky White Urine

Milky white–colored urine may be due to presence of white blood cells (pyuria), lipid, or crystals. The more concentrated the urine sample is, the more opaque it may appear. The presence of pyuria secondary to a bacterial urinary tract infection is the most common cause of milky white urine; however, pyuria may occur due to inflammation and not be associated with an infection. Lipiduria may be observed in healthy animals, but is frequently observed in cats affected with hepatic lipidosis. Crystalluria, if heavy and present in a concentrated urine sample, may also result in milky white urine color. Microscopic examination of urine sediment will aid in differentiation of these causes.

CHAPTER 40

Proteinuria

Gilad Segev

Dogs and cats may normally have small amounts of protein in their urine; however, the term *proteinuria* usually refers to the presence of an abnormal amount of protein in the urine. The term *microalbuminuria* refers to the presence of albumin in the urine in a concentration of 1 to 30 mg/dL, which is considered abnormal, but is below the detection limit of the urine dipstick.

A persistently high-magnitude proteinuria is usually an indicator of chronic kidney disease (CKD); however it may be a secondary consequence of infectious, inflammatory, metabolic, or neoplastic disorders. Thus proteinuria can serve as a sensitive indicator of both renal and extrarenal diseases, and its presence may prompt a comprehensive diagnostic evaluation even in the absence of clinical signs. Proteinuria may also serve as a prognostic marker. There is growing evidence in both the veterinary and the human literature suggesting that proteinuria is associated with a more rapid progression of CKD, a higher frequency of uremic crises, as well as an increased mortality rate.[1-3] Proteinuria has also been found to be associated with an increased risk of all-cause mortality in cats.[4] Thus, early detection of proteinuric animals should allow closer monitoring as well as early therapeutic intervention, which may decrease the magnitude of proteinuria and the disease progression rate of these patients.

For the aforementioned reasons, detection, monitoring, and treatment of persistent proteinuria in dogs and cats should not be overlooked, and urinalysis should be an integral component of the initial clinical patient evaluation when a complete blood count and serum biochemistry are performed. In addition, screening for proteinuria should be performed in any animal diagnosed with CKD or with any other disease known to be associated with proteinuria.

METHODS OF DETECTION AND INTERPRETATION OF TEST RESULTS

Cystocentesis is the recommended method of urine collection. If voided samples are used, proteinuria should be confirmed in a sample obtained by cystocentesis to exclude the genital tract or external genitalia as its origin. The most commonly used methods for detection and quantification of proteinuria include the urine colorimetric dipstick, the sulfosalicylic acid (SSA) turbidometric test, the species-specific microalbuminuria test, and the urine protein to creatinine (UPC) ratio.

The urine dipstick colorimetric test is the most commonly used method to screen for proteinuria. The urine dipstick is more sensitive to albumin compared to other proteins, and its lower detection limit is 30 mg/dL. Interpretation of any result should be done in light of the urine specific gravity. A positive result in concentrated urine reflects a smaller degree of protein loss compared to the same amount of protein in dilute urine; thus, the latter is more alarming. Both false positive and false negative results can occur using urine dipsticks. False positive reactions occur more commonly in alkaline and concentrated urine, or when an inappropriate techniques are used (e.g., contamination, prolonged urine contact with the dipstick). False negative results are more common in dilute or acidic urine, with a low-magnitude albuminuria, and with Bence-Jones proteinuria. A positive dipstick reaction can be confirmed by the more sensitive and specific SSA turbidometric test, which has a lower detection limit of 5 mg/dL. If a false negative result is suspected, the SSA test or the species-specific test for microalbuminuria can be employed. The latter has a lower detection limit of 1 mg/dL and is albumin-specific; thus, it may serve as a sensitive indicator of glomerular disease and is particularly useful when overt proteinuria is absent.

Once persistent proteinuria has been confirmed or when a high-magnitude proteinuria is suspected, it should be quantified. Although several methods are available to assess the magnitude of proteinuria, the most commonly used test in veterinary medicine is the UPC ratio. UPC results are used as a guideline for diagnostic investigation, therapeutic intervention, and monitoring response to therapy.[5] The UPC ratio has been shown to be highly correlated with 24-hour urine protein loss.[6,7] Urine protein to creatinine ratio <0.2 in dogs and cats is considered normal, and a ratio between 0.2 and 0.4 in cats and 0.2 and 0.5 in dogs is considered borderline proteinuria.

ORIGIN OF PROTEINURIA

Once proteinuria has been documented, its origin should be identified as a first step toward the diagnosis of the underlying disease (Figure 40-1).

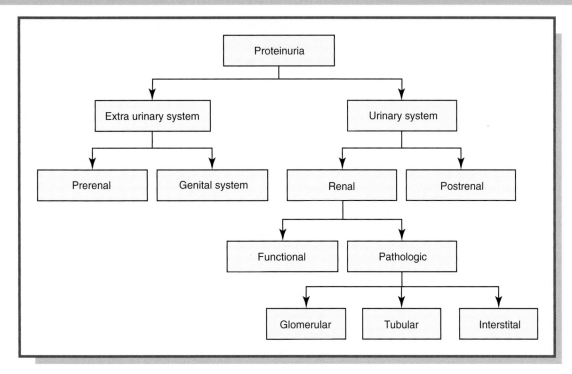

Figure 40-1   Algorithm for the origin of proteinuria. Glomerular proteinuria is the most common cause of persistent high-magnitude proteinuria.

Proteinuria can be classified as urinary system or extraurinary system in origin. Extraurinary system proteinuria may result from either prerenal or posturinary system conditions. Prerenal proteinuria results from presence of excessive amounts of normal (e.g., hemoglobin, myoglobin) or abnormal (e.g., Bence Jones) blood proteins, which can be freely filtered through the glomerulus. Thus, prerenal proteinuria can occur with normal kidney structure and function. This form of proteinuria is typically of low magnitude. Extraurinary system proteinuria can also occur with posturinary conditions, such as contamination of urine with protein arising from genital disorders.

Urinary system proteinuria can be classified as renal (functional or pathologic) or postrenal. Functional renal proteinuria represents a transient change in the permselectivity characteristics of the glomerulus, and may result from conditions such as seizures, fever, excessive exercise and stress. This form of proteinuria is transient, is typically of low magnitude, and does not require intervention. Pathologic renal proteinuria may result from glomerular (decreased permselectivity), tubular (decreased reabsorption), or interstitial (exudation of proteins to the urinary space) abnormalities. Glomerular proteinuria is the most common cause of persistent high-magnitude proteinuria. It requires close monitoring, and often warrants diagnostic evaluation and therapeutic intervention. It results from changes in the glomerular permselectivity characteristics, most commonly due to amyloidosis or glomerulonephritis. Renal proteinuria that originates from the renal tubules represents failure of the proximal tubule to reabsorb small–molecular weight proteins that are freely filtered in the glomerulus. Additional concurrent proximal tubular abnormalities, such as reabsorption of phosphorous, bicarbonate, and glucose (e.g., Fanconi's syndrome) may be present. Postrenal proteinuria relates to the entry of proteins into the urine from the renal pelvis, ureters, urinary bladder, or urethra, and results from disorders along the urinary excretory system (e.g., infection, urolithiasis, neoplasia).

DIAGNOSTIC APPROACH

The origin of proteinuria, its magnitude, and its persistency will determine the nature of diagnostic investigation warranted (Figure 40-2).

Once proteinuria has been established, follow-up measurements should be performed to classify the proteinuria as transient or persistent. Persistent proteinuria was defined in the consensus statement of the American College of Veterinary Internal Medicine as ≥ 3 positive results 2 weeks apart.[5] Recommendations of this consensus statement suggest a diagnostic work up for nonazotemic patients when the UPC ratio is ≥ 1.0. However, recent evidence suggests that even proteinuria of lower magnitude may be detrimental; therefore, diagnostic investigation should be considered even with UPC ratio values of 0.5 to 1.0.

The diagnostic workup is directed at detecting the origin of proteinuria and the underlying disease. Assessing the dog or cat with proteinuria includes a complete history and physical examination as well as diagnostic tests such as arterial blood pressure measurement, complete blood count, serum chemistry, urinalysis and urine culture, serologic testing and polymerase chain reaction for infectious diseases, diagnostic imaging, and kidney biopsy (Figure 40-2). Initially postrenal proteinuria is excluded by evaluating the urine sediment for presence of inflammation and hemorrhage. Next, extraurinary system causes should be excluded. Posturinary (genital system) proteinuria is easily excluded by performing urinalysis on urine obtained by cystocentesis, and prerenal proteinuria is ruled out by evaluating the plasma protein concentration and excluding dysproteinemia and presence of specific proteins in the urine (e.g., hemoglobinuria, myoglobinuria, and Bence Jones proteins). Glomerular proteinuria can be of any magnitude, but is particularly suspected when persistent high-magnitude (UPC ≥ 2) proteinuria is present and after ruling out extrarenal and postrenal causes. Glomerular proteinuria can be diagnosed by obtaining a kidney biopsy, which can addi-

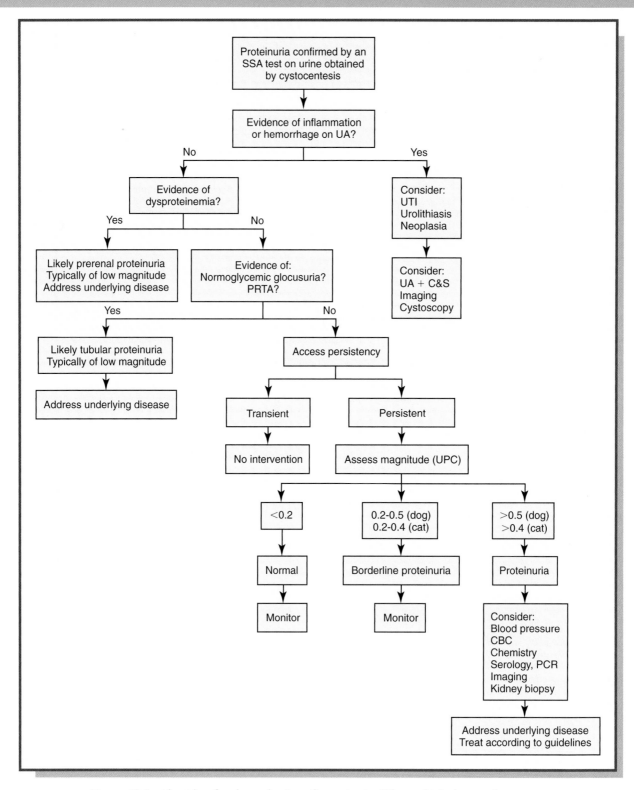

Figure 40-2 Algorithm for the evaluation of proteinuria. When a high degree of proteinuria is suspected its magnitude can be assessed even before persistency has been documented. *CBC,* Complete blood count; *C&S,* culture and sensitivity; *PCR,* polymerase chain reaction; *PRTA,* proximal renal tubular acidosis; *SSA,* sulfosalicylic acid test; *UA,* urinalysis; *UPC,* urine protein-to-creatinine ratio; *UTI,* urinary tract infection.

tionally differentiate between amyloidosis and glomerulonephritis. A combination of light microscopy, electron microscopy, and immunofluorescence allows further subclassification of the disease and may disclose the underlying etiology as well as direct therapy. Since glomerulonephritis is often a secondary complication of infectious, inflammatory, or neoplastic conditions, a diagnostic workup should be performed to identify any underlying disease. Tubular proteinuria should be suspected when concurrent tubular abnormalities such as normoglycemic glucosuria, proximal renal tubular acidosis, or abnormal electrolyte excretion are present; nevertheless, their absence does not exclude tubular proteinuria.

It should be recognized that several origins of proteinuria may coexist and their differentiation may be difficult (e.g., low-grade glomerular proteinuria versus tubular proteinuria).

TREATMENT

Therapy of proteinuria should be directed toward elimination of any underlying disease and decreasing the magnitude of proteinuria. Successful treatment of an underlying disease may resolve proteinuria; however, some dogs and cats remain proteinuric despite resolution of the disorder due to the presence of permanent glomerular damage. When proteinuria persists after elimination of the underlying disease or when the latter can neither be identified nor be eliminated, therapy is merely symptomatic. Treatment goals include decreasing the magnitude of proteinuria to the reference range to minimize progressive kidney damage, as well as preventing and treating the secondary consequences of the protein loss (e.g., thromboembolism).

Azotemic pets require therapeutic intervention at lower magnitudes of proteinuria compared to nonazotemic patients. Due to the decreased number of functional nephrons in azotemic patients, the amount of protein passing through each nephron is higher compared to patients with a normal number of functional nephrons for any given UPC ratio. Current guidelines recommend treating nonazotemic patients when UPC ratio is $\geq$ 2.0, while azotemic dogs and cats are to be treated when UPC $\geq$ 0.5 and UPC $\geq$ 0.4, respectively.[5]

Dietary modification and angiotensin-converting enzyme (ACE) inhibition are the mainstays of therapy.[8-13] Protein restriction is one of the dietary modifications recommended for protein-losing nephropathies. Even though counterintuitive, increasing dietary protein amounts is associated with increased albuminuria and may result in decreased serum albumin concentration, as has been shown in rats, dogs, and humans.[11,14,15]

Several mechanisms have been proposed for the reduction of proteinuria in response to ACE inhibitors, but decreased efferent glomerular arteriolar resistance resulting in decreased glomerular transcapillary hydraulic pressure is considered the primary mechanism. The beneficial effects of ACE inhibitors were demonstrated in both azotemic and nonazotemic patients. In a study of dogs with idiopathic glomerulonephritis and serum creatinine <3 mg/dL, enalapril (0.5 mg/kg PO q12-24h) decreased the degree of proteinuria compared to controls.[16] All dogs in this study were additionally treated with low-dose aspirin and with low-protein, low-phosphorous diets. In dogs with experimentally induced renal failure, enalapril (0.5 mg/kg PO q12h) decreased glomerular capillary pressure as well as the degree of proteinuria,[10] and in Samoyeds with X-linked hereditary nephritis, ACE inhibitors slowed the rate of increase in proteinuria and delayed the onset of increase in serum creatinine concentration.[12] Finally, a decrease in magnitude of proteinuria in response to ACE inhibitors has been also demonstrated in cats with naturally occurring CKD that were treated with benazepril (0.5 to 1 mg/kg PO q24h).[13,17]

Although there is growing evidence that ACE inhibitors have renoprotective properties in proteinuric patients, their administration should be exercised with caution, especially in severely and acutely azotemic dogs and cats. ACE inhibitors uncommonly cause a decreased intraglomerular pressure that results in a decrease in the glomerular filtration rate. Risk of this adverse effect should not be overlooked, particularly in azotemic patients or in animals prone to dehydration. In these animals, a lower daily dose of ACE inhibition should be used initially, with a gradual increase toward the target dose while monitoring kidney function.

Low-dose aspirin (0.5 mg/kg, PO, q12-24h) may also decrease proteinuria in dogs.[18] It has been shown that glomerular damage may be prevented by thromboxane release inhibition, thus preventing platelet aggregation and neutrophil chemotaxis.[19] An additional potential advantage of low-dose aspirin therapy is decreasing the risk of thromboembolism, especially in animals with a hypoantithrombinemia.

MONITORING

When persistent proteinuria has been documented, periodic monitoring should always be considered prudent. Close monitoring will discriminate patients with progressive from those with stable disease and identify those with progressive disease in a timely manner. When the degree of proteinuria is mild and therapeutic intervention is not indicated, periodic monitoring should include urinalysis, UPC ratio, and serum creatinine and albumin concentrations at least every 3 to 6 months. At each time point an assessment should be made whether diagnostic workup or therapeutic intervention is indicated. When therapy is applied, closer monitoring is indicated. In high-risk patients, their serum creatinine should be monitored 3 to 5 days after initiation of ACE inhibitor therapy to determine if a significant decrease in glomerular filtration rate has taken place. Urinary protein to creatinine ratio should be monitored periodically and therapy should be adjusted. Due to day-to-day variation not every change in UPC ratio would be considered significant. At least a 35% or 80% change should be demonstrated when the UPC ratio is high (around 12) or low (around 0.5), respectively.[20] In animals with progressive kidney disease, the magnitude of proteinuria may decrease in late stages of the disease due to a reduction in the number of remaining nephrons through which protein loss can occur.

In summary, proteinuria may be a marker of renal or extrarenal disorders as well as a prognostic marker. Once proteinuria is confirmed efforts to determine its origin and the underlying disease are warranted. Treatment is directed toward elimination of underlying diseases and decreasing the magnitude of proteinuria. Proteinuric patients should always be considered with a higher risk of developing azotemic renal failure, and should be monitored as such. Early identification of proteinuric patients will prompt close monitoring and early intervention before extensive irreversible changes have already occurred. Such intervention may slow disease progression and decrease both morbidity and mortality rates associated with CKD.

References

The reference list can be found on the companion Expert Consult Web site at *www.expertconsult.com.*

GASTROINTESTINAL

CHAPTER 41

Anorexia

Marnin A. Forman

Anorexia is a common owner concern encountered by veterinarians in small animal practice. Anorexia may be associated with multiple conditions or disease processes. This clinical sign can be both a diagnostic and therapeutic challenge (Figure 41-1), as well as a source of frustration for many owners.

Anorexia is defined as a lack or loss of appetite for food. The term *hyporexia* was recently introduced and may be a more accurate term to describe a reduction, rather than a complete loss, of appetite.[1] To further complicate understanding this clinical sign, some disease processes that classically have been described as causing anorexia more accurately produce an inability to eat, rather than a lack of appetite for food. Examples include (there are a myriad of possibilities): (1) severe dental disease; (2) a foreign body in the mouth or pharyngeal area; and (3) an inability to open the mouth due to advanced masticatory muscle myositis.

Anorexia is important because complications of prolonged inadequate nutritional intake are numerous and, for certain disease processes (e.g., feline hepatic lipidosis) can be more serious than the underlying disorder. Examples of these complications include immune system suppression (decreased cell-mediated immunity, immunoglobulin and complement production, and phagocytic activity) and secondary organ dysfunction (decreased hepatic detoxification ability and intestinal alterations).

CAUSES

Since the causes of anorexia are multiple, an organized diagnostic approach is needed to determine quickly and accurately the causative disorder (Figure 41-2; see Figure 41-1).

Obtaining a complete medical and environmental history is a mandatory first step. Many medications produce anorexia including antibiotics, antifungals, nonsteroidal antiinflammatory drugs, narcotic analgesics, chemotherapeutic agents, cardiac glycosides, and diuretics. Environmental changes, including modifications of the pet's diet (type and feeding location including establishment of physical barriers to eating) and home life (addition or absence of other dogs, cats and/or humans; change of housing location) may cause anorexia.[2]

The next step in determining the cause of anorexia is a complete general physical examination, including thorough oral, thoracic, abdominal, rectal and retinal examinations. In dogs and cats suspected of having anorexia secondary to chronic pain, an orthopedic and neurologic examination should be performed. Following these examinations, and in addition to a minimum data base (complete blood count

[CBC], biochemistry panel, and urinalysis), certain cases require imaging studies (radiography or ultrasonography) or serology. Many causes of anorexia will be identified with this initial evaluation. However, additional testing, for example cytology/histopathology, will occasionally be required. It should be understood that the purpose of the complete history and physical examination are to identify causes of anorexia that would not be obvious from blood, urine, fecal, or imaging examinations. The dog or cat with heart, liver, kidney, or any other major organ dysfunction could develop anorexia over a period of time or acutely. However, the dog or cat with an oral foreign body will likely have the same clinical problems (see Figure 41-1; Figure 41-3).

TREATMENT

Therapy of the anorectic dog or cat should always be directed at understanding and treating the underlying cause. These measures may include modification of anorexia-inducing medications or environmental stressors, instituting definitive therapy (e.g., removal of an abscessed tooth), or appropriate utilization of antiinflammatory, antiemetic or analgesic medications. During the diagnostic workup of an anorexic patient and prior to determination of the causative disorder, chemical and dietary appetite stimulants can be tried. Such stimulants provide only short-term benefit, if any. However, appetite stimulants are useful during the diagnostic workup or prior to implantation of an assisted feeding device, if one becomes necessary (Figure 41-4).

Numerous chemical appetite stimulants have been utilized including benzodiazepines (Valium), cyproheptadine (Periactin), and mirtazapine (Remeron). In the author's practice, the most commonly used stimulant is mirtazapine (feline: 1.875 to 3.75 mg total dose PO every third day; canine: 3.75 to 30 mg PO daily).[3,4]

Dietary appetite stimulation broadly involves modification of the environment or the type of food offered. Prior to discussing dietary modifications, it is important to consider learned food aversions. This condition involves the association of food with an adverse event (e.g., vomiting) and can lead to avoidance of potentially beneficial diets in the future. Warming, feeding multiple small meals, and the addition of nonnutritive flavors (e.g., garlic in dogs) may help prevent the development of learned food aversions to a new diet. Offering a new diet(s) should be avoided in nauseous pets until the nausea is resolved.

A guideline on when to initiate assisted feeding has not been established and often is dependent on patient factors. It is generally indicated when nutritional intake is less than

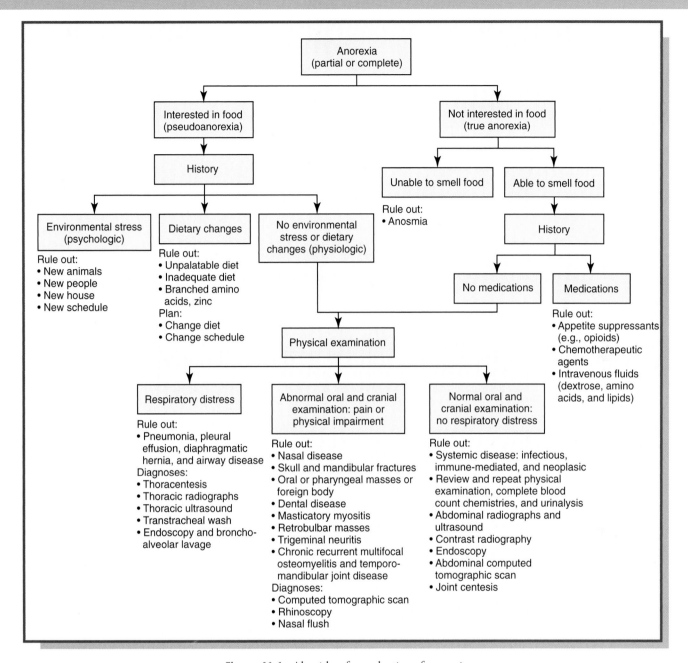

Figure 41-1 Algorithm for evaluation of anorexia.

resting energy requirements (RER) = $70 \times$ (body weight$_{kg}^{0.75}$) for 3 to 5 days. Even with identification of a causative disease process, assisted feeding can be needed during the recovery process for patient support (see Figure 41-4).

References

The reference list can be found on the companion Expert Consult Web site at *www.expertconsult.com*.

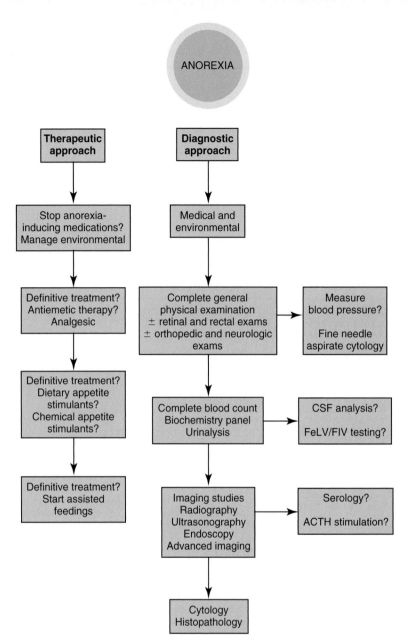

Figure 41-2 Therapeutic and diagnostic approach for feline and canine anorexia. *ACTH*, Adrenocorticotropic hormone; *CSF*, cerebrospinal fluid; *FeLV*, feline leukemia virus; *FIV*, feline immunodeficiency virus.

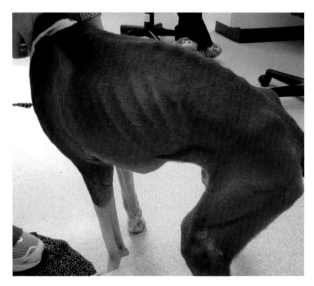

Figure 41-3 Example of prolonged inadequate nutritional intake resulting in marked vitamin deficiencies.

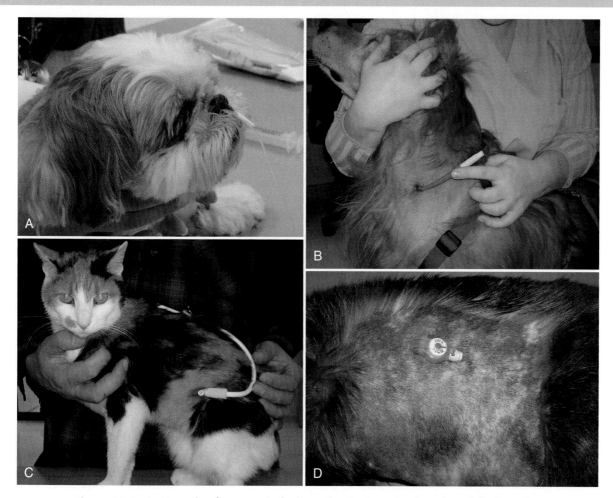

Figure 41-4 **A,** Example of nasogastric feeding tube. **B,** Example of esophageal feeding tube. **C,** Example of a percutaneous endoscopically placed gastric feeding tube (PEG). **D,** Example of a low-profile (MicKey) gastric feeding tube.

CHAPTER 42

Polyphagia

Ellen N. Behrend

Polyphagia is the consumption of food in excess of normal caloric intake. Hunger, satiety, and consequently, eating behavior are primarily controlled by certain regions in the central nervous system (CNS), but many factors affect the function of these areas. Thus polyphagia can be classified as primary (i.e., a CNS abnormality) or secondary (i.e., a systemic problem affecting the CNS). Secondary polyphagia is by far more common and is usually accompanied by clinical signs of the underlying disease.

Determining whether weight gain or loss has occurred should be the first step in formulating a list of differential diagnoses and a diagnostic plan.

PHYSIOLOGY

Food intake is controlled by a variety of factors, including gastrointestinal, environmental, and CNS phenomena. Within the CNS, key circuits regulating energy homeostasis and food intake originate in the hypothalamus and brainstem. The hypothalamus receives sensory input from the external environment plus neurologic and hormonal input from the internal environment, integrates the information, and provides output to key regulatory sites such as the pituitary, cerebral cortex, brainstem, and spinal cord. The lateral hypothalamic nuclei represent the "feeding center"; their stimulation causes an animal to eat, and their destruction results in severe, fatal anorexia. Conversely, the ventromedial nuclei are the "satiety center," as their stimulation causes a refusal to eat even highly appetizing food, and their ablation leads to polyphagia and obesity. The feeding center is constantly active unless inhibited by the satiety center (e.g., postprandially). The brainstem serves a secondary coordinating role and the nucleus of the solitary tract and area postrema have minor roles.

In the brain, melanocortin peptides, such as α-melanocyte-stimulating hormone (α-MSH), and the melanocortin-4 receptor (MC4-R), for which α-MSH is the agonist, are extremely important in food intake. Mutations in the MC4R gene are the most common monogenic form of obesity, accounting for up to 6% of severe early-onset obesity in some human cohorts. Neurons that express pro-opiomelanocortin or coexpress agouti-related protein and neuropeptide Y are also vital to food intake.

Gastrointestinal components that affect feeding include gastric distention, the rate of gastric emptying, the release of gastric hormones, and absorption of nutrients, such as fatty acids, glucose, and amino acids. The gut hormones can act locally on the gastrointestinal tract and centrally on the CNS. Secretion of insulin, glucagon, cholecystokinin and PYY, a peptide related to neuropeptide Y, and pancreatic peptide results in decreased feeding signals from the CNS. Leptin, a polypeptide released from adipose tissue, may also help to create a sense of satiety. Conversely, serum concentrations of ghrelin, a peptide secreted mainly by the stomach, decrease with meal ingestion. Concentrations of this hormone rebound to baseline before the next meal and increase with an overnight fast. Ghrelin stimulates eating. Decreased serum concentrations of glucose, amino acids, or lipid metabolites cause hunger by stimulating neural centers so as to reestablish normal levels. Feeding behavior also can be incited by increased nutrient utilization (i.e., an elevated metabolic rate).

Pathologic conditions that affect the CNS can increase feeding behavior even in the presence of normal energy stores (primary polyphagia). Secondary polyphagia exists when feeding behavior is stimulated by nonneural factors and can be caused by an increased metabolic rate or decreased nutrient supply (Box 42-1).

An augmented metabolic rate can be physiologic (e.g., pregnancy) or pathologic (e.g., hyperthyroidism). Diabetes mellitus causes an unusual condition of decreased nutrient supply. Due to an inability to respond to or a lack of insulin, the body does not recognize glucose, falsely perceiving

Box • 42-1

Differential Diagnoses of Polyphagia

Primary polyphagia
Destruction of satiety center
  Trauma
  Mass lesion (e.g., neoplasia)
  Infection
Psychogenic
  Stress
  Introduction of a more
    palatable diet

Secondary polyphagia
Physiologic increased metabolic rate
  Cold temperature
  Lactation
  Pregnancy
  Growth
  Increased exercise
Pathologic increased metabolic rate
  Hyperthyroidism
  Acromegaly
Decreased energy supply
  Diabetes mellitus
  Malassimilation syndromes
    Pancreatic exocrine insufficiency
    Infiltrative bowel disease
    Parasites
    Lymphangiectasia
  Decreased intake
    Megaesophagus (congenital)
    Low-calorie diet
    Hypoglycemia
  Unknown
    Hyperadrenocorticism
    Portosystemic shunt/
      hepatoencephalopathy
    Sudden acquired retinal
      degeneration syndrome (SARDS)

Drug-induced polyphagia
Glucocorticoids
Anticonvulsants
Antihistamines
Progestins
Benzodiazepines
Amitraz
Cyproheptadine

Reported specific cases associated with polyphagia
Feline infectious peritonitis
Lymphocytic cholangitis (feline)
Spongiform encephalopathy (feline)
Foreign body encephalitis (feline)
Disseminated *Mycobacterium avium* infection (cats)

hypoglycemia. Certain diseases (e.g., hyperadrenocorticism and liver disease) lead to polyphagia by unknown mechanisms. Secondary polyphagia can also be caused by certain drugs.

HISTORY

Change in body weight is an important differentiating feature of the various causes of polyphagia (Figure 42-1).

Primary or drug-induced polyphagia typically results in weight gain, as feeding is inappropriately increased despite consumption of adequate nutrients. Pathologic secondary polyphagia is more commonly associated with weight loss, because the nutrient supply usually does not meet physiologic demands. However, some causes, such as acromegaly, hypoglycemia caused by an insulinoma, sudden acquired retinal degeneration syndrome (SARDS), and hyperadrenocorticism (HAC), lead to weight gain. Physiologic polyphagia can result in weight gain (e.g., pregnancy, growth) or maintenance of weight (e.g., lactation, cold environment, increased exercise). An animal with HAC or in the early stages of any of these states, however, may show no weight change.

Certain causes of polyphagia may be diagnosed on the basis of the history. The possibility of feeding a low-calorie diet, exposure to a cold environment, increased exercise and, for intact females, pregnancy and lactation should be ascertained. Polyphagia is commonly associated with anticonvulsant and glucocorticoid therapy but has been observed with other medications (see Box 42-1). Psychogenic polyphagia has been noted after introduction of a more palatable diet or in response to a stressful event, most commonly introduction of a new pet into the household.

An animal with primary polyphagia caused by destruction of the satiety center may have a history of trauma or clinical signs associated with CNS disease. Depending on the extent of a hypothalamic lesion, upper motor neuron signs may be seen in all four limbs or unilaterally. A midbrain lesion often leads to incessant pacing, circling, and blindness; polyuria/polydipsia (PU/PD) may also be present. Disorders caused by diffuse or multifocal CNS disease will have other clinical signs as well, depending on the areas affected.

Perturbation of hypothalamic control of the pituitary can lead to reproductive, thyroidal, and adrenal hypofunction and associated clinical signs. Hypothyroidism secondary to pituitary dysfunction is clinically identical to primary thyroidal failure.

Historical findings associated with secondary polyphagia can be highly varied. Animals with diabetes mellitus, acromegaly, SARDS, and hyperthyroidism usually have PU/PD. It is valuable to remember that people and cats with HAC do not typically exhibit polyphagia, PU, or PD, features that are extremely common in dogs with HAC. Feline acromegaly is seen in middle-aged to older males, and naturally occurring canine acromegaly is seen almost exclusively in intact bitches. In dogs of either sex, progestin administration can lead to acromegaly. Owners may note inspiratory stridor or a change in body conformation, such as increased interdental spaces, skin folds, or head size in acromegalic animals. It should also be noted that progestin administration to dogs and cats can

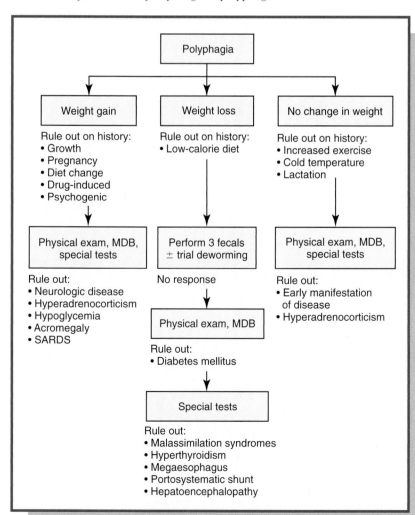

Figure 42-1 Algorithm for diagnostic approach to polyphagia. *MDB*, Minimum data base; *SARDS*, sudden acquired retinal degeneration syndrome.

increase appetite without causing acromegaly. A multitude of historical details can be associated with HAC, including abdominal enlargement, persistent panting, failure to regrow hair after clipping, lethargy, and muscle weakness. Animals with SARDS typically have the presenting complaint of sudden-onset blindness, but PU/PD and polyphagia may precede the blindness. Hyperthyroidism commonly leads to increased activity but can be associated with depression and lethargy. Gastrointestinal signs (e.g., vomiting and diarrhea) may also be present.

Hypoglycemia has a number of etiologies. Insulinoma is the most likely to lead to polyphagia, but a few other neoplasias and insulin overdose may also lead to increased appetite. Dogs and cats with hypoglycemia may exhibit weakness, trembling, ataxia, disorientation and, possibly, grand mal seizures. Malassimilation can be due to a variety of problems, e.g., parasites, pancreatic exocrine insufficiency (PEI), infiltrative bowel disease, and lymphangiectasia and generally cause large-volume, malodorous, soft stools. PEI is more common in younger dogs (i.e., those less than 2 years of age), and the German Shepherd breed shows a predisposition for this disorder. In older dogs and cats, PEI is rare but, if seen, is most commonly associated with chronic pancreatitis. The category of infiltrative disease encompasses processes such as inflammatory bowel disease, neoplasia, and infections such as histoplasmosis. Historical details vary according to the underlying disease.

Acquired esophageal disease often leads to anorexia. Animals with congenital megaesophagus are often polyphagic, especially if they have the typical history of regurgitation. Although anorexia is more common in animals with a portacaval shunt, polyphagia has been reported in approximately 10% of cases. Depression, vomiting, weight loss, polydipsia/polyuria, and neurologic signs may also be noted. Polyphagia has been reported rarely with hepatoencephalopathy; other clinical findings are the result of hepatic failure and may be similar to those in an animal with a portasystemic shunt.

PHYSICAL EXAMINATION

Physical examination findings in polyphagic animals vary, depending on the underlying disease. With primary polyphagia, neurologic abnormalities such as ataxia and proprioceptive deficits may be present. A complete neurologic and fundic examination should be performed. With acute causes of central blindness, however, the fundus appears normal.

If unclear from the history, pregnancy potentially can be diagnosed by abdominal palpation and lactation by inspection of the mammae. Approximately 80% of cats with hyperthyroidism have a palpable thyroid nodule, and approximately 50% have tachycardia or a gallop rhythm. Hyperthyroidism is much less common in dogs, and a cervical mass usually is palpable. Hyperadrenocorticism can have a variety of physical examination findings, including abdominal and hepatic enlargement, muscle wasting, bilaterally symmetric alopecia, cutaneous hyperpigmentation, areas of poor hair regrowth, or calcinosis cutis. Even when not noted by an owner, the physical changes associated with acromegaly can be documented on physical examination, but not always; a degenerative polyarthropathy may also be present.

Examination findings in a dog with SARDS may be unremarkable, because in the early stages of the disease, the retinas appear normal on examination. Dogs or cats with PEI, insulinoma, megaesophagus (a malassimilation syndrome), hepatoencephalopathy, or a portasystemic shunt may have no abnormal physical findings other than the associated weight change. In rare cases, polyneuropathies may accompany an

insulinoma. Aspiration pneumonia may accompany megaesophagus. Neurologic abnormalities may be detected in an animal with a portasystemic shunt, and ascites is noted in approximately 20% of afflicted dogs. Neurologic findings associated with hepatoencephalopathy may be episodic, and other examination findings vary with the cause of liver disease. Depending on the cause of malassimilation, the intestines may feel thickened. Lymphangiectasia may lead to ascites.

Occasionally, polyphagia may be a clinical sign of a disease with which it is not usually associated. For example, 1 cat each with feline infectious peritonitis (FIP), foreign body encephalitis, and spongiform encephalopathy have been reported as being polyphagic, as have 18 cats with lymphocytic cholangitis and a few with disseminated *Mycobacterium avium* infection. Other historical and clinical signs are present depending on the cause.

DIAGNOSTIC PLAN

The first step in diagnosis is to ascertain if there has been a change in body weight (see Figure 42-1). After as many differential diagnoses as possible have been ruled out on the basis of the history, further testing may be warranted: a minimum data base (MDB) of a serum biochemistry profile, complete blood count (CBC), and urinalysis. For dogs and cats with weight gain, pregnancy must be ruled out.

To diagnose primary polyphagia, a complete neurologic examination should be performed, any abnormalities localized, and appropriate tests obtained. A cerebrospinal fluid analysis or diagnostic imaging, such as radiography, computed tomography (CT), or magnetic resonance imaging (MRI), may be necessary. Hypoglycemia caused by an insulinoma usually can be suspected by measuring blood glucose and further supported with paired blood glucose and insulin serum concentrations when the animal is hypoglycemic. Rarely, provocative testing may be required (see Chapter 289). The diagnosis of SARDS can be made on the basis of appropriate history, physical examination findings, an MDB that rules out other causes, and, if necessary, an electroretinogram (ERG). For dogs with HAC certain changes in the MDB are typical but do not confirm the diagnosis and further adrenal testing must be performed (see Chapters 292 and 293). Diagnosis of acromegaly can be difficult because of the lack of a commercial assay for growth hormone, but measurement of insulin-like growth factor-I (IGF-I) may be helpful (see Chapter 284). The history, together with conformational changes if present, can provide evidence of the underlying disease. Many acromegalic cats have insulin-resistant diabetes mellitus, and imaging of the pituitary may reveal the growth hormone–secreting tumor.

Polyphagia, PU/PD, and weight loss are classic for diabetes mellitus. In all such animals a urinalysis and blood glucose should be determined. Diabetic dogs and cats have glycosuria and hyperglycemia. The other cause of polyphagia, PU/PD, and weight loss is hyperthyroidism—common in cats, uncommon in dogs. Hyperthyroidism can usually be diagnosed with a single serum thyroxine measurement; however, other tests, such as the free thyroxine concentration by equilibrium dialysis, may be required (see Chapter 288). Weight loss associated with polyphagia can be caused by intestinal parasitism. If parasites are suspected, the MDB should be preceded by three fecal examinations. If the results of these are negative, the MDB does not provide the diagnosis and the animal is stable, trial therapy with antiparasiticides may be warranted. If deworming does not resolve the problem, additional tests must be done.

Malassimilation syndromes cover myriad differential diagnoses (see Box 42-1). Protein-losing enteropathies can be associated with hypoalbuminemia and hypoglobulinemia. Depending on the suspected cause, measurement of serum folate or cobalamin or fecal α-1 protease inhibitor, assessment of fat absorption, abdominal radiography or ultrasonography, and/or biopsy either by endoscopy or exploratory surgery may also be considerations. For verification of PEI, serum trypsin–like immunoreactivity (TLI) should be determined. Thoracic radiographs with a positive contrast esophagram should be used to diagnose megaesophagus and may also aid in the determination of the cause. Measurement of preprandial and postprandial serum bile acid concentrations can document hepatic dysfunction, but a biopsy may be required to identify the cause. Ultrasonography or a radionuclide scan may be used to visualize a portacaval shunt.

If the disease is in the early stages, weight change may not yet have occurred, and the list of differentials may be more difficult to narrow. However, a good history and physical examination combined with an MDB can eliminate many possibilities. Although animals with HAC may not have a weight change, abdominal enlargement may create the impression of weight gain. All diseases suspected as possible differential diagnoses in this situation should be diagnosed as discussed above.

MANAGEMENT

The management of polyphagia depends on the cause. Physiologic causes of polyphagia are transient. If the condition is drug induced, the polyphagia may be temporary, as is usually seen with anticonvulsants. Psychogenic polyphagia may be corrected by removing the instigating element, if possible, or by behavioral therapy (e.g., paying more attention to the animal). If the polyphagia persists with ongoing drug therapy or if the inciting agent (stress or medication) cannot be removed, food intake should be limited to that necessary to satisfy caloric requirements. Low-calorie, high-fiber foods, such as carrots, can be added to the diet to assuage hunger and prevent obesity. Polyphagia caused by dietary factors can be managed as needed. In cases of SARDS, the polyphagia usually is self-limiting. For all other conditions, appropriate therapy should be initiated to resolve the underlying disease.

CHAPTER 43

Periodontitis

Jason W. Soukup

Periodontal disease is a broad term used to encompass a subset of two distinct conditions, gingivitis and periodontitis. Briefly, *gingivitis* is inflammation of the gingiva, while *periodontitis* is inflammation of the periodontium beyond the gingiva. A dog or cat may have periodontal disease but not periodontitis. However, all patients with gingivitis or periodontitis have periodontal disease. Periodontal disease is the most commonly diagnosed disease in dogs and cats.[1] By 2 years of age 80% of all dogs and 70% of cats are affected with periodontal disease.[2] As age increases, the incidence of periodontal disease also increases, affecting most dogs by 5 years of age.[3] Periodontal disease can affect any dog or cat but is more prevalent in small and toy breed dogs affected with malocclusions and crowding of the teeth.

ANATOMY OF THE PERIODONTIUM

The periodontium is composed of gingiva, periodontal ligament, cementum, and the alveolus (Web Figure 43-1). These tissues support the teeth and are the tissues most intimately involved in periodontal disease. The marginal, or unattached, gingiva is the terminal edge of a collar of gingiva surrounding each tooth. The gingival sulcus is a small, V-shaped crevice between the marginal gingiva and the tooth. In the healthy gingiva, the sulcus depth is 0 to 3 mm in the dog and 0 to 0.5 mm in the cat. Continuous with the marginal gingiva is a firm, resilient, and tightly bound zone of epithelium known as the *attached gingiva*. The attachment of the gingiva to the tooth at or slightly apical to the cementoenamel junction is known as the *junctional epithelium*.

Periodontal ligaments are composed of highly cellular and vascularized connective tissue that surround and attach teeth to alveolar bone. The primary components of the periodontal ligament are collagenous principal fibers that anchor each tooth, transmit occlusal forces to bone, provide a soft tissue casing for protection of associated vessels and nerves, and provide a shock-absorbing effect during mastication.[2,4,5] Cementum is a calcified, avascular tissue that forms the outer covering of the tooth root. This noninnervated tissue serves as the attachment point for the periodontal ligament fibers to the tooth. The alveolus, formed by the alveolar process of the maxilla and mandible, is composed of an inner wall of compact bone, an external plate of cortical bone, and cancellous trabeculae between the compact layers of individual alveoli.

PATHOBIOLOGY OF PERIODONTAL DISEASE

Microbiology

Plaque is a structured, resilient, yellow-to-tan biofilm composed primarily of microorganisms, salivary glycoproteins, and extracellular polysaccharides. Plaque formation is divided into three phases: (1) the formation of the pellicle, (2) adhesion and attachment, and (3) colonization and maturation. The pellicle is a saliva-derived layer of glycoproteins that coats the tooth surface within seconds after a professional cleaning.[6] Microorganisms then adhere to receptors within the pellicle to form an attachment on the tooth surface.[7] Finally, during colonization and maturation, the plaque biofilm becomes more stratified through complex bacterial interactions. This plaque biofilm serves to protect the microorganisms within the ultrastructure by increasing their resistance to antibiotics,[8-11] allowing metabolic interactions among cells of different species[12,13] and facilitating the exchange of genetic information between cells of the same species.[14] The type of bacteria present depends on the location of the tooth. Supragingival plaque is composed primarily of gram-positive cocci and rods at the tooth surface and gram-negative rods and filaments, as well as spirochetes, at the outer surface of the mature plaque mass. The subgingival microenvironment is characterized by anaerobic conditions. This microenvironment favors the establishment of gram-negative rods, gram-negative cocci, flagellated rods, and spirochetes adjacent to and within the sulcus epithelium. These bacteria are of prime importance in the tissue destruction that characterizes periodontitis. When comparing the microbial shifts from health to periodontitis, the following general shifts can be identified: from gram-positive to gram-negative species; from cocci to rods to spirochetes; from nonmotile to motile species; from facultative anaerobes to obligate anaerobes; and from fermenting to proteolytic species (Web Figure 43-2).[14]

Interactions of Microbes with the Host and Immune/Inflammatory Response

Periodontal disease is a chronic infectious disease that is determined by the interaction of microorganisms with the host. Either directly by destroying tissue or indirectly by modulating the host response, microorganisms exert a pathogenic effect. The host response serves a protective role in preventing systemic spread of the infection but can lead to significant destruction of the periodontium. Periodontal pathogens invade the tissues of the periodontium and evade the natural host defense mechanisms. They then directly cause host tissue damage through the release of metabolic byproducts, such as ammonia and volatile sulfur compounds, and the release of proteolytic enzymes.[15,16] These byproducts and enzymes lead to direct degradation of host tissues.[17,18] Pathogenic microorganisms within the plaque biofilm also stimulate an immune response that leads to the activation of complement and subsequent mast cell degranulation. Mast cell degranulation results in the release of molecules responsible for the movement of leukocytes, primarily neutrophils, into the local tissues. Mast cell degranulation and the local activity of leukocytes, fibroblasts, osteoblasts, and osteoclasts lead to the release of proteinases,[19,20] cytokines,[21-23] and prostaglandins.[24,25] These three compounds are the primary host response mediators responsible for the tissue inflammation and destruction associated with periodontal disease.

CONTRIBUTING FACTORS

Genetics

The most obvious link between genetics and periodontal disease in dogs and cats is occlusion. Patients with tooth crowding and malocclusion are at risk for early and progressive periodontal disease. Several human studies have shown that a heritable component to periodontal disease exists.[26-29]

Calculus

Calculus is a hard deposit formed by mineralization of dental plaque and has a role in maintaining and perpetuating periodontal disease (Web Figure 43-3). Calculus can create areas where removal of plaque is difficult if not impossible. It can also provide a surface that keeps plaque in close contact with the gingival tissues.

Tooth Crowding/Malocclusion

A positive correlation between tooth crowding/malocclusion and periodontal disease exists.[30-33] Mesioversion of the maxillary canine teeth, in which the canine teeth erupt in a rostral orientation, causes crowding of the canine tooth and the maxillary third incisor (Web Figure 43-4, A). This leads to a decreased ability to remove plaque in the interproximal space, which can lead to periodontal disease. Linguoversion of the mandibular canine teeth (base narrow canines) can traumatically alter the periodontium on the palatal aspect of the maxillary canine teeth, leading to progressive periodontitis (Web Figure 43-4, B).

Iatrogenic Factors

Inadequate dental procedures, such as subgingival, rough, and overhanging restoration margins can lead to periodontal disease either by altering the ecologic balance of the gingival sulcus to favor gram-negative anaerobic species or by decreasing the ability of the owner to remove plaque during routine home care.[34] Self-curing acrylics often used in fracture management and orthodontics may also be inherently injurious to periodontal tissues, leading to gingivitis (Web Figure 43-5).[35]

Xerostomia

Saliva contains numerous antimicrobial factors, antibodies, and antiproteases that help control the oral microbial population and their effect on the periodontium.[36-39] Xerostomia, or lack of salivary production, can therefore lead to an increased degree of plaque accumulation and periodontal disease. Xerostomia can be caused by sialolithiasis, radiation therapy, salivary gland disease, poorly controlled diabetes mellitus, and some medications (tricyclic antidepressants, antihistamines, antihypertensives and diuretics).

Radiation Therapy

Periodontal attachment loss has been shown to be greater in patients treated with radiation therapy.[40] Exposure to radiation induces a vasculitis that causes soft tissue ischemia, alveolar bone hypoxia, and can contribute to the destruction of the periodontium and formation of osteoradionecrosis. Radiation therapy can also cause an irreversible xerostomia.

Gingival Enlargement

Enlargement of the gingiva can contribute to periodontal disease by the formation of a gingival pocket, or pseudo-pocket. Pseudopockets are instrumental in the formation of areas that are difficult to access during oral home care. Common causes of gingival enlargement in veterinary medicine include: certain drugs, idiopathic, neoplastic, and inflammatory. Calcium channel blockers, cyclosporine, and anticonvulsants can lead to progressive gingival enlargement (Web Figure 43-6).[41,42] Idiopathic enlargement is common in Boxers, Great Danes, Collies, Doberman Pinschers, and Dalmatians and is believed to have a hereditary basis.[43] Benign and malignant tumors of the oral cavity can also cause gingival enlargement.[44] Inflammatory enlargement, a response to prolonged exposure to dental plaque, is a common cause of gingival enlargement in dogs and can also be a component of other types of enlargement.[44] Mouth breathing has also been shown to cause gingival enlargement in humans and is thought to be attributed to inflammation from surface dehydration.[45] Excessive mouth breathing may play a part in the formation of gingival enlargement in some breeds of dogs.

Systemic Health

The host's immune response, whether insufficient or exaggerated, is important and can provide some explanation as to whether the patient will or will not develop periodontal disease. Some conditions that may play a role in the progression of periodontal disease include diabetes mellitus, feline leukemia virus (FeLV), feline immunodeficiency virus (FIV), chemotherapy, and leukemias/anemias. Poorly controlled diabetes mellitus is known to cause an increased susceptibility to infections and poor wound healing. Studies have shown a propensity for gingival enlargement, periodontal abscess formation, periodontitis, and loose teeth in patients with diabetes mellitus.[46] The mechanism is thought to be secondary to diminished periodontal tissue integrity. Diabetic patients have also been shown to have impaired neutrophil function,[47] increased collagenase activity, and decreased collagen synthesis.[48]

Human immunodeficiency virus (HIV) has been linked with chronic periodontal disease and opportunistic *Candida* infections.[49,50] Similarly, FeLV and FIV can contribute to the development of oral disease. Some of the most common clinical findings in cats infected with FIV are gingivitis, stomatitis, and periodontitis.[51,52] The exact relationship is unclear, but immunosuppression and FeLV-related leukemia/anemia are likely contributing factors.

Whether occurring as a malignant neoplasia (leukemia) or secondary to FeLV or chemotherapy, leukopenia and anemia may alter natural defense mechanisms and healing of the periodontium. Poor tissue oxygenation from anemia leads to friable tissues that are susceptible to breakdown. Neutropenia may have a significant effect on the host defense mechanism considering the role of neutrophils in controlling periodontopathogens. Infiltration of leukemic cells into the gingiva can also cause gingival enlargement.[53]

PERIODONTAL PATHOLOGY

Gingivitis

Gingivitis is the first stage of periodontal disease (Table 43-1). Gingivitis begins as an inflammatory response to supragingival plaque. This stage is characterized by vasculitis; influx of macrophages, neutrophils, lymphocytes, and plasma cells; early collagen loss; increased crevicular fluid flow; erythema and bleeding upon probing.[54-60] Dogs and cats may have halitosis or they might experience minor bleeding when chewing on toys. Since no attachment loss has occurred, no radiographic abnormalities will be present. Gingivitis is the only stage of periodontal disease that may be reversible with appropriate management.

Periodontitis

In susceptible animals, gingivitis may progress to varying degrees of periodontitis (see Table 43-1). Periodontitis is defined as inflammation of the periodontal tissues beyond the gingiva, which leads to attachment loss (Web Figure 43-7). The progression of periodontitis has been shown to be cyclical with periods of active inflammation and periods of quiescence.[61] Periodontitis, therefore, can be classified as either active or nonactive based on the presence or absence of inflammation. Clinically, periodontitis may be characterized by gingival recession, alveolar bone loss, furcation exposure, tooth mobility, gingival bleeding and suppuration, severe halitosis, and the formation of periodontal pockets.[2,3] Once periodontitis has occurred, the damage to the periodontium cannot be reversed without surgical intervention, and the altered anatomy makes the disease more difficult to manage. The periodontal pocket and the pattern of bone loss can vary among patients and can have an impact on the prognosis and treatment.[62]

The Periodontal Pocket   The destruction of the periodontium associated with periodontitis leads to the formation of a periodontal pocket, which is measured from the gingival margin to the junctional epithelium. There are two types of pockets: a suprabony pocket in which the bottom of the pocket is coronal to the underlying alveolar bone and an infrabony (intrabony) pocket in which the bottom of the pocket is apical to the adjacent alveolar bone. Either type of pocket can be difficult, if not impossible, to access and clean with a home care routine.

Bone Loss Patterns   The pattern of bone loss is usually related to the type of periodontal pocket. Horizontal bone loss is typically seen with a suprabony pocket, while vertical bone loss is seen with infrabony pockets. The vertical bone loss associated with infrabony pockets is referred to as an *angular osseous defect* and is usually classified in terms of the number of osseous walls possessed (Web Figure 43-8). Determining the morphology may impact the treatment plan and prognosis.[62]

EFFECT OF PERIODONTAL DISEASE ON SYSTEMIC HEALTH

In humans, periodontal status has been shown to be a strong predictor of mortality.[63] Concentrations of proinflammatory cytokines released during the host's immune response can reach sufficient levels to cause coronary heart disease, stroke, pulmonary disease, diabetes mellitus, and preterm low–birth-

Table • 43-1

Stages of Periodontal Disease

FINDINGS	STAGE			
	I	II	III	IV
Gingival				
Inflammation	+	+ to ++	++ to +++	++ to +++
Recession	None	+/–*	+/–	+/–
Pocket formation	None	+/–* Mild	+/– Moderate	+/– Severe
Radiographic findings	None	≤25% attachment loss	25%-50% attachment loss	≥50% attachment loss
Mobility	None	None	+/–	+/–

+, Mild; ++, moderate; +++, severe.
*Attachment loss may be seen as either gingival recession, pocket formation, or a combination of the two.

weight babies.[63-69] A veterinary study showed a positive correlation between periodontal disease and histologic changes of the myocardium, renal tissues, and hepatic tissues.[70] A possible causative relationship between infective endocarditis and septicemia from a dental cleaning has also been reported in a Rat Terrier.[71]

DIAGNOSIS

Diagnosis of periodontal disease relies on clinical signs, clinical measurements, and intraoral radiography obtained under general anesthesia. Indices that have been developed to assess the periodontium include the plaque index, gingival index, calculus index, mobility index, and sulcus bleeding index.[2] Clinical attachment loss is the primary method of accurately assessing periodontal disease and is typically evaluated with intraoral radiography and measurements of pocket depth and attachment level. The pocket depth is the depth of the periodontal pocket measured from the gingival margin to the apical extent of the pocket. In the case of gingival recession, pocket depth alone does not accurately depict the degree of attachment loss, which is the distance measured from a fixed point on the tooth (cementoenamel junction) to the apical extent of the pocket. Intraoral radiography is crucial in evaluating the degree and morphology of bone loss associated with periodontal disease. Radiographically, periodontal disease may present as a break in the continuity of the lamina dura, reduced height of the alveolar crest, loss of bone density within the furcation, horizontal loss of bone, or vertical loss of bone (Web Figure 43-9). Clinical attachment loss is most helpful in determining prognosis, and therefore a treatment plan, when expressed as a percentage. When expressed as a percentage, each tooth can then be staged according to the veterinary periodontal disease index (see Table 43-1).

TREATMENT

Treatment of periodontal disease can be divided into two phases of therapy. The initial phase targets removal of the microbial etiology and contributing factors with the goal of halting the progression of the disease. The second phase, sometimes referred to as the surgical phase, is aimed at correcting anatomic conditions that favor periodontal disease, creating a maintainable state, and regenerating the periodontium. General anesthetic is required for periodontal treatment in dogs and cats. Therefore, the veterinary clinician is often forced to perform both phases of treatment during a single visit (Figure 43-1). For ease of discussion, phase I and phase II therapy are presented separately.

Phase I Therapy

Scaling and Root Planing   Scaling is the process of removing plaque and calculus from both supragingival and subgingival locations, whereas root planing is a procedure in which residual calculus embedded within the cementum is removed from the root surface. Scaling and root planing are the cornerstone of phase I therapy. This treatment alone results in a dramatic reduction in the number of spirochetes, rods, and putative pathogens[72,73] and a substantial improvement in clinical attachment levels.[74] Scaling and root planing can be performed with hand (scalers and curettes) or ultrasonic instrumentation. Hand scalers possess a sharp tip and are reserved for supragingival scaling (Web Figure 43-10, *A*). Curettes possess a rounded tip design and are intended for subgingival scaling and root planing (Web Figure 43-10, *B*). Ultrasonic instrumentation may be used as well. In

recent years, thinner ultrasonic tips have been designed that allow for safe and effective subgingival use. Ultrasonic instruments remove calculus by utilizing a mechanism known as cavitation. Cavitation is the process in which vacuum bubbles within water droplets quickly collapse and release energy. Despite the cooling water spray, the clinician should not leave the instrument in contact with the tooth for more than 5 to 15 seconds at a time in order to reduce the risk of thermal damage to the pulp. Scaling and root planing should be performed via a surgical approach with pocket depths > 5 mm.[75]

Antimicrobials

Systemic antimicrobials   Since an antibiotic strength 500 times higher than the normal therapeutic dose is needed to affect bacteria associated with periodontal disease, the widespread use of antimicrobials as a sole treatment for periodontal disease is contraindicated.[76] However, there are indications for antimicrobials as an adjunctive therapy. It is the responsibility of the clinician to use systemic antimicrobials in select cases based on the patient's health status, degree of periodontal disease and a risk/benefit analysis. Some common clinical circumstances in which the use of systemic antimicrobials may be indicated include pets with cardiovascular disease, prosthetic implants, compromised healing ability, and compromised immune systems.[77] Antimicrobials commonly used to treat oral disease include amoxicillin-clavulanic acid, clindamycin, doxycycline, and metronidazole.

Local antimicrobials   The local delivery of antimicrobials has shown benefit by reaching concentrations needed to affect the structured biofilm while limiting the concerns of antibiotic resistance.[78,79] A perioceutic gel (Doxirobe) made of a lactic acid polymer (poly[DL-lactide] dissolved in a carrier N-methyl-2-pyrrolidone) and doxycycline hyclate is available for the treatment of periodontal pockets. Studies have shown that placement of Doxirobe into periodontal pockets leads to significant reductions in gingival inflammation, gingival bleeding, pocket depths, subgingival bacteria, and clinical attachment loss in dogs.[80,81]

Host Modulation

Nonsteroidal antiinflammatory drugs   Nonsteroidal antiinflammatory drugs (NSAIDs) can alter the inflammatory cascade by inhibiting formation of prostaglandins, specifically PGE2. As previously discussed, PGE2 contributes to the destruction of the periodontium. NSAIDs have been shown to significantly reduce alveolar bone loss but must be given daily for extended periods to be beneficial.[82,83]

Bisphosphonates   Bisphosphonates, more commonly used for the treatment of osteoporosis in humans, are agents that inhibit bone resorption by disrupting osteoclast activity. They have shown promise in reducing destruction of the periodontium.[84,85] Currently, no FDA-approved products for veterinary use are available and there is some concern regarding avascular necrosis of the mandible and maxilla following oral surgical procedures in patients treated with bisphosphonates.

Subantimicrobial-dose doxycycline   Subantimicrobial-dose doxycycline (SDD) is a more recent concept in veterinary dentistry and perhaps the most promising method of host modulation. The tetracyclines, particularly doxycycline, have been shown to have significant ability to down-regulate the matrix metalloproteinases (MMPs) that cause degradation of the periodontium and to up-regulate collagen production.[86,87] SDD, at 20% of an antimicrobial dose, has been shown to

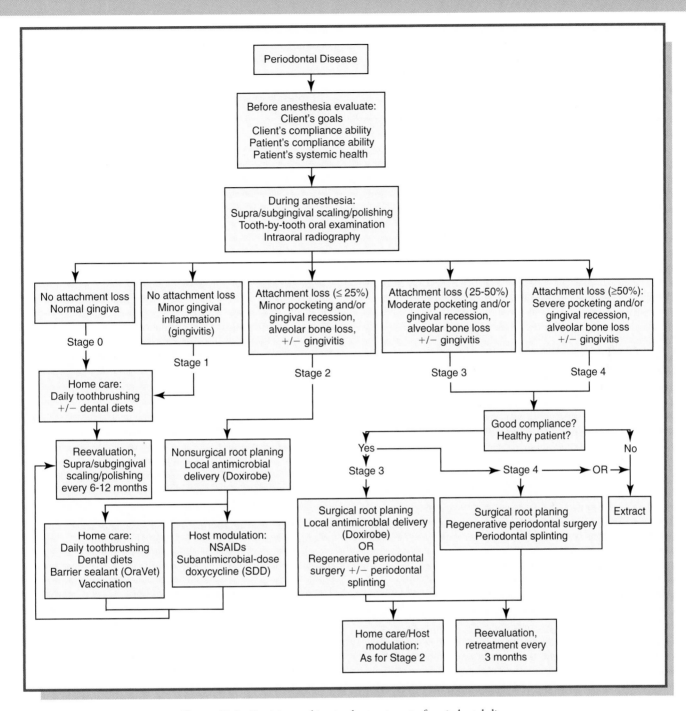

Figure 43-1 Decision making in the treatment of periodontal disease.

reduce collagenase and increase clinical attachment levels.[88-90] There have been no side effects reported from prolonged use and no evidence of antibiotic resistance.[91] SDD should not be used as a stand-alone therapy.

Treatment of Contributing Factors Any malocclusion contributing to the formation or preventing the treatment of periodontal disease should be addressed during phase I therapy. Malocclusions may be addressed with orthodontic movement, occlusal adjustment or exodontia depending on the individual case circumstances. Inadequately prepared restorative margins should be repaired or replaced. If xeros-

tomia is present and contributing to periodontal disease, the cause should be investigated and removed if possible. Any patient receiving head or neck radiation should have a thorough periodontal evaluation and treatment both prior to and after radiation therapy. Treatment of gingival enlargement is important in eliminating pseudopockets. Enlargement secondary to inflammation may resolve with routine professional and home care. Drug-induced enlargement may resolve with the removal of the inciting drug. However, surgical intervention may be necessary if the drug cannot be eliminated. Oral tumors and idiopathic gingival enlargement should also be treated with appropriate oral surgery.

Phase II Therapy

Reconstructive Periodontal Surgery   Periodontal regeneration is the ultimate goal of phase II periodontal treatment. Periodontal regeneration is defined as the true regeneration of alveolar bone, cementum, and functionally oriented periodontal ligament fibers.

Osseous grafting   Osseous grafting has been advocated for treatment of infrabony defects.[92] Graft materials can be categorized as autogenous bone grafts, allografts, and alloplasts. Autogenous grafts utilize the patient's bone, but this is no longer recommended because of the morbidity associated with the second surgery to harvest the graft.[92] Allografts are grafts transferred between individuals of the same species. The most commonly used allograft is decalcified freeze-dried bone, which has been shown to be osteoinductive.[92] Alloplasts, typically referred to as synthetic bone grafts, are implants of inert materials that are osteoconductive by providing a scaffold for osteoblasts to penetrate and form new bone.[92] An alloplast of bioactive glass (Consil) has become popular in veterinary oral surgery because it has been approved and shown to be effective for the treatment of osseous defects in the dog[93]; it can aid in periodontal regeneration by preventing migration of epithelium into the pocket[93]; and it has been shown to possess an antibacterial effect.[94]

Guided tissue regeneration   The apical migration of epithelium into the pocket is a major inhibitor of periodontal regeneration.[95] Guided tissue regeneration (GTR) is a technique utilizing a membrane to prevent apical epithelial migration along the cementum and therefore support the regeneration of functionally oriented periodontal ligament fibers. Many membranes have been developed and shown to be effective at limiting or preventing apical migration of junctional epithelium.[62,96-98] A doxycycline-impregnated bioabsorbable membrane was shown to be effective at regeneration of bone, cementum, and functionally oriented periodontal ligament fibers while preventing apical migration of epithelium.[99] There has been evidence supporting the use of Doxirobe as a GTR membrane.[99,100]

Combined techniques   Traditional GTR techniques often lead to the regeneration of periodontal ligament and cementum but not alveolar bone.[97] Therefore, most contemporary regenerative techniques use a combination of bone graft and guided tissue regeneration methodologies. Combination techniques have led to increased clinical attachment level gains over surgical debridement alone[101] and an increased percentage of cases with successful periodontal regeneration.[102] Many combination techniques have been described with good success.[97]

Prevention and Adjunctive Therapies

Mechanical Plaque Removal

Toothbrushing   Mechanical removal of plaque is the foundation of oral care and has traditionally been performed with a toothbrush. Toothbrushes of various designs, both manual and powered, are available. No one design has been shown to be advantageous.[103] The most common toothbrushing method recommended is the Bass technique[104] (Web Figure 43-11), in which the bristles are pointed toward the gingival margin at a 45° angle to the long axis of the tooth. The brush is moved in a back-and-forth motion. Fortunately, dogs and cats acquire very little plaque on the palatal and lingual surfaces of the teeth, which allows the owner to brush the buccal and labial surfaces of the teeth in a more comfortable, closed-mouth position. The teeth should be brushed at least daily. Alternatives to a traditional toothbrush include finger brushes and gauze pads. Flavored veterinary dentifrices are recommended for improving the pet's acceptance of brushing. Other dentifrice ingredients, such as chlorhexidine and antimicrobial enzymes, may be of benefit in plaque control.

Professional scaling and polishing   The true dental prophylaxis is rarely encountered in veterinary dentistry. The term *prophylaxis* suggests the absence of disease. Most patients already have some degree of periodontal disease when presented for a "dental." Some veterinary dentists have advocated the use of the terms *periodontal treatment* or *oral assessment, treatment, and prevention (ATP)* in place of obsolete terms such as *prophylaxis* and *dental*. In humans, only 40% of plaque is removed during toothbrushing. This figure is likely to be lower in dogs and cats. Residual plaque mineralizes to form calculus, which cannot be removed with toothbrushing alone. Regular professional removal of plaque and calculus is necessary to aid in prevention of periodontal disease. Supragingival and subgingival scaling can be performed with either hand or ultrasonic instrumentation. The selection of hand or ultrasonic instrumentation should be determined based on the clinician's preference and experience and the needs of each patient. The need for general anesthesia may be of concern for clients but should not prevent the clinician from making recommendations that are in the patient's best interest. Scaling should always be combined with polishing and a thorough oral examination and should be performed every 3 to 12 months based on the current periodontal status of the patient.

Dietary Methods of Plaque Removal   Various treats and complete maintenance diets are available that may be beneficial in the prevention of periodontal disease. Many studies have shown that maintenance foods designed with unique textural and size characteristics that promote chewing aid in control of plaque and calculus in dogs and cats.[105-108] These products work by mechanical disruption of plaque from the surface of the tooth. Other foods and treats contain polyphosphates, which act as mineral chelators and inhibit calculus formation by binding salivary calcium to prevent plaque mineralization. Multiple studies have shown hexametaphosphate to be effective at calculus reduction.[109,110] The Veterinary Oral Health Council (VOHC) was established to evaluate clinical evidence and recognize products effective at controlling plaque and calculus. This independent organization was established in 1997 and is run by the American Veterinary Dental College. A complete list of VOHC-approved treats and foods can be evaluated on their website.

Rinses, Gels, and Water Additives   Chlorhexidine-based oral products have been shown to reduce plaque.[111-114] A zinc ascorbate gel has also been shown to reduce gingivitis, anaerobic periodontal pathogens, and plaque accumulation in cats.[115] Xylitol-based drinking water additives may also reduce plaque and calculus scores by up to 53% in cats.[116] Many other oral hygiene products are available but few have published research backing their various claims. It is important to recognize that oral rinses, gels and water additives should be used as adjuncts, not replacements, to toothbrushing and regular professional care.

Barrier Dental Sealants   A polymer-based barrier dental sealant (OraVet) that binds electrostatically to teeth to form a protective barrier inhibiting the adherence of plaque biofilm has been developed. This product is provided in a higher-viscosity, professionally applied polymer that provides a foundation for the application of a lower-viscosity, owner-applied polymer. Application on a weekly basis has resulted in reduced mean plaque, calculus, gingival bleeding, and gingivitis indices.[117]

Vaccination A vaccine has also been developed as an adjunctive method for the prevention and management of periodontal disease. In one study,[118] a monovalent vaccine was developed from a *Porphyromonas gulae* strain previously shown to cause periodontitis. A population of mice were then immunized and subsequently challenged with the bacterial strain. The immunized population showed an 83.8% reduction in alveolar bone loss compared to the control population.[118] This study led to the development and investigation of a trivalent vaccine composed of inactivated *Porphyromonas gulae*, *Porphyromonas salivosa*, and *Porphyromonas denticanis*. This vaccine was used in a canine apical periodontitis model and shown to significantly reduce bone changes compared to a control.[119]

REFERENCES

The reference list can be found on the companion Expert Consult Web site at *www.expertconsult.com*.

CHAPTER 44

Ptyalism

Brook A. Niemiec

DEFINITION

Ptyalism is defined as a pathologic overproduction of saliva that may occur from a number of disease states.[1] *Pseudoptyalism* refers to drooling caused by an inability or reluctance to swallow a normal amount of saliva.[2] This chapter will cover both forms as they are often interrelated.

ETIOLOGY AND PATHOGENESIS

Ptyalism results from an increase in production by one or all of the salivary glands. Pseudoptyalism results from some disruption of the swallowing mechanism that can be voluntary (often pain induced) or involuntary (obstruction).

There are numerous causes for hypersalivation, and numerous locations where the inciting cause may originate. Problems can originate from the oral cavity, esophagus or alimentary tract, or within the salivary glands themselves.[3] Furthermore, hypersalivation can occur secondary to neurologic (central or peripheral), metabolic, infectious or immune-mediated disease, or to a toxic/caustic exposure or drug reaction.

CLINICAL SIGNS

Dripping (or pouring) of saliva from the oral cavity (Figure 44-1).

This drooling may be seen as mild to severe or as intermittent to continuous. Onset of signs can occur acutely or as gradual and chronic. Finally, the saliva may appear clear or mixed with sanguineous or purulent exudates (Figures 44-2 and 44-3).

Other potential clinical signs such as vomiting, regurgitation, anorexia, oral pain, and oral inflammatory lesions are related to the individual cause.

DIFFERENTIAL DIAGNOSES

Neurologic: trigeminal neuropraxia, megaesophagus, facial paralysis, neurologic diseases that result in seizures, nausea from vestibular disease; glossopharyngeal, hypoglossal, or vagus nerve lesions that result in inability to swallow

Developmental: severe brachygnathism, lip fold

Trauma: temporomandibular joint (TMJ) luxation, mandibular fracture

Postsurgical: anesthesia, mandibulectomy, mandibular canine extraction

Toxic: oroganophosphates, caustic ingestion, animal venom

Drug induced: opiates, medications with a bitter/unpleasant taste

Behavioral: associated with food (Pavlovian), contentment/mood (cats during purring), pain

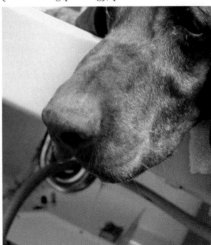

Figure 44-1 Ptyalism secondary to caustic ingestion in a dog.

 To view a video on this topic, go to **www.expertconsult.com**.

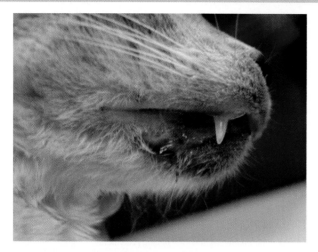

Figure 44-2 Purulent ptyalism secondary to severe periodontal disease in a cat.

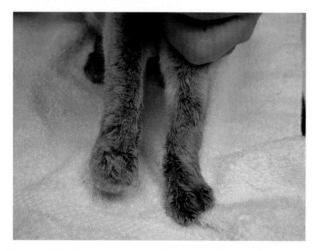

Figure 44-3 Unkempt fur on the antebrachium of a cat with significant ptyalism.

Obstructive: oral or esophageal foreign body/neoplasia
Metabolic: hepatic encephalopathy, hepatic or renal failure, hyperthermia
Gastrointestinal: nausea, hiatal hernia, megaesophagus (Figure 44-4), gastric dilatation/volvulus, gastric ulcer; esophageal stricture, neoplasia, or foreign body
Infectious: acute calicivirus or herpes virus infection, rabies, psuedorabies, tetanus, botulism, upper respiratory infection, candidiasis, severe periodontal disease
Immune mediated: CUPS in dogs, lymphoplasmacytic gingivostomatitis in cats, pemphigus, bullous pemphigoid, toxic epidermal necrolysis
Salivary: sialolith, foreign body, neoplasm, hyperplasia, infarction, sialocele, necrosis, idiopathic

DIAGNOSTIC STEPS

The most important initial steps are to obtain a complete history and perform a thorough physical exam.

HISTORY

Historical questions should include:
• General history
• Age

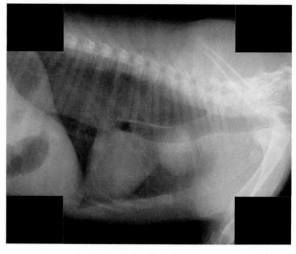

Figure 44-4 A lateral thoracic radiograph of a dog with megaesophagus.

• Acute versus chronic clinical signs
• Other gastrointestinal signs (vomiting, diarrhea, anorexia, quidding)
• Toxic exposure
• Drug administration
• Trauma

HISTORICAL SIGNIFICANCE

Age of the Patient
Young patients are more likely to have toxic exposure, foreign body, acute viral infection, or portosystemic shunts (especially small breeds such as Yorkshire Terriers and Maltese).

Mature patients are more likely to be affected by metabolic, immune-mediated, or neoplastic diseases.

Acute versus Gradual/Chronic
Acute onset of significant (pseudo) ptyalism is most often associated with a virus, toxic exposure, or oral trauma. Gradual onset is more likely to be associated with metabolic or neoplastic processes.

GI Signs
If ptyalism is associated with nausea or vomiting, a gastrointestinal (GI), systemic, or neurologic problem is more likely. Regurgitation should prompt an esophageal exam, as this is typically associated with megaesophagus. If ptyalism is noted in combination with difficulty eating or quidding (dropping food), an oral problem should be suspected and a complete oral and maxillofacial exam performed.

PHYSICAL EXAMINATION

The most important part of the physical exam is a complete oral/maxillofacial/esophageal examination. A thorough oral exam should evaluate for infection, neoplasia, fractured/abscessed teeth, periodontal status, trauma, inflammatory/ulcerative disease, and foreign bodies. Oral inspection should include the sublingual area, as this is a common place for masses and string foreign bodies. Oral ulcerative/

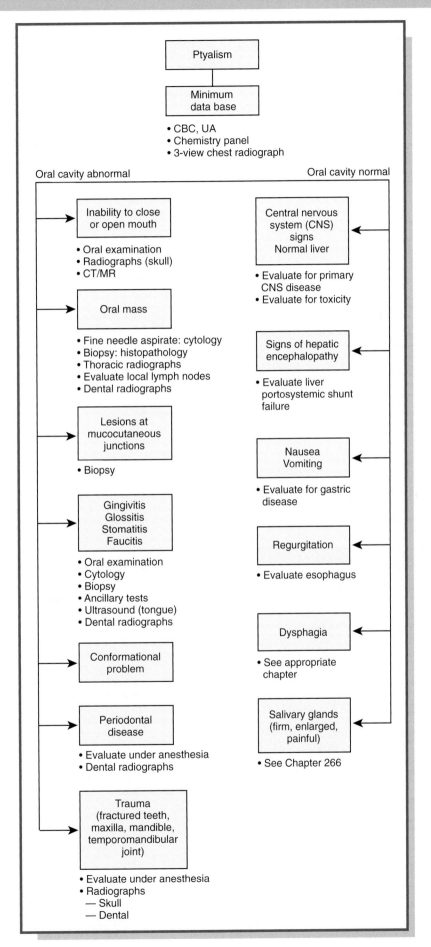

Figure 44-5 Diagnostic algorithm for diagnosing ptyalism. *CBC*, Complete blood count; *CNS*, central nervous system; *CT/MR*, computed tomography/magnetic resonance; *UA*, urinalysis.

inflammatory diseases are typically in advanced stages before ptyalism is induced, and thus in these cases abnormal oral examination findings should be readily seen. These conditions include acute calicivirus or herpes virus infection, immune-mediated diseases, caustic ingestion, and uremia. The saliva itself should be examined for consistency and any additional components.

It is important to note that a complete oral exam may not be possible without general anesthesia, and that a minimum data base should be obtained prior to an anesthetized exam.

Saliva that has a sanguineous or purulent/fetid component is usually secondary to a problem within the oral cavity, such as:
• Oral infections (including an oronasal fistula)
• Trauma
• Neoplasia
• Oral inflammatory disease
• Uremia

A maxillofacial exam should include evaluation for swellings, asymmetry, TMJ luxations, trauma, cranial nerve function, and the size and consistency of the salivary glands.

Inability to close the mouth indicates one of the following causes:
• Traumatic (TMJ/mandibular fracture/luxation)
• Neurologic (botulism or trigeminal neuropraxia)
• Obstructive (neoplastic or foreign body)

Inability to open the mouth is most commonly associated with:
• Tetanus
• Craniomandibular osteopathy

The salivary glands should be systematically evaluated. Enlargement could indicate:
• Infection
• Sialoliths
• Neoplasia

Physical examination of the esophagus is limited to external palpation for masses, pain, or foreign bodies. Complete evaluation requires radiographs and/or endoscopy.

DIAGNOSTIC TESTS

It is important to begin initial diagnostic testing with a minimum data base including a CBC/Chem/T4, and urinalysis (Figure 44-5).

For oral mucosal changes that are not obviously associated with a toxic/caustic cause or systemic disease (e.g., uremic ulcers) a surgical biopsy should be performed under general anesthesia and submitted for histopathology. When obtaining the pathology sample, ensure that it is representative of the lesion and of sufficient size for an accurate assessment. It is worthwhile to note that cytology as well as culture and sensitivity are often insufficient for an accurate assessment of disease processes in the oral cavity.[4]

In cases that clinically appear to have an oral cause but the problem cannot be readily identified on oral exam, dental radiographs should be performed. These radiographs may elucidate a subgingival cause such as a carnassial abscess or radicular cyst. Patients that present with derangements of jaw motion or maxillofacial swellings should be further evaluated with skull films or MRI/CT.

Once oral and maxillofacial causes have been ruled out, further diagnostics are indicated, initiating with thoracic and abdominal radiographs. If the cause of the ptyalism has not been identified at this point, more specific testing should be performed, where indicated, such as upper GI studies, fluoroscopy, and endoscopy. The clinician may also consider tests for botulism and rabies.

TREATMENT

Treatment is directed at the underlying cause. For example:
• Direct toxic exposures should be treated with dilutional therapy and supportive care.
• Therapy for oral inflammatory diseases should be directed toward reducing the inflammation. This can be accomplished medically (immunosuppressive agents) or surgically (extractions).
• Oral traumatic diseases are best treated surgically.
• Portosystemic shunts can be managed surgically or medically.
• Metabolic derangements should be treated as appropriate for the disease process.

In cases of idiopathic or incurable (e.g., structural, neurologic) ptyalism, treatment is directed at decreasing the flow of saliva and/or protecting the epidermis in the chronically wet area.

If one salivary gland is responsible for the increased production, it can be excised. Decreasing the overall flow of the saliva can be attempted with drug therapy (atropine, glycopyrrolate).[5] In human dentistry, injections of biotoxin into the salivary glands as well as radiotherapy, scopolamine (via a transdermal patch), and even acupuncture have been investigated options for long-term salivary control.[6-9] The practitioner must weigh the potential side effects of dry mouth (periodontal disease, caries, digestive problems) against the disease process. If chronic salivation is creating a moist dermatitis, petroleum jelly should be applied to the affected areas.

CONCLUSION

Ptyalism is not a common clinical finding, but when present, is usually secondary to a local problem such as oral/maxillofacial or GI disease. Alternatively, ptyalism may be secondary to a systemic disease problem, or less commonly may result from primary overproduction from the salivary gland(s). A thorough history and physical exam will elucidate the cause in many cases, and adding a minimum data base will identify the cause in countless more. Specific testing should be directed at the less common causes of ptyalism if the aforementioned tests have not identified a definitive diagnosis. Treatment is directed at the primary cause of the problem, and therefore varies as appropriate.

REFERENCES

The reference list can be found on the companion Expert Consult Web site at *www.expertconsult.com*.

CHAPTER 45

Gagging

William Gengler

NORMAL PHYSIOLOGY

Gagging is defined as a swallowing-vomiting reflex activity whereby elevation of the soft palate is followed by a reverse peristalsis of the upper digestive tract.[1] Swallowing is the taking in of a substance through the mouth and the pharynx and into the esophagus. It is a combination of a voluntary act and a series of reflex actions.[2] Once begun, the process operates automatically. The swallowing reflex is a rigidly ordered sequence of events that results in the propulsion of food from the mouth to the stomach while concurrently inhibiting breathing and preventing the entrance of food into the trachea (Figure 45-1).

The nerves involved with swallowing are the sensory and motor branches of the trigeminal nerve (cranial nerve [CN] V), the hypoglossal (CN XII), the facial (CN VII), and the glossopharyngeal (CN IX) nerves.[3] The afferent limb of the swallowing reflex begins with tactile receptors, most notably those near the opening of the pharynx. Sensory impulses from these receptors are transmitted to certain areas in the medulla. The central integrating areas for swallowing lie in the medulla and lower pons, called the *swallowing center*. Motor impulses

travel from the swallowing center to the musculature of the pharynx and upper esophagus via various cranial nerves.

The swallowing process is called *deglutition* and can be divided into three phases in the dog, cat, and man: (1) oral (or voluntary); (2) pharyngeal; and (3) esophageal. The oral phase is initiated by separating a bolus of food from the mass in the mouth with the tip of the tongue.[3] The bolus is moved in a dorsocaudal direction in the mouth by pressing first the tip of the tongue followed by the more caudal tongue segment against the hard palate. The bolus is forced into the pharynx and stimulates the tactile receptors that initiate the swallowing reflex. In the cat, the oral phase is much longer with the bolus accumulation in the valleculae.

The *pharyngeal* phase of swallowing occurs in less than 1 second. During this phase breathing is reflexly inhibited. The soft palate is pulled dorsally and the palatopharyngeal folds move medially preventing reflux of food into the nasopharynx. The pharyngeal passage is narrowed, directing the bolus caudally. Concurrently, the vocal cords move medially and the epiglottis covers the opening of the larynx preventing food from entering the trachea. The cranial esophageal sphincter relaxes to accept the bolus. The dorsal constrictor muscles of

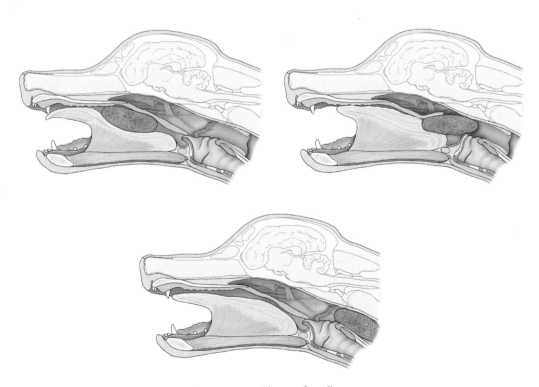

Figure 45-1   Phases of swallowing.

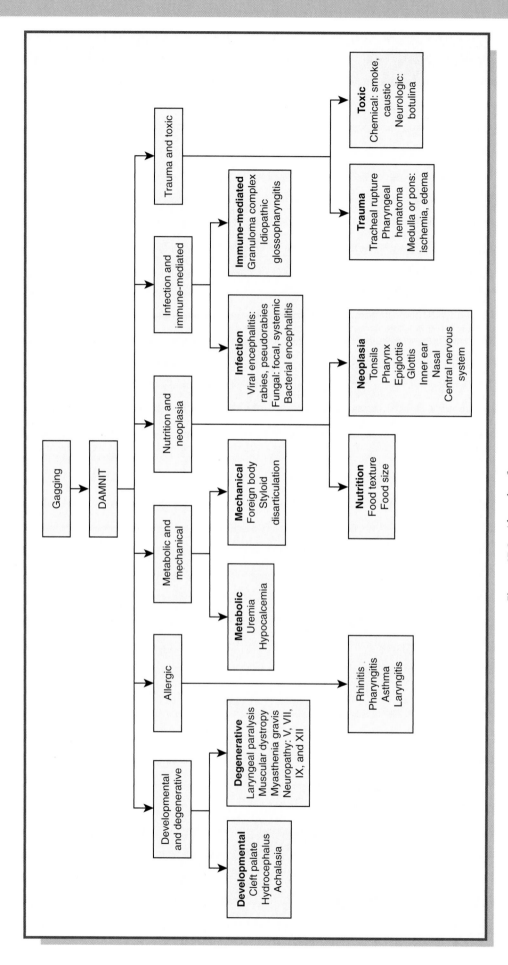

Figure 45-2   Algorithm for gagging.

the pharynx contract strongly to force the bolus deep into the pharynx. Peristalsis of these muscles initiates the movement of the bolus caudally through the cranial esophageal sphincter into the esophagus.

The *esophageal* phase of swallowing is under partial control of the swallowing center. The cranial (pharyngoesophageal) esophageal sphincter, or cricopharyngeus muscle, reflexively constricts after the bolus passes caudal to the sphincter preventing the bolus from moving back toward the mouth (regurgitation). A peristaltic wave beginning just caudal to the cranial esophageal sphincter traverses the entire esophagus in approximately 10 seconds. The initial peristaltic wave is termed *primary peristalsis* and is controlled by the swallowing center. If primary peristalsis is insufficient to clear the bolus from the esophagus, distension of the esophagus stimulates *secondary peristalsis*, which is mediated in part by the swallowing reflex and by local stretch receptors. As primary and secondary peristalsis is occurring, the caudal (gastroesophageal) esophageal sphincter relaxes to allow the bolus to continue into the stomach. In man and the dog the cranial one third of the tunica muscularis of the esophagus is predominantly composed of striated muscle and the caudal one third is predominantly smooth muscle, while the mid one third is a mixture of each. In the cat, in order to investigate the mechanism of airway defense reflex, beaded nerve terminals were studied by immunohistochemical techniques. In the supraglottic region the density of PGP 9.5-immunoreactive nerve fibers was the highest at the base of the glottic surface in the epiglottis, and in the glottic region it was the highest in the arytenoid region. These beaded nerve terminals may function as mechanoreceptors.[4] The cat esophagus changes abruptly from striated to smooth muscle at the level of the heart.[5] Somatic nerve fibers from the vagus nerve (CN X) form motor endplates on striated muscle fibers. Visceral motor nerves are preganglionic parasympathetic fibers innervating the smooth muscle cells. Gagging and sneezing in the cat has been shown to cause transdiaphragmatic pressures to reach the maximum.[6]

GAGGING

Gagging is often associated with retching. *Retching* is an involuntary and ineffectual attempt at vomiting. The causes for retching are similar to vomiting. Expulsion is induced when hypercapnia and hypoxia develop during retching, or when the oropharyngeal mucosa is irritated (the gag reflex). The central pattern generator (CPG) for expulsion has been suggested to coexist with the CPG for retching in the reticular area dorsomedial to the retrofacial nucleus, which may correspond to the Bötzinger complex (BOT). However, its participation in gagging induced by oropharyngeal irritation is unclear. To elucidate such participation, the firing patterns of BOT neurons were observed during gagging induced by stimulation of superior laryngeal afferents in decerebrate, paralyzed dogs. Only 23% of inspiratory and 34% of expiratory BOT neurons increased their firing in response to stimulation of the superior laryngeal nerve. In contrast, 75% of nonrespiratory BOT neurons showed enhanced firing with this stimulation. During gagging, each nonrespiratory, inspiratory, and expiratory BOT neuron fired with the same pattern that they exhibited during expulsion caused by changes in blood gases. These firing patterns could be classified into five types and are thought to be appropriate for generating neuronal gagging activity. These results suggest that the CPG for expulsion in the BOT produces gagging when it is activated by oropharyngolaryngeal afferents.[7]

The many causes of gagging are shown in the algorithm. Laryngeal paralysis is a frequently recognized disorder that can cause gagging. Older dogs such as the Labrador Retriever, Afghan Hound, and Irish Setter are breeds often diagnosed with laryngeal paralysis. Gagging is a common presenting sign in conjunction with exercise intolerance, inspiratory stridor, inspiratory dyspnea, coughing, and dysphonia. Two forms of laryngeal paralysis exist, hereditary and acquired. The hereditary form is found in young dogs and transmitted by an autosomal dominant gene.[8] Antibiotic administration in a solid form that is excessively large to allow passage of the esophagus has been shown to create esophageal injury and produce gagging in the cat.[9] Airway neoplasia or trauma can also be a common cause of gagging in cats.[10-12]

Retching is discussed in Chapter 46. Another physical sign similar to gagging is expectoration, which is the clearing of the airway of mucus and discharges without nausea. For cats this event can be a normal clearing of hair from the airway after grooming (Figure 45-2).

REFERENCES

The reference list can be found on the companion Expert Consult Web site at *www.expertconsult.com.*

CHAPTER 46

Dysphagia and Regurgitation

Carmenn Schaefer Woolley

Dysphagia and regurgitation may both be characterized as swallowing disorders. They may exist as separate conditions or in conjunction with each other. Localization of the disease process requires careful attention to history, clinical signs, and physical examination findings (Figures 46-1 and 46-2).

DYSPHAGIA

Dysphagia is defined as difficult or painful swallowing. The swallowing process may be divided into the oropharyngeal. esophageal, and gastroesophageal phases. *Oral dysphagia* occurs when there is difficulty with prehension and bolus

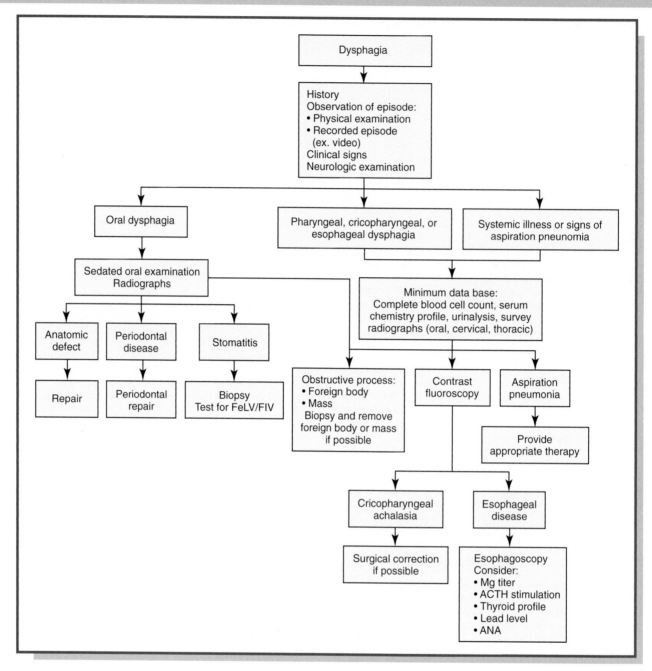

Figure 46-1 Diagnostic approach to dysphagia. *ACTH,* Adrenocorticotropic hormone; *ANA,* antinuclear antibody titer; *FeLV,* feline leukemia virus; *FIV,* feline immunodeficiency virus.

formation. *Pharyngeal dysphagia* occurs when there is impaired initiation of the involuntary passage of food through the oropharynx. *Cricopharyngeal dysphagia* occurs when there is inadequate relaxation of the cricopharyngeal muscle (achalasia), or failure of synchronization between pharyngeal contraction and cricopharyngeal relaxation (asynchrony) during swallowing. *Esophageal dysphagia* occurs when there is difficulty passing a bolus through the esophageal body. *Gastroesophageal dysphagia* occurs when there is difficulty passing a bolus through the caudal esophageal sphincter.

CLINICAL SIGNS

The clinical signs vary greatly depending on the location and severity of the swallowing disorder. Oral dysphagia results in difficult prehension of food, which can manifest as chewing

on one side of the mouth, dropping food, excessive head movements, and reingestion of dropped food. In cases of pharyngeal dysphagia prehension should be normal but there may be repeated attempts to swallow along with flexion or extension of the neck. In cases of cricopharyngeal dysphagia there are usually repeated and exaggerated attempts to swallow, gagging, coughing, or immediate regurgitation associated with swallowing. Esophageal and gastroesophageal dysphagia are associated with regurgitation. Aspiration pneumonia may result secondary to any of the above forms of dysphagia.

HISTORY

Signalment as well as onset of clinical signs may aid in a differential diagnosis. Juvenile animals are more likely to suffer

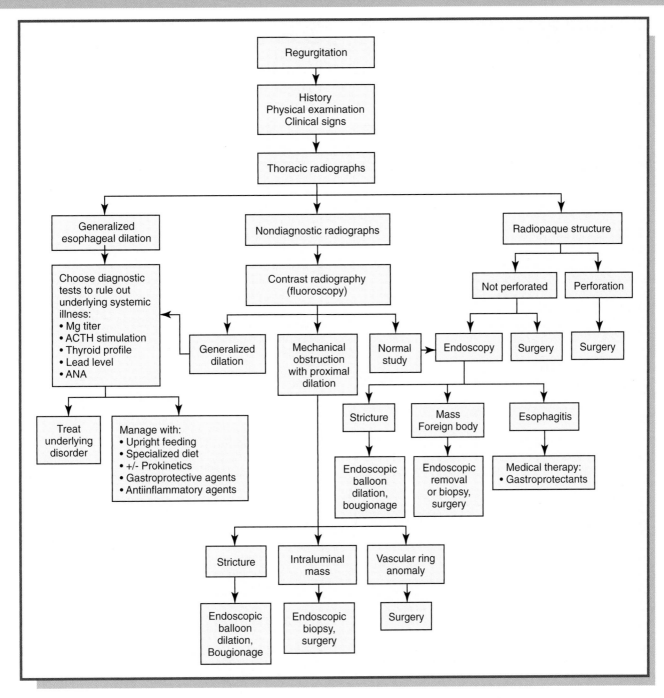

Figure 46-2 Diagnostic approach to regurgitation. *ACTH,* Adrenocorticotropic hormone; *ANA,* antinuclear antibody titer.

from congenital defects such as cricopharyngeal achalasia, which may be first observed at the time of weaning. The young to middle-aged group are more prone to mechanical obstructions (foreign bodies) or ingestion of caustic substances. Geriatric animals or those with chronic signs of disease (weight loss, anorexia) are more likely to have a systemic illness (Box 46-1).

Cricopharyngeal dysfunction has been determined to be inherited in Golden Retrievers so this breed may be overrepresented.[1]

Acute dysphagia is more likely due to an obstructive process such as a foreign body, mass, or inflammation. If other neurologic deficits coincide with dysphagia, then central nervous system diseases including neuropathies, neuromuscu-

lar junction disorders, and myopathies are likely (see Box 46-1). Hypothyroidism may be considered as a differential diagnosis in cases of cricopharyngeal achalasia.[2]

DIAGNOSIS

Complete physical examination is necessary to localize the source of dysphagia. Observation of the animal eating via recorded episode (video) or during examination may also aid in localization. A complete oral examination either under sedation or general anesthesia should be performed to identify obstructive processes (foreign body, mass) and inflammatory processes (stomatitis, periodontal disease). Neurologic exami-

Box • 46-1

Causes of Dysphagia

Obstructive Lesion (Anatomic or Mechanical)
Foreign body
Neoplasia
Inflammatory (abscess, polyp, granuloma)
Lymphadenopathy
Sialocele
Lingual frenulum disorder
Cricopharyngeal achalasia/asynchrony
Cleft palate
TMJ disorder
Trauma (fracture, luxation)

Pain
Periodontal (tooth fracture/abscess, periodontitis)
Stomatitis/glossitis/pharyngitis (viral: FeLV/FIV, immune
    mediated, caustic ingestion)
Traumatic (electric cord burn)
Retrobulbar abscess

Neurologic Disorders
Rabies
CNS disease (brainstem)
Cranial nerve disease (V, VII, IX, X, XII)

Neuromuscular Disorders
Myasthenia gravis
Inflammatory myopathy (masticatory myositis, polymyositis)
Polyradiculitis
Botulism
Tick paralysis
TMJ disease

Endocrine
Hypothyroidism

Box • 46-2

Causes of Regurgitation

Esophageal Disorder
Megaesophagus (primary or secondary)
Esophagitis
Obstructive (stricture, foreign body, vascular ring anomaly)

Alimentary Disorder
Pyloric outflow obstruction
Hiatal hernia
Gastric dilatation volvulus

Neurologic Disorder
Central nervous system (brainstem lesion, neoplastic,
    traumatic, distemper)
Peripheral neuropathy (lead, polyradiculitis, polyneuritis)
Dysautonomia

Neuromuscular Disorder
Myasthenia gravis
Botulism
Tetanus
Acetylcholinesterase toxicity

Infectious
Spirocercosis
Pythium insidiosum

Immune Mediated
Systemic lupus erythematous
Polymyositis
Dermatomyositis

Endocrine
Hypothyroidism
Hypoadrenocorticism

CNS, Central nervous system; *FeLV,* feline leukemia virus; *FIV,* feline immunodeficiency virus; *TMJ,* temporomandibular joint.

nation should also be performed (see Figure 46-1). It is important to note that since rabies is a differential diagnosis, caution should be taken during examination in any case with an index of suspicion for this disease.

Preliminary diagnostics include survey radiographs of the head, neck, and thorax. When systemic signs are present a minimum data base (complete blood cell count, serum chemistry profile, urinalysis) should be performed. Often advanced diagnostics are necessary (contrast videofluorography motion studies, endoscopy) for more definitive diagnosis (see Figure 46-1).[3]

TREATMENT

Treatment is aimed at elimination of the underlying disease process either via medical or surgical intervention. If the underlying cause cannot be treated, then management may involve dietary modification (changes in food consistency, frequency, and position of feeding) or placement of a feeding tube. Treatment of aspiration pneumonia, if present, is must also be addressed.

REGURGITATION

Regurgitation is defined as the passive expulsion of food or fluid from the esophagus or stomach. It is important to accurately distinguish regurgitation from vomiting, which is a centrally mediated reflex in which ingesta are expelled from the gastrointestinal tract (stomach, duodenum). Unlike regurgitation, vomiting is usually preceded by hypersalivation, retching, and abdominal contractions. The appearance of the expelled material along with the timing of the episode may also aid in distinguishing regurgitation from vomiting.

CLINICAL SIGNS

Regurgitation may occur immediately after eating or may be delayed for up to several hours after eating. Because ingesta may be regurgitated from the esophagus and/or stomach, the consistency of the regurgitant will vary from undigested food to digested food to clear, frothy liquid. Bilious material (yellowish-green) is not associated with regurgitation. Generalized systemic signs associated with regurgitation may include weight loss and polyphagia. Dyspnea, fever, and cough may occur if aspiration pneumonia is present.

DIAGNOSIS

Physical examination may reveal thin body condition. In severe cases of megaesophagus there may be swelling of the ventral neck due to weight loss and esophageal dilation. Thoracic auscultation may reveal harsh lung sounds if aspiration pneumonia is present. A complete neurologic examination is necessary to evaluate for the presence of neurologic deficits or neuromuscular dysfunction, which may occur with diseases such as myasthenia gravis or inflammatory myopathies (see Figure 46-2; Box 46-2).[4,5]

Survey cervical and thoracic radiographs are necessary to evaluate for generalized esophageal dilation (megaesophagus), radiopaque structures (foreign body, mass), widening of the mediastinum (thymoma), focal esophageal dilation (stricture, vascular ring anomaly), and for evidence of aspiration pneumonia. In cases where survey radiographs are nondiagnostic, contrast radiography and advanced imaging are often needed. Contrast radiography (esophagram) may be needed to better assess the size and shape of the esophagus in cases of megaesophagus and vascular ring anomalies. Endoscopic evaluation of the esophagus is useful in the evaluation of esophageal masses, foreign bodies, stricture, and esophagitis. Videofluoroscopic evaluation is used to assess motility during swallowing (esophageal dysmotility) (see Figure 46-2 and Box 46-2).

Laboratory evaluation including a minimum data base (complete blood cell count, serum chemistry, and urinalysis) is recommended any time signs of systemic illness are present with or without megaesophagus. Specialized laboratory tests may be needed depending on clinical suspicion of underlying disorders (see Box 46-2). Complete thyroid profile, adrenocorticotropic hormone (ACTH) stimulation test, acetylcholine receptor antibody test, lead level assay, and antinuclear antibody titer (ANA) should be considered (see Figure 46-2).

TREATMENT

Effective therapy is aimed at targeting the underlying disease process as well as secondary complications such as aspiration pneumonia. In cases of primary megaesophagus or esophageal dysmotility, the primary goal of therapy is to manage the regurgitation episodes. Dietary modification is a mainstay of therapy and this includes feeding small, frequent meals from an elevated position. Varying the food consistency can be very helpful and not every patient responds to liquid. Strangely, some benefit from chunky food, others soft, others liquid. Trying various formulations can help. Holding the pet upright, as if the dog's forelimbs rest across a person's legs when sitting, also can be of some help as is gentle coupage to stimulate movement of the food. Gastroprotective therapy is often warranted to prevent reflux esophagitis, especially in cases where there is gastric regurgitation. The effectiveness of prokinetic therapy (cisapride, metoclopramide) is controversial but may enhance lower esophageal sphincter pressure and tone in the esophageal body. Cisapride may be a more effective prokinetic agent in the cat due to its larger effect on cholinergically innervated muscle. A recent publication revealed a positive correlation between the cyclooxygenase-2 inhibitor celecoxib (Celebrex) on increasing lower esophageal pressure without affecting gastric emptying time in dogs.[6] Therapy with nonsteroidal antiinflammatory agents labeled as COX-2 inhibitors may warrant further consideration.

REFERENCES

The reference list can be found on the companion Expert Consult Web site at *www.expertconsult.com*.

CHAPTER 47

Vomiting

David C. Twedt

Vomiting is a common clinical sign in small animals that is frequently associated with gastrointestinal disorders but can occur with nongastrointestinal conditions as well. These possible causes for vomiting may make identifying the etiology more elusive and may result in the need for an extensive diagnostic workup in some dogs and cats.

The evolution of vomiting began as a protective means for removing toxic or noxious ingested substances from the gastrointestinal tract. This process has evolved so that when many toxic substances are absorbed into the blood stream they also initiate vomiting. Consequently, vomiting now results from both neural and humoral signals initiated by a variety of disorders including the gastrointestinal system, nongastrointestinal abdominal conditions, systemic or metabolic disease, drugs, toxins, or conditions involving the central nervous system (CNS). Our understanding of the pathophysiology of vomiting and its therapy has advanced considerably with the recognition of specific emetic receptors found throughout the body. The metabolic and physical consequences of vomiting can also be serious, potentially resulting in volume depletion, acid-base and electrolyte disturbances, esophagitis, aspiration pneumonia, and malnutrition. This chapter will cover basic pathophysiology, etiologies, and a practical clinical approach to the diagnosis and management of the vomiting patient.

PATHOPHYSIOLOGY

The physical act of vomiting can be divided into three components: nausea, retching, and expulsion of gastric contents. Nausea precedes vomiting and is associated with an episode that defies exact definition. Outward signs of nausea may include depression, shivering, hiding, yawning, and licking of the lips. Increased salivation and swallowing occur, which serve to lubricate the esophagus with bicarbonate-rich saliva that will neutralize gastric acid as stomach contents pass through. Next, there is a reduction in gastric, lower-esophageal sphincter and esophageal motility followed by increased retrograde motility of the proximal small intestine. Retching, the second phase in the vomiting process, often helps distinguish the episode from regurgitation, gagging, or coughing. Retching is the forceful contraction of the abdominal muscles and diaphragm producing negative intrathoracic pressure and positive abdominal pressure. These pressure changes cause the movement of gastric contents into the esophagus and out the mouth. The driving force is contraction of the abdominal muscles and diaphragm causing intrathoracic pressure changes from negative during retching to positive during vomiting. As the vomited material passes through the pharynx, respiration is inhibited and the nasopharynx and glottis close to prevent aspiration.

The vomiting act is initiated in the CNS. In the medulla oblongata of the brainstem are a number of nuclei that collectively have been referred to as the *emetic center*. These nuclei and their complex, integrated nerve pathways are responsible for initiating vomiting. At the present time this area is known to be abundant in serotonergic (5HT$_3$), adrenergic (α_2), and neurokinergic (NK$_1$) receptors. Activation of these receptors in the emetic center occurs either indirectly through a humoral pathway by bloodborne substances activating the chemoreceptor trigger zone (CRTZ) or by other various neural pathways leading to the emetic center (Figure 47-1).

Knowledge of likely receptors involved in the vomiting process aids in selection of specific antiemetics.

Neural stimulation of the emetic center arises through either afferent vagal, sympathetic, vestibular, cerebrocortical, or the adjacent nucleus tractus solitarius pathways. Activation of specific peripheral receptors found throughout the body initiate these stimuli. Particularly important are receptors located throughout the abdominal viscera. The duodenum contains the highest concentration of receptors and hence has been referred to as the "organ of nausea." 5HT$_3$ and NK$_1$ receptors are abundant on vagal afferent neurons, other neurons, and smooth muscle in the gastrointestinal tract. Gastrointestinal disorders directly stimulate vomiting through vagal afferent pathways. Certain inflammatory or cytotoxic factors cause the release of serotonin or substance P from local enterochromaffin cells that activate 5HT$_3$ and NK$_1$ receptors respectively on afferent vagal nerves. Receptors in the kidneys, uterus, and urinary bladder send afferent impulses via sympathetic nerves. Receptors located in the pharynx and tonsillar fossae transmit impulses thorough afferent fibers of the glossopharyngeal nerve. CNS disease will also directly activate the emetic center through pathways that lead to the emetic center. Adjacent to the emetic center in the medulla is the *nucleus tractus solitarii*, which is rich in NK$_1$ receptors. This area also plays a role in activating the emetic center.

Vomiting can also be stimulated by humoral factors in the blood. Such substances activate receptors in the CRTZ, located in the area postrema at the base of the fourth ventricle. The CRTZ is devoid of a blood brain barrier, which allows exposure to chemical stimuli found in the circulation: certain drugs, uremic toxins, electrolytes, osmolar and acid-base disorders, as well as a number of metabolic derangements. Dopaminergic (D$_2$), cholinergic (M$_1$), histaminergic (H$_1$), serotonergic (5HT$_3$), adrenergic (α_2), and neurokinergic (NK$_1$) receptors are associated with the CRTZ and act as excitatory transmitters of neurons leading to the emetic center. Enkephalinergic (ENK) receptors are also thought to occur in the CRTZ, but their exact role is poorly understood. Cats have poorly developed D$_2$ and H$_1$ receptors while their α_2 receptors are more important in vomiting but less important in the dog. Cats usually do not respond to the emetic effects of apomorphine and histamine, but xylazine, a α_2 agonist, is a potent emetic in the cat.

Vestibular stimulation passes through the CRTZ before activating the emetic center. Motion sickness, inflammation of the labyrinth, or lesions in the cerebellum result in vomiting via this pathway. Cholinergic (M$_1$), histaminergic (H$_1$) and possibly neurokinergic (NK$_1$) receptors are associated with vestibular pathways that pass through the CRTZ on the way to the emetic center.

CAUSES

Vomiting has a vast number of etiologies. Box 47-1 presents some of the more common causes of vomiting in small animals.

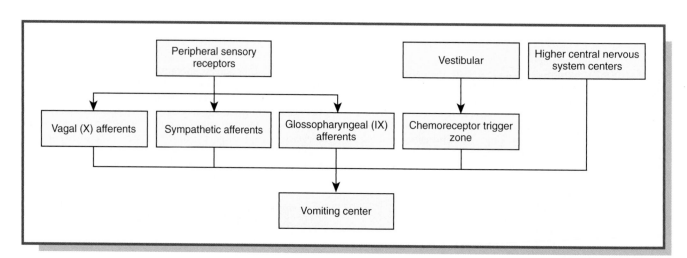

Figure 47-1 Factors that activate the vomiting center.

Box • 47-1

Common Causes of Vomiting

Metabolic/Endocrine Disorders
Uremia
Hypoadrenocorticism
Diabetes mellitus
Hyperthyroidism
Hepatic disease
Endotoxemia/septicemia
Hepatic encephalopathy
Electrolyte disorders
Acid-base disorders

Intoxicants
Lead
Ethylene glycol
Zinc
Strychnine

Drugs
Cardiac glycosides
Erythromycin
Chemotherapy agents
Apomorphine
Xylazine
Penicillamine
Tetracycline
Nonsteroidal antinflammatory drugs (NSAIDs)

Abdominal Disorders
Pancreatitis
Peritonitis
Neoplasia
Hepatobiliary disease

Dietary Causes
Indiscretions
Intolerances
Allergies

Gastric Disorders
Gastritis
Helicobacter infection
Parasites
Ulceration
Neoplasia
Foreign bodies
Dilatation-volvulus
Hiatal hernia
Obstruction
Motility disorders

Disorders of the Small Intestine
Inflammatory bowel disease
Neoplasia
Foreign body
Intussusception
Parasites
Parvovirus
Bacterial overgrowth

Disorders of the Large Intestine
Colitis
Obstipation
Parasites

CLINICAL APPROACH

A complete history is the first step in trying to establish a cause for vomiting. The signalment and history, as well as a description of the vomiting episodes, are important. First, one must determine whether the animal actually is vomiting. The veterinarian should always differentiate the owner's report of vomiting from gagging, coughing, dysphagia, or regurgitation. The description of retching is characteristic for vomiting. Signalment may also be helpful. For example, young, unvaccinated pets are more susceptible to infectious disease, such as parvovirus. Vaccination status, travel history, previous medical problems, and the medication history should be determined. Many drugs can result in vomiting, such as nonsteroidal antiinflammatory drugs (NSAIDs), which are known to cause gastrointestinal ulceration and vomiting. The clinician should also investigate the possibility of toxin or foreign body ingestion and of other concurrent signs that often arise with systemic or metabolic disease. For example, polydipsia, polyuria, and weight loss are typical of vomiting associated with diabetic ketoacidosis or chronic kidney failure.

The history should then focus on the actual vomiting episodes. The duration, frequency, and relationship of the episodes to eating or drinking should be determined. One should note a complete physical description of the vomited material. A dietary history, including the type of diet or recent dietary changes, is important because vomiting may be associated with an adverse reaction to food. Vomiting of an undigested or a partly digested meal more than 6 to 8 hours after eating, a time at which the stomach should normally be empty, suggests a gastric outflow obstruction or gastric hypomotility disorder. Gastric outflow obstructions can be caused by foreign bodies, mucosal hypertrophy, tumors, or polyps. The description of the vomit should include the volume, color, consistency, odor, and the presence or absence of bile or blood. Undigested food suggests a gastric origin, whereas vomit-containing bile makes a gastric outflow obstruction unlikely. Vomit having a fecal odor suggests a low-intestinal obstruction or bacterial overgrowth in the small intestine. The presence of blood in the vomit (hematemesis), either as fresh, bright-red blood or as digested blood with the appearance of coffee grounds, indicates gastrointestinal erosion or ulceration. Gastric ulceration is caused by metabolic conditions such as hypoadrenocorticism, reaction to certain drugs, clotting abnormalities, gastritis, or neoplasia.

A complete physical examination should include careful evaluation of the mouth and oral cavity. This examination may reveal icteric membranes with liver disease, uremic breath, and oral ulceration with kidney disease, or the presence of a linear foreign body wrapped around the base of the tongue. The presence of a fever would suggest an infectious or inflammatory process. Bradycardia or cardiac arrhythmias in a vomiting animal may be a sign of a metabolic disturbance, such as hypoadrenocorticism. The abdomen should be carefully palpated for distention or tympany (e.g., gastric dilatation–volvulus [GDV] syndrome), effusion (e.g., peritonitis), masses or organomegaly (e.g., neoplasia, intussusception, or foreign body), and pain (e.g., peritonitis, pancreatitis, or intestinal obstruction). The presence of gas- and fluid-filled intestines suggests obstruction, whereas bunching of the bowel is characteristic of intestinal plication from a linear foreign body obstruction. A rectal examination provides characteristics of colonic mucosa and feces. Melena suggests upper-gastrointestinal bleeding while the presence of foreign material in the feces supports a possible foreign body etiology. Animals that have colitis or that are severely obstipated may also vomit.

Investigation of the CNS should be considered when the cause of the vomiting is not obvious. Vomiting occurs in some animals with vestibular disease (e.g., nystagmus, head tilt, and/or ataxia). Other CNS disease may be less obvious, usually require a thorough neurologic evaluation, and occasionally imaging studies. Some dogs with intervertebral disk disease vomit due to pain or secondary intestinal ileus.

DIAGNOSTIC PLAN

Based on the history and physical examination, the animal should be classified as having either acute or chronic vomiting. The diagnostic and therapeutic approaches differ considerably based on one's clinical classification (Figures 47-2 and 47-3).

If vomiting episodes are acute and recent (<5 days in duration), they may be self-limiting. Such conditions are treated symptomatically with minimal diagnostic investigation. Most often, acute vomiting is associated with gastroenteritis secondary to dietary indiscretions and signs resolve quickly. A routine fecal examination for parasites should be performed in all animals with gastrointestinal signs to eliminate the possibility of parasitism. Investigation for environmental intoxicants is imperative. Young, unvaccinated dogs should always be evaluated for parvovirus. Parvovirus-related illness frequently begins with vomiting prior to the onset of diarrhea. Radiographic studies may be necessary to confirm GDV syndrome, gastrointestinal foreign bodies, or obstructions. Severe acute

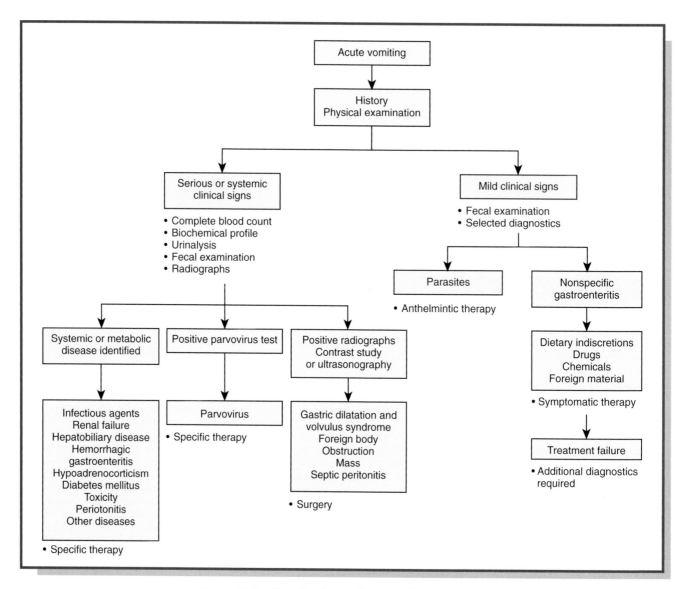

Figure 47-2   Algorithm for the diagnosis of acute vomiting.

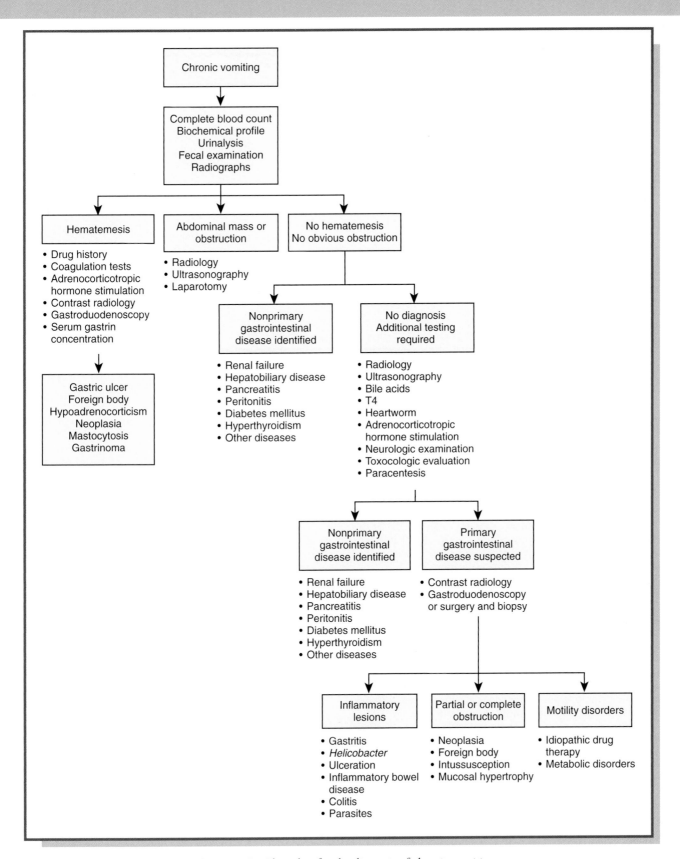

Figure 47-3 Algorithm for the diagnosis of chronic vomiting.

Table • 47-1

Classification of Common Antiemetics with Site of Action and Common Side Effects

RECEPTOR ANTAGONIST	DRUG EXAMPLES	SITE OF ACTION	COMMENT
α_2 (adrenergic)*	Chlorpromazine	CRTZ, emetic center	Sedation, hypotension
	Prochlorperizine	CRTZ, emetic center	Sedation, hypotension
D_2 (dopaminergic)†	Chlorpromazine	CRTZ	Sedation, hypotension
	Prochlorperizine	CRTZ	Sedation, hypotension
	Metoclopramide (low dose)	CRTZ	Extrapyramidal signs
$5HT_3$ (serotonergic)	Dolasetron	CRTZ, emetic center, vagal afferents	Unknown
	Ondansetron	CRTZ, emetic center, vagal afferents	Unknown
	Metoclopramide (high dose)	CRTZ	Extrapyramidal signs
NK_1 (neurokinergic)	Maropitant	CRTZ, emetic center, vagal afferents, (vestibular?)	Unknown
M_1 (cholinergic)	Chlorpromazine	CRTZ	Sedation, hypotension
	Prochlorperizine	CRTZ	Sedation, hypotension
	Scopalamine	CRTZ, vestibular	Sedation, gastrointestinal hypomotility
H_1 (histaminergic)†	Chlorpromazine	CRTZ	Sedation, hypotension
	Prochlorperizine	CRTZ	Sedation, hypotension
	Diphenhydramine	CRTZ, vestibular	Sedation

CRTZ, Chemoreceptor trigger zone.
*Possibly less important in dogs.
†Poorly developed in cats.

vomiting or vomiting with concurrent systemic signs requires laboratory diagnostic evaluation and radiographic testing. Common systemic and metabolic diseases that can cause vomiting can be identified with basic diagnostic testing. This "minimum data base" includes a complete blood count (CBC), biochemical blood screen, urinalysis, and fecal examination.

Chronic vomiting, generally characterized as vomiting that has persisted for longer than 5 to 7 days or that has failed to respond to initial symptomatic therapy, requires in-depth investigation. In the majority of dogs and cats that have chronic vomiting, routine laboratory and survey radiographs either provide an etiology or direct the next diagnostic or therapeutic step.

Vomiting may result in significant fluid, electrolyte, and acid-base alterations. The most common electrolyte disturbance from vomiting is hypokalemia. Acid-base changes generally are minimal or, if abnormal, tend toward an acidosis. However, if metabolic alkalosis is identified and is associated with hyponatremia, hypochloremia, and hypokalemia, the cause is most likely gastric outflow or high-duodenal obstruction. Rarely animals with gastrinomas or with frequent and unrelenting vomiting have a metabolic alkalosis. When routine diagnostic testing fails to identify an obvious etiology, additional tests may be required. These tests may include viral or heartworm serology, thyroid hormone testing, adrenocortical testing for hypoadrenocorticism, bile acid determination for liver disease, toxologic testing (e.g., lead poisoning), and a neurologic examination.

When testing fails to identify a nongastrointestinal cause for the vomiting, the focus should move to investigation of gastrointestinal disease as a possible etiology. The diagnostic approach includes contrast radiography, ultrasonography, endoscopy, or laparotomy. Frequently, inflammatory gastrointestinal lesions are a cause of chronic vomiting; these conditions include chronic gastritis, *Helicobacter* gastritis, inflammatory bowel disease (IBD), and chronic colitis. The diagnosis should be confirmed with gastrointestinal biopsies. Cats with inflammatory bowel disease often have vomiting as the predominate clinical sign and diarrhea as a minor clinical component. Conditions such as gastric antral pyloric mucosal hypertrophy, antral polyps, foreign bodies, or neoplasia can cause gastric outflow obstruction. These conditions cause gastric retention and vomiting. Such gastric lesions can be easily identified endoscopically or using contrast radiography. Rarely, dogs that have persistent vomiting with hematemesis that is unresponsive to standard therapy have a gastrinoma; increased serum gastrin concentrations support the diagnosis.

Obstructive intestinal lesions, such as foreign bodies, intussusception, and neoplasia, usually require radiographic contrast studies or ultrasonography for diagnosis. The diagnosis of gastrointestinal motility disorders should be considered when clinical signs support abnormal gastric retention and inflammatory or obstructive gastrointestinal lesions cannot be identified. Specialized contrast studies that evaluate motility, or possibly a clinical response to gastrointestinal prokinetic agents, would support a diagnosis of gastric hypomotility.

TREATMENT

There are a number of antiemetic agents available for treating vomiting that work directly on specific neurotransmitter receptors that have been described. Before employing such drugs, it is important to attempt determining etiology of the vomiting and to correct that underlying cause. Treating the primary disease successfully resolves vomiting in most cases. For example, the patient with acute self-limiting gastroenteritis generally improves following fluid support and withholding food for 24 hours. The indiscriminate use of antiemetics may mask the primary disease and delay diagnosis or appropriate therapy. The rational use of antiemetic therapy, which includes preventing fluid and electrolyte losses and prevention of aspiration pneumonia, improves patient comfort. Antiemetic therapy favors an early return to nutrition. Common uses include prevention of vomiting due to motion sickness, cancer chemotherapy, and vomiting from conditions such as uremia, pancreatitis, parvovirus, or acute gastroenteritis. Table 47-1 lists some of the common antiemetics used in small animals.

CHAPTER 48

Diarrhea

Michael D. Willard

Diarrhea is caused by excess fecal water that may result from decreased intestinal absorption and/or increased intestinal secretion. Small intestinal disease causes diarrhea only if the material exiting the ileum exceeds the absorptive capacity of the colon or causes colonic secretion of water. Thus, diarrhea means there is intestinal disease, but a lack of diarrhea does not eliminate significant small intestinal disease. Many dogs and cats without diarrhea experience severe morbidity or die due to small intestinal disease. In contrast, large intestinal disease commonly causes diarrhea because there is no segment of intestine distal to this area for absorption of water. Patient activity plays an important role in fecal consistency; active patients are more likely to defecate than inactive ones (e.g., those confined to a cage or crate). Thus, a patient that has not had diarrhea while confined to a hospital cage may have diarrhea shortly after going home and resuming normal activity.

DIAGNOSIS

One must first decide if diarrhea is worth the cost or effort to diagnose or treat (Figure 48-1).

Examples that should be attended to include diarrhea that (1) has a relatively small set of testable differentials, (2) is a predominant problem in the patient, or (3) is likely to cause morbidity or mortality. Diarrhea secondary to nongastrointestinal (GI) disease is usually relatively minor, and often there are historical and physical examination findings, as well as laboratory or imaging changes that are more pressing and/or more likely to quickly lead to a diagnosis. Examples of non-GI diseases causing diarrhea include acute pancreatitis, hepatic insufficiency, renal failure, and hypoadrenocorticism. Hyperthyroidism is an important non-GI cause of feline diarrhea.

The clinician should next look for and deal with "obvious" problems (e.g., heavy intestinal parasite burdens, poor-quality food, major dietary indiscretion, contagious disease). Some parasites (e.g., giardiasis) can be difficult to diagnose. Next, one should determine whether diarrhea is acute or chronic. "Acute" means nonepisodic diarrhea occurring for less than 7 to 14 days. These dogs and cats either have diarrhea that is clinically nonthreatening or they may have potentially severe diarrhea that places the patient at risk (e.g., hemorrhagic gastroenteritis; infectious, febrile gastroenteritis-like parvovirus). Most patients with acute, nonthreatening diarrhea spontaneously resolve with symptomatic/supportive therapy (e.g., anthelmintics, dietary change). Diagnostics in these patients are usually limited to fecal examinations and select laboratory tests (e.g., electrolytes, packed-cell volume [PCV]). Acute, severe diarrhea capable of causing morbidity/mortality is an indication for at least complete blood count (CBC) and serum biochemistry panel.

Diarrhea not clearly improving in approximately 14 days is considered chronic. Episodic diarrhea may also be considered chronic. Chronic diarrhea should be subdivided into large or small bowel disease. Volume and frequency of bowel movements as well as vomiting are usually not helpful in making this distinction. Weight loss, hematochezia, and fecal mucus are more reliable criteria. Small intestines absorb nutrients; therefore, loss of body weight and/or condition are expected when it is chronically and substantially diseased. Steatorrhea is infrequent and melena distinctly rare in these patients. The large intestine absorbs water and acts as a reservoir for feces until defecation. Therefore, weight loss is unexpected in large bowel disease unless the disease is severe, in which case hematochezia and fecal mucus are typical. Hematochezia and fecal mucus are uncommon when colonic disease is mild to moderate. Tenesmus may occur if the rectal area is affected.

The next decision in patients with chronic small intestinal disease is whether maldigestion (e.g., exocrine pancreatic insufficiency [EPI]) or malabsorption exists. Rare in cats, EPI is an important consideration in dogs. Serum trypsin–like immunoreactivity (TLI) is the most sensitive and specific test for EPI. Once EPI is eliminated, malabsorptive disease is diagnosed by exclusion.

Malabsorptive disease is divided into protein-losing enteropathy (PLE) and non-PLE. This distinction is important because severe hypoalbuminemia is associated with a poor prognosis, and PLE is usually an indication for an aggressive diagnostic approach. Protein-losing enteropathy is typically only considered in hypoalbuminemic patients, but PLE is a concern whenever serum albumin concentrations progressively decrease. One must measure serum albumin; serum total protein is inadequate. Panhypoproteinemia is neither sensitive nor specific for PLE, especially where hyperglobulinemia is common. Serum albumin concentrations < 2.0 g/dL are an indication for hepatic function testing and urinalysis, eliminating hepatic insufficiency and protein-losing nephropathy diagnoses PLE by exclusion. Fecal alpha-1 protease inhibitor concentrations can be helpful when PLE is suspected but cannot be diagnosed by exclusion. Most PLE and hepatic insufficiency patients are hypocholesterolemic while many protein-losing nephropathy patients are hypercholesterolemic. Imaging, endoscopy, and biopsy are usually desirable in PLE patients, but therapeutic trials (e.g., ultra–low-fat diet for lymphangiectasia) are done if anesthetic risk is too great or client constraints dictate otherwise.

Any GI disease may cause PLE, but the most common causes in adult dogs are probably lymphangiectasia, lymphoma, fungal infections (regional), and inflammatory bowel disease (IBD). Lymphangiectasia can be difficult to diagnose unless one is aware of its subtleties. Occult parasitism and chronic intussusception are important in younger dogs. In cats, IBD and lymphoma are the main causes. Other causes include ulcers/erosions, antibiotic-responsive disease, and intestinal crypt lesions.

The major causes of non-PLE malabsorptive disease in dogs are dietary-responsive disease, antibiotic-responsive disease, and parasites. IBD is often listed as an important cause. A full discussion is beyond the scope of this chapter, but there is concern that IBD has been overdiagnosed in the past because IBD is not simply a histologic diagnosis. One must find inflammation and eliminate known causes (e.g., diet, parasites, bac-

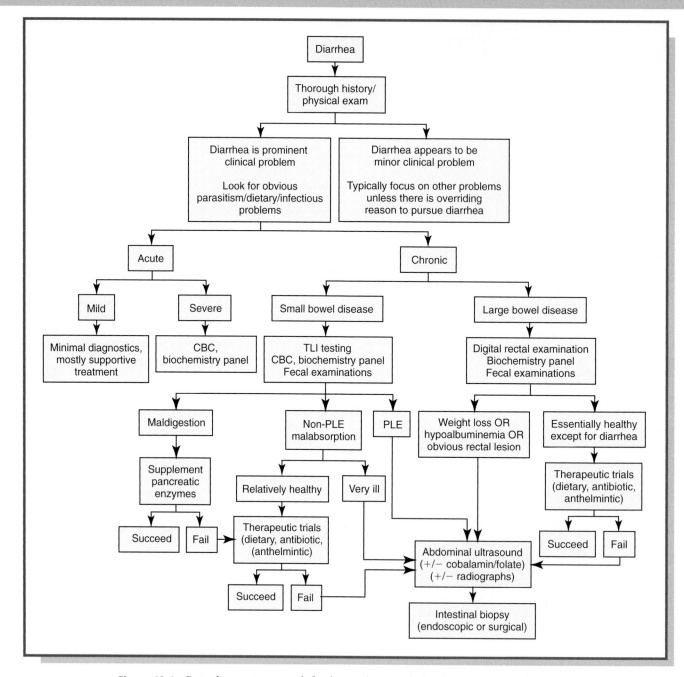

Figure 48-1   Basic diagnostic approach for dogs and cats with diarrhea. This approach may need to be modified, based upon specific situations. *CBC,* Complete blood count; *PLE,* protein-losing enteropathy; *TLI,* trypsinlike immunoreactivity.

teria). In cats, dietary-responsive disease, lymphoma, and IBD appear to be the most common causes, but hyperthyroidism closely mimics primary GI disease.

TREATMENT

The next step depends upon the patient's clinical condition. If a dog or cat is in relatively good health and not at major risk should a 2- to 3-week therapeutic trial fail, then one may elect to first treat for dietary-responsive, antibiotic-responsive, and/or parasitic disease. The first two diseases generally do not produce pathognomonic histologic lesions. If one cannot take a chance on investing 2 to 3 weeks in a therapeutic trial because of the advanced nature or rapid progression of disease,

then aggressive diagnostics are indicated. Abdominal ultrasound helps detect focal GI lesions that may be aspirated percutaneously (e.g., lymphoma, fungal infection) and may reveal whether GI disease is clearly diffuse or localized outside the reach of an endoscope. Ultrasound is specific but insensitive for GI lesions; absence of ultrasonographic changes does not eliminate serious GI disease.

Intestinal biopsy (surgical or endoscopic) is typically the next step after ultrasound. Faster, safer, and less expensive than surgery, endoscopy often allows one to find and biopsy focal mucosal lesions that cannot be seen from the serosal surface at surgery. This ability to direct biopsies enhances the chance to make a histologic diagnosis. Endoscopic biopsies of the ileum can be important in patients with GI disease; some diseases (e.g., lymphoma, IBD, lymphangiectasia) may be diagnosed there when they cannot be diagnosed with duodenal samples (even when ultrasonography does not show any obvious difference between the two sites). Endoscopy is typically more than adequate to obtain diagnostic samples if the operator has had adequate training in taking and submitting biopsies. Endoscopic biopsies should routinely include the full thickness of the intestinal mucosa (with or without muscularis mucosa). If one is not trained in taking high-quality endoscopic samples, it may be better to perform surgical biopsies or refer the patient for endoscopy. Full-thickness intestinal biopsies will not help if they are taken where there is no lesion, and intestinal disease (including severe intestinal disease) may be patchy. Diseased intestine outside the reach of the endoscope and intestines with dense, submucosal infiltrates are indications for surgical biopsy. It is rare that diagnosis requires adequate submucosal tissue in small intestinal diseases.

Chronic canine large bowel disease tends to be dietary-responsive, fiber-responsive, "clostridial" colitis (i.e., tylosin-responsive), and parasitic. Histoplasmosis and pythiosis are regionally important. Cats tend to have dietary-responsive, clostridial, parasitic (e.g., *Tritrichomonas*), and IBD colitis. Digital rectal examination should be performed in dogs to look for focal lesions (e.g., polyps) or mucosal thickening. Dogs from endemic areas should generally be treated for whipworms even if fecal examinations do not reveal ova. Dogs and cats that are otherwise normal except for diarrhea, have no rectal lesions, and have normal serum albumin may often be successfully approached with therapeutic trials because: (1) the best way to diagnose dietary-responsive disease, fiber-responsive disease, and tylosin-responsive disease is by therapeutic trial; and (2) these animals are unlikely to worsen rapidly should the trial fail. Patients from areas endemic for histoplasmosis and those having lost weight or become hypoalbuminemic should undergo testing (i.e., abdominal ultrasound, rectal scraping, colonoscopy/biopsy) because of their potential to suddenly become worse. Rectal scrapping/cytology is an easy, quick, and specific (albeit insensitive) screening test for colonic histoplasmosis. Colonic biopsy should be done endoscopically; full-thickness colonic incisions have substantial risk of dehiscence and peritonitis. Rigid biopsy forceps typically obtain large tissue samples with lots of submucosa (which is especially important in rectal lesions).

Abdominal radiographs do not commonly yield valuable information unless they detect an unsuspected radiopaque foreign body. Fecal cultures tend to be a low-yield procedure unless the history strongly suggests contagion. Furthermore, simply finding "pathogenic" bacteria does not mean that they are responsible for clinical signs. Finally, it is critical to contact the laboratory for instructions on collection and submission relative to the specific pathogen(s) being sought.

Measuring serum cobalamin and folate concentrations can be helpful in select dogs and cats. Hypocobalaminemia is relatively specific for small intestinal disease; however, sensitivity is questionable. Cobalamin and folate determinations are insensitive and nonspecific for canine antibiotic-responsive (i.e., small intestinal bacterial overgrowth) disease. Hypocobalaminemia in an animal with weight loss, but without diarrhea, is strong evidence of small intestinal disease; however, normal values are not helpful. Cobalamin supplementation can benefit hypocobalaminemic cats, and hypocobalaminemia may be prognostic in dogs.

REFERENCES

The reference list can be found on the companion Expert Consult Web site at *www.expertconsult.com*.

CHAPTER **49**

Melena and Hematochezia

Valerie L. Case

The key to evaluating a patient presenting with melena or hematochezia is a thorough history and physical examination. The results of these initials steps will help to quickly localize the source of hemorrhage and aid in the development of a diagnostic and therapeutic plan.

MELENA

DEFINITION

Melena is defined as a black, tarry stool created by the digestion of blood in the proximal gastrointestinal tract. The breakdown products of hemoglobin produce the black color (Figure 49-1).

Sources of blood to consider are the respiratory tract, where blood may be coughed up (hemoptysis) and swallowed, and the proximal gastrointestinal tract including the oral cavity, stomach, and duodenum. A black stool color may also be produced by antidiarrheal medications containing bismuth and salicylate as well as by diets containing raw meat, leading to a spurious diagnosis of melena (Figure 49-2).

A wide variety of diseases have the potential to cause melena (Box 49-1).

The majority of these conditions result in gastrointestinal hemorrhage and melena by directly or indirectly disrupting mucosal barriers to injury. Defense mechanisms utilized by the gastrointestinal mucosa include: a hydrophobic mucus layer and hydrophobic nature of mucosal cells, mucosal secretion of bicarbonate, epidermal growth factor and epithelial restitution, a high rate of mucosal blood flow, and prostaglandins. Detailed explanations of these mechanisms can be located elsewhere in the textbook.

DIAGNOSIS

Assessing a patient who presents with melena is aided first by determining the source of digested blood: respiratory or gas-

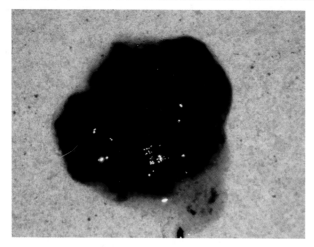

Figure 49-1 Melena. Note the dark black color created by the breakdown of hemoglobin in the proximal small intestine.

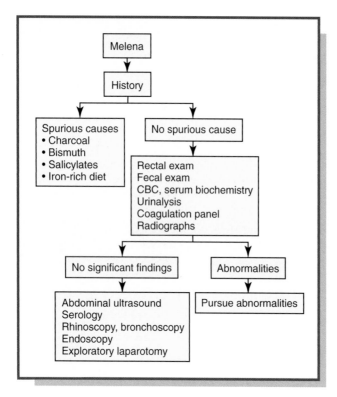

Figure 49-2 Diagnostic approach to melena. *CBC*, Complete blood count.

Box • 49-1

Causes of Melena

Ingestion of blood
 Oral lesions
 Nasopharyngeal lesions
 Pulmonary lesions
 Diet
Inflammation
 Esophagitis
 Gastroenteritis
 Inflammatory bowel disease
Infection
 Campylobacter
 Clostridium perfringens
 Salmonella
 Parvovirus
 Neorickettsia helminthoeca (salmon poisoning)
 Histoplasma
 Pythium
Parasitism
 Hookworms
Neoplasia
 Lymphoma
 Adenocarcinoma
 Mast cell tumor
 Leiomyoma/Leiomyosarcoma
 Gastrinoma
 Polyps
Trauma
 Foreign body
Drug-associated
 Nonsteroidal antiinflammatories
 Corticosteroids
Coagulopathy
 Thrombocytopenia
 Specific factor deficiencies
 Rodenticide toxicity
 Disseminated intravascular coagulation
Pancreatitis
Hypoadrenocorticism
Hepatic disease
Renal disease

---

trointestinal. The owner's history and the physical examination can most often answer this question. Owners must be asked specific questions concerning drug administration, diet, and potential for exposure to toxins. Determine immediately if the owner administered bismuth subsalicylate, or if the patient has ingested raw red meat (especially liver), spleen, or beets. By first ruling out causes for black stool other than respiratory or gastrointestinal hemorrhage, the focus can shift toward diagnosing significant pathology (see Figure 49-1). Question the owners about the presence of clinical signs other than melena. Exercise intolerance, coughing, tachypnea, or dyspnea raise suspicion for disease of the respiratory tract, while anorexia, regurgitation, vomiting, and abdominal tenderness signify a gastrointestinal origin of disease. Ask specifi-

cally about administration of corticosteroids and nonsteroidal antiinflammatory drugs (NSAIDs). Both will reduce the production of protective prostaglandins by inhibiting either cyclooxygenase (NSAIDs) or phospholipase A_2 (corticosteroids), thus leading to gastric mucosal injury through a variety of mechanisms. NSAIDs also cause direct damage to gastric cells and their protective mucus layer. The concurrent use of NSAIDs and corticosteroids appears to confer the greatest risk for gastric ulceration and erosion (GUE). Determine whether the patient had any opportunity (observed or intimated) to ingest anticoagulant rodenticides, corrosive compounds, trash containing raw or decaying meat, or foreign bodies. Be clear about the patient's origin and travel history to include appropriate infectious disease on the list of differential diagnoses.

Approach the physical examination armed with the owner's historical information, and with a focus on the respiratory and gastrointestinal systems. Thoroughly examine the nares and oral cavity for active hemorrhage or lesions with the potential to bleed and cause swallowing of blood. Patients with moderate to severe blood loss will display mucous membrane pallor, and petechiae may be noted if coagulopathy is present. Carefully auscultate the lung fields for abnormal sounds supporting the presence of pulmonary disease. Thoroughly palpate the abdomen for sites of pain, organomegaly, and masses. Patients with significant gastrointestinal pathology often display abdominal pain either focally or generally. Hepatomegaly may be palpable in patients with ulceration secondary to liver disease. Intestinal loops may be distended due to mechanical or functional ileus, and distinct masses may be palpable in cases of intestinal neoplasia or other infiltrative bowel disease. A digital rectal exam must be included to confirm the presence of melena, obtain a stool sample for fecal testing, and for assessment of mucosal abnormalities, prostatomegaly, and sublumbar lymph node enlargement. Although gastrointestinal disease causing melena primarily affects the stomach and proximal small intestine, the lower gastrointestinal tract may be involved concurrently.

After confirming the presence of true melena and the likely source of hemorrhage, diagnostic testing will provide objective support for the abnormalities discovered in the history and physical exam, with the goal of reaching a definitive diagnosis or formulating a short list of differential diagnoses. The minimum data base for a patient with melena includes a complete blood count (CBC), serum biochemistry panel, urinalysis, activated partial thromboplastin time (APTT) and one-stage prothrombin time (OSPT), fecal flotation and direct exams, and thoracic and abdominal radiographs. Anemia is the most common finding on the CBC of a patient with melena. The anemia can be mild to severe, and a regenerative response may be evident if sufficient time has elapsed. Chronic low-grade hemorrhage will result in a nonregenerative anemia. Thrombocytopenia may be present as a primary cause for melena, or as a secondary disorder due to consumption. Leukocytes may be decreased, within normal range, or increased as a result of the underlying disease. Common abnormalities on the serum biochemistry include elevated blood urea nitrogen (BUN), and hypoalbuminemia or panhypoproteinemia owing to whole blood loss and/or protein-losing enteropathy (PLE). Elevated hepatic enzymes and azotemia should raise suspicions for liver or renal disease as the primary cause for gastrointestinal hemorrhage. Hyponatremia is often a finding in cases of hemorrhage, as well as in cases of hypoadrenocorticism in conjunction with hyperkalemia. A urinalysis is performed for evaluation of concurrent disease, including differentiating cases of azotemia. Prolonged coagulation times will aid in diagnosing cases of rodenticide toxicity and disseminated intravascular coagulation (DIC). A variety of gastrointestinal parasites, enterotoxigenic bacteria, and other organisms can create melena. Fecal flotation, direct saline preparation, and stained cytologic smears are required for assessment of many of these causative agents. Radiographic imaging of the thorax and abdomen will further differentiate respiratory versus gastrointestinal sources of melena. Clearly definable lung patterns will likely be present in cases of hemoptysis. Abdominal radiographic abnormalities include radiopaque foreign bodies, abnormal size and shape of abdominal organs, mass effects, and abnormal gas and fluid patterns within the gastrointestinal tract.

Definitive diagnosis of the underlying cause of melena often requires advanced diagnostic techniques beyond the minimum data base. Specific serologic testing, fecal cultures, abdominal ultrasound, bronchoscopy, endoscopy, and exploratory laparotomy are some of the more common additional diagnostics that may be pursued. Refer to other chapters for explanations of techniques and the diagnostics required for specific disease processes.

TREATMENT

Treatment applied to patients presenting with melena will vary depending on the underlying cause. Many patients will benefit from medical therapy addressing GUE. Pharmaceuticals used in the prevention and treatment of GUE work via mechanisms that decrease intraluminal acidity and promote mucosal defense mechanisms. Histamine$_2$ (H$_2$) receptor antagonists, proton-pump inhibitors, and synthetic prostaglandin analogues are commonly used in combination as part of an overall therapeutic plan. These drugs are presented in detail in other chapters and resources.

HEMATOCHEZIA

DEFINITION

Hematochezia is defined as stool containing fresh, undigested blood originating from the colon, rectum, or anus (Figure 49-3).

Some overlap exists between the potential causes of melena and hematochezia; however, differentiating the two clinical signs is important in order to formulate the most appropriate diagnostic and therapeutic plans.

DIAGNOSIS

Similar to the approach to melena described above, thorough history taking and physical exam are paramount to successfully diagnosing hematochezia and its underlying cause (Box 49-2).

Ask questions concerning recent stress the patient may have experienced, abrupt dietary changes or indiscretion, and potential for exposure to toxins including anticoagulant rodenticides. Often owners will describe clinical signs referable to the lower gastrointestinal tract including tenesmus,

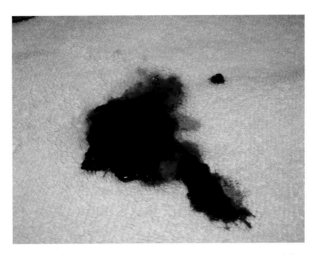

Figure 49-3 Hematochezia. Defined as the presence of fresh blood in the stool, hematochezia retains a red color more recognizable to owners as blood.

Box • 49-2

Causes of Hematochezia

Rectum and Colon
Proctitis
Rectal prolapse
Colitis
    Stress
    Dietary allergy
    Inflammatory bowel disease
    Infection
        Campylobacter
        Clostridium perfringens
        Salmonella
        Parvovirus
        Histoplasma
        Pythium
Parasitism
    Hookworms
    Whipworms
    Coccidia

Rectum and Colon—cont'd
Neoplasia
    Lymphoma
    Adenocarcinoma
    Polyps
Trauma
    Foreign body
    Pelvic fractures
    Iatrogenic
Hemorrhagic gastroenteritis

Anus and Anal Sacs
Perianal fistula
Perianal hernia
Stricture
Neoplasia (anal sac tumors)
Trauma
    Foreign body
    Bite wound
    Iatrogenic

"scooting" on the hind end, and frequent attempts at defecation producing only small amounts of stool or mucus. The animal may often be described as particularly concerned with the hind end area and may attempt to chew or scratch. If the lesion is perianal, there may be an offensive odor described as well. Additional clinical signs are often conspicuously absent.

The physical exam should be complete with particular attention paid to abdominal and rectal palpation. Abdominal pain may be noted in patients with inflammatory disease of the lower gastrointestinal tract. Goals of the digital rectal exam are to locate the presence of strictures, masses, prostatomegaly, sublumbar lymph node enlargement, pain, and crepitus indicating fracture of the pelvic floor. The anal glands should be palpated for the presence of mass lesions, severe infection, or fistula, and expressed for evaluation of their contents. A fecal sample must be obtained to confirm hematochezia and for microscopic examination.

Fecal flotation and direct exams may be the only additional diagnostic tests indicated in patients presenting with acute hematochezia and no other clinical signs. Patients with chronic hematochezia and/or other clinical signs should have a minimum data base completed as described above for patients with melena. Advanced diagnostic techniques may be indicated including specific serologic testing, fecal cultures, abdominal ultrasound, colonoscopy, and exploratory laparotomy.

TREATMENT

Treatment for patients with hematochezia will depend on the underlying cause. Initial cases that present without additional clinical signs are often successfully treated with a broad-spectrum anthelmintic, a course of metronidazole, and bland diet containing soluble fiber.

CHAPTER 50

Constipation, Tenesmus, Dyschezia, and Fecal Incontinence

Peter Foley

DEFINITIONS

Constipation is defined as infrequent or difficult evacuation of dry, hard feces. *Obstipation* is a severe form of constipation where the feces are so dry and hard, or the constipation is so longstanding, that the animal is no longer able to defecate.

Obstipation requires medical intervention. *Tenesmus* is ineffectual and painful straining at defecation or urination. *Dyschezia* is difficult or painful evacuation of feces from the rectum. In contrast to tenesmus, dyschezia is a result of disease of the anal and perianal tissues, whereas tenesmus is a result of disease of the large intestine or lower urinary tract.

Fecal incontinence is defined as defecation without conscious control.

PHYSIOLOGY OF THE LARGE INTESTINE

The large intestine or colon serves two main functions in the dog and cat: absorption of water and electrolytes and storage of feces. Absorption of water and electrolytes occurs primarily in the ascending and transverse colon, whereas the descending colon is mostly the site of storage of feces.

At rest, considerable mixing of colonic contents occurs as a result of segmental contractions of the colon. These contractions, called *haustral contractions*, are coordinated contractions of the circular and longitudinal smooth muscles of the colon that result in accumulation of colonic contents in unstimulated segments. This mixing of colonic contents increases exposure of contents to colonic mucosa for maximum water and electrolyte absorption, while slowly propelling the ingesta down the length of the colon.

In addition to haustral contractions, there are periods of intense propulsive activity down the entire length of the colon. These are called mass movements, and they serve to propel fecal matter toward the anus in preparation for defecation. These mass movements occur only a few times daily in contrast to the continuous haustral contractions. Mass movements are most common following a meal and are stimulated by the autonomic nervous system.

The anal sphincter is composed of two layers: an internal anal sphincter composed of smooth muscle, which is a direct extension of the circular smooth muscle of the rectum, and an external anal sphincter composed of striated muscle. The internal anal sphincter remains contracted most of the time and is the layer most responsible for fecal continence. The internal sphincter receives its parasympathetic nervous supply from the sacral spinal segments via the pelvic nerve. Its sympathetic innervation is from the lumbar spinal segments via the hypogastric nerve. Sympathetic stimulation results in contraction of the internal anal sphincter, whereas parasympathetic stimulation results in relaxation. The external anal sphincter is under conscious control and allows the animal to resist and prevent defecation from occurring, but it is important to remember that it is the internal anal sphincter's continuous tone that is most responsible for anal continence. The external anal sphincter is innervated by somatic efferent nerve fibers originating in the cranial sacral spinal cord segments and coursing through the pudendal nerve.

As mass movements propel feces into the rectum, the internal anal sphincter is stimulated to relax. This usually results in defecation. The animal assumes a defecation posture, the diaphragm and abdominal muscles contract to increase the intraabdominal pressure, and the external anal sphincter relaxes. The animal has the ability to override the mass movements and relaxation of the internal anal sphincter by maintaining conscious constriction of the external anal sphincter. When defecation is voluntarily prevented, the mass movements of the colon dissipate after 10 to 30 minutes, the rectum relaxes to accommodate the fecal material, the internal anal sphincter regains its tone, and the urge to defecate dissipates.

CONSTIPATION

There are several different disease states that can cause the feces to become dry, hard, and difficult to evacuate (Figure 50-1).

Diets low in fiber or high in indigestible material such as hair or bones may contribute to constipation. Lack of exercise and weakness can also be contributing factors to constipation. Good hydration status is essential for normal defecation. Animals who have had restricted access to water or who otherwise experience decreased water intake (e.g., anorexia) commonly experience constipation. Similarly, increased water loss due to polyuria or vomiting can also lead to constipation if there is insufficient water intake to replace lost body water. Colonic or rectal obstruction, either intraluminal (masses or foreign bodies) or extraluminal (mass compressing colon, pelvic fractures, perineal hernia, pseudocoprostasis), can likewise inhibit or prevent defecation and result in constipation. Neurologic abnormalities such as idiopathic megacolon or dysautonomia may likewise result in constipation due to impaired colonic motility (Figure 50-2).

Clinical Evaluation

HISTORY

Information should be gathered on the duration of the constipation and how frequently the animal is attempting to defecate. Dietary details should be collected, including how much fiber is in the diet and whether the animal is consuming significant quantities of indigestible material such as hair or bones. Anorexia or decreased access to food or water should be determined. A history of previous pelvic trauma or recent abdominal surgery may be additional contributing factors. Pets with a history of dyspnea may be reluctant to defecate as straining may worsen their respiratory distress.

SIGNALMENT

Constipation can occur in any breed or sex and at any age. English Bulldogs, Boston Terriers, and Manx cats tend to have increased incidence of constipation due to possible malformations of the sacral spinal cord. German Shepherd Dogs are predisposed to perianal fistulas that could result in dyschezia and constipation. Megacolon tends to occur more commonly in middle-aged male cats. Intact male dogs should be examined closely for prostatomegaly.

PHYSICAL EXAMINATION

The entire body should be examined closely for underlying systemic disease that may be causing weakness, anorexia, or increased water loss (e.g., polyuria) that may be contributing to the constipation. Abdominal palpation may reveal a colon distended with hard feces. The anus should be visually inspected for fecal hair mats obstructing the anus (pseudocoprostasis), masses, and perianal fistulas. The rectum and distal colon should be carefully palpated digitally for evidence of hard, dry feces; colonic or rectal masses or foreign bodies; pelvic fractures; enlarged sublumbar lymph nodes; prostatomegaly in the male dog; perianal hernias; and anal sac disease.

DIAGNOSTIC EVALUATION

A complete blood count, serum biochemistry profile, and urinalysis are useful in ruling out underlying systemic disease. Abdominal radiographs can confirm colonic distention with feces. In severe cases, the colon is so distended with feces that the feces are not able to pass through the pelvic canal. Abdominal radiographs may also reveal colonic masses, foreign bodies, sublumbar lymph node enlargement, prostatomegaly, or pelvic fractures. Abdominal ultrasound may

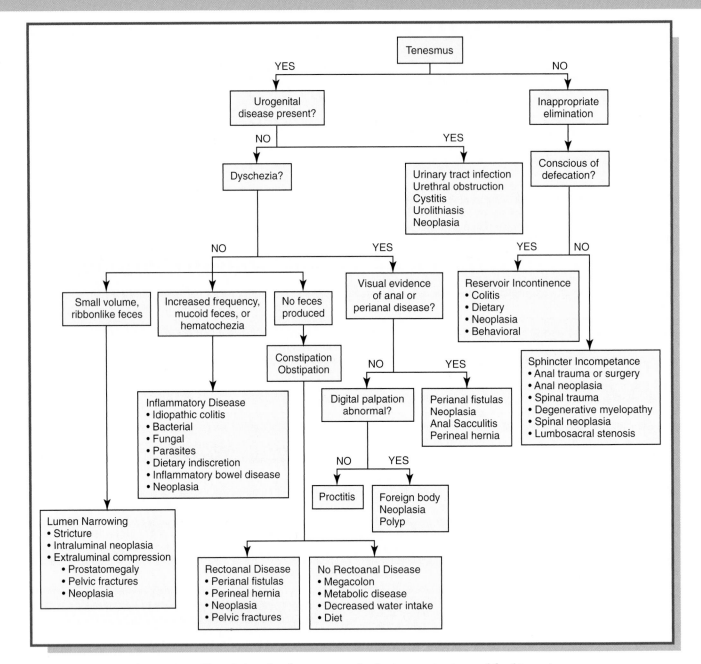

Figure 50-1   Clinical algorithm for tenesmus, dyschezia, constipation, and fecal incontinence.

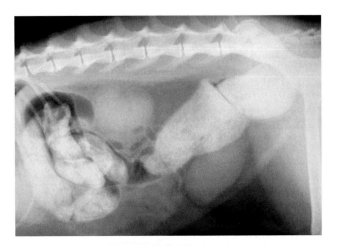

Figure 50-2   Obstipation and megacolon in a cat.

identify intraluminal or extraluminal masses, prostatomegaly, and enlarged lymph nodes. Once feces are evacuated from the colon and rectum, colonoscopy may reveal colonic neoplasia, perineal hernias, diverticula, and strictures.

TENESMUS AND DYSCHEZIA

It is important to localize the cause of straining to diseases of either the lower urinary tract or the lower gastrointestinal (GI) tract. Inflammatory and infectious diseases of the lower GI tract, such as inflammatory bowel disease, dietary indiscretion, intestinal parasitism, idiopathic colitis, pythiosis, and bacterial or fungal colitis, can cause irritation and straining at defecation. Obstructions, both intraluminal (colonic neoplasia, foreign bodies, and strictures) and extraluminal (pelvic fractures, extraluminal masses, or organomegaly), can make defecation difficult and result in tenesmus. Dyschezia results from diseases of the anus and perianal region including anal sacculitis, perianal fistulas, perineal hernia, anal/rectal neoplasia, and pseudocoprostasis.

Clinical Evaluation

HISTORY

Urination must be evaluated carefully to rule out lower urinary tract disease as a cause of tenesmus. Is the animal able to produce a normal stream of urine, and is there dripping of urine as the animal strains? Is the urine of normal appearance? Details of defecation are likewise important. Are normal feces being passed? Thin, ribbonlike feces, or small amounts of diarrhea are common with intraluminal or extraluminal obstructions. Excessive grooming of the anal/perianal region is common with disease in that location. Sometimes the owners may report the animal turning around and looking at the hind end while attempting to defecate. There may be a history of trauma and pelvic fractures. Cats with tenesmus or dyschezia commonly vocalize or defecate outside the litter box. The timing of tenesmus in relation to defecation may help localize the problem: tenesmus prior to defecation suggests an obstruction, while tenesmus after defecation suggests irritation/inflammation.

SIGNALMENT

Inflammatory diseases are more common in young to middle-aged animals, while neoplasia is more common in older animals. German Shepherd Dogs are predisposed to perianal fistulas. Boxer dogs are predisposed to histiocytic colitis.

PHYSICAL EXAMINATION

The lower urinary tract should be examined by palpation of the bladder to rule out urethral obstruction. A digital rectal palpation may sometimes reveal uroliths in the urethra or prostatomegaly in male dogs. The anus and perianal region are best inspected visually to rule out perianal fistulas, ruptured anal sacs, and fecal hair mats causing pseudocoprostasis. A digital rectal palpation should be performed to rule out rectal masses, perineal hernia, rectal polyps, anal sacculitis, sublumbar lymph node enlargement, and pelvic fractures. The rectal palpation will also allow for characterization of the feces. Absent or scant or bloody fecal material suggests an inflammatory disease.

DIAGNOSTIC EVALUATION

Complete blood count, serum biochemistry profile, and urinalysis are helpful in ruling out systemic disease. A fecal floatation can be performed to rule out gastrointestinal parasites. Abdominal radiographs and ultrasound are useful in ruling out extraluminal compression of the colon, foreign bodies, pelvic fractures, and colonic masses. Colonoscopy and proctoscopy are useful in identifying colonic masses, foreign bodies, and strictures, once fecal material is evacuated from the colon. Colonic biopsies may be necessary to evaluate the colonic wall for inflammation, infection, or neoplasia.

FECAL INCONTINENCE

Fecal incontinence can be due to damage to the anal sphincter (nonneurogenic sphincter incompetence), disruption of the nervous supply to the anal sphincter (neurogenic incompetence), or reduced capacity or compliance of the rectum (reservoir incontinence). With reservoir incontinence, the animal is aware of the urge to defecate, but conscious control of defecation is overwhelmed by the presence of colorectal disease causing irritation, decreased storage capacity of the rectum, or overwhelming fecal volume. Diseases that can damage the anal sphincter and cause nonneurogenic sphincter incompetence include anal trauma or surgery, anal neoplasia, and damage to the levator ani and coccygeus muscles. Conditions that can result in neurogenic sphincter incompetence include cauda equina syndrome; damage to the pudendal nerve; sacral spinal cord trauma, neoplasia, compressive lesions, and degenerative myelopathy.

Clinical Evaluation

HISTORY

The first thing to establish is whether the animal is consciously aware of defecation and is assuming a normal posture to defecate. Conscious awareness of defecation, and the presence of diarrhea, increased frequency of defecation, and mucus or blood in the feces suggest colorectal disease and reservoir incontinence. It is important to rule out behavioral problems when the animal is consciously defecating in inappropriate locations. With behavioral problems, there is normal posturing to defecate, normal frequency of defecation, and normal consistency of the feces. Often the location of the defecation in the home is a clue to a behavioral problem. For example, if the dog has been punished previously when defecating inappropriately in the presence of the owner, the dog may seek out locations out of sight of the owner and away from the door outside. Animals with reservoir incontinence often attempt to get outside to defecate, but are unable to retain the feces, and defecate close to the door outside.

A history of recent trauma or perianal surgery may suggest damage to the anal sphincter. With neurogenic sphincter incompetence, other neurologic dysfunction may be detected including loss of tail wagging, abnormal tail carriage, hind limb ataxia or weakness, decreased hind limb spinal reflexes, and concurrent urinary incontinence.

PHYSICAL EXAMINATION

Visual inspection of the anal sphincter may reveal trauma or neoplasia. The anal tone may be evaluated by the strength of constriction of the sphincter in response to a finger, thermometer, or hemostatic forceps stimulating the sphincter. A digital rectal exam may reveal masses disrupting the sphincter. Pain on palpating the sacrum or lumbosacral space per rectum may occur with lumbosacral stenosis. Abnormal fecal consistency, with mucus or blood, is often an indication of colorectal disease and reservoir incontinence. Neurologic examination of the hind end may reveal decreased tail tone, hind limb ataxia, decreased hopping and wheelbarrowing, decreased hind limb spinal reflexes, decreased conscious proprioception of the hind limbs, lumbosacral pain, and loss of urinary bladder tone with many cases of neurogenic sphincter mechanism incompetence as a result of spinal cord disease or damage.

DIAGNOSTIC EVALUATION

In addition to routine complete blood count, serum biochemistry profile, urinalysis, and caudal abdominal radiographs, additional diagnostic imaging of the caudal spinal cord (epidurogram, myelogram, computed tomography scan, or magnetic resonance imaging) may be required to characterize the nature of disease of the spinal cord if neurogenic causes of sphincter incompetence are suspected based on the history and physical examination.

CHAPTER 51

Flatulence

Michael E. Matz

The term *flatulence* refers to excessive accumulation of gas in the gastrointestinal tract. It may be associated with eructation, borborygmus, or flatus. *Eructation* is the expulsion of gas from the stomach. *Borborygmus* is a rumbling noise caused by the propulsion of gas through the gastrointestinal tract. *Flatus* is the anal passage of intestinal gas.

Flatulence is more commonly observed in dogs than cats and is most often noted in inactive indoor dogs. It usually results from dietary intolerances but occasionally can signal more serious gastrointestinal disease, particularly of the small bowel or pancreas. Most owners accept flatulence and borborygmus in their pets as normal and are unconcerned about its consequences.

PATHOPHYSIOLOGY

The major gastrointestinal gases are nitrogen and oxygen, which are derived from swallowed air and diffusion from blood, and hydrogen, carbon dioxide, and methane, which are primarily products of bacterial metabolism and fermentation and nonbacterial reactions (e.g., pancreatic bicarbonate interacting with acid to produce carbon dioxide) that occur in the bowel lumen. In human beings, and probably in dogs and cats, as much as 99% of flatus is composed of these odorless gases. The remaining 1% is composed of odoriferous gases, including hydrogen sulfide, methanethiol, dimethylsulfide, ammonia, skatole, mercaptans, volatile amines, and short chain fatty acids. These odoriferous gases also result from bacterial metabolism and fermentation. Sulfur-containing gases, particularly hydrogen sulfide, have been shown to be a major determinant of the malodor of canine flatus.

Most of the gas that enters the digestive tract is thought to come from swallowed air. Aerophagia mainly occurs during the ingestion of liquids and solids and can be exacerbated by rapid or competitive eating situations. Most swallowed air is subsequently eliminated by eructation from the stomach and esophagus. If not eructated, the nitrogen contained in swallowed air travels through the gastrointestinal tract with minimal absorption and subsequently is passed. It is noteworthy that the transit time for gas is considerably shorter than that for liquids or solids. Air entering the intestinal tract can be passed out the rectum rapidly (within minutes). Gases can also be removed by diffusion into blood or consumption by bacteria.

The composition and volume of flatus are affected by the quantity and variety of nutrients eaten, as well as by the type and abundance of bacterial flora. A significant amount of gas is formed from the bacterial fermentation of both dietary (e.g., fiber and poorly digestible carbohydrates and proteins) and endogenous substrates (e.g., mucin, bile acids). Foods such as legumes (soybeans, beans, peas) that contain large amounts of indigestible oligosaccharides are apt to produce large amounts of intestinal gas. The oligosaccharides are fermented to hydrogen and carbon dioxide by *Clostridium* organisms and other bacteria. Variations in the metabolic capacity of the bacteria flora may explain the different responses animals may have to nonabsorbable carbohydrates. Fiber-containing pet foods may contribute to flatulence directly, if the fibers are fermentable by colonic bacteria, and/or indirectly through reduced dry matter digestibility. Pectins and most gums are rapidly fermentable fibers found in pet foods. Sulfur-reducing bacteria convert dietary sources of sulfur, including sulfate and sulfur-containing amino acids, to the odoriferous gases hydrogen sulfide, methanethiol, and dimethylsulfide. The production of these gases usually is increased by foods containing increased amounts of sulfate (cruciferous vegetables, onions, nuts, carrageenan) or protein.

Maldigestion due to exocrine pancreatic insufficiency or malabsorption resulting from small intestinal disease often leads to excessive intestinal gas caused by the fermentation of malassimilated substrates. Lactose intolerance also can cause flatulence.

CLINICAL EXAMINATION FINDINGS

Owners may describe their dog as having frequent eructation, an increase in the frequency of flatus, an objectionable odor associated with flatus, the presence of borborygmus, or abdominal distention. Occasionally these signs are associated with concurrent abdominal pain, vomiting, diarrhea, or weight loss, any of which suggests more serious gastrointestinal disease. The owner may report that the pet has a hunched posture, exhibits unsettled behavior, or adopts a "praying position." These signs may result from excessive intestinal gas, motility disorders that disrupt the passage of gas through the bowel, or increased visceral sensitivity to bowel distention. The animal's temperament may be important. Excessive aerophagia in a nervous animal, or animals with aggressive or competitive eating habits, can increase gastric gas, although it is unclear whether ingested air contributes significantly to intestinal gas or flatus. Frequent eructation and rapid eating are risk factors for gastric dilatation/volvulus in dogs and the presence of these clinical findings should be taken seriously in "at-risk" breeds.

A complete dietary history is essential. Owners should be questioned about any recent dietary change or dietary indiscretion. An assessment of specific foods, food ingredients, treats, and supplements, as well as the potential for dietary indiscretion, should be made. In human beings, diets high in soybeans, whole wheat products, bran, and fats can cause flatulence. Similar associations appear to occur in some dogs and cats. Spoiled food and diets high in protein or fat are more likely to yield odoriferous gases. Milk products can cause flatulence in animals with lactase deficiency. The feeding method should also be thoroughly evaluated. The amount fed, feeding frequency, how the food is offered, access to other food, and the relationship of feeding to exercise should be determined.

With the exception of borborygmus, the physical examination of an animal with flatulence usually is unremarkable unless concomitant gastrointestinal disease is present. Additional diagnostic tests are warranted in the latter animals.

MANAGEMENT

The management of flatulence begins with changing the diet (Figure 51-1). Feeding a highly digestible diet reduces the food residues available for bacterial fermentation. The diet should not contain excessive amounts of rapidly fermentable fiber. Vegetarian-based diets should be avoided because these products often have sulfur-containing vegetables and legumes. Optimally, the diet should be lactose deficient. Changing sources or amounts of dietary protein, carbohydrate, and fat may benefit individual animals. Diets containing rice as the primary carbohydrate source may produce less intestinal gas than diets containing other sources of carbohydrate. Suitable commercial foods are available from most major pet food manufacturers. Dietary trials may be necessary to find a food that reduces flatulence or objectionable flatus. Vitamin-mineral supplements may increase intestinal bacterial activity and probably should be avoided.

Reducing aerophagia, by avoiding situations that provoke nervousness and discouraging rapid or competitive eating, may also be helpful. Feeding several small meals daily may alleviate some of these problems. Regular exercise also is beneficial, presumably because exercise stimulates gastrointestinal motility and defecation. In the event that dietary manipulation and regular exercise are not successful, symptomatic pharmacologic intervention can be considered.

Pharmacologic management involves reducing or controlling the amount of flatulence and/or the objectionable odor of flatus. Substances that can be used include simethicone, activated charcoal, bismuth subsalicylate, zinc acetate, *Yucca schidigera* preparations, alpha-galactosidase, pancreatic enzyme supplements, probiotics, and homeopathic remedies. These substances are preferentially used in conjunction with dietary changes

Simethicone (25 to 200 mg per dose, given every 6 hours) frequently is used as a treatment for borborygmus, gaseous colic, and flatulence in human beings. It is an antifoaming agent that reduces surface tension, allowing bubbles to coalesce so that they can be passed more easily. Simethicone is not absorbed from the gastrointestinal tract and can be safely used in dogs and cats at or near the dosage for human beings. Its effectiveness as an antiflatulent in dogs and cats is unknown. Both veterinary and human (over-the-counter) products containing simethicone are commercially available.

Activated charcoal is one of the more commonly used adsorbent antiflatulents in human beings. Its absorbency results from its porous structure, which confers a tremendous internal surface area. Charcoal is of questionable benefit for the relief of flatulence, but it may be effective in absorbing small amounts of sulfur-containing gases, which are primarily responsible for malodorous flatus. Commercial treats containing activated charcoal are available for dogs.

Zinc sulfate, bismuth subsalicylate, and *Yucca schidigera* may be effective in reducing the unpleasant odor of flatus. Poorly absorbed divalent cations (e.g., zinc, bismuth) bind sulfhydryl compounds such as hydrogen sulfide and methanethiol to form insoluble salts, and this effectively prevents the liberation of these gases. To be of benefit, bismuth subsalicylate probably needs to be given multiple times per day, which can make it impractical to use. The efficacy of *Y. schidigera* appears to be related to its ability to bind hydrogen sulfide and/or to decrease the number or activity of sulfate-reducing bacteria that generate hydrogen sulfide. Like charcoal, these agents do not appear to be particularly effective in reducing flatulence. The efficacy of the agents may be improved if administered together.

Anecdotal reports indicate that alpha-galactosidase, pancreatic enzyme supplements, probiotics, and some homeopathic remedies may be effective in reducing flatulence in some dogs and cats. Alpha-galactosidase is thought to work by improving digestion of nonabsorbable carbohydrates found in legumes. Both veterinary and human products containing alpha-galactosidase are available. Pancreatic enzyme preparations are claimed to assist the digestion of fermentable nutrients that are digested poorly by the gastrointestinal systems of monogastrics. Probiotics have been shown to reduce flatulence in human patients with functional gastrointestinal dis-

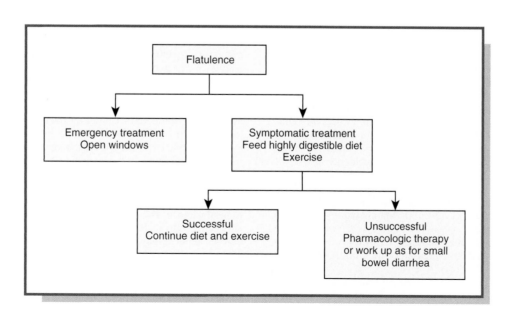

Figure 51-1 Algorithm for managing flatulence.

orders; however, their use has not been critically evaluated in small animals with flatulence. Several homeopathic remedies been recommended for the treatment of flatulence. Established doses, efficacy, and safety have not been determined.

In most dogs and cats, flatulence can be controlled successfully through dietary management alone. Relapses in controlled animals often are due to dietary indiscretion. If dietary management, exercise, and supplementary therapy are unsuccessful in reducing or controlling flatulence, an investigation similar to that for a dog or cat with small bowel diarrhea (see Chapters 48 and 270) should be considered.

NEUROLOGIC

CHAPTER 52

Neurologic Manifestations of Systemic Disease

Helena Rylander

A variety of systemic diseases can cause neurologic signs. Findings on history and physical examination may reveal abnormalities attributed to a systemic disease causing neurologic signs. Neurologic signs may be the only manifestation of systemic disease. The cerebral cortex and the peripheral nervous system are the parts of the nervous system most susceptible to systemic disease. However, white matter changes, brainstem signs, and cerebellar signs have also been documented secondary to systemic conditions. Specific neurologic signs and lesion localization are discussed elsewhere in this textbook. Once a diagnosis is confirmed, appropriate therapy can be instituted in an attempt to prevent further nervous system injury.

DISEASES CAUSING CNS SIGNS

Diseases causing central nervous system (CNS) signs are presented in Table 52-1.

Hypoxia from Systemic Disease

Hypoxic encephalopathy is the result of reduction of cerebral oxygen supply, either from decreased arterial oxygen tension or reduced cerebral blood flow. Hypoxia can occur secondary to an anesthetic accident, hematologic disorders (especially anemia), or cardiovascular and respiratory failure. Autoregulatory mechanisms provide a relatively constant cerebral blood flow despite changes in systemic arterial pressure. These mechanisms fail when blood pressure decreases below 50 mm Hg. Anesthetic accidents can result in hypotension, cardiac arrhythmia, extensive blood loss, hypercapnia, and hypoxemia. Some areas of the brain are more susceptible to energy deprivation or may contain a higher concentration of N-methyl-D-aspartate (NMDA) membrane receptors.

Increased release of the excitatory neurotransmitter glutamate in cell injury leads to increased cellular influx of calcium and neuronal death. The global ischemia results in bilateral infarcts in the "watershed zones" between areas supplied by major arteries. Changes in blood flow to the brain may occur secondary to hyperviscosity from polycythemia (relative or absolute), hypercholesterolemia/hyperlipidemia (familial hyperlipidemia, hyperadrenocorticism, hypothyroidism), immune-mediated disease, sepsis, coagulopathies, and hyperglobulinemia. Hyperviscosity can cause diffuse hypoxia or vascular accidents due to the thickness of the blood or due to embolism.[1,2] The clinical signs reflect the area of the brain affected with visual loss being a common neurologic sign in cats after anesthetic accidents.[3] Cytotoxic edema in the white matter can be detected on magnetic resonance imaging (MRI) images.[4] Treatment consists of attempting to establish normal blood flow and oxygenation in the brain. Steroids are contraindicated and may cause further brain damage. Recovery is slow, taking weeks to months, and residual neurologic signs may be present in severe injuries.

Hypertension

A rapid and sustained rise in blood pressure causes the autoregulatory mechanism for maintaining blood flow to fail and results in hypertensive encephalopathy. Neurologic signs occur at a lower blood pressure (170 mm Hg) if hypertension develops rapidly.[5] Common neurologic signs are seizures, ataxia, stupor, and blindness. Postmortem findings may include cerebral edema, caudal displacement of the vermis of the cerebellum, arteriolar hyalinosis, hyperplastic arteriosclerosis, ischemia, and necrosis (the latter two abnormalities are rare). Multiple petechial hemorrhages in the brain have been reported on both autopsy and MRI of persons with longstanding hypertension.[6] Cats may show neurologic signs due to hypertension after renal transplantation. Controlling the hypertension in these patients reduces the prevalence of seizures and neurologic complication–related deaths.[7] Dogs with chronic renal failure are more likely to develop uremic crisis if they have systemic hypertension.[8]

 To view a video on this topic, go to **www.expertconsult.com.**

Table • 52-1

Neurologic Manifestation of Systemic Disease

CENTRAL NERVOUS SYSTEM	PERIPHERAL NERVOUS SYSTEM
Energy deprivation:	Hypoxia: aortic
1. Hypoxia	thromboembolism
a) Pulmonary disease	a) Cardiovascular
b) Cardiac failure	b) Renal disease
i) Infarcts	c) Hyperadrenocorticism
ii) Hypoxia	d) Hypothyroidism
iii) Hypertension	e) Neoplasia
c) Anesthetic accident	f) Disseminated intravascular
d) Vascular	coagulation (DIC)
i) Hypertension	g) Sepsis
ii) Coagulopathies	
iii) Vasculitis	
2. Hypoglycemia	
a) Insulin producing	
neoplasia	
b) Insulin overdose	
c) Sepsis	
3. Thiamine deficiency	
Metabolic:	Metabolic:
a) Hepatic encephalopathy	a) Renal failure
b) Renal encephalopathy	b) Hypothyroidism
c) Hypothyroidism	c) Hyperthyroidism
d) Hyperthyroidism	d) Hyperadrenocorticism
e) Hyperadrenocorticism	e) Hypoadrenocorticism
f) Hypoadrenocorticism	f) Diabetes mellitus
Electrolyte abnormalities:	Electrolyte abnormalities:
a) Hypercalcemia	a) Hypokalemia
b) Hypocalcemia	
c) Hypernatremia	
d) Hyponatremia	
e) Hyperkalemia	
f) Hypokalemia	
Neoplasia:	Neoplasia:
a) Primary	a) Paraneoplastic syndrome
b) Metastatic	
c) Infarcts	
d) Paraneoplastic syndrome	

Endocrine/Metabolic Causes

Hepatic Encephalopathy Hepatic encephalopathy (HE) can be caused by portosystemic shunt (PSS), microvascular dysplasia, idiopathic noncirrhotic portal hypertension, or other causes of liver failure. Neurologic manifestations occur in 95% of dogs with PSS.[9,10] The clinical signs may be more obvious after a meal and tend to be waxing-waning. The neurologic signs are typical of diffuse cerebral disease and vary from mild—an inability to learn new things and behavioral changes—to more severe—head pressing, blindness, mentation changes and seizures. Brainstem and cerebellar signs have also been described.[11] One case report describes resolution of generalized neuromuscular weakness and regurgitation after surgical correction of a PSS.[12]

Histopathologic findings include Alzheimer type II astrocytes, degenerative leukoencephalopathy with spongy degeneration or polycavitation of brainstem, caudate nucleus, hippocampus, and internal capsule white matter. One study of two Irish Wolfhounds found spongiform changes in the neuropil and fiber bundles interspersed within the grey matter, with involvement of basal nuclei and hypothalamus, and neuronal vacuoles.[13] MRIs of dogs with PSS showed hyperintense, non–contrast-enhancing lesions in the lentiform nuclei and widened sulci.[14]

The pathogenesis of HE is not fully understood. Various endogenous toxins (amino acids, ammonia, mercaptans, γ-aminobutyric acid [GABA], false neurotransmitters) normally cleared by the liver contribute to CNS signs. There is no correlation between the severity of clinical signs and serum ammonia concentrations.[15] Hyperammonemia, >120 μmol/L, has been documented in young Irish Wolfhounds without PSS.[16] Increased cerebrospinal fluid concentration of glutamine, quinolinic acid, tryptophan, and tryptophan metabolites have been found in dogs diagnosed with a PSS as compared to control dogs.[17,18] Activation of GABA receptors by increased levels of endogenous benzodiazepines may contribute to the clinical signs of HE, and a withdrawal effect may cause postsurgical seizures.[19] Hepatic encephalopathic signs have successfully been treated with flumazenil, a benzodiazepine-receptor antagonist. Studies in people and rats have demonstrated improvement in neurologic signs after treatment with flumazenil or a benzodiazepine-receptor partial inverse agonist; these data also support a role of increased GABAergic tone in the pathogenesis of HE.[20,21]

Medical therapy is aimed at decreasing the production and absorption of toxins generated by bacteria in the gastrointestinal tract. These therapies include feeding low-protein diets and administration of antibiotics and/or lactulose.

Potassium bromide at a dose of 40 to 60 mg/kg PO, once daily, or gabapentin 20 to 60 mg/kg/day, divided TID, may aid in controlling seizures. Sodium bromide, IV, can rapidly increase serum levels. Phenobarbital should be used with caution since it is protein bound and metabolized by the liver. However, 3 to 5 mg/kg BID may effectively control seizures. Benzodiazepine (0.5 mg/kg) may prevent postsurgical withdrawal seizures.[22,23] Surgical correction of congenital PSS carries a better prognosis for postoperative survival and neurologic morbidity if done before 2 years of age according to some studies, whereas others suggest that the prognosis is similar in dogs >5 years of age.[24,25] Prophylactic phenobarbital therapy may not reduce the incidence of postsurgical neurologic signs and seizures.[26-30]

Renal Encephalopathy Toxic substances not excreted due to renal failure can cause encephalopathic signs similar to those typical of HE. Increased concentrations of parathyroid hormone (PTH) and subsequent hypercalcemia may have a major role in renal encephalopathy. Treatment can be directed at lowering PTH levels using calcitriol (although not without risk of causing hypercalcemia and hyperphosphatemia) and minimizing uptake of phosphorus through phosphate binders and low-phosphate diets. Treating high blood pressure can lower the risk for hypertension encephalopathy.[31-34]

Hypothyroidism Acute or chronic progressive central vestibular signs may be the sole clinical sign in dogs with hypothyroidism. Since thyroid hormone affects virtually every cell and organ, neurologic signs as the only evidence of hypothyroidism should be considered rare. Hypercholesterol-induced or hypertriglyceride-induced microthrombi may result in infarcts detectable with MRI. Intermittent vestibular signs may be seen with transient microthrombi, which result in transient ischemic attacks. In these cases no changes are detected on MRI or on histology of the brain. Abnormalities may also be detected on brain auditory-evoked response

(BAER) or electroencephalogram (EEG). Cerebrospinal fluid analysis may reveal an increase in protein content. Pathogenesis of hypothyroidism-associated abnormalities are likely multifactorial, and include atherosclerosis-causing infarcts or transient ischemic attacks, segmental demyelination, dysfunction of metabolic pathways within the brain, and metabolic derangement of neuronal or glial cell populations.[35,36] Treatment with thyroxin usually resolves neurologic signs.

Myxedema coma is a rare but life-threatening manifestation of hypothyroidism. Clinical signs include mentation changes, hypothermia without shivering, nonpitting skin edema, and bradycardia. Brain edema occurs. Hyponatremia and hypoventilatory hypoxia can worsen neurologic status. Treatment consists of adequate ventilation, 0.9% sodium chloride IV, passive correction of hypothermia, and levothyroxine, 5 µg/kg, IV, q12h followed by maintenance thyroid supplementation orally. Mortality is high with this condition and clinical improvement, if it is to occur, is usually seen within 24 hours.[37,38]

Congenital hypothyroidism has been described in numerous dog breeds as well as in cats. Clinical signs include disproportionate dwarfism, abnormal hair coat, lethargy, a stiff/stilted gait and abnormal mentation. Histologically, hypomyelination can be seen in the corpus callosum, corona radiata, pons, pyramids, and the lateral funiculi of the spinal cord.[39]

Hyperthyroidism Cats with hyperthyroidism may show mild CNS signs that can include hyperactivity, change in sleep/wake cycle, aggression, or obtundation. The neurologic signs improve and may completely resolve with treatment.

Hyperadrenocorticism Direct compression from a pituitary macroadenoma can cause mild to severe neurologic signs. The most common early clinical signs of macroadenoma include inappetence, mild obtundation, pacing, and disorientation. These clinical signs are typically associated with tumors that are >8 mm in greatest diameter but less than 1.5 mm. More worrisome signs are associated with masses >1.5 cm in greatest diameter that include obtundation, circling, tetraparesis, ataxia, and seizures. Blindness is more common in humans with macrotumors than in dogs or cats. Hyperlipidemia may result in infarcts. Ten of 13 dogs diagnosed with pituitary-dependent hyperadrenocorticism had a visible pituitary tumor at the time of or within a year of diagnosis, and 2 of these dogs developed neurologic signs within one year of diagnosis. Pituitary tumors cause neurologic signs in 15% to 30% of dogs before or after diagnosis and treatment for pituitary-dependent hyperadrenocorticism (PDH).[40,41]

Hypoglycemia The brain, since it cannot synthesize glucose, is dependent on blood glucose for normal cellular metabolism. It is estimated that the brain requires ~100 g of glucose per day. Persistent hypoglycemia not only impairs cellular function directly, it can also cause vascular constriction, which reduces oxygen delivery to the brain. Hypoglycemia can occur in dogs and cats secondary to a variety of conditions, including simple poor nutrition (puppy hypoglycemia, for example), insulinoma, liver failure, hypoadrenocorticism, nonislet cell tumors producing insulin-like growth factors, large metabolically active tumors (leiomyosarcoma), severe polycythemia, and sepsis (see Chapter 138). Hypoglycemia can also be associated with exogenous insulin overdose or as a paraneoplastic syndrome.[42-46]

Waxing and waning signs with episodes of obtundation and weakness, disorientation, tremors, partial or generalized seizures, blindness, and coma are seen. There is no correlation between the severity or frequency of clinical signs, degree of hypoglycemia, and survival time posttreatment. A low fasting blood glucose helps in the diagnosis. A serum insulin concentration within the midreference range or higher, in a dog or cat with a serum glucose concentration <60 mg/dL, is consistent with diagnosis of insulin-producing tumor.

Symptomatic treatment with IV glucose (2 to 4 mL/kg of 50% glucose diluted to 25% concentration) usually reverses the neurologic signs quickly. Hypoglycemia resolves if the underlying cause is removed. Medical management with prednisone to stimulate gluconeogenesis and glycogenolysis together with frequent feeding of a high-protein, high-fat, and high–complex carbohydrate diet can be used as adjuncts to surgical treatment or as a sole treatment. Median survival time in one study of dogs with insulinoma was 196 days with only medical treatment, 785 days in dogs treated with surgery and 1316 days in dogs treated medically after relapse postsurgery.[47] Diazoxide inhibits insulin secretion, stimulates production of glucose by the liver, and inhibits glucose uptake by the cell. It has been successfully used in dogs but not in cats with insulin-producing tumors.[48] Permanent brain damage from neuronal death may cause persistent neurologic signs despite normalization of blood glucose and insulin levels with treatment.[49,50]

Thiamine Deficiency Thiamine is essential for decarboxylation of pyruvic acid and other α-keto acids. Thiamine deficiency causes decreased utilization of pyruvic acid and some amino acids, increased utilization of fats, and aciduria.[51] Thiamine deficiency occurs in cats and dogs fed meat preserved with sulfur dioxide, food low in thiamine due to processing, or thiaminase-containing fish. Thiamin deficiency may result in polioencephalomalacia with bilateral symmetrical spongiosis, necrosis, and hemorrhage in the medial vestibular nuclei, caudal colliculi, cerebellar nodulus, and the subcortical grey matter.[52,53] Experimental thiamine deficiency in cats led to learning deficits likely caused by lesions in the hippocampal formation.[54] Neurologic signs of thiamine deficiency reflect lesions in the cerebrum and vestibular nuclei. Hyperintense lesions can be detected with MRI on T2-weighted and FLAIR images, and the lesions contrast-enhance postgadolinium. Oral supplementation with thiamine at 25 to 50 mg BID results in resolution of clinical signs after weeks to months.

Electrolyte Abnormalities

Hypercalcemia Hypercalcemia due to primary hyperparathyroidism or secondary to malignant neoplasm rarely has been related to seizures. The mechanism for seizures due to hypercalcemia is poorly understood. Coagulopathies in hypercalcemic dogs have been documented.[55]

Hypocalcemia Hypocalcemia due to renal failure, primary hypoparathyroidism, or lactation (eclampsia) causes increased membrane excitability in both CNS and muscle. Hypocalcemia can result in generalized weakness, tetany, and seizures. Treatment consists of 0.5 to 1.5 mL/kg 10% calcium gluconate IV over 10 to 20 minutes while monitoring the heart rate and treatment of the underlying cause to prevent recurrence (see Chapter 286).[56]

Hypernatremia/Hyponatremia Severe hyponatremia can cause cerebral edema and life-threatening, diffuse encephalopathy.[57] Overaggressive correction of hyponatremia in dogs may cause CNS signs due to cerebral edema with central pontine myelinolysis and loss of oligodendroglial cells 48 hours to several days after treatment.[58-60] MRI shows bilateral symmetrical hyperintense areas on T2-weighted images in the central thalamic nuclei. Correction of hyponatremia should not exceed 10 mEq/L during a 24-hour period to prevent these lesions. Aggressive IV saline treatment in symptomatic patients with hyponatremia of less than 24-hour duration may be successful without causing neurologic signs (see Chapter 294).

With hypernatremia, osmotic movement of water out of the brain cells results in reduction of brain volume, which may cause rupture of cerebral vessels and focal hemorrhage. Severity of neurologic signs is related to the rapidity of onset of the hypernatremia rather than the magnitude of hypernatremia. In chronic hypernatremia the brain adapts to the hypertonicity by the production of idiogenic osmoles, which prevent cellular dehydration. Rapid correction of hypernatremia results in movement of water into the cells and development of cerebral edema. Mild hypernatremia can be corrected by offering water in animals that are drinking. More severe hypernatremia can be treated with IV hypotonic saline or 5% dextrose in water. The fluid deficit is calculated using the following formula:

$$\text{free water deficit} = 0.6 \times \text{body weight (kg)} \times [(\text{plasma Na}^+/148) - 1]^{61}$$

Neoplasia

Neoplasia can cause neurologic signs from direct invasion or metastasis, or secondary to ischemic and hemorrhagic infarcts as well as transient ischemic attacks. Diagnosis is made by MRI and cerebrospinal fluid (CSF) analysis as well as by identifying the primary neoplasia.[62,63] Paraneoplastic syndromes such as hypoglycemia induced by an insulin-producing tumor and hypercalcemia secondary to lymphoma, thymoma, and apocrine adenocarcinoma directly affect the CNS.[64]

Hyperthermia

The canine brain has an intrinsic thermal resistance. The origin of neurologic dysfunction in dogs and cats with hyperthermia is usually not from effects of increased temperature directly on the brain, but from secondary changes such as hepatocellular degeneration, disseminated intravascular coagulation, respiratory alkalosis, and reduction in mean arterial pressure. Mentation changes, loss of pupillary light reflex and oculocephalic reflex, as well as tetraparesis can be seen.[65]

DISEASES CAUSING PNS SIGNS

Diseases causing peripheral nervous system (PNS) signs are listed in Table 52-1.

Hypoxia

Aortic thromboembolism, although uncommon in dogs, usually occurs secondary to an underlying disease such as cardiac disease, hyperadrenocorticism, neoplasia, disseminated intravascular coagulation, sepsis, renal disease, atherosclerosis from a condition like hypothyroidism, or autoimmune hemolytic anemia. Neurologic signs observed by owners may include chronic exercise intolerance with pelvic limb weakness, or more acute symmetric or asymmetric pelvic limb ataxia, paresis, or plegia. Such neurologic signs are due to an ischemic myopathy, neuropathy, or myelopathy.[66-68] Cats usually have peracute signs that include tachypnea, hypothermia, paraparesis, or plegia. Underlying causes are cardiomyopathy, hyperthyroidism, and neoplasia.[69]

Metabolic/Endocrine Disorders

Hypothyroidism Thyroxine (T_4) stimulates mitochondrial respiratory activity, thus facilitating production of ade-

nosine triphosphate (ATP). In hypothyroidism, ATP deficiency impairs the Na$^+$/K$^+$ pump activity, reducing axonal transport. This results in axonal degeneration and demyelination. Myopathy has also been described secondary to hypothyroidism. In rare circumstances, neurologic signs may be the only manifestation of hypothyroidism. Neurologic signs include generalized weakness and muscle atrophy, focal signs such as laryngeal paralysis, megaesophagus, facial paralysis, and peripheral vestibular signs. Lameness as the only clinical sign has been reported in four dogs.[70] (For information on diagnosing hypothyroidism, please see Chapter 287.) Electrodiagnostic abnormalities and histopathologic abnormalities on muscle and nerve biopsies may be detected before clinical signs occur.[71] The neurologic signs may resolve after several months of treatment with thyroxin supplementation.[72]

Hyperthyroidism Hyperthyroidism in cats can cause neuromuscular weakness with ventroflexion of the neck, a plantigrade stance, and exercise intolerance. The clinical signs are reversible with treatment of the hyperthyroidism.

Hyperadrenocorticism Hyperadrenocorticism is usually associated with muscle weakness. In rare cases, dogs have fibrotic myopathy or polyneuropathy. Clinical signs in fibrotic myopathy may include a stiff, stilted gait; generalized muscle atrophy; and difficulty flexing the limbs. The clinical signs with the polyneuropathy include a general weakness and muscle atrophy. Diagnosis is made on electrodiagnostic testing (electromyogram [EMG] and nerve conduction) and muscle and nerve biopsies. Type II myofiber atrophy is a common finding. In dogs with fibrosis the stiffness may only partially improve with treatment after several months.[73,74] Steroid myopathy has also been described secondary to treatment with prednisone.[75,76]

Hypoadrenocorticism Hypoadrenocorticism results in episodes of lethargy, weakness, tremors, and collapse. Painful episodes of muscle cramps are extremely rare.[77] Secondary hypoglycemia contributes to the generalized weakness. Treatment with physiologic doses of glucocorticoids (0.1 mg/kg) results in full clinical recovery.[78,79]

Diabetes Mellitus The peripheral nerves are dependent on glucose for their metabolism. A sensorimotor polyneuropathy is a late complication of diabetes mellitus (DM). The two major theories about the pathogenesis are metabolic derangement and vascular changes.[80] Clinical signs are most prominent in the pelvic limbs with a plantigrade stance, difficulty jumping, postural reaction deficits, decreased tendon reflexes, and muscle atrophy. Neuropathic signs are much more common in cats than in dogs. Horner's syndrome has been reported secondary to DM.[81,82] Abnormalities on nerve conduction studies and EMG are found in both thoracic and pelvic limbs. Histopathologic findings are demyelination, splitting, and ballooning of the myelin sheath, and axonal injury The myelin injury is associated with microvascular pathology including increase in capillary size, capillary luminal size, and increased basement membrane thickness.[83-86] Permanent deficits despite control of the DM are common.

Renal Failure Dogs and cats with chronic renal failure may have weakness associated with renal secondary hyperparathyroidism, which causes a peripheral neuropathy and myopathy. Inositol phosphates, protein kinase C, and cyclic adenosine monophosphate (AMP), among other regulatory enzymes and signal-transducing systems in muscle cells, are affected by calcitriol directly. The parathyroid hormone-mediated uremic myopathy may be reversible when treated with calcitriol. Excess PTH also partially affects the motor nerve conduction velocity. Nerve excitability is modulated by calcitriol, which also affects the synthesis of nerve growth factors. Changes can be found on electromyography and nerve conduction studies.

Electrolyte Abnormalities

Hypokalemia   Hypokalemia can be caused by reduced intake, loss associated with renal failure, and, in extremely rare situations, secondary to an adrenal tumor causing excess synthesis of aldosterone (primary hyperaldosteronism)—or, even more rare, due to adrenal-dependent hyperadrenocorticism.[87] Hypokalemia alters the muscle cell resting membrane potential resulting in muscular weakness. The neurologic signs with ventroflexion of the neck and generalized weakness are similar to any generalized neuromuscular disorder and not pathognomic for this condition. Treatment consists of supplementation via potassium IV initially, followed by oral administration. Administration of fluids with potassium IV may result in worsening of hypokalemia due to expansion of the vascular volume and increased renal loss. Oral administration of 5 to 10 mEq of KCl per day is a safe treatment. Dopamine causes a shift of potassium from the intracellular to the extracellular fluid.[88]

Paraneoplastic Syndrome   Paraneoplastic syndromes cause neurologic signs due to a remote effect of cancer, not caused by direct invasion of the nervous system by neoplastic cells or by any other mechanism related to the presence of cancer such as coagulopathy, vascular disorder, infection, and metabolic and nutritional deficits. The syndrome can affect both the CNS and the PNS. Neurologic signs can develop months to years before a tumor is detected. The lack of specific diagnostic tests makes the recognition of the syndrome difficult. Pathogenesis may be due to antibodies produced against cells of the nervous system. Removal of the tumors may result in resolution of the neurologic signs. Paraneoplastic syndrome has been documented secondary to insulinoma, adenocarcinoma, cholangiocellular carcinoma, lymphoma, melanoma, myeloma, and thymoma. Thymoma is a common cause of myasthenia gravis in humans and cats and less common in dogs. Neurologic signs can be focal (megaesophagus) or generalized. The myasthenia gravis may improve with removal of the mass; however, megaesophagus signals a poor prognosis.[89,90]

REFERENCES

The reference list can be found on the companion Expert Consult Web site at *www.expertconsult.com*.

CHAPTER 53

Movement Disorders

William B. Thomas

Movement disorders are abnormal movements affecting either overall body movement or a specific group of muscles. There is no well-recognized classification system because the neuroanatomic lesion and pathophysiology are not always known. Thus a descriptive approach provides the best categorization of these diverse disorders.

CLINICAL EVALUATION

The clinical evaluation starts with a detailed history including a description of the abnormal movement. The client's objective observations are generally more reliable than their subjective conclusions. For example, a complaint of "tremor" is less precise than reporting "the head suddenly jerks downward every second or so." For episodic abnormalities ask about the duration and frequency, as well as any factors that might precipitate the movements such as rest, excitement, or exercise. Try to determine if the patient is conscious and responsive during an episode and if the client can stop the movement

by distracting, petting, or feeding the animal. Encourage the client to videotape episodes that are infrequent. Also important are a past and current medical history including vaccination status, any previous illness, injury or toxin exposure, and other changes in between the episodes such as abnormal behavior or gait dysfunction. Perform a thorough neurologic examination to detect any persistent deficits that might help identify the neuroanatomic lesion responsible for the movement. Based on this initial evaluation and the differential diagnosis, further evaluation may be necessary such as imaging, electrodiagnostic testing, or analysis of spinal fluid.

SPASTICITY

Spasticity is an increase in muscle tone due to hyperexcitable muscle stretch (myotatic) reflexes. Muscle tone is the velocity-dependent resistance of muscle to passive stretch and is maintained by intrinsic muscle stiffness and the myotatic reflex mediated by the lower motor neurons. Descending

 To view a video on this topic, go to **www.expertconsult.com**.

upper motor neuron pathways normally attenuate the myotatic reflex. Lesions of the upper motor neuron pathway cause changes in the excitability of motor neurons, interneuronal connections, and local reflex pathways that over time lead to hyperexcitable myotatic reflexes and spasticity. The interval between injury and the appearance of spasticity varies from days to months. Once spasticity develops the chronic shortening of muscle results in enhancement of the intrinsic muscle stiffness, changes in collagen tissue, and tendons that lead to subclinical contractures and exacerbation of spasticity. Increased muscle tone predominates in the antigravity (extensor) muscles and results in a spastic gait characterized by decreased limb flexion. At rest, there is increased resistance to passive flexion of the limb and exaggerated myotatic reflexes and usually other signs of an upper motor neuron lesion such as paresis and ataxia.

Treatment of spasticity is directed at the underlying lesion, most commonly a chronic spinal cord disease. Physical therapy is helpful and usually involves strengthening of flexor muscles and stretching to maintain normal range of joint motion and minimize contracture. Benzodiazepines such as clorazepate (0.5 to 2 mg/kg orally every 12 hours) sometimes help decrease muscle tone, but in some patients spasticity actually aids weight bearing by increasing extensor muscle tone so the dose is titrated to avoid weakness.

MYOTONIA

Myotonia is prolonged contraction or delayed relaxation of a muscle after voluntary or stimulated contraction. Congenital myotonia is well characterized in the Chow Chow and Miniature Schnauzer and occurs sporadically in other breeds of dog and domestic cats. Signs are evident by 3 weeks of age and include muscle rigidity (non–velocity-dependent resistance to stretch), difficulty rising, and a stilted gait that improves as the patient moves about. Patients also have muscle hypertrophy, dysphagia, and a high-pitched bark. Tapping a muscle with a reflex hammer causes a dimple in the muscle. Diagnosis is based on clinical features. Electromyography (EMG) is useful in confirming myotonia based on finding complex repetitive discharges. In the Miniature Schnauzer, congenital myotonia is caused by a mutation in the chloride channel of the muscle and a genetic test is available. Extended-release procainamide (40 mg/kg orally every 8 to 12 hours) or mexiletine (8.3 mg/kg orally every 8 hours) improves the signs.[1]

Acquired myotonia is an uncommon complication of iatrogenic hyperadrenocorticism. Affected dogs show a stilted gait with decreased limb flexion, increased muscle tone, enlarged proximal limb muscles, percussion myotonia, and EMG evidence of myotonia. Treatment of hyperadrenocorticism partially improves the signs in some cases, but many patients have persistent myotonia. Procainamide is helpful in some patients. Myotonia is sometimes a component of other progressive myopathies.

TETANY

Tetany is sustained muscle contraction that is worsened by stimulation and lessens with relaxation. It occurs with strychnine poisoning, which blocks the inhibitory neurotransmitter glycine. A congenital syndrome characterized by stimulus-induced muscle contractions that resolve with rest has been described in a family of Labrador Retrievers.[2] Voluntary movement or stimulation induces extensor rigidity and apnea with no alterations in consciousness. Although called "reflex myoclonus," the signs are more consistent with tetany and are similar to hyperexplexia or stiff baby syndrome in children, which is caused by a glycine receptor mutation.

EPISODIC FALLING IN CAVALIER KING CHARLES SPANIELS

Episodic falling in Cavalier King Charles Spaniels, also called *hypertonicity syndrome*, is characterized by paroxysmal tetany or increased muscle tone usually starting around 3 to 4 months of age. Episodes are precipitated by excitement or variable periods of exercise and consist of sustained contraction of the muscles of the limbs and trunk, causing the dog to stand rigidly or fall over. There is no loss of consciousness and episodes last several seconds to several minutes, after which the patient recovers completely. Laboratory and electrodiagnostic testing are normal and diagnosis is based on clinical features. Clonazepam (0.5 mg/kg orally every 8 hours) is useful in minimizing the frequency and severity of attacks.[3] A similar syndrome has been reported in Springer Spaniels starting at 3 months of age, adult Wheaton Terriers, and adult Border Terriers.[4]

SCOTTIE CRAMP

Scottie cramp is inherited as an autosomal recessive trait in Scottish Terriers. Clinical signs become apparent by 6 weeks to 18 months of age. Excitement or exercise induces progressive increase in muscle tone causing lumbar kyphosis and decreased flexion of the pelvic limbs, in some cases so severe that the dog falls. There is some evidence that the disease is caused by alteration in the function of the neurotransmitter serotonin. Laboratory tests, electrodiagnostics, and muscle biopsies are normal. Treatment consists of lifestyle adjustments to avoid precipitating factors and acepromazine maleate (0.1 to 0.75 mg/kg orally every 12 hours) or diazepam (0.5 mg/kg orally every 8 hours). The disorder is nonprogressive and does not seriously compromise the dog's quality of life.[4]

CONTINUOUS MUSCLE FIBER ACTIVITY

Continuous muscle fiber activity occurs most commonly in Jack Russell Terriers but has also been reported in a Yorkshire Terrier, Border Collie, and a mixed breed dog and cat. The precise nature of this disorder is not yet clarified, so several names for the disease are used including *rippling muscle disease* and *myokymia*. Some affected Jack Russell Terriers have clinical signs of hereditary ataxia and it's unclear what, if any, role that plays in this disease. In human patients, rippling muscle disease is a myopathy characterized by muscle stiffness, mildly painful cramps, and visible rolling contractions of muscle without EMG activity. Myokymia is rolling, wormlike contractions of muscle accompanied by specific EMG activity. In affected dogs the age of onset varies from 4 months to 4 years. Episodes are often precipitated by excitement or exercise, occur several times a week to once a month, and are sometimes preceded by facial rubbing. There is increased muscle tone and visible undulating muscle contractions more obvious in proximal limb muscles. Dogs are often anxious, restless, and panting during attacks and hyperthermia is common. Episodes last from 10 minutes to several hours, but severe attacks can be fatal. Laboratory analysis may show mild increases in aspartate transaminase (AST), alanine transaminase (ALT), alkaline phosphatase, and creatine kinase. Electromyography is normal or shows myokymic discharges (spontaneous activity consisting of regularly occurring high-frequency bursts of 2, 3, or more motor unit action potentials) in muscles showing visible contractions. Procainamide (10 mg/kg every 8 hours) or mexiletine (4 mg/kg every 12 hours) is sometimes successful in decreasing the severity and frequency of attacks. Sedation or general anesthesia is necessary to abort severe attacks.[5]

TETANUS

Tetanus is sustained muscle contraction without relaxation. The most common cause is infection with *Clostridium tetani*. Under anaerobic conditions, the organism produces a toxin, tetanospasmin, that interferes with the release of the inhibitory neurotransmitters glycine and gamma-aminobutyric acid. Patients with focal tetanus present with sustained contractions in muscles close to the wound, usually the head or a limb. In generalized tetanus, patients suffer generalized muscle rigidity, trismus secondary to masticatory muscle contraction, dysphagia due to pharyngeal muscle involvement, and risus sardonicus resulting from facial muscle involvement (Figure 53-1).

MYOCLONUS

Myoclonus is a brief, shocklike contraction of skeletal muscle. Physiological myoclonus occurs in healthy animals and typically causes no disability. Familiar examples are hiccoughs (brief contractions of the diaphragm), muscle jerks during sleep, and the normal startle response, a stereotypical response to a sudden, unexpected stimulus such as a loud noise characterized by eyelid blink and brief contraction of the head, neck, and limb muscles. Epileptic myoclonus is a rare seizure disorder in which the seizures consist of focal or generalized myoclonic jerks. The cause may be idiopathic or underlying brain disease. For example, a genetic disease similar to Lafora's disease in human patients, which has been described in several breeds of dog and cat, causes intermittent myoclonic jerks of the head, neck, and thoracic limbs, often in response to visual stimuli.[6] Drug- and toxin-induced myoclonus occur due to several agents including intrathecal morphine, chlorambucil, and lead.[7-10] The myoclonus usually resolves on

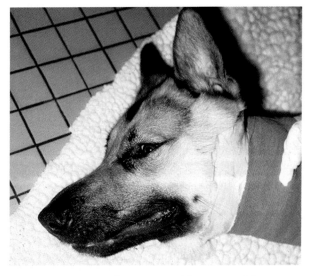

Figure 53-1 Risus sardonicus caused by tetanus. The commissures of the lips are drawn caudally and the ears are erect.

withdrawal of the offending drug or treatment of the intoxication.

ENCEPHALOMYELITIS

Encephalomyelitis caused by canine distemper virus is the most common cause of myoclonus in dogs. In older literature this movement was called *chorea*, but chorea is a more complex, nonrepetitive, irregularly timed movement, not the brief, simple muscle jerk of myoclonus. Affected dogs often have other neurologic signs of distemper such as ataxia or weakness, but myoclonus can be the only sign. The muscle contractions are most obvious at rest and can persist during sleep or even general anesthesia, usually occurring rhythmically every 1 to 3 seconds. In a few cases the myoclonus is generalized but more commonly it is restricted to a muscle or a group of muscles innervated by adjacent regions of the spinal cord or brainstem. Limb or jaw muscles are commonly involved, but any skeletal muscle can be affected including the tongue and extraocular muscles. Distemper myoclonus is often refractory to treatment although focal myoclonus is usually not terribly disabling. Procainamide (10 to 20 mg/kg orally every 8 hours) is effective in some cases. Other inflammatory diseases of the nervous system can also cause myoclonus in dogs, including granulomatous meningoencephalomyelitis, bacterial encephalitis, protozoal encephalitis, and steroid-responsive meningitis-arteritis.[11]

DYSKINESIA

Dyskinesia is a general term for various forms of abnormal movement. Paroxysmal dyskinesia is characterized by episodes of abnormal movements arising out of a background of normal movement and behavior. The clinical manifestations are variable, entailing several different movements: (1) dystonia: sustained muscle contractions resulting in twisting and abnormal posture of the face, trunk, or limbs, (2) athetosis: slow, writhing movements that tend to flow into one another, and (3) chorea: rapid, arrhythmic, brief movements of the face, trunk, or limbs. Paroxysmal dyskinesia has been reported in several related Boxer puppies and an adult Bichon Frise. Affected dogs exhibit spontaneous episodes of sustained flexion of neck or trunk muscles causing torticollis or kyphosis, respectively, unilateral facial dystonia causing a grimace, and either sustained flexion (dystonia) or rapid flexion and extension of a limb (choreoathetosis). Episodes last several minutes and evary in frequency from multiple episodes daily to once every few months. Baseline neurologic examination, brain MRI, and spinal fluid analysis are normal.[12-13]

In human patients, dyskinesia occurs as a side effect of several drugs. Those that antagonize dopamine are by far the most common, but other drugs have been implicated including metoclopramide, antiseizure drugs, anticholinergics, and antihistamines. Drug-induced dyskinesia characterized by contractions of the muscles of the face, neck, and shoulder has been reported as an adverse effect of phenobarbital in a dog.[14] Drug-induced dyskinesia should be considered in patients that develop movement disorders while taking medication. Signs typically resolve with withdrawal of the offending drug.

DANCING DOBERMAN

Dancing Doberman disease is characterized by flexion of one pelvic limb when standing, then within several months the other pelvic limb becomes affected such that the dog alternately flexes and extends each pelvic limb in a dancing motion and prefers to sit rather than stand.[15] This disorder affects Doberman Pinschers starting at 6 months to 7 years of age. There is also insidiously progressive paraparesis with decreased proprioception and atrophy of the gastrocnemius muscle. Based on electrodiagnostic testing and nerve biopsy, this may be a type of peripheral neuropathy, and the pelvic limb movements may be related to paresthesia in the paws.

OTHER ABNORMAL MOVEMENTS

Muscle spasms caused by pain, especially intervertebral disk extrusion, can be confused with movement disorders such as myoclonus. Affected animals often suffer intermittent, painful contractions of paraspinal muscles and may flex one limb. Movement often precipitates an attack. Palpation and manipulation of the spine usually identifies the painful region.

Tremor is a rhythmic oscillation of the body or body part due to alternating contractions of antagonistic muscles. It occurs with a number of disorders.

Seizures can result in variety of abnormal movements and are usually recognized by their stereotypic pattern and spontaneous onset. Seizures are often accompanied by some alteration in consciousness and there may be autonomic signs, such as urination or salivation, and postictal dysfunction such as abnormal behavior and ataxia.

Normal and abnormal movements can occur during sleep. Important features are that the movements only occur during sleep and the patient can be awakened normally during an episode with no postictal signs.

References

The reference list can be found on the companion Expert Consult Web site at *www.expertconsult.com*.

CHAPTER 54

Tremor Syndromes

Dominik Faissler

DEFINITIONS

Tremor is a common presentation in dogs and cats. The terms *tremble, shake, quiver,* and *shiver* are used interchangeably to describe this involuntary, rhythmic, and oscillatory movement. Tremor results from simultaneous or alternating contractions of agonist and antagonist muscle groups. Electromyographically, biphasic rhythmic bursts can be recorded. Clinically, tremor syndromes present with continuous, rapid, back-and-forth movements of the head, hind legs, or whole body; these movements cease with sleep.

Tremor must be distinguished from myoclonus, fasciculations, tetany, dyskinesia, and seizures. *Myoclonus* is defined as a sudden, short, jerky, shocklike, involuntary movement caused by an abrupt muscular contraction. Myoclonic jerks arise from electrical discharge of the central nervous system and can involve the head, limbs, or trunk. *Fasciculations* are arrhythmic, involuntary, visible contractions of groups of muscle fibers that indicate pathologic discharge of spinal motor neurons. *Tetany* is characterized by skeletal muscle rigidity and spasm. *Dyskinesias* are rare disorders of the central nervous system that result in involuntary, ticlike, repetitive, and episodic movements of individual muscle groups. The terms *dystonia, athetosis, chorea,* and *ballism* are used in human neurology to describe various clinical manifestations of dyskinesia.

PHYSIOLOGIC TREMOR

Physiologic tremors are difficult to see in normal animals, but they are present at low-amplitude movements, at rest, or with posture. Shivering is a normal response to hypothermia, and a fast-rising body temperature in the course of a febrile process may lead to trembling. In both cases, the caudal hypothalamus plays an important role in the induction of muscle oscillations. Fear, stress, joy, anger, and pain are the manifestations of a complex response processed in the limbic system, prefrontal cortex, and hypothalamus. These emotional conditions produce a complex pattern of reactions, including increased muscle tone, adrenergic stimulation, and physiologic muscle tremor. Trembling may also be seen after heavy exercise, hunger, or cold as a result of metabolic exhaustion and weakness.

PATHOLOGIC TREMOR

Tremor is considered pathologic when it impairs the patient's normal function. Abnormal tremor has a more synchronous activation and larger amplitude and is more easily visualized. No classification system has been devised for pathologic tremor in animals, and little information is available on the etiology and pathogenesis of this condition.

Type

A kinetic tremor with voluntary movements, commonly called an *intention tremor*, is evident when the patient performs a voluntary movement, and it is most obvious when the movement is goal oriented. Intention tremor usually presents with slow, high-amplitude, to-and-fro movements. *Resting tremor* is most visible in a relaxed condition and diminishes with voluntary movement; the amplitude of these oscillations is much lower, and the frequency is midrange. A *fine, fast*

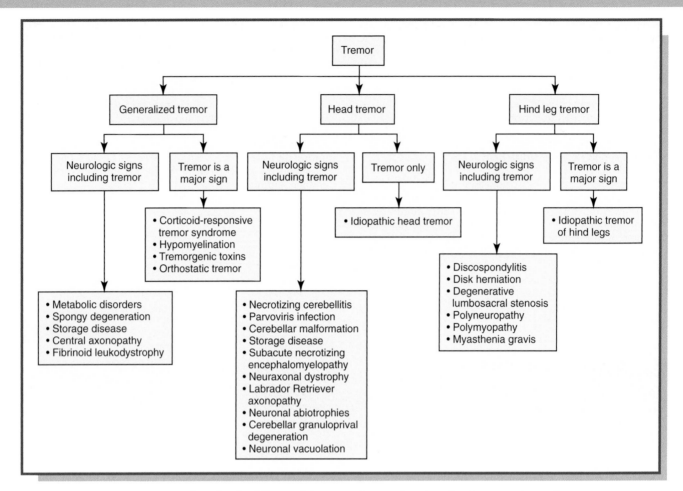

Figure 54-1   Algorithm for differential diagnosis of tremor based on distribution and neurologic signs.

action tremor occurs when parts of the body are activated in certain positions; this type of tremor may occur when the animal is attempting greater precision of movement. *Static tremor* is manifested when antigravity muscles are activated.

Distribution

Involuntary movements can be restricted to the head, and intention tremor is the most common presentation. Head bobbing in either a vertical or horizontal direction also is possible. Localized tremor may be confined to the lumbosacral area and hind legs. Generalized whole body tremors seem to be more common than focal tremors.

LOCALIZATION OF THE PACEMAKER

Lesions in the lateral cerebellar hemispheres, nucleus interpositus, and cerebellar vermis are associated with intention tremor. Experimental lesions in the rubro-olivocerebellar system of cats can induce either intention tremor or resting tremor. In general, except for intention tremor, anatomic localization of the pacemaker is uncertain in dogs and cats.

PREDOMINANCE OF CLINICAL SIGNS

Some diseases may cause trembling accompanied by other signs. A second group of selective, functional disorders presents with tremor syndromes in which shivering is the predominant complaint. An algorithm is presented in Figure 54-1.

DISORDERS IN WHICH TREMBLING IS ACCOMPANIED BY OTHER SIGNS

Metabolic Disorders

In addition to other signs, head or whole body tremors may be present in renal disease, hypoglycemia, hypocalcemia, and hypoadrenocorticism.

Intracranial Diseases

A large number of brain diseases may cause tremors, most often with cerebellar involvement. Head tremors, intention tremors and, less frequently, whole body tremors may be part of the syndrome. Other signs often are more obvious than the tremors, such as broad-based stance, ataxia, hypermetria, central vestibular dysfunction and, less frequently, paraparesis or tetraparesis, delayed proprioceptive responses, cranial nerve deficits, abnormal behavior, and seizurelike activity.

Tremors are reported to be a possible sign in multisystemic inflammatory disease in Borzois; cerebellitis caused by *Neospora caninum;* cerebellar hypoplasia due to mutation or intrauterine respectively perinatal parvovirus infection; fibrinoid leukodystrophy; the late course of neuraxonal

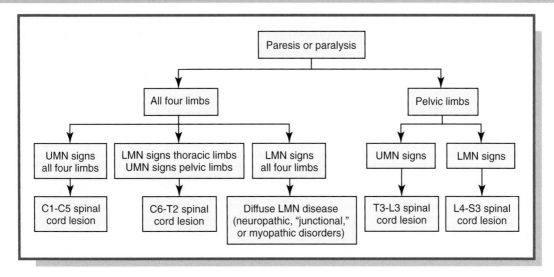

Figure 55-2 Algorithm for lesion localization in patients with paresis or paralysis. *LMN,* Lower motor neuron; *UMN,* upper motor neuron.

the lumbosacral area are present. The flexor and perineal reflexes display signs of LMN. Box 55-1 presents common diagnoses according to lesion localization.

A notable exception exists to the lesion localization within the spinal cord based on the principles of UMN and LMN. It is so-called Schiff-Sherrington phenomenon and occurs in patients with severe thoracolumbar lesions (T2-L7) damaging the propriospinal tract, which is inhibitory to the extensor muscles of the thoracic limbs. These patients are paraplegic with normal thoracic limb gait, but display, when laterally recumbent, thoracic limb spasticity.

In a paralyzed animal, it is important to establish whether or not nociception (pain perception) is intact. A noxious stimulus such as pinching at one of the toes or at the nail bed

should elicit a withdrawal of the limb accompanied by a behavioral response, such as vocalization. If the patient flexes the limb but does not have conscious perception of the painful stimulus, this indicates a severe spinal cord lesion and carries a guarded to poor prognosis, particularly if the patient had an external spinal trauma, is paralyzed for many days, and displays LMN signs.

REFERENCES

The reference list can be found on the companion Expert Consult Web site at *www.expertconsult.com.*

CHAPTER 56

Altered States of Consciousness: Stupor and Coma

Karen L. Kline

DEFINITIONS

Stupor and coma are pathologic abnormalities caused by an interruption in the structural, metabolic, and/or physiologic integrity of the brainstem or cerebral cortex. Stupor is characterized by a state in which the animal appears to be asleep or unconscious but can be aroused by a noxious stimulus. Once the stimulus is withdrawn, however, the animal may lapse back into the sleeplike state. Coma is characterized by a state of unconsciousness in which the animal cannot be aroused even by a noxious stimulus. A strong toe pinch, for example, may elicit a flexion reflex or increased extensor tone

but does not cause a behavioral response, such as crying or biting. In either case, prompt action is required to attempt to reverse these signs and correct the underlying cause.

PATHOPHYSIOLOGY

Consciousness is maintained by sensory stimuli that act through the ascending reticular activating system (ARAS) on the cerebral cortex. Decreasing levels of consciousness indicate abnormal cerebrocortical function or interference with cortical activation by the ARAS. The cerebral cortex controls the content of consciousness, whereas the brainstem controls the level of consciousness. In a sense, the cerebrum is the light bulb, and the brainstem is the rheostat that regulates its brightness. All sensory pathways have collateral input to the ARAS in the pons and the midbrain, and this information is projected diffusely to the cerebral cortex, where cholinergic synapses communicate constantly with cortical neurons. Balance is maintained between the ARAS and the adrenergic (sleep) system, which projects from the midbrain and diencephalon (thalamus). Signs ranging from hyperexcitability to coma can be observed if imbalance exists between the two systems.

The causes of stupor and coma are numerous. The three most important are (1) increased intracranial pressure, (2) cerebral edema, and (3) herniation of brain tissue. Increased intracranial pressure can occur secondary to an increase in the volume of tissue or fluid (e.g., cerebrospinal fluid, edema, or blood) within the cranial vault; even small shifts in these volumes can have dramatic consequences. Causes of increased intracranial pressure include encephalitis, meningitis, mass lesions (e.g., neoplasia, granulomas, or abscesses), vascular events, traumatic injury, or underlying metabolic disturbances, such as hypertension.

Cerebral edema is an abnormal accumulation of fluid in the brain parenchyma. It is classified into three types: (1) vasogenic, which is most commonly associated with brain masses and is due to a breakdown in blood-brain barrier integrity; (2) cytotoxic, which is most commonly associated with metabolic disturbances, such as hypoxia and neuroglycopenia, that cause cell or neuronal death; and (3) interstitial, which is most likely associated with hydrocephalus. The end result of progressively increased intracranial pressure and/or cerebral edema is brain herniation.

There are four different types of herniation, two of which can induce stupor or coma: (1) caudal transtentorial herniation, in which portions of the temporal lobe shift ventral to the tentorium cerebelli and cause midbrain compression; and (2) foramen magnum herniation, the most common form, which occurs when the caudal cerebellar vermis moves through the foramen magnum, causing a compression of the displaced cerebellum and the medulla oblongata. In these cases, injury to the respiratory center, descending motor pathway tracts, and cardiovascular centers in the caudal brainstem can lead to irreversible midbrain and cerebral hypoxia and coma.

APPROACH TO THE PATIENT WITH STUPOR OR COMA

After the pet's initial presentation, close attention must be paid to immediate life-threatening injuries and their sequelae, such as hemorrhage, hypoxia, or shock. The ABCs of critical care medicine—airway, breathing, and cardiovascular status—are paramount. Concurrently, a thorough history, including onset and progression of signs, previous illness or injury, and drug use or toxin exposure, should be ascertained. Thorough physical and neurologic examinations should be performed, with emphasis placed on the respiratory pattern as well as on cardiac rate and rhythm. Simply observing the patient for a short time can yield considerable information. An anatomic diagnosis can be ascertained on the basis of the following: (1) mental status and level of consciousness; (2) neuroophthalmologic signs (vision, pupil size and symmetry, and ocular movements); (3) alterations in respiratory pattern; and (4) skeletal motor responses. Following these trends can improve prognostication, aid the development of treatment protocols, and is essential for patient management.

Mental Status and Level of Consciousness

Consciousness is maintained by the midbrain ARAS, which acts as a rheostat, projecting diffusely to the cerebral cortex. Consequently, diffuse cerebral disease or midbrain disease can result in stupor, coma, or other alterations in consciousness, such as dementia. Differentiation between stupor and coma can be achieved with the application of a noxious stimulus, such as a hemostat or needle. Care must be taken to follow trends when evaluating the patient, and hasty prognostication should be avoided. In general, stupor has a better initial prognosis than coma, but exceptions can occur. Other factors include the patient's age, the underlying medical history, and the cause of the alteration in consciousness.

Neuroophthalmologic Signs

Pupillary Reactions   Pupil size and reactivity to light can be normal in the comatose patient; alterations in these parameters can aid in neurolocalization and prognostication. Integrity of the retinae, optic nerves, and chiasm and of the rostral brainstem is consistent with pupils that are equal in size and that respond well to light and darkness. In general, lesions of the cerebral cortex and thalamus result in normal or constricted pupils that respond to both darkness and light. Lesions in the brainstem can result in unilateral or bilateral pupillary constriction (pons) or dilatation (midbrain), depending on the location. Peripheral lesions involving cranial nerve (CN) III usually result in dilated pupils with normal vision. Pupils that are bilaterally dilated (fixed) and unresponsive to light imply a guarded to grave prognosis.

Ocular Movements   The pathways that mediate ocular movements lie adjacent to the brainstem regions responsible for consciousness, making it clinically useful to evaluate ocular movements in the stuporous or comatose patient. Physiologic nystagmus or conjugate eye movements (the oculocephalic and doll's eye reflexes) are normal and require integrity of CN VIII (vestibulocochlear nerve), the brainstem (vestibular nuclei, medial longitudinal fasciculus), the cerebellum (flocculonodular lobe), and the nuclei of CN III, IV, and VI. Any disruption in this pathway results in pathologic nystagmus (rotary, horizontal, or vertical downbeat). Ocular movements are evaluated by moving the head in a slow or rapid fashion from side to side while it is held in a fixed position. In the normal animal, this movement results in several beats of horizontal nystagmus (with the fast component toward the direction of the head movement) that stop once the head movement stops. If the nystagmus continues after the movement stops, if it occurs spontaneously, or if it changes with position, a lesion in the vestibular system is likely to exist. If there is absence of ocular movements in the comatose patient, severe brainstem injury should be suspected, and the prognosis for return to function is guarded to grave.

Alterations in Respiratory Pattern

Severe or progressive brain injury can result in changes in breathing patterns. Cheyne-Stokes respiration is characterized by hyperpnea alternating with apnea and can be an indication of a bilateral cerebral hemisphere or diencephalic lesion. Central neurogenic breathing or hyperventilation is associated with lesions in the midbrain pneumotaxic center, whereas lower pontine and medullary lesions result in apneustic or ataxic (gasping) respirations, respectively. When a change in breathing patterns is noted, aggressive therapy may need to be instituted to counteract herniation.

Skeletal Motor Responses

The examination of motor function in the comatose patient provides valuable localizing information. Trends must be monitored in order to follow the disease course. Injury to the descending motor systems can result in either increased or decreased extensor and flexor tone, depending on where the injury occurs. Involuntary movements, such as twitching or paddling, may indicate seizure activity. Decerebrate posture (all four limbs extended) indicates a lesion in the midbrain or pons and can occur primarily or secondary to cerebrocortical herniation; decerebrate posture indicates that the motor pathways that aid in flexion are damaged and stupor or coma is present. Decerebellate posture (forelimbs extended with alternating hind limb flexion and extension) indicates a rostral cerebellar lesion, and the level of consciousness may not be impaired. Flaccid paralysis due to injury to the descending motor pathways implies a grave prognosis, especially when the patient is stuporous or comatose.

DIAGNOSTIC PLAN

The causes of stupor and coma are numerous (Figure 56-1). Routine laboratory data (hemogram, serum chemistries, urinalysis) can aid in determining a metabolic cause of the

alteration in consciousness. Inflammatory, infectious, or toxic agents may cause changes in the hemogram, whereas metabolic or endocrine disorders may result in changes in the blood chemistries, which would suggest the need for other diagnostic tests, such as evaluation of blood ammonia levels and serum bile acids, adrenocorticotropic hormone (ACTH) stimulation, and thyroid profiles. Chest and abdominal diagnostic imaging (radiographs, ultrasonography) may also be indicated if metastatic or infectious disease is suspected. If minimal changes are noted in these parameters, a primary or intracranial cause of stupor or coma should be considered. Noninvasive methods used to determine the cause of intracranial disease include electroencephalography (EEG) and brainstem auditory-evoked response (BAER). These methods are useful for evaluating the integrity of the cerebral cortex and brainstem, respectively, and they can be performed without general anesthesia. Ophthalmic evaluation may help to determine whether high intracranial pressure or infectious disease is present. Computed tomography (CT) and magnetic resonance imaging (MRI) are quite useful for confirming the presence and character of intracranial lesions, such as tumors,

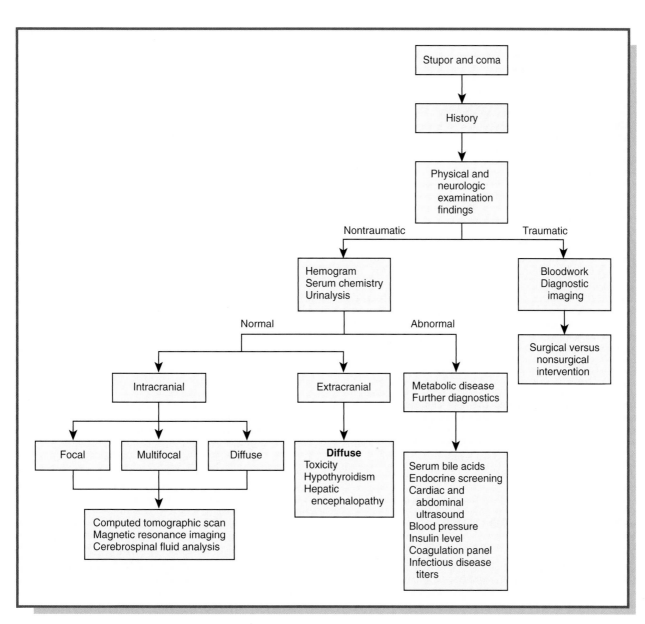

Figure 56-1 Algorithm for diagnostic approach to stupor and coma.

hydrocephalus, and vascular injuries. If the dog or cat is comatose, general anesthesia may not be necessary. Spinal fluid analysis typically is useful for determining whether the animal has an inflammatory or a neoplastic intracranial process; general anesthesia is required and does carry some risk if high intracranial pressure exists.

TREATMENT GOALS

Most dogs and cats with stupor or coma have life-threatening injuries that require immediate attention. Establishing a patent airway and maintaining respirations and cardiovascular status (in particular, blood pressure) are critical to stabilization, regardless of the underlying cause of the insult. Blood work should be evaluated, and intravenous administration of fluids, anticonvulsants, osmotic diuretics, and, in some cases, corticosteroids can be instituted to aid patient stabilization. Elevation of the head may help reduce excessive cerebral blood flow, and body temperature should be continuously monitored, especially in the case of seizures. Cerebral edema can be treated using injectable corticosteroids (once the blood pressure has stabilized), osmotic and loop diuretics (mannitol and furosemide, respectively), and hyperventilation. Seizures can be controlled using injectable anticonvulsants such as diazepam, phenobarbital, and pentobarbital. These treatments are discussed in more detail in the chapters on specific brain diseases. Intensive nursing care is paramount. Frequent turning (to avoid hypostatic lung congestion), bladder evacuation, ocular lubrication, optimal nutrition, and proper bedding are imperative.

PROGNOSIS

The prognosis for animals with stupor or coma depends on the cause of the insult, other underlying disease processes, the location of the injury, the signalment, and the response to therapy. Serial neurologic evaluations that concentrate particularly on the level of consciousness, ocular movements, pupillary size, motor tone, and breathing patterns can guide the practitioner in terms of treatment options and prognostication. Patience is necessary, especially in cases of brain trauma, and trends in improvement or deterioration need to be followed. If the patient survives the immediate injury, sequelae such as seizures, permanent neurologic deficits, and long-term nursing care should be addressed with the client.

CHAPTER 57

Seizures

Michael Podell

The approach and treatment of seizure disorders in small animals is similar in many respects to the treatment of various other ailments in veterinary medicine: An antecedent historical problem arises, a proper diagnosis is made to confirm the condition, and therapy is initiated to treat the underlying disease and/or signs of the disease. Important differences arise, however, when approaching the diagnosis and treatment of seizures in the dog and cat. First, a specific underlying etiology is often not identified. Second, the clinician must often make a therapeutic decision based on historical accounts alone. Third, treatment is often initiated when the pet is normal, with little ability to predict frequency of seizure recurrence. Finally, both the pet's and owner's quality of life during the interictal period must be balanced with the ability to limit the severity, frequency, and duration of future seizure events. This chapter is designed to help clinicians understand the variables for consideration in the treatment of seizure disorders by following 10 guiding principles of therapy.[1]

THE BRAIN IS SIMILAR TO OTHER ORGANS IN THE BODY

The brain is an organ that can get sick and recover, similar to other body systems. Epileptic seizures are a sign of a sick brain. Thus, all epileptic seizures should be taken seriously and approached in a similar fashion.

BE CERTAIN THAT EPILEPTIC SEIZURES HAVE OCCURRED

Seizures are paroxysmal in onset, have a finite duration, and are followed by a change in behavior that can last from seconds to hours. The clinical features of epileptic seizures can be separated into four components[2]: 1. The *prodrome* is the time period prior to the onset of seizure activity; 2. The *aura* is the initial manifestation of a seizure. During this time period, animals can exhibit stereotypic sensory or motor behavior (e.g., pacing, licking), autonomic patterns (e.g., salivating, vomiting), or even unusual psychic events; 3. The *ictal* period is the actual seizure event manifested by involuntary muscle tone or movement and/or abnormal behavior lasting usually from seconds to minutes; and 4. The *postictal* period occurs upon completion of the seizure and can last from minutes to hours.

Seizure types are first classified as either being self-limiting (isolated) or clustered (2 or more within 24 hours) and/or continuous (status epilepticus). Within each category, seizures are divided into being either focal or generalized. Focal seizures may be associated with a higher incidence of focal

 To view a video on this topic, go to **www.expertconsult.com**.

Table • 57-1

Antiepileptic Drug Therapy in the Dog and Cat

ANTIEPILEPTIC DRUG	CLINICAL PHARMACOLOGY				INITIAL DOSAGE		INITIAL THERAPEUTIC RANGE		ADJUSTMENT FORMULA
	DOG		CAT		DOG	CAT	DOG	CAT	
	$T_{1/2}$ (hr)	Tss (d)	$T_{1/2}$ (hr)	Tss (d)					
Phenobarbital[8] (PB)	24-40 Hepatic	10-14	34-43 Hepatic	10-14	2.5 mg/kg q12h	1-2 mg/kg/d	15-30 mg/dL	10-20 mg/dL	(Desired concentration / Actual concentration) × (# mg PB per day) = Total # mg PB/day
Bromide[9] Monotherapy with Phenobarbital	15-20 days Renal	75-100	10-13 days	28-42	50 mg/kg/d 40 mg/kg/d	NR NR	2.0-3.0 mg/mL 1.5-2.5 mg/mL	NR NR	(Target Css − Actual Css) = (2000 mg/L − Actual Css) × 0.02 = added mg/kg/day to existing dose
Felbamate[10]	5-6 Hepatic	1-2	ND	ND	20 mg/kg q8h	NR	25-100 mg/L	NR	Increase by 100-200 mg per dose every 3 days
Clonazepam[11]	1-2 Hepatic	1	ND	ND	1-2 mg q12h	0.5 mg q12-24h	20-75 µg/L	20-75 µg/L	Increase by 25% increments per dose
Diazepam	3-6 Hepatic	1	15-20 Hepatic	3-4	NR	0.5-2 mg q8-12h			
Topiramate[12]	2-4 Hepatic	1-3	ND	ND	2-10 mg/kg q12h	12.5-25 mg q8-2h	2-25 mg/L	ND	Increase by 25% increments per dose
Zonisamide (ZN)[7]	15-20 Hepatic	3-4	ND	ND	5-10 mg/kg q12h	2-5 mg/kg q12h	10-60 µg/mL	ND	(Desired concentration/Actual concentration) × (# mg ZN per day) = Total # mg ZN/day
Levetiracetam[13,14]	4-6 Renal	1-2	2-20 Renal	1-5	10-20 mg/kg q8-12h	10-20 mg/kg q8-12h	5-50 µg/mL	5-50 µg/mL	Increase from bid to tid dosing first, then increase by 20%-40% increments thereafter

Hepatic, Hepatic metabolism; *ND*, not determined; *NR*, not recommended; *Renal*, renal metabolism; $T_{1/2}$, elimination half-life; *Tss*, time to steady state concentrations.

intracranial pathology[3] and are commonly seen as facial muscle twitching or with more complex behavior patterns with impaired consciousness and/or bizarre behavioral activity (termed *complex partial*, *psychomotor*, or *automotor* seizures).[4]

Generalized seizures are subdivided into *tonic-clonic*, *clonic*, *myoclonic*, *atonic*, or *absence* types. Tonic-clonic seizures are the most common generalized seizure type described. Myoclonic epileptic seizures consist of rhythmic limb and/or head jerk–like movements, often with preservation of consciousness.

IDENTIFY THE ETIOLOGY

The most important aspect of seizure management is establishing the cause. The differential diagnoses of epileptic seizures can be divided into four main etiologic categories: *idiopathic* (most likely inherited), *symptomatic* (underlying brain pathology), *probably symptomatic* (underlying unidentified brain disease that is not suspected to be of genetic origin), and *reactive* (normal brain reacting to metabolic stresses). The differential diagnoses in terms of disease prevalence differ according the age of onset of the seizure. In general, dogs that are less than 1 or greater than 7 years of age have an initial interictal interval less than 4 weeks, and/or have initial focal seizures that should carry a higher suspicion for symptomatic epilepsy with appropriate diagnostic tests done, to include MRI scanning of the brain.[3] All cats without a metabolic cause for seizures should undergo MRI scanning of the brain and possible cerebrospinal fluid analysis.[5]

ALWAYS TREAT THE UNDERLYING DISEASE

Epileptic seizures are a sign of the disease and not the cause. Always direct specific therapy to the underlying disease, as long-term antiepileptic drug (AED) treatment of seizures may not be necessary.

START TREATMENT EARLY IN THE COURSE OF DISEASE

The earlier therapy is started, the better the potential outcome may be for seizure control. The decision to initiate therapy is based on the underlying etiology, seizure type and frequency, and diagnostic evaluation. Reasons to start therapy include: (1) identification of a structural lesion; (2) status epilepticus has occurred; (3) more than three generalized seizures occurred within a 24-hour period; (4) two or more cluster seizure events occur within an 1-year period; (5) two or more isolated seizure events occur within a 6-month period; (6) first seizure was within 1 month of head trauma; (7) prolonged ictal events (> 10 minutes), regardless of frequency; and (8) prolonged, severe, or unusual postictal periods occur.

START WITH THE APPROPRIATE AED

Limiting total AED intake is an advantageous goal in treating epilepsy. A balance exists between seizure control and quality of life afforded with all treatment. As such, monotherapy is recommended to reduce adverse effects, allow better owner compliance, and reduce overall costs. Phenobarbital and bromide are the most widely used initial AEDs (Table 57-1).

Bromide is not recommended in cats due to the high prevalence of allergic induced bronchitis.

BE PROACTIVE RATHER THAN REACTIVE

The goal to drug level monitoring is to maintain drug concentrations within a known therapeutic range to provide the best opportunity to prevent future seizures (see Table 57-1). Trough sample times are recommended to identify levels when patients are most susceptible to breakthrough seizures.

ADJUST THE DOSE ACCORDING TO DRUG CONCENTRATION

Drug dose adjustments should be made if three or more seizures occur within a 6-month period, cluster seizure activity worsens, or adverse effects are present according to current drug levels and not by weight and by established pharmacokinetic formula (see Table 57-1). Serum chemistry panels should be monitored at least every 6 months for all hepatic metabolized medications.

CONFIRM COMPLIANCE IN DOSING AND MONITORING

All owners should be sent home with a specific calendar to record seizure events, adverse effects, and changes in drug dosing. A 20% decrease in AED concentration is suspicious for poor dosing compliance.

KNOW WHEN AND HOW TO ADD OR CHANGE MEDICATIONS

Treatment should be adjusted when either no improvement in seizure control is seen despite maximal trough therapeutic serum concentration and/or when toxic effects are developing. A number of add-on AED options are now available (see Table 57-1). The selection is based on a number of factors, including mechanism of action, drug compatibility, patient tolerance, and cost. Benzodiazepines are recommended for cats in combination only with a nonhepatic metabolized AED due to the risk of acute hepatic necrosis syndrome. The most promising of the newer AED for dogs and cats is levetiracetam, which is the S-enantiomer of the ethyl analogue of piracetam that binds to SV2A, a synaptic vesicle protein, to correlate with anticonvulsant potency.[6] The drug is renal metabolized, has a relatively short elimination half-life, is available as a parenteral formulation, and has minimal adverse effects. Zonisamide is a substituted 1,2-benzisoxazole derivative that is hepatic metabolized, has a relatively long half-life, and high protein-binding affinity in dogs.[7] Broad-spectrum antiepileptic activity has been reported against a variety of seizure types, with particular improvement in the treatment of adult myoclonus epilepsy.

In summary, a logical approach of following the three "D" paradigm of diagnosis, drug selection, and dose adjustment will enhance the clinician's ability to treat epileptic patients more effectively and with overall improvement in quality of lifestyle for the patient and owner alike.

REFERENCES

The reference list can be found on the companion Expert Consult Web site at *www.expertconsult.com*.

CHAPTER 58

Peripheral Cranial Neuropathies

Dominique Paquette

Causes of cranial nerve (CN) deficits of peripheral etiology include inflammatory, infectious, neoplastic, and idiopathic. Fortunately, most of the common peripheral cranial neuropathies are idiopathic and self-limiting. Idiopathic mononeuropathies affect the cranial nerves more commonly than any other peripheral nerves. A thorough neurologic examination helps to localize the lesion either to the peripheral or central nervous system. Differentiating the two is crucial for determining treatment and prognosis. Multiple cranial nerve deficits most often imply that the problem is within the central nervous system even though specific exceptions are recognized. For instance, the combination of a head tilt, facial nerve paralysis, and a Horner's syndrome strongly suggests a lesion in the middle ear.

CN II—OPTIC NEURITIS

Optic neuritis is characterized by acute vision loss and is usually bilateral. Pupils are usually dilated and unresponsive to light stimulation. There are frequently changes on the optic disk such as swollen optic disk margins and hemorrhage. Possible causes include infectious (e.g., *Cryptococcus*, histoplasmosis, canine distemper) and inflammatory (e.g., ocular granulomatous meningoencephalitis [GME] and other immune-mediated disorders). Most of the time, no underlying cause is identified and the disease is presumed to be immune-mediated. Sudden acquired retinal degeneration (SARD) is a common cause of acute blindness in dogs and must be considered. With SARD the fundic exam can be normal initially but the electroretinogram (ERG) will be abnormal (i.e., extinguished). Optic neuritis usually responds to immunosuppressive doses of glucocorticoids. Treatment should be started as early as possible to improve prognosis for vision. Prognosis is fair (Figure 58-1).

HORNER'S SYNDROME

A lesion in the sympathetic innervation of the head causes a Horner's syndrome. Clinical signs include miosis, prolapsed nictitans, entophthalmia, and ptosis. All components are not necessarily present (i.e., partial Horner's), but miosis must at least be noted for diagnosis. Lesion localization varies from the midbrain through the spinal cord down to T1-T3 spinal segments, up the vagosympathetic trunk, and the cranial cervical ganglion next to the tympanic bulla (middle ear). A lesion at any level can cause a Horner's syndrome. Lesions are classified as first, second, or third order depending on which level is affected. Pharmacologic testing with topical phenylephrine can help to localize the lesion. The faster the response to topical phenylephrine (pupillary dilation), the closer the lesion is to the iris. Most cases are of third order and are recognized as idiopathic Horner's syndrome. Treatment is rarely necessary and is mainly aesthetic as vision is not impaired unless the problem is bilateral. Prognosis for vision is good.

CN V—TRIGEMINAL NEUROPATHY

The trigeminal nerve provides sensation of the face through three branches: the ophthalmic, maxillary, and mandibular nerves. Sensory deficits include reduced to absent palpebral and corneal reflexes as well as deficits in nasal sensation. Loss of corneal sensation can result in neurogenic keratopathy. The mandibular branch also provides motor innervation to the masticatory muscles (i.e., masseter, temporalis, pterygoid, and digastric). A dropped jaw results from a bilateral deficit in the motor function of the trigeminal nerves. A lesion affecting both trigeminal nerves implies a peripheral lesion since a lesion in the brainstem affecting both trigeminal nerves would be too extensive to be compatible with life; the trigeminal motor nucleus is located in the pons at the level of the reticular formation. It is essential to rule out other conditions that can cause inability or unwillingness to close the mouth such as temporomandibular joint disease, masticatory muscle myositis, or a retrobulbar lesion. Differential diagnoses for a dropped jaw include infectious (e.g., *Neospora*, *Toxoplasma*, *Cryptococcus*, rabies), inflammatory (immune-mediated), neoplasia (e.g., nerve sheath tumor, lymphosarcoma), and idiopathic. Idiopathic trigeminal neuritis (ITN) is the most common neurologic cause of dropped jaw in dogs. ITN mainly impairs motor function, with a variable degree of sensory loss. Treatment includes supportive care with assisted feeding. Animals usually recover within 3 weeks.

Nerve sheath tumors (NST) affecting CN V alone are also relatively common. NST are usually unilateral and cause ipsilateral muscle atrophy. Some degree of reduced facial sensation can also be noted and is manifested by reduced nasal sensation and reduced palpebral reflex. Abnormal facial sensation causing facial itchiness, rubbing, or pain can also be seen. NST are locally invasive and slow to metastasize. Treatment options include surgery, radiation, or supportive care only with glucocorticoids. Prognosis is guarded (Figure 58-2).

CN VII—FACIAL PARALYSIS

Facial neuropathy is the most common cranial neuropathy. Clinical signs associated with facial nerve deficits are acute; they include lack of palpebral closure, droopy ear, lip, and/or cheek. This condition is often associated with ptyalism. Vestibular signs are commonly seen with facial nerve deficits due to the close relationship of these nerves in two anatomic areas within the skull (i.e., brainstem and petrosal bone). Peripheral facial paralysis can be secondary to otitis media/interna, trauma/iatrogenic, neoplasia of the middle ear, metabolic (e.g., hypothyroidism, other), sulfon-

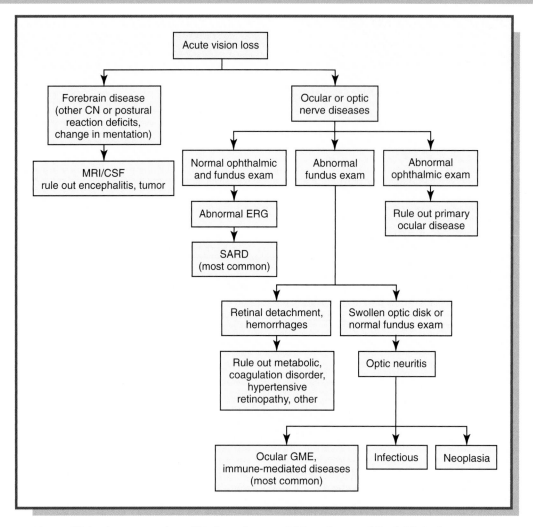

Figure 58-1 Acute vision loss. *CN,* Cranial nerve; *CSF,* cerebrospinal fluid; *ERG,* electroretinogram; *GME,* granulomatous meningoencephalitis; *MRI,* magnetic resonance imaging; *SARD,* sudden acquired retinal degeneration.

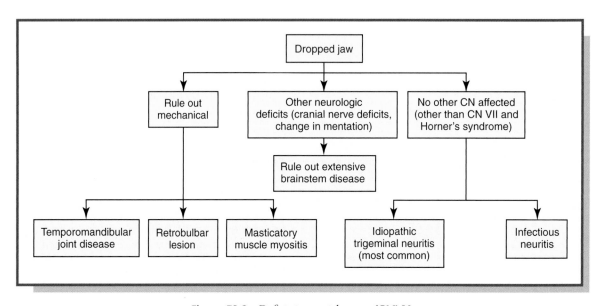

Figure 58-2 Deficit in cranial nerve *(CN)* V.

usually not different from normal dogs. Excessive daytime sleepiness, if ascertained, may provide further clues that the animal is narcoleptic.

A diagnosis of narcolepsy is most often based on EEG recordings obtained during cataplexy showing a pattern consistent with normal awake state or REM sleep. Abnormal spikes and waves typical of true seizure activity should not be observed (unless there is an associated seizure disorder). Additionally, muscles remain hypotonic or atonic during the cataplexy and autonomic signs are not observed. Myasthenia gravis and other neuromuscular disorders causing acute, profound, intermittent weakness must also be differentiated from narcolepsy-cataplexy. Extracranial diagnostic workup is within normal limits including complete blood count, serum biochemical profile, urinalysis, electrocardiography, and thoracic radiography. Routine CSF analysis is also within normal limits. The food-elicited cataplexy test (FECT) may be used to assess cataplexy as well as the efficacy of a treatment. In this test, pieces of food are laid out on the floor before the patient is released in the room. Normal dogs will eat the food quickly and usually without stopping (<2 minutes). Narcoleptic dogs, excited by the food, may have complete or partial cataplectic attacks while attempting to eat and take much longer to eat. This test is often unreliable in the clinical situation where patients are in a strange or stressful environment but may be more useful when performed in the home environment.

A cataplectic attack may be diagnosed in mildly affected animals by the use of IV physostigmine salicylate (0.025-0.1 mg/kg), a cholinesterase inhibitor that increases the chances of cataplexy occurring within 15 minutes. Starting with the lower end of the dosage range is recommended because of possible adverse effects.

Measuring CSF concentration of hypocretin-1 is a sensitive and specific diagnostic test in dogs with sporadic (hypocretin-deficient) forms of narcolepsy.[14] Low levels of hypocretin-1 (<80 pg/mL; normal = 250-300 pg/mL) may confirm a diagnosis of acquired narcolepsy. However, normal levels of CSF hypocretin do not exclude a diagnosis of narcolepsy in dogs with familial (hypocretin-receptor mutation) disease.

TREATMENT

The most important clinical sign in narcoleptic dogs is cataplexy, and treatment of narcolepsy in animals is aimed primarily at reducing frequency and duration of cataplectic attacks. Although excessive sleepiness may occur, this component has minor impact on narcoleptic dogs or their owners. In mild to moderately affected dogs, especially dogs that are confined to the house or small yard, avoidance of the inciting cause may be the best treatment. Feeding narcoleptic dogs separately

and/or at different times from other dogs in the household may significantly reduce the number of cataplectic episodes. Likewise, limiting play behaviors that stimulate the dog to cataplexy should be avoided when possible.

In dogs that are more severely affected, pharmacologic treatment, in addition to changes in routine and behavior, may be considered. Activation of adrenergic systems leading to inhibition of cataplexy is the primary focus of treatment. The following is a list of drugs that have been reported commonly to be of some benefit in treating narcoleptic animals[15,16]:

a) Tricyclic antidepressants: imipramine 1.5 to 3.0 mg/kg/day PO; clomipramine, 3.0 to 6.0 mg/kg/day PO. These drugs are the most commonly used anticataplectic drugs whose activity is correlated with their adrenergic or serotonergic reuptake inhibition and may be used long term.

b) Alpha-2 antagonists: yohimbine, 0.15 to 0.30 mg/kg BID, PO. This may be especially useful in animals that show signs of excessive daytime sleepiness and is safe for use long term.

c) CNS-like stimulants: modafinil (15 to 60 mg/kg). Stimulants are used to treat excessive daytime sleepiness and cataplexy in people and may prove to be useful in dogs.

d) Other CNS stimulants: methylphenidate (0.25 mg/kg PO SID); dextroamphetamine; pemoline. These drugs enhance dopamine activity and are more effective in treating excessive sleepiness than controlling cataplexy.

Replacement hypocretin therapy has been evaluated in narcoleptic dogs,[17] but adequate penetration of the CNS is problematic and even large doses are not sufficient to prevent cataplectic episodes in dogs with acquired narcolepsy.

PROGNOSIS

Canine narcolepsy is not a life-threatening or progressive disease, but the clinical signs remain present throughout life. With proper care and understanding by the owner, however, narcoleptic dogs may have a good quality of life. Client education about the disease is important so that the pet's environment is kept as safe as possible by use of unbreakable food bowls and furniture at the pet's level. Additionally, water should be offered in such a way that the head is elevated during drinking to prevent the possibility of aspiration should the pet have a cataplectic episode over/in the water bowl.

References

The reference list can be found on the companion Expert Consult Web site at *www.expertconsult.com*.

CHAPTER 60

Cognitive Dysfunction in Aged Dogs

Elizabeth Head
Gary Landsberg

Advanced age in dogs may be associated with behavioral changes including separation anxiety, the onset of new fears and phobias, increasing irritability and aggression, stereotypic disorders, night waking, and house soiling.[1,2] Some of these behaviors may be attributable to existing medical conditions that might be age related (including other neurologic disorders) and some may be due to primary behavior problems arising from changes in the household. Therefore to determine whether the clinical signs are related to pathologic brain aging, these other medical and behavioral signs should first be ruled out.

CLINICAL SIGNS

Until recently, clinicians had regarded the constellation of behavioral symptoms to indicate senility associated with advanced age. Cognitive dysfunction is not an inevitable consequence of aging in dogs and striking individual differences are more likely the rule than the exception. Some aged animals show little or mild behavioral decline. However, a subset of aged dogs develops severe cognitive deficits that may disrupt normal function to a level prompting euthanasia. Ruehl and collaborators have identified a more general cognitive dysfunction syndrome (CDS).[3] The clinical signs have been described using a simplified acronym DISHA—which refers to Disorientation, Interaction changes with owners or other pets, Sleep-wake cycle alterations, House soiling, and Activity changes (which might be increased, stereotypic, or reduced). Additional signs such as increasing agitation and anxiety, altered responsiveness to stimuli (which might be heightened or reduced), altered interest in food (which might be increased or reduced), and decreased ability to perform learned tasks (which might be most obvious in working dogs) may also be seen. The number of dogs affected by CDS has been assessed in a number of survey-based studies. Approximately 48% of pet owners report that their senior dogs (7 years or older) exhibit at least one clinical sign of CDS. However, only 17% of these owners reported these signs to their veterinarian. (Proprietary market research, 1999. Pet owner sample size: 150. Data on file, Pfizer Animal Health.) In another study, 180 owners of dogs aged 11 to 16 with no identifiable medical problems reported that 28% of the dogs between 11 and 12 years and 68% of the dogs between 15 and 16 years had at least one sign that might be consistent with CDS.[4] Further, CDS may be a progressive disease as aged dogs with impairments in one category were later found to have impairments in two or more categories.[5] Thus, clinical signs of cognitive dysfunction in senior and geriatric pet dogs occur in a significant number of animals and potentially signal a progressive neurologic disorder.

LABORATORY STUDIES

Questionnaire-based tools used in the clinic to identify dogs with CDS provide a measure of global brain dysfunction.

However, these behavioral checklists may be insensitive to early and subtle changes in learning and memory associated with pathologic aging in dogs. In fact, cognitive dysfunction is generally recognized as a syndrome in dogs 11 years of age and older, and signs may not be apparent until the last 18 to 24 months of a dog's life.[1] At this time, there is no biomarker for CDS in aged dogs. An alternative technique to detect cognitive dysfunction in aged dogs involves the use of neuropsychologic tests that provide quantitative measures of cognitive function without reliance on questionnaires.[6] These tests are systematic, standardized, objective, and a more sensitive measure of age-related cognitive decline. In fact, they can identify age-related deficits in learning and memory from as early as 6 years of age.[7] Although these tests are too lengthy and complex to be applicable for clinic use, a number of cognitive functions assayed with these laboratory-based tasks are also likely to be contributors to the clinical signs that might be noted by pet owners.

In studies using a battery of reward-motivated neuropsychologic tests, several cognitive domains or functions can be evaluated in aged dogs. These tests involve teaching dogs to use visual information to solve different problems. Simple learning problems include discrimination tasks that involve showing dogs two objects that are different in appearance. Dogs must learn that only one of the two objects covers a food reward. Aged dogs can learn these problems as well as younger dogs. Once dogs have learned this visual discrimination problem the reward can be switched to the previously incorrect object. This is called *reversal learning*, in which dogs must be able to change a previously learned behavior, a type of cognitive ability that depends upon the intact function of the prefrontal cortex. Aged dogs have difficulty learning to switch to selecting the previously incorrect object, suggesting a lack of ability to modify learned behaviors. These laboratory tests depend on cognitive abilities that would be involved with modifying previously learned behaviors and thus, aged dogs may be slower to modify problem behaviors. Other behaviors that are consistent with prefrontal cortex dysfunction include pacing, stereotypical behaviors, and an inability to inhibit behaviors (e.g., house soiling).

The aging process can also significantly affect memory. Spatial memory is defined as the ability of dogs to remember *where* they had last obtained a hidden food reward and is compromised in a subset of aged animals.[8] Functionally, this type of memory impairment may be reported in companion animals as disorientation, wandering, and getting lost. Dogs also show age-dependent impairments in their ability to recognize objects seen previously.[6] This type of dysfunction may be reflected in decreased recognition of familiar people or animals.

Age-related differences have also been demonstrated in behavioral reactivity tests.[9] The curiosity test, for example, allows the dogs to examine and play with a variety of toys to assess an animal's reaction to novel objects. In this brief 10-minute test, young dogs show significantly more exploration and contact with novel objects than old dogs, with cognitively impaired aged dogs showing the least object contact.[10]

Further, cognitively impaired aged dogs show higher levels of locomotion during a curiosity test than their age-matched unimpaired peers. The curiosity test measures exploratory behavior and is more amenable to clinical use because it requires brief 10-minute testing sessions and a small test area suggesting that it may be a useful clinical screen for aged animals with cognitive dysfunction.

NEUROBIOLOGIC BASIS

Cognitive dysfunction that is not attributable to other systemic or central disease may reflect underlying age-associated neuropathology. There are a number of morphologic features of aging in the canine brain.[11] For example, cortical atrophy and ventricular widening occur with age in dogs.[12] One form of pathology, the accumulation of diffuse plaques, contains a number of proteins, of which the primary constituent is the β-amyloid peptide (Aβ) (Figure 60-1).

Further, Aβ can accumulate on the membranes of neurons and on the cerebrovasculature (see Figure 60-1). Vascular Aβ may impair the ability of blood vessels to dilate or constrict and lead to subsequent hypoperfusion of the brain.[13] The extent and location of Aβ deposition in the aged dog brain is linked to the severity of cognitive deficit.[14,15] For example, aged dogs that are severely impaired on a reversal learning task have the most extensive prefrontal cortex Aβ pathology.[15] Another key feature of the aged canine brain is the progressive accumulation of oxidative damage to proteins and lipids[16] and a reduction in endogenous antioxidant activity.[17] Damaged

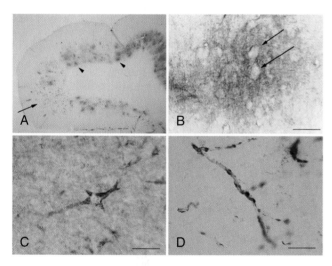

Figure 60-1 β-Amyloid (Aβ) pathology in the aged canine brain (15-year-old Border Collie). **A,** Aβ accumulates extensively in the temporal cortex as both diffuse deposits *(arrow heads)* or in on the cerebrovasculature *(arrow)*. **B,** A higher magnification of a diffuse Aβ plaque shows small fibrils accumulating in the space between neurons *(arrows)*. **C,** Aβ can also be observed on the membranes of neurons. **D,** Blood vessels within the parenchyma of the brain also can accumulate Aβ. All sections were immunostained with anti-Aβ1-42 antibody. Bars in **B-D** = 20 μm. (Brain tissue kindly provided by Carolyn Wilki.)

proteins and lipids can lead to neuronal dysfunction, which may subsequently compromise cognitive function. In support of this hypothesis, a diet rich in antioxidants and mitochondrial cofactors can significantly improve cognitive function in aged but not young dogs.[18] Aged dogs also show neuron loss in the hippocampus, a brain region thought to be important for spatial memory.[19] Interestingly, providing aged dogs with a behavioral enrichment (outdoor walks, social interaction, play toys, cognitive training) all leads to a maintenance of neuron number in this same brain region. Last, aged dogs lose the ability to generate new neurons (i.e., neurogenesis) in the hippocampus and this is linked to a loss of learning and memory ability.[20]

TREATMENT OPTIONS

Age-dependent cognitive impairments in companion animals, as mentioned previously, may reflect systemic or a CNS disease. Once other contributing factors are eliminated, the appropriate treatment can be implemented. Currently there is one pharmaceutical in North America that is approved for the treatment of cognitive dysfunction in aged dogs. Selegiline (Anipryl, Pfizer Animal Health) is a monoamine oxidase B inhibitor that can improve cognitive signs in aged dogs[21]. Its mode of action appears to be able to enhance catecholamine transmission, as well as to decrease the production and increase the clearance of toxic free radicals. Alternatively, a specially formulated senior canine food is also available, Prescription Diet Canine b/d, that contains antioxidants, mitochondrial cofactors that significantly improve cognition in both laboratory and clinical studies.[22] Combinations of ingredients that may act synergistically to improve clinical signs and slow cognitive decline such as vitamin E, pyridoxine, phosphatidylserine, and *Ginkgo biloba* have also been shown to be effective in both clinical trials and in laboratory studies.[23,24] Other pharmaceuticals that might enhance cerebral vascular blood flow or enhance cholinergic transmission and other natural combinations have also proven to have promise in preliminary trials. These are described in more detail elsewhere.[2] More recently, immunotherapy approaches have been developed for use in aged canines involving the vaccination of aged animals against the Aβ protein and this may also have future treatment potential.[25]

SUMMARY

Aged dogs, like aged humans, are vulnerable to the development of progressive brain pathology that is associated with clinical signs of cognitive dysfunction. However, it is important to rule out other contributing systemic diseases or other central nervous system disorders that can also cause cognitive impairments. Along with behavioral therapy, a variety of medical and dietary treatment options have been licensed but availability varies between countries. New treatment options are currently in development.

REFERENCES

The reference list can be found on the companion Expert Consult Web site at *www.expertconsult.com*.

CHAPTER 61

Behavioral Disorders

Andrew Urs Luescher

According to a variety of studies, the prevalence of behavior problems in dogs and cats lies between 40% and 80%. In an epidemiologic study, approximately 40% of dogs had growled at their owners, and 15% had bitten their owners. Around one third of cats appear to have at least an occasional problem with inappropriate elimination. Behavior problems jeopardize the human-animal bond and are a main cause of relinquishment and euthanasia of healthy dogs and cats. Therefore pet owners, pets, and the veterinary profession benefit from the prevention and treatment of behavior problems in patients.

Not every veterinary practice needs to offer behavior consults. Since behavior consults are lengthy (the initial appointment is normally at least 2 hours long) and do not make use of a veterinary clinic's infrastructure, they may not be cost efficient. Such cases can be referred to a veterinary behaviorist or a behaviorist can come into the clinic and perform the behavior consult. Information on veterinary behaviorists and other veterinarians that offer behavior consults can be found on the Web sites of the American College of Veterinary Behaviorists (ACVB; http://www.dacvb.org) and of the American Veterinary Society of Animal Behavior (AVSAB; http://www.avsabonline.org). In either case, in the initial appointment in which the owner raises the concern, the attending veterinarian can establish a minimum medical data base (i.e., physical exam with basic neurologic examination, complete blood count [CBC], chemistry profile including a thyroid panel, urinalysis, and additional tests as indicated). A separate and sufficiently long appointment should be set for a behavior consult.

Clinical consults should be performed methodically. Aside from the minimal medical data base, diagnosis should be based on a thorough history and direct observation and/or observation from videotapes. The history may involve collection of general information regarding early history; housing, feeding, exercising, and training the pet; the animal's behavior in various situations to assess temperament; and the specific problem. The latter information should include triggers of the behavior; the behavior itself, including body language; and consequences of the behavior. Because behavior problems often change over time, this information should be gathered for the earliest incidents in addition to the most recent. Observations need to include normal owner-pet and/or pet-pet interactions. Particular attention should be paid to behavior that is indicative of stress, motivational conflict, or frustration.

Treatment modalities include changes in management (housing, feeding, exercise, training methods, nature of owner-pet interactions, avoiding triggers), behavior modification (e.g., rewarding desired and removing the reward of unwanted behavior, counter-conditioning, response substitution, systematic desensitization), and pharmacologic treatment.

While behavior modification is being applied, exposure to the natural stimulus must be avoided. The term *counter-conditioning* involves association of a situation that previously evoked fear and/or aggression with something pleasant. The pleasant stimulus can be food or play, for example. It is unlikely that fear is reinforced by giving food or by play. Fear could easily be reinforced by picking the animal up or sheltering it, so this should be avoided.

Response substitution is a technique by which an animal is trained to perform an appropriate behavior in a situation in which it used to perform an unacceptable behavior. The animal first needs to be trained to perform the desired behavior on a cue. Then, every time the animal shows any inclination to perform the unacceptable behavior, the owner distracts it, gives the command, makes the animal do the appropriate behavior, and reinforces that behavior with a reward. The owner needs to either supervise the animal to apply response substitution on a consistent basis, or when they cannot supervise, put it in a situation in which it will not perform the inappropriate behavior. The animal should not be given any chance to perform the inappropriate behavior.

Systematic desensitization involves training a dog to assume a relaxed down-stay, and then exposing it to the stimulus at a low intensity. The patient is rewarded for staying relaxed. The stimulus intensity is increased incrementally, and at each stage the pet should be rewarded for relaxation. If the dog shows a reaction, the owners have progressed too quickly. They need to wait until the dog relaxes, reward, and then go back a few steps in the training. Systematic desensitization requires identifying the stimulus, reproducing the stimulus, and having control over the stimulus intensity. If these requirements cannot be met, or the natural stimulus cannot be avoided for the duration of behavior modification, drug desensitization may be necessary. In this case, the pet should be placed on an effective dose of an appropriate drug and exposed to the natural stimulus as often as possible, rewarded for desirable behavior, and then slowly weaned from the drug.

CANINE BEHAVIOR PROBLEMS

Aggression

Some dozen different types of canine aggression are recognized, including conflict related, dominance, possessive, territorial aggression, interdog, play induced, excitement induced, fear induced, pain induced, redirected, maternal, and predatory aggression. They fall into the two to three major groups of affective aggression, predatory behavior (part of feeding behavior), and possibly play aggression. The terms *redirected* and *learned aggression* should not be used as diagnoses as they imply a mechanism of modification.

Aggression to Humans Living in the Household   Aggression to household members is often exhibited in situations in which the dog is threatened or "challenged." This type of aggression has generally been diagnosed as dominance aggression. Dominance aggression would be expected primarily in adult dogs and intact males. Dogs would be expected to have a self-confident personality and show offensive body language when aggressive. However, the majority of cases start at young. Typically, initial aggression is shown in response to discipline or over food within the first 2 months of ownership. The affected dogs have a different disease history (severe early disease, dermatologic disease) than nonaggressive dogs. They are more excitable as puppies and more excitable and fearful (shy of people) as adults. Their body language before and during an attack is ambivalent and indicates a motivational conflict. Frequently, in the initial incidents the dog shows defensive body language, but over time it becomes more and more offensive. There is a breed predisposition; spaniels, terriers, and toy breeds are more likely to bite. Dogs most likely to be aggressive are neutered males, neutered females. Intact males are less likely and intact females are least likely to be aggressive. Intact females that are aggressive may become more aggressive when neutered. Dogs that are aggressive to their owners are also likely to be aggressive to strangers, which indicates that this aggression is not confined to the dog's social group.

The body language of aggressive dogs frequently indicates that they are in a motivational conflict (approach-withdrawal conflict) relative to people. When a person approaches, aggressive dogs' anxiety level increases and they show aggression. As the person responds by backing off, the threat diminishes. The dogs thus learn that they can resolve their conflict and reduce their anxiety by showing aggression. Thus aggression becomes conditioned through avoidance conditioning; this type of conditioning produces persistent behavior. Based on this putative pathogenesis, we have proposed the term *conflict-related aggression*. Another cause may be that dogs living in an inconsistent environment are unable to predict what is going to happen and have no control over what is happening. They are thus in a state of frustration and depending on their genetic make-up, may show aggression as a conflict behavior. They will quickly learn that aggression produces predictable results and thus provides a means for them to exert control over their environment in a predictable fashion. Highly trainable and genetically aggressive dogs are more motivated to control their environment and may be at a particular risk to develop this type of aggression.

Treatment should address the dog's basic disposition (e.g., fearfulness, hyperexcitability), the way in which the dog is managed, and the cause of conflict (i.e., the inconsistency in the environment, especially the nature of owner-dog interaction).

Recommended management changes include twice-daily meal feeding (as opposed to ad lib feeding) and regular twice-daily exercise off the property. The situations in which confrontations are likely should be avoided. This may imply that the dog needs to be confined (e.g., in a separate room or exercise pen) unless being trained. Confinement is also indicated when the owners are afraid of the dog, when smaller children are involved, or when the owner is unable to ignore the dog. A head halter with a leash attached is placed on the dog, so that the owner can control all aggression-inducing situations with response substitution in a safe, nonconfrontational, and consistent way. Toys or other assets that have caused confrontations should be removed. The dog is not to be let on furniture if that caused a problem. The dog should be reintroduced to situations in which it showed aggression only in the context of response substitution and systematic desensitization.

Owners should be instructed to avoid all casual interaction (i.e., ignore the dog most of the time) and only interact with the dog in a command-response-reward format. This ensures that all interactions with the dog are consistent and thus predictable. Highly structured obedience exercises, especially ones that desensitize the dog to owner behavior perceived as threatening, are useful. Clicker training is especially helpful when dealing with these dogs, because it is a hands-off method of training and avoids confrontations between owner and dog. No punishment, choke chain, or scolding are to be used. A head halter assists the owner in training and walking the dog. Punishment and domination procedures such as the "alpha roll-over" are not appropriate in dealing with aggression and often exacerbate the problem. Situations in which the dog still shows aggression are addressed by counter-conditioning response substitution and systematic desensitization.

Food guarding can be addressed through management (i.e., by placing the food bowl in a separate room, letting the dog in to eat, and calling the dog out of the room once it is finished eating). It can also be treated through systematic desensitization. In the latter case, the dog is tied in a different place than where it is normally fed and fed from a different food bowl (preferably a saucepan with a long handle). The ration is measured out into yet another dish that is placed out of the dog's reach. The dog is asked to sit and a few kibbles are placed into the food bowl, and the dog is offered the food as a reward for sitting. This is repeated until all the food is fed, and all meals are fed in this way for about a week. Then, the amount of food given at one time is increased. Next, the amount of food is decreased again to a few kibbles, but the owner lets go of the food bowl while the dog eats. The amount is then increased again. Eventually, a third of the food can be placed into the food bowl, and the owner adds the remainder of the ration with a ladle while the dog eats. Once this goes well, all the food can be placed in the food bowl, and the owner tosses treats into it while the dog eats. This should be done occasionally throughout the dog's life (in very mild cases, this last step may be all that needs to be done).

No drugs have been proven effective in the treatment of any type of canine aggression.

Possessive Aggression   Guarding of food and objects is a natural but unacceptable canine behavior. It becomes exacerbated if the dog is afraid of a confrontation over the item (it may therefore be regarded as a special case of conflict-related aggression). It can be addressed by management or through training. The latter option includes training "leave-it" and "drop-it" commands, or exchange exercises (a form of systematic desensitization). For exchange exercises, the dog is tied to an immovable object, initially away from where it most commonly shows aggression. The dog is asked to lie down and stay. A toy that the dog does not value much is laid down at some distance from the dog, the leave-it command is given, the toy is picked up, and the dog is rewarded for staying relaxed. At subsequent trials, the distance is reduced. The exercise is repeated with increasingly valuable toys.

Territorial Aggression   Territorial aggression is exhibited to strangers or strange dogs either on the owner's property or away from the home but in the owner's proximity. It is a normal but unacceptable canine behavior. The most simple form of treatment is to use counter-conditioning by associating the ringing of the door bell with receiving food treats. The food treats can be tossed to the dog's bed, or can be provided through a remote treat dispenser (Manners Minder; Premier). This will result in the dog going to its bed when the door bell rings. Response substitution can also be done by training the dog to sit near the door and staying while the door is opened and closed, while the doorbell is rung, and while a stranger stands at a distance and progressively closer to the door. Once the stranger can be close to the door and the dog stays sitting when the door is opened, the stranger can toss the dog treats. It is important to prevent the dog from ever showing aggression until the training program is completed.

The dog should be walked twice daily off the property on head halter and leash. Whenever a person approaches, the owner should go out of the way and keep the dog busy with fast-paced obedience, reinforcing appropriate behavior with ample food treats. We often include the "watch-me" command to keep the dog focused on the owner. Once the other person has passed, they can continue their walk. Each time, the distance to the other person can be reduced (depending on the response of the dog), until the owner can heel the dog by the other person, and then reward the dog for having passed without aggression. This method can also be used with a volunteer who stands still while the owner performs obedience training with the dog at decreasing distance. The dog can also be systematically desensitized to a stranger passing by at decreasing distance, and then approaching more and more directly.

Aggression between Dogs   Aggression to strange dogs or interdog aggression can be status related, territorial, fear based, or even predatory. Treatment is similar to that of territorial aggression and includes the same exercises on walks, counter-conditioning (making the situation when another dog is in sight pleasant), response substitution (having a helper with a dog stand still and doing obedience with the patient at decreasing distance, rewarding frequently), and systematic desensitization to a dog passing by or approaching. The dog can also be rewarded for any nonaggressive or even friendly response to another dog. Punishment is contraindicated with any form of aggression, in this case in particular because the patient would learn that the presence of another dog means it will likely get punished.

Aggression between dogs living in the same household is usually status related or related to dog overdependence on an owner (sometimes called "alliance aggression"). Fights are usually severe, especially among females.

Status-related aggression may occur between dogs that are close in social status. Fighting may also begin when a younger dog reaches adulthood, or when an older dog is no longer able to maintain its position. Treatment of status-related aggression involves deciding which dog will likely end up dominant and treat him as such (giving attention or food first, giving this dog privileges that the other dog does not have), and treating the other dog as subordinate (ignoring, cutting privileges, possibly confinement, rewarding subordinate behavior). Furthermore, counter-conditioning, response substitution and systematic desensitization (as for aggression to strange dogs) can be used. The dogs may need to be separated and/or muzzled when exposed to each other. The times the dogs are exposed to each other should be as positive as possible (counter-conditioning).

Alliance aggression is aggression to another dog in the same household shown only in the proximity of the owner. It is usually, but not always, the lower-ranking dog that initiates the aggression. The aggressive dog is usually overly dependent on the owner and becomes anxious if the other dog gets close to the owner. It may also feel much more confident in proximity of the owner.

The most important aspect of treatment is to ignore both dogs for 3 to 4 weeks, except when working with them. The dogs should be exposed as much as possible to each other. If there is any indication that the dogs will be aggressive, the owner should distract them with a loud noise (clapping hands, rape alarm) and immediately leave. Also, the aggressive dog can be rewarded for nonaggressive interactions with the other dog (clicker training). In some cases the dogs will need to be muzzled when exposed to each other. It should be determined which of the two is the dominant dog (from a videotape taken when they are on their own, without owner present) and that dog should be treated as such.

The aggressive dog can be desensitized to the owner paying attention to the other dog. While the aggressive dog is tied and in a down-stay, the owner interacts with the other dog at decreasing distance and rewards the aggressive dog frequently for staying relaxed. Dogs that exhibit alliance aggression are often not aggressive to each other in other places, or out in the yard. In this case, they can be exposed to each other initially on neutral ground, then kept together in the backyard, and then gradually allowed access to increasing parts of the house.

Predatory Aggression   Predatory aggression is highly genetically controlled and may therefore be difficult to treat. It is a particularly dangerous form of aggression because there is no warning and the bite is not inhibited. Systematic desensitization and response substitution (in combination) can be successful. The owner is instructed to do obedience training at a distance from the "prey" (e.g., horses, cars going by), using a head halter and food rewards. Gradually, the owner reduces the distance. Confinement and control, as well as a muzzle, are useful in managing the behavior. A good recall can help to control dangerous situations. Socialization of the puppy to the species that it should not consider as prey (e.g., children) is essential. Selection of a breed with little predatory behavior helps in prevention.

Separation Anxiety

Separation anxiety is a common problem, especially among dogs obtained from shelters. Affected dogs are usually friendly and more highly trained than dogs with other behavior problems. Their type of owner attachment may be different from that of dogs without separation anxiety. Affected dogs become anxious when separated form their owner (i.e., when the owner is either not home with the dog, or not accessible to the dog) and express this anxiety in a variety of ways (e.g., by destroying property, barking, salivating, pacing, urinating or defecating, self-mutilation). Diagnostically it is important to note that anxiety-related behaviors start within a short time of the owner leaving. First line treatment may include two daily walks to reduce anxiety; ignoring the dog for approximately 30 minutes before leaving and after coming home until the dog settles; giving a hollow toy containing food treats some 5 to 10 minutes before leaving; and ignoring attention-getting behavior at any time. In addition, owners may want to train the dog to a long down-stay and then use that command to prevent the dog from following all the time, and when doing planned departures (see below). Mixing up the order of predeparture cues disassociates these cues from departures, and desensitization to these same cues (by presenting them frequently without leaving) will reduce the dog's response to them. Drug treatment concomitant with behavior treatment is often indicated. Clomipramine (Clomicalm, Novartis) and fluoxetine (Reconcile, Lilly) are the only drugs licensed in the United States for the treatment of separation anxiety. Treatment with Dog Appeasement Pheromone (DAP, CEVA Sante Animale) can be provided either via plug-in dispenser or collar.

If necessary, the owner can do planned departures, leaving the dog for initially short and increasingly longer times, while giving the dog a safety cue (e.g., the sound of the radio). If at all possible, dogs with separation anxiety should not be confined when left alone, because usually this makes the anxiety worse. If the owners keep the dog confined and do not want to risk leaving him loose, they may want to use the planned departure technique with the dog loose in the house during practice departures. In this way they can find out without great risk if it is safe to leave the dog loose (if done this way, being loose becomes a safety cue for the dog).

Fear

Fear is a combination of physical, emotional, and physiologic responses to a threatening stimulus or situation that, in the wild, would protect the animal from harm. In a domestic situation, strong fear reactions are usually undesirable. Fear may become a maladaptive "phobia" when the response is out of proportion to the threat. The dog may be afraid of specific stimuli or be globally fearful. The cause of fearfulness may be genetic, or early experience (lack of socialization and exposure before 14 weeks of age, or an adverse experience in the fear period 8 to 10 weeks of age). Specific fears are usually learned later in life.

Learning can exaggerate any fear. Reinforcement is most easily achieved through avoidance or escape conditioning. However, it is difficult to reinforce fear with food. Giving food to a fearful dog is therefore not contraindicated, but recommended, because it makes the situation more pleasant (counter-conditioning).

Specific fears can usually be treated effectively with systematic desensitization, counter-conditioning, and response substitution. For fear caused by early experience, generalized fear or when fear-evoking stimuli cannot be avoided, controlled or replicated (e.g., thunderstorms), drug desensitization is indicated. The dog is given a large enough dose of a drug with anxiolytic effects to reduce fear to the point at which the dog is capable of habituation to the stimuli (behavior modification should be used simultaneously). Once the dog functions well at that dose, the dose is slightly reduced. When the dog no longer shows fear on the lower dose, the dose is further reduced, and the dog is thus gradually weaned off the drug. Throughout the procedure, the dog should be rewarded for acting confidently. Even after successful treatment, the dog should be periodically exposed to the fear-inducing stimuli and rewarded for not responding fearfully, to prevent spontaneous recovery of the fear response. A fear response is not ever to be punished.

Hyperexcitability

A high level of activity may be normal for a certain breed and age of dog. Although there are various physiologic (e.g., similar to ADHD in children) and environmental reasons (large groups of dogs, hyperactive children in the household) for abnormally high activity, reactivity, or inability to focus, the most common cause is inadvertent conditioning with owner attention. Consequently, the first treatment strategy is to ignore the dog, especially when excitable. Relaxed, calm behavior should be rewarded. Obedience training, especially a long, relaxed down-stay, and regular twice-daily walks will also help in most cases. Dogs that are hyperactive due to physiologic reasons usually need to be treated pharmacologically with drugs such as methylphenidate or fluoxetine.

Canine House Soiling

Before a diagnosis of house soiling is made, medical causes, urine marking, separation anxiety, and other anxiety-related disorders have to be ruled out. Behavioral causes of house soiling include insufficient initial house training, long periods of cage confinement during puppyhood so that the dog learned to soil its bed, age-related cognitive dysfunction, and various other factors that can result in the loss of house training.

To treat house soiling, the factors that affect elimination have to be understood. Elimination is most likely after rest, eating, and physical activity. It is also stimulated by the smell of previous elimination. The dog should be fed two to three times a day (depending on its usual number of stools per day) and walked thereafter to the same location. The dog should also be taken to that location when first waking from sleep, after play, and frequently in between. When the dog eliminates at that location, it should be rewarded. If it does not eliminate this time, it can be brought back to the house but should be taken out again within 10 minutes or so. Indoors, the dog should be under constant supervision (crate confinement or on leash with the owner). The soiled areas should be treated with an effective cleaner and can then be made aversive with biweekly application of pine oil or citrus-scented liquid, or small amounts ($\frac{1}{4}$ teaspoon) of mothball powder brushed into the pile of the carpet (mothball crystals are toxic).

Canine Urine Marking

Canine urine marking can be a territorial behavior, greatly facilitated by testosterone in intact males (especially in the presence of other intact dogs or bitches in heat), or related to anxiety. It involves deposition of small amounts of urine in specific places, usually on or near vertical objects. The strongest stimulus is environmental competition of other males and freshly voided urine from other dogs.

Stimuli that elicit urine marking should be identified and, if possible, eliminated. If urine marking is anxiety related, then the cause of the anxiety has to be addressed. The marked areas should be cleaned and deodorized as described for house soiling. Castration reduces leg lifting in the house in about 60% of cases.

Behavior modification involves constant supervision in the house, possibly with the dog tied to the owner with a leash (umbilical cord technique). Whenever the dog shows any signs of wanting to mark a place, the leave-it command (it will have to be taught in advance) or response substitution should be used. Punishment generally does not work as it is usually not applied consistently, and because the dog may learn to lift the leg only when the owner is absent.

Stereotypies and Compulsive Disorder in Dogs

Compulsive and stereotypic behaviors are repetitive or sustained, apparently abnormal behaviors performed out of context. Compulsive behaviors include fixation on a goal, while stereotypic behaviors are repetitive motor patterns. These behaviors could be categorized as related to locomotion, oral activity and grooming, aggression, vocalization, and hallucinatory behaviors. In dogs, locomotory behaviors include circling, tail chasing, pacing, jumping in place, chasing light reflexes, and freezing. Oral behaviors and behaviors related to grooming manifest, among others, as leg or foot chewing, licking, flank sucking, scratching, chewing objects, pica, and snapping in the air ("fly-snapping"). Compulsive behaviors related to aggression include self-directed aggression, attacking inanimate objects, and possibly unpredictable aggression to people. Vocalization may be rhythmic barking or whining. Hallucinatory behaviors may be staring at "shadows," chasing light reflexes, and waking up suddenly without any discernible trigger.

Stereotypies and compulsive behaviors may be considered an expression of stress, frustration, and/or motivational conflict. Stress that leads to these behaviors frequently relates to an unpredictable and uncontrollable environment. Frustration refers to the situation in which an animal is motivated to perform a behavior, but prevented from doing so. Motivational conflict results from two opposing, similarly strong motivations (such as approach and withdrawal). Prolonged and particularly repeated conflict situations may result in normal conflict behaviors developing into compulsive or stereotypic behavior. A genetic predisposition is probably present in any case. Physical lesions or irritations, such as ones caused by allergy, may trigger this disorder in some dogs by increasing stress and by directing the abnormal behavior towards a particular body site. Owner attention may reinforce existing compulsive or stereotypic behaviors, or condition normal conflict behaviors to the extent that they appear stereotyped. Disease that increases stress and/or irritability may contribute to this condition, as may other stressful behavioral problems (e.g., interdog aggression or separation anxiety) or certain temperament traits (e.g., fearfulness).

A diagnosis is based primarily on a detailed history and on ruling out other possible behavioral and medical causes for the observed behavior. One aspect of the history that is particularly important for the diagnosis is the development of the problem. In many cases (especially locomotory behaviors), the behavior is first shown in a specific conflict situation but later may generalize to other contexts in which the animal experiences a high level of arousal. Once established, these abnormal behaviors are displayed outside of their natural context and are often excessive. The animal is in full consciousness while performing the behavior and aware of its surroundings (although in some cases they may not respond to any stimuli in their environment, and may even run into furniture, etc.). The behavior can usually be interrupted, albeit often with difficulty, and the animal does not exhibit a postictal phase. Their performance is not dependent on the owner's presence.

The differential diagnosis has to consider various behavioral, neurologic, dermatologic, and other medical conditions. To exclude other possible causes for the behaviors, a minimal medical data base consisting of a physical exam including a basic neurologic exam, CBC, chemistry profile, possibly thyroid panel, and urinalysis should be obtained. Additional tests may be needed in specific cases.

Behavioral differentials include acute conflict behavior only shown in specific contexts, and conditioned behavior only shown in a person's presence. Neurologic rule-outs are seizures, forebrain and brainstem lesions, lesions of the vestibular system (circling), lumbosacral stenosis (tail chasing), hydrocephalus, sensory neuropathies, and neuromas (self-mutilation).

Any dermatologic lesion or other condition that results in itching or pain can cause licking. Preexisting wounds or pressure point granulomas can also direct compulsive licking towards a particular area.

Treatment is directed at identifying and removing the cause of conflict, frustration, and stress. In cases in which the cause of stress cannot be removed, it may be possible to desensitize the animal to the stressful situation.

Drug therapy may prove necessary or will at least facilitate treatment. Pharmacologic intervention is most likely achieved with serotonin reuptake inhibitors such as clomipramine (Clomicalm, Novartis Animal Health US, Greensboro, N.C.) at 3 mg/kg b.i.d., or fluoxetine (Reconcile, Eli Lilly, Indianapolis) or paroxetine (Paxil, GlaxoSmithKline, Pittsburgh) at 1 mg/kg s.i.d.-b.i.d. It may take more than 4 weeks to see a drug effect. The drug needs to be given for some time beyond apparent improvement of the signs, and then weaned gradually over at least 3 weeks. Weaning is important to avoid a rebound effect.

The above behavioral treatment with or without drug treatment is likely to reduce the frequency of the behavior. Now that the dog performs the behavior less frequently, consistent response substitution can be practical and highly effective for the treatment of compulsive disorder.

Cognitive Dysfunction Syndrome

Over 60% of dogs over 11 years of age have abnormal cognitive decline not wholly explainable by changes in health, or cognitive dysfunction syndrome (CDS). This syndrome can be recognized by a range of signs, and can go along with other behavioral problems (increased anxiety, separation anxiety, loss of house training).

Signs of CDS include: *D*isorientation, reduced social *I*nteraction, changes in *S*leep-wake cycle, *H*ouse soiling (the so-called DISH signs), and decreased activity. Diagnosis is largely based on owner reports. The disorder is not easily visible in the veterinary clinic. Therefore, the veterinarian *asking about the DISH signs should be part of the routine* at every visit of dogs 7 years and older.

Physical changes in the CDS brain include ventricular dilation, vascular changes, decreased cell number, meningeal fibrosis, cerebral and cerebellar white matter degeneration, and diffuse β-amyloid plaques (β-amyloid is neurotoxic). These plaques occur mostly in the cerebral cortex and hippocampus, i.e., brain structures involved in cognition and memory. Changes in neurotransmitter levels, especially a depletion of dopamine and norepinephrine, have been implicated as well. Increase in MAO-B, an enzyme that breaks down dopamine, has been suspected to play a role in CDS. Toxic free radicals are a consequence of MAO-B activity in many species and cause cell damage and neuronal death.

The diagnosis is made based on the history and by ruling out primary medical illness (e.g., neurologic, urinary tract, PUPD [polyuria/polydipsia], cardiovascular) and other behavior problems (e.g., phobias, separation anxiety, compulsive disorder, loss of house training, urine marking). However, since many medical problems and some behavior problems may be age related, the presence of CDS should be evaluated independently even if primary medical or other behavioral disease is identified. A behavioral check list is useful for that.

Management includes changing the environment, mental stimulation (exercise off property and training), drug treatment (Anipryl [Pfizer]: selegiline hydrochloride, an MAO-B inhibitor), and diet change (Science Diet BD: diet high in antioxidants). It must be emphasized that selegiline hydrochloride is metabolized to amphetamines. Therefore, increased activity after administration of this drug should not be considered a positive response; rather, it is a simple and direct side effect.

FELINE BEHAVIOR PROBLEMS

Inappropriate Urination and Defecation

Inappropriate elimination includes voiding of urine and feces, and marking in inappropriate areas. When marking, a cat eliminates usually on vertical objects, whereas a house-soiling cat tends to empty its bladder on a horizontal surface. Some cats mark with full urination and/or defecation on human's concentrated body odor (e.g., beds, bath mats, dirty clothes).

Cats may stop using their litter-box for a variety of reasons. They may have developed an aversion to the litter, the pan, an odor, or the location; they may have developed a preference for certain substrates or locations; they may be under some environmental stress; or they may have underlying disease, most commonly urinary tract infection or cystitis, and in older cats also arthritis or cognitive dysfunction.

The first step in treatment is to identify which cat of a multicat household is the culprit (Box 61-1).

To differentiate disease-related from behavioral house soiling, a physical exam, CBC, profile, urinalysis, and urine culture are indicated. Then litter-box factors need to be addressed. The number of boxes should equal the number of cats plus one. Owners should scoop the box daily and wash

PUPPY CLASSES

Puppy classes are designed to prevent future problems through socialization, training, and owner education. They are also likely to strengthen the human-animal bond. Enrolment in puppy class should be strongly encouraged as soon as the puppy has begun its vaccination program (10 days after its first vaccination). The class should be using nonaversive training methods.

Classes should include socialization and play periods with other puppies, children, and adults. The puppies should learn to be handled and touched by adults and children, and be desensitized to veterinary examination and handling. Puppy classes should include desensitization to obstacles, surface textures, sights, and sounds that the puppy is likely to encounter in its later life.

Basic training should include sit, down, come, and stay. In addition, the puppies should learn the off command, bite inhibition, and food bowl safety. The class should be conducted in an atmosphere of fun and happiness. Absolutely no physical punishment should be used. No choke chains should ever be used in puppy class! Rewards should be used liberally.

KITTEN CLASSES

Kitten classes are less popular. The socialization period of kittens ends at around 7 weeks of age. Kittens should not be taken from the mother until 8 to 10 weeks of age. Thus, kitten classes cannot take advantage of this early sensitive period. However, kittens can be desensitized to various stimuli, to handling, grooming, restraint, and veterinary procedures. They can be trained basic commands including going in and out of a carrier, and can be taught a claw and bite inhibition.

OBEDIENCE CLASSES

Veterinary practices might offer obedience classes at the clinic, especially for adolescent dogs that went through the puppy class. Alternatively they should have a good working relationship with trainers in the area that use humane and effective training methods, and refer their clients to them. Clicker training that goes beyond traditional obedience training (i.e., includes training for everyday situations at home, such as behavior at door, etc.) is recommended. Support of the owner during the adolescent period is particularly important since this is the time when most problems start to develop and dogs are most likely to be relinquished.

BEHAVIOR WELLNESS APPOINTMENT

Around the time the pet is 6 to 10 months old is when most owners experience some behavior-related problems. It has therefore been suggested to schedule a routine behavior appointment around that time. Information is collected to identify risk factors for relinquishment:
- Is the owner unwilling to neuter their pet for financial reasons?
- Did they acquire the animal for little money?
- What expectations do owners have of the pet? Does the pet fail to meet the owners' expectations?
- Does the owner not allow the pet in the living area of the house?
- Are there any behavior problems, especially house training status, but also chewing/destructiveness, aggression, running away, jumping up, scratching, etc.?

- Are there problems with excitability, fearfulness and disobedience?
- Are the owners unwilling to walk their dog; do they allow their cat outside?
- Are they reluctant to spend money on their animal (preventive health care, yearly veterinary visits, quality of food, etc.)?
- Are there problems with training and obedience?
- Do they use aversive stimuli to correct or discipline their pet?
- Where do they get their information about behavior? Not from the veterinarian? (Relying on their veterinarian for information on behavior reduces the risk of relinquishment.)
- Is there weak owner attachment? Owner attachment can be assessed using a validated scale (Lexington attachment scale).

Problems are identified, discussed with the owner, and corrective action is initiated. Easy behavior modification techniques can be demonstrated, head halters may be fitted if appropriate, etc. Some problems may warrant referral to a behaviorist.

BEHAVIORAL INTERVENTION

Since problems with behavior or human-animal interaction can occur at any age, and the clients frequently do not approach veterinarians about them, veterinarians should take an active role in bringing up behavior in their discussions with clients. Unfortunately, many veterinarians do not take the initiative to talk about behavior. In a recent study, only about 11% of veterinarians agreed that it was the veterinarian's responsibility to initiate discussion about behavior. Over half of the respondents in the study talked about behavior only rarely at annual checkups. However, since behavior problems are a frequent reason for euthanasia, why is asking about problem behavior any less important than asking about eating, drinking, and eliminating? We suggest that at every visit of a pet to the veterinary clinic, the veterinarian should collect information relative to the most common behavior problems and the most important risk factors for relinquishment (similar to the behavior wellness appointment). Without it, behavior problems go untreated, and the bond is unnecessarily weakened or broken. An example of a common behavior problem that usually remains untreated is separation anxiety: It is estimated that only about 10% of cases get diagnosed and treated, presumably resulting in distress to the owners, broken bonds, and euthanasia, and a significant loss of business to the veterinary practice.

Another reason for talking about behavior is that patients are often presented to veterinarians for physical problems that are caused by a behavioral problem such as phobia, anxiety, pica, interdog/cat aggression, compulsive disorder, etc. It is important that such underlying behavioral problems be recognized and addressed, and not just the resulting surgical or medical diagnosis. In cases of disease-induced inappropriate urination, the behavioral component should be addressed to prevent continuation of the problem after treatment of the medical cause.

SENIOR BEHAVIORAL EXAM

Asking behavior questions is also important at geriatric visits, since cognitive decline that is not treated commonly results in behavior problems that result in premature euthanasia. The clinician should collect some of the same information as during the annual visits or during the behavior wellness appointment. In addition, special emphasis needs to be placed on how much the dog or cat is still involved in family activities, and the so-called DISH signs (*D*isorientation, lack of *I*nteraction, changes in the *S*leep-wake cycle, and *H*ouse soiling) that might indicate cognitive decline, a common and debilitating disease frequently resulting in unnecessarily early euthanasia.

Because most veterinarians do not ask about signs indicative of cognitive dysfunction, only about one third of cases of this disorder are diagnosed and treated.

SENIOR DOG CLASSES

Classes for senior dogs to stimulate mental activity (similar to learning another language in older people) are now occasionally offered. These classes obviously differ from regular obedience classes in that the tasks need to accommodate geriatric and likely arthritic dogs. Tasks such as scent discrimination or searching for hidden treats or toys may lend themselves for senior dogs.

GRIEF COUNSELING

Managing the human-animal bond also means to help dissolve the bond if necessary, and to support the owner during the time of euthanasia and grief. Veterinarians should recognize signs of pathologic grief, know how to react to a grieving client, and have a support service to which they can refer a client in need.

REFERENCES

The reference list can be found on the companion Expert Consult Web site at *www.expertconsult.com*.

CARDIORESPIRATORY

CHAPTER 63

Coughing

Kelly Anderson-Wessberg

A cough is a sudden, forceful expiration against a closed glottis. Sudden opening of the glottis and turbulent airflow create the noise identified as a cough. Coughing may occur as a conscious action or as a reflex. The coughing reflex is stimulated by mechanical or chemical irritation of the pharynx, larynx, trachea, bronchi, and smaller airways. Less commonly, disease processes involving the pleura, pericardium, diaphragm, nose, nasal sinuses, and mediastinum may also stimulate the coughing reflex.

Coughing may be the first indicator of a serious disease. On the other hand, coughing may be confused with other symptoms such as sneezing, gagging, panting, labored breathing, reverse sneezing, retching, and vomiting. The presence of a terminal retch is often misinterpreted as vomiting. Reverse sneezing has a characteristic sound with audible inspiratory and expiratory components. Failure to differentiate a cough from these other signs results in misdiagnosis and treatment failure.

The causes of coughing in small animals may be divided into the following categories (Box 63-1): inflammatory, neoplastic, cardiovascular, allergic, traumatic and physical factors, parasitic, and fungal.

DIAGNOSTIC APPROACH

Signalment and Historical Findings
The age and breed of the animal will influence the likelihood of certain conditions. Puppies and kittens are more likely to suffer from infectious respiratory diseases. Toy and miniature breeds such as Chihuahuas, Pomeranians, Toy Poodles, Yorkshire Terriers, Shih Tzus, and Lhasa Apsos are predisposed to collapsing trachea. Lungworm typically occurs in dogs less than 2 years of age, although it may occur in older animals. Cats do not typically cough with heart disease and are more likely to have lower airway disease, neoplasia, or other respiratory-related disorder. The history should focus on the general health of the pet, previous medical problems, recent diagnostics performed (heartworm testing, general blood profile, fecal examination, radiographic studies), vaccination status, heartworm prevention, exposure to other animals, and other symptoms the pet is experiencing. The history should include all recent and current medications, dosages, length of treatment, and response to each medication. Environmental history may provide important additional information. Exposure to dog parks, grooming facilities, kennels, and stray animals increases the likelihood of contagious disease. Any changes in the animal's environment should be noted along with the health of the other pets in the household. An accurate travel history should be obtained. Certain respiratory diseases are common in specific geographic areas and unlikely to occur in others.

Nature of the Cough
A description of the cough provides additional diagnostic clues. Specific questions regarding the cough should include the following: How does the cough sound, is it productive or nonproductive, what stimulates the cough, when does it

Box • 63-1

Causes of Coughing in Small Animals

Allergic/Inflammatory
Pharyngitis
Tonsillitis
Tracheobronchitis
Chronic bronchitis
Bronchiectasis
Granuloma
Chronic pulmonary fibrosis
Bronchial asthma
Eosinophilic pneumonitis
Eosinophilic pulmonary granulomatosis
Pulmonary infiltrate with eosinophilia (PIE)
Sinusitis (?)

Physical/Traumatic Factors
Collapsed trachea
Hilar lymph node enlargement
Secondary to esophageal dysfunction
Foreign body
Tracheal stenosis
Left atrial enlargement (mainstem bronchial compression)

Neoplastic
Primary
Mediastinal
Metastatic
Tracheal
Laryngeal
Ribs, sternum, muscle
Lymphoma

Cardiovascular
Left heart failure—pulmonary edema
Cardiomegaly—especially left atrium
Pulmonary emboli
Pulmonary edema—vascular origin

Infectious
Larval migration (*Toxocara* spp., *Ancylostoma caninum*, *Strongyloides stercoralis*), *Filaroides* spp. (dog), *Aelurostrongylus abstrusis* (feline lungworm), *Paragonimus kellicotti* (dog, cat), *Dirofilaria immitis* (dog, cat), *Capillaria aerophilia* (dog, cat), *Crensoma vulpis* (dog)
Toxoplasmosis (cat)
Pneumocystis (dog)
Blastomycosis
Histoplasmosis
Coccidiomycosis
Cryptococcosis
Aspergillosis
Pneumonia—bacterial, viral
Abscess

occur, how often does it occur, is the cough worse at night or during the day, is it stimulated by exercise, is the timing of the cough related to eating or drinking, and does the cough respond to diuretics or other medications? Cardiac disease initially results in nocturnal coughing, but advanced cardiac disease may result in coughing during any time of day or night. Tracheal collapse typically produces a characteristic "goose-honk" sound easily recognized by most owners and experienced clinicians. Coughing due to tracheal collapse or tracheal irritation is stimulated by excitement, drinking water, and by pulling on the collar. A productive cough may be produced by the following conditions: chronic bronchitis/ bronchiectasis, pneumonia, pulmonary edema, esophageal dysfunction, and hemoptysis. A nonproductive cough may be produced by the following conditions: bronchitis, early cardiac disease, left atrial enlargement without pulmonary edema, lymphadenopathy, allergic lung disease, and tracheal irritation or collapse. These lists are not meant to be all-inclusive and some diseases may produce both types of cough. Also, some animals may be experiencing more than one disease process at a time, thus having multiple reasons for a cough.

Physical Examination

As with other body systems, a thorough physical examination is required for obvious reasons. Emphasis is placed on the cardiorespiratory system. Careful auscultation will reveal the presence or absence of a murmur, arrhythmia, gallop, crackles, wheezes, rales, upper airway noises, nasal discharge, or evidence of pleural effusion. Some physical examination findings may help exclude specific differentials. For example, the presence of a respiratory sinus arrhythmia makes heart failure very unlikely. On the other hand, pulmonary crackles are less specific and may occur due to chronic pulmonary disease or due to pulmonary edema.

Radiographs

Thoracic radiographs may provide essential information leading to a diagnosis. Radiographs should be analyzed for evidence of cardiac enlargement, congested pulmonary veins, pulmonary disease, pulmonary edema, and narrowing of the trachea. If pulmonary edema is identified, left heart enlargement and venous congestion is expected. Right heart enlargement alone does not typically result in a cough. It is important to distinguish coughing due to cardiac enlargement and coughing due to pulmonary edema. Left atrial enlargement may result in compression of the mainstem bronchi. Although some findings may be obvious, it may be impossible to distinguish between neoplasia, fungal infection, and pneumonia on radiographic examination alone. An algorithm for a general approach to interpreting thoracic radiographs in the presence of a cough is presented in Figure 63-1.

Further Diagnostics

In some cases, it may be necessary to perform further diagnostics in an effort to obtain a diagnosis and proper treatment plan. A complete blood cell count, general chemistry profile, and heartworm test (in endemic regions or when there is a travel history that might suggest exposure in nonendemic regions) should precede further diagnostics. Descriptions of further diagnostics involving the cardiac and respiratory systems can be found elsewhere in this textbook and may include: blood gas analysis, electrocardiogram, echocardiogram, thoracic ultrasound, bronchoscopy, fluoroscopic examination of airways, transtracheal wash or bronchoalveolar lavage, titers for infectious disease, fecal Baermann, fine

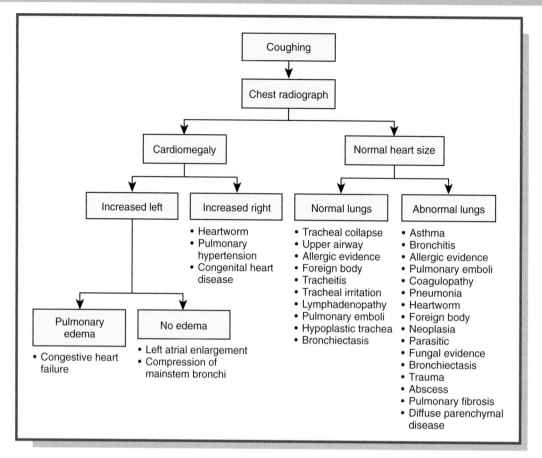

Figure 63-1 Algorithm for interpretation of thoracic radiographs in the presence of a cough.

Table • 63-1

Drugs Commonly Used for Canine and Feline Coughing

GENERIC NAME	TRADE NAME	DOSAGE
Antitussive		
Codeine	Multiple	1-2 mg/kg PO q6-12h
Hydrocodone	Hycodan	Dog: 0.22 mg/kg PO q6-12h
Hydrocodone/Homatropine	Tussigon	Dog: 0.22mg/kg PO q6-12h
	Hydromet Syrup	(Dose based on hydrocodone)
Hydrocodone/Chlorpheniramine (extended release)	Tussionex	Dog: 1 cc per 20 lbs PO q12h
Butorphanol	Torbutrol	Dog: 0.5 mg/kg PO q6-12 h
Tramadol	Ultram	Dog: 1-2 mg/kg PO q8-12h
Bronchodilator		
Aminophylline	Multiple	Dog: 10 mg/kg PO, IV q8h
		Cat: 5 mg/kg PO q12h
Theophylline	Multiple	Dog: 6 mg/kg PO q8h q12h
Theophylline slow release	Theochron (Inwood Labs)	Dog: 10 mg/kg PO q12h
	Theocaps (Inwood Labs)	Dog: 10 mg/kg PO q12h
Albuterol	Multiple	Dog: 0.05 mg/kg PO q8h
Terbutaline	Brethine	Dog: 0.625 (small dog)–5 mg (large dog) PO q12h
		Cat: 0.312-0.625 mg per cat PO q12h
Prednisone/trimeprazine	Temaril-P	Dog: 1 tablet/20 lbs PO q12h
Expectorant/Antitussive		
Guaifenesin/dextromethorphan	Robitussin-DM	Dog: 1-2 mg/kg PO q6-8h
	Cough Tabs	(Dose based on dextromethorphan)

needle aspiration of lung, cytologic evaluation of masses or effusions. Cardiac biomarkers such as NT-pro ANP and NT-pro BNP and troponin may be particularly helpful to distinguish cardiac from noncardiac disease.

Treatment Goals

The ideal treatment for a cough is based on a definitive diagnosis and treatment of the underlying problem. However, it is not always possible to obtain a definitive diagnosis, and in such cases, treatment options must be based on clinical assumptions or a preliminary diagnosis. If no specific diagnosis has been made, there is no underlying problem identified, or the cough persists despite treatment of the underlying problem, the use of antitussives should be considered. Table 63-1 outlines medications commonly used for coughing.

As a general rule, antitussive agents are contraindicated in cases when suppressing a cough masks important clinical symptoms or when a cough is actually encouraged as part of therapy. Specific treatment of underlying disorders can be found elsewhere in this textbook.

CHAPTER 64

Dyspnea and Tachypnea

Scott Forney

DEFINITIONS

Dyspnea is defined as difficult or labored breathing. Dyspnea is caused by insufficient oxygenation in the blood or hypercapnia, which is sensed in the peripheral and central chemoreceptors, respectively. *Tachypnea* is defined as an increased rate of respiration. *Panting* is often a normal thermoregulatory response in dogs but is almost always abnormal in cats. Inappropriate or persistent panting in dogs may be an indication of pathology including fever, anxiety, pain, metabolic disease, cardiovascular disease, endocrine disease, and hypertension. *Orthopnea* is defined as difficulty breathing unless in an upright position.

INITIAL APPROACH TO THE DYSPNEIC PATIENT

Recognition and quick assessment are crucial in any patient presenting with respiratory distress. Transportation to the veterinarian, unfamiliar surroundings and noises, physical examination or restraint, and diagnostic testing may all result in sudden decompensation of the patient's clinical condition. Oxygen supplementation should be administered in the least stressful and most effective manner possible while initial assessment is performed. Flow-by or mask oxygen, nasal oxygen, and oxygen cages can be considered depending upon the situation and availability. Oxygen cages tend to be the least stressful; however, this may be the least effective at delivering the highest oxygen content. This method does not allow the clinician to perform a physical examination without compromising the oxygen content delivered to the patient. Nasal oxygen may provide the highest amount of delivered oxygen but is often the most stressful and should not be attempted if any resistance is encountered.

Historical information useful in the initial assessment of the patient includes onset of respiratory signs (acute or chronic), recent trauma or electrical cord bites, toxic exposure (rat bait), current medications, and previous signs referable to a particular area of the respiratory system including coughing, sneezing, and nasal discharge. History of vomiting or regurgitation could indicate aspiration pneumonia. Other symptoms noted by owners may be associated with metabolic or systemic conditions.

Patients should be quickly evaluated on initial presentation. Should imminent respiratory arrest be evident, all efforts should be focused on the need for endotracheal intubation and resuscitation. Intubation may provide useful and occasionally diagnostic information. Upper airway obstruction may be noted and bypassed during the intubation process. Serosanguineous fluid evident in the endotracheal tube suggests pulmonary edema (cardiogenic or noncardiogenic), fluid and food particles aspiration pneumonia, and frank blood indicates pulmonary hemorrhage. There are situations where sedation and intubation (and occasionally tracheotomy) may be the only means by which a clinician can gain control of the situation. In general, these are patients with airway obstruction due to laryngeal paralysis, collapsing trachea, neoplasia, or a foreign body. Patients with airway obstruction may become hyperthermic, and often times cooling techniques must be employed. If it is determined by the clinician that immediate intervention is not necessary, physical examination is the clinician's best tool to localize the cause of the respiratory distress.

PHYSICAL EXAM FINDINGS

Initial examination of any patient, especially a dyspneic one, does not require the clinician to touch the patient. Many times the source of the respiratory distress may be evident based on respiratory sounds and the nature of the breathing. The rate and depth of respiration, abdominal movement, inspiratory, expiratory, or mixed respiratory effort, patient posture, and breathing noises can all provide important clues (Figure 64-1).

Auscultation, palpation, and percussion may further narrow down the differentials and provide useful information for diagnosis and treatment. If the patient is stable, full evaluation of other organ systems should be performed and may provide valuable information as to the underlying cause of the respiratory distress.

Upper Airway

The upper airway consists of the nasal passages, pharynx, larynx, and trachea. Patients with upper airway disease have inspiratory dyspnea only unless complicated by another condition. *Stertor* refers to a snoring sound that is generally due to partial obstruction of the nasal passage and/or nasopharynx. Stenotic nares, nasal foreign bodies, neoplasia, or rhinitis are all possible causes. *Stridor* is defined as a harsh, shrill sound that results from an upper airway obstruction, generally laryngeal in nature, but that can be due to pharyngeal, cervical tracheal, or nasal disease. Laryngeal paralysis, neoplasia, polyps, brachycephalic syndrome, foreign bodies, inflammation, and tracheal collapse are the more common causes of upper airway dyspnea. These patients can become acutely dyspneic and decompensate within a matter of minutes. Sedation and active cooling procedures (if hyperthermic) may be enough to make the patient more comfortable. Anesthesia and intubation to bypass any obstruction may actually be required. It is in these cases where oxygen supplementation is inadequate. Auscultation of the thorax usually reveals very harsh and loud sounds that are referred from the upper airways. Auscultation of louder sounds over the cervical trachea allows the clinician to differentiate between increased pulmonary versus referred upper airway sounds. Of importance is the fact that these abnormal sounds are usually observed without physically touching the patient and are often heard even before entering the examination room.

Small Airway

Small airways refer to the bronchi and bronchioles. Respiratory patterns of small airway disease are usually a quick/shortened inspiratory period and prolonged expiration, occasionally with an expiratory push. There can be an increase in abdominal effort. Auscultation may reveal very harsh bronchovesicular sounds including rhonchi (wheezes) and rales (crackles) on inspiration or expiration. These sounds are the result of partial lower airway obstruction, either secondary to bronchoconstriction and/or secretions. Feline asthma is one of the more common small airways conditions encountered. Other diseases include bronchitis (allergic or chronic), smoke inhalation, bronchopneumonia, and chronic obstructive pulmonary disease. Another description of these sounds is sibilant or whistling rales that mimic a high frequency whistling sound on deep inspiration or during the expiratory wheeze.

Pleural Space

Respiration with pleural space disease is often referred to as a *restrictive pattern of breathing*. Due to the pleural pathology, the respiratory rate is increased while the depth of inspiration is decreased due to the lungs inability to expand. There may be increased intercostal contraction resulting in cranial motion of the diaphragm and inward motion of the abdomen. This is referred to as paradoxical abdominal motion. Auscultation findings depend upon the degree and type of pleural pathology. Types of pleural disease include pneumothorax, mass effects, idiopathic chylothorax, pyothorax, hemothorax, neoplastic and cardiogenic effusions, and diaphragmatic hernia. Effusions can result in muffled heart and lung sounds, or the lung sounds may only be heard in the dorsal fields due to displacement by fluid. Percussion of the thorax reveals dull sounds in the ventral lung fields. Pneumothorax also results in decreased lung sounds but increased resonance on percussion. Cats usually have compressible chest walls, so patients with cranial thoracic masses may have decreased compliance. In any patient presenting with decreased lung sounds, a restrictive breathing pattern, and suspicion of air or fluid in the pleural space, a diagnostic pleural tap is indicated. When considered safe, a radiograph of the thorax is recommended first to ascertain tap position and other abnormalities.

Lung Parenchyma

Dyspnea due to lung parenchymal disease tends to have a mixed (inspiratory and expiratory) component. Oftentimes there are increased bronchovesicular lung sounds and/or crackles. Changes in these sounds can be very useful for monitoring progression or improvement of an individual; however their presence does not indicate the underlying pathology. There are numerous causes of parenchymal disease including both cardiac and noncardiac pulmonary edema. Noncardiogenic pulmonary edema may be caused by upper airway obstruction or strangulation, head trauma, seizures, and electrocution. Presence of a loud heart murmur or gallop rhythm should increase suspicion of cardiogenic pulmonary edema. Pneumonia (bacterial, viral, fungal) is another common cause of parenchymal disease. In any patient with a history of vomiting, regurgitation, or recent anesthesia, aspiration pneumonia should be suspected. Other causes include hemorrhage or contusions (trauma or coagulopathy), metastatic or primary neoplasia, parasitic, or pulmonary thromboembolism (heartworm disease, Cushing's, PLN/PLE, other).

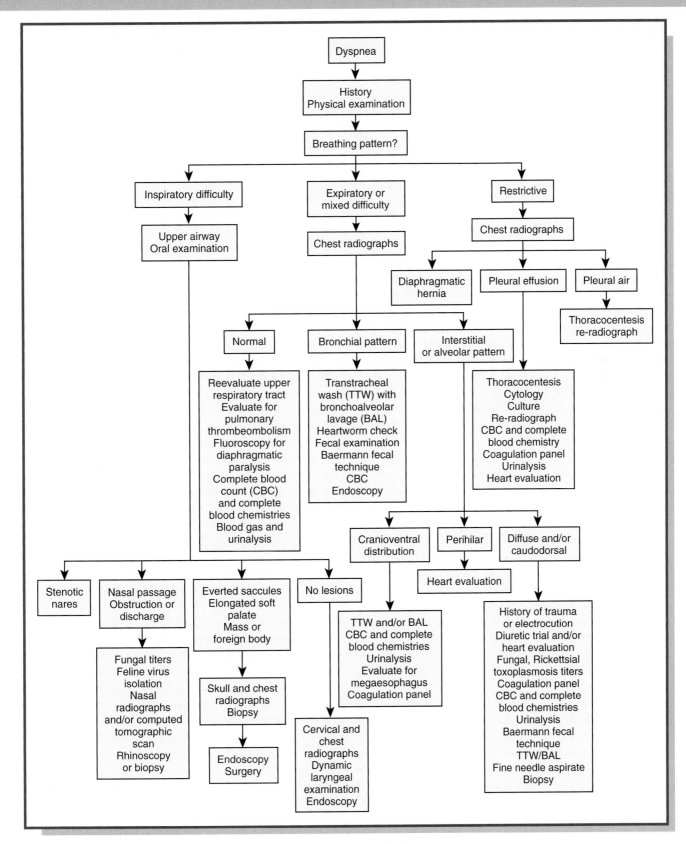

Figure 64-1 Algorithm for dyspnea.

CHAPTER 65

Innocent Heart Murmurs

Marie-Claude Bélanger
Etienne Côté

The auscultation of a heart murmur in a puppy or kitten can represent a diagnostic challenge for any practicing veterinarian. Pathologic murmurs must be differentiated from innocent heart murmurs, because correctly identifying the location, timing, and quality of a heart murmur makes it possible to formulate proper recommendations for the patient's owners.

Innocent heart murmurs are sounds made by the blood circulating through a structurally normal heart's chambers or valves, or through normal blood vessels near the heart. Although the exact nomenclature remains debated in human cardiology,[1,2] an "innocent" murmur can occur in a healthy heart due to systemic disturbances such as anemia (sometimes referred to as a *physiologic murmur*), or due to normal growth (sometimes referred to as a *juvenile murmur*). For the purposes of this chapter, the terms *innocent murmur* and *juvenile murmur* are considered equivalent, and denote heart murmurs of normal puppies and kittens <6 months old.

On auscultation, innocent murmurs are typically pure in character as opposed to coarse; low- to medium-frequency in children and any frequency, low or high, in puppies; short (early- or midsystolic); and sometimes intermittent (Figure 65-1).

These murmurs are variably audible according to body position, heart rate, or conditions associated with an increased cardiac output such as exercise or stressful events. Most innocent heart murmurs in children increase in intensity with exercise,[3,4] in contrast to puppies, where an innocent murmur

may increase or decrease in intensity when the heart rate increases. Innocent heart murmurs are present in 8% to 60% of all children of school age.[5] This prevalence can be increased to 87% after vigorous exercise,[4] and in human pediatric cardiology, it is said that innocent heart murmurs are so frequent during childhood that even in a well child, the absence of a murmur rather than its presence occasions a surprise.[6] Innocent murmurs are generally soft in intensity (grade III/VI or less) and therefore are not associated with a palpable thrill. They are always systolic in timing, and never cause signs of congestive heart failure or syncope since, by definition, they are not associated with cardiac disease.

GENESIS OF INNOCENT HEART MURMURS

Heart murmurs are the audible expression of turbulent blood flow. The factors that determine whether flow is laminar or turbulent are described by a dimensionless quantity known as the Reynolds number[7,8]:

$$Re = V \times D \times \rho / \eta$$

where V = mean linear average flow velocity (cm/s), D = tube diameter (cm), ρ = fluid density (no units), and η = fluid viscosity (unit: poise). The higher the Reynolds number, the greater the likelihood of turbulence. In the normal circulation, the Reynolds number may rise above 200 to 400, causing small amounts of turbulence at vessel bifurcations, for example, and a Reynolds number >2000 is almost invariably associated with turbulence.[7,8] As the formula shows, the possibility of turbulence increases as blood flow velocity increases, blood viscosity decreases, or the area of the vessel increases abruptly.

The term "innocent murmur" was introduced by Evans in 1943.[1,9] This broad term in fact encompasses a number of different specific murmurs of growing juvenile patients. The identification of specific subtypes of innocent murmurs is clearly recognized in human pediatric medicine but not in small animal medicine.[10-18] In children, murmurs that are considered to be part of the "innocent" category include the vibratory innocent murmur (Still's murmur), the pulmonary systolic ejection murmur, the supraclavicular arterial bruit, and the cervical venous hum.[2,19] The first two are the most common, and innocent murmurs in puppies likely are similar or identical to these two types.

The first and most common innocent heart murmur, Still's murmur, is a short, buzzing or musical, pure, and medium-frequency sound that is typically heard between the lower left sternal edge and apex.[2,20] Carotid pulse tracings, echocardiography, and intracardiac phonocardiography indicate that it originates from the left heart.[21] Specifically, it has been associated with high-velocity aortic flow caused by a larger left ventricular stroke volume, with[22-24] or without[25] a relatively

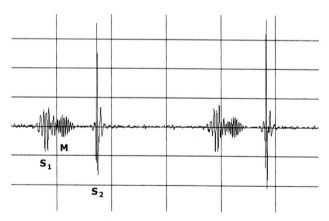

Figure 65-1 Phonocardiogram demonstrating a typical physiologic murmur in a healthy dog with a normal echocardiogram. The reader should note that the murmur *(M)* is short, early-systolic (beginning after the first heart sound *[S₁]* and occupying less than half of systole), crescendo-decrescendo or "diamond-shaped," and low-to-moderate in intensity. The same features are seen on the second heartbeat *(unlabeled).* S_2, Second heart sound.

WWW. To view a video on this topic, go to **www.expertconsult.com.**

smaller aortic valve and ascending aorta; intraluminal left ventricular bands[25]; fibrous bands in the aortic arch[26]; ventricular false tendons[5,27-30]; relative bradycardia[25]; and intraventricular periodic vibrations.[25] The result on auscultation can be a characteristic twanging sound, analogous to the sound made by twanging a piece of string (see Figure 65-1) (Web Figure 65-1).

The second type of innocent heart murmur represents an exaggeration of normal ejection vibrations within the pulmonary trunk. It occurs in the first part of systole, when the velocity of systolic ejection is maximal. This normal pulmonary systolic murmur is short, relatively impure, or coarse.[31] Innocent heart murmurs are better heard in pediatric patients than in adults due to a thin chest wall in youth, more angulated great vessels, and more dynamic circulation.[19]

In the dog, it has been hypothesized that young animals have a larger stroke volume compared to the size of the great vessels than do older animals. This can result in an increase in flow velocity to the point of producing turbulence, either in the aorta or in the pulmonary artery, and a resultant innocent heart murmur.[14,17] The increase in the velocity and associated turbulence is usually mild, so the heart murmur is soft (i.e., grade I/VI to III/VI). The innocent heart murmur generally disappears before 4 to 6 months of age, when the great vessels enlarge in diameter with growth. A notable exception is the Boxer breed, where a smaller left ventricular outflow tract is associated with systolic murmurs in otherwise normal adults.[32]

DIFFERENTIATION OF INNOCENT MURMURS FROM PATHOLOGIC MURMURS

A heart murmur is a common finding on routine examination of puppies. When murmurs are due to congenital heart defects, corrective intervention is indicated as soon as appropriate because repair may substantially improve long-term outcome.[33,34] Therefore, as a first step, innocent heart murmurs should be differentiated from pathologic heart murmurs associated with congenital heart defects. This task is sometimes difficult to achieve in some very active young animals! Some useful auscultation tips include the following: panting should be minimized by having the mouth of any puppy held closed during auscultation; even so, some puppies whine or sniff relentlessly, and this interference, or purring in kittens, can be minimized by intermittently occluding the patient's mouth and nostrils with the hand for 1 to 3 seconds at a time (imposed breath-holding); patients in whom this technique is not tolerated sometimes can be distracted into brief silence by performing the auscultation while "scruffing" (Figure 65-2)—elevating the skin of the nape of the neck such that the forepaws are almost off the exam table (in dogs, this technique is generally only useful for pups 10 weeks or younger); or by cradling a pup in a sitting position in the practitioner's right arm and auscultating the pup while walking around the exam room (Figure 65-3).

The latter technique works best in small (<15 kg), cooperative puppies, and the procedure seems particularly distracting to the pup—and therefore effective—if the examiner walks with tight, abrupt turns. Heavy-coated young dogs that pant continually may be auscultated more successfully outdoors, where fresh air can reduce panting.

ASSESSMENT OF MURMURS THAT MAY BE PHYSIOLOGIC OR PATHOLOGIC

Web Figure 65-1 illustrates the intensity profile of the murmurs caused by the most common heart defects in

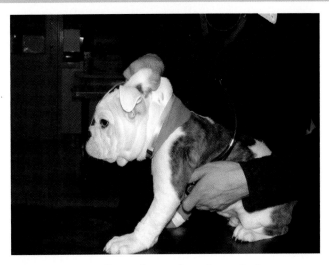

Figure 65-2 Scruffing technique for reducing body movement and respiratory noise during auscultation of kittens or very young puppies.

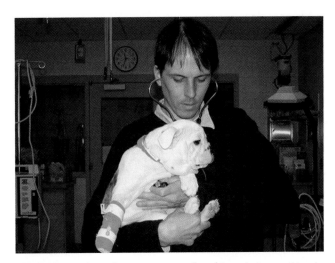

Figure 65-3 Auscultating a puppy placed in a sitting position in the examiner's right arm. Moving in tight circles and abrupt turns distracts the puppy and briefly reduces whining, sniffing, and other interference. The hindlimbs are held securely.

puppies. Although the relative prevalence of pathologic versus physiologic murmurs is not known in small animal medicine, physiologic murmurs are more common than pathologic murmurs in children[5] and veterinary clinical experience likewise is consistent with the widespread occurrence of innocent murmurs in puppies and, to a lesser degree, in kittens. Knowing the breed predisposition for common congenital cardiac disorders is helpful in diagnostic decision making in a puppy with a heart murmur (Web Table 65-1), although such prevalence information at best provides a rough index of suspicion when examining an individual patient.

In dogs and cats, innocent murmurs are systolic in timing, usually occurring early in systole and being of short duration (ejection type, and less than holo/pansystolic). Innocent heart murmurs are typically I/VI or II/VI in intensity, rarely III/VI but not louder unless a systolic whoop is also present. A systolic whoop is a loud, high-pitched vibration resembling the call of a seagull and is thought to represent periodic vibra-

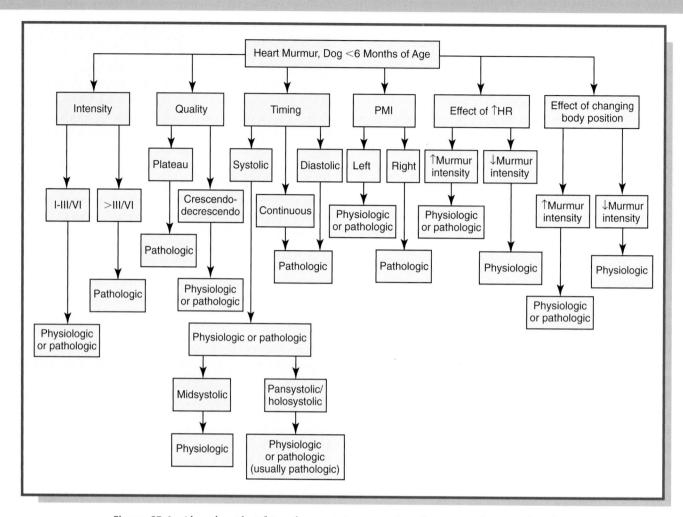

Figure 65-4 Algorithm identifying characteristics suggestive of murmurs that are physiologic, pathologic, or either. *HR,* Heart rate; *PMI,* point of maximal intensity.

Table • 65-1

Auscultatory Characteristics of Congenital Defects in Puppies

DEFECT	TIMING OF MURMUR	QUALITY OF MURMUR	PMI
PDA	Continuous	Wind tunnel, machinery-type	Cranial to the left base
SAS	Systolic	Crescendo-decrescendo	Left base or right base
PS	Systolic	Crescendo-decrescendo	Left base
VSD	Systolic	Holosystolic or pansystolic plateau	Cranial to or at right apex, sternum, left base
ASD	Systolic	Soft	Left base
MD	Systolic	Holosystolic or pansystolic	Left apex
TD	Systolic	Holosystolic or pansystolic plateau	Right apex
TF	Systolic	Crescendo-decrescendo	Left base
AR	Diastolic	Soft, blowing, decrescendo,	Left base

AR, Aortic regurgitation/aortic insufficiency; *ASD,* atrial septal defect; *MD,* mitral dysplasia; *PDA,* patent ductus arteriosus; *PS,* pulmonic stenosis; *SAS,* subaortic stenosis; *TD,* tricuspid dysplasia/Ebstein's anomaly; *TF,* tetralogy of Fallot; *VSD,* ventricular septal defect.

tions of the mitral valve leaflets or other structures.[35] A systolic whoop is striking due to its loudness but does not necessarily indicate a cardiac lesion; it occurs rarely in puppies and virtually never in cats. Innocent murmurs often have a vibrating or musical quality that novice auscultators describe as surprising or "funny-sounding." Since they are ejection-type murmurs, they are usually crescendo-decrescendo in nature, and they are best heard along the left sternal border and do not radiate to the rest of the thorax. Overall, the sound of innocent murmurs may give the impression of a "puff" (low or medium frequency) or a wheeze or "cooing" (high frequency, "musical") that occupies part—but not all—of systole. The bell of the stethoscope is particularly useful to identify the lower "twanging" vibratory frequencies that may be present in some innocent heart murmurs. Vagal maneuvers usually decrease the intensity of an innocent (or a pathologic) heart murmur. Increases in heart rate, such as those induced by exercise, invariably increase the intensity of murmurs associated with congenital heart malformations, but increases in heart rate may increase or decrease the intensity of innocent heart murmurs in dogs. In other words, a soft-grade systolic heart murmur that decreases in intensity immediately after exercising the puppy is most likely innocent, but a murmur that increases in intensity with exercise may be innocent or pathologic.

In general all murmurs that are diastolic, holosystolic (pansystolic), late systolic, or continuous, or are loud (grade >III/VI), are considered pathologic and should prompt further diagnostic procedures (Figure 65-4).[19]

Correctly identifying the location, timing, and quality of a pathologic murmur makes it possible to formulate a tentative list of possible diagnoses (Table 65-1).

Indications for proceeding to diagnostic testing include any of the following: the clinician's suspicion of a pathologic murmur on initial examination, the persistence of a murmur previously thought to be physiologic and which has not disappeared several weeks after initial detection and/or by age ≥6 months, the clinician's uncertainty regarding the nature of a murmur, client/owner anxiety or wishes, and the presence of signs of decompensation such as manifestations of congestive heart failure.[19] Such diagnostic testing typically consists of thoracic radiographs and echocardiography, including complete two-dimensional, M-mode, spectral Doppler, and color Doppler studies.

REFERENCES

The reference list can be found on the companion Expert Consult Web site at *www.expertconsult.com*.

CHAPTER 66

Abnormal Heart Sounds and Heart Murmurs

Robert Prošek

Cardiac auscultation is an important tool in the clinician's armamentarium. Interpretation of heart and lung sounds is predicated on the clinician's understanding of their genesis in health and a variety of clinical disorders. Cardiovascular sounds of short duration are referred to as *transient heart sounds* and include the normally heard first heart sound (S_1) and second heart sound (S_2).

Heart murmurs are auditory vibrations of longer duration created when laminar flow is disrupted.

Implementing good technique with a quality stethoscope is fundamental. During auscultation the animal should be standing or sitting in a quiet environment. Both sides of the thorax should be carefully auscultated with the stethoscope's diaphragm and bell with special attention to the areas overlying the cardiac valves. The clinician should correlate the various heart sounds to the events of the cardiac cycle. A good orientation is palpation of the precordial impulse (left apex beat) that occurs just after S1, and the arterial pulse that is felt between S_1 and S_2.

TRANSIENT HEART SOUNDS

The First (S_1) and Second (S_2) Heart Sounds
The first heart sound is associated with closure and tensing of the atrioventricular valves (mitral and tricuspid) at the onset of systole coinciding with the QRS complex on the electrocardiogram. S_1 is longer, louder, and lower pitched than the second heart sound. Causes of increased intensity of S_1 include thin chest wall, tachycardia, high sympathetic tone, systemic arterial hypertension, and anemia. Diminished intensity of S_1 may be auscultated in animals with obesity, pleural or pericardial effusion, diaphragmatic hernia, dilated cardiomyopathy, hypovolemia, emphysema, or a prolonged P-R interval. Splitting of S_1 is occasionally auscultated at the cardiac apex in healthy, large-breed dogs or may result from electrical disturbances (ectopic beats, bundle branch blocks, cardiac pacing) or mechanical factors (tricuspid or mitral stenosis).

The second heart sound is associated with closure of the semilunar valves (aortic and pulmonic) at the end of systole following the T wave on the electrocardiogram. In dogs and cats, pulmonic valve (P_2) closure follows aortic valve (A_2) closure by a very short interval, which causes S_2 to be heard as a single sound. On occasion an audible split-second heart sound may be seen in healthy, large-breed dogs during inspiration due to a longer right ventricular ejection period. Pathologic splitting of S_2 occurs with heartworm disease and right-to-left patent ductus arteriosus.

Delayed closure of P_2 also occurs with left-to-right intracardiac shunts (atrial septal defects), pulmonic stenosis, right bundle branch block, ectopic beats, and ventricular pacing. Premature A_2 closure can on occasion be noted with mitral insufficiency and mitral stenosis. Paradoxic splitting of S_2 results from delayed closure of the aortic valve and is sometimes audible in dogs with aortic stenosis, left bundle branch block, ectopic beats, and systemic hypertension.

WWW. To view a video on this topic, go to **www.expertconsult.com**.

The Third (S₃) and Fourth (S₄) Heart Sounds

The third and fourth heart sounds occur during diastole and are not audible in normal dogs and cats. S_3 and S_4 heart sounds are of lower frequency than S_1 and S_2 and are usually best heard with the bell of the stethoscope. When heard, S_3 and S_4 may sound like the triple cadence of a galloping horse.

The term *gallop rhythm* should probably be avoided because the presence of an audible S_3 or S_4 has nothing to do with the heart's underlying electrical rhythm. Rapid ventricular filling generates the S_3 sound, also known as S_3 *gallop, protodiastolic gallop,* or *ventricular gallop.* An audible S_3 is most commonly heard with diastolic volume overloading as in dilated cardiomyopathy, patent ductus arteriosus, and mitral insufficiency. In dogs with mitral insufficiency, the S_3 gallop may be mistaken for the second heart sound if a loud pansystolic murmur extends through the second heart sound. Protodiastolic gallop sounds in cats are most commonly associated with dilated cardiomyopathy, anemia, and hyperthyroidism.

The presystolic gallop, also called S_4 *gallop* or *atrial gallop,* is heard just before S_1 and occurs just after the P wave on the electrocardiogram. This low-frequency sound is generated by blood flow into the ventricles during atrial contraction; hence the absence of S_4 gallops with atrial fibrillation. An audible S_4 in the cat and dog is usually associated with increased ventricular hypertrophy and stiffness and is sometimes audible in animals with third-degree atrioventricular block.

At fast heart rates, rapid ventricular filling and atrial systole transpire very close together, which makes differentiation between S_3 and S_4 impossible. The resulting single accentuated sound is referred to as a summation gallop.

Ejection Sounds, Systolic Clicks, Opening Snaps, and Pericardial Knocks

Ejection sounds are left basilar high-frequency sounds generated by opening of the semilunar valves or dilatation of the great vessels during early systole. These sounds are occasionally noted in pulmonic stenosis, aortic stenosis, tetralogy of Fallot, and heartworm disease. Systolic clicks are mid to late high-frequency sounds usually heard best over the mitral valve area. Systolic clicks are occasionally associated with degenerative valvular disease, mitral valve prolapse, and mitral dysplasia. The genesis of the sound in dogs is uncertain but is likely caused by the sudden tensing of redundant valve leaflets or elongated chordae tendineae as they buckle into the left atrium. A systolic click should be differentiated from a split or gallop heart sound. Pericardial knocks are uncommon early diastolic sounds caused by restrictive pericardial disease. Timing of the sound is similar to S_3 and appears to be generated by abrupt restriction to ventricular filling by a diseased

Figure 66-1 Murmur shapes and descriptions with some common examples. Also depicted are normal and abnormal transient heart sounds and their location within the cardiac cycle. *Proto,* Early; *meso,* mid; *tele,* late; A_2, aortic valve closure; P_2, pulmonic valve closure; S_1, first heart sound; S_2, second heart sound; S_3, third heart sound; S_4, fourth heart sound.

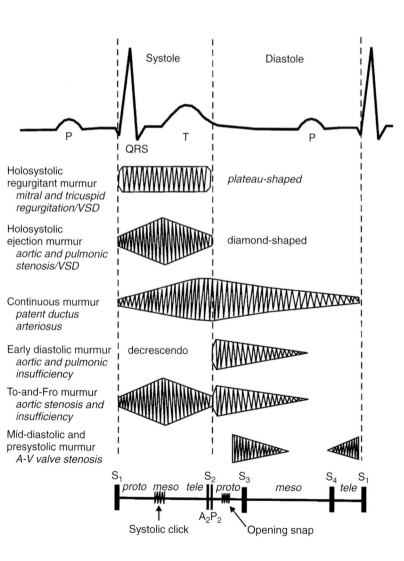

pericardium. (See Figure 66-1 for timing of transient heart sounds and description of murmurs.)

Cardiac Murmurs

Cardiac murmurs represent sounds of longer duration than the transient heart sounds. Cardiac murmurs are caused by turbulent blood flow in the heart or adjacent blood vessels created upon disruption of normal laminar flow. The development of turbulent blood flow can be created by high-velocity flow, flow from narrow restricted area into a larger area, or low blood viscosity. The relationship of cardiac murmurs with flow velocity, vessel size, and blood viscosity is defined by the Reynold's number. When the number reaches a critical high level, blood flow becomes turbulent.

Reynold's number = (Radius)(Velocity)(Density) ÷ Viscosity

Murmurs can be characterized and described by their timing within the cardiac cycle (systolic, diastolic, portions thereof), location (point of maximal intensity), radiation, intensity (loudness), shape, and frequency (pitch).

Timing

Systolic murmurs may start immediately at the first (S_1) heart sound and last through the second (S_2) heart sound (pansystolic murmur), may start immediately after S_1 and last until S_2 (holosystolic), or may occur in early (protosystolic), mid (mesosystolic), or late (telesystolic) systole. Diastolic murmurs most commonly occur in early diastole (protodiastolic), throughout diastole (holodiastolic), or can occasionally be audible only at the end of diastole (presystolic).

Location and Radiation

The location of a murmur refers to the valve area at which the murmur is heard best (point of maximal intensity). Alternatively, location can be described simply by the terms *apex* or *base* (e.g., left apex or mitral valve area). Some murmurs may also radiate to other areas, yielding important clues as to the source of the murmur. For example, the murmur of subvalvular aortic stenosis (PMI at left heart base) may radiate to the ventral neck area due to turbulence in the carotid arteries and may also be heard on the right cranial thorax.

Intensity (Loudness)

The intensity of the murmur is commonly graded on a 1 to 6 scale, with grade 1 murmur the softest and grade 6 the loudest (Box 66-1).

A grade 1 murmur is the faintest murmur and is heard in a quiet environment with particular effort, whereas grade 5 and 6 murmurs are associated with palpable vibrations on the chest wall (palpable thrill). The intensity of the murmur at its origin is determined by blood flow velocity and the rate of flow (velocity × flow = force). The intensity of the murmur at the body surface is affected by direction of the turbulent jet, character of tissue between auscultation area and the turbulent jet, and the frequency of the murmur. Often the intensity of a heart murmur is not directly correlated with the severity of a lesion. However, describing the loudness of a murmur is important for serial examinations, and in certain heart diseases at least a rough correlation exists.

Pitch (Frequency)

A murmur's quality and pitch relate to its frequency components, which may be high, medium, low, or of mixed frequency. Most murmurs consist of midrange mixed-frequency sounds. On occasion high-frequency musical tones or low-frequency "honks" are auscultated. Musical murmurs are most commonly identified in dogs with modest mitral valve disease.

Box • 66-1

Grading of Cardiac Murmurs

Grade 1
Very soft, localized murmur detected in a quiet room after intently listening for a few minutes

Grade 2
Soft murmur but easily heard after a few seconds

Grade 3
Moderate-intensity murmur

Grade 4
Loud murmur but not accompanied by a palpable thrill (vibration)

Grade 5
Loud murmur accompanied by a palpable thrill

Grade 6
Very loud murmur that produces a palpable thrill still audible after stethoscope is removed from the chest

---

Shape

Heart murmurs are often described by their frequency profile within the cardiac cycle in relation to their shape on a phonocardiogram. Terms that are commonly used include *plateau-* or *band-shaped murmurs* for those murmurs of equal intensity throughout their duration; *decrescendo* for murmurs that gradually taper off from an initial peak; and *crescendo decrescendo* (diamond-shaped, ejection murmur) for murmurs that build up to a peak intensity and then taper in intensity.

SYSTOLIC HEART MURMURS

Mitral Insufficiency

The murmur of mitral insufficiency is best heard at the left apex (mitral valve area) and commonly radiates dorsally and to the right thorax making reliable diagnosis of tricuspid regurgitation difficult.

The characteristic murmur is plateau (band-shaped) and holosystolic; however, in its early stages the murmur may be protosystolic, and with mitral valve prolapse the murmur may develop in mid- to late-systole. Mitral insufficiency murmur is typically of mixed frequency and harsh sounding, but it may be high-pitched or musical (whooping) in quality.

Mitral insufficiency can be caused by chronic degenerative valvular disease (endocardiosis), endocarditis, hypertrophic obstructive cardiomyopathy, congenital malformations, and diseases that cause left heart enlargement and dilation of the mitral annulus (e.g., patent ductus arteriosus, dilated cardiomyopathy).

Tricuspid Insufficiency

The murmur of tricuspid insufficiency sounds similar to that of mitral insufficiency but is loudest over the right apex (tricuspid valve area). It is often difficult to distinguish tricuspid insufficiency from a radiating murmur of mitral insufficiency. Tricuspid murmurs might be a different pitch compared with a radiating mitral murmur and can be accompanied by jugular pulsations. Tricuspid insufficiency can result from congenital malformations of the valve, chronic degenerative valve disease, or any disorders that cause marked right heart enlargement and valve annulus distention, such as pulmonary hypertension and arrhythmogenic right ventricular cardiomyopathy. Tricuspid valve endocarditis is extremely rare in dogs and cats.

Aortic Stenosis

Valvular and subvalvular aortic stenosis (SAS) produce a systolic ejection (crescendo-decrescendo) murmur that is usually best heard at the left heart base.

The murmur is usually of mixed frequency and harsh, and it sometimes radiates towards the right cranial thorax and up the neck along the carotid arteries. Mild obstructions cause soft murmurs that are difficult to distinguish from innocent or functional murmurs. Murmurs that vary dramatically in intensity with exercise or excitement should prompt consideration of a dynamic left ventricular outflow tract obstruction. Dynamic outflow tract obstruction is the most common type of ejection murmurs in cats with hypertrophic cardiomyopathy and its onset and duration coincide with systolic anterior motion of the mitral valve. Dynamic left ventricular outflow tract obstruction occurs uncommonly in dogs as an isolated abnormality or in association with mitral valve dysplasia or hypertrophy of interventricular septum.

Pulmonic Stenosis

Pulmonic stenosis murmur is typically a high-frequency crescendo-decrescendo (ejection) holosystolic murmur, best heard at the left heart base over the pulmonic valve.

The murmur can be very similar to aortic stenosis murmur described above but should not radiate along the carotid arteries. As the pressure gradient between the right ventricle and pulmonary artery increases, the murmur intensity becomes louder and peaks later in systole.

Ventricular Septal Defect

Ventricular septal defects (VSDs) produce murmurs that vary tremendously in shape and quality. Most often the murmur is a harsh, mid- to high-frequency holosystolic murmur best heard on the right cranial thorax.

Murmur intensity may be reduced when the VSD is large and as pulmonary hypertension develops. With severe pulmonary hypertension, the murmur may be entirely absent and splitting of the second heart sound is noted.

Atrial Septal Defect

Heart murmurs in dogs and cats with an atrial septal defect (ASD) result from increased flow across the pulmonic valve as a result of the left to right shunting. This murmur resembles that of mild pulmonic stenosis but is often accompanied by a fixed splitting of the second heart sound. Flow across the atrial septal defect is usually not audible.

Physiologic and Innocent Murmurs

Functional (physiologic) murmurs are usually caused by decreased blood viscosity or increased cardiac output. Physiologic murmurs are most often noted in animals with anemia, fever, pregnancy, hyperthyroidism, and increased sympathetic tone. These murmurs usually are proto- to mesosystolic, soft to moderate intensity (grade 1/6 to 3/6), and loudest at the left heart base. They tend not to radiate extensively.

Innocent murmurs should disappear as the dog matures and appear to be the result of larger stroke volumes in puppies for the size of their great vessels in comparison with adult dogs.

In some cats, turbulent blood flow can be noted in the region of the right ventricular outflow tract, often causing a soft systolic apical sternal murmur ranging in grades from 1 to 3/6, with no evidence of structural heart disease and little clinical consequence.

DIASTOLIC HEART MURMURS

Aortic Insufficiency

The murmur of isolated aortic insufficiency is typically a decrescendo murmur starting at the time of S_2 and extending variably into diastole.

In young dogs, aortic insufficiency can occur as an isolated defect or in combination with subaortic stenosis or a ventricular septal defect. Detection of aortic insufficiency in an adult dog or cat should prompt consideration of bacterial endocarditis.

When the regurgitant volume is large, the diastolic murmur is often accompanied by a soft mesosystolic ejection murmur, creating a distinct "to-and-fro" murmur.

The systolic ejection component tapers off in late systole and allows recognition of S_2 and differentiation from a continuous murmur. Other causes of "to-and-fro" murmurs include ventricular septal defects that cause loss of aortic root support and pulmonic valve stenosis and significant pulmonic insufficiency (rare). Occasionally massive aortic regurgitation causes premature closure of the mitral valve producing functional mitral stenosis and a diastolic murmur referred to as an *Austin Flint murmur.*

Pulmonic Insufficiency

The murmur of pulmonic insufficiency is similar to that of aortic insufficiency; however, clinically significant pulmonic insufficiency is uncommon. It is sometimes detected in animals with pulmonary hypertension, pulmonic valve dysplasia, or idiopathic dilation of the pulmonary artery.

Mitral Stenosis

The diastolic murmur of mitral stenosis is difficult to recognize in dogs and cats.

This low-frequency murmur begins in mesodiastole and has presystolic accentuation due to atrial contraction. Mitral stenosis might be accompanied by other cardiac malformations, which cause murmurs such as valvular or subvalvular aortic stenosis. In dogs, mitral stenosis may be more common in breeds that are prone to congenital mitral valve malformations such as the Bull Terrier breed, in which it is often associated with aortic stenosis.

CONTINUOUS MURMURS

The most common cause of a continuous murmur at the left heart base is patent ductus arteriosus (PDA). This classic "machinery-like" murmur of a PDA is usually audible throughout the cardiac cycle with peak intensity near S_2.

The intensity of the murmur is diminished in late diastole in dogs with very slow heart rates and the diastolic component can also disappear with the development of pulmonary hypertension. Less common causes of continuous murmurs include aorticopulmonary windows, ruptured aneurysms of sinus of Valsalva, and coronary arteriovenous fistulas.

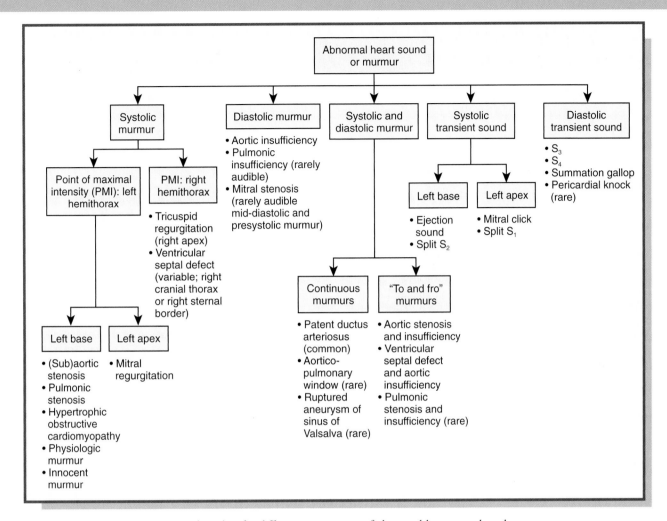

Figure 66-2 Algorithm for differentiating causes of abnormal heart sounds and murmurs.

AUSCULTATION AND BEYOND

Historical findings may suggest underlying heart disease; however, a thorough auscultation with identification and understanding of abnormal heart sounds and their genesis will permit recognition of the most likely cause (Figure 66-2).

As important a tool as cardiac auscultation is, it should be one part of a complete physical exam that integrates evalua-tion of lung fields, jugular veins, arterial pulses, and peripheral circulation. Increasingly the affordability and availability of next-generation electronic stethoscopes will allow the clini-cian to pick up difficult-to-hear heart sounds and other body sounds.

Additionally, other diagnostic tests might be needed to further classify and define the animal's abnormality, and in some cases differentiate a pathologic from a physiologic murmur (especially cats).

CHAPTER 67

Pulse Alterations

Anna Tidholm

ARTERIAL PULSES

Arterial pulse qualities, such as rate, rhythm, symmetry and strength, provide important information regarding cardiac output and perfusion (Figure 67-1).

The intensity of the arterial pulse, termed the *pulse pressure*, depends on the difference between the systolic and diastolic blood pressure, which may be assessed by digital palpation of artery. However, body condition affects the perceived strength of the arterial pulse, as it is usually more prominent in lean animals as opposed to obese animals. Three physiologic factors are important in determining arterial pulse pressures as follows: (1) heart rate, (2) stroke volume, and (3)

peripheral vascular resistance. An increased heart rate may be accompanied by a weak peripheral pulse, as the decreased duration of diastole may increase the diastolic pressure, which will decrease the pulse pressure. Bradycardia, on the other hand, may lead to excessive run-off during diastole as well as a greater strength of contraction due to greater diastolic filling, causing a strong pulse. A decrease in stroke volume, as found in patients with left-sided heart failure, hypovolemia, or cardiac tamponade, will produce a *hypokinetic pulse* (i.e., decreased pulse pressure). However, due to compensatory increase in arterial resistance, a hypokinetic pulse will only be found when the stroke volume becomes markedly reduced. If peripheral vascular resistance is decreased, or if arterial

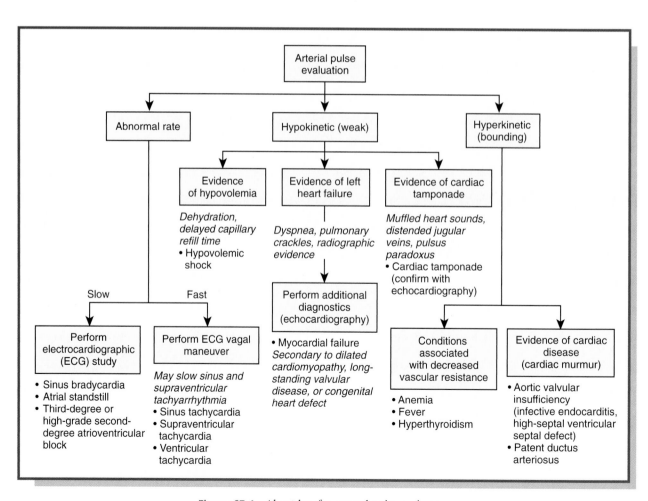

Figure 67-1 Algorithm for arterial pulse evaluation.

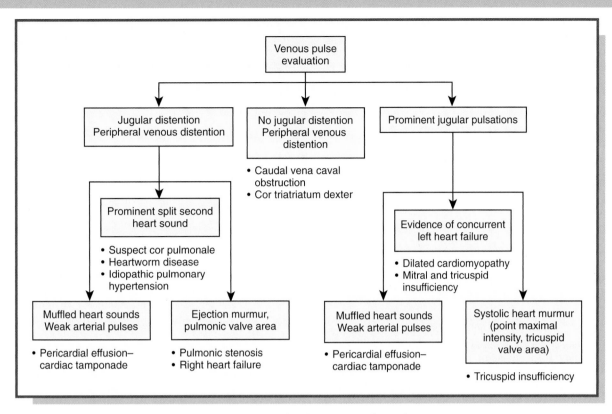

Figure 67-2   Algorithm for venous pulse evaluation.

compliance is increased, pulse pressure may also decrease. *Hyperkinetic pulses* may be caused by increased systolic blood pressure and/or decreased diastolic blood pressure, and are most prominent in aortic insufficiency and in left-to-right shunting PDA, leading to a bounding pulse. Bounding pulses can also be found in animals with fever, anemia, hyperthyroidism, severe bradycardia, and arteriovenous fistulas.

Pulsus paradoxus denotes an exaggerated decrease in systolic, mean, and pulse pressure on inspiration, and an exaggerated increase on expiration. This phenomenon is strongly suggestive of cardiac tamponade. *Pulsus alternans* refers to alternating strong and weak pulses that may occur when the left ventricle is severely dysfunctional, such as in dilated cardiomyopathy. Pulse deficit occurs in tachyarrhythmias where diastole is not long enough to allow adequate filling of the left ventricle to result in ejection of enough blood. Systemic thromboembolism secondary to feline cardiomyopathy or hypercoagulable states may result in a complete loss of arterial peripheral pulsations. Altered pulse conformation may also occur. Dogs with severe aortic stenosis may have a weak pulse or may have a pulse pressure that has a later-than-normal peak in systole due to prolonged ejection time (pulsus parvus et tardus). Dogs with mitral valve insufficiency may have a rapidly rising and declining pulse due to a shorter ejection time.

VENOUS PULSES

Jugular venous distension occurs when right atrial pressure is increased, as jugular venous pressures correlate with right atrial and ventricular pressures. Distended jugular veins indicate increased systemic venous pressure or occlusion of the venous system between the jugular veins and the right atrium. An increase in systemic venous pressure is most commonly observed secondary to an increase in right ventricular diastolic pressure. Animals with right-sided heart failure of any cause may have distended jugular veins (Figure 67-2).

When jugular waveforms are analyzed, the following components can be detected: The *A wave*, corresponding to right atrial contraction, is the most prominent wave. During right atrial relaxation there is a slight dip in pressure, the *Z point*. The following *C wave*, corresponding to right ventricular isovolumetric contraction, is produced by bulging of the tricuspid valve into the right atrium. During right ventricular ejection, the downward displacement of the tricuspid valve produces a prominent negative deflection, the *X decent*. A third positive deflection, the *V wave*, occurs late in systole and is caused by increased blood volume and pressure in the right atrium. A second prominent dip in jugular venous pressure, the *Y decent*, occurs when the right atrium empties as a result of right ventricular relaxation.

Jugular venous pulsations occur when tricuspid regurgitation is present. In normal animals, the jugular pulsations should not extend more than one third the distance up the neck from the thoracic inlet. Pulsations in the underlying carotid arteries may mimic jugular venous pulsations. Occlusion of the jugular vein by manual compression will help differentiate venous pulsations from arterial pulsations. Performing the *hepatojugular* or *abdominojugular reflux test*, by applying abdominal pressure for 30 to 60 seconds, may enhance jugular venous distention, as increased venous return in the presence of right-sided heart disease may elevate right atrial pressure and thus impede jugular venous return. Jugular vein pulsations may be caused by exaggerated A waves, "cannon A waves," or prominent V waves. Exaggerated A waves may occur secondary to severely decreased right ventricular compliance, as may be present in right ventricular hypertrophy, restrictive right ventricular disease, and constrictive pericarditis, resulting in increased right ventricular diastolic pressure. "Cannon A waves" may also occur in third-degree A-V block and other forms of A-V dissociation, when the atria contract against closed tricuspid valves. Prominent V waves may occur secondary to tricuspid regurgitation as the right atrial volume is increased.

CHAPTER 68

Pleural Effusion

O. Lynne Nelson

DEFINITION

The pleura surround the lung lobes (visceral pleura) and line the thoracic cavity (parietal pleura). Normally, the pleural space contains 3 to 5 mL of a low-protein fluid that lubricates the pulmonary tissue to allow for respiratory motion. The fluid is essentially an ultrafiltrate of blood, and is continually being added to and removed from the pleural cavity. The same Starling forces that determine fluid movement across capillary walls are responsible for fluid movement in and out of the pleural space. Abnormal accumulations of pleural fluid may occur due to increased capillary hydrostatic pressure or capillary permeability, decreased intravascular oncotic pressure, or impaired lymphatic drainage. The mediastinum of the dog and cat is fenestrated or incomplete; therefore pleural effusions are usually bilateral. Pleural effusion is typically a secondary phenomenon; therefore recognition of pleural effusion is not analogous to diagnosis of a dog or cat's underlying condition. A thorough investigation should reveal the primary disease (Figure 68-1).

CLINICAL SIGNS

Clinical signs associated with pleural effusion are most often related to the respiratory system. Severity of signs is deter-

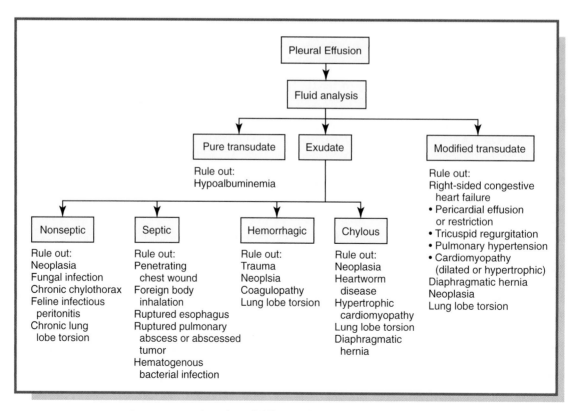

Figure 68-1 Algorithm of differential diagnosis of pleural effusion.

mined by the amount of the effusion and how quickly the effusion developed. The respiratory pattern caused by pleural effusion results from the interference of normal lung expansion. This observed pattern of ventilation is often called a restrictive pattern of respiration. The respiratory pattern is characterized by a pronounced inspiratory phase and a rapid expiratory phase, often with a prominent abdominal component. The increased inspiratory effort associated with pleural effusion can be difficult to differentiate from the inspiratory effort of airway disease by observation alone. As a general rule, dogs and cats with pleural effusion have significant tachypnea compared to animals with uncomplicated airway disease and often manifest decreased lung sounds ventrally on thoracic auscultation. The presence of a fluid line may be determined by auscultation of a definitive point on the chest wall, where respiratory sounds shift from muffled to normal or slightly increased. By contrast, dogs and cats with airway disease often have abnormal inspiratory airway sounds such as crackles and wheezes. Most animals with significant pleural effusion are tachypneic as a compensatory measure because total lung expansion capacity is reduced. Coughing is occasionally noted with pleural effusion. Depending upon the underlying cause, systemic signs of disease may also be present.

DIAGNOSTIC EVALUATION

A thorough physical examination often provides clues to the underlying cause of pleural effusion. For example, the presence of uveitis may alert the clinician to possible systemic inflammatory conditions such as viral disease (e.g., feline infectious peritonitis), rickettsial disease, fungal infection, or sepsis or systemic neoplasia (e.g., lymphosarcoma). Lymphadenopathy may suggest systemic inflammatory process or lymphosarcoma. Jugular distension and pulsation suggests increased right heart filling pressures that may be associated with cardiomyopathy, pericardial effusion, tricuspid regurgitation, pulmonic stenosis, or any of the many causes of pulmonary hypertension (e.g., heartworm disease, thromboembolic disease, parenchymal lung disease). Jugular distension without pulsation is more likely to be associated with occlusion of right heart inflow, due to mediastinal masses or severely increased intrapericardial pressures. Many cats with large mediastinal masses will have decreased compressibility of the cranial (anterior) thorax. A thorough palpation of the skeleton and the abdomen may uncover masses or painful regions associated with inflammatory disease. Abdominal effusion may be present with cardiac disease, hepatic disease, neoplasia, or hypoalbuminemia.

Dogs and cats with severe respiratory distress from pleural effusion may be quite fragile. Unnecessary handling should be avoided until the animal is sufficiently stable. In these cases, oxygen therapy may be provided and thoracocentesis should be performed before additional diagnostics are planned. Although thoracocentesis is invasive, the potential therapeutic benefit far outweighs the small chance of complications. Patients that present in stable condition may have chest radiographs taken to confirm presence of pleural effusion before thoracocentesis.

Thoracic radiography can confirm pleural effusion and often identifies the underlying cause (e.g., cardiac disease, mediastinal mass). In many cases, critical evaluation of the chest cannot be performed because the fluid silhouettes the normal thoracic structures, which obscures their borders. Repeating chest radiographs after thoracocentesis may aid in identification of thoracic pathology.

Fifty to 100 mL of fluid must be present for pleural effusion to be recognized radiographically. A minute amount of effusion may be detected as pleural fissure lines on the radiograph. These radio-opaque lines arc from the periphery toward the hilar region and outline individual lung margins. As effusions progress, lung lobes retract from the chest wall and lung borders become rounded. With large volumes of effusion, the lungs appear to float on the fluid line and the trachea is displaced dorsally on the lateral radiograph, which mimics cardiomegaly or cranial mediastinal mass. The fluid often obscures cardiac margins, interfering with cardiac size interpretation. The cardiac silhouette is not visualized at all on the dorsoventral radiograph in significant pleural effusion. A ventrodorsal radiograph may provide a better view of the cardiac silhouette in these cases (Figure 68-2).

Lung lobes may appear abnormally dense due to incomplete expansion, collapse, or lung lobe torsion. Pockets of fluid accumulation or unilateral effusions should alert the clinician to the possibility of inflammatory lesions and pleural adhesions.

A thoracic ultrasound exam may be performed before thoracocentesis if the patient is stable. In contrast to thoracic radiography, the fluid provides a good acoustic window and enhances examination of thoracic structures. In addition, ultrasound is more sensitive in detecting small volumes of fluid that are uncertain radiographically. Ultrasound may be used to guide fluid or mass aspiration. Echogenic fluid detected by ultrasound is more likely to be cellular or exudative in nature.

Analysis of the pleural fluid obtained by thoracocentesis provides important clues in determination of the cause. The thoracocentesis technique is described in detail elsewhere in this text. Figure 68-3 demonstrates one technique used for thoracocentesis in a cat.

Samples should be placed into anticoagulant tubes (EDTA) for cell counts, clot tubes for possible biochemical analysis, and culture devices in the event septic processes are identified by cytologic evaluation. Measurement of protein concentration, a total cell count, and cytologic analysis may reveal a specific diagnosis or, by categorizing the effusion, assist in directing the next diagnostic steps. Pleural effusions can generally be categorized as transudates and modified transudates; septic and nonseptic exudates; or chylous, hemorrhagic, or neoplastic effusions.

TRANSUDATES AND MODIFIED TRANSUDATES

Pure transudates are fluids characterized by low protein concentration (less than 2.5 g/dL) and low nucleated cell counts (less than 1000/μL). Macrophages, lymphocytes, and mesothelial cells are the primary cell types. Modified transudates have slightly higher protein concentration of up to 3.5 g/dL and cell counts of up to 5000/μL. In addition to the above cell types, neutrophils are a common finding. Pure transudates are classically transparent, whereas modified transudates may have very slight turbidity.

The most common cause of a pure transudate is decreased oncotic pressure from hypoalbuminemia. The finding of a pure transudate should alert the clinician to assess serum albumin concentration and to screen for underlying causes of hypoalbuminemia (impaired hepatic production, or albumin loss via gastrointestinal or renal lesions). Occasionally, pleural effusions of hypoalbuminemia will be modified transudates in long-standing cases.

The most common cause of modified transudates is increased hydrostatic pressure of the vascular system or lym-

Figure 68-2 Thoracic radiographs of a dog with mild to moderate pleural effusion. The different projections reveal the typical radiographic findings. **A,** The lateral radiograph demonstrates increased opacity ventrally with scalloping of the lung margins as fluid opacity outlines the individual lobes. **B,** The dorsoventral projection reveals the classic "disappearing heart" especially in the cardiac apical regions as heart opacity silhouettes with the fluid collecting in the ventral thorax. Lung lobe retraction from the chest wall and pleural fissure lines are present. **C,** In the ventrodorsal projection, the cardiac silhouette is better visualized as fluid has now settled in the dorsal thorax, away from the heart. Lung lobe retraction and pleural fissure lines are also present.

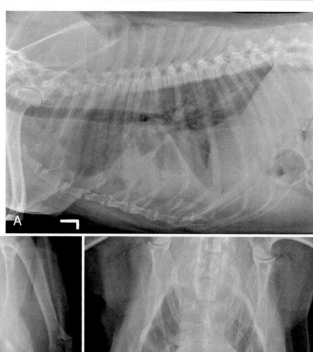

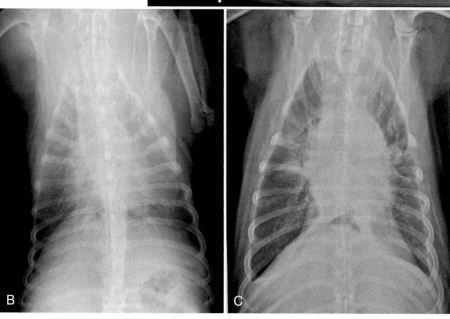

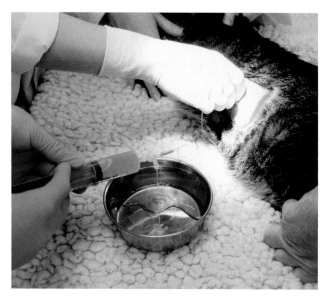

Figure 68-3 Thoracocentesis performed on an 8-year-old Domestic Shorthair cat presenting for tachypnea and anorexia. The fluid was classified as a modified transudate. Ultimately lymphosarcoma was diagnosed.

phatics. Pleural effusion due to increased intravascular hydrostatic pressure is typically referred to as *right-sided congestive heart failure*. Cardiomyopathy (dilated and hypertrophic), severe tricuspid regurgitation, pulmonary hypertension, and pericardial effusion or restriction are some common examples of diseases that may result in right heart failure. Pleural effusion from lymphatic obstruction can be caused by neoplasia, lymphangitis, or strangulation of intrathoracic tissue such as with diaphragmatic hernia or lung lobe torsion.

SEPTIC AND NONSEPTIC EXUDATES

Exudates are usually the result of inflammation and increased vascular permeability. Exudates have a higher protein content and cell count than transudates. Protein concentrations are classically greater than 3 g/dL and cell counts are greater than 5000/μL. These fluids appear turbid as a result of the higher cellular content. The cell types are similar for septic and nonseptic exudates (neutrophils, macrophages, eosinophils, lymphocytes), but septic processes usually have extremely high nucleated cell counts, that is, greater than 50,000/μL. In septic exudates, degenerate neutrophils predominate and bacteria can also be observed within the neutrophils or free fluid. However, the absence of bacteria does not rule out an infectious process and all exudative fluids should be submitted for Gram stain and aerobic/anaerobic culture. Prior antibiotic therapy can alter the cellular concentration of the pleural fluid and diminish bacterial numbers; therefore cytology (and culture) should ideally be performed prior to initiation of treatment. In some cases the septic exudates will have a foul odor. Septic pleural effusions are also called *pyothorax*. Penetrating chest wounds, penetrating esophageal or airway lesions, migrating foreign material such as grass awns, and extension of bacterial pneumonia are relatively common causes of pyothorax in the dog and cat.

Nonseptic exudates may be difficult to differentiate from septic processes. The cell count is usually lower for nonseptic effusions. Although macrophages and lymphocytes may appear activated, neutrophils are typically nondegenerate. As stated earlier, the absence of obvious bacteria in fluid does not guarantee a nonseptic process. Culture and sensitivity testing should be performed. Differential diagnoses for patients with nonseptic exudates include neoplasia, resolving sepsis, chronic diaphragmatic hernia and lung lobe torsion, fungal infection, feline infectious peritonitis, and long-standing chylothorax.

HEMORRHAGIC EFFUSIONS

Hemorrhagic effusions are grossly red with red blood cells and may appear similar to frank blood. A packed cell volume (PCV) should be determined on the fluid and compared with a peripheral blood sample. PCV of similar values suggest active bleeding into the chest cavity, whereas effusions with lower PCV than the peripheral blood suggest other factors are responsible for the bloody effusion. Hemorrhagic effusions due to active inflammatory causes often have increased numbers of neutrophils and macrophages compared with the peripheral blood sample, and erythrophagocytosis is commonly present. Hemorrhagic effusions may result from trauma, neoplasia, lung lobe torsion, and systemic coagulopathies such as rodenticide ingestion.

CHYLOUS EFFUSIONS

Chylous pleural effusion (chylothorax) results from leakage of material from the thoracic duct. These effusions may occur from increased lymphatic hydrostatic pressure or obstruction. Common causes include cardiac disease, pericardial disease, dirofilariasis and pulmonary hypertension, lung lobe torsion, diaphragmatic hernia, neoplasia, and trauma. Idiopathic cases of chylothorax are suspected to be secondary congenital or acquired defects of the thoracic duct.

Chylous effusion is usually milky white due to the presence of chylomicrons, but it may be clear if the animal has fasted. Occasionally, the effusions are blood tinged and resemble tomato soup. These fluids must be differentiated from exudative processes, as protein concentration and cell counts are similar. The predominant cell type in chylous effusion is the mature lymphocyte. With chronic effusions, increasing numbers of nondegenerate neutrophils and macrophages may be seen. A definitive diagnosis of chylothorax may also be made by comparing the triglyceride content of the effusion to that of serum. The triglyceride content of chyle is classically greater. Occasionally, this test may need to be repeated if an animal has been anorectic. Fibrosing pleuritis can be a complication of chronic chylothorax.

NEOPLASTIC EFFUSION

Thoracic neoplasia can cause any type of pleural effusion with the possible exception of pure transudates. Neoplastic cells may or may not exfoliate into the effusion for cytologic identification. Most commonly seen are lymphosarcoma, mast cell tumor, carcinoma, and mesothelioma. Differentiating carcinoma from mesothelioma and reactive mesothelial cells from neoplasia can be extremely difficult cytologically. Repeat thoracic radiography after thoracocentesis (particularly with mediastinal neoplasia), thoracic ultrasonography, or computed tomography may uncover masses, but definitive diagnosis requires fine needle aspiration or biopsy.

TREATMENT AND PROGNOSIS

Recognition of pleural effusion is not analogous to diagnosis of the patient's underlying condition. A thorough investigation should reveal the primary disease process. Initial treatment for patients with respiratory distress from pleural effusion is thoracocentesis. Thoracocentesis provides therapeutic as well as diagnostic benefit. The prognosis for pleural effusion is directly related to the underlying condition.

CHAPTER 69

Sneezing and Nasal Discharge

Narelle Lila Brown

Sneezing refers to the explosive release of air from the lungs through the nasal cavity and mouth. It is a protective reflex designed to rapidly remove both chemical and physical irritants from the nasal epithelial surface. Disorders characterized by sneezing are frequently accompanied by nasal discharge. These clinical signs generally result from diseases of the nose, sinuses, and nasopharynx, but may be secondary to diseases of the lower airways (Box 69-1).

They may also reflect a systemic disease or process (Box 69-2).

Box • 69-1

Nasal and Paranasal Causes of Sneezing and Nasal Discharge

Congenital
Cleft palate
Ciliary dyskinesis
Nasopharyngeal stenosis
Choanal atresia

Inflammatory
Lymphocytic-plasmacytic rhinitis
Allergic rhinitis
Nasopharyngeal stenosis
Nasopharyngeal polyp (C)
Polypoid rhinitis

Infectious
Viral
Feline calicivirus (C)
Feline herpesvirus 1 (C)
Bacterial
Mycoplasma spp. (C)
Bordetella bronchiseptica (C)
Fungal
Aspergillus (D, C)
Penicillium (D)
Rhinosporidium (D, C)
Cryptococcus (C)
Parasitic
Pneumonyssus caninum (D)
Eucoleus boehmi (D, C)
Cuterebra sp. (D, C)
Linguatula sp. (D, C)
Capillaria sp. (D, C)

Neoplastic
Adenocarcinoma
Squamous cell carcinoma
Chondrosarcoma
Osteosarcoma
Fibrosarcoma
Lymphosarcoma
Transmissible cell carcinoma
Neuroendocrine carcinoma

Foreign Body
Trauma
Oral Disease
Tooth root abscess
Oronasal fistula

Vascular Malformation

Box • 69-2

Systemic Causes of Sneezing and Nasal Discharge

Hemostatic Disorder
Thrombocytopenia
Thrombocytopathia
von Willebrand disease (vWD)
Coagulation factor deficiency
    Congenital (hemophilia A and B, others)
    Acquired (anticoagulant rodenticide toxicity, disseminated
        intravascular coagulation [DIC], liver failure)

Vasculitis
Toxic
Inflammatory
Immune-mediated
    Systemic lupus erythematosus (SLE)
Neoplastic
Infectious
    Ehrlichiosis
    Feline infectious peritonitis (FIP)
    Rocky Mountain spotted fever
    Leishmaniasis

Hyperviscosity
Multiple myeloma
IgM (Waldenstrom's) macroglobulinemia
Chronic lymphocytic leukemia (CLL)
Lymphosarcoma
Ehrlichia canis
FIP (rare)
Amyloidosis
Plasma cell leukemia

Hypertension
Primary or essential (rare)
Secondary
    Acute or chronic renal failure
    Pheochromocytoma
    Hyperadrenocorticism
    Hyperthyroidism
    Hypothyroidism
    Acromegaly
    Polycythemia
    Diabetes mellitus
    Overhydration

Infections
Infectious tracheobronchitis
Distemper
Bacterial bronchopneumonia

C, Cats; D, dogs.

Generally a diagnosis cannot be made from clinical signs alone and ancillary diagnostics are mandatory. These include advanced imaging, rhinoscopy, nasopharyngoscopy, cytology, mycology, and nasal biopsy/histology.

CLINICAL PRESENTATIONS

Stertor

This term refers to a coarse snoring/snorting respiratory sound and generally indicates an obstruction to airflow at the level of the nasopharynx. It is classically heard in brachycephalic breeds with elongated soft palates, excessive nasopharyngeal tissue, and airway stenoses. It also occurs with nasopharyngeal swellings or mass lesions that cause airway narrowing.

Reverse Sneezing

This is a loud inspiratory noise that generally occurs in paroxysms and is usually initiated by nasopharyngeal irritation. The purpose is to move secretions and foreign material to the oropharynx where they can be swallowed. Causes include excitement, foreign bodies, the nasal mite *(Pneumonyssus caninum)*, viral infections, and epiglottic entrapment of the soft palate. Reverse sneezing is usually idiopathic, nonprogressive, and commonly recognized in small dogs.

Nasal Discharge

Nasal discharge can be unilateral, bilateral, or initially unilateral and become bilateral. Unilateral disease is commonly associated with foreign bodies, oronasal fistulas, and neoplasia. Bilateral discharge is more typical of inflammatory and infectious diseases. Character of a nasal discharge may help the clinician formulate a list of appropriate differential diagnoses, although it must be recognized that there is extensive overlap between types of discharge and underlying diseases. The discharge is usually classified as: serous, mucoid, mucopurulent, purulent, sanguinous (ranging from blood tinged to frank hemorrhage), or food containing.

Serous discharge is watery and clear. It can be a normal finding but if excessive may indicate noninfectious inflammatory disease (either species) or an upper respiratory tract viral infection (cats). It may transition into a different type of discharge.

Mucopurulent discharge is thicker and usually a white or yellow color. It may accumulate within the nasal passages and obstruct airflow and/or drainage from the frontal sinuses. It is nonspecific and can be present with any nasal disease that causes inflammation and secondary bacterial infection.

A bloody nasal discharge (epistaxis) may be associated with any disease that causes significant nasal turbinate destruction or erosion of nasal vascular structures, such as mycotic infections or neoplasia. It may also be a manifestation of a systemic disease such as hypertension or a hemostatic disorder (i.e., thrombocytopenia, thrombocytopathia, vasculitides, or a coagulopathy). Craniofacial trauma may also result in epistaxis.

The presence of food material within the nasal cavity in a young animal suggests a congenital abnormality such as a cleft palate or a dysphagic condition. In older animals this may be seen with an oronasal fistula.

DIAGNOSTIC APPROACH

Clinical signs associated with nasal disease are variable and depend not only upon the nature of the underlying disease but also on the extent and duration of the disorder. Although some signs are highly suggestive of particular etiologies, none are pathognomonic. Consider also the inaccessibility of the nasal cavity, and it is easy to understand how determining the cause of nasal disease can be challenging. To select an appropriate diagnostic plan, the clinician must consider the patient's signalment, clinical signs, and physical examination findings. Even with a systematic approach, however, many cases of chronic nasal disease remain undiagnosed. One study of dogs with nasal disease reported no specific diagnosis in 36.3% and nonspecific inflammatory rhinitis in another 23.7%.[1] It is likely that at least some of these dogs had underlying undiagnosed early neoplasia or foreign bodies. In cats with chronic nasal disease, nonspecific inflammatory rhinosinusitis is commonly diagnosed. One study reported this diagnosis in 64% of affected cats and a definitive diagnosis was found to be more likely in older cats.[2] This large proportion of undiagnosed cases most likely results from the adverse effects of upper respiratory tract viruses on normal nasal anatomy—altering local defense mechanisms, predisposing to secondary bacterial infections, and promoting abnormal immune responses.

Signalment

Infectious causes of nasal disease are more likely to occur in young animals, in situations where animals are housed together (shows/kennels), or with the introduction of new animals to a household. Young animals are also more likely to have congenital abnormalities such as a cleft palate or ciliary dyskinesia. Conversely, neoplasia and dental disease occur more frequently in older animals.

Brachycephalic breeds commonly have conformational causes of upper airway disease and less commonly nasal neoplasia.[3] This may be related to more pulmonary exposure to pollutants because of less effective nasal air filtration. Brachycephalic cats have been found to be at an increased risk of fungal rhinitis *(Aspergillus/Penicillium)*.[4] Dolichocephalic breeds in general are overrepresented with respect to nasal disease, which may be related to their greater mucous membrane surface area and increased exposure to inhaled irritants and allergens. They have a higher incidence of fungal rhinitis and are about 2.5 times more likely to develop nasal tumors.[3] Outdoor/hunting breeds have a greater opportunity to inhale foreign material and sustain head trauma compared to indoor dogs.

History

Important considerations include: travel history (allergic rhinitis?), attendance at shows/kennels (infectious diseases), nature of the pet's daily activities (hunting and outdoor pursuits), history of trauma, previous or concurrent medical conditions, and vaccination history (intranasal vaccine reaction or inadvertent mucous membrane exposure to a modified live parenteral vaccine in cats). Exposure to certain environmental factors may be associated with particular diseases, such as eucalyptus trees or pigeon manure with *Cryptococcus* spp. infections. Consider recent dental treatment (oronasal fistula) or anesthesia (possibility of nasopharyngeal gastric reflux).

The onset of clinical signs (peracute, acute, chronic) can also help diagnostically. For instance, an acute onset of sneezing in cats is generally associated with a viral upper respiratory tract infection or a nasal foreign body. Admittedly, the latter is more common in dogs and the pathogenesis appears to be different in cats. Instead of inhaling them (a more difficult endeavor as the opening to the external nares is much smaller), feline nasal foreign bodies tend to result from vomiting or regurgitation into the nasopharynx—explaining why they are frequently grass blades or fur balls. In dogs an acute onset of sneezing with or without pawing at the face, suggests a foreign body or the inhalation of irritant aerosols. The most common nasal foreign body in dogs is some type of plant material—particularly grass awns.

Physical Examination

A thorough physical examination can help to confirm a clinical suspicion of nasal disease, although it is important to remember that significant pathology can exist in the absence of any abnormalities. Areas of particular interest, apart from the nose, include the oral cavity, eyes, lymph nodes, and thorax.

The nose should be examined for the presence of discharge (noting the type of discharge and whether it is unilateral or bilateral), ulceration/crusting around the nares, depigmentation of the external nares (nasal aspergillosis), asymmetry of the nose and/or face (nasal neoplasia, *Cryptococcus*), evidence of pain over the dorsum of the nose (nasal aspergillosis/nasal neoplasia) or presence of abnormal tissue or material occluding or protruding from the external nares (*Cryptococcus*/rhinosporidiosis/neoplasia/foreign body).

The patency of the nasal passages should be assessed. This can be done by occluding one nostril while keeping the mouth closed. In dogs with normal nasal passages, this maneuver should not compromise respiration. Alternatively, a glass slide may be placed in front of the nares and the resultant condensation on the slide examined as evidence of airflow. A wisp of cotton wool can be held in front of each nare and observed for movement associated with inspiration and expiration.

An oral examination may reveal mucosal ulceration (feline calicivirus), fractured teeth, oronasal fistulae, ventral displacement of the soft palate (nasopharyngeal tumors/polyps/foreign bodies), periodontal disease, or a cleft palate. The soft palate should be palpated as nasopharyngeal mass lesions or erosions may be appreciated. Halitosis is often associated with nasopharyngeal foreign bodies, dental disease, or oronasal fistulas. General anesthesia is required for proper assessment of this region.

A retrobulbar mass may be suspected if there is exophthalmos, prolapse of the nictitans, deformity of the facial bones or hard palate, or an inability to retropulse the eyes. Epiphora may be noted with nasal disease that occludes the nasolacrimal duct (neoplasia, cryptococcosis). Chorioretinitis may occur with cryptococcosis, ehrlichiosis, and lymphosarcoma.

The submandibular lymph nodes should be palpated as a lymphadenopathy may result from metastatic neoplasia or from reactivity to local disease (including nasal or oral disorders).

An assessment of mentation should be made as central nervous system involvement can occur with extension of nasal disease beyond the cribriform plate (neoplasia/aspergillosis).

Nasal signs can also occur secondary to primary thoracic disease as secretions may be coughed into the nasopharynx, causing secondary involvement of that region. Systemic diseases such as thrombocytopenia, hypertension and vasculitis, can also cause nasal signs. If the primary lesion is crusting of the nares with an absence of sneezing/nasal discharge, keratoconjunctivitis sicca (KCS), or primary dermatoses such as discoid lupus erythematosus (DLE) should be considered.

If epistaxis is the main clinical sign, the dog or cat should be examined for evidence of a hemostatic disorder such as petechiae, ecchymoses, or melena. Systemic hypertension can also cause epistaxis and may be recognized by fundic examination findings of tortuous retinal vessels, retinal hemorrhages, or detachment. Epistaxis is the most common clinical sign associated with thrombocytopenia.

DIAGNOSTIC PLAN

After consideration of signalment, history, and physical examination findings, the clinician should be in a position to tailor an appropriate diagnostic plan (Figure 69-1).

It should be remembered, however, that even with obvious unilateral signs such as nasal discharge or obstruction of airflow, both sides of the nose should always be examined. Nasal disease can also cause signs of nasopharyngeal disease or coughing without the more usual signs of discharge and sneezing. This is more common with caudal nasal cavity abnormalities.

With the notable exception of cryptococcal serology, clinical pathology (complete blood count [CBC], chemistry panel, urinalysis) is not usually helpful in determining the etiology of nasal disease. There are no specific changes noted on the CBC for most nasal diseases although an anemia may be present with severe or chronic epistaxis. An inflammatory leukogram may be seen with a concurrent systemic disease such as bronchopneumonia. Similarly the biochemistry panel is often unremarkable. It should be remembered, however, that the investigation of nasal disease requires general anesthesia and these tests give an overall evaluation of health status and may be useful if a systemic disease with predominantly nasal signs is present.

Aspergillus serology has traditionally been considered unhelpful although a recent paper showed the agar gel immunodiffusion (AGID) test designed to detect antibodies to *Aspergillus* spp. was highly specific (98%) but not sensitive (i.e., a negative result did not rule out the disease).[5] Serology has also been supportive with other types of fungal rhinitis.

In cases of epistaxis, a buccal mucosal bleeding time (BMBT), platelet count, coagulation times (PT, APTT) or PIVKA levels may be indicated. Blood pressure should also be assessed.

Oropharyngeal or conjunctival swabs for virus isolation (feline calicivirus, feline herpesvirus-1) by immunodiffusion, ELISA, or PCR may be helpful in cases of acute upper respiratory signs in cats. PCR is the most sensitive of these tests, though specificity is lowered by the high prevalence of feline upper respiratory tract viruses.

Cytologic examination of nasal secretions usually reveals nonspecific inflammation. Samples may be obtained by means of flushing, swabbing, brushing, fine needle aspiration, or by impression smears prepared from tissue fragments. It is generally only helpful with fungal rhinitis or, occasionally, neoplasia. The submandibular lymph nodes and any palpable facial or nasal swellings may be aspirated or biopsied (needle core [Tru-Cut]/punch). Ultrasound guidance may be helpful.

The use of nasal swabs for bacterial culture (from nasal discharge or deep within the nasal cavity) is somewhat controversial but generally considered to be of little value. Primary bacterial rhinitis is rare in dogs, and bacterial invasion generally occurs secondary to some other disease process that impairs normal host defense mechanisms (e.g., viral, fungal, parasitic, neoplasia, dental disease, bacterial bronchopneumonia). The combination of inflammation and mucosal injury promotes the proliferation and invasion of normal commensal microflora. Without resolution of the initial insult, a chronic inflammatory state may ensue. Bacterial cultures are therefore difficult to interpret as they normally yield a mixed growth of bacteria similar to that of the normal nasal flora. Despite this, some authors still advocate cultures of tissue biopsies although the significance of such isolates remains unknown. The main exceptions to this are infections in cats with *Bordetella bronchiseptica* and *Mycoplasma* spp. Both of these are considered to be potential primary respiratory pathogens in cats.[6,7]

For most pets with chronic nasal disease, it is recommended to adopt a systematic approach to the investigation. This includes (in this order), a basic oral examination under general anesthesia, radiographs of skull or CT (computed tomography) of the nasal cavities and frontal sinuses, nasopharyngoscopy and rhinoscopy with biopsies of both nasal passages. Dental probing should be the last procedure performed as it may result in hemorrhage within the nose, a situation that would adversely affect any

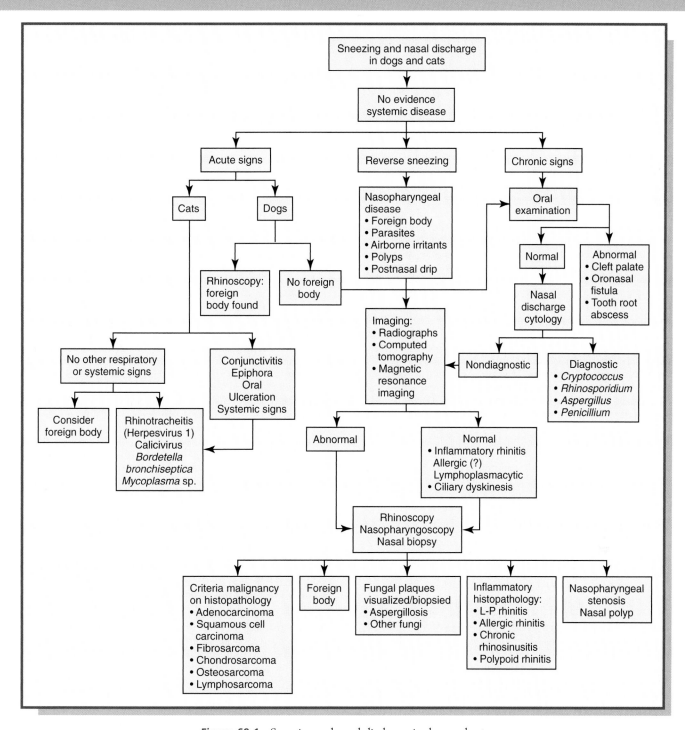

Figure 69-1 Sneezing and nasal discharge in dogs and cats.

imaging studies and impede visualization during endoscopic procedures.

Skull Radiographs

Radiography of the nose has the advantage of being relatively inexpensive and is a diagnostic modality to which most practitioners have access. It does, however, require general anesthesia and proper patient positioning to provide useful information. The main disadvantage of this form of imaging is the inability to detect subtle changes within the nasal cavities as a result of the inevitable superimposition of structures in that region. Any fluid accumulation within the nasal cavity will also potentially obscure abnormalities because of radiographic silhouetting. For this reason, imaging is always performed prior to any other procedures that could result in hemorrhage within the nasal cavity (rhinoscopy or dental probing).

Changes that may be detected include turbinate destruction, deformation of the vomer bone, frontal sinus opacification (fluid/tissue), radiolucency at the tips of the tooth roots (abscessation), nasopharyngeal opacification (foreign body/fluid/tissue), changes associated with the tympanic bullae (otitis media/polyps/neoplasia), large or radio-opaque foreign bodies (rarely), evaluation of soft palate position and length, and osteolytic/osteoproductive changes within the bones of the skull (neoplasia). Bone sequestra and foreign bodies may be evident as a focal radiodensity surrounded by a rim of lysis. Standard views include a right or left lateral, intraoral, dorsoventral, ventrodorsal open mouth, and rostrocaudal (for frontal sinus evaluation). Lateral oblique views are required to evaluate the dental arcades.

Computed Tomography (CT)

The main advantage of this advanced form of imaging is the ability to obtain detailed images of the nasal cavity and associated structures, without the problem of superimposition. It provides information regarding the extent of the disease and reasonably accurate differentiation of neoplastic versus nonneoplastic disease and identifies areas that should be targeted for rhinoscopic evaluation and biopsy. It is the best imaging technique for the detection of cortical bone lesions, and although it will detect soft tissue lesions, it cannot determine the nature of the abnormal soft tissue. A particular pattern of change identified on CT is often so characteristic of a particular disease that a presumptive diagnosis can generally be made, helping to direct the ongoing investigation. One study compared CT findings in dogs with nasal disease with rhinoscopy and histopathology and found that neoplasia was typically associated with a soft tissue density and extensive turbinate destruction. Inflammatory rhinitis was associated with either normal turbinate structures or mild to moderate turbinate destruction, with or without the presence of soft tissue densities within the nasal cavities. Fungal rhinitis was associated with extensive turbinate destruction and hyperlucency of the nasal passages.[8] Integrity of the cribriform plate can also be assessed with CT, important when planning therapeutic strategies for fungal rhinitis or neoplasia.

Although CT scans are becoming more readily available, access can still be an issue for some practitioners. Like radiography, it requires general anesthesia and is relatively expensive—shortcomings that are more than offset by the superior images obtained.

Magnetic Resonance Imaging (MRI)

This form of advanced imaging is currently not part of the routine investigation of chronic nasal disease. It is expensive, requires prolonged general anesthesia, and is less readily available than CT. It has the advantage of being able to differentiate between thickened nasal mucosa and secretions or fungal colonies. One study suggested that the value of CT and MRI for the diagnosis of nasal aspergillosis was similar.[9] Although the benefits of MRI do not appear to outweigh the disadvantages currently, this may change in the future given the high proportion of chronic nasal disease cases that remain undiagnosed.

Rhinoscopy/Nasopharyngoscopy

These procedures allows for direct visualization of the nasal cavities, nasopharynx, and, in some cases, the frontal sinuses. The equipment required is moderately expensive and some expertise with these techniques is required. A small endoscope, patience, careful guidance, and suctioning are needed to allow adequate visualization of the nasal cavities. It can be diagnostic (e.g., visualization of fungal plaques, foreign bodies, nasal polyps, mass lesions) as well as therapeutic (removal of foreign bodies, fungal plaques, flushing/suctioning excessive secretions). Either flexible or rigid endoscopes can be used. The rigid scopes have better optics and are easier to maneuver while flexible scopes are better for more inaccessible parts of the nose, especially the frontal sinuses. Flexible scopes are associated with less mechanical trauma to the tissue.

Retroflexion of flexible scopes behind the soft palate enables examination of the nasopharynx—traditionally a difficult area to access. Mass lesions may be biopsied (neoplasia), polyps visualized, foreign bodies removed, nasal mites and nasopharyngeal stenosis identified, and secretions suctioned from the area. A study of animals with signs of respiratory disease that underwent examination of the choanae showed 26 of 34 animals with nasal neoplasia were correctly identified by biopsies obtained in this area. As the biopsies are relatively small, however, an erroneous diagnosis may result if a representative sample is not obtained—as was the case with five dogs in this study.[10] Trephination and sinuscopy may be required if disease is limited to the frontal sinus. One study identified this scenario in 8 of 46 dogs with nasal aspergillosis.[11]

Nasal Biopsy

A nasal biopsy should be obtained in all dogs and cats with chronic nasal disease. Even if the etiology appears obvious (nasal foreign body) or unilateral, several biopsies from each nasal cavity should be obtained. This is especially true in cats where there is a reasonably weak correlation between gross rhinoscopic mucosal findings and histologic evidence of inflammation. Many conditions that begin unilateral later become bilateral, and different diseases may occur concurrently (e.g., fungal rhinitis secondary to a chronic FB).

Nasal tissue specimens may be obtained via traumatic nasal flush, rhinoscope-guided biopsy (preferred technique), blind biopsy, or biopsy via rhinotomy. Mass lesions, fungal plaques, and specific mucosal lesions should be biopsied with visualization, if possible, to ensure obtaining a representative sample. Approximately 75% of nasal tumors were visible on rhinoscopy in one study.[1] Impression smears can be made from these samples prior to fixation as cytology may provide a quick initial impression pending histology results. Blind biopsies may also be collected. In this instance, however, the clinician should measure the distance from the tip of the nose to the medial canthus of the eye and ensure the biopsy instrument does not pass beyond this distance in order to avoid inadvertent penetration of the cribriform plate. Complications that should be anticipated include hemorrhage (which can be life threatening) and aspiration of blood.

TREATMENT/OUTCOME

In many cases of chronic nasal discharge and sneezing, despite a systematic and extensive investigation, an etiologic diagnosis remains elusive. More often a descriptive diagnosis, such as nonspecific rhinitis, or no diagnosis is made, and management is based on symptomatic therapies designed to alleviate clinical signs. Such outcomes have been reported in up to 60% of dogs and even more frequently in cats. Specific treatment options are available for neoplasia, fungal rhinitis, foreign bodies, most congenital abnormalities, parasites, and dental disease. Nonspecific rhinitis remains problematic. It is unclear what the significance of the different inflammatory infiltrates is and whether they are different manifestations of the same disease. It is likely that inflammatory infiltrates within the nasal mucosa is a nonspecific response to many different insults and as such is likely to reflect a spectrum of different diseases rather than just one—similar to inflammation of the gastrointestinal tract. Client education is therefore paramount prior to undertaking such an investigation to avoid unrealistic expectations and potential frustration.

REFERENCES

The reference list can be found on the companion Expert Consult Web site at *www.expertconsult.com*.

CHAPTER 70

Syncope

Kristine Yee

SYNCOPE

Syncope, from the Greek *syn* ("with") and *koptein* ("to interrupt"), is a transient loss of consciousness and muscle tone caused by inadequate cerebral oxygenation or perfusion to the reticular activating system of the brainstem. Onset and recovery are generally rapid and spontaneous, without the long duration and preictal and postictal period of seizures.[1-6] While unconscious, the syncopal animal may urinate, have a short duration of myoclonus, or even have tonic spasms that may be confused with seizure activity. The animal may not lose full consciousness and may experience presyncope. However, the diagnostic approach to presyncope is the same as that for syncope.[7] Syncope is a clinical sign; it is not itself a disease entity. In humans, syncope is classified into five different pathophysiologic causes: (1) cardiac arrhythmias, (2) structural cardiac and pulmonary causes, (3) reflex-mediated syncope, (4) orthostatic hypotensive syncope, and (5) cerebrovascular disorders. Of these, the first four are described in the veterinary literature; cardiac arrhythmias are the most common cause of syncope in dogs and cats. A sixth reported class is severe and abrupt hypoxemia, described in dogs with laryngeal paralysis or other severe upper respiratory obstruction.[8] Syncope must be differentiated from other conditions such as seizures, narcolepsy, cataplexy, vestibular disease, hypoglycemia, prolonged muscle weakness, and drug intoxication. Differentiation between syncope and these other conditions can be difficult to impossible. Sometimes the cause for syncope remains elusive. In humans, up to 30% of syncopal cases remain undiagnosed.[9]

CAUSES OF SYNCOPE

It should be noted that one disease might cause syncope through one or more of the pathophysiologic causes above (e.g., aortic stenosis and hypertrophic obstructive cardiomyopathy can cause syncope due to arrhythmias, structural outflow obstruction, or neurally mediated reflexes) (Figure 70-1).

Cardiac Arrhythmias

Bradyarrhythmias or tachyarrhythmias cause syncope by markedly decreasing cardiac output for greater than 6 to 8 seconds. Bradyarrhythmias achieve this by pausing electrical activity, while tachyarrhythmias produce syncope by increasing heart rate to approximately 300+ beats/min, causing inadequate ventricular filling in diastole.[10] These arrhythmias include high-grade (advanced Mobitz type II) second-degree AV block, third-degree AV block, sick sinus syndrome (bradycardia-tachycardia syndrome), severe sinus bradycardia, ventricular preexcitation,[11] supraventricular tachyarrhythmias, atrial fibrillation, and ventricular tachyarrhythmias.

Sudden death is common in high-grade (advanced Mobitz type II) second-degree AV block and third-degree AV block; it is uncommon in sick sinus syndrome. Ventricular tachyarrhythmias are more likely to result in sudden death compared with supraventricular tachyarrhythmias. Therefore, diagnosis of the arrhythmia and underlying disorder with appropriate treatment is vital. Diseases associated with arrhythmias are sinus nodal disease, atrioventricular nodal disease, dilated cardiomyopathy, arrhythmogenic right ventricular cardiomyopathy, hypertrophic cardiomyopathy, restrictive cardiomyopathy, chronic degenerative valvular disease, cardiac neoplasia, abdominal neoplasia, systemic or metabolic disorders (e.g., electrolyte disturbances), sepsis, coagulopathies causing myocardial changes, myocarditis, or drug-induced (e.g., digitalis intoxication).[12] Infectious diseases reported in the veterinary literature causing myocarditis or other conduction disturbances include *Blastomyces dermatitidis*,[13] *Trichinella spiralis*,[14] *Citrobacter koseri*,[15] *Bartonella* spp., and *Borrelia burgdorferi*.[16] Stokes-Adams syndrome, originally described in children with heart block, is described in humans where the syncopal episode is accompanied by brief tonic/clonic activity that occurs after 10 to 20 seconds of asystole. These episodes can be mistaken for seizures, but are cardiac in origin.[7] These are seen commonly in syncopal dogs and cats.

Structural Cardiac and Pulmonary Causes

Structural cardiac or cardiopulmonary diseases cause syncope when the circulatory demands of the body outweigh the heart's ability to increase cardiac output. Diseases associated with this class include aortic stenosis, pulmonic stenosis,[17] tetralogy of Fallot, atrial septal defect,[18] hypertrophic obstructive cardiomyopathy, cardiac neoplasia causing obstruction to blood flow,[19-21] pericardial effusion/tamponade causing decreased venous return, pulmonary embolism, and pulmonary hypertension with or without *Dirofilaria immitis* or *Angiostrongylus vasorum* infestation.[22] Heart failure by itself is not a cause of syncope; by definition, syncope is transient and self-limiting. The weakness and collapse seen with heart failure is not transient nor self-limiting since it can only be alleviated with medical intervention.[8]

Reflex-Mediated Syncope (Neurally Mediated, Vasovagal, Vasodepressor, Neurocardiogenic Syncope)

Reflex syncope is a response that, when triggered, results in reflex vasodilation with or without bradycardia; this leads to hypotension and subsequent transient loss of consciousness. It is characterized by sudden autonomic nervous system failure: withdrawal of sympathetic tone with abrupt increase in vagal tone.[23] The exact mechanisms underlying neurally mediated syncope remain controversial.[24] The triggering events are variable and determined by which afferent nerve or receptor is stimulated.[25] Types of reflex syncope include carotid sinus syncope—triggered when the carotid sinus is manipulated or during carotid sinus massage in patients with an exaggerated baroreceptor-mediated reflex; situational syncope—triggered when vagal neurons are stimulated by coughing, vomiting, sneezing, micturition, defecating, swallowing, or visceral pain, and; glossopharyngeal neuralgia—where pain associated with the ninth cranial nerve causes activation of a vagal reflex in the neighboring tenth cranial nerve that mimics carotid sinus baroreceptor activation.[3,26] Of these reflex triggers, only cough syncope is well recognized though ill defined. It is seen in geriatric small-breed dogs with chronic degenerative valvular disease or chronic pulmonary disease. There are a few other proposed mechanisms to cough syncope in addition to reflex-mediated causes. One mechanism involves increased intrathoracic and intraabdominal pressures from coughing that cause increased venous pressure with resultant increase in intracranial pressure. A reflex transient decrease in cerebral perfusion results causing syncope.[27] Animals with aortic stenosis or hypertrophic obstructive cardiomyopathy can also be syncopal for neurally mediated reasons. The Bezold-Jarisch reflex[28] is the primary mechanism for neurally mediated syncope in these patients. This reflex originates in cardiac sensory receptors with nonmyelinated vagal afferent C fibers in the left ventricle. When the receptors are stimulated by increased left ventricular pressure due to outflow obstruction, the increased pressure is perceived as hypertension; reflex vasodilation, bradycardia, and syncope result. Interestingly, this reflex is also triggered in animals suffering rapid, severe hemorrhage. With vigorous contraction of the left ventricle around an almost empty ventricular chamber, an abrupt paradoxical increase in firing of these receptors results in reflex bradycardia and vasodilation.[29]

Orthostatic Hypotensive Syncope

This type of syncope, rarely reported in animals, is also caused by a failure of the autonomic nervous system to maintain blood pressure in an upright, bipedal posture. This type of syncope encompasses syncope in these patients that is exacerbated by major volume depletion, decreased circulating blood volume, and drug-induced causes. It has been described anecdotally in one dog, and in dogs with canine dysautonomia.[8,30]

Cerebrovascular Disorders

This type of syncope, known as *vascular steal syndrome*, is not documented in animals and is rare in humans. It involves diversion of blood supply from the brain to another organ. The most common example is the subclavian steal syndrome in patients where the subclavian artery delivers a disproportionate amount of perfusion to the arm at the expense of the brain during exercise of that limb.[17]

Severe, Acute Hypoxemia

This is rare, and has been described in dogs with severe laryngeal paralysis[31] or upper airway obstruction. Transient, abrupt hypoxemia results in syncope.[8]

DIAGNOSTIC WORKUP

A thorough history and physical examination are essential in making a diagnosis of syncope. Questions should focus on the activities leading up to the event, activities during the event, length of the episode, and activities following the event. Onset of the episode may occur with exercise or excitement. The description of the episode itself may include complete or transient flaccidity, tonic spasms, vocalization, opisthotonus, myoclonus, urination, or defecation. The episode is by definition short and transient. After the episode, the animal should generally return to normal consciousness and function within a few seconds. In contrast, seizure episodes can have a preictal period of anxiety or increased hiding behaviors. Second, seizures can last for longer durations of time and may be associated with hypersalivation, foaming at the mouth, generalized

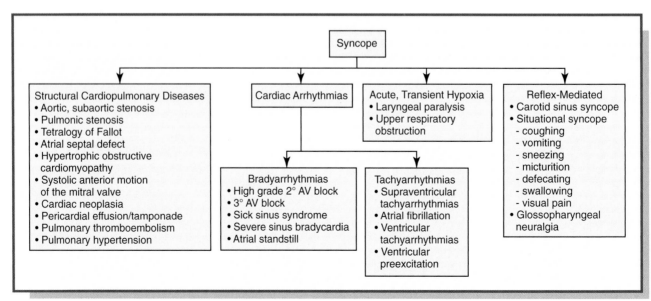

Figure 70-1   Differential diagnosis for syncope in dogs and cats (neurologic and metabolic causes for diseases that mimic syncope have been ruled out). *AV,* Atrioventricular.

tonic-clonic movements, or chattering of the teeth. Lastly, seizures can be followed by a postictal period of up to hours where the animal may be confused, anxious, or display localizing neurologic signs.

Physical examination with emphasis on the cardiovascular and neurologic systems may be completely normal, or may reveal cardiovascular abnormalities such as arrhythmia, heart murmur, or pulse abnormalities. Localizing neurologic deficits may be detected, increasing the suspicion for seizure activity.

CBC and serum chemistries may reveal evidence of conditions that mimic syncope or episodic muscular weakness (e.g., anemia, hypoglycemia), or give additional information as to underlying etiologies for detected arrhythmias (e.g., electrolyte abnormalities).

A resting 6-lead electrocardiogram (ECG) should be evaluated for at least one minute, preferably longer. If a bradyarrhythmia is present, an atropine response test is indicated (0.04 mg/kg IV, IM, or SQ). Expected response in the dog is elevation of ventricular rate to 140 to 220 beats/min.[8]

If the resting ECG is normal, or if the arrhythmia cannot be definitively related to the syncopal event, then a continuous recording of the ECG is indicated. This way, the ECG can temporally implicate a cardiac rhythm to a syncopal event. Ascertaining this confirmation can be like finding a needle in a haystack. However, the ECG can still prove useful even if the patient does not have a documented event during the monitoring period; arrhythmias may provide clues as to the origin of the syncopal events. A Holter monitor is a 24-hour ambulatory ECG monitor that can be connected to a dog, recording the dog's ECG for 24 consecutive hours. This monitor can later be reviewed and analyzed, in coordination with a log of the patient's activities during those 24 hours. Alternatively, a cardiac event recorder or intermittent loop recorder is an ambulatory ECG monitor that can be connected to a dog or cat for one to several weeks. During that time, the recorder continually records and erases the patient's ECG. If the patient has an event, the owner presses a button that activates the recorder to save the current loop of ECG. Therefore, the patient's ECG from immediately before and immediately after the event is saved. This information can later be reviewed and analyzed. Lastly, in-hospital telemetry can be performed to provide 24 hours or more of continuous ECG monitoring. The decision as to which ECG monitor is used depends on frequency of events, clinical judgment, veterinarian preference, and availability. Insertable loop recorders are implantable event recorders that must be surgically placed[32] and are not commonly used in veterinary practice.

Radiography and echocardiography with Doppler can identify structural and functional cardiopulmonary abnormalities.

Other tests used in humans such as head up tilt testing, exercise/stress testing, electrophysiologic testing, and recording a signal-averaged ECG are generally impractical and of limited use in veterinary medicine. These tests are used to identify or exacerbate arrhythmias.

TREATMENT

Treatment of syncope is dependent on the underlying cause of syncope:

Sick sinus syndrome and third-degree AV block: Pacemaker implantation.

Other bradyarrhythmias, including those that are responsive to an atropine response test as well as reflex-mediated bradyarrhythmias: Vagolytic agents (e.g., atropine 0.04 mg/kg PO q8-12h diluted 1:10 in corn syrup), beta agonists (e.g., terbutaline), or pacemaker implantation. Dogs that do not respond to medical treatment should be treated with pacemaker implantation. However, reflex-mediated syncope can still occur after pacemaker implantation if the syncope is due to vasodilation and not bradycardia, which is often the case.[33]

Atrial tachyarrhythmias: Appropriate antiarrhythmic therapy (e.g., digoxin, beta blockers, calcium channel blockers).

Ventricular tachyarrhythmias: Appropriate antiarrhythmic therapy (e.g., mexiletine, amiodarone, sotalol).

Cough syncope: Treat the underlying disease that is causing the cough; if ineffective, then use cough suppressants (e.g., hydrocodone, butorphanol).

Outflow obstruction due to aortic stenosis (Holter monitor should be evaluated to confirm that syncope is not due to arrhythmia): Beta blockers to prevent the initial increase in sympathetic tone, thus decreasing the reflex increase in contractility, theoretically preventing or alleviating the reflex trigger (e.g., atenolol).

PROGNOSIS

Prognosis is dependent on the underlying cause of syncope. Generally, cardiac causes are associated with greater mortality rate. Cough syncope and sick sinus syndrome rarely cause sudden death.

REFERENCES

The reference list can be found on the companion Expert Consult Web site at *www.expertconsult.com*.

HEMATOLOGIC/CHEMICAL

CHAPTER 71

Pallor

Theresa Ortega-Simpson

Tissue or mucous membrane color is determined by the amount of oxygenated hemoglobin in the blood, the degree of tissue blood flow (or perfusion), and by the presence of other serum pigments such as bilirubin or myoglobin. *Pallor*, defined as the paleness of a tissue,[1] is caused by two main categories of disease: disorders that cause *anemia* (low red blood cell count) and disorders that cause decreased tissue *perfusion* ("shock" or severe pain); oftentimes, both mechanisms are responsible for pallor in an individual. During physical examination, pallor is usually identified on examination of the oral mucous membranes. In some dogs and cats, pallor can also be identified on examination of non-pigmented lips, nose, nares, skin, or urogenital mucous membranes.

EVALUATION

To determine the cause for pallor, a systematic evaluation should be pursued. The owner history can be helpful in determining whether the cause may be acute or chronic, and can sometimes provide direct clues as to cause. During physical examination, a dog or cat's capillary refill time (CRT), hydra-

tion status, heart/pulse rate and rhythm, and pulse quality should be evaluated. CRT is determined by pressing on the buccal mucosa to blanch the mucosa and observe the time (in seconds) it takes for prior mucous membrane color to return. Normal CRT is 1.0 to 2.0 seconds; prolonged CRT is >2.0 seconds and is diagnostic for poor tissue perfusion.[2]

Since dehydration can lead to poor tissue perfusion by causing hypovolemia, hypotension, and vasoconstriction, it is always important to evaluate a patient's hydration status. In a normally hydrated dog or cat, oral, nasal, and/or ocular mucous membranes are usually moist and the interscapular skin quickly returns to normal position when pulled upwards and released (skin turgor). A review of the characteristics of increasing degrees of dehydration has been summarized.[3]

Normal heart rates in dogs and cats have been previously published.[2] An increased heart rate is commonly seen with pallor regardless of its cause. Severe anemia may increase heart rate to compensate for poor oxygen-carrying capacity of the blood, while almost all causes for poor tissue perfusion increase heart rate. An abnormal brady- or tachyarrhythmia can be either the sole cause or a contributing cause for pallor by causing poor tissue perfusion. Femoral pulses are palpable on the medial aspect of the proximal hind limbs and are evalu-

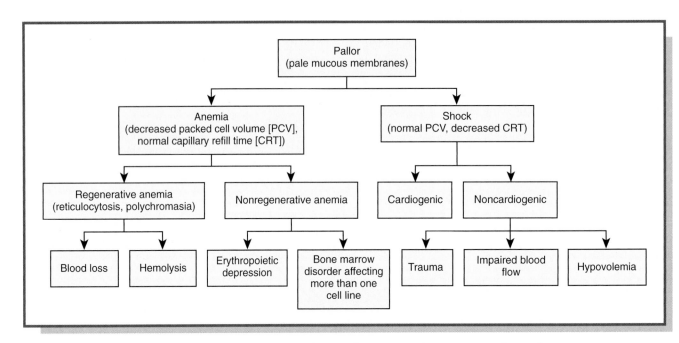

Figure 71-1   There are numerous, varied causes for anemia and poor tissue perfusion, the main determinants of pallor. The above algorithm illustrates how the *initial* evaluation of a patient with pallor helps determine the cause, and how pallor may have more than one cause.

ated for symmetry, rate, strength, and synchronicity with the auscultated heart rate. Pulse strength will be reduced in animals that are dehydrated, that have a tachyarrhythmia, or that are hypovolemic. These are all causes for poor tissue perfusion.

In addition to the physical examination, packed cell volume (PCV) or hematocrit (HCT) measurement helps to further determine the basic cause for pallor. If all of the above physical exam parameters are normal and the PCV is low, then anemia is likely the sole mechanism for pallor. If any of the above physical exam parameters are abnormal, then abnormal tissue perfusion may be the sole or a contributing cause (Figure 71-1).

DIAGNOSTIC TESTS

Baseline diagnostic tests for dogs and cats with pallor should include thorough history, complete physical examination, CBC, chemistry panel, and urinalysis. In an emergency, these tests may not be immediately available. Therefore, in an emer-

gency PCV, total solids (TS), blood glucose, BUN, electrolytes, and blood smear evaluation along with a thorough history and physical examination are indicated. Additional baseline tests that may be indicated based on history and physical examination findings include: electrocardiogram (EKG), blood pressure, pulse oximetry, blood gases, lactate, saline slide-agglutination, coagulation tests (PT/PTT/PIVKA), thoracic or abdominal radiographs, abdominal/cardiac ultrasounds, and fecal occult blood. Additional tests that may ultimately be indicated to determine a definitive diagnosis may include: serum iron assays, bone marrow aspiration cytology/biopsy, direct Coombs' test, ACTH stimulation test, blood or urine cultures, serum insulin level, tissue biopsy and others.

REFERENCES

The reference list can be found on the companion Expert Consult Web site at *www.expertconsult.com*.

CHAPTER 72

Polycythemia and Erythrocytosis

Urs Giger

DEFINITIONS

In contrast to anemia, polycythemia is a relatively rare clinical presentation. *Polycythemia*, denoting literally many cells in blood, describes an increase in the total volume of red blood cells or red cell mass without referring to blood leukocytes and platelets. However, an increase in the concentration of erythrocytes, whether measured as number of red blood cells (RBCs), hemoglobin (Hb), or packed cell volume (PCV), is best termed *erythrocytosis*. Indeed, erythrocytosis may result either from a reduced blood volume, so-called relative erythrocytosis, or from a true expansion of the red cell mass, known as *absolute polycythemia* or *erythrocytosis*. Nevertheless, the terms erythrocytosis and polycythemia are often applied interchangeably, and clinically polycythemia is more frequently used in veterinary medicine.

PATHOPHYSIOLOGY

The above explanation of terms implies that varied causes and mechanisms lead to erythrocytosis and/or polycythemia; this has major implications for its diagnostic approach and clinical management. The classification of polycythemias is shown in Figure 72-1.

Diminished fluid intake and/or rapid severe loss of body fluids reduce the plasma volume and produce a *relative erythrocytosis* (spurious polycythemia). Hemoconcentration may result from water deprivation, severe diarrhea or vomiting, postoperative complications, shifts of vascular fluid into the interstitial space, heat stroke, and burns. Clinical manifesta-

tions of severe dehydration are generally readily evident aside the history of a site of fluid losses and/or a lack of fluid intake.

In contrast, *absolute polycythemia* reflects an increased red cell volume, and as the red cell mass rises, the total blood volume also expands. Absolute polycythemia reflects an increased erythropoiesis, while the erythrocyte survival in polycythemic states is generally normal. Absolute (or true) polycythemia is divided into primary and secondary polycythemias based upon "independent" and "erythropoietin (EPO)-driven" erythropoiesis, respectively. Much has recently been learned about the molecular mechanisms of erythropoiesis that now explains the different forms of polycythemia.

Erythropoiesis involves the staggering production of a few billion erythrocytes per kilogram body weight and day, which is primarily regulated by renal oxygenation and the hormone EPO. Indeed, EPO production and secretion is tightly controlled by a classic feedback loop mechanism. Renal hypoxia, and not the actual red cell count or mass, stimulates EPO synthesis in the interstitial renal cells in the inner cortex lying in immediate proximity to the proximal tubules. Factors affecting the delivery of oxygen to the kidney such as anemia, low atmospheric oxygen tension, cardiopulmonary dysfunction, and impeded renal blood flow can stimulate EPO production and erythropoiesis. Conversely, any adequate or excessive supply of oxygen to the kidneys diminishes EPO production. Normally, plasma EPO concentrations show an inverse relationship with the blood's oxygen-carrying capacity. A rise in plasma EPO level is dependent on *de novo* synthesis rather than the release of preformed stores, and EPO has a plasma half-life of ~10 hours.

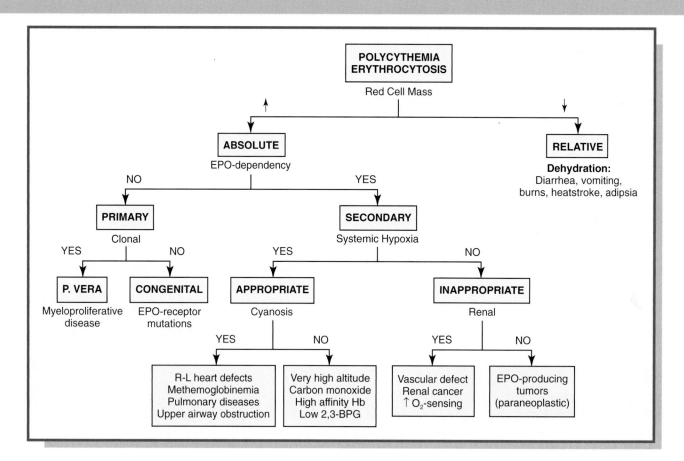

Figure 72-1 Algorithm showing the diagnostic approach and classification of polycythemia. *2,3-BPG*, 2,3-Biphosphoglyceride; *EPO*, erythropoietin; *Hb*, hemoglobin; *P. vera*, polycythemia vera.

Renal oxygen sensing involves complex regulatory mechanisms. An oxygen-dependent propylhydroxylase regulates the stability of hypoxia-inducible factor (HIF). In hypoxia the HIF-1α remains unhydroxylated, binds to HIF-β, and is translocated to the nucleus, where it stimulates expression of EPO, while in normoxia HIF-1α is hydroxylated, which ultimately leads to its degradation.

The EPO effects are mediated through the cell surface EPO receptors, which are expressed as early as the more mature burst-forming units–erythroid (BFU-E) but particularly the colony-forming units–erythroid (CFU-E) and which decline after the proerythroblast stage. Upon EPO binding, the dimeric EPO receptor undergoes conformational changes, which activate tyrosine phosphorylation via major signaling pathways involving JAK2 and signal transducers and activators of transcription, the phosphatidylinositol 3 kinase-Akt, and the mitogen-activated protein kinase pathways.

Primary polycythemia is associated with low serum EPO concentrations and may be congenital or acquired. *Polycythemia vera* (P. vera) is an acquired myeloproliferative disorder leading to clonal expansion of a single hematopoietic stem cell and is characterized by EPO-independent hematopoietic colony formation, proliferation and complete differentiation into the three bone marrow cell lines, and maturation into blood cells. Hence, human patients with P. vera may exhibit not only erythrocytosis but also thrombocytosis and leukocytosis. Moreover, their disease can progress to leukemia and myelofibrosis. Recently, the amino acid substitution V117F in JAK2, leading to constitutive activation of

JAK2 and the downstream signaling pathways, has been found in a large proportion of human patients with P. vera. Dogs and cats with erythrocytosis are often presumed to have P. vera, but their clonality, EPO-independent proliferation, and molecular basis have never been conclusively studied.

Primary congenital polycythemia (erythrocytosis) in humans may be caused by several dominant mutations in the EPO receptor and more recently in JAK2 that lead to EPO receptor hypersensitivity and downstream signaling pathway activation, respectively. Some of these were previously placed into the idiopathic polycythemia group. These patients neither have a completely EPO-independent nor clonal disorder. Companion animals with isolated persistent erythrocytosis documented in early adulthood that have never been shown to develop thrombocytosis and/or leukocytosis, and never progressed to myelofibrosis and/or leukemia even after years, may well have had EPO receptor or JAK2 mutations rather than P. vera. Further studies of polycythemic companion animals may be warranted.

Secondary polycythemias may also be associated with congenital or acquired conditions that result in increased EPO production and secretion. Further classification into appropriate and inappropriate secondary polycythemia is based upon whether or not there is chronic systemic hypoxia present that drives EPO production. The most common causes of *secondary appropriate polycythemia* are congenital heart defects with right-to-left shunting of blood such as reversed patent ductus arteriosus (rPDA), ventricular septal defects, and tetralogy of Fallot, while acquired heart failure very rarely results in a marked erythrocytosis. Chronic pulmonary diseases (e.g., pulmonary infiltrates with eosinophils) and upper airway obstruction (as seen in Bulldogs with sleep apnea) may cause hypoxia due to abnormal ventilation or ventilation-perfusion mismatch, but are rarely a cause of severe erythrocytosis. The author followed a young polycythemic mildly tachypneic cat with eosinophilic bronchitis secondary to dirofilariasis that resolved after a couple of years. Hypoxemia due to high altitude can mildly increase the hematocrit in animals but does not cause clinical signs of erythrocytosis, at least at the elevations we practice at.

However, chronic or recurrent exposure to carbon monoxide may lead to severe erythrocytosis as the author observed in a cat living near a defective furnace and exhaust system. Similarly, defects affecting the oxygen-carrying capacity of Hb can rarely cause polycythemia in cats and in dogs. Methemoglobin reductase deficiency has been documented in several canine breeds and also Domestic Shorthair cats, and due to the inability of methemoglobin to bind oxygen, these animals can develop a moderate erythrocytosis. Hemoglobin mutations resulting in M-Hb, which is unable to bind oxygen, or high-affinity Hb, as well as defects in the generation of 2,3-biphosphoglyceride (2,3-BPG) in erythrocytes affecting the Hb-oxygen dissociation curve, have not been described in dogs and cats. It should be noted that feline Hb's oxygen release is not 2,3-BPG dependent and has no BPG. And although phosphofructokinase-deficient dogs have low erythrocytic 2,3-BPG concentrations, they do not become polycythemic because of their chronic and alkaline-induced hemolytic disease.

Secondary inappropriate polycythemia refers to conditions leading to elevated serum EPO levels without systemic hypoxia. Renal disorders such as renal neoplasia (e.g., carcinoma, nephroblastoma, lymphoma) may cause local hypoxia and thereby trigger EPO production (rather than EPO being produced by tumor cells). Similarly, renal amyloidosis, infection, and inflammation may induce renal hypoxia and erythrocytosis. One cat exhibiting inappropriately high EPO levels following renal transplantation has been reported, which represents a known complication in human patients. Moreover, EPO production may be part of a paraneoplastic syndrome of other extrarenal malignancies which has been documented in dogs with cecal leiomyosarcoma and hepatoma.

Regardless of the cause of absolute polycythemia, the consequence of an increased PCV is an increase in blood viscosity. The rise in viscosity becomes much more pronounced at a PCV >60%, and viscosity is twice normal at a PCV of 70% (for dogs). Furthermore, because it is known that the smaller the RBC size the higher the blood viscosity, companion animals may be exposed to significantly higher viscosity in polycythemia than humans due to the normally very small feline RBCs and microcytic RBCs produced in iron-deficient canine patients. Depending on the degree of viscosity and local or systemic vascular hindrance, capillary blood flow diminishes leading to local hypoxia, sludging of blood cells, vessel injury, and thrombosis. Impaired microcirculation and arterial thrombosis of the brain is considered a leading cause for the neurologic signs—a common presentation in polycythemic animals.

CLINICAL SIGNS

The manifestations of *relative polycythemia* are usually obvious and depend on the severity of dehydration and the underlying disease process. As the treatment of relative erythrocytosis (polycythemia) is so different from that of absolute polycythemia, every effort has to be made to detect signs of dehydration based upon prolonged capillary refill time, decreased skin turgor, tachycardia, and hypotension. Moreover, a history of

diarrhea or vomiting as well as signs of heat stroke or burns may be noted.

The clinical features of *absolute erythrocytosis* are related in part to the underlying disorder in addition to manifestations associated with the increased blood volume and increased blood viscosity, which affect blood flow and oxygen delivery. While absolute polycythemia develops slowly and some patients are incidentally discovered to be polycythemic by routine complete blood cell count screening, clinical signs often occur acutely when a certain PCV and degree of hyperviscosity have been reached.

In patients with *absolute primary polycythemia*, signs are mainly related to hyperviscosity with the conjunctival blood vessels injected and torturous. Mucous membranes appear hyperemic, like red brick, although on occasion they may be a little ruddy due to impaired blood flow. More than half of the cases with primary polycythemia are presented for neurologic complications such as seizures, ataxia, blindness, tremor, or behavior changes. Due to the hyperviscosity, hemorrhage may occur such as epistaxis, hyphema, or gastrointestinal bleeding. Thrombotic events have also been reported in humans. Splenomegaly may also be present.

The clinical hyperviscosity features of *absolute secondary polycythemia* are similar to cases of primary polycythemias, but they may also have signs referable to the underlying disease process. Clinically helpful, they can be divided into patients with hyperemic versus cyanotic mucous membranes. Polycythemic animals with cyanosis may have congenital heart disease due to right-to-left cardiac shunting and very rarely pulmonary diseases or methemoglobinemia, which is often referred to as chocolate-brown discoloration. Noteworthy, animals with a rPDA have differential cyanosis of the caudal body parts (anus and prepuce or vulva) and no murmur, while other cardiac right-to-left shunting (typically with a heart murmur) and pulmonary diseases cause generalized cyanosis. All other secondary polycythemias have red and injected mucous membranes. In fact animals with carbon monoxide poisoning have cherry red mucous membranes. Other clinical signs may relate to a specific cause of secondary polycythemia such as a heart murmur (none with a rPDA), respiratory distress, and renal or other masses.

DIAGNOSTIC TESTS

Both polycythemia and erythrocytosis depict conditions in which the PCV, Hb concentration, and/or RBC count exceed the upper limit of normal. All of these values refer to concentrations and are therefore dependent on plasma volume as well as circulating red cell mass. It is important to recognize that normal upper values of these erythrocyte parameters for dogs are different from those for cats. Upper limits for dogs versus cats are PCV of 55% versus 48%, RBC count of $8.5 \times 10^6/\mu L$ versus $10 \times 10^6/\mu L$, and Hb concentration of 18 versus 15 g/dL. Certain breeds such as Greyhounds and some other sight hounds as well as some Dachshunds have higher PCV values (sometimes slightly exceeding 60%) than other breeds. Splenic contraction can lead to a temporary increase of circulating RBCs in dogs (but not in cats), which is generally slight (except in case of splenomegaly) and never exceeds 60%. Canine hyperadenocorticism and feline hyperthyroidism can also result in slightly increased PCV.

With relative polycythemia the PCV is generally mildly increased (i.e., in dogs 56% to 65% and 49% to 60% in cats) and returns to normal with fluid therapy. Depending on the amount of fluid versus concomitant protein loss (due to diarrhea, vomiting, or burns) or extravascular shift, the plasma protein concentration will be often high but can sometimes be in the normal to low range. In the case of acute hemorrhagic gastroenteritis, dogs may not only be severely hypoproteinemic but also become anemic after fluid administration.

Among absolute polycythemias P. vera is a diagnosis by exclusion in animals; therefore all diagnostic steps are used to identify a secondary cause of polycythemia (see Figure 72-1) before a diagnosis of P. vera is reached and at this time P. vera cannot be differentiated from congenital polycythemias in animals. When presented with an animal with absolute polycythemia a complete blood cell count, reticulocyte count, chest and abdominal radiographs, abdominal ultrasound, echocardiography, blood gases, blood methemoglobin and serum EPO determinations are often indicated, albeit one or the other finding may sway and simplify the diagnostic approach (e.g., discovering met- or deoxyhemoglobin).

While a PCV or complete blood cell count may provide the first evidence of polycythemia, a reticulocyte count, a chemistry panel, and urinalysis belong to the minimal data base as for any sick animal. This generally enables the clinician to further distinguish absolute from relative polycythemia, to assess the degree of polycythemia, and to determine the effects of therapeutic interventions. In clinical practice it is rarely necessary or feasible to determine total red cell mass. On the other a hand, a reticulocyte count is an inexpensive method to gauge the degree of erythropoietic activity in absolute polycythemia. The absolute reticulocyte count is generally mildly to moderately increased (50 to 250,000/μL) and if only relative reticulocyte counts are determined they need to be corrected upwards for polycythemic animals rather than downward as typically done for anemic animals.

In cyanotic patients it is prudent to first differentiate deoxy- from methemoglobin. This can be quickly accomplished by exposing venous blood to air by gently rotating an aerated EDTA blood tube or placing a drop of blood on a filter paper. Deoxyhemoglobin rapidly turns bright red on exposure to air, while methemoglobin remains dark brown. In the latter case methemoglobin can be quantified by some veterinary reference laboratories (10% to 55%; >65% fatal; normal <1%), but determination of blood carbon monoxide levels are restricted to human hospital or special toxicology laboratories. Although an arterial blood gas value should detect systemic hypoxia, the high viscosity can hamper sampling and interpretation. Hence it is recommended to stabilize the patient first and repeat measurements when initially low after phlebotomy. Normal values are expected in all but appropriate polycythemia with cardiopulmonary disease (theoretical exception: hemoglobinopathies where pO2 is normal). If hypoxia is the cause of polycythemia, the changes are usually marked and venous blood gases parallel these changes. Pulse oximetry can be used if arterial blood gas determination is not available. A low saturation (<90%) with a reliable recording and repeatability suggests hypoxia.

Abdominal ultrasound is used to detect renal disease, abdominal neoplasia, or both. Unspecific signs such as hyperechoic kidneys may be found in primary polycythemia possibly secondary to hyperviscosity. Thoracic radiographs and echocardiogram (with Doppler) examinations are directed toward identifying pulmonary and cardiac abnormalities and have mostly replaced angiographic radiology. Mild changes such as myocardial hypertrophy or bronchointerstitial changes can be found in primary and secondary noncardiogenic polycythemia, again resulting from hyperviscosity.

Contrary to the general belief, examination of routine bone marrow aspirate or core biopsy cannot distinguish P. vera from other primary and secondary polycythemia and hence is generally not helpful. In either case erythroid hyperplasia with complete maturation is observed. The subtle differences in bone marrow cell morphology and colony formation noted by experts in humans with P. vera have not been reported in animals. Growth performance of erythroid precursors in EPO-free culture medium can be helpful because erythroid cells of patients with P. vera show normal growth, whereas erythropoiesis in secondary polycythemia is EPO-dependent. However, this method, just like the clonality assay, is restricted to research laboratories and not generally available.

As primary and secondary polycythemia are principally classified based upon serum EPO levels, it would appear that measurement of serum EPO concentrations is generally helpful. However, it appears that only an increased EPO value is clinically helpful. And although an increased serum EPO level is diagnostic for secondary polycythemia and values up to fiftyfold elevation have been found in secondary polycythemia, a low or normal serum EPO value can also be found in animals with secondary polycythemia. Thus far, only few human test kits using an enzyme-linked immunosorbent assay (ELISA) have been validated for animals with normal ranges below 20 mU/mL. As of this writing, no veterinary laboratory is offering a validated serum EPO assay for dogs and cats, as previously used ELISA assays are no more available.

THERAPEUTIC AND PROGNOSTIC CONSIDERATIONS

Treatment of a polycythemic animal is very much dependent on the cause; most importantly relative polycythemias have to be differentiated from absolute polycythemias as their treatments are opposite. Relative polycythemia is treated with rapid intravenous fluid administration, while absolute polycythemia is initially treated with phlebotomy.

In the case of absolute polycythemia serial phlebotomies are performed and 10 to 20 mL/kg blood is withdrawn until clinical signs have resolved or the target hematocrit is reached. In primary polycythemia the target hematocrit is below 55% for dogs and below 50% for cats. In cases of secondary appropriate polycythemia the aim of treatment is resolving clinical signs of polycythemia and a higher hematocrit (60% to 70%) can be acceptable. A slightly higher than normal hematocrit might provide higher oxygen-carrying capacity without causing hyperviscosity complications. Alternatively repeated bloodletting may be accomplished by leeching (each leech may suck 5 to 10 mL). Care should be given to maintaining the blood volume as rapid and large blood withdrawal or massive fluid administration can further compromise these patients. Moreover, anticonvulsive drugs are not effective in controlling seizures in polycythemic animals without correction of the erythrocytosis and maintenance of blood volume.

Most treated polycythemic animals will continue to have a lifelong tendency to become polycythemic. This may be readily accomplished by serial phlebotomies every 4 to 8 weeks with regular monitoring of PCV and total protein. Myelosuppressive drug therapy with hydroxyurea should only be used in cases where the underlying cause cannot be corrected and repeated phlebotomies are not well tolerated or are required too frequently. Multiple-dose regimens have been suggested in the literature, but none have been well established. It is advisable to first reduce the PCV by phlebotomy to the target value before initiating treatment with hydroxyurea. Some regimens use a loading dose starting with 30 to 50 mg/kg orally once a day; after 1 week the dose is reduced to 15 mg/kg/day, then titrated to effect. Other regimens propose using a maintenance dose such as 50 mg/kg every other day and titrating to effect. Side effects are reversible and include myelosuppression (thrombocytopenia and granuocytopenia), hair loss, and gastrointestinal upsets. Hence patient's clinical course and complete blood cell count need to be monitored.

The prognosis for primary polycythemia is guarded, but some have remained asymptomatic for years and survival for more than 6 years has been achieved in treated animals. The prognosis for secondary polycythemia depends on the underlying cause. In cases of congenital heart defects, survival of up to 5 years has been reported. Animals with hereditary methemoglobin reductase deficiency generally do not require any specific treatment and have a good life expectancy as long as they are not exposed to oxidative agents.

CHAPTER 73

Cyanosis

Justin Allen

Cyanosis is blue discoloration of the mucous membranes and/or skin (*cyan* = blue, Greek); it is the visible result of increased amounts of deoxygenated *(reduced)* hemoglobin in the blood. This is a subjective property, and depends on lighting, pigmentation of mucous membranes or skin, and the observer. Cyanosis is a clinical sign observed in many different disease processes, and is typically categorized as *central* or *peripheral*.

Central cyanosis is caused by a global deoxygenation of arterial blood, most commonly due to cardiovascular, pulmonary, or other diseases resulting in ventilation-perfusion abnormalities. It is generally indicative of a severe and potentially life-threatening condition. Less common causes include methemoglobinemia and polycythemia. Peripheral cyanosis is caused by a local reduction in oxygenated hemoglobin; it can be secondary to obstructive causes (e.g., thromboembolism), vasoconstriction (e.g., shock, hypothermia), or any of the causes of central cyanosis; peripheral cyanosis may indicate a severe underlying condition, but is not itself life-threatening. Central cyanosis is generally most evident in the oral mucous membranes (the tongue may be the earliest and most visible indicator), whereas peripheral cyanosis is most evident at the foot pads and nail beds of the affected limb(s).

PHYSIOLOGY AND PATHOPHYSIOLOGY

Partial pressure of a gas is the molecular pressure of that gas in a mixed gas environment (alveoli) or in fluid (blood). Normal partial pressure of oxygen in the alveolus (PAO_2) at room air (~20% oxygen) averages 104 mm Hg. Normal partial pressure in the arterial blood (PaO_2) is also ~100 mm Hg, due to nearly complete oxygen exchange by normal pulmonary tissue. Approximately 97% of oxygen is carried by hemoglobin of red blood cells, with the remaining oxygen dissolved in water.

Cyanosis is generally observed when deoxygenated hemoglobin exceeds 5 g per 100 mL blood within capillary beds. In animals with normal hemoglobin levels (approximately 10 to 20 g/dL), oxygen saturation must decrease to levels below 80% to produce consistently visible cyanosis. As a result, it is an insensitive indicator of blood oxygen content. *Polycythemia* is a condition characterized by an elevated red blood cell (RBC) count; in small animal medicine, it is most commonly due to conditions resulting in chronic hypoxia. Polycythemic animals have higher total hemoglobin levels, making it easier for reduced hemoglobin to accumulate. For example, in an animal with a PCV of 65%, 5 g/dL of deoxygenated hemoglobin may be present if oxygen saturation (SaO_2) drops below 89%. Conversely, in anemic animals, cyanosis is rarely present; an absolute reduction in hemoglobin means that SaO_2 must decrease to levels incompatible with life to produce cyanosis.

Central cyanosis is most commonly due to cardiovascular or pulmonary diseases that result in arterial deoxygenation (hypoxemia). A decrease in PaO_2 results in a decrease in SaO_2 according to the oxygen-hemoglobin dissociation curve (Figure 73-1).

Causes of hypoxemia can be categorized by the type of pathophysiology present (Box 73-1).

Ventilation-perfusion mismatch is probably the most common cause of hypoxemia encountered in clinical practice. In diseases causing pulmonary infiltration (e.g., edema, pneumonia) alveolar ventilation and oxygen exchange are impaired, so that blood flowing to those areas is inadequately oxygenated. This creates a "physiologic shunt," as the deoxygenated blood mixes with the oxygenated blood returning from better-ventilated areas of lung.

Hypoventilation is another potential cause of decreased PaO_2; in these cases, alveoli are not ventilated due to elevated pleural pressure (pleural effusion or pneumothorax), depressed respiratory drive (neurologic disease, drug overdose), or respiratory muscle failure. Obstructive causes of hypoxemia, such as laryngeal paralysis or tracheal foreign body, result in decreased oxygen availability. Venous-to-arterial shunts ("right-to-left" congenital cardiac or extracardiac shunts) cause deoxygenated venous blood to mix with oxygenated arterial blood, which can result in hypoxemia and cyanosis. If cyanosis is present in a young animal, congenital heart disease must be suspected. A right-to-left patent ductus arteriosus (PDA) results in *differential cyanosis* due to the location of the shunt. Deoxygenated blood from the pulmonary artery is shunted through the PDA to the aorta distal to the brachiocephalic and subclavian arteries; this produces cyanosis of the caudal portion of the body without cranial cyanosis. Other cyanotic congenital heart defects (e.g., tetralogy of Fallot) result in central cyanosis, as the shunt occurs at the cardiac level.

Peripheral cyanosis is due to a local reduction of oxygenated blood. Any cause of slowed capillary blood flow will result in increased oxygen extraction by tissues, resulting in deoxygenated hemoglobin. Clinically, this is most commonly

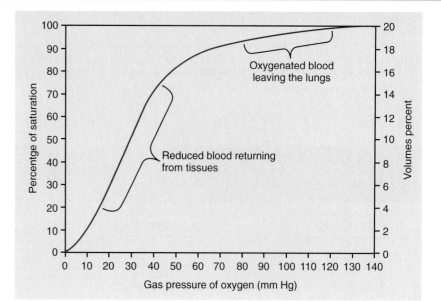

Figure 73-1 Transport of oxygen and carbon dioxide in the blood and body fluids.

due to arterial thromboembolism (saddle thrombus) and/or shock; other causes include occlusion to venous drainage (such as a tourniquet) and hypothermia (Table 73-1).

Methemoglobin is a normal product of hemoglobin oxidation, which is maintained at low levels (~1%) by the red blood cell enzyme methemoglobin reductase. When this enzyme is overwhelmed, or congenitally absent (rare), methemoglobin levels can rise to clinically significant levels. As methemoglobin is incapable of carrying oxygen, hypoxia may occur. Common oxidants resulting in methemoglobinemia include acetaminophen (Tylenol), benzocaine, and nitrites; when levels of methemoglobin exceed 10%, a brown discoloration to blood is grossly visible.

INITIAL EVALUATION/CLINICAL SIGNS

Despite a low sensitivity and specificity, cyanosis is a valuable and recognizable clinical sign. All levels of hospital staff, from receptionist to veterinarian, can readily identify cyanosis as an indicator of a potentially life-threatening condition that requires immediate attention. Once central cyanosis is identified, oxygen therapy should be initiated as soon as possible. Signalment should be noted, as age and breed will help stratify differential diagnoses. A brief assessment of the patient's respiratory pattern (tachypnea, dyspnea, orthopnea) should be made, as well as assessment of airway patency. Stridor, if noted, is usually indicative of upper airway obstruction, which may necessitate emergency tracheostomy or endotracheal intubation. Auscultation is essential; noting the presence or absence of abnormal heart sounds (murmur, gallop, arrhythmia) or lung sounds (crackles, wheezes) is important to determine the most appropriate diagnostic and therapeutic approach to the cyanotic patient.

History is often helpful in determining the cause of central cyanosis. Exposure to toxicants (such as acetaminophen or sedatives) may be determined. The duration of clinical signs is important in identifying chronic pulmonary or cardiac conditions. Peripheral cyanosis may present with signs of acute lameness. Physical examination of these patients may reveal signs of thromboembolism (pain, pulselessness, pallor, and

paresis), a mass or foreign body (i.e., rubber band) causing venous occlusion, or generalized peripheral cyanosis due to vasoconstriction that may respond to warming or massage of the extremities.

DIAGNOSTIC PLAN

Cyanotic patients are frequently presented in critical condition. In those cases, most diagnostics should be delayed until the animal is more stable. A working diagnosis can usually be obtained from physical examination, history, and signalment. For example, older dogs are more prone to chronic cardiopulmonary disease, whereas younger animals with cyanosis are more likely to have a congenital cardiac defect or airway obstruction.

Blood work can be helpful if the patient is stable enough for venipuncture. Polycythemia may indicate congenital heart disease or chronic hypoxia; a presumptive diagnosis is usually based on signs and signalment. Gross inspection of the blood may reveal a brownish color, indicating methemoglobinemia. *Thoracocentesis* can be both diagnostic and therapeutic for pleural effusion and pneumothorax; if a strong index of suspicion exists for either condition, thoracocentesis should be performed prior to other diagnostic tests. *Radiographs* can be essential to differentiate the many causes of cyanosis, such as pulmonary edema, pneumonia, pleural effusion, pneumothorax, or bronchial disease. Unfortunately, due to stress and limited resources, this can also be a lethal diagnostic test, so the necessity of radiography must be weighed against patient stability. *Echocardiography* may be extremely helpful in identifying cardiac disease, pulmonary hypertension, and pleural or pericardial effusion. Bubble studies can help determine if right to left shunting lesions are present. *Arterial blood gas* (ABG) analysis may be helpful in determining the etiology of central cyanosis (see Table 73-1).

ABG should be evaluated on room air and 100% inspired oxygen; unfortunately, this typically requires anesthesia, which is problematic in many patients with cyanosis. Pulse oximetry, which approximates SaO_2, can be performed in

Prehepatic Hyperbilirubinemia

In cases of autoimmune processes (primary or secondary) leading to hemolytic anemia (IMHA), immunosuppressive doses of glucocorticoids are the mainstay of therapy. They are fast acting, effective, and inexpensive. Some additional immunosuppressive therapy (cyclosporine, azathioprine, etc.) is often instituted in these disease processes. These drugs tend to have significantly longer onsets of action. They are important in the long-term management of these diseases by maintaining immunosuppression and allowing for more rapid steroid reductions. This limits the adverse side effects of ongoing immune suppressive doses of steroids. These medications are significantly more costly than steroids, but are not typically cost prohibitive. RBC destruction regardless of the etiology often causes secondary systemic inflammation and antiinflammatory doses of glucocorticoids are often beneficial in short-term management. These should be used with caution, or avoided in cases suspected of having a primary infectious etiology. Infectious causes of hemolytic anemia and secondary hyperbilirubinemia should be treated by appropriate antimicrobial therapy.

Hepatic Hyperbilirubinemia

Treatments for hepatic causes of hyperbilirubinemia are dictated by the underlying etiology. Infectious etiologies should be treated with appropriate antimicrobials. Intoxicants should be treated with appropriate antidotes (if and when available). Autoimmune etiologies should be treated with appropriate immunosuppressive therapies (as above). Congenital etiologies should be addressed as best possible. Regardless of the etiology, hepatocellular inflammation often leads to increased oxygen free radicals and inflammatory cytokines.

A variety of antioxidants/hepatobiliary supportive medications including ursodiol, adenosyl, vitamin E, and silymarin are available to help treat the side effects of these diseases. Although these medications are nonspecific, they are often used as "liver support" in both hepatic and posthepatic diseases. Many of these neutraceuticals do not have clearly detailed mechanisms of action or entirely proven benefits. However, there are many indications and preliminary research papers that are suggestive of benefits. Additional information regarding these medications, their proposed mechanisms, and their potential benefits are reviewed in other resources. Generally, side effects are manageable and most commonly related to gastrointestinal upset. They typically have excellent safety margins. Vomiting caused by ongoing primary disease versus the administration of antioxidant neutraceuticals may be difficult to differentiate.

Posthepatic Hyperbilirubinemia

Several reports and texts have documented and advocated medical management of biliary diseases. Partial gallbladder obstruction can resolve over time without surgical intervention. Spontaneous resolution, or resolution with medical management, is more likely to occur with particular etiologies (pancreatitis) than with others (cholelithiasis, neoplastic disease, and mucocele). The potential choleretic properties of ursodiol may be beneficial in partial gallbladder obstructions, but are theoretically contraindicated in complete obstructions. Differentiating between partial and complete gallbladder obstructions is often challenging and this can lead to frustration and incomplete response to medical management.

Cholecystitis can also be treated medically, but poor perfusion of an inflamed gallbladder will often inhibit antibiotic penetration and may cause poor response to medical management.

There are a variety of surgical procedures (cholecystectomy, cholecystoduodenostomy, cholecystojejunostomy, and biliary stents and tube placements) to address the variety of problems that may result in partial and complete biliary obstructions. Outcomes are different for the various surgical procedures and are also often dependent upon the etiology of the biliary obstruction, severity of disease at the time of surgery, and the immediate postoperative recovery period.

Surgical intervention not only allows more complete evaluation of the biliary system, but also aids in histopathologic diagnosis of the underlying etiology. Expression or removal of the gallbladder also often provides significant therapeutic benefits and will often lead to reduced hyperbilirubinemia following surgery.

It is this author's opinion that surgical intervention in biliary disease often provides better definitive diagnosis and long-term clinical outcome than medical management. However, acute disease, particularly in the case of pancreatitis, can be significantly worsened in the immediate postoperative period.

Primary Treatment of Hyperbilirubinemia

Extracorporeal hemoperfusion has been documented in dogs. Plasma diafiltration has been documented to primarily remove bilirubin from human blood. These procedures may be theoretically beneficial in cases of severe hyperbilirubinemia although it does not correct the underlying etiology and is not readily available to most clinicians.

There is a clinical syndrome of icterus or jaundice without hyperbilirubinemia. Chronic and/or severe hyperbilirubinemia will lead to bilirubin irreversibly bound to albumin and body tissues. This "dyeing" effect may cause clinical jaundice, long after resolving the hyperbilirubinemia. This tissue dyeing effect may be prolonged, but is not clinically significant.

REFERENCES

The reference list can be found on the companion Expert Consult Web site at *www.expertconsult.com*.

CHAPTER 75

Bleeding Disorders: Epistaxis and Hemoptysis

Tracy Gieger

EPISTAXIS

Epistaxis is defined as hemorrhage originating from the nose. The following areas should be emphasized when evaluating a dog or cat with epistaxis (Figure 75-1).

SIGNALMENT

Pets allowed to roam are susceptible to trauma, parasitic, rickettsial, and fungal infections, rodenticide toxicity, intranasal transmissible veneral tumor (TVT), and foreign body (FB) inhalation. Purebred dogs are more commonly affected with immune-mediated diseases, von Willebrand disease (vWD), or congenital coagulation factor deficiencies. Nasal tumors are more common in older animals, although nasal lymphoma occurs in younger cats. Nasopharyngeal polyps occur more often in young cats, while brachycephalic felines are more susceptible to chronic viral respiratory infections.

HISTORY

Nasal trauma results in acute-onset and often severe bleeding that resolves with supportive measures and does not recur. Historical bleeding after tooth loss or elective neutering may indicate a congenital coagulation factor deficiency or platelet disorder. FB inhalation, most commonly wood splinters or grass awns, often causes an acute onset of epistaxis, sneezing, and pawing at the face; however, if foreign objects remain lodged in the nasal cavity, chronic nasal discharge secondary to granuloma formation may result. Allergic rhinitis may cause seasonal epistaxis. Chronic or intermittent epistaxis is more common with oronasal fistulas, fungal rhinitis, and nasal tumors; often these diseases begin with mucoid nasal discharge that progresses to epistaxis later in the course of disease. The owner should be questioned about the pet's history of travel to areas endemic for fungal and rickettsial organisms, leishmaniasis, and hepatozoonosis. Drug and vaccine administration may result in sequelae such as inhibition of platelet function (nonsteroidal antiinflammatory drugs [NSAIDs]), immune-mediated platelet destruction (drugs, vaccines), and thrombocytopenia (estrogen, phenylbutazone, chemotherapy drugs), which may be an underlying cause of epistaxis.

Characterization of Epistaxis

Many intranasal diseases such as nasal tumors begin with unilateral epistaxis that can become bilateral as the disease progresses and the nasal septum is disrupted. Although bilateral epistaxis may indicate "extranasal" causes such as coagulopathies, hypertension, thrombocytopenia, and thrombocytopathia (a defect in platelet function), such systemic abnormalities can also cause unilateral epistaxis.

PHYSICAL EXAMINATION

The clinician should examine the face for visual or palpable asymmetry, which is most commonly secondary to neoplasia. A glass slide may be held close to the nose to document airflow through the nostrils by the presence of condensation on the slide. (Some veterinarians favor the use of cotton or other tools to assess nasal air flow.) Ulceration and depigmentation of the nasal planum may be seen with aspergillosis, immune-mediated disease, lymphoma, or squamous cell carcinoma. Polypoid masses extending from the nares are seen with rhinosporidiosis and cryptococcosis. Cats with nasal cryptococcosis often have a characteristic convexity of the nose ("Roman nose"). The mouth should be examined for palate deformity, masses, oronasal fistulas, or loose teeth. Nasal tumors often cause facial or hard palate deformity, inability to retropulse the globe, or epiphora. A fundic examination may reveal chorioretinitis or signs of hypertensive retinopathy or hyperviscosity. Regional lymph nodes should be aspirated and examined for infectious organisms, inflammation (i.e., reactive lymph nodes), or metastatic neoplasia. Animals with petechia, mucosal bleeding, melena, or fundic hemorrhages are likely to have a defect of primary hemostasis (platelets), whereas those with hemarthrosis, hematomas, or bleeding into body cavities are likely to have a defect of secondary hemostasis (coagulation factors). Melena and hematemesis may occur when blood from the nasopharynx is swallowed. Central nervous system (CNS) dysfunction may occur with hyperviscosity syndromes or nasal tumors invading the brain. The external genetalia should be examined for masses since intranasal TVT is a rare cause of epistaxis.

DIFFERENTIAL DIAGNOSIS

The differential diagnosis for epistaxis can be divided into systemic and local causes (Box 75-1). Local diseases may progress and develop systemic complications that can exacerbate bleeding.

Systemic Conditions Causing Epistaxis ("Extranasal" Causes)

Mechanisms of epistaxis include hemostatic defects or increased capillary fragility. Primary hemostatic defects (platelet plug formation) include thrombocytopenia or thrombocytopathia. Mechanisms of thrombocytopenia include decreased production, increased destruction, sequestration, and increased consumption. Spontaneous bleeding is uncommon unless the platelet count is less than or equal to $50,000/\mu L$, and usually is associated with counts $<30,000/\mu L$. Decreased production of platelets can occur secondary to infections (viral, rickettsial, protozoal, parasitic, or bacterial), neoplasia (resulting in myelophthisis), drug administration, or immune-mediated phenomena. Increased destruction of platelets may be immune mediated or related to microangiopathy (seen with

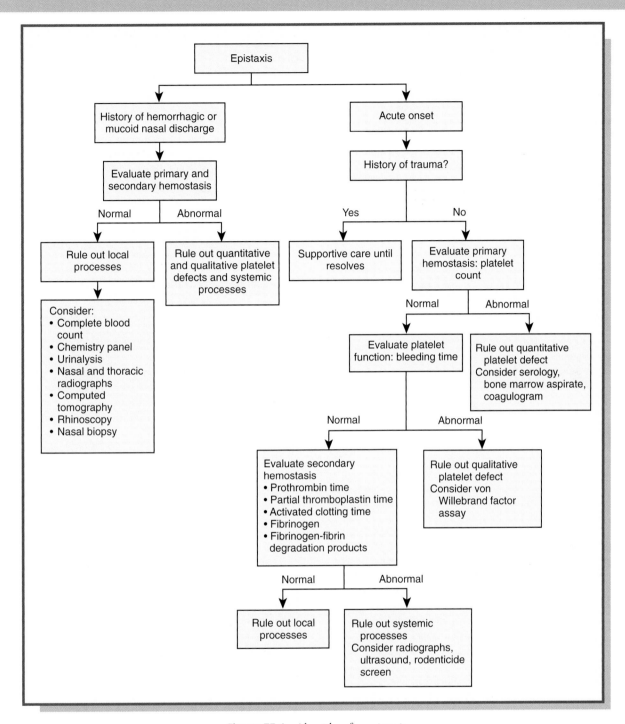

Figure 75-1 Algorithm for epistaxis.

hemangiosarcoma). Sequestration of platelets in the spleen, liver, or large vascular tumors results in peripheral thrombocytopenia. Increased platelet consumption is seen with disseminated intravascular coagulopathy (DIC), vasculitis, and hemorrhage. Thrombocytopathia may be primary (vWD), or secondary to uremia, dysproteinemias (secondary to ehrlichiosis, multiple myeloma, etc.), or drugs such as NSAIDs. Coagulation factor defects such as hemophilia A and B are uncommon congenital abnormalities that vary in severity. Acquired coagulopathies include anticoagulant rodenticide toxicity and decreased coagulation factor production second-

ary to hepatic failure. Increased capillary fragility and rupture can result from hypertension, neoplasia invading blood vessels, hyperviscosity syndromes, hyperlipidemia, and thromboembolic disease.

Localized Conditions Causing Epistaxis ("Intranasal" Causes)

Local processes are the most common cause of epistaxis. Bacterial rhinitis is almost always secondary to inflammation or damage to the nasal mucosa, although *Bordetella*, *Pasteurella*, and *Mycoplasma* spp. may be primary pathogens. Asper-

Box • 75-1

Causes of Epistaxis

Extranasal (Systemic) Causes of Epistaxis
Thrombocytopenia (quantitative platelet abnormality)
  Decreased production
    Infectious: Ehrlichiosis, feline leukemia virus (FeLV), feline
      immunodeficiency virus (FIV), Rocky Mountain
      spotted fever, hepatozoonosis, septicemia,
      endotoxemia, leishmaniasis, *Bartonella* spp. infections
    Drugs: Cytotoxic drugs, modified live virus vaccines,
      estrogens
    Neoplasia: Myelophthisis secondary to myeloproliferative
      or lymphoproliferative diseases
    Immune-mediated: Antibodies against megakaryocytes
    Other: Bone marrow aplasia, cyclic thrombocytopenia,
      myelofibrosis, hyperestrogenism (secondary to Sertoli
      cell and granulosa cell tumors), myelodysplasia,
      toxins, osteosclerosis, idiopathic
  Increased destruction
    Immune-mediated: Idiopathic or secondary to drugs,
      neoplasia, infection
    Microangiopathy: Shearing of platelets; associated with
      hemangiosarcoma
  Sequestration
    Neoplasia: Large vascular tumors
    Splenomegaly or splenic torsion
    Hepatomegaly
  Increased consumption
    Disseminated intravascular coagulopathy (DIC)
    Vasculitis: Rocky Mountain spotted fever, endotoxemia,
      neoplasia, heartworm disease, bacteremia, *Bartonella*
      spp. infections
    Hemorrhage-induced thrombocytopenia
Thrombocytopathia (qualitative platelet defect)
  Congenital: von Willebrand disease (vWD), platelet
    procoagulant activity deficiency in German Shepherd
    Dogs, Glanzmann's thrombasthenia in Great Pyrenees,
    Basset Hound thrombopathia
  Acquired: vWD (associated with hypothyroidism), uremia,
    dysproteinemia (associated with multiple myeloma,
    ehrlichiosis, leishmaniasis), drugs (NSAIDs)
Coagulation factor deficiency
  Congenital: Hemophilia A and B, others

Acquired: Anticoagulant rodenticide toxicity, liver failure,
  DIC
Increased capillary fragility
  Hypertension: Primary or secondary to chronic renal failure,
    glomerulonephropathies, pheochromocytoma,
    hyperadrenocorticism, hyperthyroidism, heart disease
  Hyperviscosity syndrome: Secondary to multiple myeloma,
    ehrlichiosis, polycythemia (primary or secondary to
    hypoxia or neoplasia), leukemias
  Hyperlipidemia
  Thromboembolic disease
  Neoplasia invading blood vessels

Intranasal (Localized) Causes of Epistaxis
Trauma
Benign nasal polyps (cats)
Neoplasia
  Epithelial: Adenocarcinoma, undifferentiated carcinoma,
    squamous cell carcinoma
  Mesenchymal: Chondrosarcoma, fibrosarcoma,
    hemangiosarcoma, osteosarcoma, melanoma
  Round cell: Lymphoma, transmissible venereal tumor, mast
    cell tumor
Infection
  Fungal: *Cryptococcus, Aspergillus, Penicillium,
    Rhinosporidium, Exophiala jeanselmi,*
    phaeohyphomycosis
  Parasitic: *Pneumonyssus, Eucoleus, Cuterebra, Linguatula,
    Capillaria*
  Bacterial: Primary *(Bordetella, Pasteurella, Mycoplasma)* or
    secondary
  Viral: Canine infectious tracheobronchitis, canine distemper,
    feline viral rhinotracheitis, calicivirus
Inflammation
  Lymphoplasmacytic: Primary or secondary
  Eosinophilic: Allergic rhinitis
Dental disease
  Tooth root abscess
  Oronasal fistula
Foreign body (FB)
Vascular malformation

---

gillosis is more common in dogs, and nasal cryptococcosis is seen more frequently in cats. Animals with oronasal fistulas may have nasal discharge or epistaxis. Nasal parasites are highly irritating and can cause severe epistaxis and intractable head rubbing and itching. Viral diseases rarely result in epistaxis in dogs, and cats with upper respiratory infections uncommonly develop chronic nasal discharge and sneezing that results in intermittent epistaxis. Allergic (eosinophilic) and lymphoplasmacytic rhinitis are uncommon immune-mediated phenomena that are often steroid responsive. Arteriovenous malformations can rupture, causing sudden-onset epistaxis. Nasal tumors are the most common cause of epistaxis in older pets.

DIAGNOSTIC PLAN

Complete Blood Count Including Platelet Count
Regenerative anemia indicates a bone marrow response to blood loss, but with chronic epistaxis, iron deficiency and a nonregenerative anemia may occur. Schistocytes are observed with microangiopathies that occur with hemangiosarcoma and DIC. Leukocytosis is anticipated with chronic inflammation or infection, and leukopenia suggests chronic ehrlichiosis, cytotoxic drug administration, or sepsis. Thrombocytopenia is the result of increased destruction or consumption, sequestration, or decreased production of platelets. Evaluation of a blood smear may be useful while awaiting laboratory results:

drugs have been evaluated for adverse effects on platelet function in dogs and cats. Platelet dysfunction induced by aspirin,[5] carprofen,[5,6] cephalothin,[7] and hydroxyethyl starch[8] has been documented in vitro in the dog, but the in vivo effects of these drugs on platelet function are less clear. Nevertheless, it would seem prudent to avoid use of such drugs in dogs with known bleeding disorders.

Von Willebrand Disease

Von Willebrand disease (vWD), the most common inherited bleeding disorder in the dog, results from a reduction in the amount of functional plasma von Willebrand factor, leading to impaired platelet-vessel adhesion. vWD rarely causes petechiae, although ecchymoses may be observed in some dogs with vWD following trauma and surgical procedures. As with other primary hemostatic defects, typical signs of vWD include bleeding from mucosal surfaces (e.g., epistaxis, melena, hematuria) and excessive bleeding following surgery or trauma.

Vascular Disorders

In the absence of a quantitative or qualitative platelet abnormality, the presence of purpura suggests a vascular disorder. Vasculitis, secondary to infectious, inflammatory, immune-mediated, or neoplastic diseases or drug reactions, is the most common cause of vascular purpura. Some dogs with Cushing's disease also are prone to develop ecchymoses following minor trauma (e.g., cystocentesis), possibly as a result of increased protein catabolism leading to dermal and connective tissue atrophy and thus altered dermal vascular support.

PATIENT HISTORY AND PHYSICAL EXAMINATION

In a dog or cat with petechiae, ecchymoses, or both, the history may provide important clues as to the cause of the disorder. Given the many possible effects of various drugs on primary hemostasis (bone marrow suppression, immune-mediated thrombocytopenia, platelet dysfunction, and vasculitis), a complete medication history is imperative. Likewise, recent vaccinations, tick exposure, and previous or concurrent medical problems are relevant. A history of previous episodes of mucosal surface bleeding or purpura in an otherwise healthy animal or a family history of similar bleeding may be suggestive of an inherited thrombopathia.

Given that thrombocytopenia, thrombopathia, and vascular disorders may be associated with an underlying disease, a complete physical examination is essential. Peripheral lymphadenopathy, hepatomegaly, or splenomegaly (or a combination of these abnormalities) may indicate an underlying infectious, inflammatory, or neoplastic disease. Petechiae are most readily found on mucous membranes of the gingiva, prepuce, and vulva, as well as on sparsely haired skin of the ventral abdomen (Web Figure 76-1) and pinnae (Web Figure 76-2).

After phlebotomy, ecchymoses are commonly observed around the venipuncture site.

DIAGNOSTIC APPROACH

Because thrombocytopenia is the most common cause of petechiae and ecchymoses, the initial laboratory evaluation should always include a platelet count (Figure 76-1).

Spontaneous bleeding is not typically noted unless the platelet count is <30,000/µL, and platelet counts are often less than 10,000/µL in dogs with IMT. Electronic particle counters can quickly and accurately perform platelet counts in the dog. However, cell counting instruments with a threshold function to separate platelets and red blood cells (RBCs) by volume may not be accurate in the cat (considerable overlap exists between erythrocyte and platelet volumes), resulting in spuriously low platelet counts. In addition, feline platelets tend to clump. Evaluation of a blood smear is recommended for all cats and for dogs in which the automated platelet count is low. In an emergency situation, evaluation of a blood smear to obtain an estimate of platelet number is sufficient; 10 to 20 platelets per oil immersion field are deemed adequate. In addition to providing an estimate of platelet number, evaluation of a blood smear may reveal evidence of RBC regeneration (polychromasia, anisocytosis, and macrocytosis), blood parasites, RBC agglutination, spherocytosis, or RBC fragments.

If the dog or cat is thrombocytopenic, evaluation of the complete blood cell count (CBC) to determine if other cytopenias are present will aid in formulation of a list of differential diagnoses and a focused diagnostic plan. Pancytopenia is most suggestive of bone marrow disease, whereas concurrent anemia and thrombocytopenia may be the result of blood loss anemia due to thrombocytopenia, immune-mediated destruction of both RBC and platelets, or bone marrow disease. Newly synthesized or reticulated platelets can be identified using the ribonucleic acid (RNA)–binding fluorescent dye thiazole orange and flow cytometry. Reticulated platelets lose RNA within 24 hours after entering the peripheral circulation. The percentage of reticulated platelets is typically increased in dogs with IMT.[9] However, the absolute numbers may be within reference range because of the low total number of platelets.[9] The assay for measurement of reticulated platelets is rapid and less invasive than obtaining bone marrow samples to evaluate thrombopoiesis, although it is not routinely available through commercial diagnostic laboratories.

Assessment of coagulation is indicated in the evaluation of a thrombocytopenic patient to rule out a combined hemostatic disorder (e.g., disseminated intravascular coagulation). Point-of-care coagulation analyzers (e.g., IDEXX Coag Dx Analyzer) are now readily available to provide quick and accurate measurements of prothrombin time (PT) and activated partial thromboplastin time (aPTT). Alternatively, an activated clotting time (ACT), which assesses the intrinsic and common pathways of the coagulation cascade and thus provides similar information to the aPTT, may be performed. Normal ACT in the dog is 60 to 110 seconds and in the cat is 50 to 75 seconds. In dogs and cats with severe thrombocytopenia (<10,000/µL), the ACT may be slightly prolonged by approximately 10 seconds because of decreased availability of platelet phospholipid to support coagulation.

A bone marrow aspirate or biopsy is indicated in dogs and cats with pancytopenia, nonregenerative anemia and thrombocytopenia, persistent thrombocytopenia despite therapy, or atypical cells noted in the peripheral blood. A bone marrow aspirate is not necessary in all patients with IMT, but should be considered when the platelet count has not increased within 5 to 7 days of initiating immunosuppressive therapy. Despite severe thrombocytopenia, excessive bleeding is rarely a complication of bone marrow aspiration or biopsy.

The buccal mucosal bleeding time (BMBT) evaluates only primary hemostasis or the platelet-vessel interaction. A BMBT is indicated in animals presenting with petechiae and ecchymoses that are not thrombocytopenic. The BMBT is performed using a spring-loaded device that is standardized to produce uniform incisions. Bleeding time templates are available with one or two blades and produce uniform incisions

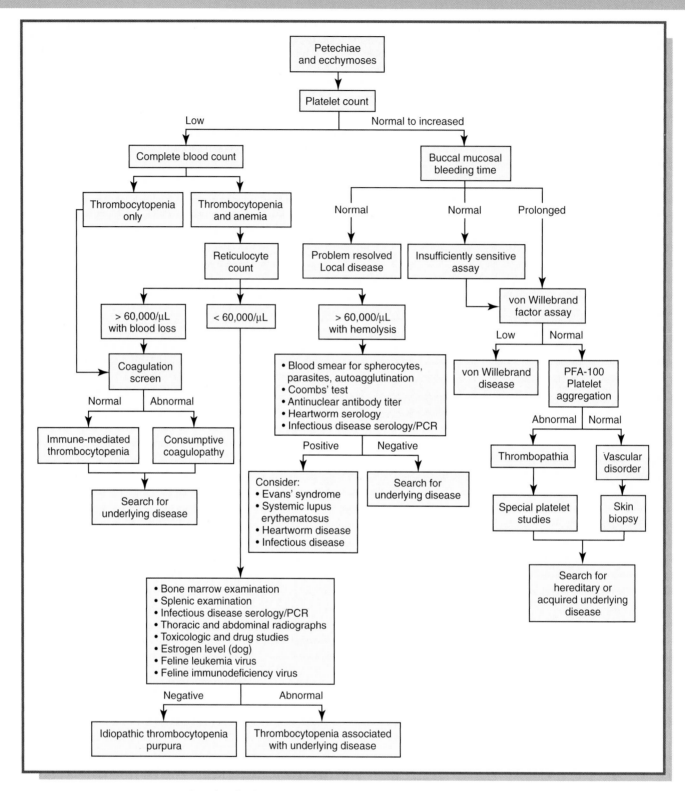

Figure 76-1 Algorithm for diagnostic approach to petechiae and ecchymoses. *PCR,* Polymerase chain reaction; *PFA,* platelet function analyzer.

approximately 5 mm long and 1 mm deep (clinicians should not use blades with only 0.5 mm depth). Single-blade devices are recommended for cats and small dogs. Normal BMBT in the dog is less than 4 minutes and in the cat is less than 2 minutes. The effect of a low hematocrit (HCT) on bleeding time is often neglected, but ample evidence in the literature

indicates an inverse relationship between HCT and bleeding time (the lower the HCT, the more prolonged the bleeding time) in humans.[10] Altered rheological properties of the blood and a reduced source of adenosine diphosphate (ADP) (RBCs release ADP) to activate platelets are mechanisms proposed for the prolongation of bleeding time in severely anemic patients. A prolongation of the BMBT in an animal with a normal platelet count and HCT suggests a thrombopathia, vWD, or a vascular disorder. Because vWD is much more common in the dog than intrinsic platelet function defects or vascular disorders, measurement of plasma von Willebrand factor concentration is recommended before platelet function testing, particularly in dogs being evaluated for development of ecchymoses following surgery (Web Figure 77-3) rather than spontaneous formation of petechiae.

A point-of-care platelet function analyzer, the PFA-100 (Dade Behring, Miami, Fla.), assesses platelet adhesion and aggregation under conditions of high shear forces in citrated whole blood (800 µL per test sample) and provides results in less than 10 minutes. As with the BMBT, results of the PFA-100 are dependent on platelet count and HCT. This instrument, now available at a few veterinary teaching hospitals, has been useful in quickly identifying dogs with vWD and some thrombopathias.[11] Measurement of plasma vWF concentration is necessary to differentiate vWD, a platelet adhesion defect, from a platelet aggregation disorder. However, replacement of the test dog's citrated plasma with normal canine plasma will correct the PFA-100 closure time in dogs with vWD but not a thrombopathia, allowing clinicians to make timely medical management decisions while awaiting confirmatory test results.[12]

While specialized tests of platelet function necessitate a dog or cat traveling to one of the few veterinary institutions offering such diagnostics, recent identification of the mutations causing several hereditary thrombopathias in the dog has greatly simplified the process. DNA testing (using 1 mL EDTA blood) is now available through Auburn University for diagnosis of thrombopathias in the Great Pyrenees, Otterhound, Bassett Hound, Spitz, and Landseer.

TREATMENT

Medical management of patients with petechiae and ecchymoses varies widely. Treatment is aimed at the underlying disorder (e.g., rickettsial infections, neoplasia, immune-mediated diseases). Because IMT is the most common cause of severe thrombocytopenia in dogs with resultant formation of petechiae and ecchymoses, most thrombocytopenic dogs should be initially treated with doxycycline and prednisone pending results of diagnostic tests. In some cases, discontinuation of medications (e.g., methimazole, sulfonamides) may be all that is necessary to resolve the primary hemostatic disorder.

Dogs and cats presenting with petechiae and ecchymoses as the sole form of bleeding rarely require blood transfusion support. However, if concurrent mucosal surface bleeding exists, particularly into the gastrointestinal tract, leading to anemia, transfusion of packed RBCs may be indicated to provide additional oxygen-carrying support. Platelet transfusions in the form of fresh whole blood, platelet-rich plasma, or platelet concentrate are indicated in life-threatening or uncontrolled bleeding. A small amount of bleeding into the brain, myocardium, lungs, or oropharynx could have devastating consequences without resulting in anemia. Platelet transfusions are generally not recommended in patients with IMT (unless uncontrolled or life-threatening bleeding occurs) because the transfused platelets have a short life span (typically destroyed within minutes to hours).

REFERENCES

The reference list can be found on the companion Expert Consult Web site at *www.expertconsult.com*.

CHAPTER 77

Electrolyte Disorders: Sodium (Hyper/Hyponatremia)

Noemi Benitah

TERMINOLOGY AND NORMAL PHYSIOLOGY

Total body water represents about 60 percent of body weight and is about two thirds intracellular and one third extracellular. The extracellular fluid (ECF) is divided into the interstitial fluid ($3/4$ of the ECF), the blood plasma or intravascular fluid ($1/4$ of the ECF), and the transcellular fluid (e.g., synovial fluid). The ECF volume is directly dependent on body sodium content. A disruption in water balance results in hypernatremia or hyponatremia.

Osmolality refers to the concentration of osmotically active particles in a solution.[1] *Tonicity* refers to the ability of a solution to initiate movement of water and can be thought of as *effective* osmolality.[2] Plasma osmolality can be measured using an osmometer or the approximate osmolality can be estimated using the following equation:

$$\text{Calculated plasma osmolality (mOsm/kg)} = 2(Na^+[mEq/L]) + [\text{Blood urea nitrogen (mg/dL)}/2.8] + [\text{Glucose (mg/dL)}/18]$$

Normal plasma osmolality ranges from 290 to 310 mOsm/kg in dogs and 290 to 330 mOsm/kg in cats.[3, 4]

HYPERNATREMIA

ETIOLOGY

Hypernatremia is defined as a rise in the plasma sodium concentration to a value exceeding reference limits, usually approximately 155 mEq/L (in dogs) or 162 mEq/L (in cats).[1] Hypernatremia may result from water loss or an excessive sodium intake (Box 77-1, Figure 77-1).

Box • 77-1

Causes of Hypernatremia

Pure Water Loss (Normovolemia)
Diabetes insipidus (central or nephrogenic)
Inadequate water intake (hypodipsia, adipsia)
   Neurologic disease
   Altered set-point in the osmoreceptors in the
      hypothalamus affecting antidiuretic hormone (ADH)
      release
   Defect in the thirst mechanism
Increased insensible fluid losses (respiratory losses (panting)
   due to heat stroke, fever, exercise, seizures)
Inadequate access to water

Hypotonic Fluid Loss (Hypovolemia)
Extrarenal causes
   Gastrointestinal loss (vomiting, diarrhea)
   Third space loss (peritonitis, pancreatitis)
   Cutaneous loss (burns)
Renal causes
   Osmotic diuresis (diabetes mellitus)
   Diuretic use (corticosteroids, furosemide)
   Renal disease (polyuric acute, postobstructive diuresis,
      chronic)

Sodium Gain (Hypervolemia)
Excessive salt ingestion (salt poisoning)
Iatrogenic
   Hyperosmolar intravenous solutions administration
      (hypertonic saline, sodium bicarbonate, parenteral
      nutrition)
   Sodium phosphate–containing enemas
Primary hyperaldosteronism
Hyperadrenocorticism

Modified from DiBartola SP: Disorders of sodium and water: hypernatremia and hyponatremia. In DiBartola SP, editor: Fluid, electrolyte and acid-base disorders in small animal practice, ed 3, Philadelphia, 2006, Saunders, p 47.

A deficit of pure water (uncommon) may occur with diabetes insipidus (central[5-9] or nephrogenic[10-12]), inadequate water intake (primary hypodipsia,[13-19] essential hypernatremia[20]), or increased insensible fluid losses. Hypernatremia due to pure water loss rarely occurs in a conscious animal with normal thirst mechanism and access to water. Loss of hypotonic fluids (common) can result from extrarenal or renal causes.[1] Sodium gain (uncommon) may result from excessive salt ingestion,[21-25] sea water ingestion,[26] administration of hyperosmolar solutions (hypertonic saline,[27] sodium bicarbonate, sodium phosphate–containing enemas[28]), primary hyperaldosteronism,[29] and hyperadrenocorticism.[30,31]

CLINICAL SIGNS

The brain is the organ most obviously affected by hypernatremia. Hypernatremia and hyperosmolality cause water to move out of the brain cells into the extracellular space causing a rapid decrease of brain volume (neuronal dehydration). This can result in rupture of cerebral vessels causing focal intracerebral hemorrhage. Severity of neurologic signs may be related more to the rapidity of the rise in sodium than to the magnitude of hypernatremia.[1] When hypernatremia is gradual and develops slowly, the brain cells can produce osmotically active solutes (called idiogenic osmoles) to adapt to hypertonicity, which, in turn, minimizes dehydration of the brain. Clinical signs of hypernatremia are usually observed when the sodium concentration exceeds 170 mEq/L (plasma osmolality > 350 mOsm/kg).[21,22,32] These include lethargy, disorientation, muscle weakness and fasciculations, behavior changes, ataxia, seizures, coma, and death in severe cases.* If hypernatremia is due to hypotonic losses, clinical signs of hypovolemia can be noted on physical exam. If hypernatremia is due to sodium excess, clinical signs of hypervolemia may be noted.

TREATMENT

The first goal in treating a hypernatremic dog or cat is to restore the ECF volume toward normal slowly to avoid neurologic complications. Correction of the serum sodium concentration at a rate of less than 0.5 mEq/L/hr, minimizes the fluid shift from the ECF to the ICF, reducing the risk of brain cell swelling, cerebral edema, and increased intracranial pressure.[35] Oral water administration is preferable for correcting water deficits. Fluid administered intravenously is necessary when oral administration is not possible. If a patient's neurologic status deteriorates after initiating treatment to correct hypernatremia, cerebral edema should be suspected and the rate of fluid administration should be reduced. The use of mannitol and/or furosemide may be warranted for their osmotic and diuretic effects, respectively. If a dog or cat is hypovolemic due to hypotonic losses, isotonic replacement fluid should be used first to restore ECF volume and correct hypovolemia. If poor perfusion persists despite crystalloid therapy, a colloid can be administered.

Once the ECF volume has been expanded, hypotonic fluids can be administered to provide maintenance fluid needs. Free water deficit can be replaced by giving 5% dextrose in water (D5W) intravenously. Typically, glucose is metabolized once it enters cells. Therefore, giving D5W is equivalent to administration of water. The formula for determining the volume of any water deficit is:

$$\text{water deficit (L)} = 0.6 \times \text{lean body weight (kg)} \times [(\text{plasma Na}/140) - 1]$$

Serial monitoring of the patient's serum sodium concentration is essential. Dogs and cats with sodium overload are difficult to treat because hypernatremia needs to be corrected without further increasing the ECF volume and causing pulmonary congestion and edema. Administration of a loop diuretic can promote natriuresis and minimize the risk of pulmonary and cerebral edema.

HYPONATREMIA

ETIOLOGY

Hyponatremia is defined as a decrease in the plasma sodium concentration to a value below reference limits (usually less than 137 mEq/L). Hyponatremia may result from increased water gain, or an excessive sodium loss, or both (Box 77-2, Figure 77-2).

Hyponatremia can be classified according to hydration state, plasma osmolality, and plasma volume status.

---

*References 13, 17, 21, 22, 26, 32-34.

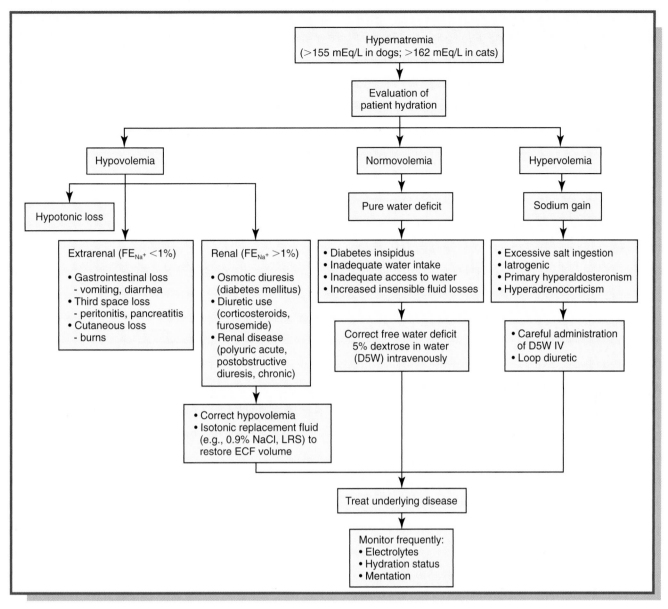

Figure 77-1 Algorithm for the clinical approach to the diagnosis and treatment of hypernatremia. *ECF,* Extracellular fluid; *FE$_{Na^+}$,* Fractional excretion of sodium = (Urine sodium/Plasma sodium) × (Plasma creatinine/Urine creatinine) × 100; *LRS,* lactated Ringer's solution.

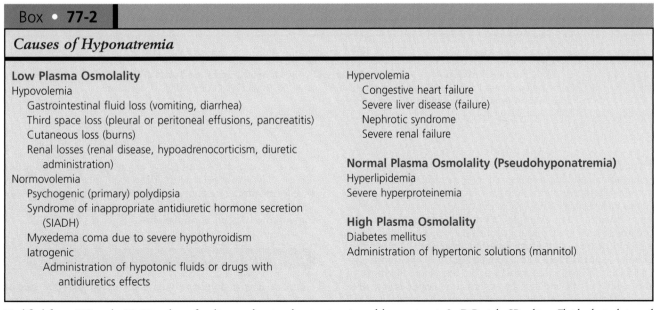

Box • 77-2

Causes of Hyponatremia

Low Plasma Osmolality
Hypovolemia
   Gastrointestinal fluid loss (vomiting, diarrhea)
   Third space loss (pleural or peritoneal effusions, pancreatitis)
   Cutaneous loss (burns)
   Renal losses (renal disease, hypoadrenocorticism, diuretic administration)
Normovolemia
   Psychogenic (primary) polydipsia
   Syndrome of inappropriate antidiuretic hormone secretion (SIADH)
Myxedema coma due to severe hypothyroidism
Iatrogenic
   Administration of hypotonic fluids or drugs with antidiuretics effects

Hypervolemia
   Congestive heart failure
   Severe liver disease (failure)
   Nephrotic syndrome
   Severe renal failure

Normal Plasma Osmolality (Pseudohyponatremia)
Hyperlipidemia
Severe hyperproteinemia

High Plasma Osmolality
Diabetes mellitus
Administration of hypertonic solutions (mannitol)

Modified from DiBartola SP: Disorders of sodium and water: hypernatremia and hyponatremia In DiBartola SP, editor: Fluid, electrolyte and acid-base disorders in small animal practice (fluid therapy in small animal practice), ed 3, Philadelphia, 2006, Saunders, p 47.

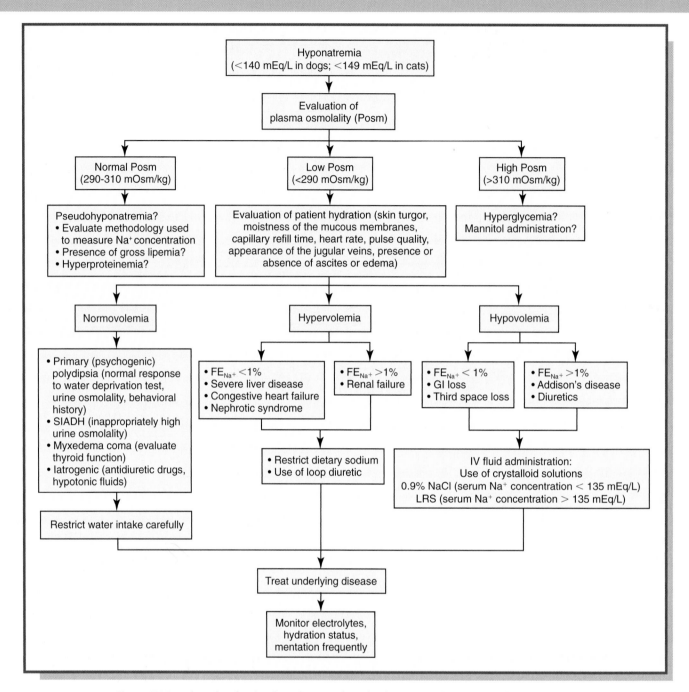

Figure 77-2 Algorithm for the clinical approach to the diagnosis and treatment of hyponatremia. FE_{Na^+}, Fractional excretion of sodium = (Urine sodium / Plasma sodium) × (Plasma creatinine / Urine creatinine) × 100; *GI*, gastrointestinal; *LRS*, lactated Ringer's solution; *SIADH*, syndrome of inappropriate antidiuretic hormone secretion.

Hyponatremia must be differentiated from pseudohyponatremia, which is a measured hyponatremia (as a result of certain laboratory methodologies) in the presence of normal plasma osmolality. With severe hyperglycemia caused by diabetes mellitus, for example, dilutional hyponatremia with measured increased plasma osmolality can be noted due a water shift from the intracellular compartment to the extracellular compartment.[36] Hyponatremia and hypoosmolality can occur if losses are replaced by hypotonic fluids or if the ability of the kidneys to excrete free water is impaired due either to secretion of antidiuretic hormone (ADH)

despite serum hypoosmolality or impaired renal diluting ability. Hyponatremia with decreased plasma osmolality (<290 mOsm/kg) may occur in a patient with hypovolemia,[37-42] hypervolemia due to a decreased effective circulating volume,[43,44] and normovolemia.[45-51]

CLINICAL SIGNS

Clinical signs of hyponatremia are variable but are mainly neurologic. The signs include lethargy, anorexia, vomiting, weakness, incoordination, disorientation, seizures, and coma.[52,53] These CNS signs are due to cerebral edema developing as changes in plasma osmolality cause fluid to shift from the extracellular to the intracellular space.[54] The onset and severity of clinical signs vary and depend on the rate of decrease of the sodium, but also on the degree of hyponatremia. Clinical signs are usually observed when the sodium concentration falls below 125 mEq/L. With mild or chronic hyponatremia, signs are often absent. With acute hyponatremia, the decrease in plasma osmolality is more rapid then the brain's ability to compensate for the shift of water into the neurons and so clinical signs are noted.

TREATMENT

The diagnosis and management of the underlying cause should be a priority. Use of crystalloid solutions is recommended as a fluid replacement for the dehydrated, hypovolemic patient.

To avoid neurologic complications such as myelinolysis, hyponatremia correction should not exceed 12 mEq/L during the first 24 hours.[55-59] The following formula can be used to calculate serum sodium deficits:

$$0.6 \times \text{body weight (kg)} \times$$
$$[\text{normal serum Na}^+ \text{ (mEq/L)} -$$
$$\text{patient's serum Na}^+ \text{ (mEq/L)}]$$

Serial monitoring of serum sodium concentration is necessary. Water intake should be carefully restricted to a volume less than urine output in normovolemic patients with hyponatremia. A loop diuretic and dietary sodium restriction can be considered in overhydrated patients.

REFERENCES

The reference list can be found on the companion Expert Consult Web site at *www.expertconsult.com*.

CHAPTER 78

Electrolyte Disorders: Potassium (Hyper/Hypokalemia)

Edward C. Feldman
David Buchanan Church

Dogs and cats have approximately 50 mEq of potassium per kilogram of body weight within their systems. About 98% of this potassium is intracellular and a small amount is extracellular. In health, serum potassium concentrations are exquisitely maintained at about 3.6 to 5.6 mEq/L. The large concentration gradient between intracellular and extracellular potassium favors transfer from cells, opposite to that which exists for sodium. Maintenance of high intracellular potassium and high extracellular sodium concentrations is accomplished with sodium-potassium "pumps" located in cell membranes. This is vital for normal health. Serum potassium excess or deficiency may cause abnormalities in many biologic processes, including cell volume; acid-base status; electrophysiologic properties of cells; and synthesis of RNA, protein, and glycogen. Too much or too little potassium in the vascular space is worrisome and, if severe and untreated, will result in death. Direct assay of serum electrolyte concentrations is specific and sensitive for diagnosing hyperkalemia or hypokalemia.

HYPERKALEMIA

Recognizing the Problem
There are no consistently obvious clues to the presence of hyperkalemia on history or physical examination. One must assume that all ill dogs and cats have serum electrolyte abnormalities and that serum chemistry analysis can reveal potentially life-threatening conditions. An alternate to serum chemistry analysis for rapid identification of severe hyperkalemia is with an electrocardiogram. If P waves are not seen on an electrocardiogram taken on an ill pet, and the heart rate is

slow, severe hyperkalemia should be suspected. Invariably, the serum potassium concentration in a dog or cat without P waves is >7.5 mEq/L.

DIFFERENTIAL DIAGNOSIS (Figure 78-1)

Dogs and cats with nonadrenal causes of hyperkalemia must be distinguished from those with hypoadrenocorticism (Addison's disease). However, the acute management of hyperkalemia is similar regardless of cause, except that an animal with urinary obstruction or anuria must have either of those specific problems relieved. Clinicians must be certain before diagnosing hypoadrenocorticism and pursuing lifelong therapy.

Hypoadrenocorticism (Addison's Disease) The classic electrolyte alterations in Addison's disease are hyponatremia, hypochloremia, and hyperkalemia. These abnormalities are due primarily to aldosterone deficiency, causing failure of the kidneys to conserve sodium and excrete potassium. Deficiency in adrenocortical hormones allows greater amounts of sodium to pass into the intracellular compartment as intracellular potassium concentrations decrease. Hyperkalemia results from a shift of potassium from intracellular to extracellular compartments and from a decrease in renal excretion. The former condition results from a loss of aldosterone effects on the sodium-potassium pump. In addition to the aldosterone deficiency, acidosis also enhances shift of potassium from the intracellular to the extracellular space. Decreased potassium exchange for sodium in the distal renal tubule leads to decreased urinary potassium excretion

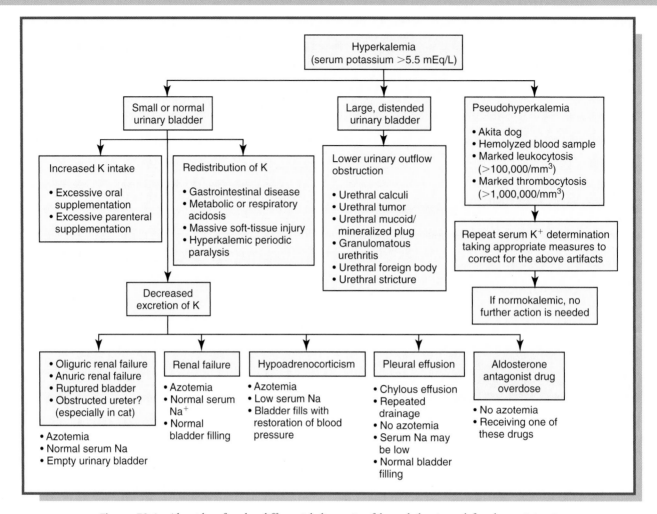

Figure 78-1 Algorithm for the differential diagnosis of hyperkalemia and for determining its cause. (From Feldman EC, Nelson RW: Canine and feline endocrinology and reproduction, ed 3, St Louis, 2004, Saunders.)

and increased sodium excretion. The shift in electrolytes between body compartments may be partly corrected by the administration of cortisol, but aldosterone, or another mineralocorticoid, must be given to prevent renal loss of sodium and retention of potassium.

Serum potassium concentrations in dogs at the time hypoadrenocorticism is diagnosed vary from normal to extremely increased values that induce clinically obvious cardiac rhythm disturbances. More than 90% of hypoadrenal dogs have serum potassium concentrations greater than 5.5 mEq/L at the time of diagnosis. Dogs with ACTH deficiency should not have hyperkalemia. The sodium-to-potassium ratio has frequently been used as a diagnostic tool to aid in gaining a suspicion or in specific identification of dogs with adrenal insufficiency. The normal ratio varies between 27:1 and 40:1. Values are often below 27:1 and may be below 20:1 in dogs with primary hypoadrenocorticism. Ratios are nonspecific and are not recommended for confirming a diagnosis. However, determination of serum electrolyte concentrations from dogs or cats that are extremely ill and/or suspected of having adrenal insufficiency is of paramount importance.

Urinary Tract Disorders   The most common nonadrenal causes of hyperkalemia are renal failure, urethral obstruction, rupture of the bladder, or avulsion of a ureter. These problems prevent excretion of potassium. Hyperkalemia is not common in chronic renal failure unless the dog or cat

is severely dehydrated, anuric, or oliguric. After rupture or avulsion of any component within the urinary system, urine leakage into the peritoneal cavity or into the sublumbar space prevents potassium and urea excretion, two parameters that quickly become severely increased.

Gastrointestinal Disease   Gastrointestinal disorders can cause serum electrolyte abnormalities consistent with Addison's disease. These disorders include intestinal parasitism (trichuriasis, ancylostomiasis), intestinal infection (salmonellosis), perforated duodenal ulcers, and gastric torsion. Similar serum electrolyte abnormalities have been encountered in some puppies with parvovirus infection or canine distemper. Severe malabsorption syndromes occasionally cause hyperkalemia or hyponatremia or both. Dogs with trichuriasis, hyponatremia, and hyperkalmeia do not have decreased serum concentrations of aldosterone.

Acidosis, Pancreatitis, and/or Trauma   Rapid cellular release of potassium and resultant hyperkalemia may occur as a result of severe acidosis or tissue destruction after surgery, crush injury, or extensive infection. Although not commonly associated with hyperkalemia, examples of disorders that can cause this disturbance are pancreatitis, diabetic ketoacidosis (although total body concentrations are usually decreased), aortic thrombosis in cats, and rhabdomyolysis secondary to heat stroke or prolonged exercise in dogs or cats. These conditions may also be associated with impaired renal excretion of potassium.

Pleural Effusions Hyperkalemia and hyponatremia have been identified in some dogs with chylous pleural effusion after repeated pleural drainage procedures. The incidence of this complication in dogs with pleural effusion appears to be low because only 2 of 17 dogs with experimentally induced chylothorax had hyperkalemia and hyponatremia. Hyperkalemia and hyponatremia may result from the failure of renal tubular sodium to enter cells in the distal nephron, thereby diminishing sodium resorption and subsequently decreasing potassium excretion into the renal tubule.

Miscellaneous Disorders Low sodium:potassium ratios have been described in dogs with pyometra, perhaps as a result of acidosis, gastrointestinal disturbance, and/or severe dehydration. Hyperkalemia and hyponatremia have also been described in a few near-term pregnant Greyhounds, in several dogs with disseminated neoplasia, rarely in dogs with congestive heart failure, and in one dog with mushroom toxicity. Liver failure could cause similar electrolyte abnormalities, perhaps secondary to interference with the renin-angiotensin-aldosterone system, because angiotensin I is synthesized in the liver.

Iatrogenic and/or Nonadrenal Drug Therapy Excess potassium intake is an uncommon cause of hyperkalemia except in dogs or cats with renal insufficiency. Hyperkalemia can develop with overzealous potassium supplementation in IV fluids, using salt substitutes, or giving parenteral feeding solutions high in potassium. Potassium-sparing diuretics, angiotensin-converting enzyme inhibitors, and nonsteroidal anti-inflammatory drugs also have the potential to cause mild hyperkalemia.

Adrenocortical Destruction Secondary to Mitotane (o,p'-DDD) or Trilostane Therapy Dogs with hyperadrenocorticism (Cushing's syndrome) overdosed with o,p'-DDD or trilostane can develop hypocortisolemia. This may be the most common cause of hypocortisolemia in veterinary practice. Clinical signs include depression, anorexia, vomiting, and diarrhea. Serum electrolyte concentrations are usually (but not always) within reference ranges. The zones of the adrenal cortex (zonae fasciculata and reticularis), which produce cortisol, are more sensitive to the cytotoxic effects of o,p'-DDD than is the zona glomerulosa, which is responsible for producing aldosterone. Classic "Addison's disease" (including hyperkalemia) secondary to destruction of all three adrenocortical zones can develop from o,p'-DDD or trilostane overdose.

Artifact (non-Akita) Severe hypernatremia may falsely increase potassium measurements performed with dry-reagent analysis. Hypertonicity has been suggested as a cause for hyperkalemia. Extreme leukocytosis (>100,000 mm^3) or thrombocytosis (>1,000,000 mm^3) may allow sufficient amounts of potassium to be released into the serum during clotting to falsely elevate the serum potassium concentration. In the latter situation, potassium increases in the serum as blood is clotting, an in vitro phenomenon.

Artifact (the Akita) The Akita breed appears to have unusually high red blood cell concentrations of potassium. In one study, six of eight Akitas had high erythrocyte potassium concentrations and plasma from these dogs displayed pseudohyperkalemia after being refrigerated in contact with red cells for longer than 4 hours. The rise in serum potassium concentration (pseudohyperkalemia) correlated with duration of red cell contact and was accompanied by a decrease in serum sodium concentration.

TREATMENT

Background The finding of the classic "Addisonian" electrolyte abnormalities or of hyperkalemia without a decrease in the serum sodium concentration or vice versa (decreases in serum sodium without an increase in the serum potassium concentration) should prompt immediate therapy. The assumption that a dog or cat may have Addison's disease is warranted and may be lifesaving. If the provisional diagnosis of hypoadrenocorticism, based on serum electrolyte concentrations, is incorrect, emergency therapy is rarely harmful.

Aggressive management of hypoadrenocorticism is not significantly different from that for life-threatening renal or gastrointestinal diseases. However, the limitations of a diagnosis based solely on serum electrolyte determinations must be realized. Reliance on serum electrolyte concentrations as the sole criterion for diagnosing adrenal insufficiency can be misleading because there are situations associated with normal serum electrolyte concentrations or with nonadrenal hyperkalemia/hyponatremia. First, primary adrenal insufficiency may be slowly progressive and initially associated with normal serum electrolyte concentrations; second, dogs with pituitary failure continue to secrete aldosterone (normal electrolytes); and third, hyperkalemia and hyponatremia are not pathognomonic for adrenal insufficiency (see Figure 78-1).

Specific Therapy for Hypoadrenocorticism Therapy need not be overzealous when serum potassium concentrations are less than 6.5 mEq/L, whereas intensive therapy may be vital in dogs and cats with serum potassium concentrations greater than 7.5 mEq/L. Intravenous 0.9% normal saline is a reliable treatment for attempting to lower the serum potassium concentrations rapidly. Virtually every dog in hypoadrenocortical crisis that we have treated has received only rapid administration of 0.9% normal saline (with or without glucose) during the first hour of treatment. This approach *alone* has resulted in dramatic clinical, biochemical, and ECG improvement. IV saline rapidly corrects the life-threatening complications of hypoadrenocorticism (e.g., hyponatremia, hypochloremia, hypovolemia, hypotension, hyperkalemia, and azotemia). The serum potassium concentration decreases, in part, because of the dilutional effect provided by saline (which contains no potassium) and by improved renal perfusion. Increased renal blood flow allows further excretion of potassium into the urine. If sodium bicarbonate therapy is used, it will increase the serum sodium concentration and help shift potassium ions into the intracellular space. The other therapeutic mainstay for this condition is mineralocorticoid. For this, desoxycorticosterone pivalate (DOCP) is given at a dose of 2.2 mg/kg IM or SQ. Neither insulin nor calcium therapy has been employed for dogs or cats in hypoadrenal crisis, but may be of value in treating severe, acute hyperkalemia of urinary obstruction and some other conditions.

Nonspecific Methods for Decreasing Serum Potassium Concentrations Hyperkalemia may be treated by antagonizing the effects of excess potassium on cell membranes. Such measures are most often employed in dogs and cats with severe hyperkalemia secondary to urinary obstruction. Calcium gluconate drives potassium into cells. One can administer 2 to 10 mL of a 10% solution IV, slowly. This begins to have effect within minutes and lasts less than an hour. Hyperkalemia decreases cellular electrical *resting* potential. Calcium decreases the *threshold* potential, thus normalizing the difference between the two potentials. This may transiently protect against cardiac disturbances associated with hyperkalemia. The electrocardiogram must be monitored for arrhythmias induced by overzealous therapy.

Both glucose and bicarbonate also have the potential to drive potassium from the extracellular to the intracellular space. Administered glucose stimulates insulin secretion. Insulin, in turn, drives glucose into cells. Potassium follows glucose into cells, decreasing its extracellular concentration. The effect of administering 5%, 10%, or even 50% dextrose begins within an hour and may last several hours. Some have recommended administering insulin to cats with severe hyperkalemia secondary to urethral obstruction (0.5 to 1.0 U/kg, IM, regular insulin plus 2 g dextrose per unit of insulin, IV) to ensure potassium lowering. Administration of insulin certainly is more dangerous than that of glucose alone, since iatrogenic hypoglycemia can follow. This is not a concern if only glucose is given. Sodium bicarbonate (1 to 2 mEq/kg, IV) works by driving potassium ions into cells as hydrogen ions leave cells to titrate administered bicarbonate. Bicarbonate begins to work within an hour and lasts several hours. Atropine has been given to increase the pace of the sinoatrial node if a slow sinoventricular rhythm is present and due to hyperkalemia.

HYPOKALEMIA

Recognizing the Problem
Hypokalemia, defined as a serum potassium concentration of less than 3.6 mEq/L, may occur with an increased, normal, or decreased total body potassium.

DIFFERENTIAL DIAGNOSIS AND EVALUATION

Anorexia, vomiting, and diarrhea cause depletion of body potassium and account for many cases of hypokalemia in dogs and cats. Decreased intake of potassium is unlikely to be the sole cause for this disturbance in any dog or cat. Polyuric disorders (e.g., diabetes mellitus, chronic renal insufficiency) may cause hypokalemia. Long-term therapy for chronic renal failure is commonly associated with hypokalemia in cats, more so than dogs. Serious hypokalemia may occur in dogs or cats being treated for diabetic ketoacidosis (DKA). In treating a dog or cat for DKA, IV fluids, glucose, insulin, and bicarbonate can each cause hypokalemia. Together, these therapies can cause life-threatening hypokalemia.

Hypokalemia has been documented in hypothermic animals and after rattlesnake envenomation. A syndrome that includes muscle weakness and hypokalemia has been reported in related 4- to 12-month-old Burmese cats. Some forms of renal tubular acidosis are associated with hypokalemia. Rarely, dogs and cats have been diagnosed as having an adrenocortical tumor secreting excess aldosterone (mineralocorticoid excess) and causing secondary muscle weakness due to hypokalemia as well as hypertension due to sodium retention that increases water load and blood volume. Pituitary- or adrenal-tumor—dependent hyperadrenocorticism is not typically a cause of hypokalemia. Hypokalemia commonly occurs, if not treated, during diuresis after relief of urinary obstruction in dogs, but even more often in cats. A history of diuretic administration (loop, osmotic, or volume) may be noted in hypokalemic pets. History and physical examination findings depend on specific cause, but severe potassium depletion usually causes muscular weakness. It may also cause ileus. Polydipsia-polyuria may occur due to a defect in renal concentrating ability. Laboratory evaluation of a hypokalemic pet usually depends

on the cause of the disorder. A hemogram, serum biochemical profile, and urinalysis are indicated. As previously mentioned, acid-base status may affect extracellular potassium concentrations. Measurement of blood gases and pH, or plasma total CO_2, may help in the interpretation of hypokalemia. Alkalosis causes reduction of serum potassium and acidosis the opposite. Frequent measurement of serum potassium is necessary to assess response to treatment and to avoid continuing hypokalemia or iatrogenic hyperkalemia.

TREATMENT

Correction of hypokalemia depends on whether body potassium is decreased or normal (redistribution of potassium). Since 98% of body potassium is located intracellularly and is not practically available for measurement, determining whether or not a "whole-body potassium deficit" is present is difficult. However, it is the extracellular potassium concentration that is vital. Although mild cellular potassium depletion can occur with a normal serum potassium concentration, especially in acidotic animals, most dogs and cats with significant body potassium depletion will become hypokalemic. Hypokalemia usually indicates cellular potassium depletion but can also be caused by redistribution of potassium from extracellular to intracellular fluid (as seen in alkalosis and insulin therapy).

The rate and route of potassium replacement will depend on the severity of clinical signs and cause of potassium loss. Remember that IV saline and dextrose in water (D5W) solutions contain no potassium while the 4 mEq/L of potassium found in lactated Ringer's solution is virtually the same as that found in saline and D5W. Maintenance fluid therapy should contain 20 to 30 mEq/L of potassium. Before administering potassium, one should make certain that urine production is adequate. It may be safer to rehydrate a pet with low potassium fluids and establish the presence of urine production prior to administering potassium-enriched solutions. Life-threatening hypokalemia is rare; therefore, aggressive IV potassium replacement is usually not necessary and is potentially dangerous (it can lead to hyperkalemic cardiotoxicity).

Table • 78-1

Guidelines for Potassium Supplementation in IV Fluids

SERUM K⁺ (mEq/L)	TYPICAL GUIDELINES K⁺ SUPPLEMENT/LITER OF FLUIDS	GUIDELINES FOR DKA K⁺ SUPPLEMENT/LITER OF FLUIDS
>5.0	Wait	Wait
4.0-5.5	10	20-30
3.5-4.0	20	30-40
3.0-3.5	30	40-50
2.5-3.0	40	50-60
2.0-2.5	60	60-80
<2.0	80	80

From Feldman EC, Nelson RW: Canine and feline endocrinology and reproduction, ed 3, St Louis, 2004, Saunders.
Total hourly potassium administration should not exceed 0.5 mEq/kg body weight.

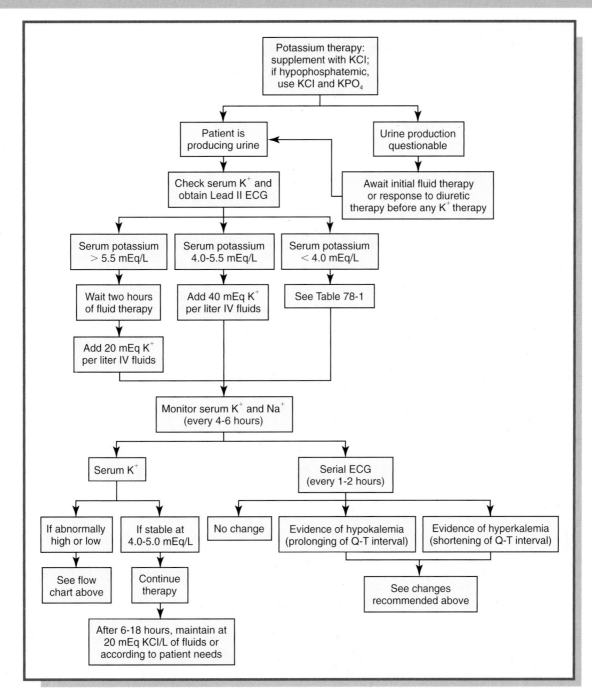

Figure 78-2   Potassium therapy in the management of diabetic ketoacidosis. (From Feldman EC, Nelson RW: Canine and feline endocrinology and reproduction, ed 3, St Louis, 2004, Saunders.)

Potassium given IV should be administered at a rate not exceeding about 0.5 mEq potassium/kg/hr. However, aggressive IV potassium therapy is warranted in conditions such as diabetics being treated for ketoacidosis (Table 78-1). This challenge presents an example for managing severe and life-threatening hypokalemia (Figure 78-2).

Oral potassium replacement is preferred whenever vomiting is not a problem. Most commercial dog and cat foods contain sufficient potassium to correct mild potassium deficiencies. For moderate and severe potassium depletion (such as the cat with chronic renal failure), potassium-containing tablets and liquids for oral use are commercially available.

Liquids are preferred over tablets because of more dependable absorption. Subcutaneous administration of polyionic, isotonic fluids, such as Ringer's or lactated Ringer's solutions enriched with 30 mEq of potassium chloride per liter, is another safe method of potassium replacement. Total daily potassium dosage is estimated based upon suspected severity of potassium depletion. Acid-base disturbances should be corrected, and the primary disorder should be treated appropriately. Hypokalemia due to redistribution of potassium may be corrected by appropriate treatment of the cause (e.g., correction of alkalosis or reduction of insulin dosage).

CHAPTER 79

Electrolyte Disorders: Ca-P and Mg

Patricia A. Schenck

CALCIUM

Normal Regulation of Calcium Metabolism

Calcium in serum or plasma exists in three fractions: ionized (free), complexed (to phosphate, bicarbonate, sulfate, citrate, and lactate), and protein-bound.[1] In normal dogs, protein-bound, complexed, and ionized calcium accounts for 34%, 10%, and 56% of total serum concentration,[2] and these fractions show a similar distribution in cats (40%, 8%, and 52%, respectively).[3] Ionized calcium (iCa) is the biologically active fraction of calcium, and is important for many physiologic functions.

Calcium ions directly bind to iCa-specific cell membrane receptors,[4] and the iCa concentration is maintained within a narrow range by interactions among iCa, phosphorus, parathyroid hormone (PTH), vitamin D metabolites, and calcitonin. The intestine, kidney, and bone are the major target organs involved in calcium regulation, and the skeleton provides a major source of calcium when intestinal absorption and renal reabsorption are inadequate to maintain normal iCa concentration. Parathyroid hormone is secreted by the parathyroid glands in response to a decrease in iCa concentration. PTH acts to increase the tubular reabsorption of calcium (by decreasing loss of calcium in the urine), to increase bone resorption, and to increase the formation of 1,25-dihydroxy-vitamin D (calcitriol) by the kidney. The net effects of increased PTH are to increase iCa and decrease serum phosphorus concentration. Calcitonin is synthesized within the thyroid gland and is secreted in response to hypercalcemia; its role in calcium homeostasis is minor.

25-Hydroxyvitamin D and calcitriol are the most important vitamin D metabolites involved in calcium homeostasis. Dogs and cats are dependent on vitamin D in their diet; hydroxylation of vitamin D occurs in the liver to produce 25-hydroxyvitamin D. The 25-hydroxyvitamin D is then again hydroxylated, to calcitriol, in the proximal tubules of the kidney. Calcitriol is the only active metabolite of vitamin D, and acts to increase serum iCa and phosphorus concentrations by stimulating the resorption of bone; increasing calcium, phosphorus, and magnesium absorption from the intestine; and increasing renal tubular resorption of calcium and phosphorus by the kidney.[1]

Assessing Ionized Calcium Concentrations

The calcium status of any dog or cat is usually based on assessment of serum total calcium (tCa) concentration. Reliance on tCa has been based on the assumption that tCa is directly proportional to the iCa concentration. Use of tCa alone can lead to erroneous interpretation of calcium status in some clinical conditions, with the most important exception being the high percentage of disagreement between tCa and iCa in both dogs and cats with renal disease.[5,6]

Adjustment formulas to correct tCa based on serum total protein or albumin were developed for dogs years ago.[7] These corrections seemed reasonable at the time because of the substantial binding of calcium to protein and the lack of a readily available commercial iCa assay. Subsequent attempts to verify these formulas as correctly predicting iCa measurement failed.[5] In fact, the adjustment formulas to predict iCa status showed a higher diagnostic discordance than did measurement of serum tCa alone. Adjustment formulas perform poorly because they only take into account the protein binding of calcium and ignore the complexed calcium fraction, which can vary, especially in pets with renal disease.[8] The use of adjustment formulas to predict iCa status is not recommended. Accurate measurement of any dog or cat's calcium status should be determined by specifically assaying iCa directly.[9]

Accurate determination of iCa concentration requires that samples be collected and processed correctly. Silicone separator tubes are not recommended, as serum iCa concentration may increase due to release of calcium from the silicone gel.[10] Protein binding of calcium is influenced by pH. For example, an alkaline pH develops with the loss of CO_2. This, in turn, favors calcium binding to protein and decreases the amount of calcium that would be ionized.[11] Similarly, mixing serum with air results in an increased pH and a decrease in iCa concentration. Anaerobic collection of serum is technically difficult; therefore, accurate aerobic methods for iCa measurement have been developed. Species-specific correction formulas have been developed by laboratories to correct the measured iCa concentration of aerobically handled samples to a pH of 7.4, with excellent correlation to iCa measured in anaerobically handled samples. Typically serum is used for iCa measurement, though heparinized plasma or whole blood can also be used. The amount and type of heparin used can impact iCa measurement[12]; therefore it is imperative that when using portable clinical analyzers that utilize heparinized whole blood, a rigid protocol for collection be established. Results using heparinized whole blood cannot be directly compared to serum results, as iCa concentrations are typically lower in heparinized whole blood.[13]

Disorders of Hypercalcemia

Approximately 60% of dogs and cats evaluated for calcium disorders are hypercalcemic.[14,15] In hypercalcemia, the interaction of calcium with phosphorus is important. Whenever the product of the tCa (mg/dL) multiplied by the phosphorus concentration exceeds ~70, tissue mineralization is likely. This is critical since the tissues that most often mineralize are nephrons. Mineralized nephrons die, reducing the ability of that individual to excrete phosphorus which, in turn, further increases the Ca × Phosphorus product.

Clinical signs of hypercalcemia are usually present if tCa concentration is >15 mg/dL or if iCa is >1.8 mmol/L; the patient is typically critically ill if tCa is >18 mg/dL or iCa is >2.2 mmol/L. About 60% of dogs with primary hyperparathyroidism (PHPTH) that have a tCa >12 mg/dL have clinical signs. About 40% of PHPTH dogs do not have signs, as observed by owners. Dogs with this condition only rarely become critically ill, regardless of their serum calcium concentration. Hypercalcemic dogs that are critically ill typically have a serious underlying illness (e.g., malignancy, hypoadrenocorticism) and do not have primary hyperparathyroidism. Polyuria, polydipsia, weakness, and decrease in appetite are the most common clinical signs of hypercalcemia in dogs; vomiting, depression, and constipation can occur. Cats most often exhibit anorexia, and do not exhibit polyuria, polydipsia, or vomiting as often as dogs.

In dogs, neoplasia (e.g., lymphosarcoma, apocrine carcinoma of the anal sac, multiple myeloma) is the most common cause of hypercalcemia. Other causes include hypoadrenocorticism, primary hyperparathyroidism, and renal failure. Renal failure is characterized by an elevation of tCa but not usually iCa (Box 79-1).

In cats, hypercalcemia is most commonly idiopathic or secondary to neoplasia. Anticipated changes in calcemic hormones and serum biochemistry results associated with disorders of hypercalcemia are summarized in Table 79-1.

An algorithm for the clinical approach to diagnosis of hypercalcemic disorders is presented in Figure 79-1.[16]

Therapeutic options for the management of hypercalcemia are presented in Table 79-2.

Volume expansion, diuretic administration, glucocorticoid therapy, and bisphosphonate therapy can improve or normalize hypercalcemia.[17] Definitive therapy involves treatment of the underlying disorder.

Disorders of Hypocalcemia

Common clinical signs of hypocalcemia include muscle tremors, fasciculations, facial rubbing, muscle cramping, stiff gait, seizures, restlessness, aggression, hypersensitivity, and disorientation.[18] Other clinical signs may include panting, pyrexia, lethargy, depression, anorexia, tachycardia, prolapse of the third eyelids (in cats), polyuria, polydipsia, hypotension, respiratory arrest, and death. Clinical signs are usually present when the serum tCa is <6.0 mg/dL, or iCa is <0.8 mmol/L. A tCa <4.5 mg/dL is often life-threatening. Hypocalcemia associated with either chronic renal failure or secondary hyperparathyroidism rarely causes clinical signs. The most common causes of hypocalcemia include chronic or acute renal failure and eclampsia. Less common causes include acute pancreatitis, hypoparathyroidism, rhabdomyolysis, ethylene glycol intoxication, intestinal malabsorption, and hypovitaminosis D (Box 79-2).

Anticipated changes in calcemic hormones and serum biochemistry results associated with disorders of hypocalcemia are summarized in Table 79-3.

An algorithm for the clinical approach to diagnosis of hypocalcemic disorders is presented in Figure 79-2.[18]

Treatment of hypocalcemia involves a combination of parenteral and oral calcium, with vitamin D supplementation, depending on the underlying condition (Table 79-4).

In patients with renal disease, iCa concentration should always be evaluated. In one study, the serum tCa was increased in 22% of 490 dogs with chronic renal failure, yet iCa was increased in only 9%.[5] This discrepancy in tCa versus iCa can be explained by an increase in complexed calcium in dogs with chronic renal failure.[8] With renal disease, even if serum tCa and/or iCa concentrations are within reference limits, derangements in calcium homeostasis can be occurring and should be evaluated. Secondary hyperparathyroidism (characterized by normal to low iCa and increased serum PTH concentrations) occurs as the number of functional renal proximal tubules decrease and calcitriol synthesis is impaired. Excess PTH is secreted in the attempt to maintain iCa concentration within a normal range.[1]

Box • 79-1

Conditions Associated with Hypercalcemia

Nonpathologic Conditions
Hyperlipemia
Nonfasted serum samples
Young growing dogs
Laboratory error or improper handling of sample

Transient Conditions
Hemoconcentration
Hyperproteinemia

Pathologic Conditions
Parathyroid-dependent hypercalcemia (primary hyperparathyroidism)
Parathyroid-independent hypercalcemia
 Malignancy-associated hypercalcemia
  Lymphoma
  Adenocarcinoma of the apocrine glands of the anal sac
  Multiple myeloma
  Metastatic bone tumors
  Miscellaneous tumors (lymphocytic leukemia, mammary carcinoma, fibrosarcoma, pancreatic adenocarcinoma, testicular interstitial cell tumor, lung carcinoma, squamous cell carcinoma, thyroid adenocarcinoma, and osteosarcoma)
Hypoadrenocorticism
Renal failure
Hypervitaminosis D
 Cholecalciferol (rodenticide) toxicity
 Dovonex ingestion
 Iatrogenic due to dietary supplementation
 Houseplants (Cestrum diurnum, Solanum malocoxylon, Triestum flavescens)
 Granulomatous disease—blastomycosis, schistosomiasis
Grape toxicity
Bone lesions—sepsis, disuse osteoporosis
Severe hypothermia
Idiopathic hypercalcemia in cats

PHOSPHORUS

Phosphorus Metabolism

Phosphorus is important in maintaining the structure of bones and teeth, maintenance of cell membranes, and in the supply of energy. Most inorganic phosphorus is within bone. Less than 1% is in serum. The majority of phosphorus is in the organic form within phospholipids. Phosphorus is absorbed in the small intestine and excreted by the kidneys. Phosphorus absorption and excretion is regulated with calcium; calcitriol increases phosphorus absorption, and PTH decreases phosphorus reabsorption in the kidney. The kidney is the most important regulator of phosphorus, as 80% to 90% of filtered phosphorus is typically reabsorbed by the proximal tubules.

Table • 79-1

Anticipated Changes in Calcemic Hormones and Serum Biochemistry Associated with Disorders of Hypercalcemia

DISORDER	tCa	iCa	alb	Corr tCa	Pi	PTH	PTHrP	25(OH)-D	1,25(OH)₂-D	PTG (ULS, SURGERY)
1-HPTH	↑	↑	N	N	↓N	↑N	N	N	N↑	Single ↑
2-HPTH, nutritional	N↓	N↓	N	N↓	N↑	↑	N	↓N	N↓	Multiple ↑
2-HPTH, renal	N↓↑	N↓	N	N	↑N	↑	N	N↓	N↓	Multiple ↑
3-HPTH	↑	↑	N	↑	↑	↑	N	N↓	↓N	Multiple ↑
Malignancy associated										
Humoral hypercalcemia	↑	↑	N↓	↑N	↓N	↓N	↑N	N	↓N↑	↓
Local osteolytic	↑	↑	N↓	↓N	N↑	↓N	N↑	N	N	↓
Hypervitaminosis D										
Cholecalciferol	↑	↑	N	↑	↑N	↓	N	↑	N↑	N↓
Calcitriol	↑	↑	N	↑	N↑	↓	N	N	↑	↓N
Calcipotriene	↑	↑	N	↑	↑N	↓	N	N	↓N	↓N
Hypoadrenocorticism	↑	↑	N↓	↑	↑N	↓N	N	N	↓N	N
Hypervitaminosis A	↑	↑	N	↑	N	↓	N	N	N↓	↓N
Idiopathic (cat)	↑	↑	N	↑	N↑	↓N	N	N	N↓↑	↓N
Dehydration	↑	N↑	↑N	↑N	N↑	N↓	N	N	N	N
Aluminum exposure (renal failure)	↑	↑	N	↑	↑N	↓N	N	N	N↓	N↑↓
Hyperthyroidism (cat)	↑	↑	N	↑	N↑	↑N↓	N	N	N↓	N↑
Raisin/grape toxicity (dog)	↑	—	N	↑	N↑	—	—	—	—	—

From Schenck PA, Chew DJ: Diseases of the parathyroid gland and calcium metabolism. In Birchard SJ, Sherding RG, editors: Saunders manual of small animal practice, ed 3, St Louis, 2006, Saunders, pp 343-356.
1,25(OH)₂-D, 1,25-dihydroxyvitamin D₃; *25(OH)-D*, 25-hydroxyvitamin D₃; *alb*, albumin; *Corr tCa*, corrected total calcium; *iCa*, ionized calcium; *N*, normal; *Pi*, phosphorus; *PTG*, parathyroid glands; *PTH*, parathyroid hormone; *PTHrP*, parathyroid hormone-related protein; *tCa*, total calcium; *ULS*, ultrasound.

Table • 79-2

Treatment of Hypercalcemia

TREATMENT	DOSE	INDICATIONS	COMMENTS
Volume Expansion			
SQ Saline (0.9%)	75-100 mL/kg/day	Mild hypercalcemia	Contraindicated if peripheral edema is present
IV Saline (0.9%)	100-125 mL/kg/day	Moderate to severe hypercalcemia	Contraindicated in congestive heart failure or hypertension
Diuretics			
Furosemide	2-4 mg/kg BID-TID; IV, SQ, PO	Moderate to severe hypercalcemia	Volume expansion is necessary prior to use of this drug
Glucocorticoids			
Prednisone	1-2.2 mg/kg BID; PO, SQ, IV	Moderate to severe hypercalcemia	Use prior to identification of etiology may make definitive diagnosis difficult
Dexamethasone	0.1-0.22 mg/kg BID; IV, SQ		
Inhibition of Bone Resorption			
Calcitonin	4-6 IU/kg SQ BID-TID	Vitamin D toxicity	Short acting; vomiting may occur
Bisphosphonates		Moderate to severe hypercalcemia	Expensive, use in dogs and cats limited
EHDP-Etidronate	5-15 mg/kg SID-BID		
Alendronate	10 mg/cat once weekly; PO		Limited data available
Pamidronate	1.3-2.0 mg/kg in 150 mL 0.9% saline a 2-hr IV infusion; can repeat in 1-3 weeks		Very expensive

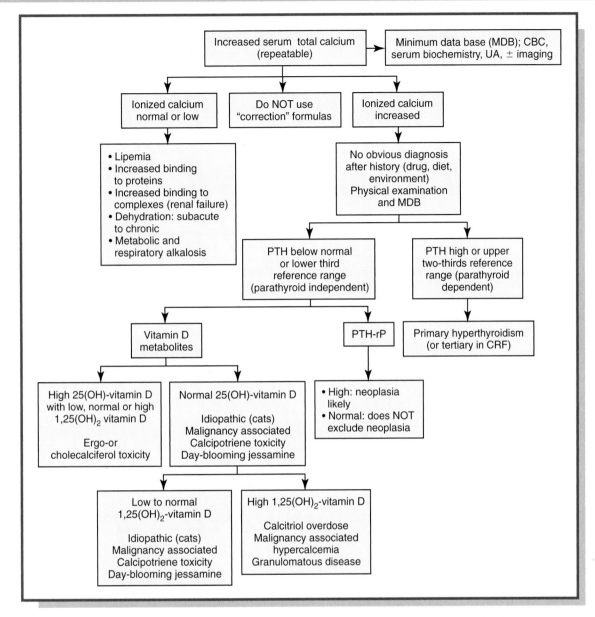

Figure 79-1 Algorithm for diagnosis of hypercalcemic disorders. *CBC,* Complete blood count; *CRF,* chronic renal failure; *PTH,* parathyroid hormone; *UA,* urinalysis. (From Schenck PA, Chew DJ: Hypercalcemia: a quick reference. Vet Clin North Am Small Anim Pract 38:449-453, 2008.)

Box • 79-2

Conditions Associated with Hypocalcemia

Causes of Severe Symptomatic Hypocalcemia
Puerperal tetany/eclampsia
Hypoparathyroidism (spontaneous, iatrogenic, postoperative)
Phosphate enemas (acute hyperphosphatemia causes reciprocal
    calcium decrease)

Causes of Mild Asymptomatic Hypocalcemia
Hypoalbuminemia (most frequent cause of hypocalcemia)
Primary renal disease (CRF, ARF due to obstruction or ethylene
    glycol toxicity)

Pancreatitis
Intestinal malabsorption syndromes
Chelating agents that bind calcium (EDTA, citrates, oxalates,
    phosphates)
Rhabdomyolysis due to soft tissue trauma
Nutritional secondary hyperparathyroidism
Dilutional with infusion of calcium-free fluids
Laboratory error/artifact
Idiopathic (unexplained)

ARF, Acute renal failure; *CRF,* chronic renal failure; *EDTA,* ethylenediaminetetraacetic acid.

Table • **79-3**

Anticipated Changes in Calcemic Hormones and Serum Biochemistry Associated with Disorders of Hypocalcemia

DISORDER	tCa	iCa	alb	Corr tCa	Pi	PTH	PTHrP	25(OH)-D	1,25(OH)$_2$-D	PTG (ULS, SURGERY)
1-HypoPTH	↓	↓	N	↓	↓N	↓N	N	N	N↓	Multiple ↓
PseudohypoPTH	↓	N↓	N	↓	↑N	↑	N	N	N↑	N↑
Sepsis/critical care	↓N	↓	N	↓N	N↑	↑N	N	N	N	N
Ethylene glycol tox	↓	↓	N	↓	↑N	↑	N	N	↓N	N
Paraneoplastic	↓	↓	N	↓	↓	↑N	N	N	N	N↑
Phosphate enema	↓	↓	N	↓	↑	↑	N	N	N↓↑	N
Eclampsia	↓	↓	N	↓	↓	Mild ↑, N	N	N	N↓	N
Hypoalbuminemia	↓	↓N	↓	N	N	N↑	N	N	N↑	N↑

Schenck PA, Chew DJ: Diseases of the parathyroid gland and calcium metabolism. In Birchard SJ, Sherding RG, editors: Saunders manual of small animal practice, ed 3, St Louis, 2006, Saunders, pp 343-356.

1,25(OH)$_2$-D, 1,25-dihydroxyvitamin D$_3$; *25(OH)-D,* 25-hydroxyvitamin D$_3$; *alb,* albumin; *Corr tCa,* corrected total calcium; *iCa,* ionized calcium; *N,* normal; *Pi,* phosphorus; *PTG,* parathyroid glands; *PTH,* parathyroid hormone; *PTHrP,* parathyroid hormone-related protein; *tCa,* total calcium; *ULS,* ultrasound.

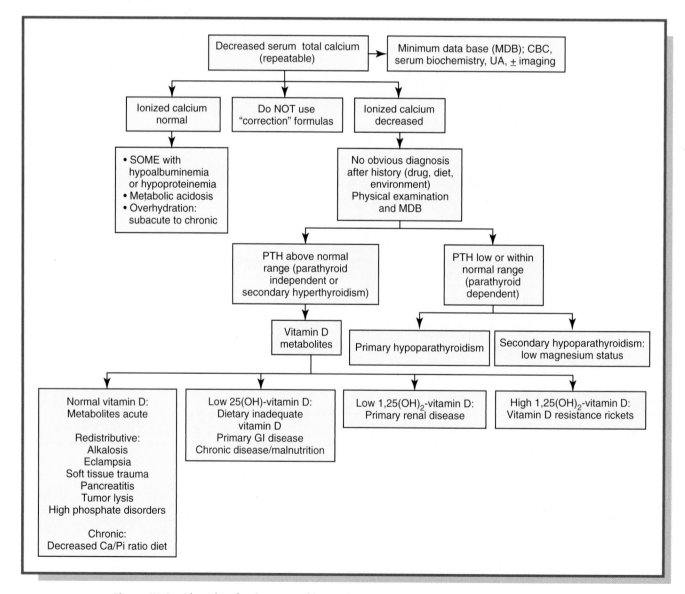

Figure 79-2 Algorithm for diagnosis of hypocalcemic disorders. *CBC,* Complete blood count; *GI,* gastrointestinal; *PTH,* parathyroid hormone; *UA,* urinalysis. (From Schenck PA, Chew DJ: Hypocalcemia: a quick reference. Vet Clin North Am Small Anim Pract 38:455-458, 2008.)

Table • 79-4

Treatment of Hypocalcemia

DRUG	PREPARATION	CALCIUM CONTENT	DOSE	COMMENT
Parenteral Calcium*				
Calcium gluconate	10% solution	9.3 mg of Ca/mL	a. Slow IV to effect (0.5-1.5 mL/kg IV)	Stop if bradycardia or shortened QT interval occurs
			b. 5-15 mg/kg/h IV	Infusion to maintain normal Ca SQ calcium salts—not recommended. Can cause severe skin necrosis/ mineralization.
Calcium chloride	10% solution	27.2 mg of Ca/mL	5-15 mg/kg/h IV	Only given IV; extremely caustic perivascularly
Oral Calcium†				
Calcium carbonate	Many sizes	40% tablet	25-50 mg/kg/day	Most common calcium supplement
Calcium lactate	325 and 650 mg tablets	13% tablet	25-50 mg/kg/day	
Calcium chloride	Powder	27.2%	25-50 mg/kg/day	May cause gastric irritation
Calcium gluconate	Many sizes	10%	25-50 mg/kg/day	
Vitamin D				*Time for maximal effect to occur:* *Time for toxicity effect to resolve:*
Vitamin D_2 (ergocalciferol)			Initial: 4000-6000 U/kg/day Maintenance: 1000-2000 U/kg once daily to once weekly	5-21 days 1-18 weeks
$1,25\text{-}(OH)_2\ D_3$ (calcitriol)			Initial: 20-30 ng/kg/day for 3-4 days Maintenance: 5-15 ng/kg/day	1-4 days 2-14 days

*Do not mix calcium solution with bicarbonate-containing fluids as precipitation may occur.
†Calculate dose on elemental calcium content.

Hyperphosphatemia

Phosphorus concentrations are typically higher in young, growing dogs. Increased serum phosphorus concentrations can be caused by enhanced gastrointestinal (GI) absorption, decreased excretion of phosphorus, or transcellular shifts.[19] An increase in GI absorption is typically the result of an increase in calcitriol or calcitriol-analogue (calcipotriene) concentration (vitamin D toxicity). Hyperphosphatemia is dangerous in this instance since serum calcium is also elevated, increasing the risk of soft tissue mineralization as previously discussed. Decreased excretion of phosphorus can occur in renal disease, uroabdomen, urinary tract obstruction, hypoadrenocorticism, hypoparathyroidism, acromegaly, and hyperthyroidism. Transcellular shifts can be seen with tumor cell lysis, rhabdomyolysis, or hemolysis. Hyperphosphatemia may also be seen in hyperlipidemic samples, or with hyperproteinemia. Hyperphosphatemia does not usually cause clinical signs. However, hyperphosphatemia can induce hypocalcemia (mass law effect) with clinical signs.

Hypophosphatemia

Hypophosphatemia results from decreased intestinal absorption, increased renal excretion, or from transcellular shifts.[19] Decreased intestinal absorption occurs in vitamin D deficiency, malabsorption, vomiting and diarrhea, and with phosphate binders. Increased renal excretion occurs with diabetes mellitus, primary hyperparathyroidism, renal tubular defects, diuretic administration, hyperadrenocorticism, eclampsia, and hyperaldosteronism. Transcellular shifts occur with insulin, bicarbonate, or parenteral glucose administration, hypothermia, refeeding syndrome, and respiratory alkalosis. Hypophosphatemia is not usually associated with clinical signs and, if present, signs are vague. Concentrations of phosphorus <1 mg/dL are life-threatening, with hemolysis, respiratory failure, seizures, and death.

MAGNESIUM

Magnesium Metabolism

Magnesium is an important cofactor in many enzymatic reactions. Like calcium, magnesium exists in three fractions: ionized, protein-bound, and complexed. Ionized magnesium (iMg) accounts for approximately 65% of the serum total magnesium concentration in healthy dogs and cats.[20] The ionized fraction is biologically active, and cannot be predicted from the total magnesium concentration, especially in disease states. As with calcium, iMg should be directly measured to provide an assessment of magnesium status.

Hypomagnesemia

Hypomagnesemia is common in the critical care setting. In one study on sick dogs and cats, 30% had low serum iMg concentrations.[21] Causes of hypomagnesemia include GI malabsorption, renal loss, concurrent electrolyte disorders, and drug administration (gentamicin, carbenicillin, ticarcillin, cyclosporin, cisplatin). GI disorders resulting in hypomagnesemia include reduced intake, chronic diarrhea, malabsorption, short bowel syndrome, and colonic neoplasia. Renal loss occurs with diabetes mellitus, diuretic administration, osmotic agents, postobstructive renal diuresis, hyperaldosteronism, hyperthyroidism, and renal tubular acidosis.[22]

In animals with suspected calcium abnormalities, 34% of cats and 12% of dogs were hypomagnesemic based on serum iMg concentration. In association with calcium disorders, hypomagnesemia is most commonly seen in primary hypoparathyroidism; 32% of dogs (n=794)[14] and 85% of cats (n=80)[15] with hypoparathyroidism exhibited hypomagnesemia. Depletion of magnesium impairs PTH secretion, impairs calcitriol synthesis, and increases organ resistance to PTH. With low serum iMg concentrations, cell membrane receptors also have reduced sensitivity to iCa.[1] The association of hypomagnesemia and hypoparathyroidism is important, as some patients with hypoparathyroidism may be refractory to calcium and vitamin D therapy if they are also hypomagnesemic. Ionized magnesium concentration should be evaluated in any dog or cat that appears refractory to therapy, and magnesium supplementation (oral magnesium sulfate 1 to 2 mEq/kg/day) should be considered in those with low iMg.

Hypomagnesemia enhances renal loss of potassium and the potential for secondary hypokalemia. Clinical signs are related to the hypokalemia in addition to hypomagnesemia, and include neuromuscular signs (hyperexcitability, tremors, ataxia, tetany) and cardiac arrhythmias. Other causes of hypomagnesemia include excessive loss from lactation, acute myocardial infarction, acute pancreatitis, insulin administration, or catecholamine excess.[22]

Hypermagnesemia

Hypermagnesemia can be seen if urinary excretion of magnesium is compromised, such as in chronic renal failure. Approximately 20% of dogs (n=2112)[14] and 9% of cats (n=1491)[15] with secondary hyperparathyroidism due to chronic renal failure exhibited elevated iMg. Clinical signs of hypermagnesemia are rare unless the serum iMg is greater than 1.2 mmol/L. Clinical signs of hypermagnesemia include paresis, paralysis, cardiovascular depression, hypotension, nausea, and vomiting. Therapy involves treatment of the underlying condition.

References

The reference list can be found on the companion Expert Consult Web Site at *www.expertconsult.com.*

SECTION **III**
Techniques

GENERAL

CHAPTER **80**

Venous and Arterial Puncture

Harold Davis

VENIPUNCTURE

The most commonly used veins for venipuncture are the cephalic (dog and cat), lateral saphenous (dog), medial saphenous (cat), and jugular (dog and cat). The ear veins (dog and cat), sublingual veins (dog and cat), and abdominal veins (dogs) have also been used. Any visible vein is an option for venipuncture.

The most important aspects of any venipuncture technique are the proper restraint of the animal and proper distention and immobilization of the vessel. These objectives are most easily accomplished when the procedure is done as a two-person project. The phlebotomist should only attempt the venipuncture when the vessel can be clearly delineated. Blind venipuncture attempts, in the hopes of accidentally "skewering" the vein, are doomed to failure and create unnecessary patient discomfort. If the phlebotomist is unable to locate the vessel (by visual inspection or digital palpation), the manner in which the vessel is distended and immobilized must be changed.

Awake animals need to be restrained for any of these procedures, but excessive restraint should be avoided because it may incite more resistance from the animal than the venipuncture procedure itself. All venipunctures (and arterial punctures) must be done aseptically. The hair should be clipped and the skin prepared with antiseptic solutions as if for surgery.

CEPHALIC VEIN VENIPUNCTURE

The dog or cat may be positioned in sternal or lateral recumbency. The restrainer leans over the top of the animal and grasps the leg of interest at the elbow. The other hand or arm can be used to restrain the animal's head if the animal is awake, to prevent an aggressive response to the skin puncture. If the animal is in sternal recumbency, the restrainer should lean on his or her elbow to help prevent the animal from withdrawing its leg at some critical time during the procedure. The thumb or forefinger is wrapped around the leg at the level

of the elbow. Pressure at this point occludes the cephalic vein. The skin is then rotated outward to roll the vein to the top (anterior) of the leg.

The phlebotomist grasps the leg with one hand at the level of the metacarpus and further extends the leg. In loose-skinned animals, it may be necessary to flex the carpus. The objective is to tether the vein between the two points of traction (at the elbow and at the carpus) so that the vein is both distended and does not roll from side to side. It should not be necessary for the phlebotomist to use his or her thumb to help immobilize the vein; this may only serve to collapse the vein, making venipuncture more difficult.

The needle is directed, as much as possible, along the longitudinal axis of the vein. The needle is inserted through the skin with the bevel facing up. It is not necessary to achieve both skin and vein puncture in the first movement. The skin puncture is the painful part, and animals will often move in response to it. Once the animal has settled down, the needle can be directed into the vein. If blood does not spontaneously flow into the hub of the needle, the phlebotomist should gently aspirate to determine if the needle is or is not in the vein. If it is not in the vein, the needle should be advanced a bit further and the process repeated. The needle can be advanced to its full length. If at this point the venipuncture has not been successful, the needle will have to be withdrawn to its subcutaneous position (it should not be removed entirely, because another skin puncture will then be necessary). It is most important to withdraw the needle slowly, while gently aspirating. The deep wall of the vein may have been inadvertently penetrated, and the lumen will thereby be found as the needle is withdrawn.

Once the blood sample is taken or the drug is administered, the needle is withdrawn from the vein and digital pressure applied over the venipuncture site for at least 30 seconds. The site should be monitored for bleeding or hematoma formation for an additional several minutes.

Lateral Saphenous Venipuncture
Dogs are usually positioned in lateral recumbency for this procedure (Figure 80-1, *A*).

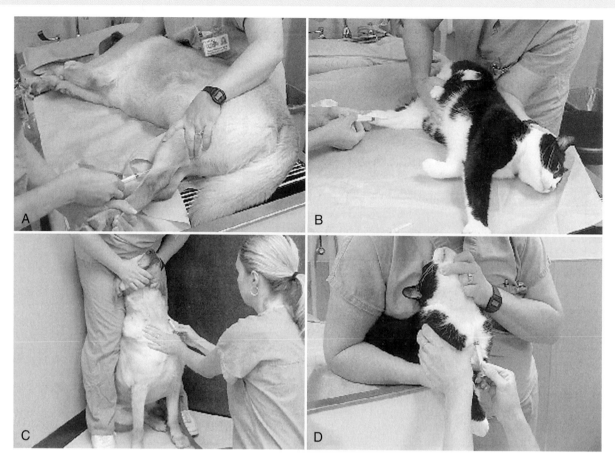

Figure 80-1 The various positions used for dog and cat venipuncture. **A,** Dog positioned for venipuncture of the lateral saphenous vein. **B,** Cat positioned for venipuncture of the medial saphenous vein. **C,** Dog positioned for venipuncture of the jugular vein. **D,** Cat positioned for venipuncture of the jugular vein.

The restrainer grasps the upper leg at the stifle. The other hand or arm can be used to restrain the animal's forelegs and head if the animal is awake. Circumferential pressure is applied at the stifle to occlude and distend the vein. The phlebotomist grasps the leg with one hand at the level of the metatarsus. In loose-skinned animals it may be necessary to extend the leg and flex the tarsus to better tether and immobilize the vein. It should not be necessary for the phlebotomist to use his or her thumb to help immobilize the vein. The venipuncture is performed as described previously.

Medial Saphenous Venipuncture
Cats are usually positioned in lateral recumbency for this procedure. The restrainer grasps the lower leg at the stifle while reflecting the upper leg caudally with the forearm. The other hand or arm can be used to restrain the animal's forelegs and head if the animal is awake. Circumferential pressure is applied at the stifle to occlude and distend the vein. Alternatively, in the cat, the phlebotomist should grasp it by the scruff of the neck and place in lateral recumbency (Figure 80-1, *B*). The upper hind leg is abducted and flexed to expose the medial surface of the bottom leg. Applying pressure with the edge of the hand that abducts and extends the upper leg distends the vein. The phlebotomist grasps the leg with one hand at the level of the metatarsus. In loose-skinned animals it may be necessary to extend the leg and flex the tarsus to better tether and immobilize the vein. It should not be necessary for the phlebotomist to use his or her thumb to help

immobilize the vein. The venipuncture is performed as described previously.

Jugular Venipuncture
Dogs and cats may be positioned in sternal or lateral recumbency for this procedure. In sternal positioning, one convenient technique includes backing the animal into a corner, between the legs of the holder (Figure 80-1, *C*). Alternatively, the dog or cat can be restrained on a table in sternal recumbency (Figure 80-1, *D*). One hand grasps the legs at the carpel joint and stretches the legs over the edge of the table. In any position the head will need to be extended. Either the restrainer or the phlebotomist occludes the vein by applying occlusive pressure at the thoracic inlet. Care must be taken not to compress the trachea or impair breathing. Vein distention and immobilization can be maximized by pressing into the thoracic inlet in a caudal direction and by further extending the head. Extensive longitudinal traction, however, can collapse the vein. With optimal positioning, the vein is easy to palpate (or visualize) and does not roll much from side to side. In sternal positioning, the venipuncture is usually done in a cephalad direction; in lateral positioning the venipuncture is generally done is a caudal direction. The venipuncture is performed as described previously.

Arterial Puncture
The dorsal metatarsal (pedal) and femoral arteries are most commonly used for arterial blood sampling. The dorsal meta-

tarsal is smaller, but the interstitial connective tissues around it are tight (compared with the femoral artery), which facilitates vessel positioning and minimizes postpuncture hematoma formation. The radial, brachial, aural, and sublingual arteries have also been used.

Arterial puncture is usually done with the animal in lateral recumbency; however, it can be accomplished when the animal is standing if it resents the lateral recumbent positioning. The pulse is palpated with one or two fingers of one hand. The needle is inserted through the skin but not into the artery. Once the animal settles down from the skin puncture, the needle is aligned with the longitudinal axis of the artery (bevel up). The tip of the needle and the artery are simultaneously palpated with the one finger, and the needle inserted into the artery. Blood should spontaneously flow into the hub of the needle in an animal with normal blood pressure; however,

gentle aspiration on the plunger may be required in animals with low blood pressure or when small needles are used. If the arterial puncture is unsuccessful, the needle can be inserted a bit further. As for venipuncture, when the needle is withdrawn, it should be done slowly and with gentle aspiration applied to the plunger in case the deep wall of the artery was inadvertently punctured during needle introduction. The needle is withdrawn to its subcutaneous position and the arterial puncture is reattempted.

Once the sample collection is complete, the clinician should withdraw the needle and apply digital pressure over the puncture site for at least 1 minute; then the animal should be monitored for bleeding or hematoma formation for another 4 minutes. If blood gas measurements cannot be done immediately, the sample should be stored in ice water to minimize in vitro metabolic changes in the measured parameters.

CHAPTER 81

Jugular Catheterization and Central Venous Pressure

Darlene L. Riel

Catheterization of the jugular vein is a common method of achieving central venous access. Of the four general categories of intravenous (IV) access devices (winged needle, over-the-needle, through-the-needle, and multilumen catheters), the through-the-needle and multilumen catheters are favored for jugular catheterization. These catheters are available in a variety of lengths and diameters.

THROUGH-THE-NEEDLE CATHETERS

Through-the-needle catheters are as stated. The catheter is packaged in a protective plastic sleeve to prevent contamination. After catheter placement, the needle is withdrawn and a needle guard is applied to prevent trauma to the dog or cat and to protect the catheter from shearing.

MULTILUMEN CATHETERS

Multilumen catheters have two to five separate lumens in one catheter and are available in both the over-the-needle and through-the-needle designs. They are useful for administering two or more continuous infusions at the same time and/or for monitoring central venous pressure. Catheter placement is accomplished with the aid of a guide wire and a vein dilator.

JUGULAR CATHETERIZATION

Supplies and Patient Preparation for All Catheters

The catheterization supplies (Box 81-1) are gathered and arranged so as to be ready for use on a clean tray or countertop close to the patient.

An appropriate-size catheter for the dog or cat is selected. The tip of the jugular catheter should reach the vena cava, close to the right atrium. The length to which the catheter

---

Box • 81-1

Jugular Catheterization Supplies

Clippers and antiseptic preparation solutions
Through-the-needle catheter or multilumen catheter kit
Antimicrobial ointment
Sterile 2 × 2 gauze sponge
Heparinized saline syringes
Surgical drapes, if necessary
Sterile gloves
Small utility surgical set
Suture material
Injection cap (or caps) or T-port
Bandage material
Tape

---

should be inserted is determined by measuring from the expected catheter insertion site to the caudal edge of the triceps muscles.

Proper positioning of the dog or cat, usually in lateral recumbency, is crucial. An assistant should extend the patient's head and direct the front limbs caudally. The assistant should hold off the vein by pressing into the thoracic inlet. Placement of a bag of fluids, a sandbag, or rolled towels under the neck may help stabilize the vein. If the vein is not properly stabilized, it may roll laterally or crumple longitudinally. Hair should be clipped wide enough to prevent contamination during the catheterization procedure. Aseptic technique is used, and the site is prepared as would be a surgical site. Sterile drapes are rarely necessary.

Through-the-Needle Catheterization Technique

The operator should first inspect the through-the-needle catheter to make sure the catheter is retracted back into the needle and is not visible at the needle bevel. Grasping the needle firmly, with the needle bevel up, the operator inserts the needle through the skin and advances it subcutaneously parallel to the vein for at least 1.25 cm before it is introduced into the vein. Venipuncture is confirmed when a flash of blood is seen within the catheter. The operator then advances the needle well into the vein, holds the needle with one hand, and threads the catheter with the other hand by pushing the catheter hub within the protective plastic sleeve until the catheter hub is advanced into the needle hub. Pressure is applied at the catheter puncture site; the needle is backed out from the skin, and the plastic sleeve is disconnected from the needle. The needle is secured with a needle guard. If a wire stylet is present, it is removed from the catheter. The catheter then is capped with an injection cap or T-port. Placement is confirmed by successful aspiration of blood, and the catheter is then flushed with heparinized saline. The catheter is sutured close to the insertion site, and care is taken not to kink the catheter. The insertion site is covered with a sterile dressing. Finally, the catheter is secured with a stabilizing wrap.

Multilumen Catheter Technique

All the "pigtail" ports of the multilumen catheter are flushed with sterile heparinized saline, and injection caps are applied to all the ports except the most distal one. A No. 11 scalpel blade is used to make a full-thickness stab incision large enough to accommodate the vessel dilator (too small an incision makes it difficult to pass the dilator). The catheter introducer (usually an over-the-needle style catheter) is inserted, and the guide wire is fed through the catheter introducer and into the jugular vein. A length of wire is left exposed that is equivalent in length to the multilumen catheter. It is important that the operator control the wire so as to prevent contamination outside the sterile field and to prevent the wire from slipping down the jugular vein. The catheter introducer is then withdrawn from the vein over the guide wire, leaving the guide wire in the vein. The vein dilator is threaded over the guide wire and advanced into the jugular vein to its full length. Some resistance is expected, and the dilator may need to be rotated or twisted to insert it into the jugular vein. Digital pressure is applied to minimize bleeding, and the dilator is removed from the vein and then withdrawn over the guide wire. Care must be taken not to remove the guide wire! The catheter is threaded over the guide wire until the operator can grasp the guide wire from the open pigtail injection port. The operator holds the guide wire and advances the catheter into the jugular vein to the predetermined length. Once the catheter is in place, the guide wire is removed, leaving the multilumen catheter in the vein. An injection cap is placed on the pigtail of the distal port, air is aspirated, and the port is flushed with heparinized saline. The catheter is then sutured in place, and the insertion site is covered with a sterile dressing. Finally, the catheter is secured with a stabilizing wrap.

CENTRAL VENOUS PRESSURE MEASUREMENT BY WATER MANOMETER

Central venous pressure (CVP) is a luminal pressure measurement taken from the intrathoracic portions of the cranial vena cava. The accepted normal range for CVP is 0 to 10 cm H_2O.

Supplies Needed for Central Venous Pressure Measurement

A catheter with the tip properly placed in the intrathoracic vena cava is required. The materials needed include a sterile bag of fluids with an attached fluid administration set, an IV fluid extension set, a three-way stopcock, and a water manometer.

Procedure

The dog or cat should be positioned in lateral or sternal recumbency. A water manometer is placed in the fluid line via a three-way stopcock and the extension set (Figure 81-1).

The fluid administration set and the extension set are primed with sterile fluids from the fluid bag while the stopcock is in the "Off" position to the water manometer. There must be no air bubbles in the fluid lines. The primed extension set is attached to the patient's catheter. The stopcock at the bottom of the manometer should rest on the table or cage floor. The administration set is opened, again with the stopcock in the "Off" position to the manometer, to allow fluid to flow into the patient's catheter, thus ensuring that the catheter is patent. If fluid does not flow freely into the patient's catheter, a valid CVP measurement will not be obtained. Next, the stopcock is turned so that the "Off" position is now to the patient. The fluid will now fill the manometer, which is allowed to fill about three-quarters full. The stopcock then is turned "Off" to the fluids, allowing a pathway only from the fluid-filled manometer and the patient's catheter.

The level of fluid in the manometer falls until the hydrostatic pressure of the column of fluid reaches equilibrium with the hydrostatic pressure of the blood at the end of the catheter. Therefore it is essential to know where the catheter tip lies in relation to the manometer fluid column. When the animal is in lateral recumbency, the cranial vena cava lies near the midline, and the manubrium is a good reference point. When the animal is in sternal recumbency, the cranial vena cava is about at the level of the point of the shoulder or the scapulohumeral joint. With the stopcock resting on the tabletop or cage floor, a zero reference point is determined by a horizontal line drawn between the manometer and the appro-

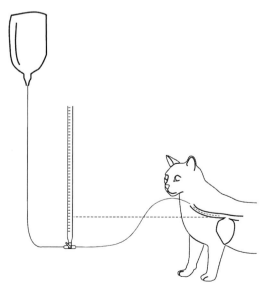

Figure 81-1 Setup for central venous pressure (CVP) assessment.

priate external anatomic landmark (manubrium or scapulo-humeral joint). The centimeter mark where the horizontal line intersects the manometer is the zero reference point. A carpenter's level fastened to a taut string is an excellent guide for the horizontal line from the anatomic landmark to the manometer. The difference between the equilibrium point reading and the zero reference point is the CVP measurement. For example, if the initial reading is 15 cm H_2O (where the fluid level stopped falling) and the zero reference point is 10 cm H_2O (horizontal line drawn between the external ana-tomic landmark and the manometer), the CVP is 5 cm H_2O. The presence of a well-placed, unobstructed catheter can be verified by the fluid column in the manometer, which will slightly oscillate up and down as the animal's heart beats or as the animal breathes. Readings are taken between ventilatory excursions. Trends in central venous pressure are more inform-ative than single values. Each time a CVP measurement is obtained, the patient should be in the same recumbent posi-tion. The goal is to be consistent in taking the readings and to monitor the trends.

CHAPTER 82

Veterinary Diagnosis of Bacterial, Fungal, and Viral Disease

Janet E. Foley

INDICATIONS FOR TESTING

Indications for testing of infectious disease are common. For example, animals may have nonspecific localized or systemic signs consistent with infection or inflammation, follow-up may be required on a dog or cat with an earlier infectious diagnosis, an isolate may be required for further testing (such as for antibiotic susceptibility), or it may be necessary to determine the risk of transmission of an infection to other animals or to people. Depending on the clinician's intent, the recommended tests and methods of interpretation may vary considerably; therefore it is helpful to clarify the purpose for testing in each case. For example, if the goal is to determine whether an animal poses a risk to an immunocompromised human in a household, it would be important to document active infection; thus culture or antigen-based tests would be used, not serology. Moreover, it is important to evaluate test results in the context of the whole patient evaluation; docu-menting the presence of of exposure to a pathogen does not prove that the pathogen is the cause of the animal's clinical signs.

TYPES OF TESTS: PROS, CONS, AND LIMITATIONS

In general, there are two classes of tests for infectious agents: either direct or indirect (Figure 82-1).

Direct tests detect a pathogen, its nucleic acids, or its anti-gens and document an active or at least recent infection. These tests include culture, polymerase chain reaction (PCR), antigen tests, and direct visualization. Culture definitively documents that the infection is active at the time of sample acquisition, while cytology and histology can strongly suggest active infection. PCR or antigen tests may remain positive for a brief period after effective treatment has been initiated or after the target agent has died. For example, the blood of a bacteremic animal could be PCR positive for bacterial DNA for a few days after administration of antibiotics and after the animal has become culture negative. Indirect tests seek evi-dence of exposure to a pathogen by evaluating host response; these tests consist primarily of serology for host antibodies specific to a pathogen.

Good tests should be sensitive (high likelihood of detecting an infectious agent if it is present) and specific (low likelihood of a positive result if the agent is not present). Culture often is insensitive but highly specific. Bacterial culture often is negative in samples from animals recently started on antibiot-ics, and some agents may require days to weeks to grow in vitro. However, culture should be highly specific, depending on how well "positives" are further characterized in the labora-tory. Culture has the additional advantages of providing an isolate for testing antibiotic, antifungal, or antiviral agents, molecular epidemiologic studies, and possible experimental infections. Culture sensitivity depends on sample handling (discussed below). Many agents cannot be cultured; therefore alternative methods for these organisms are critical and may be useful for improving sensitivity even for agents that can be cultured.

Direct visualization of a pathogen varies in sensitivity and specificity. Sometimes direct visualization is like looking for a needle in a haystack. Inflammation may be helpful in directing the attention of the clinical pathologist or micro-biologist to the area containing organisms. Gram stains are useful in bacterial processes, because culture virtually always underestimates the number and diversity of bacteria, whereas a semiquantitative Gram stain can reveal both. Special stains, such as silver-based stains or calcofluor white (a fluorescent stain), can enhance spirochetes, some bacteria, fungi, and other organisms. Immunohistochemical stains use monoclonal or polyclonal antibodies raised against the pathogen to target areas in tissue where a pathogen is present, coupled with a technique for flagging the pathogen (usually either a fluorescent dye or a chemical chromogen). However, stain and tissue artifacts may make it difficult to find pathogens, and pathogen load may be low and undetectable by visualization.

PCR is emerging as a powerhouse for the diagnosis of infectious diseases. PCR is an iterated biochemical reaction performed in a thermal cycler, a machine that cycles repeat-edly through a series of temperatures, with the end result that a few target DNA fragments in a sample can yield millions of copies. Millions of same-size DNA fragments can be visualized

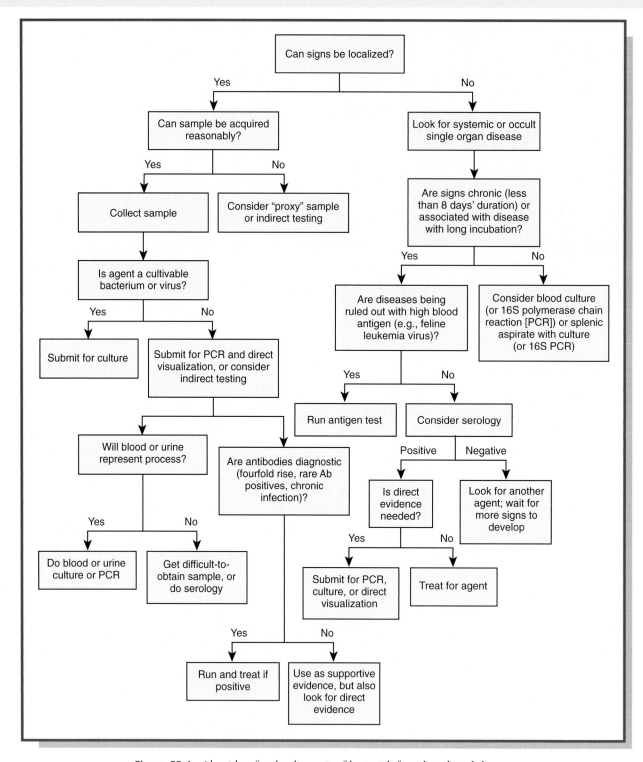

Figure 82-1 Algorithm for the diagnosis of bacterial, fungal, and viral diseases.

on an electrophoretic gel. Alternatively, newer real-time PCR technologies perform the same chemical reaction but quickly (within a few hours), and results are output directly to a computer. A key factor in the sensitivity and specificity of PCR is primers to start the reaction that anneal to a particular target and only that target. Thus *Hemobartonella felis* (now *Mycoplasma hemofelis*) primers should anneal only to *M. hemofelis* DNA and *Anaplasma phagocytophilum* primers only to *A. phagocytophilum* DNA. In several instances, it is

valuable to use more generalized primers and follow-up with a secondary test that will increase specificity. For example, there are primers that will amplify most or all known *Rickettsia* spp., and then cloning and DNA sequencing can be performed on any positive products to further identify which rickettsia was present. Similarly, eubacteria have conserved regions in some genes, such as the 16S rRNA gene, which may be amplified by PCR. After PCR is performed, the resulting fragment can be sequenced and the results checked against a database to identify the bacterium present in the sample.

Even carefully designed PCR reactions occasionally have been found to amplify nontargets (when by chance, some other organism has a region of DNA to which the primers anneal); therefore it is important to verify PCR results with DNA sequencing, a DNA probe, a second PCR in another region of DNA, or some other method. Two other limitations of PCR are the feasibility of obtaining sufficient quality RNA or DNA from the clinical sample and inhibitors in the sample. RNA in viruses such as FECV, canine distemper, and others is prone to the effects of RNA-degrading enzymes and must be kept as cold as possible and processed rapidly in a laboratory using special techniques to protect the RNA. Delays in sample handling increase the rate of false-negative PCR results. DNA is more stable and can be shipped dried, frozen, at room temperature, in paraffin-embedded tissue, and so forth. Some pathogens are harder to "crack" in terms of obtaining DNA, particularly mycobacteria and many fungi. Blood, feces, ascitic fluid, ticks, and other samples have inhibitors that can make the reaction less sensitive. Also, PCR can become cross-contaminated with DNA in the laboratory; therefore positive results should be trusted only if the laboratory has excellent quality control and makes stringent use of negative controls.

Antigen tests are available for a few veterinary pathogens for which there are high levels of antigen in a sample; some of these pathogens are feline leukemia virus (FeLV), *Cryptococcus neoformans*, and canine parvovirus. In other infections, such as feline immunodeficiency virus (FIV), antigen load is generally insufficient to make such a diagnostic modality feasible.

Antibody testing has several advantages. The sample typically is serum, which may be easier to obtain than, for example, tissue, and animals may remain seropositive for months after exposure, providing a larger window for testing. However, this large window may be a drawback as well, because the animal remains seropositive long after infection has resolved. In diseases that do not resolve (e.g., FIV), antibody testing documents infection; however, in other diseases, such as ehrlichiosis, serology only documents previous exposure. Serology has two

other drawbacks: there is no detectable immunoglobulin G (IgG) early in infection (up to 10 to 14 days), and vaccines induce cross-reacting seropositivity in some diseases, such as feline herpesvirus, calicivirus, and canine parvovirus. Twofold or fourfold rises in titer over 2 to 4 weeks are helpful for documenting recent infection in some diseases (and are part of the human case definition for ehrlichiosis) but are not helpful in others (e.g., feline infectious peritonitis [FIP]). Negative titers in a disease process that has been ongoing for at least 2 weeks are extremely informative in terms of ruling out some infections.

SAMPLE COLLECTING, HANDLING, AND SUBMISSION

The packaging and transport of samples depend on the tests to be run. The requirements are:
- Direct visualization, pathology, or immunohistochemistry: Rapid transport, a cool but not frozen temperature, and room air (unless formalin fixed). If samples are frozen, some of the architecture can be lost.
- Virus isolation, PCR, or antigen and antibody tests: Frozen. For PCR with RNA viruses, special transport media can be obtained, which helps protect the sample from degradation.
- Aerobic bacterial and fungal culture: Cooled with room air. Do not use viral culture media as this often contains antibiotics.
- Anaerobic or microaerophilic bacteria: Cooled with special atmospheres. This often can be provided with a swab that comes with an oxygen scavenger to prevent the bacteria from encountering what is to them toxic air.

Although each institution has a different configuration of laboratories, infectious disease diagnosis could involve clinical pathology, virology, immunology, microbiology, parasitology, biochemistry, and/or molecular biology. Clinicians should verify, through contact with the laboratory, how much sample and what paperwork are required to route the sample to all desired laboratories.

CHAPTER 83

Fecal Examination

Byron L. Blagburn
Jennifer A. Spencer

Internal parasites are prevalent and important disease agents in companion animals, and potential causes of zoonotic disease in pet owners.[1,2] Fecal detection of internal parasites is an important component of veterinary practice. Techniques include direct smear (wet mount), sedimentation, flotation (both centrifugal and standing), Baermann procedure, and fecal immunologic and molecular biologic techniques. Although the latter are not yet used commonly in the veterinary hospital, they are available at some diagnostic and reference laboratories, or can be requested from academic laboratories. Failure to employ "best practices"

techniques when conducting fecal examination procedures can result in failure to detect parasite stages in fecal specimens.[2-4] Following is an overview of common techniques and procedures used to recover eggs, larvae, and cysts from fecal specimens.

COLLECTING AND STORING FECAL SPECIMENS

The accuracy of fecal procedures often depends on amount and quality of the fecal specimen. For most procedures, we recommend the use of at least 2 g of feces. Two grams of firm, normal feces will form a cube approximately ½ to ¾ of an inch on a side. Occasionally, it is necessary to use a sample obtained with a fecal loop or a rectal thermometer. In these cases, a negative result can be meaningless; a positive result on the other hand can imply a high level of parasitism. The specimen size should be increased as the amount of water in the sample increases. Ironically, diarrheic fecal specimens from animals with a large burden of parasites may contain fewer fecal parasite stages because of this dilution effect.

Only fresh fecal specimens should be collected, immediately after defecation, if possible. Specimens collected from the ground may contain eggs, larvae, or other stages of free-living organisms that can confound a diagnosis. Feces should be stored in a container that will exclude air. A plastic bag or container with a tightly secured lid will suffice. Specimens should be held in a cool, dry location, out of direct sunlight. Storage in a standard refrigerator would be ideal, although most clients are reluctant to place such samples in a refrigerator with food. Samples can be refrigerated for several days to a week without affecting most parasites. Trophozoites of *Giardia* and *Tritrichomonas*, and certain nematode larvae, will not survive storage. When these parasites are suspected, the specimen must be examined immediately. Most other parasite stages can survive storage under the above conditions for days to weeks. It is always good practice to examine specimens as soon as possible after submission for reasons mentioned above. It is important to note that if fecal specimens are maintained at room temperature for more than a day or two prior to examination, many eggs and oocysts will begin to embryonate or sporulate. Recognition of partially embryonated or sporulated eggs or oocysts can be a challenge, particularly for the novice. Fecal specimens can be fixed in 5% to 10% buffered formalin if a sample is to be submitted to another laboratory. If molecular or immunologic techniques are to be used by the reference laboratory, it is always a good idea to inquire as to how best to submit the specimen.

GROSS EXAMINATION OF THE FECAL SPECIMEN

Fecal specimens should be examined grossly for consistency (formed, semifluid or pulpy fluid), and for the presence of fresh blood (hematochezia), mucus, or intact parasites. Parasite-induced damage to the small intestine often results in dark, tarry feces (melena), indicative of the presence of partially digested blood. Color, consistency, and the presence of mucus or froth (air bubbles) are often indicators of gastrointestinal disease that may be caused by parasites.

FECAL SMEAR

The direct fecal smear or "wet mount" technique is used to detect motile protozoa such as *Giardia*, *Tritrichomonas*, *Pentatrichomonas*, amoeba, or larvae that may be damaged by flotation solution. Many diagnosticians presume that if only a small amount of feces is available, the direct smear should be the procedure of choice. This is not true. Selection of techniques should not be dictated by amount of feces. For example, if an overall assessment of a sample for parasites is intended, the best technique would likely be a centrifugal flotation. If the sample is fluid, it is probably best to examine the specimen using both direct smear and centrifugal flotation, even though the size of specimen may be small for each.

The direct smear is performed by placing a small amount of feces (some say peppercorn size), using an applicator stick, into a small amount of warm or room temperature 0.85% to 0.9% saline or lactated Ringer's solution (Web Figures 83-1, 83-2).

Do not use tap water; tap water is not an isotonic solution and will usually rupture most fragile protozoa. We use 22 × 22 mm coverslips, but some parasitologists use 22 × 40 mm coverslips and claim that they make the specimen layer thinner and easier to read. The most common mistake made in preparing a direct smear preparation is to use too much fecal sample. Specimens should be prepared so that newsprint can be read when placed under the specimen (see Web Figure 83-1). Always adjust the contrast on the microscope for adequate visualization of small, motile parasites. Do this by rotating the substage iris diaphragm. Do not lower the substage condenser to increase contrast; this will lower the performance of the lens by decreasing its functional numerical aperture. We often add a drop of Lugol's or D'Antoni's iodine to the saline on the slide prior to adding the specimen, or we "wick" it under the edge of the applied coverslip (see Web Figure 83-2). This will increase detail to allow for better visualization of internal structures. Keep in mind that although iodine may increase detail in the specimen, it will also kill the organisms so that they are no longer motile. Also be aware that other parasite stages, such as hookworm eggs and coccidial oocysts, will also stain brown and may not be recognized. Smears may also be stained with methylene blue.

FECAL FLOTATION TECHNIQUES

Fecal flotation is the most common clinical parasitology procedure performed in veterinary clinics and laboratories. Fecal flotation is employed to separate parasites from other objects and debris based on their different densities. Density is the weight of a parasite or other object per unit volume. Density is usually expressed as specific gravity, which is the ratio of a parasite's density to the density of water (density of tap water is 1.0). A parasite with a density of 1.10 would be 1.10 times denser than tap water. Successful fecal flotation is based on the principle that when a fecal specimen is placed in a sugar or salt solution, those parasites (and other objects) that are less dense than the prepared flotation solution will move to the top of the solution; those that are more dense will eventually settle to the bottom. A buoyant force, resulting from the differences in density of the parasite and the flotation solution, acts to force the parasite upward, while gravity and the viscosity (thickness) of the solution tend to retard upward movement. If the buoyant force exceeds the forces of gravity and viscosity, the parasite eventually moves to the surface. Successful recovery of parasites depends on the parasite's density, the density and viscosity of the flotation solution that is used, and how these factors interact. These factors will determine how long we centrifuge or allow flotation preparations to stand before we examine the coverslip for parasites. The densities of some common parasites and flotation solutions are given in Table 83-1.

In preparing fecal specimens for flotation, it is desirable to eliminate as much large debris as possible. This can be achieved by preparing the sample as described in Web Figure 83-3 and Figures 83-1 through 83-3.

First, the fecal specimen is added to an amount of flotation solution that will fill the tube into which the mixture will be poured to about 80% of its capacity. The mixture is stirred to distribute the fecal material throughout the flotation solution. If sucrose is used, do not stir the mixture too vigorously. This will minimize the formation of air bubbles. The mixture is then poured through a strainer or one to two layers of gauze into another clean container, and then into a centrifuge

Table • 83-1

Densities of Common Parasites and Flotation Solutions*

FLOTATION SOLUTION	DENSITY (SPECIFIC GRAVITY)	PARASITE EGG	DENSITY (SPECIFIC GRAVITY)
Sodium nitrate (338 g/L of water)	1.18-1.20	*Toxocara canis*	1.09
Zinc sulfate (331 g/L of water)	1.18-1.20	*Toxocara cati*	1.10
Sheather's sucrose† (454 g/355 mL of water, 6 mL of formaldehyde)	1.25-1.27	*Ancylostoma* spp.	1.06
Sodium chloride (350 g/L of water)	1.18-1.20	*Trichuris vulpis*	1.15
Magnesium sulfate (450 g/L of water)	1.20	*Taenia* spp.	1.23
		Physaloptera spp.	1.24

*Modified from references 2 and 4.
†Heat the water to near boiling. Add the granulated sugar and stir until it is dissolved. Allow the mixture to cool before adding the formaldehyde. Check the specific gravity and adjust to 1.27 by adding either water or sugar.

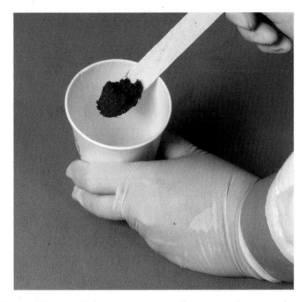

Figure 83-1 Add fecal specimen to flotation solution and mix thoroughly.

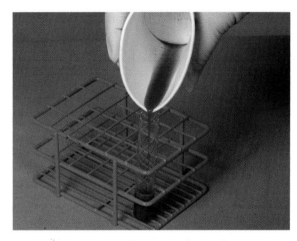

Figure 83-3 Pour filtrate into a centrifuge tube.

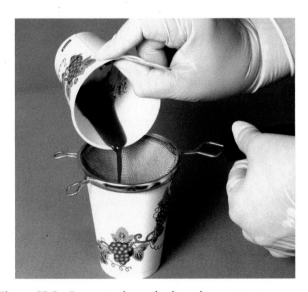

Figure 83-2 Pour mixed sample through a strainer to remove large debris.

tube. The filtrate is ready for flotation. In our laboratory, we use disposable paper cups, disposable tongue blades, and washable tea strainers (Figure 83-4).

FLOTATION SOLUTIONS

Common fecal flotation solutions are presented in Box 83-1. The density (specific gravity) of the different solutions is determined by the concentration of salt or sugar in tap water. The densities of most of the solutions are between 1.18 and 1.20. The densities of most of the common parasites listed in Table 83-1 are less than 1.18, indicating that they would likely be recovered using those solutions. We are presuming that the flotation procedure is conducted properly with an adequate amount of feces. We are often asked why flotation solutions are not prepared at the highest density possible. Couldn't we recover even the heavier parasite stages (i.e., *Taenia* and *Physaloptera* in Table 83-1)? The answer is yes. We could prepare the solutions at densities often approaching 1.35. The problem with very dense flotation solutions is that they not only float the heavier parasites, they also float the heavier debris. The presence of too much debris on the slide can make the slide preparation more difficult to read, or interfere with the rise of parasites of interest. Also, very high flotation densities often damage or distort certain eggs or oocysts. We recommend specific gravities between 1.18 and 1.27 for optimal recovery of parasites.[2] Research suggests that a sucrose solution mixed

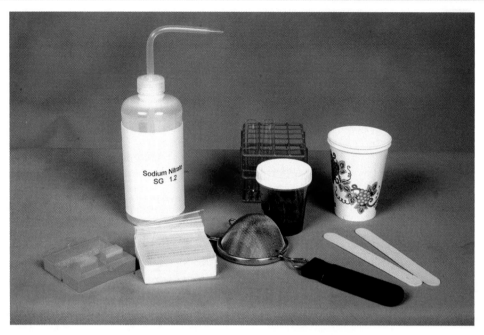

Figure 83-4   Materials needed for fecal flotation.

to a specific gravity of 1.27 and combined with centrifugal flotation results in the highest parasite recovery rates (see Table 83-1).[3] Regardless of the flotation solution that is used, it is important to monitor the density of the solution with an appropriate hydrometer on a regular basis (Table 83-2, Web Figure 83-4).

Solutions should be tested each time they are prepared and at weekly intervals. We are often asked whether instruments used to measure specific gravity of urine or salt water fish tanks can be used to test the specific gravity of fecal flotation solutions. These instruments measure specific gravity in ranges that are far below those used in veterinary practice and are not suitable for testing flotation solutions.

CENTRIFUGAL FLOTATION VERSUS STANDING FLOTATION?

Centrifugal flotation is more sensitive than standing flotation in detecting parasites in fecal specimens. The reason is simple—the buoyant and centrifugal forces that we can apply to the solution containing the parasites when the tubes spin in the centrifuge are much greater than the forces of buoyancy and gravity that concentrate parasites during standing flotation. Research has confirmed that centrifugal flotation is more effective than simple flotation in recovering parasites from fecal specimens.[2-5] Recovery rates were particularly improved for heavier eggs such as *Trichuris vulpis* (whipworms), *Taenia* spp. (tapeworms), and also for *Eucoleus (Capillaria)* spp. and *Isospora* (coccidia) spp. when centrifugal flotation was used. Given that well–cared-for pets are more likely to harbor a lower burden of parasites, it is more important to employ centrifugation to increase the parasite recovery rates.[2,3]

Contrary to most presumptions, swinging bucket and fixed angle centrifuges require little hospital bench space. Many are less than 16 inches square. Most centrifuges are reasonably priced and can be used for decades with minimal service and often little or no repair. Also, a variety of rotors are available to suit the needs of the busiest of practices. Examples of

---

Box • 83-1

Common Fecal Flotation Solutions

Magnesium Sulfate
($MgSO_4$: SG=1.20)
Add 450 g of $MgSO_4$ to 1000 mL of warm tap water

Zinc Sulfate
($ZnSO_4$: SG=1.18-1.20)
Add 331 g of $ZnSO_4$ to 1000 mL of warm tap water

Sodium Nitrate
($NaNO_3$: SG=1.18-1.20)
Add 338 g of $NaNO_3$ to 1000 of warm tap water

Sodium Chloride
($NaCl$: SG=1.18-1.20)
Add 350 g of $NaCl$ to 1,000 mL of warm tap water

Sheather's Sucrose Solution (SG=1.27)
454 g granulated sugar
355 mL tap water
6 mL formaldehyde
1. Heat the water to near boiling.
2. Add the granulated sugar and stir until it is dissolved.
3. Allow the mixture to cool to room temperature before adding the formaldehyde.
4. Check the specific gravity. Adjust to 1.27 using either tap water or sugar.

commercially available centrifuges are given in Tables 83-3 and 83-4.

STANDING FLOTATION

Standing flotation (sometimes called *passive, simple,* or *table-top* flotation), depends on the force of gravity to move heavier objects (debris) to the bottom of the tube, and the buoyant force to move lighter objects (parasites) to the top. The procedure is detailed in Web Figure 83-5.

Specimens are prepared as described above and in Web Figures 83-1 and Figures 83-1 through 83-3. The fecal specimen is mixed with flotation solution and passed through a tea strainer or gauze sponge. The filtrate is added to a tube, a reverse meniscus is formed, and a coverslip is placed. The preparation is allowed to stand for a minimum of 15 minutes. The coverslip is then removed and examined for parasites.

CENTRIFUGAL FLOTATION

Centrifugal flotation is the procedure of choice for concentration of parasites from feces.[5,6] It is considered by most to be the gold standard for fecal examination.[6] Centrifugal flotation can be performed using either a swinging bucket or fixed angle centrifuge (Figure 83-5).

We prefer the swinging bucket centrifuge because it decreases the number of times that the specimen is handled. When using a swinging bucket centrifuge, place the specimen into a tube holder (bucket) in the centrifuge. Add flotation solution to form a reverse meniscus at the top of the tube. Gently place a coverslip on the tube. It is important to avoid trapping air bubbles under the slide. This can be prevented by placing one side of the coverslip in contact with the tube and then slowly "layering" the remainder of the coverslip over the meniscus of the specimen (Figures 83-6 through 83-8).

The next step is the most important when using a swinging bucket centrifuge. The speed of the rotor should be increased gradually to a maximum of 600 to 800 rpm (Web Figure 83-6).

This is only possible if the centrifuge is equipped with a dial, knob, or digital entry button that will allow you to increase the speed incrementally. If the rotor speed is increased gradually to the target speed, the centrifuge bucket will move slowly to a horizontal position and the coverslip will remain in place. If the speed of the rotor is increased too rapidly, the coverslip may be dislodged from the specimen tube. If the centrifuge does not have variable speeds, or the initial speed is too fast, follow the instructions below for the fixed angle centrifuge. After the required centrifuge time of 10 minutes, turn off the centrifuge and allow the rotor to come to a complete stop. Do not touch the rotor or use the centrifuge "brake" to slow it. Remove the coverslip in one deliberate upward motion and place it on a microscope slide. Place one side of the coverslip on the slide first and "layer" it onto the glass slide as described previously to prevent entrapped air bubbles. We are often asked whether it is best to allow the specimen to stand an additional 5 minutes after placement of the coverslip. Although there is data to suggest that an additional 5 minute incubation time may increase parasite recovery rates, we suggest that if extra time is going to be added to the procedure, the extra time should be included in the time that the specimen is allowed to spin in the centrifuge.

Centrifugal flotation using a fixed angle centrifuge requires a change in procedures after spinning the sample (Web Figure 83-7).

Because the specimen is placed in the centrifuge at an angle, it is not possible to form a meniscus at the top of the centrifuge tube or to place a coverslip on the tube. Also, since the tube is not topped with a coverslip, the final speed at which the specimen is centrifuged is not as important, nor is it necessary to start the centrifuge at a slower speed. The specimen should be centrifuged at approximately 1200 rpm for 5 minutes. However, faster centrifuge rates can be used without adversely affecting the result. We do not suggest reducing the centrifuge time to less than 5 minutes. Allow the centrifuge to stop as described above. Remove the centrifuge tube, place it in a holder, and add flotation solution to form a reverse meniscus (Figure 83-9).

Follow the same procedure for placing the coverslip as described previously. Allow the specimen to stand for a minimum of 10 minutes before removing the coverslip to a slide and examining it for parasite stages. If sucrose is used as a flotation solution, we have found that it may be necessary to allow the tube and coverslip to stand for 15 to 20 minutes to recover all of the parasites' stages. It is not necessary to wait longer than 10 minutes when all other flotation solutions are used.

Table • 83-2

Examples of Commercially Available Hydrometers*

SUPPLIER	CONTACT INFORMATION	CATALOG #	DESCRIPTION	CURRENT PRICE
Fisher	1-800-766-7000 www.fishersci.com	11-522A	1.000-1.225 SG 185 mm long	$40.31
Fisher	1-800-766-7000 www.fishersci.com	11-522B	1.200-1.425 SG 160 mm long	$40.31
VWR	1-800-932-5000 www.vwrsp.com	34623-106	1.000-1.250 SG 165 mm long	$36.35
VWR	1-800-932-5000 www.vwrsp.com	34623-150	1.200-1.450 SG 165 mm long	$36.35
Cole Parmer	1-800-323-4340 www.coleparmer.com	C-08291-10	1.000-1.225 SG 150 mm long	$29.00
Cole Parmer	1-800-323-4340 www.coleparmer.com	C-08291-20	1.200-1.425 SG 150 mm long	$29.00

*These hydrometers are given as examples. Other suitable models are also available.
SG, Specific gravity.

Table • 83-3

Examples of Commercially Available Centrifuges with Swinging Bucket Rotors*

MANUFACTURER	MODEL	SPEED	DISTRIBUTOR†	CATALOG #	SIZE (INCHES) L × W × H	COST	ROTOR	TOTAL COST
IEC/Thermo Electron	Centra CL2 Mfr #426	1000-8500 rpm	Fisher 1-800-766-7000 www.fishersci.com	05-101-7	15 .75 × 13.25 × 10.75	$2166	Swing-out system— includes rotor, shields, and cushions 6 × 15 mL 05-155-18 $824	$2990
Eppendorf	Centrifuge 5702 Mfr # 22-62 600-1	100-4400 rpm	Fisher 1-800-766-7000 www.fishersci.com	05-400-300	16 × 12.5 × 9.5	$2045	Swing-out 8 × 15 mL 05-400-301 $278 Mfr # 22-63 950-1	$2323
Cole-Parmer	Compact Variable Speed Universal Centrifuge	6000 rpm max	Cole-Parmer 1-800-323-4340 www.coleparmer.com	EW-17306-01	14.6 × 11 × 10.25	$1560	Swing-out 6 × 5 mL EW-17306-54 $480 (note: this rotor only holds 5-mL tubes)	$2040
LW Scientific	Straight-8 3K Centrifuge	0-3000 rpm	Lab Essentials 1-888-522-7226 www.labessentials.com	LE-S8-3K	15.4 × 12.6 × 14	$599	Swing-out rotor included	$599
LW Scientific	C-3 Select Centrifuge	3000 rpm (blood) 1600 rpm (urine and semen) 1300 rpm (fecals)	Lab Essentials 1-888-522-7226 www.labessentials.com	LE-C3S-15	18 × 14.5 × 12	$695	Swing-out rotor included	$695
LW Scientific	C-5 Centrifuge	800-5000 rpm	Lab Essentials 1-888-522-7226 www.labessentials.com	LE-C5-15	15.5 × 13.75 × 14.25	$1375	Swing-out rotor included	$1375

*These centrifuges are given as examples. Other models are also available.
†Other distributors may also carry these products.

Table • 83-4

Examples of Commercially Available Centrifuges with Fixed Angle Rotors*

MANUFACTURER	MODEL	SPEED	DISTRIBUTOR†	CATALOG #	SIZE (INCHES) L × W × H	COST	ROTOR	TOTAL COST
Fisher	Centrific Model 225	5100 max rpm (with manual dial)	Fisher 1-800-766-7000 www.fishersci.com	04-978-50Q	16 dia. × 14	$1427.26	24 place fixed angle rotor—$517.49 04-978-52Q	$1944.75
LW Scientific	EW-79000-12 Clinical Centrifuge	Variable, max 3300 rpm	Cole-Parmer 1-800-323-4340 www.coleparmer.com	EW-79000-12	13 × 13 × 9	$395	Included, 8 × 15 mL	$395
LW Scientific	EW-79000-14 Clinical Centrifuge	Variable, 4-speed 800, 1500, 1800, 3300 rpm	Cole-Parmer 1-800-323-4340 www.coleparmer.com	EW-79000-14	13 × 13 × 9	$480	Included, 8 × 15 mL	$480
Labnet	Labnet Z100A Clinical Centrifuge	Variable, 1000-4000 rpm	Denville Scientific 1-800-453-0385 www.denvillescientific.com	C 0100	10.5 × 13.4 × 9.8	$495	Included, 6 × 15 mL	$495

*These centrifuges are given as examples. Other models are also available.
†Other distributors may also carry these products.

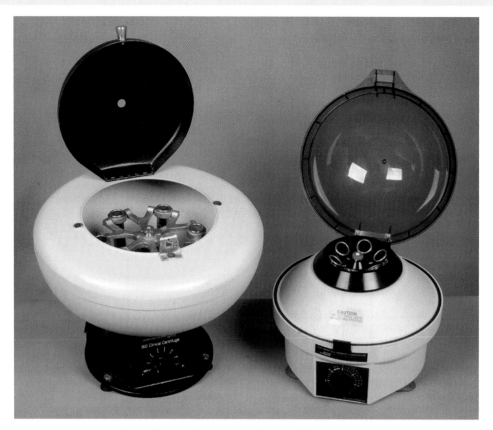

Figure 83-5 Centrifuges fitted with a swinging bucket *(left)* and a fixed angle rotor *(right)*.

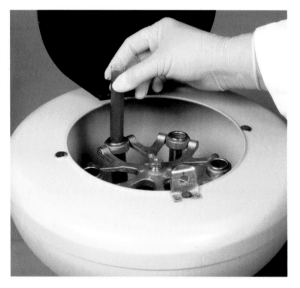

Figure 83-6 Place specimen in the centrifuge bucket.

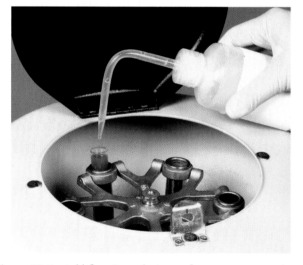

Figure 83-7 Add flotation solution to form a reverse meniscus.

PROPER EXAMINATION OF THE COVERSLIP

The coverslip should be examined systematically and thoroughly. It is important to remember that a prepared fecal slide is three dimensional, meaning that it has length, width, and depth. The latter is the most important. We tell students and veterinarians to focus on dust on the top of the coverslip and then move downward. The smaller parasites (e.g., *Giardia, Cryptosporidium,* small coccidia) will be found in the first or topmost layer. The next layer down will contain the large eggs (roundworms, hookworms, whipworms), oocysts, and larvae (if present). To examine the coverslip, start at one corner and move systematically through the specimen as shown in Web Figure 83-8.

Focus up and down as you move through the specimen, unless a parasite of particular size is suspected. If this is the case, you may concentrate your efforts at the layer in which that parasite is found. The entire coverslip should be examined using the 10× objective (total magnification 100×). Small parasites or other objects should then be examined using the

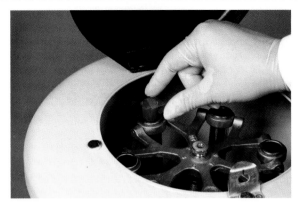

Figure 83-8 Apply a coverslip to the centrifuge tube.

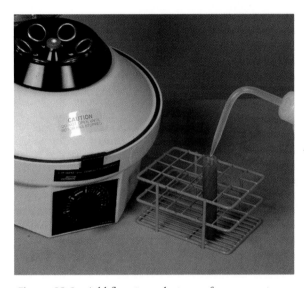

Figure 83-9 Add flotation solution to form a meniscus.

40× objective (total magnification of 400×). The 100× (oil immersion) objective should not be used to examine fecal flotation slides. Some laboratories will "spot-check" 5 to 10 fields in the center of the slide using 400× magnification to ensure that very small parasites are not overlooked. This certainly is a viable option, although we do not recommend it as a routine procedure.

FECAL SEDIMENTATION

Sedimentation is often employed to concentrate eggs or larvae that are too dense to float in flotation solutions. Sedimentation can be performed using either the standing or centrifugal procedure, but without flotation solution. We prefer to use a centrifuge because it results in faster movement of particulate material to the bottom of the tube. To perform the procedure, mix the fecal specimen after removal of large particulate debris with either saline, water, or 0.1 to 1.0% soap in water solution and add the mixture to a centrifuge tube (Web Figure 83-9).

Centrifuge the specimen (speed is less important, although some suggest 2 minutes at 1000 rpm) or allow the tube to stand undisturbed for 30 minutes to force parasites and debris to the bottom of the tube. Most of the supernatant is then removed and the entire sediment is examined microscopically. Some parasitologists recommend resuspending the sediment

a second time in solution used previously and then repeating the above steps.

BAERMANN PROCEDURE

The Baermann procedure is used to isolate larvae of parasites such as *Aelurostrongylus* and *Strongyloides* from fecal specimens. Larvae of these and similar parasites must be alive for successful recovery. Therefore, this procedure must be performed on fresh feces. The Baermann apparatus is a glass or plastic funnel with a piece of clamped flexible rubber or plastic tubing attached to the stem. Three to 10 g of fresh feces is enclosed in two layers of gauze or cheesecloth that is tied or secured with rubber bands and placed on a wire mesh platform inside the funnel. Warm water (not hot water) is placed in the funnel until it covers the fecal specimen. The apparatus is allowed to stand undisturbed for approximately 6 hours (some allow the specimen to stand overnight). Any larvae that are present are collected by slowly opening the clamp and allowing 5 to 10 mL of liquid to flow into a centrifuge tube. The tube is centrifuged gently for a few minutes to sediment any larvae. The supernatant is removed and the sediment is examined for larvae.

FECAL CULTURE FOR *TRITRICHOMONAS FOETUS*

Numerous techniques have been used to culture protozoa such as *Giardia*, *Tritrichomonas*, and *Pentatrichomonas* from canine or feline feces. Generally, these procedures require resources that are not readily available in the veterinary hospital. Veterinarians should submit samples either to reference or academic laboratories if fecal culture is to be attempted. One exception might be *Tritrichomonas foetus*. This agent causes large bowel diarrhea in cats and can be grown with relative ease in a commercially available culture system (In Pouch TF, Biomed Diagnostics, White City, Ore.). A very small amount of freshly voided feces (approximately 0.05 g) or feces contained on a moistened cotton-tipped rectal swab can be added to the In Pouch. The In Pouch is incubated for 24 hours at 37° C and then held at room temperature and examined every 2 days for 10 days. Media in the In Pouch system allows the few organisms that may be present to reproduce, thus increasing the likelihood of visualizing the motile trophozoites. The In Pouch can be maintained at room temperature if an incubator in not available. However, organisms are likely to appear in higher numbers sooner following preliminary incubation at 37° C.

IMMUNOLOGIC AND MOLECULAR TECHNIQUES

Several techniques have been developed to identify specific proteins or DNA from parasites in fecal specimens.[7-14] Immunologic techniques include enzyme-linked immunosorbent assays (ELISA) and fluorescent antibody tests. ELISA is a biochemical technique used to detect the presence of either an antibody or an antigen in a fecal sample. An indirect ELISA is usually used to detect antibodies to known antigens produced by the host. In this type of ELISA, specific antigens are bound to wells of microtiter plates and are used to capture antibodies present in test samples. These antigens are often synthesized or are recombinant expressed proteins, either from the surface of a parasite, or parasite secretions or excretions. A second species-specific antibody conjugated to an enzyme is added and will bind to any antibodies present in the test system. A substrate is then added and the presence of any bound enzyme-linked antibody will change the color of the substrate. When attempting to detect parasite antigens, a sandwich ELISA is the preferable method. This type of ELISA involves immobilizing an antigen-specific antibody to the wells of a microtiter plate or solid substratum. These antibodies can be polyclonal, or more specifically, monoclonal, detecting immunodominant antigens on parasites. The antigen-containing fecal samples are then added to the plate followed by the addition of another specific antibody conjugated to an enzyme. A substrate is then added and the presence of any bound enzyme-linked antibody will change the color of the substrate. Alternatively, if an enzyme conjugated antibody is not available, the available antibody can be covalently bound to a biotin molecule. Commercially available streptavidin conjugated enzyme is added. Because of the natural affinity of avidin to biotin, an antibody-biotin/avidin-enzyme complex is formed. Reaction of the enzyme with a substrate subsequently added to the mixture results in a detectable color change. Perhaps the best known fecal ELISA procedure is SNAP *Giardia* (IDEXX Laboratories, Westbrook, Me.). This test uses a unique method of capturing *Giardia* cyst wall proteins (CWP) present in the feces of *Giardia*-infected animals. To conduct the assay, a small sample of feces is mixed with an antibody/enzyme conjugate in a bulb. The bound antigen-antibody/enzyme mixture formed in the fecal/reagent emulsion is transferred to the snap device. Additional specific antibodies located on the solid substratum of the SNAP device trap the CWP/antibody/enzyme conjugate as it moves across the result window. When the cassette is snapped, wash solutions and substrate are released. The wash solution eliminates nonbound CWP, and the substrate is converted to a visible blue product by the enzyme. The SNAP *Giardia* test is an excellent method of confirming *Giardia*-induced cases of diarrhea in dogs and cats. Currently, the test is recommended only for testing samples from animals with clinical signs consistent with *Giardia* infection. Testing should not be conducted as a screening procedure on healthy animals.

A direct fluorescent antibody assay is also commercially available for diagnosis of *Giardia* and *Cryptosporidium*. The Merifluor *Cryptosporidium*/*Giardia* assay (Meridian Diagnostics, Inc, Cincinnati, Ohio) contains a fluorescein isothiocyanate (FITC)-labeled monoclonal antibody specific for cyst wall antigens. The Merifluor test requires the presence of cysts in feces to achieve a positive result. Consequently, this test is not as sensitive as the SNAP *Giardia* assay, which detects free CWP. The Merifluor test also requires an epifluorescence microscope, which is usually not available in veterinary hospitals. Assays designed for use in humans, such as the ProSpecT Microplate ELISA for *Giardia* and *Cryptosporidium*, are also available, but are not used with great frequency in veterinary medicine.

There are many examples of the application of molecular techniques to fecal diagnosis of parasitic infections. Application of molecular techniques is particularly helpful in instances of low parasite shedding or low worm burdens. These techniques are currently available only in academic and reference laboratories. It is possible that commercialized, user friendly versions of these tests will be available in the not-too-distant future.

POLYMERASE CHAIN REACTION (PCR)

PCR is a widely used technique that derives its name from one of its key components, DNA polymerase, an enzyme used to amplify a piece of DNA (amplicon). DNA primer sets are available commercially that are capable of binding to and amplifying target parasite DNA sequences. As the PCR reaction progresses, the DNA generated is itself used as template for replication. This results in a chain reaction in which the target parasite DNA template is amplified exponentially. Eventually, copies of the DNA are so numerous that they are easily visualized on an agarose gel. PCR is particularly helpful when parasites are present in feces in very low numbers or are very slow to replicate. PCR has been used to detect numerous fecal parasites including *Cryptosporidium*, *Giardia*, and *Tritrichomonas*.

Variations on the standard PCR technique have been developed that have abundant applications.

MULTIPLEX PCR

Multiplex PCR uses multiple, unique primer sets within a single PCR mixture to produce amplicons of varying sizes specific to different segments of the DNA sequences. By targeting multiple genes, additional information may be gained from a single test run that otherwise would require several times the reagents and more time to perform. An important requisite for multiplex PCR is that amplicons generated must have sufficient size differences so that their base pair length can easily be differentiated when visualized by gel electrophoresis. A more widespread use of this technique has been in the simultaneous detection of numerous organisms in a single sample.

NESTED PCR

Nested PCR increases the specificity of DNA amplification by reducing background due to nonspecific amplification of DNA. Two sets of primers are used in two successive PCR reactions. In the first reaction, one pair of primers is used to generate DNA products, which, in addition to the intended target, may consist of nonspecifically amplified DNA fragments. These product(s) are then used in a second PCR with a set of primers whose binding sites are completely or partially different from each of the primers used in the first reaction. Nested PCR is often more successful in specifically amplifying longer DNA fragments than in conventional PCR, but it requires more detailed knowledge of the target sequences. Nested PCR has been used in the identification of *Tritrichomonas foetus* infections in cats

QUANTITATIVE REAL-TIME PCR

This is a laboratory technique used to simultaneously amplify and quantify a targeted DNA molecule. It enables both detection and quantification (as absolute number of copies or relative amount when normalized to DNA input or additional normalizing genes) of a specific sequence in a DNA sample. Real-time PCR is a technique growing in popularity in veterinary medicine. Its uses include the blood detection of *Babesia* species, *Leishmania*, and the simultaneous detection of multiple fecal helminth infections.

DIAGNOSTIC RESOURCES

Several diagnostic manuals can assist diagnosticians in identifying internal parasites. These resources are listed in the reference section.[15-18]

REFERENCES

The reference list can be found on the companion Expert Consult Web site at *www.expertconsult.com*.

CHAPTER 84

Ear Vein Blood Glucose Monitoring

Melanie D. Thompson

In dogs and cats with diabetes mellitus, owner observation of clinical signs and in-hospital evaluation of serial blood glucose curves are common methods for assessing glycemic control. These parameters are also used as aids in determining both dose and type of insulin to be used as well as frequency of administration. Diabetic dogs and cats are typically hospitalized for glucose monitoring and blood samples are collected at 1- or 2-hour intervals by means of direct venipuncture of a peripheral vein. Hospitalization, restraint for blood sample collection, and venipuncture have all been associated with stress hyperglycemia (especially in cats), and some hospitalized pets may not eat. This can complicate interpretation of the resulting blood glucose curve.

Most human diabetics perform self-monitoring of blood glucose concentrations using a portable blood glucose meter (PBGM) and capillary blood, which is collected by pricking a fingertip with a lancet device. Portable blood glucose meters are being used more frequently to generate serial blood glucose curves in diabetic dogs and cats. These meters are inexpensive, require only a single drop of blood for analysis, and provide results rapidly. In addition, the results obtained with these meters have been shown to correlate with those obtained by reference laboratories. When only a small amount of blood is required for analysis, use of an ear vein for blood sampling can minimize patient discomfort, preserve the integrity of peripheral veins, and decrease need for physical restraint during sample collection. Studies have shown that the marginal ear vein nick technique is a reasonable alternative to venous blood collection for serial measurement of blood glucose concentrations. Studies have also shown good correlation between the glucose concentration of capillary and venous blood. Two methods of capillary blood sampling from the ear of dogs and cats are described here. Both methods are quick and easy to perform.

CAPILLARY BLOOD SAMPLING WITH CONVENTIONAL LANCET DEVICE

The first technique utilizes conventional lancet devices designed for pricking the fingertips of human beings. A device with a variable needle depth should be chosen. This allows the appropriate depth to be selected in order to provide an adequate amount of blood for the test (dogs usually require greater depth compared to cats). Although any portion of the inner pinna can be sampled, use of the marginal ear vein (MEV) usually results in the best sample. First the MEV is identified, then a warm, damp gauze sponge (or warm washcloth) is applied to it to increase perfusion as needed (Figure 84-1, A).

A thin film of Vaseline can be placed over the sampling site in longhaired pets to allow the drop of blood to form without dissipating into the fur. The automatic lancing device should then be placed over the vein (Figure 84-1, B); the

ejected needle will nick the ear, causing a drop of blood to form (Figure 84-1, C). The person performing the test should place a folded gauze sponge between the ear and the individual's finger to avoid an inadvertent finger nick. The PBGM with the test strip already inserted is then applied to the drop of blood to measure the blood glucose concentration (Figure 84-1, D and E).

CAPILLARY BLOOD SAMPLING WITH VACUUM LANCING DEVICE

The second technique utilizes a vacuum lancing device, the Microlet Vaculance (Bayer Diagnostics, Tarrytown, N.Y.), to facilitate collection of an adequate drop of blood (Figure 84-2, A).

The device was designed to allow blood collection from body sites other than the fingertips in human beings. It also has variable needle depth. This technique allows sampling of the inner pinna in dogs and cats. The tip of the ear is held between the thumb and index finger, and the surface of the pinna is held flat by the rest of the fingers (Figure 84-2, B). The lancet device then is set on a nonhaired area of the ear. An airtight seal between the device and the ear is obtained by pushing the outer ear against the device with the tip of one finger. The entire edge of the endcap must be in contact with the skin (Figure 84-2, C). The site is lanced by pressing the plunger cap down until it comes to a complete stop. While pressure is maintained between the endcap and the skin, the plunger is slowly released. This creates a negative pressure, and the skin slightly bulges up into the endcap. The negative pressure is maintained until there is an adequate drop of blood (Figure 84-2, D). When an adequate drop of blood has formed, the plunger is pressed three fourths of the way down to release the vacuum and remove the device. The PBGM with the test strip already inserted is then applied to the drop of blood to measure the blood glucose concentration.

Clinicians should be aware that there are some important limitations to the use of a PBGM. In particular, several factors can affect the accuracy of the blood glucose concentrations obtained with these meters, including the level of training of the user, whether the meter is properly maintained, whether appropriate quality control checks are performed, whether the animal has any concurrent diseases, and the hematocrit of the animal. All PBGMs overestimate the blood glucose concentration of anemic animals. Dehydration results in falsely lower blood glucose concentrations. Other factors may also affect results, such as altitude, environmental temperature and humidity, hypotension, hypoxia, and the triglyceride concentration. Abbot has introduced a veterinary glucometer (AlphaTRAK) that has been shown to be superior to 5 meters marketed for human use. The meter has been validated and calibrated for cats and dogs.

WWW. To view a video on this topic, go to **www.expertconsult.com.**

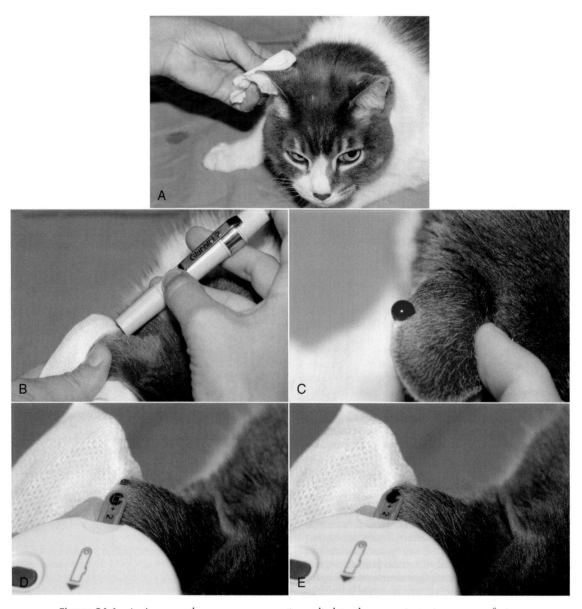

Figure 84-1 **A,** A warm, damp gauze sponge is applied to the ear vein to increase perfusion. **B,** The automatic lancing device is placed over the ear vein. Note that the gauze is folded so that the individual performing the test does not inadvertently get nicked. **C,** After the ejected needle nicks the ear, a drop of blood will form. **D,** The portable blood glucose meter with the test strip already inserted is applied to the drop of blood. **E,** The drop of blood is aspirated by capillary action into the reaction chamber after contact with the test strip.

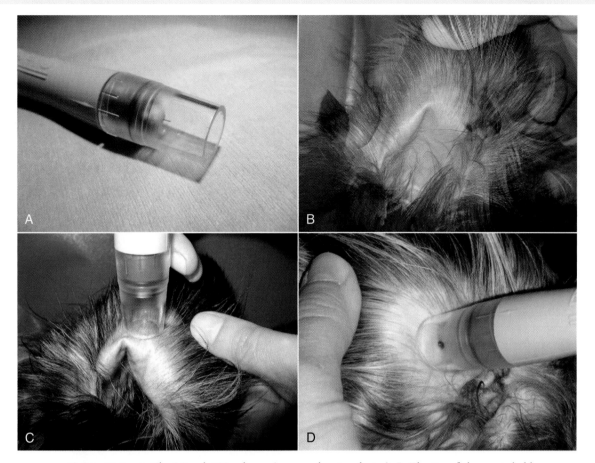

Figure 84-2 **A,** The Microlet Vaculance (vacuum lancing device). **B,** The tip of the ear is held between the thumb and index finger. The surface of the pinna is held flat by the rest of the fingers. **C,** The lancet device is set on a nonhaired area of the ear. The outer ear is pushed against the device to form an airtight seal. **D,** After lancing the ear, pressure is maintained and the plunger is slowly released. Negative pressure causes the skin to bulge up into the endcap.

A PBGM that is simple to operate should be chosen. Portable blood glucose meters are constantly being improved, and the result is greater precision, faster measurement, decreased blood volume, and decreased operator dependence. It is important to become familiar with the PBGM and perform routine maintenance. With practice, veterinarians, veterinary technicians, and veterinary students can become proficient in the techniques outlined here, and errors can be minimized.

Ear vein sampling can become the routine method of generating serial blood glucose curves in the hospital. These techniques can also be taught to clients for home monitoring of blood glucose concentrations.

Owners also can be directed to Web sites dedicated to diabetic pets, which contain information on home monitoring of glucose. In the search field, type "home monitoring of diabetic pets."

CHAPTER **85**

Nasoesophageal, Esophagostomy, Gastrostomy, and Jejunal Tube Placement Techniques

Stanley L. Marks

Enteral feeding is indicated in animals that cannot ingest adequate amounts of calories but have sufficient gastrointestinal (GI) function to allow digestion and absorption of feeding solutions delivered into the gastrointestinal tract via an enteral feeding device. Many techniques for obtaining enteral access are available, and the approach used depends on several variables: anticipated duration of enteral support, aspiration risk, integrity of the GI tract, the animal's temperament, the clinician's expertise, and the animal's tolerance to anesthesia.

ENTERAL FEEDING ACCESS DEVICES

Most feeding tubes are made of polyurethane or silicone. The main shortcoming of silicone is related to its stiffness and flexibility. Silicone feeding tubes require thick side walls to obtain tube wall integrity or stiffness; therefore, their internal diameter is smaller than the internal diameter of a similar-sized polyurethane tube.[1] The flexibility and decreased internal diameter of silicone tubes may lead to clogging or kinking. In addition, silicone is known for notch sensitivity that is associated with propagation of a defect in the material when the silicone gets a nick or a tear.[1] New feeding tube materials are being developed that are copolymers of silicone and polyurethane and other polymer end groups in an effort to mimic the softness of silicone and the durability and wall thickness of polyurethane. The French (F) unit measures the outer lumen diameter of a tube (each French unit is equal to 0.33 mm).

Nasoesophageal Tubes

Nasoesophageal tubes are a simple and efficient choice for short-term (less than 10 days) nutritional support of most anorectic hospitalized animals that have a normal nasal cavity, pharynx, esophagus, and stomach.[2,3] Nasoesophageal tube feeding is contraindicated in animals that are vomiting, comatose, or lack a gag reflex. Polyvinylchloride (Infant Feeding Tube, Argyle Division of Sherwood Medical, St. Louis, Mo.) or red rubber tubes (Robinson catheter, Sherwood Medical, St. Louis, Mo.) are the least expensive for dogs and cats, although the polyvinylchloride tubes may harden within 2 weeks of insertion and cause irritation or ulceration of the pharynx or esophagus. Tubes made of polyurethane (MILA International, Inc., Erlanger, Ky.) or silicone (Global Veterinary Products, Inc., New Buffalo, Mich.) are more expensive, less irritating, more resistant to gastric acid, and allow prolonged usage. An 8-French, 91 cm tube with or without a tungsten-weighted tip is suitable for dogs weighing more than 15 kg. A 5-French tube is more comfortable for cats and smaller dogs.

The length of tube to be inserted into the distal esophagus is determined by measuring the distance from the tip of the nose to the seventh or eighth intercostal space. This helps verify correct placement of the tube in the distal esophagus rather than the stomach, and decreases likelihood of reflux esophagitis.[4] Place a tape marker on the tube once the appropriate measurement has been made. Desensitization of the nasal cavity with 0.5 to 1 mL of 0.5% proparacaine hydrochloride is recommended. Tilt the head up to encourage the local anesthetic to coat the nasal mucosa. Lubricate the tip of the tube with 5% lidocaine viscous prior to passage, maintain the animal's head in the normal angle of articulation (avoid hyperflexion or overextension of the head and neck), and gently direct the tube tip in a caudoventral medial direction. The tube should move with minimal resistance through the ventral meatus and nasopharynx and into the esophagus. Nasoesophageal intubation is more difficult to perform in dogs because of their long, narrow nasal passages and extensive turbinate structures. In addition, the presence of a small ventral ridge at the proximal end of the nasal passage in dogs necessitates directing the tip of the tube dorsally initially to allow passage over the ventral ridge and into the nasal vestibule[2] (Figure 85-1). The tube is then directed in a caudoventral and medial direction while pushing the external nares dorsally.[5] This maneuver opens the ventral meatus and guides the tube into the oropharynx.

If the tube is unable to be passed with minimal resistance into the oropharynx, it should be withdrawn and redirected because it could be positioned in the middle meatus with its tip encountering the ethmoid turbinate. Once the tube has been passed to the level of the tube marker, it should be

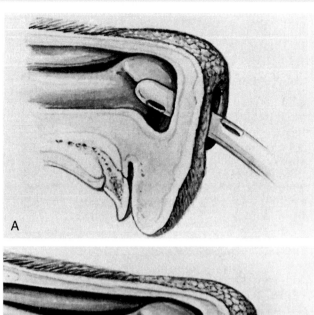

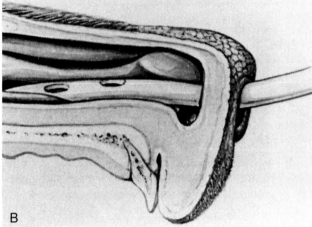

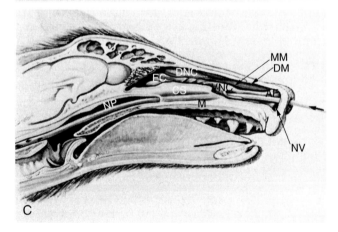

Figure 85-1 Parasagittal section showing stepwise insertion of a nasoesophageal tube through the ventral meatus of a dog. **A,** The presence of a small ventral ridge at the rostral end of the nasal passage necessitates directing the tip of the tube dorsally to clear the protuberance. **B,** Once past the protuberance, the tube is aimed medially and ventrally and advanced into the ventral meatus. **C,** Tube through ventral meatus and nasal pharynx *(NP).* Structures identified: nasal vestibule *(NV),* cartilaginous septum *(CS),* maxilla *(M),* dorsal meatus *(DM),* middle meatus *(MM),* ethmoidal conchae *(EC),* ventral nasal conchae *(VNC),* dorsal nasal conchae *(DNC),* and alar fold *(AF).* (Reprinted with permission from Crowe DT: Clinical use of an indwelling nasogastric tube for enteral nutrition and fluid therapy in the dog and cat. J Am Anim Hosp Assoc 22:675-682, 1986.)

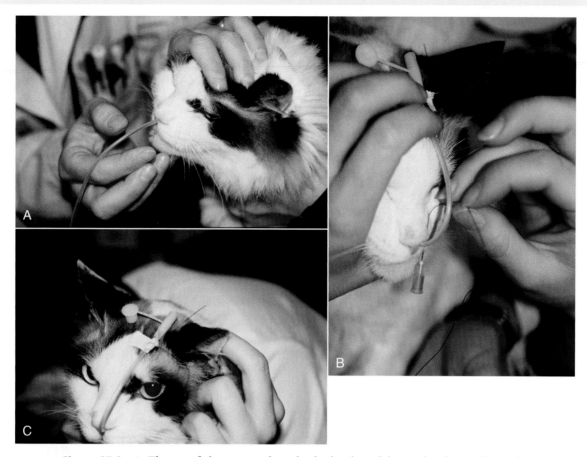

Figure 85-2 A, The tip of the nasoesophageal tube has been lubricated and passed into the ventral meatus by positioning the animal's head in a normal angle of articulation. **B,** The tube should be secured as close to the nostril as possible, with either suture material or glue. **C,** The nasoesophageal tube can be secured to the skin on the dorsal midline between the eyes with tape "butterflies."

secured as close to the nostril as possible, with either suture material (Figure 85-2, *A*) or glue (Superglue, Loctite Corp., Cleveland, Ohio). A second tape tab should be secured to the skin on the dorsal midline between the eyes (Figure 85-2, *B* and *C*). In the cat, the tube must not exit laterally nor come in contact with the whiskers. An Elizabethan collar is usually required for dogs to prevent inadvertent tube removal; however, most cats do not require such a device. Removal of the tube is facilitated by clipping the hair that is attached to the glue.

After placement, the tube position is checked by injecting 5 to 10 mL of air while auscultating the cranial abdomen for borborygmus, by infusing 3 to 5 mL of sterile saline or water through the tube and observing for a cough response,[2] or by obtaining a lateral survey thoracic radiograph. Verification of placement can also be done with an end-tidal CO_2 monitor. Tubes placed within the esophagus or stomach should yield no CO_2 when checked with an end-tidal CO_2 monitor. The most common complications associated with the use of nasoesophageal tubes include epistaxis, dacrocystitis, rhinitis, tracheal intubation (pneumonia), and vomiting.[2] A major disadvantage of nasoesophageal feeding tubes is their small diameter, necessitating the use of liquid enteral formulas. Commercially available canned pet foods that are diluted with water invariably clog feeding tubes. The caloric density of most human and veterinary liquid enteral formulas varies from 1.0 to 2.0 kcal/mL. Diets are fed full strength on continuous (pump infusion) or bolus feeding schedules.

Esophagostomy Tubes

Esophagostomy feeding tubes are easily inserted, only requiring light general anesthesia with isofluorane or heavy sedation, and intubation with a cuffed endotracheal tube. The technique is minimally invasive and no specialized endoscopic equipment is needed. The patient should be placed in right lateral recumbency, and the left lateral cervical region clipped and aseptically prepared for tube placement.[6-8] Placement of the feeding tube in the left side of the neck is preferred because the esophagus lies slightly left of midline. A 14- to 20-French red rubber catheter, (Robinson catheter, Sherwood Medical, St. Louis, Mo.), silicone catheter (Global Veterinary Products, Inc., New Buffalo, Mich.), or polyurethane catheter (MILA International, Inc., Florence, Ky.) should be premeasured from the midcervical esophagus to the seventh or eighth intercostal space, and marked with a permanent marker to ensure the distal end of the catheter terminates in the distal esophagus.[4] Aseptically prepare the left midcervical area from the angle of the mandible to the thoracic inlet. Three basic techniques for placement of a midcervical esophagostomy tube have been described.[6-8]

Technique Using Curved Carmalt, Mixter, or Schnidt Forceps   Advance the right-angle forceps into the midcervical esophagus from the oral cavity. Use the angle of the jaw and the point of the shoulder for landmarks to help ensure that the tip of the forceps can be palpated externally in the midcervical region. Push the curved tips of the forceps laterally at the midcervical esophagus, so they can be palpated below the skin. Use a No. 11 scalpel blade to make a stab incision through the skin only, exposing the subcutaneous tissue and muscle layers of the esophagus. Be careful to avoid the jugular and maxillofacial veins when selecting the stoma site. Exteriorize the tip of the forceps from the esophageal lumen through the skin incision. Guide the advancing forceps through the esophageal muscle layers and carefully dissect the esophageal mucosa off the tip of the forceps with a scalpel blade. Use the tip of the forceps to grasp the distal end of the feeding tube and draw the tube out of the oral cavity. Secure the distal end of the feeding tube using the forceps to ensure that the tube remains exteriorized while the proximal end of the tube is pulled out of the animal's mouth. Retroflex the proximal tip of the feeding tube and advance it in an aboral direction across the pharynx and down the esophagus, while slowly retracting on the external end of the tube 2 to 4 cm. A wire guide can be used to facilitate pushing the proximal tip of the feeding tube into the esophagus. The exteriorized portion of the tube will be observed to rotate in a cranial direction as the tube moves down the esophagus, indicating correct placement of the tube in the esophagus. Retention sutures (Chinese finger-trap suture) using 2-0 polypropylene are used to secure the distal end of the tube to the skin. An additional method of securing the tube involves passing a heavy suture on a taper needle through the skin next to the tube and into the periosteum of the wing of the atlas. Antibiotic ointment and gauze dressing are placed at the incision site, and the tube and entrance site is loosely bandaged with conforming gauze wrap. The correct placement of the tube in the mid to distal esophagus should be confirmed radiographically. It is important to ensure that the tube does not traverse the lower esophageal sphincter, as the tube can cause irritation and predispose the patient to gastroesophageal reflux. Feeding can be instituted immediately following full recovery of the patient from anesthesia. The tube esophagostomy-skin interphase should be examined at least daily during the first week for evidence of infection or leakage of food or saliva. The stoma site can be kept clean with a topical antiseptic solution (1:100 Betadine solution in 0.9% saline). The tube can be easily removed once nutritional support is no longer needed by cutting the Chinese finger-trap anchoring suture and

pulling the tube. The wound should be allowed to heal by second intension.

Percutaneous Feeding Tube Applicator Technique   An alternative tube esophagostomy technique utilizing an Eld percutaneous feeding tube applicator or similar device can be used.[8] The applicator is inserted into the midcervical esophagus via the oral cavity, the distal tip is palpated, and an incision is made through the skin and subcutaneous tissue over the tip of the Eld. Activate the spring-loaded instrument (Figure 85-3, *A*) to advance the trocar through the esophageal wall and incision (Figure 85-3, *B*) The distal end of the feeding tube is secured to the eyelet of the trocar with suture material. The Eld device and attached feeding tube are retracted into the esophagus and exteriorized out of the oral cavity. The feeding tube is redirected into the midcervical esophagus after inserting a wire stylet into the distal tip of the feeding tube. The tube is secured to the skin as mentioned above.

Percutaneous Needle Catheter Technique   This method incorporates the use of an esophagostomy introduction tube (Van Noort esophagostomy tube set, Global Veterinary Products, Inc., New Buffalo, Mich.) (Figure 85-4) that is introduced into the midcervical esophageal area. The slot in the distal portion of the tube is palpated, and a Peel-Away sheath needle (Global Veterinary Products) is introduced into the distal portion of the tube. The needle is removed from the sheath and a 10-French catheter is introduced through the sheath to the distal third of the esophagus. The sheath is peeled away and the esophagostomy tube carefully removed. The feeding tube is secured as described. This technique has limitations as the small diameter of the feeding tube (10 French) only allows for the administration of fluids and liquid enteral formulas.

Despite the potential for esophageal scarring and stricture formation, esophageal stricture or a persistent esophagocutaneous fistula has not developed. The most common minor complication is peristomal inflammation, with peristomal abscessation occurring infrequently.[6-9] Most inflammatory reactions are mild and respond to cleansing with topical antibiotics. Other, less common, complications include vomiting the tube into the oral cavity and tube obstruction.[6-9]

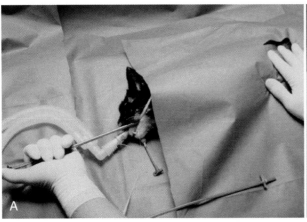
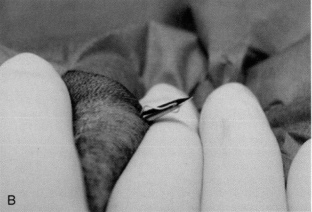

Figure 85-3   A, Demonstration of the Eld device for placement of an esophagostomy tube or blind percutaneous gastrostomy technique. Activation of the spring-loaded instrument advances the trocar through the esophageal or gastric wall. **B,** Suture material is attached to the exteriorized eyelet of the trocar which is retracted into the lumen of the instrument, and carefully removed out of the esophagus and out the mouth of the animal. The exteriorized suture material is attached to a feeding tube.

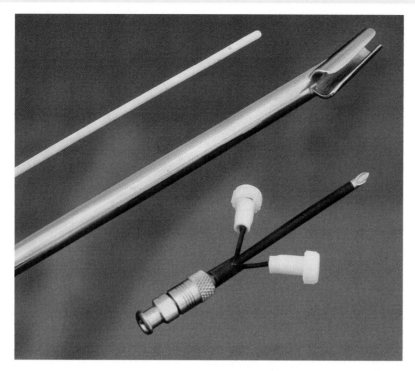

Figure 85-4   Photograph of the esophagostomy tube set, illustrating the esophagostomy introduction tube; 10-gauge, 5.0-cm-long needle with Peel-Away sheath needle; and a 10-French silicone catheter.

Gastrostomy Tubes

Gastrostomy tube feeding is indicated for long-term (weeks to months) nutritional support of anorectic or dysphagic animals that have adequate gastrointestinal function to allow digestion and absorption of feeding solutions. Gastrostomy feeding tubes are of comparatively large diameter (20 to 24 French), allowing the economic use of blended pet foods and the direct administration of medications. Gastrostomy tube feeding is contraindicated in animals with persistent vomiting, decreased consciousness, or GI obstruction. Caution should be exercised in conditions under which the stomach cannot be apposed to the body wall (severe ascites, adhesions, space-occupying lesions).

Gastrostomy tubes can be placed percutaneously or during laparotomy. Placement is usually accompanied via a percutaneous endoscopic gastrostomy (PEG) technique,[10,11] or a blind percutaneous gastrostomy (BPG) technique.[12,13] There are a variety of feeding tubes that can be utilized for gastrostomy feeding including latex, polyurethane, and silicon tubes with French-Pezzer mushroom, balloon, bumper, or silicone dome tips (Figure 85-5). The silicone catheters can be purchased from Global Veterinary Inc., New Buffalo, Kentucky, and from US Endoscopy, Mentor, Ohio; polyurethane from MILA International, Inc., Erlanger, Kentucky; and latex catheters from BARD Urological Division, Murray Hill, New Jersey. One can modify the catheters by cutting off and discarding the flared open end of the catheter and cutting off two 2-cm pieces of tubing (to be used as internal and external flanges) from the same end of the catheter. The end of the catheter opposite the mushroom tip is trimmed to facilitate its introduction into the larger opening of a disposable plastic micropipette. Make a small stab incision through the center of each flange and fit one flange over the cut end of the catheter, sliding it down until it rests against the mushroom tip. The other 2-cm piece of tubing will be used as an external flange that lies against the abdominal wall. Cutting the small nipple on the mushroom tip to enhance the flow of food through the tube is not recommended because it compromises the integrity of the mushroom and hinders percutaneous removal of the tube.

Percutaneous Endoscopic Gastrostomy (PEG) Technique   Endoscopic and blind placement of gastrostomy tubes necessitates brief anesthesia. The animal should be placed in right lateral recumbency so that the stomach tube can be placed through the greater curvature of the stomach and the left body wall. Patient preparation for both percutaneous procedures is identical and involves a surgical prep of the skin caudal to the left costal arch. The endoscope is introduced into the stomach and the stomach is carefully inflated until the abdomen is distended but not drum tight. The left body wall is transilluminated with the endoscope to ensure that the spleen is not positioned between the stomach and body wall. An appropriate site for insertion of the tube is determined by endoscopically monitoring digital palpation of the gastric wall. A small incision is made in the skin with a scalpel blade, and an intravenous catheter (16 to 18 G, 1.5 to 2 inch) is stabbed through the body wall into the lumen of the stomach (Web Figure 85-1, *A*). The stylet is removed and nylon or polyester suture is threaded through the catheter into the lumen of the stomach. The suture material is grasped with the endoscopic biopsy forceps (Web Figure 85-1, *B*), and the endoscope and forceps are carefully withdrawn through the esophagus and out of the mouth. The suture material is secured to the feeding tube and gentle traction is applied to the suture material at its point of exit from the abdominal wall (Web Figure 85-1, *C*). The feeding tube is pulled out through the body wall, allowing the mushroom end to draw the stomach wall against the body wall (Web Figure 85-1, *D*). The feeding tube is anchored in this position by the external flange placed over the catheter at the skin surface (Web Figure 85-1, *E*). The

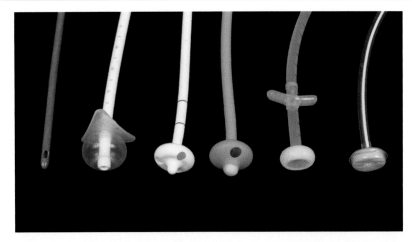

Figure 85-5 Gastrostomy tubes illustrating the various materials and catheter tips; *from left to right*, French red rubber catheter, silicone balloon catheter, silicone mushroom catheter, latex mushroom catheter, silicone catheter with dome, polyurethane catheter with bumper.

endoscope is then reinserted into the stomach to verify the correct placement of the mushroom against the gastric mucosa. If blanching of the mucosa is observed, less tension should be applied to the tube, otherwise necrosis of the gastric wall may ensue as a result of ischemia. A plastic clamp is placed over the tube and the tube is capped with a Y-port connector. A jacket made from stockinette (San Jose Surgical Supply, Inc., San Jose, Calif.) is fitted to protect the tube (Web Figure 85-1, *F*).

Complications related to PEG tubes include those associated with placement of the tube (splenic laceration, gastric hemorrhage, and pneumoperitoneum), and delayed complications such as vomiting, aspiration pneumonia, tube extraction, tube migration, and stoma infection.[10,11,14] Splenic laceration can be minimized by insufflating and transilluminating the stomach prior to placement of the needle or catheter into the abdominal wall. A discordant number of large-breed dogs have had major complications caused by the stomach falling off the silicone dome at the end of the gastrostomy tube. The stoma appeared normal in all dogs, with the unfortunate consequence that several dogs were fed through the gastrostomy tube. This complication occurred despite the placement of an internal flange between the dome and the gastric mucosa. For this reason, it is recommended that all dogs heavier than 30 kg, particularly those that have delayed wound healing secondary to malnutrition, uremia, or chemotherapy administration, do not have a PEG procedure, and instead have a gastrostomy tube placed surgically or placement of an esophagostomy tube. Minor complications include pressure necrosis at the stoma site and cellulitis.[10,11,14]

Blind Percutaneous Gastrostomy Technique   An alternative technique for nonendoscopic and nonsurgical gastrostomy tube placement has been described.[12,13] The gastrostomy tube placement device can be prepared with a length of vinyl or stainless steel tubing (diameter 1.2 to 2.5 cm) purchased from a hardware store, or an Eld Gastrostomy Tube Applicator (Jorgensen Laboratories, Loveland, Colo.) or gastrostomy tube introduction set (Global Veterinary Inc., New Buffalo, Ky.). The Eld Gastrostomy Tube Applicator is the only device that utilizes an internal trocar, whereas the Cook gastrostomy tube introduction set contains a wire that is threaded through an introduction needle. The distal tip of a stainless steel tube can

be flared and deflected 45 degrees to the long axis of the tube to help displace the lateral body wall. The lubricated tube is passed through the mouth into the stomach and advanced until the end of the tube displaces the stomach and lateral abdominal wall. Positioning the animal with its head over the edge of the table and lowering the proximal end of the tube will facilitate identifying the tube tip through the body wall.

For the Cook gastrostomy introduction set or similarly prepared device, a percutaneous needle is introduced into the tube while an assistant firmly holds the distal tip of the tube between two fingers. A skin nick is made over the end of the tube and a 14-gauge needle advanced into the lumen of the introduction tube (Web Figure 85-2, *A*). Proper positioning of the needle is confirmed by moving the hub from side to side and feeling the needle tip strike the inside of the tube. A guide wire included in the kit is threaded through the lumen of the needle, into the tube, and out the mouth. The introduction tube is removed and the threaded end of the guide wire is secured to an adapter that fits snugly into the end of a feeding tube (Web Figure 85-2, *B* and *C*). Gentle traction is applied to the guide wire at its point of exit from the abdominal wall, facilitating the placement of the mushroom end of the feeding tube against the gastric mucosa. The feeding tube is secured in an identical fashion to the PEG tube procedure described above.

The reported complication rate for BPG is similar to that of PEG; however, the risk of penetrating the spleen, stomach, or omentum is greater when the stomach is not insufflated with air prior to positioning the tube against the lateral abdominal wall.[15] Contraindications to using the "blind" technique include esophageal disease and severe obesity, which precludes accurate palpation of the tube against the abdominal wall. In either case, gastrostomy tubes should be placed surgically.

Jejunostomy Tubes

Jejunostomy tubes are indicated for dogs and cats unable to tolerate intragastric or intraduodenal feeding, despite having normal distal small intestine and colon function.[16] Specific indications for feeding via jejunostomy tube include gastric outlet obstruction, gastroparesis, recurrent/potential aspiration, proximal small bowel obstruction, and partial gastrectomy. Jejunal tube feeding minimizes the stimulation of pancreatic secretion and is a viable route for patients with severe pancreatitis.[16]

Surgically placed jejunostomy tubes are the most widely used and familiar method for long-term feeding of the small intestine directly. An alternative approach to the surgical jejunostomy technique is the placement of a feeding tube via percutaneous techniques. This includes both percutaneous jejunostomy and percutaneous gastrojejunostomy (PEG-J) tubes placed under fluoroscopic or endoscopic guidance. The advantage of the PEG-J technique is that it allows ready access to the stomach for aspiration of gastric luminal contents.

Successful placement of PEG-J tubes has been demonstrated in healthy dogs and cats,[17] according to the method described by Leichus et al.[18] Four sequential steps are followed: (1) routine PEG placement; (2) deep guide wire passage into the small intestine; (3) endoscope retraction leaving the guide wire in place; and (4) jejunostomy feeding tube placement over the guide wire. Briefly, the animal is anesthetized and placed in right lateral recumbency. A PEG tube is routinely placed, and the external portion of the tube trimmed to a length of 6 inches to maximize the amount of jejunostomy tube that can be passed into the small intestine. Placement of a 65-cm jejunostomy tube (Gastro-Jejunal Feeding Tube, Wilson-Cook Medical Inc., Winston-Salem, N.C.) works well in cats, whereas a jejunostomy feeding tube ≥95-cm is recommended for most dogs. A standard loop snare is passed through the PEG tube into the stomach using an endoscope. The snare is opened and the endoscope advanced through the open snare toward the pylorus. The animal is then positioned in left lateral recumbency and the endoscope is advanced as far down the small intestine as possible. The accessory channel of the endoscope is flushed with water to facilitate rapid passage of a guide wire that is passed down the biopsy channel into the small intestine. As the endoscope is carefully retracted into the stomach, the tip of the endoscope is pulled past the open snare, which is then closed snugly on the guide wire. The endoscope is then removed from the animal with the resultant extension of the guide wire out of the oral cavity. The closed snare is then pulled out through the gastrostomy tube, facilitating the exit of a portion of the guide wire from the opening of the gastrostomy tube. The snare is then released and an assistant gently pulls on the proximal end of the guide wire. The oral end of the guide wire is pulled through the gastrostomy tube, leaving the distal (aboral) end in the small intestine. The jejunostomy tube is flushed with water, which activates a lubricant on its inner diameter. The jejunostomy tube is threaded over the guide wire under endoscopic guidance until its proximal end is seated in the gastrostomy tube. The guide wire is then removed from the PEG-J tube, and abdominal radiographs are taken to confirm adequate placement of the jejunostomy tube 40 to 60 cm distal to the pylorus. Passage of the jejunostomy tube deeply into the jejunum is deemed critical to prevent retrograde catheter migration into the stomach.

Esophagostomy, Gastrostomy, and PEG-J Tube Removal

Unlike gastrostomy tubes, an esophagostomy tube can be removed the same day it is placed if necessary without concern for leakage and development of secondary complications. The dressing and sutures are removed while the tube is held in place. The tube is then occluded by kinking and pulled out using gentle traction. The ostomy site should be cleaned, antibiotic ointment applied, and a light dressing placed around the neck. The dressing should be removed in 24 hours and the ostomy site inspected. The ostomy site should close within 24 to 36 hours. Skin sutures are not needed for closure of the ostomy site. For PEG tubes and PEG-J tubes, it is recom-

mended that the PEG tube be left in place for a minimum of 14 days. Animals receiving immune-suppressive therapy or patients that are severely debilitated may require longer for a peritoneal seal to form. The tube should only be removed when oral food intake is sufficient to meet the patient's caloric requirement. One of two methods of Pezzer PEG tube removal can be applied. The tube can be cut at the body wall and the mushroom tip pushed into the stomach to be passed in the feces. This method is safe in medium- to large-size dogs, because the mushroom and internal flange should be easily passed in the stool. Alternatively, a stylet can be inserted into the tube to flatten the mushroom tip, while exerting firm traction on the tube. This method is recommended for cats and small dogs, because the mushroom can cause intestinal obstruction. Removal of the MILA catheter is accomplished by deflating the bumper, which occurs once the Y-port adapter is removed. Catheters with a dome (US Endoscopy) are removed by gentle but firm traction on the tube. The gastrocutaneous tract should seal with minimal or no leakage within 24 hours.

Gastrostomy and Esophagostomy Tube Replacement

The PEG tube may malfunction or be prematurely removed by the patient, requiring replacement. If the gastrostomy tube is removed within 14 days of placement (before establishment of the gastrocutaneous tract), a PEG procedure should be performed to evaluate the gastric mucosa and verify correct positioning of the replacement gastrostomy tube. If the tube is inadvertently removed once the gastrocutaneous tract is well healed, one can replace the original catheter with a balloon-type catheter (Flexiflo Gastrostomy Tube, Ross Laboratories, Columbus, Ohio)[19] or a low-profile gastrostomy device (LPGD) (Bard Interventional Products Division, Murray Hill, N.J.) (Web Figure 85-3, A). Neither catheter type requires an endoscopic procedure or anesthesia for placement. The gastrostomy "button" is a small, flexible silicone device that has a mushroom-like dome at one end and two small wings at the other end that lie flush with the outer abdominal wall (Web Figure 85-3, B). A one-way antireflux valve prevents reflux of gastric contents through the top of the tube. There are two types of LPGDs: obturated and non-obturated. The obturated device has an enlarged mushroom tip that must be stretched for placement in the stomach by using a special introducer[20] (Web Figure 85-3, C). The non-obturated tube works like a Foley catheter and does not require forceful entry into the gastrostomy stoma. The length of the gastrocutaneous fistula must be precisely determined to guide correct selection of the appropriate "button" shaft length. This is accomplished with a special stoma-measuring device provided with the kit. The main advantages of the LPGDs include their durability due to their silicon material, decreased likelihood of inadvertent removal by the patient, and their aesthetically pleasing appearance to the owners.[21]

COMPLICATIONS OF ENTERAL FEEDING

Gastric Pressure Necrosis

Gastric pressure necrosis can occur from either the mushroom of the PEG tube or flange eroding the mucus layer of the stomach due to excessive tension being exerted on the PEG tube during placement. In addition, overzealous traction of the PEG tube followed by placement of the external flange flush against the skin of the patient can also cause pressure necrosis characterized by redness, swelling, and moistness of the skin. To minimize the chance of this problem occurring, ensure that the PEG tube can be rotated following its placement and leave a 1-cm space between the external flange and the skin.

Feeding Tube Displacement

This is a relatively common problem, particularly with naso-esophageal and PEG-J tubes. Displacement of the tube can lead to aspiration, diarrhea, or, in the case of gastrostomy tubes, peritonitis. Gastrostomy tubes should be marked with tape or a marking pen at the level of the skin to help verify the position of the tube. Detachment of the stomach from the abdominal wall with consequent intraperitoneal leakage of gastric contents can occur in large-breed dogs, and an internal flange should be placed in these animals to minimize dislodgement of the tube.

Tube Obstruction

Obstruction of the feeding tube is one of the most common complications of enteral feeding.[22] Most obstructions are secondary to coagulation of formula, although obstruction by tablet fragments, tube kinking, and precipitation of incompatible medications can also result in tube obstruction. Naso-esophageal tubes are prone to obstruction because of their small diameters, and obstruction also occurs up to three times more frequently in patients fed by continuous versus bolus feedings.[23] Sucralfate and antacids have been reported to precipitate with enteral formulas and cause tube obstruction.[23] Several "remedies" have been advocated to relieve tube obstruction. Warm water injected with gentle pressure and suction will relieve most obstructions. For more unyielding obstructions, carbonated water is instilled into the tube and allowed to sit for 1 hour before applying gentle pressure and suction. Pancreatic enzyme infusions[22] and meat tenderizer have also been advocated to dissolve tube obstructions. On rare occasions, the passage of an angiographic wire down the lumen is needed to unclog the tube. Tube obstructions can be minimized by flushing the feeding tube with warm water before and after administering medications or enteral feedings. The tube should also be flushed after checking for gastric residuals, because the acid pH will cause the formula to coagulate in the tube. Elixir forms of medication should be used rather than crushed tablet forms whenever possible. Tablets should be crushed and dissolved in water prior to administration through the feeding tube, if no alternative form of medication is available.

Leakage through Ostomy Sites

Mild leakage at the stoma site can occur for the first few days following placement of the feeding tube. Persistent leakage may indicate tube dysfunction, peristomal infection, or a stoma site larger than necessary for the tube. Signs of inflammation with or without discharge or fever may indicate infection of the stoma site. This must be differentiated from fasciitis as a simple wound infection can usually be treated locally with dilute Betadine solution, topical Betadine anti-bacterial ointments, and more frequent dressing changes. Systemically administered antibiotics are usually reserved for patients with systemic signs of infection.

Aspiration

Pulmonary aspiration is a common complication of enteral feeding, although the actual incidence of this complication is difficult to determine due to the lack of consistency in how aspiration is defined. Risk factors for aspiration include impaired mental status, neurologic injury, absence of a cough or gag reflex, mechanical ventilation, and previous aspiration pneumonia.[24] The source of the aspirated material should be identified because withholding gastrostomy feedings or placing a jejunostomy feeding tube in a patient will have no benefit if the patient aspirated oropharyngeal secretions. Although controversial, most authors agree that postpyloric feeding reduces the risk of aspiration.[25] In addition, the use of continuous versus bolus feedings has been shown to induce less gastroesophageal reflux than bolus feedings.[26]

Diarrhea

Diarrhea is the most commonly cited complication associated with tube feeding in human and animal patients, with an incidence ranging from 2.3% to 63%.[27] The clinical implications of enteral feeding–related diarrhea are significant. Severe diarrhea leads to fluid, electrolyte, and nutrient loss, and can cause considerable distress to the patient. Diarrhea in tube-fed patients occurs due to multiple factors, including hypoalbuminemia, hyperosmolar or high-fat diets, infected diets, and concomitant antibiotic therapy.[28] The incidence of diarrhea in enterally fed patients taking antibiotics far exceeds the incidence in normally fed patients taking the same antibiotics. Antibiotic-associated diarrhea may arise from overgrowth of enterobacteria (*Klebsiella, Proteus, Pseudomonas*) or from proliferation of *Clostridium difficile*. Antibiotic administration is also associated with decreased concentrations of fecal short-chain fatty acids, occurring as a result of decreased colonic carbohydrate fermentation.[29]

REFERENCES

The reference list can be found on the companion Expert Consult Web site at *www.expertconsult.com*.

CHAPTER 86

Veterinary Nuclear Medicine

Brian A. Poteet

Nuclear imaging (scintigraphy) has been used in veterinary medicine as a primary or secondary modality to aid in the diagnosis of disease processes and for therapy. The utility of nuclear medicine procedures lies in the fact that they enable the imaging of physiologic processes.

Nuclear medicine is to physiology as radiographs are to anatomy. Table 86-1 lists six nuclear medicine studies and their primary indications for use.

Although these studies and others have been used in animal patients, the thyroid scan, portal scan, bone scan, and glomerular filtration rate (GFR) scan are the most commonly performed scans in a clinical setting. The *Handbook of Veterinary Nuclear Medicine*[1] further describes these and other types of scans.

Nuclear imaging differs from radiographic imaging in that the instrumentation (a gamma camera) emits no radiation. Instead, the patient emits gamma radiation after a dose of radiation has been intravenously administered. The most common radionuclide used for diagnostic purposes is ^{99m}Technetium (^{99m}Tc, Tc, Tech, or pertechnetate). ^{99m}Tc is eluted using sterile saline in liquid form from its parent isotope, ^{99}Molybdenum (^{99}Mo), in a lead-encased generator system (also known as the "cow"); the whole process is commonly referred to as "milking the cow." The eluate (^{99m}Tc suspended in saline) is then placed in a small lead-encased dosing bottle (known as the "pig") and kept for use either alone (as a radionuclide) or it tagged to a pharmaceutical (to form a radiopharmaceutical). The amount of radioactivity obtained with each elution is variable and will depend on the size of the generator system, its age, and the timing of each elution. The most common unit of a dose of radioactivity is the Curie (Ci), with most fresh eluates being around 1 Ci in strength. Most patient doses are in the millicurie (MCi) range (1 Ci = 1000 MCi). An individual or institution must have a radioactive materials license (RML) from either the state in which it practices (an "agreement state") or from the Nuclear Regulatory Commission (NRC). Qualifications and experience required to obtain an RML vary, but it generally requires proven experience and training in nuclear medicine procedures and radiation safety. The regulations concerning the use of radioactive materials in veterinary patients are often different from that of human patients. The major differences usually pertain to patient release criteria and safety requirements. For example, human patients are allowed to leave the hospital if they have been administered 30 MCi or less, as compared with animal patients, who must typically be hospitalized for 24 hours until their exposure levels are below a specific level that the state has set (typically 0.5 mR/hour at 1 m). The overall dose of radiation that a patient is exposed to from a typical nuclear medicine procedure is minimal, and adverse side effects are rarely seen.

The site and method of tissue localization depend on several factors, the more important of which are blood flow, the type of radiopharmaceutical used, and individual species differences. When administered intravenously to a patient as a radionuclide (pertechnetate ion), localization will mimic that of halogenated compounds, such as iodine, and occurs in glandular tissues, such as the thyroid gland, choroid plexus, salivary glands, and mucosal glands that line the stomach. When administered as a radiopharmaceutical, the method and site of localization depend on the physical or chemical characteristics of the radiopharmaceutical itself. Table 86-2 lists commonly used radiopharmaceuticals, their various sites and methods of tissue localization, and their various uses.

Instrumentation required in a basic veterinary nuclear medicine lab will vary, but includes a gamma camera, an interfaced computer with acquisition and processing software, an exposure meter, safety equipment including a radioactive materials spill containment and clean-up kit, shielding material such as lead bricks, and a properly shielded and ventilated radiation isolation ward. New gamma cameras and computers are expensive, but good-quality used and refurbished equipment is available.

Radiation safety is extremely important when performing nuclear medicine procedures. The word "nuclear" often conjures up thoughts of nuclear weapons, mushroom clouds, and genetic defects. In fact, many owners are surprised to find out that their animals will not "glow in the dark" after a scan. Four basic premises to radiation safety are considered universal. The first is the as low as reasonably achievable (ALARA) concept, which states that individuals should never allow themselves to be exposed to any more radiation than is absolutely required to do their jobs. The last three radiation safety guidelines that should be remembered are time, distance, and shielding. One should always minimize the time exposed to a radiation source, maximize the distance from it, and when possible place protective shielding (lead, cement walls) between him

Table • 86-1

Commonly Performed Nuclear Medicine Studies in Veterinary Medicine

SCAN NAME	INDICATIONS FOR USE
Thyroid scan	Feline hyperthyroidism, occult hyperthyroidism
Portal scan	Macroscopic portosystemic shunt detection
Bone scan, three-phase bone scan	Occult lameness, differentiate septic arthritis or osteomyelitis vs. severe chronic degenerative joint disease (DJD), metastatic bone disease
Glomerular filtration rate (GFR) scan	Quantitative evaluation of differential renal function
Perfusion lung scan	Pulmonary thromboembolic disease
Multigated acquisition cardiac scan (MUGA)	Subjective and objective evaluation of cardiac performance

Table • 86-2

Commonly Used Radiopharmaceuticals

RADIOPHARMACEUTICAL OR RADIONUCLIDE	SITE OF LOCALIZATION	METHOD OF LOCALIZATION	TYPICAL USE
^{99m}Tc-Methylene diphosphate	Hydroxyapatite	Chemiadsorption	Bone scan
^{99m}Tc-Diethylene triamine pentaacetic acid	Glomerular filtrate	Active transport	GFR scan
^{99m}Tc-Macroasgregated albumin	Pulmonary capillary bed	Capillary blockade	Perfusion lung scan
^{99m}Tc-HIDA xxx	Hepatocytes and bile	Active transport	Hepatobiliary scan
^{99m}TcO$_4$ xxx	Glandular tissue		Thyroid scan
^{67}Gallium xxx	Sarcoma tissue, abscess	Transferring analog	Sarcoma imaging, FUO
$^{123 \text{ or } 131}$MIBG xxx	Neuroendocrine cells	Active transport	Pheochromocytoma

FUO, Fever of unknown origin; *GFR*, glomerular filtration rate.

or herself and the radiation source. For nuclear medicine procedures performed in veterinary medicine, the users should always wear disposable exam gloves, a lab coat, and should be monitored (properly wearing a radiation exposure detection device) with a film badge, thermoluminescent dosimeter (TLD) badge, or pocket dosimeter. For most institutions, employees working strictly with nuclear medicine patients will have about one tenth the dose of other employees who work in radiology sections.

THYROID SCINTIGRAPHY

Introduction and Basic Techniques

The thyroid scan is the most commonly performed diagnostic scan in veterinary nuclear medicine and is used to confirm and diagnose feline hyperthyroidism. The diagnostic thyroid scan is considered to be the "gold standard" means of diagnosing feline hyperthyroidism. Because technetium behaves as a halogen (iodine) when administered, it is actively trapped by thyroid cells. However, unlike iodine, technetium is only trapped and does not progress through the remaining steps of thyroid hormone synthesis (organification, coupling, storage, and release).[2,3] The trapping of technetium is competitive with iodine (recent administration of iodinated contrast material may hinder the uptake by the thyroid) and is also influenced by thyroid-stimulating hormone (TSH) levels. Adenomatous hyperplasia of the feline thyroid results in a hyperfunctional gland in two ways. First, the gland synthesizes and releases too much thyroxine, resulting in an elevated T4 value, and (more fundamentally) the gland has increased ability to trap iodine (and therefore technetium). This is not always true in the canine species as will be discussed later.

Although the thyroid scan can be performed with either ^{123}I or ^{99m}Tc, technetium has the advantages of being more economical, readily available, and it has a shorter half-life. If disparate imaging between the two radionuclides occurs, they are typically insignificant.[4] The dose of ^{99m}Tc used for a feline patient is typically 4 MCi (+/− 2 MCi) and is administered intravenously into a cephalic or medial saphenous vein. It has been shown that the maximal uptake by thyroid cells is at 45 to 60 minutes after injection[5]; although approximately 90% of cats will demonstrate positive scans in just seconds after injection. Normal salivary gland–to–thyroid gland ratios are 1:1.2 or less[6] and can be obtained by calculating the count density within a region of interest (ROI) encircling the respective glands. For practical purposes, however, the zygomatic salivary glands and thyroid gland should have very similar degree of uptake in normal cats. In hyperthyroid cats, a portion or all of one or both of the thyroid lobes will have significantly more uptake than that seen by the salivary glands.

Indications for Performing a Thyroid Scan

A thyroid scan should be performed for several reasons. The scan can be used to confirm suspect hyperthyroidism in feline patients that have elevated circulating thyroxine levels prior to administration of radioiodine. The majority of centers routinely perform thyroid scans on all patients prior to administration of radioiodine (^{131}I), thus preventing wrongful treatment of normal patients that have a false-positive elevated T4 or fT4 assays. Negative results of a thyroid scan will prevent an unnecessary surgery or inappropriate administration of radioiodine. The amount of uptake and size of the glands may also aid the clinician in determining the dose of radioiodine to be used, thus allowing some degree of individual tailoring of the dose of radioiodine. Lastly, by routinely performing a diagnostic thyroid scan on all patients, one may be able to exclude a patient whose scan suggests an aggressive thyroid carcinoma, the presence of which may change the owner's decision-making process.

Thyroid scanning may also diagnose patients with "occult" hyperthyroidism. In these cases a diagnostic thyroid scan can quickly diagnose hyperthyroidism in a patient that may otherwise be missed.

A thyroid scan can also be used before or after attempts at surgical resection of one or both lobes of the thyroid in clinically persistent hyperthyroid cats. In these cases, foci of ectopic thyroid tissue can be easily localized within the cervical region (incomplete resection) or within the cranial mediastinum. Once located, the persistent hyperfunctional thyroid tissue can be removed or ablated with radioiodine.

Image Acquisition

A minimum of three views should be taken during acquisition of a routine feline thyroid scan (Figure 86-1). The first image

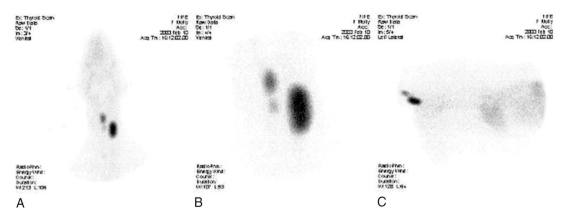

A   B   C

Figure 86-1 Thyroid scan. Hyperfunctional thyroid adenoma, bilateral, in a 14-year-old male castrated Domestic Shorthair, technetium injected with 4 MCi of [99m]Tc. Images shown are 200,000-count static images with pinhole collimation. **A,** Ventral neck view. Focal intense activity is seen by both lobes of the thyroid glands, more so than that seen by the salivary glands. The right thyroid has a "hot" nodule in the cranial and caudal pole. **B,** Ventral thyroid view. Both glands exhibit benign scanning characteristics (intense center, homogeneous uptake, tapering margins, no evidence of regional tissue invasion). **C,** Left lateral thorax view. No abnormal areas of uptake in the thorax are seen.

should be a ventral view, which includes both lobes of the thyroid gland and the mandibular and zygomatic salivary glands. This view is used to confirm the diagnosis of hyperthyroidism because the amount of uptake by the thyroid glands can be easily compared with that of the salivary glands, either by drawing ROIs around the individual glands and comparing count density or by subjective comparison. The second ventral view should be a close-up view of just the thyroid gland itself, taking care to include any area of uptake. This view is important in evaluation of the morphology of the thyroid itself. The last view that should be acquired is a lateral view (right or left), including the entire thorax. To ensure that the entire thorax is included, the thyroid should be seen on one side of the image and stomach uptake on the opposite side. This view is important in evaluating for possible uptake within the cranial mediastinal region and lung fields. If uptake is seen in these regions, a ventral view of the thorax and opposite lateral should also be obtained. All images should be acquired on a count basis (as opposed to a time acquisition) for approximately 200,000 counts using pinhole collimation.

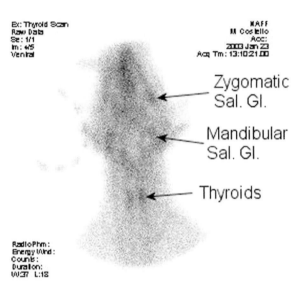

Figure 86-2 Normal feline thyroid scan. The amount of uptake by the thyroid gland is similar to that seen by the salivary glands.

Each image acquisition should take approximately 3 minutes, giving a total scan time of about 10 minutes (assuming a ^{99m}Tc dose of 4 MCi).

Interpretation and Analysis
In normal cats (not hyperthyroid) the amount of uptake seen by the salivary glands and thyroid gland is very similar. Placement of ROIs around the salivary glands and thyroid tissue with comparison of the amount of uptake should yield a thyroid to salivary gland ratio of less than 1.2 in normal animals. In most cases the placement of ROIs is not needed to confirm the diagnosis of hyperthyroidism, and subjective evaluation of significantly more uptake within the thyroid tissue versus that of the salivary gland tissue is all that is needed (Figure 86-2).

False-positive ^{99m}Tc thyroid scans can be seen in hyperthyroid cats secondary to recent administration of methimazole because it may cause false increased uptake by the thyroid tissue due to stimulation by an elevated TSH concentration.[7] This same phenomenon has not been evaluated in normal euthyroid cats. False-negative thyroid scans are extremely rare but may be due to severe thyroiditis, recent intake of iodinated contrast material, or ingestion of excess dietary or administered iodine[8] overlying and attenuating soft tissues or malfunctioning nuclear medicine equipment.

Several classifications of feline hyperthyroidism exist based on the location of uptake. Unilateral uptake by one lobe with complete suppression of the contralateral lobe is reportedly seen in approximately one third of patients[3] (Figure 86-3, *A*). Bilateral uptake in both lobes is seen in the remaining two thirds[3] (Figure 86-3, *B*). Bilateral uptake is defined as uptake, regardless of the amount, seen in both thyroid lobes. It is common for one lobe to have more uptake, be larger than the contralateral lobe (incomplete suppression), or both; however, this is still considered to be bilateral because a normally functioning thyroid should demonstrate no evidence of autonomous function and be completely suppressed (thus not seen at all) (Figure 86-3, *C*).

Hyperfunctional ectopic tissue can occur anywhere from the base of the tongue to the base of the heart; the incidence is estimated to be as high as 10%[9] (Figure 86-4). The presence of ectopic hyperfunctional thyroid tissue does not imply malignancy. It is also very common to detect adenomas with intense focal uptake by very small (2 to 3 mm), nonpalpable, thyroid nodules (Figure 86-5).

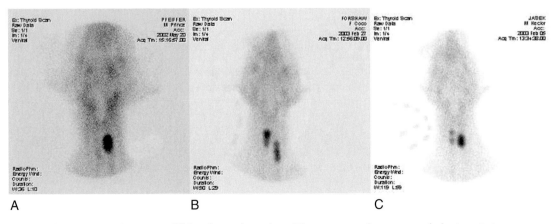

Figure 86-3 Variations of feline hyperthyroidism. Three commonly seen morphologic variations of feline hyperthyroidism exist. **A,** Unilateral with complete suppression of normal contralateral thyroid lobe. **B,** Bilateral hyperthyroidism. **C,** Bilateral hyperthyroidism with incomplete suppression of one thyroid lobe.

A thyroid scan can also be used to help differentiate benign adenomatous hyperplasia versus a malignant thyroid carcinoma. Close examination of the morphologic scanning characteristics of each thyroid lobe may give clues that help distinguish nonaggressive disease versus an infiltrative carcinoma. Pinhole collimation is very helpful in evaluating the morphology of thyroid disease because it magnifies the appearance of the otherwise small lobes. Characteristics of a simple adenoma (benign) include round to oval shape, smooth or homogeneous uptake, margins that taper uniformly, and no evidence of regional tissue invasion. Malignant thyroid carcinomas often exhibit very abnormal shapes with poorly defined, irregular margins, heterogenic uptake, and evidence of invasion into surrounding tissue facial planes (Figure 86-6).

Common findings that occur in adenomas that can be confused with a carcinoma include nodular to multinodular uptake, photopenic areas caused by thyroiditis, follicular cyst or parathyroid adenoma, or ectopic hyperfunctional tissue within the thoracic inlet or cranial mediastinum. In these cases it is important to examine each focal area of uptake individually for evidence of benignancy or malignancy. If the cat has undergone previous attempts at thyroidectomy, caution must be exercised because the surgical intervention can cause a very abnormal morphologic appearance of the persistent or recurrent thyroid tissue that can mimic a thyroid carcinoma (Figure 86-7).

In cats with suspected thyroid carcinoma, ultrasound is often the next step because it can often detect the reason for photopenic areas caused by follicular cysts or an enlarged parathyroid gland and evaluate if the thyroid appears to be well encapsulated. If none of the aforementioned are true, if

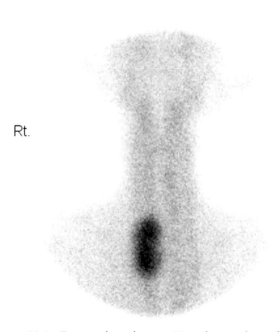

Rt.

Figure 86-4 Ectopic thyroid tissue. Ventral view shows focal intense uptake in functional thyroid tissue located within the cranial mediastinum on the right.

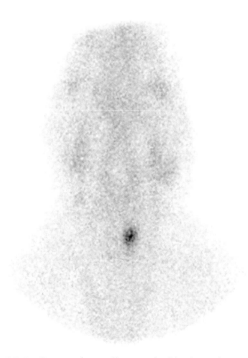

Figure 86-5 Extremely small, nonpalpable thyroid tissue. Focal intense uptake is evidenced by a very small foci of thyroid tissue on the left side. This nodule was not palpable even in retrospect after the scan localized it.

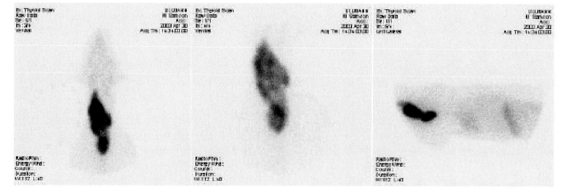

Figure 86-6 Feline thyroid adenocarcinoma. The right thyroid lobe shows very heterogeneous uptake with irregular margins. Extension of functional malignant tissue can be seen into fascial planes and into the cranial mediastinum. Numerous photopenic areas are present.

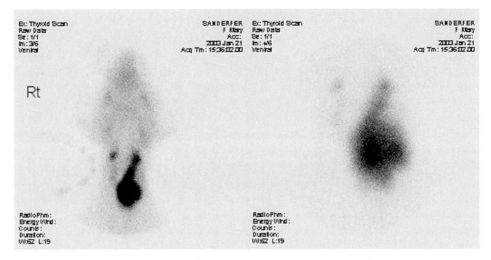

Figure 86-7 Postsurgical thyroid. Fifteen-year-old Domestic Shorthair, female spayed. Patient is persistently hyperthyroid despite two attempts at bilateral subcapsular thyroidectomy. The left thyroid lobe is irregular in shape and bulbous in appearance secondary to previous surgical intervention (left-sided subcapsular thyroidectomy) and subsequent recurrence. The right thyroid lobe is incompletely suppressed.

the thyroid gland appears of mixed echogenicity, or if it appears invasive into surrounding tissues, surgical intervention usually follows.

After a diagnostic thyroid scan using ^{99m}Tc, the feline patient must be housed in a radiation isolation ward until it clears the individual clinic's release criteria, which is typically set by the issuer of the RML (the author's practice requires 0.5 mR/hour at 1 m). This is measured using an appropriate monitoring device such as a Geiger counter or "Cutie Pie" exposure meter. Once the animal returns home, the owner is instructed on how to care for the pet physically, told to minimize time holding the cat for the next week or so, and instructed how to handle the very small amount of radioiodine that will still be excreted in the cat's urine. (The specifics of these requests often vary from state to state.)

Radioiodine Therapy for Feline Hyperthyroidism

Three treatment options exist for feline hyperthyroidism: (1) medical therapy with methimazole, (2) surgical removal of the thyroid glands, and (3) radioiodine therapy. All methods have pros and cons, which will be discussed.

Radioiodine therapy using ^{131}I also has both advantages and disadvantages. Radioiodine therapy is extremely targeted in that, once injected, the iodine is preferentially trapped and organified by the hyperfunctional thyroid cells (little to no uptake is seen by normally suppressed thyroid cells) and once there, the high-energy beta particles that are emitted during the decay process cause irreparable damage to the cells. The distance of beta particle travel, and therefore the area of tissue damage, is confined to 1 to 2 mm; thus concurrent damage to adjacent parathyroid tissue is not seen. Administered radioiodine is taken up by all hyperfunctional thyroid tissue, regardless of its anatomic location. Because feline hyperthyroidism is not an autoimmune form of thyroid disease (human Graves disease) and most closely resembles toxic nodular goiter (multinodular goiter), the great majority of cats that are diagnosed with hyperthyroidism retain some suppressed (but otherwise normal) thyroid cells. The advantage is that approximately 95% of cats treated with radioiodine will be euthyroid after treatment, requiring no supplementation. It is relatively common for cats to have subnormal total thyroid hormone levels immediately after radioiodine therapy, but it is extremely rare for any of these cats to demonstrate any signs

of hypothyroidism. In these cats, a recheck of the thyroid hormone levels in 1 to 3 months after therapy will often demonstrate normal values.

Care must be taken regardless of the form of therapy chosen if the patient has concurrent renal compromise. Readers are encouraged to review the many studies that pertain to the correlation of the treatment of hyperthyroidism and renal disease.[10-12] In general, cats that have normal renal function based on normal serum blood urea nitrogen (BUN) and creatinine (CR) values should have few problems with any form of therapy for hyperthyroidism. In patients that are both hyperthyroid and show equivocal or definitive evidence of renal failure (azotemia and inability to concentrate urine), a 3- to 4-week trial period using methimazole is recommended. If at the end of this time the BUN and CR levels are not increased, the animal is not showing signs of renal failure, and the total T4 values have dropped to within the normal range, a more definitive form of therapy can be safely considered. In these patients a lower dose of radioiodine may be used in an effort to minimize any effects on the kidneys and, at the same time, control hyperthyroidism. Radioiodine itself is not toxic to the kidneys. The cause of the worsening of renal disease that can accompany any form of hyperthyroid therapy is unknown but may relate to changes in hemodynamics within the kidney and glomerular filtration. Supplementation of thyroid hormone in cats that experience manifestation of renal failure after definitive thyroid therapy may be of benefit; however, no such studies have been undertaken to prove this theory.

Thyroid Scan and Canine Thyroid Disease

The parotid salivary glands in dogs demonstrate much more uptake compared with those of cats; however, the amount of uptake by the salivary glands and thyroid should be very similar in individual animals of either species (Figure 86-8).

The indications to perform thyroid scans in dogs are fewer than in cats but may include presurgical evaluation of the degree of regional tissue invasion (which may aid the surgeon in evaluating the degree to which one rejects the cervical mass). A thyroid scan can also confirm that a cervical mass is indeed thyroid in origin and identify functional distant metastasis. Canine thyroid carcinoma is different from that seen in cats in that approximately one third of affected patients will

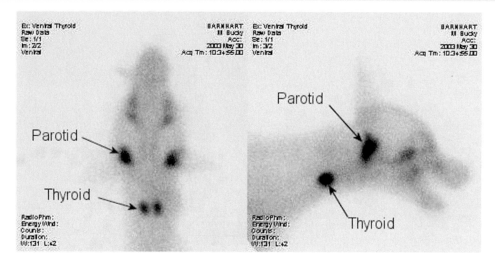

Figure 86-8 Normal canine thyroid scan. Similar amounts of uptake of the radionuclide by the parotid salivary glands and the thyroid tissue occur. Both thyroid lobes are normal in size, shape, and location.

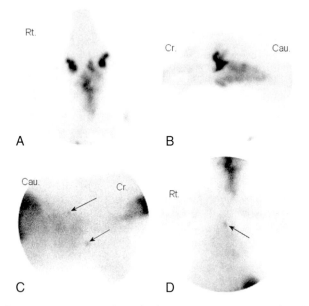

Figure 86-9 Canine thyroid adenocarcinoma. **A,** Ventral neck view shows heterogeneous, ill-defined uptake associated with the left thyroid lobe. Invasion into the caudal and cranial neck region and into fascial planes is seen. **B,** Lateral view of neck. **C,** Right lateral view of the thorax showing two functional pulmonary metastatic lesions *(arrows).* **D,** Dorsal view of the thorax with a visible functional metastatic pulmonary nodule *(arrow).*

demonstrate decreased or no uptake (inability to trap ^{99m}Tc), one third of patients will have relatively normal amounts of uptake (normal ability to trap ^{99m}Tc), with the last third demonstrating increased uptake (increased ability to trap ^{99m}Tc). Uptake by distant metastasis appears to have similar patterns. The same scanning characteristics of malignancy can be applied to the canine patient in that most carcinomas will demonstrate heterogeneous uptake, very irregular gland shapes, and often evidence of regional tissue invasion (Figure 86-9). Thoracic radiographs are more sensitive than a thyroid scan for the detection of pulmonary metastasis, and as such

they should always be obtained whenever thyroid carcinoma is suspected.

Radioiodine Therapy for Canine Thyroid Carcinoma
^{131}I has also been used as therapy for canine thyroid carcinoma.[13,14] Radioiodine therapy is best suited for therapy for micrometastatic disease in cases where the primary carcinoma is proven to retain the ability to trap iodine (technetium); as such a diagnostic thyroid scan using ^{99m}Tc or ^{123}I should be performed prior to surgical intervention. The thyroid-associated mass should be removed or debulked surgically followed by radioiodine therapy. Presurgical external beam radiation therapy may also be used in certain cases in an attempt to shrink the primary tumor prior to intervention. If the primary tumor exhibits no ability to concentrate iodine, then conventional chemotherapeutics may be preferential for potential or known micrometastatic disease in combination with external beam radiation therapy for any incompletely resected margins. The dose used for canine thyroid carcinoma varies widely but may range from 20 MCi to 100 MCi or more. The dose is usually administered intravenously through a preplaced catheter. After administration, the animal must be kept in a radiation isolation ward until it has cleared release criteria. Strict radiation safety practices must be instituted during the entire stay, and it is not uncommon for these patients to contaminate their exterior surfaces with iodine. The typical hospital stay for these patients in the author's practice ranges from 10 to 21 days. Side effects seen with large-dose radioiodine therapy are rare but may include transient neutropenia that lasts only a few days.

PORTAL SCINTIGRAPHY

Background and Basic Techniques
Nuclear portography (portal scan) has been used as first introduced in the canine by Caride.[15] A portal scan greatly aids in the diagnosis of a macroscopic portosystemic shunt. The scan can rarely differentiate the types of portal shunts (it typically cannot differentiate if the shunt is intrahepatic versus extrahepatic or if a shunt is a single-vessel extrahepatic shunt or from a multivessel extrahepatic shunt). Hepatic microvascular dysplasia will result in a normal portal scan because the radioactive bolus is transported in normal fashion to the liver prior to the cardiac ROI.

Indications for Performing a Portal Scan

The usefulness of a portal scan appears to be in patients that are suspected of having a portosystemic shunt based on clinical signs and high bile acid levels. The portal scan is performed to confirm the existence of a macroscopic shunt prior to surgical exploratory and subsequent ligation or coil placement.

Image Acquisition

A portal scan is performed on a tranquilized or (preferably) anesthetized animal in right lateral recumbency with the diaphragm centered over a gamma camera. The field of view (FOV) should include the entire heart and liver region. Although the scan can be performed without the aid of an interfaced nuclear medicine acquisition computer system, one is highly recommended and is necessary for any type of quantitative analysis and subsequent storage. To help localize the position of the heart and liver, an external source of activity (μCi point sources or the ends of a flexible cobalt ruler) are placed ventral to the animal, directly below the point of maximum intensity (heart) and level of the xiphoid (liver).

A red rubber catheter is placed into the descending colon and inserted to the level of the cranial-most aspect of the ilial wings. Careful placement of the tip of the catheter along the ventral aspect of the colon is helpful in preventing a "fecal-o-gram." It is preferable to perform a portal scan with an empty colon, and administration of a cleansing enema 2 to 3 hours prior to the scan is recommended by some[16]; however, it is not routinely required. A dose of approximately 3 to 8 MCi of ^{99m}Tc is used in a volume of 0.5 to 1.0 mL of saline. The higher the dose used, the more accurate the results will be owing to better counting statistics. A three-way stopcock is attached to the preplaced catheter, the dose syringe, and a 12-mL syringe filled with room air. A $\frac{1}{8}$-inch thick piece of lead is placed between the camera top (imaging table) and the

patient, directly under the tip of the catheter and caudal abdomen. Care must be taken to avoid placement of the lead under the liver region or too caudally, which can create a "bloom" artifact from the radioactive bolus within the colon. The bolus of radiation is injected first, followed by a small amount (3 to 10 mL) of room air at a slow to moderate rate. A dynamic acquisition should be obtained, starting just prior to injection of the bolus of radiation and continued at 4 seconds per frame for a total of about 3 minutes. Once the pertechnetate is placed within the colon, a small percentage (10% to 20%) is absorbed across the colonic mucosa and is taken up within the portal venous system.

Interpretation and Analysis

In normal patients, activity should be seen within the liver ROI prior to activity seen within the cardiac ROI (Figure 86-10). In animals with macroscopic shunts, the cardiac ROI is seen at the same time or preceding the liver ROI (Figure 86-11). With the aid of a computer and appropriate software, percent shunt fractions can also be obtained using the following formula:

$$\frac{\left(\sum \text{ total heart counts over time i}\right)}{\left[\sum (\text{total heart counts} + \text{total liver counts})\text{over time i}\right]} \times 100$$

Normal animals will have a shunt fraction of less than 20%. A positive scan is considered to be one with a shunt fraction of greater than 50%. Values obtained between 20% and 50% are considered to be abnormal and may be caused by a less severe shunt. In these cases the scan should be repeated or the animal should be explored. A shunt fraction of 0% is not physiologic, owing to the hepatic arterial blood supply. Calculation of a shunt fraction is not necessary for the diagnosis of the existence of a shunt. False-negative scans may be caused

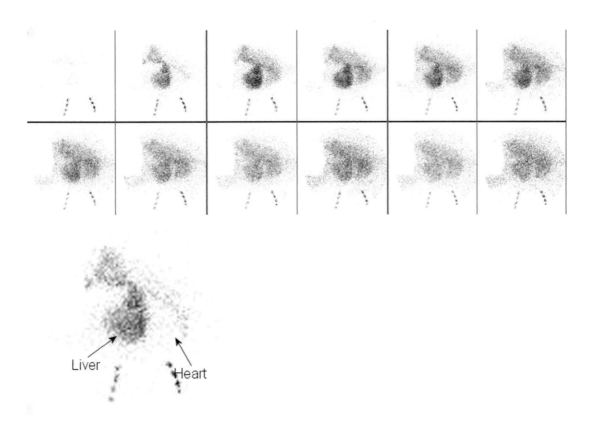

Figure 86-10 Normal portal scan. Dynamic image acquisition shows uptake within the liver region of interest (ROI) preceding that seen within the cardiac ROI.

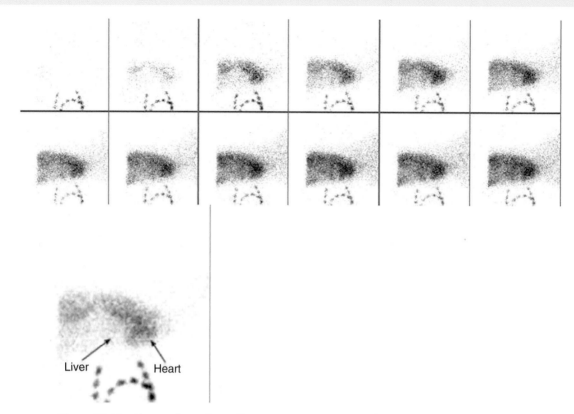

Liver   Heart

Figure 86-11 Abnormal portal scan. Dynamic image acquisition shows uptake within the cardiac region of interest (ROI) preceding that seen within the liver ROI.

by improper placement of the radionuclide bolus in the colon cranial to the level of the shunt, incomplete absorption of the bolus across the colonic mucosa due to infiltrative disease of the colonic wall itself, or if the bolus is lodged in a ball of feces. Incorrect results (falsely elevated shunt fraction) may be seen if the bolus is administered too far cranially within the colon, where a bloom artifact may overlie the liver ROI. This is commonly seen if the colon is filled with liquid, such as just after administration of an enema. The majority of the technetium is excreted in the feces (that which remains in the colon) and in the urine (that which was absorbed systemically) within the first 12 hours after the scan.

Portal streaming, as reported by Daniel,[17] is a phenomenon seen in a small portion of animals that causes only one or two lobes of the liver to scintillate. Portal streaming is caused by abnormal patterns of blood flow within the extrahepatic or initial portion of the intrahepatic vasculature that results in a "steering" of the radioactive bolus into only a section of the liver.

In the author's facility, animals with a positive portal scan accompanied by high preprandial and postprandial bile acids are subsequently ultrasounded to help rule out the possibility of an intrahepatic shunt or multivessel extrahepatic shunt. If the ultrasound is negative for an intrahepatic shunt and no evidence of a multivessel extrahepatic shunt is seen, the patient proceeds to surgery for definitive localization and repair. Only in rare cases are intraoperative mesenteric portograms required for definitive identification of the shunt vessel.

BONE SCINTIGRAPHY

Background and Basic Techniques
Bone scans are highly sensitive and equally highly nonspecific. Evaluation of the extent, pattern, and anatomic origin of an

area of abnormal uptake, coupled with other factors such as the animal's age, sex, breed, history, physical examination, and radiographic findings can increase the specificity; in many cases a diagnosis can be made. Most images are acquired with the gamma camera head placed underneath a Plexiglas scanning table. Care should always be taken to ensure that the camera face is placed as close as possible to the underside of the imaging table and is exactly parallel to the tabletop. Imaging from under the animal makes positioning easier and allows the patient to feel less threatened than if the camera were placed above it. Dorsal and ventral dynamic or static images can be easily obtained on most, if not all, small animals. Using a large FOV gamma camera, a whole-body bone scan can be obtained on a large-breed canine in approximately 30 to 45 minutes.

Indications for Performing a Bone Scan
Bone scintigraphy has multiple uses in small animals. These include evaluation for primary and metastatic disease, septic arthritis, osteomyelitis, prosthetic implant loosening or infection, soft tissue and bone viability, occult lameness, and fracture healing. Bone scanning can often localize subtle lesions not seen radiographically until days or weeks later.

Image Acquisition
In small animals, all static images should be acquired on a count basis, as opposed to a timed acquisition. Timed acquisitions often result in images with low count densities and poor target-to-background ratios, which renders less-than-optimal image quality. The count density and target-to-background ratio images that are obtained using count acquisition parameters are usually of much higher quality than those obtained on a time acquisition basis. The longer scan time needed per image (1 to 3 minutes) is only significant if the animal is not under general anesthesia and patient movement is likely.

Patient preparation prior to scanning is not needed. The radiopharmaceutical ^{99m}Tc-MDP is used commonly and results in high-quality images with good target-to-background ratios. Nonradioactive ("cold") MDP is sold in a kit form and is easily made using a fresh eluate of reduced (Sn) ^{99m}TcO$_4$, which allows the labeling ("tagging") of the short chain polyphosphate. Because little binding of the radiopharmaceutical to plasma proteins takes place, urinary excretion is rapid, with 59% of the dose excreted within 24 hours.[18] Adequate blood flow is necessary for delivery of the radiopharmaceutical; however, once delivered, skeletal uptake is not a function of perfusion.[19] The exact mechanism of binding is not well understood, but it is known that the phosphate itself is merely the delivery vehicle for the ^{99m}Tc; once arriving at the hydroxyapatite surface, the ^{99m}Tc is released and then chemiadsorbs to the hydroxyapatite surface as ^{99m}Tc-oxide.[19,20] Uptake of the MDP is directly proportional to osteoblastic activity and can be affected by decreased perfusion and regional sympathetic tone.[21] Maximum bone uptake is at 65 minutes postinjection, with the maximum target-to-background ratio (highest activity in the bone and lowest activity in the soft tissues) occurring at 6 hours postinjection.[22]

Radiopharmaceutical dose ranges from approximately 5 MCi to 30 MCi, depending on the animal's size (Web Table 86-1).

Dosing of small animals for nuclear medicine procedures will vary; however, small-breed canines (e.g., Toy Poodles) and cats are administered 5-MCi doses, medium-sized canines (e.g., Beagles) are given 10- to 15-MCi doses, large-breed dogs (e.g., Labradors) are given 20-MCi doses, and giant-breed dogs are given 30-MCi doses. As with all radiopharmaceuticals, intravenous routes of administration are used. If the dose is injected through a preplaced catheter, the catheter should be flushed well after the dose is given. Even a small amount of extravasated dose will result in an injection site hot spot on subsequent imaging. Because injection site hot spots occur, it is recommended to inject in a limb that is not in question for diagnosis or to inject into a rear limb if imaging a front limb, for example. For single-phase scans, bone phase images should be acquired no earlier than 3 hours after administration. During this incubation time, care should be taken to minimize external contamination of the animal by urine. When possible, the urinary bladder should be emptied just prior to scanning by passing a urinary catheter, manually evacuating the urine, and safely disposing of the radioactive waste when done. Emptying of the bladder should be done in a careful manner to minimize contamination in the surrounding area. Clinicians should adhere to the ALARA concept in all cases; personnel who will handle the patient or urine should wear examination gloves to avoid exposure.

Routine bone scan images should be obtained using a general all-purpose (GAP) parallel hole collimator with a 20% window centered over the 140 keV gamma photo peak of ^{99m}Tc. Occasionally, a pinhole collimator is helpful in acquiring high-resolution images of small parts, such as the coxofemoral joints (Legg-Calve-Perthes disease), elbows, carpi, and sesamoid bones associated with the extremities. If a pinhole collimator is used, the number of acquired counts will need to be decreased because the acquisition time becomes prohibitively long.

As with thyroid imaging, all static images should be acquired on a count basis. Generally speaking, the more counts that can be acquired, the higher quality the image will be. Web Table 86-2 provides suggestions regarding recommendations for static acquisitions for different body parts.

During acquisition, the animal should not be allowed to move. Movement associated with respiration cannot be avoided; however, panting artifact can be minimized by manually holding the animal's muzzle closed.

Positioning of the animal for a particular body part to be imaged can be critical in obtaining a high-quality scan that is free of artifact. Web Table 86-3 lists recommendations that can aid in positioning.

Two methods for accurately comparing two similar ROIs (e.g., the elbows) are available. The easier way is to place both limbs or ROIs in the middle of the camera in the same field of view. Care must be taken to ensure that both limbs are positioned exactly and not rotated. It is also very important to make sure that both limbs or ROIs are equally distant from the camera face, ideally in contact with the camera face. If one limb is farther from the camera than the other, it will appear artifactually more intense. The second method for comparison of similar ROIs is to image the areas separately. This is accomplished by imaging one ROI for a preset number of counts and recording the time of acquisition. The contralateral ROI should then be imaged for the amount of time it took to acquire the first ROI image and the total number of counts then recorded. For this method to be accurate it is very important to make sure that the two images used for comparison appear exactly the same on the field of view.

Interpretation and Analysis

Without experience the normal bone scan in small animals can be difficult to interpret. Skeletally immature animals have very focal intense uptake in metaphyseal regions of long bones and at costochondral junctions (Web Figure 86-1). Normal areas of increased skeletal uptake in all (immature and mature) small animals include areas of thick bone (ends of long bones), temporomandibular joints (TMJs), occiput, the first cervical vertebrae (on the lateral image), sinuses, and costochondral junctions (Web Figure 86-2). Normal areas of soft tissue accumulation include kidney and urinary bladder. Activity in the kidneys can be minimal to marked. Activity in the bladder is marked, requiring evacuation prior to imaging or lead shielding.

Nonskeletal distribution of bone-seeking radiopharmaceuticals include calcinosis cutis, pulmonary mineralization, renal infarcts, acute rhabdomyolysis, lymph node uptake (after extravasation of the dose),[23] thyroid uptake of free pertechnetate, or dystrophic mineralization of soft tissues.[24] Tracer uptake has also been reported in lactating breast tissue of women[25-27] and the pregnant uterus.[28]

Several reasons exist for generalized poor skeletal uptake that results in poor image quality. These include decreased cardiac output, an increased overlying mass of soft tissue (edema formation), renal failure, or simple old age.

Neoplastic Disease

Bone scanning is the most common nuclear medicine procedure performed at many human hospitals, making up more than half of the nuclear medicine caseload. By far, the most common indication to order a bone scan is for evaluation of possible or known metastatic bone disease.[29] Bone scanning has been shown to be a sensitive indicator for the detection of skeletal metastasis.[30,31] The majority of these patients have primary prostatic or breast cancer. In these patients, a whole-body bone scan is obtained using a moving gamma camera (or moving patient gantry) that acquires a static image of the entire human body in less than 30 minutes. If an abnormal area of uptake is seen, additional "spot" images can be obtained. In veterinary medicine, overall rate of occurrence of skeletal metastasis is not known but is considered low (<10%).[32] Tumors that have shown a propensity for bone metastasis include prostatic adenocarcinoma, transitional cell carcinomas, primary bone osteosarcoma, thyroid adenocarcinoma, and mammary carcinomas (Web Figure 86-3).[32,33] Bone scans have been shown to be 30% to 50% more sensitive for the detection of metastatic bone disease than radiographs.[34]

Because of this, the bone scan may pick up metastatic disease before the animal shows skeletal pain.[33] In many cases, bone scans allow for earlier detection of metastatic bone disease, which can significantly alter the owner's decision to proceed with further therapy or change treatment options. Several patterns of metastatic bone disease have been described, the most common of which is variably sized, multiple, focal, intense hot spots, randomly distributed throughout skeleton.[35] The axial skeleton is most commonly affected (skull, vertebral bodies, ribs, and pelvis), followed by the femur and humerus.[36] In the skull the metastatic lesions are usually associated with suture lines. Rib uptake should be randomly distributed—uptake at the same level on adjacent ribs is most often due to previous trauma, not metastatic disease. If this is seen, a careful history should be obtained from the owner and radiographs of the ROI should be obtained. In the ribs the normal increased uptake of costochondral junctions should also be differentiated from metastatic bone disease. If the appendicular skeleton is involved, metastatic bone disease will typically spread to the diaphyseal portions of long bones, especially at the sites of nutrient foramen. False-negative bone scans are uncommon but can be due to the fact that up to 5% of bone metastasis are "cold," showing little to no uptake.[37] In most cases multiple myeloma or other purely lytic tumors are generally negative (although ^{99m}Tc-Sestamibi or ^{201}Tl may be positive), owing to the fact that little osteoblastic activity takes place. Other benign lesions that may have similar focal intense uptake include sepsis, osteophytes, enthesiophytes, spondylosis deformans, and chronic healed fractures. These lesions can usually be differentiated based on the location of uptake (metaphyseal, diaphyseal, or within a joint space) and the history, signalment, and physical examination findings.

A persistent problem in both human and veterinary medicine is that of a solitary focus of increased uptake in a patient known to have a primary tumor elsewhere. Although a similar study does not exist in veterinary medicine, Tumah and colleagues[38] reported only 10% of solitary rib lesions were due to metastatic disease in a group of patients with known breast cancer. In these cases radiographic correlation is essential, and demonstration of benign radiographic features can sometimes answer the question definitively. In some cases histologic confirmation may be required.

Primary bone neoplasia such as osteosarcoma, chondrosarcoma, fibrosarcoma, or synovial cell sarcoma most commonly is seen first on radiographs. Scanning characteristics associated with primary bone tumors include metaphyseal location, extremely intense uptake, and extension toward the diaphyseal portion of the involved bone; many may have photopenic centers or heterogeneous uptake (Web Figure 86-4).[39,40] The usefulness of a bone scan in these patients is to rule out the presence of metastatic bone disease prior to costly amputation, chemotherapy, radiation therapy, or limb-sparing techniques. Magnetic resonance imaging (MRI) has proven to be superior to radiography, computed tomography (CT), and scintigraphy in evaluating the extent and degree of invasiveness of neoplastic bone tumors.[41-43] Bone scans tend to overestimate the extent of primary bone tumors due to the "bloom" effect (Web Figure 86-5).[39] Pulmonary metastasis may demonstrate a faint blush on bone scans, and areas of mineralized soft tissue (metastatic or dystrophic mineralization) will also be positive (Web Figure 86-6).

In rare cases a "super scan" is seen (Web Figure 86-7).[44,45] Although the exact mechanism is not clear, these scans are felt to be related to paraneoplastic hypercalcemia. Such scans will have marked, diffuse, symmetrical skeletal uptake; the kidneys are not seen; little-to-no soft tissue uptake occurs; and obvious bone activity is seen on soft tissue phase images. The significance of the "super scan" is not known, and it does not appear to be correlated to one particular tumor type.

Nonneoplastic Disease

In small animals, acute hematogeneous osteomyelitis is relatively rare; however, septic arthritis, physitis, and discospondylitis are more common. Hematogeneous osteomyelitis will typically demonstrate intense linear cortical uptake within 24 to 48 hours[46] (radiographs are positive at 10 to 21 days).[47] The bone scan will often remain positive for weeks to months after the infection has resolved.[48] Because of this, bone scanning cannot confirm presence of active disease, but a negative scan excludes it. Septic arthritis (Web Figure 86-8), septic physitis, and discospondylitis will all demonstrate extremely focal intense uptake on bone phase images and in some cases may be positive prior to radiographs.[49,50]

Occult lameness can be defined as a persistent, often subtle, undiagnosed lameness that cannot be localized on physical or orthopedic examination. If anatomic localization is possible, radiographs are often normal or inconclusive. Causes for an occult lameness often include mild panosteitis, fragmented medial coronoid processes, partial tear of the cranial cruciate ligament, meniscal injury, stress fractures, fractures of the sesamoid bones, and small avulsion fractures (Web Figure 86-9). Both single-phase and three-phase bone scanning may be useful in definitively localizing these conditions.

Panosteitis appears on bone scans as intense linear uptake within the medullary cavity of the diaphysis on bone phase images, as well as minimal-to-marked uptake on the soft tissue phase images (Web Figure 86-10). Bone scans can often diagnose panosteitis on animals with subtle, nonlocalizable lameness or may be helpful when radiographic findings are equivocal.

Although radiography is typically the primary imaging modality to assess abnormalities associated with the medial coronoid process, radiographs can often be inconclusive in the early stages of this developmental disease because many of the Roentgen signs include degenerative changes associated with the anconeal process and ulnar trochlear notch.[51-53] CT has also been shown to have excellent sensitivity in diagnosis of fragmented medial coronoid processes; however, the availability of CT may be limited.[52] Bone scan findings that suggest a fragmented medial coronoid process are dependent on the animal's age. In puppies the medial coronoid process overlies the proximal radial physis on the lateral view. Because this physis demonstrates typical physeal uptake, a focal intense "hot spot" in this region may be due to either a fragmented medial coronoid process or the proximal radial physis. In these dogs, however, comparison of the amount and pattern of uptake bilaterally can be helpful in diagnosing a unilateral fragmented medial coronoid process. Focal intense uptake associated with the proximal radial physis should be symmetrical. Asymmetrical uptake suggests a diagnosis of fragmented medial coronoid process. Because the diagnosis is dependent on asymmetrical activity in these young dogs, the scintigraphic diagnosis of bilateral fragmented medial coronoid processes may be insensitive using bone scan findings alone. Although rare, fragmented medial coronoid processes can occur in middle-aged to older dogs (Shetland Sheepdogs). In these animals the scintigraphic diagnosis is often easier because no focal increased uptake of the proximal radial physis occurs. In skeletally mature animals, the amount of uptake by the radial head and medial coronoid process region should be similar to that of the distal humeral condyles (in the lateral projection). Focal increased uptake by the region of the medial coronoid process that is significantly more than that seen by the distal humeral condyles is highly suggestive of a fragmented medial coronoid process (Web Figure 86-11).[54] In both young and older animals, anterior-posterior (AP) views or pinhole collimation (or both) may also be helpful in differentiating uptake by the radial head and the medial coronoid process.

Three-phase bone scans may also be helpful in diagnosing partial (incomplete) tears of the cranial cruciate ligament (Web Figure 86-12).[55] In these cases the soft tissue phases may be helpful in differentiating acute (active) synovitis from chronic (inactive) intracapsular soft tissue swelling. In the normal canine stifle, a distinct photopenic area is seen within the cranial aspect of the stifle joint that corresponds with the shape and location of the infrapatellar fat pad. In animals with active synovitis, this area demonstrates a faint uptake (blush). Comparison to the contralateral stifle is usually helpful. This same "blush" is not seen in animals with chronic effusion or joint capsule thickening. Bone phase images are not typically helpful in evaluating potential acute cruciate disease.

Stress fractures result from repetitive, prolonged muscular action on bone that is unaccustomed to such stress. Typical symptoms include mild to marked lameness, bone pain, and minimal soft tissue swelling that are relieved by discontinuing the exercise. In dogs, stress fractures are seen in athletic and working species and most commonly occur within the diaphyseal portions of long bones, particularly the tibia (Web Figure 86-13). Bone scintigraphy has proven to be highly sensitive in the early detection of stress-related bone disease[56-58] and is often positive prior to radiographic abnormalities.

In human beings the incidence of bipartite sesamoid bones is approximately 10% to 33%. Although the incidence in small animals is unknown, breeds such as Rottweilers, Greyhounds, Dobermans, and Labradors may have higher incidence of sesamoid disease.[59,60] A bone scan can also differentiate bipartite sesamoid bones from fractured sesamoid bones. Bipartite sesamoids will have no abnormal uptake, whereas recently fractured sesamoid bones will have marked focal uptake (Web Figure 86-14).

Evaluation of fracture and fracture healing can also be performed using bone scanning. Bone phase images are very sensitive to fracture, and it can be difficult to differentiate acute pathologic conditions from healed previous fracture. It has been reported that bone scans (bone phase images) are 80% positive by 24 hours, 95% positive by 72 hours, and 98% positive by 7 days.[61] It has also been shown that 90% of patients with previous fracture are negative on bone phase images at 2 years.[21] Bone scans may also be helpful in the evaluation of the nonunion fracture (lack of progressive healing at 6 months postfracture). Focal intense uptake at fracture ends indicates viable tissue and shorter time to union, whereas little uptake at fracture ends indicates nonunion is likely.[62]

Avascular necrosis of the femoral head (Legg-Calve-Perthes disease) has a unique appearance, depending on the maturation of the disease. Within 12 to 48 hours after injury, a focal photopenic area within the femoral head is seen, which is then followed by a rim of moderately focal intense activity around a central photopenic core at 1 to 3 weeks. As the condition becomes chronic, the photopenic central core will fill in and have similar activity to the remainder of the femoral head.[63]

Three-Phase Bone Scanning

Multiphase bone scanning is extremely helpful in differentiating active septic from nonseptic conditions.[64] The three-phase bone scan (Web Table 86-4) consists of an initial "arterial phase" dynamic study (2 seconds/frame for 30 frames) of blood flow (Web Figure 86-15). The imaging sequence is started immediately upon injection of the radiopharmaceutical into a peripheral vein. The injection should be made as far away from the area of interest as possible to minimize any injection site hot spots that would interfere with interpretation. It is recommended that the dose be injected in bolus fashion (within 2 seconds) into a preplaced intravenous catheter followed by 12 mL of saline flush. The use of an extension set and three-way stopcock is preferred. Because of the dynamic acquisition, the arterial phase is limited to one ROI. Because of the number of images that are acquired over a short period of time, matrix sizes (in pixels) of 64 × 64 or 128 × 128 are used. Postprocessing of these images includes viewing a cine loop and summing pertinent images together to render a high–total count static image.

Phase two is termed the *blood pool phase* and is obtained by acquiring static images over the ROI at minutes postinjection (Web Figure 86-16). Blood pool (sometimes called *venous phase*) images include 1 to 2 static, 500-K images over the ROI and contralateral area for comparison.

Phase three represents the "bone phase" images. Static spot bone phase images of the ROI, as well as comparison views of the contralateral side and remaining skeleton, are obtained at 3 to 4 hours postadministration. A matrix size (in pixels) of 256 × 256 is recommended for both the blood pool phase and bone phase images.

The three-phase bone scan helps to differentiate noninflammatory versus inflammatory conditions. The technique can be helpful in differentiating a loosened versus a septic total hip prosthesis. The typical appearance of a loosened femoral component includes a normal vascular and blood pool phase with focal increased activity of moderate intensity seen at the level of the distal tip of the metallic stem, usually in the mid-diaphyseal region on the bone phase images (Web Figure 86-17). Loosening of the acetabular component is seen as curvilinear area of focal, moderately intense uptake in the acetabulum on bone phase images and normal soft tissue phase images. A septic prosthesis is suspect when moderate to marked uptake occurs on all three phases in and around the acetabular component or diffusely surrounding the femoral component (Web Figure 86-18).[65] When comparing with the contralateral limb on the same dorsal image, close attention to symmetrical positioning should be paid to ensure both acetabuli and femoral shafts are equidistant to the camera face and that no foreshortening of the limb occurs.

Three-phase bone scanning is also helpful in assessing tissue viability secondary to injury such as gunshot[66] and frostbite.[67] Decreased perfusion (soft tissue phase images) and uptake (bone phase images) indicate nonviable tissue, which usually necessitates amputation. Decreased perfusion but normal to slightly decreased uptake on bone phase images can often be successfully treated with débridement surgery and medical therapy.

For more information on this topic, please visit the companion Expert CONSULT Web site at www.expertconsult.com.

References

The reference list can be found on the companion Expert Consult Web site at *www.expertconsult.com*.

CHAPTER 87

Digital Radiology: DICOM, PACS

Brian A. Poteet

Digital radiography systems have been commonplace in human medicine for at least 15 years, but only since approximately 2004 have they started to invade the veterinary market. Initially, only university teaching hospitals and large specialty referral centers were interested in this technology. Currently, however, due to several factors (probably most importantly a trend towards decreasing price of these systems) many general veterinary practices are now starting to jump on board the digital bandwagon.

Digital radiography offers many advantages over conventional film screen radiology. In most cases, the biggest advantage is that the image quality is greatly improved. However, the advantages of digital radiography are by no means limited to increased film quality. When a switch to digital radiography is made, the films are obtained more quickly and there are significantly fewer retakes due to exposure problems. There is no need for a film processor (or processor maintenance expense) or even a darkroom, no need for a place to store film jackets and no need to order developing chemicals or film. Other advantages that are related to electronic images include no film degradation over time, no lost films/film jackets, easy transfer or duplication of films, as well as the ability to send images by electronic means to other practitioners or specialists. Many of the advantages of digital radiography will also result in a cost savings over time, which of course can be used to help pay for the initial capital outlay when the system is purchased.

In this author's opinion, digital radiographic systems are one of the major advantageous technical changes introduced in veterinary medicine in years. I have not met a veterinarian who has purchased a high-quality digital radiography system and regretted doing so. The key, however, is to purchase a high-quality system initially. This is not as easy as it sounds, as it can be a very confusing process.

The purpose of this chapter is to introduce the reader to digital radiography, types of digital radiographic systems, electronic image transfer and storage (DICOM and PACS) and potential integration with existing practice management (or hospital information system [HIS]) software.

DIGITAL RADIOGRAPHY

A digital radiograph is an electronic radiographic image that is produced without hard copy film. The digital radiograph is viewed on a computer monitor as opposed to a traditional backlit view box. A digital radiograph should not be confused with a digitized radiographic image. A digitized radiographic image is produced from hard copy film, which is then digitized in some manner, typically by means of a dedicated radiographic film scanner or a digital camera. A digitized radiograph will suffer from decreased quality and dynamic range compared to a digital radiograph. Another disadvantage is that a veterinary clinic that chooses to digitize its radiographs will not realize the inherent cost savings that accompany a digital radiography system (i.e., you are still obtaining hard copy films).

Digital radiography, in general, will offer substantially improved image quality. As opposed to conventional screen-film technology, the image detectors used for digital radiography are linear in their response to radiation. Thus these systems are much more sensitive to low exposure levels and also more sensitive to higher exposure settings. This results in an imaging system with far greater dynamic range than film-screen technology can provide. Although beyond the scope of this article, image preprocessing, processing, and postprocessing techniques can provide enhancements in image quality. Image preprocessing refers to the initial steps that are applied to the raw imaging data and are generally out of the hands of the end user. Preprocessing corrects for imperfections in the detector device (bad pixels, etc.) and detector nonuniformity. Thus preprocessing eliminates errors introduced by the digital radiography system hardware. Image processing further modifies the radiographic image to make the image more appealing to the human eye. This is typically accomplished by improving image contrast ("unsharp masking"), optimizing spatial resolution, and suppressing image noise. Image postprocessing is performed by the end user at the imaging review workstation and usually involves image rotation and flipping, additional modification of image brightness and contrast, as well as edge enhancement or smoothing. Postprocessing manipulation can aid the diagnostician but does not change the stored image data set.[1]

DIGITAL RADIOGRAPHIC SYSTEMS

The first step when deciding to make the analog to digital conversion is to select the appropriate digital radiography system, a very daunting and confusing task. Unfortunately, the terminology used by vendors to describe these systems can be somewhat misleading as one specific term or acronym used by one company may have a different meaning when used by another company. When deciding on which system is right for your practice, a few "rules of thumb" should be adhered to. First, "you usually get what you pay for" will almost always hold true. If you purchase the most inexpensive system available, you are nearly guaranteed to regret your decision to convert to digital radiography. You will constantly be fighting a losing battle involving poor image quality, numerous artifacts, and problems associated with storage and transmission of images. Secondly, "doing your homework before selecting a system" is critically important. Ask your colleagues if they would purchase their digital radiographic system again. Often it is best to ask the practice manager or a senior technician, as the practice owner may not want to readily admit he/she made a bad purchasing decision. And lastly, "always read the fine print of the buyer's order/contract." Watch out for hidden charges associated with forced DICOM compatibility, approved LUTs (Look Up Tables), software update charges, etc., as well as determine who has rights to your image database.

There are two basic types of digital radiography systems: computed radiography (CR) and digital radiography (DR).[2-6] To complicate the issue, there are two distinctively different types of DR systems: flat panel DR detector systems and CCD (charge coupled device) DR systems. This basic classification has more to do with the time of image acquisition and display than anything else. In general CR systems will display a radiographic image on a computer monitor in about 1 to 1.5 minutes. In contrast, DR systems (both flat panel and CCD systems) will display the image in 6 to 10 seconds after exposure. To complicate the matter even more, there are two subclassifications of flat panel DR systems—direct flat panel DR and indirect flat panel DR. A brief discussion of these different types of systems as well as some advantages and disadvantages for each follows.

CR was first developed by the Fuji Corporation in the early 1980s.[7] A CR system will consist of a conventional x-ray machine, special CR x-ray cassettes, an image reader device, and an interfaced computer system. In order to obtain an image, the x-ray machine is used to expose the CR cassette in a standard manner. Inside the CR cassette, the film and screen have been replaced with a photostimulable phosphor detector. These phosphor detectors are similar in appearance to the screen, which is normally mounted on the inside of a conventional x-ray cassette; however, they are thicker (about 1 to 2 mm) and are flexible. Among other properties, the phosphor detectors used for CR applications have the ability to store a "latent image" for a period of time (hours). Thus, a "latent x-ray image" is stored within the CR phosphor plate after each exposure. The CR cassette is then placed in an image-reading device where the phosphor plate is automatically removed from the cassette (in some cases, the phosphor plate is manually removed from the cassette and loaded onto a reading device). The "latent image" is extracted as a helium-neon laser beam passes the phosphor storage plate, releasing energy from "trapped" high-energy electrons. The image is then transferred to the interfaced computer and displayed on a monitor. Not all energy stored in the phosphor plate is read out in this process, and the remaining energy must be erased (or "blanked") by flooding the phosphor plate to intense white light. Once erased, the phosphor plate then is reused to obtain another image. The typical CR phosphor plate will last for up to 10,000 images; however, this is variable.

Advantages with CR systems are that they are typically less expensive than flat panel DR systems, horizontal beam radiography is possible, and the image quality can be high. Disadvantages include a longer waiting period between x-ray exposure and image display (compared to DR systems), less "technique forgiveness," and often times increased exposure settings. Although the actual reading/processing time (about 60 seconds in most cases) is comparable to that of most conventional x-ray film processors, the total process can be substantially longer due to the fact that you must also wait for the CR phosphor plate to be erased and ejected from the reader and that the CR reader can only process one plate at a time (you cannot load one film in after the other as you can with a conventional x-ray film processor). For example, if one were to shoot three views of a thorax in a patient with conventional film-screen, it might take a total of 3 minutes of actual processing time. With a "60-second" CR system, it would most likely take a total of 5 to 6 minutes—and that is assuming you have several CR cassettes available.

CCD DR systems use a small (typically 2-cm) photo detecting/storage chip (the CCD chip) similar to that found in a modern digital camera used for photography. CCD technology has been used in radiography, mostly in fluoroscopic systems, for years.[7] CCD chips have the advantage of being small and relatively inexpensive to manufacture. A CCD-based digital x-ray system consists of a phosphor plate (again similar to that found in a conventional x-ray cassette), optics to reduce the large aerial image so it can fit on the small CCD detector(s), the CCD detector itself, and often an image intensifier. X-rays excite the photostimulable phosphor scintillator plate, which in turn emits a flash of light proportional to the x-ray exposure. The light then must be minified and concentrated on the small CCD chip (i.e., the 14 × 17 inch image must be minified to fit on a 2-cm CCD chip) by using optics, such as mirrors and lenses. Unfortunately, up to 90% of the light photons can be lost as the image data is passed through these optical devices. This can result in a grainy appearance to the final image that can only be countered with increased x-ray exposure. Because the optics associated with a CCD-based DR system must be factory coupled with the x-ray machine, scintillator phosphor plate, and the CCD chip itself, these systems are always sold with a new x-ray machine. To many veterinarians, this sounds advantageous, but often this is not the case. CCD technology has improved tremendously over the years and undoubtedly will continue to do so.

Flat panel DR digital x-ray systems are considered to offer the highest image quality.[7] Flat panel x-ray detectors are rigid plates made up of thousands of individual light-detecting devices, each of which has an integrated readout mechanism. The flat panel detector is generally mounted in a fixed position in or near where the Bucky tray is found, under the x-ray table top. When an x-ray is exposed, the detectors in the plate convert the x-ray energy into a digital image in one of two ways. Flat panel detectors that take x-ray energy and first convert it to light, which in turn is converted to electrical energy, are termed "indirect" flat panel detectors (they indirectly convert x-ray energy to electrical energy). On the other hand, "direct" flat panel detectors take x-ray energy and "directly" convert it to electrical energy (no light-emitting intermediate stage). Again, the physics of both methods is beyond the scope of this article and the reader is advised to consult the references.

Once the digital image is stored on the computer system (whether it arrives from a CR system, CCD-based DR system, or indirect or direct DR system), the images undergo preprocessing, processing, and postprocessing as discussed previously. These processing steps are normally proprietary and the types and quality of such vary widely among manufacturers.

Which system type to purchase is dependent on multiple factors including financial resources, caseload in your particular practice, expectations of incorporating other modalities (such as ultrasound [US]) in the same database (see PACS to follow), and of course, image quality. Buyers should be aware that most veterinary vendors do not actually manufacture the equipment themselves, but often purchase pieces of equipment from manufacturers and assemble the digital x-ray system that is to be sold. This company may then sell the equipment directly or rely on local distributors to sell for them. When service or application questions are needed, it can be difficult to locate the person who can actually address your specific question or service issue. Other considerations pertaining to support and service should also be considered, including uptime guarantee, loaner equipment program, real 24/7 support, and initial and extended warranty options. In the author's opinion, proven DICOM compatibility is extremely important and will be discussed in more detail later in this article. It is highly recommended that a knowledgeable veterinary radiologist be consulted prior to making a purchase decision.

INTRODUCTION TO DICOM, PACS, AND HIS

DICOM is an acronym for *Digital Image COmmunication in Medicine* (www.medical.nema.org). DICOM is a method of electronic image transmission and storage.[2,8] An imaging system (CR, DR, DX, US, computed tomography [CT], magnetic resonance [MR], etc.) that is "DICOM compliant or compatible" will be able to seamlessly transmit any DICOM image from one DICOM site to another DICOM site, regardless of the brand name of the imaging device. In other words, a GE brand can send images to a Toshiba brand, which in turn can send images to a Philips brand, and all can send to any independent DICOM picture archival and communication (PACS) server. DICOM eliminates the need for individual viewing workstations each with proprietary software. DICOM also allows the transmission of images to anyone of your choosing, not of the supplying companies' choosing. DICOM is the worldwide, proven, and accepted standard means of medical image transmission. DICOM is so accepted by the medical and veterinary community, it is ubiquitous and there is no real alternative. DICOM communication between systems not only involves the transmission of digital images but also of the pertinent data that is stored along with each image (so-called DICOM tags). Examples of DICOM tags include patient first name, last name, date and time of image acquisition, modality, manufacturer, etc.

There are many parts of the "DICOM standard." Examples include the ability to print to a DICOM film printer, DICOM storage, DICOM query/retrieve, DICOM modality work list, etc. Unfortunately, for a vendor to claim its product is "DICOM compliant," it need only satisfy one component of the DICOM standard. Thus a "DICOM-compliant" DR system may be able to print to a DICOM printer, but it may not be able to send images via DICOM or search a DICOM database. The buyer is strongly urged to prove DICOM compliance themselves with any piece of imaging equipment they are considering to purchase. This can only be done by actually sending DICOM-stored images (and the associated DICOM tags) to an independent DICOM-viewing computer system (Efilm, Osirix, etc.). Unfortunately, there are no DICOM "police," and adherence to the DICOM standard is voluntary.

PACS is an acronym for *Picture Archival and Communication System*. A PACS system consists of all of the technologies that participate in the creation, storage/retrieval, distribution, presentation, and archiving of medical images and associated data. Typically a PACS consists of one or more modalities (digital radiology, US, CT), broadband network, storage server, diagnostic workstations, software, and interplay with the HIS commonly called *Practice Management Software* in veterinary medicine. The integration of PACS and DR will eliminate hard copy film, a film processor and its associated expenses, and the need for physical storage of film jackets. PACS will also allow remote access (via the Internet) of your images. A PACS system is not just a picture viewer. A "real" PACS system should seamlessly support multiple imaging modalities (such as US, CT, and MR, as well as DR). The advantage of this is that when a patient's radiographic images are retrieved for a particular day, all of the previous images on that patient, from all modalities, are automatically retrieved for comparison at the same time. PACS should also support multiple DICOM service class objects (DICOM print, DICOM query/retrieve, DICOM modality work list, etc.) and as such should seamlessly communicate with other PACS systems, regardless of brand or manufacturer. Ideally, PACS should also interface with the HIS portion of the practice, which allows for a single portal of entry of patient demographic information when the patient is first admitted. Entering patient information only once and having all subsequent electronic links (such as digital radiographs) automatically prepopulated with the same demographic information will facilitate a much more streamlined workflow and greatly reduce errors that occur when having to retype patient information. The ideal PACS should also offer a means of temporary image backup (to another hard drive) either on site or, preferably, off site with user-selectable methods and amounts of image compression, a method of permanent image storage (usually to optical media such as CD or DVD), maintenance of all DICOM header information, and a searchable database based on the same DICOM header information. An ideal PACS should also offer user-configurable and user-updatable electronic orthopedic templates, be secure from computer hackers, and have standard, intuitive ways to flip, rotate, mirror, window level, annotate, and measure, as well as allow the user to view a written image report while viewing the study, have user-configurable screen layouts and hanging protocols, access the DICOM log (commonly referred to as a "DICOM dump"), and output "key" images.

In order to transfer a DICOM image to and from a PACS, three pieces of information are needed:
1. AE (Application Entity) Title—typically a combination of letters and numbers, no spaces and all CAPS
2. Port Number—the route the data exits and enters your computer
3. IP Address—unique electronic address for you computer

Each piece of digital equipment (whether it be a digital radiology unit or ultrasound machine) must have a UNIQUE AE Title.[9] This is similar to a fingerprint in that no other machine anywhere in the world should have the same AE Title. Thus when images are transferred to a radiologist or other specialist, they will always be able to tell where the images originated from and there will be no "DICOM collisions" (this happens when images arrive from two different sources but the AE Titles are the same). When assigning an AE Title during installation, it is recommended to have a part of the clinic name included.

IMAGE DISPLAYS

The display of medical images can be much more difficult than the display of photos. Most medical images are grayscale and the images can be very large (especially digital radiographs).[10] Image display quality can be evaluated by describing the luminescence, resolution and contrast ratios. Monitor luminescence is measured in foot-lamberts (ft-L) and should be a minimum of 50 ft-L. Recommended monitor resolution should be no less than 2 megapixels. The contrast ratio (or dynamic range) is the ratio of luminescence between the whitest and the blackest pixel. The higher the contrast ratio, the better. Medical grade, monochrome (grayscale) monitors are ideal; however, they are costly. There have been numerous studies comparing the diagnostic accuracy of medical grade, monochrome monitors versus consumer grade color LCD monitors. In general, a high-quality consumer grade, color monitor is considered adequate for medical image viewing as long as software tools (such as magnification, window leveling, etc.) are used correctly.

References

The reference list can be found on the companion Expert Consult Web site at *www.expertconsult.com*.

CHAPTER 88

Interventional Endoscopy/Interventional Imaging

Albert E. Jergens
Kristina G. Miles

Interventional endoscopy/imaging has ushered in new diagnostic and treatment options for clinicians wishing to offer alternatives to traditional medical procedures, such as open jejunostomy catheter placement, excisional biopsy, and surgical therapy for tracheal collapse. The advantages of interventional procedures include their effectiveness, lack of morbidity, and shortened (sometimes outpatient) hospitalization periods with reduced patient costs. A spectrum of interventional procedures (Table 88-1) may now be employed depending upon the clinical disorder, technical expertise of the operator, and the in-house availability of specialized imaging equipment.

This chapter presents current information regarding guidelines and practical techniques for performing interventional endoscopic/imaging procedures in dogs and cats.

INTERVENTIONAL ENDOSCOPIC PROCEDURES

Percutaneous Endoscopic Gastrojejunostomy (PEG/PEJ) Tube Placement

Acute pancreatitis, hepatobiliary disease, and proximal gastrointestinal tract disorders are well-recognized clinical situations where delivery of nutrients via jejunostomy tube may be preferable to a feeding gastrostomy.[1] Animals are anesthetized and positioned in right lateral recumbency. An endoscope is passed into the stomach and an appropriate gastrostomy site position verified by transillumination. A 24-F percutaneous endoscopic gastrostomy set and a 12- to 24-F jejunal (PEJ) feeding set (Wilson-Cook Medical Inc., Winston-Salem, N.C.) are then placed according to methods previously described for use in humans. In brief, a snare is inserted through the gastrostomy tube and correctly positioned in the proximal stomach using endoscopic guidance. The snare is opened and the endoscope is passed through the open snare and advanced into the small intestine. A 0.035-mm curved-tip guide wire is then passed through the endoscope accessory channel deeply (approximately 250 cm) into the jejunum. Correct placement of the guide wire may be confirmed by fluoroscopy. The endoscope is then slowly withdrawn as the guide wire continues to be fed into the endoscope channel. As the endoscope is brought back into the stomach, it is pulled past the open snare, which then is closed snugly on the guidewire. The endoscope may now be removed and the oral end of the guide wire held by the endoscopist. An assistant pulls the closed snare out of the gastrostomy tube and the grasped guide wire, which is now shaped like a U, is observed exiting the orifice of the gastrostomy tube. The snare is released and the proximal (oral) and distal ends of the wire are identified by the assistant. The oral end of the wire is pulled through the gastrostomy tube while the distal end is left positioned in the intestine. The PEJ tube is next flushed with copious amounts of water, which activates a lubricant on its inner diameter, and then threaded over the guide wire until its proximal end is seated in the gastrostomy tube. The guide wire is then removed from the endoscope. Postprocedural abdominal radiographs confirm the distal end of the jejunostomy tube to be correctly positioned 40 to 60 cm distal to the pylorus. Jejunostomy catheter lengths vary and it is recommended that a minimum length of 65 cm and 95 cm be used in the cat and dog, respectively.

Several high-quality enteral diets are commercially available for jejunostomy feeding use. It is important to accurately calculate caloric requirements prior to enteral feeding. Both

Table • 88-1

Interventional Endoscopic/Imaging Procedures of Potential Utility in Dogs and Cats

INTERVENTION PROCEDURE	PRIMARY MODALITY	COMMENT
PEG/PEJ feeding tube placement	Endoscopy	Fluoroscopy/radiographs confirm correct tube placement
Balloon dilatation of strictures	Endoscopy	Treat for esophagitis postdilatation
Removal of foreign bodies	Radiography/endoscopy	Postprocedure thoracic radiographs for esophageal FB
Image-guided sample collection	Radiography/ultrasound/CT	Prebiopsy coagulation profile may be required
Choledochal stents for EHBO	Ultrasound/radiography	Stent placement requires duodenotomy; monitored via radiographs
Nitinol stents for tracheal collapse	Radiography/fluoroscopy	Palliative procedure with terminal tracheal collapse
Amplatz duct occlusion for PDA	Ultrasound/angiography	Residual duct flow monitored with Doppler echocardiography

CT, Computed tomography; EHBO, extrahepatic biliary obstruction; FB, foreign body; PDA, patent ductus arteriosus; PEG/PEJ, percutaneous gastrojejunostomy.

 To view a video on this topic, go to **www.expertconsult.com.**

body condition score (BCS) and maintenance energy requirements (MER) are used to initially estimate a patient's daily caloric requirements. Additionally, it may be necessary to factor in an illness factor of 1.1-1.3 × MER to maintain body weight and BCS in sick dogs and cats. Jejunostomy catheter feeding is initiated within 4 to 6 hours of catheter placement using the following schedule: Day 1, $\frac{1}{3}$ of daily energy requirements (DER) divided into three separate feedings; Day 2, $\frac{2}{3}$ of DER divided into three feedings; and Day 3, full DER via PEJ tube divided into three feedings. Routine maintenance of PEJ tubes (i.e., bandage change, E-collar, tube flushed prefeeding and postfeeding) is identical to that used for conventional gastrostomy tubes. Published studies indicate that this feeding regimen is well tolerated by most dogs and cats.[1] Complications of PEJ tubes are uncommon but may include tube blockage, retrograde tube migration, localized infection at the skin exit site, and iatrogenic removal.

Balloon Dilatation of Esophageal Strictures

Esophageal strictures result from severe esophagitis secondary to gastroesophageal reflux (anesthesia-associated or secondary to vomiting), retained foreign bodies, neoplasia (rare), or the ingestion of caustic substances.[2,3] Treatment for esophageal strictures has previously included surgery and bougienage with reported success rates for cats and dogs of <50% and <75%, respectively. Stricture dilatation using a balloon catheter is simple, fast, and very effective in comparison to these other treatment modalities. This procedure may be performed using a variety of commercial balloon catheters, which are constructed of a strong plastic that becomes nondeformable when maximally inflated. The Rigiflex Balloon Dilator (Microvasive Inc., Watertown, Mass.) is one such instrument, and it has a balloon diameter (fully inflated) of 18 mm and is 8 cm in length. This size catheter is ideal for dilating strictures in most dogs and cats. Note that larger balloon catheters (>30 mm OD) will be required for dilatation procedures in large and giant breed dogs. A pressure gauge, also purchased from the manufacturer, is recommended to avoid balloon overdistension and inadvertent rupture during maximum dilatation.

With the patient under general anesthesia, the stricture is identified by esophagoscopy and its diameter and length is determined. The diameter of the stricture may be estimated by comparing the lumen to the open jaws of a biopsy forceps (~ 5 mm) to that of the stricture.

The balloon catheter and pressure gauge are then assembled. The balloon catheter (with balloon collapsed) is passed alongside the insertion tube and positioned directly through the center of the stricture using endoscopic guidance. The balloon is slowly distended with water while directly visualizing the stricture. An assistant monitors dilatation pressure on the pressure gauge. Maximal dilatation is maintained for 2 to 3 minutes and then the balloon is deflated. It is best to use three separate but progressively greater dilatation procedures per each anesthesia.

Typically, a total of two to three balloon dilatations (each requiring a separate anesthesia) are performed q48h over a 7-day period.[2] Those animals having active esophagitis with stricture may require a greater number of dilatations. Mucosal hemorrhage is often marked and is to be expected following most procedures. The major advantages of this technique are direct visualization of the stricture during dilatation, less risk for esophageal perforation, fewer repeated dilatations, and longer remission of clinical signs between dilatation procedures.

Complications of balloon dilatation include mucosal hemorrhage, perforation, and restricturing. Postdilatation medical therapy for esophagitis should be performed in all patients to alleviate further esophageal injury. Consideration should also be given to the nutritional needs of the patient, and placement of a gastrostomy tube may be necessary for nutritional support and to provide esophageal rest.

Removal of Gastrointestinal Foreign Bodies

Foreign bodies are commonly encountered in clinical practice and are most common in young dogs and cats. Endoscopy provides minimally invasive visual assessment of the retained object and permits adept retrieval in comparison to surgical removal.[2] Bones, fishhooks, sewing needles, and linear foreign bodies may lodge in any part of the gastrointestinal tract, but most endoscopic interventions involve objects found within the esophagus and stomach. Survey radiographs of the cervical neck, thorax, or abdomen should be first performed to localize radiopaque objects to an anatomic region. A variety of instruments are available for foreign body retrieval with flexible endoscopes. The diameter of the accessory (working) channel of the endoscope will significantly influence the type and size of grasping instruments that can be used. A working channel diameter of 2.8 mm is ideal for accommodating those retrieval instruments which are most commonly utilized. Interventional procedures will require that the patient be maintained under general anesthesia in left lateral recumbency in most instances.

Esophageal foreign bodies generally require prompt attention since the incidence of complications (e.g., respiratory distress, mucosal trauma, motility disturbance) associated with retained objects increases over time. Bones may be problematic if they are angular and thoroughly wedged against the esophageal mucosa. Sturdy forceps, such as a two-pronged rat-tooth instrument, are essential to dislodge these objects. Fishhooks may be carefully removed from the esophageal mucosa and pulled retrograde up the esophagus. Alternatively, treble hooks may be advanced into the stomach and repositioned with grasping instruments to have their barbs pointing caudal as the hook is carefully pulled toward the mouth. The esophageal mucosa may be damaged from retained objects and it should be carefully inspected for excessive trauma following foreign body retrieval. Postprocedural survey radiographs will confirm esophageal perforation. Gastric foreign bodies (e.g., coins, rocks, bones, small toys) are less problematic since the operator has more room to maneuver objects around and to firmly grasp them for endoscopic removal. Duodenal foreign bodies are more difficult to remove than gastric objects since there is limited space for maneuvering. Soft, pliable objects that lodge in the proximal duodenum may be removed endoscopically.

INTERVENTIONAL IMAGING PROCEDURES

Image-Guided Sample Collection

Percutaneous image-guided sample collection is used to obtain needle aspirates and tissue-core biopsy specimens for a more definitive diagnosis. These techniques offer real-time visualization of needle placement for precise sampling of a selected portion of an organ or focal mass lesion. Common clinical indications include evaluation of hepatopathy, splenic masses, protastomegaly, mesenteric lymphadenopathy, and increased intestinal wall thickness. For fine needle aspiration (FNA) specimens, an 18- to 20-gauge spinal needle is inserted into the tissue or lesion under ultrasound guidance and aspirated, most commonly using a free-hand technique. Alternatively, the needle may be repeatedly repositioned within the tissue

CHAPTER 90

Constant Rate Infusions

Tim Hackett
Eileen Sullivan Hackett

Intravenous (IV) administration of a drug allows immediate and complete absorption and minimizes delay between administration and desired effect. For some drugs, it is preferable to maintain constant plasma and tissue levels in order to achieve the desired pharmacologic effect. Infusions minimize fluctuations in plasma drug levels seen with multiple dose regimens. Drugs with a narrow therapeutic spectrum, and those with rapid onset and elimination, can be titrated to meet the needs of an individual dog or cat with continuous IV administration. Constant rate infusions (CRI) can be administered using an IV drip set or infusion pump system. In small animal hospitals, infusion pumps allow the most precise and controlled drug administration. Volumetric infusion pumps that deliver fluid at a continuous flow are preferred. Pumps are commonly equipped with safety alarms to alert operators to occlusion, air in line, and end of infusion. In many small animal hospitals both syringe pumps (Medfusion Syringe pump, Smiths Medical International Limited, Kent, United Kingdom) and infusion pumps (Alaris Gemini Infusion Pump, Cardinal Health, Dublin, Ohio) are used and allow flexibility in application.

Drugs are given at constant rate infusions to provide sedation, analgesia, anesthesia, pressor and inotropic support, antiarrhythmic treatment, and primary disease therapy. In some instances, these drugs are mixed into the animals' daily maintenance fluids, simplifying administration. Mathematical formulas can be used to calculate infusions doses. Careful attention to units is necessary to ensure accuracy.

To convert µg/kg/min infusion rate to mL/hr pump rate:

$$\mu g/kg/min \times Body\ Wt\ (kg) = \mu g/min \times 60\ min/hr$$
$$= \mu g/hr \div \mu g/mL\ of\ solution$$
$$= mL/hr$$

To incorporate infusion into mL/hr total fluid requirements:

$$\mu g/kg/min \times Body\ Wt\ (kg) = \mu g/min \times 60\ min/hr$$
$$= \mu g\ added\ to\ known\ volume\ of$$
$$crystalloid\ fluid\ administered$$
$$by\ pump\ each\ hour$$

To convert concentration per volume to an equivalent drug dose in a larger dilution volume:

$$Volume_1\ (mL) \times Concentration_1\ (mg/mL) =$$
$$Volume_2\ (mL) \times Concentration_2\ (mg/mL)$$

Excel spreadsheets or web-based CRI calculators can be used to minimize errors in drug calculation of commonly used infusions.[1-5] Upon starting an IV CRI, drug levels in plasma begin to rise. A plateau of plasma drug concentration is reached when rate of administration matches the rate of elimination. This plateau in plasma drug level is known as *steady state*. A drug reaches steady state between 5 and 7 elimination half-lives, with 5 corresponding to 95% of the steady state drug concentration and 7 corresponding to 99% of the steady state drug

concentration. Many clinicians consider onset of drug action to occur at 3⅓ half-lives, a time that corresponds to 90% of the steady state drug concentration. If a drug has a long elimination half-life or an immediate onset of pharmacologic effect is desired, a combination of IV bolus and CRI is used. The aim of the bolus dose is to reach the target concentration more rapidly. Regardless of the size of the IV drug bolus that is selected, steady state drug concentration will still be achieved at 7 elimination half-lives, as steady state concentration is directly dependent on the infusion rate (Figure 90-1). The half-life also determines the time to reach a new steady state concentration when the rate of infusion is changed following patient response. When the IV infusion is discontinued, the drug concentration falls by one half every half-life. The decision to use an initial IV bolus prior to beginning a constant rate drug infusion depends on drug, patient, and personnel factors. The ideal bolus drug dose is therapeutic, with the CRI adjusted to maintain therapeutic levels. This is best demonstrated when the bolus dose and infusion dose are complementary (see Figure 90-1).

Drug bolus administration is primarily determined by volume of distribution, not half-life. Volume of distribution of drugs is affected by patient factors such as obesity, overhydration, dehydration, and altered circulation. In some instances, time to reach steady state can be used as a guide for whether to use an initial bolus administration (Table 90-1).[6-50]

If clinicians are concerned about drug toxicity resulting from bolus drug administration, the bolus can be divided into small fractions given at multiple time intervals or adminis-

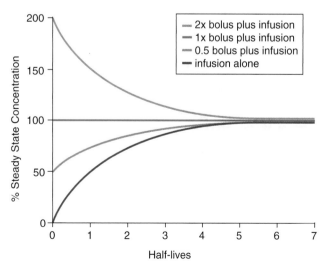

Figure 90-1 The effect of bolus drug administration on plasma concentration prior to reaching steady state concentration. (Adapted from Rowland M, Tozer TN: Clinical pharmacokinetics: concepts and applications, ed 3, Baltimore, 1995, Lippincott Williams and Wilkins, with permission.)

tered as an infusion over a longer period than that required to push the drug IV (10 to 15 minutes).

Little is currently known about the effect of critical illness, disease states, and drug interaction on pharmacokinetics in small animals. Renal and hepatic organ systems are commonly affected in critically ill animals. If drug elimination is delayed by disease, the half-life is prolonged and bolus drug dose will need to be adjusted. Until further research can be undertaken, the lowest drug dosage that achieves the desired effect should be used. This requires astute observation by well-trained staff. Alternatively, therapeutic drug monitoring may allow dose adjustment on a "case by case" basis. Therapeutic drug monitoring allows measurement of plasma drug concentration at steady state and adjustment of the infusion to achieve the desired drug concentration.

Many drugs are eliminated through hepatic metabolism. If hepatic function is decreased secondary to disease, drugs eliminated in this manner will accumulate. Decrease in clearance is of particular concern with drugs that have a narrow therapeutic index. With drugs such as lidocaine and verapamil, significant increases in half-life have been documented in people with hepatic dysfunction; therefore a twofold to threefold decrease in dosage is recommended.[51,52] Dose reduction of drugs eliminated through hepatic metabolism should be commensurate with degree of hepatic impairment. Dosage reduction may also be required when hepatic perfusion is decreased, as in animals with cardiovascular disease or portosystemic shunt.[53]

Renal impairment may result in decreased elimination and subsequent plasma accumulation of drugs and their metabolites cleared by this route. Drugs and their metabolites commonly affected by renal disease include those that are highly water soluble. Serum creatinine or creatinine clearance can be used to estimate proportional dose adjustment of drugs whose clearance is decreased in renal disease. In humans with chronic renal failure, even pharmacokinetics of drugs primarily cleared by the liver can be affected. Some theorize that accumulated metabolites or uremic toxins directly impact the metabolizing enzymes responsible for drug disposition. An example of this is lidocaine, whose half-life doubles and clearance is cut in half in patients with severe renal insufficiency.[54]

With limited routes of vascular access, it is common for two or more drugs to be administered through the same IV line.[55] When mixing multiple drugs IV, always consider compatibility. Drug incompatibility can result from the preservatives, buffers, degree of dilution, stand time, light, temperature, pH, or carrier solution.[56] Use caution when mixing drugs that have known compatibility issues such as furosemide, heparin, midazolam, diazepam, and mannitol. For example, furosemide will form visual precipitate when mixed with phenylephrine or vasopressin.[57] Conversely, fentanyl and ketamine mixture results in a stable solution.[58]

With careful planning and patient monitoring, constant rate drug infusions can be incorporated into small animal hospital practice. Infusion system type, drug pharmacokinetics, initial bolus administration, animal fluid requirements, presence of critical illness or organ dysfunction, and drug compatibility in multidrug regimens are all important considerations.

CASE EXAMPLE

A 15-kg dog admitted for trauma after being hit by a car has multiple lacerations and a long bone fracture. Once stable, the dog is hospitalized overnight with surgery planned the next day. The clinician plans to treat the dog's pain with a fast-acting, short-acting narcotic. The dog is given a bolus dose of 3 μg/kg (45 μg) of fentanyl:

$$45\,\mu g \div \text{the fentanyl concentration of } 50\,\mu g/mL = 0.9\ mL \text{ intravenously}$$

Following the bolus, the dog is started on a CRI at a dose of 3 μg/kg/hr (0.05 μg/kg/min) with a range prescribed by the clinician of 2 to 5 μg/kg/hr (0.03 to 0.08 μg/kg/min):

$$3\,\mu g/kg/hr \times 15\ kg = 45\,\mu g/hr$$

$$45\,\mu g/hr \div 50\,\mu g/mL = 0.9\ mL/hr$$

The dog's pain seems poorly controlled and during the night the dose is increased from 3 to 5 μg/kg/hr:

$$1.5\,mL/hr \text{ of } 50\,\mu g/mL \text{ fentanyl: } 5\,\mu g/kg/hr \times 15\ kg = 75\,\mu g/hr \div 50\,\mu g/mL = 1.5\,mL/hr$$

With the fentanyl dose near the clinician's upper limit it is decided to add other analgesic drugs to provide multimodal therapy allow them to decrease the total narcotic dose. They settle on lidocaine (at a dose of 30 μg/kg/min) and ketamine (at a dose of 2 μg/kg/min). They could use separate syringe pumps to administer the lidocaine and ketamine:

Lidocaine:

$$30\,\mu g/kg/min \text{ of } 20\,mg/mL \text{ lidocaine} \times 15\ kg = 450\,\mu g/kg/min$$

$$450\,\mu g/kg/min \div 20{,}000\,\mu g/mL = 0.0225\,mL/min \times 60\,min/hr = 1.35\,mL/hr$$

Ketamine:

$$2\,\mu g/kg/min \text{ of } 100\,mg/mL \text{ ketamine} \times 15\ kg = 30\,\mu g/kg/min$$

$$30\,\mu g/min \div 100{,}000\,\mu g/mL = 0.0003\,mL/min \times 60\,min/hr = 0.018\,mL/hr$$

Since the volume of ketamine is so small, it would be easier to add the drug directly into the patient's maintenance fluids. For this example the dog is receiving 0.9% NaCl at a maintenance rate of 60 mL/kg/day:

$$60\,mL/kg/day \text{ of } 0.9\% \text{ NaCl} \times 15\,kg = 900\,mL/day \div 24\,hr/day = 37.5\,mL/hr$$

Since we want the dog to receive 0.018 mL/hr of ketamine for analgesia, we can calculate the amount of drug to add to the maintenance fluids:

$$0.018\,mL/hr \text{ of } 100\,mg/mL \text{ ketamine} \div 37.5\,mL/hr \text{ maintenance fluids} = 0.00048\,mL \text{ ketamine/mL maintenance fluids}$$

$$0.00048\ mL \text{ ketamine} \times 1000\,mL/1\text{-L bag of } 0.9\% \text{ NaCl} = 0.43\ mL \text{ ketamine}$$

Therefore if 0.43 mL of 100 mg/mL ketamine is added to the 15-kg patient's bag of 0.9% NaCl, which is then delivered at 37.5 mL/hr, the dog will receive 2 μg/kg/min continuous infusion dose of the ketamine.

REFERENCES

The reference list can be found on the companion Expert Consult Web site at *www.expertconsult.com*.

Table • 90-1

Approximate Dosage, Half-Life, and Time to Steady State of Drugs Commonly Administered as a Constant Rate Infusion (CRI) in the Dog*

DRUG	CRI DOSAGE (µg/kg/min; UNLESS†, THEN U/kg/min)	ELIMINATION HALF-LIFE (hr)	TIME TO STEADY STATE 7 HALF-LIVES (hr)
Atracurium	4-9	0.33[6,7]	2.33
Buprenorphine	0.017-0.05	5.9[8]	41.3
Butorphanol	1.7-16.7	1.53[9]	10.71
Diazepam	1.7-16.7	0.25[10]	1.75
Digoxin	0.08-0.18	28[11]	196
Diltiazem	5-20	*5*[12]	*35*
Dobutamine	2-20	*0.04*[13]	*0.29*
Dopamine	1-20	*0.11*[13,14]	*0.82*
Epinephrine	0.005-1	0.03[15]	0.21
Esmolol	20-200	*0.15*[16]	*1.05*
Fenoldopam	0.1-0.6	*0.08*[17,18]	*0.58*
Fentanyl	0.03-0.3	2.6[19]	18.3
Furosemide	2-15	1[20]	7
Heparin (UF)	0.17-0.42†	*Nonlinear*[21]	*Nonlinear*
Hydromorphone	0.17-0.83	0.57[22]	3.99
Insulin (regular)	0.0015†	*0.28*[23]	*1.98*
Isoproterenol	0.04-0.08	0.05[24]	0.35
Ketamine	0.83-33.3	1.02[25]	7.15
Lidocaine	15-80	1.73[26]	12.13
Mannitol	1000-2000	1.19[27]	8.35
Medetomidine	0.008-0.05	0.96[28,29]	6.72
Metaclopramide	0.04-0.3	1.5[30]	10.5
Midazolam	1.7-8.3	*2.5*[31]	*17.5*
Milrinone	1-10	1.7[32]	11.9
Morphine	0.83-16.7	0.6[33-35]	4.2
Nicardipine	0.5-5	*4.75*[36,37]	*33.25*
Norepinephrine	0.05-2	*0.004*[13,38]	0.03
Pentobarbital	1.7-83	5[39]	*35*
Phentolamine	5-30	*3.17*[40]	*22.17*
Procainamide	20-40	2.43[41]	17
Propofol	50-400	1.33[42,43]	9.33
Pyridostigmine	0.17-0.5	*1.87*[44,45]	*13.1*
Sodium nitroprusside	1-3	72[46]	*504*
Sufentanil	0.1	*3.4*[47,48]	*23.8*
Terlipressin	167-667	*0.83*[49]	*5.83*
Vasopressin	0.0005-0.004†	0.09[50]	0.63
Verapamil	2-10	*5*[12]	*35*

*Half-lives listed in italics are extrapolated from other species.

CHAPTER 91

Buccal Mucosal Bleeding Time

Catharina Brömel

EVALUATION OF HEMOSTASIS

Examination of a dog or cat suspected of having a bleeding disorder includes assessment of vascular response and platelet function with formation of the platelet plug (primary hemostasis) and of the coagulation cascade leading to formation of fibrin and stabilization of the plug (secondary hemostasis). Persistent hemorrhage from superficial cutaneous injuries and mucosal surfaces (nasal, gingival, gastrointestinal, genitourinary) and formation of petechiae or ecchymoses are characteristic indicators of abnormalities in primary hemostasis. Primary hemostasis can be evaluated through quantitative measures (platelet estimate from blood smear, platelet count, mean platelet volume) and qualitative measures (von Willebrand factor [vWF] concentration and in vitro platelet function tests, such as optical aggregometry, aperture closure time, and flow cytometry). The buccal mucosal bleeding time (BMBT) is an in vivo, easily performed screening test for evaluation of primary hemostasis in dogs and cats.

The traditional coagulation pathway has been updated so that it more accurately reflects the in vivo mechanisms of secondary hemostasis (modern coagulation cascade). Abnormalities in secondary hemostasis can cause hematomas, hemarthrosis, and bleeding into the pleural and peritoneal cavities. These abnormalities are identified by coagulation screening tests (prothrombin time, activated partial thromboplastin time, activated coagulation time, fibrinogen), proteins induced by vitamin K absence or antagonism (PIVKA), and individual coagulation factor assays.

DETERMINATION OF THE BMBT

Determination of the BMBT requires two people and can generally be performed without sedation in dogs. The materials needed are: (1) a bleeding time device, such as the Surgicutt (ITC, Edison, N.J.), shown in Figure 91-1; (2) a gauze strip approximately 5 cm wide; (3) circular filter paper; and (4) a stopwatch.

The animal should be placed in lateral recumbency. The upper lip facing the examiner is everted to expose the buccal mucosa, and the gauze strip is tied around the maxilla and mandible to cause moderate venostasis of the buccal mucosa (in sedated cats, the gauze strip can be tied through the open mouth around the cranium). The safety clip (see Figure 91-1) of the single- or dual-blade spring-loaded bleeding time device is removed. The device is placed evenly against the exposed mucosal surface rostral to the gauze, with care taken to avoid visible blood vessels. The trigger is depressed, resulting in one or two standardized 5 mm by 1 mm mucosal incisions. The stopwatch is started at the time of trigger activation, and the device is removed from the mucosa. The filter paper is used to blot the blood in 5- to 10-second intervals about 2 mm

from the incision; care is taken to avoid disrupting platelet plug formation by touching the incision itself (Figure 91-2).

Blood should be prevented from reaching the animal's mouth, because this causes agitation. Blotting and the stopwatch are stopped upon complete cessation of hemorrhage, when blood is no longer absorbed by the filter paper. The BMBT is the time elapsed between mucosal incision and cessation of hemorrhage. If two incisions are made, bleeding generally stops at the same time at both sites. If not, the time should be recorded when the first incision ceases to bleed.

Published reference ranges for the BMBT are 1.4 to 3.5 minutes in dogs and 1.5 to 2.5 minutes in cats. For clinical purposes in dogs, a BMBT of less than 4 minutes is considered normal.

BMBT measurement is not indicated in animals with thrombocytopenia (less than 70,000/μL), because an abnormal result would be expected. Other causes of a prolonged

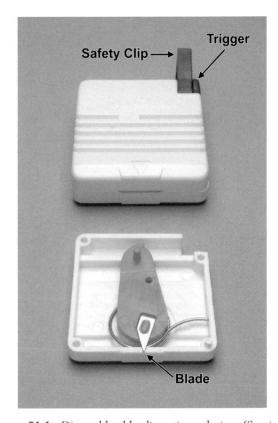

Figure 91-1 Disposable bleeding time device (Surgicutt). *Top,* Entire device. *Bottom,* Device with front cover removed, after safety clip has been removed and trigger pressed and removed.

 To view a video on this topic, go to www.expertconsult.com.

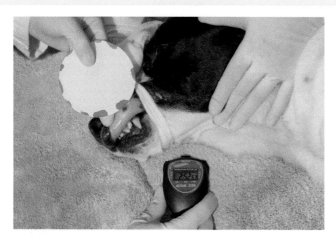

Figure 91-2 Determination of the buccal mucosal bleeding time in a dog.

BMBT are von Willebrand disease (vWD), thrombocytopathies, and vascular disorders. Impaired platelet adhesion and aggregation are present in vWD, a hereditary deficiency of vWF that is reported in various dog breeds but is rare in cats. In a dog with a normal plasma vWF concentration and absence of thrombocytopenia, a prolonged BMBT suggests a defect in platelet function that can be congenital or acquired. Inherited thrombocytopathies (intrinsic platelet function defects) are rare. They include disorders of platelet membranes (e.g., Glanzmann's thrombasthenia in Otterhounds and Great Pyrenees dogs) and disorders of platelet secretion (e.g., Spitz and Basset Hound thrombopathy and platelet granule storage pool deficiency in American Cocker Spaniels and feline Chédiak-Higashi syndrome). These defects have been associated with a prolonged BMBT. However, not all conditions or agents that cause a platelet dysfunction are reported to result in an abnormal BMBT.

Acquired thrombocytopathies are seen in uremic animals, in whom the prolonged BMBT is primarily due to defective platelet adhesion. Platelet aggregation is not consistently altered in uremic animals. Uremic toxins are thought to play a role in the pathogenesis of this condition. A prolonged BMBT compared with pretreatment measurements was noted after intravenous infusion of dextran 70 in dogs. Nonsteroidal antiinflammatory agents interfere with platelet function through inhibition of cyclooxygenase 1 (COX-1), leading to decreased synthesis of thromboxane A_2, a platelet-aggregating and vasoconstricting factor. Aspirin was found to prolong the canine BMBT. Carprofen and meloxicam both have COX-1–sparing properties and did not prolong the BMBT in dogs, although platelet aggregation in response to adenosine diphosphate (measured by use of an aggregometer) was decreased after treatment with carprofen, meloxicam, and aspirin in dogs with osteoarthritis. Administration of etodolac, firocoxib, or indomethacin also did not affect the BMBT in healthy dogs. Reports on ketoprofen have been conflicting. Acquired thrombocytopathies associated with dysproteine-

mias and with disseminated intravascular coagulation are thought to result from platelet coating by paraproteins and fibrin degradation products. Other causes of a prolonged BMBT include infectious diseases (e.g., feline retrovirus-induced thrombocytopathy, canine leishmaniasis, infections with *Ehrlichia canis* or *Anaplasma platys*), myeloproliferative diseases, and vasculopathies (e.g., vasculitis and inherited vascular defects). Coagulation factor deficiencies do not produce an abnormal BMBT because functional primary hemostasis leads to the formation of an unstable platelet plug; however, rebleeding can occur.

The BMBT is a quick, useful cage-side test for evaluation of primary hemostasis. It requires minimal preparation and few materials, and it is fairly noninvasive, safe, cost-effective, and easy to perform. Results are available immediately, which allows efficient presurgical screening and repeated evaluation to assess response to treatment. The test can be used as a complement to in vitro function tests, which may not fully reflect platelet function in vivo. However, the BMBT procedure is affected by iatrogenic variables that could normalize the result. Reports on sensitivity and specificity for the detection of primary hemostatic disorders vary, and some studies question the sensitivity of the BMBT measurement. A normal result does not eliminate a diagnosis of vWD or a platelet function defect, especially if the degree of dysfunction is mild. No correlation was found between the BMBT and plasma vWF concentration in dogs. The BMBT test is not standardized (e.g., degree of venostasis) and not reproducible. For any two readings in the same dog, the BMBT may vary by up to 2 minutes with one observer or between two observers.

Bench-top platelet function analysis and thromboelastography are gaining clinical importance in the diagnosis of hemostatic disorders, especially in dogs. One point-of-care instrument (PFA-100) that has been investigated in dogs evaluates platelet adhesion and aggregation in vitro by measurement of the closure time (time required for occlusion of an aperture by a platelet plug). It provides a tool for sensitive and rapid evaluation of primary hemostasis in nonanemic dogs. Thromboelastography is a technique that allows global assessment of hemostasis (precoagulation, coagulation, and fibrinolysis). It is a quick bench-top technique that provides a graphic representation of clot formation and lysis in real time (thromboelastogram).

In clinical practice, determination of the BMBT is a valuable and inexpensive tool for the initial assessment of the patient with a suspected bleeding disorder, together with the signalment, medical history (e.g., congenital versus acquired thrombocytopathy), medication history, physical examination findings, and results of other hemostatic, biochemical, and hematologic parameters.

REFERENCES

The reference list can be found on the companion Expert Consult Web site at *www.expertconsult.com*.

SKIN

CHAPTER 92

Ear Flushing

Kinga Gortel

Acute otitis externa in cats and dogs can usually be managed with topical medications and ear cleaning administered by owners. There are, however, frequent instances in which in-clinic ear flushing is essential for the successful resolution of otitis. The most common indication for in-clinic ear flushing is the failure of owner-administered therapy to clear an infection within a reasonable period (2 to 4 weeks). Ears containing exudate that cannot be removed by simple cleaning respond incompletely to topical medications and are prone to recurrences of infection (Figure 92-1). Another common indication for ear flushing is the presence of purulent exudate associated with gram-negative bacteria such as *Pseudomonas*. Ear flushing is also recommended when there is a suspicion of otitis media, a foreign body, or otic neoplasia. Ear flushing allows evaluation of the ear canal and tympanic membrane, as well as myringotomy if necessary. It permits cleaning of the tympanic cavity and its sampling for culture and cytology. It also facilitates removal of foreign bodies and visualization and sampling of masses.

COMPLICATIONS FROM EAR FLUSHING

Complications from ear flushing are infrequent in dogs but appear to be more common, though usually transient, in cats. Complications include vestibular symptoms, deafness, Horner's syndrome, and facial nerve paralysis. The possible need for myringotomy to fully evaluate and treat the ear disease should be explained to the owner prior to flushing. The explanation should include the fact that the tympanic membrane usually heals after myringotomy. Healthy tympanic membranes heal within 3 to 5 weeks. Unplanned ear flushing during another anesthetic procedure should be avoided unless the owner has been forewarned of possible side effects. It is important to understand the anatomy of the external and middle ear, since it may be severely altered by chronic inflammation. If ear canal stenosis, glandular hyperplasia, or edema prevent passage of an otoscope tip, ear flushing should be postponed until the canal can be rendered more accessible by a 1- to 2-week course of topical and systemic corticosteroids (e.g., prednisone 1 mg/kg PO daily for dogs) (Figure 92-2).

If severe stenosis persists, surgical intervention is more likely to result in a favorable outcome than ear flushing and medical therapy.

EAR FLUSHING TECHNIQUE

General anesthesia is required for full cleaning or myringotomy (Figure 92-3).

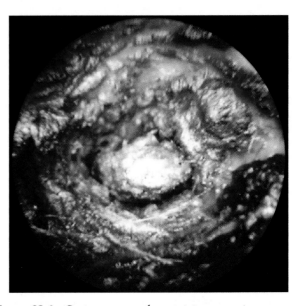

Figure 92-1 Canine ear canal containing excessive cerumen viewed through MedRxInc video otoscope. (Courtesy Dr. Louis N. Gotthelf.)

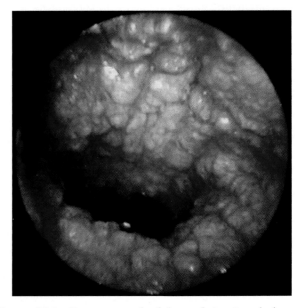

Figure 92-2 Ceruminous gland hyperplasia viewed through MedRxInc video otoscope. (Courtesy Dr. Louis N. Gotthelf.)

 To view a video on this topic, go to **www.expertconsult.com.**

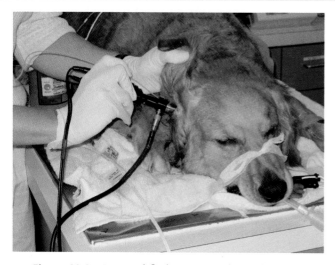

Figure 92-3 Ear canal flushing in anesthetized patient.

An endotracheal tube with an inflated cuff is used to prevent lower respiratory tract contamination via the auditory tubes. With either lateral or sternal recumbency, positioning the patient with a slight downward tilt of the nose allows fluids to escape rostrally from the nares. If bulla radiographs or computed tomography are to be performed, they should precede the ear flush. These imaging studies are helpful in assessing otic structures including the bullae. Various ear flushing techniques utilizing hand-held and video-otoscopes have been described. The procedure should allow removal and sampling of exudate in the outer ear canal, a myringotomy if needed, and sampling and cleaning of the tympanic cavity.

Ear flushing in dogs utilizing a hand-held otoscope may be performed as follows. A surgical otoscope is preferred for the procedure as it allows passage of catheters and other instruments. Once the dog is anesthetized, the ears are examined otoscopically and swabs for culture and cytology are collected from each ear. It is imperative that cytology is collected from every patient to correlate with the culture results, assess for organisms that may not grow on culture (such as yeast), and assess the degree of inflammation. The ear canals may then be filled with a mild ceruminolytic ear cleaner if the otic exudate is tenacious and waxy. The dog is then placed into lateral recumbency. An ear bulb syringe is used to gently remove exudate, using isotonic saline solution warmed to body temperature. At least 1 L of saline solution should be warmed and available for flushing. Addition of other substances to the fluid is not usually necessary. All of the ceruminolytic agent must be removed from the ear canal to prevent irritation and possible ototoxicity. To protect the tympanic membrane from undue pressure, the ear canal must not form a tight seal with the bulb syringe. A new bulb syringe should be used for each patient. Once the flushing yields clear fluid, the canal is suctioned using a catheter (such as an 8-French polypropylene catheter cut to desired length, an open-ended tomcat catheter, or a red rubber feeding tube) attached to a 12-mL syringe introduced through the otoscope. The tip of the polypropylene catheter may be heated over a flame to reduce sharp edges. The ear is examined and flushing continues via the catheter until the canal appears clean. Repeated flushing, suctioning, and reevaluation are usually needed. An ear curette can be used to remove tenacious exudates. Grasping tools such as alligator forceps should be used to remove hair, wax balls, or foreign bodies. Finally, the ear canal is thoroughly suctioned. The procedure for myringot-

omy and middle ear flushing is described below. Ear flushing in cats is performed similarly. Pretreatment with a ceruminolytic agent is not recommended due to higher susceptibility to complications from ear flushing in this species.

Video-otoscopy greatly facilitates ear flushing procedures, permits documentation of findings, and provides greater magnification and illumination as compared with hand-held units. A major advantage of these instruments is that their working channel allows simultaneous flushing and visualization, and clear fluid introduced during flushing actually improves the image. This is in contrast to hand-held otoscopes, with which instruments and fluids obscure the visual field and repeated suctioning is needed to assess progress. Placing patients in sternal recumbency is most convenient, but lateral recumbency is preferred by some. It is important to monitor the orientation of the otoscope, which may rotate during the procedure and confuse assessment of ear anatomy.

With video-otoscopy, the stream of saline from the flushing catheter can be directed effectively at adherent material. Pretreatment with a ceruminolytic agent and cleaning with an ear bulb syringe are still helpful time-saving processes. A simple technique for flushing uses a long 5-French polypropylene urinary catheter attached to a 20- to 35-mL syringe. An assistant flushes warmed saline solution in pulses while the tip of the catheter is moved by the operator within in the ear canal. Fluid exits the ear canal around the otoscope tip. A more convenient approach that does not require the repeated filling of syringes is the use of a combined suction and lavage instrument. Both the Earigator (MedRx) and the Vetpump (Karl Storz Veterinary Endoscopy, Inc.) are instruments that can be attached to irrigation catheters and combine suction and lavage control in one hand-piece. Various other methods of combining lavage and suction have been described, including a three-way stopcock attached to an assistant-operated syringe (or intravenous bag of saline under pressure) for flushing, and to a syringe or suction apparatus for removing saline from the ear.

After thorough cleaning, the area of the tympanic membrane can be evaluated. Its obliteration in cases of chronic otitis is common. Even with experience, observing the normal location of this structure can at times be difficult. If the otoscope tip is advanced as far as possible and the tympanum is not seen, rupture should be suspected. The intense light source in video-otoscopy may make the lining of the tympanic cavity appear reflective and white, confusing the operator in its similarity to the tympanum. If the tympanum is absent or partially ruptured, material from the middle ear is obtained by passing two sterile swabs into this area, preferably through a sterile otoscope cone. The first swab is cultured and the second used for cytologic evaluation. The middle ear cavity should be gently but thoroughly flushed through a catheter to remove exudate or ceruminolytic agent. It is preferable to direct catheters and other instruments ventrally within the tympanic cavity. Often, inspissated material is seen to exit the tympanic cavity in surprisingly large pieces with repeated flushing. It is normal to see flushing solution exiting the nares during a flush of the tympanic cavity if the nose is tilted slightly downward.

MYRINGOTOMY

Diagnostic and therapeutic myringotomy should be performed if otitis media is suspected, as the tympanum may be intact despite a middle ear infection. Otitis media should be suspected in cases of chronic, relapsing, or unremitting otitis, if the tympanum appears abnormal, if neurologic signs are present, or if suggestive radiographic evidence is present. Myringotomy allows collection of samples from and thorough flushing of the middle ear. After cleaning and drying the ear canal, the myringotomy incision may be made using a 5-French polypropylene catheter cut at an angle. Other instruments used to perform myringotomy include a spinal needle, an open-ended tomcat catheter, a small calcium alginate swab, or a short CO_2 laser pulse. The incision is made in the ventral portion (preferably the caudoventral quadrant) of the tympanic membrane to minimize the damage to the tympanic germinal epithelium and middle ear structures. If a swab is used, it may be submitted for culture, with a second swab collected for cytology. If a catheter or needle is used, aspiration is attempted to sample fluid material. If none is present, the middle ear may be instilled with a small amount (0.5 mL) of sterile saline solution and then aspirated. The collected fluid is used for culture and cytologic examination. This is followed by repeated flushing of the tympanic cavity as described above, though the myringotomy incision. Flushing is continued long enough to dislodge any firm, inspissated exudate. Flushing of the middle ear may be followed by administration of therapeutic nonototoxic agents directly into this structure.

FOLLOW-UP

Essential to the successful outcome of the ear flush is the ability to keep the ear clean, so topical and oral antimicrobial agents should immediately be initiated based on cytology. Once- to twice-daily ear cleaning by owners is prescribed, and a 1-week follow-up is scheduled. Saline solution may be used in an ulcerated ear or immediately following myringotomy. Alcohol-containing solutions should be avoided. Oral corticosteroids are recommended to facilitate at-home treatment and to reduce the production of inflammatory exudate in painful or ulcerated ears. At 1-week follow-up topical and oral antimicrobial agents may be changed based on culture, and a more effective ear cleaner prescribed.

CHAPTER 93

Skin Scrapings and Skin Biopsies

Ralf S. Mueller
Sonya V. Bettenay

GETTING THE MOST FROM SKIN SCRAPINGS

In veterinary dermatology, skin scrapings to diagnose cutaneous ectoparasites are classified as either superficial or deep. They aim at identifying different parasites and differ substantially in their procedural approach.

Superficial Skin Scrapings

Indication   Superficial skin scrapings detect mites living on the skin surface or burrowing within the stratum corneum. *Cheyletiella* spp. or *Otodectes cynotis* are typically surface dwellers. Female *Sarcoptes scabiei* (SS) or *Notoedres cati* dig tunnels in which to lay their eggs, but all stages of the life cycle can be found walking on the surface. Both *Cheyletiella* and *Sarcoptes* mites can be difficult to find; between 50% and 70% of SS cases yield positive results on skin scrapings.[1,2] Cats with *Notoedres cati* typically have an abundant number of mites. The preferred anatomic sites vary with the ectoparasite and this determines the sites to be scraped. In the dog with scabies, the elbows, ear margins, hocks, and ventrum are commonly affected. In cats, *Notoedres cati* affects the head. In both dogs and cats, *Cheyletiella* mites inhabit the dorsal trunk and typically cause scaling. *Otodectes cynotis* is most frequently associated with otitis externa, but may produce a head and neck pruritus and rarely a generalized dermatitis.

Superficial skin scrapings should thus be performed in any scaly or pruritic dog or cat.[3]

Procedure   Mineral oil is applied to the scalpel blade AND affected skin as this facilitates the gathering of debris and increases the chance of positive results.[1] Select nonexcoriated scaly and/or papular sites and scrape over a large area (at least 5 × 5 cm). Hairy dogs with suspected scabies should be clipped first—without removing the surface scale or crust that may be present, as *Sarcoptes* mites may be dislodged with such cleansing. Clipping is not indicated in pets that might have cheyletiellosis. The oil is gently scraped off the surface, using a "buttering bread" motion (Web Figure 93-1) in the direction of hair growth. The oil is then transferred onto a glass microscope slide.

With this technique, there is a larger volume of oil to be collected and thus more slides to examine, but a higher change of success. When evaluating a sample microscopically for ectoparasites, a coverslip is applied to distribute the debris evenly. This minimizes the chance of missing mites covered by debris and enables a rapid yet thorough scanning at low magnification without the need for continuous adjustment of focus. Lowering the condenser of the microscope increases the contrast. Skin scrapings for ectoparasites should be examined under the microscope within a few hours of sample collection. Mites can actually move from the slide during the course of a day.

Interpretation   One mite or egg is diagnostic and should be considered reason to initiate miticidal therapy. A negative scraping does not rule out presence of these mites and trial therapy may still be indicated. Occasionally, a short-bodied *Demodex* mite may be found on superficial skin scrapings. These short-bodied mites live in the epidermis rather than the follicles, but can occur in combination with a proliferation of follicular *Demodex* mites; thus their detection should trigger deep skin scrapings.

Deep Skin Scrapings

Indication Deep skin scrapings are performed to detect *Demodex* mites. In the dog, *Demodex canis* lives in the hair follicle, a longer-bodied *Demodex* mite *(Demodex injai)* is suspected to live in the sebaceous glands.[4-6] Canine demodicosis is characterized clinically by alopecia, comedones, papules, pustules, scales, and crusts and is on the list of differential diagnoses for almost any dog with skin disease. A deep skin scraping is one of the most common diagnostic procedures performed in veterinary dermatology. Demodicosis in the cat is less common, typically secondary to systemic disease and affecting the head.[7,8] A ventral alopecia pattern has also been reported.[9]

Procedure The site for scraping (especially follicular papules or pustules) is chosen so that it allows an area of at least 1cm² to be sampled. Mite counts are higher when the skin is squeezed (prior to and during scraping) in an attempt to push the mites out from the depths of the follicles.[10] Sedation may be necessary when the face and paws are affected. Using a blade covered with mineral oil, the skin is scraped in the direction of hair growth until capillary bleeding is observed. Trichograms (hair plucks, placed in mineral oil on a glass slide for examination) provide an alternative test particularly useful in pets with periocular or pedal lesions. Trichograms are almost as reliable as deep skin scrapings, if sufficient hair shafts over the same area of 1 to 2 cm² are plucked.[10,11]

Interpretation *Demodex canis* is a normal component of the cutaneous fauna and an occasional mite can be found on the skin scraping of normal dogs. Nevertheless, it would be quite rare for more than one *Demodex* mite to be seen on a dog not affected by demodicosis. If only one mite is found, but clinical signs are compatible, further scrapings, trichogram, or a biopsy are indicated.[3] When evaluating deep skin scrapings, it is important to assess and to note in the record the site of scraping and the relative numbers of adults, larvae, nymphs, and eggs per LPF. In subsequent monthly visits, assessment of response to therapy should be based on comparison of such numbers after the same sites have been sampled.

GETTING THE MOST FROM A SKIN BIOPSY
(Web Box 93-1)

While skin biopsies are recommended as a useful pathologic test, they do not always yield a specific diagnosis. Site and biopsy methodology can make the difference between obtaining and failing to obtain a specific diagnosis.[3,12] Even "inconclusive results" can rule out a number of differential diagnoses.

Site Selection

The selection of a biopsy site requires a careful examination of the entire animal for the most representative range of lesions. Lesions have "lives." Disease is a dynamic process and the biopsy site can be analogous to a single frame taken from a roll of movie film. Because it reveals only this "snapshot," the clues as to the cause of the disease may simply not be present at that point in time. Taking multiple samples from well-chosen clinical sites exhibiting a variety of lesions will broaden the pathologist's perspective and help to avoid inconclusive results. In a pustular disease, erythematous macules develop into papules, then pustules and finally crusts/erosions. Sampling each of these stages and several of the most exciting lesions, the pustules, supplies the widest range of lesions. If present, pustules or vesicles should always be

sampled. Depigmenting lesions should be biopsied in an area of active depigmentation (i.e., gray color) rather than the final stage (i.e., white). Alopecic areas should be sampled in the center of the most alopecic area as well as in junctional and normal areas. When submitting these samples, it can be extremely helpful if the pathologist knows which sample came from which site. This can be achieved by either placing samples in separate, carefully labeled, bottles of formalin, or through the use of tissue dyes to mark each piece with a different color (Web Figure 93-2).

If possible, avoid the glabrous (nonhaired) areas of the body as they contain fewer hair follicle units and smaller sebaceous glands.

Ulcerated areas should be avoided, unless deep dermal, vascular, or pannicular pathology is suspected. When sampling an ulcerated lesion, use an elliptical incision and include the area of transition between affected and adjacent "normal or intact" skin within the biopsy as this may contain a clue as to the reason for the ulceration. Orientation is based on the long axis running from the center of the ulcer, across the border, and into the healthy skin.

Include normal skin. In the case of a severe inflammatory disease, clues with regard to the follicular growth characteristics may be present only in adjacent normal skin.

Surgical preparation of the site should not be performed at all. Crusts should be left on the skin and included in the biopsy as they may contain microorganisms, inflammatory or acantholytic cells, that will help establish a diagnosis. Write "please cut in crusts" on the submission form. Infection resulting from a lack of surgical preparation is almost never seen. After formalin fixation, the sample usually looks uniformly gray. A line drawn—prior to biopsy—on the skin in the direction of the hair growth using a waterproof pen helps the technician to orient the tissue appropriately (Figure 93-1, Web Figure 93-3).[13]

Surgical Technique

Overlying hair should be clipped and gently removed to preserve any scale and crusts. No aseptic preparation is performed, except when excising solitary nodules. General anesthesia is indicated for facial or paw biopsies and may also be necessary for larger excisional biopsies. Local anesthesia, with or without sedation, is a practical alternative for many pets with truncal biopsies. The subcutaneous injection of 1 or 2 mL of Xylocaine without adrenaline will usually provide

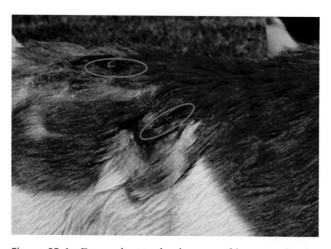

Figure 93-1 Draw a line in the direction of hair growth. This technique has revolutionized the interpretation of follicular pathology. Do not draw over fragile lesions like pustules, which may rupture with pressure.

adequate local anesthesia. The maximum amount of Xylocaine to be used will depend on the body size of the animal. Keep the needle entry point outside the proposed biopsy area to avoid disruption to the tissue in the biopsy and mark the site to enable easy relocation.[13]

Wedge/Ellipse versus Punch Biopsy

The punch biopsy is quick, relatively atraumatic, and is typically employed when infectious, inflammatory, and endocrine dermatoses are suspected. Disposable 8-mm punches are preferred, but 6-mm punches should be used with extremely small dogs and cats. Four-mm punches are reserved for biopsies of footpads, nasal planum, mucocutaneous junctions, or eyelids.

Punch Biopsy Sampling   Hold the punch at a 90° angle to the surface of the skin, firmly brace the surrounding skin, and rotate the punch in one direction with continuous, but relatively little, pressure. When the skin no longer tries to "turn" with the rotation of the punch, a sufficient depth has been reached to free the dermis from its underlying attachment. The punch is removed and any blood is carefully blotted. It is critical to remove the punched out plug of tissue without squeezing it. Grasp the tissue gently at the base—which should be the panniculus—and sever the subcutaneous attachments. Under no circumstance should the dermis or epidermis be squeezed as this leads to "crush artefact" and may result in a sample that is unreadable or misinterpreted as scarring. The use of fine instruments such as iris scissors and forceps used in ophthalmology can be helpful. The punch technique is not suitable when lesions of the panniculus or deep dermis are suspected.

Excisional/Incisional Sampling   The wedge or elliptical biopsy should be employed as an excisional technique when a deep dermal or panniculus lesion is clinically suspected. This method should also be used when removing solitary nodules or fragile lesions (such as vesicles). It is used when complete excision is not possible or desirable. This method is also indicated when an area of skin exhibits a range of changes radiating from the center to the edge of a lesion (e.g., ulceration or alopecia and adjacent normal tissue can be included in the ellipse). In general, it is best not to use a punch in the margin of a lesion (Figure 93-2, *A* and *B*).

In the case of a suspected neoplasm, an incisional biopsy may be indicated. This allows an accurate diagnosis without the potential of contaminating surrounding tissue and without compromising any subsequent wide excisions. Cytology may diagnose malignancy without the need for a biopsy, but it cannot replace the prognostic information obtained from the assessment of margins that histology allows.

Once the biopsy has been taken, the wound should be closed routinely.

Fixation of Tissue   The biopsy sample surface should be gently blotted prior to placing it in formalin. A minimum volume of formalin of (approximately) 10 times the volume of the sample is recommended for adequate fixation. Inadequate fixation results in necrotic, unreadable samples. In cold climates, the addition of one part alcohol to nine parts formalin will prevent the possibility of freezing during shipping. Large nodules should be sectioned into 1-cm thick pieces to allow adequate penetration of the formalin into the center of the lesion. However, do not section through the skin nodule completely—leave the sections attached at the base (adipose tissue) so that they are held together in the original orientation. Multiple impressions for cytology of

the freshly excised surface is a valuable adjunctive test to perform.

Shave Biopsies   On the pinnae, cartilage is found directly under an extremely thin dermis and the panniculus is absent. With punch and wedge techniques, cartilage may inadvertently be damaged and a permanent change in the shape of the pinna may result. Many diseases of the pinnae, such as lupus erythematosus, pemphigus complex, and infections with bacteria or yeast, are diseases of the epidermis, dermoepidermal junction, and superficial dermis. Deep biopsies of such lesions are not necessary. The shave biopsy is a fast technique, but it needs to be performed under general anesthesia. The outside of the ear will need to be clipped; the inside may not. A scalpel blade is held in one hand; the pinna is bent over the index finger of the other hand (Web Figure 93-4).

On the stretched and bent convex surface, the scalpel blade should be used to cut into the skin at an angle of approximately 20° only to a depth where capillary bleeding is observed. At that particular depth, the incision should be continued parallel to the surface of the skin until a specimen

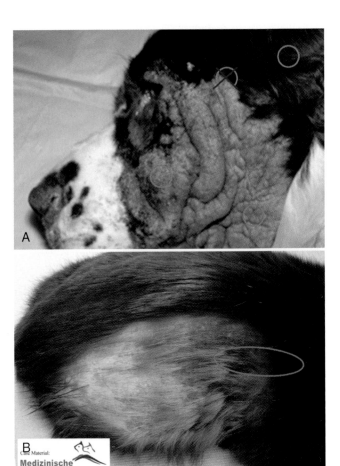

Figure 93-2 A, Rule of thumb—include 100% lesional or nonlesional skin when sampling with a punch biopsy. **B,** The histopathology technician will usually section the elliptical biopsy specimen along the midline of the long axis of the ellipse. Orientation of the ellipse across the junction between abnormal and normal tissues will allow the pathologist to view the skin from affected, through active, to nonaffected areas and so gain the best possible appreciation of the stages of the disease and hence the etiology.

of about 5 × 5 mm (0.25 × 0.25 inches) is obtained. This sliced-out specimen is typically an extremely thin piece of skin and needs to be placed with the dermal surface down on a piece of a tongue depressor or cardboard to avoid distortion during fixation (Web Figure 93-5).

A piece of lens paper may be draped around the specimen and cardboard to ensure that the technician can find it. Three minutes of firm digital pressure or use of a silver nitrate stick typically stops hemorrhage and no suturing is usually necessary. There is typically no scarring. Although this technique sounds easy, it takes a little experience to determine the depth of the "shave." Histology will reveal changes in the epidermis and upper dermis, as the depth of the specimen with proper technique will reach the midfollicular level (Web Figure 93-6). Deep dermal changes such as vasculitis and pathology of the cartilage cannot be evaluated.

Interpretation—Making a Diagnosis

One of the major reasons to perform a skin biopsy is to obtain a diagnosis. The second aim, and one which is still extremely useful even in the absence of a confirmed diagnosis, is to rule out differential diagnoses. In order for the pathologist to look for subtle clues and to interpret unusual changes, it helps if a differential diagnosis list with details of the clinical lesions has been included with the submission. Choose a pathologist with an active interest in dermatopathology or a dermatologist with advanced dermatopathology training.

REFERENCES

The reference list can be found on the companion Expert Consult Web Site at *www.expertconsult.com*.

CHAPTER 94

Cytology of the Skin and Subcutaneous Tissues

Deborah C. Bernreuter

Cytology should be regarded as a rapid screening test to determine if a biopsy, culture, or surgical excision is necessary. Quite often cytologic examination is the only test needed to arrive at a diagnosis, prognosis, and treatment plan. A representative cytologic sample at least can yield a short list of possible diagnoses. If the cytologic evaluation is not completely diagnostic, a biopsy is required to rule out or to confirm various differential diagnoses. When the cytologic results are considered in conjunction with the patient's history; the location, description, and duration of the lesion; the physical examination results; diagnostic imaging findings; and other laboratory determinations, the list of differential diagnoses becomes quite short.

REQUIRED EQUIPMENT

The following equipment is required for obtaining an adequate representative sample for cytologic evaluation:
- Needle: 21-gauge for dogs, 22-gauge for cats is best
- 12-mL syringe
- Unused glass slides, preferably with frosted ends for ease of labeling
- Lavender-top tube (for fluid)
- Sterile swab (for fistulous tracts and mucous membranes) and saline
- Paper towel (for impression smears)

If the cytologic evaluation is to be done in-hospital, a good-quality, well-maintained binocular microscope, a "quick" type of Romanowsky stain, and distilled water are also required.

PROCEDURE FOR SAMPLE COLLECTION

Samples from Solid Masses or Fluid-Filled Lesions

For solid masses and fluid-filled lesions, a 21- or 22-gauge needle on a 12-mL syringe is usually used to collect and transfer cells or fluid (or both) to several glass slides. Sedation or anesthesia can be used if required to reduce risk and unnecessary pain. Local anesthesia is not used on superficial lesions, because the pain associated with aspiration of a sample is no greater than the pain felt during injection of the local anesthesia. Skin preparation is the same as that required for a venipuncture or an injection. If the lesion will also be sampled for microbiologic culture, surgical preparation should be done on the collection site.

Before the sample is collected, four glass slides should be made ready to receive it. This minimizes clotting of the sample in the needle, which can occur while slides are located to receive the sample. It is not necessary to submit more than four smears; even a single smear can be adequate if it is representative.

The needle is attached to the syringe while the plunger is depressed. One hand is used to grasp the lesion firmly to stabilize it, and the other hand is used to insert the tip of the needle deep into the mass. Inserting the needle deeply into the mass yields a larger sample than inserting the needle only superficially. When the tip of the needle is in a representative location, the plunger of the syringe is pulled back as far as possible and held for a few seconds. The plunger is never pumped! The pumping action that is useful in the collection of bone marrow samples is harmful for cells in all other anatomic sites. It causes excessive tissue damage, and encourages hemodilution and clotting (release of tissue thromboplastin). The direction of the needle within the mass should be changed only when the needle has been almost completely withdrawn so as to avoid excessive tissue destruction and subsequent lysis of cells, which would occur with an attempt to change the direction of the needle while it is still embedded in the mass. Aspiration can be done in two or three different orientations in the mass to collect the most representative sample. The hub of the needle where it is attached to the syringe must be watched; blood must not be allowed to flow into the syringe. Blood dilutes a previously representative sample and causes clotting. If blood appears in the needle hub while the plunger is withdrawn, the plunger (and thus the vacuum pressure) is released immediately. A needleful of cells is sufficient to make a dozen smears if necessary.

Only after the vacuum in the syringe has been released is the needle removed, first from the lesion and then from the syringe. A small amount of air is then drawn into the syringe, the needle is reattached, and the plunger is rapidly advanced while the needle's tip is close to a glass slide (i.e., not from a great height). In this way, the sample is expelled onto the slide intended, and it does not inadvertently shed a few cells onto the adjacent slide. On several occasions this author has identified misdiagnoses made because a few tumor cells or organisms were inadvertently sprayed onto adjacent slides, which, because they grossly appeared to be unused slides, were then used to prepare smears from a different patient. When slides are prepared to receive cytology samples, they should not be placed close to each other, to avoid overspray.

Liquid Samples

If the sample is liquid, only one drop of sample should be placed on each slide so that when the sample is smeared rapidly to make a feathered edge (and thus a monolayer of cells), the entire smear will be one half to three fourths the length of the slide. If too large a drop is accidentally expelled onto a slide, the excess is immediately reaspirated into the syringe. It is helpful if an assistant who can make a feathered edge is available to smear out the drop of sample as soon as one is placed on a slide, while additional drops are being placed on additional slides. If the sample consists of a large amount of fluid, a couple of feathered edge smears are made, and the remaining fluid is expelled into a lavender-top tube. Watery fluid is smeared correctly by raising the angle between the sample slide and the spreader slide to 40 to 45 degrees and smearing very quickly. Thick fluid is smeared to a monolayer by lowering the angle to 15 to 20 degrees and smearing slightly more slowly. Normal blood or fluid is smeared with a 30-degree angle. Any remaining fluid should be expelled into a lavender-top tube and mixed well to avoid clotting so that accurate cell counts can be attained and smears of concentrated cells can be prepared. The ethylenediamine tetraacetic acid (EDTA) in the lavender-top tube is the preservative of choice for accurate cell morphology. Heparin can distort cells. Both the fresh smears and the fluid are submitted to the laboratory. At the laboratory, some of the fluid can be placed in a cytocentrifuge for production of concentrated smears. Cytocentrifuges concentrate the cells directly onto a small area of a glass slide, which is especially useful with fluids of low cellularity. In addition, some of the fluid can be centrifuged and a drop of sediment (or buffy coat smear, if the sample is very hemorrhagic) can be prepared, stained, and examined.

Semisolid Samples

If the sample is semisolid, another slide should be placed flat on top of the sample and the two slides should be gently and quickly pulled apart to make monolayers on both slides. With either the direct smear or the "pull" technique, all smears should be thin enough to air dry within 1 minute. The smears should be double-checked to ensure that they are completely dry before they are encased in a slide holder for transportation to a laboratory.

An impression smear can be useful with a biopsy sample. Before the biopsy sample is placed in formalin, its cut surface can be blotted with a paper towel to remove surface blood and tissue fluid and then touched to a glass slide several times to make an impression smear. Always submit slides and biopsy jars in separate bags (see item 9 in list of common mistakes).

Samples from Mucous Membranes of the Vagina, Conjunctiva, and Mouth and from Fistulous Tracts

For sampling the mucous membranes of the vagina, conjunctiva, or mouth or for sampling fistulous tracts, a sterile swab moistened with saline can be used to swab the lesion. If the lesion is already moist, the saline is not needed. The tissue is swabbed, and the swab then is rolled onto a glass slide. Never rub the swab on the slide; it causes disruption of the cells.

COMMON MISTAKES TO AVOID IN COLLECTION AND PREPARATION OF CYTOLOGY/FLUID SAMPLES

The following common mistakes should be avoided in sample collection and preparation:

1. Pumping the syringe plunger during collection. This causes tissue destruction and lysis of cells, as well as hemodilution. It also increases the risk of clotting due to release of tissue thromboplastin.
2. Using a syringe with a capacity of less than 10 mL. If the syringe is too small, the vacuum pressure it creates is too weak, and the sample is often too small for adequate evaluation.
3. Placing too large a sample on one slide. If the drop of sample is too large, the consequences are: (1) the largest cells are pushed off the end of the smear, resulting in a nonrepresentative sample; (2) a monolayer is not formed, and the smear will be too thick for evaluation; and (3) thick smears dry slowly, causing cell lysis and distortion. If too much sample is inadvertently placed on a slide, just reaspirate the extra back into the syringe and transfer it to an additional slide.
4. Failing to smear out the sample. A drop of sample left in one place on the slide dries slowly, causing lysis, and forms a thick jumble of cells, which cannot be evaluated. If two cells are on top of each other, neither can be evaluated. If excessive cell fragility is present (this can be one criterion of malignancy), the cells might not be able to survive smearing, and a biopsy would be necessary for evaluation.
5. Refrigerating the smears. When smears are placed in slide holders and then refrigerated, the ambient humidity from the room air in the slide holder condenses, causing droplets of water to fall onto the smears. Water is hypotonic and causes cell lysis; only a homogeneous, proteinaceous background is observed on cytology.
6. Placing the slides in the slide holder before they are completely dry. Slow drying causes lysis of cells. If cells are lysed and then placed near an ice pack while liquid, the cells crystallize into shapes of long spears, preventing evaluation.
7. Submitting samples for cytology or fluid analysis without including the signalment, patient history, and other physical findings, as well as the anatomic location, a description, and the duration of the lesion. Without these other parameters, only a description, not an interpretation, is possible.
8. Submitting fluid without anticoagulant. Fluid is always submitted for analysis in an EDTA tube, and in addition a fresh smear is submitted for accurate cell counts (without clots).
9. Submitting cytology smears in the same laboratory bag with a biopsy jar. Formalin fumes from the jar can fix the cytology cells and prevent subsequent adequate staining.

DETERMINING THE CHOICE OF CYTOLOGY OR BIOPSY

The choice of cytology or biopsy depends on the type and location of the lesion. For discrete masses in the intradermal and subcutaneous tissues, a fine needle aspiration biopsy is often diagnostic. It is useful for identifying the mass as a site of inflammation, a cyst, or a solid tumor. In addition, if the lesion is a site of inflammation, the etiology (e.g., bacteria, fungal elements, yeast, parasites, or keratin debris from a ruptured epithelial cyst) can often be observed. Bacteria can be identified as cocci, rod-shaped, spirochetes, possible anaerobes, mycobacteria, or a mixed population, which can be helpful in choosing an appropriate class of antibiotic while awaiting results of a culture and susceptibility test. If Gram's stain is also available, additional unstained smears can be used to determine gram positivity or negativity. If the lesion is a

solid tissue tumor, an experienced cytologist can further classify it as epithelial or mesenchymal in origin, and list any criteria of malignancy observed. If it is a discrete round cell tumor, cytology is often sufficient for diagnosis.

If the lesions are vesicular, however, such as pemphigus lesions, cytology is not useful. Instead, an intact vesicle (or at least the edge of a vesicle if none is intact) is gently excised, and the tissue is placed in formalin for biopsy. For other superficial flat lesions (e.g., ulcers) that are not associated with a mass, a biopsy of the entire lesion or the edge of the lesion is usually more helpful than cytology. If a dermal mass has an ulcerated surface, impression smears of the lesion will contain only the secondary inflammatory cells and organisms; they will not be representative of the primary lesion underneath. For this reason, an aspirate of the deeper layers of the mass would probably be more representative (Figure 94-1).

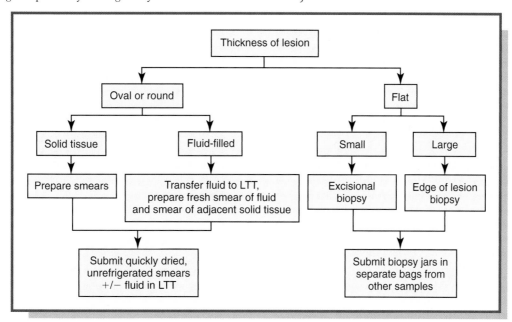

Figure 94-1 Decision tree and sample selection for lesions in the skin and subcutaneous tissues. *LTT,* Lavender top tube.

ABDOMEN

CHAPTER 95

Abdominal Ultrasonography

Rachel E. Pollard
Eric J. Herrgesell

Abdominal ultrasound is rapidly becoming a major component in the diagnostic arsenal for small animal practitioners. A fundamental understanding of ultrasound physics and imaging principles can allow the user to make basic diagnoses. Moreover, a consistent and repeatable methodology for performing an abdominal ultrasound examination will minimize errors, omissions, and missed lesions.

ULTRASOUND PHYSICS

Medical ultrasound functions in a way similar to sonar. A sound beam of a specific frequency (megahertz [MHz]) is sent into the area of interest by the transducer. The transducer waits for the returned echoes and "listens" for their amplitude (intensity) and location (directly related to how long it takes

 To view a video on this topic, go to **www.expertconsult.com.**

for the echo to return). Once the ultrasound beam enters the area of interest, it can be absorbed, refracted, or reflected. If the beam is absorbed, no ultrasound waves will return to the transducer and, consequently, no information becomes available for generating an image. Similarly, if the ultrasound waves are refracted, their pathway is altered such that they do not return to the transducer. Thus, only ultrasound waves that enter the body, encounter an object (tissue), and are reflected directly back to the transducer are used to generate an image. Highly reflective structures will appear bright (gas, mineral), whereas parenchymal organs will be variable in their reflectivity and appear as shades of gray.

TISSUE CHARACTERISTICS

Most organs are described according to their size, shape, echogenicity (brightness) and echotexture (parenchymal pattern). Size and shape are self-explanatory terms and will not be further discussed. Echogenicity is assessed on a relative scale in comparison to other organs and to what is anticipated as normal. An object or tissue that is anechoic has no echogenicity and is black. An object that is bright in comparison to other objects or the anticipated norm is hyperechoic. An object that is dark in comparison to other objects or the anticipated norm is hypoechoic.

A relative scale of normal tissue echogenicity can be established (Table 95-1).

It is essential to compare tissues to one another in order to establish true echogenicity since tissue brightness can also be affected by machine settings. However, using this scale of relative echogenicities, one can define pathologic changes. For example, a fibrotic or fat-infiltrated liver will become more hyperechoic than it should be in comparison to other organs because it has been infiltrated by more hyperechoic tissue. Similarly, an edematous or congested spleen will become more hypoechoic than it should be in comparison to other organs since it contains more fluid than it should.

The assessment of tissue echotexture is more subjective. Most normal organs have a smooth and homogenous echotexture. Changes in echotexture result in a heterogeneous appearance to the tissue, either focally or diffusely, and often accompany a change in echogenicity. Terms to describe diffuse changes in echotexture might include *coarse, mottled,* or *nodular* while focal lesions would be described as *complex, mixed echogenicity,* or *mass*.

Table • 95-1

A List of Tissues in Order of Relative Echogenicity from Darkest (Fluid) to Brightest (Mineral, Gas)

TISSUE	ECHOGENICITY
Water/fluid	Anechoic
Renal medulla	Hypoechoic
Renal cortex	Medium echogenicity
Liver	Medium echogenicity
Spleen	High echogenicity
Prostate	Hyperechoic
Fibrous tissue, fat	Very hyperechoic
Mineral, gas	Most hyperechoic

PERFORMING THE COMPLETE ABDOMINAL ULTRASOUND EXAMINATION

Preparation

Before the ultrasound evaluation begins one must ensure that the animal is comfortable. It is recommended that the ultrasound exam be performed in a dimly lit room with as little traffic as possible. The ultrasound machine is placed adjacent to and to the left of the dog's and cat's head, and the transducer is held in the right hand. Restraint of the pet is typically accomplished by having technicians hold the animal's legs and head while performing the exam. A foam pad cut into a wedge (V-trough) is used as a comfortable positioning device to hold an animal on its back during the examination. In the event that an animal is highly stressed or aggressive or that the ultrasound examination is lengthy, chemical restraint may be indicated.

For adequate ultrasound scanning, hair needs to be clipped from the ventral abdomen to reduce artifacts and provide better visualization of abdominal organs. The hair should be clipped from the xiphoid caudally to the inguinal region with the lateral margins of the clip following the costal arch and extending roughly half way up the flank. Alcohol or a water solution should then be applied to moisten the skin, displace air associated with the hair follicles, and remove the surface layer of grease, which can be present on the skin surface. The final preparation includes applying liberal amounts of coupling gel to the abdomen. This sonographic gel should be manually worked into the shaved skin surface for optimal acoustic coupling.

Getting Started

The image orientation dot or symbol on the screen should be positioned on the left side of the image display. This dot correlates to a mark, line, dot, or light on the transducer. This indicator should be directed toward the head of the animal for the longitudinal scan plane and directed toward the animal's right side (toward the machine and sonographer) for the transverse scan plane. When performing the ultrasound scan, the transducer should not be lifted from the skin when moving to another region; instead slide the transducer along the abdomen until the next area of interest is encountered.

Region 1: The Liver

To begin the scan the transducer should be placed in a longitudinal orientation adjacent to the xiphoid process with the transducer angled craniodorsally at 60°. This position will give the sonographer a longitudinal image of the liver. Beginning the evaluation with the liver allows images of the liver to be obtained before the dog or cat has an opportunity to swallow air into the stomach. Air has the potential for blocking out some or all of the liver. Additionally, the liver resides in the deepest portion of the abdomen and is normally relatively homogenous. Machine depth, time gain compensation (TGC), and the overall gain can be set appropriately.

Once an adequate longitudinal image of the liver is obtained, the transducer should be angled back and forth from the left to the right to "interrogate" the liver. The gall bladder is best visualized by pointing the transducer toward the animal's right elbow with the transducer just to the right of the xiphoid process. For transverse scanning of the liver, the transducer is rotated counterclockwise so the indicator is toward the animals' right. As with the longitudinal plane, it is recommended to use a "fanning" motion to interrogate the liver instead of making large sliding movements with the transducer. The transducer should then be moved with a sliding motion toward the left to visualize the stomach. Complete evaluation of the stomach is usually not attainable due to the variable amounts of gas present within the gastric lumen.

Region 2: Left Pancreatic Limb, Spleen, Left Kidney

With the transducer in the longitudinal orientation the stomach is positioned to the left (cranial) of the display. The area on the caudalmost aspect of the stomach represents the greater curvature and fundic portion of the stomach and is one of the landmarks for the left pancreatic limb. Other landmarks include the splenic vein, spleen, and transverse colon. In the normal animal the pancreas is not usually visualized.

As the transducer is moved to the animal's left across the abdomen in a caudal and lateral direction, the spleen should be visible in the "near" field. The dorsal extremity of the spleen lies adjacent to the lateral surface of the gastric fundus and can extend into the far field along the left lateral body wall (dorsally). After the dorsal aspect of the spleen is assessed, the display depth can be reduced so as to allow the sonographer to evaluate the more superficial body and tail of the spleen. Either the transverse or the longitudinal plane can be used to evaluate the spleen with equal effectiveness.

The transducer should then be moved caudally in the longitudinal imaging plane along the lateral surface of the abdomen until the left kidney is visualized. Once the left kidney is located, imaging the organ in the longitudinal plane initially is usually easiest and most informative. This plane allows the sonographer to evaluate kidney size and shape along with visualization of the corticomedullary definition. The transducer can then be rotated counterclockwise to produce a transverse kidney image. The transverse plane of the kidney is the most sensitive image for detecting renal pelvic dilation.

Region 3: The Left Adrenal

The landmarks used for the left adrenal are the medial aspect of the left kidney, the left renal vessels, and the abdominal aorta. To locate the adrenal one must first locate the left kidney in a longitudinal plane and then aim medially to look for the aorta in the far field. By dropping or lowering the proximal portion of the transducer toward the table, the aorta will come into view. The normal adrenal gland lies in close proximity to the lateral wall of the aorta. The renal artery and vein are seen adjacent to the caudal surface of the adrenal and act as the most caudal landmark. When the abdominal aorta is identified in a longitudinal plane, the adrenal can be located by fanning the sound beam dorsally or ventrally. In most animals it is necessary to increase the hand pressure placed on the transducer to obtain adequate visualization of the adrenal.

Region 4: Urinary Bladder, Prostate/Uterus, Sublumbar Lymph Nodes

The transition to this region requires the transducer to be drawn down the left side of the abdomen in a caudal and medial manner. The descending colon and multiple loops of small intestine (jejunum) are seen during the transition. The urinary bladder is usually easiest to identify in the longitudinal plane; however, in some animals with a small bladder, or a large, gas-filled descending colon, the transverse plane may be the easiest. The complete evaluation of the bladder requires both the longitudinal and transverse planes to be acquired because small bladder lesions such as polyps or early tumors can be easily missed. In the male dog it is recommended to scan the bladder from both sides of the prepuce in both imaging planes for a complete evaluation. It is best to image the urethra in the longitudinal plane initially and then move to the transverse plane. Hand pressure should be increased slightly as compared to that used for the urinary bladder and the transducer should be kept as close to midline as possible. In most animals the transducer must be angled in the caudal direction 10° to 40° to obtain images dorsal to the pubis. In the intact male, the prostate is hyperechoic (see Table 95-1),

symmetrical on either side of midline, oval in shape, with the urethra in its center. The prostate in neutered males is usually quite small and hypoechoic. The remnant of the prostate can be somewhat difficult to visualize in dogs that were neutered at an early age.

The body of the uterus, unlike the uterine horns, is usually visible adjacent to the urinary bladder. The location of the uterine body is somewhat variable but usually dorsal and lateral to the bladder. It is advantageous to locate the uterine body in the transverse plane and then rotate the scanhead to image the uterus in the longitudinal plane.

The iliac (sublumbar) lymph nodes are identified deep (dorsal) to the urinary bladder where the abdominal aorta branches to become the external iliac vessels and terminal aorta. Visualization of these nodes is inconsistent in the normal animal and depends on technique and machine settings. It is easiest to find the nodes using the transverse plane because this gives the sonographer the best opportunity to visualize the aortic branches. The sublumbar lymph nodes can usually be visualized cranial to and between the vascular branches. The bifurcation of the caudal vena cava is also apparent in the caudal lumbar region on the right side of the aorta and can be identified based the ability to compress its lumen with increased transducer pressure.

Region 5: The Right Kidney, Duodenum/Right Pancreatic Limb

During the transition from the region of the bladder to the right kidney one is usually able to visualize more small intestine and the ascending colon. The small intestine lies medial to the region of the right kidney as does the ileocolic junction. The right kidney lies in a more cranial and lateral location than one would expect. In the dog, the best way to visualize the right kidney is to place the transducer medial to the 13th rib and direct the sound beam cranially and perhaps a bit laterally. In the cat the right kidney is usually easily seen and can be imaged directly from the right side without the interference of the ribs and the associated costal arch. Complete evaluation of the right kidney consists of both the longitudinal and transverse projections. Transducer pressure should be moderate for evaluation of the kidney, as the overlying small intestine needs to be displaced to limit imaging artifacts secondary to intestinal gas.

The descending duodenum and associated right pancreatic limb are in close proximity to the right kidney. Transducer pressure should be decreased from that used to image the right kidney and the depth of the display can often be decreased to increase resolution. The duodenum is located by fanning laterally from the kidney in the longitudinal plane. The right pancreatic limb is inconsistently visualized in the normal animal and lies adjacent to the medial aspect of the descending duodenum.

Region 6: The Right Adrenal

As with the left adrenal, in order to locate the right adrenal the sonographer must locate the kidney and the great vessels. Landmarks utilized in visualizing the right adrenal gland include the right kidney and the caudal vena cava. Adequate imaging of the adrenal requires the transducer to be directed in a dorsal and medial direction starting from a longitudinal view of the right kidney. This adrenal gland lies parallel to the vena cava and is often seen in the far field adjacent to the wall of the vessel.

Region 7: The Mid Abdomen

Evaluation of the mid abdomen includes the mesenteric lymph nodes and the small intestine along with the associated omentum. The technique for the mid abdomen includes variations in transducer pressure and imaging planes. One should attempt to visualize loops of the small intestine in both a transverse and longitudinal plane.

The mesenteric or jejunal lymph nodes lie in clusters associated with the mesenteric vessels in the mid abdomen. These nodes are inconsistently visualized in the normal dog but often can be seen in the cat. They are usually in close association with the cranial mesenteric artery adjacent to the body of the second lumbar vertebra. The lymph nodes can be either round or fusiform in shape and often will have the same echogenicity as the spleen. In the young animal the mesenteric nodes are sometimes easily visualized and can appear prominent.

CONCLUSION

As with radiographic interpretation, a good abdominal ultrasound examination requires a solid knowledge of anatomy and a systematic approach. A basic knowledge of physics and tissue characteristics is also useful. The assessment of organ size, shape, echogenicity, and echotexture coupled with an understanding of what causes alterations in these four factors is the basis of all ultrasound diagnoses.

CHAPTER 96

Abdominal Ultrasound: Aspirations and Biopsies

Wendy D. Fife

Use of abdominal ultrasonography has the potential ability to detect parenchymal changes within organs and to define both origin and extent of lesions. Abnormalities detected with ultrasonography are often nonspecific, with a great deal of overlap in the appearance of various disease processes. Ultrasound-guided fine needle aspirates or tissue-core biopsies are therefore often required for cytology or histology to aid in reaching a definitive diagnosis. The use of ultrasound guidance when obtaining samples allows for real-time monitoring of needle placement so that a selected portion of an organ or a focal mass lesion may be sampled. Ultrasonography allows for the assessment of nearby vessels or other structures to be avoided and can be used to reassess the dog or cat after a biopsy procedure for evidence of complications, such as hemorrhage. Ultrasonography and ultrasound-guided biopsies are relatively noninvasive and rarely require general anesthesia.

INDICATIONS

Percutaneous ultrasound guidance may be used to obtain samples or to provide therapeutic intervention. Fine needle, large-gauge–needle, or tissue-core biopsies are chosen based on the size and type of lesion to be sampled. Biopsy samples of a specific organ may be warranted in cases of diffuse parenchymal abnormalities, focal loss of parenchymal homogeneity, or mass lesions, or in the case of a normal ultrasonographic appearance of an organ when the results of other diagnostics indicate organ dysfunction. Therapeutic uses of ultrasonography include the drainage of intraabdominal or intrathoracic cysts, abscesses, or fluid, or to instill local chemotherapeutics or other chemical therapy.

MATERIALS

Sector or linear-array transducers may be used, depending on the depth of the structure to be biopsied. Linear-array transducers provide superior resolution for more superficial structures, whereas sector transducers are used to biopsy deeper tissues. The lesion to be biopsied should be placed within the focal zone of the transducer to allow for the best resolution. Some transducers are equipped with biopsy guides, and separate guides are available for attachment to conventional transducers. The guides function to keep the needle in the plane of the ultrasound beam (Figure 96-1).

Dedicated biopsy transducers and those equipped with biopsy guides often display electronic markers on the display screen. The lesion or tissue to be biopsied can then be placed between the markers and a needle inserted with its position continuously monitored. Dedicated biopsy transducers are more expensive and specialized than conventional transducers or transducer biopsy guides and are rarely used in veterinary medicine.

The size and type of needle to be used depends on the size of the lesion being sampled and the type of sample desired. The smallest needle that will provide a diagnostic sample should be used because larger needles may be associated with higher complication rates, such as hemorrhage. Fine needle samples most commonly yield samples for cytology, whereas histologic evaluation requires a tissue-core biopsy. Fine needle samples are commonly obtained when the organ being sampled has a diffusely abnormal appearance, when a small lesion (<1 cm) is being sampled, or when the tissue being sampled is relatively vascular. Tissue-core biopsies may be preferred in the case of a large mass or when histology is necessary. In many cases, a fine needle aspiration may be obtained first and a tissue-core biopsy pursued if the sample is inconclusive or nondiagnostic.

For fine needle aspiration, 20- to 25-gauge needles are typically used. In the case of the freehand technique, standard injection needles are used. A longer needle (e.g., 3½ inch) is required if a transducer guide is used. This needle length is necessary to pass it through the biopsy guide and into the target tissue. In the case of a tissue-core biopsy, a 14- to 18-gauge needle is usually recommended. Manual and automated biopsy devices are available. A manually operated Tru-Cut needle requires two hands to operate, so two people are required for the procedure: one to place the transducer and another to operate the biopsy device. The operator is able to control the depth of the needle and the length of tissue to be sampled. Several types of semiautomatic and automatic biopsy devices have been developed. The inner cutting needle is manually advanced to the desired depth with a semiautomatic device. The outer cutting shaft, which is spring loaded, is then triggered. The exact depth of tissue biopsied is manually controlled. The inner cutting needle and outer shaft of an automatic device are initially advanced manually, 1.5 to 2.0 cm superficial to the tissue to be biopsied. Automatic biopsy guns automatically advance the cutting needle and external shaft when triggered. Caution is advised when using an automatic biopsy gun; the inner cutting shaft advances a specific distance (15 to 20 mm) beyond the external shaft to acquire the tissue sample when it is triggered. Most automatic biopsy guns accept disposable needles of varying sizes, and the distance the cutting shaft will advance can be adjusted to control the length of tissue sampled. This is particularly useful in cats and in the case of small lesions. This gun is reusable and can be sterilized. Individual disposable spring-loaded automatic and semiautomatic biopsy needles are available in various sizes.

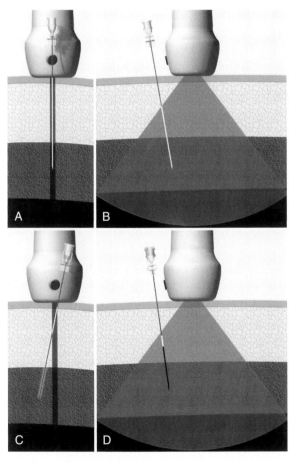

Figure 96-1 The angle of the biopsy instrument relative to the plane of the ultrasound beam is essential to visualize the tissue being sampled with the freehand method. **A** and **B,** Proper alignment of the biopsy instrument and ultrasound beam, with the two remaining parallel the entire length of the needle. **C** and **D,** Improper alignment of the needle relative to the ultrasound beam. Only a small segment of the length of the needle can be seen as it intersects the plane of the beam. The tip of the needle and therefore the tissue being sampled cannot be seen. The white portion of the needle represents that which transects the path of the scanning plane and is therefore visualized.

TECHNIQUE

Needles should never enter more than one organ or pass completely through an organ. A separate needle should be used for each organ sampled. Multiple samples of an organ or lesion are usually obtained. The freehand technique can be used, in which case the transducer is operated with one hand and the needle with the other (Figure 96-2). This allows for greater flexibility in the approach to the structure of interest but requires hand-eye coordination and practice. The entire length of the needle must be kept within the ultrasound beam, and the tip must be visualized (Web Figure 96-1).

Moving the needle gently up and down while fanning the region with the ultrasound probe may aid in locating the needle tip. Under no circumstances should the location of a needle be determined by moving the needle side to side within an organ. This causes unnecessary tissue trauma. Roughening the outer needle shaft prior to introduction will create an irregular interface to increase sound reflection and sonographic visualization. Commercially available Teflon or other highly reflective coated needles are available to enhance visualization. Use of larger-gauge needles usually facilitates visualization but may also increase risk of complications. The needle tip should be placed at the focal zone of the transducer to enhance resolution. Injection of a small amount of air or sterile saline may help localize the needle tip. After needle placement, and stylet removal in the case of a spinal needle, a syringe or extension tubing with syringe are attached to the needle. If the lesion is fluid filled, that fluid should be aspirated. If large amounts of fluid are to be aspirated, a three-way stopcock is attached. For cytologic samples, aspiration is performed as the needle is moved slightly up and down within the tissue or lesion. Some individuals prefer to simply move the needle up and down within the tissue, without aspiration, to obtain a cytologic sample. This technique may provide less blood contamination within the sample and has been shown to yield diagnostic results. When using a spinal needle to obtain a sample, the stylet may be left in place as the needle is advanced. Once the needle is placed at the desired depth, the stylet is removed and the sample is acquired. This may be particularly useful in the case of traversing fat within the falciform ligament to obtain a liver aspirate in the cat. Without a stylet, the sample may consist of fat only, which may be improperly interpreted as hepatic lipidosis.

Use of a needle guide requires less dexterity, but once the needle enters the skin, the probe cannot be moved. Transducer guides also cause the angle of the needle relative to the ultrasound beam to be fixed, thereby limiting the angle at which the surface of the dog or cat can be approached and prohibiting biopsy of superficial structures.

Patient Preparation

The patient is usually placed in dorsal recumbency on a padded trough. An intravenous catheter is placed in the case of a tissue-core biopsy so that intravenous sedatives can be administered. In the case of a very small lesion or a lesion in close proximity to large vascular structures, general anesthesia may be required. The use of some drugs should be avoided, including those that cause splenic enlargement or panting.

Depending on the tissue being sampled, the patient's clinical status, and the type of biopsy being performed, screening of the dog or cat's coagulation status is recommended. For fine needle aspirations, coagulation screening profiles are not routinely performed unless the lesion to be sampled is extremely vascular or the pet is at an increased risk of bleeding.

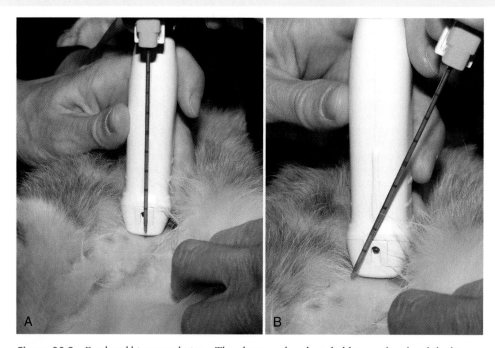

Figure 96-2 Freehand biopsy technique. The ultrasound probe is held in one hand and the biopsy instrument in the other hand. The biopsy instrument must be maintained within the plane of the ultrasound beam. **A,** Proper alignment of biopsy instrument relative to ultrasound beam. **B,** Improper alignment, with the biopsy instrument angled relative to the ultrasound beam. This will not allow proper visualization of the biopsy instrument within the scan plane.

Specific Biopsy Sites

Fine needle aspiration and tissue-core biopsies of the liver are commonly done. Fine needle aspiration is performed when sampling focal masses that are complex or highly vascular, whereas a tissue-core biopsy is preferred in the case of a focal solid-appearing mass. In cases of diffuse hepatic disease, a fine needle aspirate may yield a diagnosis in cases of specific diseases, such as lymphoma or hepatic lipidosis. Other diffuse hepatic diseases require a tissue-core biopsy for a definitive diagnosis. The left-lateral aspect of the liver is generally the safest area to sample because it is the largest and the gallbladder and hilar vessels can be avoided. If a focal lesion is in a different location, or if the liver is small, sampling of another portion of the liver may be warranted. If the liver is small or located cranially, an intercostal approach is sometimes used, being cautious to avoid lung tissue. General anesthesia and positive pressure ventilation may also be used to displace the liver caudally for easier access. Multiple biopsies are routinely obtained.

The gallbladder may be sampled in cases of acalculous cholecystitis for culture and cytology. A transhepatic approach and a 22-gauge needle are used. The transhepatic approach is reported to decrease the risk of bile leakage.

Diffuse infiltrative splenic diseases, such as lymphoma and mast cell disease, and focal splenic masses are common indications for aspiration. Needle biopsy without aspiration may decrease the potential for blood contamination in splenic samples. If the aspiration technique is used, aspiration should be discontinued if blood appears in the hub of the needle. Complications due to splenic aspirates are extremely rare, but caution should be used when sampling complex, cavitary masses, such as those seen in splenic hemangiosarcoma. If fine needle samples of the spleen are nondiagnostic, a tissue-core biopsy of a solid mass lesion or the solid portion of a complex lesion may be indicated.

Renal biopsy may be performed in cases of diffuse renal disease or focal renal masses. Fine needle aspirates are usually performed if diffuse disease such as lymphosarcoma is suspected, whereas tissue-core biopsies are required to diagnose glomerular and tubular diseases and renal mass lesions. Sampling of the left kidney is preferred in cases of diffuse bilateral renal disease due to its relatively caudal location and easier access. The caudal cortex of the kidney should be sampled (including glomeruli but avoiding the medulla and hilar vessels). The biopsy plane should be directed laterally to avoid puncturing the renal hilus, caudal vena cava, or aorta. Feline renal biopsies are commonly done by manually stabilizing the kidney close to the ventral or lateral skin surface while performing a core biopsy of the lateral cortex with or without direct ultrasound guidance. Complications are rare and in most cases self-limiting but may include intraabdominal hemorrhage or hemorrhage manifested as hematuria. Small dogs and cats may have an increased risk of hemorrhage and cats with hypertension are at particular risk. The animal's packed cell volume (PCV) should be monitored for several hours after the procedure. Renal biopsies should not be performed indiscriminately because fatal hemorrhage can occur.

Urinary bladder masses are commonly identified ultrasonographically. They are usually readily accessible for aspiration with a 21- or 22-gauge needle. In cases of transitional cell carcinoma, percutaneous biopsy often yields a diagnostic sample, but seeding of the tumor into the abdomen and subcutaneous tissues can occur. Ultrasound-guided urinary catheter placement and vigorous suction is a viable diagnostic alternative and avoids the potential for seeding of tumor cells.

Percutaneous biopsy of the prostate may be indicated when parenchymal abnormalities or prostatomegaly are identified. Fine needle aspiration of fluid-filled cysts or cavities within the prostate may be obtained for culture and cytology.

These lesions may occur in association with prostatitis or neoplasia. If prostatic neoplasia is suspected, a fine needle aspirate may provide a diagnosis; a tissue-core sample can be obtained if a larger sample is necessary. The biopsy is obtained from the caudal abdomen, lateral to the prepuce. Adjacent vascular structures, such as the aorta and caudal vena cava, should be avoided. If the prostate is small or caudally located, the pubic bone may interfere.

The pancreas may be aspirated to differentiate between pancreatitis and pancreatic neoplasia. Secondary pancreatitis is an uncommon complication. Infection may develop in conjunction with pancreatic neoplasia, so false-negative diagnoses may occur.

Other abdominal structures that may be aspirated or biopsied include enlarged intraabdominal lymph nodes and gastrointestinal (GI) masses. Aspiration of adrenal masses has been reported in veterinary medicine but is uncommonly performed; blood pressure alterations and severe hemorrhage may occur in the case of pheochromocytoma. Close proximity to the caudal vena cava and aorta are additional risks.

Ultrasound-guided percutaneous drainage of intraabdominal abscesses may be performed as an alternative to surgical treatment. With the patient under sedation, the abscess cavity is drained using a 20-gauge or larger needle. Samples are submitted for culture and cytology. Drainage may be followed by alcoholization with the injection of ethanol. Follow-up ultrasound examinations, possibly in conjunction with repeated abscess drainage, can be done. The procedure may reduce morbidity and mortality associated with abdominal abscesses treated surgically.

CONTRAINDICATIONS AND COMPLICATIONS

Complications related to ultrasound-guided biopsy procedures are uncommon. The risk of complication varies based upon the size of the needle being used and the location of the lesion. A 22- to 25-gauge needle should be used when possible, and larger gauge and tissue-core biopsies pursued if samples are nondiagnostic. Hemorrhage is minor and self-limiting in most instances. The results of physical examination and laboratory testing when necessary will identify patients at increased risk for hemorrhage. Color Doppler imaging is recommended when available to assess the vascularity of tissues and adjacent structures before the biopsy is performed and to monitor for hemorrhage in the postbiopsy period (Web Figure 96-2).

The risk of peritonitis associated with penetration of the bowel is small in cases of fine needle aspiration, but bowel should be avoided with larger-gauge needles and tissue-core biopsies. Seeding of a tumor along a needle tract is also rare but has been reported in cases of transitional cell carcinoma in the canine urinary bladder. As with any procedure, adequate restraint and sedation are necessary to minimize risk to the patient.

CHAPTER 97

Abdominocentesis and Diagnostic Peritoneal Lavage

Elke Rudloff

PATIENT PREPARATION

There should be no gross evidence of an intraabdominal mass and the urinary bladder must be empty before the procedure. If the animal is unable to void voluntarily, careful manual expression or urinary catheterization should be performed.

SURGICAL SCRUB REQUIRED

The ventral abdominal skin from the xyphoid to pubis region should be clipped free of hair and surgically prepared.

CONSCIOUS SEDATION

The clinician should use intravenous butorphanol 0.4 mg/kg or hydromorphone 0.2 mg/kg and diazepam or midazolam 0.2 mg/kg; this is more important for diagnostic peritoneal lavage (DPL) than for centesis.

LOCAL ANESTHESIA REQUIRED

Up to 4 mg/kg of lidocaine should be used in the region where the needle or catheter is to be placed, infused to the level of the peritoneum.

ABDOMINOCENTESIS

If a blind abdominocentesis is to be performed, the animal can be standing or in lateral recumbency. Ultrasound-guided centesis of any fluid pocket is the preferred method for fluid collection and is performed in lateral or dorsal recumbency. If ultrasound is unavailable, a four-quadrant tap can be performed. In each of the four abdominal quadrants, an 18- to 22-gauge 1-inch needle or over-the-needle catheter should be percutaneously inserted. Sample yield is maximized if fluid is allowed to flow out of the needle under the influence of gravity and not aspirated. A negative tap does not rule out the presence of intraabdominal pathology.

 To view a video on this topic, go to **www.expertconsult.com.**

DIAGNOSTIC PERITONEAL LAVAGE

If a DPL is to be performed, the animal should be placed in left-lateral recumbency or in a ventrodorsal position to avoid traumatizing the spleen.

CATHETER PLACEMENT FOR DPL

The entry site is at, or a few centimeters caudal to, the umbilicus, and on the midline, or a few centimeters lateral to the midline. When using an over-the-needle catheter (Figure 97-1), the clinician should make a small skin incision at the site of the skin block and insert the catheter just through the body wall.

There will be a slight pop as the peritoneum is penetrated. The catheter should then be rotated and advanced over the needle until it is fully inserted. If the catheter does not advance easily, it may still be in the subcutaneous tissue or against an organ and should be repositioned.

Peritoneal lavage catheters (Figure 97-2) are usually placed using a Seldinger technique, with instructions contained in the kit.

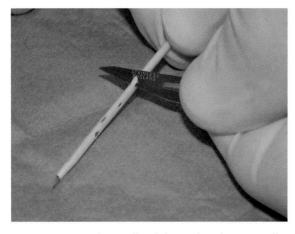

Figure 97-1 Over-the-needle abdominal catheter. Small side holes (two to four) are carefully cut into a 14- to 18-gauge 2-inch catheter 2 mm apart with a scalpel blade. The edges of the holes are kept smooth to prevent the catheter from barbing and possibly breaking.

The kits contain all the materials necessary (except for the fluid to be infused), including local anesthetic, drapes, and disinfectants.

When placing a catheter, the following points should be kept in mind:

- If fluid freely drains from the catheter, samples should be collected.
- If no fluid drains, the clinician should infuse 20 mL/kg of warmed isotonic replacement crystalloid (e.g., 0.9% sodium chloride, Ringer's lactate solution) and clamp the infusion set. Then the animal should be gently rolled back and forth (to thoroughly bath the abdominal organs) and turned on its side. The infusion set should then be opened, and the first few milliliters allowed to drain out of the catheter before collecting samples.
- If an abdominal bleed is suspected, the catheter can be sutured in place to permit evaluation of followup samples. If septic peritonitis is suspected, the catheter can be left in place until surgical intervention to permit periodic lavage to dilute and drain septic material. If an aseptic peritonitis or pancreatitis is suspected, the catheter can be left in place to permit periodic lavages to dilute and drain inflammatory mediators.
- Complete removal of the infused fluid is not always possible or necessary; it may be used to partially replace calculated fluid deficits when peritonitis is not present.
- If the catheter is to be removed, the skin is pinched around the catheter while it is removed and a temporary dressing is placed on the area.
- Cytology: The presence of vegetable or meat fibers, intracellular bacteria, or toxic neutrophils is an indication for surgical exploration and culture submission.
- Special laboratory tests required: The packed cell volume (PCV) of the undiluted abdominal fluid can be compared with the peripheral PCV and serially monitored if abdominal hemorrhage is suspected. A white blood cell (WBC) count greater than $1000/mm^3$ is diagnostic for peritonitis. If chemical analysis reveals that the creatinine or potassium level (or both) in the abdominal fluid is higher than in the peripheral blood, a urinary tract rupture is suspected. If the total bilirubin of the fluid is greater than that of peripheral blood, a leaking biliary system is suspected. In the dog, if the glucose of undiluted abdominal fluid is 20 mg/dL or less than the plasma glucose, and/or if peritoneal fluid lactate is >2.5 mmol/L, and/or a blood–to–peritoneal fluid lactate difference is <–2.0 mmol/L, then septic peritonitis is suspected.

Figure 97-2 Manufactured abdominal drains. *Top,* Abdominal drainage catheter. *Bottom,* Peritoneal lavage catheter (Teleflex, Reading, Pa.).

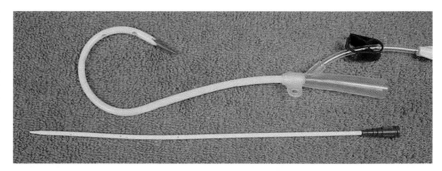

CHAPTER 98

Laparoscopy

Keith Richter

The use of laparoscopy for diagnostic and therapeutic purposes has increased tremendously in human and veterinary medicine during the last 10 years. This acceptance of laparoscopy stems from technologic advances in equipment, improved access and training, and superior results for many procedures achieved with this noninvasive modality. Though many procedures performed in human beings will have little applicability in veterinary medicine, many of the procedures will gain acceptance due to their ease, effectiveness, and lack of morbidity. Advantages of laparoscopy over open surgery include less postoperative pain, a lower infection rate, improved visualization in many cases, and a shorter hospitalization time. Laparoscopy also has some advantages over other minimally invasive procedures, such as ultrasound and ultrasound-guided biopsy.

EQUIPMENT

Light is transmitted from a remote light source via a fiberoptic light cable to the rigid fiberoptic laparoscope (telescope). Size and viewing angles of laparoscopes vary. A forward-viewing (0°), 5.0-mm outer diameter, 35-cm long scope is preferred for most dogs and cats. Since most laparoscopic instruments are also 5-mm, this provides more versatility by allowing the scope and instruments to be interchangeable with the same cannula. Smaller scopes have a smaller image with less field of view. In addition, a greater light intensity is needed for smaller scopes. Scopes up to 10-mm diameter can also be used. Though these have slightly better image quality and allow more light than 5-mm diameter scopes; the difference is small and they only provide an advantage in very large dogs. Scopes are available in various degrees of angulation of view, including 0° (direct forward viewing) up to 70°. The 0° angle is easier to use and generally preferred for most procedures. A 30°-angle scope can be used to view structures to the side of the tip, and through rotation, to expand the field of view. Angled scopes are more difficult for inexperienced operators with regards to spatial orientation. Most scopes have no biopsy channel. Operating scopes have a 5- or 6-mm channel, with an eyepiece extending from the proximal end. These scopes allow introduction of instruments through the same puncture as the scope. The disadvantage of operating scopes is the limited ability to manipulate instruments passing through the channel. Usually the accessory or secondary puncture technique is preferred (see below).

Video capabilities can be achieved with a handheld charged coupling device (CCD) video camera mounted on the eyepiece. These cameras have high resolution, magnify images 5 to 15 times, and provide a clear image. The use of video is essential for operative laparoscopy. A bright light source (usually 150 to 300 watts) is required to adequately illuminate the abdomen.

To visualize abdominal structures, a pneumoperitoneum must be created to lift the abdominal wall away from the viscera. This is accomplished by insufflating gas through tubing attached to a Veress needle. The latter has a spring-loaded blunt inner portion and an outer cannula with a sharp point. The sharp point is used to penetrate the abdominal wall; then the inner blunt portion is protruded past the sharp point and left in that position to avoid traumatizing abdominal viscera. Gas can then be continually insufflated as needed throughout the procedure. Carbon dioxide is recommended because it has the advantage of being rapidly absorbed, and thus the risk for air embolism is minimized. The latter is a reported complication of laparoscopy using room air (the gas absorbed most slowly). The disadvantage of CO_2 is that it is slightly more irritating to the peritoneal surface and therefore requires a slightly higher plane of anesthesia. Gas is infused with an automatic insufflator. These devices regulate flow rate and intraabdominal pressure. Initial infusion of gas should be slow (1 L/min) to allow gradual accommodation to the increased intraabdominal pressure. Once optimal insufflation pressure is reached, a higher flow rate can be used to maintain the desired pressure. Ideally, intraabdominal pressure should not exceed 10 mm Hg (cats and small dogs) to 15 mm Hg (large dogs). Excessive pressure decreases venous return to the heart and causes decreased ability to ventilate.

The laparoscope is introduced into the abdomen with the use of a trocar/cannula assembly. The cannula is a metal or hard plastic sleeve with a one-way valve that permits passage of instruments (such as the trocar, laparoscope, and accessory instruments) and prevents the escape of gas. The trocar is a sharp-pointed stylet that is used to penetrate the abdominal wall. It is then removed, leaving the cannula in place so that the laparoscope can then be introduced. Accessory puncture sites are made for introduction of additional trocar/cannula assemblies. This allows the introduction of blunt metal probes, suction tips, cautery instruments, grasping forceps, "spoon," or "clamshell" style (oval cup) biopsy forceps, and a wide variety of surgical instruments. These instruments are elongated, narrower versions of standard surgical instruments. The use of stapling equipment has enabled surgeons to perform procedures such as vessel ligation and bowel resection.

INDICATIONS FOR LAPAROSCOPY

Common indications for laparoscopy are for hepatobiliary evaluation. Laparoscopy allows procurement of large specimens (similar in size to surgical biopsies) using a 5-mm "spoon" or "clamshell" forceps. This has been shown to obtain tissue with a superior diagnostic yield compared to needle biopsies, with the latter having only an approximate 50% concordance with histologic findings from surgical biopsies.[1] Furthermore, the ability to visualize the liver gives the

 To view a video on this topic, go to **www.expertconsult.com.**

clinician a better feel for pathologic processes. Laparoscopy can be also used to examine and biopsy the pancreas, an organ that can be difficult to image with radiographs and ultrasound. Other organs that can be biopsied via laparoscopy include the kidney, spleen, prostate, intestine, mesentery, omentum, and the parietal peritoneum. Laparoscopy can be used to diagnose and stage abdominal tumors through direct visual assessment and allowing directed biopsies. Laparoscopy can detect lesions less than 1 mm in diameter on the surface of organs. It can guide aspiration of the gallbladder, loculated ascites, and abdominal cysts or abscesses. Laparoscopy can guide transabdominal intrauterine artificial insemination. Laparoscopy can also be used in evaluation of abdominal trauma. Such injuries as hepatic and splenic laceration, diaphragmatic hernia, bladder rupture, renal rupture, and abdominal hernia can be assessed. There are also a variety of surgical procedures than can be accomplished laparoscopically.

TECHNIQUE

It is preferred to perform laparoscopy with the animal under general anesthesia. The position of the dog or cat and location of the various puncture sites will depend on the procedure, size of patient, and organ being examined. Because the liver is the most common organ examined and biopsied, this procedure will be described in detail.

LAPAROSCOPY-GUIDED LIVER BIOPSY

The main advantage of laparoscopy-guided biopsy is the ability to obtain large biopsy samples and to visualize the liver, biliary tree, and other abdominal organs. With experience, the gallbladder can be examined, palpated with a blunt probe, and the bile duct traced to its entry into the duodenum. In this manner it can be determined whether a common bile duct or cystic duct obstruction exists. In addition, because focal lesions of the liver can be directly visualized, an appropriate biopsy site can be selected while avoiding other intrahepatic structures (gallbladder and portal vessels). Hemorrhage can be observed and, when excessive, controlled with direct compression with a blunt probe over the biopsy site. Alternatively, electrocautery or application of a hemostatic material (Gel-Foam) can be used to control hemorrhage. Compared with laparotomy, much less anesthetic time exists. A complete laparoscopic examination can be completed and multiple hepatic biopsies obtained in 10 to 15 minutes. Because only a 0.5- to 1.0-cm incision is made, less risk exists for wound dehiscence and infection.

The animal is placed in left dorsal oblique recumbency at a 45° angle. This position allows visualization of both sides of the liver, gallbladder, bile duct, pancreas, duodenum, and much of the abdominal viscera, and avoids the falciform ligament (which may be encountered with a midline approach). The puncture sites should be surgically prepared and draped. The Veress needle (for insufflation) is inserted through a small stab incision (using a No. 11 blade) on the midline just to the right of the umbilicus. Prior to insufflation, the Veress needle is aspirated to confirm that no viscus has been entered. Saline (6 to 8 mL) is then infused to ensure free flow into the abdominal cavity. The abdomen is then insufflated with gas to an appropriate pressure as determined by a pressure gauge on an automatic insufflator (see above) or when the abdominal wall is tympanic to the touch. Overdistention should be avoided so as not to decrease venous return or cause impairment in ventilation. Once the desired degree of pneumoperi-

toneum is reached, a 0.5- to 1.0-cm skin incision is made on the right lateral abdomen between the last rib and the flank. The incision is adjusted in a cranial direction for larger animals, in a caudal direction for smaller animals, and should take into account the size of the liver. The trocar and cannula assembly is then "popped" into the abdominal cavity with a twisting motion. Extending the forefinger down the shaft of the cannula or grasping the cannula ~3 cm from the tip with the free hand will prevent inadvertent insertion of the assembly too far into the abdomen. The trocar is removed and laparoscope inserted into the abdominal cavity through the cannula. The remote light source is connected to the laparoscope with a fiberoptic cable and the liver examined. If a video camera is available, this should be placed on the eyepiece of the laparoscope. The insufflation line is then switched from the Veress needle to this cannula. The Veress needle is removed, its incision extended to 0.5 cm, and a second cannula is introduced under direct visualization. This allows introduction of a blunt probe, which can be used to palpate the liver and gallbladder. The probe should also be used to lift up each lobe of the liver to examine the dorsal surface and to get the omentum out of the way so the bile duct can be traced to its entry into the duodenum. The right limb of the pancreas should also be examined.

Once the abdomen has been examined, a suitable place on the liver is selected for a biopsy site. The author prefers using a laparoscopic "spoon" or "clamshell" type of biopsy instrument. This can be placed through the same accessory cannula as the blunt probe, thus avoiding an additional puncture site. This type of instrument results in less hemorrhage than biopsy needles and obtains much larger specimens. Repeated twisting of the shaft or retracting the closed jaws into the advanced cannula will prevent ripping of liver tissue and result in less bleeding. The number of biopsies obtained depends on the risk of bleeding and the anticipated need of adequate tissue. Multiple samples from various areas of the liver are recommended (observing for hemorrhage after each sample). If excessive bleeding occurs, the blunt metal probe is used to put direct compression over the biopsy site. Suction can also be applied to clear the field if bleeding cannot be adequately assessed. If bleeding is not controlled, an electrocautery probe can be used to stop the bleeding. Alternatively, laparoscopic forceps can be used to place a piece of a hemostatic material (Gel-Foam) on the bleeding biopsy site. Once the biopsy samples are obtained, the clinician completes the procedure by removing all instruments, evacuating all the gas through opened cannula valves, and suturing the puncture sites. More detailed descriptions of laparoscopic techniques have been previously described.[2,3]

Potential complications of the procedure include those related to a general anesthetic, excessive bleeding, inadvertent organ damage during instrument introduction, overdistention of the abdomen with gas, air embolism, and a tension pneumothorax if the diaphragm is inadvertently punctured (as abdominal gas enters the thoracic cavity). Meticulous attention to details of technique together with experience will minimize the probability of these complications. Postoperative pain should be anticipated, and this should be addressed with appropriate analgesics.

LAPAROSCOPIC SURGERY

Many laparoscopic surgical procedures are currently being performed on dogs and cats. These include ovariectomy and hysterectomy, adrenalectomy, bile duct exploration, gastropexy, cystotomy with calculus removal, crypt orchid removal, jejunostomy tube placement, splenoportography, cholecystectomy, and others. Limitations of laparoscopic surgery include the two-dimensional image, restricted freedom of movement of the instruments, restricted sense of touch, limited opportunity to move the position of instruments once cannulae have been placed, and the need for extensive training. Controlled studies are necessary to substantiate the role of all laparoscopic procedures in veterinary medicine. As clinicians and equipment manufacturers address technical limitations, many surgical procedures performed within a body cavity should be amenable to laparoscopic surgery.

REFERENCES

The reference list can be found on the companion Expert Consult Web site at *www.expertconsult.com.*

GENERAL CENTESIS AND BIOPSY

CHAPTER 99

Techniques for Bone Marrow Aspiration and Biopsy

Leo J. "Ty" McSherry

Peripheral blood abnormalities are the most common indications for the evaluation of bone marrow. These include poorly or nonregenerative anemia, persistent or unexplained neutropenia, unexplained thrombocytopenia, or any combination of peripheral cytopenias. A persistent leukocytosis or thrombocytosis, dysplastic changes, or the inappropriate presence of immature hematopoietic cells in the peripheral circulation are additional indications for bone marrow evaluation. Bone marrow can be used to stage neoplasia, evaluate lytic bone lesions, or determine the cause of unexplained hypercalcemia or hyperproteinemia, especially hyperglobulinemia, as may relate to lymphoma, multiple myeloma, or some systemic infections. Less commonly, bone marrow can be evaluated to help determine the cause of fever of unknown origin or evaluate total body iron stores.

Contraindications to bone marrow aspiration or biopsy are few and are generally related to the use of sedation or restraint. Hemorrhage is an uncommon complication, even in severely thrombocytopenic animals, and severe or unexplained thrombocytopenia is a common indication for marrow evaluation. Peripheral neutropenia is also a common indication for marrow evaluation; however, infection is unlikely because the aspirate and/or biopsy is performed as a sterile procedure. The potential complications associated with hemorrhage or infection are minimal and should not dissuade the clinician from evaluating the marrow if indications to do so are present.

With the possible exception of a Petri dish or watch glass, most hospitals will have the necessary materials for bone marrow aspiration and biopsy. These include aspiration or biopsy needle, sedation or anesthesia, microscope slides, anticoagulant, scalpel blade (No. 11, No. 13), Petri dish or watch glass, 12-mL syringe, hematocrit capillary tubes, 2% lidocaine, and surgical scrub.

BONE MARROW ASPIRATION

Three types of aspiration needles are available: (1) the Illinois sternal, (2) the Jamshidi, and (3) the Rosenthal.

These are available in 15- and 18-gauge sizes, 1 to ½ inches in length. The 18-gauge needles are typically used in cats and small dogs, whereas the 15-gauge needles are reserved for dogs greater than 20 pounds. The Illinois sternal needles have a removable plastic cap (designed to hold the stylet in place during placement of the needle) and a removable needle guard. However, the plastic cap and needle guard necessitate the use of gas sterilization. The Jamshidi needles are stainless steel, durable, and may be heat sterilized; however, they lack a removable cover or needle guard.

The use of adequate sedation or general anesthesia will greatly facilitate the collection of bone marrow. Many authors describe collection with nothing more than a local anesthetic, and this may be all that is necessary or permissible in stoic animals or those at a high risk of anesthetic complications. Aspiration is a painful procedure, however, and a struggling or anxious animal will likely interfere with collection of an adequate sample. Sedation or anesthesia is suggested.

The use of an anticoagulant, although not necessary, is recommended and allows for the preparation of high-quality slides. It also allows time to complete the procedure before slides need to be prepared. Anticoagulant can be prepared by injecting 0.35 mL of sterile saline into a 3-mL lavender-top tube containing EDTA, withdrawing the solution, and then reinjecting it into a second EDTA tube. This should yield approximately 0.5 mL of a 2.5% EDTA solution. Alternatively, an aqueous solution of EDTA (Sequester-Sol) is available in 35 mL or 1.25 fl oz bottles from many medical supply companies. This is a practical and recommended alternative for hospitals that regularly perform bone marrow aspiration. A volume of 0.3 to 0.5 mL is recommended per collection.

Three sites are commonly used for the collection of bone marrow: (1) the proximal humerus, (2) the iliac crest, and (3) the trochanteric fossa. The proximal humerus is an easily accessible site in dogs and cats of all sizes. It has little overlying tissue and provides a fairly large area for placement of the needle. Its disadvantages include its proximity to the head and the thick, rounded cortex. The greater tubercle is easily palpated, and the needle is inserted into the flat area of the craniolateral aspect of the humerus distal to the greater tubercle. The needle is inserted perpendicular to the long axis of the humerus (Figure 99-1).

The iliac crest is easily accessible in thin dogs or those in good body condition, as well as in large cats. It should be avoided in large or obese animals because it may be difficult to palpate or to seat the needle due to a large amount of overlying tissue. The iliac crest is the widest and most dorsal aspect of the wing of the ilium.

The trochanteric fossa may be used in cats or small dogs. The trochanteric fossa is medial to the greater trochanter. The greater trochanter is palpated, and the needle inserted medial to it (into the trochanteric fossa). The needle is inserted parallel to the long axis of the femur (Figure 99-2). The trochanteric fossa is generally avoided in well-muscled or obese animals due to a significant amount of overlying tissue.

After sedation the animal is placed in lateral recumbency for collection from the proximal humerus, or it can be placed in either lateral or sternal recumbency for collection from the iliac crest. In nonsedated animals, lidocaine is used to block the surgically prepared site, beginning with the periosteum. The needle is then slowly withdrawn while blocking the overlying tissues and finally the skin. The sterile aspiration needle, scalpel blade, and 12-mL syringe are placed on the sterile glove field. Sterile gloves are worn, and 0.3 to 0.5 mL of anticoagulant is drawn into the 12-mL syringe, which is then placed again on the sterile field. A small stab incision is made in the skin. The incision only need be wide enough for the aspiration needle.

The site of collection can be localized using one hand. The aspiration needle should be firmly seated in the palm of the hand and the needle held securely between the thumb and index finger. The plastic needle guard on the Illinois sternal needle has a small lip on which the thumb and index finger can be placed to grip the needle securely and to apply firm pressure. A tendency exists to hold the needle as if it were a pen. This should be avoided because it does not allow sufficient pressure to be applied to advance the needle through the cortex. In addition, if using the Jamshidi aspiration needle, pressure should be applied to the top of the stylet to prevent it from being dislodged while placing the needle. This is accomplished by holding it firmly in the palm of the hand.

The aspiration needle is placed through the stab incision down to the periosteum. With the needle seated on the bone, firm clockwise-counterclockwise rotational pressure is applied to advance the needle. Frequently a slight decrease in resistance occurs when the needle enters the marrow cavity. When approaching the proximal humerus in cats, the needle may suddenly "pop" into the marrow cavity. When the needle has been properly positioned, it should feel very firmly seated, as might a nail in a block of wood. During advancement, the needle may occasionally and suddenly slide off the cortex into the surrounding soft tissue. This is especially common when approaching the proximal humerus and to a lesser degree the iliac crest. The needle will be freely movable in the subcutaneous tissues and not be firmly seated. Should this occur, the clinician should simply withdraw the needle to the level of the cortex, again seat the needle, and begin rotational pressure. When approaching the iliac crest, it is useful to have an assistant place counterpressure against the distal femur at the level of the stifle.

Once the needle is seated, the clinician should remove the top (if using an Illinois sternal needle) and stylet and place them on the sterile field. Next, the 12-mL syringe should be attached. While holding both the aspiration needle and syringe

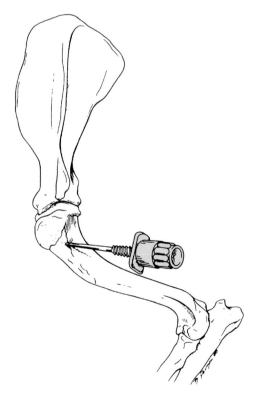

Figure 99-1 The needle is inserted perpendicular to the long axis of the humerus. (From Grindem CB: Bone marrow biopsy and evaluation. Vet Clin North Am Small Anim Pract 19:669, 1989.)

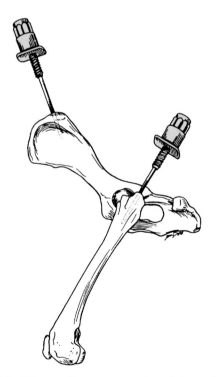

Figure 99-2 The needles are inserted medial to the greater trochanter and parallel to the long axis of the femur. (From Grindem CB: Bone marrow biopsy and evaluation. Vet Clin North Am Small Anim Pract 19:669, 1989.)

with one hand, the clinician should make several firm aspirations by rapidly pulling the plunger back. Marrow can appear after the first attempt at aspiration; however, several attempts could be necessary before marrow appears in the syringe. A total volume of 1 or 2 mL is collected if possible. If anticoagulant has been used, the syringe is removed from the needle and gently rocked to mix the marrow and anticoagulant. The sample may then be set down and the needle removed before preparing slides. Should no marrow appear in the syringe after vigorous aspiration, the syringe is removed from the needle and the stylet replaced. The needle is then advanced slightly using the same pressure with which it was placed, and aspiration is reattempted. Occasionally while approaching the iliac crest, the needle may be advanced too far into the opposite cortex. Unsuccessful attempts at aspiration will result. The needle should then be slightly withdrawn before again attempting aspiration.

After mixing the marrow and anticoagulant, the sample is expelled into a Petri dish or watch glass. The Petri dish or watch glass may be gently shaken or tilted to allow visualization of the marrow spicules. Marrow spicules appear as small, irregular white or gray particles that may adhere slightly to the dish or glass.

These are collected using a hematocrit capillary tube or pipette. Only a small amount of sample needs to be collected in the capillary tube to prepare an adequate slide. The sample is placed on one end of a glass slide. A second slide is overlain on the bottom slide and the sample permitted to spread briefly between the slides.

Digital pressure on the top slide is typically not necessary and is discouraged because cell lysis can result. The top slide is then smoothly but rapidly pulled down the length of the bottom slide and the sample rapidly air-dried.

If anticoagulant is not used, the slide must be prepared immediately after successful aspiration. Bone marrow clots very rapidly, and a clotted sample will not allow adequate slides to be prepared. As soon as marrow appears in the syringe, negative pressure is released and both the aspiration needle and syringe are removed. It is important to have several clean glass slides laid out prior to collection. The clinician should rapidly place a few drops of sample near the top of each of the slides. An assistant should then follow closely, preparing slides as the clinician goes down the row. It is difficult to prepare several slides by oneself because the marrow is likely to clot before the smears can be prepared. Several slides should be prepared and submitted. The preparation of 12 to 15 slides should result in several diagnostic slides and would permit additional testing or special staining should this be necessary to identify a poorly differentiated leukemia. In addition, accurate interpretation of the marrow is dependent upon the findings of a concurrent complete blood count (CBC), and a CBC (or current CBC results) should always be submitted with the aspirates.

BONE MARROW BIOPSY

Bone marrow biopsy is indicated if repeated attempts at aspiration are unsuccessful, if evaluating for metastatic neoplasia, or if evaluating lytic bone lesions resulting from neoplasia, inflammation, or infection. Unsuccessful aspiration resulting in a dry tap may result from myelofibrosis, myelophthisis, hypoplasia or aplasia, or technical error. Bone marrow can be collected immediately after aspiration and can be collected from the same site or a distant site. Collection from separate sites can increase the likelihood of identifying metastatic neoplasia. Concurrent aspiration and biopsy is beneficial in that aspirated samples can occasionally be insufficient, necessitating histologic evaluation. Additionally, marrow biopsy immediately after aspiration may prevent the need for an additional anesthetic procedure should the aspirates be insufficient for a diagnosis.

Patient preparation, sites of collection, and approach are similar to those described for aspiration. Biopsy is considerably more painful, and good sedation or (preferably) anesthesia should be used. Jamshidi bone marrow biopsy needles are 11 to 13 gauge and 3 to 4 inches long.

The 13-gauge needles are typically used in cats and dogs less than 20 lb. Due to the larger size of these needles, the wing of the ilium can be too thin to be used in cats or very small dogs.

The biopsy needle is seated on the cortex and advanced using the same clockwise-counterclockwise rotational pressure that is used to place the aspiration needle. It is beneficial to lay the index finger along the shaft of the needle while advancing the needle to stabilize it while it is rotated. With the needle firmly imbedded, the stylet is removed and the needle is advanced an additional inch or more using the same rotational pressure to collect an adequate sample. The biopsy fragment must be broken loose using several 360° twists in both directions, and the needle is withdrawn. This step is not necessary if the clinician is using a newer, specimen-capturing Snarecoil biopsy needle. The biopsy fragment is pushed out the top of the needle in a retrograde fashion using the wire that accompanies the needle. The biopsy needle is tapered, and attempting to push the sample out the tip will crush it and damage the sample. The collection of a sufficient sample will allow the core to be sectioned and part submitted for culture if an infectious process is suspected. The biopsy fragment is typically submitted in formalin; however, consulting the surgical pathology service may be beneficial because other fixatives are occasionally preferred. Biopsy samples should not be submitted in the same packaging as cytology preparations because the formalin vapors can interfere with the staining quality of cytologic preparations.

ADDITIONAL SOURCES OF INFORMATION ON TECHNIQUES FOR BONE MARROW ASPIRATION AND BIOPSY

EDTA solution: Sequester-Sol 35-mL bottle
Cambridge Diagnostic Products, Fort Lauderdale, Florida
800-525-6262
Illinois bone marrow aspiration needle: 15 gauge and 18 gauge
VWR Scientific Products
800-932-5000
www.vwrsp.com
Jamshidi bone marrow biopsy needle: 11 gauge and 13 gauge
VWR Scientific Products
800-932-5000
www.vwrsp.com
Goldenberg snarecoil bone marrow biopsy needle
Ranfac Corporation
800-272-6322
www.ranfac.com

REFERENCES

The reference list can be found on the companion Expert Consult Web site at *www.expertconsult.com*.

CHAPTER 100

Cytology of Internal Organs

Amy L. MacNeill
A. Rick Alleman
James F. Naughton

Cytologic evaluation of internal organs is a powerful diagnostic technique that can provide valuable clinical information in a short period of time. This chapter briefly describes proper sampling and handling of aspirates from internal organs. Cytologic characteristics of selected disease processes are also described.

ASPIRATE COLLECTION AND PREPARATION

Diagnostic cytology of internal organs is most useful in conjunction with ultrasonography to guide aspiration of nodules, masses, or diffuse disease in an organ. B-mode and Doppler ultrasonography can also be used to monitor the dog or cat for bleeding after tissue aspiration. If generalized organ enlargement is detected, blind aspiration can be performed; however due to potential complications, this is not recommended. Ultrasound-guided fine needle aspiration can usually be performed without sedation. The animal should be positioned for optimal visualization and access to the target tissue and the skin adjacent to the target organ surgically prepared for aseptic collection of samples. Thoracic aspiration should be approached with extreme caution.

For abdominal organ cytology, a 6- to 12-mL syringe is attached to a 22-gauge, 1.5-inch needle. One or two cubic centimeters of room air is introduced into the syringe. The tissue of interest is ultrasonographically localized and the needle introduced into the target tissue using the ultrasound probe and image for guidance. Gentle aspiration of the syringe by pulling back on the plunger two to three times, releasing the plunger, and withdrawing the needle is a reliable method of obtaining samples from most organs. However, in highly vascular organs such as the liver and spleen, blood contamination caused by aspiration may interfere with cytologic interpretation. An alternate method is fenestration of the tissue. With this method, the plunger is not moved; instead the needle is gently directed into and out of the lesion several times. Fenestration should not be used for thoracic cytology. If ultrasound guidance is not being utilized, the needle should be introduced into the caudodorsal aspect of the spleen or liver to avoid piercing the diaphragm. The organ can then be aspirated.

The sample is placed near one edge of a clean slide and smeared by placing a second slide flat onto the sample slide. The top slide is then pulled from the edge on which the sample had been placed to the open edge of the bottom slide in one continuous, smooth motion. The weight of the second slide is sufficient to smear the sample. It is important not to pull the sample off the end of the slide. Once a sample has been collected, it should be air-dried and stained for cytologic examination; Romanowsky-type stains are commonly used. If a slide is sent to a laboratory, it should be shipped separately from histology samples to avoid exposure of the cells to formalin fumes.

It is important to take multiple samples so that different areas of the lesion are represented. The center of large masses is often necrotic and should be avoided. If fluid is collected, some should be smeared directly onto a slide, and the rest should be saved in a sterile tube for determination of cell count, protein concentration, and culture, if indicated. If the fluid is bloody, a portion of the fluid should be placed in an ethylenediamine tetraacetic acid (EDTA) tube. It is important to keep a small amount of fluid in a sterile container without EDTA to be sent for culture and sensitivity if cytology results are suggestive of sepsis.

Cytologic examination of touch preparations from non-fixed biopsy samples can also be informative. Ultrasound guidance is highly recommended for collection of samples with biopsy needles. If large enough, the biopsy can be handled with forceps by grasping the edge of the sample to avoid damaging the tissue architecture. The biopsy is blotted on absorbent tissue to minimize hemodilution, then pressed against a clean slide multiple times to create cellular imprints. If the sample is too small to handle with forceps, it can be gently rolled along the length of a slide. The biopsy can then be placed in formalin for histopathologic examination and the impression smear can be stained for cytologic evaluation.

THORACIC ORGAN CYTOLOGY

Pulmonary Aspirates

Aspirates from normal pulmonary tissue tend to be hemodilute and contain low numbers of respiratory epithelial cells and macrophages. Bacterial infection is typically associated with purulent inflammation, whereas fungal infections tend to cause pyogranulomatous disease. Several specific fungal diseases can be diagnosed cytologically, including blastomycosis (Figure 100-1).

Carcinomas tend to exfoliate as sheets of epithelial cells with visible cell junctions, basophilic cytoplasm that often contains punctate cytoplasmic vacuoles, and round to polygonal nuclei (Web Figure 100-1). Acinar structures may be observed with adenocarcinomas (Figure 100-2).

Metastatic carcinomas can rarely be distinguished from primary lung tumors. As with most malignant lesions, features such as anisocytosis, anisokaryosis, prominent nucleoli, an increased nuclear-to-cytoplasmic ratio (N:C), mitotic figures, coarse chromatin, and multinucleation must be observed for diagnosis. Also, inflammation can cause epithelial cells to have characteristics of malignancy. Therefore neoplasia cannot always be reliably diagnosed if inflammation is observed.

Heart-Based Tumors

Echocardiography and anesthesia are necessary to obtain aspirates of heart-based masses. Hemangiosarcomas exfoliate poorly and are hemorrhagic with low numbers of basophilic,

 To view a video on this topic, go to **www.expertconsult.com.**

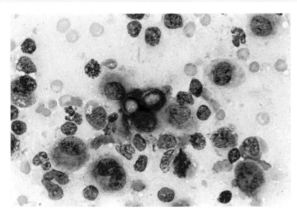

Figure 100-1 Blastomycosis, canine lung. Two round organisms, approximately 15 μm in diameter with a nonstaining capsule and broad-based budding, are characteristic of *Blastomyces dermatiditis* organisms. Infiltrating macrophages and lymphocytes are also noted. (Wright-Giemsa stain, ×250.)

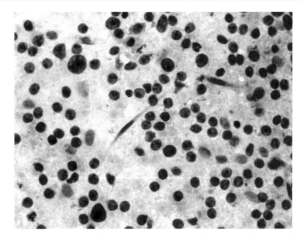

Figure 100-3 Heartbase tumor (chemodectoma) from a dog. Neuroendocrine-type tumors appear as free nuclei arranged in a background of cytoplasm with no defined cytoplasmic boarders between individual cells. (Wright-Giemsa stain, ×100.)

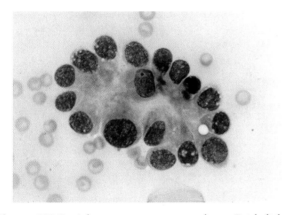

Figure 100-2 Adenocarcinoma, canine lung. Epithelial cells arranged in an acinar structure are pictured. Note the marked anisokaryosis and prominent nucleoli. (Wright-Giemsa stain, ×250.)

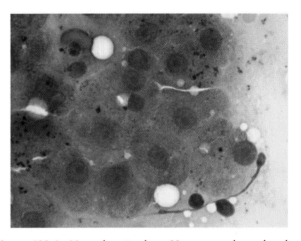

Figure 100-4 Normal canine liver. Hepatocytes have abundant cytoplasm, round nuclei, and single prominent nucleoli. (Wright-Giemsa stain, ×500.)

spindle-shaped cells with large pleomorphic nuclei, multiple prominent nucleoli, and other features of malignancy. Erythrophagia may be noted within neoplastic cells and macrophages. Neuroendocrine tumors, including chemodectomas and aortic body tumors, contain aggregates of pale blue cytoplasm with indistinct cell borders that are associated with round "naked" nuclei (Figure 100-3).

Thymus
Thymic enlargement can be caused by a thymoma or thymic lymphoma. Thymomas contain clusters of thymic epithelial cells, large numbers of small lymphocytes, low numbers of intermediate to large lymphocytes, and mast cells (Web Figure 100-2).

Thymic epithelial cells have a moderate amount of blue-gray cytoplasm and single round nuclei. Thymic lymphomas have a predominant population of intermediate or large lymphocytes with scant, deeply basophilic cytoplasm, round to pleomorphic nuclei, and prominent nucleoli.

ABDOMINAL ORGAN CYTOLOGY

Liver
Normal hepatocytes are large cells that occur in clumps with distinct cytoplasmic borders and abundant, basophilic cyto-

plasm that may contain eosinophilic granules (Figure 100-4). The nuclei are round and contain a single, round, prominent nucleolus. Due to the focal nature of many inflammatory lesions, cytologic identification of inflammatory liver disease may be difficult.

Vacuolar degeneration is a common cytologic finding that can be caused by glycogen or lipid accumulation. Glycogen accumulation appears as diffuse, pinpoint cytoplasmic vacuoles that are most prominent in the periphery of the cytoplasm (Figure 100-5). Glycogen accumulation is seen in dogs with steroid hepatopathy, nodular hyperplasia, or idiopathic vacuolar degeneration. Hepatocytes with lipid accumulation contain discrete, clear cytoplasmic vacuoles (Figure 100-6). Lipid degeneration is typically a secondary response to diseases such as diabetes mellitus, pancreatitis, and cholangiohepatitis.

Hepatic cholestasis is characterized by the presence of dark blue bile pigment in casts between adjacent hepatocytes (Web Figure 100-3). This is a common finding in hepatobiliary disorders and precedes the onset of icterus.

Tumors commonly found in the liver include hepatocellular carcinoma (HCC), bile duct carcinoma, lymphoma, and hemangiosarcoma. The diagnosis of HCC is made when anaplastic cells with differentiation toward mature hepatocytes are aspirated from a hepatic mass (Web Figure 100-4). Bile

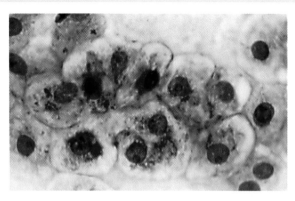

Figure 100-5 Vacuolar degeneration, canine liver. Indistinct cytoplasmic vacuoles concentrated at the borders of hepatocytes typify excess glycogen storage in the liver. (Wright-Giemsa stain, ×250.)

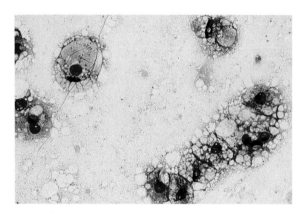

Figure 100-6 Vacuolar degeneration, feline liver. Large, distinct cytoplasmic vacuoles are observed with lipid accumulation in the liver. (Wright-Giemsa stain, ×125.)

duct carcinomas contain dense clusters of epithelial cells that are smaller than hepatocytes and have scant, basophilic cytoplasm with a very high N:C and other nuclear features of malignancy.

Spleen

Aspirates from normal spleen are hemodilute with clusters of splenic reticular elements, large numbers of small lymphocytes, moderate numbers of intermediate to large lymphocytes, and low numbers of plasma cells and mast cells. Common cytologic diagnoses associated with generalized splenomegaly are extramedullary hematopoiesis (EMH) and lymphoma. EMH is commonly observed and all lineages of hematopoietic precursors can be present (Web Figure 100-5).

Splenic lymphoma is difficult to diagnose due to the mixed population of lymphocytes in a normal spleen. If a monomorphic population of either intermediate or large lymphocytes makes up greater than 70% of the cells, splenic lymphoma can be suspected. The most common cause of splenic nodules is nodular hyperplasia, which may contain markedly increased numbers of large lymphocytes that can mimic lymphoma (Figure 100-7).

Hemangiosarcomas, hemangiomas, or hematomas cause large hemorrhagic nodules that can be difficult to differentiate cytologically.

Intestinal Tract

Intestinal aspirates tend to be poorly cellular with low numbers of epithelial cells. Lymphocytes may be seen due to lymphoid tissue associated with the intestine, inflammatory bowel

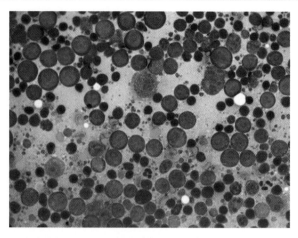

Figure 100-7 Nodular hyperplasia, canine spleen. Several large lymphocytes with deeply basophilic cytoplasm, round nuclei, and one to four prominent nucleoli are present. Moderate numbers of small and intermediate-sized lymphocytes are also depicted. (Wright-Giemsa stain, ×500.)

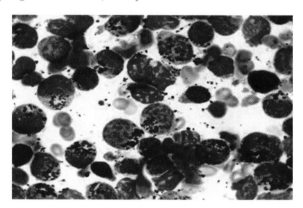

Figure 100-8 Large, granular lymphoma, feline intestine. Large lymphoblasts are seen with a scant amount of cytoplasm that contains a focal accumulation of large cytoplasmic granules. The large size of the lymphocytes, along with the cytoplasmic granules, allows easy distinction between large, granular lymphoma and lymphocytic/plasmacytic enteritis using cytology alone. (Wright-Giemsa stain, ×100.)

disease, or intestinal lymphoma. In all of these cases, small lymphocytes can predominate, which prevents cytologic differentiation of these processes (Web Figure 100-6). However, large granular lymphoma is easily diagnosed cytologically due to the presence of cytoplasmic granules (Figure 100-8).

Intestinal carcinomas contain dense clusters of epithelial cells with deeply basophilic cytoplasm, round to pleomorphic nuclei, prominent nucleoli, an increased N:C, and other features of malignancy. Infectious diseases may also be observed. Web Figure 100-7 is an example of intestinal pythiosis.

Kidney

Aspirates of enlarged kidneys require anesthesia and ultrasonography. Renal aspirates are hemodilute with rare clusters of renal tubular epithelial cells that have abundant blue cytoplasm, distinct cell borders, and round nuclei. Clear cytoplasmic vacuoles may be seen. In animals with renal lymphoma, the neoplastic lymphocyte population is usually composed of large lymphoblasts, allowing easy cytologic distinction between a neoplastic and a reactive lymphocytic infiltrate (Web Figure 100-8).

Inflammatory lesions should be cultured. Renal carcinomas are rare.

CHAPTER 101

Arthrocentesis and Arthroscopy

Mark C. Rochat

ARTHROCENTESIS

Synovial fluid is a dialysate of plasma combined with hyaluronic acid produced by type 2 (B) synoviocytes in the inner synovial membrane of the joint capsule. The viscosity of normal synovial fluid provides lubrication, shock absorption, and joint stability. Arthropathy results in loss of integrity of the synovial membrane and introduction of inflammatory mediators into the joint. Inflammatory cells and infectious agents release hyaluronidase and other matrix metalloproteinases, resulting in breakdown of hyaluronic acid. Loss of normal hyaluronic acid leads to loss of synovial fluid viscosity, improper cartilage nutrition, and decreased shock absorption, culminating in development of osteoarthritis.

Arthrocentesis is the process of withdrawing synovial fluid from a joint by use of a hypodermic needle and syringe. Arthrocentesis is a secondary diagnostic tool that should be preceded by a thorough history, physical and orthopedic examinations, and, depending on the preceding results, diagnostic imaging studies. Diagnostic imaging studies should be performed prior to arthrocentesis because artifacts such as hematomas may be created by needle insertion into a joint, leading to difficulty in interpreting radiographic images.

Arthrocentesis is indicated for characterizing the nature of arthropathies. The source of lameness can usually be isolated to a specific joint by history, as well as physical and orthopedic examination. Rarely, joint effusion, pain, or other signs of arthropathy cannot be readily identified, and the animal has vague and often diffuse lameness or stiffness or systemic signs such as cyclic fever.[1] This is common in immune-mediated polyarthropathies. In these situations, arthrocentesis is indicated as a screening tool when historical information is suggestive of a diagnosis of polyarthropathy. Multiple joints should be aspirated to enhance the likelihood of identifying the arthropathy.

Arthrocentesis rarely yields a definitive diagnosis. An example would be the presence of *Ehrlichia morulae* in intraarticular monocytes, typical of joint sepsis due to ehrlichiosis. More often, arthrocentesis reveals the general cellular pattern and characteristics of the synovial fluid and joint environment, allowing confirmation that an arthropathy does exist and broad classification of the arthropathy. Arthrocentesis is also the primary method of monitoring response to therapy for immune-mediated polyarthropathies.

Arthrocentesis may require brief heavy sedation or anesthesia to allow safe aspiration of synovial fluid while minimizing the risk of injury to intraarticular structures or articular cartilage if the animal is fractious, painful, or energetic or if the shoulder or hip are to be aspirated. Aseptic technique is required. The aspiration site should be clipped and aseptically prepared with chlorhexidine gluconate. If palpation of the site is required to identify the proper point of entry into the joint, sterile gloves should be worn.[2] Draping is not necessary. To perform arthrocentesis, the animal is positioned in lateral recumbency with the affected limb uppermost. A 22- to 25-gauge needle attached to a 3- to 5-mL syringe is inserted with the clinician's dominant hand, while the opposite hand stabilizes the limb and joint if necessary. Proper orientation of the needle to safely enter the joint is facilitated by palpation of the joint during flexion and extension, reviewing diagrams illustrating proper needle placement (Figure 101-1), or by viewing skeletal specimens.[3,4]

The needle is inserted and gentle vacuum applied with the hand that inserts the needle and syringe. The needle is advanced until synovial fluid enters the syringe. In small joint spaces, a short beveled spinal needle may facilitate entry into the joint with less risk of iatrogenic cartilage injury.[5] Use of a 3- to 5-mL syringe allows the operator to achieve an adequate degree of suction using only the hand inserting the needle. Only gentle suction should be applied to the plunger to avoid iatrogenic hemorrhage. The needle should be withdrawn if blood is encountered, and a new needle and syringe should be used for a second aspiration attempt. Hemarthrosis secondary to trauma does occur in small animals but is uncommon. Aspirated blood is usually a contaminant and should clot whereas blood present due to hemarthrosis should yield a yellow to red supernatant following centrifugation and decreased fluid viscosity.[6] Generally as much as 1 to 2 mL of fluid should be aspirated if possible, but the application of excessive negative pressure or aspiration of large volumes of fluid may increase the risk of aspirating blood, thereby ruining the sample. After the fluid is collected, negative pressure is released and the needle withdrawn. If no synovial fluid is obtained, the needle is redirected after reviewing the angle of placement. Occasionally, osteophytes or redundant synovium may interfere with fluid aspiration. If the needle is properly aligned but little or no synovial fluid is obtained, the needle may be plugged with soft tissue or hematomas or there may be insufficient fluid for aspiration as occurs in normal joints.

Aspirated fluid should be immediately transferred to an EDTA tube if a sufficient amount of fluid was aspirated (0.5-mL fluid for a 3-mL EDTA tube). Smears of the synovial fluid should also be made and air-dried prior to submission. If sufficient synovial fluid remains for bacterial culture and susceptibility, it can be inoculated at room temperature for 24 hours in a sterile red-tube top with blood culture media at a 1:9 ratio. If only a small amount of fluid (1 drop) remains in the needle hub, 0.5 mL of blood culture media can be aseptically aspirated in a separate syringe, the needle with residual synovial fluid placed on the syringe, and the media flushed through the needle into a sterile red-top tube and incubated as previously described.

Proper preparation of slides requires the smearing slide to be drawn slowly across the opposite slide when synovial fluid is of normal viscosity. Although the loss of viscosity typical of arthropathy reduces the risk of improper slide preparation, caution should still be exercised to not make smears too rapidly.[7] Prepared slides and the EDTA tube should be sub-

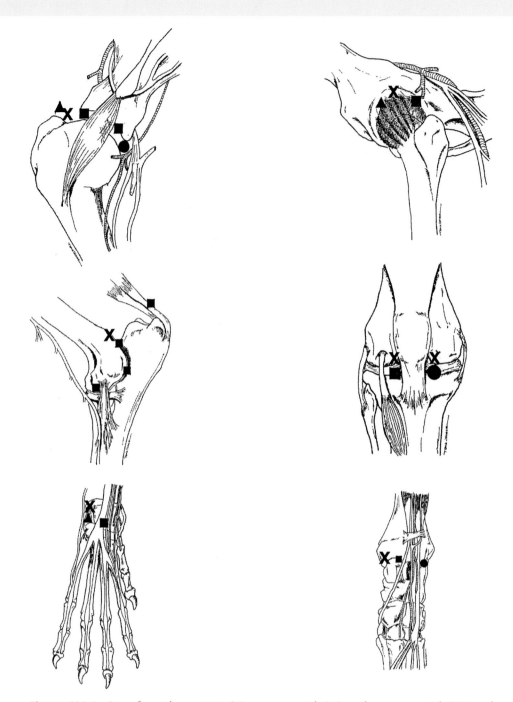

Figure 101-1 Sites for arthrocentesis **(X)**, egress portal (▲), arthroscope portal (■), and instrument portal (●) for the large joints of the appendicular skeleton.

mitted to a clinical pathology laboratory for evaluation. Synovial fluid characteristics that should be evaluated include volume, color, turbidity, total protein, total cell count, cell differential, viscosity, mucin clot test, and cytologic exam for cellular characteristics, infectious organisms, neoplastic cells, crystals, and other abnormalities (Table 101-1; Figure 101-2).

Synovial fluid characteristics for cats are extrapolated from dogs.[8] If immediate results are needed or only a drop or two of fluid are aspirated, some aspects of synovial fluid analysis can be determined in the clinical setting. Some appreciation of color, turbidity, and viscosity can be made when the fluid is expelled onto the glass slide. Synovial fluid with normal hyaluronic acid content will be viscous and tend to "string out" for 3 to 5 cm as it is expelled from the syringe onto a slide. Loss

of hyaluronic acid due to arthropathy results in a more aqueous fluid that doesn't "string out" for as long a distance, but this highly subjective test may not allow detection of mild arthropathies. Cytologic examination of the fluid will provide a rough estimate of the cellularity of the sample, the types of cells present, and specific cellular characteristics such as inclusions or organisms, cytoplasmic granules, nuclear changes, phagocytosed cellular debris, and vacuolation. A rough estimate of the number of white blood cells per cubic millimeter can be made by multiplying the number of white blood cells per high-powered field by 1000. Other findings such as crystals may be identified. Cytologic examination is the single best test for determining the nature of the arthropathy if the amount of fluid obtained limits the extent of the fluid analysis. The wide

Table • 101-1

Synovial Fluid Characteristics for General Classes of Arthropathies[1,2,4]

CONDITION	APPEARANCE	PROTEIN	VISCOSITY	MUCIN CLOT TEST	NUCLEATED CELL COUNT	CELL DIFFERENTIAL	COMMENTS
Normal	Clear; colorless to straw colored	<2.5 g/dL	High	Good	<3000/mm^3	<5% neutrophils >95% mononuclear cells	Small amounts present (<0.5 mL or less)
Osteoarthritis	Clear; colorless to light yellow	<2.5 g/dL	Varies	Good to fair	<5000/mm^3	<10% neutrophils >90% mononuclear cells	
Septic	Cloudy; off-white to yellow	>2.5 g/dL	Decreased	Fair to poor	40,000-250,000/mm^3	>90% neutrophils <10% mononuclear cells	Large volume usually present; infectious agents may be seen
Nonerosive Immune-mediated	Cloudy; off-white to yellow	>2.5 g/dL	Decreased	Fair to poor	4400-350,000/mm^3	>85% neutrophils <15% mononuclear cells	Moderate to large volume present
Rheumatoid	Cloudy; off-white to yellow	>2.5 g/dL	Decreased	Fair to poor	4400-350,000/mm^3	20%-80% neutrophils	LE cells, ragocytes may be seen rarely
Traumatic	Clear; yellow to slightly blood-tinged	Varies	Decreased	Unreported	2500-3000/mm^3	<25% neutrophils >75% mononuclear cells	Iatrogenic blood will clot

LE, Lupus erythematosus.

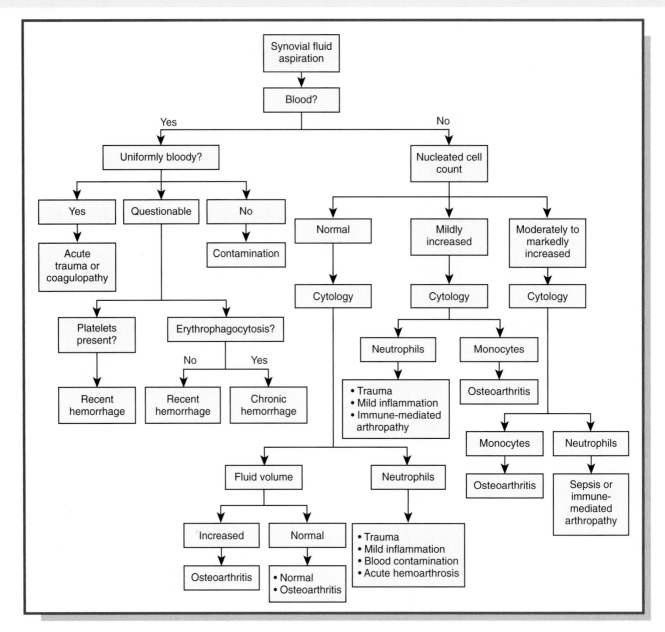

Figure 101-2 Algorithm for synovial fluid aspiration.

variety of neutrophil morphology can make accurate differentiation between immune-mediated and septic arthropathies difficult, and caution should be exercised when making a definitive diagnosis based solely on cell characteristics in the absence of infectious organisms.[9] Complications associated with arthrocentesis are rare and generally limited to articular cartilage injury, hemorrhage, and iatrogenic infection.

ARTHROSCOPY

Arthroscopy is the process of examining and treating joint disorders by use of a small fiberoptic telescope. The advantages of arthroscopy are a minimal degree of invasiveness, decreased recovery times from surgery, visualization of a greater percentage of the joint surfaces than what is possible by arthrotomy, and improved visualization of joint pathology. The disadvantages of arthroscopy are the expense of the associated equipment, steep learning curve required to master the

technique, and general limitation of the technique to the shoulder, elbow, carpus, hip, stifle, and hock joints of medium- to large-breed dogs.

Arthroscopy is indicated for characterizing ill-defined arthropathies of the previously mentioned joints by synovial biopsy and visualization of the pathology. Arthroscopy is also indicated in the treatment of joint diseases such as osteochondritis dissecans, bicipital tendinitis, fragmented medial coronoid process disease, cranial cruciate ligament disease, and stifle meniscal injury. As the science and instrumentation of arthroscopy improves, other techniques for addressing various and often less common arthropathies are being treated by arthroscopic methods.

The basic principles of surgery are observed whenever arthroscopy is performed. Canine and feline arthroscopy must be performed with the patient under general anesthesia. The patient is clipped and prepared in the same fashion as for an arthrotomy. Strict adherence to principles of aseptic technique should be observed throughout the procedure. Perioperative antibiotics are unnecessary due to the minimally invasive nature of the procedure, generally brief operative periods, and the continuous irrigation of the joint surfaces. The instrumentation required for arthroscopic surgery in dogs and cats is not extensive but it is delicate and expensive. A complete discussion of arthroscopic instrumentation and technique is presented elsewhere.[10]

Complications observed with arthroscopy include failure to properly create an arthroscopic or instrument portal, damage to intraarticular structures, premature dislodgement of the arthroscope, collapse of the joint capsule secondary to excessive fluid extravasation, hemorrhage from inadvertent puncture or injury of periarticular vessels or the stifle intraarticular fat pad, damage to the arthroscope from excessive bending forces, neurologic injury, infection, and inability to adequately explore or treat the joint disease. The incidence of complications is, generally, directly related to the experience of the arthroscopist.

REFERENCES

The reference list can be found on the companion Expert Consult Web Site at *www.expertconsult.com*.

CHAPTER 102

Lymph Node Aspiration and Biopsy

Cecile T. Siedlecki

Lymph node aspirate and biopsy is indicated when these structures are enlarged, suspected, or assessed to be involved in a disease process, or to assess remission status. When staging a patient for metastatic disease, the draining lymph node(s) should be sampled even if they are normal in size. Palpation of lymph nodes alone has been shown to be an insensitive indicator of nodal metastasis.[1,2] When patients present with generalized lymphadenopathy, multiple lymph nodes should be sampled. The superficial cervical and popliteal lymph nodes are easily accessible for both aspiration and biopsy. The mandibular lymph nodes drain the oral cavity and, as a result, often yield a reactive population of lymphocytes that may not be representative of a disease process. Very large lymph nodes should be sampled towards the periphery as central areas are more likely to contain necrosis.

The sampling technique chosen depends on several factors, which include the lymph node size, anatomic location, suspected disease process under investigation, patient's health status including coagulation parameters and suitability for sedation or anesthesia, and the clinician's personal preference.

Advantages of lymph node aspirate for cytology include ease of obtaining a sample, low cost, rapid interpretation, and low risk for complications such as hemorrhage and infection. Sedation or anesthesia is not usually required unless sampling an intracavitary lymph node or for fractious patients. Evi-

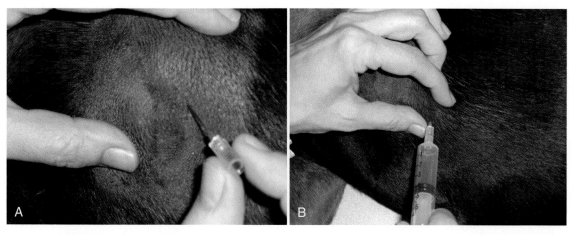

Figure 102-1 Nonaspiration techniques to obtain lymph node cytology using the needle alone **(A)** and the needle attached to a syringe **(B).**

 To view a video on this topic, go to www.expertconsult.com.

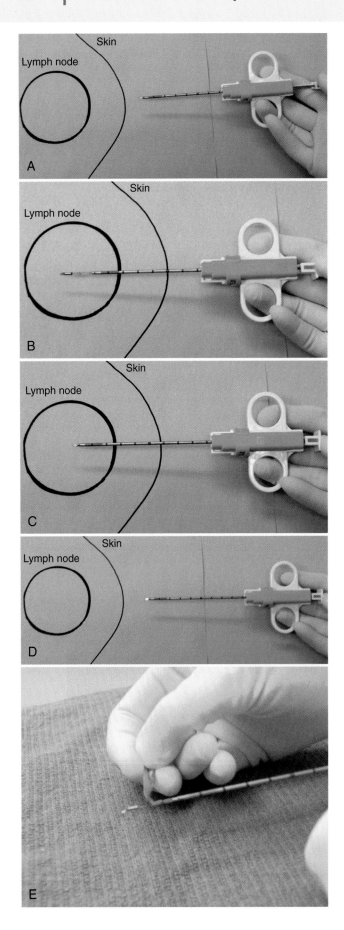

Figure 102-2 Lymph node biopsy using needle-core biopsy. **A,** With the instrument closed (the outer cannula covering the specimen notch), and, in the case of automatic instrument, "cocked," the needle is advanced through a small skin incision until the outer capsule of the lymph node is penetrated. **B,** The inner cannula is advanced into the lymph node driving tissue into the specimen notch. **C,** The outer cannula is advance either by trigger or manually. **D,** With the tissue contained within the closed unit, the instrument if removed from the skin. **E,** The inner cannula is advanced to expose the tissue, which is gently lifted from the specimen notch.

dence suggests that lymph node cytology is both sensitive and specific for detecting nodal metastasis compared to the "gold standard" of excisional biopsy.[1] Disadvantages include small sample size and lack of information regarding tissue architecture, both of which may lead to erroneous or nondiagnostic results.

Lymph node biopsy methods yield larger tissue samples for histopathologic examination. Methods include incisional techniques such as needle-core and wedge biopsy, and excisional techniques involving removal of the entire lymph node. Excisional lymphadenectomy affords the most complete examination of nodal architecture, which may be advantageous in differentiating diseases with similar cytologic appearances such as low-grade lymphoma and reactive lymphadenopathy. Excisional biopsy requires general anesthesia, a knowledge of the regional anatomy, and proficiency with basic surgical techniques. The reader is referred to other sources for further explanation. Needle-core biopsies are simple to obtain, inexpensive, and can usually be obtained with only sedation and local anesthesia. A procedure for obtaining a needle-core biopsy is outlined below.

While slides made from aspiration or impression smears of biopsy samples allow in-house examination of the submitted samples and may provide a preliminary diagnosis, the author encourages submission to a veterinary reference laboratory for interpretation by a board-certified veterinary pathologist.

LYMPH NODE CYTOLOGY TECHNIQUES

Samples for cytologic examination of lymph nodes can be obtained using aspiration and nonaspiration techniques. Required materials include 20- to 22-gauge needles, 3- to 12-cc syringes, and microscope slides. Surgical preparation of overlying skin should be performed for percutaneous aspiration of intracavitary lymph nodes or when submitting for a sample culture.

One nonaspiration technique can be performed using a needle alone as shown in Figure 102-1, *A*. Holding the needle hub between the thumb and forefinger, the needle is placed within the lymph node and then redirected four to five times in different directions without withdrawing it from the nodal tissue. The needle is removed and attached to an air-filled syringe to expel the contents onto a microscope slide.

Both nonaspiration and aspiration techniques can be accomplished with the needle attached to a syringe. In the aspiration technique shown in Figure 102-1, *B*, the syringe plunger is drawn back to fill the syringe with air prior to attaching the needle.

The technique is similar to the needle-only technique in that negative pressure is not utilized to obtain the sample. The air-filled syringe allows for rapid expulsion of the sample onto a microscope slide.

When using the aspiration technique, the needle with syringe attached is inserted into the lymph node and negative pressure is applied by rapidly pulling the plunger back while redirecting the needle within the lymph node. Negative pressure is released prior to removing the needle from the lymph node to avoid aspiration of the sample within the needle into syringe. The needle is detached and the syringe is filled with air. The needle is reattached and the sample is expelled onto a microscope slide. Caution should be used when using aspiration for lymph node cytology as aggressive suction may result in hemodilution of the sample and rupture of the fragile cells.

Aspirate smears are prepared by expelling the sample near the top of the slide. A second slide is promptly placed over the specimen. The weight of the slide spreads the sample. Then the second slide is gently pulled across the length of the first slide with one continuous motion. Certain cell types, such as immature lymphocytes, are fragile and should be spread gently to avoid rupturing of the cells. Slides are air-dried prior to placing them into containers for transport. Slides should be shipped separately from histologic samples to avoid contamination with formalin fumes that can result in poor staining and loss of cytologic detail.

LYMPH NODE INCISIONAL (NEEDLE-CORE) BIOPSY TECHNIQUE

Needle-core biopsy instruments may be operated manually or by automatic spring-loaded or pneumatically powered instru-ments. Automatic instruments such as the E-Z Core (Products Group International, Inc.) device have an automatic spring-operated Tru-cut biopsy needle that can be operated with one hand, leaving the other hand free to manually isolate and stabilize the lymph node of interest between the thumb and forefinger.

The need for sedation or general anesthesia will depend on the patient's demeanor, size of the lymph node, and anatomic location to be biopsied. In awake patients, local anesthetic block is used to include the overlying dermis.

The skin over the lymph node is clipped and aseptically prepared. A 1- to 2-mm, stab incision through the skin with a No. 11 blade will allow for smoother advancement of the biopsy instrument. Multiple samples are taken from this entry hole as outlined in Figure 102-2.

The tissue obtained is gently lifted off of the instrument using a sterile hypodermic needle or scalpel blade and placed into formalin. Closure of the stab incision is usually not required unless there is excessive hemorrhage.

REFERENCES

The reference list can be found on the companion Expert Consult Web Site at *www.expertconsult.com.*

CHAPTER 103

Rhinoscopy, Nasal Flushing, and Biopsy

Mark J. Acierno
Mary Anna Labato

INDICATIONS

Clinical signs of acute and chronic nasal disorders vary but often include an obstruction of one or both nasal passages and a discharge that can be clear, mucoid, or hemorrhagic. Some cases respond to empirical therapy while others take a progressive and insidious course. Further diagnostic procedures are indicated for these pets.

Nasal flushing and rhinoscopy are only part of the diagnostic workup for nasal diseases. Diagnostic imaging (radiographs, computed tomography [CT], or magnetic resonance imaging [MRI]) should precede any invasive diagnostic procedure. Imaging is important not only because it may reveal a characteristic lesion but because it can also be used to direct the nasal flush and rhinoscopy. Although skull radiographs are sometimes helpful, CT and MRI are significantly more sensitive in detecting and characterizing intranasal lesions. Historical questions of interest include the onset and duration of the condition, whether one or both nostrils are involved, and the clinical progression of the disorder. The physical examination should include both the general physical and a detailed examination of muzzle, nasal planum, and nares. Looking at the condensation that forms on a glass slide placed in front of the nares is a convenient way to assess airflow. When used together, the history, physical examination, blood work, and diagnostic imaging provide an important foundation for more invasive procedures.

ANATOMY

A basic understanding of nasal anatomy is essential if consistently rewarding diagnostic procedures are to be performed (Figure 103-1).

The left and right nasal cavities are separated by the bony nasal septum. The vestibule, located just within the nostril, contains the cartilaginous alar fold. The rostral aspect of each cavity is then divided into four airways (dorsal, middle,

 To view a video on this topic, go to **www.expertconsult.com.**

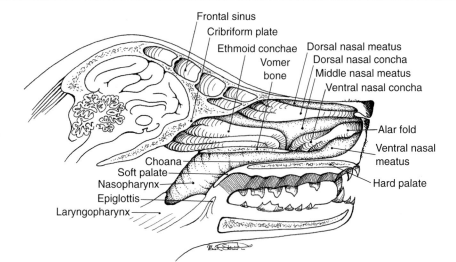

Figure 103-1 Nasal anatomy of canine. (Drawn by Mariah Steinwinter.)

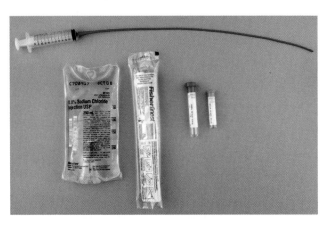

Figure 103-2 Setup for a nasal flush.

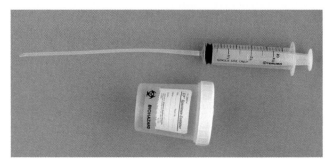

Figure 103-3 Setup for a modified nasal flush with a polypropylene catheter cut with an angled tip.

ventral, and common meatus) by the simple dorsal nasal concha and the more complex scroll-like ventral nasal concha. These conchae are primarily composed of cartilage rostrally and become increasingly calcified caudally. Nasal conchae are covered with a ciliated pseudocolumnar mucosal lining that serves to warm, humidify, and filter air as it travels through the meatus. The caudal aspect of the nasal cavities is filled with ethmoid conchae. These delicate, mucosa-covered, scroll-like structures arise from the ethmoid bone; they extend to the cribriform plate and up to the sinuses. The cribriform plate, which also arises from the ethmoid bone, separates the nasal cavities from the cranial vault. Although dogs and cats have a complex arrangement of sinuses, these are rarely visualized during endoscopic procedures. All inspired air leaves the nasal cavity by passing from the ventral meatus to the nasopharynx via the choanae. The choanae is dorsal to the hard palate and funnels air from the two nasal sinuses into the common nasopharynx. The nasopharyngeal space, which is delineated ventrally by the soft palate and dorsally by the vomer bone, directs the flow of air into the oropharynx and eventually the trachea.

NASAL FLUSH (Figure 103-2)

The nasal flush is the least invasive method of obtaining diagnostic samples from the nasal cavity; however, this procedure has several limitations. Samples collected are obtained by infusing saline into the caudal aspect of the nasal cavity and collecting it as it leaves the nares. Therefore only cells and debris that are easily dislodged are collected. Many tumors will not exfoliate sufficient cells to permit diagnosis. In addition, no attempt is made to visualize the structures of the nasal cavity. This allows for gross abnormalities to escape detection. Lastly, although sterile saline is infused into the nasal cavity, it is collected as it flows out of the nares, allowing for contamination by bacteria from outside the nasal cavity.

The anesthetized patient is placed in sternal recumbency with its nose pointed toward the floor. A cuffed endotracheal tube should always be used to prevent possible aspiration. A mouth gag is placed and a soft catheter (red rubber) is inserted into the nasopharynx so that its tip is pointed rostrally and the end of the catheter exits via the mouth. Sterile saline is then forcibly injected into the end of the catheter and fluid is collected as it leaves the nares. Depending on the size of the patient, 5 mL to 60 mL of infused saline should be sufficient to obtain samples for bacterial culture, fungal culture, and cytologic study. The flush can be repeated several times to improve diagnostic yield.

MODIFIED NASAL FLUSH (Figure 103-3)

A second technique for nasal flushing has been described. Briefly, the tip of a polypropylene urinary catheter is cut to form a jagged edge. The distance from the nares to the eyes is measured and then marked on the catheter. This line estimates the distance from the nares to the cribriform plate;

the catheter should never be advanced beyond this distance. The patient is then positioned as described previously and the catheter is inserted into the nares and advanced into the nasal cavity. While using the syringe to both flush saline into the nasal cavity and then suction the fluid back out, the sharpened catheter tip is used to scrape the nasal mucosa. Although this procedure has the theoretic advantage of active exfoliation of cells and larger samples, it is still performed blindly and has not been proven to provide greater diagnostic sensitivity. Some samples collected in this fashion may be suitable for histopathology.

RHINOSCOPY AND BIOPSY

A thorough examination of the upper respiratory tract requires direct visualization of each nasal cavity, nasopharynx, oropharynx, and larynx. The oropharynx and larynx can be examined in a sedated patient using only a laryngoscope, whereas visualization of the nasal cavities and nasopharynx requires general anesthesia and specialized equipment and techniques. Although no currently available endoscopic system will allow visualization of the entire nasal cavity and nasopharynx, the combined use of carefully selected rigid and flexible scopes will allow examination of most of the nasopharynx and nasal cavity.

Bacterial and fungal cultures should always be collected prior to rhinoscopy because the procedure is likely to introduce contamination. Once the patient is anesthetized, a nasal flush is performed and the sample submitted for culture. Alternatively, culture swabs are carefully inserted into the nasal cavity and then removed; contact with the external nares is avoided. Additional samples can also be retrieved during the rhinoscopy procedure if bacterial or fungal infection is suspected.

Examination of the nasopharynx is best achieved using a small, flexible endoscope. Two commonly used instruments are the 5-mm bronchoscope and the 2.5-mm cystoscope. In this procedure the anesthetized patient is placed in sternal recumbency with the nose pointed slightly toward the floor. A cuffed endotracheal tube should always be used to prevent the aspiration of secretions, blood, or saline. In addition, a mouth gag is always used to prevent possible damage to the scope and facilitate proper scope placement. The scope is flexed to 180°. With the tip of the retroflexed scope parallel to the lower jaw, the scope is inserted into the oral cavity and advanced. Once past the caudal aspect of the soft palate, the scope is rotated so that the tip is pointing up and perpendicular to the lower jaw. By moving the scope slightly rostrally, the tip "hooks" the nasopharynx and proper placement of the scope is achieved.

Once inside the nasopharynx, a careful examination of the relevant structures can begin. It is important to remember that because the scope is flexed, the image will be inverted; therefore the soft palate will be viewed dorsally. The entire nasopharynx should be examined by moving the tip of the scope rostrally until the choanae can be clearly visualized. The nasopharynx and choanae should be assessed for texture, contour, and patency. The soft palate should be pink, smooth, and flexible, whereas the dorsal wall of the nasopharynx is smooth, dome shaped, and rigid. A cobblestone appearance to the mucosa may be evidence of lymphoid follicular hyperplasia (inflammation) or lymphoma. Fungal colonies will often appear as gray or yellow plaques. Large masses or polyps can protrude into the airway. Chronic inflammation, infectious diseases, or surgery all can result in scarring and stenosis of the nasopharynx, whereas a membranous obstruction of the choanae (atresia) can be caused by a congenital abnormality. Foreign material that has been vomited into the nasophar-

ynx resulting in inflammation and obstruction may be visualized.

Any deviation from the normal anatomic structure should be investigated by biopsy and histopathology or culture. A biopsy instrument should not be passed through the scope's instrument channel when it is maximally flexed because the scope may sustain permanent damage. Therefore it is recommended that the scope be removed from the nasopharynx and straightened before the instrument is passed through the channel. The biopsy instrument should be positioned so that its forceps lie at the tip of the scope. Once in this position, the scope can be retroflexed and reinserted as described previously. This maneuver must be repeated for each biopsy sample.

It is possible to examine the rostralmost aspect of the nasal cavity by inserting a nasal speculum or flexible endoscope into the nares; however, an examination of the turbinates necessitates the use of a small-diameter rigid endoscope. One such instrument is the 2.7-mm universal telescope (Karl Storz Veterinary Endoscopy). This scope provides the user with a 16.5-cm working length and a 5-French (F) biopsy channel, which also allows for irrigation. The primary advantage of this system is that it allows direct visualization of a large portion of the nasal cavity and guided placement of biopsy forceps. For cats and small dogs the 1.9-mm telescope with a 4-French working channel is a more appropriately sized scope.

The anesthetized patient is placed in sternal recumbency with the nose pointed slightly toward the floor. The use of a cuffed endotracheal tube is essential to prevent aspiration. In addition, the placement of gauze sponges in the oropharynx may provide additional protection to the airway. Although the bleeding associated with rhinoscopy and biopsy can sometimes be a source of concern, instilling the nasal cavity with 0.25 to 0.5 mL of a dilute (1:10) mixture phenylepinephrine and lidocaine just prior to the procedures can be helpful in minimizing hemorrhage. The scope is inserted into the nasal cavity by lifting the flap of the nasal planum laterally and directing the scope over the alar fold. The scope can then be directed into the dorsal, middle, or ventral meatus. Warm saline should be infused through the biopsy channel. This assists in visualizing the nasal structures by keeping the lens free of blood, mucus, and debris. The scope is directed caudally to examine both the turbinates and meatus; however, the clinician should never advance the tip of the scope past the level of the eyes. The preliminary diagnostic workup may provide important information in regards to the location of a nasal lesion, yet a thorough examination of the entire nasal cavity is always recommended so as not to miss more subtle lesions.

The turbinates should be examined for color, texture, and contour. They should be smooth, scroll-like, and covered with a shiny pink mucosa. Each meatus should be patent, free of debris, and contain minimal mucous. In addition, the air passages will gradually taper in the caudal aspect of the nasal cavity, and sudden widening or narrowing is evidence of a lytic or proliferative lesion. Abnormal findings include increased mucus production, swelling of the turbinates, changes in the color or texture of the turbinates, foreign bodies, destruction or proliferation of the turbinates, fungal colonies, polyps, or tumors.

Increased mucus production, swelling of the turbinates, and changes in the appearance of the turbinates are nonspecific inflammatory findings that can be associated with allergic rhinitis, lymphoplasmacytic rhinitis, foreign bodies, bacterial infections, fungal infections, dental disease, and neoplasms. Destruction of the turbinates is often associated with fungal rhinitis (*Aspergillus, Penicillium*), bacterial rhinitis, viral rhinitis (cats), foreign bodies, and malignancies. The appearance of masses in the nasal passage is variable but usually causes some degree of turbinate destruction, mucous production, and tissue proliferation, which obstructs the meatus. It is important to note that some fungal organisms, including *Rhinosporidium* and *Cryptococcosis*, can induce masslike formations rather than turbinate destruction. Biopsies of affected tissues should be submitted for histopathologic examination as well as bacterial and fungal culture. It is important to

remember that the source of the nonspecific inflammatory changes may be the result of dental disease. Therefore a complete dental examination should always be performed while the patient is anesthetized. It cannot be overemphasized that any deviation in the normal appearance is sufficient reason to obtain a biopsy specimen for histopathology as well as bacterial and fungal cultures.

CARDIOVASCULAR/PULMONARY

CHAPTER 104

Diagnostic Blood Pressure Measurement

Rebecca L. Stepien

Acute blood pressure (BP) measurement is required to diagnose hypertension or hypotension or to exclude these diagnoses as a cause for clinical signs in a patient. Multiple BP measurement techniques are available; each is associated with advantages and disadvantages.

PATIENT SELECTION

Blood pressure measurements are assessed as one part of a clinical evaluation that includes the patient history, physical examination findings, results of other diagnostic testing, and evaluation of concomitant medications, including anesthetics and sedatives. Many BP measurement techniques have test characteristics that require low diagnostic cutoff values for maximum sensitivity to hypertension (maximum opportunity to correctly identify an abnormally high value). Unfortunately, low diagnostic cutoff values also are associated with increased numbers of false-positive diagnoses. As a result, many BP measurement techniques are best able to correctly identify truly hypertensive patients as abnormal when the test is applied to patient populations with clinical signs or diseases likely to be associated with systemic hypertension. Routine "screening" BP measurements in clinically normal patients may assist the clinician in establishing a typical baseline BP value for an individual patient, but abnormally high BP values obtained from clinically normal patients must be viewed with caution due to the high incidence of false-positive readings in this patient population.

INDICATIONS FOR BLOOD PRESSURE ASSESSMENT

Blood pressure measurement should be part of the diagnostic evaluation for any feline or canine patient with clinical signs associated with systemic hypertension, known or suspected systemic diseases known to be associated with systemic hypertension, or both. Clinical signs of systemic hypertension occur when there is hypertensive damage to various organ systems ("target organ damage"). The organ systems most frequently affected include the eyes, kidney, brain, and heart. Damage

to these systems may be overt (e.g., retinal detachment or seizures) or may be subtle, requiring the clinician to have a high index of suspicion for systemic hypertension when examining patients with subtle or vague clinical abnormalities. Overt and more subtle clinical signs of target organ damage are outlined in Table 104-1.

Blood pressure assessment is indicated when any of the overt or subtle signs of end-organ damage are detected. Conversely, if systemic hypertension is diagnosed, these body systems should be carefully evaluated for damage in conjunction with further diagnostic testing for causative diseases. In cases of renal disease, diagnostic testing for causative disease and target organ damage involve the same testing.

CATS

The most common reason for clinical presentation of hypertensive cats is ophthalmologic abnormalities. Although other causes of intraocular hemorrhage (e.g., coagulopathy) and retinal detachment (e.g., inflammatory disease) should be ruled out, immediate measurement of systemic BP guides the course of the diagnostic evaluation in these patients. For cats with neurologic signs in addition to ophthalmologic signs, diagnosis of critical levels of hypertension and immediate therapy can lead to rapid improvement in BP and relief of clinical signs.

Suspicion or diagnosis of diseases proven to be associated with systemic hypertension in cats (renal insufficiency or thyrotoxicosis) should lead to BP assessment. Other findings that may indicate BP assessment is warranted include palpable goiter or unexplained left ventricular hypertrophy. Systemic BP should be assessed in cats whenever auscultatory cardiac abnormalities (e.g., gallop rhythms, left-sided systolic murmurs) and radiographic, electrocardiographic, or echocardiographic findings are consistent with hypertrophic myocardial disease involving the left side of the heart. Systemic hypertension (and hyperthyroidism in cats over 8 years of age) should be excluded by appropriate testing before a diagnosis of idiopathic hypertrophic cardiomyopathy is made. Early recognition of abnormal BP typically leads to

Table • 104-1

Overt and Subtle Signs of Target Organ Damage with Recommended Testing Required to Assess Extent of Damage

ORGAN SYSTEM AFFECTED	OVERT CLINICAL SIGNS	SUBTLE CLINICAL SIGNS	RECOMMENDED TESTS
Eyes	• Acute blindness • Complete or near complete retinal detachment • Hyphema	• Behavior changes related to unrecognized vision loss • Bullous retinal detachment • Retinal hemorrhages • Tortuous retinal arteries • Periarterial subretinal infiltrates • Papilledema	• Detailed direct or indirect funduscopic exam
Kidneys	• Weight loss/inappetence • Polyuria/polydipsia • Palpable renal abnormalities • Azotemia • Increased urine protein/creatinine ratio	• Decreased urine-concentrating ability with normal creatinine/BUN • Increased urine protein/creatinine ratio with normal creatinine/BUN	• Assessment of creatinine and serum urea nitrogen concentrations • Urinalysis, with particular attention to urine specific gravity and protein content • Urine culture if required to rule out infection as a cause of proteinuria • Urine protein/creatinine ratio or other assessment of urine protein loss • Imaging, typically ultrasound, ± renal biopsy
Brain	• Seizures • Changes in mentation • Obtundation/coma	• Focal facial seizures • Depression • Photophobia • Behavioral changes (e.g., hiding)	• Detailed neurologic examination • Serum chemistry to rule out electrolyte and glucose abnormalities • Brain imaging (e.g., MRI)
Heart	• New murmur • New gallop rhythm	• Acute heart failure after fluid administration • Left ventricular hypertrophy on echocardiogram	• Echocardiographic examination

BUN, Blood urea nitrogen; MRI, magnetic resonance imaging.

evaluation for other systemic diseases, especially renal insufficiency.

DOGS

Ophthalmologic abnormalities are less common in dogs with systemic hypertension than cats. Systemic hypertension in dogs is most often diagnosed when BP is evaluated as part of the clinical workup of dogs with systemic disease known to be associated with hypertension. In dogs, the diseases most frequently associated with elevations in BP are protein-losing renal disease, acute or chronic renal failure of any etiology, hyperadrenocorticism, diabetes mellitus, and pheochromocytoma. In the case of renal disease, signs of renal dysfunction may be subtle (e.g., proteinuria without azotemia). Renal disease cannot be completed excluded based on a normal creatinine or serum urea nitrogen concentration, and a urinalysis should be performed to assess concentrating ability and protein loss. As with cats, systemic hypertension should be ruled out as a cause of left ventricular thickening of unknown etiology. Lastly, BP should be evaluated in dogs with any type of intracranial neurologic signs.

Hypotension
Dogs and cats that are presented with clinical signs of low cardiac output (e.g., weak peripheral pulses, cold extremi-

ties), shock, blood loss, or obtundation should be evaluated for hypotension. In some cases, hypotension is diagnosed clinically based on the constellation of history, presenting signs, and suspected clinical diagnosis (see Chapters 139 and 153). Accurate measurement of BP is important in any hypotensive patient to confirm the diagnosis and to provide baseline data for monitoring the response to therapy. BP evaluation methods differ in their sensitivity to low BP. Automated noninvasive techniques (i.e., oscillometric techniques) may fail to detect a pulse when hypotension is present, and operator-reliant techniques for pulse detection (e.g., Doppler sphygmomanometry) can be unreliable if the pulse signal is difficult to discern. Of the methods typically used in acute BP measurement, arterial cannulation is the most accurate method of documenting and monitoring hypotension.

CHOOSING A BLOOD PRESSURE MEASUREMENT TECHNIQUE

Acute Diagnostic Blood Pressure Measurement
Detection of systemic hypertension may prompt additional testing for an underlying disease condition. Therefore, it is often preferable to measure BP acutely (i.e., during a clinical examination or diagnostic evaluation), rather than hospitalizing patients and placing indwelling arterial catheters. When

a technique to measure BP in a particular animal is chosen, specific issues to be considered include the availability of equipment, the availability of "normal" values to use for comparison, the skill and experience of the person making the measurement, and specific issues related to the animal (e.g., size, obesity, temperament).

The accuracy and usefulness of the measurement technique chosen ultimately depends more on attention to detail and use of applicable normal values (i.e., generated with the same technique as the one in use) than on which technique is used. Although multiple studies have addressed correlation or lack of correlation between invasive and noninvasive techniques in both dogs and cats, few studies address the ability of these techniques to discern "normal" from "abnormal" in a conscious clinical population. Therefore assessment of BP values obtained may involve comparisons with normal values or comparison with values known to be associated with clinical signs.

Continuous Blood Pressure Monitoring: Conscious Patients

The monitoring of BP over time requires either continuous measurement (arterial catheterization) or repeated measurements, recorded automatically (oscillometric methods) or manually (Doppler sphygmomanometric methods). Arterial catheterization has the greatest number of advantages in conscious patients. Blood pressure obtained via arterial cannulation is accurate when the technique is used correctly and the values obtained are objective and repeatable (no manual pulse detection is required). A particularly important advantage is that the system can be secured to continue BP measurement when the animal moves. The major disadvantages are the technical skills and equipment required to maintain an arterial catheter and transducer system. Noninvasive methods are commonly used to take serial BP measurements in conscious animals. Although noninvasive BP measurements appear to be technically simple to obtain, they are subject to marked inaccuracy with animal movement, poor pulse pressure, arrhythmia, or inconsistent technique. When repeated BP measurements are obtained using these methods for monitoring, cuff size and positioning, as well as limb position, should be identical for the repeated recordings.

Continuous Blood Pressure Monitoring: Anesthetized Patients

Blood pressure monitoring by most clinical methods is accurate and repeatable in anesthetized animals. The primary confounding problem of patient movement is absent in these patients, which renders them ideal subjects for BP measurement. Nonetheless, differences between values obtained by invasive methods (arterial catheterization) and noninvasive methods have been documented in numerous studies of dogs and cats. These studies indicate that numeric values obtained by means of noninvasive methods often underestimate true BP. In the case of anesthetized animals, this may result in an erroneous diagnosis of hypotension, but it seldom leads to the more dangerous error of overestimating BP in these patients. In any case, the marked hypotensive effects of many anesthetic agents should be taken into account when assessing BP in an anesthetized patient.

BLOOD PRESSURE MEASUREMENT TECHNIQUES

Arterial Puncture or Arterial Cannulation ("Invasive" or "Direct" Technique)

Direct BP measurement involves advancing a needle attached to a pressure transducer directly into an artery to measure BP. This procedure may be performed acutely to obtain instanta-neous BP readings, or BP can be measured over time through the use of an indwelling arterial catheter instead of a needle. Invasive BP measurements are typically used during anesthetic procedures, in critical care patients when ongoing BP information is desired, or to document or exclude hypertension acutely as a clinical diagnosis in dogs. Acute arterial puncture is seldom used for clinical diagnosis of hypertension in cats.

Direct BP measurement is usually performed by means of puncture of the femoral artery in dogs. Use of local anesthesia is strongly recommended for this procedure and when used, the procedure is well tolerated by most dogs. The patient is gently restrained in lateral recumbency. Approximately 5 minutes prior to arterial puncture, 1 to 2 mL of 2% lidocaine hydrochloride is injected subcutaneously over the area in which the femoral pulse is palpated. A 22-gauge, 1-inch needle is attached to a transducer and flushed with heparinized saline, ensuring that no bubbles remain in the transducer. The transducer is zeroed at the level of the sternum in the laterally recumbent dog. The femoral pulse is palpated in the femoral triangle, and the needle is carefully advanced into the femoral artery (Figure 104-1) until a satisfactory pressure waveform is recorded on the monitor screen.

A sample of the tracing is recorded, and the needle is withdrawn. Firm pressure is applied to the area of arterial puncture for a minimum of 5 minutes after measurement. The patient should be monitored closely for at least 1 hour after the procedure for any complications related to hematoma formation. Systolic, diastolic, and mean BP values from five consecutive cardiac cycles during normal sinus rhythm are averaged to obtain a representative value for the patient. When use of an arterial catheter is preferred, the catheter is usually inserted into the dorsal pedal artery. A local anesthetic may be used as described previously.

Oscillometric Technique

Oscillometric BP measurement involves the use of an automated detection system and a cuff that is wrapped around a limb or tail over an artery. The cuff is inflated automatically to a pressure that causes occlusion of the artery and then slowly deflated. The machine detects oscillations in the vessel

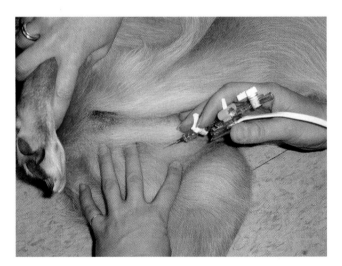

Figure 104-1 Invasive blood pressure measurement via direct arterial puncture in a dog. A 22-gauge needle (with an attached pressure transducer, previously flushed with heparinized saline and zeroed) is advanced into the femoral artery at the level of the palpable pulse in the femoral triangle.

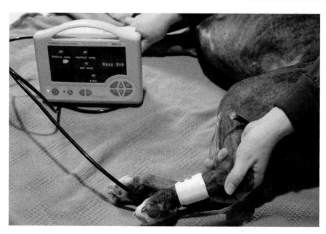

Figure 104-2 Correct cuff placement for oscillometric measurement of blood pressure (BP) via the dorsal pedal artery in a dog. The cuff tubing is attached to the oscillometric BP monitor for readings and the patient is gently restrained in lateral recumbency.

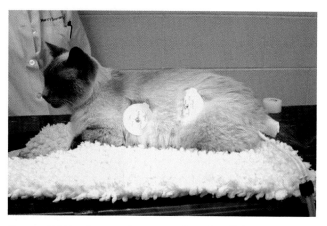

Figure 104-3 Correct placement of a tail cuff for oscillometric readings in a cat. The cat is relaxed and minimally restrained in sternal recumbency.

wall as the occlusion is eased, and the pressure at which oscillations are maximal is recorded as the mean arterial pressure. Systolic and diastolic pressures are then calculated by the monitor using algorithms specific to the technique. This technique uses data from many cardiac cycles to render a single reading and is therefore unsuitable for use in animals with rapidly changing BP.

Oscillometric BP measurement methods are more accurate in dogs than in cats. This measurement method may return inaccurate results if the patient is not motionless (e.g., trembling), has a weak or irregular pulse, or has a small artery (i.e., most cats). Use of a cuff of appropriate size is extremely important to ensure accurate measurements. Cuff width should be approximately 40% of the circumference of the limb or tail in dogs and approximately 30% of the appendage circumference in cats. When used on the tail, the cuff is wrapped snugly high on the tail head with the dog in sternal or lateral recumbency. Although tail cuffs can be used in standing animals, animal movement often interferes with accurate measurement. Limb cuffs are wrapped around the forelimb distal to the elbow or around the midmetatarsus at the level of the superficial plantar arterial arch (Figure 104-2).

To maximize accuracy, the cuff should be at the level of the heart during readings; therefore lateral or sternal recumbency is preferred, and use in standing patients is not recommended. In cats, tail cuffs return more repeatable measurements than limb cuffs. Typically, the cat rests in sternal recumbency during readings (Figure 104-3).

In all cases, best results are obtained when the patient is minimally restrained and soothed during the procedure. A short acclimation period prior to measurement is recommended to allow the cat to become more calm. A series of at least five readings are obtained at approximately 1-minute intervals. Any readings that are clearly erroneous are discarded. The multiple readings are then averaged to obtain a representative result.

Oscillometric techniques are valuable in anesthetized dogs and cats to monitor trends in BP. Because the animal is immobilized and BP shows less variability over time, repeatable and accurate readings can be obtained over time in both dogs and cats.

Doppler-Ultrasonic Technique (Doppler Sphygmomanometry)

Doppler ultrasonic flow detection through the use of a piezo-electric crystal allows detection of flow in a peripheral artery. Hair is clipped just proximal to the palmar metacarpal pad at the level of the superficial palmar arterial arch for forelimb measurement; over the dorsal pedal artery for hindlimb measurement; or on the ventral aspect of the tail for tail measurement. An occluding cuff (sized as outlined for oscillometric techniques) is placed proximal to the point of flow detection (midradius in the forelimb, proximal to the hock in the hindlimb, or proximal to transducer placement on the tail), and measurements are obtained with the cuff at the level of the heart. Ultrasonic coupling gel is placed on the concave surface of the Doppler transducer, and the transducer is held in position during measurements (Figure 104-4) or fixed in position using adhesive tape.

An audible pulse signal is obtained, and the cuff is inflated with a bulb attached to a pressure gauge. The cuff is inflated to a pressure no less than 40 mm Hg above the audible cutoff point of the signal. The cuff is then slowly deflated, and the pressure at which the Doppler signal is again audible is recorded as the systolic pressure. The cuff is deflated further, and the pressure at which the audible signal abruptly changes in pitch or becomes muffled is recorded as the diastolic pressure.

The Doppler flow detection system of BP measurement is considered the most accurate and repeatable of studied noninvasive BP measurement techniques in conscious cats. It is frequently used in dogs but may provide spurious high readings in some individuals. When abnormal readings are obtained by this method from dogs, care should be taken to make sure the abnormal readings are repeatable over multiple measurement periods. The advantages of this technique include flexibility with regard to motion, low pressure, small vessels, or the presence of arrhythmias, as well as speed of measurement. The rapidity of the measurement techniques allows for prompt assessment of changing BP, but meticulous attention must be paid to obtaining strong, audible signals in order to obtain the most accurate BP readings. This technique is also the most operator dependent of the techniques discussed. Accurate identification of diastolic pressures improves with operator practice, and BP measurement using Doppler ultrasonic flow detection techniques is most accurate if a few well-trained individuals in a practice are responsible for this diagnostic test and perform the test frequently.

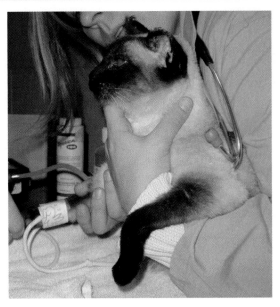

Figure 104-4   Measurement of blood pressure via Doppler sphygmomanometry from the forelimb of a cat with acute blindness due to retinal detachment. Note that the inflatable cuff is at the same level as the heart in the sitting and comfortably restrained animal.

CHAPTER **105**

Pulse Oximetry

Peter J. Pascoe

A pulse oximeter is a device designed to measure the percent saturation of arterial hemoglobin with oxygen. The value calculated is usually referred to as SpO_2 to differentiate it from a value obtained by direct measurement from arterial blood (SaO_2). To understand the likelihood of this device producing an accurate result it is important to understand how it works.

PRINCIPLES

The basis for this technology is that oxygenated hemoglobin and deoxygenated hemoglobin have different light absorption characteristics and hence different colors. Light absorption is usually measured as an extinction coefficient (ε), which was originally defined as the thickness of the material that was required to decrease the intensity of light passing though it to one tenth of the incident light.[1] This is depicted in Figure 105-1 showing ε for hemoglobin (Hb), oxyhemoglobin (HbO_2), methemoglobin (MetHb), and carboxyhemoglobin (HbCO) over a spectrum of light wavelengths from orange (600 nm) through to infrared (>700 nm).

Pulse oximeters generally use two light-emitting diodes (LEDs) that produce light at 660 nm and 940 nm and a silicone photodiode that can detect light at either wavelength, with a quantitative output proportional to the intensity of the light. At 660 nm, εs for MetHb and Hb are similar and greater than those for HbO_2 and HbCO. At 940 nm, εs are different for each species of Hb with that of HbCO being low. However, the important issue for pulse oximetry is that the ε for HbO_2 is now higher than that for Hb—the opposite of what happens at 660 nm. Given these facts the absorption of the light at each wavelength is going to depend on the relative concentrations of Hb and HbO_2. The εs are measured in Hb solutions and these do not appear to vary much across species.[2] However, the absorption of light may be different between species because of differences in red cell numbers and morphology.

Pulse oximeters cycle each individual LED on and off and record the transmitted light with the silicone photodiode, so they have a signal at each wavelength. The cycling rate varies from manufacturer to manufacturer but it is done rapidly enough (e.g., 75 to 480 Hz) that the relative absorptions can be taken over the whole pulse cycle, and waveforms can then be built that reflect the changes in light absorption over each pulse. The signal is put through a high-pass filter to remove the nonvarying part of the signal, and once these waveforms have been normalized for background light intensity, relative absorptions at the peak of each wave can be compared (Figure 105-2).

The pulse oximeter then must rely on empirically derived values in order to convert relative absorption to SpO_2 because there is no way of calculating saturation directly. These values have been determined in healthy people by plotting the

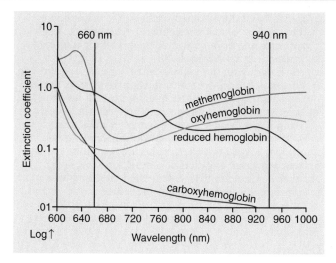

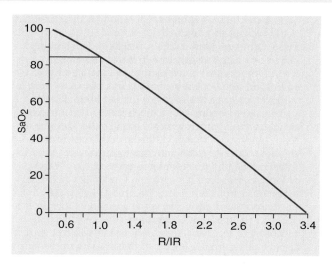

Figure 105-1 Extinction coefficients shown over a range of wavelengths for reduced hemoglobin, oxyhemoglobin, carboxyhemoglobin, and methemoglobin. The lines at 660 and 940 nm represent the red and infrared wavelengths, respectively, used by most pulse oximeters.

Figure 105-3 This curve is constructed from empiric data in people to correlate the differential absorption of red *(R)* and infrared *(IR)* light at different hemoglobin saturations. The data are generated in the 70% to 100% saturation range and the rest of the curve is a projection from these data. The line at R/IR = 1 is the neutral point and corresponds to a hemoglobin saturation of ~85%.

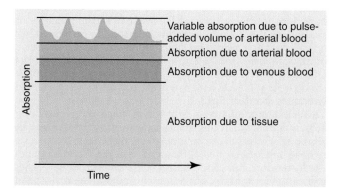

Figure 105-2 Sources of absorption of light as it passes through tissue. The pulse oximeter is able to recognize the change in absorption associated with a pulse and can then calculate the difference in absorption of red and infrared light at the peak of each pulse.

numeric ratio of the red to infrared absorption against the measured SaO_2 using co-oximetry (Figure 105-3).

The fact that this has been done in people means that the real "calibration" curve for most pulse oximeters only extends from 70% to 100% saturation because of the concerns of exposing people to PO_2s less than ~40 mm Hg (SaO_2 = 70%)! Despite the fact that pulse oximeters are widely used in various species, none of the manufacturers appear to have generated these data in the species for which the device is targeted, using a more extended range of SaO_2. The pulse oximeter uses the equation describing this relationship to do the final calculation for SpO_2.

From this description of operation principles, a number of issues arise that may alter the reading accuracy or the ability of the machine to obtain a reading.

1. The tissue used for the initial calibration versus the tissue that is being measured may affect the final reading. Background absorption from tissue will vary according to the nature of the tissue—if a pulse oximeter is placed on a human finger, the light may be shining through skin, a nail bed, bone, and muscle whereas on a tongue it will be passing through a mucous membrane and then mainly muscle. This could alter the relative absorption of the light and may affect the "calibration" of the pulse oximeter.

2. The presence of HbCO or MetHb. The HbCO at the lower wavelength cannot be distinguished from HbO_2 and so the pulse oximeter might report values that are in the "reference" range in an animal with significant quantities of HbCO.[3] For MetHb the absorption is roughly equal at the two wavelengths of light used and the reported saturations tend to be falsely low above SaO_2s of 85% and falsely high below 85%.[4,5]

3. The presence of Hb-based oxygen carrier molecules (e.g., Oxyglobin) may interfere with the reading because it has different light absorption properties from normal Hb. This is a dose-dependent alteration.[6]

4. The presence of other dyes such as methylene blue, indocyanine green, isosulfan blue, indigo carmine, nitrobenzene, and patent blue may alter the absorption of these two light frequencies and hence the resultant SpO_2.

5. From Figure 105-3, note that the absorption of red versus infrared light is equal at about 85% saturation. This is sometimes referred to as the *neutral point* and is the value that the pulse oximeter will read when it is trying to read from an Hb-free solution. This can be readily demonstrated by taking a rubber glove and filling it with water. If a pulse oximeter probe is place on a finger of the glove and a "pulse" created by alternately squeezing and relaxing pressure on the glove, the pulse oximeter will generally read ~85%! We have seen this happen when the probe has fallen off the

animal and there is sufficient vibration on the table that it still recognizes a "pulse."

6. Pulse oximeters need to use sophisticated electronics driven by computer software in order to arrive at a result. The circuitry must control the cycling of the LEDs, and some of the manufacturers have also built in variable power to the LEDs so that an optimal light signal can be obtained for a given tissue. The incoming signal has to be processed to recognize the background tissue absorption, to adjust for the amplitude of the signal, and to recognize and transform the waveform to calculate the differences in absorption and try to recognize artifacts. This signal processing is where the different manufacturers have the most significant impact on the result because the algorithms they use to program the device will determine the sensitivity and reliability of the device (e.g., whether it will recognize a signal coming from a relatively thin tissue with a low pulse amplitude such as from a cat's tongue), how versatile it might be in terms of being used on different animals (e.g., whether it will recognize a heart rate >250 beats/min), and whether it can cope with some degree of motion or arrhythmia artifact. Given these factors it is not surprising that two different pulse oximeters placed on the same animal might give a different result![7]

7. The placement of the probe and how it is fixed to the animal will play a significant role in how well the instrument works.

   a. If the tissue is quite thin, there might not be enough light absorption for the detector to register a difference. This is typically the case when a probe is placed on the ear, where a pulse oximeter often fails to read SpO_2. This can sometimes be fixed by putting some gauze or paper towel (colored towels might interfere with the reading!) over the ear to increase the absorption of light and allow the device to read.[8]

   b. If the tissue is too thick or is heavily pigmented, the light signal may not penetrate the tissue adequately to give a reading. In people with heavily pigmented skin, pulse oximeters work but the readings may be erroneously high.[9] The density of black pigment in many dogs and cats is such that it is often impossible to get a reading from these tissues.

   c. If the probe is applied and the device holding the probe is too tight, or it has been taped in place, or someone is holding it in place, the increased pressure on the tissue might eliminate the pulse oximeter's ability to detect a waveform and reduce the likelihood that it will give an accurate reading.

8. Since the sensor is responding to light, it is possible that ambient light may interfere with the reading it is receiving from the LEDs. Some manufacturers include a time when the LEDs are both off during the cycle so that the sensor can recognize background input. This still may not prevent erroneous reading or failure to read under high-light conditions. A ray of sunshine or a powerful surgical light shining on the probe can easily cause such a problem. Once recognized, this is easily corrected by covering the probe with a cloth or other material to blot out the external incident light.

9. The signal generated must be strong enough to allow for the machine to recognize the difference in absorption. Since the amount of Hb present will have a role in this, the effect of anemia has been investigated.[10] This study found that the incidence of failing to give an accurate reading increased dramatically once the hematocrit decreased below 10% and the bias and precision of the obtained readings also became worse. However, at hematocrits above 10%, readings were accurate and in most anemic animals the pulse oximeters appear to work well.[11]

10. Hypoperfusion, due to low cardiac output, compression of a vessel to an extremity, intense vasoconstriction, or a decreased peripheral temperature can all lead to a signal that has insufficient amplitude for the pulse oximeter to be able to interpret it. In a laboratory setting, hypotension induced with nitroprusside to 40 mm Hg did not alter the accuracy of pulse oximeters. However, in a clinical setting[11] or when using phenylephrine to vasoconstrict and increase blood pressure, the ability to obtain a reading was affected.[12]

CLINICAL USES

Pulse oximeters are a standard of care in human anesthesia and critical care. There is some controversy over the true benefit of this requirement but it would be difficult to get an estimate of its impact since it would now be almost impossible to eliminate access to this technology.[13-16] Most veterinary practices have at least one pulse oximeter, but it appears that understanding the information provided by the device is deficient.[17] It is important to recognize that pulse oximeters do not measure the amount of Hb present or the quantity of blood flow. It is quite possible for saturation to be normal but oxygen delivery inadequate if Hb concentration and/or cardiac output are low.

Measurement of SpO_2

This is the prime function of the device and can be useful in any animal in which there is a suspicion that SaO_2 might be abnormal. In the awake animal, probe placement to obtain a reliable reading can be difficult. There are 2 probe types used—transmission and reflectance. Transmission probes come in an array of conformations. Digital probes are designed for human fingers but can work well on the tongue or on small cat paws; ear lobe probes usually consist of a clip that holds the sending and receiving diodes on opposite sides and these are the most widely used type in veterinary medicine. There are also disposable, stick-on probes that have been designed for specific uses in people and can be adapted for animals. Once in place, these probes are less likely to move and may be more reliable than the clip-on probes. Transmission probes rely on placing the LED on one side of a piece of tissue and the receiving diode opposite that site so that the light is transmitted through the tissue to the receiver. For this to work an area of tissue needs to be found that is neither too thin nor too thick, that is not densely pigmented, that is not too hairy/furry (hair/fur may need to be clipped away to make it easier for the probe to work), and that has sufficient circulation to provide an adequate signal. Sites such as the ear, the lip, the tongue, the prepuce, the vagina, a toe, the skin between the Achilles tendon and the tibia, or the inguinal and axillary skin folds have all been used for this purpose with variable success.[7,11,18] In general it has been more difficult to obtain good readings from cats as compared with dogs.[18] Although some of the most technically advanced pulse oximeters can cope with patient motion, many older monitors consistently fail if an animal does not remain still, making it difficult to get reliable readings. Reflectance probes have the LEDs and receiving electrode on the same surface so the light is shone into the tissue and reflected back to the receiver. Rectal, esophageal, and skin surface probes have been developed using this approach. The skin surface probes will still fail with hairy/furry or densely pigmented skin, and the rectal and esophageal probes may fail because of insufficiently close contact with the mucosa[19] or, in the case of rectal probes, due to pigments in the rectum. The development of a reflectance probe that could be stuck to an animal's leg or body, had sufficient power to get a signal on pigmented skin, and could read while the animal was in motion would represent a significant advance for the application of pulse oximetry in awake animals. Pulse oximeters come in a variety of shapes and sizes and, as for other monitoring devices, it is best if the machine displays the waveform that it is using to estimate SpO_2. This allows the observer to ensure that the generated wave correlates with the pulse and is not full of artifactual peaks and valleys. Some monitors display a series of LEDs that light up according to the strength of the signal (often referred to as a "bouncing bar") that is less interpretable but better than having no display of the signal. Many pulse oximeters link the pitch of the pulse beep to the saturation, providing an immediate auditory cue to the person monitoring the patient.

Pulse oximetry in anesthetized animals would appear to be good for monitoring desaturation. However, when one examines the oxyhemoglobin dissociation curve (Figure 105-4), it is clear that Hb becomes almost fully saturated at a PaO_2 of about 100 mm Hg, which is achievable when breathing room air.

When an animal is breathing a high concentration of oxygen and has a PaO_2 of 500 mm Hg, the pulse oximeter should read 99% to 100%, and if something significant happens to the animal (e.g., pneumothorax, pulmonary edema, atelectasis) that decreases the PaO_2 to ~250 mm Hg, the pulse oximeter will likely continue to read 99% to 100%, and it will not get to an SpO_2 of 95% until PaO_2 gets to about 90 mm Hg.[20] This makes the tool a crude monitor for healthy

animals breathing >90% O_2, and the problem is compounded by the lack of reliability of the technology. It is common to see pulse oximeters giving SpO_2 values of <90% even when animals have SaO_2 values of 100%, and this leads the clinician or technician to distrust the readings to the extent that they try to fix the problem (e.g., move the probe to another site) without actually looking at the animal to see if there really is a low SaO_2 (cyanosis). On the other hand a pulse oximeter provides a continuous, noninvasive method of reading SpO_2, and in patients with the potential to desaturate (e.g., thoracotomy, bronchoscopy, animal breathing an FiO_2 <0.4), it is an essential component of being able to deliver safe care. The SpO_2 gives an indication of how much oxygen can be carried by the available Hb but it does not indicate how available that oxygen is to the animal. If the Hb dissociation curve is shifted to the left or the right, the actual PaO_2 at that saturation may be different than expected and consequently its availability to the tissues would vary (see Figure 105-4).

Measurement of Pulse Rate

Pulse oximeters count the heart rate off the pulse generated by the LEDs and diode system.[12] This can also be prone to artifact (venous pulses, rhythmic movement, panting) and so it is important to check that the indicated pulse rate matches the real pulse rate, because if the machine is not generating

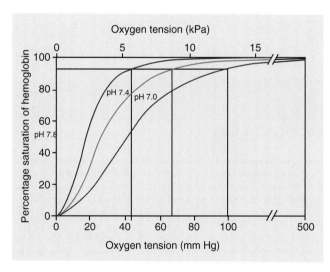

Figure 105-4 Oxyhemoglobin dissociation curves at three different pH values. At normal pH hemoglobin is ~97% saturated at a PO_2 of 100 mm Hg (e.g., breathing room air). When an animal is breathing 95% oxygen, its PaO_2 might be 500 mm Hg or higher and the graph indicates that, at normal pH (7.4), saturation will only decrease from 100% to 97% with a decrease in PO_2 from 500 to 100 mm Hg, showing that SpO_2 is a very insensitive monitor of these significant changes. The line at ~93% saturation shows that the PO_2 can vary significantly (~43 to 100 mm Hg) depending on the position of the dissociation curve.

Table • 105-1

Causes of Inaccurate Readings or Failure to Report a Value with Pulse Oximetry

CAUSE	SpO₂ vs. SaO₂
HbCO	Higher
MetHb	Falsely low at SaO₂s >85% and falsely high below 85%
HBOC	Dose-dependent increase in difference between SpO₂ and SaO₂
Skin pigment or fur/hair	No reading or higher
Motion	No reading with older machines. Newer machines can cope with some motion.
Hypoperfusion	No reading
Insufficient thickness of tissue	No reading
Anemia	No reading or readings become less accurate at packed cell volume <10%
High ambient light	No reading
Methylene blue, indocyanine green, isosulfan blue, indigo carmine, nitrobenzene and patent blue	Decreased
Probes misaligned or dirty	No reading or low value
Electrosurgical interference	False pulse rates and decreased SpO₂
Pressure on the probe	No reading or decreased SpO₂

HbCO, Carboxyhemoglobin; HBOC, hemoglobin-based oxygen carrying compound; MetHb, methemoglobin.

the correct value for this, it may also not be measuring the SpO$_2$ correctly.

Measurement of Blood Pressure

Since the pulse oximeter can display a pulse signal, it can be placed on a distal extremity and a cuff placed above this site to occlude blood flow. The cuff can be inflated to a point above systolic arterial blood pressure and then deflated while watching the plethysmographic trace on the pulse oximeter. Systolic pressure should be the pressure in the cuff where the trace returns. In one study, in cats, the pressure measured by this method had a greater correlation to mean pressure than to systolic pressure.[21] In dogs using the tongue as the measurement site the technique was neither accurate nor precise.[22]

COMPLICATIONS

Inaccurate Readings

Due to the fact that this is an indirect technique of measurement that is highly dependent on sophisticated technology,

there are many reasons why the readings obtained may be inaccurate. These are summarized in Table 105-1.

Burns

The diodes do not generate a lot of heat, but if circulation is poor and they are left at one location for a long time, the patient may be burned.[23,24] Other causes for burns associated with pulse oximeters have been by connection of probes by one manufacturer to a unit from another manufacturer[25] or when the skin has been sensitized to light (photodynamic therapy).[26]

REFERENCES

The reference list can be found on the companion Expert Consult Web Site at *www.expertconsult.com.*

CHAPTER **106**

Transtracheal Wash and Bronchoscopy

Brian C. Norman

Transtracheal wash and bronchoscopy are diagnostic procedures used in the diagnosis of bronchopulmonary airway disease. The transtracheal wash is used to obtain tracheobronchial cells and secretions for cytology and microbiologic evaluation. The bronchoscope is a more specific procedure that allows visualization of the trachea and airways while obtaining samples. The choice of procedure should be based on stability of the patient, diffuseness of disease, and operator skill level.

TRANSTRACHEAL WASH

A transtracheal wash can be performed in animals with a diffuse disease that cannot undergo prolonged sedation. The ventral portion of the patient's neck is clipped and aseptically prepared. The patient is then placed in sternal recumbency with an assistant holding the head and pointing the nose up. Sedation with propofol (Diprivan) or a short-acting barbiturate anesthetic is preferred. In dogs, a 16-gauge through-the-needle jugular catheter is inserted between proximal tracheal rings or the cricothyroid membrane and advanced down the airway. In cats, an open-end polypropylene urinary catheter or 5-F red rubber catheter can be placed through a sterile endotracheal tube. The catheter is slowly advanced down the trachea. Warm sterile saline is infused through the catheter: 5 mL is infused for cats and small dogs up to a maximum of 20 mL in large dogs. After 5 to 10 seconds, the operator attempts to retrieve the sample by applying gentle negative pressure several times with the syringe. Generally, 50% of the

original volume will be retrieved. Several drops of the sample should be placed on a culture swab for culture and sensitivity, and the remainder should be placed in a sterile tube or container for cytology.

Pneumomediastinum and subcutaneous emphysema are complications of this procedure that may need to be addressed.

BRONCHOSCOPY

Bronchoscopy is best performed with a flexible fiberoptic or video bronchoscope. The patient is anesthetized with propofol and maintained on a drip or gaseous anesthesia. In larger animals, an endotracheal tube may be placed and the bronchoscope can go through the tube. In smaller animals, the bronchoscope may be too large to pass through the endotracheal tube. After the animal is lightly anesthetized, the bronchoscope is inserted through the arytenoids and into the trachea. Inspection of the trachea should include the appearance of the mucosa, the amount of secretions, and any evidence of collapse. The carina should then be identified, and each lung lobe should be systematically examined (Figures 106-1 and 106-2). The operator must note the presence of mucus plugs, foreign bodies, dynamic collapse of airways, masses or nodules, and parasites.

The bronchoscope offers several options to sample the airways. The first method uses a bronchoscope brush. The brush is covered by plastic that can be pulled back once the brush is in its desired location. With the bronchoscope

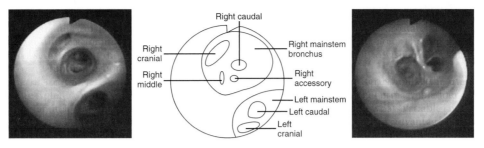

Figure 106-1 Diagram of normal bronchoscopic image of the division of the carina, demonstrating the position of the right and left main stem bronchi.

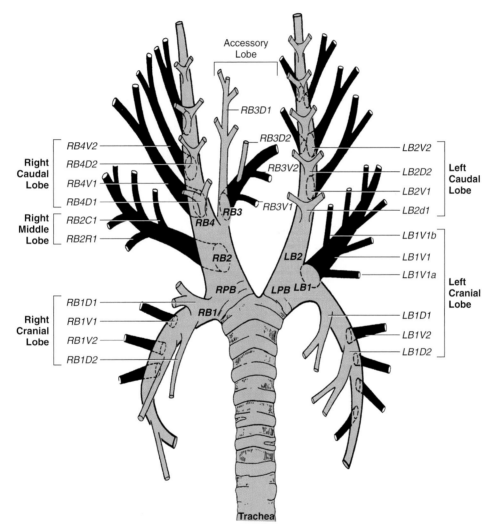

Figure 106-2 Diagram of normal bronchial anatomy in dogs. Each lobar bronchus is subdivided into segmental bronchi: *V1,* first ventral segmental bronchus; *V2,* second ventral segmental bronchus; *D1,* first dorsal segmental bronchus; *D2,* second dorsal segmental bronchus; *C1,* first caudal segmental bronchus; and *R1,* first rostral segmental bronchus. Segmental bronchi are subdivided into subsegmental bronchi: *V1a,* first subsegmental bronchus; *V1b,* second subsegmental bronchus. *LB1,* Lobar bronchus of left cranial lung lobe; *LB2,* lobar bronchus of left caudal lung lobe; *LPB,* left main stem bronchus; *RB1,* lobar bronchus of right cranial lung lobe; *RB2,* lobar bronchus of right middle lung lobe; *RB3,* lobar bronchus of accessory lobe; *RB4,* lobar bronchus of right caudal lung lobe; *RPB,* right main stem bronchus. (From Amis TC, McKiernan BC: Systematic identification of endobronchial anatomy during bronchoscopy in the dog. Am J Vet Res 47:2649, 1986.)

in the desired location, a small sampling brush is passed through the sampling channel. When the brush is visualized, the brush is extended and gently scraped against the airway. The brush is then pulled back into its casing and removed from the scope. The brush can be cultured and then gently rubbed on a glass slide for cytology.

The second sampling method uses a biopsy instrument. In a similar method, the bronchoscope is placed in the desired location and then the biopsy instrument is inserted into the sampling port. The bronchoscope is then used to guide the instrument to the desired location and the biopsy is taken. The sample can be submitted for culture and histopathology.

The third sampling method is bronchial or bronchoalveolar lavage. This is performed after all lobes have been inspected. The bronchoscope is directed into the desired lung and then advanced until it is wedged or is occluding the airway. The clinician should instill 10 to 30 mL of warm sterile saline into the sampling port, and (5 to 10 seconds later) aspirate the sample using a syringe. Approximately 40% to 50% of the sample should be retrieved. It is helpful if the patient is not heavily sedated. The lightly sedated animal will cough, producing a better sample. This procedure can be repeated several times. Several drops of the sample should be cultured, and the rest should be placed in sterile tubes for cytologic evaluation.

CHAPTER 107

Thoracic and Pericardial Taps and Drains

Jean-Paul Petrie

THORACOCENTESIS

Thoracocentesis is a simple procedure used to remove pleural air or fluid. If a significant amount of pleural effusion is identified by a combination of physical examination and radiographs or ultrasound, thoracocentesis should be performed (Figure 107-1).

If the patient is severely dyspneic and thoracic radiographs cannot be obtained safely, the clinician may observe a marked inspiratory effort, which is commonly observed in animals with a large volume of effusion. Thoracocentesis can be used for both diagnostic and therapeutic purposes. Potential contraindications to performing this technique include a severe coagulopathy, small volume effusions, and uncooperative patients. Potential complications include iatrogenic pneumothorax, hemothorax, and laceration of intrathoracic organs.

The two most common techniques are the "butterfly" catheter or fenestrated plastic catheter. The technique utilized depends on the size and body condition of the patient, the presence of air versus fluid, quantity of the pleural effusion, and the clinician's preference. In cats and small dogs, the "butterfly" technique is recommended. A 19- to 23-gauge

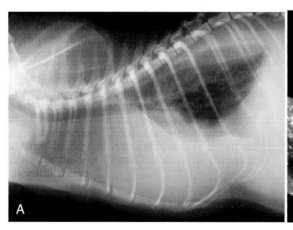
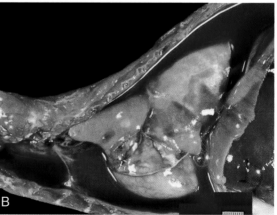

Figure 107-1 **A,** Right lateral radiograph of a cat that presented for dyspnea showing a large amount of pleural effusion. The intrathoracic structures are obscured by the pleural fluid. Thoracocentesis would be indicated in this patient. **B,** A gross pathology specimen of a cat with a large volume of pleural effusion. The orientation of the specimen corresponds to the radiograph shown in **A.** This picture illustrates the distribution of the fluid relative to the intrathoracic structures.

lobectomy. General anesthesia with endotracheal intubation is used, and close anesthetic monitoring is required because a moderate pneumothorax is induced during the procedure. VATS is performed more commonly in dogs than cats because of their larger body size. This technique requires specialized rigid telescopes, trocars, and endoscopic instruments, a light source, and a video monitor. Formal training is required to develop expertise in this procedure. Peripheral biopsies of a distal lung segment can be obtained with a stapling instrument or an endoscopic loop ligature. Alternatively, a lung lobe can be resected.

Lung biopsy of a peripheral segment can also be obtained through a modified (keyhole) thoracotomy. The animal should be placed under general anesthesia and surgically prepared. An intercostal thoracotomy is performed, and a wedge of lung is exteriorized. A biopsy sample is obtained by applying loop ligatures around the segment or by using a stapling device.

In an animal with a solitary mass lesion, consolidated lung lobe, central pulmonary infiltrate, or focal abnormality, exploratory thoracotomy with lung biopsy, partial lobectomy, or lung lobectomy may be required to obtain a diagnosis. A lateral intercostal approach on the side of the lesion provides the best access to structures in the immediate area and usually has the advantage of an uncomplicated approach and closure. The technique is associated with less postoperative discomfort than a sternotomy; however, it does not allow access to the entire contents of the chest cavity. Median sternotomy is performed when a complete thoracic cavity exploratory is required, but it is difficult to perform lung

lobectomy by this approach. In addition, access to hilar structures through a median sternotomy is limited in large, deep-chested dogs.

COMPLICATIONS

The most common complications of fine needle lung aspiration and percutaneous lung biopsy are pneumothorax and hemorrhage, although seeding of the pleural cavity with neoplastic cells is also of theoretical concern. Complications can occur when the technique is done either blindly or with ultrasound guidance, but the occurrence rate is substantially lower when small-gauge needles are used. Proper patient selection is also of critical importance, because animals with marked tachypnea and/or pronounced respiratory distress are more likely to develop pneumothorax. Highly agitated or fractious dogs or cats that are difficult to restrain are prone to hemorrhage, as are animals with coagulopathies or pulmonary hypertension. Sedation or anesthesia of fractious animals might improve the safety of the procedure.

The most serious complication of thoracoscopic lung biopsy is hemorrhage, which may require transition to an open thoracotomy. Complications of open lung biopsy are those associated with duration of anesthesia or respiratory depression. Chest tubes are placed after surgery, thus limiting the occurrence of pneumothorax. Hypotension, hypoxemia, and poor ventilatory recovery are potential postoperative problems.

CHAPTER 109

Electrocardiographic Techniques

João S. Orvalho

The electrocardiogram (ECG) is a recording of the electrical activity generated in the heart that is measured at the body surface. During the cardiac cycle the averaged electrical potentials of the myocardial cells result in a vector that acts as a dipole. The electrocardiograph (galvanometer) is able to record this dipole when a negative and a positive electrode are placed in or on the body, separated by a small distance containing the dipole. Most commonly these electrodes are positioned on the limbs of the animal, which represent an extension of the electrical field created by the heart.

LEAD SYSTEMS

The ECG records the average wavefront, which is seen as one large dipole and is constituted by multiple dipoles. The magnitude and direction of this wavefront can be determined by using multiple leads. A lead parallel to the direction of the wavefront will be represented as the largest deflection, and the one perpendicular to the wavefront will have the lowest or no deflection. For a point in time the cardiac electrical activity remains constant, but the positive and negative electrode changes from lead to lead. Each pair of electrodes is called a *lead*, and each lead illustrates the view from a different angle.

Standard Bipolar Leads
The standard leads (I, II, and III) are the most extensively used in veterinary electrocardiography and were the first fixed lead system to be proposed by Willem Einthoven, in 1902. This system consists of three bipolar leads that result from the placement of three electrodes: one on the right front leg, one on the left front leg, and another on the left hind leg. These leads provide information on frontal plane and form a triangle, named *Einthoven's triangle*.

The placement of the electrodes for the standard bipolar leads is shown in Table 109-1.

Augmented Unipolar Leads
The unipolar augmented leads are additional leads that use the same electrodes as the standard leads. These leads are generated by a positive electrode and a neutral reference point, which is the average of the other two electrodes. The unipolar leads record half of the voltage of the standard leads, and the electrocardiograph amplifies the deflections in order to make them comparable with the other leads. Therefore, these are augmented leads and an *a* precedes the designation (aVR, aVL, and aVF) (see Table 109-1).

Unipolar Precordial Chest Leads
The unipolar precordial chest leads use electrodes that record the electrical activity from the dorsal and ventral planes. A

Table • 109-1

Electrode Position for Standard and Augmented Leads

LEAD	POSITIVE	NEGATIVE/NEUTRAL
I	Left arm	Right arm
II	Left leg	Right arm
III	Left leg	Left arm
aVR	Right arm	Left arm, left leg
aVL	Left arm	Right arm, left leg
aVF	Left leg	Right arm, left arm

Table • 109-2

Electrode Position for Unipolar Precordial Chest Leads

LEAD	CHEST LOCATION
CV_5RL (V_1)	Fifth intercostal space, near sternum, right side
CV_6LL (V_2)	Sixth intercostal space, near sternum, left side
CV_6LU (V_4)	Sixth intercostal space, costochondral junction, left side
V_{10} (V_6)	Seventh thoracic vertebra, over spinous process

positive electrode is placed on the chest and is associated with another electrode (indifferent electrode) that generates a V lead. In humans six different V leads have been described (V_1 through V_6), which were modified for veterinary medicine (CV_5RL, CV_6LL, CV_6LU, and V_{10}). In animals these leads are especially useful for detecting p waves and right and left ventricular enlargement as well as identifying bundle branch blocks (Table 109-2).

Modified Orthogonal Lead Systems

The orthogonal lead system uses three leads perpendicular to each other (X, Y, and Z) that view the heart in three planes (frontal, sagittal, and transverse), creating a three-dimensional perspective of the cardiac electrical activity.

This system can be used to create a vectorcardiogram, which is a more accurate graphic representation of the cardiac vector. This is a cumbersome system that does not provide additional information and requires the use of multiple electrodes at very precise sites. Consequently, it is not commonly used in veterinary medicine.

ELECTROCARDIOGRAPHIC RECORDING

The patient should be placed on a nonconductive surface in right lateral recumbency. The limbs must be perpendicular to the body and slightly separated. The handler should rest the right arm over the patient's neck and the left arm over the hindquarters, as shown in Figure 109-1.

In a dyspneic or tachypneic patient, the ECG can be recorded in sternal or standing position. This recording can still be used for detection of rhythm abnormalities.

The electrodes are attached directly to the skin with alligator clips, electrode patches, or metal plates. The forelimb electrodes are placed proximal to the olecranon (elbow), and the hindlimb electrodes are attached to the patellar ligament

Table • 109-3

Electrocardiograph Color-Coded Cables

CABLE COLOR	LIMB
White	Right arm (RA)
Black	Left arm (LA)
Red	Left leg (LL)
Green	Right leg (RL)

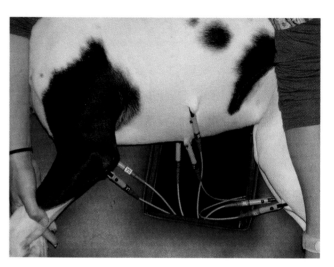

Figure 109-1 Patient in right lateral recumbency with standard leads and precordial chest leads.

(stifle). The skin and the electrodes should be moistened before the electrodes are placed, with alcohol or ECG paste. The limb electrodes are color coded and must be placed as illustrated in Table 109-3. The chest leads are placed over the patient's thorax in their specific sites (see Table 109-2).

Once the patient is positioned and the electrodes are appropriately attached, the ECG can be recorded. The electrocardiograph is usually calibrated so that a 1 mV signal generates a 10 mm deflection (standard calibration). This calibration can be changed to produce larger (double sensitivity: 1 mV corresponds to 20 mm) and smaller (half sensitivity: 1 mV corresponds to 5 mm) complexes.

An ECG can be recorded at any paper speed, but the most commonly used speeds are 25 mm/sec and 50 mm/sec. Measurements of intervals, wave duration and segments should be performed in lead II at 50 mm/sec, and rhythm recordings can be obtained at 25mm/sec. A minimum recording of three complexes is usually recommended for each lead, and if a dysrhythmia is observed a longer recording is advised. Filters can be applied to reduce baseline artifact, but should not limit high-frequency deflections. In dogs 50-Hz filters are usually appropriate, and 150-Hz filters should be used in cats. Technical and mechanical artifacts can lead to erroneous ECG interpretation; therefore it is very important to minimize potential artifacts caused by inappropriate patient positioning, electrical interference (60-Hz cycle), or respiratory, muscle tremor and movement artifacts.

REFERENCES

The reference list can be found on the companion Expert Consult Web site at *www.expertconsult.com*.

CHAPTER 110

Echocardiography

Marie-Claude Bélanger

Echocardiography is a unique noninvasive tool that provides a great deal of information about cardiac anatomy and function. Since its introduction in Sweden in 1953, clinical echocardiography has matured into new techniques and applications like tissue Doppler imaging, contrast, and transesophageal and three-dimensional (3-D) imaging. The following chapter focuses on the basics of transthoracic echocardiography in small animals.

PRINCIPLES OF ULTRASOUND PHYSICS

Propagation of sound waves is favored by fluids and soft tissue and inhibited by bone, metal, and air. The basic idea of any ultrasound is that the probe emits a pulse of sound that penetrates the target tissue. A portion of that emitted ultrasound will go through the organ and will be lost, whereas another portion of the ultrasound will be reflected back to the probe. If a lot of sound is reflected back, as from the myocardium for example, the structure is said to be *hyperechoic* and will appear on the screen as a whiter image. When very little of the sound is captured back, as in blood or blood vessels, the structure is called *hypoechoic* and appears dark on the screen.

The echocardiographic ultrasound beam is generated by a phased array transducer that consists of a series of small piezoelectric crystals that produce sound waves that travel in cycles. Sector scanning probes are usually preferred in echocardiography because of the necessity to use probes with small footprints that will allow imaging of the heart through narrow intercostal spaces (Figure 110-1).

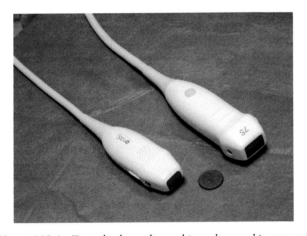

Figure 110-1 Typical echocardiographic probes used in cats and dogs. Small footprints allow imaging through narrow intercostal spaces of our small patients.

The frequency of a probe is determined by the number of cycles sent out per minute. High-frequency transducers emit more cycles per time unit and thus have shorter wavelengths. These transducers reflect sound from smaller structures and therefore produce a better image definition and resolution but less tissue penetration than low-frequency transducers. The choice of the transducer is determined by the size of the patient since tissue penetration is inversely proportional to the frequency of the probe. In other words, the higher the frequency of the probe, the less tissue penetration. Cats and small dogs usually require a 7.0-MHz transducer. A 5.0-MHz probe is appropriate for most dogs. Very large dogs may require a 3.5-MHz transducer to obtain optimal tissue penetration.

EQUIPMENT

The quality of images obtained from echocardiographic studies depends on the sophistication and technology of the ultrasound machine, skill and experience of the operator, as well as the individual patient characteristics. Better quality images are usually obtained with the animal in lateral recumbency. A special table with an opening that allows examination from beneath the animal is used to create a large and stable acoustic window (Figure 110-2, *A*).

This position allows gravity to improve the degree of contact between the cardiac structures and the chest wall. Echocardiograms can also be obtained from a standing position in giant-breed dogs.

TECHNIQUE

In animals, hair is usually clipped to improve skin contact and image quality and coupling gel is applied over the right or left precordial thoraces. Shaving is sometimes unnecessary in dogs with very short hair. Always warn breeders before shaving a show dog! The application of alcohol or water can sometimes replace the coupling gel since it provides good but briefer contact. The animal is gently restrained in lateral recumbency on a special table with an imaging opening (Figure 110-2, *B*). Sandbags can be placed over the caudal limbs to limit the need of an additional technician. The patient's forelimbs should be pulled cranially by a technician in order to keep the elbows out of the area of great interest. The probe is placed on the prepared area and twisted, tilted, or slid as needed to find a good window in order to optimize the quality of images from the cardiac structures.

An echocardiogram can usually be performed in dogs and cats without chemical restraint since the procedure is painless, quiet, and peaceful. On the other hand, sedation has the

WWW. To view a video on this topic, go to **www.expertconsult.com.**

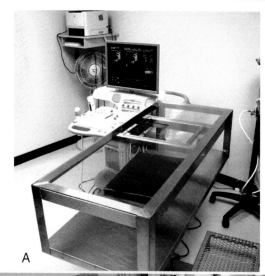

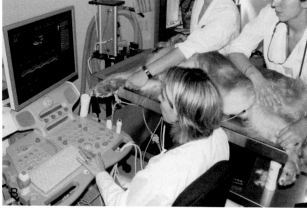

Figure 110-2 **A,** Typical examination setting for echocardio-graphic studies in veterinary medicine. Rectangular or circular cutouts allow the transducer to be introduced from the bottom of the scanning table. **B,** The animal is held in lateral recumbency with the shaved thoracic window over the hole. The examiner is scanning from the right parasternal location.

advantage of minimizing stress, examination time, and poor image quality in squirmy patients. Truly uncooperative, anxious, or aggressive animals in which an underlying cause of discomfort has not been found (e.g., painful joint disease or respiratory pathology) may require sedation. Animals with overt clinical signs of congestive heart failure should be clinically relieved with diuretics before the echocardiogram is performed. Table 110-1 describes different sedation protocols used for echocardiography.

THE NORMAL ECHOCARDIOGRAM: IMAGE ACQUISITION, STANDARD VIEWS AND SEQUENCE

A comprehensive echocardiography study includes two-dimensional (2-D), M-mode, and finally, Doppler imaging. The examination always starts with the 2-D study, which provides orientation, reference, and diagnostic clues to the M-mode and Doppler imaging. The most important information given by an echocardiogram often does not appear on the screen of the machine. It is essential to combine the echo

Table • 110-1

Suggested Sedation Protocols for Echocardiography

SITUATIONS	DRUGS
Canine Sedation Protocols	
Most asymptomatic dogs needing sedation	Hydromorphone 0.05 mg/kg + midazolam 0.2 mg/kg IM or IV
Aggressive asymptomatic dog	Hydromorphone 0.1 mg/kg + midazolam 0.2 mg/kg IM in the same syringe
If sedation needed rapidly	Butorphanol 0.3 mg/kg + diazepam 0.3 mg/kg IV (do not mix together and flush between drugs)
Puppies	Acepromazine 0.005 mg/kg (avoid in Boxers) + buprenorphine 0.01 mg/kg IV
	Or
	Hydromorphone 0.05 mg/kg + midazolam 0.2 mg/kg IM
Dog with congestive heart failure	Butorphanol 0.2 mg/kg + midazolam 0.2 mg/kg IM (treat with furosemide before ultrasound if dyspnea)
Feline Sedation Protocols	
Most asymptomatic cat needing sedation	Midazolam 0.2 mg/kg + hydromorphone 0.1 mg/kg IM in the same syringe
Aggressive asymptomatic cat	Acepromazine 0.05-0.1 mg/kg + hydromorphone 0.1 mg/kg SQ or IM
	Or in very aggressive cats: Medetomidine 20 µg/kg IM then reverse with atipamezole 100 µg/kg IM
Kittens	Hydromorphone 0.05 mg/kg + midazolam 0.1 mg/kg IM
Cat with congestive heart failure	Butorphanol 0.2 mg/kg + midazolam 0.2 mg/kg (or acepromazine 0.05 mg/kg if very uncooperative) IM (treat with furosemide before ultrasound if dyspneic)

findings with the observation of the patient itself. An accurate diagnosis combines a good physical examination and thorough history with an echocardiographic examination.

2-D ECHOCARDIOGRAPHY

2-D echocardiography is used to evaluate the cardiac structural changes resulting from congenital defects or cardiac diseases. It produces a real-time anatomic evaluation of the heart throughout the cardiac cycle. A complete 2-D study includes the imaging of all valves, great vessels, and relative size and wall thickness of the cardiac chambers.

COMMON 2-D ECHOCARDIOGRAPHIC POSITIONS

Most of the heart is covered by impenetrable structures such as bones (ribs and sternum) and lungs. However, the right lung does not cover the heart completely, and there is an area just dorsal to the sternum at the fourth or fifth intercostal space where the pericardium lies directly beneath the chest wall. This region is termed the *right parasternal window* or location. For most patients, placement of the probe over the thoracic area, where the heartbeat is palpable, is generally the best starting point. For canine brachycephalic breeds, where the thorax is ventrally compressed, the best acoustic window is obtained by placing the probe closer to the sternum or more ventrally than usual. The marker of the probe should be pointing toward the animal's shoulder in order to obtain a standard long-axis, four chamber view (Figure 110-3, *A*).

The views that are routinely performed from the right parasternal location are the long-axis four chamber view, the long-axis left ventricular outflow view, and the different short-axis views as described in Figures 110-3 and 110-4.

Conventionally, echocardiographic views are named from the positioning of the transducer and the structures that are examined (e.g., right parasternal long-axis view). The right parasternal, left cranial parasternal, left apical, and subcostal positions are used most often, but a multitude of planes can

be obtained to better visualize a distinct part of the heart. The subcostal or subxiphoid position is used to specifically evaluate the left ventricular outflow tract (LVOT) in the dog (Figure 110-5).

The image obtained from the subcostal view can often be improved by having the dog inhale after occluding its mouth and nostrils for 5 to 10 seconds. Inspiration lowers the diaphragm and pulls the heart down toward the transducer. The long-axis view is obtained by an imaging plane that transects the heart parallel to its long axis from apex to base, whereas a perpendicular imaging plane will be performed to obtain the short-axis view (see Figures 110-3 and 110-4). Technically, this means that the short-axis views can be obtained from the long-axis views by a 90° rotation of the probe. The echocardiographer must always adjust the depth and gain settings to optimize the image on the monitor. By convention, the heart, on a 2-D view, should occupy two thirds to three fourths of the screen.

The second half of the echocardiographic study consists of the left-sided views. One should ALWAYS perform the echocardiogram on both sides of the thorax. Evaluating only the right side is similar to the auscultation of only one lung; some information is gained but much information is missed! As opposed to the right parasternal location, there are two acoustic windows on the left side. The left cranial parasternal views are obtained at the level of the fourth intercostal space,

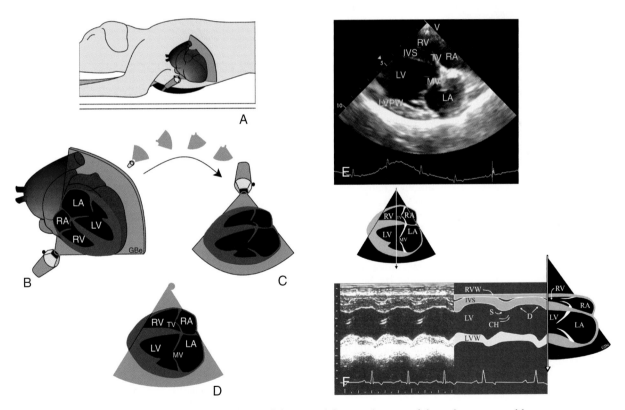

Figure 110-3 **A,** Typical positioning of the animal for visualization of the right parasternal long-axis view. In the dog, the long-axis of the heart is parallel to an imaginary line connecting the shoulder to the xiphoid. **B,** Spatial orientation of the right parasternal location, long-axis four chamber view. **C,** Spatial orientation of the right parasternal location, long-axis four chamber view as observed on the ultrasound monitor. **D,** Illustration of the different cardiac structures observed by this window. **E,** Real-time two-dimensional image of the right parasternal location, long-axis four chamber view. **F,** Corresponding M-mode image obtained from this window. The heart is seen as it fills and empties (diastole and systole). *IVS,* Interventricular septum; *LA,* left atrium; *LV,* left ventricle; *LVPW,* left ventricular wall; *MV,* mitral valve; *RA,* right atrium; *RV,* right ventricle; *RVW,* right ventricular wall; *TV,* tricuspid valve.

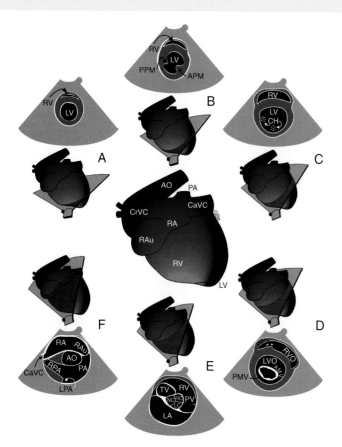

Figure 110-4 Standard two-dimensional echocardiographic study obtained from the right parasternal transducer location, short-axis views at the level of **(A)** the apex **(B)** the papillary muscles **(C)** the chordae tendineae *(CH)* **(D)** the mitral valve **(E)** the aorta **(F)** the pulmonary arteries. *AMV,* anterior mitral valve cusp; *APM,* anterior papillary muscle; *AS,* atrial septum; *CaVC,* caudal vena cava; *CrVC,* cranial vena cava; *IVS,* interventricular septum; *LA,* left atrium; *LC,* left coronary aortic cusp; *LPA,* left pulmonary artery; *LV,* left ventricle; *NC,* noncoronary aortic cusp; *PA,* pulmonary artery; *PMV,* posterior mitral valve cusp; *PPM,* posterior papillary muscle; *PV,* pulmonary valve; *RA,* right atrium; *RAu,* right auricle; *RC,* right coronary aortic cusp; *RPA,* right pulmonary artery; *RV,* right ventricle; *RVO,* right ventricular outflow; *S,* systole; *TV,* tricuspid valve. (Modified from Thomas WP, Gaber CE, Jacobs GJ: Recommendations for standards in transthoracic two-dimensional echocardiography in the dog and cat: Echocardiography Committee of the Specialty of Cardiology, American College of Veterinary Internal Medicine. J Vet Intern Med 7:247-252, 1993.)

whereas the left caudal (apical) parasternal views are best visualized from the fifth to sixth intercostal space of the animal (Figure 110-6).

M-MODE ECHOCARDIOGRAPHY

M-mode refers to real-time *motion-mode.* M-mode echocardiography is used to evaluate the phasic motion of the cardiac structures during the cardiac cycle. M-mode echocardiography is complementary to the 2-D echocardiogram since it has a higher sampling rate, allowing good resolution of rapidly moving structures. It is especially useful to record subtle changes in wall and valve motion and to perform accurate measurements of chamber diameters and wall thicknesses. The M-mode image is viewed on a video screen, where depth

of the structures is plotted on the Y axis and time is shown on the X axis. Only the structures transected by the cursor are seen on the M-mode images. The steerable cursor scrolls across the heart, and the associated changes in thickness or position of the structures are recorded on the screen as the heart fills and contracts (Figure 110-7; see Figure 110-3, *F*).

In veterinary medicine, M-mode echocardiography is generally performed only from the right parasternal location. The usual M-mode echocardiogram includes an evaluation of the left ventricle (see Figures 110-3, *F,* and 110-7), mitral valve, and aortic root (Figure 110-8).

As recommended by the American Society of Echocardiography (ASE), end-diastolic measurements are taken at the onset of the QRS complex and end-systolic measurements are made at the level of the maximum excursion of the interventricular septum. The *leading edge* method is used (i.e., the measurements of each echo line are made beginning at the edge that is closest to the transducer). The sonographer should be aware that a tremendous potential exists for artefactual measurements when the M-mode image is obtained in a suboptimal plane (e.g., tangential slices).

The left ventricular M-mode study provides absolute measurements of the left ventricular walls and chamber during systole and diastole (Tables 110-2 through 110-5). It can be performed using the right parasternal long-axis four chamber view or the right parasternal short-axis view at the level of the papillary muscles (see Figure 110-7). These M-mode measurements are also used to calculate the ejection phase indices as described in the section on the evaluation of systolic function.

DOPPLER ECHOCARDIOGRAPHY

Spectral and color flow Doppler imaging are used to evaluate blood flow velocity and direction within the heart and great vessels. The first description of the physical principles used in Doppler echocardiography was made by the Austrian mathematician Johann Christian Doppler during the 19th century. The Doppler principle relies on the fact that the transducer generates ultrasound waves that are reflected by the red blood cells. The change in frequency between sound transmitted by the transducer and sound received by it is called the *Doppler shift* (Δf). Since velocity = frequency × wavelength, the magnitude of the Doppler shift is directly proportional to red blood cell (RBC) velocity:

$$\Delta f = \frac{2f_0 \times V \times \cos\Theta}{C}$$

Where f_0 is the frequency transmitted by the transducer; V is the flow velocity of RBC (m/sec); Θ is the intercept angle; and C is the speed of sound in blood (1540 m/sec).

One experiences the Doppler effect every day. For example, when standing on an overpass, we hear the sound of a car approaching toward us at a higher pitch than the sound we hear when the same car is moving away from the overpass. The engine is emitting the same sound when passing under the overpass, but we hear a change in pitch dependent upon the speed and the direction of the car (Figure 110-9).

When the transmitted sound waves encounter red blood cells moving toward the transducer, they are reflected back at a frequency higher than that at which they were sent, producing a positive Doppler shift or positive deflection on the screen (Figure 110-10).

The opposite effect occurs when the sound waves hit red blood cells moving away from the transducer, producing a negative Doppler shift. Doppler echocardiography assesses direction and velocity of blood flow. Blood moving toward

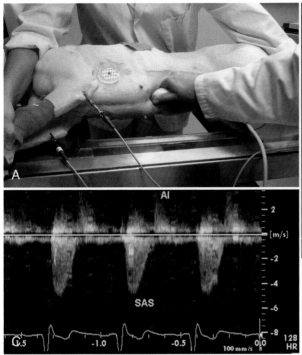

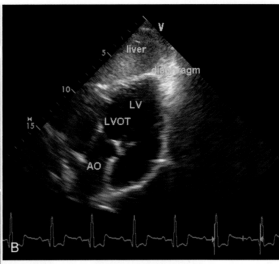

Figure 110-5 **A,** Positioning for the probe for the subcostal view. **B,** Real-time two-dimensional imaging of the subcostal view. **C,** Left ventricular systolic outflow velocity is measured with continuous wave Doppler from the subcostal view, in a dog with severe subaortic stenosis. *AI,* Aortic insufficiency; *AO,* aorta; *LV,* left ventricle; *LVOT,* left ventricular outflow tract; *SAS,* subaortic stenosis.

the transducer creates a positive frequency shift encoded in red on color Doppler and is displayed above the baseline of spectral Doppler. Blood flow moving away from the transducer is blue and is inversely displayed as a negative flow profile under the baseline (see Figure 110-10).

Spectral Doppler

Cardiac spectral Doppler study uses imaging planes that align the sound beam along the blood flow. A marker is represented on the cursor line that corresponds to the sampling volume or *gate* where the flow is interrogated. The parallel beam positioning is in contrast to the M-mode, in which the beam is oriented in a perpendicular manner to visualize the cardiac structures. When performing Doppler studies, care should be taken to align the Doppler beam with the jet flow (intercept angle <20°) in order to minimize the underestimation of flow velocity. Parallel alignment of the ultrasound beam measures the true or maximum velocity of the blood flow. In contrast, perpendicular alignment to flow will give a velocity of zero. Therefore, a wider angle of interrogation will result in a false reduction in the measured velocity as compared to the real velocity (Figure 110-11).

Flow signals are displayed with time on the horizontal axis and velocity on the vertical axis. Two types of spectral Doppler are used clinically: pulsed wave Doppler (PW) and continuous-wave Doppler (CW). An intermediate between PW and CW Doppler, called *high pulse-repetition frequency* (HPRF), is another type of spectral Doppler that is used less frequently. Spectral Doppler is helpful in the assessment of pressure gradients, intracardiac chamber pressure, regurgitant fractions, shunt ratios, valve area/effective orifice area, and cardiac output.

In veterinary medicine, spectral Doppler is often used to calculate *instantaneous pressure gradients* (ΔP) across a stenotic area or regurgitant valve. The maximum pressure gradient is calculated from the maximum flow jet velocity (v) using the modified Bernoulli equation:

$$(\Delta P) = 4v^2$$

The peak pressure gradient is used in combination with the determination of the effective orifice area and other 2-D and M-mode echocardiographic findings in the clinical assessment of stenosis severity (see specific section on aortic and pulmonary stenoses).

Pulsed Wave Doppler

PW Doppler uses a single crystal transducer that transmits and receives the Doppler signal. Short pulses of ultrasound are produced and the returning echoes from a small sample segment (called *sample volume*) along the ultrasound beam are analyzed (Figure 110-12).

The main advantage of PW Doppler is the possibility of interrogation of direction, velocity, and spectral characteristics (laminar versus turbulent) of the blood flow from a distinct anatomic region of the heart or blood vessels. Laminar flows are characterized by the similarity of the red blood cell velocities within the blood vessel or heart, which creates a Doppler signal with less disparity in velocity and little spectral broadening, as shown in Figure 110-13.

Due to friction, blood flow is always slightly slower near the walls of a vessel, which gives the signal a typical parabolic profile. Flow across the cardiovascular system is normally laminar and rarely exceeds 2 m/sec in dogs and cats. Turbulent flow profiles are broad, and the area under the curve is filled in because the transducer is receiving many frequency shifts associated with variable velocities (Figure 110-14).

Turbulence is present where there is some obstruction resulting in alteration of the laminar profile. Red blood cell

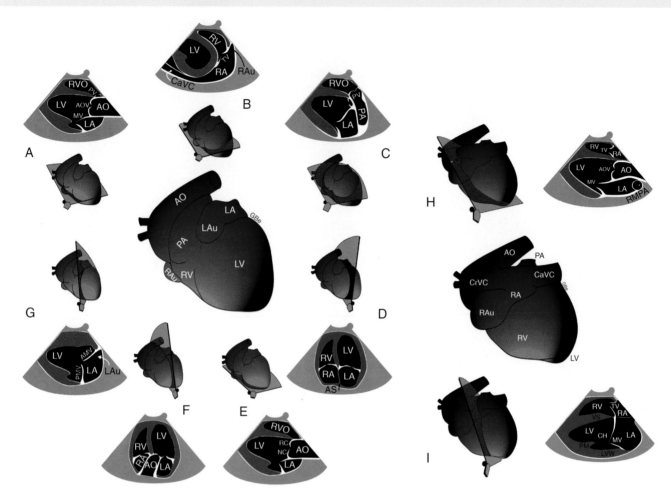

Figure 110-6 Standard two-dimensional long-axis views. **A,** Left cranial parasternal view optimized for the aortic root. **B,** Left cranial parasternal view optimized for right atrium and auricle. **C,** Left cranial parasternal view optimized for the right ventricular outflow tract and main pulmonary artery. **D,** Four chamber inflow view from the left caudal (apical) parasternal position. **E,** Left caudal (apical) parasternal view optimized for visualization of the left ventricular outflow tract. **F,** Five chamber left ventricular outflow view from the left caudal (apical) parasternal position. **G,** Left caudal (apical) parasternal location, two chamber view optimized for visualization of the left ventricular inflow and left auricle. **H,** Left ventricular outflow view from the right parasternal position. **I,** Four chamber right parasternal long-axis view. *AO,* Aorta; *AOV,* aortic valve; *AMV,* anterior mitral valve cusp; *AS,* atrial septum; *CaVC,* caudal vena cava; *CH,* chordae tendineae; *LA,* left atrium; *LAu,* left auricle; *LV,* left ventricle; *LVW,* left ventricular wall; *MV,* mitral valve; *NC,* noncoronary aortic cusp; *PA,* pulmonary artery; *PM,* papillary muscle; *PMV,* posterior mitral valve cusp; *PV,* pulmonary valve; *RA,* right atrium; *RAu,* right auricle; *RC,* right coronary aortic cusp; *RMPA,* right pulmonary artery; *RV,* right ventricle; *RVO,* right ventricular outflow; *TV,* tricuspid valve. (Modified from Thomas WP, Gaber CE, Jacobs GJ: Recommendations for standards in transthoracic two-dimensional echocardiography in the dog and cat: Echocardiography Committee of the Specialty of Cardiology, American College of Veterinary Internal Medicine. J Vet Intern Med 7:247-252, 1993.)

motion becomes disorganized and produces various eddies and whirls or different velocities and directions. Turbulent flow is usually indicative of an underlying pathology.

The disadvantage of PW Doppler is that it relies on a maximum measurable velocity called the *Nyquist limit*, which cannot be exceeded because of a limited pulse repetition frequency. In other words, PW Doppler is only accurate when measuring low velocities. A simple change of probe can sometimes overcome this limitation. It is important to realize that the Nyquist limit is determined by the frequency of the transducer used. A lower frequency probe increases the ability to record higher velocities at any given range. The main drawback of this trick is a reduction in the quality of the output. Interrogation of a high velocity, as seen in stenotic valvular

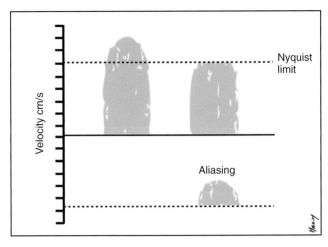

Figure 110-15 Illustration of the "aliasing phenomenon" caused by the interrogation of a flow velocity exceeding the maximum recordable velocity (or Nyquist limit) with a given probe using pulsed wave Doppler.

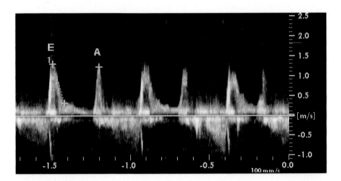

Figure 110-16 Spectral Doppler recording of a normal mitral flow obtained from the left apical position with the pulsed wave Doppler gate located in the left ventricular inflow tract. The E point represents the rapid ventricular filling. The A wave corresponds to the atrial contraction.

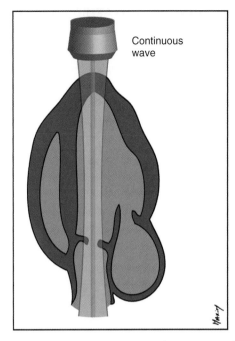

Figure 110-17 Continuous wave Doppler measures all velocities along the cursor line.

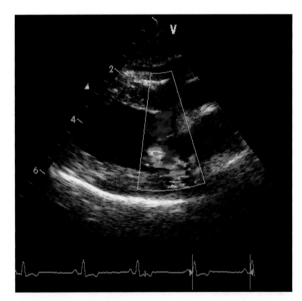

Figure 110-18 Color-flow Doppler recording from the mitral valve of a dog with chronic mitral valve disease, showing a jet of mitral regurgitation.

Table • 110-6

Normal Values for Spectral Doppler Velocities in Dogs and Cats (m/sec)

	CANINE	FELINE
Mitral Valve		
Peak E wave	0.8-1.0	0.55-0.77
Peak A wave	0.5-0.7	0.44-0.60
Aortic Valve		
Peak systolic velocity	≤2.0	≤1.2
Pulmonic Valve		
Peak systolic velocity	≤1.5	≤1.2
Tricuspid Valve		
Peak E wave	0.8-0.9	—
Peak A wave	0.5-0.6	—

These guidelines are based on the author's experience and published data.

tial imaging of cardiac structures is a common pitfall of the echocardiographic study. Some artefactual images can be mistaken as masses or pseudomasses. A simple way to differentiate a real mass from an artefact is to examine the perpendicular plane where that mass is seen. If the mass cannot be confirmed in the perpendicular plane, then it is not real. Again, the most common cause of a false-negative echocardiogram is failure to examine the heart completely (i.e., from multiple windows). Many publications describing common echocardiographic artefacts in animals are available elsewhere.

SPECIAL ECHOCARDIOGRAPHIC TECHNIQUES

Other echocardiographic techniques can provide useful information in the imaging of the canine and feline heart. These techniques include tissue Doppler imaging, contrast, and transesophageal and three-dimensional echocardiography. Although very useful in the clinical setting, some of these imaging methods have a limited application in veterinary medicine since they require expensive equipments. Transesophageal echocardiography necessitates general anesthesia, which increases the time and cost (and a potential danger) of the procedure.

Doppler Tissue Imaging (DTI)

DTI assesses the velocity of the myocardium tissue motion rather than conventional Doppler evaluation of blood flow velocity. DTI is especially useful in evaluating diastolic function because the diastolic velocity of the heart muscle is much less dependent on preload conditions than transmitral flow. The pattern of myocardial motion is similar but inverted and slower than the transmitral flow (Figure 110-20).

LV myocardial Doppler tissue signals are recorded on the left apical four chamber view using PW Doppler. The sample can be located at the levels of the mitral annulus, basal ventricular wall, and apex. DTI is now commonly used in veterinary cardiology, particularly in the evaluation of feline hypertrophic cardiomyopathy.

Transesophageal Echocardiography (TEE)

TEE uses a specialized transducer mounted on a flexible, steerable endoscope tip. The heart is imaged through the esophageal wall (Figure 110-21).

TEE is considered a complementary technique that allows better imaging of cardiac structures above the atrioventricular node such as the atria and pulmonary veins. The image quality is improved with TEE because of closer proximity of the cardiac structures to the transducer and the lack of intervening lung and bone structures. TEE is also very helpful in assisting many interventional cardiology procedures (Figure 110-22).

Three-Dimensional Echocardiography (3-DE)

3-DE is not yet a standard part of the routine clinical examination in animals and humans. It provides a more detailed anatomic description of cardiac defects and masses (Figure 110-23) and more accurate quantification of chamber volumes (Figure 110-24).

During 3-DE, the cardiac structures are shown in relationship to each other in all three spatial dimensions. Four-dimensional echocardiography has recently become available and refers to 3-DE performed in real-time display.

Contrast Echocardiography

Contrast echocardiography is another useful imaging method in the clinical evaluation of the cardiovascular system. It has four main applications: detection of shunts, enhancement of Doppler signals, left ventricular opacification, and myocardial perfusion.

The microbubble technique was the first contrast echocardiography to be performed. Microbubbles obtained from the agitation of two connected syringes filled with 3 to 10 mL of physiologic saline can be injected in a peripheral vein to confirm right-to-left intracardiac shunting. Microbubbles reflect ultrasound and do not cross pulmonary or systemic capillaries. They are reabsorbed by the pulmonary capillaries.

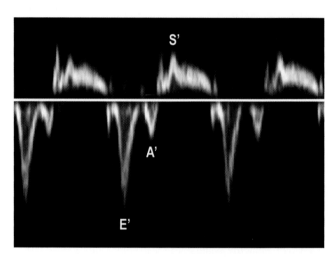

Figure 110-20 Doppler tissue imaging display of the lateral mitral valve annulus. *E'* and *A'* represent the diastolic motion, and *S'* corresponds to the systolic motion.

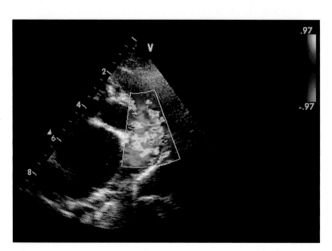

Figure 110-19 Turbulent mosaic in the pulmonary artery of a puppy with patent ductus arteriosus.

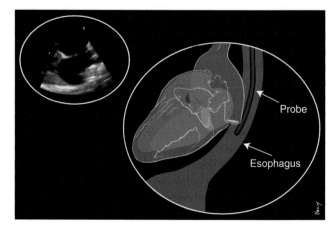

Figure 110-21 Illustration of transesophageal echocardiography with a two-dimensional real-time imaging of an atrial septal defect in a dog.

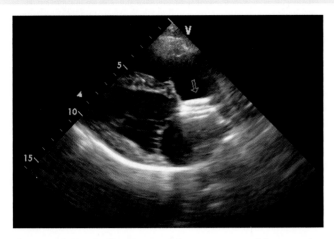

Figure 110-22 Right parasternal long-axis view of the same dog after amplatzer prosthesis insertion to correct the atrial septal defect.

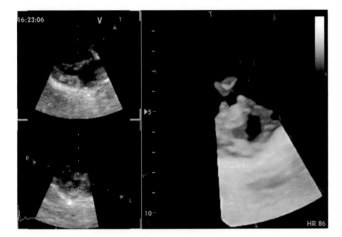

Figure 110-23 Three-dimensional echocardiogram from a dog with chronic mitral valve disease showing a thickened valve *(arrow)*.

Therefore, the microbubbles injected in the cephalic vein will stay on the right side of the heart in a normal patient. When right-to-left shunting is present, microbubbles will also be observed in the left side of the heart. Agitated saline is still the preferred contrast agent for the right side of the heart.

Recently, real contrast agents have been used in echocardiography to improve diagnostic accuracy. These agents are injected into the bloodstream producing an opacification of the cardiac chambers or increasing the echo density of the myocardium. Contrast agents are mostly used for left-sided studies and consist of low-solubility fluorocarbon gas in stabilized microbubbles encapsulated with denatured albumin.

EVALUATION OF CARDIAC STRUCTURES AND FUNCTION

Cardiac Size and Chamber Dilation

Cardiac chamber dimensions are determined by M-mode echocardiography and sometimes 2-D echocardiography. Table 110-7 summarizes the most common etiologies for anomalies in chamber size.

The *left atrial–to-aortic ratio* (LA:Ao ratio) is used to estimate the degree of left atrial enlargement. The M-mode method compares the diameter of the left atrium in systole to the diameter of the aorta in diastole. This ratio is best obtained from the right parasternal short-axis view, but it may also be evaluated from the right parasternal long-axis view. The M-mode LA:Ao ratio is criticized because of the subjectivity of the cursor placement. This method underestimates the left atrial size when the cursor does not reach the body of the left atrium. Conversely, it overestimates the relative left atrial size when a tangential plane of the aorta is performed. The reported M-mode LA:Ao ratio in normal dogs and cats is <1.3. A more accurate 2-D echocardiographic method has been described by Rishniw for estimation of left atrial size in adult dogs. This method measures the LA:Ao ratio from the right parasternal short-axis view of the aorta and left atrium when the aortic valve is closed. The internal diameter of the aorta is measured along the commissure

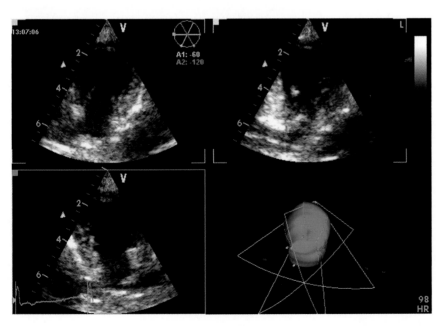

Figure 110-24 Three-dimensional evaluation of the left ventricular systolic and diastolic volumes using Simpson's rule from the left apical view.

Table • 110-7

Common Causes of Chamber Anomalies

	DILATION	REDUCTION	HYPERTROPHY
LV	Volume overload	Volume depletion	Pressure overload
	Mitral regurgitation	Severe dehydration	Aortic stenosis
	Right-to-left shunting	Hypoadrenocorticism	Hypertension
	Aortic insufficiency	Hypovolemic shock	Hypertrophic cardiomyopathy
	Dilated cardiomyopathy	Inadequate blood return to the left heart	Infiltrative myocardial disease
	High output stage	Dirofilariasis	
	Hyperthyroidism	Tetralogy of Fallot	
	Anemia		
RV	Volume overload	Cardiac tamponade	Pressure overload
	Tricuspid regurgitation	Volume depletion	Pulmonic stenosis
	Atrial septal defect		Tetralogy of Fallot
	Dilated cardiomyopathy		Cor pulmonale
			Pulmonary hypertension
			Dirofilariasis
			Feline hypertrophic cardiomyopathy
			Feline restrictive cardiomyopathy
LA	Chronic degenerative mitral valve disease		
	Dilated cardiomyopathy		
	Left-to-right shunting		
	Mitral stenosis		
	Mitral dysplasia		
RA	Tricuspid regurgitation/dysplasia		
	Dilated cardiomyopathy		
	Dirofilariasis		
	Right-to-left shunting		
	Tricuspid stenosis		
	Cor pulmonale		
	Pulmonary hypertension		

LA, Left atrium; *LV,* left ventricle; *RA,* right atrium; *RV,* right ventricle.

between the noncoronary and right coronary aortic valve cusps after aortic valve closure (Figure 110-25).

The left atrial internal diameter is measured from a line parallel to the commissure between the noncoronary and left coronary aortic valve cusps to the distant margin of the left atrium. A LA : Ao ratio >1.6 in dogs and >1.5 in cats suggests left atrial dilation.

Systolic Function

Virtually all forms of cardiac disease are associated with a certain degree of systolic and diastolic dysfunction. Evaluation of these dysfunctions provides valuable prognostic information. Systolic function in all cases should be part of the routine echocardiogram. Many techniques to indirectly assess systolic dysfunction have been described in the literature. The following parameters are those that are frequently used in clinical veterinary cardiology.

The ejection phase indices are often used to evaluate LV performance. They are calculated from linear M-mode measurements and include the *fractional shortening*, the *velocity of circumferential fiber shortening*, the *stroke volume*, and the *ejection fraction*. The *end-systolic diameter* is also by itself a good indicator of LV performance and it is a more specific index of myocardial contractility than the fractional shortening. M-mode methods of volume determination have a poor cor-

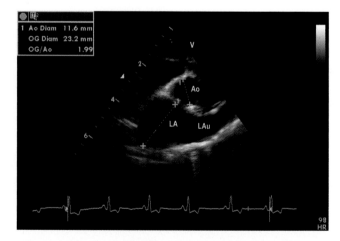

Figure 110-25 Two-dimensional measurement of the left atrium–to-aortic root ratio from the right parasternal short-axis view of the aorta *(Ao)* and left atrium *(LA)*. The calculated ratio of 1.99 indicates a significant LA dilation in this dog with chronic mitral valve disease. *LAu,* Left auricle.

relation with more invasive methods, so these indices should rather be calculated from 2-D–specific evaluations. Also, the examiner should always remember that these indices are significantly influenced by ventricular loading conditions (preload and afterload).

Fractional shortening Fractional shortening (FS) is the percent change in diameter of the ventricular cavity from diastole to systole. It provides a rough index of cardiac function. The FS is the clinical index used most commonly in the evaluation of global inotropism and systolic function in veterinary medicine. Normal values in dogs range from 27% to 48%, but there is a great variation among breeds. FS is calculated as follows:

$$FS(\%) = \frac{EDD - ESD}{EDD} \times 100$$

where *EDD* is the left ventricular internal dimension at the end of diastole and *ESD* is the left ventricular internal dimension at the end of systole.

Velocity of circumferential fiber shortening The velocity of circumferential fiber shortening (V_{cf}) measures the rate of change in the circumference (circ) of the LV during systole. It is calculated as follows:

$$V_{cf}(circ/sec) = \frac{EDD - ESD}{EDD \times LVET}$$

where *LVET* is the LV ejection time (see Systolic Time Intervals, below). Normal values for V_{cf} are 1.6 to 2.8 circ/sec in dogs and 1.3 to 4.5 circ/sec in cats.

Left ventricular volumes Determination of left ventricular volumes (LVV) and derived ejection fraction is essential to evaluate the systolic function. Many experimental models and formulas have been described in the canine patient to assess LVV by use of M-mode and 2-D echocardiography. Left ventricular end-diastolic volume (LVV_{ED}) and end-systolic volume (LVV_{ES}) can be estimated by the Teichholz method, the bullet method, and the disc summation method (i.e., Simpson's rule). The latter is considered the more accurate echocardiographic method in veterinary medicine. As discussed above, M-mode–derived Teichholz's method is less accurate since many of the volumetric estimates are calculated from only one dimension, which is certainly not ideal in a diseased heart. The Teichholz method calculates the end-systolic and end-diastolic volumes as follows:

$$LVV_{ES} = \frac{7(ESD^3)}{2.4 + ESD} \quad LVV_{ED} = \frac{7(EDD^3)}{2.4 + EDD}$$

This formula takes into consideration that the short axis of the left ventricle widens more than the long axis when the heart dilates. The ASE recommends the use of 2-D methods involving fewer geometric assumptions, such as in the disk summation method (Figure 110-26).

This method is especially more accurate when the heart has an irregular, enlarged, or asymmetrical shape as in many of the canine and feline cardiomyopathies.

Stroke volume The *stroke volume* (SV) and, ultimately, the cardiac output can be calculated from the LV end-systolic and end-diastolic volumes. SV is computed as follows:

$$SV(mL) = LVV_{ED} - LVV_{ES}$$

Ejection fraction The *ejection fraction* (EF) is a rough index of LV cardiomyocyte shortening, since it is the percentage of the LVV_{ED} ejected with each heart beat. It also corresponds to the 3-D volumetric equivalent of the FS. The EF is the ratio of the left ventricular SV to the LVV_{ED} as calculated here:

$$EF(\%) = \frac{LVV_{ED} - LVV_{ES}}{LVV_{ED}} \times 100$$

E-point to septal separation *E-point to septal separation* (EPSS) is also a useful parameter in the assessment of left ventricular dilation and systolic dysfunction. EPSS measures the distance from the maximum opening of the mitral valve (E point) to the endocardial aspect of the interventricular septum (Figure 110-27).

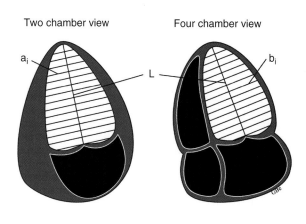

$$V = \frac{\pi}{4} \sum_{i=1}^{n} a_i b_i \frac{L}{n}$$

Figure 110-26 Disk summation method to estimate left ventricular volumes.

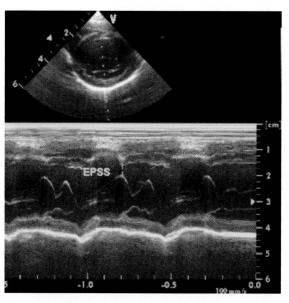

Figure 110-27 E-point to septal separation *(EPSS)* measurement. A line is drawn between the interventricular septum and the maximum initial opening of the mitral valve (E point).

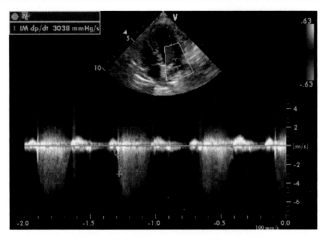

Figure 110-28 Measurement of LV dP/dt from a continuous wave Doppler tracing of a dog with mitral regurgitation.

In the normal heart, the mitral valve opens in diastole and its anterior leaflet almost contacts the interventricular septum. In dilated hearts, where there is decreased contractility (such as in dilated cardiomyopathy), the mitral valve does not reach the septum. Reports in human medicine have shown that the size of the left ventricle alone does not alter the EPSS unless systolic dysfunction is present.

LV dP/dt   The calculation of *LV dP/dt* has proven to be a sensitive and accurate method to assess LV systolic function. It represents the rate of increase in the LV pressure. When measured during the isovolumetric contraction, it is a relatively load-independent measure of ventricular inotropy. LV dP/dt is often calculated from the spectral display of a mitral regurgitation signal (Figure 110-28).

To determine dP/dt, one calculates the time difference from the point at which the velocity is 1 m/sec and 3 m/sec. The time between these two time points represents the period during which a known amount of pressure (usually 32 mm Hg) is gained in the LV. A reduced dP/dt indicates a decreased contractility. dP/dt is calculated as follows:

$$dP/dt = 32 \text{ mm Hg} \div time(seconds)$$

Systolic time intervals   Systolic time intervals (STI) are other indices used in the assessment of global LV function. They are obtained by simultaneous recording of the ECG and M-mode echocardiogram of the aortic valve (Figure 110-29).

Three intervals are routinely measured during systole. The preejection period (PEP) is the time between the ventricular depolarization (initial deflection of the QRS) and the onset of LV ejection, which corresponds to the opening of the aortic valve. PEP represents the isovolumetric contraction time. LVET is the time length of aortic valve opening, which is measured from the aortic valve opening to its closure. LVET is determined by the SV and the rate of flow. Generally, improvement of LV systolic performance is characterized by a shortening of the PEP or decreased isovolumetric contraction time and a prolongation of the LVET, which corresponds to an improved SV. Total electromechanical systole (QAVC interval) is the interval of time between the beginning of the Q wave and the aortic valve closure. In other words, QAVC is the sum of PEP + LVET. One should remember that the STI are affected by heart rate (HR) and preload or afterload variations. The PEP/LVET index is therefore recommended

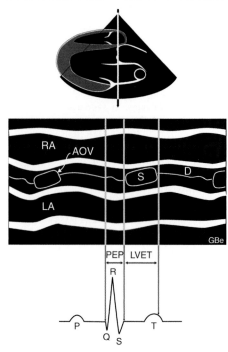

Figure 110-29 Illustration of the method used to evaluate the systolic time intervals. *AOV*, Aortic valve; *D*, diastole; *LA*, left atrium; *LVET*, left ventricular ejection time; *PEP*, preejection period; *RA*, right atrium; *S*, systole.

Table • 110-8

Normal Values for Left Ventricular Systolic Time Intervals (STI) in Dogs and Cats

STI (ms)	CANINE*	FELINE†
PEP	54 ± 7	44 ± 9
LVET	159 ± 15	116 ± 11
PEP/LVET	0.34 ± 0.05	0.38 ± 0.08
QAVC	214 ± 18	—

LVET, Left ventricular ejection time; *PEP*, preejection period; *QAVC*, total electromechanical systole.
*From Atkins JE, Snyder PS: Systolic time interval and their derivatives for the evaluation of cardiac function. J Vet Intern Med 6:55-63, 1992.
†From Fox PR, Bond BR, Peterson ME: Echocardiographic reference values in healthy cats sedated with ketamine hydrochloride. Am J Vet Res 46:1479-1484, 1985.

since it is less influenced by these loading parameters. Normal values for STI are shown in Table 110-8.

Cardiac output   2-D and Doppler echocardiography can be used to calculate the *cardiac output* (CO), which ultimately reflects global LV performance. The *cardiac index* is the CO indexed for body surface area (BSA) in order to take into account body size variation between animals. BSA is calculated from body weight using the formula:

$$BSA = (10.1 \times w^{2/3}) \times 10^{-4}$$

where *w* is body weight in grams. CO is product of HR and SV:

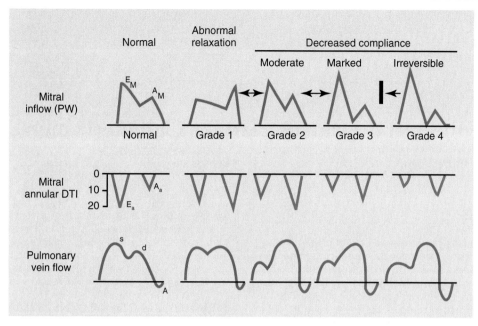

Figure 110-30 Schematic representation of various mitral inflow, mitral annular Doppler tissue imaging *(DTI)*, and pulmonary vein flow profiles. *PW,* Pulsed wave. (Modified from Feigenbaum H: Feigenbaum's echocardiography, ed 6, Philadelphia, 2005, Lippincott Williams and Wilkins, p 170.)

$$CO = HR \times SV$$

CO can be calculated from the SV determined by the assessment of LVV by Simpson's rule. The continuity equation can also be used to evaluate the CO by use of Doppler. It is based on the theory of conservation of mass applied to fluids, which specifies that flow through a given area of a conduit must equal flow through an adjacent area over a given time. Accordingly, SV ejected through a valvular orifice during systole is equal to the flow that passes through the valve as expressed by this equation:

$$SV = A \times VTI$$

where *A* is the cross-sectional area of the orifice calculated from the diameter measured by 2-D echocardiography and *VTI* is the velocity-time integral of the pulsed-Doppler signal across the valvular orifice.

$$A = D^2 \times (\pi/4)$$

$$CO = HR \times D^2(\pi/4) \times VTI$$

Virtually any valve or area in the heart can be used to estimate the CO, but the left ventricular outflow tract and the aortic valve are used most often.

Diastolic Function

There are many echocardiographic techniques described in the contemporary literature to assess diastolic function. Currently in veterinary medicine, Doppler techniques evaluating transmitral flow profiles (E and A waves) or pulmonary vein flow profiles (S, D, A waves) and DTI of the mitral annulus are the most useful in the clinical setting (Figure 110-30).

In general, when a decreased ventricular compliance is present, the passive filling velocity, or E wave, is decreased and the active atrial contraction velocity, or A wave, is increased, making the E/A ratio less than 1 and causing a delayed relaxation pattern in diastole. When faster than 160 beats/min, the E/A ratio is difficult to evaluate since it causes fusion of the E and A waves. A *restrictive pattern* has also been described in some cardiomyopathies, when the peak E wave velocity is increased in combination with a decreased A wave velocity.

Evaluation of pulmonary vein flow is typically performed via the left apical view. The sample volume of the PW Doppler is placed in the pulmonary vein and the flow signal is recorded. Normal pulmonary vein flow profile consists of a diastolic (D), systolic (S), and atrial reversal (A) wave (see Figure 110-30).

NORMAL VALUES

M-mode measurements vary with body size, body surface area, breed, and sedative drugs. They are also modified by situations like fear and stress, which significantly affect the heart rate and contractility of our patients. Therefore, reported normal values should always be regarded as approximate. Kienle collected values from the literature to establish mean normal M-mode values from dogs ranging from 3 to 68 kg. Normal dogs generally have values within a range of 10% of either side of the mean.

RENAL/URINARY

CHAPTER 111

Cystocentesis and Urinary Bladder Catheterization

S. Dru Forrester
David C. Grant

CYSTOCENTESIS

Cystocentesis is usually performed to collect urine for diagnostic evaluation but is occasionally used to temporarily decompress the urinary bladder in dogs or cats with urethral obstruction. Obtaining urine from the urinary bladder bypasses contamination from the lower urogenital tract and is the preferred technique when samples are to be submitted for bacterial culture. When performed correctly, cystocentesis is a safe, easy, and practical procedure. In most dogs and cats, a 22-gauge, 1.5-inch needle attached to a 12-mL syringe is used. For large or obese dogs, a 22-gauge, 3-inch spinal needle may be needed. If the urinary bladder cannot be palpated, ultrasound guidance usually allows correct needle placement.

Cystocentesis can be done with dogs standing or in dorsal or lateral recumbency; for most cats it is easiest to perform cystocentesis when they are in lateral recumbency. The urinary bladder should be palpated to determine the site for puncture, to immobilize the bladder, and to provide a simple "target" for needle placement. Usually the needle is inserted into the ventral or ventrolateral aspect of the urinary bladder. Hair can be clipped over the site and the skin prepared aseptically; however, in most situations simply using alcohol to wipe the skin over the puncture site is all that is needed. The urinary bladder can be immobilized with one hand, and the other hand is used to guide the needle through the abdominal wall and into the target. If the urinary bladder contains a small amount of urine or if cystocentesis is done therapeutically, the needle should be inserted near the urinary bladder neck, rather than at the apex, so that urine can be removed continuously as the urinary bladder becomes smaller. Urine is aspirated by pulling back gently on the plunger to create negative pressure. If urine is not obtained, the needle should not be redirected; rather, the needle should be removed from the abdomen and the procedure begun again. Excessive pressure on the urinary bladder during and immediately after aspiration should be avoided to prevent leakage of urine into the abdominal cavity.

If the urinary bladder cannot be palpated and ultrasound is not available, cystocentesis can be done "blindly." Although this technique may not be consistently effective, it can be attempted if a dog or cat cannot be hospitalized for a period of time to allow the bladder to fill or if the pet is likely to void frequently due to pollakiuria. "Blind" cystocentesis is performed with the dog or cat positioned in dorsal recumbency, and a puncture site is selected on the midline, halfway between the umbilicus and pelvic brim (this is often the point where alcohol pools when dripped onto the area in female dogs) (Figure 111-1).

In male dogs, the penis and prepuce should be retracted laterally so that the needle can be inserted into the abdomen on the midline. Urine should be aspirated as described above. If a sample is not obtained, the needle is removed and aspiration is attempted at a site just cranial or caudal to the original puncture. If urine is not obtained after a total of three attempts, cystocentesis should be delayed until the urinary bladder can be palpated or ultrasound guidance is possible.

URINARY BLADDER CATHETERIZATION

Urethral catheterization is indicated to collect urine for analysis or bacterial culture (primarily in male dogs), to measure urine output, to inject radiographic contrast material, and to relieve urinary retention secondary to functional or anatomic urethral obstruction. Potential complications include iatrogenic urinary tract infection (more likely in females) and urethral or urinary bladder trauma. Catheterization should always be performed aseptically using a sterile catheter. Flexible catheters (e.g., rubber) are appropriate for the collection of urine for diagnostic purposes and are less traumatic than polypropylene catheters. Urethral catheters with an inflatable balloon near the tip (e.g., Foley catheters) are useful for indwelling catheterization. Catheters are available in a variety of sizes and lengths. Catheter diameter is most often expressed in French (F) units (3 F = 1 mm). For male dogs, depending on the patient's size, catheter diameters of 3.5 to 5 F (<10 kg), 8 to 10 F (10 to 25 kg), and 10 to 12 F (>35 kg) are appropriate. Catheters ranging from 5 to 14 F are adequate for most female dogs.

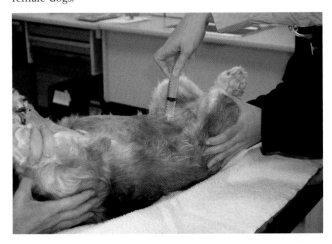

Figure 111-1 Cystocentesis may be performed with the patient in dorsal recumbency, particularly if the procedure is being done when the urinary bladder cannot be palpated. The site for needle insertion is generally at a point midway between the umbilicus and the pelvic brim.

WWW. To view a video on this topic, go to **www.expertconsult.com.**

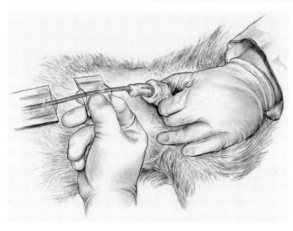

Figure 111-2 Urethral catheterization of a male dog. A portion of the catheter's package is used to aseptically advance the catheter through the urethra.

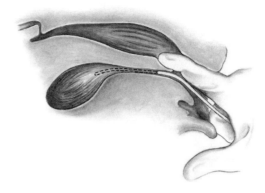

Figure 111-3 Urethral catheterization of a female dog. An index finger is placed over the urethral orifice to guide the catheter ventrally into the urethra.

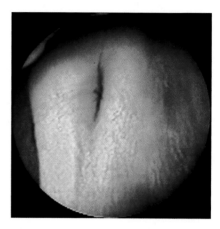

Figure 111-4 Appearance of urethral orifice in a female dog as visualized during endoscopic examination.

Male dogs should be restrained in lateral recumbency and an assistant should retract the prepuce to expose the penis. The tip of the penis should be cleansed with a mild antiseptic solution. The length of catheter needed to reach from the distal end of the penis to the neck of the urinary bladder should be estimated. Estimating the necessary length of the catheter helps avoid overinsertion of the catheter. Inserting too much catheter could damage bladder mucosa or, much worse, cause the catheter to loop upon itself and create a knot. If a knot is created, it usually will require surgery to remove the catheter. The tip of the catheter should be lubricated with a sterile, water-soluble lubricant from a single-use packet. The urinary catheter should be maintained in sterile condition during catheterization; this may be accomplished by using a sterile hemostat, wearing sterile gloves, or using a cut portion at the end of the catheter package to advance the catheter (Figure 111-2).

The tip of the catheter should be inserted into the external urethral opening and gently advanced. Some resistance may occur as the catheter is advanced through the area of the os penis and again at the ischial arch. If the catheter has been inserted to the appropriate level and urine is not observed in the lumen, a syringe can be attached to the catheter to aspirate urine. After urine collection, the catheter should be gently removed.

Urethral catheterization is more technically difficult in female dogs, and sedation may occasionally be helpful in some cases (e.g., with small or fractious dogs). Catheterization may be performed using a speculum (e.g., human nasal speculum, otoscope cone) to visualize the urethral orifice or blindly, with or without digital palpation. Selection of technique depends on the preference and experience of the clinician and the temperament of the dog or the size of the vagina. It is helpful to insert a lubricated, sterile, metal stylet or 3.5-F polypropylene catheter through the lumen of the Foley catheter to increase its rigidity and facilitate its passage. The stylet should be advanced to the tip of the Foley catheter to prevent it from exiting the eye of the catheter and causing urethral damage during placement.

Female dogs are most easily catheterized while standing or in sternal recumbency with the rear legs hanging over the end of a table; an assistant should hold the tail to one side. Excessive hair around the vulva should be clipped, if necessary, and the area should be cleansed with antiseptic soap. A lubricated tuberculin syringe can be inserted into the vagina, and 0.25 to 0.5 mL of local anesthetic (e.g., 0.5% lidocaine or topical ophthalmic anesthetic) instilled in the area of the urethral orifice (approximately 3 to 5 cm cranial to the vulvar opening). While sterile conditions are maintained, the tip of the catheter is lubricated with water-soluble lubricant.

For the visual technique, the vaginal speculum is lubricated and the tip is gently inserted dorsally through the vulva and then directed cranially to avoid the clitoral fossa. The blades of the speculum are opened gently so that the urethral orifice can be visualized. The handles of the speculum should be directed dorsally so that they do not interfere with visualization. A sterile glove is worn to pick up the catheter; the tip is inserted through the urethral orifice, and the catheter then is gently advanced through the urethra into the urinary bladder. If the catheter is to remain in place, air or saline is injected to inflate the balloon near the catheter tip.

For the digital technique, the person passing the catheter should wear sterile gloves. A lubricated index finger is inserted into the vagina, and the urethral orifice is palpated. The other hand is used to insert the catheter ventral to the finger in the vagina; the catheter is guided ventrally on the midline so that it enters the urethral orifice (Figures 111-3 and 111-4).

If a finger cannot be inserted into the vagina, the catheter can be passed blindly. After the catheter has been inserted through the vulva, it is directed ventrally along the midline of the vestibular floor and advanced cranially. If resistance is encountered, the catheter has most likely advanced cranial to the urethral orifice to the cervix. If this occurs, the catheter is withdrawn and the procedure is repeated. If urine is not noted from the catheter, a syringe is attached and urine is obtained through aspiration.

CHAPTER **112**

Unblocking the Urethra of the Male Cat

Mary H. Bowles

The male cat may have an obstructed urethra due to inflammation, spasms, trauma, congenital defects, urethral or periurethral masses, foreign bodies, uroliths, and urethral plugs. The length and narrow diameter of the urethra predisposes male cats to obstruction. Urethral plugs and idiopathic disease have been the causes most frequently linked to obstruction.[1]

Cats with feline lower urinary tract disease often display similar clinical signs regardless of the cause or the presence or absence of obstruction. Dysuria, hematuria, and frequent attempts to urinate are common but not exclusive signs of urethral obstruction. However, when these signs are combined with vocalization, licking the prepuce or penis, or systemic evidence of illness (e.g., depression, loss of appetite), it is likely that the animal has a urethral obstruction. Palpation of a distended bladder that is difficult to express is a key feature of urethral obstruction. Applying excessive pressure to an obstructed bladder should be avoided due to the possibility of causing a rupture or potentially forcing bacteria into the ureters.

When urethral obstruction is suspected, a thorough assessment of the cat's physical condition is indicated prior to catheterization, especially if the cat is systemically ill. In addition to establishing further evidence of urethral obstruction by bladder palpation and inspection of the distal penis, special attention should be paid to the cardiac status because hyperkalemia-related arrhythmias may be present that affect the treatment plan. Quick assessment tests (QUATS) (e.g., blood urea nitrogen [BUN], glucose, packed cell volume [PCV], electrolytes, and electrocardiogram to look for presence or absence of P waves, if a serum potassium concentration is not immediately available) are indicated in any cat prior to catheterization to evaluate both anesthetic risk and overall condition. Appropriate blood samples should be saved for subsequent complete blood count (CBC) and biochemistry profile evaluation, especially in systemically ill cats. Bladder decompression by cystocentesis provides optimal samples for urinalysis and culture, alleviates distress, and may facilitate flushing obstructive material back into the bladder when necessary. Urethral catheterization usually requires general anesthesia unless the cat is moribund. Anesthetic agents requiring renal excretion should be used with caution.

UNBLOCKING TECHNIQUE AND INDWELLING CATHETER PLACEMENT (Figure 112-1)

If manual expression of the bladder and manipulation of the distal penis do not result in free flow of urine, the cat should be anesthetized or sedated and placed in lateral or dorsal recumbency. The clinician should then clip the hair in the perineal area and surgically scrub the prepuce and tip of the penis, taking care to avoid undue trauma to the penis. The tail and hindlimbs can be drawn forward toward the head to provide better exposure of the preputial area. Using sterile technique, the prepuce should be pushed back toward the body, exposing the distal end of the penis. Because urethral plugs often lodge near the external urethral orifice, the exposed distal penis should be gently massaged to loosen any obstructing material present and extrude it from the urethra. The lubricated tip of an open-ended tomcat catheter (3.5 F polypropylene, 4.5 to 5.5 inches in length), a Minnesota olive-tipped feline urethral catheter (22 gauge × ½ to 1½ inch E-JAY International, Inc., Glendora, Calif.), or an open-ended, 3.5-F, 4- to 6-inch, polytetrafluroethylene catheter with a silicone hub (Slippery Sam urethral catheter, Smiths Medical, Waukesha, Wis.) should then be inserted into the external urethral orifice, extending the penis caudally and dorsally until it is parallel to the spine to facilitate advancement of the catheter (Figure 112-2).

A pair of small hemostats may be used to lightly grasp the penile sheath to aid in extension if difficulty is encountered accomplishing extension with the fingers alone. Once the obstruction has been reached, the clinician should attach a syringe (>20 mL) filled with saline or lactated Ringer's solution to the catheter either directly or by an intravenous extension set. A liberal amount of flushing solution should then be injected into the urethral lumen, allowing fluid to run back out of the urethral orifice. The clinician should periodically attempt to cautiously advance the catheter toward the bladder, noting evidence of relief of obstruction, such as debris emerging from the orifice or a decrease in reflux of flushing solution. Applying moderate pressure to the bladder wall and occasionally repeating gentle massage of the extruded penis between flushings may facilitate dislodgement of a urethral plug or urolith.

If the previously described technique does not result in relief of obstruction, the clinician should continue to flush while manually occluding the urethra around the catheter tip, attempting to dilate the urethral lumen and force the obstructive material back into the bladder. As pressure builds up in the obstructed urethra, the clinician should try to carefully advance the catheter toward the bladder. To prevent iatrogenic damage to the urethra, excessive force should be avoided when advancing the catheter and when flushing solution from the syringe into the manually occluded urethra.

If the urethra is successfully unblocked, a catheter should be inserted into the bladder lumen and the majority of urine aspirated from the bladder, saving a portion for urinalysis and culture, if not obtained previously by cystocentesis. The bladder should be flushed repeatedly with saline or lactated Ringer's solution until aspiration of the flushing solution appears relatively free of blood and particulate material. Agitating the bladder manually through the abdominal wall may facilitate the removal of sediment. If a urethral plug or urolith was obtained during the unblocking procedure, it should be

WWW. To view a video on this topic, go to **www.expertconsult.com.**

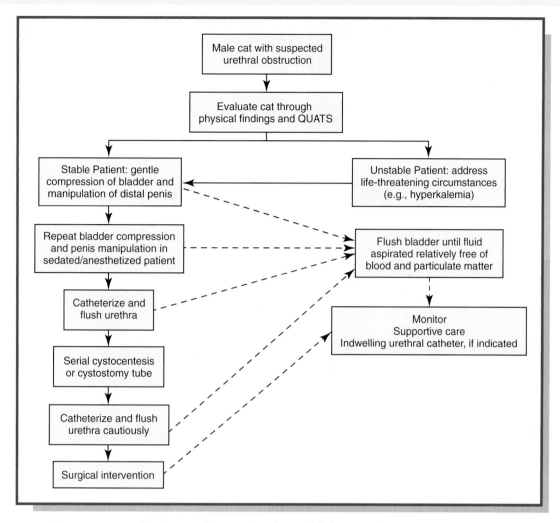

Figure 112-1 Unblocking technique algorithm. *Solid line,* Urethral obstruction unresolved. *Dotted line,* Urethral obstruction resolved.

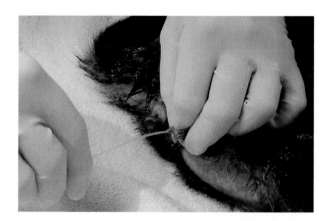

Figure 112-2 Proper positioning of the feline penis for urethral catheterization with a 3.5-F polypropylene catheter. The cat is positioned in lateral recumbency with the penis extended caudally and parallel to the spine while the tail and hind limbs are drawn forward toward the head.

saved for analysis. Urethral plugs can be examined cytologically, and uroliths can be submitted for quantitative analysis and culture.

If the unblocking techniques previously described are unsuccessful, the bladder can be serially decompressed by cystocentesis, or a cystostomy tube can be placed for temporary urine diversion. These procedures provide relief while the cat receives supportive therapy. The veterinarian can then consider the need for diagnostic imaging to further define the source and location of any obstruction. In addition, alternative treatment plans, such as surgery, may need to be developed if the obstruction cannot be relieved. Catheterization attempts can also be continued, remembering that vigorous flushing and manipulation of the bladder should be avoided postcystocentesis or post–cystostomy tube placement.

Monitor urination for at least 24 hours after relief of obstruction. Express the bladder manually at least three times daily if the cat is not voiding regularly or large amounts of urine are retained in the bladder after voiding. Use of an alpha blocker such as prazosin (0.25 to 0.5 mg/cat q12h) may enhance the passage of urine through urethral relaxation. Place an indwelling catheter immediately after the unblocking procedure if a strong urine stream is not present on expression, the cat is systemically ill, excessive hematuria exists, or relief of obstruction was difficult. An indwelling catheter may be placed up to several hours later if the cat reobstructs or has difficulty urinating due to an atonic bladder. Ideally, a 5-French (F) (the 3.5-F size may be used but becomes obstructed more easily) red rubber (polyvinyl) or Foley catheter should be used because these catheters are more pliable than the polypropylene variety and may be less likely to cause injury to the urethral and bladder mucosa. Placement of these

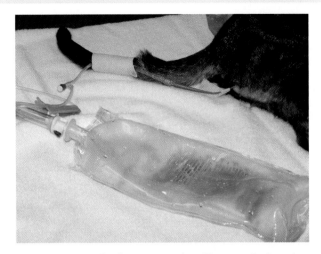

Figure 112-3 Indwelling 5-F red rubber urethral catheter attached to a sterile, closed urine collection system. Elastic wrap attaches the urine collection system to the tail, and an elastic wrap flange is loosely sutured to the preputial area to reduce the tension on the urethral catheter and help keep it in place.

catheter types may require the use of a wire guide due to their pliability. The application of a generous amount of lubricant is often required to facilitate passage, especially for the balloon portion of the Foley catheter. To minimize bacterial contamination after insertion into the bladder lumen, the clinician should attach the indwelling catheter to a sterile, closed collection system available as a commercial product (Cook Urological, Spencer, Ind.) or constructed from a recently emptied intravenous (IV) fluid bag attached to a sterile IV administration set. The clinician can reduce tension placed on the indwelling catheter by the collection system by using elastic wrap and suture to attach the apparatus to the cat (Figure 112-3).

Indwelling catheters should be removed as soon as possible, generally within 1 to 3 days after placement. Although indwelling catheters predispose the cat to urinary tract infection, antibiotic therapy is not recommended unless evidence of urinary tract or systemic infection exists. Pain management should be incorporated into the postobstruction treatment plan.

REFERENCES

The reference list can be found on the companion Expert Consult Web site at *www.expertconsult.com.*

CHAPTER 113

Peritoneal Dialysis

Cathy Langston

Peritoneal dialysis is used to treat acute renal failure, occasionally poisoning by a dialyzable toxin (i.e., ethylene glycol, phenobarbital, ethanol), or chronic renal failure. Some peritoneal dialysis techniques can also be applied for peritoneal drainage (i.e., uroabdomen) or peritoneal lavage (i.e., pancreatitis, hypothermia, hyperthermia).

PERITONEAL DIALYSIS CATHETERS

Access to the peritoneal cavity is accomplished via a peritoneal catheter. The general design of percutaneously placed catheters includes multiple fenestrations at the tip of the catheter to allow fluid ingress and egress. A variety of catheters are available that are made specifically for this purpose: the Peritoneal Lavage Catheter (Cook Veterinary Products, Spencer, Ind.), a fenestrated chest tube, or a Jackson Pratt suction drain. For percutaneous placement, local anesthesia in conscious animals or a short-acting injectable anesthetic may be used. The urinary bladder should be emptied to avoid perforation. The dog or cat should be placed in dorsal recumbency, and the abdomen is sterilely prepped and draped. A stab incision through the skin lateral to the midline at the level of the umbilicus allows introduction of a trocar threaded through the dialysis catheter. The trocar should be tunneled under the skin for 1 to 2 cm before puncturing the abdominal musculature and then directed toward the opposite hip. Having the abdomen slightly distended with fluid facilitates

percutaneous placement. After the trocar has been introduced, the catheter should be advanced off the trocar. The tip of the catheter should rest near the urinary bladder to facilitate fluid drainage. If a trocar is not provided with the catheter, the tip of the catheter can be grasped with curved hemostats, which can be used to tunnel the catheter under the skin and then puncture the abdomen.

Coaxial catheters (Cook Veterinary Products, Spencer, Ind.) and fluted-T catheters (Ash Advantage Peritoneal Dialysis Catheter, Medigroup, Inc., Aurora, Ill.) are less likely to occlude with omentum. The fluted-T catheter has two limbs, each with channels extending the length of the catheter, to minimize chances of complete occlusion. These catheters are placed surgically or via laparoscopy. Both have a Dacron cuff that allows attachment of fibroblasts to the subcutaneous portion of the catheter to enhance stability and diminish leaks and infection. With surgical placement, the catheter is placed in the abdomen via a small caudal abdominal incision. The catheter should exit the ventral body wall through a separate stab incision (not through the abdominal incision) and tunnel under the skin lateral to the midline. Again, the catheter tip should rest near the urinary bladder. A partial omentectomy should be performed to diminish chances of catheter occlusion. If omentectomy is not desired due to recent intestinal surgery, an omentopexy should be performed.

Both the percutaneous and surgically placed catheters should be secured to the skin at the exit site via a purse-string suture. A sterile dry bandage is placed over the catheter.

pate in CRRT procedures. Since patients typically require 24-hour care for days or weeks, staffing issues can become challenging. A doctor and a technician or trained veterinary student should always be by the patient's side.

SUMMARY

CRRT provides a new set of tools for treating patients suffering from acute kidney injury, toxin exposure, and cardiac-related fluid overload. Although resource- and time-intensive, there has been good success treating patients with these new tools.

REFERENCES

The reference list can be found on the companion Expert Consult Web site at *www.expertconsult.com*.

GASTROINTESTINAL

CHAPTER 115

Gastric Lavage

Roger Gfeller[†]
Jennifer J. Devey

Gastric lavage is widely used as a gastrointestinal (GI) decontamination technique in small animals poisoned by ingestion of toxins. Removal of the stomach contents by gastric intubation and irrigation can be performed rapidly by trained staff members and does not require a cooperative patient. Experts are beginning to question the value of gastric lavage and it is recommended as a procedure to be done rarely if at all in human medicine since studies fail to confirm its value as a practical clinical procedure. In addition, administration of activated charcoal without lavage has shown very similar outcomes in people with many different types of toxin ingestion. Even when gastric lavage can be performed within minutes of ingestion, recovery of the toxin is limited. If the procedure is not completed within an hour of ingestion, recovery of many toxins is less than 15%. In small animal veterinary medicine, it is rare that gastric lavage would be completed within this period.

The volume of lavage fluid has also become a focus of attention. Using previously recommended volumes often results in gastric distention and complications (including fluid and electrolyte imbalances). Currently a volume of 5 to 10 mL/kg of fluid is recommended, and it is advisable to have one staff member responsible for monitoring the amount of distension. Although visual observation of the abdomen is acceptable, it is better if one repeatedly palpates the stomach during lavage.

One study found that when the volume administered resulted in gastric distention, as much as 25% of the lavage fluid passed into the small intestine carrying the ingested toxin with it, although these results were later refuted. Concern that this might be occurring, however, led to the suggestion that there may be benefit in administration of activated charcoal prior to lavage as well as following lavage. The length of time the charcoal would need to remain in the stomach prior to lavage to ensure adsorption of the toxin varies with the type of charcoal and the toxin ingested.

Reported complications of gastric lavage include hypernatremia when large volumes of saline were used and hyponatremia when water was used as the lavage solution. Additional complications include aspiration pneumonia; traumatic injury of the oropharynx, esophagus, or stomach; hypoxemia; hypercapnia; and hypothermia. Gastric lavage is contraindicated in patients with an unprotected airway. Ingestion of caustic or corrosive toxins (e.g., acids, alkalis) or toxins with a high risk of aspiration (e.g., hydrocarbons) is also a contraindication to gastric lavage. A relative contraindication to gastric lavage is ingestion of a foreign body that could cause physical damage to the alimentary tract.

Gastric lavage has risks, it is messy, and it may not decontaminate the GI tract as efficiently as once thought. Inducing emesis, which may remove up to 40% to 60% of an ingested toxin, is far more effective at decontaminating the patient than gastric lavage.

PROCEDURE

The patient must be anesthetized and intubated with a cuffed endotracheal tube (Box 115-1).

Box • 115-1

Materials Needed for Gastric Lavage

1. Large-bore stomach tube with additional fenestrations in one end (egress tube) and small-bore stomach tube (ingress tube) or integrated two-tube system
2. Lubricant
3. Stomach pump or funnel
4. Activated charcoal if desired
5. Lavage solution (water or saline)
6. Container appropriate for laboratory submission of gastric contents, if desired
7. Disposal area for large quantities of lavage solution

[†]Deceased.
Dr. Devey has updated this chapter in view of the goals and thoughts of Dr. Gfeller.

The cuff should be inflated just enough to create a seal between the tube and the trachea. The pop-off valve should be closed, and the rebreathing bag squeezed to a pressure of approximately 15 cm of water while the cuff is inflated. The clinician should listen for air escaping around the cuff and stop inflating the cuff immediately when no further leakage of air occurs. The patient is maintained on an appropriate gas or injectable anesthetic. If injectable anesthesia is used instead of gaseous agents, the patient should be maintained on oxygen. Ideally blood pressure, capnography, and pulse oximetry should be monitored and appropriate measures should be taken if abnormalities are seen. It is not uncommon for patients to hypoventilate during this procedure and positive pressure ventilation may be required.

The clinician should prepare two tubes for use or use a commercial lavage system that consists of two tubes. The first tube is the egress tube. The egress tube should be as large as possible to allow rapid and complete removal of stomach contents. Additional side fenestrations near the end that will be inserted into the stomach may be useful. The tube should be marked with a piece of tape or an indelible marker at a distance equal to the distance from the incisors to the thirteenth rib. The second tube is the ingress tube, through which lavage solution and activated charcoal (if desired) will be instilled into the stomach. This tube should be smaller in diameter to allow the egress tube to be as large as possible.

The patient is secured in right lateral recumbency. The patient's head should be positioned approximately 20 degrees lower than the chest. The clinician should apply an appropriate lubricant (e.g., KY Lubricating Jelly, Johnson & Johnson, Arlington, Tex.) and insert the egress tube into the esophagus. The tube should be advanced into the stomach but not farther than the mark established previously. Excessive force must not be used to pass the tube into the stomach; if there is difficulty passing the tube through the lower esophageal sphincter, a twisting motion often allows the tube to pass. If this does not work, a separate smaller tube (the ingress tube if a two-tube system is being used) can be passed alongside the larger one and into the stomach first. This opens the lower esophageal sphincter and permits the larger tube to pass. As much of the stomach contents as possible should be allowed to drain from the tube. If nothing drains from the stomach, the clinician should confirm that the tube is in the stomach. This can be done by several methods. In small animals, direct observation of the tube entering the esophagus and advancement of the tube to the measured distance is usually sufficient. Alternatively, one can push air through the tube while listening over the stomach. A gurgling sound can be heard in the stomach if the tube is properly positioned. Rarely a radiograph may be required for confirmation.

If nothing comes from the egress tube after it has been confirmed to be in the stomach, the clinician should lubricate and insert the ingress tube if a two-tube system is being used. At this point the patient can be lavaged. If so desired, the manufacturer's recommended dose of activated charcoal can be instilled and allowed to mix with the stomach contents. Gentle external agitation of the stomach will help. If charcoal is administered, this should be drained first before starting the lavage.

Whether water or saline is to be used as the lavage solution, it should be warmed. Warming the lavage solution will slow gastric emptying and help prevent patient hypothermia. If a passive system is being used, the fluid source should be attached to the ingress tube and approximately 5 to 10 mL/kg of fluid should be infused while the stomach is being observed for distention. If a stomach pump system is being used, the clinician should attach the stomach pump to the ingress tube, infuse the approximately 5 to 10 ml/kg of the lavage solution slowly, and monitor gastric distension. Gentle external agitation of the stomach will help mix and remove stomach contents. If the egress tube does not allow free flow of fluid from the stomach, the tube should be withdrawn slowly a maximum of 2 to 3 inches in case the tube is against the wall of the stomach. If flow begins, the lavage should continue. If no flow can be established, a small amount of water or air should be infused through the large bore tube to dislodge material. If flow is still not established, the clinician should remove the tube and check for a plug, then gently reinsert the tube to establish flow.

The procedure should be continued until the effluent is clear, which usually takes a minimum of 15 to 20 exchanges, but in some cases this may take extremely large volumes of lavage solution and a great deal of time. At no time should the patient's stomach be distended. The patient should be lavaged in both left and right lateral recumbency. In some cases it is helpful to move the egress tube gently back and forth to help mix and dislodge stomach contents. If this is necessary, it must be done gently to avoid trauma to the pharynx, esophagus, and stomach.

When the stomach is emptied, the clinician should crimp or clamp the egress tube and remove it. He or she should ensure that the endotracheal tube is still properly placed and sealed and instill activated charcoal through the remaining tube, if indicated. Then the ingress tube should be crimped or clamped and removed.

To minimize the chances of aspiration, the patient should be recovered with the endotracheal tube in place and the cuff inflated until the swallowing reflex returns. The patient's head and neck should be elevated approximately 30 degrees. The oropharynx should be carefully checked for fluid, activated charcoal, or stomach contents and suctioned clean before the endotracheal tube is removed. If there has been reflux of gastric contents around the stomach tube, irrigation and suction of the oropharynx and esophagus may be indicated.

CONCLUSION

Gastric lavage is a procedure that is rarely indicated; however, if inducing vomiting is contraindicated and the patient ingested a massive amount of toxin, if the toxin is associated with delayed gastric emptying, or if there is no effective antidote, then gastric lavage should be performed. The clinician should be aware that only very small quantities of the toxin may be removed if the gastric lavage is performed more than 15 minutes following ingestion, and continued symptomatic and supportive care along with any antidotes if available will usually be required in these patients. When performed carefully, there should be minimal complications.

CHAPTER 116

Endoscopic Procedures for Evaluation of the Gastrointestinal Tract

Michael E. Matz
David C. Twedt

ENDOSCOPIC PROCEDURES

Gastrointestinal (GI) endoscopy is a minimally invasive, atraumatic technique that permits direct visualization of the mucosa of the esophagus, stomach, small bowel, and colon. Diagnostically, it allows clinicians to obtain samples for cytologic and histologic examination with relative ease. Therapeutically, it can be used for the removal of foreign bodies, dilation of esophageal or colonic strictures, and placement of gastric or jejunal feeding tubes. These endoscopic procedures offer an alternative to surgical intervention.

ENDOSCOPIC EQUIPMENT

Both rigid and flexible endoscopes can be useful in GI endoscopy. Rigid endoscopes are available in several sizes, inexpensive, and easy to use. Rigid endoscopes are most valuable for performing proctoscopy and colonoscopy. Poor visualization, limited maneuverability, and relatively short length compared with flexible endoscopes limit the use of rigid endoscopes for other diagnostic procedures. A number of flexible endoscopes of different makes, lengths, diameters, and functions are available. Fiberoptic endoscopes use fiberoptic bundles to deliver bright light to the tip of the endoscope and transmit the image to the eyepiece. The quality of the image is dependent on the number, size, and quality of the fibers. Numerous, small-diameter fibers produce a better image than larger, less numerous fibers. Video endoscopes replace the image fiber bundle with a computer chip camera that transmits an electronic signal to a processor, where it is converted to a video image and displayed on a high-resolution monitor. Image quality is superior with video endoscopes.

Versatility is important because dogs and cats vary so much in size. A flexible endoscope to be used for GI endoscopy in dogs and cats should possess the following characteristics: a working length of at least 110 cm (ideally 125 cm); an insertion tube diameter of less than 9.8 mm, optimally less than 8.5 mm; a minimum instrument channel diameter of 2.0 mm, with the ideal size being 2.8 mm; four-way distal tip deflection with at least 180° to 210° in one direction and 90° to 100° in the other three directions; automatic air-water insufflation; suction capabilities; a forward direction of view; an angle of view of 90° to 120°; a depth of field of 3 to 100 mm; and comfortable handling. Light sources for the endoscope should be halogen or preferably xenon. An external vacuum source (portable or central) is necessary.

Additional instrumentation required for flexible diagnostic endoscopy includes biopsy forceps and cytology brushes. A wide variety of different biopsy forceps are available. Larger cupped forceps tend to obtain samples with a larger surface area, but there is little difference in the depth of the tissue acquired. Forceps with central spikes or bayonets allow more than one specimen to be obtained without removing the instrument and may improve the ease of biopsying lesions tangential to the endoscope tip. Many forceps contain fenestrated cups that may minimize crush artifact and facilitate removal of tissue from the instrument. In general, the final decision of what type of forceps to use is a matter of personal preference. There are no data supporting a major advantage of one forceps over another, although many endoscopists prefer a fenestrated ellipsoid cupped biopsy forceps without a central spike. For rigid endoscopes, alligator biopsy forceps (punch-type preferred) are necessary.

ENDOSCOPIC TECHNIQUE

Upper Gastrointestinal Endoscopy

Diagnostically, upper GI endoscopy is indicated for evaluation of dysphagia, persistent regurgitation, acute vomiting with hematemesis, chronic vomiting, chronic small bowel diarrhea, melena, and unexplained salivation, weight loss, or anorexia. It is essential for the animal to be fasted to prevent ingesta from interfering with the examination. In most cases an 8- to 12-hour fast is sufficient; however, a longer fast may be necessary if evidence of delayed gastric emptying exists. Upper GI endoscopy should not be performed within 24 hours of a barium contrast study. This allows for clearing of residual barium that often adheres to mucosal surfaces even when radiographically it may appear that the barium has been cleared from the GI tract. Appropriate preparation is essential for maximizing examination efficiency and for ensuring safety.

General anesthesia with placement of a cuffed endotracheal tube is necessary for upper GI endoscopy. The choice of anesthetic regimen should be made based on the animal's general condition and suspected disease processes. Narcotics (morphine, meperidine, butorphanol) increase antral motility and may increase pyloric tone, potentially interfering with the passage of the endoscope into the duodenum. The animal should be positioned in left lateral recumbency with a mouth speculum placed to protect the endoscope.

The insertion tube of the endoscope is passed initially over the endotracheal tube and through the oropharynx and upper esophageal sphincter. Once the endoscope is in the esophagus, air is insufflated until the esophagus is adequately distended to visualize the lumen. The endoscope is centralized in the esophageal lumen and then slowly advanced toward the gastroesophageal junction. The endoscope should only be advanced when the lumen is clearly visible. It is important to examine the esophagus completely during the insertion of the endoscope because it may become traumatized during passage

WWW. To view a video on this topic, go to **www.expertconsult.com.**

of the endoscope. Normal esophageal mucosa is smooth, pale, and glistening. Submucosal vessels are not normally visualized in dogs, but are easily observed in cats. Little or no fluid is normally found in the esophageal lumen. In the proximal esophagus, an impression of the trachea can be seen. Pulsations of the heart and aorta are visualized in the thoracic esophagus. In the distal one third of the esophagus of cats, concentric circular rings are observed because of the presence of smooth muscle. The gastroesophageal sphincter (GES) is usually closed in the normal animal. The bright pink to red color of the gastric mucosa may be visible at the GES, creating an irregular rosette appearance. At the GES, a slight directional change is necessary to align the tip of the endoscope with the center of the sphincter. Insufflation of air, while gently advancing the endoscope, should result in passage into the stomach. When the endoscope is properly directed, there should be minimal resistance to advancing it into the stomach.

The large lumen of the stomach means the endoscopist must develop and maintain a systematic approach to gastroscopy so that completeness and reproducibility are ensured. During initial examination of the stomach, it is important to obtain at least a cursory view of the mucosa as the endoscope is advanced to avoid misinterpreting endoscope-induced trauma as an abnormality during endoscope withdrawal. Normal gastric mucosa is smooth, glistening, and pink. Submucosal vessels are not normally observed, except in the cardia. The presence of ingesta or fluid, ease of distensibility of the gastric wall during insufflation, and the appearance of the rugal folds should also be evaluated.

Upon entry into the stomach, the endoscope will lie along the greater curvature. The stomach will be collapsed, and prominent longitudinal rugal folds will be visible. Air should be insufflated into the stomach only until spatial orientation is achieved. Care must be taken not to overinflate the stomach. Overdistension of the stomach can occur quickly in cats and small dogs because of their relatively small stomach size. The endoscope should continue to be advanced along the greater curvature until the junction between the antrum (characterized by the lack of rugal folds) and the body comes into view. A frontal view of this area is usually accomplished in dogs, but in cats the antrum is often hidden behind the incisura angularis, a narrow shelf of tissue that separates the pyloric antrum from the lesser curvature of the gastric body. To enter the antrum the endoscope is advanced farther along (dogs), or deflected off (cats), the greater curvature.

Once in the antrum, the endoscope can be slowly advanced toward the pylorus. The pylorus in most dogs and cats is readily visible. The appearance and location of the pylorus will vary. In general, it has clean margins and is not obscured by excessive folds. It may be closed or open. Passing the endoscope tip through the pylorus into the duodenum can be the most difficult portion of upper GI endoscopy; however, with experience, the pylorus can be passed in nearly every case. If gastric distension is minimized, the pylorus is usually in a more relaxed state, facilitating duodenal intubation. Passage into the duodenum is most easily accomplished by gradually advancing the endoscope while subtle and continuous adjustments are made to keep the pylorus aligned in the center of the field of view. Rapid and forceful advances of the endoscope should be avoided. If the endoscope is not properly oriented, with the axis parallel to the pyloric lumen, the endoscope will slide into the antrum. If this occurs, the endoscope should be withdrawn and the pylorus revisualized. Passage should again be attempted, making a greater effort to obtain proper alignment. If the pylorus cannot be properly aligned, repositioning of the dog or cat (dorsal or right lateral recumbency) may help to improve alignment.

Just beyond the pylorus is the cranial duodenal flexure. To negotiate this sharp turn, the tip of the endoscope should be deflected downward and to the right while insufflating and gently advancing the endoscope. During this advancement the mucosa will be seen sliding by the viewing lens. Once the tip of the endoscope has successfully negotiated the flexure, center the tip of the endoscope within the lumen. Normal intestinal mucosa is paler, more granular, and more friable than the gastric mucosa. The major duodenal papilla is observed on the medial wall of the duodenum in most dogs and in some cats. Careful examination may reveal the minor duodenal papilla in dogs. The papillae may be best visualized as the endoscope is slowly retracted back into the proximal duodenum because of their close proximity to the duodenal flexure. In dogs, Peyer's patches are often observed as shallow, pale craters on the lateral aspect of the nondistended descending duodenal wall. The endoscope should be advanced until it reaches its full working length, as long as only minimal resistance is encountered.

A more thorough evaluation of the duodenal and gastric mucosa is often best accomplished as the endoscope is withdrawn. Diagnostic procedures are also performed at this time. Once the endoscope has been retracted into the stomach, the pylorus, antrum, and incisura angularis are examined carefully. A frontal view of the angularis can usually be obtained while the endoscope is removed from the antrum. The endoscope is then withdrawn along the greater curvature and retroflexed 180° to allow visualization of the lesser curvature, fundus, and cardia—the latter region being defined by the location of the entrance of the endoscope into the stomach and the presence of submucosal vessels. Torquing the endoscope at this point will provide complete (360°) evaluation of this area. Once the proximal stomach has been thoroughly evaluated, the scope tip is straightened and the endoscope is slowly retracted. At this point, insufflation of the stomach should be sufficient to cause flattening of the rugal folds without causing overdistention, facilitating observation of the entire gastric mucosa. Before retraction of the endoscope into the esophagus, all air or residual fluid is suctioned from the gastric lumen. The esophagus should be carefully reexamined as the endoscope is removed.

Proctoscopy and Colonoscopy

Proctoscopy and colonoscopy are relatively easy to perform in dogs and cats because their large intestines are anatomically simple. For this reason, clinicians with an appreciation of normal and abnormal endoscopic anatomy can become proficient in performing proctoscopy and colonoscopy within a relatively short period of time. Endoscopic examination of the rectum and colon can be accomplished with either a rigid or flexible endoscope. Rigid endoscopes limit visualization to the rectum and descending colon. Flexible endoscopes allow evaluation of the rectum, entire colon, cecum, and possibly, distal ileum.

Indications for proctoscopy and colonoscopy include chronic large bowel diarrhea, obstipation or tenesmus, dyschezia, or hematochezia that accompanies formed feces. Because most inflammatory diseases of the large intestine in the dog and cat are diffuse, their presence is usually detected in the descending colon, allowing rigid endoscopy to be a valuable procedure.

One of the keys to successful proctoscopy or colonoscopy is adequate patient preparation. Various protocols can be used depending on the extent of the examination to be performed, the availability of support staff to complete the necessary work, and the degree of patient cooperation. Proper preparation for colonoscopy requires complete evacuation of fecal material from the colon and production of a clear ileal effluent. Food should be withheld for a minimum of 24 to 36 hours before the procedure. If flexible endoscopy is to be used, use of an oral GI lavage solution is recommended, such as one containing polyethylene glycol as the main nonabsorbed solute (Golytely, Nulytely, Colyte). These are isosmotic solutions that result in a severe diarrhea with virtually no net absorption or secretion of electrolytes, bicarbonate, or water. This method has been shown to result in superior colonic preparation compared with multiple enemas in dogs. Disadvantages are that fairly large volumes of the colon electrolyte lavage solution need to be used and administration via orogastric or nasoesophageal intubation is usually necessary. Although dose guidelines have not been firmly established for the dog and cat, two doses of a lavage solution are recommended at 30 to 60 mL/kg via orogastric (dog) or nasoesophageal (cat) tube 2 to 4 hours apart in the afternoon prior to the examination. In addition, a warm-water enema (20 mL/kg body weight) should be given after the first dose of lavage solution and the morning before colonoscopy. The well-lubricated enema tube should be inserted a length equal to that from the anus to the last rib. Enemas should be avoided in animals with rectal pain.

For rigid endoscopy, patient preparation does not have to be as vigorous as the protocol outlined previously. Preparation may be limited to withholding food for an appropriate time (usually 36 to 48 hours) and administering multiple warm-water enemas 1 to 2 hours apart on the afternoon before the procedure. Enemas should be given until the water exiting the rectum is repeatedly clear. A final enema is given 2 to 4 hours before the procedure is begun. These and similar protocols generally result in adequate rectal and colonic cleansing. It is essential that the rectum and colon be as clean as possible before endoscopy to avoid missing lesions.

General anesthesia is usually recommended for colonoscopy, although heavy sedation may be adequate for proctoscopy or rigid colonoscopy. Passage of a flexible endoscope into the transverse and ascending colon and cecum may cause painful stretching of mesenteric attachments.

Before performing endoscopy, a digital rectal examination should be done to rule out the possibility of anal and rectal lesions or perineal hernias. Insertion of a digit is also useful for straightening the rectal lumen, making it easier to insert the endoscope into the colon.

Rigid endoscopy is usually performed with the animal in right lateral recumbency to reduce gravitational flow of fluid and fecal material into the distal colon. The well-lubricated rigid endoscope is advanced into the rectum. Rigid endoscopes have a smooth obturator that facilitates advancement of the endoscope through the anal sphincter. The obturator is removed after entering the rectum and the hinged viewing lens is closed tightly over the end of the endoscope. Air is insufflated to distend the colon and the endoscope advanced under direct visualization until its entire length has been inserted. With a rigid endoscope, air insufflation is done manually with a bulb-pumping device. Normal colon should have a pale pink, smooth, glistening mucosa with visible submucosal blood vessels. Lymphoid follicles, seen as 2- to 3-mm plaques (often with humiliated surfaces) are normally observed in descending colon and cecum.

Flexible endoscopy is performed with the animal in left lateral recumbency to prevent compression of the area of the ileocolic valve by abdominal viscera. After the endoscope is inserted into the rectum, air is insufflated. It is often necessary, especially when small-diameter flexible scopes are used, to have an assistant apply digital pressure around the anal orifice to prevent insufflated air from escaping from the colon. Insufflation distends the colon and flattens out mucosal folds, which are most prominent in the rectum and distal descending colon. The endoscope tip is then centralized and advanced slowly. The endoscope should only be advanced if the lumen is clearly in view. At the junction of the descending and transverse colon the splenic flexure will be observed. The tip of the endoscope should be deflected around the flexure and advanced slowly along the mucosa. The mucosa should be seen sliding freely across the viewing lens. After passing the flexure, the tip of the endoscope can again be centralized within the lumen of transverse colon. The transverse colon is short in the dog and cat. The hepatic flexure will be encountered at the junction of the transverse and ascending colon. This flexure can be passed in a manner similar to the splenic flexure. In the cat, distinct flexures delineating the boundaries between the sections of the colon are generally not observed as clearly as in the dog. Upon entering the ascending colon, the ileocolic junction is visualized. The ileocolic sphincter often protrudes into the lumen. If the ileum is to be entered, centralize the tip of the endoscope within the lumen of the sphincter and advance the endoscope using gentle pressure combined with air insufflation. If the scope cannot be advanced into the ileum, blind biopsy specimens can be obtained by passing the biopsy forceps through the ileocolic sphincter. Using this blind biopsy technique does, however, increase the risk of perforation. The cecocolic junction may be partially open or, if closed, appear as a flat sphincter. The cecum usually can be entered. In the dog, the scope should be advanced into this spiral structure (8 to 30 cm in length) until the blind end is reached. The cecum of the cat is comma shaped and short (2 to 4 cm).

A more thorough evaluation of the colon should be performed as the scope is withdrawn. Diagnostic procedures are performed at this time. The endoscope should be slowly retracted while making necessary directional adjustments to ensure that the entire circumference of the colon is carefully evaluated. As the rectum is approached in dogs larger than 15 kg, the flexible endoscope should be retroflexed 180° to allow better visualization of the terminal rectum.

DESCRIPTIVE ENDOSCOPIC TERMINOLOGY

The esophageal, gastric, duodenal, jejunal, and colonic mucosa should be described using the following terminology: hyperemia, friability, granularity, erosion or ulceration, degree of luminal narrowing, stricture, and visibility of submucosal vessels. The presence of an intraluminal mass, polyp, or foreign body should be noted. Mucosal hyperemia should be carefully interpreted because it can be affected by a number of factors, including anesthesia, warm-water enema, and mild trauma from the endoscope. The amount of insufflation can alter the appearance of the mucosa (e.g., its granularity) and should be considered during evaluation. A shallow mucosal defect is termed an *erosion*. If there is perceived depth to the defect, it should be termed an *ulcer*. A description of the location, extent, severity, and size of any lesion(s) should be recorded. Size of a lesion can be roughly estimated by comparing the lesion to an open biopsy forceps. With experience, the endoscopist will learn to detect subtle GI mucosal abnormalities.

TISSUE SAMPLING

Tissue analysis is most frequently performed by obtaining pinch biopsy samples through the instrument channel of the endoscope. Flexible endoscopic biopsy samples are small (2 to 3 mm). In view of the small size of these biopsy samples, multiple biopsies and good technique are essential to provide diagnostic material. It is important to remember biopsy forceps mainly recover specimens of mucosa and occasionally fragments of submucosa. To obtain a biopsy sample with the flexible scope, the tip of the endoscope should be placed in close proximity to the intended biopsy site and directed as perpendicular to the mucosal surface to be biopsied as possible. Removing a majority of luminal air will facilitate attaining a perpendicular orientation of the tip in narrower tubular lumens such as the small intestine. A biopsy forceps is advanced through the instrument channel until it protrudes from the endoscope tip and is clearly visible. The endoscopic assistant opens the forceps, and the endoscopist advances the forceps towards the mucosa. The forceps should be advanced with gentle pressure until resistance is met. The assistant then closes the forceps, and the endoscopist pulls the biopsy instrument back into the biopsy channel. This avulses the mucosa, capturing a small tissue sample for examination.

As previously noted, biopsy specimens are obtained while the endoscope is gradually withdrawn from the area of the GI tract being investigated. In instances where a focal mucosal lesion is identified, multiple directed biopsy specimens should be taken. In instances where the abnormality is diffuse or where no gross abnormalities are visualized, multiple biopsy specimens should be obtained from various anatomic sites. For upper GI endoscopy, these sites include the duodenum/jejunum (minimum of 10 to 12 biopsies), and antrum, incisura angularis, lesser curvature, greater curvature, and cardia of the stomach. For colonoscopy, these sites include the cecum, ascending colon, transverse colon, and proximal, middle, and distal descending colon.

To obtain biopsy specimens with a rigid endoscope, the tip of the endoscope should be placed 1 to 2 cm from the area to be sampled. The viewing lens is then opened, allowing the colon to collapse as air moves out. The area to be sampled should be visible in the tip of the endoscope. Alligator biopsy forceps are advanced through the endoscope, opened, and the area to be biopsied gently grasped. Before the tissue is pinched off, the biopsy forceps should be gently moved back and forth. If only mucosa or submucosa has been grasped, the tissue should be freely movable and the biopsy cups can be clamped down to obtain the sample. However, if the grasped tissue remains firmly attached to the colonic wall, this indicates that the forceps has gathered muscular tunics and colonic perforation is possible. In this event the forceps should be opened and a new site, at least 1 cm away, selected. A total of four to five samples should be obtained from the descending colon while the endoscope is progressively withdrawn.

Endoscopic biopsy specimens are delicate and easily damaged. Biopsy specimens should be handled gently and not allowed to dry. Placing the biopsy specimens on some form of support minimizes tissue contraction and preserves orientation. Transfer of the biopsy specimen directly from the biopsy forceps onto a moistened (normal saline) histopathology cassette sponge is recommended. Teasing the biopsy specimen from the biopsy forceps with a needle may damage the tissue. The sponge is placed in a labeled cassette and immersed in 10% formalin.

CONTRAINDICATIONS

Other than anesthetic considerations, GI endoscopy has no absolute contraindications. Endoscopic procedures are discouraged in inadequately prepared animals and in animals with bleeding disorders. Food within the stomach increases the risk of aspiration.

COMPLICATIONS

Complications of GI endoscopy include perforation of the GI wall, with resultant mediastinitis, pleuritis, or peritonitis. Perforation can result from forceful insertion of the endoscope or biopsy forceps. The endoscope should only be advanced if the lumen is visible. Underlying disease in the bowel wall may predispose to perforation. Perforation usually results in the immediate development of air-filled body cavities (e.g., pneumoabdomen). Overdistension of the stomach can cause cardiopulmonary compromise by impeding venous return, limiting tidal volume, and inducing vagal stimulation. Vagovagal reflexes can be induced by excessive traction on the mesentery. Significant hemorrhage can occur after biopsy procedures, but is rare. Enteropathogenic bacteria may be transmitted by poorly disinfected endoscopes. Gastric dilatation and volvulus can occur because of the inadequate removal of insufflated air.

CYTOLOGIC PROCEDURES

Cytologic samples can be used for the diagnosis of inflammatory, infectious, and neoplastic disorders of the GI tract of dogs and cats. Appropriate samples can be obtained manually (fecal smear, rectal scraping) or endoscopically. The clinician should prepare fecal smears by obtaining a fleck of mucus or a sample of feces from stool surface and smearing the sample thinly on a microscope slide. To obtain a rectal scraping for cytologic evaluation, a gloved finger or small curette can be inserted into the rectum and scraped along the mucosal surface. The sample collected should be thinly smeared on a microscope slide. After staining with new methylene blue or Wright's stain, fecal smears and rectal scrapings can be evaluated for the presence of inflammatory or neoplastic cells and pathologic organisms (e.g., *Histoplasma capsulatum*, *Prototheca* spp., *Campylobacter jejuni*, *Clostridium perfringens*).

Cytologic examination of exfoliative specimens obtained endoscopically can be a useful adjunct to mucosal biopsy for the diagnosis of GI inflammation and malignancy in dogs and cats. It can also be useful for identification of *Helicobacter* in the gastric mucosa. Cytologic preparations can be obtained by brush or touch cytologic techniques (or both). The basic technique of brush cytology involves advancing a single-use guarded brush through the instrument channel, extending the brush beyond its protective sheath, and vigorously brushing the area of interest under direct visualization to exfoliate cells. The brush is then retracted into its sheath and removed from the endoscope. Finally, the brush is extended from its sheath and gently rolled across a glass slide. Theoretically, brush cytology offers the advantage of allowing for sampling of a larger surface area than biopsy. The touch cytology technique involves the transfer of an endoscopic mucosal biopsy to a glass slide. The clinician then makes multiple cytologic imprints by placing a second slide on top of, and at right angles to, the first slide and applying gentle pressure. Proper cytologic evaluation of samples obtained using these techniques requires an experienced GI cytopathologist.

NEUROLOGIC

CHAPTER 117

Cerebrospinal Fluid Collection, Myelography, Epidurography, and Discography

P. Filippo Adamo

CEREBROSPINAL FLUID COLLECTION

Cerebrospinal fluid (CSF) analysis is an important component of the diagnostic evaluation of patients with neurologic diseases, and abnormalities in the color, cellularity, and protein level of the CSF may contribute to or confirm the diagnosis. Cerebrospinal fluid abnormalities have to be viewed in the context of the neurologic examination, historical complaints, clinical findings, advanced imaging, and any laboratory abnormalities.

Spinal Needles
Spinal needles with a 22-gauge stylet are commonly used; 20-gauge needles may be acceptable in larger dogs. Spinal needles 1½ inches long are appropriate in most of dogs for cisternal tap and in cats for both lumbar and cisternal tap. Spinal needles 2½ inches long may be used in large dogs for both cisternal and lumbar tap. The 3½-inch-long needles are usually reserved for the lumbar tap in large and obese dogs.

Sample Stability
The CSF should be collected in a sterile plain glass tube without anticoagulant. Usually, 1 to 2 mL are collected; 1 mL per 5 kg body weight of CSF can be safely removed for analysis. Since cell morphology and cell recognition in the CSF are time dependent, the sample should be analyzed immediately, or no later than 4 to 8 hours, after collection. If a longer delay is expected, adding 50% hydroxyethyl starch (hetastarch) improves the stability of the sample for up to 48 hours.

COLLECTION TECHNIQUES

Collection Sites
Two sites are available for CSF tap: the cerebellomedullary cistern (cisternal tap) and the lumbar region (lumbar tap). Cisternal tap is easier, and a sample taken from this area is less likely to be contaminated with blood. CSF flows in a cranial to caudal direction, and cisternal tap is appropriate to investigate intracranial diseases. For diseases affecting the spinal cord, a lumbar tap is more likely to be diagnostic. Collection of CSF in dogs and cats is performed under general anesthesia. Patients should be intubated, and ventilator support must be available. The site of collection must be clipped and prepared aseptically, and sterile surgical gloves should be worn.

Cisternal Tap
Because the neck will be severely flexed when cisternal tap is performed, the patient should be intubated with a kink-proof endotracheal tube to avoid occluding airflow. The patient is positioned in right lateral recumbency for the right-handed

operator. The head and entire spine is positioned close to the edge of the table facing the operator. The head is held by an assistant in 90° flexion with the nose parallel to the table. Placing some form of support under the neck (foam wedge or rolled-up towel) to support the nose will help maintain the alignment between the spine of the axis and the external occipital protuberance. The assistant holding the head of the patient, being careful not to block access to the landmarks for CSF collection, is instructed to "tuck in the animal's chin" and push the occipital protuberance toward the operator (Figure 117-1).

The proper location for needle insertion can be estimated in several ways. It is the author's preference to locate the caudal aspect of the occipital protuberance with the index finger of the left hand while simultaneously locating the wings of the atlas with the thumb and the middle fingers. Pressing firmly with the index finger tip as the finger is simultaneously moved caudally, just behind the occipital protuberance, allows palpation of a slight depression in the muscle, and the caudal edge of this depression is the point of needle insertion. The

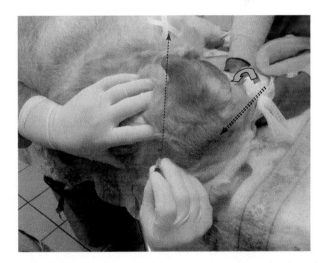

Figure 117-1 Cisternal tap. The patient is positioned in lateral recumbency with the entire spine and the head close to the edge of the table. The assistant, maintaining the head parallel to the table, is flexing the neck *(green arrow)* and pushing the occipital protuberance toward the operator *(double-dotted arrow)*. The needle is inserted in the muscle depression caudal to the occipital protuberance, at about a 30° angle along the midline, and is directed toward the tip of the shoulder joint *(single-dotted arrow)*. To facilitate recognition of the shoulder joint during collection, this landmark may be marked with bandage tape.

needle is inserted at approximately a 30° angle along the midline, and it is directed toward the tip of the shoulder joint. The skin is punctured first, and the needle is slowly advanced into the underlying muscle and fascia. In many instances, a slight sudden loss of resistance (slight "pop") may be felt as the atlanto-occipital membrane and dura mater are penetrated simultaneously. However, this sensation is not consistent, and in small dogs and cats this may be difficult to feel. Often the clinician must rely on the length of the needle used and on his/her tridimensional reconstruction of the anatomic area. The needle is usually advanced with the stylet in place and in small increments; the stylet can be removed between each movement to check whether CSF is present in the needle. Advancing the needle without stylet increases the chance that the needle will become obstructed with tissue or blood clot Additionally, there will be less damage if the nervous tissue is penetrated with the stylet in place. If the tip of the needle hits bone, the needle is slightly withdrawn and redirected slightly cranially or caudally to the original trajectory. When the desired level has been reached, the palm of the left hand is placed on the skull for support and the hub of the needle is grasped with the thumb and index finger. The stylet is removed with the right hand and is observed for fluid flow. If fluid is not seen, the stylet is replaced, and the needle is further advanced 1 to 2 mm at a time. After each advancement the stylet is removed to observe for fluid flow. When the desired level has been reached but no fluid has emerged, a slight rotation of the needle may be enough to dislodge any obstruction and allow the CSF to flow. To increase CSF flow, pressure can be applied to the jugular veins. If whole blood flows from the needle, the needle should be withdrawn and the procedure repeated using a fresh needle. This indicates that a venous sinus has been penetrated. Because these structures are in the extradural space, the CSF is not contaminated with blood and

the procedure can be repeated. If CSF is tinted with blood, either a dural vessel has been penetrated or the blood may be part of the disease process. In the first case, the CSF may clear as the CSF drips from the needle, and the CSF may then be collected. Rotating the needle may also help to clear this type of bleeding. Centrifugation of the fluid may be used to differentiate hemorrhage from contamination or from a disease process. If hemorrhage is part of the disease process, centrifugation of the CSF will result in a yellow color (xanthochromia) from the hemoglobin breakdown products from the erythrocytes present; in the case of contamination, the supernatant will be clean and colorless (Figure 117-2).

Small amounts of iatrogenic hemorrhage do not interfere significantly with evaluation of the CSF.

Lumbar Tap

Lumbar tap is usually more difficult, and blood contamination tends to occur more often. Collection is usually from L5-L6 or L4-L5 in dogs. In cats, L6-L7 can also be used. Lumbar collection can be obtained with the animal in lateral or ventral recumbency. It is the author's preference to collect the fluid with the animal in ventral recumbency. In this position is easy to align the spine and to maintain the hind limbs cranially extended. This widens the interarcuate space, which facilitates the needle penetration in the vertebral canal (Figure 117-3).

For a collection at the L5-L6 site, the tip of the L6 spinous process is palpated. The needle is inserted just lateral to the midline alongside the caudal edge of the L6 spinous process. The needle is inserted at approximately a 45° angle (caudally) from an imaginary line perpendicular to the long axis of the spine; it is then directed cranially and ventrally through the ligamentum flavum into the vertebral canal. After the interarcuate space is passed, the needle penetrates the dura and enters the subarachnoid space. Due to the mechanical stimu-

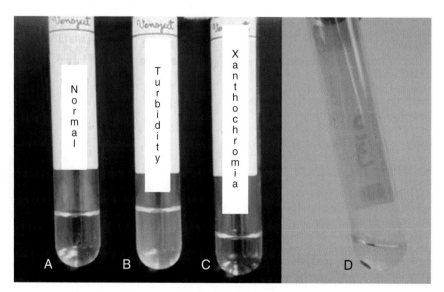

Figure 117-2 Cerebrospinal fluid (CSF) appearance. **A,** Normal CSF has a waterlike appearance. **B,** Turbidity is usually due to an increased number of cells (more than 200 white blood cells/µL, more than 400 red blood cells/µL) and occasionally is due to an increased protein level. Elevated protein levels will also cause increased viscosity. A marked increase in the protein level often causes the CSF to clot. **C,** Xanthochromia (yellowish color) is indicative of recent hemorrhage as part of the disease process; xanthochromia is the result of the hemoglobin breakdown products from the erythrocytes. Xanthochromia after centrifugation of the CSF sample differentiates between iatrogenic and ongoing hemorrhage in the subarachnoid space as part of the disease process. **D,** In case of iatrogenic blood contamination after centrifugation, the supernatant will be clear and colorless.

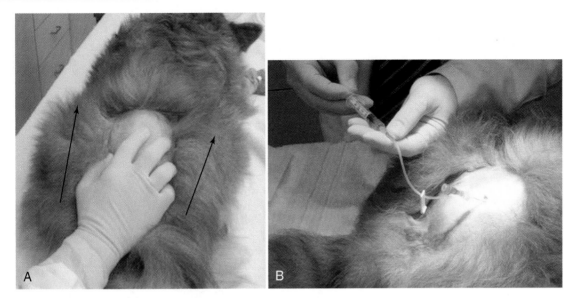

Figure 117-3   Lumbar tap. **A,** With the animal in sternal recumbency it may be easier to maintain the spine in alignment while opening the interarcuate space by extending the hindlimbs cranially *(arrows).* This may facilitate the needle placement in the vertebral canal. **B,** After the needle is in the proper position, to facilitate collection a 2.5-mL syringe with a short injection set is connected to the needle and gentle suction is applied to complete the cerebrospinal fluid collection.

lation of the spinal cord and/or nerve roots at this level, a twitch of the pelvic limbs and/or tail it is usually noted. The needle is advanced to the floor of the vertebral canal and then slightly retracted 1 to 2 mm. At this point the stylet is withdrawn. CSF tends to flow more slowly in lumbar collection than in cisternal collection. To facilitate collection it is the author's preference to connect a 2.5-mL syringe with a short injection set to the needle and to apply gentle suction to complete the CSF collection. If the collection fails, the operation may be repeated on the contralateral side first, and then at the more cranial L4-L5 site.

Risks and Complications
Inadvertant needle penetration of the parenchyma at the cerebellomedullary angle may cause brainstem dysfunction ranging from temporary vestibular abnormalities to cessation of voluntary respiration and death. Foramen magnum herniation, with the cerebellar vermis herniating caudally and compressing the brainstem, may also be a lethal complication. This risk has been decreased by the use of MRI, which should be performed before CSF collection. MRI may identify patients where the cerebellum is already herniated or prone to herniation (Figure 117-4).

In these patients mannitol and hyperventilation may be used to decrease intracranial pressure (ICP) before CSF collection. To avoid puncturing an already herniated cerebellum, a lumbar tap is the preferred method for CSF collection.

MYELOGRAPHY

Myelography may be performed by either cervical or lumbar injection. With the patient in lateral recumbency the needle is placed as described above for CSF collection. Ideally, lumbar myelography injection should be made at L5-L6 as the incidence of complications increases with injections at sites cranial to this. To study lesions in the lumbosacral area, cisternal myelography is advised, which may decrease the risk of contaminating the area with an epidurography. In the cervical

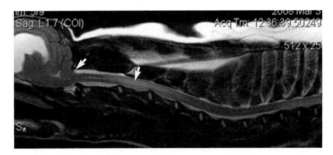

Figure 117-4   Contraindications for cisternal tap. MRI T2 sagittal plane of a dog with obstructive hydrocephalus causing cerebellar herniation *(left arrow)* and syringomyelia *(right arrow).* In this patient, the needle placement in the cerebellomedullary cistern would likely puncture the herniated cerebellar vermis; therefore, cisternal tap is contraindicated in this case.

injection the bevel of the needle should be directed caudally and in the lumbar injection cranially. Injection should be performed by connecting the syringe to the spinal needle with a short injection set prefilled with contrast medium. Cervical injection is easier but lumbar injection is usually preferred. Cervical injection is usually associated with the accumulation of contrast medium into the cerebral ventricular system, which may increase the risk of postmyelographic seizures. This may be alleviated by maintaining (just after the injection) the patient tilted at about 30° with the head elevated. However, a lesion causing severe cord swelling or severe spinal cord compression may not allow the contrast medium to flow caudally to the lesion, resulting in equivocal interpretation of the study that will require a subsequent lumbar myelogram. Lumbar injection can be performed under pressure, forcing the contrast medium to pass the lesion outlining the cranial and the caudal edge of the spinal cord lesion. Serial radiographs may help to locate the needle in the desired spot. Fluoroscopic guidance can also facilitate proper needle placement.

CSF should be collected before the injection of the contrast since the most common contrast mediums used (iohexol or iopamidol, 240 to 300 mg/mL) tend to induce an inflammatory reaction. A test injection (with 0.5 to 1.0 mL, depending on patient size) of contrast medium should be performed, and after radiologic confirmation (by radiographs or fluoroscopy) that the contrast is in the subarachnoid space, the remainder of the calculated dose can be injected. The volume of contrast to inject varies from 0.3 mL/kg to 0.45 mL/kg body weight; this depends on the site of the injection and the expected location of the lesion. For cervical myelogram with lumbar injection, the higher dose is recommended. After the contrast medium is injected, a series of radiographs in lateral and ventrodorsal position are taken. Additional oblique views are often needed in dogs with herniated disc to further identify the site of the lesion. Stress view radiographs in linear traction, dorsiflexion, and ventriflexion are usually performed in dogs with caudal cervical spondylomyelopathy, and stress view radiographs with maximum flexion and extension (both in lateral and ventrodorsal position) of the lumbosacral junction are usually performed in dogs with lumbosacral diseases. Transient exacerbation of neurologic signs may be seen after myelography; this is usually caused by transient chemical myelitis secondary to contrast injection. This risk may be higher in patients affected by an inflammatory myelopathy or chronic spinal cord compression. This usually resolves within a few days. Accidental injection of the contrast medium within the spinal cord parenchyma or within the central spinal canal may cause worsening of the neurologic status. In most cases, patients recover when iatrogenic trauma occurs in the lumbar region, but contrast medium injection in the cervical region may be fatal (Figure 117-5).

Intracranial subarachnoid hemorrhage is also a rare but fatal complication associated with lumbar myelography.

EPIDUROGRAPHY

Epidurography is usually combined with myelography and discography to help visualize diseases of the cauda equine. However, MRI has largely replaced the use of these two studies. Epidurography is particularly indicated in dogs where the dural sac does not extend to the sacrum and is usually performed after myelography. With the area aseptically prepared and the patient in lateral recumbency, the spinal needle is inserted between the spinal process of L7 and S1, between the sacrum and the first coccygeal vertebra, or between one of the caudal intervertebral spaces. The volume of contrast to inject is 0.1 to 0.2 mL/kg body weight.

DISCOGRAPHY

Discography is usually used in conjunction with epidurography for evaluation of L7-S1 disk diseases. The contrast is injected directly into the nucleus pulposus of the L7-S1 disk and radiographs in lateral and dorsoventral projection are taken. The volume of contrast is 0.1 to 0.3 mL/kg of body weight. In a normal disc, it is very difficult to inject contrast and usually no more then 0.1 mL may be injected. In a degenerated and/or herniated disc 2 to 3 mL may be easily injected and the contrast may also flow out in the spinal canal through

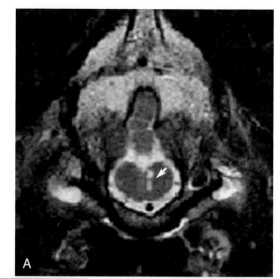

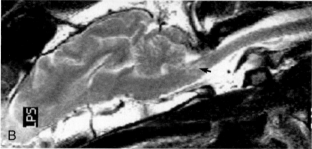

Figure 117-5 Fatal complication of improper needle placement during myelography. T2-weighted MRI of a German Shepherd Dog presented with depressed mental status, poor gag reflex, reduced tongue movement, and reduced sensation of the mandibular and maxillary branches of the trigeminal nerve. Myelography to rule out compressive spinal disease was attempted at a different facility 3 days prior to this MRI. The dog never recovered properly from the myelography and the owner elected euthanasia 3 weeks later. **A,** Transverse plane: the hyperintense line traversing almost the entire caudal brainstem in a dorsoventral direction is the damage created by the needle tract *(arrow).* **B,** The diffuse hyperintensity in the caudal brainstem *(arrow)* is most likely edema secondary to the intraparenchymal needle placement. (Courtesy Dr. Rodolfo Cappello and Dr. Annette Wessmann.)

the degenerated disc. The combination of discography/ epidurography may be performed using a single needle puncture. Discography is performed and radiographs are taken first; the needle is withdrawn to the epidural space and additional contrast is injected, followed by radiographs.

References

The reference list can be found on the companion Expert Consult Web site at *www.expertconsult.com.*

CHAPTER 118

Muscle and Nerve Biopsy

Peter J. Dickinson
Richard A. LeCouteur

Biopsy of muscle and/or nerve can be an essential aid in the diagnosis and therapy of suspected neuromuscular disease of small animals. Examination of the specific components of the motor unit, as well as of sensory and autonomic nerves, permits definition and classification of the underlying pathology.

MUSCLE BIOPSY

Conventional biopsy and formalin fixation techniques, as used with most organ systems, severely limit the quality of information that may be obtained from muscle specimens. Development of specialized enzyme histochemical techniques, using frozen specimens, has greatly increased the understanding both of normal muscle and of the underlying pathologic processes of many neuromuscular diseases.

Selection of Muscle
The selection of a muscle for biopsy is guided by a number of criteria:
1. The muscle should be affected by the disease process but should not be end-stage. This choice may be based on electrophysiologic data, including abnormal electromyographic (EMG) results, and on clinical abnormalities suggesting muscle involvement (atrophy, hypertrophy, apparent pain, weakness).
2. The muscle should be easily identified surgically, with low associated morbidity, and with fibers oriented in a single direction.
3. Specimens should be harvested from muscles for which there is previous interpretive experience. Standard muscles include the lateral head of the triceps brachii (distal third), vastus lateralis (distal third), cranial tibial (proximal third), and temporalis muscles. Biopsy specimens from both a thoracic and a pelvic limb muscle, or other distant locations, and from a proximal and a distal muscle, are necessary for optimal diagnosis of generalized neuromuscular disease.
4. Muscle biopsy specimens should be harvested from a site remote to tendinous insertions and aponeuroses.
5. Specimens should be free of artifact induced by previous disease, intramuscular injections, and EMG needle insertion.
6. Some specialized procedures may require biopsy specimens from specific muscles or regions within muscles. For example, diagnosis of congenital myasthenia gravis is based on the demonstration of decreased numbers of acetylcholine receptors in biopsies of external intercostal muscle.

Open Muscle Biopsy Procedure
Open biopsies are done most often under general anesthesia following an electrodiagnostic study. After routine surgical preparation, the skin and fascia overlying the muscle are incised, allowing visualization of myofiber orientation. A specimen for fixation is harvested first. Two incisions are made with a No. 11 scalpel blade, parallel to the direction of the myofibers and approximately 2 cm long, 0.25 cm apart, and 0.5 cm deep. Specialized muscle clamps are placed at either end of the incised strip of muscle (to minimize myofiber contraction), and the isolated muscle is freed from the surrounding muscle with a scalpel blade or scissors. The specimen should be immediately immersed in fixative, usually glutaraldehyde (either sodium phosphate–buffered glutaraldehyde or Karnovsky's fixative). Clamps may be removed 24 hours following fixation. If a specialized muscle clamp is not available, the specimen may be sutured to the wooden stem of a cotton-tipped applicator. Specimens for freezing and routine histochemical staining (approximately 0.5 to 1 cm in cross section and 1 to 1.5 cm long) may be harvested from adjacent muscle. It is not necessary to maintain these specimens in a stretched position. To reduce artifact, handling of the specimen should be kept to a minimum. Wound closure is routine. External dressings are not necessary. Complications (infection, hematoma) are uncommon and usually are the result of animals interfering with the biopsy site. Collection of a muscle biopsy specimen may be contraindicated in dogs or cats with coagulopathy.

Percutaneous Muscle Biopsy Procedure
Percutaneous needle or punch muscle biopsy is not recommended routinely due to the limited size and poor orientation of the biopsy specimens obtained.

Specimen Processing and Transport
Ideally, muscle biopsy specimens should be frozen immediately following harvesting or transported to specialized laboratories for processing and interpretation. Specimen blocks are mounted on thin cork squares using tissue-embedding medium, with the muscle fibers oriented vertical to the cork, and frozen for approximately 20 seconds in isopentane (2-methylbutane) cooled to approximately −150° C in liquid nitrogen. Rapid freezing of the specimen is critical for preservation of morphologic detail and prevention of artifacts. Frozen blocks may be stored in airtight containers at −80° C or in liquid nitrogen storage vessels. For biopsy specimens that are to be transported to specialized laboratories for processing, one fact cannot be overemphasized: *The quality of the information that will be obtained depends on the quality of the biopsy specimen that arrives at the laboratory.* Before a biopsy procedure is completed, the destination laboratory's specific instructions for selection, handling, and transportation of the specimen should always be obtained. Nonfrozen specimens should be wrapped in saline-moistened swabs that have been thoroughly wrung dry; the specimens then should be placed in an airtight container and maintained at 4° C using cold packs. The specimen container should be wrapped in a layer of newspaper to insulate it from the cold packs to prevent partial freezing of the specimen. Specimens should be shipped in order to reach the laboratory within 30 hours and should not arrive at the laboratory during a weekend.

Muscle specimens to be used for biochemical analysis (such as carnitine quantitation) and glutaraldehyde-fixed specimens may be transported in a container separate from the chilled biopsy specimen. Many laboratories request that 5 mL of the animal's serum be shipped with the muscle biopsy specimen.

NERVE BIOPSY

Selection of Nerve

As with muscle selection, certain guidelines should be followed in the selection of a nerve for biopsy:

1. The nerve should be affected by the disease process, as evidenced by abnormal results on electrophysiologic investigations or by neurologic abnormalities in areas innervated by the nerve (atrophy, hypotonia, hyporeflexia, paresis, sensory deficits).
2. If the disease process is generalized, a nerve should be selected that (1) is easily biopsied with low morbidity, (2) has established normal electrophysiologic and morphometric data available, and (3) innervates a muscle that may be routinely biopsied.

Biopsy of the mixed (motor/sensory/autonomic) common peroneal nerve is recommended when generalized neuromuscular disease is suspected. This nerve is relatively easy to identify and biopsy because it is flat and contains prominent fascicles. Other mixed nerves that may be biopsied easily are the tibial nerve (pelvic limb) and the ulnar nerve (thoracic limb). When a predominantly sensory neuropathy is suspected, biopsy of cutaneous sensory nerves, such as the caudal cutaneous antebrachial nerve or the caudal cutaneous sural nerve, may be appropriate. Biopsy of nerve roots via laminectomy may be necessary when pathologic changes are restricted to the most proximal portions of the peripheral nervous system. If both dorsal and ventral nerve roots are affected, biopsy of the dorsal nerve root is preferred. Biopsy of cranial nerves is infrequently done, largely due to the inaccessibility of these nerves.

Nerve Biopsy Technique (Common Peroneal)

The common peroneal nerve may be palpated on the lateral aspect of the distal femur just caudal to the proximal tibia. A 6- to 8-cm incision is made over this region, exposing the fascia of the biceps femoris muscle. After the nerve has been palpated through the fascia, a small incision (4 to 5 cm) is made in the fascia while the fascia is elevated with a pair of rat-toothed forceps to prevent inadvertent damage to the nerve. The nerve may be seen as it passes over the lateral head of the gastrocnemius muscle. A 5-0 or 6-0 silk suture is placed through the caudal one fourth to one half of the nerve at the proximal end of the biopsy site, allowing minimal gentle traction as a 3- to 4-cm fascicular biopsy is excised using fine iris scissors. Severely diseased nerves may be markedly reduced in size and may appear almost translucent. Care should be taken to dissect as much fat and fascia from around the nerve as possible. Wound closure is routine. External dressings normally are not required. Some animals may exhibit proprioceptive deficits, with knuckling of the distal pelvic limb on the side of the biopsy. This usually resolves within 3 to 4 days, and long-term deficits are uncommon.

Nerve Specimen Processing

The nerve should be placed immediately into fixative (usually glutaraldehyde). Contraction artifact is minimized by (1) pinning the nerve at either end to a piece of balsa wood; (2) suturing the nerve at either end onto the wooden stem of a cotton-tipped applicator; or (3) suspending the nerve in fixative with a stainless steel weight. The sample then may be transported to the laboratory in a sealed screw-top bottle. Specimens collected in this manner may be used for plastic embedding, teased fiber preparations, or electron microscopy. A nerve specimen also may be frozen in liquid nitrogen if specialized biochemical analysis is required.

CHAPTER 119

Electromyography and Nerve Conduction Velocity Studies

Paul A. Cuddon

Electrophysiology is one of the most important diagnostic tools for animals suspected of having disease of peripheral nerves, muscles, or neuromuscular junctions. It provides invaluable information about the severity, distribution, and character of the disease process and guides the clinician to the most appropriate site for muscle and peripheral nerve fascicular biopsies.

ELECTROMYOGRAPHY

Electromyography (EMG) is the recording and study of insertional, spontaneous, and voluntary muscle electrical activity.[1] Due to the difficulty of patient compliance, awake EMG is not routinely performed in small animals. Therefore, voluntary muscle contraction and assessment of myofiber recruitment and interference patterns usually are not evaluated. Most patients are tested under general anesthesia, where insertional and spontaneous muscle activities are primarily assessed. All EMG testing is subject to technical difficulties due to external noise from other electrical outlets (60-cycle interference) or anesthesia-related equipment in the same room. The animal should be placed on a padded surface, grounded to the machine, and be in a warm environment to prevent artifacts.[2]

The most commonly used EMG recording electrodes in veterinary medicine are the concentric needle electrode and use of two monopolar needle electrodes.[3] The concentric (coaxial) needle electrode detects less background noise than monopolar needles, although it does cause increased tissue injury. Monopolar needle electrodes are less electrically stable and "noisier" than concentric needle electrodes, although they do produce less pain and record a considerably larger potential from the same source than the concentric needle. The monopolar electrodes are also able to detect distant potentials due to their substantial interelectrode distance.[3]

EMG assesses the initial insertional activity of a muscle during placement of the recording electrode into the muscle. This normally consists of brief bursts of electrical activity, producing a crisp, static sound that arises from mechanically stimulated or injured myofibers. In normal muscle, insertional activity should have an abrupt onset and termination, lasting a few hundred milliseconds, without waxing and waning. Insertional activity can be utilized to determine muscle excitability, measuring muscle fibrosis as decreased electrical excitability and denervation or myositis as increased electrical excitability.[1]

Normal resting muscle is generally electrically silent once the inserted recording electrode is at rest. However, there are three types of normal muscle activity that can be observed. These include miniature endplate potentials (MEPPs), endplate spikes, and motor unit action potentials (MUAPs). These waveforms are associated with the recording electrode being placed near a muscle endplate zone. MEPPs represent low-amplitude activity produced by sustained, random, spontaneous release of single ACh quanta, causing postsynaptic membrane depolarization. Endplate spikes are always associated with MEPPs and represent a single discharging myofiber that is excited by nerve terminal and junctional activity. MUAPs are only seen in awake or lightly anesthetized animals, representing a compound action potential of myofibers in the electrode's recording range.[1] Although assessment of normal muscle activity and muscle recruitment patterns can be difficult in the awake dog or cat, one valid area of application is in the assessment of traumatic peripheral nerve injury, most commonly associated with the brachial plexus. The lack of any MUAPs in extensor muscles with weight bearing or in flexor muscles with assisted flexion of a joint would indicate severe nerve injury.

There are four abnormal spontaneous muscle activity patterns with EMG—fibrillation potentials, positive sharp waves (PSWs), complex repetitive discharges (CRDs), and myotonic potentials.[4-7] Fibrillations (biphasic or triphasic waves) and PSWs (large downward spikes followed by short upward peaks) represent the same underlying pathologic changes and differ only in their orientation to the recording electrode. They both arise from spontaneously firing, single hypersensitive myofibers, caused by destabilization of the sarcolemmal membrane seen with denervation and inflammatory or degenerative myopathies (muscular dystrophy). They have the classic sound of frying eggs or the wrinkling of tissue paper. CRDs are uniform, polyphasic repetitive waveforms produced from the spontaneous discharge of multiple myofibers that are firing in near synchrony. These are usually associated more with chronic denervation or with certain muscle disorders, such as Cushing's associated myopathy. Myotonic potentials are repetitive waxing and waning discharges, representing independent repetitive discharges from single injured myofibers. These, and only these, are characteristic of myotonia congenita. The waxing and waning nature of these potentials produces the classic "dive-bomber" sound.[4-7]

It is important to remember that EMG changes associated with denervation are not detected in small animals for a minimum of 4 to 5 days after the trauma or disease onset, with maximum changes being delayed until 8 to 10 days.[5,8] The shorter the distance from the site of injury to the tested muscle, the earlier the spontaneous activity occurs. Serum creatinine kinase levels are also not significantly affected by performing EMGs. Even though serum CK has been shown to increase, the values are usually within the normal range.[9]

MOTOR AND SENSORY NERVE CONDUCTION STUDIES

Motor and sensory nerve conduction are the most common peripheral nerve evaluation modalities in small animals. Independent of whether motor or sensory nerve conduction is being evaluated, certain principles need to be followed to obtain the most accurate recordings for interpretation. The cathodal (negative) stimulating electrode should always be placed closer to the recording electrode than the anode to prevent anodal block.[10] Distance measurements between individual sites of stimulation must be from cathode to cathode. In addition, to accurately evaluate action potential amplitudes, all waveforms should be recorded at supramaximal stimulus strength. To diminish stimulus artifact, the ground electrode should be positioned between the stimulating and the recording electrodes.[5,10]

In motor nerve conduction studies, many mixed and motor nerves can be readily accessed. The most commonly used nerves are the radial, ulnar, and median nerves in the thoracic limb and the peroneal and tibial nerves in the pelvic limb.[11,12] Although needle recording electrodes record only a small percentage of the potentially recordable compound muscle action potentials (CMAPs) and need more critical placement than surface recording electrodes, they are much easier to manipulate and adjust.[10] Typically, CMAPs are recorded from at least two sites along the length of the tested nerve, and the resultant motor nerve conduction velocities (MNCVs) are calculated by dividing the distance between each of the consecutive stimulation sites (mm) by the latency (time) difference between the onset of each of the corresponding recorded CMAPs (msec). MNCVs are measured in meters/second.[5,11-13] To avoid inaccuracies in surface distance measurement, the distance between two consecutive sites of stimulation should be at least 100 mm.[5] Measurement of MNCVs reflects the degree of myelination along a segment of nerve, whereas CMAP amplitude and area measurements represent the volume of functional axons as well as the number of responding myofibers to an electrical stimulus. Normal values for canine and feline MNCVs and CMAP amplitudes/areas have been published elsewhere.[11-18] MNCVs and CMAP amplitudes can be influenced by nonpathologic factors such as the age of the patient, the limb temperature, and the limb length. Increasing age will decrease MNCV, as will decreasing limb temperature and increasing limb length.[10,12,18-21] Cats have faster MNCVs compared to dogs.[5,16] Utilizing motor nerve conduction techniques, supramaximal repetitive stimulation can assess neuromuscular junction diseases, such as botulism and myasthenia gravis.[22-25]

The major pathologic abnormalities associated with motor nerve conduction studies are demyelination, axonal degeneration, or a combination of the above. Demyelination classically will produce a decrease in MNCVs without a decrease in CMAP amplitudes, although severe demyelination can produce CMAP temporal dispersion and/or polyphasia. If there is a segmental demyelination involving two or more sequential internodes, a decreased proximal versus distal CMAP amplitude will result, which represents an effective blockade of impulses attempting to cross this region even though more distal internodes may still be conductile. This is termed *conduction block*. Axonal involvement will produce a generalized decrease in CMAP amplitudes and areas without temporal dispersion. However, CMAP amplitude decrease can also reflect primary myopathy or neuromuscular junction disease (botulism).[5]

Sensory nerve conduction studies are more technically challenging to perform due to the small size of the waveforms and the difficulty in distinguishing them from background noise. To minimize background noise and muscle contraction artifact, signal averaging is utilized and often the animal is chemically paralyzed while under anesthesia.[26-28] Only one stimulation site is necessary since the sensory nerve action potential (SNAP) is recorded directly from the nerve, thus avoiding unknown time delays at the neuromuscular junction seen with motor nerve conduction.[10,13] Since SNAP amplitudes are variable between animals and even between sides in the same animal, only SNCVs are of consistent diagnostic value. SNCVs are calculated by dividing the surface distance (mm) from the cathodal-stimulating electrode to the recording electrode by the latency (time) measurement from the stimulus artifact to the first positive (downward) peak of the recorded SNAP. Both sensory and mixed nerves can be assessed by this technique.[26-28] The abnormalities discussed for MNCVs apply in principle to sensory nerve conduction studies.

MOTOR AND SENSORY NERVE ROOT STUDIES

Direct stimulation and recording from dorsal and ventral nerve roots and the most proximal portions of peripheral nerves are difficult due to their inaccessibility. By using antidromic and orthodromic conduction properties of motor nerves and the ability to record over the dorsal horn of the spinal cord, these otherwise inaccessible regions can be indirectly assessed.

F waves, long-latency motor action potentials, are an excellent assessor of the proximal motor nerve, ventral nerve roots, and the spinal cord ventral horn cells.[5,29-31] Since the conduction pathway is considerably longer than it is in MNCV measurements, borderline conduction abnormalities are magnified, resulting in a more sensitive assessment of motor nerve function. F waves are also more accurate in detecting subtle nerve and nerve root pathology since latency measurements have a much narrower normal range.[5,29-31] To circumvent the F wave latency variation between dogs with different limb lengths, regression equations are utilized for the ulnar and sciatic-tibial nerves.[32] In cats, normal values for F wave latencies do not have to use regression equations due to similar limb lengths in this species.

Cord dorsum potentials (CDPs) represent purely sensory events and are recorded from the dorsal horn of the spinal cord.[33,34] They are an excellent means of assessing the most proximal portion of sensory nerve roots as well as their entry into the dorsal horn of the spinal cord. The active electrode is placed in the interarcute foramen of C7-T1 for the ulnar and radial nerves and generally in the interarcute foramen of C4-C5 for the peroneal and tibial nerves.[33] Normal CDP onset latency predictive values have been established in the dog for the distal tibial and superficial radial nerves, using regression equations.[33] Normal latency measurements have also been established for the cat. CDP recordings appear to be a more accurate and sensitive measurement of peripheral sensory function than SNCVs.

References

The reference list can be found on the companion Expert Consult Web site at *www.expertconsult.com*.

CHAPTER 120

Brain Biopsy

Richard A. LeCouteur
Peter J. Dickinson

Neoplastic, vascular, infectious, or inflammatory diseases of dogs and cats can result in focal brain involvement. In affected animals, results of ancillary diagnostic investigations, such as cerebrospinal fluid (CSF) analysis and electroencephalography, may be within normal limits or may provide only "indirect" evidence of the presence of a brain lesion. The use of computed tomography (CT) and magnetic resonance imaging (MRI) has enabled accurate detection of many focal brain lesions. Although CT and MRI are sensitive in determining location, extent, and relationships to adjacent structures of brain lesions, both have limited specificity. Non-neoplastic lesions (such as those seen in association with infectious, inflammatory, or vascular diseases) may mimic the CT or MRI appearance of a neoplasm. In most instances, results of CT or MRI provide only a broad list of differential diagnoses for a focal brain lesion. Accurate histologic diagnosis of an intracranial lesion is critical before recommending a specific management or treatment strategy.

OPEN BRAIN BIOPSY

Open brain biopsy may be appropriate in certain clinical situations in which cortical architecture needs to be preserved, for leptomeningeal sampling, for superficially located lesions, and when a decompressive craniectomy with good cortical visualization may be helpful in addition to obtaining a biopsy sample.

For superficial brain lesions, a craniectomy is performed, the dura is opened, the lesion is located, and a specimen of affected brain is excised using a No. 11 scalpel blade. For more deep-seated brain lesions, freehand fine needle (22-gauge) aspiration, or Tru-Cut biopsy (using a 14-gauge Tru-Cut biopsy needle, Travenol Laboratories Inc., Deerfield, Ill.), CT-guided freehand Field-Lee needle biopsy (using a 13-gauge Field-Lee brain biopsy needle, V. Mueller, Chicago, Ill.), or ultrasound-guided Menghini needle brain biopsy techniques (using a 16-gauge Menghini biopsy needle, Miltex Corp., Lake Success, N.Y.) have been reported for use in dogs after a limited craniectomy.

Although open brain biopsy techniques usually are accompanied by low morbidity and mortality, these techniques no longer are recommended for deep-seated brain lesions. Stereotactic brain biopsy procedures are preferred, as they have been shown to be safe, effective, and consistent in cats and dogs.

STEREOTACTIC BRAIN BIOPSY

With the advent of CT and MRI and the development of CT-guided stereotactic frames, closed stereotactic brain biopsy has become the standard of care. Essentially all closed methods rely on the three-dimensional CT-generated coordinates identifying the lesion location. These coordinates are used to plot the optimal trajectory and depth needed for a biopsy needle to reach a target and obtain a diagnostic tissue sample.

Technical impediments exist to the direct application of most human stereotactic systems to dogs and cats. Most commercially available systems use a cumbersome head frame and localizing system, designed specifically for the human skull, and require dedicated, expensive computer software for the planning phase. Several different systems for image-guided stereotactic brain biopsy have been reported for use in dogs and cats.

Stereotactic biopsy begins with proper patient selection. The possibility of nonneoplastic disorders such as infection, cerebral infarction, or vasculitis must be considered and investigated prior to biopsy. When the differential diagnosis includes neoplasms and inflammatory lesions, the appropriate handling of tissue samples should be discussed with a neuropathologist in advance of the procedure. All pets should be tested for coagulation parameters (prothrombin time [PT], partial thromboplastin time [PTT]) prior to the procedure and should have a platelet count greater than 100,000. Neither dogs nor cats should receive aspirin products the week before surgery.

General anesthesia is required for stereotactic brain biopsy. Biopsy generally is done on the CT scanner table. For those lesions not well identified on CT images, MRIs that demonstrate a lesion may be used to localize the lesion on CT images, using well-defined anatomic landmarks (e.g., lateral ventricles). Axial CT images are used to define the CT coordinates of reference markers and the biopsy target. Dorsal or sagittal images may be used for trajectory planning. An entry point should be selected that is associated with a low risk for neurologic deficit or hemorrhage (e.g., avoidance of dorsal sagittal sinus). Ependymal puncture should be avoided where possible. A small craniotomy (2-mm diameter) is made by means of a twist drill, the dura mater is punctured with an 18-gauge needle, and biopsies can be done with a side-cutting aspirator biopsy needle (Nashold Biopsy Needle, Integra Radionics, Burlington, Mass.) with a 10-mm side opening. On average, two or three specimens are harvested. It is important to biopsy several regions of the intracranial lesion using a single trajectory.

The intraoperative goal should be to confirm by means of smear or touch preparations whether tissue satisfactory for an eventual diagnosis has been obtained. A specific histologic diagnosis may require routine formalin fixation and paraffin embedding of the biopsy tissue. At the conclusion of the biopsy procedure, the needle is withdrawn in increments to assess any possibility of hemorrhage. In the case of hemorrhage, blood should be permitted to egress from the needle until the bleeding stops. An immediate postoperative CT scan should be obtained to assess hemorrhage, whether or not bleeding was observed. Although stereotactic brain biopsy is minimally invasive (compared with open biopsy techniques), complications rarely may occur. Morbidity may include seizures, hemorrhage, new neurologic deficits, brain infection, tumor seeding, and lack of a definitive diagnosis.

Handling the Intraoperative Specimen

The intraoperative specimen must be processed rapidly and carefully to provide timely and accurate diagnostic information. For large specimens, cytologic analyses (touch imprints, smears) may be done in conjunction with frozen sections. Cytologic analyses alone may be done in situations where access to frozen sections is difficult or when the biopsy specimen is small.

The clinician can make a smear (or "squash") preparation by placing a small fragment of tissue at one end of a standard glass microscope slide. The end of another glass slide should be placed over the tissue with mild pressure applied to both slides. The slides are then gently and rapidly pulled apart to produce a smear. The slides are fixed immediately in 95% alcohol and stained with a rapid hematoxylin and eosin stain. Other techniques include fixation of the specimen in alcohol followed by toluidine blue, Giemsa, or Papanicolaou staining, or air-drying the specimen prior to Romanovsky or Wright's staining.

The clinician may take touch imprints by pressing a glass slide briefly to the surface of the fresh (unfixed) biopsy specimen. Small fragments first may be blotted to remove excess blood or fluid. The slides are fixed and stained in a similar manner to the smear preparations.

Frozen sections provide superior architectural detail for the intraoperative interpretation of biopsy specimens. They are done by placing carefully oriented tissue fragments on a cryostat chuck and freezing them in a viscous freezing medium (such as OCT), either within the cryostat with use of coolant spray and a metal heat extractor, or by snap freezing in supercooled isopentane or 2-methylbutane. Frozen sections are cut and thaw mounted on glass slides. They may be fixed either immediately in alcohol or air-dried before fixation. The sections then are stained with a rapid hematoxylin and eosin stain.

With results of one of the rapid tests outlined previously, a decision may be made regarding the need for further biopsy specimens to define the exact nature of the lesion (e.g., if results from an initial specimen are inconclusive) or the need for additional specimens for completion of specialized techniques (e.g., culture and sensitivity testing for a suspected inflammatory or infectious disorder).

Most intracerebral biopsy specimens may be safely fixed in 10% neutral buffered formalin and processed for hematoxylin and eosin staining. Small samples (1 to 2 mm) can be adequately fixed in 1 to 2 hours, whereas larger specimens may require overnight fixation. If any doubt exists as to the appropriateness of the fixative, a neuropathologist should be consulted immediately. Although technical improvements in immunohistochemical staining permit accurate assessment of samples after formalin fixation and paraffin embedding, immunohistochemical staining assessment of ultrastructural detail using electron microscopy requires fixatives containing glutaraldehyde.

CHAPTER 121

Imaging Neurologic Patients

Peter V. Scrivani

SELECTING THE EXAMINATION

The goals of any imaging examination are any or all of the following: to make a diagnosis or at least to reduce diagnostic uncertainty to a level where it is appropriate to take the next step, define the extent of disease sufficiently to plan treatment (e.g., radiation therapy, surgery), and monitor response to treatment or track disease progression. Neuroimaging is a special category of imaging that deals with diseases of the brain, spinal cord, peripheral nerves, and supporting structures (e.g., the skull and vertebral column). Neuroimaging may be further divided into two broad categories: structural and functional imaging. Structural imaging deals with diseases that produce morphologic changes in the nervous system (e.g., tumor, abscess, malformation). Functional imaging is used for metabolic diseases (although some metabolic diseases produce morphologic changes) and studying how the brain processes information by detecting changes in blood flow associated with neural activity. Functional imaging in animals mostly is performed at research institutions and currently has limited clinical applicability. Therefore, in veterinary medicine, most neuroimaging examinations are directed toward detecting morphologic changes.

The first step in imaging the neurologic patient is determining which imaging examination should be performed. This decision is based on neuroanatomic localization of the lesion, suspected disease for which one wants to test, accuracy and availability of imaging modalities, cost, and risk. For example, if the neuroanatomic localization is the prosencephalon and a neoplasm is suspected because of the patient's older age and recent onset of signs, then brain magnetic resonance imaging (MRI) is recommended because of its greater ability to meet the goals of an imaging examination. If MRI is not available, the next best option would be brain computed tomography (CT) because this examination is reasonably accurate for tumors in dogs. If CT also is not available or declined by the owner, no imaging examination and symptomatic treatment are recommended. One could perform skull radiography, but detecting signs of disease during radiography is rare and often too insensitive and nonspecific to be justifiable (unless evidence of a mass is seen or palpated during physical examination). Also, if the results of imaging would not alter treatment, the cost of the examination is prohibitive, or the risk of general anesthesia is too great, no imaging is necessary.

Radiography
Radiography often is too insensitive to diagnose soft-tissue lesions in the brain, spinal cord, or peripheral nerves. Radiography, however, is affordable and available at most veterinary hospitals and is indicated when the following conditions are suspected: trauma (especially bone), atlantoaxial subluxation, discospondylitis, vertebral physitis, vertebral osteomyelitis, vertebral neoplasm, or some congenital malformations. For these conditions, characteristic changes of the bone (versus soft tissue) often are detected when the disease is sufficiently advanced. Negative results, however, do not exclude these conditions. Therefore, selection of this imaging modality should be made when there is a reasonable chance to make a

diagnosis and missing a treatable or diagnosable condition would result in mismanagement of the patient. Frequently, a diagnosis of one of these conditions during radiography is sufficient to make patient management decisions. Often, however, radiography is only the first step in fully evaluating the patient and additional imaging is performed subsequently.

Myelography is a contrast radiographic procedure where a nonionic, iodinated contrast agent is injected into the spinal subarachnoid space. Myelography is performed less frequently in some hospitals today in lieu of cross-sectional imaging (e.g., CT myelography or MRI). Myelography, however, is still a common procedure in veterinary medicine and may be used to test for extramural spinal cord compression (e.g., intervertebral disk herniation, vertebral neoplasm, subluxation), intradural extramedullary spinal cord compression (e.g., meningioma, nerve sheath neoplasm, nephroblastoma), or intramedullary spinal cord compression (e.g., spinal cord neoplasm, edema, inflammation). Myelographic signs are considered reasonably accurate for these conditions, but CT myelography and spinal MRI are both more accurate.

Cross-Sectional Imaging
CT and MRI are noninvasive methods of examining the nervous system. Both modalities provide cross-sectional imaging and improved ability to differentiate various tissue types, which are limitations of radiography. For most diseases of the brain or spinal cord, MRI is preferred because of increased accuracy (both in sensitivity and specificity). For diseases of the skull or vertebral column, either CT or MRI may be preferential. Indeed, it should be considered that CT and MRI are competitive and complementary modalities because they provide similar and unique information. Both modalities typically require general anesthesia unless the patient is comatose. Modern multislice CT scanners and some MR pulse sequences allow for examination under heavy sedation.

CT has certain advantages related to technical considerations and cost. For example, CT generally has shorter imaging times, which is an important consideration when patient motion may cause substantial artifacts or critical care is needed. CT often is more affordable and does not require specialized monitoring equipment or personnel training as with MRI. Additionally, whereas certain implants may cause important artifacts that degrade the image during CT or MRI, they do not preclude the examination because of patient safety considerations. During MRI, certain life-supporting implants may not function, may move and compress adjacent tissues, or may generate excessive heat. CT also has additional benefits related to diagnosis. For example, CT is more sensitive to detecting small areas of mineralization, gas accumulation, and early hemorrhage. When these attributes are important differentiators of the disease, CT is recommended. For most of neuroimaging, however, MRI is the preferred imaging modality. MRI is more sensitive for detecting small brain lesions, white matter disease, and non–contrast-enhancing diseases. MRI also is very sensitive for detecting hemorrhage or infarcts, does not have beam-hardening and cupping artifacts that preclude complete evaluation of the soft-tissue structures dorsal to the caudal fossa (as in CT), and does not expose patients and personnel to ionizing radiation.

Sometimes both modalities are recommended because they provide unique and complementary information. For example, CT has superior spatial resolution, and MRI has superior contrast resolution. Spatial and contrast resolution refers to the ability to detect two structures as two different structures. With spatial resolution, the issue is how close two tissues can be and still be recognized as different structures. Picture two lines: How close can you draw them and still differentiate them as two lines? With contrast resolution, the issue is differentiating dissimilar tissues based on subtle changes in tissue composition. Because of these differences between CT and MRI regarding spatial and contrast resolution, CT often provides unique information when subtle changes in bone structures are part of the disease process. MRI more often provides unique information when there are subtle changes in soft tissues. That being said, a common misinterpretation of these points is an oversimplification that CT is good for bone and MRI is good for soft tissue. MRI is great for examining bone, especially when there are changes in the bone marrow. The two examinations provide complementary information.

MR scanners are broadly classified as low-field (<1.0 T) and high-field (≥1.0 T). There are minimal data to suggest that one is diagnostically more accurate than the other for particular diseases, but there are pros and cons to each one and there is certain information that can be gained from a high-field scanner that is not possible with a low-field scanner. The rationale for low-field MRI systems is to avoid the high costs associated with high-field MRI, but flexibility in diagnostic applications is limited. Some low-field MR scanners have optimized protocols that allow use of the machine by individuals without specialized training in MR technology. Therefore, they provide a cost-effective solution for some practices.

TECHNICAL CONSIDERATIONS

The rest of the chapter deals with clarifying certain aspects of neuroimaging that may be confusing to individuals unfamiliar with CT or MRI. The topics discussed are: T1 and T2, pulse sequences, anatomic planes, and windowing and leveling. Only the most basic descriptions are provided so that individuals new to the subject can understand the role of these topics in the overall picture of imaging the neurologic patient.

T1 and T2
Understanding what is meant by T1 and T2 often is complicated by complex mathematical explanations, but a more simple understanding is useful for clinical application. T1 and T2 simply are tissue characteristics. All tissues have characteristics such as size, shape, color, weight, smell, texture. They also have characteristics called T1 and T2. Therefore, just as a tissue may be very large, very small, or very red, a tissue also may be very T1 or not so much. Frequently, it is difficult to comprehend this notion because T1 and T2 are intangible and unfamiliar. In order to sense T1 and T2, you must do MRI because that is what a MR scanner does—it measures how much T1 and T2 are in tissues. (This is where the math comes into descriptions—to explain how and what is being measured during MRI.) Suffice it to say that T1 and T2 are two different descriptions of how protons in the body behave in a strong magnetic field. Note that all tissues have a characteristic T1 signal and a characteristic T2 signal that are independent of each other. Therefore, a tissue may have a lot of T1 and a lot of T2, very little T1 and very little T2, a lot of T1 and little T2, little T1 and a lot of T2, or intermediate combinations. For example, normal cerebrospinal fluid (CSF) has a low T1

signal and high T2 signal. Cortical bone has low T1 and low T2 signals. Recognizing disease during MRI is based in part on recognizing changes in the normal T1 and T2 signals of tissues. Therefore, it is important to be familiar with the T1 and T2 signals of various tissues.

An MRI scan can only display either the T1 or T2 characteristics of the tissues at one time. Therefore, during the examination, multiple scans are obtained to display at one time the T1 characteristics and at another time the T2 characteristics. During MRI, the T1 and T2 characteristics are measured in small bits of the body called *voxels* (e.g., a voxel may be a 3-mm cube of tissue), and each voxel is represented on the MRI scan as a small square called a *pixel*. The pixels are located on the image in the same orientation as they are in the body. Therefore, all the pixels together represent a cross section of the body. Whereas it is possible to display the numerical value of T1 or T2 for each voxel, that grid of numbers would not make as much sense as an image of the body. Therefore, the numerical values are assigned a shade of gray, which produces an image. If the scan displays tissues that have a lot of T1 signal as white and tissues that have little T1 as a black (and shades of gray in between the extremes), the scan is referred to as a *T1-weighted image* because the image is "weighted" to show you the T1 characteristics of the tissues as being white. If the scan displays tissues that have a lot of T2 signal as white and tissues that have little T2 as a black, the scan is referred to as a *T2-weighted image*. Whereas all tissues have T1 and T2 characteristics, only one characteristic can be displayed at a time and multiple scans are needed to see both the T1 and T2 characteristics (Figure 121-1).

Pulse Sequence and Anatomic Planes
A pulse sequence is the method by which the MR signal is produced and used to generate a T1-weighted or T2-weighted image. The MR signal can be produced using several different techniques (e.g., spin echo, gradient echo), and the resulting pulse sequences often are named by the technique and the weighting of the signal (e.g., T1 spin echo). These techniques, along with other parameters that can be changed on the MR scanner, are chosen to optimize the image by making compromises between signal strength, acquisition time, and artifacts. Two parameters that may be changed on the MR scanner are time to echo (TE) and time to repeat (TR). These terms often are confused with T1 and T2. The terms TE and TR refer to settings that may be made on the MR scanner to produce a

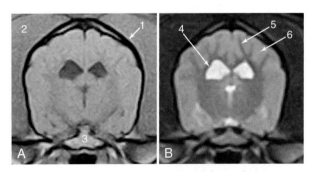

Figure 121-1 T1-weighted **(A)** and T2-weighted **(B)** transverse MR scans of the same dog at the same level in the brain. On the T1-weighted scan, tissues with a high T1 signal are displayed as white and those with a low T1 signal as black. On the T2-weighted scan, tissues with a high T2 signal are displayed as white and those with a low T2 signal as black. The same anatomic structures are seen on both scans; compare the T1 and T2 signals of cortical bone *(1)*, muscle *(2)*, marrow *(3)*, cerebrospinal fluid *(4)*, white matter *(5)*, and gray matter *(6)*.

pulse sequence that will generate a T1-weighted or T2-weighted image. Therefore, TE and TR refer to machine settings and T1 and T2 refer to tissue characteristics. Several different types of pulse sequences are used in addition to the most basic ones mentioned. For example, the FLAIR (fluid attenuation inversion recovery) is a special type of sequence used commonly for neuroimaging to produce T2-weighted images that displays CSF as black (although a T1-weighted FLAIR is possible). This sequence is used to look for periventricular lesions (i.e., to differentiate a white lesion when it is adjacent white CSF) or increase lesion conspicuity.

As mentioned, one reason why multiple scans are obtained during an MR examination is to determine both the T1 and T2 signal characteristics of tissues. Another reason is to evaluate lesions in multiple anatomic planes, which helps in understanding the extent of the lesion and planing treatments. Whereas CT scans only display transverse sections of the body because of the construction of the scanner and because of the way the body fits into the scanner, MRI can display any anatomic plane (transverse, sagittal, dorsal, oblique) without repositioning the patient. This limitation of CT is overcome in modern multislice CT scanners by performing isotropic imaging, which allows for computer reconstruction of the data into any anatomic plane or three dimensions.

Windowing and Leveling

In CT, windowing and leveling are the processes of using the calculated HU to make an image. The Hounsfield unit (HU) is a measure of how many x-rays are stopped by a voxel of tissue. Tissues that stop more x-rays have a higher HU. Since it is easier to look at an image than a grid of HUs, these numerical values can be assigned a shade of gray and displayed as a two-dimensional, cross-sectional image of the body (i.e., the CT scan). During CT, thousands of different HUs are possible, but computer monitors generally only display up to 256 different shades of gray at one time. Therefore, it is not possible to display one shade of gray for each HU and some compromise must be made about how to divide up the number of HUs between the available 256 shades of gray. Alternatively, not all 256 shades are needed to optimize display of a tissue. Therefore, a rule for relating HUs to shades of gray is defined. For example, one shade of gray may be used for each HU, but then only 256 HUs can be represented—above a certain value all HUs are white; below a certain value, black. Alternatively, 3 HUs may be used for each shade of gray and, since there are still only 256 shades of gray, the image represents 768 HUs. This spread of HUs is referred to as a *window*. Smaller windows produce more contrast in the image, which is better for soft-tissue structures (versus bone). A window also could be less than 256 HUs. Changing or setting the window width to a certain range of HUs is what is meant by *windowing*.

To understand leveling, consider a range of the window to be 70 HUs. *Leveling* is the task of picking which 70 HUs to

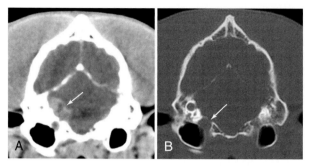

Figure 121-2 Contrast enhanced, transverse, CT scans of the same dog at the level of the tympanic bulla using a soft-tissue window **(A)** and bone window **(B)**. When using a soft-tissue window (window width = 200; level = 50), note that the tumor *(arrow)* may be differentiated from the brain, and the bone is completely white with minimal detail. When using a bone window (window width = 4095; level = 400), note that all the soft tissues are the same homogeneous shade of gray and there is better spatial resolution of bone, including trabecular markings and tumor extending into bone *(arrow)*.

look at out of the thousands available. For example, let's say that the HUs ranged from −1000 to +1000. We can set the center of the 70 HUs window (i.e., the level) to −200, +30, +400 or any other value and produce different depictions of the same anatomy. If we pick +30 as the level, the window would extend from −5 to +65. Setting the level optimizes viewing of the tissue of interest (e.g., lung, bone). For example, if you want to look at bone, you set the level close to the HU characteristic of bone (e.g., +400). To further confuse the situation, people will talk about a "soft-tissue window" or "bone window." In this context, the term *window* means that the windowing, leveling, and other properties related to acquiring the image are optimized for the specified tissue (Figure 121-2).

SUMMARY

Effective neuroimaging is based on selecting the best imaging method to optimally affect patient care. The selection should be based on the goals of the imaging examination, which may be to make a diagnosis or at least to reduce diagnostic uncertainty to a level where it is appropriate to take the next step, define the extent of disease to plan treatment (e.g., radiation therapy, surgery), or to monitor response to treatment or track disease progression. Ultimately, the decision is based on neuroanatomic localization, suspected disease for which one wants to test, accuracy and availability of imaging modalities, cost, and risk.

REPRODUCTIVE

CHAPTER 122

Artificial Insemination in the Dog

Catharina Linde Forsberg

Success using artificial insemination (AI) in dogs is dependent on a number of factors: the health and fertility of the bitch, when in relation to ovulation and how many times during the estrous cycle the AI is performed; the quality of the freshly ejaculated semen and how it has been handled; and the quality of the AI technique. This chapter will deal only with AI techniques.

AI TECHNIQUES IN THE DOG

Methods for AI in bitches include vaginal deposition of the semen, transcervical intrauterine deposition using the Scandinavian catheter or with the aid of an endoscope, intrauterine insemination by laparoscopy, and surgical intrauterine insemination. In several countries surgical AI is not considered ethically acceptable and in some it is illegal.

The anatomy of the canine vaginal tract is shown in Figure 122-1. It consists of the vulva, the vestibulum, the vagina with its narrow paracervical region, the cervix, and the fornix.

Significantly higher whelping rates are obtained when fresh (by 30%), chilled (by 44%), and frozen-thawed (by 51%) semen is artificially inseminated using intrauterine as opposed to intravaginal techniques. Litter size using intrauterine AI of frozen-thawed semen is also significantly larger than by vaginal AI (by 80%). It has been estimated that 10 times as many

spermatozoa are required to obtain similar results by vaginal AI as by intrauterine AI in the dog.

Palpation of the Cervix

To obtain good results by AI in the bitch it is absolutely essential to learn to locate the cervix by abdominal palpation so that the semen can be deposited in the correct place and the bitch is not injured during the insemination procedure. The bitch should have an empty stomach and bladder to facilitate the palpation. In order to palpate the cervix, a rigid single-use plastic canine AI catheter (Figure 122-2) is introduced into the vagina. The introduction of the catheter is facilitated if the vulva is elevated to just below the anus (like when the bitch stands for the male dog).

By inserting the catheter along the left or right side of the vestibulum, the centrally located urethral opening can be avoided. Because the urethral opening of the bitch is located at the pelvic brim, it is surprisingly easy for the plastic AI catheter, or a thin, rigid endoscope, to be unintentionally introduced into the urinary bladder. Apart from the hazards of perforating the bladder with the catheter, it is obvious that no pregnancy would follow after an AI if this occurs. Thus, the position of the catheter should always be checked by palpation before depositing a semen dose. If the catheter is in the urinary bladder, the cranial part of the vagina and the cervix can be palpated above the catheter. The walls of the urinary bladder usually are thinner than those of the vagina and the tip of the catheter stands out more distinctly than if it were in the vagina.

When the tip of the catheter is advanced to a point immediately cranial to the pelvic brim, its position should be checked by palpation. Cranially the vagina in most bitches slopes slightly downward. However, in some breeds (especially the sight hounds, many of which have an arched loin), the vagina may have a more dorsal direction (see Figure 122-1). The cranial end of the catheter should now be lowered closer to the abdominal wall to make it more accessible to palpation. When the catheter tip can be palpated and its correct position in the vagina thus checked, it is carefully introduced further, under continued palpatory control, until it reaches the paracervical area. This is the narrow, cranial portion of the vagina created by the dorsal, median postcervical fold and can be palpated as a 1- to 2-cm long, usually somewhat firm structure. It ends at the cervix, which in a bitch in estrus is a 0.5- to 1.5-cm, hard, rounded to ovoid, freely movable structure (see Figure 122-1).

The rigid plastic AI catheter, which has a diameter of 5 mm, may be too wide to be introduced into the paracervical area in some bitches, especially those of the smaller breeds or those that have not given birth to a litter of pups. Consequently, it is hardly ever possible to pass the outer protecting sheath of the Scandinavian catheter, which has a diameter of 10 mm, into the paracervical area. Once the cervix has been identified, the corpus uteri and the uterine horns can be palpated in front of this structure. This can be achieved by lower-

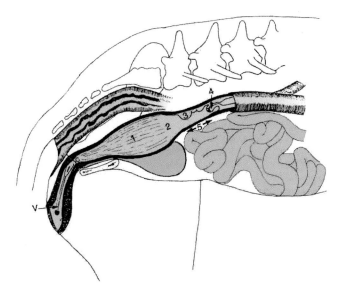

Figure 122-1 A schematic drawing of the canine paracervical region and the cervical canal. *v*, Vulva; *1*, vagina; *2*, cranial vagina; *3*, caudal tubercle of the median dorsal fold; *4*, cervical canal; *5*, paracervical region. (From Lindsay 1983, JSAP with permission.)

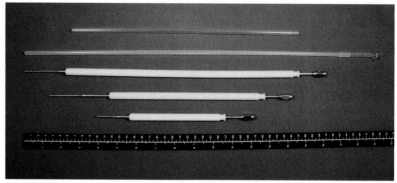

Figure 122-2 The three sizes of the Scandinavian AI catheter for dogs, and the two sizes of rigid plastic single-use vaginal AI catheters.

ing the tip of the catheter and closing the tip of the thumb against that of the index finger above the catheter, then lifting the cranial end of the catheter in such a way that the cervix and the uterine horns are pulled upward between the fingers. Their size and consistency then become evident. (This method of palpating the uterus is also useful for early pregnancy detection and to examine bitches with suspected endometritis or pyometra.)

VAGINAL INSEMINATION

Vaginal AI is usually done using a rigid plastic single-use catheter (20 to 45 cm long and 5 mm in diameter) (see Figure 122-2), which is introduced into the cranial vagina and as close to the cervix as possible, as previously described. With the catheter in place in the cranial vagina, a syringe containing the semen is attached and the hindquarters of the bitch then elevated before infusing the semen. After deposition of the semen dose, the catheter is withdrawn and the bitch is held with elevated hindquarters for 5 to 10 minutes to facilitate the transport of spermatozoa toward the oviducts. The bitch should also be "feathered" around the vulva and perineal region to stimulate uterine contractions. Spermatozoa may reach the tip of the uterine horn within 30 seconds to 1 minute during a natural mating and within about 30 seconds to 2 minutes after a vaginal AI if the bitch is held with elevated hindquarters. Vaginal AI with the bitch standing horizontally may prevent the transport of spermatozoa into the uterus and oviducts.

INTRAUTERINE INSEMINATION USING THE SCANDINAVIAN CATHETER

The Scandinavian catheter (see Figure 122-2) consists of a 1- to 2-mm-wide steel catheter with a 0.75- to 1-mm diameter tip (Figure 122-3) and comes in three different lengths: 20, 30, or 40 cm. It is used together with a 10-mm diameter outer protecting nylon sheath. The medium-sized catheter fits most small and medium-sized bitches.

Intrauterine AI with the Scandinavian catheter is performed with the bitch standing on the floor or on a table. Sedation is rarely needed; on the contrary, most bitches in estrus freely accept this type of handling. In case light sedation should be required (in a large, obese, or nervous bitch), 1 to 3 mg/kg xylazine IM or IV can be used. The nylon sheath is first introduced into the vagina as far as possible. If lubrication should prove necessary, a small amount of liquid paraffin or Vaseline (neither of which are spermicidal) can be used. If the nylon sheath is introduced together with the inner steel cath-

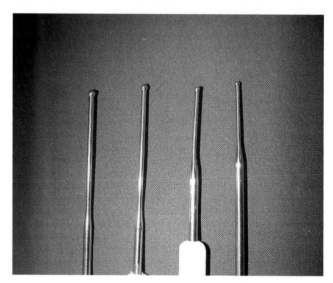

Figure 122-3 Close-up picture of the different sizes of tips of the Scandinavian catheters.

eter, the tip of the steel catheter must be placed so that it is completely protected by the nylon sheath. The cranial end of the nylon sheath is palpated in front of the pelvic brim as previously described. If the tip of the sheath is lowered closer to the abdominal wall, the cervix usually can be palpated a few centimeters in front of and above the catheter. The steel catheter then is introduced through the sheath until its tip reaches the ventral fornix. To achieve this there must be an alignment between the catheter and the cervix.

The cervix is then fixed between the thumb and the index finger, taking care not to squeeze it so that it is canal is closed and, by applying a slightly downward traction at the corpus uteri, it is tilted so that the angle of the cervical canal becomes more horizontal. The tip of the steel catheter is then carefully withdrawn while pushing it repeatedly against the surface of the cervix in search of the opening of the cervical canal. The sensation when this opening is found can in many cases be described as if touching cartilage (i.e., "crispy"). Once the opening has been found, fix the catheter and start working the cervix against the catheter. The cervical canal is 5 to 10 mm long and not always completely straight (see Figure 122-1). Thus, a slight pressure may have to be applied while rotating the catheter to ease it through. In most bitches, the tip of the catheter easily can be felt in front of the cervix in the corpus uteri. In some bitches, however, the sensation is not as distinct, and in a few bitches the catheter can only be introduced halfway through the cervix, which, however, is often sufficient.

The syringe containing semen is firmly connected to the catheter and the semen slowly infused into the uterus, while pressure is applied with thumb and index finger around the cervix to prevent backflow. Sometimes there is resistance to infusion if the opening of the catheter is pressed too hard against the endometrial mucosa. A slight downward traction at the corpus uteri or of the cervix usually alleviates the situation and allows semen infusion. (To check that the catheter really is in the uterus of the bitch, 1 to 2 mL of physiologic saline can be infused. If the catheter is in the right position in the uterine body, the fluid can easily be infused. If, on the other hand, the catheter is in the paracervical region, there will be an almost immediate backflow of saline between the catheter and the nylon sheath.) After intrauterine deposition of the semen, the catheter is withdrawn. To minimize backflow of semen and to facilitate uterine transport of spermatozoa toward the oviducts, the bitch should be held with elevated hindquarters for 5 to 10 minutes after the AI while being feathered around the vulva and perineal region to stimulate uterine contractions and sperm transport.

To learn this technique requires some practice, but once learned it is a quick procedure, usually being accomplished within minutes and generally fewer than 5% of attempts are unsuccessful. It is recommended that, initially, organ specimens be obtained for training purposes and anatomic study. It is also an advantage if the first attempts are made in medium-sized, calm, nonobese bitches that have given birth to one or more litters, as they are usually considerably easier to catheterize. Perforations may occur if the catheter is introduced blindly or with force. Provided that the catheterization is performed under careful palpatory control, however, the technique is completely safe for the bitch. Some bitches are more difficult to catheterize, particularly those belonging to some of the giant breeds, as well as obese or nervous animals. (This technique can be used for other infusions—for instance, for intrauterine infusion of contrast medium for hysterographic examinations of the bitch with suspected pyometra.)

INTRAUTERINE INSEMINATION USING ENDOSCOPIC VISUALIZATION OF THE CERVIX

Transcervical intrauterine insemination on the standing, nonsedated bitch can also be accomplished with the aid of a rigid fiberoptic endoscope, i.e., a cystourethroscope, 30 cm in length and 4 mm in diameter with an oblique viewing angle of 25°, together with a stainless steel sheath with a working length of from 23 to 29 cm and a diameter of 4 mm. The endoscope can be used together with a camera and monitor and with or without a deflector (Figures 122-4 to 122-6).

A 6- to 8-F dog urinary catheter is passed through the operating channel of the sheath. The endoscope is introduced into the vagina and advanced until the external os of the cervix can be visualized, and the urinary catheter is then manipulated into the cervical opening and further into the uterus. To guide the endoscope through the often tortuous vaginal vault, it can be quite helpful to let the urinary catheter lead the way by a few centimeters, thus indicating the right direction. Similar to when using the Scandinavian catheter, it can also be established by abdominal palpation whether the tip of the endoscope is correctly positioned in relation to the cervix. If the opening of the cervical canal is directed away from the endoscope and thus out of sight, the cervix can be manipulated by pushing it with the tip of the endoscope or with the catheter while moving the instrument from side to

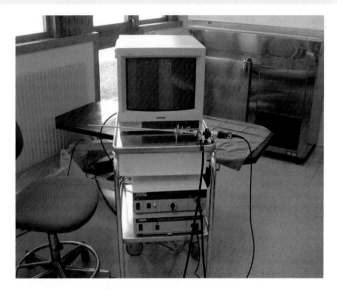

Figure 122-4 Transcervical intrauterine insemination can also be accomplished with the aid of a rigid fiberoptic endoscope, with or without a camera and monitor, and a canine 6- to 8-F urinary catheter.

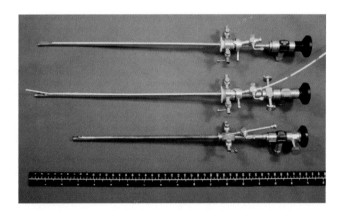

Figure 122-5 The endoscopes come in 23- or 29-cm working length, and with or without a deflector.

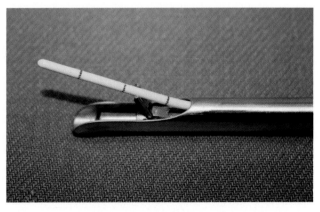

Figure 122-6 A close-up of the deflector with which the urinary catheter can be directed toward the cervical os.

side below the cervix. When the semen has been inseminated into the uterus, the catheter and the endoscope are removed and the bitch is kept with elevated hindquarters for 5 to 10 minutes, as previously described.

A significant advantage of this technique is that it allows direct visualization of the cervical opening. Still, it involves manipulation of the scope and catheter and requires some practice. In addition, to be able to catheterize bitches of all sizes with this method, several endoscopes of varying width and length may be required. Although the equipment is expensive, for practitioners specializing in canine reproduction and AI it should be a good investment to obtain at least one endoscope of medium size that fits most average-sized breeds. The endoscope is also a great help when training to perform transcervical catheterization with the Scandinavian catheter.

INTRAUTERINE INSEMINATION USING SURGERY

Surgery to effect intrauterine insemination is still widely used. The bitch is under general anesthesia and in dorsal recumbency. The ventral abdomen is clipped, and after routine surgical preparation a 4- to 6-cm incision is made midway between the pubis and the umbilicus, through the linea alba. The uterus is elevated through the incision, and the needle of the syringe containing the semen is inserted into the lumen of the uterine body at a 45° angle with the bevel of the needle up. The semen is slowly injected into the uterus. It should flow easily with obvious distention of the uterine horns, or else the needle should be repositioned. A saline-moistened gauze should be held over the injection site after the needle is withdrawn. After 1 minute the gauze is removed, the uterus replaced into the abdomen, and the wound closed using routine methodology. To avoid backflow of semen the bitch should be positioned with its rear elevated as she recovers from anesthesia. Whether it is ethically acceptable to resort to surgery to achieve pregnancies is debatable. The method, although advocated by some, is considered by many to be unethical and unacceptably stressful for the bitch. The risks for infection associated with surgery in general and the limited number of surgical AIs that can be performed in a given bitch are two obvious disadvantages. The method is also costly and time consuming.

INTRAUTERINE INSEMINATION USING LAPAROSCOPY

Abdominal laparoscopy should offer a somewhat more acceptable alternative to full surgery for AI in the dog, but this method has not met with acceptance from practitioners, most likely because they are more accustomed to the surgical technique.

CHAPTER **123**

Transcervical Catheterization in the Bitch

Autumn P. Davidson

The normal anatomy of the vagina and cervix in the bitch has traditionally hampered transcervical access to the canine uterus. Historically, both intrauterine diagnostic sampling (for endometrial biopsy, cytology, and culture) and intrauterine insemination have required an invasive procedure (laparotomy or laparoscopy) in the bitch. In addition to being an invasive approach, laparotomy requires general anesthesia, factors many clinicians and clients find objectionable for an elective procedure such as artificial insemination (Figure 123-1).

A laparoscopic approach to the canine uterus has not been used frequently, especially in the private practice setting, because of its invasive nature (multiple incisions, insufflation) and because it requires special equipment, expertise, and anesthesia. Cryopreservation and subsequent thawing diminish semen quality, necessitating special insemination technology. The process and resultant quality of canine cryopreservation have improved with time; however, insemination techniques remained challenging until transcervical intrauterine access was developed.

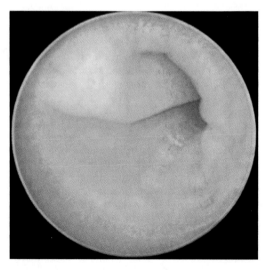

Figure 123-1   The dorsal median fold is seen extending cranially toward the cervix.

 To view a video on this topic, go to **www.expertconsult.com.**

SECTION IV
Critical Care

CHAPTER 124

Acid-Base, Oximetry, and Blood Gas Emergencies

Marie E. Kerl

Acid-base and oxygenation disorders are common in dogs and cats in response to respiratory or metabolic abnormalities secondary to trauma, intoxication, or naturally occurring disease. Advances in point-of-care testing have made rapid initial assessment and repeat monitoring of blood gas parameters accurate, practical, and affordable. Correct identification of abnormalities and appropriate therapeutic response relies on maintaining a working knowledge of both acid-base and respiratory physiology and pathophysiology.

Blood gas testing may be performed using either arterial or venous blood; however, only arterial blood can be used to assess oxygenation. Acid-base parameters other than partial pressure of oxygen (PO_2) may be evaluated using either arterial or mixed venous samples. In most emergencies, venous blood is easier to obtain. Samples should be drawn into syringes that are coated with 1:1000 heparin to prevent clot formation, or into specialized blood gas syringes (Vital Signs, Englewood, Colo.) containing pelleted heparin (Figure 124-1, A and B). Immediately after sample acquisition, the syringe should be made airtight to prevent contamination with room air, which could alter gas measurements. The sample should be analyzed within 15 minutes or placed on ice.

BASIC ACID-BASE PHYSIOLOGY

An acid is a hydrogen ion (H^+) (i.e., proton) donor, and a base is a proton acceptor. Hydrogen ions are nonvolatile or fixed acids produced by normal metabolism of proteins and phospholipids. They are excreted by the kidneys. Acids are represented by the notation HA, which signifies a hydrogen ion and any negatively charged particle. When placed in solution, HA dissociates into H^+ (acid) and A^- (base). A base combines with an acid to lower the amount of acid in solution, or to buffer the solution.

Carbon dioxide (CO_2) is a volatile acid, or fat-soluble gas, that can combine with water in the presence of carbonic anhydrase to form carbonic acid (H_2CO_3). Carbon dioxide is formed during normal carbohydrate and fat metabolism and is excreted via the respiratory system. These two sources of acid (H^+ and CO_2) are interrelated, as is shown in the carbonic acid equation:

$$H^+ + HCO_3^- \leftrightarrow H_2CO_3 \leftrightarrow H_2O + CO_2$$

This chemical reaction can go either direction, depending on the availability of substrate on either side of the equation. The enzyme carbonic anhydrase catalyzes this reaction; therefore, any cell containing carbonic anhydrase is capable of this reaction.

By definition, *pH* is the negative log of the hydrogen ion concentration. An acid gain results in a decrease in blood pH (acidemia), whereas an acid loss results in an increased pH (alkalemia). Acid can be gained systemically from reduced renal elimination of a naturally occurring compound or from ingestion of an exogenous acid source. Changes in CO_2 influence the H^+ concentration, as evidenced by the carbonic acid equation. As CO_2 is eliminated by increasing respiratory rate and alveolar ventilation, carbonic acid dissociates to form more CO_2. In turn, H^+ and bicarbonate (HCO_3^-) combine to form more carbonic acid. This effectively lowers the H^+ concentration and increases pH. Conversely, as CO_2 increases from ventilation impairment, pH decreases.

Buffers act to bind H^+, preventing large fluctuations in pH. A variety of buffer systems exist in the body, including nonbicarbonate buffers (proteins and phosphates), which are primarily intracellular, and HCO_3^-, which is the primary extracellular buffer. Bicarbonate is an effective buffer because it exists in relatively large concentrations compared with other buffers, and it participates in the carbonic acid equation to produce CO_2 gas, which can be eliminated through ventilation. The HCO_3^- buffer system, therefore, is considered an open system that can continue to buffer as long as the respiratory system is functional. In disease states causing HCO_3^- to be lost excessively from the urinary or gastrointestinal (GI) system, CO_2 and H_2O combine to form carbonic acid, which dissociates to increase H^+ and cause acidemia. For more in-depth discussion, readers are referred to more in-depth references.[1-3]

ACID-BASE DISORDERS

According to the Henderson-Hasselbalch equation, which is

$$pH = 6.1 \times \log\{HCO_3^-/0.03 PCO_2\}$$

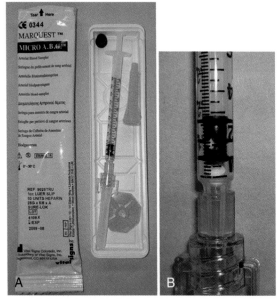

Figure 124-1 **A,** Arterial blood gas sampling kits contained a heparinized syringe and devices to render the syringe impervious to air. The advantage of these syringes is that arterial pressure will cause blood to fill the syringe chamber to the level at which the plunger is drawn. **B,** The syringe in the arterial blood gas sampling kit contains pelleted heparin as an anticoagulant in a sufficient amount to anticoagulate the maximum quantity of blood in the syringe.

pH can be characterized by changes in HCO_3^- and partial pressure of carbon dioxide (PCO_2). Because a predictable change in HCO_3^- occurs with gain or loss of H^+ ions, HCO_3^- can be used to correctly identify acid-base abnormalities arising from metabolic disorders. Acidemia or alkalemia resulting from a primary respiratory disorder should show a corresponding change in PCO_2. Increases in PCO_2 result in respiratory acidosis, and decreases in PCO_2 result in respiratory alkalosis. In metabolic acidosis, an H^+ increase shifts the carbonic acid equation to result in a decrease in HCO_3^-; and in metabolic alkalosis, an H^+ decrease has the opposite effect. Commonly available commercial blood gas analyzers typically measure pH and PCO_2 and calculate HCO_3^-.

This equation can also be used to predict how compensatory mechanisms engage to lessen the degree of change in the pH. When metabolic acidosis develops, the respiratory system is stimulated to increase the respiratory rate to eliminate CO_2 from the lungs and create respiratory alkalosis. Likewise, with a primary respiratory disorder, the opposite metabolic disorder is generated. The respiratory system provides rapid compensation, changing with the onset of a metabolic disorder in minutes. Metabolic compensation occurs more slowly, taking days before becoming maximally effective. With either system, compensatory mechanisms should slow as the pH approaches normal, and compensation should never completely normalize the pH.

Base excess, which is expressed in milliequivalents per liter (mEq/L), is the amount of base above or below the normal buffer base, a value calculated by taking into account the expected change in HCO_3^- secondary to acute changes in PCO_2. The general rule of thumb is that the HCO_3^- concentration rises about 1 to 2 mEq/L for each acute 10 mm Hg increase in $PaCO_2$ above 40 mm Hg to a maximum increase of 4 mEq/L, and that the HCO_3^- concentration falls 1 to 2 mEq for each acute 10 mm Hg decrease in $PaCO_2$ below

40, to a maximum decrease of 6 mEq/L. This negative base excess may be referred to as a *base deficit*.

By convention, a simple acid-base disorder is limited to the primary disorder and the appropriate compensatory response. A mixed disorder is one in which at least two separate abnormalities occur simultaneously. These abnormalities may both result in acidosis (i.e., metabolic acidosis and respiratory acidosis), may both result in alkalosis (i.e., metabolic alkalosis and respiratory alkalosis), or may be a combination of acidosis and alkalosis (e.g., metabolic acidosis and respiratory alkalosis). It takes cautious examination of a patient and blood gas results to avoid attributing the latter scenario to simple compensation. Normal values at sea level for venous blood gas interpretation are pH, 7.35 to 7.45; PCO_2, 40 to 45 mm Hg; and HCO_3^-, 19 to 24 mEq/L. Base excess normally should be −5 to 5 mEq/L. An algorithm for interpretation of blood gas values is provided in Figure 124-2.

Respiratory acidosis results from an increased partial pressure of CO_2 in the blood (hypercapnia). Hypercapnia can be caused by any condition that prevents normal pulmonary gas exchange, including impaired circulation, reduced respiratory rate or effort, circulation of blood to nonventilated portions of the lung, or impaired gas diffusion. Diffusion impairment is the least likely cause of hypercapnia, because CO_2 is approximately 20 times more diffusible than oxygen. Therefore, profound diffusion impairment is necessary before hypercapnia results. Disorders that can cause respiratory acidosis include circulatory failure from cardiopulmonary arrest, nervous system disease (central, spinal, or neuromuscular junction), respiratory muscle failure (e.g. severe hypokalemia), physical impairment of ventilation (e.g., pleural space disease, pain, thoracic wall disease, external constriction), or primary pulmonary disease (e.g., alveolar flooding, interstitial disease, pulmonary thromboembolism).[4] Iatrogenic respiratory acidosis results from inadequate ventilatory monitoring and assistance under general anesthesia.

Clinical signs of hypercapnia are consistent with the underlying disorder. Situations that might cause respiratory acidosis must be anticipated since there are no specific clinical signs that would clue the clinician in to its presence. End-tidal CO_2 can be monitored noninvasively in animals with endotracheal tubes in place on closed-circuit breathing loops under general anesthesia or on mechanical ventilation. In animals with regular respirations in which alveolar gas exchange is occurring, end-tidal CO_2 approximates $PaCO_2$.[5]

Treatment for respiratory acidosis involves correcting the underlying disorder by increasing alveolar ventilation. Chronic respiratory acidosis should be corrected slowly. Sodium bicarbonate should not be administered to treat respiratory acidosis because this drug exacerbates hypercapnia by donating substrate for the carbonic acid equation. Increasing the inspired oxygen concentration may be lifesaving; however, with severe hypercapnia, stimulation for respiration becomes driven by hypoxia. In those situations, administration of oxygen therapy and resolution of the hypoxia may result in decreasing the rate of voluntary respiration, which may in turn promote hypercapnia. The hypoxic drive for respiration remains adequate below a dissolved oxygen content of arterial blood (PaO_2) of 60 mm Hg. It is not necessary to administer supplemental oxygen with a goal of normalization of oxygenation.

Respiratory alkalosis results from an increase in ventilation through which more CO_2 is eliminated than is produced by normal metabolic function. Hypocapnia develops, and alkalemia ensues. Causes of respiratory alkalosis include hypoxemia produced by pulmonary or circulatory abnormalities that result in hyperventilation, primary pulmonary diseases that stimulate ventilation independent of hypercapnia, central nervous system disorders, and iatrogenic tachypnea/

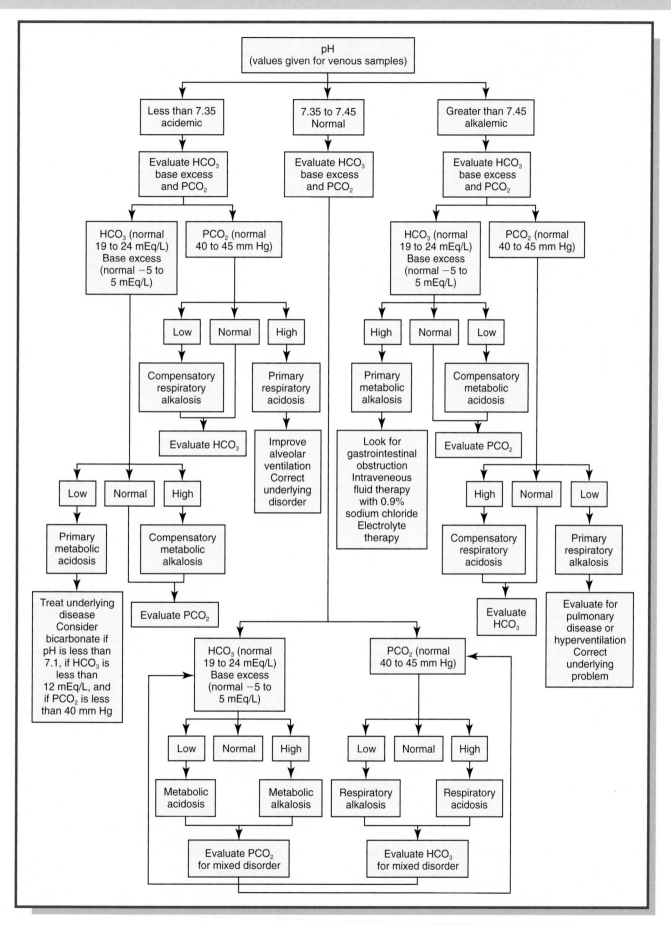

Figure 124-2 Algorithm for evaluating blood gas results.

hyperpnea in animals receiving assisted ventilation. Chronic respiratory alkalosis is usually well compensated.

Treatment of animals with respiratory alkalosis is primarily aimed at the underlying cause of tachypnea or hyperpnea (e.g., treatment for bacterial pneumonia, resolution of anxiety-associated tachypnea with sedation). As with respiratory acidosis, there are few if any clinical signs suggesting this specific acid-base disorder. Again, oxygen supplementation can be useful in support of these animals while the underlying disease is addressed.

Metabolic acidosis results commonly from a gain of H^+ through ingestion of an acid into the body, increased production of an endogenous acid, or failure to eliminate an acid load by the renal tubular cells. Metabolic acidosis can also be caused by a loss of HCO_3^- buffering ability. Differentiating these two causes of metabolic acidosis is important both for diagnosis of the underlying disorder and for determining correct therapeutic intervention.[6]

Dissociation of acid into the H^+ ion and the corresponding anion occurs in the circulation. When acid accumulates, HCO_3^- combines with H^+ to buffer the acid load, while the anion remains in solution. Because electroneutrality must be maintained as anions accumulate following acid dissociation, some other circulating anion must decrease correspondingly. Anion gap (AG), the difference between measured cations and measured anions, is useful in the classification of disorders causing metabolic acidosis. Anion gap, which is calculated from four common cations and anions measured on a serum chemistry profile, is stated:

$$AG = [Na^+ + K^+] - [Cl^- + HCO_3^-]$$

Although ranges for anion gap can vary somewhat based upon the reference ranges of electrolytes for various laboratories, a reference value of 16 ± 4 is typical. When metabolic acidosis exists with an increased anion gap, there has usually been a gain of organic acid. Causes of anion gap metabolic acidosis include ethylene glycol intoxication, uremia, tissue hypoxia (e.g., lactic acidosis), diabetic ketoacidosis, salicylate intoxication, and other unusual intoxications (e.g., drugs, alcohol). Metabolic acidosis characterized by a normal anion gap is caused by loss of bicarbonate buffers or a failure to excrete H^+ ions, with a corresponding increase in chloride to maintain electroneutrality. This is often referred to as a *hyperchloremic metabolic acidosis*. Hyperchloremic metabolic acidosis occurs less commonly than metabolic acidosis with an increased anion gap and is caused by renal tubular acidosis (failure of the renal bicarbonate buffer or hydrogen excretory system) or by severe diarrhea and loss of intestinal bicarbonate.[7] Iatrogenic hyperchloremic metabolic acidosis can also occur with administration of an alkali-free chloride-containing crystalloid solution, such as 0.9% sodium chloride (0.9% NaCl) for intravenous volume replacement.

Abnormalities associated with metabolic acidosis include lethargy, decreased cardiac output, decreased blood pressure, and decreased hepatic and renal blood flow. These changes may be referable to the acidemia, to the underlying cause of the acid-base disorder, or both. Unless the patient has some impairment of normal ventilatory ability, compensatory mechanisms cause an increase in the respiratory rate, which allows the animal to eliminate CO_2 generated by carbonic acid formation, mitigating acidosis.

Treatment should be aimed at correcting the underlying disorder. This might involve improving tissue perfusion (e.g., appropriate intravenous fluid therapy), eliminating ingested toxin, or correcting metabolic, renal, or GI disease. With severe metabolic acidosis (pH of <7.15 and HCO_3^- <12 mEq/L), injectable sodium bicarbonate may be administered judiciously according to the following formula:

$$\text{Bicarbonate dose} = (0.3)(\text{Body weight [kg]})(\text{Base deficit})$$

Half of this dose should be administered slowly intravenously over 6 hours, and the acid-base status should be reevaluated prior to continuation of therapy. Rapid correction of metabolic acidosis can cause a number of undesired side effects, including hyperosmolarity, hypernatremia, and hypokalemia. Hypocalcemic tetany may be caused by shifting of calcium from the ionized to the protein-bound form after bicarbonate administration. Paradoxical central nervous system acidosis occurs when CO_2 generated following bicarbonate administration crosses the blood-brain barrier and takes part in the carbonic acid equation, essentially fueling acid production in the CNS. Iatrogenic metabolic alkalosis can also occur after administration of bicarbonate.

Metabolic alkalosis is generated by loss of chloride in excess of extracellular fluid volume, which often occurs as a result of upper GI fluid loss or sequestration. Additionally, administration of a thiazide diuretic may cause chloride wasting. Rarely, metabolic alkalosis may be caused by overzealous administration of sodium bicarbonate or another organic anion or by hyperaldosteronism (i.e., Conn's syndrome), which causes sodium retention in excess of chloride. The most common clinical problem associated with metabolic alkalosis in small animal practice is gastric outflow obstruction. During gastric outflow obstruction, appropriate renal compensation prevents an acid-base disorder until hypovolemia induced by vomiting results in aldosterone release. Aldosterone increases renal uptake of sodium. Normally, sodium is reabsorbed with bicarbonate or chloride or is exchanged for potassium. Because gastric fluid has high chloride and potassium concentrations, animals with gastric outflow obstruction become systemically depleted of these electrolytes so that renal reabsorption of sodium can only occur with concurrent bicarbonate uptake.

As with other acid-base disorders, clinical signs of metabolic alkalosis are dictated by the underlying disorder generating the acid-base abnormality. Muscle twitching and seizures have been reported in animals with metabolic alkalosis. Signs associated with concurrent potassium depletion may include weakness, cardiac arrhythmias, renal dysfunction, and GI motility disturbances.

Treatment of metabolic alkalosis is directed at resolving the underlying cause. Intravenous 0.9% NaCl is the fluid of choice to replace volume deficits and normalize chloride concentrations since these patients are often chloride-depleted. Fluids should not contain buffer (e.g., not lactated Ringer's solution). Pyloric outflow obstruction is often addressed surgically, or by removal of an obstructing foreign body. In animals with profuse vomiting unassociated with obstruction, drug therapy to minimize gastric hydrochloric acid (HCl) excretion may be warranted (e.g., famotidine, omeprazole). Because animals with metabolic alkalosis often have concurrent hypokalemia, cautious intravenous potassium chloride supplementation is often indicated.

OXYGENATION

Hypoxemia may occur as a result of a low concentration of inspired oxygen, hypoventilation, diffusion impairment, ventilation-perfusion mismatch, or pulmonary shunting.[8] Two methods are available to assess oxygenation in an emergency setting: measurement of PaO_2 and measurement of peripheral oxygen saturation (SpO_2) by pulse oximetry. A pulse oximeter is a noninvasive device that calculates hemoglobin oxygen saturation by measuring differences in absorption of two wavelengths of light (red and infrared) by oxygenated and deoxygenated hemoglobin. The measured light absorption values are applied to a preset nomogram, and a value for SpO_2

is determined. If tissue perfusion is adequate, SpO_2 approximates arterial hemoglobin saturation (SaO_2).[5]

The advantage of oximetry as a monitoring tool is that it provides continuous, noninvasive determination of hemoglobin oxygen saturation. Technical aspects that help ensure accuracy include placing the probe on nonpigmented, moist skin with adequate perfusion (usually the tongue, the buccal, vaginal, or preputial mucosa, or the ear pinna), avoiding probe movement and light pollution, and monitoring the pulse rate to ensure accurate pulse signal transmittance. In poorly perfused tissues, the SpO_2 may be falsely low compared with the SaO_2. If inaccuracy of oximetry is suspected, the arterial blood gas PaO_2 may be obtained to evaluate oxygenation. In patients with alterations of hemoglobin concentration causing increased carboxyhemoglobin or methemoglobin, oximetry may be normal despite severe patient hypoxemia. Oximetry does not evaluate the PCO_2 and cannot be used to determine ventilation status.

The hemoglobin saturation of oxygen and partial pressure of oxygen (PaO_2) both contribute to arterial oxygen content (CaO_2) according to the following formula:

$$CaO_2\,(mL\,O_2/dL) = \{SaO_2\,(\%) \times Hemoglobin\,(g/dL) \\ \times 1.34\,(mL\,O_2/g)\} + \{PaO_2\,(mm\,Hg) \\ \times 0.003\,(mL\,O_2/dL/mm\,Hg)\}$$

Therefore, SpO_2, which approximates SaO_2, provides an estimation of hemoglobin saturation, whereas PaO_2 estimates dissolved oxygen in blood. According to the formula listed, hemoglobin saturation is the biggest determinant of arterial oxygen content. Increasing the PaO_2 by increasing the inspired oxygen concentration has a minimal effect, whereas increasing the SaO_2 has a greater potential effect. In an anemic patient, increasing the arterial oxygen content would best be accomplished by increasing hemoglobin by transfusion of a product containing red blood cells or purified hemoglobin.

By the oxyhemoglobin dissociation curve, an SaO_2 of 90% corresponds to a PaO_2 of 60 mm Hg. This value is clinically important in that small decreases beyond this point in either partial pressure of oxygen or oxygen saturation of hemoglobin may have tremendous clinical consequences for oxygenation. The goal of treatment for hypoxemia is to maintain the SpO_2 above 90% and the PaO_2 above 60 mm Hg. Sometimes this can be accomplished through supplemental oxygen therapy. Methods of increasing the inspired oxygen content include use of an oxygen chamber, tent or mask administration, placement of an indwelling nasal oxygen catheter, or mechanical ventilation with an increased fraction of inspired oxygen. Other methods to correct hypoxemia are related to correcting the underlying cause. For instance, hypoxemia in an animal with severe pneumothorax or pleural effusion would be accomplished through thoracic drainage while hypoxemia related to airway obstruction would be addressed by relief of the obstruction.

REFERENCES

The reference list can be found on the companion Expert Consult Web site at *www.expertconsult.com*.

CHAPTER 125

Acute Abdomen

Jennifer J. Devey

Acute abdomen can be defined as a condition characterized by an acute onset of abdominal pain. All acute abdomen patients have the potential of having a life-threatening condition, one that may require rapid surgical intervention, and although a thorough diagnostic workup must be completed in a timely fashion, patient treatment must take priority. While many patients present in a critical condition, some are more stable. Once resuscitation measures have been initiated and analgesics have been administered, the focus can be switched to ensuring a complete history has been taken, a thorough physical exam has been performed, and a diagnostic plan has been instituted with the goal of determining the underlying cause. Definitively diagnosing the cause of acute abdomen can be challenging. The goal of early and aggressive treatment is to minimize the impact of the systemic inflammatory response syndrome (SIRS), sepsis and to avoid multiple organ dysfunction syndrome (MODS).

The abdominal pain characteristic of this condition is typically caused by inflammation, especially of the peritoneal lining, stretching of or traction on a hollow viscus such as a gall bladder or loop of intestine, stretching of or traction on the capsule of a solid organ such as the liver, or ischemia. Typically the pain is severe, although the degree of pain detected on palpation may vary depending on the underlying disease as well as the nature of the patient. Patients that present collapsed in a state of hemodynamic shock may not exhibit signs of pain until resuscitation has been instituted.

Extraabdominal causes of abdominal pain that need to be ruled out include conditions such as intervertebral disc disease, steatitis and myositis.

INITIAL SURVEY

On presentation a primary survey examination (evaluation of level of consciousness, airway, breathing, and circulation) should be completed within 30 to 60 seconds. Altered levels of consciousness, collapse, tachycardia with weak or absent peripheral pulses, tachypnea, and pale mucous membranes with delayed capillary refill time and cool extremities indicate serious perfusion abnormalities and the need for immediate fluid resuscitation. Findings of fever, tachycardia with bounding pulses, and injected mucous membranes with capillary refill times of less than 1 second are consistent with a hyperdynamic phase of shock. These patients usually have a relative hypovolemia due to decreased systemic vascular resistance and also need immediate fluid resuscitation. A very brief history is obtained at this time if possible; however, resuscitation should not be delayed in the critical patient while a complete history is obtained. Diagnostic tests are frequently required in order to determine the extent of the disease and to confirm the diagnosis; however, resuscitation of the critical patient should not be delayed while tests are being performed unless those tests are absolutely required to guide resuscitation.

IMMEDIATE TREATMENT

The goal of resuscitation is to reverse the signs of shock and provide effective oxygen delivery to the cells. Efforts should be aimed at maximizing hemoglobin levels (oxygen-carrying capacity), blood volume, and cardiac function. Oxygen and intravenous fluid therapy should be provided. Patients presenting in extremis may require rapid intubation and ventilatory support. Hypoglycemic patients should be treated with dextrose. Antibiotics may not be indicated in all cases; however, in general the patient should be started on broad-spectrum antibiotics to cover both aerobic and anaerobic gram-positive and gram-negative bacterial infections. The use of corticosteroids remains somewhat controversial; however, increasing evidence suggests no improvement or a worsening of outcome unless the corticosteroids are administered prior to the insult or prior to the onset of a reperfusion injury.

If there is sufficient distention of the abdomen to interfere with ventilation, measures should be taken immediately to relieve the distention and dorsal recumbency should be avoided. Gastric distention with air can be relieved using transabdominal trocarization, insertion of a nasogastric tube, or orogastric intubation. Orogastric intubation should only be performed if the animal is intubated due to the risk of regurgitation around the tube and subsequent aspiration. Ideally the stomach should not be decompressed until fluid resuscitation has been addressed since rapidly relieving pressure on the vena cava may cause acute hemodynamic collapse; however, if the patient cannot ventilate effectively, the stomach should be trocarized immediately. Severe abdominal distention secondary to fluid may need to be addressed by emergent drainage.

ANALGESIA

Analgesia is an essential part of the early therapeutic plan. Nonsteroidal antiinflammatory drugs should be avoided due to their negative effects on splanchnic organs. Opioids such as butorphanol, hydromorphone, morphine, and fentanyl are recommended. Pure mu agonists are preferred, although butorphanol can be useful in the cat due to side effects of some of the pure mu agonists in this species. Drugs should be given intravenously since absorption from subcutaneous or intramuscular sites may be unpredictable. Because constant-rate infusions provide constant analgesia and can be titrated to effect, they are ideal in patients with significant pain, in patients who will need to go to surgery (since the constant-rate infusion can be continued intraoperatively and postoperatively), and in patients where it is anticipated significant pain may last a day or more. Providing analgesia via the epidural route is also very effective. Doses may need to be reduced to 25% to 50% of normal since critical patients are often sensitive to the sedative and negative cardiorespiratory effects. For those patients who do not respond to systemic analgesics, a peritoneal lavage with or without local anesthetic may be useful, especially in patients with pancreatitis or serositis.

SIGNALMENT AND HISTORY

Acute abdomen can affect patients of any age and breed; however, the signalment of the patient may help narrow down the underlying cause. For example, foreign bodies are more common in young animals, prostate disease is more common in older intact male dogs, and torsions are more common in deep-chested dogs.

A complete history should be obtained when time permits. Close attention should be paid to the possibility of exposure to high-fat table scraps, garbage, toxins, and foreign bodies along with the animal's predilection for ingesting foreign material. The owner should be questioned about any preexisting medical conditions and any medication the animal may be receiving, especially nonsteroidal antiinflammatory drugs. The history often includes nonspecific signs such as lethargy or depression, anorexia, retching, vomiting, diarrhea, and abdominal distention, which may have been peracute in onset or may have been more insidious in nature. On occasion the signs are more subtle and include restlessness, abnormal posture, or vocalizing. The owner should be asked to characterize any abnormal signs. Nonproductive retching is often associated with gastric dilatation and volvulus and should be suspected no matter what breed or age the dog is. The character of any vomiting noted may assist in diagnosing the location of the problem and the possibility of obstruction. Stool consistency, frequency, and color should be noted. Patients with significant gastrointestinal ulceration will typically have evidence of blood in the stool, although the absence of blood does not rule out ulceration, especially if the ulceration is peracute or is not associated with significant hemorrhage. Tenesmus usually indicates a colonic disorder but can be associated with urogenital tract abnormalities including prostate disease and calculi. The presence of dysuria, stranguria, pollakiuria, and hematuria indicates a urogenital problem.

PHYSICAL EXAMINATION

A secondary survey, or complete physical examination including an objective assessment of the five vital signs, is completed once the primary survey is completed and resuscitation is instituted. Temperature, respiratory rate, heart rate, and blood pressure are measured and a score should be assigned to the pain. Fever suggests an infectious or inflammatory process and is a nonspecific finding while hypothermia indicates a more serious condition. Patients may have concurrent conditions such as pneumothorax, aspiration pneumonia, and metastatic disease, and close attention should be paid to the ventilatory pattern and thoracic auscultation.

The abdomen should be palpated, ausculted, percussed, and balloted with the goal of localizing pain and detecting the presence of fluid waves, gas-filled organs, enlarged organs, or solid masses. Auscultation should precede palpation since palpation can cause gut sounds to diminish. Increased gut sounds are usually associated with diffuse gastrointestinal disease such as inflammatory, infectious, or toxic enteritis. Absent gut sounds suggest ileus, which can be associated with hypovolemic shock, chronic intestinal disease (inflammatory or obstructive), or peritonitis. Percussion can help determine the presence of free air as well as the location and extent of gas accumulation within the gastrointestinal tract. Ballottement permits detection of free intraabdominal fluid unless the animal is very obese, in which case movement of the extraabdominal fat can be mistaken for fluid.

Palpation should proceed in a systematic fashion. Palpation of the cranial abdomen can be facilitated in deep-chested breeds by elevating their thoracic limbs above floor level. Pressure should be applied gently initially in order to evaluate for any abnormal swelling, masses, or accumulation of subcutaneous fluid followed by more deep palpation as the animal permits. Foreign bodies may be able to be directly palpated in rare situations. Bunched-up intestines may suggest a linear foreign body. A thick, tubular structure may indicate a foreign body or an intussusception. A prominent spleen with a very sharp caudal border is consistent with splenic congestion, which is characteristic of an acute splenic torsion.

A rectal exam should be performed to assess the feces, including the presence of blood, the pelvic canal, the prostate in male dogs, the urethra, and the sublumbar lymph nodes. The abdomen may need to be clipped if the animal is a victim of penetrating trauma to ensure wounds are not overlooked. Petechiation or ecchymoses may indicate wounds, thrombocytopenia, or a coagulopathy. Periumbilical hemorrhage may be seen with a hemoabdomen, and periumbilical masses may be seen with pancreatic carcinoma. Distended abdominal veins are consistent with increased intraabdominal pressure.

DIAGNOSTIC TESTS

Blood tests including packed cell volume, total solids via refractometer, blood urea nitrogen, and glucose should be part of a STAT database. Ideally the STAT database should also include electrolytes and a blood gas (venous or arterial) and albumin, since total solids often do not correlate with albumin in the critically ill or injured patient. The blood gas provides useful information regarding ventilation and perfusion. A complete blood count with microscopic evaluation of a blood smear in order to complete a manual differential, estimate the number of platelets, and evaluate both white and red cell morphology should be performed. A complete biochemical profile and urinalysis is indicated in every patient as part of a more complete workup. Coagulation parameters should be evaluated in patients with suspected liver dysfunction, SIRS, or sepsis. A fecal examination including a fecal occult blood, direct smear, fecal flotation, *Giardia*, and parvovirus cite tests may be indicated. Ultimately the choice of tests will vary based on the presenting complaint.[1]

A lead II electrocardiogram is indicated in any patient with an auscultable arrhythmia, audible arrhythmia via Doppler, or suspicion of splenic disease. The electrocardiogram should be assessed for both the presence of arrhythmias and signs consistent with myocardial hypoxia/ischemia.

Chest radiographs should be evaluated preoperatively in every trauma patient and in any patient in which pneumonia or metastases are a potential concern. Abdominal radiographs are indicated to assess organ size and location, free air, gas bubbles within solid organs, foreign bodies, and loss of detail. The intestine should be evaluated for obstructive patterns and linear foreign bodies. If findings are not definitive, a radiograph can be repeated in 3 to 4 hours to determine if the gas and/or foreign body is moving. Unless a patient has had surgery within the previous 3 weeks or is suffering from a penetrating abdominal injury, free air indicates a rupture of the gastrointestinal tract. Air bubbles within solid organs often indicate a necrotizing process and the presence of gas-forming bacteria. A loss of detail on the x-rays suggests the possibility of peritonitis, and an abdominocentesis is indicated immediately. If a gastric volvulus is suspected but compartmentalization is not visible on the right lateral, a left lateral view should be taken. Contrast studies including barium series, intravenous urography, cystography (single and double contrast), and angiography may be required. Water-soluble contrast material should be used instead of barium if there is any concern regarding gastrointestinal perforation or aspiration.

Abdominal ultrasound can be extremely useful for diagnosing many causes of acute abdomen, especially when there is a significant volume of fluid in the peritoneal cavity, which can make radiographic evaluation difficult, although significant amounts of air within the gastrointestinal tract can interfere with interrogation. Cytologic and biochemical evaluation of ultrasound-guided aspirates of fluid, masses, or abnormal organs can often provide valuable diagnostic information.

Results of abdominal fluid examination are extremely useful not only in diagnosing a condition but also in determining the need for exploratory surgery in cases where the diagnosis is uncertain. Abdominal fluid should be evaluated cytologically as well as biochemically. A packed cell volume, protein level, white blood cell count, and microscopic examination of the fluid for evidence of septic peritonitis (plant fibers, intracellular bacteria, mixed population of extracellular bacteria with or without degenerative neutrophils) should be performed. Cultures are indicated if bacteria are present. Biochemical analysis also can be performed. In the dog a blood glucose concentration that is at least 20 mg/dL more than that in the abdominal fluid is strongly supportive of septic peritonitis.[2] A blood-to-fluid lactate difference of less than 2 mmol/L is also suggestive of septic peritonitis in the dog.[2] Concentrations of abdominal fluid amylase or alkaline phosphatase that are higher than serum suggest pancreatitis or intestinal disease. Concentrations of bilirubin that are higher in the abdominal fluid than serum indicate a disruption of the biliary tract. High potassium concentrations are consistent with urinary tract rupture. Urea nitrogen will equilibrate rapidly between the serum and peritoneum, but in an acute bladder rupture the peritoneal urea concentration will be higher than serum.

Abdominocentesis should be performed in 4 quadrants (unless ultrasound-guided centesis is available). Abdominocentesis has a high incidence of false-negative results. Ultrasound-guided abdominocentesis significantly improves the yield over standard abdominocentesis, but it may still produce false-negative results if the disease process is focal or if the disease is peracute and minimal effusion is present. Diagnostic peritoneal lavage has an extremely low rate of false results and should be performed if a confirmation of the diagnosis is required.

DIAGNOSTIC PERITONEAL LAVAGE

For a diagnostic peritoneal lavage the animal is placed in left lateral recumbency, which generally causes the spleen to fall away from the midline. Ideally the urinary bladder is emptied. A clip and surgical prep is performed of a 4-cm² area approximately 2 cm distal to the umbilicus on the midline. A local block is placed in the skin and peritoneum 2 cm caudal to the umbilicus either on the midline or just lateral to the midline. Sedation may be indicated. Surgical gloves are worn and ideally a drape is placed. A stab incision is made in the skin and a multiholed catheter is inserted into the abdomen in a caudodorsal direction. In cats and small dogs an 18-G, 2-inch (5-cm) catheter is ideal. In medium and larger sized dogs a 16- or 14-G, 5.25-inch (13-cm) catheter is inserted. Side holes should be added to standard over-the-needle catheters using a No.15 scalpel blade. Alternatively a commercial diagnostic peritoneal lavage catheter can be used. If fluid is retrieved a sample is collected aseptically for analysis. To complete the lavage 20 mL/kg of warm (body temperature) isotonic crystalloid fluid is infused. Since infusion of this volume of fluids will increase pressure on the diaphragm, the respiratory rate and effort should be watched closely and infusion stopped if the animal starts to show signs of respiratory distress. Once the fluid has been infused, the animal is gently rotated to mix the fluid around and then fluid samples are collected for analysis. If the catheter is being used to monitor intraabdominal hemorrhage, it can be sutured in place and serial samples can be taken or serial lavages can be performed. If the catheter is removed, a dressing is placed over the incision. A suture or staple can be placed if desired.

THE DECISION TO GO TO SURGERY

Some acute abdomen patients can, and should, be managed medically, and some require emergency surgery (within minutes to hours of presentation); therefore, it is important to be able to determine rapidly whether surgery is indicated (Figure 125-1). Some patients cannot be completely resuscitated until surgery is performed. In some situations the need for surgical intervention is obvious; however, in some cases the decision to go to surgery may not be so straightforward. If there is any doubt, it may be better to perform an exploratory laparotomy rather than wait and have the patient deteriorate. Even if surgery is indicated, a decision to delay the operation may be appropriate if surgery is not required as part of resuscitation and if it is determined that a delay will help decrease the likelihood of morbidity or mortality. Acute abdominal conditions requiring emergency surgery include conditions such as trauma-related disease, gastrointestinal obstruction, gastrointestinal accident, peritonitis, torsion, abdominal masses, and vascular accident (Table 125-1).[3]

ONGOING CARE

Once the patient has been stabilized, a plan for ongoing care should be formulated. Specific treatment should be directed at the underlying cause whenever possible at the same time that supportive care is being provided.[4] Close monitoring and intensive care are often essential in order to minimize patient morbidity and mortality. The frequency and type of

Table • 125-1

Differential Diagnoses for the Acute Abdomen

BODY SYSTEM CAUSE OF ACUTE ABDOMEN	TREATMENT	BODY SYSTEM CAUSE OF ACUTE ABDOMEN	TREATMENT
Gastrointestinal Digestive System		**Reproductive System**	
Gastric dilation-volvulus	DS, DE	*Female*	
Gastric or intestinal ulceration	NS	Acute metritis	PS, PE
Gastric or intestinal perforation	DS, DE	Pyometra/uterine rupture	DS, DE
Gastric or intestinal rupture	DS, DE	Uterine torsion	DS, DE
Gastric or intestinal dehiscence	DS, DE	Dystocia	PS, DE
Gastroenteritis	NS	Ovarian cyst	PS, PE
Hemorrhagic gastroenteritis	NS	Ovarian neoplasia	DS, PE
Intestinal obstruction	DS, PE	*Male*	
Intestinal obstruction: functional (ileus)	NS	Acute prostatitis	NS
Intestinal volvulus	DS, DE	Prostatic abscess	DS, PE
Cecal inversion	DS, PE	Prostatic cysts	DS, PE
Obstipation	NS	Prostatic neoplasia	DS, PE
Colitis	NS	Testicular torsion	DS, DE
Hepatobiliary Digestive System		**Hematopoietic System: Spleen**	
Acute hepatitis	NS	Splenic mass	DS, PE
Hepatic abscess	DS, PE	Splenic rupture (mass, trauma)	DS, DE
Hepatic trauma	PS, PE	Splenic torsion	DS, DE
Hepatic rupture	PS, PE		
Hepatobiliary neoplasia	PS, PE	**Peritoneum and Mesentery**	
Biliary obstruction	PS, PE	Peritonitis septic	DS, DE
Biliary rupture	DS, DE	Peritonitis: chemical (bile, urine, pancreatic)	PS, PE
Cholecystitis	PS, PE	Parietal peritoneal trauma: blunt	NS
Cholangiohepatitis	NS	Parietal peritoneal trauma: penetrating	DS, DE
		Mesenteric traction: large masses	DS, PE
Pancreatic Digestive System		Mesenteric lymphadenopathy	PS, PE
Acute pancreatitis	NS	Mesenteric lymphadenitis	NS
Pancreatic abscess	DS, PE	Mesenteric volvulus	DS, DE
Pancreatic neoplasia	DS, PE	Mesenteric avulsion	DS, DE
		Mesenteric artery thrombosis	DS, DE
		Adhesions with organ entrapment, internal hernia	DS, PE
Urinary System			
Acute nephrosis, nephritis/pyelonephritis	NS	**Abdominal Wall**	
Urinary calculi (renal, ureteral, cystic, urethral)	PS, PE	Trauma: blunt	PS, PE
Trauma-avulsion-rupture	DS, PE	Trauma: penetrating	DS, DE
Obstruction (ureter, urethra)	DS, PE	Abscess	DS, PE
Renal artery thrombosis	PS, PE	Strangulated hernia	DS, DE
Renal neoplasia	PS, PE		

Modified with permission from Mann FA: Acute abdomen. In Bonagura JD, Twedt DC, editors: Kirk's current veterinary therapy XIV, St Louis, 2009, Saunders, pp 67-72.

DE, Definitely requires emergent surgery; *DS*, definitely surgical; *NS*, nonsurgical (some nonsurgical emergent cases may eventually require surgery); *PE*, potential requires emergent surgery; *PS*, potentially surgical.

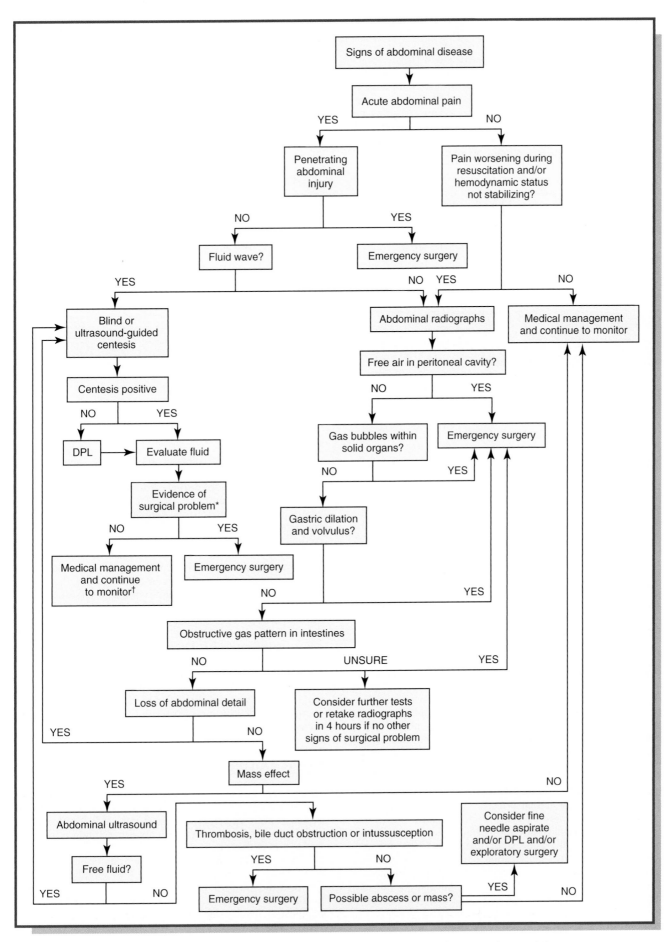

Figure 125-1 Algorithm to determine whether a patient has a medical or surgical acute abdominal condition. *, See text for further detail; †, possible exception to monitoring if high index of suspicion for gastric perforation; *DPL,* diagnostic peritoneal lavage.

monitoring will vary with each patient and with the treatments that were started during resuscitation. Vital signs including blood pressure and an assessment of pain should generally occur no less frequently than hourly during at least the first 6 to 12 hours. Serial physical exams also may be important in some patients, especially when the diagnosis is still open. Adjustments to the treatment plan should be made according to findings. Pain should be aggressively managed, and drugs should be given on an "as-needed" basis in addition to the regularly scheduled doses. Fluid therapy may consist of a combination of crystalloid and colloid fluids and should be guided by blood pressure and blood volume measurements, measured ins and outs, as well as hemoglobin, albumin, and electrolyte concentrations, and blood gases. The patient's level of dehydration should be estimated, and the calculated

deficit should be replaced over 6 to 12 hours unless there are concerns for fluid overload. Nasogastric decompression may be required along with antiemetics for the persistently vomiting patient. Gastric protectants are indicated in those with evidence of upper gastrointestinal ulceration. Antibiotics should be continued in at-risk and septic patients pending cultures. Early enteral feeding should be considered to help maintain gastrointestinal function and integrity.

REFERENCES

The reference list can be found on the companion Expert Consult Web site at *www.expertconsult.com*.

CHAPTER 126

Cardiac Emergencies

Kirstie A. Barrett

The management of cardiac emergencies can be very rewarding if a prompt diagnosis is made and if the proper treatment is instituted without delay. Sometimes patients are not stable enough to handle extensive diagnostics, and treatment decisions must be made quickly. In such cases, an insightful history and physical examination are critically important because the choice of further diagnostics may be limited.

Cardiac emergencies commonly seen in veterinary patients are arrhythmias, acute congestive heart failure, pericardial effusion, and arterial thromboembolism. Other cardiac emergencies or potential cardiac emergencies, described elsewhere in detail, include cardiopulmonary resuscitation (CPR), shock, syncope, hypertension, and hypotension.

ARRHYTHMIAS

Arrhythmias, which occur in a high percentage of critical patients, represent a disturbance in the rate, regularity, or site of cardiac electrical impulse formation. Their clinical significance is a result of a heart rate that is either too slow or too rapid, depressing cardiac output and potentially leading to heart failure or circulatory collapse. Cardiac arrhythmias are particularly ominous if they have the potential to deteriorate into an electrically unstable form, causing or exacerbating circulatory failure or cardiac arrest.

A correct electrocardiographic (ECG) diagnosis is essential to appropriate management and therapy and should always be interpreted in the context of the patient's history and current clinical status. Identification and correction of precipitating factors (e.g., cardiopulmonary disease, metabolic derangements, acid-base and electrolyte imbalances, current drug therapy) are equally essential to successful management of cardiac arrhythmias and to the clinician's decision on whether to initiate antiarrhythmic therapy.

Arrhythmias that cause clinical signs generally warrant therapy. Clinical signs that reflect decreased cardiac output may be acute or progressive and include weakness, exercise

intolerance, syncope, collapse, ataxia, pulse abnormalities, congestive heart failure, and sudden death.

Arrhythmias present during cardiopulmonary arrest (CPA) include asystole (complete absence of QRS-T complexes), ventricular fibrillation (chaotic depolarization of the ventricles characterized by a lack of QRS-T complexes with unorganized fibrillation waves), and electromechanical dissociation (little or no myocardial contractile activity with a normal ECG tracing). All these arrhythmias require immediate intervention using standard CPR recommendations. Other potentially lethal arrhythmias include continuous (sustained) or intermittent (paroxysmal) ventricular tachycardia, ventricular flutter, paroxysmal or sustained supraventricular tachycardia, sick sinus syndrome (SSS), complete or high-grade second-degree atrioventricular block, and sinus standstill. Sinus bradycardia frequently precedes CPA in critically ill patients. Antiarrhythmic therapy should be initiated if treatment of the underlying disorder does not improve the arrhythmia, if hemodynamic impairment is identified, or if the risk of sudden death exists. Identification of the above arrhythmias and treatment options are discussed in detail elsewhere.

HEART FAILURE

Heart failure is a clinical syndrome caused by cardiac disease that results in systolic or diastolic cardiac dysfunction or both. Systolic failure describes decreased myocardial performance, and diastolic failure results from abnormal filling of the ventricles during diastole.

Decompensated heart failure manifests either as congestion/edema (backward heart failure) or circulatory failure (low-output, forward heart failure). Right-sided congestive heart failure results in systemic venous congestion and may manifest as jugular distention, subcutaneous edema, hepatic congestion, ascites, and/or pleural effusion. Left-sided congestive heart failure presents as pulmonary edema.

Because the clinical signs of left-sided congestive heart failure can mimic those of pulmonary disease, it is important to determine accurately which condition is truly present. The signalment, history, and response to treatment can be helpful in making this distinction. The single most useful test for confirming congestive heart failure is a thoracic radiograph. However, the potential stress of any diagnostics must be seriously considered because the anxiety associated with even minimal handling of a severely dyspneic animal can be life-threatening.

The immediate goals of medical therapy in acute congestive heart failure are the reduction of pulmonary venous pressure (use of a diuretic to reduce total blood volume and a vasodilator to redistribute intravascular fluid volume), inotropic support, and adjunct therapy (oxygen, anxiolytics). Furosemide is the diuretic of choice for relieving acute pulmonary edema and normalizing cardiac filling pressures. High doses of furosemide (up to 4 mg/kg given intravenously or intramuscularly every 2 hours) may be used initially to induce diuresis. Intravenous furosemide acts within 5 minutes, peaks within 30 minutes, and dissipates after 2 to 3 hours. Use of the intravenous route is preferred, but this must be weighed against the potential stress of administration. Lasix can also be given using a constant rate infusion (CRI) (0.5 to 1.0 mg/kg/hr) after an initial loading dose is given.

Intramuscular administration of furosemide is an alternative to the IV route. The dose is highly variable and depends on the response desired. The dose and frequency should be reduced as a clinical response (diuresis, respiratory rate reduction, and respiratory character improvement) is achieved. Cats tend to be more sensitive to furosemide than dogs and respond to lower doses (2 mg/kg).

Nitroglycerin, a venodilator, may further reduce congestion, although information in the veterinary literature is merely anecdotal. Nitroglycerin paste can be applied to the inner surface of the pinna of the ear (¼ to 1 inch every 6 hours in the dog; ⅛ to ¼ inch every 6 hours in the cat). Nitroglycerin is typically used for only 48 hours due to the drug tolerance that develops.

Hydralazine, a potent arteriolar dilator, can be used in the emergency management of a normotensive congestive heart failure patient (0.5 to 2.0 mg/kg given orally). Nitroprusside is both a potent venodilator and a potent arteriolar dilator for use in severe, refractory congestive heart failure (1 to 2 μg/kg/min given intravenously initially). Continual blood pressure monitoring is essential with nitroprusside.

Augmentation of systolic performance is important with acute congestive heart failure due to DCM and severely decompensated mitral regurgitation. The positive inotropic agents most commonly used increase cytosolic cyclic adenosine phosphate (cAMP). As a result, there is enhanced ventricular contraction (a result of increased calcium entry into the cell), ventricular relaxation, and peripheral vasodilatation. Dobutamine and dopamine are sympathomimetic agents that bind to B1 receptors, thereby increasing production of cAMP. Dobutamine increases contractility with little effect on heart rate or afterload. It is administered by CRI (5.0 to 15 μg/kg/min). Dopamine stimulates B1 receptors and at high doses also releases norepinephrine. At low doses (<5 μg/kg/min) dopamine causes arteriolar dilatation in renal, mesenteric, coronary, and cerebral vascular beds. Systemic arteriolar vasoconstriction occurs at higher doses (10 to 20 μg/kg/min). Dopamine is therefore administered by CRI at a dose of 2 to 8 μg/kg/min. Amrinone and milrinone are potent positive inotropes with direct-acting arterial vasodilator properties. These bipyridines increase cAMP by phosphodiesterase inhibition. Amrinone and milrinone are available as IV preparations. Unfortunately, both the sympathomimetics and the bipyridines can promote tachycardia and ventricular arrhythmias.

Pimobendan is a benzimidazole-pyridazinone derivative approved for the treatment of congestive heart failure due to DCM and MVI in dogs. Pimobendan is classified as an inodilator (i.e., positive inotrope and arteriovenous dilator). The positive inotropic effects are primarily through sensitization of the cardiac contractile apparatus to intracellular calcium. This is done with little or no increase in myocardial oxygen consumption. There is improved efficiency with limited arrhythmogenic side effects seen with other positive inotropes. The vasodilating properties of pimobendan are due to the phospodiesterase inhibition.

Pimobendan has a rapid onset of action and can be used in the treatment of acute congestive heart failure when a positive oral inotrope is needed. Following oral administration (0.1 to 0.3 mg/kg q12h) peak hemodynamic effects are achieved in 1 hour and last 8 to 12 hours.

A low dose of morphine (0.05 to 0.1 mg/kg given subcutaneously or intramuscularly) can reduce the anxiety associated with pulmonary edema and provide mild venodilatation.* The dose is repeated up to four times a day, as necessary, to achieve the desired effect. The primary adverse consequence of using morphine is respiratory depression; therefore, it must be used with caution in hypoxic animals. Acepromazine (0.05 to 0.1 mg/kg given subcutaneously) is an anxiolytic that does not depress respiration. Acepromazine is an alpha-adrenergic blocker that decreases peripheral vascular resistance, which may also be beneficial.

Strict cage rest and prevention of stress are critically important to the management of a congestive heart failure patient. Additional measures that may benefit the patient are thoracocentesis and oxygen therapy. Cats with congestive heart failure can present with pulmonary edema, pleural effusion, or both. When congestive heart failure results in pleural effusion of significant quantity and the animal is dyspneic, thoracocentesis often results in prompt and dramatic improvement (the technique is described elsewhere in this text).

Dogs and cats with severe pulmonary edema are hypoxic due to the decreased ability of oxygen to diffuse from the alveoli into the pulmonary capillaries. Supplemental oxygen increases this pressure gradient, resulting in an increase in arterial oxygen tension. Therefore, it is of critical importance that patients with severe edema have supplemental oxygen. This can be achieved using an oxygen cage (40% oxygen) adjusted to maintain a normal temperature (20° to 22° C [68° to 72° F]) and appropriate humidity (45% to 55%). Oxygen cages are generally better tolerated and less stressful than other means of administration. In a larger dog, oxygen can be administered through a nasal cannula. An oxygen mask is an alternative but should not be used if the animal is struggling against the mask.

Endotracheal intubation may be required in animals with extreme respiratory distress and fulminant pulmonary edema to provide controlled ventilation and 100% oxygen administration. In addition, copious amounts of pulmonary edema may be removed physically by suction or postural drainage. Intravenous fluids are rarely indicated in the treatment of acute, cardiogenic pulmonary edema because they often exacerbate the edema.

PERICARDIAL EFFUSION

Pericardial effusion is an abnormal accumulation of fluid in the pericardial sac. The hemodynamic effects of pericardial effusion depend on the rate and volume of the fluid accumula-

---

*Notably, morphine can cause agitation and aggression in cats.

tion and the compliance of the pericardium itself. If the effusion develops slowly, the pericardium will expand and the intracardiac pressure will not increase enough to compromise cardiac filling. In contrast, acute cardiac tamponade is characterized by rapid accumulation of fluid in the pericardial space, leading to a rise in intrapericardial pressure. The results are restriction of ventricular filling, decreased cardiac output, and arterial hypotension. Clinical signs of right-sided congestive heart failure or reduced cardiac output predominate and include anorexia, lethargy, syncope, dyspnea, weakness, exercise intolerance, and abdominal distention (hepatomegaly, ascites). Common physical examination findings are muffled heart sounds, jugular venous distension, sinus tachycardia, and weak femoral pulses. Pulsus paradoxus (an exaggerated decline greater than 10 mm Hg in systemic arterial pressure during inspiration) is a valuable clinical sign that may also be appreciated in cardiac tamponade.

Although thoracic radiography typically demonstrates an enlarged, globoid cardiac silhouette, echocardiography is the most sensitive and specific noninvasive means of diagnosing pericardial effusion. The therapeutic goal for patients with pericardial effusion is to reduce the intrapericardial pressure quickly. Pericardiocentesis is the treatment of choice for initial stabilization of dogs and cats with pericardial effusion and cardiac tamponade. Attempts to lower venous pressures with medical therapy (i.e., diuretics) should be avoided because the patient's cardiac preload depends on these elevated pressures. The result can be a significantly reduced cardiac output, manifested as hypotension or syncope or both.

ARTERIAL THROMBOEMBOLISM

Arterial thromboembolism is a common sequela to all types of feline myocardial disease (hypertrophic cardiomyopathy, dilated cardiomyopathy, and restrictive cardiomyopathy); it is uncommon in the setting of a structurally normal or mildly abnormal heart. Arterial thromboembolism results in significant morbidity and mortality. Systemic thromboembolism is rarely reported in the dog and is usually associated with neoplasia, sepsis, Cushing's disease, protein-losing nephropathy, or other hypercoagulable states. Distal aortic embolization (saddle thrombus at the distal aortic trifurcation) occurs in more than 90% of feline cases. Corresponding clinical signs may occur with embolization of other organs, such as the lungs (respiratory distress), kidneys (acute renal failure), brain (central nervous system signs), gastrointestinal tract (bowel ischemia), and right (more commonly than left) brachial artery (pain and paresis).

A distal aortic embolism presents as peracute paresis or paralysis with vocalization due to intense pain. The clinical consequences depend on the site, extent, and duration of the embolization, as well as the degree of functional collateral circulation. The *four Ps* characterize the clinical signs of changes observed in the extremities: *p*aralysis, *p*ain, *p*ulselessness (lack of palpable femoral pulses), and *p*allor (cold, pale distal extremities and pads). Absence of bleeding from a cut nail on the affected limb may also be seen. Ten to 12 hours after the embolization, the anterior tibial and gastrocnemius muscles often become firm as a result of ischemic myopathy. In most cases these muscles become softer after 24 to 72 hours. Respiratory distress is commonly associated with systemic thromboembolism in cats because most have concurrent congestive heart failure. Acute aortic blockade by the thromboembolus increases afterload to the left ventricle. The clinician must differentiate the respiratory changes seen with congestive heart failure from those seen with pain.

A variety of therapeutic measures can be used to offset the consequences of a thromboembolism. These range from attempts to limit thrombus growth or formation and pain control to supportive care and treatment of accompanying congestive heart failure.

Although heparin has no effect on established thrombi, it is commonly administered in hopes of limiting thrombus growth.* Heparin can be administered at an initial dose of 220 U/kg given intravenously, followed by a maintenance dose of 70 to 200 U/kg given subcutaneously every 6 hours. Thrombolytic agents such as streptokinase, urokinase, and tissue plasminogen activator (t-PA) are used extensively in humans and infrequently in cats. These agents are expensive, have not been studied extensively, and are associated with high mortality and poor outcomes. Risks of bleeding complications, death from reperfusion syndrome (hyperkalemia, metabolic acidosis), and rethrombosis are common.

During the initial stages of the disease, most cats experience intense pain. The pain subsides as sensory nervous function is lost. Common choices for pain control include oxymorphone (0.05 to 0.15 mg/kg given intramuscularly or intravenously every 6 hours), butorphanol (0.1 mg/kg given intravenously or 0.02 to 0.4 mg/kg given intramuscularly or subcutaneously every 4 hours), and/or acepromazine (0.05 to 0.1 mg/kg given intravenously). Euthanasia should be considered as an option when severe, unrelenting pain is present.

General supportive care consists of maintaining hydration and normal electrolyte status, massaging firm muscles, expressing the bladder as necessary, and preventing self-mutilation. Management of concomitant congestive heart failure is discussed above.

---

*Heparin has never been proven to limit thrombus growth.

CHAPTER 127

Cardiopulmonary Arrest and Resuscitation

Efrat Kelmer
F.A. (Tony) Mann

Cardiopulmonary cerebral resuscitation (CPCR) has been used in clinical practice since the 1960s as a method for treating cardiopulmonary arrest (CPA). In general, the prognosis for dogs and cats suffering CPA is poor, with reported survival to discharge rates varying between 0% to 4% in dogs and 2% to 22% in cats.[1-3] Despite the low success rate, CPCR can be undoubtedly lifesaving if performed promptly and effectively on a select patient population, and therefore veterinarians should strive to be proficient in it. A retrospective study evaluating 15 dogs and 3 cats that survived CPCR reported long-term neurologic deficits in only 1 dog.[4]

The most recent American Heart Association (AHA) guidelines for human CPCR were published in 2005.[5] Because no controlled studies have been reported in veterinary medicine, guidelines for companion animals are largely extrapolated from human data. The AHA recommendations for CPCR are divided into classes based on the level of evidence supporting the use of each specific treatment. The different classes are summarized in Table 127-1, and class recommendations are mentioned throughout this chapter.

DEFINITIONS

Cardiopulmonary arrest is defined as the cessation of effective ventilation and circulation. Cardiopulmonary resuscitation (CPR) provides artificial ventilation and circulation to restore spontaneous cardiopulmonary function and includes basic life support (BLS), advanced life support (ALS), and prolonged life support (PLS). The term *cardiopulmonary cerebral resuscitation* was coined in recognition of the severe central nervous system complications of prolonged CPR. CPCR is aimed at restoration of blood flow to the brain, not only the heart and the lungs, to avoid cases in which return of spontaneous circulation (ROSC) results in a poor neurologic outcome such as a vegetative state.

PREPAREDNESS

Preparedness includes ascertaining that each patient has a code status upon hospitalization, the presence of a fully equipped crash cart (Table 127-2), a minimum of three people trained in CPCR, a ready area, and a routine plan of action.

All hospitalized patients should have one of three code assignments: do not resuscitate (DNR or no code), closed chest code (external compressions only), or open chest code (internal compressions). The code status should be discussed

The author would like to acknowledge Ms. Misty Bailey for editing this chapter.

at the time of admission, and owner's wishes should be clearly stated on the chart. The ready area and the crash cart should be inspected and stocked daily.

RECOGNITION OF CPA

In general, patients experiencing CPA can be divided into three broad categories: (1) those who succumb to an underlying terminal or multisystemic illness—a DNR code status may be appropriate for these patients for ethical reasons and since their prognosis is generally grave; (2) those suffering from a severe, but potentially reversible, medical condition such as trauma (e.g., hemorrhage, pneumothorax, diaphragmatic hernia), upper respiratory obstruction, or electrolyte abnormalities—this population has a slightly higher chance for ROSC, assuming the underlying cause can be quickly reversed; and (3) those with anesthetic complications, drug reactions, and accidental drug overdoses. Three retrospective studies published in veterinary medicine concluded that the last group has the highest survival rates as they are usually witnessed arrests and in some cases already have an endotracheal tube in place.[1-3]

Prior to initiation of CPCR, the senior person on the scene should take a few seconds to confirm full CPA. Respiratory arrests alone carry a better prognosis and do not necessitate chest compressions. In addition, the animal may not be pulseless but rather bradycardic, which will alter the order of drugs used during ALS such that atropine is given prior to epinephrine. Signs that precede CPA include bradycardia or other cardiac arrhythmias, hypotension, hypothermia, irregular respiratory pattern, and vagally mediated activities such as vomiting or urination in a critically ill patient.

BASIC LIFE SUPPORT

Basic life support is the foundation of CPCR (class I AHA recommendation) and follows the mnemonic of ABC (*a*irway, *b*reathing, *c*irculation). It should be initiated immediately upon recognition of CPA to establish an airway, ensure adequate ventilation, and generate blood flow. Basic life support includes endotracheal intubation, ventilation with an Ambu bag or an anesthesia machine connected to 100% oxygen (with the inhalant anesthetic turned off), and external or internal cardiac compressions. Time should be taken to ensure that the endotracheal tube is in place, secured, and inflated. If intubation is not possible due to upper airway obstruction, emergency tracheostomy is performed. The mouth and trachea should be suctioned if secretions are present.

Respiratory rate is aimed at 10 to 24 breaths/min, a tidal volume of 10 to 15 mL/kg, and a peak inflation pressure of 20 cm H_2O. Some animals may require a higher respiratory rate, but hyperventilation should be avoided. The volume

 To view a video on this topic, go to www.expertconsult.com.

Table • 127-1

Class Recommendations of the 2005 American Heart Association Guidelines for CPCR

CLASS	INTERPRETATION	DEFINITION	EXAMPLE
I	Benefit >>> Risk	Treatment should be performed/ administered	ABC Defibrillation for VF
IIa	Benefit >> Risk	It is reasonable to perform or administer treatment	Atropine for sinus bradycardia Minimize interruption of chest compressions
IIb	Benefit ≥ Risk	Treatment can be considered and may be helpful	Epinephrine for CPA
Intermediate	Unknown	Research underway, cannot recommend for or against	Vasopressin for asystole Routine administration of IV fluids during CPA
III	Risk ≥ Benefit	Treatment should not be performed/ administered. It is not helpful and may be harmful.	Cardiac pacing for asystole

ABC, Airway, breathing, circulation; *CPA,* cardiopulmonary arrest; *CPCR,* cardiopulmonary cerebral resuscitation; *IV,* intravenous; *VF,* ventricular fibrillation.

delivered should produce a *visible* chest rise of approximately 25% to 30% of resting state, but should not be too forceful to avoid barotrauma. If an anesthesia machine or Ambu bag is not available, mouth-to-tube or mouth-to-nose ventilation can be performed. For chest compressions, the animal is positioned in right lateral recumbency, and compression rate is aimed for 100 to 120 compressions/min. If the animal is already in dorsal recumbency, such as during a surgical procedure, it may remain this way. If the first recorded arrest rhythm is ventricular fibrillation (VF), defibrillation should be performed as soon as possible, but BLS should not be delayed. In anesthetic-related incidents, inhalant anesthetics should be turned off immediately, and anesthetics, sedatives, or analgesics should be reversed if possible.

ADVANCED LIFE SUPPORT

Advanced life support consists of drug administration, electrocardiography (ECG) interpretation, and electrical defibrillation (D and E). Drug and defibrillation doses are listed in Table 127-3.

Drug Administration and Access

Establishing access for drug administration is vital during CPCR. A central line is the preferred route because of short circulation times, but if not already in place, time should not be wasted on establishing a central line during CPCR.[6] Peripheral catheterization using a large-bore catheter should be established as soon as possible, and if not feasible, an intraosseous catheter may be placed (class IIa). Drug administration via a peripheral catheter should be followed by large flush volumes to facilitate drug delivery to the central circulation.[7] If intravenous (IV) access is not possible, drugs can also be given intratracheally (IT). Epinephrine, atropine, lidocaine, naloxone, and vasopressin are all absorbed via the trachea but may result in lower blood concentrations and a less predictable drug delivery and pharmacologic effect than the same dose given IV.[8-16] The optimal endotracheal dose of most drugs is unknown, but typically the dose given is twice the recommended IV dose. Endobronchial administration of epinephrine diluted with water for injection, instead of sterile saline, was shown to achieve the highest blood concentrations.[17] In summary, if IT administration is used, drug doses should be doubled; the drug should be diluted with a few

milliliters of water for injection and administered via a red rubber or polypropylene tube that is passed through the endotracheal tube to the level of the carina.[5] Sodium bicarbonate and calcium gluconate should not be given IT.

Epinephrine is the drug of choice for all types of CPA (class IIb). Epinephrine is a potent catecholamine with strong affinity to both α- and β-adrenergic receptors. Administration causes immediate peripheral vasoconstriction mediated by its alpha effects; however, the β-adrenergic activity may cause significant tachycardia, which will shorten diastole and decrease myocardial perfusion. Atropine is a parasympatholytic agent that acts to increase heart rate by antagonism of muscarinic receptors. If sinus bradycardia is present on initial auscultation, atropine should be administered before epinephrine (class IIa). Otherwise, atropine is given following epinephrine.

Amiodarone affects sodium, potassium, and calcium channels as well as α- and β-adrenergic blocking properties. It can be considered for the treatment of VF or pulseless VT unresponsive to shock delivery, CPR, and vasopressors (class IIb). Intravenous amiodarone is rarely maintained in most veterinary hospitals, is expensive, and is not a drug that an inexperienced individual should probably use. Lidocaine, a sodium channel blocker, is an alternative antiarrhythmic with fewer immediate side effects than may be encountered with other antiarrhythmics. Lidocaine, however, has no proven short-term or long-term efficacy in cardiac arrest (class indeterminate). In addition, lidocaine should not be used in cats. Magnesium can effectively terminate torsades de pointes (irregular/polymorphic VT associated with prolonged QT interval).

Electrocardiography (ECG)

Changes in ECG throughout CPCR dictate the type of interventions that should be implemented and serve as a monitoring tool. The three recognized arrest rhythms are asystole, pulseless electrical activity, and VF (Figure 127-1). Asystole is the most common arrest rhythm in companion animals, while VF is more common in humans. Ventricular fibrillation has the highest likelihood of being converted with the aid of defibrillation and CPCR, which is most likely one of the reasons for the higher success rates reported in some human studies.

Although the most common initial arrest rhythm in companion animals is asystole, this rhythm can often change as CPCR progresses, and defibrillation may be indicated. ECG

Table • 127-2

Equipment List for Stocking a "Crash Cart"

EQUIPMENT	COMMENTS
Laryngoscopes	Straight (Miller) and curved (Macintosh)
Cuffed endotracheal tubes and tracheostomy tubes	Sizes 3-12
Oxygen source	Already connected with tubes that can connect to an Ambu bag
Ambu bags	Large and small
Gauze ties	To secure endotracheal tubes
Syringe	1-20 mL for inflating endotracheal cuffs, drug administration, and flushing
Suction apparatus with Yankauer and rubber tips	To suction mouth and endotracheal tube
Sterile saline flushes	3 mL and 20 mL
Red rubber or polypropylene catheters	5-8 F, for intratracheal drug administration
Needles	23-18 gauge
Drugs	Listed in Table 127-3 plus dopamine, dobutamine, dexamethasone, atipimazole, furosamide, sterile saline, water for injection, 50% dextrose
Defibrillator, ECG paste	External and internal handles
Intravenous and intraosseous catheters	For animals weighing less than 5 kg, an 18-gauge needle can be placed intraosseous
Thoracotomy pack for open-chest CPCR	Scalpel blade and handle, rib retractors, Mayo scissors, DeBakey tissue forceps, right-angle forceps, vascular and hemostatic forceps, and Rumel tourniquets
Monitoring equipment	Stethoscope, ECG monitor, capnograph, pulse oximeter, Doppler blood pressure monitor
Tracheostomy pack	Scalpel blade and handle, Metzenbaum scissors, Gelpi retractor
Thoracocentesis kit	21-19–gauge butterfly catheters attached to a stopcock and a 60-mL syringe in a sterile bag
Pericardial effusion pack	14-16–gauge catheters, scalpel blade, stopcock, extension set, 60-mL syringe, ACT tube

ACT, Activated clotting time; *CPCR*, cardiopulmonary cerebral resuscitation; *ECG*, electrocardiography.

interpretation should be performed concurrently to auscultation, as pulseless electrical activity can appear as a normal rhythm on the ECG screen with no audible pulse or heart rate. Pulse palpation should also be interpreted with caution, as it is the pulse pressure that determines the blood pressure and not the pulse quality.

Fluid Therapy

Administration of large fluid boluses during CPCR should not be performed routinely because it may decrease coronary perfusion pressure (CPP), which represents the difference between aortic pressure and right atrial pressure during diastole. Large fluid volumes may decrease CPP as they increase right aortic pressure. In animals suffering CPA due to congestive heart failure, fluid therapy should be avoided. If the animal is euvolemic, conservative fluid therapy may be considered. However, large fluid volumes should be reserved for those cases suffering CPA due to hypovolemic shock.

MONITORING DURING CPCR

Monitoring tools for CPCR include a stethoscope, ECG, Doppler blood pressure monitor, pulse oximeter, and capnograph. ECG monitoring was discussed earlier. A capnograph is one of the most important monitoring tools during CPCR. Higher end-tidal carbon dioxide ($ETCO_2$) levels during CPCR are associated with increased myocardial perfusion pressure and increased success rates in human beings and dog models of CPCR, whereas a low $ETCO_2$ represents ineffective elimination of CO_2 due to low flow.[18] Rising levels of $ETCO_2$ during a successful CPCR indicate tissue perfusion and ROSC. However, arterial blood gases should be interpreted cautiously during CPCR, as they may not provide a reliable indicator of the severity of tissue hypoxemia, hypercarbia, or tissue acidosis.

PROLONGED LIFE SUPPORT

PLS refers to the time period following ROSC and the measures required to support continued perfusion, maintain adequate circulation and oxygenation, and treat underlying conditions. As the likelihood of recurrence of CPA in an animal that already suffered one is high, intensive monitoring is required in post-CPCR patients. The following parameters should be monitored: pulse rate, rhythm, and character, mental status, ECG, pulse oximetry, body temperature, lung sounds, mucous membrane color, capillary refill time, urine output, electrolytes, blood gases, PCV and total solids, blood glucose concentration, serum lactate concentration, central venous pressure, neurologic function, and patient comfort. Oxygen supplementation should be provided initially. Some patients may need mechanical ventilation to maintain adequate oxygenation. Positive inotropes and vasopressors (e.g., dobutamine, dopamine, or vasopressin) may need to be used to support circulation and maintain blood pressure. Mannitol (0.5 to 1 g/kg over 20 minutes administered via a filter) may be considered in patients with suspected cerebral edema or neurologic dysfunction.

OLD CONTROVERSIES AND NEW RECOMMENDATIONS FOR CPCR

Open- versus Closed-Chest CPCR

As no prospective randomized studies of open-chest CPCR for resuscitation have been published, performing it remains controversial and largely depends on clinician and owner preference. In humans, open-chest CPCR is considered a class IIa recommendation only for patients with cardiac arrest in the early postoperative period after cardiothoracic surgery and when the chest or abdomen is already open.[5] In addition, several retrospective studies suggest there may be a role for open thoracotomies in patients with penetrating thoracic and cardiac trauma. In veterinary medicine, open-chest CPCR is

Table • 127-3
Drugs Commonly Used during CPCR*

DRUG (CONC.)	DOSE†	WEIGHT (lb) 5 / WEIGHT (kg) 2.5	10 / 5	20 / 10	30 / 15	40 / 20	50 / 25	60 / 30	70 / 35	80 / 40	90 / 45	100 / 50	COMMENTS
		mL OR JOULES											
Epinephrine low (1:10,000 or 0.1 mg/mL)	0.01 mg/kg	0.25	0.5	1	1.5	2	2.5	3	3.5	4	4.5	5	Repeat dose q3-5min
Epinephrine high (1:1000 or 1 mg/mL)	0.1 mg/kg	0.25	0.5	1	1.5	2	2.5	3	3.5	4	4.5	5	High dose no longer recommended in human CPCR
Atropine (0.54 mg/mL)	0.04 mg/kg	0.25	0.5	1	1.5	2	2.5	3	3.5	4	4.5	5	
Lidocaine (20 mg/mL)	2 mg/kg (dogs) 0.2 mg/kg (cats)	0.25	0.5	1	1.5	2	2.5	3	3.5	4	4.5	5	Use cautiously in cats
Sodium bicarbonate (1 mEq/mL)	1 mEq/kg	2.5	5	10	15	20	25	30	35	40	45	50	Should not be used IT
Calcium gluconate (100 mg/mL)	50 mg/kg	1	2.5	5	7.5	10	12.5	15	17.5	20	22.5	25	Should not be used IT
Magnesium (4 mEq/mL)	0.2 mEq/kg	0.1	0.25	0.5	0.75	1	1.25	1.5	1.75	2	2.25	2.5	Indicated for torsades de pointes
Vasopressin (20 U/mL)	0.1-0.8 U/kg	0.1	0.2	0.4	0.6	0.8	1	1.2	1.4	1.6	1.8	2	Can replace one dose of epinephrine; Potent vasoconstrictor
Amiodarone (50 mg/mL)	5 mg/kg	0.25	0.5	1	1.5	2	2.5	3	3.5	4	4.5	5	Indicated for refractory VF
Naloxone (0.4 mg/mL)	0.04 mg/mL	0.25	0.5	1	1.5	2	2.5	3	3.5	4	4.5	5	Opioid reversal agent
Flumazenil (0.1 mg/mL)	0.02 mg/mL	0.5	1	2	3	4	5	6	7	8	9	10	Benzodiazepine reversal agent
External defibrillation	2-10 J/kg	20	30	50	100	200	200	200	300	300	300	360	
Internal defibrillation	0.2-1 J/kg	2	3	5	10	20	20	20	30	30	30	50	

CPCR, Cardiopulmonary cerebral resuscitation; IT, intratracheally; VF, ventricular fibrillation.
*Many of the common drug doses (e.g., epinephrine, atropine, and lidocaine) are given 1 mL per 10 kg.
†Drugs given IT should be diluted with 2-3 mL of water for injection and given at the level of the carina using a red-rubber or polyethylene catheter.

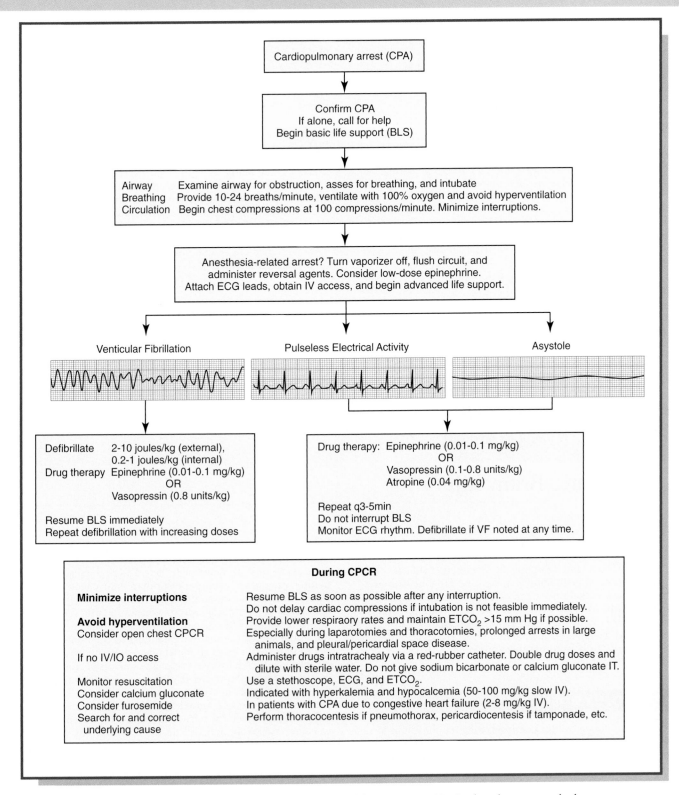

Figure 127-1 Algorithm for basic and advanced life support. *CPCR,* Cardiopulmonary cerebral resuscitation; *ECG,* Electrocardiography; *ETCO₂,* end-tidal carbon dioxide; *IO,* intraosseous; *IV,* intravenous; *VF,* ventricular fibrillation.

recommended for patients in which external compressions are unlikely to be effective, such as very large dogs and patients with pleural or pericardial effusion, pneumothorax, diaphragmatic hernia, or thoracic trauma, or if the thoracic or abdominal cavities are already open.

Epinephrine Dosage

Although epinephrine has been used universally in resuscitation, there is a paucity of evidence to show that it improves survival in humans. Administration of high dose epinephrine (0.1 to 0.2 mg/kg, IV) has been called into question, as the β-adrenergic properties of epinephrine cause significant tachycardia, decreased diastolic filling, and decreased coronary perfusion and have been associated with decreased survival. Based on several clinical trials, the 2005 AHA guidelines recommend the use of low-dose epinephrine (0.01 to 0.02 mg/kg, IV). For in-hospital witnessed CPA, the author is in favor of using low-dose epinephrine in veterinary patients.

Vasopressin versus Epinephrine

Vasopressin is a potent noradrenergic vasopressor, acting through direct stimulation of vasopressin (V1) receptors in vascular smooth muscle. As opposed to catecholamines, its vasoconstrictive effects are not blunted in the presence of acidosis and, following ROSC, there is no increase in myocardial oxygen demand. In a recent human clinical trial comparing IV vasopressin (two doses of 40 IU) with epinephrine (two doses of 1 mg) in 1219 out-of-hospital cardiac arrests, patients with VF, asystole, and pulseless electrical activity did not have survivability differences compared to patients with only VF or pulseless electrical activity; however, vasopressin was superior to epinephrine in asystolic patients.[19] In addition, recovery from CPA has been reported in one case in veterinary medicine using vasopressin with no epinephrine.[20] The single use of vasopressin, at a dose of 0.1 to 0.8 U/kg IV, has otherwise been anecdotally used in veterinary CPCR. A CRI of 0.01 to 0.08 U/kg/hr can be used for the postresuscitation period. The authors have successfully resuscitated patients with vasopressin in conjunction with epinephrine; however, more studies are needed to confirm the role of vasopressin in veterinary CPCR.

Hyperventilation and Interruptions during CPCR

An observational study found that emergency medical service personnel consistently hyperventilated human patients in the arrest scene,[21] and several small case series in humans showed that during CPR, health care providers delivered an inadequate number and depth of compressions, interrupted compressions frequently, and provided excessive ventilation.[22-24] The 2005 AHA guidelines stress the importance of early initiation of chest compressions with minimal interruptions and a 50:50 compression/relaxation rate to allow diastolic filling of the heart and maximize myocardial perfusion. Although establishing an airway is the first step in CPCR, chest compressions should not be delayed if an airway cannot be captured immediately.

References

The reference list can be found on the companion Expert Consult Web site at *www.expertconsult.com*.

CHAPTER 128

Traumatic Brain Injury

Rebecca S. Syring

Traumatic brain injury (TBI) is an important cause of morbidity and mortality in veterinary medicine. The severity of brain injury can be quite variable, with neurologic signs ranging from minor deficits to life-threatening impairments. An understanding of the pathophysiologic changes that occur following TBI and the appropriate diagnostic and therapeutic interventions for a dog or cat with head injury can help to optimize outcome in these critically ill patients.

PATHOPHYSIOLOGY

TBI can be caused by blunt or penetrating trauma. Blunt force to the head, resulting from vehicular trauma, falls from a height, crush injury, and inadvertent or purposeful harm from others, is the most common category of TBI. With blunt trauma, the kinetic energy from the impact is diffusely dissipated across the surface of the body. Head injury may be overtly obvious in these patients or overshadowed by more severe injuries elsewhere in the body. While less common, penetrating injuries to the head, such as gunshot, stab, or bite wounds, are more likely to result in isolated trauma to the brain, as the kinetic energy from the trauma is focally dissipated along the penetrating tract.

Primary versus Secondary Injury

There are two described phases following TBI: primary and secondary injury. *Primary injury* refers to pathologic changes that take place at the time that injury is sustained—it is complete at the time of trauma and there is little that can be done to alter its course. Examples of primary injury include direct axonal damage and vascular disruption. *Secondary injury* refers to a variety of pathologic processes that occur after the primary insult, resulting in progressive neuronal damage, not only at the initial site of trauma but extending to the brain globally. Because the brain has high metabolic requirements, decreased cerebral oxygen delivery or hypoglycemia can rapidly result in adenosine triphosphate depletion, cell membrane pump failure, and loss of ion homeostasis. This can lead to excitotoxicity, oxidative stress, cytotoxic and vasogenic cerebral edema, inflammatory mediator release, activation of the coagulation cascade, vasospasm, and cell death. With ongoing anaerobic metabolism, hyperglycemia has been documented to exacerbate neurologic damage by increasing lactic acid accumulation in the brain, resulting in neuronal and glial cell death. Since secondary injury occurs after the initial insult and has a progressive nature, medical intervention should focus on preventing the development of this type of injury. Two factors that have significant impact on the perpetuation of secondary injury are systemic hypoxia and hypotension, both of which can be easily recognized and treated clinically.

Intracranial Pressure and Cerebral Perfusion Pressure

In the healthy brain, pressure autoregulation ensures that cerebral blood flow (CBF) is maintained within an acceptable range over a wide spectrum of systemic mean arterial blood pressures (50 to 150 mm Hg). In response to changes in blood pressure, parallel changes in cerebral vascular resistance occur to maintain blood flow to the brain. Pressure autoregulation is often impaired (either globally or regionally) in pets with TBI, at which time CBF becomes linearly dependant upon systemic blood pressure.

Intracranial pressure (ICP) is defined as the pressure exerted between the skull and its intracranial contents. The components of ICP are the volume of blood, brain tissue, and cerebrospinal fluid (CSF) within the cranial vault. In TBI, intracranial volume will increase with hemorrhage or edema. Compensatory decreases in CSF production, shunting of CSF into the cisterna magna, or by arterial vasoconstriction to lower blood volume attempt to maintain ICP within a normal range (4 to 12 mm Hg in cats and dogs). ICP increases when changes in intracranial volume exceed the ability for compensatory decreases in the other components.

Cerebral perfusion pressure (CPP) is the primary determinant of CBF in patients with TBI. With intracranial hypertension, CPP is equal to systemic mean arterial blood pressure (MAP) less ICP (CPP = MAP − ICP). Maintaining CPP at or above a 50 to 70 mm Hg is recommended to optimize oxygen and nutrient delivery to the brain. Since ICP is infrequently measured in veterinary medicine, determination of CPP is not always possible. However, an understanding of this equation stresses the importance of optimizing blood pressure in head trauma patients. Small increases in ICP can result in inadequate CPP with a normal MAP.

PATIENT ASSESSMENT

When evaluating patients with TBI, it is imperative to assess all body systems rather than focusing solely on the brain, as head trauma often occurs coincident with trauma to other body systems. Common systemic injuries following blunt trauma, such as pulmonary contusions, pneumothorax, and hemoabdomen, can impair systemic oxygenation and perfusion and perpetuate secondary injury if not rapidly addressed. A systematic approach to the traumatized patient should focus on evaluation of major body systems, cardiovascular and respiratory stabilization, and then a secondary assessment and definitive medical therapy (see Chapter 132). A full neurologic examination is not necessary, and may not be in the dog or cat's best interest, during initial assessment. An abbreviated neurologic assessment should focus upon three main categories: level of consciousness, brainstem reflexes, and motor activity/posture.

An altered level of consciousness indicates abnormalities in the cerebral cortex or brainstem (reticular activating system). Level of consciousness can be divided into four main categories: alert, depressed/obtunded, stuporous, and comatose. An obtunded animal should still respond to noise or touch. Stupor indicates a severely impaired level of consciousness, with response only to noxious stimuli. A comatose animal exhibits no response to stimuli, including repeated noxious stimuli. Using standardized categories allows for uniform comparison of neurologic function over time in patients. It is important to remember that shock (decreased tissue oxygen delivery) can cause moderate alterations in consciousness that should improve with restoration of tissue perfusion.

Brainstem reflex assessment should focus on pupil size, symmetry, and position, pupillary light responses, and physiologic nystagmus. Miotic pupils indicate a lesion above the brainstem, leaving the oculomotor nerve intact and unopposed from higher centers. Mydriatic pupils are seen with brainstem lesions affecting the oculomotor nerve on the side of the injury. Anisocoria may indicate a neurologic lesion affecting one side exclusively or more than the other. In the absence of an underlying ophthalmologic disorder, the lack of a pupillary light response indicates disruption of the oculomotor nerve tracts ipsilateral to the injury. Physiologic nystagmus refers to the normal tracking movements of the eye in response to turning the head from side to side. The absence of this reflex indicates injury to the central region of the brainstem, as may be seen with hemorrhage or compression caused by swelling or herniation.

Abnormalities in any of these brainstem reflexes can help localize neurologic lesions and grade severity. Pupils that are of normal size but not responsive to light represent significant brainstem dysfunction, and are only one step less severe than a fixed and dilated pupil. Serial evaluation of these reflexes assists in monitoring of progression or improvement of neurologic function. For example, if midrange or mydriatic pupils without a pupillary light reflex are present on initial examination and no progression is noted, one may suspect brainstem hemorrhage. These signs, in conjunction with a comatose state and loss of physiologic nystagmus, are associated with a grave prognosis. Alternatively, a gradual progression of pupils toward mydriasis or loss of pupillary light response may indicate the development of cerebral edema that may respond to therapy to lower ICP.

Notation of the patient's motor activity and posture may help to localize neurologic lesions. Following TBI, the presence of ataxia, hemiparesis, or tetraparesis may be the result of lesion in the cerebral cortex or brainstem. The evidence of other cranial nerve abnormalities will help differentiate intracranial from cervical lesions. Decerebrate rigidity (extension of all four limbs and opisthotonus) indicates a rostral brainstem lesion and is often associated with brainstem compression secondary to marked intracranial hypertension and/or herniation. Decerebellate rigidity (extension of the front legs with hindlimb flexion) indicates a cerebellar lesion, as may be seen with cerebellar herniation. Patients with decerebrate posturing will have markedly altered levels of consciousness while those with decerebellate posturing are usually alert and aware of their surroundings.

The Cushing (or CNS ischemic) response is a compensatory mechanism that can be seen with markedly elevated ICP. Intracranial hypertension results in decreased CBF. In response to CO_2 accumulation from decreased blood flow, the vasomotor center emits a sympathetic discharge, resulting in peripheral vasoconstriction, which elevates MAP to maintain CPP. The increased blood pressure sensed at baroreceptors results in a reflex bradycardia. The combination of hypertension and bradycardia in a patient with a decreased level of consciousness should alert the clinician to the possibility of increased ICP and prompt aggressive treatment.

THERAPEUTICS AND PATIENT CARE

Extracranial Stabilization

In patients with TBI, it is essential that extracranial organ systems be assessed and stabilizing therapy be instituted before initiating therapy directed at lowering ICP. The goals of extracranial stabilization should focus on early optimization of systemic oxygenation, ventilation, and tissue perfusion to minimize perpetuation of secondary neurologic injury. Hypoxemia should be avoided with TBI, as desaturation worsens outcome in humans with head trauma. Oxygen supplementation should be provided to maintain a hemoglobin saturation above 97% or a PaO_2 >90 mm Hg. When in doubt, supplemental oxygen should be given to avoid any potential adverse consequences. Intranasal and intratracheal routes should be avoided, as they can cause sneezing or coughing, which transiently increases ICP.

Hypoventilation, resulting in an elevated partial pressure of arterial carbon dioxide ($PaCO_2$), can occur with TBI secondary to direct damage to the respiratory center, sedatives, thoracic trauma causing pain or pleural space disease, and mechanical airway obstruction. Acute hypercarbia (respiratory acidosis) is sensed at the central chemoreceptors and results in cerebral vasodilation, increasing CBF and exacerbating elevations in ICP. $PaCO_2$ should be maintained below 40 mm Hg with TBI. If $PaCO_2$ cannot be maintained within a normal range, intubation alone or in combination with mechanical ventilation is required.

The primary goal of fluid therapy with TBI is rapid restoration of tissue perfusion and blood pressure, such that CPP is maintained above 50 mm Hg. Fluid restriction should be avoided, as it will achieve only minimal decreases in ICP and will place the animal at greater risk for hypovolemia and decreased CPP and exacerbate cerebral ischemia. There are a variety of fluids for intravascular volume replacement in the head trauma patient, including isotonic crystalloids, hypertonic saline, and artificial colloids (see Chapter 129). No one fluid type can be deemed optimal for every situation. Hypotonic solutions (5% dextrose in water, 0.45% sodium chloride) should be avoided for resuscitation of head trauma patients, as these fluids preferentially expand the intracellular space and may exacerbate cerebral edema. Hypertonic saline (7.5%) is considered by many to be a superior fluid for resuscitation with TBI because of its ability to rapidly restore euvolemia due to its hyperosmolarity, allowing very small volumes (3 to 5 mL/kg over 10 to 15 minutes) to be used for resuscitation. Additional attractive properties of hypertonic saline include the ability to lower of ICP via its osmotic effect and its abilities to minimize vasospasm, excitotoxicity, and the inflammatory response in the brain.

Intracranial Stabilization

Once the cardiovascular and respiratory systems have been addressed, steps toward stabilization of the brain may ensue. The goals of intracranial stabilization are to limit intracranial hypertension, by decreasing cerebral edema and optimizing intracranial blood volume, and minimize elevation in cerebral metabolic rate. Cerebral edema is a common problem with TBI that can cause progressive elevation of ICP. Mannitol has traditionally been the drug of choice to decrease cerebral edema. In addition, mannitol may scavenge free radicals involved in oxidative stress and improve microvascular flow within the injured brain. The concern that mannitol may exacerbate intracranial hemorrhage is unfounded, and the global beneficial effects of its use far outweigh this potential risk. Mannitol (0.5 to 2.0 g/kg) should not be administered until euvolemia has been restored, as its diuretic effect will contract intravascular volume and potentially worsen CPP. Hypovolemic animals may respond better if hypertonic saline (7.5%) is used, as this fluid will both restore intravascular volume and exert osmotic effects on the brain. Corticosteroids are not indicated, as multiple prospective clinical trials in human head trauma patients have shown no benefit. This, in combination with the many adverse effects of corticosteroids (hyperglycemia, immunosuppression, gastric ulceration, delayed wound healing, and exacerbation of a catabolic state), precludes its recommendation for use in animals with TBI.

Elevating the head and neck uniformly 15° to 30° above the rest of the body facilitates venous drainage from the brain, thereby decreasing ICP. Angles higher than 30° and kinking of the neck such that the jugular veins become occluded should be avoided, as arterial inflow and venous outflow can be compromised, respectively. Hyperventilation can be used as a short-term method to decrease intracranial blood volume as a result of cerebral vasoconstriction. Excessive hyperventilation ($PaCO_2$ no lower than 30 mm Hg) should be avoided, as this can worsen cerebral ischemia. Space-occupying masses (e.g., subdural hematomas) may require surgical evacuation if there are static or worsening neurologic problems. Computed tomography (CT) scanning is the diagnostic tool of choice for early TBI (compared to MRI), as it provides good detail for bone, cerebral edema, and acute hemorrhage, is more readily available, and allows for greater patient access during the scan (Web Figure 128-1, *A* and *B*).

Minimizing elevations in cerebral metabolic rate is another important concern with TBI. Seizures should be tightly controlled with anticonvulsants. Hyperthermia, secondary to trauma to the thermoregulatory center, excitement, paddling, iatrogenic causes (heating pads) or pain, should be avoided.

Ancillary Therapeutics and Patient Monitoring

Analgesia and nutrition are important treatment concerns with TBI. Provision of adequate analgesia is essential, utilizing drugs that minimize cardiovascular and respiratory depression, such as butorphanol or hydromorphone. Barbiturates, propofol, and etomidate are acceptable anesthetic agents as they do not adversely affect CBF or cerebral metabolic rate. For these reasons, ketamine, acepromazine, and xylazine should be avoided. Immediately following head injury, a hypermetabolic state develops that persists for many days. Early institution of nutritional support is crucial to minimize protein catabolism.

Frequent physical examination parameters assessing tissue perfusion should be employed. Oxygenation and blood pressure should be monitored either continuously or as often as is feasible in the early phase of treatment, with goals to maintain oxygen saturation above 97% (PaO_2 >90 mm Hg) and mean arterial blood pressure above 80 mm Hg. Likewise, $PaCO_2$ should be monitored to assess for adequate ventilation. Blood glucose, hematocrit, and total protein concentrations should be checked at least twice daily to ensure adequate fuel, oxygen-carrying capacity, and oncotic pressure. Sampling from the jugular vein should be avoided, as temporary occlusion of this vessel can result in a rapid elevation in ICP. Since mannitol can cause excessive free-water loss through the kidneys, daily electrolyte monitoring (particularly sodium) should be performed and urine output should be quantified. Fluid input should be adjusted to account for ongoing losses. Nursing care should focus on provision of adequate bedding, frequent turning, and passive range of motion physical therapy on the limbs to prevent pressure sores and limb contraction. Neurologic status should be evaluated and recorded hourly initially to assess response to treatment. The Small Animal Coma Scale, a modification of the Glasgow Coma Scale, has been developed for animals to quantitatively score severity of neurologic injury. Serial scores can provide an objective measure over time.

Successful management of severe TBI can be a rewarding. The animal can be discharged when neurologic signs have improved or reached a static level and the patient is able to maintain hydration and nutritional requirements (voluntarily or with a feeding tube). Neurologic recovery may be complete or residual deficits may persist. Owners need to be dedicated and educated to the fact that they may need to provide substantial caretaking when their pet is sent home.

References

The reference list can be found on the companion Expert Consult Web site at *www.expertconsult.com*.

CHAPTER **129**

Crystalloid and Colloid Fluid Therapy

Jennifer J. Devey

Fluid therapy forms the cornerstone of treatment of most ill or injured small animal patients. Patients who are moderately or significantly dehydrated or showing signs of poor perfusion should receive fluid therapy in hospital. Understanding the difference between perfusion abnormalities and dehydration is extremely important. The approach to fluid therapy, including the type of fluids administered, fluid rates, and choice of parameters to be monitored to ensure the appropriate end goal has been reached, depends on whether the patient is dehydrated or has perfusion abnormalities or both. Inappropriate fluid therapy can lead to both patient morbidity and mortality. An in-depth review of fluid therapy is beyond the scope of this chapter and the reader is referred to other sources.[1]

DISTRIBUTION OF FLUIDS

Approximately 60% to 70% of body weight is water, of which one third is extracellular and two thirds is intracellular. Of the water that is extracellular, 75% to 80% is interstitial and 20% to 25% is intravascular. The movement of fluid between compartments is dependent upon the permeability of the membranes separating the compartments as well as the osmotically active particles in each compartment. The colloid osmotic pressure (COP), or oncotic pressure, is one of the major forces governing fluid movement. Larger proteins that do not readily move between compartments generate this pressure. Approximately 80% of the oncotic pressure is produced by albumin. This effect is enhanced by the negative charge of the protein, which attracts cations such as sodium that then attract water.

There are four forces that govern fluid movement across capillary membranes: capillary hydrostatic pressure, interstitial hydrostatic pressure, plasma oncotic pressure, and interstitial oncotic pressure. Movement of molecules also depends to some extent on the size of the molecule. The *filtration coefficient* represents the ability of water and small molecules to pass through membrane. The *reflection coefficient* represents the ability of macromolecules (generally plasma proteins) to pass through membranes. Starling's equation on diffusion of fluids across membranes is stated below.

$$Q = K\left[(P_c - P_i) - \sigma(\pi_p - \pi_i)\right]$$

where Q = fluid flux, P_c = intravascular hydrostatic pressure, P_i = interstitial hydrostatic pressure, π_p = plasma oncotic pressure, π_i = interstitial oncotic pressure, K = the filtration coefficient, and σ = the reflection coefficient.

Fluid flux varies in the different organs. In general intravascular hydrostatic pressure and plasma oncotic pressure are the key forces in regulating fluid balance, with the net movement of fluid being toward the interstitial space. The remaining fluid is moved back into the circulation via the lymphatics. The lung is far more permeable to albumin than are other organs. This means that hydrostatic forces play a much larger role in the lung than in other tissue beds and also that the pulmonary lymphatics are extremely effective at preventing accumulation of fluid. This explains why patients with hypoalbuminemia do not regularly develop pulmonary edema, even in the face of peripheral edema, but patients with increased hydrostatic pressure, such as fluid overload, do. Clinically insignificant changes in extravascular lung fluid have been noted in research animals subjected to significant changes in COP. This is due to the ability of the lymphatics to dramatically increase the fluid uptake (as much as sevenfold).

ALBUMIN

Albumin plays a vital role in the body, of which maintaining oncotic pressure is only a part. It plays an important role as a free radical scavenger, it reduces microvascular permeability, and it reduces endothelial cell apoptosis. It is important as a carrier of drugs and other endogenous substances and affects acid-base status and metabolic functions and has anticoagulant effects. Current recommendations suggest maintaining the albumin concentration at or above 2.0 g/dL in patients with acute hypoalbuminemia. Approximately 60% of the albumin is within the interstitial space, so replenishing albumin levels often requires significant volumes of plasma, especially in large dogs.

POOR PERFUSION (SHOCK)

Perfusion is defined as the flow of blood through an organ. Poor perfusion indicates some degree of cellular shock exists associated with inadequate blood supply and delivery of oxygen to the cells. Waste products (primarily CO_2) accumulate as well. The combination leads to anaerobic metabolism and acidosis/acidemia. This can lead to a breakdown in the cellular functions and ultimately cell death. Patients presenting in shock often are hypovolemic from fluid loss (hemorrhage) or decreased vascular resistance (sepsis) leading to decreased venous return, but they may have poor cardiac output (congestive heart failure) poor blood flow due to circulatory disturbances (saddle thrombus). Hypovolemic shock is the most common and is usually secondary to trauma (e.g., whole blood loss), third spacing of fluids (e.g., vasculitis, idiopathic hemorrhagic gastroenteritis, peritonitis), or acute severe dehydration (e.g., severe vomiting and/or diarrhea). Understanding the cause helps determine the appropriate treatment.

Altered levels of consciousness, weakness, tachycardia (not typically seen in the cat) or bradycardia with weak or absent peripheral pulses, tachypnea or severe bradypnea, pale mucous membranes with delayed or absent capillary refill time and cool extremities all indicate a state of poor perfusion or shock.

BLOOD VOLUME

Approximately 10% of the blood volume is in the arteries, 20% is in the capillaries, and 70% is in the veins. If the blood volume is normal, preload and blood pressure should be normal, assuming the animal is healthy. If a healthy animal's blood volume is low, the animal is hypovolemic, although a combination of changes in systemic vascular resistance and shunting of blood from various tissue beds means blood pressure may be normal. This can be misleading, since these patients actually require fluids to expand the intravascular space. Patients with hypervolemic states (e.g., congestive heart failure, advanced liver disease, oliguric renal failure) that require fluid therapy often present a significant challenge since continued expansion of the intravascular space can easily lead to fluid overload.

In clinical terms *preload* is the volume returning to the right side of the heart. It is assessed most effectively by measuring central venous pressure (CVP) (normal, 1 to 3 cm H_2O). If no central catheter is present, the jugular veins should be clipped and examined for distention and filling. Patients with hypovolemic shock will have flat jugular veins and poor filling when the vein is held off at the thoracic inlet. Patients with diseases that interfere with return of blood to the right side of the heart (e.g., pericardial tamponade, tension pneumothorax) may have distended jugular veins in the face of hypovolemia. Patients with right-sided heart failure and advanced liver disease generally will have elevated CVP.

DEHYDRATION AND INTERSTITIAL VOLUME

Dehydration is caused by inadequate fluid intake for the animal's fluid output leading to a decrease in the fluid level in the interstitial and intracellular spaces. Dehydration is often defined by evaluating clinical parameters such as moistness of mucous membranes, skin turgor, and eye position (Table 129-1); however, these are very subjective and can be difficult to evaluate. At less than 5% dehydrated the patient may not have any physical exam abnormalities. Changes become more evident as dehydration worsens: at 10% to 12% dehydration signs of shock will be evident, and dehydration greater than 15% is associated with impending death.

Animals that are salivating from nausea may have moist oral mucus membranes but be significantly dehydrated. In these patients assessing vulvar membranes or performing a digital rectal examination using a nonlubricated digital examination may be helpful in determining the level of dehydration. Geriatric animals have decreased skin elasticity and emaciated animals have depleted fat stores, which can lead to findings of decreased skin turgor and sunken eyes in the face of normal hydration.

History often plays a major role in helping assess a patient's level of dehydration. For instance an animal that has been vomiting several hundred milliliters every 2 hours for the past 12 hours and has not been drinking has to be significantly dehydrated even if the physical exam does not confirm this. Owners should be closely questioned to determine frequency of fluid losses (vomiting, diarrhea, salivation, panting) and approximate size of puddles noted at home as well as recent oral intake. This also will help in estimating potential ongoing losses the patient may experience regardless of whether the animal is discharged to home care or hospitalized.

Laboratory tests may help with the assessment of dehydration as long as the patient was normal initially.[2] For example an elevated total solids often indicates dehydration but can be confounded by the presence of hyperglobulinemia. An elevated blood urea nitrogen is consistent with prerenal azotemia as long as the patient did not have preexisting renal disease or does not have gastrointestinal hemorrhage. A urine specific gravity above the high range of normal for the species and hyperalbuminemia are always consistent with dehydration.

FLUID TYPES

Fluids administered to patients are characterized frequently by their osmolality and are considered *hyperosmolar, isosmolar,* or *hypoosmolar.* Fluids are also referred to as being *hypertonic, isotonic,* and *hypotonic* to the patient's serum based on the number of effective osmoles in a solution. Osmolality is the concentration of osmotically active particles in a kilogram of solution. It is dependent solely on the number of particles and is not affected by size, weight, or charge of the particle. Osmolarity is the number of particles per litre of solvent. Normal osmolality for dogs is 290 to 310 mOsm/kg and 308 to 335 mOsm/kg in cats. Osmolality can be calculated by the formula:

$$Osmolality = 2(Sodium) + BUN/2.8 + Glucose/18$$

Osmoles may be effective or ineffective. Effective osmoles generate osmotic pressure—the ability to cause water to shift from one compartment to another. If the membrane separating the two compartments is permeable to the solute in question, the osmole is ineffective. Urea is an osmole but is generally ineffective since it is permeable across most membranes. Glucose is an effective osmole since it will not pass across most membranes without the addition of insulin. *Tonicity* refers to the effective osmolality.

Crystalloids

Crystalloids are aqueous solutions of mineral salts (usually predominantly sodium and chloride) or other water-soluble molecules that are capable of distributing to all fluid compartments. They include replacement fluids, maintenance fluids, and fluids such as 5% dextrose in water. Crystalloids are generally isosmolar; however, they become hyperosmolar once other medications or supplements are added to the fluids. This may be important to patient therapy. All of the replacement fluids, except for 0.9% saline, are hypotonic in the cat.

Replacement crystalloids have electrolyte concentrations that resemble the extracellular fluid. Commonly used replace-

Table • 129-1				

Clinical Signs of Dehydration

	APPEARANCE	EYES	MUCOUS MEMBRANES	SKIN TENT
3%-5%	Normal	Normal	Normal	<2 sec
6%-8%	Mildly depressed	Mildly sunken	Sticky/dry	>3 sec
10%-12%	Depressed	Deeply sunken	Dry ± cold	Persists
>15%	Moribund			

Table • 129-2

Characteristics of Crystalloids

	GLUCOSE						BUFFER			
	g/L	Na	Cl	K	Ca	mg	mEq/L	mOsm/L	Cal/L	pH
5% dextrose	50	0	0	0	0	0	0	252	170	4.0
2.5% dextrose in 0.45% saline	25	77	77	0	0	0	0	280	85	4.5
5% dextrose in 0.9% saline	50	154	154	0	0	0	0	560	170	4.0
0.45% saline	0	77	77	0	0	0	0	154	0	5.0
0.9% saline	0	154	154	0	0	0	0	308	0	5.0
Lactated Ringer's solution	0	130	109	4	3	0	28 (L)	272	9	6.7
5% dextrose in lactated Ringer's	50	130	109	4	3	0	28 (L)	524	179	5.0
2.5% dextrose in half-strength LRS	25	65.5	55	2	1.5	0	14 (L)	263	89	5.0
Normosol-M in 5% dextrose	50	40	40	13	0	3	16 (A)	364	175	5.5
Normosol-R	0	140	98	5	0	3	27 (A) 23 (G)	296	18	6.4
Plasmalyte-A	0	140	98	5	5	3	27 (A) 23 (G)	296	18	7.4
Plasmalyte-M in 5% dextrose	50	40	40	16	5	3	12 (A) 12 (G)	376	178	5.5
Plasma	1	145	105	5	5	3	24	300	—	7.4

A, Acetate; G, gluconate; L, lactate.

ment fluids are 0.9% saline, lactated Ringer's solution, and Normosol-R or Plasmalyte-A (Table 129-2).

Since approximately 75% of extracellular fluid is in the interstitial space, crystalloids will rapidly redistribute, and after as short a period of time as 20 to 60 minutes only approximately 25% of the administered volume will remain in the circulation. This number may be even smaller in the face of increased vascular permeability. The remainder of the fluid will be in the interstitium minus a small amount that will have been lost via the urine. This increase in interstitial fluid can lead to tissue edema, which decreases the ability of oxygen to diffuse to the cells. Interstitial edema may be extremely detrimental in cases of cerebral edema and pulmonary edema. On a short-term basis crystalloids will expand the intravascular space, but this effect will be temporary. Replacement crystalloids should be thought of as interstitial rehydrators, not intravascular volume expanders.

All of the replacement crystalloids except for 0.9% saline contain a buffer. Buffered solutions usually contain lactate, gluconate, or acetate, which when metabolized produce bicarbonate. Lactate must be metabolized in the liver. Significant liver dysfunction must be present in order for the lactate in lactated Ringer's solution to cause a clinically significant problem. Solutions buffered with acetate and gluconate (e.g., Plasmalyte-A, Noromsol-R) have theoretical advantages over lactated Ringer's solution in that muscle can metabolize the acetate and gluconate and the amount of buffer present in these solutions is almost double the amount in lactated Ringer's solution. Concerns have been raised about the routine use of lactated Ringer's solution due to the adverse effects of the lactate, including neutrophil priming and worsening of cellular apoptosis. Buffered solutions are usually indicated for resuscitating patients in shock as well as routine use in patients that require a replacement fluid.

Due to its acidifying nature, 0.9% saline should generally be reserved for patients with gastric outflow obstructions,

patients with hypoadrenocorticism, and patients with hypercalcemia. It is important to note that electrolyte abnormalities cannot be corrected in patients with any of these three conditions without infusion of saline.

Maintenance crystalloids contain electrolyte concentrations designed to match normal daily electrolyte losses in urine and feces. They contain much less sodium (40 to 60 mEq/L) and more potassium (15 to 30 mEq/L) than a replacement crystalloid (see Table 129-2). Maintenance fluids are isotonic in the bag due to the added dextrose; however, the dextrose is rapidly metabolized to free water, making the solution hypotonic. Maintenance crystalloids should be used in patients who are unable to drink, and, therefore, have a free-water requirement, but only have ongoing electrolyte losses through normal urine and feces production. Maintenance fluids should also be used in those who will not tolerate the sodium load of a replacement fluid such as patients with heart failure, severe liver disease, or oliguric renal failure.

Dextrose 5% in water is a nonelectrolyte fluid and should not be used for fluid resuscitation. It is hypotonic and may cause fluid shifts and red cell lysis. It is typically used to replace free-water deficits or as a diluent for medications that need to be administered via constant rate infusion. It should never be given as a large volume bolus since the rapid decrease in osmolality can lead to life-threatening cerebral edema. Dextrose 5% in water only contains 200 kcal/L and does not contain sufficient energy to keep up with patient caloric requirements.

Hypertonic saline is a hyperosmolar crystalloid fluid. It is usually given as a 7.5% solution (2600 mOsm/L). The hyperosmolarity leads to extremely rapid intravascular volume expansion by drawing fluids from the interstitial and intracellular space into the intravascular space. It can produce an intravascular volume expansion equivalent to that of colloids but at one fourth the volume. Because it is a crystalloid it will rapidly redistribute, similar to all other sodium chloride–based solutions; however, its effects can be prolonged by concurrent administration of a colloid. It also appears to have immunomodulatory effects including decreasing mesenteric lymph production and eliminating neutrophil priming, which decreases susceptibility to sepsis following hemorrhagic shock.[3] It is used in resuscitation of severe hypovolemic shock and is the fluid of choice in patients who are in extremis due to its rapid onset of action as well as efficacy. It should be used with caution in patients with uncontrolled internal hemorrhage since the rapid rise in volume and blood pressure can worsen the hemorrhage.

Colloids

Colloids are effective intravascular volume expanders. They are fluids containing high–molecular weight substances that generally are not able to pass through capillary membranes. The colloid osmotic pressure they exert is related to the size of the molecule: the smaller the size of the molecule the higher the initial oncotic pressure since more smaller particles fit in a volume of fluid than larger molecules.[4] The larger the molecule, the longer it lasts. Examples include synthetic colloids such as the gelatins, dextrans, hydroxyethyl starches, and hemoglobin-based oxygen-carrying solutions, and natural colloids such as whole blood, plasma, and human serum albumin (Table 129-3).[5]

Colloids are usually isosmolar. Most have the potential to cause allergic reactions; however, clinically this appears to be limited to exposure to the gelatins. All synthetic colloids have the potential to cause a dilutional coagulopathy if doses higher than 20 mL/kg are given daily.

Gelatins are hyperosmolar fluids produced from bovine gelatin. Their average molecular weight is 30,000 Daltons. They are very potent colloids but are short acting, with a plasma half-life of 2 to 4 hours. They have no direct effects on coagulation or platelets.

Dextrans are polysaccharides produced by the bacterium *Leukonostoc* in a sucrose media. Dextran 40 has an average molecular weight of 40,000 Daltons, and dextran 70 has an average molecular weight of 70,000 Daltons. Because of the larger number of particles per unit volume in dextran 40 than in dextran 70, dextran 40 has the larger oncotic pull and will

expand the intravascular volume by approximately 1.8 to 2.1 times the volume infused; however, because molecules of 40,000 Daltons are freely filtered in the urine, the effect is short-lived. Dextran 70 expands the fluid volume by approximately 1.4 times and has a slightly longer duration of effect of approximately 4 to 8 hours versus 2 to 6 hours for dextran 40. Since albumin has a molecular weight of 69,000 Daltons, any disease associated with a vascular leakage of albumin is likely to lead to loss of dextran 70 equally quickly. With dextran 70 a coagulopathy may occur secondary to dilution, coating of platelets, change in the function of factor VIIIR:Ag, and destabilization of the clot through polymerization with fibrin. Dextran 70 can cause red blood cell cross-linking; this leads to rouleaux formation, which may interfere with cross matching. In dehydrated patients the dextran 40 molecules that are filtered may precipitate and cause renal tubular obstruction and subsequent renal failure.

Hydroxyethyl starch is a molecule made from maize or sorghum that is primarily an amylopectin. Hetastarch and pentastarch are the two main types of hydroxyethyl starches available.[6] Both expand the volume by about 1.4 times the volume infused. Hetastarch has an average molecular weight of 450,000 Daltons and has a half-life of 25 hours. Because of its size and half-life, hetastarch provides an effective means of expanding the intravascular volume for an extended time. Hetastarch has properties that are of value in treating patients with sepsis.[7] Research with hetastarch in endotoxic shock has shown that it has a significant antiinflammatory effect with a subsequent improvement in capillary permeability.[8] Through down-regulation of endothelial surface adhesion molecules, it inhibits the accumulation of neutrophils, cytokine-induced neutrophil chemoattractant protein, nuclear factor-kappaB, and leukocyte diapedesis.[9,10] Similar to dextran 70, hetastarch can interfere with factor VIII and von Willebrand factor but does so to a lesser extent. Doses greater than 20 mL/kg/day have been associated with an increased incidence of bleeding problems, which may be due to dilution, increased microvascular perfusion, or decreased platelet aggregation.

Pentastarch is a slightly lower molecular weight hydroxyethyl starch with an average molecular weight of 264,000 Daltons. This makes it a more potent colloid than hetastarch but it has a shorter half–life, with about 70% being eliminated within 24 hours.

Synthetic colloids are indicated when the patient is hypovolemic and has a low colloid osmotic pressure. Conditions including acute hemorrhage or loss of albumin ("third-spacing") due to increased vascular permeability such as SIRS (systemic inflammatory response syndrome) and sepsis frequently lead to low oncotic pressure. Since most patients in shock require sustained intravascular volume expansion, colloids are indicated frequently during fluid resuscitation. Sequential volumes of 5 mL/kg to a maximum of 20 mL/kg in the dog and 15 mL/kg in the cat are given during resuscitation. Synthetic colloids can be given as a slow intravenous push in dogs but should be given over 15 to 20 minutes in cats because hypotension will worsen temporarily in some cats following a rapid infusion. Patients with SIRS or sepsis with ongoing losses of albumin frequently require constant rate infusions of a synthetic colloid until the inflammation has subsided. Hetastarch typically is infused because of its large molecular size at a dose of 20 mL/kg/day (0.8 mL/kg/hr). During constant rate infusions of colloids crystalloid infusion volumes are decreased by 40% to 60% of what would be calculated if crystalloids alone were being used. If volumes greater than 20 mL/kg/day are infused, the patient should be monitored for the possible onset of a dilutional coagulopathy.

Table • 129-3

Mean Molecular Weight (MW) and Colloid Osmotic Pressure (COP) of Selected Colloids

FLUID	MEAN MW (kDa)	COP (mm Hg)
Dextran 70	70	61.7 ± 0.5
6% hetastarch in 0.9% saline	450	32.7 ± 0.2
6% hetastarch in balanced electrolyte solution	670	37.9 ± 0.1
10% pentastarch	200	32 ± 1.4
HBOC—Oxyglobin	200	43.3 ± 0.1
25% human serum albumin	69	200
Canine fresh frozen plasma	69	17.1 ± 0.6

Data from Chan DL, Freeman LM, Rozanski EA, et al: Colloid osmotic pressure of parenteral nutrition components and intravenous fluids. J Vet Emerg Crit Care 11:269, 2001.
HBOC, Hemoglobin-based oxygen carrying solution.

Hemoglobin-Based Oxygen Carriers

The only hemoglobin-based oxygen-carrying (HBOC) solution currently approved for use in veterinary medicine is Oxyglobin (Biopure, Cambridge, Mass.), which is a purified, polymerized bovine hemoglobin that is in a modified lactated Ringer's solution. It has many properties that make it a valuable fluid during resuscitation.[11] It is isosmotic and has an average molecular weight of 200,000 Da, making it a very effective colloid, and a pH of 7.8. Its oxygen affinity is dependent upon the chloride ion concentration not the concentration of 2,3-diphosphoglycerate (2,3-DPG). This provides a distinct advantage over canine blood that has been stored longer than 1 week, which may have significantly depleted 2,3-DPG levels lead to increased oxygen binding and decreased oxygen delivery at the tissue level. In addition, the normal oxygen affinity of Oxyglobin is lower than that of normal canine blood, which enhances delivery of oxygen to the tissues. It has a lower viscosity than canine blood, which may improve microvascular flow. Because it is a smaller molecule than red cells, it is able to perfuse vasoconstricted tissue beds that red cells cannot pass through. It has vasoconstricting properties that are of benefit in shock; however, concerns have been raised about excessive vasoconstriction in some tissue beds—especially the lung, where pulmonary hypertension may result.

Oxyglobin can be administered via standard intravenous administration sets, and standard intravenous infusion pumps can be used for delivery. Because it contains no antigens, cross-matching is not required and there is no possibility of transfusion reactions. Filters are not required. It can be kept at room temperature and has a 3-year shelf life, which makes it useful for hospitals that cannot keep blood products readily available. Once opened, the bag must be discarded within 24 hours due to the production of methemoglobin.

Oxyglobin is up to 10 times more effective than blood when given during fluid resuscitation to animals in hemorrhagic shock. For this reason, low volumes of Oxyglobin can be used effectively to treat hemorrhagic shock. It has a short half-life (30 to 40 hours); however, the length of clinical benefit is currently unknown. Primary effects last about 24 hours, and 90% of the Oxyglobin is eliminated in 5 to 7 days.

HBOCs are indicated during resuscitation when increased oxygen delivery to tissues is desired. Administration of HBOCs also is indicated in anemic patients but must be used with caution in patients that are euvolemic (e.g., those with immune-mediate hemolytic anemia), and should be used with extreme caution in patients that are hypervolemic (e.g., patients with congestive heart failure or oliguric/anuric renal failure) because of its potent onconotic pressure. Since cats appear to be more predisposed to rapid onset of pulmonary edema when fluid overload occurs, Oxyglobin should be infused over a minimum of 8 hours in euvolemic cats.

Low-volume resuscitation with Oxyglobin may restore aerobic metabolism, although hypovolemia, hypotension, and low cardiac output persist. The hemoglobin is dissolved in the plasma, and some is able to diffuse into the interstitium, which makes it a very effective oxygen-carrying solution. Therefore, the amount of Oxyglobin administered should be based on clinical signs rather than a specific target hemoglobin concentration. Doses of Oxyglobin as low as 3 to 5 mL/kg may be effective in improving tissue oxygen delivery in moderate shock, and doses as low as 7 to 8 mL/kg may be all that is indicated in severe hemorrhagic shock.[12] The daily volume administered should not exceed 30 mL/kg/day.

Side effects include discoloration of mucous membranes, sclera, and urine, which affects patient monitoring. Measurements of many serum tests are affected for at least 24 to 72 hours after administration of Oxyglobin. A list of which tests are accurate with different analyzers is available. Packed cell volumes do not correlate with hemoglobin; therefore, hemoglobin levels should to be measured directly if an accurate measurement is indicated. Mild gastrointestinal effects have been reported but are very rare.

Human Albumin

Human albumin, made from pooled human plasma, is a concentrated source of albumin. At a 25% concentration the COP is 200 mm Hg, making it a very potent colloid that is able to expand the intravascular volume by 4 to 5 times the volume infused. It is also hyperosmolar at 1500 mOsm/L. Because of these combined effects, the risk for fluid overload in a patient that is only mildly hypovolemic or euvolemic is high. It provides all the beneficial effects of albumin (see above). The fluid infusion should be considered a transfusion with all the potential for both acute reactions such as facial swelling, fever, vomiting and anaphylaxis and delayed immune-mediated reactions such as polyarthritis and vasculitis that may not show up for several weeks. Whenever possible a species-specific source of albumin should be transfused to avoid the risk for a transfusion-related reaction; however, this can be cost prohibitive or a source of feline or canine albumin may not be available, in which case human serum albumin can be a cost-effective means of reducing morbidity and even mortality in the critical patient. The half-life is approximately 16 hours. Doses of 2.5 to 5.0 mL/kg have been recommended with a maximum dose of 2 g/kg/day.[13] It is recommended that, once the bottle is spiked, the infusion be completed over 4 to 6 hours; however, infusions over a slower period of time have been reported. Continuous or intermittent transfusions over 24 to 72 hours have also been reported. Once patients have been exposed to the human serum albumin, they will develop antibodies and transfusions should never be administered again during the life of the patient (severe allergic reactions may make human albumin a product to be used only if no other options are available).

Natural Colloids

Natural colloids include whole blood (fresh, stored, or autotransfused), packed red blood cells (although the oncotic pressure of packed red blood cells is very low), and plasma. (The reader is referred to Chapter 142 for further information.) If the patient is acutely anemic, administration of red blood cells may be required. In the critical acutely anemic patient the goal should be to maintain a hematocrit of approximately 30% in the dog and 27% in the cat.

Autotransfused blood is the simplest to give but has a potential for significant side effects. Blood should be collected aseptically into sterile containers and administered with a filter. The need to anticoagulate is somewhat controversial since blood collected from body cavities tends to lack platelets and fibrin and is not able to clot. If a large volume of autotransfused blood is administered, fresh frozen plasma should be transfused to minimize the likelihood of disseminated intravascular coagulation developing. Ideally blood from the abdomen should not be used until it has been determined that there is no gross contamination (e.g., from a ruptured bowel). In emergency situations only, the blood may have to be used without aseptic collection or knowing whether it is contaminated, and may be delivered without a filter.

Unless the blood type of the recipient and donor are known, all recipients of a red cell–containing transfusion ideally should have a major and minor crossmatch. Dogs who are in danger of dying and have never received a transfusion usually can be transfused without a crossmatch, but the patient should be monitored closely for any immune-mediated reactions including delayed reactions that may not show up for several weeks. Since cats have naturally occurring alloantibodies, they must be typed or ideally crossmatched prior to transfusing since even a few drops of type A blood given to a type B cat can cause death. If a large volume of anticoagulated blood was infused, calcium levels should be closely monitored. The citrate will bind the serum calcium causing a clinically significant hypocalcemia.

Patients with acute hypoalbuminemia (less than 2.0 g/dL) should receive a source of albumin to maintain the albumin as close to 2.0 g/dL as possible. It takes approximately 15 to 20 mL/kg of plasma to raise the albumin 0.5 g/dL assuming no ongoing losses. Known coagulopathic patients should receive coagulation factors (fresh blood or fresh frozen plasma depending on the situation) as soon as possible. Patients with SIRS or sepsis are often at risk for becoming coagulopathic, and transfusion should be considered as soon as signs of coagulation abnormalities are noted. Plasma also provides a source of α-macroglobulin, which binds the activated and liberated proteases in patients with pancreatitis and therefore has some as yet clinically unproven benefits in these patients.

Blood and blood products are typically infused over 2 to 6 hours; however, they can be infused as fast as necessary to restore perfusion parameters in patients who need rapid volume resuscitation.

ADMINISTRATION

The ideal route of fluid administration restores the patient's fluid balance to normal as quickly as possible. Fluids should be administered intravascularly in all patients with perfusion deficits. Typically this involves placement of a peripheral catheter; however, central catheters may be indicated in some patients, and intraosseous access may be the only accessible route in very small patients, reptiles, birds, and rodents. The intraosseous route typically can be used safely to administer any fluid that would be administered via a central catheter. The exception to this is hypertonic saline, which should not be infused intraosseously until further data are available since it has been shown experimentally to cause myonecrosis.

Rapid fluid administration is indicated in most patients in shock. Based on Poiseuille's law, flow is directly proportional to the radius to the fourth power and indirectly proportional to length; therefore, a large-gauge, short catheter will allow the most rapid administration rates. General guidelines are as follows: 18 gauge in cats and smaller dogs, 16 gauge in medium-sized dogs (10 to 30 kg), and 14 gauge in larger dogs (greater than 30 kg). A large-bore catheter should be placed in every patient that might be at risk for developing shock, such as an animal undergoing any type of abdominal surgical procedure.

If slower rates of fluids are acceptable, catheter size becomes less important. Ideally, significantly hyperosmolar fluids (greater than approximately 550 mOsm/L) should be infused via a central catheter. If this is not possible, the smallest gauge catheter possible should be inserted. The small gauge of the catheter encourages blood flow around the catheter, which helps dilute the hyperosmolar fluid and prevent phlebitis.

Fluids can be administered via several routes in the dehydrated patient, although the intravenous route usually is preferred. Since dehydrated patients do not absorb fluids well from the subcutaneous space, this is not an ideal route unless the dehydration is very mild. In addition skin elasticity often limits the amount of fluid that can be given. Prior to injecting fluids subcutaneously, a calculation of the fluid deficit should be performed based on estimated percent dehydration and a decision should then be made as to whether the calculated volume of fluid can realistically be given subcutaneously. If it

cannot, the fluids should be given by an alternative route. Subcutaneous fluids should be given with caution in cats with occult cardiomyopathy since the sudden absorption of a large volume of fluid can precipitate congestive heart failure. Moderate to large volumes of subcutaneous fluids should also be given with caution in patients with polyuric renal failure and hypokalemia since the ensuing diuresis can lead to a hypokalemia severe enough to cause severe muscle weakness. Irritating or hypertonic fluids should not be given subcutaneously.

Fluids can be administered to dehydrated patients via the gastrointestinal tract if it is functional. Feeding tubes may be indicated in these patients to ensure the patient receives adequate fluids. For instance, infusing fluids via a nasoesophageal tube can be a very effective means of keeping a cat with an upper respiratory infection well hydrated.

Fluids can be given intraperitoneally to smaller patients, but this route is generally avoided due to the slow uptake and, depending on the type of fluid being administered, the potential for peritoneal irritation. Blood can be administered intraperitoneally but is not absorbed for up to 48 to 72 hours.

FLUID PLANS

Fluids should be chosen based on the desired end goal of the therapy (Figure 129-1). The fluid choices are usually based on the underlying disease process and type of fluid the patient has already lost, as well as to some extent anticipation of future losses. Fluids are chosen based more on an understanding of the pathophysiology behind a disease process than on a diagnosis. Significant volumes of whole blood loss ideally should be replaced with whole blood. Patients with protein-losing enteritis should ideally receive a combination of electrolyte-containing fluids and albumin-containing fluids. Patients with pure water and electrolyte loss should receive a fluid that replaces the water and electrolytes. Evaluation of recent laboratory tests such as hematocrit, albumin, glucose, electrolytes, urea, creatinine, and blood gases also can help guide the choice of fluid. Often the ideal fluid is not feasible due to lack of hospital resources or lack of client resources (finances). In these situations the next best fluid is chosen, but the clinician should be aware that there might be negative side effects of a treatment that is less than ideal. The side effects should be monitored in an attempt to minimize their negative impact on the patient.

FLUID ADDITIVES

Fluid additives are often required as a part of patient therapy. The most common are potassium (Table 129-4) and dextrose. The amount of potassium to be added to the fluid should be adjusted based on the fluid being administered, the patient's underlying disease, the patient's pH and serum potassium concentration, and the rate of fluid administration. A rate of 0.5 mEq/kg/hr ideally should not be exceeded without close cardiac monitoring. Potassium along with other electrolytes should be checked daily—more frequently if the potassium supplementation rate is high or there are concerns for severe, ongoing losses.

The addition of medications increases the osmolality of the fluids. This is rarely a problem but should be evaluated on a patient-by-patient basis. Additives should always be checked for compatibility with the fluid being used as a diluent to ensure the pH or the constituents of the fluid will not inactivate the medication or cause it to precipitate. Compatibility with other medications or fluids that are being infused through the same intravenous line also should be checked. For instance, calcium-containing fluids should not be administered concur-

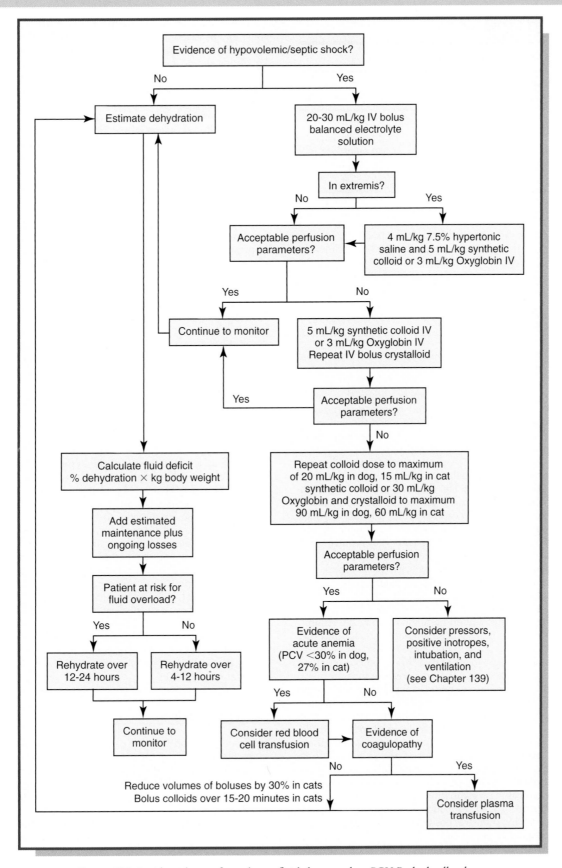

Figure 129-1 Algorithm to formulate a fluid therapy plan. *PCV,* Packed cell volume.

Table • 129-4

Potassium Supplementation

SERUM POTASSIUM CONCENTRATION	RECOMMENDED CONCENTRATION IN FLUID
3.5-5.5 mEq/L	20 mEq/L
3.0-3.5 mEq/L	30 mEq/L
2.5-3.0 mEq/L	40 mEq/L
2.0-2.5 mEq/L	60 mEq/L
<2.0 mEq/L	80 mEq/L

rently through the same line as blood products anticoagulated with citrate since the resultant precipitate may be detrimental to the patient. Additives should be checked carefully for light stability.

RESUSCITATION: EARLY GOAL-DIRECTED THERAPY

The amount of fluid to be administered during resuscitation is based on the objective of attempting to restore tissue perfusion with the goal of restoring normal oxygen delivery and waste removal (primarily in the form of carbon dioxide).[14] Often a combination of crystalloids and colloids is required.[15] The smallest volume of fluid possible to reach the end goals should be infused to avoid complications from excessive fluid administration. Fluid should be infused until signs of perfusion have normalized. In an ideal situation this would mean that the heart rate is normalized, blood pressure (systolic pressure of 100 to 120 mm Hg, diastolic pressure of 60 to 80 mm Hg) and CVP (6 to 9 cm H_2O) are normalized, mucous membrane color and capillary refill time are normalized, temperature (toe web and central) is normalized, and urine output is normalized. Most patients that require fluid resuscitation have confounding problems such as pain that can increase the heart rate or underlying sepsis, which makes it difficult to achieve a normal blood pressure or underlying renal dysfunction, which in turn makes it difficult to know what "normal" urine output is for the individual patient. However, every attempt should be made to bring the parameters to as close to normal as possible taking into account the patient's underlying disease. Blood pressure should be measured, not estimated, since estimation based on pulse palpation is notoriously inaccurate. If blood pressure measurement is not available, the strength of peripheral pulses (dorsal metatarsal) should be assessed rather than femoral pulses. Ideally, blood gas values and/or lactate concentrations should also be used to help determine the effectiveness of resuscitation. Although it is unlikely the metabolic parameters will normalize immediately due to oxygen debt at the cell level, they should be trending towards normal and ideally should be close to normal within the first 12 to 24 hours. If blood volume has been maximized based on estimation of jugular venous distention, measurement of CVP, or evidence of fluid overload, but the patient is still hypotensive, positive inotropes or vasopressors may be required.

More specific goals recently defined for septic human patients in order to reduce morbidity include achieving a mean arterial pressure of greater than 65 mm Hg, a CVP of 6 to 9 cm H_2O, a urine output greater than 0.5 mL/kg/hr, and a central venous oxygen saturation of 70%. These goals remain untested in dogs and cats; however, they may prove to be of value.

The maximum fluid volume to be infused is chosen to some extent based on the blood volume of the patient, which in the dog is approximately 80 mL/kg and in the cat is 60 mL/kg. Fluids should be given as fast as necessary to resuscitate the patient. Because of the rapid redistribution rate of crystalloid fluids, very rapid boluses are required in order to determine if the patient is responding to volume infusion. Resuscitation is usually started with a bolus of 20 to 30 mL/kg of a buffered, balanced electrolyte solution. This volume is reduced by approximately 30% in cats. Doses of 4 mL/kg of a 7.5% saline solution are given to dogs and 2 to 4 mL/kg to cats for patients in extremis. If the patient is suspected—based on clinical presentation, lack of response to an initial bolus of crystalloids, or initial lab work—of having a low colloid osmotic pressure, synthetic colloids are used during initial resuscitation with sequential boluses of 5 mL/kg to a maximum of 20 ml/kg in the dog and 15 mL/kg in the cat to improve the blood volume and blood pressure to the desired end point. Doses of Oxyglobin of 3 to 5 mL/kg can be given in lieu of other synthetic colloids.

The patient must be monitored closely once goals have been reached to ensure the goals are maintained. Patients that appeared stable can rapidly destabilize secondary to conditions such as ongoing hemorrhage, ongoing losses through vomiting, diarrhea, polyuria, or third-space losses, as well as movement of crystalloids out of the vascular space.

HYPOTENSIVE RESUSCITATION

Hypotensive resuscitation refers to a controversial form of resuscitation provided to trauma patients that may still be actively hemorrhaging internally.[16] It involves the use of limited fluid resuscitation until the hemorrhage is controlled. The systolic blood pressure is maintained between approximately 80 and 100 mm Hg with the goal being to avoid increased hemorrhage from normotension or hypertension that might cause fragile clots to be disrupted. This not only helps prevent loss of hemoglobin but also other plasma proteins including albumin and clotting factors. Dilution of clotting factors from excessive administration of crystalloids or synthetic colloids also is avoided. There is danger of maintaining inadequate perfusion to various organs, especially the gastrointestinal tract, kidneys, muscles, and skin, since the patient is not being adequately resuscitated. The advantage is that severe hemorrhage may ultimately be controlled without requiring administration of multiple units of blood products and the patient's life may be saved. Hypotensive resuscitation can be particularly helpful in patients with significant intraabdominal hemorrhage.

REHYDRATION

Mild dehydration rarely causes severe problems other than making the patient feel unwell; however, if the patient has other underlying diseases such as renal insufficiency, even mild dehydration can lead to serious problems. If severe enough, dehydration can lead to perfusion problems.

In dehydrated patients perfusion deficits should be dealt with using intravenous fluids according to the guidelines above (see Table 129-1). The degree of dehydration should always be estimated and a calculation performed to estimate the volume deficit of the patient. The body weight in kilograms is multiplied by the estimated percent dehydration (as a decimal). This will indicate fluid deficit in liters of fluid. For instance a 5-kg patient estimated at 8% dehydrated has a fluid deficit of 0.4 L, or 400 mL. Fluid deficits should always be calculated since estimating fluid rates by placing an animal on two or three times maintenance rates will almost always significantly underestimate fluid requirements, which can lead to significant patient morbidity. Along with assessment of physical examination parameters, monitoring urine specific gravity (assuming renal function is normal) can help determine if adequate volumes of fluid are being administered.

Fluids should be given more slowly to restore dehydration since the fluids need to have time to redistribute. Patients with no underlying disease that could lead to volume overload (advanced heart disease, liver or oliguric renal failure) should be rehydrated over 4 to 12 hours. Shorter time frames are used in patients who became dehydrated very acutely or if there are concerns for severe, ongoing losses. Older patients or patients with concurrent disease process may need to be rehydrated over 24 hours.

CALCULATING DAILY REQUIREMENTS

Daily fluid requirements will vary based on maintenance requirements and ongoing losses. Recommendations for daily maintenance requirements vary considerably from 40 to 60 mL/kg/day or 2 mL/kg/hr. These formulas may underestimate for smaller patients and overestimate for much larger patients. Some advocate using a volume based on the daily energy requirement formula of (30 × body weight [kg]) + 70 in dogs and 50 × body weight (kg) in cats. Puppies and kittens will generally have much higher fluid requirements than adult animals, and recommendations are to double the adult fluid requirement in these patients. Polyuric patients, especially those with renal dysfunction (e.g., renal failure, postobstructive diuresis), can have extremely high fluid requirements. Some cats will need as much as 100 mL/hr. Fluid rates should be adjusted to match measured urine production and to ensure elevated serum urea nitrogen and creatinine concentrations are continuing to decrease. An increase in renal blood tests may be in indication of pending oliguric and anuric renal failure but more commonly is associated with inadequate fluid therapy, especially if the potassium concentrations are not rising. In renal failure patients it is almost impossible to maximize fluid diuresis without measuring CVP without causing fluid overload. Regardless of the formula chosen, the patient must be monitored clinically every 4 to 8 hours for signs of dehydration, normal hydration, and overhydration, and based on findings the fluid plan should be adjusted accordingly.

FLUID OVERLOAD

Normal patients are quite tolerant of excessive volume administration; it is removed by the kidneys in the form of increased urine production. The sick patient may not be so tolerant. If the intravascular space is expanded too rapidly, the patient may develop signs of pulmonary edema. This is a late sign and indicates the earlier signs were overlooked or the patient had unrecognized cardiac disease. Central venous pressure or jugular filling will increase followed by an increase in respiratory rate and effort (often more easily monitored in the cat than the dog) before auscultable or radiographic signs of pulmonary edema develops.

If excessive crystalloids are administered, patients will typically develop signs of overhydration before they develop signs of hypervolemia. If the kidneys are functioning normally again, increased urination will usually be noted. Signs of pathologic overload include chemosis and serous nasal discharge. Weight gain also will be noted although accurate weights in animals often can be complicated by variations based on how the animal sits on the scales. If the patient is hypooncotic the first sign may be peripheral edema. In recumbent dogs this most commonly occurs in the distal pelvic limbs, usually the downside limb. If "fat face" occurs the patient has significant fluid overload; this is often a poor prognostic finding.

MONITORING THE PATIENT

Once a fluid therapy plan has been instituted—whether it is to resuscitate a patient, rehydrate a patient, or just keep up with daily losses—the patient must be monitored to ensure goals are being achieved and maintained. Physical examination parameters relating to the fluid therapy should be assessed at least three times daily—more frequently (every 1 to 4 hours) in more critical patients—including vitals signs, ins and outs, and body weight. Jugular venous distention and blood pressure should be monitored similarly in patients that are not hemodynamically stable and every 8 hours in patients that are stable. Jugular catheters should be placed for monitoring of CVP in patients where estimation of blood volume needs to be more objective. Disposable pads can be placed under the patient and weighed in order to get a more accurate assessment of urine production. When close monitoring of outs is required, a urinary catheter should be placed. As a rule of thumb a patient without underlying renal dysfunction should be producing 1 mL/kg/hr or urinating every 4 to 6 hours when receiving intravenous fluid therapy. Sodium, potassium, and chloride, as well as ionized calcium and phosphorus if applicable, should be monitored daily in stable patients, more frequently in unstable patients. The same applies for blood gases, hematocrit and total solids, albumin, coagulation parameters, and urine specific gravity.

FLUID THERAPY PRECEPTS

Infusion of excessive volumes of crystalloids should be avoided since patients who are given large volumes of crystalloids during resuscitation will develop interstitial edema, which will worsen oxygen delivery at the cellular level.

Synthetic colloids, not plasma, should be used for volume resuscitation if the patient has an albumin less than 2 g/dL.

Synthetic colloids are not a replacement for albumin or clotting factors, and patients who need synthetic colloids frequently need plasma.

Ideally, serum albumin levels should be maintained as close to 2 g/dL as possible using species-specific albumin sources.

The patient's hematocrit should be maintained at or above 27% to 30% in the case of acute hemorrhage and below 48% in hemorrhagic gastroenteritis patients to maintain good rheology and oxygen delivery.

Infusion of whole blood or HBOC to anemic patients that are euvolemic can rapidly cause fluid overload and should be avoided or given very slowly.

Colloids should be avoided in patients with chronic hypoalbuminemia because they are not always hypovolemic and it is easy to fluid overload them.

When rehydrating patients, the degree of dehydration should always be estimated and a fluid deficit calculated and replaced over 6 to 12 hours unless the patient is at risk for fluid overload. This deficit needs to be added to the maintenance requirements as well as estimated ongoing losses.

Fluids should be given based on the needs of the patient. Polyuric patients may produce far more urine than anticipated and providing "three times maintenance" may severely underestimate their requirements.

It is difficult to maximize fluid administration without assessing central venous pressure.

Fluids should be infused to achieve a desired end point.

REFERENCES

The reference list can be found on the companion Expert Consult Web site at *www.expertconsult.com.*

CHAPTER 130

Diabetic Ketoacidosis and Hyperglycemic Hyperosmolar Syndrome

Michael Schaer

Dogs and cats afflicted with either diabetic ketoacidosis (DKA) or hyperglycemic hyperosmolar syndrome (HHS) can become acutely ill and benefit from prompt diagnosis and treatment. These disorders usually occur in middle-aged to old pets, often after a variable period of time characterized by polydipsia, polyuria, and weight loss. Alternatively, they can occur as acute metabolic complications of other conditions, such as acute pancreatitis or sepsis. The primary pathophysiology, clinical signs, and medical management of these interesting and challenging disorders are discussed in this chapter. Certain clinical findings shared by the two syndromes are discussed in the section on ketoacidosis.

PATHOPHYSIOLOGY OF KETOACIDOSIS

Hyperglycemia and accelerated ketogenesis occur when there is an absolute or relative deficiency of insulin and a relative excess of glucagon and other "counter-regulatory hormones" such as cortisol, growth hormone, and epinephrine. Consequently, glucose and ketoacids are both overproduced and underutilized. Ketoacidosis can occur as a result of insulin deficiency, but coexisting glucagon excess will accelerate the process. Because the pathophysiologic details of DKA are discussed elsewhere in this text and throughout the medical literature, only those germane to the care of the critically ill patient are mentioned in this section.

The nitroprusside reaction is used to detect and semiquantitate plasma, serum, and urinary ketones. The test detects acetone and acetoacetate but does not react with beta hydroxybutyrate. This characteristic has clinical importance in situations in which shocklike states promote the production of beta hydroxybutyrate, thereby disabling clinical detection of ketoacidosis with the nitroprusside test.

After institution of insulin treatment, the beta hydroxybutyrate–to-acetoacetate (B:A) ratio decreases as a result of the metabolism of beta hydroxybutyrate to acetoacetate. Although acetoacetate concentrations eventually decrease, the shifting B:A ratio explains the clinical paradox occasionally encountered in which test results may initially be negative for ketones, but the same test performed on the second and third days of treatment may, occasionally, be positive despite clinical improvement. A lingering ketonuria can also occur as a dog or cat improves because of the delayed clearance of acetone. Therefore, it is not uncommon for ketones to persist well into

the third or fourth hospital day while the pet shows signs of improvement. It is for this reason that the calculation of insulin dosages should depend solely on the blood glucose concentration.

DIAGNOSIS

History and Physical Examination

Owner observations regarding a dog or cat with either DKA or HHS often indicate that anorexia, depression, weakness, and vomiting may have been seen for only 1 to 3 days. Oliguria or anuria should be suspected if the owner reports polyuria for days or weeks and then no urine for 1 to 2 days prior to the examination. A complete physical examination is essential to detect any concurrent disorders that can significantly affect the outcome. It has been suggested that both conditions are invariably associated with concurrent disorders. The term *diabetic coma* is frequently used to describe the mental effects of the ketoacidotic and hyperosmolar conditions, but only a small percentage of dogs or cats actually have profound decreases in consciousness.

DIAGNOSTIC EVALUATION

Medical evaluation of a sick diabetic dog or cat should be thorough and should include thoracic and abdominal radiographs, abdominal ultrasound scan, hematology, serum chemistry, and urinalysis. The acquired information creates an important data base for subsequent medical and sometimes surgical management.

Because hepatic production of glucose is increased in diabetic dogs or cats, the degree of hyperglycemia is determined by the severity of plasma volume depletion. Therefore, extreme levels of hyperglycemia tend to occur only when extracellular fluid volume and blood pressure have decreased so much that urine flow is impaired. This is most obvious in dogs or cats that have extreme increases in blood glucose concentrations with minimal glucosuria, which will usually signify oliguria.

Metabolic acidosis is mainly attributed to ketoacid buildup, but acidosis can be enhanced by coexisting disease, such as renal failure and lactic acid production. The metabolic acidosis often is accompanied by a large anion gap (AG) (greater than 30 mEq/L) that can be calculated using the following formula:

$$AG = (Na^+ + K^+) - (HCO_3^- + Cl^-)$$

Hyponatremia in both syndromes can be factitious (attributable to hypertriglyceridemia) or real (due to urinary or gastrointestinal loss of sodium ions). Spurious hyponatremia can also occur when any rapid increases in the plasma glucose concentration draw water into the extracellular space, there by diluting plasma constituents and allowing for cellular dehydration.

The serum potassium concentration in DKA and HHS can range from less than the reference range to normal to greater than the reference range. Hyperkalemia can result from a shift of potassium from the intracellular to the extracellular space as a consequence of acidemia, insulin deficiency, and increased plasma hyperosmolarity. It may also be associated with oliguric or anuric acute renal failure. Pseudohyperkalemia can accompany any patient that has a thrombocytosis as can be found with coexisting hypercortisolism.

Hypokalemia is the most common and most serious electrolyte disturbance. This is usually a reflection of a substantial reduction in total body potassium stores. Even dogs and cats with normokalemia can have life-threatening deficits of total body potassium; because 98% of total body potassium is intracellular, these concentrations are not easily assessed. Potassium losses occur with vomiting and osmotic diuresis and can be further complicated by therapy. Serum dilution from rehydration, continued urinary losses, correction of acidosis, and increased cellular uptake can "unmask" hypokalemia. A coexisting ketoalkalosis can also cause hypokalemia, usually caused by losses through excessive vomiting.

Phosphorus is an integral component of lean body mass. The enhanced catabolism of muscle and fat that invariably occurs in diabetes mellitus results in increased urinary phosphorus excretion and phosphorus wasting.

Increased serum liver transaminase (ALT) and alkaline phosphatase (SAP) activity is commonly attributable to the hepatic lipidosis that occurs in patients with DKA. Hypovolemia-induced central lobular necrosis can also increase liver enzyme values as can cholangiostasis due to coexisting acute pancreatitis. These hepatic changes are completely reversible, and serum liver enzyme activity moves toward normal after successful treatment. Because diabetic dogs and cats almost always have abnormal liver enzyme values, it is common for these test results to completely "normalize" within a week or two so long as the hepatic lipidosis does not progress.

Azotemia can be either prerenal or renal in origin. Extensive primary renal dysfunction is characterized by isosthenuria (fixed urine specific gravity of 1.008 to 1.012) in a dehydrated patient and an accompanying azotemia that does not readily resolve with rehydration. It should be remembered, however, that both glycosuria and hyperosmolarity can raise a urine specific gravity that remains "isosthenuric" (a specific gravity of 1.020 when the serum osmolality is 400 does not indicate good renal function). Urine sediment should be screened for any signs of infection such as pyuria and bacteriuria. Urine output should be monitored to detect oliguria or anuria.

A leukocytosis with a mature neutrophilia in the 20×10^3 range can be due to the stress associated with both disorders. Detection of bands and toxic cell changes should prompt a search for an inflammatory focus, which may or may not be accompanied by an infection.

TREATMENT

Fluid and Electrolytes

Disturbances in hydration and electrolyte balance are of great importance in both DKA and HHS. Such fluid deficits require expedient correction (Figure 130-1).

Calculated fluid requirements should include the patient's dehydration deficits, the 24-hour maintenance needs, and extra losses that result from vomiting or diarrhea. The dehydration status can be approximated on a scale ranging from mild (5%) to extreme (12%). The needed isotonic crystalloid fluid replacement volume can be calculated using either of the following equations:

- Dehydration volume deficit $(mL) =$ Dehydration $(\%)$
  $\times$ Body weight (kg)
  $\times 1000$

- Dehydration $(\%) \times$ Body weight $(lb) \times 500$

The 24-hour maintenance volume is roughly estimated (assuming adequate urine output) at 66 mL/kg (30 mL/lb). Therefore, the first 24-hour total fluid volume is the sum of the dehydration and the maintenance volumes plus any ongoing losses from vomiting or diarrhea.

If the animal is 8% to 12% dehydrated, half of the estimated dehydration deficit should be administered intravenously over the first 2 to 4 hours of hospitalization; the remaining replacement and maintenance volumes, given over the following 20 to 22 hours, should be accompanied by any adjustments necessitated by changes in urine volume. Oliguria and anuria call for major parenteral fluid reductions to where the amount infused will include measured urine output, insensible fluid losses, and any ongoing losses.

Hydration alone can substantially decrease the blood glucose level and hyperosmolarity. Hypovolemia in DKA and HHS is corrected with isotonic solutions, such as lactated Ringer's solution or 0.9% saline. Recommended maintenance solutions include 0.45% saline or half-strength lactated Ringer's solution so long as hyponatremia does not occur. Dextrose solutions (2.5% to 5%) are used when the patient's blood glucose declines to 250 mg/dL or less in the setting of continued insulin administration. Hyponatremia for both disorders is corrected with intravenous 0.9% saline solution to avoid any plasma hypoosmolality that might occur when the hyperglycemia is reduced with insulin treatment. Plasma hypoosmolality can cause a reversal of osmotic gradients and overexpansion of the intracellular compartment with resultant potentially fatal cerebral edema.

Potassium supplementation is best provided by adding potassium chloride solution to the parenteral fluids. If concurrent hypophosphatemia is present, one third of the potassium supplement can be in the form of potassium phosphate. Potassium supplementation is best begun after the first 2-hour period of fluid replacement, when hydration, blood pressure, and urine output are improved. If the patient is initially hypokalemic, potassium chloride (KCl) can be added to the hydrating solution; however, the infusion should be slowed so that half the dehydration replacement volume is delivered over an additional 1 to 3 hours. Although most texts list the maximum rate of potassium ion administration as 0.5 mEq per kilogram of body weight (BW) per hour, the author's experience has shown that this rate can be safely doubled when the patient is severely hypokalemic (serum potassium level less than 2.5 mEq/L) as long as electrocardiographic and urine output monitoring is done. The recommended amount of potassium that can be added to the parenteral fluids *over a 24-hour period* is shown, using two different but equally effective methods.

- *Mild hypokalemia* (serum K$^+$ of 3.0 to 3.5 mEq/L): Administer 2 to 3 mEq/kg *or* add 30 to 40 mEq KCl per liter of replacement fluid.
- *Moderate hypokalemia* (serum K$^+$ of 2.5 to 3.0 mEq/L): Administer 3 to 5 mEq KCl/kg *or* add 40 to 60 mEq KCl per liter of replacement fluid.

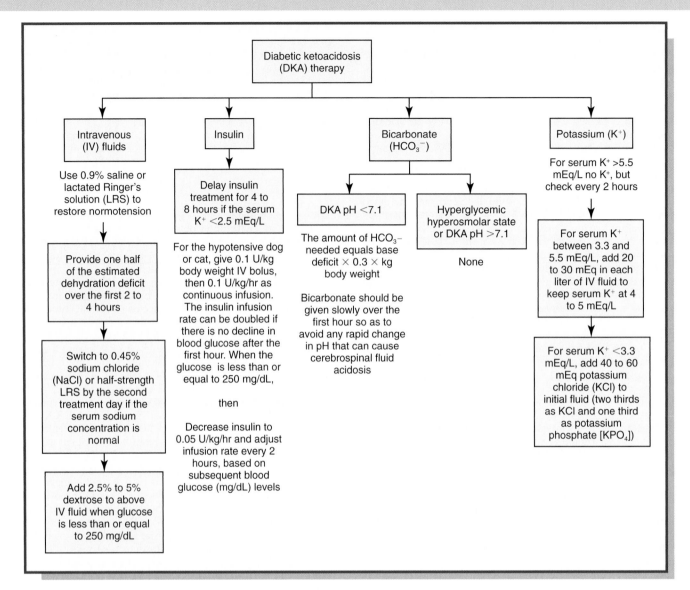

Figure 130-1 Algorithm for the management of the critically ill dog and cat with diabetic ketoacidosis and hyperglycemic hyperosmolar syndrome. (Modified from Umpierrez GE, Kelly JP, Navarrete JE, et al: Hyperglycemic crises in urban blacks. Arch Intern Med 157:669, 1997.)

• *Severe hypokalemia* (serum K⁺ below 2.5 mEq/L): Administer 5 to 10 mEq KCl/kg *or* add 60 to 80 mEq KCl per liter of replacement fluid.

Daily serum electrolyte determinations and the necessary treatment adjustments are made until normal values are obtained. In some dogs and cats, serum electrolyte concentrations should be assessed 2, 3, 4, or more times in a 24-hour period to better understand and respond to abnormalities. Intravenous fluids are discontinued when serum biochemistry values are normal, hydration is normal, and the dog or cat is able to eat and drink without vomiting.

Any needed phosphate replacement can be given as potassium phosphate solution at the recommended dose of 0.01 to 0.03 mmol/kg BW/hr, with repeat serum phosphorus determinations every 6 hours. Attention should be given to avoiding iatrogenic hyperphosphatemia and hypocalcemia. These complications can be avoided if the phosphate replacement is discontinued when the serum level is restored to 2.5 mg/dL.

Hypomagnesemia has been shown to cause specific problems, especially cardiac arrhythmias, in diabetic humans; however, its association with any particular dysfunction in diabetic dogs and cats has not yet been demonstrated. The ionic and total bound forms of magnesium can be measured. The total bound form for the dog ranges from 1.7 to 2.5 mg/dL and that for the cat ranges from 1.8 to 2.5 mg/dL. The ionized serum magnesium for dogs ranges from 1.07 to 1.46 mg/dL while that for the feline ranges from 1.09 to 2.08 mg/dL.

Sodium bicarbonate treatment for DKA is controversial. Advocates of this treatment cite concern that severe acidosis (blood pH less than 7.0) can adversely affect cardiovascular function; opponents base their concern on the treatment's causal relationship with paradoxical cerebrospinal fluid acidosis, hypokalemia, and worsened intracellular acidosis with overshoot alkalosis and delayed ketoanion metabolism.

The use of sodium bicarbonate should be restricted to dogs or cats with a blood pH below 7.1 or those with a serum total carbon dioxide (CO_2) concentration less than 10 to 12 mEq/L. During most treatment courses, metabolic acidosis reverses without bicarbonate treatment because of the cessation of ketogenesis, the metabolic conversion of ketones to bicarbonate after initiation of insulin treatment, improved renal function, and conversion of the lactate in lactated Ringer's solution to bicarbonate. In severe cases of metabolic acidosis (i.e., an anion gap greater than 30 mEq/L and an arterial pH less than 7.1), sodium bicarbonate ($NaHCO_3$) can be given according to the following equation:

$$NaHCO_3 \, (mEq) = Base \; deficit \; (mEq) \times 0.3 \\ \times Body \; weight \; (kg)$$

Subsequent alkali treatment depends on the results of repeat plasma pH measurements; it should be discontinued when the blood pH has been restored to 7.2 or higher or until the serum total CO_2 concentration is greater than 10 to 12 mEq/L.

Mixed acid-base disorders can also occur. Ketoalkalosis can occur from excessive vomiting of gastric secretions. Combined metabolic acidosis and respiratory acidosis can occur when severe hypokalemia impairs respiratory muscle function.

Insulin

The cornerstone of management of a sick DKA or HHS dog or cat is insulin administration. Regular crystalline insulin is used when the pet has signs of depression, dehydration, anorexia, and vomiting. Regular insulin has several advantages, including its various routes of administration (intravenous, intramuscular, and subcutaneous), rapid onset of action, and short duration of action. These properties allow adequate insulin titration throughout the day according to the animal's needs. The clinician must remember that the blood glucose concentration declines much earlier than ketones, allowing for the persistence of ketonuria for the first 48 to 96 hours.

Regular insulin given intravenously by slow constant rate infusion (CRI) is the preferred method of treatment for the critically ill hypotensive pet. The patient's hypovolemia should be partially corrected with isotonic fluids over the first 2 hours, before the insulin is administered.

A separate intravenous cannula is usually necessary for the insulin infusion. The CRI insulin solution is prepared by adding 5 U of regular insulin to a 500-mL bottle of 0.9% saline or lactated Ringer's solution to make up a solution that provides 0.01 U of insulin per milliliter. The infusion is delivered by an automatic injection syringe, an intravenous infusion pump, or a pediatric intravenous infusion set to deliver a therapeutic insulin dose of 0.1 U/kg BW/hr. To prevent binding of insulin to the intravenous lines, some clinicians prefer to run some of the diluted insulin infusion through the line before attaching it to the patient. Before this slow infusion is begun, the patient can receive an initial intravenous insulin bolus at a dose of 0.1 U/kg. To avoid any complicating osmotic disequilibrium effects on the brain, the rate of decline in the blood glucose level should not exceed 75 to 100 mg/dL/hr. When the blood glucose level has declined to 250 mg/dL after several hours of the CRI insulin infusion, the rate should be decreased to half the initial amount (i.e., 0.05 U/kg/hr), and dextrose should be added to the intravenous fluid to achieve a 2.5% to 5% dextrose concentration. The blood glucose level subsequently should be determined every 2 hours, using glucose oxidase reagent strips or a reflectance meter. Thereafter, the rate of insulin infusion should be adjusted to maintain a blood glucose range of 150 to 250 mg/dL to avert hypoglycemia.

The disadvantages of the CRI insulin administration technique are the frequent need for a separate intravenous cannula, intensive care monitoring, and frequent monitoring of the blood glucose and serum potassium concentrations. If the patient initially is hypokalemic, the clinician can begin treatment with isotonic fluids containing added potassium chloride and delay insulin treatment for the first 4 to 8 hours.

Low doses of regular insulin also can be given intramuscularly. Initially, 2 U are injected into the thigh muscles of cats and dogs weighing less than 10 kg. For dogs weighing more than 10 kg, the initial dose is 0.25 U/kg BW. Subsequent hourly injections of 1 U for cats and small dogs and 0.1 U/kg BW for larger dogs are given until the blood glucose level is less than 250 mg/dL, at which time the subcutaneous route can be used to administer the insulin every 6 hours or as needed. The low doses used in this technique can be accurately measured with a special low-dose calibrated syringe.

Subcutaneous administration of regular insulin is a suitable alternative to the intravenous and intramuscular methods when intensive care monitoring is unavailable and when the patient is alert and normotensive. The initial dose is 0.5 U/kg BW, with subsequent doses given every 6 to 10 hours, depending on the need.

The patient is regarded as stable when normal hydration has been restored, blood glucose levels are below 250 mg/dL, serum and urine ketones are minimal to absent, and eating resumes. Subsequent insulin treatment can be changed to the intermediate-acting or the ultra–long-acting type.

COMPLICATIONS

The main complications surrounding DKA treatment include hypoglycemia, hypokalemia, cerebral edema, metabolic alkalosis, and paradoxical cerebrospinal fluid acidosis. Most of these problems are avoidable with meticulous medical management geared toward avoiding overtreatment of the patient.

HYPERGLYCEMIC HYPEROSMOLAR SYNDROME

The hyperglycemic hyperosmolar syndrome (HHS) is characterized by extreme dehydration, renal dysfunction, abnormal brain function, marked hyperglycemia, and the lack of significant ketoacidosis. The incidence of this disorder in the dog and cat has not been reported; however, isolated case reports can be found in the veterinary literature spanning the past 25 to 30 years. Underlying renal disease and a precipitating condition, such as an infection or pancreatitis, can often be found.

PATHOPHYSIOLOGY

Only the main pathophysiologic mechanisms are covered in this section. The development of HHS is attributed to three main factors: (1) decreased insulin utilization and glucose transport, (2) increased hepatic gluconeogenesis and glycogenolysis, and (3) impaired renal excretion of glucose.

Two concepts have been advanced to reasonably explain the pathophysiology of HHS. The first suggests that an insulinized liver (reflecting residual beta cell secretory activity) coexists with a diabetic periphery, resulting in inactivation of intrahepatic oxidation of incoming free fatty acids, which are directed largely along nonketogenic metabolic pathways, such as triglyceride synthesis. This could account for the absence of hyperketonemia. The absence of hyperketonemia can also occur when the primary ketone body is beta hydroxybutyrate, which will not be detected with the nitroprusside reagent that is used for body fluid ketone detection. The second proposal suggests that enhanced gluconeogenesis occurs in the liver due to the prevailing elevated portal vein ratio of glucagon to insulin. This effect plus those due to severe dehydration (greater than 8%) and reduced urine production are responsible for the development of marked hyperglycemia.

The decrease in consciousness and the onset of the associated neurologic abnormalities that characterize HHS result from the direct effects of the serum sodium concentration and hyperosmolarity-induced dehydration on the brain parenchyma. A direct pathogenetic role, independent of osmotic diuresis, for hyperglycemia in causing coma is difficult to establish. Although acute, massive intravenous administration of glucose can cause a transient reduction in brain water in animals, over longer periods hyperglycemia does not appear to dehydrate the brain. The reasons for this include that the brain is relatively permeable to glucose, even in the absence of insulin, and that brain tissues restore their intracellular water content in response to hyperglycemia by accumulating electrolytes and "idiogenic osmols" over several hours or days when the hyperglycemia occurs gradually.

One hypothesis that explains why some extremely hyperglycemic animals show neurologic deterioration rests on the serum sodium concentration. Although marked hypernatremia does not occur in most cases of HHS, the "corrected" serum sodium level is often quite elevated. This is calculated by increasing the serum sodium concentration by 1.3 to 1.6 mEq/L for every 100 mg/dL increase in the serum glucose concentration. When tending to a patient with HHS, both the serum osmolality and the serum sodium concentration should be assessed. A normal or elevated serum sodium implies that substantial cellular dehydration has taken place and that the risk of neurologic abnormalities is high, whereas hyponatremia suggests that cellular dehydration has not occurred or has occurred to only a limited extent.

DIAGNOSTIC EVALUATION

Several clinicopathologic abnormalities characterize the HHS. The blood glucose levels are often elevated above 800 mg/dL. Serum osmolality is elevated (normal serum osmolality is 290 to 310 mOsm/kg body water) and can be determined by the freezing point depression method with an osmometer, or it can be calculated using the following formula:

$$sOsm = 2(Na^+ + K^+) + \frac{Glu}{18} + \frac{BUN}{2.8}$$

where Na^+ is serum sodium, K^+ is serum potassium, Glu is serum glucose, and BUN is blood urea nitrogen.

Most dogs and cats with HHS are azotemic, a condition that may be renal or prerenal in origin. The disturbances in serum electrolyte concentrations were described in the DKA section, above. It should be noted that an elevated serum sodium level during severe hyperglycemia can be explained only by significant plasma volume contraction caused by large water losses associated with hypotonic urine excretion. Parenteral fluid therapy in this situation can be harmful if the solution is hypotonic or free of sodium because this would favor a rapid influx of water into the brain cells, which would be harmful if the brain cells were dehydrated. The adverse effect caused by this cerebral edema can be prevented by administering a sodium-containing solution and by administering insulin in such a way as to avoid lowering the blood glucose any faster than 75 to 100 mg/dL per hour.

TREATMENT

The main treatment objectives with HHS include reestablishment of normal hydration and adequate urine output, judicious use of insulin to avoid a precipitous decline in blood glucose levels, and ample potassium supplementation to make up the total body potassium deficit. Treatment techniques were described in the previous section. The regular insulin dosage requirements for the hyperglycemic hyperosmolar diabetic are often less than those needed to treat diabetic ketoacidosis, but the technique for delivery is the same.

The diabetic ketoacidotic and hyperglycemic hyperosmolar syndromes pose noteworthy challenges to the practicing clinician. A sound understanding of the underlying pathophysiology, along with logical and timely therapeutic intervention, can usually lead to a remarkably optimistic outcome.

REFERENCES

The reference list can be found on the companion Expert Consult Web site at *www.expertconsult.com*.

CHAPTER **131**

Gastrointestinal Emergencies

Elke Rudloff
Rebecca Kirby

Shock, dehydration, collapse, acute pain, electrolyte imbalances, respiratory distress, and cardiac arrhythmias are potential life-threatening consequences of gastrointestinal (GI) emergencies. The history, physical examination findings, and clinical signs attributed to the GI tract (e.g., vomiting, diarrhea, abdominal pain or distention) direct the investigation for either primary GI disease or pathology in other organs that manifests with GI signs.

Primary pathology involving the GI tract (i.e., the esophagus, stomach, small intestines, large intestines, cecum, rectum, and/or anus) can be a result of distention, inflammation, obstruction, hypoxia, and/or ischemia of affected GI tissues

 To view a video on this topic, go to **www.expertconsult.com**.

(Box 131-1). Inflammatory mediators are released locally, causing local arteriolar and venous dilatation and increased capillary permeability. Severe inflammation results in loss of blood, fluids, electrolytes, and proteins from the capillaries into the GI tract (third body fluid spacing). Distension or inflammation of the GI tract can cause peripheral receptor stimulation of the vomiting center in the brainstem (Figure 131-1). Alterations in GI motility, secretory function, or permeability can result in diarrhea. In addition, vomiting and diarrhea can have life-threatening consequences such as increased vagal tone, aspiration pneumonia, bacterial translocation, and malnutrition.

Gastrointestinal signs can be secondary to disease of other organs or a consequence of systemic diseases (see Box 131-1).

Stimulation of receptors associated with the vomiting center and chemoreceptor trigger zone, as well as stimulation of peripheral GI receptors, can be caused by organ inflammation or distention, drugs or toxins in the circulation, and central nervous system pathology (see Figure 131-1). Alterations in nerve conduction and smooth muscle action of the GI tract can occur as a result of toxins, electrolyte disturbances, or acid-base imbalances, any of which could alter GI function.

The life-threatening consequences of vomiting and diarrhea can be similar regardless of cause (primary or a secondary GI disease), making initial stabilization crucial prior to diagnostic testing. The animal should first be assessed for life-threatening conditions (called primary survey) and resuscitated as needed. Diagnostic tests are then performed to determine underlying cause and whether emergency surgical intervention is required.

Box • 131-1

Causes of Gastrointestinal Emergencies

Primary

Gastrointestinal Obstruction
Foreign body*
Neoplasia*
Pyloric hypertrophy
Intestinal stricture*
Functional ileus
Infection (bacterial, fungal,
　viral, protozoal)
Trauma
Gastrointestinal inflammation
Diffuse neoplasia
Adverse reaction to food
Inflammatory bowel disease
Hemorrhagic gastroenteritis
Drugs/toxins
Ulcerative disease*
Lymphangiectasia

**Gastrointestinal Hypoxia/
Ischemia**
Gastric dilatation-volvulus*
Mesenteric torsion*
Intestinal volvulus*
Intussusception*
Mesenteric thromboembolic
　disease*

Secondary
Organ dysfunction
Pancreatic disease
Urinary tract disease
Hepatobiliary disease
Pyometra/metritis*
Adrenocortical insufficiency
Diabetic ketoacidosis
Central nervous system
　disorder
Increased intracranial
　pressure
Meningoencephalitis
Vestibular disease

Systemic Disorders
Electrolyte disorders
Acid-base disorders
Peritonitis*
Toxemia/sepsis

Toxin/Drug Reaction

*May require emergency surgical intervention for correction.

Careful monitoring is required throughout treatment and recovery for early detection of potential complications.

PRIMARY SURVEY

The primary survey is a rapid evaluation of the patient's history and physical parameters to detect life-threatening complications that require immediate intervention. The history may reveal vomiting, diarrhea, abdominal pain or distension, collapse, or respiratory distress. Airway, breathing, and circulation are rapidly assessed at presentation. Upper airway obstruction can occur from aspiration of gastric contents and manifest as labored, loud breathing (heard without the aid of a stethoscope), and/or cyanosis. When aspiration pneumonia causes lung parenchymal pathology, physical evidence of a labored, synchronous breathing pattern (chest and abdomen moving together) with moist or harsh lung sounds may be heard on lung auscultation.

Circulatory problems are evidenced by poor perfusion and can result from rapid fluid loss, organ hypoxia, or endotoxemia. Any of these problems can result from GI pathology. Poor perfusion is seen as pale mucous membranes, a prolonged capillary refill time, poor pulse quality, and tachycardia (in the dog) on physical examination. Dehydration is detected by dry mucous membranes, increased skin tenting, and, when severe, dry corneas. An altered level of consciousness or the presence of a dysrhythmia can suggest electrolyte and/or acid-base imbalances, hypoglycemia, circulating toxins, or hypoxia. Bradycardia may be a primary problem or the result of excessive vagal stimulation, severe hyperkalemia, or late-stage decompensatory shock. Abdominal pain or distension or a fluid wave alerts the clinician to shock, dehydration, and serious primary GI pathology.

RESUSCITATION

Life-threatening problems should be immediately resuscitated. Breathing abnormalities warrant immediate flow-by oxygen administration. An intravenous (IV) catheter is placed, and analgesia is provided as fluids are being administered, if pain is present. When upper airway obstruction is suspected, the oropharynx is suctioned, and, when necessary, an airway is established with oxygenation and ventilation provided. Poor perfusion and dehydration are treated with fluid therapy. Balanced isotonic crystalloids (dogs: 20 to 50 mL/kg; cats: 5 to 10 mL/kg) should be infused IV and repeated as necessary to reach desired end points. Synthetic colloids such as hetastarch (15 mL/kg dogs; 5 mL/kg cats) are infused simultaneously with initial crystalloid therapy, with the colloid dosage (5 mL/kg) repeated as necessary to improve flow to the tissues and reach desired end points of resuscitation.

Gas distention of the stomach, as seen with dilatation-volvulus or severe aerophagia, that compromises breathing and circulation warrants immediate careful percutaneous decompression of the stomach to relieve the pressure enough to improve ventilation. It is ideal for this to occur after initiating fluid resuscitation and will relieve pain and pressure on the diaphragm and vena cava. Hypoglycemia is treated with IV dextrose (0.5 g/kg). Life-threatening bradycardia is treated with atropine (0.02 mg/kg) IV and a rapid assessment of the serum potassium level is made.

SECONDARY SURVEY

Once the patient's condition has been stabilized, information is obtained from a more thorough history and physical exami-

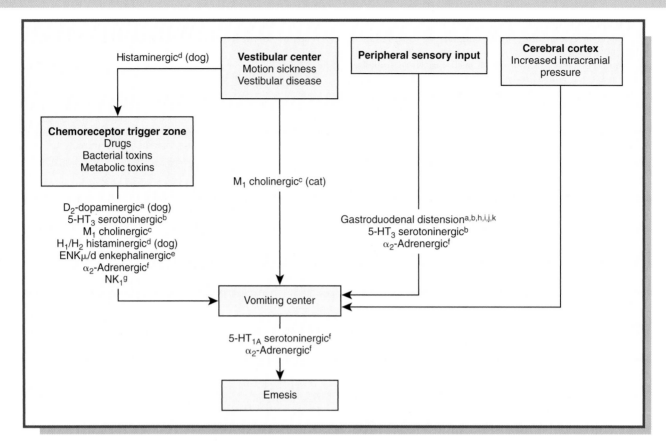

Figure 131-1 Vomiting reflex and antiemetics. Receptors located in the vomiting center and chemoreceptor-trigger zone (CRTZ) in the brainstem can be triggered by sensory and chemical input from multiple sources. Targeting the different neurotransmitters is the basis of antiemetic therapy. Specific antiemetic therapy should be selected based on the most likely mechanism initiating the stimulus to vomit. *5-HT*, 5-Hydroxytryptamine; *ENK*, enkephalin; *NK*, neurokinin. (For a complete list of antiemetic drugs, please see this figure on the companion Expert Consult Web site at www.expertconsult.com.)

nation to determine the origin of the GI signs. Historical information should be obtained regarding the vaccination and internal parasite history, recent or chronic administration of medications (e.g., nonsteroidal or steroidal antiinflammatory agents); changes in appetite; sudden changes or excessive fat content in the diet; access to garbage, bones, or moldy food; and the availability of string, toys and balls, corncobs, socks, and other potential foreign bodies (FBs) or toxins. Vomiting (active abdominal contractions preceeding expulsion of gastric contents) must be differentiated from regurgitation (passive expulsion of food contents). Nonproductive vomiting or retching may indicate the presence of a gastric dilatation-volvulus. Vomiting and/or diarrhea should be characterized by color, consistency, and frequency (Table 131-1).

The rectal temperature can reveal fever associated with inflammation or hypothermia from poor perfusion. Digital examination demonstrates the consistency of the stool. Careful abdominal palpation can detect abdominal pathology associated with organ distension, thickening, masses, FBs, free fluid, or fluid in the bowel. Physical signs that increase the likelihood of needing emergency surgical intervention include: gas distention of the stomach or bowel; nonresponsive shock with evidence of intraabdominal pathology; progressive abdominal distension; palpation of intestinal placation, painful mass, or FB; and persistent, severe vomiting unresponsive to therapeutic intervention.

TESTS

Blood, urine, and fecal samples are evaluated. An immediate data base (packed cell volume, total protein, blood glucose, electrolyte panel, acid-base panel, blood urea nitrogen, lactate, platelet estimate, and activated partial thromboplastin time and prothrombin time) may be useful in detecting the presence of hemorrhage, a coagulopathy, protein depletion, hypoglycemia (supporting sepsis), hypoxemia, or a gastric outflow obstruction (hypochloremia with a metabolic alkalosis). In addition, a complete blood count, serum biochemistry profile (including amylase and lipase), pancreatic lipase immunoreactivity testing, microscopic fecal examination, parvoviral fecal antigen test, fecal cultures, fecal pathogen profile, urinalysis, and coagulation profile may aid in determining the underlying cause, as well as secondary complications or additional organ dysfunction. Hyperphosphatemia may reflect intestinal ischemia or severe intestinal inflammation. Specific diagnostic tests to identify secondary GI disease are performed as indicated (e.g., adrenocorticotropic hormone [ACTH] stimulation, preprandial and postprandial bile acids).

Two-view abdominal radiography (Table 131-2), as well as abdominal ultrasonography, may help identify the cause of GI signs. A lateral thoracic radiograph may show a gas-dilated esophagus indicative of megaesophagus or right middle lung lobe consolidation suggestive of aspiration pneumonia. When

Table • 131-1

Character and Origin of Vomiting and Diarrhea

CHARACTER OF VOMIT OR VOMITING EPISODE	LESION	DIFFERENTIAL CAUSES
Occurs shortly after eating	Gastric inflammation Gastric obstruction	Gastric ulceration Foreign body (FB) Toxin ingestion Infection
Large amounts of undigested food up to 6 hours postprandial	True vomiting: Pyloric outflow obstruction Gastric atony Regurgitation: Esophageal outflow obstruction	Pyloric hypertrophy Pyloric mass Foreign body Electrolyte imbalance Megaesophagus Esophagitis Esophageal FB/mass/stricture Persistent right aortic arch Hiatal hernia
Projectile vomiting	Pyloric or upper duodenal outflow obstruction Upper duodenal ileus	Pyloric hypertrophy Mass Foreign body Pancreatitis Infiltrative bowel disease
Blood in vomit in the absence of nasal or oral disease Streaks of blood White or mucoid fluid	Esophageal hemorrhage Gastric hemorrhage Duodenal hemorrhage Gastric mucosal damage Gastric fluid Swallowed saliva from true regurgitation	Ulceration Coagulopathy Severe inflammation Persistent vomiting Gastritis Megaesophagus Esophagitis Gastric dilatation-volvulus Gastric outflow obstruction
Yellow Green Fetid brown fluid	Gastric fluid Upper duodenum Lower duodenum Jejunum	Gastritis Foreign body Duodenal ileus/obstruction Pancreatitis Intestinal obstruction

CHARACTER OF DIARRHEA	LESIONS	DIFFERENTIAL CAUSES
Watery	Small bowel inflammation	Infectious disease Partial small intestinal obstruction Pancreatitis Toxin/drug reaction
Mucoid	Large bowel inflammation	Infectious disease Partial large intestinal obstruction Toxin/drug reaction
Presence of digested blood (black stool) in the absence of nasal or oral disease	Esophageal hemorrhage Gastric hemorrhage Small bowel hemorrhage	Ulceration Coagulopathy Severe inflammation Ischemia
Presence of frank (bright red) blood	Large bowel hemorrhage	Ulceration Coagulopathy Severe inflammation Ischemia

Table • 131-2

Radiographic Changes Noted during Gastrointestinal Emergencies

RADIOGRAPHIC CHANGE	INDICATION	CAUSE
Generalized loss of radiographic detail	Intraabdominal fluid	Ascites
		Peritonitis
		Hemorrhage
Diffuse gas dilatation of the small and large intestines	Ileus	Enteritis
		Mesenteric volvulus
Severe segmental gas dilatation of the small intestine	Obstruction	Foreign body
		Mass
		Mesenteric volvulus
Intestinal bunching, plication, "string of pearls"		Intussusception
		Linear foreign body
Severe segmental gas dilatation of the large intestine ± colonic displacement	Colonic obstruction	Colonic torsion
Severe gas dilatation of the stomach without pyloric displacement	Gastric outflow obstruction	Foreign body
		Pyloric mass
		Pyloric hypertrophy
		Motility disorder
with pyloric displacement		Gastric dilatation-volvulus
Free intraabdominal gas	Gastrointestinal (GI) rupture	Rupture of GI tract
		Growth of gas-forming bacteria
		Abdominal wall perforation
	Infection	
Radioopacities involving the GI tract	Foreign body	Foreign body
	Mass lesion	Neoplasia
Duodenal loop sign or loss of contrast in right upper abdominal quadrant	Duodenal ileus	Pancreatitis
	Focal inflammation	

the pathology is likely intraabdominal and the definitive cause cannot be determined by radiographs or ultrasound, advanced imaging with computed tomography or abdominal paracentesis and/or diagnostic peritoneal lavage are indicated (see Chapter 97). Emergency surgical intervention becomes part of the diagnostic and therapeutic plan when primary GI pathology is suspected to be associated with ischemia, severe ongoing hemorrhage, or sepsis or when a diagnosis is lacking in a dog or cat whose condition is deteriorating.

MEDICAL INTERVENTION

Fluid therapy is adjusted to meet ongoing fluid, electrolyte, and acid-base abnormalities. Definitive treatment of the underlying pathology is initiated as soon as possible. When GI integrity is compromised, injectable antibiotics are administered effective against gram-positive, gram-negative, and anaerobic bacteria that translocate from the bowel into the bloodstream. Cefazolin or ampicillin (20 mg/kg IV every 8 hours), in addition to metronidazole (10 mg/kg given via slow IV every 8 hours), can provide broad-spectrum coverage. Signs of pain are treated with opioid drugs (for mild pain: butorphanol, 0.4 mg/kg IV, followed by a constant-rate infusion of 0.1 mg/kg/hr; for moderate or severe pain: fentanyl, 5 μg/kg given IV followed by a constant-rate infusion of 5 μg/kg/hr). Analgesia can be augmented with concurrent administration of antianxiolytic and sedative medication (e.g., midazolam, 0.2 to 0.5 mg/kg given IV).

The selection of antiemetic agent is based on the anticipated mechanisms of vomiting (see Figure 131-1). Motility inhibitors (e.g., Centrine) are not used as antiemetics/antidiarrheals because motility inhibition can allow toxins to accumulate and can affect nutrient delivery and absorption. A nasogastric tube allows for continued gastric decompression, cold water lavage for severe intragastric hemorrhage, and trickle flow feeding of the gastric mucosa. Promotility agents are administered only after GI obstruction has been ruled out.

When esophageal or gastric ulceration is suspected, H2-blockers (famotidine 0.5 mg/kg IV every 12 hours in the dog or SC in the cat every 24 hours) or H-pump inhibitors (omeprazole, 1 mg/kg up to 20 mg given orally every 24 hours, or pantoprazole 1 mg/kg IV every 24 hours) are administered to reduce acid secretion and reflux and promote mucosal healing. Liquid sucralfate (1 g/10 kg given orally every 4 to 8 hours) is administered to protect the area of ulceration once vomiting has been controlled.

SURGICAL INTERVENTION

When emergency surgery is indicated, perfusion and hydration are stabilized prior to anesthetic induction. However, stabilization may be difficult to achieve when there is ongoing large-volume fluid loss, organ ischemia (gastric or intestinal volvulus/torsion, intussusception, necrosis), or uncontrolled hemorrhage. Rapid induction of anesthesia using injectable anesthetics is recommended since ventilation may be impaired with significant abdominal distension, aspiration pneumonia, or analgesic medication. Oropharyngeal and esophageal suctioning may be required if gastric fluid has refluxed during anesthetic induction. Placement of a nasogastric tube for suction prior to induction of anesthesia can reduce the incidence of and complications associated with reflux and aspiration.

Surgical intervention for acute GI emergencies may require the use of specific equipment, such as access to a GI stapling device, to reduce the surgical time. Clinicians are referred to surgical texts for detailed surgical techniques for specific GI problems.

Gastric dilatation-volvulus requires decompression, derotation, and gastropexy. Gastric necrosis requires resection of compromised tissue. If a gastric FB is palpated or gastric ulcers are present, a gastrotomy is performed. Ulcerative mucosal lesions should be resected and submitted for histologic evaluation. When a GI foreign body is present, an attempt can be made to gently pull it from the intestines and out through the gastrotomy site. If resistance is felt, the FB is transected at the level of the pylorus. An attempt is then made to massage the remaining FB through the intestines to the distal colon, where it can be removed by digital rectal examination. When a linear FB is present, the gastric portion is cut and the remaining portion is sutured to a red rubber feeding tube, which can be massaged out through the colon. If the FB cannot be milked through the intestines into the distal colon, one or more enterotomies may be required to remove the object.

Ischemic or perforated bowel requires debridement or resection prior to closure. The most difficult regions to resect are the descending duodenal flexure (where the duodenum is fixed to the parietal peritoneum) and the ileocecal region (where various vascular supplies feed the region). When multiple ischemic sites in proximity are discovered, en bloc resection may prove more efficient and pose less risk of complications. Either simple interrupted or continuous closure can be performed, provided there is good apposition and minimal restriction of blood flow. GI stapling can also be used for rapid anastomosis.

Placement of a nasogastric, nasoesophageal, nasojejunal, esophagostomy, gastric, gastrojejunal, or jejunal feeding tube is considered if injury to the GI tract is significant or if a prolonged time to voluntary oral nutrition (longer than 2 days) is expected. A gastrostomy tube can help maintain gastric decompression when motility disorders are present. When gastric or proximal intestinal tract dysfunction or procedures are a factor (e.g., pancreatitis, peritonitis, Billroth procedures), placement of a nasojejunostomy, gastrojejunostomy, or jejunostomy tube allows immediate initiation of enteral feeding. The intraabdominal tubes are placed prior to abdominal wall closure.

When bowel or peritoneal perforation has occurred, a decision must be made regarding the placement of abdominal drains. If the peritoneal wall and serosal surfaces appear only mildly hyperemic and the repair is considered curative, copious saline lavage and suctioning may be all that is required.

If inflammation of the peritoneal wall or serosal surfaces is localized to the surgical site or there is abdominal contamination or inflammation, placement of abdominal suction drains is recommended. Aerobic and anaerobic culture samples are collected when abdominal fluid is present.

Tissue samples should be obtained from the liver, stomach, duodenum, jejunum, and mesenteric lymph nodes. Fluid from the duodenum is evaluated for *Giardia* organisms. Samples of the spleen, pancreas, and kidney, as well as fluid from the gallbladder and urinary bladder, are taken for histologic evaluation and/or culture at the discretion of the surgeon. Intensive care and monitoring are required during all phases of treatment of GI emergencies.

RECOVERY

An organized, systemic approach is required during the recovery phase of the GI emergency. The Rule of 20 provides a checklist of critical parameters that must be monitored and treated for an optimal outcome (Box 131-2).

Box • 131-2

Rule of 20

Monitoring and treatment of the following critical parameters help ensure the best outcome for the recovery phase of a gastrointestinal (GI) emergency:

Fluid balance
Colloid osmotic pressure
Serum albumin
Blood pressure
Heart rate and rhythm
Electrolytes and acid/base balance
Oxygenation and ventilation
White blood cell count, immunity and antibiotic therapy
Red blood cell and hemoglobin concentration
Mentation
Drug dosages and interactions
Liver function and drug metabolism
GI motility and integrity
Nutrition
Renal function
Coagulation
Wound care
Nursing care
Body temperature
Pain control

CHAPTER 132

Global Approach to the Trauma Patient

Kenneth J. Drobatz

*T*rauma is defined as a "wound or injury" caused by an "accident." Severity of injury secondary to any trauma can range from undetectable to fatal. Trauma may affect only one organ system or multiple organ systems, either directly or indirectly. Therefore, a global and thorough approach is required to improve survival and decrease morbidity in traumatized dogs and cats. The initial approach to a critically ill traumatized pet often makes the difference in the eventual outcome. The veterinary staff should be well versed in the evaluation and therapy of a traumatized dog or cat. Initial trauma assessment includes evaluation of tissue oxygen delivery (respiratory and cardiovascular systems), the central nervous system, and the urinary system. This primary survey should be followed by complete examination of all other systems.

PRIMARY SURVEY

The first goal with a critically injured trauma patient is to optimize oxygen delivery to the tissues. All initial assessments and therapeutics are oriented toward this goal. Emphasis on early detection and aggressive reversal of impaired tissue perfusion or oxygen delivery improves survival and minimizes multiorgan dysfunction. Oxygen delivery depends on the blood oxygen content and tissue perfusion (Figure 132-1).

BLOOD OXYGEN CONTENT

Maintaining oxygen saturation of hemoglobin through assessment and treatment of respiratory abnormalities is one of the first goals of the critical care team in maintaining oxygen delivery. Pale, cyanotic, or gray mucous membranes; signs of respiratory distress, such as increased respiratory rate and effort, extended head and neck, and open mouth breathing; and loud upper airway sounds and abnormal or diminished breath sounds on auscultation are all potential indicators of inadequate oxygen saturation of hemoglobin. More objective assessments of the oxygenation of blood include pulse oximetry and arterial blood gas analysis. Supplemental oxygen should be provided to any critically ill traumatized animal until it is proved that oxygen supplementation is not necessary.

A variety of conditions associated with trauma can result in respiratory distress and decreased oxygenation of hemoglobin (Figure 132-2; also see Chapter 141), but the most common are pneumothorax and pulmonary contusions. In animals suspected of having pleural space disease (decreased lung sounds with signs of respiratory distress), thoracocentesis should be performed even before thoracic radiographs are taken. If done correctly, benefit far outweighs risk (see Chapter 107). Tension pneumothorax is rare but represents an acute, life-threatening pleural space abnormality. It is characterized by extreme respiratory distress, poor tissue perfusion and, rarely, a "barrel chest" appearance. Rapid thoracocentesis is immediately indicated. A small incision in the intercostal space may release the air more quickly in animals in whom death or collapse is imminent.

Increased bronchovesicular sounds in a traumatized animal are commonly a result of pulmonary contusions. Pulmonary contusions often worsen before they improve. Intravenous fluid therapy for other conditions should be given with caution

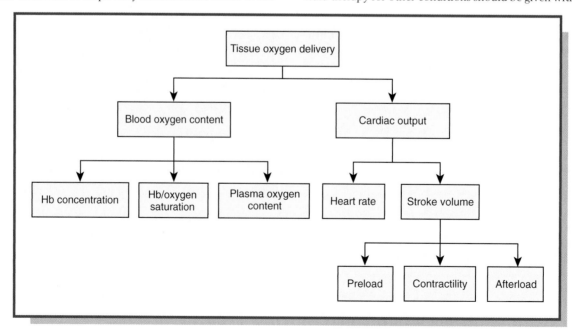

Figure 132-1 Determinants of tissue oxygen delivery. *Hb,* Hemoglobin.

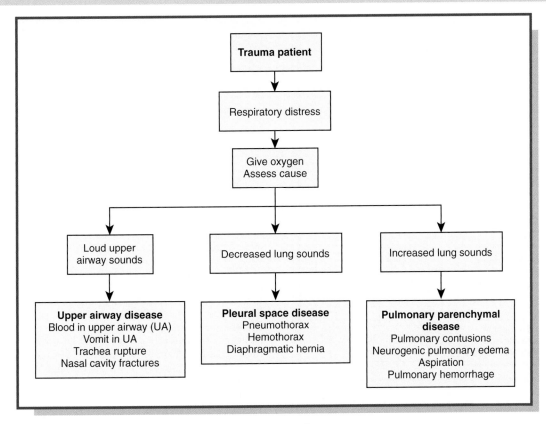

Figure 132-2 Causes of respiratory distress in a trauma patient.

in these dogs and cats. There is no specific therapy for pulmonary contusions. Supportive care with oxygen supplementation and pain relief are the mainstays of treatment. Most dogs and cats with pulmonary contusions begin to improve 24 to 36 hours after the initial insult (see Chapter 141).

Other respiratory conditions include open chest wounds, flail chest, and rib fractures. Open chest wounds should be covered and sealed as soon as possible. Once accomplished, the closed pneumothorax should be resolved by thoracocentesis. Treatment of an animal with a flail chest or rib fractures involves oxygen supplementation and pain management. Surgical repair is rarely necessary.

Neurogenic pulmonary edema occurs rarely but is most often associated with severe head trauma. This form of pulmonary edema can range from mild to severe enough to require mechanical ventilation. Most of these pets can be managed successfully with supportive care, such as oxygen supplementation and judicious diuretic therapy. Generally, respiratory problems in animals with neurogenic pulmonary edema caused by head trauma improve substantially within 48 hours, or death ensues due to the severe respiratory compromise.

An adequate amount of hemoglobin in the vascular space is essential to maintenance of tissue oxygen delivery. Decreased hemoglobin content severely limits the oxygen-carrying capacity of the blood and can contribute to decreased tissue oxygen delivery. The packed cell volume (PCV) provides the most rapid estimate of the hemoglobin concentration in a traumatized dog or cat, but it should be interpreted in conjunction with assessment of the vascular volume status (see Tissue Perfusion, below) to get a complete assessment of the total hemoglobin content of the vascular space. Typically, acute blood loss is not reflected by the initial PCV measurement because of splenic contraction in the dog and the length of time it takes for interstitial fluid to shift into the vascular

space to dilute the PCV. Initial total solids (TS) and serial measurements of both PCV and TS as intravenous fluids are administered can be more sensitive indicators of acute blood loss. There is no specific PCV at or below which transfusion is required. Transfusion therapy should be based on whether the animal is affected by the decreased hemoglobin content, which is indicated by clinical signs such as pale mucous membranes, tachycardia, tachypnea, bounding or weak pulses, depressed mentation, or cardiac arrhythmias. As with any animal in critical condition, it is best to anticipate and treat problems before they cause physiologic compromise. For example, if the PCV is dropping rapidly, it is best to start a blood transfusion or administer hemoglobin solutions before the hemoglobin content drops to a life-threatening level.

TISSUE PERFUSION

Physical assessments of tissue perfusion on the first examination include mucous membrane color, capillary refill time, and pulse rate and quality (Figure 132-3).

The arterial blood pressure should be measured directly or indirectly by Doppler or oscillometric techniques when possible. The most common clinical signs indicative of poor tissue perfusion are pale or gray mucous membranes, a prolonged capillary refill time, a rapid heart rate, and weak pulses. The most common cause of poor tissue perfusion after a traumatic event is hypovolemia secondary to hemorrhage.

Administration of a balanced electrolyte solution at a rate of 90 mL/kg body weight/hr in the dog (40 to 60 mL/kg body weight/hr in the cat) is indicated with physical evidence of poor tissue perfusion. Two separate, large-bore, intravenous catheters may be required in large dogs (i.e., body weight exceeding 20 to 30 kg). Mucous membrane color, capillary refill time, pulse quality, heart rate, and blood pressure (if

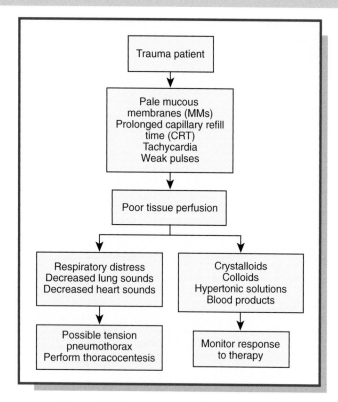

Figure 132-3 Assessment of tissue perfusion.

available) should be assessed continuously and the intravenous fluid rate adjusted as perfusion parameters improve or worsen. In most uncomplicated situations, improvement in tissue perfusion often is seen by the time one half of a vascular volume of fluid (45 mL/kg in the dog, 20 to 30 mL/kg in the cat) has been administered. As mentioned above, aggressive fluid therapy should be applied cautiously to animals known or suspected of having pulmonary contusions.

If clinical perfusion parameters or the blood pressure has not significantly improved after this volume of fluid has been administered, an investigation into causes of nonresponsive cardiovascular shock should be pursued. Such causes include ongoing intravascular volume loss (most commonly due to ongoing hemorrhage) or, less commonly, cardiogenic causes, such as arrhythmias, pericardial effusion, myocardial depression or failure, electrolyte abnormalities, decreased venous return (e.g., tension pneumothorax), or ischemic organs. The peritoneal space represents the most common location of substantial hemorrhage that can lead to hypovolemia. Less common locations are the pleural space and retroperitoneal space, external hemorrhage, and hemorrhage into the muscles surrounding the femur.

Abdominal binding may help control ongoing intraabdominal hemorrhage. However, this is no substitute for adequate intravascular volume supplementation. In human beings, some physicians advocate delayed resuscitation. In animals with severe hemorrhage, the fluid of choice is whole blood, packed red blood cells and plasma, hemoglobin substitutes (e.g., Oxyglobin), and/or colloid supplementation, such as hydroxyethyl starch or dextran 70 (see Chapter 129). Hypertonic solutions can be considered after head trauma if a dog or cat is hypovolemic (see Chapter 128) or if an animal appears to be in severe hypovolemic shock and may die before an adequate amount of balanced electrolyte solution can be administered (see Chapter 139).

Traumatized animals are physiologically dynamic and should be continuously monitored until physiologic parameters are stable. Close monitoring of cardiovascular and respiratory trends allows early detection of problems, before they become life-threatening.

CENTRAL NERVOUS SYSTEM AND URINARY TRACT

The central nervous system (CNS) (brain and spinal cord) and the renal system are two other organ systems that should be assessed and supported as priorities. Compromise of either of these systems can result in irreversible damage. After the initial assessment and treatment of the cardiovascular and respiratory systems, the clinician should complete a thorough neurologic examination, including assessment of mentation and of cranial nerve and spinal cord function. The results of such an evaluation establish a baseline for further monitoring and therapy. Brain dysfunction may be a result of poor oxygen delivery, direct tissue damage, intracranial hemorrhage, cerebral edema, ischemia, and/or increased intracranial pressure. Therapeutic considerations with head trauma and brain dysfunction include optimization of tissue perfusion, administration of mannitol (0.5 to 1.5 g/kg given intravenously), mild elevation of the head (avoiding flexion of the neck and occlusion of the jugular veins), and maintenance of oxygenation (see Chapter 128). Spinal cord assessment should include palpation of the spine and assessment of spinal function, including voluntary motor movement, conscious proprioception, ambulation, spinal reflexes, and pain sensation.

Neurologic function should always be evaluated in light of how well the central nervous system is perfused. In most animals, head trauma is obvious. However, those with severely compromised perfusion may have severely depressed mentation, as well as diminished pain sensation. The mentation and sensation abnormalities may normalize with correction of the poor tissue perfusion.

Manifestations of urinary tract injury or dysfunction may not be immediately evident and may not be detected until several hours of continuous monitoring have passed. Potential renal system abnormalities include direct kidney damage (e.g., contusions, hematomas, avulsion), ureteral rupture, bladder rupture, and urethral trauma. Any animal that has been traumatized may have experienced renal system trauma. Serial assessment of the blood urea nitrogen, creatinine, and serum potassium concentrations, as well as of urine output, should be considered. It should be remembered that animals with a ruptured urinary bladder might still urinate. Ureteral rupture may result in urine accumulation in the retroperitoneal space, a situation in which abdominocentesis fails to obtain fluid. Abdominal radiographs, abdominal ultrasound scans, and intravenous contrast studies may be necessary to diagnose ureteral rupture. If free abdominal fluid is present, it should be analyzed for the creatinine and potassium concentrations, which should be compared to the concentrations in peripheral blood. If the abdominal fluid is urine, its creatinine and potassium concentrations are higher than that of blood.

SECONDARY SURVEY

After assessment of tissue oxygen delivery, CNS function, and renal function, a full physical examination should be performed. Limb function should be evaluated and should include palpation of the entire appendicular and axial skeletal system. The eyes and oropharyngeal area should be examined for evidence of trauma. The mouth should be manually opened and closed to assess for malocclusion, pain, or crepitus. The roof of the mouth should be checked for split palate, a common finding in cats that have fallen from heights. A rectal examination should be performed, and attention should be paid to palpation of the pelvic canal for fractures or instability and evidence of blood in the rectum. The skin should be thoroughly examined for lacerations, abrasions, and bruising.

MONITORING

After the initial assessment, all the above systems should be monitored for at least 24 to 48 hours, despite how well the animal looks when first examined. In general, if problems are going to occur, they usually occur within this time frame.

The intensity and duration of the monitoring should be proportional to the degree of compromise. Owners should also be warned that rarely complications may arise several days later. For example, clinical signs of a ruptured gallbladder are not often manifested until several days after the traumatic injury.

SUMMARY

Assessment of tissue oxygen delivery should be performed at presentation and treated appropriately. Assessment should also include the CNS and renal systems, as well as the musculoskeletal, cutaneous, and peripheral nervous systems. A global approach, with emphasis on the most life-threatening conditions first, optimizes the outcome.

CHAPTER **133**

Heatstroke

Elisa M. Mazzaferro

Hyperthermia is defined as a severe elevation body temperature from 104.9° to 109.4° F after an animal has been exposed to elevated ambient temperatures or has performed strenuous activity.[1,2] Pyrogenic hyperthermia is associated with the body increasing the hypothalamic thermoregulatory center set point in response to a variety of endogenous or exogenous pyrogens and in most cases is a normal physiologic process.[2,3] Nonpyrogenic hyperthermia, however, is abnormal: an inability to dissipate heat.[1] Exertion or exercise in animals in locations with high environmental temperature and elevated ambient humidity can cause hyperthermia in as little as 30 minutes, particularly in animals without access to shade or opportunity to cool down and rest.[2,4,5] This can result in exertional heat stroke or exertional hyperthermia when animals cannot dissipate heat.

PATHOPHYSIOLOGY

Body temperature is maintained by the thermoregulatory center in the hypothalamus. Thermoregulation allows the core body temperature to remain constant despite exposure to a wide range of environmental and physiologic conditions.[3] Heat balance occurs through the actions of heat gain and dissipation mechanisms. Heat gain occurs through oxidative metabolism of foodstuffs, exercise or increased metabolic activity, and elevated environmental temperature.[2,3] Heat-dissipating mechanisms help prevent the excessive gain of heat and include behavioral changes such as seeking a cooler location, changes in circulation that include peripheral vasodilation, evaporative cooling primarily in the form of respiratory heat exchange, radiation, and convection.[2] When environmental temperature increases and approaches body temperature, evaporative heat loss becomes important to maintain normothermia.[2,3] Animals, who lack sweat glands, depend primarily on the dissipation of heat from evaporative cooling from the respiratory system in the form of panting.[2,6] When body temperature increases, the thermoregulatory center in the hypothalamus is activated and sends a relay of signals to the panting center. This is a basic reflex mechanism by which an animal responds to heat excess and dissipates heat to prevent hyperthermia. As air comes in contact with the mucous membranes of the upper airways, evaporative cooling occurs.[6] If high ambient humidity is present, however, evaporative cooling mechanisms are not as effective and body temperature can continue to rise despite the body's efforts to cool itself.[2,7] As core body temperature rises, metabolic rate also increases and results in further heat accumulation. A second method of cooling can occur by convection, in which an overheated animal lies on a cooler surface and the body heat is passively transferred to the cooler surface.

A number of factors can increase the risk of heatstroke, including high ambient humidity, upper airway obstruction, laryngeal paralysis, brachiocephalic airway syndrome, collapsing trachea, obesity, and a previous history of hyperthermia or heat-induced illness.[4] Additionally, lack of shade and a lack of a cooling down period after exercise can predispose an animal to developing exertional heat stroke or exertional hyperthermia. Any animal that works or exercises in a hot, humid climate without acclimation must be allowed time to rest in a cool, shady place with plenty of water every 30 to 60 minutes.

The differential diagnosis of heat stroke or hyperthermia must be considered in any animal with a rectal temperature greater than 104.9° F and no other signs of infection. Pyrogenic hyperthermia results from the hypothalamic thermoregulatory center increasing its set point in response to any number of endogenous or exogenous pyrogens. Nonpyrogenic hyperthermia, however, results from the body's inability to adequately dissipate heat. Therefore, antipyretic agents are often ineffective in reducing body temperature in animals with heat-induced illness and are actually contraindicated due to potentially adverse side effects. Differential diagnoses in patients with rectal temperatures greater than 104.9° F include inflammatory diseases of the central nervous system such as meningitis and encephalitis and hypothalamic mass lesions that affect the thermoregulatory center. Other potential differential diagnoses include malignant hyperthermia in affected animals, particularly Labrador Retrievers, and unwitnessed seizure activity. Toxins such as metaldehyde, strychnine, and neurogenic mycotoxins can also cause seizures and muscle fasciculations to such an extent that core temperature rises.

As body temperature rises, the thermoregulatory center in the hypothalamus detects changes in temperature and increases neural signals to the panting center.[6] The animal responds by panting, increasing dead space ventilation and increasing evaporative cooling mechanisms in an attempt to dissipate heat. If ambient humidity is high or temperature rises too quickly, adaptive cooling mechanisms become ineffective and the body's core temperature continues to rise. Early in hyperthermia, increase in dead space ventilation occurs, with little effect on carbon dioxide elimination.[6] As hyperthermia progresses, however, metabolic alkalosis can occur.[3] The effects of prolonged hyperthermia override the body's normal adaptive mechanisms, and cerebrospinal fluid hypocapnia and alkalosis, factors that normally decrease panting, are no longer effective, and panting continues. Additionally, as core body temperature increases, the body compensates by peripheral vasodilation.[3,6] Increased blood flow to the skin and periphery can help to decrease heat by convective mechanisms. To help maintain adequate blood pressure, splanchnic vessels constrict to maintain adequate circulating volume.[6] Further, circulating catecholamines increase heart rate and cardiac output in an attempt to increase peripheral circulation.[3] Early in hyperthermia, there is an increase in cardiac output and decrease in peripheral vascular resistance.[6] As hyperthermia progresses, however, blood pressure and cardiac output decrease.[6] There is also a decrease in circulating plasma volume that can result in hypovolemia. As perfusion to vital organs is decreased, widespread organ damage can result.

As body temperature rises, widespread thermal injury occurs to neuronal tissue, cardiac myocytes, hepatocytes, renal parenchymal and tubular cells, and gastrointestinal barrier function.[3] Additionally, oxidative phosphorylation and enzyme activities are reduced, causing a decrease in energy production. The combined effects of decreased organ perfusion, enzyme dysfunction, and uncoupling of oxidative phosphorylation are a decrease in aerobic glycolysis and an increase in tissue oxygen debt, both of which contribute to increased lactate production and lactic acidosis.[3] Lactic acidosis can occur within 3 to 4 hours of initial heat-induced injury.

The kidneys are affected by direct thermal injury to tubular and parenchymal cells. Additionally, decreased renal blood flow and hypotension cause hypoxic damage to the tubular epithelium and cell death. With disease progression, thrombosis of renal vessels can occur with disseminated intravascular coagulation (DIC). Consistent findings in severely hyperthermic pets are renal tubular casts and glycosuria. Both factors indicate severe renal injury. Rhabdomyolysis can also be associated with severe myoglobinuria and pigment-associated damage to the renal tubular epithelium.[3]

The gastrointestinal tract is a key player in multiorgan failure associated with hyperthermia.[3] Decreased perfusion to the mesentery and thermal injury to enterocytes often results in a disruption of the gastrointestinal mucosal barrier and subsequent bacterial translocation. Bacteremia and elevation of circulating bacterial endotoxin can lead to sepsis, systemic inflammatory response (SIRS), and multiorgan failure.[3] Patients with severe hyperthermia often present with hematemesis and severe hematochezia, and often slough the lining of their intestinal tract.

Thermal injury to hepatocytes results in decreased hepatic function, with elevations of hepatocellular enzyme activities, increased ALT, AST, and total bilirubin.[1,4] Necropsy findings in one retrospective study of 42 dogs with hyperthermia found centrilobular necrosis, widespread tissue congestion, hemorrhagic diathesis, and pulmonary infarction.[4] Persistent hypoglycemia in affected patients may be associated with hepatocellular dysfunction and glycogen depletion. Decreased hepatic macrophage function and portal hypotension can also predispose the patient to sepsis with associated bacteremia and SIRS.

Hyperthermia also induces widespread endothelial damage, one of the key players in the development of DIC.[8] All elements of Virchow's triad, which consists of vascular endothelial injury, venous stasis, and a hypercoagulable state, occur during hyperthermia. Sluggish blood flow during periods of hypotension and decreased production of clotting factors due to hepatic injury both contribute to DIC. Exposure of subendothelial collagen and tissue factor cause widespread platelet activation, consumption of clotting factors, activation of the fibrinolytic pathway, and subsequent DIC. Massive global thrombosis associated with DIC can result in multiorgan failure and death. Although one study demonstrated no significant outcome associated with treatment for DIC, many authors advocate empiric therapy to prevent DIC in all patients with hyperthermia.

Finally, hyperthermia can cause direct damage to neurons, neuronal death, and cerebral edema. Thrombosis or intracranial hemorrhage can also occur with DIC. Damage to the hypothalamic thermoregulatory center, localized intraparenchymal bleeding, infarction, and cellular necrosis can all lead to seizures. Altered levels of consciousness are among the most common clinical signs of heat-induced illness. As hyperthermia progresses, severe central nervous system depression, seizures, coma, and death may occur. The potential for reversal of cerebral edema is related to the duration of the neurons' heat exposure. Severe mentation abnormalities are associated with a negative outcome. In one retrospective study of dogs, the only presenting clinical sign that was negatively associated with outcome was the animal being comatose.[4] A unfavorable outcome was also associated with the development of stupor, coma, or seizures within 45 minutes of presentation.[4]

CLINICAL SIGNS

Patients with heat-induced illness or hyperthermia often have a history of excessive panting, collapse, vomiting, ataxia, hypersalivation, seizures, or diarrhea. Listlessness, muscle tremors, altered level or loss of consciousness, hematuria, cyanosis, epistaxis, swollen tongues, head tremors, vocalizing, stridor, and dilated pupils are less frequently described. Changes in mentation, oliguria, vomiting, hematemesis, diarrhea, dyspnea, icterus, and petechiation can occur almost immediately after heat-induced illness, or may become apparent 3 to 5 days after the inciting event. Therefore, all animals that have sustained heat stroke and hyperthermia should be watched carefully during this period of time.

LABORATORY CHANGES

Animals with hyperthermia should have serial complete blood counts, biochemical analyses, coagulation profiles, arterial blood gases, venous lactates, and urinalyses performed. In many cases, prerenal and renal azotemia is present, with elevated BUN and creatinine concentrations.[1,4] BUN and creatinine elevate secondary to renal tubular necrosis. Serum creatinine greater than 1.5 mg/dL has been associated with a higher fatality rate.[1] Alterations and elevations in hepatocellular enzyme function secondary to hepatocellular thermal injury or hepatic thrombosis are also demonstrated with elevated ALT, AST, alkaline phosphatase, and total bilirubin.[1,4] However, hypocholesterolemia, hypoalbuminemia, and hypoproteinemia were associated with a less favorable outcome. Total bilirubin and creatinine were higher in nonsurvivors than survivors. Elevations in creatine kinase (CK) and AST are secondary to rhabdomyolysis. Blood glucose is inconsistently decreased. In patients whose blood glucose remains low despite aggressive supplementation, or is less than 47 mg/dL, a less favorable outcome is observed.[1,4] Packed cell volume and total solids may be increased secondary to hypovolemia and dehydration with subsequent hemoconcentration.[1] Thrombocytopenia, prolonged prothrombin time and activated partial thromboplastin time and elevated fibrin degradation products may be observed if DIC is present. Destruction or consumption of clotting factors can occur. In some dogs and cats, thrombocytopenia may not become apparent for several days after the initial insult. Thrombocytopenia is one of the most common clinicopathologic abnormalities observed in animals with heat-induced illness.[1] However, there was no significant difference in platelet counts of survivors versus nonsurvivors.[1] The presence of coagulation abnormalities may or may not be associated with an increased risk of mortality.[1] In one study, a calculated discomfort index, but not environmental temperature, was significantly associated with the development of DIC.[1] Arterial blood gas analyses can be variable, as respiratory effort may be increased in heat stroke, producing a respiratory alkalosis. However, metabolic acidosis, with increased circulating lactate, can produce a metabolic acidosis, thus a mixed acid-base disturbance can occur. The need for administration of sodium bicarbonate is a negative prognostic indicator.[3,4]

TREATMENT

Treatment goals are to manage the hyperthermia, provide cardiovascular support, and to treat any complications associated with hyperthermia. Cornerstones of therapy include restoration of circulating blood volume, improving glomerular filtration and renal blood flow, stabilizing electrolyte balance, and providing broad-spectrum antibiotics to minimize complications of bacterial translocation and sepsis. Early recognition of hyperthermia and instituting early cooling measures are important. First, move the animal to a cool area in the shade or indoors, away from direct sunlight. Next, spray the animal with cool but not cold water. Cool packs can be placed in the axillary and inguinal regions. Air conditioning or cool fans can also help dissipate heat and improve convective cooling mechanisms. It is important to cool the patient to 103° F within 30 to 60 minutes of initial presentation but to avoid overcooling. As the thermoregulatory center becomes deranged in animals with heat-induced illness, overcooling past 103° F will cause a rapid drop in core temperature. Animals brought to a veterinarian within 90 minutes of the inciting event have a more favorable prognosis than animals seen later.[1] Animals cooled prior to presentation by their owners may or may not have a more favorable prognosis and decreased risk of mortality than animals not cooled at the time of initial injury.[1,4] Overcooling can also be injurious, as patients who presented with hypothermia were more likely to die.[4] As cooling progresses to less than 103° F, shivering can occur, which will increase metabolic rate and further increase core body temperature. Immersion in ice baths or cold water is absolutely contraindicated, as cold water immersion causes peripheral vasoconstriction and prevents vasodilation, one of the animal's primary methods of cooling. Vasoconstriction results in further elevation of core body temperature and thus should be avoided at all costs. Massaging the skin can increase peripheral circulation, improve peripheral blood flow, and improve heat loss. Other methods of cooling that have been described but offer no real advantage or improvement of clinical outcome include administration of cool intravenous fluids, gastric lavage, cold-water enemas, and cool peritoneal lavage. Placing alcohol on the footpads has been described, but can further complicate overcooling and thus should not be performed.

Intravenous fluid administration should be tailored to each patient's individual needs, and can be administered based on central venous pressure, acid-base and electrolyte status, blood pressure, thoracic auscultation, and colloid oncotic pressure. A balanced electrolyte fluid such as Normosol-R, Plasmalyte-M, or lactated Ringer's can be given as determined by calculated dehydration deficits. If a free water deficit is present, as evidenced by hypernatremia, the clinician should calculate the free water deficit and replace it slowly over a period of 24 hours, to prevent further cerebral edema from occurring. Experimental evidence has also suggested that the use of hydroxyethyl starch may be superior to the use of saline alone to resuscitate animals with hyperthermia.[9] Oxygen should be administered in animals with signs of upper airway obstruction. If laryngeal paralysis is present, sedative and anxiolytic agents such as acepromazine should be considered. In cases of severe upper airway obstruction and laryngeal edema, glucocorticoids can also be administered to decrease airway edema. General anesthesia and airway intubation should be considered. The use of empiric glucocorticoids in patients without signs of airway obstruction is controversial, as they can further impair renal perfusion and predispose to gastrointestinal ulceration. Their empiric use is not justified and is not advised. Broad-spectrum antibiotics such as a second generation cephalosporin (cefoxitin 30 mg/kg IV q8h), ampicillin (22 mg/kg IV q6h) with enrofloxacin (10 mg/kg IV q24h), and sometimes metronidazole (10 mg/kg IV q8h) should be administered to decrease bacteremia. Nonnephrotoxic antibiotics should be administered, as compromised renal function is a serious concern in patients with hyperthermia. Antipyretic agents such as dipyrone, flunixin meglumine, carprofen, and etodolac are contraindicated for a number of reasons. First, these agents act to decrease the set point of the thermoregulatory center in patients with a fever, not hyperthermia, and are therefore ineffective. Antiprostaglandins are only effective on lowering body temperature in dogs with a true fever. Their use may also worsen hypothermia, if present. Second, in high doses these agents have been shown to decrease renal perfusion and can predispose the patient to gastrointestinal ulceration. Therefore, their use is contraindicated in patients with hyperthermia. Urine output should be quantitated and calculated to observe if oliguric or anuric renal failure is present. After volume resuscitation, urine output should be 1 to 2 mL/kg/hr. If urine output is less, a constant rate infusion of dopamine at 3 to 5 µg/kg/min can be started to increase renal perfusion and urine output. The presence of persistent oliguria or anuria can potentially be treated with peritoneal or hemodialysis. Ventricular dysrhythmias should be monitored via ECG and treated when necessary.[5] Seizures should be controlled with diazepam.

PROGNOSIS

Severe hyperthermia can result in widespread organ failure and must be recognized and treated promptly. In most cases, prognosis is guarded to grave, depending on the presence of underlying diseases and complications. Mortality rates are directly associated with the duration and intensity of hyperthermia. In one study, mortality rate was 50%.[1] Obesity, renal failure, and DIC all increase the risk of death associated with

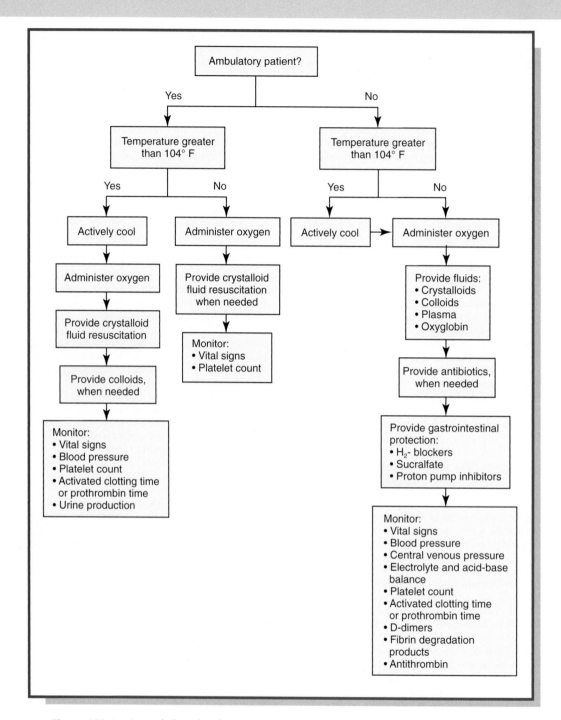

Figure 133-1 General algorithm for approach to the patient with heatstroke. Approach can be tailored to the individual patient, with more aggressive monitoring in the most critically ill animals.

hyperthermia.[1] Permanent damage to kidneys, liver, and brain can occur, including permanent changes in the hypothalamic thermoregulatory center that can predispose the patient to further hyperthermic episodes.[3] In most cases, the clinician must give a guarded prognosis. If death is going to occur, it usually happens within the first 24 hours of the incident.[1,4] If an animal survives past 48 hours of hospitalization, the outcome is generally good.[4] Animals who present with coma or hypothermia after a hyperthermic event generally have a very grave prognosis, even with extremely aggressive therapy (Figure 133-1).

REFERENCES

The reference list can be found on the companion Expert Consult Web site at *www.expertconsult.com*.

CHAPTER 134

Hepatic and Splenic Emergencies

Susan W. Volk
David Holt

Diagnosis and treatment of splenic, hepatic, or biliary emergencies require a thorough history and physical examination. However, further diagnostics are vital to elucidate and confirm any underlying etiology and to define appropriate medical and/or surgical management. Life-threatening conditions associated with splenic or liver disease arise due to hemodynamic instability associated with blood loss from these organs, torsions of their vascular pedicles, peritonitis (focal or generalized) due to abscessation, leakage of bile from the extrahepatic biliary system, or loss of significant hepatic function.

HEPATIC AND SPLENIC EMERGENCIES ASSOCIATED WITH HEMOPERITONEUM

Traumatic injury to the liver or spleen, or rupture of splenic or hepatic masses can cause life-threatening intraperitoneal hemorrhage. Trauma to these organs is often associated with motor vehicle accidents, falls, and accidental or malicious blunt abdominal injuries. The most common nontraumatic cause of hemoperitoneum in dogs is rupture of splenic hemangiosarcoma.[1] Less commonly, hemorrhage can occur from other vascular intraabdominal masses, including splenic hematomas and hepatic tumors. Hemorrhage from hepatic and splenic neoplasms accounts for approximately 50% of feline nontraumatic hemoperitoneum.[2]

Animals with traumatic injuries usually present with an appropriate history. These animals have often sustained severe injuries to other organs. A rapid initial examination is performed focusing on the central nervous, respiratory, and cardiovascular systems and life-threatening issues should be addressed immediately. Common clinical findings in animals with traumatic hemoperitoneum include depressed mentation, pale mucous membranes, delayed capillary refill time, a rapid heart rate, and poor peripheral pulse quality. The abdomen may or may not be visibly distended. Once potentially life-threatening conditions are addressed, a more thorough and detailed examination is necessary to identify other consequences of trauma (e.g., fractures, urinary tract rupture, wounds) that will affect prognosis and expense.

Animals with nontraumatic, bleeding splenic or hepatic masses are typically older and have either acute collapse or more chronic problems, such as lethargy, anorexia, weight loss, or vomiting, that have acutely worsened. Physical examination findings associated with poor tissue perfusion are similar to those of animals with traumatic hemoperitoneum; however, a mass can often be detected on abdominal palpation.

Intravenous (IV) access is mandatory in animals with either traumatic or nontraumatic hemoperitoneum. At least two large-bore IV catheters should be placed, samples drawn for a minimum data base, and resuscitation commenced. The rate and type of IV fluid resuscitation is based on the veterinarian's assessment of the animal's perfusion deficits and the presence of concurrent injuries. This can then be adjusted according to the patient's response to initial treatment. Full shock doses

(60 to 90 mL/kg/hr IV in the dog; 45 to 60 mL/kg/hr IV in the cat) of crystalloids or hypertonic saline and dextran (5 to 7 mL/kg IV given over 5 minutes) followed by crystalloids may be necessary. Opinions on the volume and rate of fluid resuscitation vary. Increasing blood pressure with crystalloid or colloid resuscitation may promote rebleeding,[3] but limited volume resuscitation with hypertonic saline and/or colloid did not restore or sustain systemic hemodynamics in a canine hemorrhagic shock model.[4] Fluid resuscitation should be limited (10 to 20 mL/kg IV for the first hour) in animals with suspected pulmonary contusions. The temporary application of a tight abdominal bandage ("abdominal counterpressure") can slow or arrest bleeding due to parenchymal or venous bleeding by raising intraabdominal pressure. Increasing intraabdominal pressure for prolonged periods can adversely affect renal and hepatic blood flow.[5]

Response to therapy and ongoing requirements for crystalloids and colloids should be continually assessed from repeated clinical and laboratory monitoring (urine output, EKG, blood pressure, pulse oximeter, arterial blood gas, and lactate). Blood component therapy is often required to maintain the animal's packed cell volume (PCV) above 25. Autotransfusion can be a life-saving source of red blood cells in cases where fresh whole or stored blood is not available. Contraindications to autotransfusion include intraabdominal sepsis or neoplasia; hence, animals with no history of trauma should not be autotransfused. Peritoneal fluid should be evaluated cytologically before autotransfusion.

Hemoperitoneum is often suspected based on historical and physical examination findings. A focal or generalized loss of serosal detail on abdominal radiographs indicates free peritoneal fluid. The diagnosis of hemoperitoneum is confirmed by peritoneal fluid evaluation. A sample is obtained by abdominocentesis with or without ultrasound guidance. In animals with hemoperitoneum, the peritoneal fluid sample should not clot unless the spleen has been inadvertently aspirated, in which case the PCV of the fluid is greater than or equal to that of the peripheral blood. Unfortunately, peritoneal fluid cytology is rarely helpful in diagnosing neoplastic causes of hemoperitoneum. In animals with either a palpable abdominal mass or no history of trauma, splenic neoplasia is a distinct possibility. Obvious pulmonary metastatic disease should be ruled out by taking high-quality lateral and dorsoventral thoracic radiographs. Abdominal ultrasonography is useful to define an intraabdominal mass and evaluate other abdominal organs for evidence of metastatic disease.

Definitive treatment varies depending on the underlying cause of the hemoperitoneum and the response to medical stabilization. Some cases of traumatic splenic or hepatic hemorrhage will stabilize with fluid resuscitation, blood transfusion, and abdominal counterpressure. Surgery is indicated in animals with traumatic hemoperitoneum that continue to hemorrhage in spite of appropriate medical treatment. In humans, such cases would initially be investigated with interventional radiologic techniques and obvious bleeding arteries embolized. Such techniques are currently investigational. Survival rates of small animals treated medically and those requiring surgical intervention have been 75% and 67% respectively, with larger animals having an increased survival rate.[6]

In animals with hemoperitoneum secondary to a bleeding splenic or hepatic mass, the aims of surgery are to stop ongoing hemorrhage, remove the mass, obtain a histopathologic diagnosis, and perform a complete exploratory to rule out gross metastatic disease. The prognosis for these animals depends on the tumor type. The two most common splenic masses in dogs are hemangiosarcoma and hematoma.[1] Dogs have an excellent prognosis after hematoma removal; dogs with splenic hemangiosarcoma have only a 6- to 8-month average survival time even with chemotherapy. Splenectomy alone results in median survival times of 19 to 65 days.[7-9] In contrast to a 31% 2-month postoperative survival rate for dogs with hemangiosarcoma, the 2-month survival rate for dogs with non–neoplastic-related hematomas was found to be 83%.[9] Feline visceral hemangiosarcoma is an uncommon tumor that involves the spleen and liver in greater than 50% of cases and has a poor prognosis: euthanasia was chosen in 77% of cats within 1 day of diagnosis and a median survival of only 77 days was documented in the remaining cats.[10]

Splenic and Liver Lobe Torsion

Although uncommon, splenic torsion should be considered in any dog with either chronic gastrointestinal (GI) signs or signs of acute abdominal disease. The pathogenesis of splenic torsion and predisposing factors for this condition are not completely understood, but Great Danes and German Shepherd Dogs are at increased risk compared to other dog breeds.[11] In many dogs, the history includes chronic signs of abdominal discomfort and GI disease such as depression, anorexia, vomiting, and weight loss. However, many dogs with splenic torsion will present as true emergencies with signs of acute, worsening abdominal disease. Physical examination findings will depend on the degree of cardiovascular instability and may include pale mucous membrane color, poor capillary refill time, and poor peripheral pulse quality. Splenomegaly is usually detected on abdominal palpation and should increase the clinician's suspicion for splenic disease.

The differential diagnosis for such animals should include gastric dilatation-volvulus syndrome, GI foreign body obstruction, mesenteric torsion, peritonitis, neoplasia, and other causes of splenomegaly. A complete blood count, serum biochemical screening, and abdominal imaging are indicated to further define underlying disease. Radiographs show splenomegaly in all affected dogs; some can also have a loss of abdominal detail associated with peritoneal effusion or hemorrhage. In addition, splenic location or shape (including the appearance of the spleen folded into a "C" shape) or gas accumulation within the spleen may also be evident. Abdominal ultrasound findings of a hypoechoic pattern in the splenic parenchyma and decreased blood flow through the splenic veins strongly supports a diagnosis of splenic torsion.

Animals should be stabilized with IV fluid resuscitation prior to anesthesia. Some animals with moderate to severe anemia may require preoperative or intraoperative transfusions. Many dogs with splenic torsion have evidence of abnormal coagulation; therefore, a coagulation screen and blood type are indicated prior to surgery. A crossmatch should be performed if the animal has previously received blood products or if a full medical history is unavailable. A protocol of balanced anesthesia with minimal cardiovascular depression is used. Ventricular arrhythmias commonly develop intraoperatively or postoperatively; electrocardiographic and blood pressure monitoring is vital. At surgery, the spleen is removed without untwisting the splenic pedicle. Partial pancreatectomy may be necessary if twisting of the splenic pedicle has involved the pancreatic branch to the left limb from the splenic artery. Concurrent gastropexy is recommended by many surgeons to prevent subsequent gastric volvulus. The prognosis is good for dogs with splenic torsion when appropriate emergency resuscitation and critical care management is combined with prompt diagnosis and surgical treatment.[11]

Liver lobe torsion occurs rarely in dogs and cats.[12] Clinical signs and laboratory data are nonspecific. A distended abdomen or a palpable abdominal mass can sometimes be detected on physical examination. The diagnosis is confirmed at exploratory laparotomy. The affected liver lobe is resected either manually or with stapling equipment and submitted for histopathology.

Splenic Infarction

Splenic infarction in dogs occurs rarely and is often associated with altered blood flow and coagulation secondary to other diseases. Hypercoagulable states associated with hepatic and renal disease, hyperadrenocorticism, thrombosis secondary to cardiovascular disease, or neoplasia have been associated with splenic infarcts.[13] It is key to identify and treat the underlying disease(s) associated with splenic infarction. Emergency surgical management is reserved for those patients with life-threatening complications such as hemoabdomen or sepsis.

Hepatic and Splenic Abscesses

Hepatic and splenic abscesses are both uncommon clinical entities in dogs but may present as true emergencies.[14] The clinical signs and physical examination findings in dogs with these conditions are nonspecific. Dogs most commonly have a history of anorexia and lethargy that may be accompanied by vomiting and diarrhea. They are often febrile, and have pain and hepatomegaly or splenomegaly on abdominal palpation. Occasionally, dogs with hepatic abscess have evidence of epistaxis, ecchymosis, or hematochezia, indicating abnormal blood clotting function.

A complete blood count, serum biochemical profile, coagulation screen, and abdominal imaging studies are logical diagnostic steps in animals with these physical examination findings. Historically, all dogs with hepatic abscessation have had elevated serum alkaline phosphatase (ALP) and alanine aminotransferase (ALT) levels and the majority have a leukocytosis, thrombocytopenia, and hypoalbuminemia.[8] Results of abdominal radiography are often unrewarding; in one study of dogs with hepatic abscesses, the majority of dogs radiographed had hepatomegaly; one third had splenomegaly and one third had a loss of abdominal detail.[5] Abdominal ultrasound is useful in these cases and shows either hypoechoic or anechoic changes in one or multiple liver lobes. Samples can be obtained from affected lobes for cytology and aerobic and anaerobic culture and sensitivity testing using ultrasound guidance. Where ultrasound is not available, peritoneal lavage or exploratory laparotomy may be required for definitive diagnosis.

The etiology of hepatic and splenic abscesses is debated and probably multifactorial. However, given that hematogenous bacterial spread is one potential cause, once a diagnosis is established, possible reservoirs of bacterial infection such as the urinary tract and heart valves should be investigated. Affected animals should also be evaluated for concurrent conditions associated with hepatic and splenic abscessation, such as biliary tract disease, diabetes mellitus, pancreatitis, neoplasia, and endogenous or exogenous glucocorticoid excess. Thoracic radiographs are indicated to rule out pneumonia; radiographic evidence of alveolar infiltrates consistent with pneumonia were found in nearly half the cases examined in one study.[14]

Initial stabilization in affected animals involves cardiovascular support with IV fluids and administration of broad spectrum, bacteriocidal antibiotics with gram-positive, gram-negative, and anaerobic coverage pending the results of culture and sensitivity tests. Bacteria cultured from canine hepatic abscesses include *Escherichia coli, Klebsiella pneumoniae, Staphylococcus epidermidis, Enterococcus* sp., and *Clostridia* sp. Treatment involves surgical resection of the abscessed liver lobe(s) or splenectomy. In cases with diffuse hepatic involvement, percutaneous, ultrasound-guided drainage of abscesses may be appropriate. Ultrasound-assisted drainage and alcoholization of hepatic abscesses has been used in five dogs and one cat with success.[15] All animals are treated with long-term (6 to 8 weeks) antibiotic therapy. Follow-up ultrasound evaluations are recommended to monitor the response to treatment.

Rupture of the Biliary System

Rupture of the biliary system is more commonly seen in dogs than cats and is usually caused by abdominal trauma or associated with severe cholecystitis and rupture of the gall bladder.[16,17] Rupture has also been reported in dogs secondary to gall bladder infarction.[18] In animals with trauma-associated biliary leakage, there is usually a lag time of days to weeks between the initiating trauma and the development of clinical signs associated with bile peritonitis. Animals with underlying cholecystitis may have chronic or intermittent clinical signs associated with the hepatic and GI systems. Once substantial bile leakage occurs, clinical signs of peritonitis develop, thus prompting owners to seek veterinary attention.

The severity of clinical signs varies depending on the extent (local vs. general) of the peritonitis and the presence or absence of secondary bacterial infection of the bile and peritoneal fluid.[16,17] Clinical signs may include lethargy, anorexia, vomiting, and diarrhea. On physical examination, the mucous membranes may be icteric; parameters indicating perfusion such as capillary refill time, heart rate, and pulse quality will be variably altered depending on the severity of the peritonitis. The abdomen is often distended and painful. Plain abdominal radiographs show a local or generalized loss of abdominal detail. In cases of necrotic cholecystitis, choleliths and/or free gas may be visible in the cranial abdominal quadrant. Blood work often shows a leukocytosis, elevated serum bilirubin concentration, and elevations of serum ALP and ALT. A diagnosis of bile leakage is made from an analysis of peritoneal fluid samples. The finding of free bile crystals on cytology or a peritoneal fluid bilirubin level higher than that of the serum should prompt exploratory surgery. It should be noted that these changes may not be seen in patients with bile peritonitis secondary to a ruptured gallbladder mucocele because the gelatinous bile often fails to disperse throughout the abdomen.

Prior to surgery, the animal is rapidly and aggressively stabilized with IV crystalloids and possibly colloids. Broad spectrum, bactericidal antibiotics are administered as bile peritonitis often has gram-negative bacterial contamination.[16] A preoperative coagulation screen is mandatory in these cases as the absence of bile salts in the duodenum and jejunum precludes the absorption of fat and fat-soluble vitamins such as vitamin K. Fresh frozen plasma is required to prevent excessive surgical hemorrhage secondary to lack of coagulation factors. Vitamin K supplementation is given immediately (1 to 2 mg/kg subcutaneously). In cases of traumatic biliary leakage, the biliary system is either directly repaired or bile is diverted via a cholecystoenterostomy. In cases of gall bladder rupture secondary to cholecystitis, a cholecystectomy is performed. Samples are taken from the liver and peritoneal cavity for bacterial culture and sensitivity testing. The liver is biopsied. The peritoneal cavity is copiously lavaged with sterile isotonic fluid and either closed or left open. The reader is referred to Chapter 34 for a more detailed description of the management of peritonitis.

The prognosis in small animals with extrahepatic biliary disorders is varied and depends on underlying pathology and presence of an infectious process (primary or secondary). Extrahepatic biliary obstruction and trauma in dogs is associated with a high rate of mortality and prolonged hospitalization. Bacterial contamination appears to be a key factor in mortality associated with bile peritonitis since only 27% to 45% of animals with septic biliary effusion survived compared to 72% to 100% with nonseptic effusions in two studies.[16,17] Other prognostic indicators identified to negatively impact survival include elevated serum creatinine concentrations, prolonged partial thromboplastic time (PTT), and a lower postoperative mean arterial pressure. Furthermore, a separate study identified increasing age, gamma-glutamyltransferase (GGT) activity, blood urea nitrogen, phosphorus and bilirubin concentrations, preanesthetic heart rate, and the use of biliary diversion procedures as risk factors for death.[19] This study also concluded that the overall prognosis was guarded for dogs requiring biliary surgery; however, a good long-term prognosis can be given to patients that survive the early postoperative period. In one study focusing on cats with extrahepatic biliary obstruction, only 60% of cats with non-neoplastic lesions survived longer than 1 week after surgical intervention.[20] Feline extrahepatic biliary obstruction associated with neoplasia was associated with 100% mortality within 72 hours of presentation in this study.

Acute Hepatic Failure

Peracute hepatic failure has many potential causes in small animals including chemical agents, biotoxins, anesthetics and other drugs, viral, bacterial and other infectious agents, neoplasia, copper storage disease, and hepatic lipidosis in cats.[21] Hepatic failure is diagnosed in humans who have hepatic encephalopathy (HE) and a concurrent coagulopathy. Hepatic encephalopathy is a complex syndrome of neurologic alterations seen in association with moderate to severe liver disease. The cause of the neurologic signs seen in HE is multifactorial; elevations in serum and central nervous system (CNS) ammonia levels alter the glutamate, gamma-aminobutyric acid, and serotonin neurotransmitter systems. Changes in the central and peripheral benzodiazepine receptor systems also occur. Affected small animals often have clinical signs of weakness, depression, collapse, anorexia, vomiting, and diarrhea. Physical examination findings are rarely specific; signs of spontaneous hemorrhage including ecchymosis, icterus, and cranial organomegaly increase suspicion for liver disease but do not differentiate between an acute hemolytic crisis and extrahepatic biliary obstruction. Owners should be questioned carefully about possible drug or toxin exposures.

A diagnosis is suspected based on the history and physical examination findings and the results of serum biochemical and liver function tests, including a coagulation profile (see Chapter 192). Abdominal ultrasound is helpful to visualize the liver and obtain either aspirates or biopsy specimens for cytology, culture, and histopathology. Treatment is largely supportive and involves cardiovascular support with crystalloid and colloid fluids, correction of electrolyte and acid-base imbalances, lowering serum ammonia levels, and treating any seizure activity. The clinician should pay particular attention to hypokalemia and alkalosis as both of these conditions increase ammonia uptake to the CNS. Serum ammonia is lowered by administering lactulose, a nondigestible disaccharide that acidifies the colon, decreasing ammonia production and converting ammonia into nonabsorbable ammonium ions. In comatose animals, lactulose is administered as an enema (10 to 80 mL). In some instances, administration of flumazenil, a benzodiazepine receptor antagonist (0.01 to 0.02 mg/kg IV or SQ) may ameliorate clinical signs. In animals with HE and seizurelike activity, propofol is administered as a bolus (0.5 to 1 mg/kg IV), then as an infusion (0.05 to 0.1 mg/kg/min IV). Although surgical or minimally invasive radiologic intervention for identified single intrahepatic and extrahepatic shunts may be indicated, it is important that these animals be medically managed and stabilized for signs of hepatic dysfunction prior to addressing the underlying etiology.

REFERENCES

The reference list can be found on the companion Expert Consult Web site at *www.expertconsult.com*.

CHAPTER 135

Oxygen Therapy

Kate Hopper

Oxygen therapy increases the concentration of inspired oxygen in an attempt to increase the content of oxygen in the arterial blood. Oxygen therapy is an essential supportive care measure routinely administered to critically ill or injured pets and is required for most animals in respiratory distress. In order to provide appropriate oxygen therapy, it is necessary to be able to measure or estimate the concentration of oxygen provided and to monitor the effects of therapy. The concentration of oxygen delivered to patients is quantified as the fraction of inspired oxygen (F_IO_2) and may be recorded as a percentage (21% to 100%) or a decimal (0.21 to 1.0). The concentration of oxygen in room air is always 21%. Supplemental oxygen can provide an F_IO_2 of 30% to 100% depending on the technique and equipment utilized.

INDICATIONS

Oxygen therapy aims to increase the delivery of oxygen to the tissues. The determinants of oxygen delivery are hemoglobin concentration, arterial blood oxygenation, and cardiac output as described by the equation in Box 135-1.[1]

There are three main indications for oxygen therapy: significant anemia, hemodynamic compromise, and decreased blood oxygen concentrations (hypoxemia). Hypoxemia maybe suspected based on the patient's clinical signs or it may be documented directly with pulse oximetry and/or arterial blood gas measurement. Clinical signs suggestive of hypoxemia include respiratory distress, apnea, and cyanosis. Unfortunately, clinical assessment of hypoxemia is insensitive. An uncommon but important indication for oxygen therapy is carbon monoxide poisoning. Oxygen therapy will both attenuate tissue hypoxia and accelerate the elimination of carbon monoxide binding to hemoglobin.[2] All emergency patients should be given the benefit of supplemental oxygen until they are adequately stabilized and their requirement for ongoing oxygen administration can be fully assessed.

GOALS OF OXYGEN THERAPY

The goal of oxygen therapy will depend upon the reason for its administration. In patients with anemia, hemodynamic compromise, or carbon monoxide poisoning, the goal is to maximally increase arterial oxygen content in an attempt to increase oxygen delivery to the tissues until more definitive therapy can be instituted. To this aim, the highest possible F_IO_2 should be provided. In most pets that require oxygen therapy beyond the initial stabilization period, the goal is to correct hypoxemia. Hypoxemia is defined as a partial pressure of arterial oxygen (PaO_2) less than 80 mm Hg or an arterial oxygen saturation of less than 95%. Severe hypoxemia is present when the PaO_2 is less than 60 mm Hg or the arterial oxygen saturation is less than 90%.[1] Ideally, oxygen therapy is adjusted as needed for the patient to maintain a PaO_2 of 80 to 120 mm Hg. This will maintain hemoglobin saturation between 95% and 100%. A higher PaO_2 is of little clinical benefit assuming the patient has an adequate hematocrit and stable cardiovascular status. Animals with a normal hematocrit and normal cardiovascular function will often tolerate mild to moderate hypoxemia (PaO_2 of 60 to 80 mm Hg). In animals with severe disease, acceptance of mild to moderate hypoxemia may be preferable to the use of higher F_IO_2 levels for prolonged periods of time, in an attempt to avoid oxygen toxicity.

TECHNIQUES

Oxygen therapy requires a source of oxygen, either from an oxygen tank, an in-wall system, or via an anesthetic machine. There are numerous ways in which this oxygen can be delivered to the patient. The oxygen therapy technique chosen is based on availability of equipment, patient demeanor, and the severity of disease.

Flow-by Oxygen
The simplest way to administer oxygen is by directing oxygen gas flow toward the patient's mouth and nose (Web Figure 135-1). Tubing or a Bains circuit connected directly to a regulator and flow meter on an oxygen source is ideal for this

---

Box • 135-1
Oxygen Delivery (DO₂)
$$DO_2 = CO \times CaO_2$$ $$CaO_2 = ([Hb] \times 1.34 \times SaO_2) + (0.003 \times PaO_2)$$

CaO₂, Arterial blood oxygen content; *CO*, cardiac output; *Hb*, concentration of hemoglobin in g/dL; *PaO₂*, partial pressure of oxygen in the arterial blood; *SaO₂*, arterial saturation of hemoglobin.

technique. A Bains circuit or circle system (with anesthetic gases flushed out) attached to an anesthetic machine will also be effective. An oxygen flow rate of 2 to 3 L/min will provide an F_IO_2 of approximately 25% to 40%.[3] This technique is most suitable for short-term administration of oxygen during initial triage and stabilization of emergency patients. This is an easy mode of administration and patients generally tolerate it well. The disadvantages are that it is labor intensive, wastes oxygen, and the exact F_IO_2 delivered cannot be determined. Some pets resent the direct gas flow directed at their face.

Mask Oxygen

A face mask will allow administration of a higher F_IO_2 than can be achieved with simple flow-by oxygen, but close-fitting masks may not be well tolerated by many pets with respiratory distress. It is possible to deliver 60% or higher F_IO_2, and the exact F_IO_2 can be measured by placing an oxygen sensor in the mask alongside the animal's nose (Web Figure 135-2).[3] Disadvantages include the possibility for heat and carbon dioxide to accumulate in tight-fitting face masks, and animals in respiratory distress often resent the placement of a face mask. Care must be taken when using a face mask to avoid causing corneal trauma with the edge of the mask.

Elizabethan Collar

An Elizabethan collar with an oxygen source secured inside and the front covered with clear plastic wrap is a cheap, readily available method by which reasonably high levels of oxygen can be administered (Web Figure 135-3). It is important to make a window in the top of the plastic wrap to prevent accumulation of heat and carbon dioxide. Flow rates of 0.5 to 1 L/min can provide an F_IO_2 of 30% to 40%.[4] At higher oxygen flow rates an F_IO_2 of 60% to 70% may be delivered and oxygen therapy for long periods of time is feasible. It maybe difficult to tightly control the F_IO_2 with this approach, and some animals with respiratory distress will not tolerate the placement of the collar.

Nasal Prongs

A simple method of oxygen administration is placement of human nasal prongs (Figure 135-1). These are only practical in medium-sized dogs or larger. The advantages of the nasal prongs are their ease of placement and ready availability. The disadvantages include the ease in which they can be dislodged and the fact that the exact F_IO_2 delivered cannot be measured. It can be assumed that the F_IO_2 delivered would be less than that achieved with a nasal oxygen catheter at a similar flow rate (Table 135-1).

Nasal Oxygen Catheter

A nasal oxygen catheter is generally well accepted by most pets and can supply an F_IO_2 of 37% to 58% with oxygen flow rates of 50 to 200 mL/kg/min. Bilateral nasal oxygen catheters can provide an F_IO_2 of up to 77% (see Table 135-1).[5] Nasal oxygen catheters have the advantage of allowing hands-on patient assessment and management without interruption to

the oxygen therapy. Unfortunately, most severe respiratory distress patients will not tolerate the restraint required for placement, and some individual animals are extremely adept at removing the catheters. Other disadvantages include nasal mucosal irritation and difficulty in determining the actual F_IO_2 delivered (although it can be approximated from the information in Table 135-1). In order to reduce nasal irritation, the administered oxygen should first pass through a bubble humidifier and local anesthetic should be administered as required.

The nasal oxygen catheter should be a soft, smooth-tipped catheter such as an infant feeding tube or red rubber catheter. Such catheters should be placed in the ventral meatus of the nose after application of local anesthetic with the tip advanced to the level of the medial canthus of the eye, (Figure 135-2). The catheter should be secured as close to the nares as possible and then across the top or side of the head with sutures, staples, and butterfly tape or cyanoacrylate adhesive (see Figure 135-2).

Transtracheal Oxygen

Transtracheal oxygen delivery requires the placement of a catheter into the trachea. An oxygen source is then connected directly to the catheter and flow rates of 50 to 200 mL/kg/min used. Transtracheal oxygen therapy will provide a higher F_IO_2 for the same oxygen flow rate compared to nasal oxygen administration. A flow rate of 50 mL/kg/min is reported to provide and F_IO_2 of 40% to 60%.[6] A transtracheal catheter

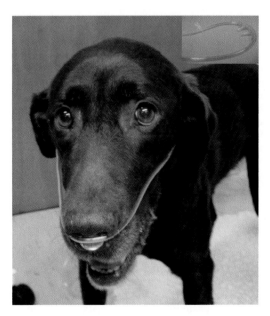

Figure 135-1 Nasal prongs are a simple method of oxygen therapy suitable for medium- and large-breed dogs.

Table • 135-1

F_IO_2 Reported for Unilateral and Bilateral Nasal Oxygen Catheters at Varying Oxygen Flow Rates

mL/kg/min	UNILATERAL 50	UNILATERAL 100	UNILATERAL 200	BILATERAL 50	BILATERAL 100	BILATERAL 200
F_IO_2 %	29.8 ± 5.6	37.3 ± 5.7	57.9 ± 12.7	36.4 ± 5.9	56 ± 11.9	77.3 ± 13.5

From Dunphy ED, Mann FA, Dodam JR, et al: Comparison of unilateral versus bilateral nasal catheters for oxygen administration in dogs. J Vet Emerg Crit Care 12:245-251, 2002.

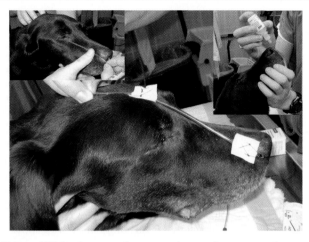

Figure 135-2 Prior to placement the nasal oxygen catheter is premeasured to the level of the medial canthus *(upper left)*. Following instillation of local anesthetic *(upper right)*, the catheter is guided into the ventral meatus to the premeasured length. It is then secured with sutures, staples, and/or suitable adhesive.

can be placed percutaneously or via a key hole incision in the trachea. Both techniques require some operator skill, and strict aseptic technique is required. This technique can be useful for the mobile animal and those intolerant of other oxygen administration methods. It may also be indicated when other less invasive methods of oxygen administration have not been successful. The placement of a transtracheal catheter requires animal restraint and/or general anesthesia, which may be contraindicated in an animal with respiratory distress. This technique can also be utilized as a short-term life-saving procedure in pets with a complete upper airway obstruction. Aggressive gas flow rates in this setting should be avoided to prevent barotrauma.

Oxygen Cage

An oxygen cage allows administration of a known F_IO_2 to patients in a low-stress, noninvasive manner. It is particularly effective for cats in respiratory distress as they may quickly decompensate when handled. The advantages include patient comfort, the ability to control F_IO_2 accurately, and the ability to provide very high F_IO_2 levels when required. Oxygen cages are expensive and require high oxygen flow rates, so they are a more expensive method of oxygen delivery compared to most other methods. It has been suggested that monitoring and treatment may necessitate interruption of oxygen delivery when using an oxygen cage. However, this problem is rare if the small patient-handling doors are used and if constant oxygen flow and/or addition of flow by oxygen is utilized during animal handling. Large dogs can become overheated in oxygen cages, and the temperature should be monitored closely. If a homemade oxygen cage is utilized, there is also a concern that carbon dioxide can accumulate and adequate cage ventilation is essential.

Positive Pressure Ventilation

When hypoxemia cannot be corrected with oxygen therapy or if a patient requires F_IO_2 levels of greater than 60% for long periods of time (24 to 48 hours), positive pressure ventilation is indicated. Positive pressure ventilation will often allow correction of hypoxemia at a lower F_IO_2.

Humidification

Inspired gases are normally humidified by the upper airways. The delivery of dry gas to the nose, trachea, or lower airways can cause irritation, inflammation, and thickening of airway secretions. For this reason any oxygen administration method that delivers high gas flows intranasally or intratracheally should use humidified gas.[7] This is especially important if oxygen therapy is provided for more than a few hours. Humidification is most simply achieved by use of a bubble humidifier attached to the oxygen source (Web Figure 135-4). The reservoir should be kept filled with sterile water. The entire unit can be sterilized between patients.

MONITORING

Patient monitoring is essential to determine when oxygen therapy is indicated, to ensure that sufficient oxygen supplementation is provided, and to avoid excessive oxygen supplementation. The first priority of oxygen administration should be the resolution of life-threatening hypoxemia and the relief of respiratory distress. As effective monitoring is often impossible during acute respiratory compromise, high F_IO_2 levels should initially be used.

Monitoring pets receiving oxygen therapy includes physical examination, arterial blood gases, and/or pulse oximetry. Respiratory rate and effort, heart rate, and anxiety levels are usually easily evaluated and can be useful in assessing response to oxygen therapy in pets with respiratory distress.

Arterial blood gas measures the PaO_2 and is the gold standard for evaluation of arterial oxygenation. Assessment of arterial blood gases requires an arterial blood sample and a blood gas analyzer. The normal or "expected" PaO_2 is dependent on the F_IO_2 and the barometric pressure. A useful rule of thumb is that the normal PaO_2 in a patient at sea level is approximately 5 times the F_IO_2 measured in percent. For example, for 21% room air at sea level, the normal PaO_2 is approximately 100 mm Hg while the normal PaO_2 on an F_IO_2 of 100% at sea level is approximately 500 mm Hg. The expected PaO_2 for a given F_IO_2 when at a high altitude is lower due to the decrease in barometric pressure. As previously mentioned, the goal of oxygen therapy is to maintain a PaO_2 of 80 to 120 mm Hg. If the PaO_2 is less than 80 mm Hg, the F_IO_2 should be increased; if the PaO_2 is greater than 120 mm Hg, the F_IO_2 should be decreased. Reevaluation of oxygenation status following any change in F_IO_2 is always important.

In the absence of arterial blood gas analysis, pulse oximetry can be utilized. Pulse oximetry evaluates the arterial saturation of hemoglobin with oxygen (SpO_2). Hemoglobin saturation is determined by the PaO_2 and this relationship is defined by the oxygen-hemoglobin dissociation curve. A PaO_2 of 80 mm Hg correlates to a SpO_2 of approximately 95%, while a PaO_2 of 60 mm Hg correlates to an SpO_2 of approximately 90%. Consequently the aim of oxygen therapy is to maintain a SpO_2 of greater than 95%. When the SpO_2 is 99% to 100% consistently, the F_IO_2 should be gradually decreased until the F_IO_2 at which the SpO_2 decreases is identified. The F_IO_2 should then be set at or just above this point in an attempt to avoid the use of unnecessarily high F_IO_2 levels.

OXYGEN TOXICITY

Intensive oxygen therapy is frequently required for patients with significant hypoxemia and places these animals at risk of oxygen toxicity. The lung is the organ most vulnerable to oxygen toxicity, and the associated damage is often severe and irreversible.

Guidelines for Oxygen Administration

Oxygen toxicity is not just a function of the level of oxygen administered, it is also related to the duration of oxygen exposure. The general recommendation for dogs and cats is to avoid the administration of 100% oxygen for longer than 12 to 24 hours and in situations of long-term oxygen therapy the fraction of inspired oxygen should be maintained at less than 60%.[7,8] Critical illness is commonly associated with depletion of endogenous antioxidant levels; for this reason it is possible that inspired oxygen levels of less than 60% could be potentially toxic. In addition, there is no way to predict an individual animal's susceptibility to toxicity. This leads to the

recommendation that the F_IO_2 should always be titrated to the lowest level a patient can tolerate.[9]

REFERENCES

The reference list can be found on the companion Expert Consult Web site at *www.expertconsult.com*.

CHAPTER 136

Renal Emergencies

Jennifer Prittie
Cathy Langston

ACUTE KIDNEY INJURY

Acute kidney injury (AKI) can vary from mild damage that does not elevate commonly measured renal parameters (such as creatinine) to complete anuria. Early suspicion and prompt recognition of mild AKI may allow measures to decrease or reverse the damage, whereas intervention is predominantly supportive in severe AKI. AKI can result from prerenal, intrinsic renal, or postrenal causes, and AKI can be superimposed on chronic kidney disease.

When faced with a patient who is not excreting an adequate amount of urine (1 to 2 mL/kg/hr), immediate action is necessary. The patency of the urinary tract should be evaluated for obstruction or rupture. To restore adequate urine flow, the structural problem must be alleviated or bypassed.

ACUTE RENAL FAILURE

Insufficient blood flow to the kidney from prerenal causes can substantially decrease GFR, and longstanding ischemia may lead to intrinsic renal failure. A wide variety of factors can cause acute intrinsic renal failure, which may exist as oligo-anuria (<0.25 mL/kg/hr), nonoliguria (0.25 to 2 mL/kg/hr), or polyuria (>2 mL/kg/hr). Patients with chronic kidney disease presenting in a decompensated uremic crisis are initially managed as nonoliguric acute renal failure (ARF).

Owners may present the pet with a known history of potential renal insult (e.g., ingestion of nephrotoxic drug or antifreeze, recent ischemic event) or with signs suggestive of ARF (recent onset of polyuria and polydipsia, vomiting, anorexia). Physical examination may reveal renomegaly or pain, uremic ulcers or halitosis.

CLINICAL SIGNS

In the initial stages of ethylene glycol intoxication (½ to 12 hours after ingestion), clinical signs may include central nervous system (CNS) depression, incoordination, ataxia, somnolence, seizures, or coma. Hypothermia and vomiting are also common. Marked polydipsia occurs in dogs, and both

dogs and cats initially become polyuric. These signs may resolve, followed by signs of ARF after 24 to 72 hours in dogs and as early as 12 hours after ingestion in cats.

With leptospirosis, clinical signs commonly encountered include fever, musculoskeletal pain, severe and persistent vomiting and diarrhea, oculonasal discharge, hemorrhagic diathesis, peripheral lymphadenopathy, or dyspnea. The presence of icterus in a patient with ARF is suggestive of leptospirosis, although not all serovars are associated with hepatic involvement. Leptospirosis is a zoonotic disease, and appropriate precautions should be utilized when handling any dog that is suspected to have leptospirosis.

Obstructing ureterolithiasis in cats is increasing in frequency. Hydronephrosis can usually be identified with ultrasonography; intravenous or antegrade pyelography may be required to determine the location and extent of obstruction. If the obstructing urolith does not pass within 24 hours, physical removal (surgery or lithotripsy) or bypass (ureteral stenting) are recommended. In addition to standard medical management of ARF, percutaneous placement of a nephropyelostomy tube helps to determine intrinsic renal function and helps alleviate uremic signs if the azotemia was predominantly due to the obstruction, making the patient more stable for anesthesia for definitive repair.

Cage-side tests that suggest ARF include presence of a high–anion gap metabolic acidosis, hypocalcemia, or hyperkalemia. Ethylene glycol toxicity may cause hyperglycemia. In addition to isothenuria, urinalysis may reveal proteinuria, glucosuria, hematuria, pyuria, or cylindruria. Oxalate crystals may be present with ethylene glycol toxicity. Abdominal radiographs will typically show either normal or enlarged kidneys; the contours should be smooth with ARF. With ethylene glycol toxicity, the kidneys may appear more radiopaque than surrounding soft tissue structures. In many cases of ARF, abdominal ultrasonography shows normal to enlarged kidneys with normal architecture. Ethylene glycol toxicity will frequently cause hyperechoic cortices compared to liver. Thoracic radiographs may show an interstitial pattern with leptospirosis, or an interstitial to alveolar pattern if volume overload has led to pulmonary edema.

Serum chemistry panel will document azotemia and hyperphosphatemia. Liver enzymes may be elevated with leptospirosis, with peak liver involvement occurring about 6 to 8 days after the onset of renal involvement. Changes in the complete blood count are usually nonspecific. Dogs with leptospirosis may have a mild nonregenerative anemia, leukocytosis, or thrombocytopenia. Urine culture may reveal bacterial growth in cases of bacterial pyelonephritis.

Specific tests available for ARF include an ethylene glycol test to confirm exposure. However, due to limits of detection of the test, cats can have nephrotoxic ethylene glycol levels with a negative test, and the test may be negative in both dogs and cats 12 hours after ingestion, due to metabolism of ethylene glycol. Leptospirosis serology is not available on an emergency basis.

TREATMENT

Fluid therapy is one of the first considerations for treatment of renal emergencies. Rehydration should occur over 4 to 24 hours, depending on the cardiovascular status. Most ARF patients should be rehydrated over a short time (4 to 6 hours). If the patient appears hydrated, a fluid volume equal to 3% to 5% of body weight should be administered to account for clinically undetectable dehydration. Urine output should be assessed after rehydration and fluid therapy should be tailored to fluid output (ins-and-outs). Administered fluid should be at a base rate equaling insensible loss (22 mL/kg/day) plus the volume of sensible loss (urine production) over the previous time period. If vomiting is profuse, an estimate of this volume is added to measurements of urine output. This method is appropriate for both oliguric/anuric patients, to avoid overhydration, and for polyuric patients, who frequently have volumes of urine exceeding the clinician's estimate. Plasma or colloids (e.g., hetastarch, dextran) may be indicated.

If urine output remains low (<0.25 mL/kg/hr) in a hydrated patient with blood pressure adequate to perfuse the kidneys (>80 mm Hg MAP), diuretics are indicated. Mannitol (0.5 g/kg administered IV over 20 minutes) is an osmotic diuretic, but is contraindicated in dehydrated or overhydrated patients. Furosemide, a loop diuretic, may induce urine flow in 20 to 30 minutes after an initial IV bolus of 2.2 mg/kg. If not, the dose can be doubled, up to 10 mg/kg. Higher doses may lead to ototoxicity. Furosemide does not improve the renal outcome. Furosemide and mannitol can be given together. Dopamine is no longer recommended for treating oliguric acute renal failure.

Treatment of metabolic acidosis is recommended when the blood pH is below 7.2 or the serum bicarbonate concentration is less then 16 mEq/L. Sodium bicarbonate is dosed according to the formula: body weight (kg) $\times$ 0.3 $\times$ (20 − patient bicarbonate concentration). One quarter to $\frac{1}{3}$ of the calculated dose can be administered as an IV bolus, and an additional $\frac{1}{4}$ to $\frac{1}{3}$ of the dose administered over the next 4 to 8 hours. Rapid administration, excessive dosing, or administration to a patient with impaired respiratory function can lead to paradoxical CNS acidosis.

Hyperkalemia may cause cardiac or ECG abnormalities, characterized by bradycardia, wide, flattened or absent P waves, peaked T waves, wide QRS complex, atrial standstill, idioventricular rhythm, ventricular fibrillation, or asystole. Regular insulin (0.1 to 0.25 U/kg IV) with dextrose to prevent hypoglycemia (1 to 2 g/unit of insulin as an IV bolus, followed by 1 to 2 g/unit over the next 4 to 8 hours) or bicarbonate (0.5 to 2 mEq/kg IV) temporarily shifts potassium intracellularly, with an effect occurring within about 20 to 30 minutes. If more immediate effect is needed, 10% calcium gluconate (0.5 to 1.0 mL/kg IV) can be administered as a slow IV bolus for its cardioprotective effect, although it does not decrease plasma potassium concentration. These emergency treatments need to be followed by procedures that remove potassium from the body (e.g., inducing urine flow or dialysis).

Uremia may induce gastritis or gastric ulceration. Histamine (H_2 receptor) blockers are commonly used to treat gastritis and include famotidine (0.5 to 1 mg/kg IV q24h), ranitidine (2.2 mg/kg IV q24h), or cimetidine (2.5 to 5 mg/kg IV q12h). Because of significant renal excretion of ranitidine and cimetidine, this is a reduced dosage. Sucralfate (0.25 to 1 g PO q6-8h) aids in healing of uremic ulcers. It should be given at least 30 to 60 minutes prior to oral antacids. Uremic toxins can induce nausea by stimulation of the chemoreceptor trigger zone. Metoclopramide (0.2 to 0.5 mg/kg IV or IM, q6-8h or 0.25 to 0.5 mg/kg/day as IV constant infusion) is a centrally acting antiemetic. Metoclopramide is a dopamine receptor antagonist and should not be administered concurrently with dopamine. Cerenia (1 mg/kg SQ q24h) can be used to treat vomiting in dogs. Anecdotally, 5-HT3 serotonic receptor antagonists, like ondansetron or dolasetron, seem more effective than metoclopramide.

Hyperphosphatemia is common in both acute and chronic renal failure as a result of decreased renal excretion. An acute increase in phosphate concentration will cause a compensatory decrease in calcium concentration. The ionized calcium concentration is usually maintained within normal limits, so signs of hypocalcemia tetany are infrequently observed. Oral phosphate binders (e.g., aluminum hydroxide) should be used once vomiting is controlled and the patient is being fed enterally.

Respiratory compromise from pleural effusion caused by volume overload may require thoracocentesis. No effective method of addressing pulmonary edema exists in the anuric patient other than ultrafiltration via dialysis. Careful attention to fluid therapy and urine output is crucial to avoiding this complication.

Hypertension may accompany either acute or chronic renal failure, and excessive volume expansion (particularly in the face of oliguria or anuria) can exacerbate the condition. Therapy may not be necessary if the hypertension is mild and the renal failure is resolving rapidly. However, emergency therapy may be necessary to prevent catastrophic effects in more severe cases.

Anorexia is common with acute renal failure. Because of the highly catabolic state associated with ARF, nutritional support should be started early in the course of the illness. If vomiting can be adequately controlled pharmacologically, enteral feeding with a feeding tube should be started. If enteral feeding is not possible, partial or total parenteral nutrition should be instituted. Although feeding a restricted quantity of high-quality protein is established therapy for chronic kidney disease, the need for protein restriction in ARF is less clear.

Uremia induces a thrombocytopathy, and the risk of bleeding should be considered when planning invasive procedures (e.g., renal biopsy, feeding tube placement). Because coagulation parameters and platelet numbers may be normal, a buccal mucosal bleeding time is the preferred method of assessment.

For ethylene glycol toxicity, specific antidotes are indicated. Four-methylpyrazole (4-MP, fomepizole, Antizol-Vet, Orphan Medical, Minnetonka, Minn.) is effective in dogs if given within 8 hours of ingestion. Standard doses are not effective in cats. Dosing for dogs is 20 mg/kg IV initially, then 15 mg/kg at 12 and 24 hours, followed by 5 mg/kg at 36 hours. If 4-MP is not available, 20% ethanol can be used to competitively inhibit alcohol dehydrogenase. A dose of 5.5 mL/kg every 4 hours for five treatments, then every 6 hours for four treatments can be given as an intermittent IV bolus, but is better as a constant rate infusion. In cats, 20% ethanol can be dosed at 5 mL/kg every 6 hours for five treatments, then every 8 hours for four treatments. Drinking alcohol (50% ethanol [100 proof]) can be diluted with saline. Respiratory depression can be profound with alcohol. Neither 4-MP nor alcohol is effective if started more than 8 hours after ingestion.

Antibiotics should be administered if leptospirosis or pyelonephritis is suspected or documented. High doses of penicillin are effective at clearing leptospiremia. Doxycycline (2.5 mg/kg q12h) is effective at clearing leptospiremia and possibly leptospiruria. The most common cause of bacterial pyelonephritis is *Escherichia coli*. Empiric antibiotic choice should have a good gram-negative spectrum and not be nephrotoxic.

MONITORING

Adequate monitoring of patients with acute renal failure is essential. These are acutely, severely ill patients whose status can change rapidly and dramatically. Urine output should be monitored in all patients with renal failure. This is most accurately accomplished with an indwelling urinary catheter with a closed collection system. Changes in body weight over the

course of hospitalization primarily reflect changes in body water content and hydration. Other parameters, such as blood pressure, central venous pressure, and packed cell volume, should be monitored as needed.

DIALYTIC THERAPY

If conventional medical management fails to induce diuresis in an oliguric or anuric patient, if life-threatening complications are present (e.g., hyperkalemia, volume overload), or if azotemia fails to improve after 24 hours of therapy, dialytic therapy (i.e., intermittent hemodialysis, continuous renal replacement therapy, or peritoneal dialysis) should be considered.

OUTCOME

The outcome of acute renal failure is poor. Approximately 60% of cases will die or be euthanized. Renal trauma may require emergency surgery to control massive hemorrhage.

CHAPTER 137

Reproductive Emergencies

Saralyn Smith-Carr
Andrew Lee McGraw

Reproductive emergencies of the dam are common and usually occur during the periparturient period. Reproductive emergencies of the sire are usually due to trauma or are idiopathic. The goal of this chapter is to detail how each disease should be approached as an emergency. Common reproductive emergencies of periparturient dam are dystocia, eclampsia, and metritis. Those of the sire are fractured penis, priapism and paraphimosis.

REPRODUCTIVE EMERGENCIES OF THE DAM

Dystocia is the inability of the female to expel the fetus through the birth canal at birth. Primary uterine inertia is the most common cause of dystocia.[1-3] Clinical signs vary from overdue parturition date to labor without success for ≥4 hours. Treatment is based on the initial presentation and diagnostics needed (Figure 137-1).

A good history is central to determine owner's knowledge, breeding practices, and whether the due date has truly passed. A physical examination should be performed to determine if signs of maternal or fetal distress exist. Presence of the fetal body parts on digital vaginal palpation, brownish-green vaginal discharge, and existence of straining are all indications that labor has commenced and possibility of maternal or fetal distress. Abdominal radiographs are critically important to determine if fetal number, size, or presentation are causative of the dystocia.[4,5] Abdominal ultrasound is best used to determine decreased fetal heart rate (normal, 180 to 200 beats/

min), which is the best indicator of fetal distress.[4,5] Parenteral administration (IV or IM) of 1.1 to 2.2 U/kg of oxytocin with or without prior treatment with 1 to 3 mL 10% calcium gluconate (IV or SQ) can be tried if fetal obstruction is not present.[5,6] The oxytocin usually causes uterine contraction and expulsion of the fetus in ≤30 minutes but can be repeated if minimal effects are seen (do not exceed 20 units). The majority of pregnant dams with dystocia require a Cesarean section.[1-3,5,6] The choice of anesthesia is an important consideration for both the dam and fetus.[5,7] Anesthetics that should be avoided are ketamine hydrochloride and thiobarbituates.[7] Supplemental oxygen during anesthesia induction, along with intravenous fluid administration and tilting the surgery table toward the surgeon during surgery, are recommended.[8] Trained technical personnel should be available for fetal resuscitation. Fetuses may require removal of membranes surrounding their bodies, they may benefit from removal of fluid from airways using gentle suction of the mouth and/or nares, they may need gentle stimulation to encourage breathing, and proper umbilical cord clamping and cutting might be necessary.

Eclampsia is a condition of low blood calcium secondary to high lactation demands. The most common presentation is in week 2 to 3 after whelping.[5,8,9] Clinical signs include nervousness, panting, salivation, stiff gait, ataxia, and clonic-tonic muscle contractions that can proceed to seizure activity. Low serum calcium and/or ionized calcium are diagnostic of this condition, although it is not recommended to wait for test results before initiating therapy. Treatment consists of a 10%

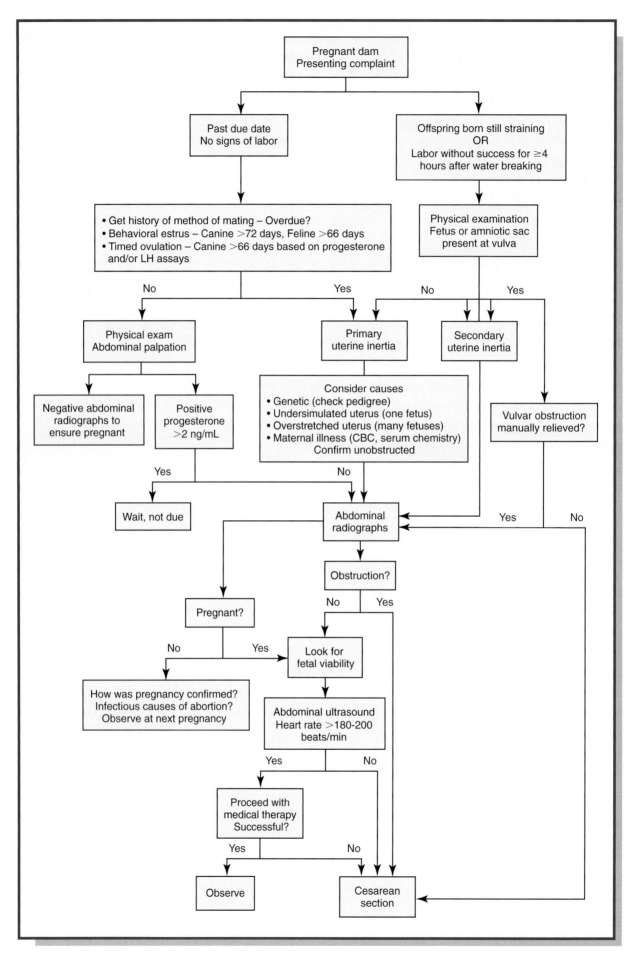

Figure 137-1 Algorithm for diagnosis and treatment of dystocia based on clinical findings. *CBC,* Complete blood count; *LH,* luteinizing hormone.

to 20% calcium gluconate solution administered by slow intravenous infusion in 5 to 10 mL increments with heart monitoring via stethoscope or electrocardiogram for bradycardia or an arrhythmia. The infusion should be stopped should either occur. Once acute signs have discontinued, subcutaneous (SQ) calcium gluconate diluted with saline (do NOT use calcium chloride as it is quite caustic) may be given at 8-hour intervals with daily monitoring of calcium levels to ensure normalcy. Most veterinarians recommend using the same total dose of calcium needed IV to control clinical signs as the starting dose for SQ therapy. Oral calcium supplementation should be given for the remainder of their lactation period with weaning of the neonate should signs recur.

Metritis is bacterial infection of the uterus secondary to obstetric manipulations, retained fetus, fetal membranes and/or placenta.[5,9,10] Clinical signs usually occur within week 1 to 2 postpartum and consist of anorexia, lethargy, vomiting, disinterest in the nursing offspring, and hemorrhagic-brown fetid vaginal discharge. A palpably enlarged uterus may be found on physical examination along with fever, poor capillary refill, dehydration, and lethargy. Abdominal radiographs may confirm the enlarged uterus, presence of fetal skeletal remains, or loss of serosal detail secondary to peritonitis. Ultrasound may confirm an enlarged, fluid-filled uterus, peritonitis, and thin, weakened uterine walls. A complete blood count (CBC), serum chemistry, and urinalysis should be performed prior to treatment and for correction of fluid and electrolyte abnormalities. Laboratory values may reveal a neutrophilia with left shift CBC, elevated blood urea nitrogen, total protein, alanine aminotransferase, and alkaline phosphatase and low glucose. The uterine infection is usually due to gram-negative bacteria. Treatment with fluid therapy and broad-spectrum antibiotics should be administered at the time of medical therapy and/or prior to surgical therapy. Antibiotics should be chosen with the nursing neonate in mind. Antibiotics to avoid in the neonate are gentamicin, amikacin, tetracycline, chloramphenicol, and enrofloxacin. Medical treatment consists of oxytocin or other ecbolic agents if uterine walls are not thin and there is no evidence of peritonitis. Surgical therapy consists of ovariohysterectomy and is recommended if the dam will not be used for breeding. Other reasons for surgery are worsening of condition or failure to improve despite medical therapy. Surgery may be a life-saving procedure and may be considered the first line of therapy in severe cases.

fence, but such a finding is not typical.[11-14] Clinical findings are typical of lower urinary tract disease such as dysuria, pollakiuria, and stranguria. Physical examination may reveal an awkward ventral angular deviation of the penis, crepitus of the os penis, and an enlarged urinary bladder in the event of obstruction.[12-14] Radiographs confirm the diagnosis.[13] Consequences of a fractured os penis are urethral laceration and callus formation that may result in urethral obstruction and uremia. Immediate care after acute injury consists of cage rest with urinary catheterization for 5 days to provide minimal stabilization and urine diversion in the event of a urethral laceration.[11] Comminuted or chronic nonhealing fractures may necessitate surgical intervention to realign the fragments, bone plating with a finger plate, or a urethrostomy proximal to the affected site.[11,12]

Priapism is an inappropriate and persistent erection not associated with coitus, which may result in pain and stranguria.[13-16] The pathophysiology involves excessive parasympathetic stimulation or impairment of normal venous drainage from the corpus cavernosum. Potential etiologies are trauma while mating,[16] chronic distemper encephalomyelitis, penile thromboembolism, mass impeding venous drainage, and idiopathic. A delay in treatment may lead to ischemic necrosis and gangrene resulting in penile amputation and scrotal urethrostomy as the only viable therapeutic option.[17]

Paraphimosis is the inability of the male dog to retract a flaccid or erect penis into the preputial sheath.[13,14] Causes include entrapment of the penis due to strangulation by hair ring, malicious placement of a string or rubber band, or a narrow preputial opening; neurologic causes (intervertebral disk disease or encephalitis), excessive grooming of the penis, fracture of the os penis, trauma, ineffective preputial or retractor penis muscles, or idiopathic.[14,17] Necrosis and trauma are possible with prolonged desiccation or self-mutilation. Treatment consists of removing the underlying cause along with cleaning and lubricating the penis before replacing with placement of purse string sutures in acute cases. Chronic cases may require surgery to advance the prepuce and shorten preputial musculature.[13,17] As with priapism, failure of these therapies or extensive damage to the penis will necessitate amputation with scrotal urethrostomy.

REPRODUCTIVE EMERGENCIES OF THE SIRE

Fractured os penis can be seen in dogs with a history of an injurious event such as dog fight or incompletely clearing a

REFERENCES

The reference list can be found on the companion Expert Consult Web site at *www.expertconsult.com*.

CHAPTER 138

Sepsis and the Systemic Inflammatory Response Syndrome

Amy DeClue

The *systemic inflammatory response syndrome (SIRS)* refers to the complex clinical response to a nonspecific insult of either infectious or noninfectious origin. Heart rate, respiratory rate, body temperature, and white blood cell count are the clinical criteria used to categorize patients with

SIRS in veterinary medicine (Table 138-1). These criteria have been used to determine the severity of illness and prognosis in critically ill animals. In one study of 500 dogs, mortality was significantly associated with the number SIRS criteria fulfilled.[1]

Table • 138-1

SIRS Criteria in Dogs and Cats[1,7]

SIRS CRITERIA	DOG	CAT
Temperature	>103.5° F or <100° F	>103.5° F or <100° F
Heart rate	>60	>225 or <140
Respiratory rate; PCO_2	>40; <32 torr	>40
White blood cell count	>12,000/µL or <4000/µL or >10% bands	>19,500/µL or <5,000/µL or >5% bands

SIRS, Systemic inflammatory response syndrome.

Box • 138-1

Definitions Pertaining to Sepsis and SIRS[3]

- *Bacteremia:* the presence of viable bacteria in the bloodstream
- *Systemic inflammatory response syndrome (SIRS):* a clinical syndrome caused by systemic inflammation of infectious (i.e., sepsis) or noninfectious origin. In dogs, the diagnosis of SIRS is based on fulfillment of at least two of four criteria—tachycardia, tachypnea, hypothermia or hyperthermia, and either leukocytosis, leucopenia, or bands.
- *Sepsis:* the systemic inflammatory response to infection
- *Severe sepsis:* the systemic inflammatory response to infection associated with organ dysfunction and manifestations of hypoperfusion or hypotension
- *Septic shock:* the systemic inflammatory response to infection with hypotension despite adequate fluid resuscitation along with the manifestations of hypoperfusion
- *Multiple organ dysfunction syndrome (MODS):* altered function of two or more organs secondary to SIRS such that homeostasis cannot be maintained without intervention
- *Acute respiratory distress syndrome (ARDS):* a pulmonary inflammatory disorder characterized by noncardiogenic pulmonary edema, neutrophilic inflammation, and hypoxemia

Sepsis is a Greek work meaning "decomposition of animal or vegetable organic matter in the presence of bacteria."[2] In the clinic, sepsis has come to mean infection with concurrent clinical evidence of the systemic inflammatory response (i.e., SIRS because of infection). At one time, sepsis and bacteremia were considered synonymous terms. However, as our knowledge of sepsis has grown we have realized that the clinical manifestations of sepsis relate to widespread inflammation and not necessarily widespread infection. Terminology used to describe the severity of sepsis and SIRS is listed in Box 138-1.[3]

In dogs and cats, bacterial infections are the most common cause of sepsis with *Escherichia coli* being the most common isolate.[4-13] However, any microbial organism (e.g., fungus, parasite, virus) may cause sepsis. Sepsis most commonly originates from the abdomen followed by the respiratory tract in dogs.[4-6] In cats, sepsis is commonly associated with septic peritonitis, pyothorax, and hepatic abscessation.[9-14]

PATHOGENESIS

The sequence of events leading to sepsis is complex and incompletely understood. In the initial phases of infection, microbial products (e.g., endotoxin from gram-negative bacteria; exotoxins, peptidoglycans, and superantigens from gram-positive bacteria; and fungal cell wall material) induce systemic inflammation through activation of immune cells. The induction of systemic inflammation may start at a local site like an abscess on the limb. For sepsis to develop from a local infection, inflammatory mediators and/or microbial products must enter into the systemic circulation and activate inflammatory cells throughout the body. Since *E. coli* bacterial infection is the most common cause of sepsis, the focus of this chapter is on the interaction of gram-negative bacteria and the immune system.

During gram-negative sepsis, lipopolysaccharide (LPS), the glycolipid component of the cell wall of gram-negative bacteria, is released. Upon release, the lipid A portion of LPS binds to LPS-binding protein. The LPS–LPS-binding protein complex is recognized via macrophage cell surface receptors like CD14. The main function of CD14, which lacks a transmembrane domain, is to transfer LPS to toll-like receptor-4 (TLR4) and MD-2 for subsequent cellular activation. Once LPS binds to these cell surface receptors, the macrophage becomes activated and intracellular signaling through activation of nuclear factor kappa-B (NF-κB) is initiated. Activation and nuclear translocation of NF-κB results in the transcription of multiple inflammatory mediators that have been implicated in the induction and maintenance of sepsis. Interestingly, many physical and chemical stimuli are capable of activating NF-κB. This may be one explanation for why, although there is a plethora of inciting causes for SIRS, the inflammatory outcome is similar in many cases.

There are many inflammatory mediators involved with sepsis and SIRS. Tumor necrosis factor-α (TNF-α), interleukin-6 (IL-6), nitric oxide, and leukotrienes are examples of important mediators contributing to the pathology of sepsis in dogs and cats.[15-21] Sepsis is not simply the induction of inflammation, but rather it is induction of proinflammatory components of the immune system to the extent that they overwhelm normal antiinflammatory counter-regulatory mechanisms allowing inflammation to go unchecked. Ultimately, the unchecked proinflammatory cascade leads to inflammatory cell infiltration, altered thermoregulation, vasodilation, vascular leakage, coagulation, hemodynamic instability, and multiple organ failure (Web Figure 138-1).

Multiple organ dysfunction syndrome (MODS) is a devastating consequence of sepsis. Pathogenesis of organ failure (e.g., renal failure) during sepsis is multifactorial but centers around the development of mitochondrial dysfunction. Circulatory collapse, microcirculatory changes, hypoxemia, and inflammation lead to tissue ischemia, reduced mitochondrial and then cellular function. The resultant organ damage may be permanent, or may resolve when sepsis is resolved. Some forms of organ dysfunction, like acute respiratory distress syndrome (ARDS), are the result of inflammation, not circulatory collapse and mitochondrial damage. During the initiation of ARDS, inflammatory mediators and microbial products activate pulmonary macrophages resulting in vasodilation, vascular leak, pulmonary edema, and neutrophilic inflammation.[22]

CLINICAL ASPECTS

Clinically, dogs can have either a hyperdynamic or hypodynamic response during sepsis. The hyperdynamic response is characterized by fever, brick-red mucous membranes, tachycardia, and bounding pulses. As the disease process progresses, a hypodynamic response characterized by hypotension, pale mucous membranes, and hypothermia may be observed. Often dogs will have gastrointestinal (GI) or respiratory signs associated with endotoxemia. Hyperglycemia or hypoglycemia, hypoalbuminemia, azotemia, hyperbilirubinemia, increased alanine aminotransferase and/or alkaline phosphatase, leukocytosis, neutrophilia with a left shift or a leukopenia, anemia, and thrombocytopenia are clinicopathologic abnormalities that have been recognized during sepsis. Evidence of coagulopathy including decreased protein C and antithrombin concentrations, prolonged prothrombin time, partial thromboplastin time, and increased D-dimer concentrations have been documented in dogs with naturally acquired sepsis.[4,23] Many dogs with sepsis will have myocardial dysfunction and vasodilation leading to hypotension. Poor perfusion, tissue hypoxia, and cellular metabolic derangement can lead to metabolic acidosis.

Cats with sepsis may develop clinical signs and clinicopathologic abnormalities that are similar to those of dogs during sepsis with a few exceptions. Bradycardia, hypothermia, and abdominal pain are frequent, unique findings in cats with sepsis.[7,12,14] Cats also appear to develop septic shock more readily than dogs, and typically the hyperdynamic phase is not recognized during feline sepsis. The mechanisms by which these unique manifestations develop are unknown.

Sepsis commonly results in MODS in humans. The incidence of sepsis-induced MODS is not known in dogs or cats with sepsis although cardiovascular, GI, hepatic, renal, endocrine, and respiratory dysfunction/failure have been recognised.[24-29]

DIAGNOSIS

History, physical examination, blood pressure, complete blood count (CBC), serum biochemical profile, urinalysis, blood gas analysis, coagulation profile, and appropriate diagnostic imaging should be performed in any critically ill dog or cat. The diagnosis of sepsis is accomplished by demonstrating evidence of infection and systemic inflammation (i.e., SIRS). Infection may be identified via culture, cytology (Figure 138-1), histopathology, or serology.

In dogs and cats where bacterial infection is suspected, culture and sensitivity should always be performed so that antibiotic selection can be tailored to the particular organism. Based on the clinical findings, specimens should be collected from blood, urine, wound exudate, peritoneal fluid, bronchoalveolar lavage fluid, and/or synovial fluid prior to antibiotic administration. For patients with suspected bacterial peritonitis, glucose concentration of the blood can be compared to the peritoneal fluid to achieve a rapid diagnosis. A difference of >20 mg/dL between blood and peritoneal fluid glucose concentrations is diagnostic for septic peritoneal effusion.[6] In some cases, identification of infection is difficult and/or delayed and a presumptive diagnosis of infection based on the clinical picture will be necessary. However, it is important to remember that there are many causes of the SIRS that are noninfectious in origin (e.g., acute pancreatitis,

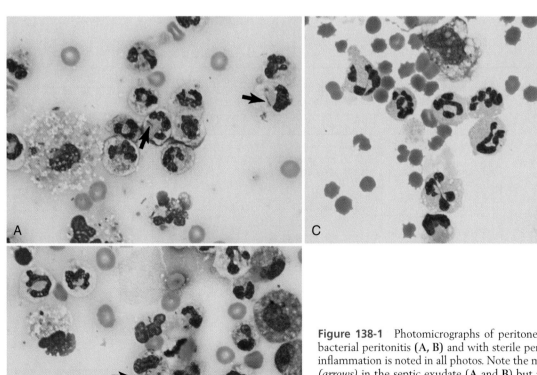

Figure 138-1   Photomicrographs of peritoneal fluid from a dog with bacterial peritonitis (**A, B**) and with sterile peritonitis (**C**). Suppurative inflammation is noted in all photos. Note the many intracellular bacteria *(arrows)* in the septic exudate (**A** and **B**) but not in the sterile exudate (**C**). (Courtesy Dr. Linda Berent, University of Missouri.)

autoimmune disease, envenomation). Care should be taken to consider noninfectious differentials for SIRS when appropriate.

TREATMENT

The most important aspect of treating sepsis centers on the identification and eradication of the inciting cause. Although stringent effort should be made to identify the cause of sepsis, early antimicrobial treatment is critical for survival and should not be withheld pending culture results. Broad spectrum, bactericidal antimicrobial agents (e.g., fluoroquinolone + beta-lactam antibiotic) administered IV should be instituted as quickly as possible in patients with suspected sepsis. Antibiotic therapy should be selected based on the most likely type of organism given the site of infection. Depending upon

the source of infection, surgical debridement may be necessary for infection control. Once culture-specific antibiotic sensitivity is determined, the antibiotic with the narrowest spectrum of activity should be chosen and administered until there is complete clinical resolution. The remainder of therapy centers on maintenance of tissue perfusion, management of organ failure, and aggressive supportive care (Figure 138-2).

Most pets with sepsis will have a relative or absolute hypovolemia, hypotension, and/or poor tissue perfusion. Isotonic crystalloids (dog, 80 to 90 mL/kg in 20 mL/kg increments, IV to effect; cat, 40 to 60 mL/kg in 10 mL/kg increments, IV to effect) or colloids (dog, 10 to 20 mL/kg in 5 mL/kg increments, IV to effect; cat, 5 to 10 mL/kg in 1 to 5 mL increments, IV to effect) can be used for rapid initial volume resuscitation and administered based on evaluation of end points (e.g., heart rate, blood pressure, central venous pressure). Then, fluid therapy should be tailored to the needs of

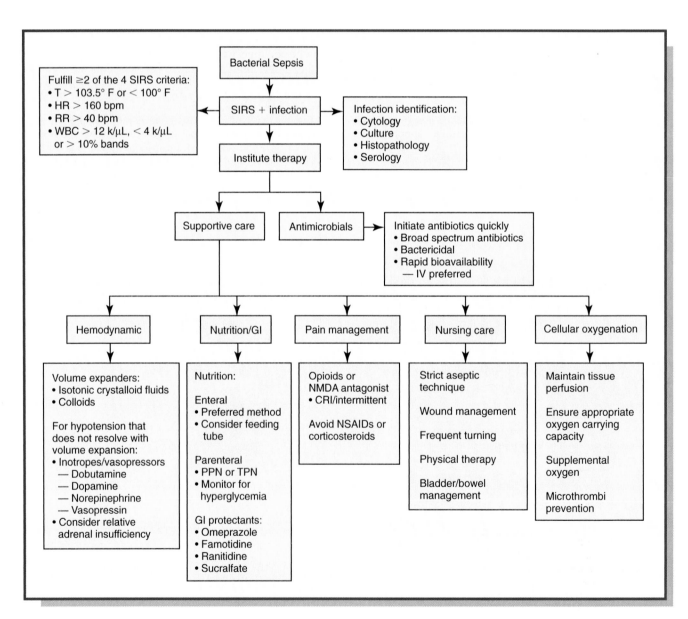

Figure 138-2 Algorithm for the diagnosis and treatment of sepsis in dogs. *CRI*, Constant rate infusion; *GI*, gastrointestinal; *HR*, heart rate; *NMDA*, N-methyl-D-aspartic acid; *NSAIDs*, nonsteroidal antiinflammatory drugs; *PPN*, partial parenteral nutrition; *RR*, respiratory rate; *SIRS*, systemic inflammatory response syndrome; *T*, temperature; *TPN*, total parenteral nutrition; *WBC*, white blood cell.

the patient. Patients with sepsis will have a propensity to develop interstitial edema because of increased vascular permeability and decreased blood colloid osmotic pressure. Colloids (e.g., hetastarch) may help prevent interstitial edema and should be considered for volume resuscitation and during maintenance of sepsis patients.

Despite aggressive volume resuscitation, some patients will require additional support to maintain normal blood pressure and perfusion. The most efficacious, safest treatment for septic shock has not been determined in dogs or cats. Prior to administration of any sympathomimetic drug, care should be taken to ensure that a dog or cat is not hypovolemic. Since the goal of treating septic shock is to maintain tissue perfusion, medications that cause vasoconstriction should be used only if absolutely necessary. Positive inotropic drugs (e.g., dobutamine) may be a good initial management choice for septic shock since they help combat decreased cardiac output caused by myocardial dysfunction without inducing peripheral vasoconstriction. If volume resuscitation and positive inotropic support has failed to restore blood pressure, a vasopressor agent (e.g., dopamine, norepinephrine, epinephrine, or vasopressin) could be added. Although there are no clinical trials evaluating these drugs, epinephrine was found to adversely affect organ function, systemic perfusion, and survival compared to the use of norepinephrine or vasopressin[30] and had detrimental effects on gastric mucosal pH and plasma lactate concentrations compared to dobutamine and norepinephrine[31] in experimental canine sepsis. Relative adrenal insufficiency has been documented in dogs with sepsis and refractory hypotension[27] and should be considered in any dog requiring vasopressor therapy during sepsis.

Bacterial translocation from the GI tract can contribute to systemic inflammation during sepsis. Early placement of a feeding tube and initiation of enteral or, in patients with vomiting, parenteral nutrition will help maintain GI barrier function. Additionally, medication aimed at maintaining normal GI protective mechanisms (e.g., omeprazole, famotidine, sucralfate) could be considered. Hyperglycemia can be a complication of nutritional therapy, especially parenteral nutrition. Hyperglycemia has been associated with increased inflammation and a poorer prognosis in people with sepsis and SIRS. Although the importance of glucose homeostasis in dogs and cats with sepsis is unknown, iatrogenic hyperglycemia should be avoided.

Oxygenation, acid-base status, CBC, and organ function should be closely monitored. Along with maintaining good tissue perfusion, maximizing cellular oxygenation will help maintain tissue viability and avoid multiple organ dysfunction. This may be accomplished by ensuring good oxygen-carrying capacity, providing supplemental oxygen when indicated, and preventing microthrombi formation. For the majority of patients, acid-base abnormalities are related to lactic acidosis secondary to poor tissue perfusion. Typically these abnormalities will resolve once perfusion is restored. Therefore, bicarbonate administration is rarely needed. When organ dysfunction is recognized, specific therapy aimed at maintaining homeostasis should be considered. In some cases, peritoneal or hemodialysis, plasma or blood transfusion, positive inotropic agents, and mechanical ventilation may be necessary.

Finally, care should be taken to ensure adequate patient comfort including management of pain, careful catheter maintenance, bladder/bowel care, and frequent patient turning/movement to prevent decubital ulcers. Almost all patients with sepsis will require analgesic administration for pain management. Although many analgesics like ketamine[32] and buprenorphine[33] may offer specific antiinflammatory advantages during endotoxemia, some may be detrimental. Morphine, for instance, augments the inflammatory response to endotoxin, has a detrimental effect on mean arterial pressure, and increases mortality in endotoxemic rats.[33,34] It is not known if morphine is detrimental during canine or feline sepsis.

Since sepsis is a systemic inflammatory disease, it is logical that strategies aimed at halting inflammation or the consequences of inflammation have been proposed as novel therapies for sepsis. Many antiinflammatory therapies have been evaluated in human clinical trials with little success. For example, despite their strong antiinflammatory properties, the use of corticosteroids for the treatment of sepsis has fallen out of favor due to their lack of efficacy combined with their immunosuppressive, ulcerogenic, and prothrombotic nature.[35,36] One exception may be the use of low or physiologic doses of corticosteroids for management of relative adrenal insufficiency during sepsis.[37] Although relative adrenal insufficiency is recognized in dogs with sepsis, the administration of corticosteroids in this subset of patients has not been studied.[27]

Activated protein C and administration of regular insulin to maintain tight glycemic control are two antiinflammatory treatments that have been shown to be beneficial in human clinical trials. Human recombinant activated protein C has antithrombotic, profibrinolytic, and antiinflammatory actions and has been shown to decrease the risk of death during sepsis in people.[38] No work has looked at activated protein C administration in dogs, and the hefty cost will likely prohibit its use in veterinary medicine. Hyperglycemia has been linked to increased inflammatory cytokine production and an increased risk of mortality in people.[39] Intensive insulin therapy to maintain tight glycemic control has decreased mortality in critically ill adults by as much as 40% in clinical trials.[40] This management strategy has not been evaluated in dogs or cats. Regardless, good glycemic control should be a consideration in septic patients.

The only antiinflammatory therapy with some positive benefit that has been tested in canine clinical trials is polymyxin B. Polymyxin B binds to endotoxin from gram-negative bacteria, preventing the interaction between endotoxin and the immune system. In a placebo-controlled clinical trial, dogs treated with polymyxin B (12,500 IU/kg, IM q12h) had significantly improved dehydration, capillary refill time, pulse quality, and significantly lower plasma TNF concentrations than the control group.[41] Polymyxin B may be a potential treatment for gram-negative sepsis in dogs and further study is warranted.

PROGNOSIS

Mortality rates for dogs and cats with sepsis range from 48% to 79% despite aggressive management.[12,23,27,42-44] Hypotension, anemia, hypoalbuminemia, acidemia, coagulopathy, increased ALT, and inflammatory mediators such as TNF and IL-6 have been associated with a poorer prognosis in some studies of canine sepsis. As our understanding of sepsis grows, new therapies aimed at more aggressive supportive care and restoring a normal proinflammatory and antiinflammatory balance may help decrease morbidity and mortality.

REFERENCES

The reference list can be found on the companion Expert Consult Web site at *www.expertconsult.com*.

CHAPTER 139

Shock

Elise Mittleman Boller
Cynthia M. Otto

Shock is not a disease but a complex physiologic state. Historically, shock was described as the effect of generalized circulatory abnormalities that led to inadequate tissue perfusion. Although this classic description still holds important clinical relevance, it has been recognized that the complexity of shock states result not from the initial insult per se, but the host's systemic response to that insult. Furthermore, the ultimate result of shock is decreased cellular energy metabolism and adenosine triphosphate (ATP) production. It is recognized that these abnormalities may occur despite normal tissue perfusion. Utilizing this definition of shock, one may consider a functional classification system whereby shock is defined as decreased cellular energy production and shock categories are expanded to include types other than the classic hypovolemic, distributive, and cardiogenic types (Figure 139-1).[1]

Etiologies of shock with this system include syndromes that are clinically apparent causes of shock but that do not fit into the traditional classification scheme; for example, severe anemia, methemoglobinemia, and bromethalin exposure are often associated with clinical shock states, yet the patient has normal blood volume, cardiac function, and systemic vascular resistance.

TYPES

Hypovolemic shock is defined as a life-threatening decrease in circulating blood volume and is the most common form (see Figure 139-1). It leads to inadequate delivery of oxygen and nutrients to tissues and an accumulation of byproducts of cellular metabolism due to insufficient circulating blood volume. Intravascular volume depletion can result from hemorrhage (internal or external), nonhemorrhagic fluid losses (e.g., gastrointestinal, urinary, third spacing), or decreased intake of fluid.

Cardiogenic shock results predominantly from failure of adequate forward blood flow. The dysfunction can occur in either the diastolic or systolic phase or can result from an obstruction of flow. Systolic or forward flow failure results from an overt failure of contractility (e.g., intrinsic heart disease, drug overdose) or severe tachyarrhythmias. Diastolic failure can result from primary cardiac disease such as hypertrophic or restrictive cardiomyopathy. Obstructive shock is the result of occlusion of either forward flow or venous return, as seen in pericardial tamponade, tension pneumothorax, thromboembolic disease, tumors, or distended organs (e.g., gastric dilatation and volvulus). Obstructive disease and systolic and diastolic dysfunction all lead to decreased cardiac output, hypotension, and reduced coronary blood flow. Neurohormonal compensatory mechanisms such as catecholamine release and salt and water retention worsen the situation by increasing myocardial oxygen demand and afterload, thus creating a downward spiral of cardiac function and systemic perfusion.

Distributive shock is a condition in which the systemic vascular resistance (SVR) is abnormal causing a maldistribution of blood flow. Distributive shock is most commonly associated with decreased SVR; however, there may also be regional vasoconstriction and endothelial dysfunction that cause sluggish capillary blood flow and arteriovenous shunting, both of which are forms of maldistribution of blood flow. The classic example of distributive shock (commonly referred to as *vasodilatory shock*) is septic shock. Other vasodilatory states, however, can also lead to distributive shock, such as systemic inflammatory response syndrome (SIRS), adverse drug reactions or overdose, anaphylaxis, heat stroke, and neurogenic shock. Sepsis and heat stroke are both complicated by a vigorous systemic inflammatory response and further compromise of tissue oxygenation due to maldistribution of blood flow (i.e., arteriovenous shunting) and microcirculatory and mitochondrial dysfunction.

Hypoxemic shock is caused by decreased blood oxygen content. Examples of diseases associated hypoxemic shock include anemia, methemoglobinemia, carbon monoxide poisoning, hypoventilation, and pulmonary parenchymal disease. Despite normal blood volume and blood pressure, an animal can display cardinal signs of shock secondary to severely decreased blood oxygen content.

Metabolic shock is caused by deranged cellular metabolism that, as in all shock states, leads to decreased cellular energy production. Examples of altered cellular metabolism might include cyanide and bromethalin toxicity (both cause direct interference with mitochondrial function and ATP production), severe hypoglycemia, relative adrenal insufficiency, and severe pH derangements. In addition to the vasomotor abnormalities of septic shock, there is a component of metabolic shock, and it is thought that there is an acquired defect in oxidative phosphorylation that causes decreased cellular energy production (called *cytopathic hypoxia*).[2]

The categories of shock are not mutually exclusive, and many animals with distributive shock will also have some degree of hypovolemia, particularly as SIRS leads to increased vascular permeability and fluid loss. Mediators of SIRS and ischemia reperfusion injury include substances that contribute to cardiac dysfunction. Thus progression of both distributive and hypovolemic shock can lead to cardiogenic shock. Cardiogenic shock can cause hypoxemic shock when complicated by pulmonary edema. Any animal with inadequate intestinal perfusion may develop bacterial translocation and sepsis. Unrecognized, untreated shock initiates a cascade of doom. Therefore, early recognition based on index of suspicion, aggressive monitoring of patients at risk, and appropriate interventions are essential for successful treatment of shock states.

HOST RESPONSE

To a large degree, the host's systemic response to the inciting cause of shock determines the course of the syndrome.[3] There may be genetic and immune factors that play a role in how the host responds to the insult. This is most clearly demonstrated in septic shock, where the cascade of events that leads

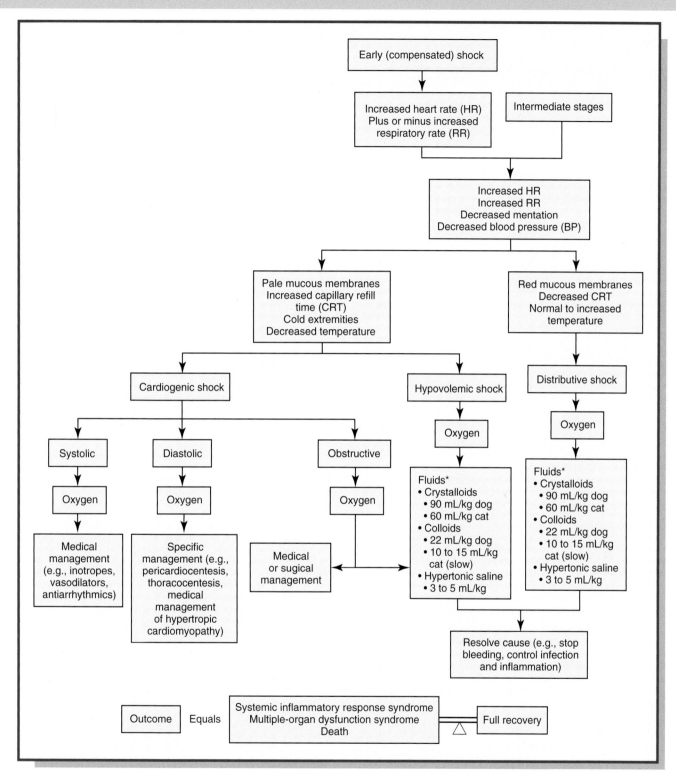

Figure 139-1 Algorithm for assessment and treatment of shock. *, When administering fluids for shock, ¼ to ⅓ a shock volume is administered over 5 to 15 minutes, with repeated evaluations of cardiovascular response.

to irreversible cardiovascular collapse is the systemic inflammatory response initiated by products of infectious agents. It has been recognized that SIRS can also be triggered by noninfectious insults including tissue hypoxia, tissue acidosis, pancreatitis, trauma, and major surgery. Similarly, although hypovolemia can be reversed, reperfusion of ischemic tissues leads to inflammation and production and release of inflammatory mediators. These complex cascades confound the treatment of shock, since reversing the perfusion abnormalities may not stop the progression once the inflammatory cascade has been initiated. Treatment directed at the downstream cellular mediators of shock has not proven beneficial either. No matter what type, one of the most successful approaches to the treatment of shock is early recognition and correction of the inciting cause before the cascade of inflammation is triggered.

STAGES AND CLINICAL SIGNS

Shock is a dynamic state and the clinical condition can change quickly. The normal physiologic response to shock is to increase sympathetic tone, which causes vasoconstriction and increases in both heart and respiratory rates. In the early (sometimes called *compensated*) stages of shock, tachycardia may be the only clinical sign. Patients in the early, compensated stages of shock may also show normal or mildly decreased mentation; normal, pale, or hyperemic mucous membranes; tachypnea; strong pulse quality; and normotension. Early stages of shock may not be clinically obvious, as compensatory mechanisms are recruited to maintain cardiac output and tissue perfusion. With time and progression to the intermediate stages (also referred to as *early decompensated shock*), profound vasoconstriction results from the attempt to increase venous return and maintain stroke volume. In the intermediate stages, additional compensatory mechanisms trigger an increase in salt and water retention (i.e., the renin-angiotensin-aldosterone system and antidiuretic hormone) and release of vasoconstrictors (e.g., vasopressin) in an effort to increase cardiac output and redistribute blood flow to vital organs. Organ dysfunction appears, and most patients in this progressive stage of shock will die without intervention. Patients in the intermediate stages of shock will show pale mucous membranes and prolonged capillary refill time (CRT); tachycardia, poor pulse quality, and hypotension; decreased mentation and weakness; tachypnea; cool extremities; and decreased rectal temperature. In late stages of shock (also referred to as late *decompensated* or *irreversible shock*), compensatory mechanisms fail and systemic inflammation leads to multiple organ failure and death. Successful clinical intervention is uncommon. Patients in the late stages of shock will show stupor or coma; pale mucous membranes with prolonged or absent CRT; bradycardia; hypothermia; and poor to absent pulse quality. This chapter will focus on the clinical presentations associated with the major types of shock in the early and intermediate stages.

With the exception of early distributive shock, clinical signs of shock (as described above) are similar regardless of the type or its etiology. A hallmark clinical sign of all types of shock is mental dullness, especially as shock progresses beyond the early compensated state. In contrast, the hallmark of distributive shock is the failure of effective vasoconstriction, secondary to circulating mediators that interfere with vascular tone. This failure leads to relative hypovolemia; this is most commonly seen with distributive shock secondary to sepsis. Accordingly, the clinical signs include red mucous membranes, rapid CRT (<1 second), normal or increased rectal temperature, tachycardia, tachypnea, bounding pulses, hypotension, and depressed mentation. Distributive shock that is complicated by concurrent fluid loss (due to changes in vascular permeability and fluid compartment shifts or the underlying etiology) may initially be associated with clinical signs more typical of hypovolemic shock, but upon resuscitation, clinical signs of distributive shock may develop. One other unique feature of septic shock is that cats frequently become bradycardic rather than tachycardic.

In order to differentiate cardiogenic shock from all other forms of shock that would require fluid therapy, careful heart auscultation, an electrocardiogram, and a thorough physical examination are required. Chest radiographs and cardiac ultrasound are beneficial; however, animals in shock are frequently not stable enough to obtain extensive diagnostic tests.

Emergency treatment can (and should) be initiated based on physical examination and historical findings.

TREATMENT AND MONITORING

The goal of treatment in early shock is to restore effective tissue perfusion and oxygenation.[4-6] In later stages of shock, restoration of perfusion alone is usually insufficient to halt the progression of the inflammatory cascade. Aggressive support of organ function and prevention of additional proinflammatory stimuli (including hypotension, hypoxia, and infection) are critical. At all stages, correction of the inciting cause is necessary.

Oxygen is universally administered regardless of the type of shock. Additional therapy depends on the etiology of the shock. For most forms of shock, except systolic and diastolic forms of cardiogenic shock, fluid therapy is essential and the goal is to increase the effective circulating volume. The choice of fluids depends on the cause of shock; however, crystalloids (isotonic-balanced electrolyte solutions) or colloids are typically used for initial treatment. The fluid rate and the actual volume given should be tailored to each individual animal. A shock volume of isotonic crystalloid fluid is considered to be equivalent to a blood volume of approximately 90 mL/kg in the dog and 60 mL/kg in the cat. Typically, $\frac{1}{4}$ to $\frac{1}{3}$ of a shock volume is provided within the first 5 to 15 minutes, with repeated evaluation of the cardiovascular response (e.g., heart rate, mucous membrane color, pulse quality, blood pressure, and CRT). Colloids should be used for shock resuscitation of hypoproteinemic animals; they may also be used to hasten resuscitation of large animals where the time taken to administer the required large volume of crystalloid fluids may be too long and, therefore, life-threatening. The same general principles apply to resuscitation using colloids (i.e., giving fractions of shock doses at a time) but the volumes are smaller (5 to 20 mL/kg bolus in dogs, and 3 to15 mL/kg bolus in cats). Synthetic colloids have been associated with prolongations in clotting times at doses of greater than 20 mL/kg in 24 hours but this effect is unpredictable.

Hypertonic solutions (e.g., 7.2% to 7.5% saline) are quite effective at rapidly expanding the intravascular space; however, this crystalloid fluid rapidly redistributes to the extravascular space and should be combined with a colloid to lengthen the effect on the intravascular space. In order to make a hypertonic solution that contains colloid, 23% saline is diluted with a synthetic colloid such as hydroxyethyl starch to a final concentration of 7.2% to 7.5%, which can be given as a 3- to 5-mL/kg (dog) or 2- to 3-mL/kg (cat) bolus over 5 to 15 minutes. Never administer undiluted 23% saline to a patient because it will cause hemolysis and phlebitis. As with colloids, the small volumes of hypertonic solutions required may be particularly beneficial in larger animals in which volumes of crystalloid fluids are rate limiting. Because of the recruitment of water from the intracellular to the intravascular space, hypertonic saline may also be beneficial in animals with hypovolemic shock and concurrent brain injury. It is relatively contraindicated in patients who are interstitially dehydrated or are already hypernatremic (which signifies intracellular dehydration). It is contraindicated in patients with preexisting hyponatremia due to the risk of the rapid rate of serum sodium rise causing osmotic demyelinization syndrome.

The resuscitative fluid of choice for hemorrhagic hypovolemic shock is blood. Administration of 1 mL/kg of packed red blood cells or 2 mL/kg of whole blood will raise the hematocrit by approximately 1%. Massive transfusions (greater than one blood volume in 24 hours or greater than

½ blood volume in 3 hours) may be required in some cases (see Chapter 142). Expected side effects of massive transfusions include thrombocytopenia, ionized hypocalcemia, and coagulopathy.

In systolic and diastolic forms of cardiogenic shock and in hypoxemic shock due to lung injury, aggressive fluid therapy may be fatal. Treatment of cardiogenic shock relies on correction of the underlying cause. Treatment with antiarrhythmics, diuretics, vasodilators, or inotropes may be required (see Chapter 126). In obstructive shock, fluid therapy is often required. Resolution of obstruction to flow may require physical intervention (e.g., surgery for tumors and gastric dilation and volvulus) or medical management (e.g., thrombolytics for thromboembolic disease). Prior to intervention, adequate circulatory volume and optimal perfusion must be established.

Specific therapy should be directed at the cause of shock. For example, in hemorrhagic hypovolemia, bleeding must be controlled, and in septic shock the source of infection must be eliminated. Vasopressors may be required when hypotension persists despite adequate volume repletion. Detailed discussion of sepsis can be found in Chapter 138. Despite over 30 years of investigation, most specific antiinflammatory therapies have generally failed in clinical trials of shock and sepsis. Although long touted for beneficial effects in shock, there is absolutely no clinical evidence to support the use of pharmacologic doses of glucocorticoids in the treatment of any form of shock; however, there may be a place for physiologic replacement in cases where relative adrenal insufficiency is suspected or diagnosed.[7]

Monitoring is critical during the resuscitation of shock. In addition to monitoring routine physical cardiovascular parameters (e.g., heart rate, mucous membrane color, pulse quality, CRT, respiratory rate, temperature, mentation), monitoring blood pressure, hematocrit, electrolytes, blood gases, urine output, central venous pressure, body weight, blood pH, base excess, and lactate provides invaluable information to aid in determination of volume status and guide fluid resuscitation. More advanced macrohemodynamic monitoring that may be beneficial in managing the shock patient includes invasive or noninvasive cardiac output monitoring to derive more direct information about volume status, oxygen delivery, and oxygen extraction. It is important to note that microcirculatory abnormalities (arteriovenous shunting, uneven tissue oxygen extraction, platelet and leukocyte aggregation) may be present despite the macrohemodynamic parameters being normal. This may result in pathologic oxygen supply limitation and further tissue hypoxia. It is possible to visualize the microcirculation (e.g., using side stream darkfield imaging); further understanding and characterization of microcirculatory abnormalities may, in the future, help to direct treatments aimed at resuscitation of the microcirculation.

In humans, the use of venous oximetry (i.e., continuous monitoring of mixed [SvO_2] or central [$ScvO_2$] venous oxygen saturation) has proven to be a useful guide to resuscitative therapy, because it can be seen as a global reflection of the tissue oxygen supply-to-demand relationship. SvO_2 is pathologically decreased (below 65% to 70%) when oxygen delivery is decreased (e.g., decreased cardiac output, anemia, hypoxemia) or when oxygen consumption is increased. Mixed venous oxygen saturation can be pathologically increased in states of decreased tissue oxygen consumption (e.g., cytopathic hypoxia, microvascular shunting) or increased oxygen delivery (e.g., increased cardiac output in the hyperdynamic phase of septic shock).

REFERENCES

The reference list can be found on the companion Expert Consult Web site at *www.expertconsult.com*.

CHAPTER **140**

Systemic Anaphylaxis

Lori S. Waddell

Systemic anaphylaxis is an acute, life-threatening allergic reaction resulting from massive, generalized release of mast cell mediators, including histamine. Anaphylaxis can be triggered by venoms from insects and reptiles; medications such as hormones, antibiotics, nonsteroidal antiinflammatory drugs, anesthetics, and sedatives; parasiticides; and other miscellaneous drugs and foods (Box 140-1). Immediate recognition and treatment of anaphylaxis in a dog or cat is essential for a successful outcome.

PATHOGENESIS

Hypersensitivity reactions are classified as one of four types, depending on immunologic response: type I, immediate (immunoglobulin E [IgE] dependent); type II, cytotoxic (IgG, IgM dependent); type III, immune complex (IgG or IgM complex dependent); and type IV, delayed (T lymphocyte dependent). Anaphylaxis can be caused by either an anaphylactic or anaphylactoid reaction. Anaphylactoid and anaphylactic reactions have exactly the same clinical appearance and are treated identically. Anaphylaxis is defined as a type I, IgE-mediated hypersensitivity reaction with an interaction of antigen and IgE antibody on the surface of sensitized mast cells. This interaction causes the release of histamine and other inflammatory mediators. Sensitization requires previous exposure to an antigen or hapten, which can range in size from a protein to a small, low–molecular weight drug. Proteins act directly as an antigen, while the smaller drugs will bind to cells and act as haptens. IgE is produced by and bound on the surface of mast cells and basophils by high-affinity receptors (FcεRI) for the Fc portion of the immunoglobulin. When an antigen causes cross-linkage of two surface IgE molecules, the mast cell is activated and primary and secondary mediators are released (Table 140-1).

The cross-linking of the FcεRI receptors activates tyrosine kinases, which cause activation of phospholipase C, leading to production of diacylglycerol and inositol triphosphate. These mediators increase intracellular calcium concentrations

Box • 140-1

Causes of Anaphylaxis

Venoms
Insects of the Hymenoptera order—bees, wasps, ants
Spiders—black widow, brown recluse
Lizards—Gila monster, Mexican beaded lizard
Snakes—pit vipers (rattlesnakes, copperheads, water moccasins),
    coral snakes

Hormones
Insulin
Corticotropin
Vasopressin
Parathyroid hormone
Betamethasone
Triamcinolone
Glucocorticoids

Antibiotics
Penicillins—amoxicillin, ampicillin, procaine penicillin
Chloramphenicol
Lincomycin
Gentamicin
Tetracycline
Sulfonamides
Cephalosporins
Polymyxin B
Doxorubicin hydrochloride

Nonsteroidal Antiinflammatory Drugs
Aspirin
Ibuprofen

Anesthetics and Sedatives
Acepromazine maleate
Ketamine hydrochloride
Barbiturates
Lidocaine and other local anesthetics
Narcotics
Diazepam

Parasiticides
Dichlorophen
Levamisole hydrochloride
Piperazine
Dichlorvos
Diethylcarbamazine
Thiacetarsemide

Miscellaneous
Blood products
Aminophylline
Asparaginase
Calcium disodium edetate
Iodinated contrast media
Neostigmine
Amphotericin B
Vaccines
Allergen extracts—pollens, molds, foods
Enzymes—chymotrypsin and trypsin
Vitamins—vitamin K, thiamine, and folic acid
Dextrans and gelatins

Foods
Milk
Egg white
Shellfish
Legumes
Fruits—citrus
Chocolate
Grains

Physical Factors
Cold
Heat
Exercise

and activate multiple protein kinases. Phosphorylation of myosin, found in intracellular filaments, causes granules to move to the cell surface, fuse, and release the primary mediators of anaphylaxis: histamine, heparin, tryptase, kallikreins, proteases, proteoglycans, eosinophilic chemotactic factor of anaphylaxis (ECF-A), and neutrophil chemotactic factor of anaphylaxis (NCF-A). Cross-linking of the FcεRI receptors also activates phospholipase A_2, which produces arachidonic acid from membrane phospholipids, resulting in release of the secondary mediators: leukotrienes, prostaglandins, thromboxanes, and platelet-activating factor. The protein kinases also alter gene expression, causing synthesis and secretion of other cytokines (interleukin-4 [IL-4], IL-5, IL-6, IL-13, tumor necrosis factor-α, macrophage inflammatory protein-1α), responsible for the late-phase inflammatory response. Release of the inflammatory mediators is rapid: granule exocytosis occurs within seconds to minutes, activation of the arachidonic acid cascade in minutes, and cytokine synthesis and secretion within 2 to 24 hours.

Anaphylactoid reactions cause anaphylaxis without IgE, either through directly activating mast cells to release histamine or, more commonly, by activating the complement pathway. They do not require previous exposure and sensitization. Activation of complement results in production of C3a and C5a, the anaphylatoxins, which causes degranulation of mast cells and release of histamine and other primary mediators, activation of the arachidonic acid cascade, and gene expression and synthesis of the inflammatory mediators.

Both anaphylactoid and anaphylactic types of reactions result in hypovolemia and vasodilation, potentially leading to severe hypovolemic shock. Histamine and the leukotrienes are potent vasodilators and increase vascular permeability, allowing leakage of protein and fluid into the interstitial space. There are three types of histamine receptors that contribute to the signs seen during anaphylaxis. Activation of H_1 receptors results in pruritus and bronchoconstriction and stimulates endothelial cells to produce nitric oxide, a potent vasodilator

Table • 140-1

Mediators of Inflammation in Anaphylaxis

MEDIATORS	EFFECTS
Primary	
Histamine	Increased vascular permeability, vasodilation, constriction of smooth muscle of bronchi and GI tract, increased mucus production
Proteases	Kinin production, activation of complement, initiation of disseminated intravascular coagulation
Heparin	Anticoagulation, urticaria, immune modulation
ECF-A	Eosinophil chemotaxis
NCF-A	Neutrophil chemotaxis
Secondary	
Prostaglandin E_2	Vasodilation, increased vascular permeability
Prostaglandin D_2	Bronchoconstriction, increased vascular permeability, pulmonary vasconstriction, peripheral vasodilation
Prostacyclin	Vasodilation, inhibition of platelet aggregation
Leukotrienes	Bronchoconstriction, increased vascular permeability, vasodilation, increased WBC chemotaxis
Thromboxane A_2	Increased platelet aggregation, smooth muscle contraction
Platelet-activating factor	Platelet aggregation, platelet sequestration, increased platelet thromboxane production, increased vascular permeability, vasoconstriction, and bronchoconstriction

ECF-A, Eosinophilic chemotactic factor of anaphylaxis; *GI*, gastrointestinal; *NCF-A*, neutrophil chemotactic factor of anaphylaxis; *WBC*, white blood cell.

that significantly contributes to hypotension. H_1 receptors also mediate coronary artery vasoconstriction and cardiac depression. H_2 receptors stimulate gastric acid production, as well as cause coronary artery and systemic vasodilation and increase heart rate and contractility. H_3 receptors are located on presynaptic terminals of sympathetic effector nerves that innervate the heart and systemic vasculature and inhibit endogenous norepinephrine release from sympathetic nerves.[1] Activation of the H_3 receptors results in worsened signs of anaphylactic shock because it inhibits normal compensatory sympathetic responses.

CLINICAL MANIFESTATIONS

Anaphylaxis can result in hypotension, bronchospasm, urticaria, erythema, pruritus, pharyngeal and laryngeal edema, arrhythmias, vomiting, and hyperperistalsis. Clinical signs are dependent on species and method of exposure. In dogs, the liver is considered the shock organ, and clinical signs result

from hepatic vein congestion and portal hypertension. Initial signs may include excitement, vomiting, defecation (often diarrhea), then progress to respiratory distress, collapse secondary to hypovolemic shock, and death within 1 hour if not treated. A dog with anaphylaxis may have generalized wheals, angioedema (particularly of the face), pruritus (Web Figure 140-1), pale mucous membranes, poor capillary refill time, tachycardia, poor pulse quality, and appear depressed or even collapsed. Severe cases may result in respiratory distress secondary to upper airway obstruction from laryngeal and pharyngeal edema.

In cats, the lungs are considered the shock organ, and respiratory distress is the first sign in cats with systemic anaphylaxis. Respiratory distress results from airway obstruction secondary to laryngeal edema, bronchoconstriction, and increased mucus production. Other signs in cats include severe pruritus, vomiting, diarrhea, depression, and death. On physical examination, a cat in anaphylactic shock usually will be in severe respiratory distress, have wheezes on auscultation, and have pale mucous membranes, poor capillary refill time, and poor pulse quality.

The most severe anaphylactic reactions are generally seen if the antigen is given by parental injection. Oral ingestion often causes vomiting, diarrhea, urticaria, and angioedema. Inhalation can result in rhinitis and bronchospasm. Topical administrations can cause conjunctivitis and urticaria with or without systemic signs. In general, patients that have the most rapid onset of clinical signs after exposure to an antigen develop the most severe signs of anaphylactic shock.

DIAGNOSIS

Diagnosis of systemic anaphylaxis is based on the history of exposure and peracute onset of clinical signs. Clinical signs often occur within seconds to minutes of exposure. Oral exposure can cause a delay of up to 30 minutes or longer before clinical signs appear.

TREATMENT

Initial treatment of a dog or cat with anaphylaxis consists of the basics of emergency medicine and the administration of epinephrine. These basics include ensuring that the dog or cat has a patent airway and is effectively breathing/ventilating. The veterinarian should address cardiovascular dysfunction and treat with drugs and/or fluids as indicated. Dogs or cats having an anaphylactic reaction may have respiratory distress resulting from upper airway obstruction. The clinician should be prepared to intubate with an endotracheal tube or perform a tracheostomy if intubation is not possible. If respiratory distress without airway obstruction is present, oxygen should be administered by mask or flow-by during initial assessment and stabilization, and then by nasal catheter or oxygen cage. Vascular access is essential for treatment, both for fluid administration and medications. Hypovolemic shock is a significant contributor to morbidity and mortality in anaphylaxis. Hypovolemia occurs secondary to increased vascular permeability and venous pooling. Fluid therapy, often starting with a shock bolus of crystalloids at a dose of 90 mL/kg in dogs and 60 mL/kg in cats, is indicated. Ongoing crystalloid therapy will be necessary at rates higher than maintenance to keep up with ongoing losses and will need to be tailored to the individual patient. Additional fluid therapy may include a synthetic colloid such as hetastarch, given in small, incremental boluses of 5 to 10 mL/kg in dogs and 3 to 6 mL/kg in cats. A constant rate infusion (CRI) of synthetic colloids of 1 mL/kg/hr may also be used once the patient has been resuscitated. If a coagulopathy is present, blood products, especially fresh frozen plasma, may be necessary. This should be given at a dose of 10 to 20 mL/kg over several hours (or faster if needed for volume resuscitation). Fluid therapy is guided by clinical parameters including heart rate, pulse quality, mucous membrane color, capillary refill time, respiratory rate and effort, and packed cell volume (PCV) and total solids.

Epinephrine is the mainstay of therapy for treatment of systemic anaphylaxis. Traditionally, a dose of 0.01 mg/kg of the 1:10,000 solution given slowly IV is recommended, although 0.02 mg/kg can be given into the trachea if the patient is intubated and IV access cannot be obtained. Epinephrine can also be administered SQ or IM at a dose of 0.01 mg/kg in less severe cases. Epinephrine is useful because of its inotropic and chronotropic effects on the heart. Epinephrine also causes bronchodilation and increased intracellular concentrations of cyclic adenosine monophosphate, which decreases synthesis and release of inflammatory mediators of anaphylaxis. A single dose of epinephrine given IV, IM, or SQ after maximal hypotension had developed did not produce a sustained improvement in hemodynamic parameters in a study on dogs with induced anaphylactic shock. Only the IV dose produced a transient improvement (less than 15 minutes) in mean arterial pressure, stroke volume, and pulmonary wedge pressure.[2] A recent study of induced anaphylaxis in dogs showed that administration of epinephrine by CRI was the only route that caused sustained improvement in hemodynamic parameters compared to the nontreatment group and the groups that received a bolus given IV, SQ, or IM.[3] The dose used for the CRI was 0.05 μg/kg/min. These studies suggest that epinephrine is acting primarily as a pressor rather than specifically improving immunologic recovery. Consideration should be given to administering epinephrine as a CRI rather than an IV bolus, but further studies need to be completed. Heart rate, rhythm, and blood pressure should be monitored when giving epinephrine, especially IV, because of its ability to cause arrhythmias and hypertension (at high doses). Epinephrine and fluid therapy should begin to improve clinical signs within minutes. Dogs and cats ideally will be fully stabilized within an hour.

Other medications that may be useful in the treatment of systemic anaphylaxis include pressors, glucocorticoids, antihistamines, aminophylline, and atropine. Dopamine at a dose of 4 to 10 μg/kg/min or other pressors may be used if refractory hypotension is present. Aminophylline may be used if bronchoconstriction is refractory to epinephrine. It will cause bronchodilation, increase respiratory drive, and increase con-

tractility of the muscles of respiration. A dose of 10 mg/kg IV for dogs and 5 mg/kg IV for cats is recommended. Atropine at a dose of 0.02 to 0.04 mg/kg IV or IM should be used if bradycardia is present despite epinephrine administration. Glucocorticoids are useful in blocking the arachidonic acid cascade and reducing the severity of the late-phase anaphylactic reactions. Doses of 1 to 2 mg/kg IV for dexamethasone have been recommended unless the patient has developed anaphylaxis from administration of one of the glucocorticoids, as cross-reaction may occur. It is essential that glucocorticoids not be used in place of epinephrine in the emergency situation because they have little effect on the immediate stages of anaphylaxis. Antihistamines competitively bind at the histamine receptors and block its effects. Diphenhydramine, an H_1 blocker, should be administered at 0.5 to 1.0 mg/kg slow IV or IM to reduce pruritus and angioedema. The H_2 blockers such as ranitidine at 1 mg/kg IV or famotidine at 0.5 mg/kg IV can be used to decrease gastric acid secretion stimulated by histamine. These antihistamines are not very useful in the acute, life-threatening stage of anaphylaxis, but may be helpful after a dog or cat has been stabilized. In one study, pretreatment of dogs with the experimental H_3 blocker thioperamide maleate resulted in increased heart rate and improved left ventricular stroke work, but its clinical usefulness in naturally occurring anaphylaxis after the onset of signs remains to be determined.[1]

Intense monitoring of a dog or cat for at least 12 to 24 hours after the anaphylactic episode is essential. This should include respiratory rate and effort, heart rate and rhythm, blood pressure, pulse oximetry and/or arterial blood gases, coagulation parameters, renal and hepatic function, PCV, total solids, and glucose. Other supportive care, such as ventilatory support, should be provided as needed. Avoidance of the trigger for anaphylaxis is prudent in the future. Careful questioning of the owner about recent exposure to insects, reptiles, foods, topical therapies, and medications and prevention of reexposure is essential. Prognosis for a patient presenting with systemic anaphylaxis is variable. The earlier the patient receives appropriate therapy, the better the prognosis. This is especially important since death can ensue in 1 hour or less from time of exposure.

REFERENCES

The reference list can be found on the companion Expert Consult Web site at *www.expertconsult.com*.

CHAPTER 141

Thoracic Trauma

Matthew W. Beal

Trauma to the thorax can be classified as blunt or penetrating. Blunt thoracic trauma commonly occurs after motor vehicle accidents, falls from a height, human–animal interactions, and dog bites. Dog bites are also a commonly recognized cause of penetrating thoracic trauma along with gunshot wounds and impalement injuries. Independent of the cause of the trauma, it is critical for veterinarians to

recognize that trauma is most commonly a multisystemic problem (polytrauma). This necessitates attention to the entire animal. Similarly, injuries to the thorax are rarely isolated and more commonly are identified in combination (e.g., pneumothorax and pulmonary contusion). Keys to maximizing the likelihood of a positive outcome in dogs and cats with thoracic trauma include thorough physical examinations, anticipation of common injuries, understanding the pathophysiology of those injuries, and a proactive method to their identification and treatment.

TRAUMA-ASSOCIATED PLEURAL SPACE PATHOLOGY

Trauma-associated pleural space pathology includes pneumothorax, hemothorax, and diaphragmatic hernia. As a group, these injuries are most likely to manifest with varying degrees of dyspnea accompanied by muffled lung and heart sounds on auscultation of the thorax. Differentiating these injuries will be largely based on a thorough physical examination and aided by thoracocentesis and diagnostic imaging techniques.

Pneumothorax is the accumulation of air in the pleural space between the parietal and visceral pleurae and is one of the two most commonly recognized results of traumatic injury to the thorax. Traumatic pneumothorax is classified as "closed" or "open." Closed pneumothorax most often results from rapid compression of the thorax (and lungs) against a closed glottis resulting in alveolar disruption. Additional causes of closed pneumothorax include laceration of the lung by a broken rib, rupture of bullae or blebs, or pneumomediastinum. Air enters the pleural space from an injury to the thoracic wall in cases of "open" pneumothorax. Tension pneumothorax occurs due to a one-way–valve effect, in which air enters the pleural space during inspiration and cannot be evacuated during expiration. The resultant increase in intrapleural pressure results in hypoventilation and decreased venous return, manifesting with signs of severe respiratory and cardiovascular compromise.

Appropriate management of the traumatized small animal necessitates the assumption that *pneumothorax is present until proven otherwise. Clinically significant pneumothorax is a physical examination diagnosis.* Most animals with pneumothorax prefer to stand or to position themselves in sternal recumbency. In this position, on auscultation, decreased lung sounds are most likely to be noted dorsally and in both hemithoraces. Temporary relief and definitive diagnosis of pneumothorax is based on oxygen administration and bilateral thoracocentesis (see Chapter 107). Radiography for the diagnosis of clinically significant pneumothorax may jeopardize the stability of a traumatized dog or cat and should be avoided until patient stability has been achieved (Figure 141-1).

Often, bilateral thoracocentesis is sufficient treatment for traumatic closed pneumothorax. However, if pneumothorax recurs (sometimes rapidly), thoracostomy tube placement and continuous pleural space drainage are recommended (see Chapter 107). Closed traumatic pneumothorax is rarely a condition that requires surgical intervention. Open pneumothorax warrants immediate anesthetic induction using cardiovascular-sparing agents to facilitate intubation. Positive pressure ventilation (PPV) is then initiated to support the respiratory system while injuries are managed. Alternatively, the wound may be covered with an occlusive dressing and the thorax evacuated by thoracocentesis or thoracostomy tube placement. Once stability has been achieved, open pneumothorax is always managed surgically (see Penetrating Thoracic Injury).

Hemothorax is the accumulation of blood in the pleural space. Hemothorax results from disruption of pulmonary, thoracic wall, or mediastinal blood vessels. Hemothorax can also be seen in dogs and cats with diaphragmatic hernia and concurrent hemoabdomen. *Clinically significant hemothorax (although uncommon) is a physical examination diagnosis.* Hemothorax results in decreased lung and heart sounds ventrally to diffusely and concurrent signs of hypovolemic shock

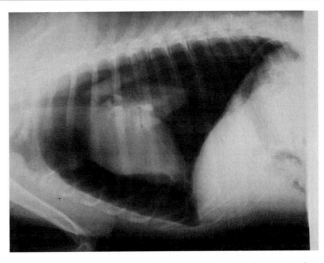

Figure 141-1 Radiograph of a dog with pneumothorax. Radiographic evidence of pneumothorax includes retraction of the lung from the chest wall (loss of vascular markings in this space), consolidation of lung lobes, and on lateral radiographs, the appearance of the heart "floating" on a cushion of air. The latter radiographic finding is due to collapse of the heart to the side of the atelectatic lung lobe.

(pale mucous membranes, slow capillary refill time [CRT], high pulse rate, weak pulses) and dyspnea. Diagnosis of a clinically significant hemothorax, much like pneumothorax, is based on thoracocentesis. In addition, oxygen support and vigorous volume expansion techniques are always indicated as part of the initial treatment strategy for dogs and cats with hemothorax. Thoracostomy tube placement (see Chapter 107) and continuous pleural drainage is indicated when greater than 5 mL/kg of blood is retrieved from the pleural space. Continuous drainage allows quantification of ongoing blood loss, prevention of atelectasis, and autotransfusion of shed blood. Radiographs may be performed after patient stabilization and evacuation of the pleural space (Web Figure 141-1).

Diaphragmatic hernia is most often recognized after blunt thoracic trauma and is thought to result from rapid compression of the abdomen with the majority of the force directed cranially. Penetrating thoracic and abdominal injuries can also cause diaphragmatic hernia. The dog or cat with diaphragmatic hernia may not show clinical signs or may have dyspnea, decreased lungs sounds ventrally to diffusely, borborygmi on auscultation of the thorax, an "empty" abdominal palpation, or a combination thereof. Diaphragmatic hernia is commonly associated with pleural effusion. Some dogs and cats may develop clinical signs of diaphragmatic hernia months to years after the initial trauma. Oxygen support will be beneficial in the initial stabilization of animals with diaphragmatic hernia. In addition, positioning the pet with the chest slightly higher than the abdomen may promote movement of mobile abdominal viscera back into the abdomen. Diaphragmatic hernia may be suspected on physical examination but is confirmed through diagnostic imaging techniques (survey radiographs [Web Figure 141-2], positional radiographs, positive contrast peritoneography, upper gastrointestinal contrast studies, ultrasound, or computed tomography).

Diaphragmatic hernia is a surgical problem that necessitates elective repair as soon as the respiratory and cardiovascular systems have been stabilized. Indications for immediate surgical intervention include fever, small bowel obstruction, biliary obstruction, protracted vomiting, or a distended stomach within the pleural space. In the latter clinical syndrome, transthoracic gastrocentesis or orogastric intubation are indicated prior to anesthesia to relieve signs of dyspnea. Prognosis for survival of dogs and cats with diaphragmatic hernia is approximately 90%.[1]

TRAUMA-ASSOCIATED PULMONARY INJURIES

Pulmonary contusion (PC) refers to lung lesions that occur after a compression-decompression injury. Subsequent hemorrhage and edema lead to alveolar collapse and lung consolidation.[2-4] Hypoxemia results from ventilation: perfusion mismatch, shunt, diffusion impairment, and in severe cases, hypoventilation. Much like pneumothorax, pulmonary contusion is common after trauma. *All dogs that have sustained trauma have PC until proven otherwise. The presence of clinically significant PC (severe enough to cause clinical signs) is a physical examination diagnosis.* On auscultation of the thorax, increased lung sounds distributed unevenly between the hemithoraces are most commonly recognized. However, exceptions include the presence of concurrent pleural space disease and complete lobar consolidation, both of which may result in decreased lung sounds. Coughing and hemoptysis may be seen in dogs with moderate to severe PC. Small animals with rib fractures or flail chest often have concurrent PC. Radiographic evidence of PC includes interstitial to alveolar infiltrates and lobar consolidation (Web Figure 141-3). Initial therapy for PC is oxygen support to maintain oxygen saturation above 92%. Severity of PC can be quantified through arterial blood gas analysis and calculation of alveolar-arterial oxygen gradient and the $PaO_2:FiO_2$.

Treatment of PC is largely supportive.[2-4] The cornerstones of therapy include oxygen delivery by cage, hood, or nasal cannulae to maintain SpO_2 greater than 92% on FiO_2 less than 0.60 without severe increases in respiratory effort. Often overlooked is the importance of frequent changes in position of the animal. Standing and short walks may prevent and combat atelectasis. PPV is indicated if oxygenation or ventilation requirements cannot be met or if they can only be met with severe increases in respiratory effort. Fluid therapy in the animal with PC is challenging. Basic guidelines include maintenance of euvolemia in light of concurrent injuries, maintenance of hydration, and efforts to avoid fluid overload. Despite numerous opinions, there is no clear answer to the question of whether crystalloid or colloid therapy is most appropriate for dogs with PC. In one study, corticosteroids were not shown to decrease duration of hospitalization or oxygen support.[2] Because PC is associated with increased vascular permeability, furosemide is unlikely to be of benefit unless iatrogenic fluid overload has taken place. Bronchodilators are also unlikely to be of benefit because PC is not a reactive small airway disease, and antibiotics are not indicated because of the exceedingly low incidence of bacterial pneumonia in dogs with PC. Prognosis for dogs with PC is based on severity of pulmonary injury but is generally good.[2] Dogs that require PPV to maintain oxygenation and adequate ventilation have a more guarded prognosis.[2,5]

TRAUMA-ASSOCIATED THORACIC WALL INJURIES

Thoracic wall trauma is most often associated with a host of concurrent thoracic injuries such as pneumothorax and pulmonary contusion.

Penetrating Thoracic Injury
Wounds to the thorax should be immediately covered with an occlusive sterile dressing. Broad-spectrum antibiotic therapy should be initiated as soon as possible to combat bacterial infection. Antibiotic therapy should be empirical, based on likely contaminants while cultures (acquired during surgery) are pending. Following stabilization and management of concurrent injuries (please see discussion of pneumothorax above) and radiography, the dog or cat should be placed under general anesthesia and the wounds explored. Simple probing is *not* adequate to determine whether wounds have penetrated the pleural space. Penetrating thoracic wounds should be explored, debrided, lavaged, cultured, and reconstructed with use of appropriate drainage techniques. The external wound in animals with penetrating thoracic injury is often the "tip of the iceberg" and necessitates an aggressive, proactive approach to maximize the likelihood of a favorable outcome.

Rib Fractures
Rib fractures happen with variable frequency after trauma and are diagnosed based on physical examination and/or thoracic radiography. Pain is the primary problem induced by rib fractures; however, penetration of the visceral pleura by a broken rib could result in pneumothorax and/or hemothorax. The chest wall is a resilient structure that requires significant force to cause a fracture. When such forces are applied across the thorax, intrathoracic injury is common. *Rib fractures are commonly associated with pulmonary contusion.* Pain associated with rib fractures can be controlled with regional anesthesia (opioid epidural), systemic analgesics, or local intercostal blockade with bupivacaine (dogs: 0.75% solution diluted to 0.25% infiltrated as a small bleb caudal to the rib and dorsal and ventral to rib fractures; block single nerves cranial and caudal to the injured rib or segment; total dose should not exceed 1.5 mg/kg and extreme caution should be exercised not to compromise ventilation by blocking too many intercostal nerves). *Flail chest* refers to the fracture of multiple adjacent ribs in multiple locations, which creates a floating thoracic segment that moves paradoxically to the remainder of the chest wall. Flail chest is a diagnosis based on physical examination. The combination of pendulous airflow, underlying pulmonary trauma, concurrent pleural space injuries, and pain predispose to hypoxemia and hypoventilation.[6] Treatment of flail chest should initially be directed towards pain control and management of concurrent thoracic injury (e.g., pulmonary contusion, pneumothorax). Surgical fixation of flail chest is frequently unnecessary.[7] When needed, it should be performed after the animal is stable.

TRAUMA-ASSOCIATED MYOCARDIAL INJURY

Arrhythmias
Cardiac arrhythmias, most commonly of ventricular origin, are often diagnosed 12 to 36 hours after trauma. These arrhythmias, often referred to as *traumatic myocarditis* and *myocardial contusion*, may result from direct injury to the heart or decreased myocardial oxygen delivery resulting from shock, with subsequent ischemia and later reperfusion injury. Physical examination may reveal pulse deficits, high pulse rate, and/or weak pulses. Severe arrhythmias may cause signs of shock. Common arrhythmias include isolated premature ventricular contractions, accelerated idioventricular rhythms, and ventricular tachycardia. Much debate exists as to when or if trauma-associated ventricular arrhythmias need to be treated. Definite indications for treatment of ventricular arrhythmias include heart rate greater than 180 beats/min, R on T phenomena, and any arrhythmia that is causing signs of decreased tissue perfusion. It is recommended that treatment be based on heart rates greater than 140 beats/min to decrease myocardial (and thus whole body) oxygen consumption. Prior to use of antiarrhythmic agents, blood pressure should be

normalized (if possible), SpO$_2$ should be greater than 93%, and electrolyte and acid-base status should be normalized. Packed cell volume (PCV) should be greater than 20% and accompanied by euvolemia. Subsequent treatment with lidocaine (2 to 4 mg/kg bolus followed by 50 to 80 µg/kg/min constant rate infusion in dogs) will abolish most ventricular arrhythmias. Refractory arrhythmias causing clinical signs of decreased perfusion of the tissues may be treated with procainamide. Most trauma-associated arrhythmias will resolve over 2 to 4 days.

Pericardial Effusion

Pericardial effusion is a rare complication of trauma in the dog and cat; however, it should be considered as a differential diagnosis in animals with clinical signs of shock. Clinically significant pericardial effusion should be suspected from physical examination findings and confirmed through echocardiographic assessment. Physical examination findings consistent with pericardial effusion include pale mucous membranes, slow CRT, muffled heart sounds, pulsus paradoxus (waxing and waning pulse pressure with respiratory cycle), and distended jugular veins. In the trauma situation, however, these physical examination findings may be complicated by concurrent injuries and hypovolemia. In this situation, echocardiography is the most appropriate diagnostic test (Web Figure 141-4).

Thoracic radiography may be helpful, but in acute pericardial effusion, the cardiac silhouette may not appear significantly enlarged although it may be more round than normal. Clinically significant pericardial effusion should be relieved by pericardiocentesis (see Chapter 107). Definitive surgical intervention may be necessary.

TRAUMA-ASSOCIATED MEDIASTINAL INJURY

Pneumomediastinum

Pneumomediastinum is defined as an accumulation of air within the mediastinal space and, like rib fractures, should serve as a "flag" for concurrent injuries. Pneumomediastinum may result from injury to the large airways (see below), esophagus, alveoli (with subsequent tracking of air back into the mediastinum), and the skin in the cervical region. In the cervical region, air can track along the trachea and vascular structures of the neck into the mediastinum. Pneumomediastinum is rarely of clinical consequence. Pneumomediastinum can be definitively diagnosed on thoracic radiographs. An effort should be made to identify and definitively treat concurrent and causative injuries.

Tracheal Avulsion

Tracheal avulsion is thought to occur due to a rapid and extreme hyperextension injury to the head or neck and is more common in cats than in dogs. Tracheal avulsion may affect the intrathoracic or extrathoracic trachea. Both intrathoracic and extrathoracic tracheal avulsion can be associated with subcutaneous emphysema, signs of respiratory distress, and airway obstruction on initial physical examination. Radiographic examination will illustrate pneumomediastinum and may or may not reveal discontinuity of the tracheal silhouette (Web Figure 141-5). Frequently, clinical signs will abate as the airway is maintained by a thin mediastinal reflection. However, within the following 1 to 2 weeks, dyspnea usually develops secondary to fixed airway obstruction as the ends of the avulsed trachea begin to stenose. Subsequent radiographic evaluation will better illustrate lack of continuity of the tracheal silhouette. Treatment is tracheal anastomosis. The prognosis for cats with tracheal avulsion managed surgically is good.[8]

REFERENCES

The reference list can be found on the companion Expert Consult Web site at *www.expertconsult.com*.

CHAPTER 142

Blood Transfusions, Component Therapy, and Oxygen-Carrying Solutions

Ann E. Hohenhaus

Blood transfusions can play an essential role in the management of diseases of nearly every body system. Transfusion's critical role in replenishing red blood cells, coagulation factors, platelets, and albumin can provide lifesaving supportive treatment until a primary disorder can be controlled or resolved. A wide variety of clinical conditions require blood transfusions and multiple factors must be considered in determining a transfusion protocol. The decision to transfuse an anemic dog or cat is usually based on the "transfusion trigger," commonly defined as the packed cell volume (PCV, or hemoglobin [Hb] or hematocrit [Hct]) below which a transfusion is considered needed to sustain life. Although the PCV (or Hb concentration or Hct) provides information about the oxygen-carrying capacity of the blood and serves as a general guideline for the initiation of transfusion in patients, it is inadequate as the sole criterion for instituting red blood cell transfusion (Table 142-1). Additional factors considered in the decision to administer a red blood cell transfusion to a dog or cat include the perfusion status, the ability of the lungs to oxygenate the blood, the chronicity of the anemia, and the regenerative capacity of the bone marrow.

Perfusion status is reflected by the state of volume repletion and cardiac output. Chronicity of anemia determines the impact of physiologic compensatory mechanisms. These mechanisms include the ability of tissues to increase their oxygen extraction ratio, the ability of the heart to increase cardiac output, and adaptations in the Hb's ability to uptake oxygen from the lungs and download oxygen to the tissues.[1]

Table • 142-1

Factors to Be Considered When Determining Transfusion Protocols

STEPS TO DETERMINE A TRANSFUSION PROTOCOL	ANEMIA	COAGULOPATHY

Determine transfusion need	• Oxygen-carrying capacity of blood (PCV, Hct, Hb)
	• Perfusion status
	  ○ Volume
	  ○ Cardiac output
	• Ability of lungs to oxygenate blood
	• Acute versus chronic anemia
	• Bone marrow regenerative capacity
	• Physiologic compensatory mechanisms
	  ○ Oxygen extraction
	  ○ Cardiac output
	  ○ Hb adaptations
		• Severity of hemorrhage
		• Severity of resulting anemia
		• Need for invasive procedure

Select blood product	• Identify optimal *available* product of correct species • Consider volume status during selection process	
Perform pretransfusion testing	• Obtain transfusion history • Measure physical examination parameters • PCV, Hb, Hct • Blood type/crossmatch	• Obtain transfusion history • Measure physical examination parameters • Coagulation parameter
Consider administration issues	• Route • Rate • Temperature of product administered	
Monitor posttransfusion	• PCV, Hb, Hct • Monitor physical examination parameters	• Coagulation parameters • Monitor physical examination parameters

Hb, Hemoglobin; *Hct*, hematocrit; *PCV*, packed cell volume.

Potential improvements in a patient's clinical status following transfusion must be weighed against the potential adverse effects of transfusion. Recently, conservative transfusion triggers (Hb <7 g/dL versus >9g/dL) have resulted in lower mortality in critically ill humans. In a model of acute anemia in dogs, the compensatory mechanisms appeared to fail when the PCV reached 20%. Thus, 20% is often used as the transfusion trigger in dogs with anemia due to acute hemorrhage.[2] Higher or lower PCVs may be chosen as the transfusion trigger depending on the condition affecting an animal. Pneumonia, pulmonary edema, myocardial failure, or sepsis may require more liberal transfusion strategies while more restrictive transfusion criteria may be applied in chronic anemia due to retroviral infection, bone marrow failure, or chronic renal failure. When the PCV reaches approximately 10%, the myocardium exhausts its ability to compensate for anemia and becomes hypoxic, and providing increased oxygen-carrying capacity becomes imperative.[3]

Typically the "transfusion trigger" is discussed in relationship to transfusion for anemia; however, similar criteria should be utilized when a plasma transfusion is considered as a component of the treatment for coagulopathy. Prior to initiation of a plasma transfusion for coagulopathy, the underlying condition should be confirmed as an abnormal coagulation profile and not hemorrhage from loss of vascular integrity. Identification of the disorder as one of primary or secondary hemostasis allows the appropriate blood product, platelets, or plasma product to be transfused. The presence of abnormal coagulation tests in the absence of hemorrhage is not an absolute indication for platelet or plasma transfusion; however, if an invasive procedure such as an ultrasound-guided biopsy is required, a prophylactic platelet or plasma transfusion may be administered.

TRANSFUSION IN ANEMIC DOGS AND CATS

Epidemiologic data regarding red blood cell transfusions for anemia are limited in veterinary medicine. In one survey of over 1000 consecutive reference laboratory submissions, 31% of dogs over 8 years of age had a PCV below the reference range, indicating anemia is moderately frequent in dogs.[4] Red blood cells can be provided via whole blood transfusion or by transfusion of packed red blood cells. A 1992 survey of American Animal Hospital Association member practices[5] found most practices used whole blood to treat anemia in dogs. Since that time, there has been an increase in the use of component therapy for treatment of anemia. Increased usage of canine packed red blood cells in a veterinary school clinic was recognized following institution of a transfusion medicine curriculum designed to promote component therapy.[6] Commercial veterinary blood banks predominantly provide blood components, making this form of therapy more common. Component therapy is considered optimal since it conserves a limited resource by providing only the component of blood the patient requires for its clinical condition. In contrast to these therapeutic trends in dogs, whole blood continues to be the dominant product administered to anemic cats. Commercially available blood bag systems are not designed for the small volume of blood that is collected from cats, and commercial blood banks frequently provide whole blood. Both of these factors contribute to the continued usage of whole blood in cats.

Anemia is often categorized based on its cause: hemolysis, blood loss, or erythropoietic failure. Blood loss anemia is the most common anemia category for which red blood cells are transfused in both dogs and cats (Table 142-2). Dogs and cats with coagulation disorders often require treatment of anemia

Table • 142-2

Percentage of Dogs and Cats Receiving Transfusions by Anemia Category

SPECIES	BLOOD LOSS ANEMIA	HEMOLYTIC ANEMIA	ERYTHROPOIETIC FAILURE	REFERENCE
Dog	70%-72%	14%-22%	8%-14%	31, 35
Cat	27%-52%	10%-14%	25%-38%	32, 34, 90

in addition to coagulopathy treatment. Because each of these categories of anemia is different with regard to transfusion needs, the following sections of this chapter will discuss the transfusion needs for each category. Regardless of the category of anemia being treated, the goals of a red blood cell transfusion are to reduce morbidity, mortality, and functional impairment caused by inadequate delivery of oxygen.

PRETRANSFUSION TESTING IN ANEMIC DOGS AND CATS

Prior to transfusion of red blood cells, data should be collected to ensure compatibility, safety, and efficacy. Pretransfusion compatibility testing prior to transfusion of a red blood cell–containing component should include a blood type if a cat has not previously been transfused to ensure the recipient and donor are the same blood type. Feline blood types A, B, and AB can be determined by card typing, gel tube typing, or slide typing. If these methods are not available, crossmatching can be performed prior to the first transfusion to determine red blood cell compatibility. Blood typing or crossmatching prior to the first transfusion is not necessary in dogs. Blood-typing cards or gel tube typing can determine the dog erythrocyte antigen (DEA) 1.1 status of a dog. Blood typing is useful in dogs even if the recipient has not previously been transfused if the donor blood is DEA 1.1–positive. DEA 1.1–positive blood administered to a DEA 1.1–negative dog causes production of antibodies against DEA 1.1 and may cause an acute hemolytic transfusion reaction if DEA 1.1–positive blood is administered in subsequent transfusions.[7] DEA 4 alloantibodies can also cause an acute hemolytic transfusion reaction if a DEA 4– dog is transfused with DEA 4+ blood and an anti–DEA 4 antibodies are produced.[8] Subsequent transfusions of DEA 4+ blood are likely to cause an acute hemolytic transfusion reaction. Recently, two new blood groups have been identified, one in dogs (Dal) and one in cats (Mik).[9,10] Dal appears to be common in dogs and transfusion of Dal– dogs with Dal+ blood results in antibody production that may lead to an acute hemolytic transfusion reaction. The Dal antigen appears to be lacking in some Dalmatians. Mik– cats appear to have a naturally occurring anti-Mik alloantibody that may cause transfusion incompatibility without prior transfusion. The prevalence of these antigens in the general pet population is unknown, and their significance in transfusions is not known. When a second transfusion is administered more than 4 days after the first transfusion, a crossmatch should be performed in both dogs and cats to determine compatibility of the red blood cells to be transfused. If Oxyglobin is the product being used to treat anemia, blood typing and crossmatching are not necessary.

In order to assess the effect of a red blood cell transfusion on the dog or cat, a Hct, PCV, or Hb should be measured prior to and following administration of red blood cells. The choice can be based on test availability, except in the case of Oxyglobin administration. Oxyglobin is a hemoglobin-based oxygen carrier (HBOC), and although it is used to treat anemia, it does not contain red blood cells. Measurement plasma Hb and total Hb should be used to determine the response to administration of Oxyglobin.

Body temperature, respiratory rate, heart rate, and blood pressure should be monitored prior to red blood cell transfusion and intermittently during and for several hours after a transfusion to promote early identification of a transfusion-related adverse event. A transfusion should be discontinued if vomiting, diarrhea, collapse, or urticaria are noted.

TRANSFUSION FOR BLOOD LOSS ANEMIA

The transfusion trigger is variable in cases of blood loss anemia. Acute blood loss resulting in hemodynamic instability despite volume replacement requires red blood cell transfusions at a higher PCV than does chronic blood loss. If blood loss is internal, approximately 50% of the hemorrhaged red blood cells will reenter the circulation over 24 hours.[11] In those cases, red blood cell dosage can be more conservative than in cases of external hemorrhage. If blood loss has been slow, allowing for physiologic compensation, a PCV of greater than 15% may be adequate for routine diagnostic testing, but if anesthesia is required, if a pet has cardiac or respiratory disease, or if blood loss from an invasive procedure may occur, red blood cell transfusion is indicated. Chronic blood loss may result in erythropoietic failure. Transfusion issues for erythropoietic failure are discussed in a later section.

Several products are available to increase oxygen-carrying capacity in blood loss anemia (Table 142-3). Whole blood is the least appropriate since it contains plasma, which is unnecessary for the treatment of anemia. Although Oxyglobin does not contain red blood cells, it is recommended for treating reduced oxygen-carrying capacity when appropriate blood products are not available. Oxyglobin should be used cautiously in dogs and cats with cardiovascular disease and circulatory overload states.

Massive transfusion is defined as transfusion dose greater than 1 blood volume in a 24-hour period. In the dog, this had been defined as 90 mL/kg in 24 hours or 45 mL/kg in 3 hours.[12] The large volume of citrate-based anticoagulant administered with the red blood cells results in hypocalcemia and hypomagnesemia. Dilutional coagulopathy results if the blood administered has been stored and does not contain active coagulation factors. Acid-base abnormalities may also occur after a massive transfusion. Therefore, after any dog or cat is given a massive transfusion, electrolytes, coagulation parameters, and acid-base status should be monitored.

TRANSFUSION FOR IMMUNE-MEDIATED HEMOLYTIC ANEMIA

Red blood cell transfusion is a common treatment for dogs and cats with immune-mediated hemolytic anemia (IMHA).[13-15] Historically, red blood cell transfusion was discouraged because of the fear it would promote hemolysis and worsen

Table • 142-3

Suggested Blood Components for Treatment of Various Anemias

TYPE OF ANEMIA	OPTIMAL COMPONENT	ALTERNATE COMPONENT	ALTERNATE COMPONENT
Blood loss anemia (hypovolemic)	Packed red blood cells* and crystalloid or colloid solutions	HBOC	Whole blood
Blood loss anemia (normovolemic)	Packed red blood cells*	HBOC	Whole blood
Anemia of chronic renal failure	Packed red blood cells*	Whole blood	
Anemia of bone marrow failure	Packed red blood cells*	Whole blood	HBOC
Hemolytic anemia	Packed red blood cells*	HBOC	Whole blood

HBOC, Hemoglobin-based oxygen carrier.
*Packed red blood cells include: packed red blood cells, packed red blood cells in additive solution, leukoreduced packed red blood cells.

the patient's condition.[16] This has largely been refuted in recent years.[13,17] Determining the patient's requirement for increased oxygen-carrying capacity has become the major factor influencing the transfusion trigger in IMHA, as it should be for animals with other conditions. If clinical signs indicate need for increased oxygen-carrying capacity, withholding transfusion risks progressive hypoxic damage to the heart, liver, and kidneys.[18]

A reasonable recommendation is to transfuse DEA 1.1–negative red blood cells in the smallest volume necessary to improve a dog or cat's clinical status.[18] Any of the packed red blood cell products are appropriate selections in IMHA (see Table 142-3). Daily transfusions may be required until immunosuppressive therapy arrests the hemolytic process and the pet is able to maintain its own oxygen-carrying capacity. Concerns of inducing accelerated hemolysis have led to the recommendation to use a HBOC (Oxyglobin) for increasing oxygen-carrying capacity in IMHA because the antigenic red blood cell membranes have been removed during manufacturing. This theoretical recommendation not been confirmed in clinical trials, but individual cases of IMHA respond well to transfusion of HBOC.[19]

IMHA may represent a unique situation where blood typing and crossmatching are not possible due to autoagglutination of the patient's sample; however, blood from most dogs and cats with this disorder can successfully be crossmatched to a donor.[17,18]

TRANSFUSION FOR ANEMIA OF ERYTHROPOIETIC FAILURE

Because anemia caused by erythropoietic failure typically takes weeks to resolve, red blood cell–containing products are optimal. The half-life of red blood cell–containing products depends on the storage medium but ranges from 21 to 35 days.[20-26] The half-life of Oxyglobin is 18 to 43 hours when it is administered at a dose of 10 to 30 mL/kg.[27] Packed red blood cell products have an advantage over both whole blood and Oxyglobin in the treatment of anemia caused by erythropoietic failure. Animals with this type of anemia are usually normovolemic or hypervolemic, and packed red blood cells have the same amount of oxygen-carrying capacity in a smaller volume than either whole blood or Oxyglobin.

ADMINISTRATION CONSIDERATIONS IN TRANSFUSION FOR ANEMIA

The initial dosage of red blood cell–containing blood products varies based on the product selected and the type of anemia

Table • 142-4

Initial Dosage of Red Blood Cell–Containing Components

DISEASE	DOSAGE
Packed red blood cells*	6-10 mL/kg
Packed red blood cells in additive solution	10-15 mL/kg
Leukoreduced packed red blood cells	15 mL/kg
Whole blood	10-20 mL/kg

*0.9% saline may be added to this product to decrease viscosity and facilitate transfusion.

being treated (Table 142-4). Chronic and nonregenerative anemia may require a smaller increase in oxygen-carrying support, and thus a lower dosage to alleviate clinical signs, than acute and regenerative anemia since the body will have responded to chronic anemia through compensatory mechanisms. The rate of administration of oxygen-carrying products will be influenced by the volume status of the pet, which depends on the concurrently administered intravenous solutions as well as the type of anemia.

Initially, 1 to 3 mL of red blood cells can be administered over a period of about 5 minutes while the pet is observed for adverse reactions. Following the initial transfusion, normovolemic patients and those with chronic anemia can be transfused at a rate of 10 to 20 mL/kg/hr.[28] Hypovolemic patients with acute anemia may be given as much as 60 mL/kg/hr. Slow transfusion rates are indicated in dogs or cats with cardiac disease.

Regardless of the disease being treated, an attempt should be made to administer any transfusion in less then 4 hours. If the patient's clinical condition dictates the transfusion be administered for longer than 4 hours, the unit should be split into smaller aliquots and one aliquot refrigerated while the other is administered. The recommended rate of Oxyglobin administration is up to 10 mL/kg/hr.[27] Higher dosages place the patient at risk for circulatory overload. Red blood cell–containing products are typically administered intravenously, but can successfully be administered interosseously.[29] Any intravenous catheter commonly used in veterinary medicine is appropriate. All blood products should be administered through a blood administration set with a filter or a filter added to the intravenous line. Warming is not required, but may be advantageous if large volumes are being administered, if the recipient is hypothermic, or if the pet is small.[30]

POSTTRANSFUSION MONITORING IN DOGS AND CATS TRANSFUSED FOR ANEMIA

In order to assess the effect of the red blood cell transfusion on the patient and determine if additional transfusion is required, Hct, PCV, or Hb should be measured following administration of red blood cells. Measurement of Hb is the appropriate test to determine the response to administration of Oxyglobin.

Body temperature, respiratory rate, heart rate, and blood pressure should be monitored after any transfusion. Changes in any of these parameters during or immediately following transfusion are an indication of a transfusion-associated adverse event. Extra emphasis should be placed on monitoring respiratory rate, heart rate, and thoracic auscultation when Oxyglobin is administered because this product increases the risk of circulatory overload.

ADVERSE EVENTS ASSOCIATED WITH RED BLOOD CELL ADMINISTRATION

The most serious adverse effect of administration of any red blood cell–containing component is acute hemolytic transfusion reaction due to recipient antibodies against the donor red blood cells.[31-37] Transfusions also carry risk of circulatory overload, Type I hypersensitivity reactions, vomiting, and fever. The most common reaction, fever, is believed to be due to cytokines contained in the transfused blood or from antibodies against red blood cells, white blood cells, or platelets. Fever also occurs with bacterial contamination of blood.[38] An increase in body temperature of 1° C should be considered a transfusion-associated fever.

Adverse events associated with Oxyglobin are different than those related to transfusion of red blood cell–containing products and are due to the unique properties of Oxyglobin. Oxyglobin does not contain antigenic red blood cell membranes and will not cause an acute hemolytic transfusion reaction. The most common adverse event associated with Oxyglobin administration is circulatory overload, manifested as pulmonary edema or pleural effusion.[39] Posttransfusion monitoring should focus on assessment of parameters, such as blood pressure or central venous pressure, either of which could aid in identifying development of circulatory overload. Oxyglobin has strong colloid effect because its colloid osmotic pressure (COP) is 43 mm Hg and it also causes transient discoloration of mucus membranes (muddy pink, icteric orange, or brown), skin, and urine (pigmenturia).[19,27] Vomiting and diarrhea are less commonly seen adverse effects.

POTENTIAL LONG-TERM PROBLEMS AFTER TRANSFUSIONS FOR ANEMIC DOGS AND CATS

Diseases where multiple transfusions are given over a prolonged period of time are uncommon in veterinary transfusion medicine; consequently, long-term problems caused by transfusion are rarely described. One such adverse event is posttransfusion purpura.[40] In this transfusion complication, thrombocytopenia occurs 1 to 2 weeks following transfusion. The recipient, sensitized by transfusions containing platelet antigens, can produce antibodies against platelets which, in turn, can cause thrombocytopenia. The syndrome usually naturally resolves in 1 to 4 weeks. A second long-term problem caused by transfusions in dogs is hemochromatosis.[41] Iron from senescent transfused red blood cells accumulates in the liver, ultimately resulting in liver failure from transfusional hemochromatosis.

All transfusions carry the risk of infectious disease transmission. Of greatest concern in veterinary patients are canine and feline vector-borne diseases and feline retroviral diseases.[42] Blood donor screening recommendations have been made to minimize the risk of disease transmission, but transmission of infectious disease via transfusion does cause morbidity and mortality.[43-47]

TRANSFUSION IN COAGULOPATHIC DOGS AND CATS

Deficiencies of coagulation factors and platelets can be treated with fresh frozen plasma and its related products, cryoprecipitate and cryosupernate plasma, platelet-rich plasma, or platelet concentrates. These products are not appropriate for the treatment of nutritional deficiencies, hypoalbuminemia, or as colloid supplementation. Treatment of decreased colloid osmotic pressure will be discussed in a following section. Cats frequently have abnormal coagulation tests despite the absence of spontaneous hemorrhage. Coagulation test results are commonly abnormal in cats with liver disease, neoplasia, and infectious diseases.[48,49] In dogs the most common inherited coagulation disorder is von Willebrand disease (vWD) and the most common acquired coagulation disorder is immune-mediated thrombocytopenia.

PRETRANSFUSION TESTING IN COAGULOPATHIC DOGS AND CATS

Prior to transfusion of plasma products for the treatment of coagulopathy, safety and efficacy testing should be performed. Compatibility testing, which is critical in red blood cell transfusions, is not routinely performed in the dog, but blood type–compatible plasma must be given to cats since Type A cat plasma contains anti-B antibodies and Type B cat plasma contains anti-A antibodies. Compatibility can be determined by crossmatching or blood typing using card, gel tube, or slide-typing methods. Both anti-A and anti-B antibodies can cause a hemolytic transfusion reaction if plasma is given to a cat with a different blood type. The availability of point of care coagulation testing has made possible pretransfusion testing to assess efficacy of plasma transfusions for coagulation disorders. A dog or cat with hemorrhage should be evaluated for coagulopathy using a prothrombin time (PT) and either an activated partial thromboplastin time (aPTT) or activated clotting time. Platelet count should be determined by reviewing a blood smear or by automated methods. Once an abnormality in one or more of these parameters has been identified as the cause of hemorrhage, a diagnosis can be made and the appropriate transfusion initiated.

Correcting abnormal coagulation tests or thrombocytopenia is not necessary in the absence of hemorrhage unless an invasive procedure is planned. Major bleeding complications are more common when platelet counts are lower than 80,000/μL. Kidney biopsies are associated with more bleeding complications than liver biopsies.[50] Human plasma transfusion guidelines recommend plasma transfusion be administered prior to an invasive procedure if the PT is elevated 1.5 times or more above the midpoint of the normal range or aPTT is elevated 1.5 times the upper limit of normal.[51]

ADMINISTRATION AND MONITORING OF PLASMA PRODUCT TRANSFUSIONS

Body temperature, respiratory rate, heart rate, and blood pressure should be monitored prior to plasma transfusion to establish baseline monitoring criteria. Frozen plasma products must be thawed prior to administration, but warming is not usually required. Warming may be advantageous if large volumes of cold products are being administered, if the recipient is hypothermic, or if the animal is small.[30] A blood transfusion administration set with an integral filter should be used to administer all plasma products. Plasma products are typically administered intravenously, but can successfully be administered interosseously or intraperitoneally. Any intravenous catheter commonly used in veterinary medicine is appropriate. The rate of administration varies with the product being administered (Table 142-5).

TRANSFUSION FOR SPECIFIC COAGULOPATHY

Anticoagulant rodenticide intoxication is a significant cause of morbidity and mortality in dogs and cats.[52,53] Although dogs appear to be more commonly affected, anticoagulation rodenticide intoxication in cats does occur, resembling the disorder in dogs both in clinical signs and laboratory abnormalities. Vitamin K is the antidote for the rodenticide-induced depletion of coagulation factors. In pets with life-threatening hemorrhage, central nervous system hemorrhage, pulmonary or pleural hemorrhage, or hemorrhage resulting in severe anemia, replacement of coagulation factors by transfusion should be initiated in addition to administration of vitamin K. Cryosupernatant plasma is the ideal product for treatment of anticoagulant rodenticide intoxication because it contains factors II, VII, IX, and X (Table 142-6).

Table • 142-5

Suggested Rates of Administration for Plasma Products

PRODUCT	ADMINISTRATION RATE	REFERENCE
Fresh frozen plasma	4-6 mL/min	91
Cryoprecipitate	Over 1 hour	92
Platelet concentrate (frozen)	Over 1-2 hours	92
Platelet-rich plasma	1-2 mL/min cats 3-6 mL/min dogs	64
Cryosupernatant plasma	Over 2-4 hours	92

Although fresh whole blood can be used to treat anticoagulant rodenticide toxicity, if the pet is not anemic from hemorrhage, the red blood cells contained in the whole blood transfusion are not necessary. Administration of one plasma dose often stops hemorrhage and improves coagulation test results.

Deficiency of von Willebrand factor (vWF, FVIIIR:a) results in vWD, which is a common inherited bleeding disorder in dogs.[54-56] It is rarely reported in cats.[57] Spontaneous hemorrhage occurs in severe conditions; however, dogs with 30% or less of the normal level of vWF are usually at risk for surgical hemorrhage.[58]

Control of spontaneous hemorrhage or prevention of interoperative hemorrhage is often required in dogs with vWD. Treatment has predominantly been empiric with either fresh frozen plasma or cryoprecipitate. Cryoprecipitate is rich in the hemostatically active high–molecular weight multimers of vWF. Evidence suggests using cryoprecipitate prepared by treating donors with arginine vasopressin (1 μg/kg SQ) prior to blood donation for the treatment of vWD results in higher plasma levels of vWF and improved buccal mucosal bleeding times when compared with treatment using fresh frozen plasma[56,59] (see Table 142-6). The recommended dosage of cryoprecipitate does not always result in control of hemorrhage, and additional cryoprecipitate may be required. Plasma levels of vWF remain elevated for approximately 2 hours following infusion. Additional infusions of cryoprecipitate may be required 4 hours after initial infusion. Because vWD is rare in the cat, little is known about treatment, and canine treatment recommendations should be adapted for cats with vWD.

Disseminated intravascular coagulation (DIC) is a secondary syndrome provoked by a primary disease and resulting in excessive consumption of coagulation factors and platelets. In veterinary patients, most pets with DIC are recognized when consumption of platelets and coagulation factors exceed their production and hemorrhage occurs. Coagulation testing in these patients typically shows thrombocytopenia, prolonged coagulation times, and evidence of increased fibrinolysis (increased fibrin degradation products, or D-dimer). Treatment of DIC with blood products is empiric and symptomatic. Fresh frozen plasma is used concurrently with treatment of the primary disease to replace coagulation factors and to control hemorrhage. A commonly recommended dosage of plasma is 6 to10 mL/kg TID[60] (see Table 142-6).

A dosage of 12-15 mL/kg BID resulted in improvement of prolonged aPTT and PT in critically ill dogs.[61] Additional units of plasma should be administered based on daily reevalu-

Table • 142-6

Suggested Blood Components for Treatment of Various Coagulopathies

TYPE OF COAGULOPATHY	OPTIMAL COMPONENT	DOSAGE	ALTERNATE COMPONENT
Anticoagulant rodenticide intoxication	Cryosupernatant plasma	6-10 mL/kg until hemorrhage stops	Fresh frozen plasma
Disseminated intravascular coagulation	Fresh frozen plasma	6-10 mL/kg TID until coagulation times improve	
von Willebrand disease	Cryoprecipitate	1 U/10 kg until hemorrhage stops	Fresh frozen plasma
Hemophilia A Factor VIII deficiency Fibrinogen (factor I) deficiency	Cryoprecipitate	1 U/10-15 kg until hemorrhage stops	Fresh frozen plasma
Hemophilia B Factor IX deficiency Factor II, VII, X, IX deficiency	Cryosupernatant plasma	6-10 mL/kg until hemorrhage stops	Fresh frozen plasma
Liver disease coagulopathy (hepatic synthetic failure)	Fresh frozen plasma	6-10 mL/kg up to TID until coagulation times improve	
Thrombocytopenia/thrombocytopathy	Platelet-rich plasma	1 U/1 kg	

ation of the clinical status, platelet count, and coagulation times.

Liver disease is a common cause of coagulation abnormalities.[32,48,60,62,63] Liver disease–associated coagulation disorders include hepatic synthetic failure, vitamin K deficiency, and DIC. Treatment of DIC is described above. Pets with hepatic failure can be treated with fresh frozen plasma if spontaneous hemorrhage is recognized or if a liver biopsy is required (see Table 142-6). Plasma can be administered as often as TID until coagulation times normalize.

Congenital factor deficiencies other than canine vWD are rare in veterinary patients.[64-66] Clinical signs of hemophilia appear in puppies and kittens associated with normal activity, during teething, or following neutering. Deficiencies of fibrinogen (factor I) and hemophilia A (factor VIII) necessitate transfusion of cryoprecipitate or fresh frozen plasma. Fresh whole blood can be administered if the patient is also anemic. Deficiencies of other factors, such as factor IX (hemophilia B), factor II, VII, X, or XI are treated with cryosupernatant or stored plasma. Stored whole blood can be administered to these patients if they are also anemic.

Thrombocytopenia is the most common acquired coagulation disorder in the dog.[67] Immune-mediated thrombocytopenia (ITP) is relatively common in dogs but rarely occurs in cats. Red blood cell transfusion is common in cases of ITP; if the patient requires an increase in oxygen-carrying capacity guidelines can be found in the previous section on blood loss anemia.[68] In cases of ITP with life-threatening hemorrhage, central nervous system hemorrhage, pulmonary or pleural hemorrhage, or hemorrhage resulting in severe anemia, transfusion of platelet-containing products should be considered; however, the efficacy of platelet transfusions in this disease (where platelets are destroyed) remains unproven.[69] Some evidence indicates transfusion of platelets is of little benefit in increasing the platelet count in ITP.[64] Fresh platelets, either as platelet concentrate or platelet-rich plasma have a shelf life of 48 hours. Frozen platelets have a 6-month shelf life, but lose function as a result of cryopreservation.

POSTTRANSFUSION MONITORING IN DOGS AND CATS TRANSFUSED FOR COAGULOPATHY

In order to assess the effect of the plasma transfusion on the patient and to determine need for additional plasma transfusions, coagulation parameters should be measured following completion of the plasma transfusion. In addition to observational assessment of ongoing hemorrhage, Hct, PCV, or Hb should also be measured following administration of plasma to determine if hemorrhage has abated as a result of the plasma transfusion.

Body temperature, respiratory rate, heart rate, blood pressure, and physical status should be monitored after transfusions. Changes in any of these parameters during or immediately following transfusion may be indicative of a transfusion-associated adverse event. Emphasis should be placed on monitoring respiratory rate and heart rate and performing thoracic auscultation to identify circulatory overload, especially if the patient has received large volumes of crystalloids, colloids, or other blood products.

ADVERSE EVENTS ASSOCIATED WITH TRANSFUSION FOR COAGULOPATHY

Physical examination parameters should be monitored intermittently during and for several hours after the transfusion to promote early identification of a transfusion-related adverse event. The occurrence of vomiting, diarrhea, collapse, or urticaria during a transfusion should result in the discontinuation of the transfusion and investigation of its cause. The most common adverse event associated with administration of plasma-containing transfusions is urticaria.[65] Slowing the rate of transfusion and administering antihistamines and glucocorticoids are adequate in most cases. Circulatory overload is another potential complication of plasma transfusion and is especially common in patients receiving large volumes of crystalloids and colloid solutions in addition to blood products. The use of cryoprecipitate, when appropriate, as opposed to fresh frozen plasma, lessens the risk of this complication because cryoprecipitate is contained in a smaller volume of plasma (30 to 40 mL) compared to fresh frozen plasma, which has a volume of approximately 250 mL.

TRANSFUSIONS IN PATIENTS WITH DECREASED COLLOID OSMOTIC PRESSURE

The serum albumin concentration contributes 60% to 70% of the vascular COP component of Starling's forces and is critical in maintaining fluid homeostasis. In daily clinic practice, hypoalbuminemia is a common finding on routine laboratory testing.[4] Although hypoalbuminemia is a negative predictive indicator for survival in diseases such as histiocytic sarcoma, IMHA, and chronic enteropathy, the impact on survival by repairing the albumin deficiency with human albumin supplementation, species-specific plasma, or increased colloid osmotic pressure with synthetic colloids is unknown.[14,70,71] Treatment of the underlying disease is critical to long-term control of hypoalbuminemia, but supplementation may be necessary to control clinical signs of edema, effusion, and hypotension. In addition to treating the cause of hypoalbuminemia and administering agents to increase the COP, enteral or parenteral nutrition should be considered in severely hypoalbuminemic patients who are unable to voluntarily maintain adequate nutritional intake. Repair of hypoalbuminemia with 25% human albumin has been described in critically ill dogs and cats with hemorrhage, protein-losing enteropathy and nephropathy, liver failure, malnutrition, and septic peritonitis.[72-74] Administration of 25% human albumin results in an increase in total solids, albumin concentration, and blood pressure, but should be reserved for those patients with hypoalbuminemia where standard therapy has failed to improve the clinical condition. The PCV, total protein concentration, serum albumin concentration, or the COP should not be the sole criterion for administration of colloid supplementation. Patients with hypoalbuminemia but lacking clinical signs of hypoalbuminemia should not automatically be administered colloid support. For patients requiring surgery, the recommendation has been made to keep the total protein above 3.5 g/dL and in those not requiring surgery to keep the albumin between 2.0 and 2.5 g/dL and the COP between 13 and 20 mg Hg.[75]

The choice of synthetic colloid, species-specific plasma, or heterologous albumin depends on the underlying disease, cost, and product availability. Species-specific plasma requires administration of a large volume to increase the albumin. One calculation suggests 45 mL of plasma per kilogram of body weight is required to increase the albumin 1 g/dL.[76] The limited availability of plasma and the large volume required to increase albumin concentration restricts its utility for treatment of hypoalbuminemia. In protein-losing nephropathy and enteropathy, administration of albumin-containing colloid solutions is likely to only transiently increase the albumin concentration and hydroxyethyl starch may be more appropriate since the large molecules in this product are less likely to be lost through the kidney or intestine. Prior to administration of species-specific plasma or heterologous albumin, testing

Table • 142-7

Intravenous Immunoglobulin Dosage in Various Disease States

DISEASE	DOSAGE	RATE
Immune-mediated hemolytic anemia	0.5-1.0 g/kg	Once over 6-8 hours
Immune-mediated thrombocytopenia	0.28-0.76 g/kg	Once over 6-8 hours
Cutaneous adverse drug reactions	1 g/kg	Over 4 hours on two consecutive days

should include COP, total protein concentration, and serum albumin concentration as well a measurement of vital signs to establish a baseline for the recipient. Monitoring blood pressure is critical with administration of albumin since it has been shown to increase blood pressure.[72] A suggested dosage for administering 25% human albumin solutions is 2 mL/kg.[75] The albumin dosage can also be calculated using the following formula:

Albumin dosage in grams = ([Desired albumin – patient albumin] × plasma volume [40 mL/kg in dogs] × 2) ÷ 100[77]

Albumin can be administered as a slow bolus (recommended maximum dosage of 4 mL/kg) or as a continuous rate infusion (0.1 to 1.7 mL/kg/hr).[72]

ADVERSE EVENTS ASSOCIATED WITH TRANSFUSION FOR DECREASED COLLOID OSMOTIC PRESSURE

Clinical investigations of administration of both human to *normal* dogs unexpectedly resulted in anaphylactoid and Type III (delayed) hypersensitivity reactions.[78,79] In a few dogs these reactions were fatal; however, the adverse reactions to administration of albumin to hypoalbuminemic dogs and cats have been minor.[72,73] Dogs without a history of prior human albumin administration appear to have IgG antibodies against human albumin and may have a hypersensitivity reaction in response to an initial albumin infusion. Dogs administered human albumin develop a pronounced IgG response following exposure; consequently, repeated administration appears to result in adverse reactions.[74,79]

During albumin administration, dogs and cats should be carefully monitored for signs of an anaphylactoid reaction. When the pet is discharged, the owners should be advised to monitor for signs of delayed hypersensitivity reactions, which have been described to occur as late as 14 days after human albumin administration. Facial edema and urticaria with vomiting, inappetence, and lethargy appear to be the common clinical signs.

TRANSFUSIONS IN PATIENTS WITH MISCELLANEOUS DISORDERS

Failure of Passive Transfer

Neonatal puppies and kittens that have failed to receive adequate colostrum may benefit for replacement of immunoglobulin through transfusion. Fresh plasma, fresh frozen plasma, frozen plasma, or serum may all be used as the source of immunoglobulin; the choice depends on the most readily available product. Pretransfusion testing is not recommended.

Plasma or serum can be administered intravenously, but the intraosseus or intraperitoneal routes work well and may be more practical in neonates.

In kittens with failure of passive transfer, a dose of 150 mL/kg of serum administered SC or IP has raised serum IgG to normal levels.[80] A dose of 22 to 40 mL/kg of serum has been recommended in puppies with passive transfer, but normalization of IgG levels was not attained.[81] Adverse reactions have not been reported but would be anticipated to be the same as for any plasma transfusion.

Immune-Mediated Disorders

Using the traditional definition of blood transfusion, transfusions replace a missing component of blood—for example, red blood cells in an anemic patient. Purified human immunoglobulin is transfused not to replace immunoglobulin deficiency but as an immunomodulatory agent in disorders of the immune system such as IMHA, ITP, and some immune-mediated dermatologic disorders.[82-88] Laboratory investigation demonstrates the mechanism of action of human intravenous immunoglobulin occurs via binding to the Fc receptor of canine lymphocytes and monocytes and through inhibition of Fc-mediated phagocytosis of antibody-coated red blood cells.[89]

The use of intravenous immunoglobulin has been recommended in the treatment of immune-mediated diseases because of its apparent rapid onset of immunosuppression. When the drug is effective in IMHA, hemolysis abates within 7 days and sometimes as soon as 2 days following infusion.[82,83] A similar rapid response has been seen in cases of ITP and cutaneous manifestations of adverse drug reactions.[85-88] It is not used frequently for long-term management of these diseases because of the risk of anaphylaxis due to antibody formation following repeated administrations, its cost, and the concern that a single administration of the drug does not result in long-term immunosuppressive effects. Blood typing and crossmatching are not necessary prior to administration. Multiple different doses of intravenous immunoglobulin have been recommended (Table 142-7).

The patient's volume status should be monitored closely during and following administration since these dogs typically have received multiple transfusions and large volumes of crystalloids or colloids and are at risk for circulatory overload. Reported adverse events following administration of intravenous immunoglobulin for the treatment of IMHA include thrombosis and thrombocytopenia; however, these adverse events are common complications of IMHA and may not be associated with administration of intravenous immunoglobulin.[82,83]

REFERENCES

The reference list can be found on the companion Expert Consult Web site at *www.expertconsult.com.*

CHAPTER **143**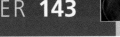

Initial Evaluation of Respiratory Emergencies

Carol R. Reinero
F.A. (Tony) Mann

A common and serious clinical sign in dogs and cats with respiratory disease is respiratory distress. Understanding the causes of respiratory distress is critical for prompt and effective treatment. One scheme to classify the causes of respiratory distress involves the following eight categories: (1) upper airway obstruction, (2) lower airway obstruction, (3) flail chest, (4) abdominal enlargement, (5) pulmonary parenchymal disease, (6) pleural cavity disorders, (7) pulmonary thromboembolism (PTE), and (8) "look-alike" syndromes. This classification system is useful because the first four causes can be usually be recognized quickly at the time of initial assessment. Each of these four conditions can be distinguished by the physical appearance of the dog or cat, the cycle of respiration predominantly affected, and audible sounds that might be heard resulting from certain disorders (to be discussed later). The remaining four causes will require additional diagnostic testing to establish a definitive diagnosis.

EIGHT MAJOR CATEGORIES OF RESPIRATORY DISTRESS

Upper airway obstruction is due to mechanical or functional obstruction of the large airways (pharynx, larynx, or trachea cranial to the thoracic inlet) and includes intraluminal or extraluminal masses (neoplasia, granuloma, abscess, blood clots, polyps), foreign bodies, laryngeal paralysis, laryngeal collapse, elongated soft palate, everted laryngeal saccules, tracheal collapse, tracheal stenosis, or tracheal stricture. Obstruction of the trachea within the thoracic cavity is included in the category of lower airway obstruction. Lower airway obstruction also arises from narrowing of the bronchial lumen due to bronchospasm, accumulation of mucus or other exudate, bronchial wall edema, or diffuse bronchomalacia. The classic example of a disease associated with the first three of these changes is feline asthma. Asthma in dogs is an exceedingly rare diagnosis, but lower airway obstruction in dogs can be seen with severe chronic bronchitis due to bronchomalacia, which allows for passive collapse of the airways on exhalation. Flail chest results from trauma to the thoracic cavity, where there is destabilization of a portion of the rib cage (i.e., multiple ribs are fractured at two different locations, leaving a segment that is detached from the rest of the rib cage). Paradoxical respiration is seen so that, as an animal inhales, the chest wall segment is sucked inward, and as it exhales, the segment is blown outwards. Severe abdominal enlargement can put pressure on the diaphragm and make it more difficult for the thoracic cavity to expand on inhalation. Examples of conditions associated with abdominal enlargement include ascites, gastric dilatation, hepatosplenomegaly, neoplastic abdominal masses, pregnancy, or pyometra. Pulmonary parenchymal diseases are disorders affecting the terminal and respiratory bronchioles, interstitium, alveoli, or vasculature. They may be associated with infiltration by infectious microorganisms, inflammatory cells, or neoplastic cells; the airspaces may be filled with edema fluid or foreign material; or lung tissue may be replaced with fibrotic tissue. Examples of conditions affecting the pulmonary parenchyma include infectious pneumonia (bacterial, fungal, viral, protozoal, and parasitic), aspiration pneumonitis, aspiration pneumonia, interstitial lung diseases, pulmonary edema (cardiogenic or noncardiogenic), hemorrhage, neoplasia, and acute lung injury (ALI) or acute respiratory distress syndrome (ARDS). Pleural cavity disorders arise when the space between the parietal and visceral pleura, which normally contains just a small amount of fluid for lubrication, fills with fluid (pleural effusion), air (pneumothorax), a mass, or abdominal organs (e.g., diaphragmatic hernia). Pulmonary thromboembolism refers to obstruction of blood flow in the pulmonary vasculature by a thrombus or embolus formed in the systemic venous system or right side of the heart. Any condition causing an abnormality in blood flow, endothelial damage, or hypercoagulability can predispose to thromboembolism. Finally, look-alike syndromes are conditions that result in apparent difficulty in breathing due to nonrespiratory causes, such as pain, severe anemia, hyperthermia, acidosis, drugs (e.g., opioids), and hypotension.

Evaluation of the pattern of breathing (Figure 143-1) can be useful to help localize the region of the respiratory tract that is affected. In an emergency situation, the first four causes of respiratory distress (upper and lower airway obstruction, flail chest, and abdominal enlargement) should be discernable on initial examination of a patient. Dogs and cats with upper respiratory obstruction will have a characteristic stridorous or squeaking noise that is readily audible, even without a stethoscope. Additionally, respiratory distress will occur on inhalation. Dogs and cats with a lower airway obstruction should have an audible wheeze (although sometimes a stethoscope is required to hear quieter wheezes). In these cases, respiratory distress will occur predominantly on exhalation, the so-called expiratory push. Visual examination will reveal if a flail chest (with paradoxical respiration) or abdominal enlargement (with increased inspiratory effort and no audible noise) is present.

For the remaining four causes of respiratory distress, physical examination may provide additional useful clues. Thoracic auscultation may reveal absent or quiet lung sounds, which are compatible with pleural cavity disease; crackles, which support pulmonary parenchymal disease; and murmurs or arrhythmias, which may indicate underlying cardiac disease that may be associated with pulmonary parenchymal disease (cardiogenic pulmonary edema), pleural cavity disease (especially in cats), and PTE. Physical examination may increase the index of suspicion for look-alike diseases if very pale/white mucus membranes are seen (severe anemia), substantially elevated body temperature is measured, or pain is elicited on palpation. Additional diagnostics are commonly required to discriminate these four causes of respiratory distress.

In an emergency situation, if there are decreased pulmonary or cardiac sounds on auscultation, it is prudent to proceed directly to thoracocentesis both as a diagnostic and therapeutic measure. Removal of any air or fluid will help stabilize the patient for further diagnostics.

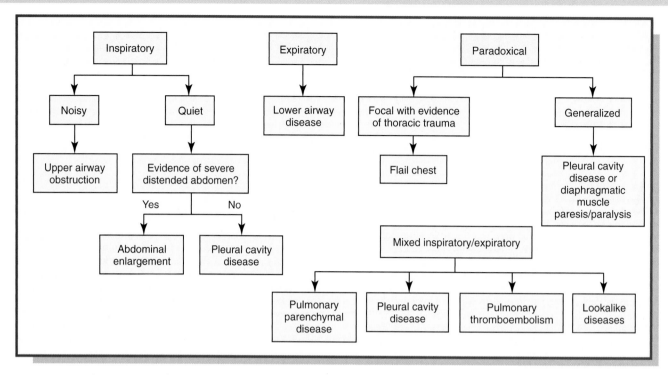

Figure 143-1 Flow chart to localize the cause of respiratory distress based on the pattern of breathing.

RADIOGRAPHY

Radiography is likely the single most important diagnostic tool for patients in respiratory distress. It is important to attempt to localize the cause of respiratory distress as described above, because if disease is localized to the upper airways, cervical and thoracic radiographs should be performed. For suspected dynamic collapse, both inspiratory and expiratory cervical and thoracic radiographs are required to highlight the obstructed area during the different cycles of respiration. Even with upper airway obstruction, it is still important to perform thoracic radiography to evaluate for noncardiogenic pulmonary edema (which can result from severe upper airway obstructions) and for metastatic disease if the airway obstruction is due to a mass. Significant thoracic radiographic changes may include intrathoracic tracheal narrowing (collapse or obstructive mass), a bronchial pattern as evidence of hyperinflation (lower airway disease), an interstitial or alveolar pattern (pulmonary parenchymal disease), evidence of pleural cavity disease (pleural effusion, pneumothorax, pleural mass, loss of a clear border of the diaphragm, or a blunted tortuous vessel with uneven vascular diameters and distribution of blood flow between lung lobes [PTE]). Other nonspecific thoracic radiographic findings may include cardiomegaly, pulmonary nodules, or atelectasis.

ADDITIONAL DIAGNOSTICS

Additional diagnostics beyond the scope of this chapter can be planned based on results of radiographic examination to more precisely identify the underlying disease process. Other useful diagnostics may include some of the following: complete blood counts, serology for infectious diseases, fecal examination, heartworm testing, advanced thoracic imaging (ultrasound or computed tomography), abdominal imaging (looking for related disease in the abdominal cavity), fundic examination, arterial blood gas, fine needle aspiration for cytology/culture, laryngeal examination, transtracheal wash, endotracheal wash, bronchoalveolar lavage, bronchoscopic examination, bronchial mucosal or mass biopsies, and biopsies obtained by a key-hole procedure, thoracoscopy, or thoracotomy (see Chapters 82, 87, 100, and 106-108).

It is crucial to keep in mind that many diagnostic tests must await appropriate patient stabilization. Any dog or cat with respiratory distress should benefit, to some degree, from the provision of supplemental oxygen. In patients with suspected upper airway obstruction, sedation may minimize struggling. Securing an airway by oral intubation or tracheostomy may be required. In dogs monitoring body temperature and cooling as needed is an important aspect of medical management since panting to dissipate heat is impaired. Finally, an antiinflammatory dose of corticosteroids may help reduce swelling in the upper airways. For cats with lower airway obstruction, minimal handling, bronchodilators (injectable or inhaled) to relieve bronchoconstriction, and corticosteroids can provide symptomatic relief. Bronchodilators are likely of less benefit to dogs with lower airway obstruction, as the most common diseases in this category are intrathoracic tracheal collapse and diffuse bronchomalacia—neither of which is associated with smooth muscle constriction of the bronchi. Sedation and an antiinflammatory dose of corticosteroids may be useful in the short term. For animals with flail chest in the emergent situation, placing the affected side down with the patient in lateral recumbence and pain management are important. For patients with abdominal distension, addressing the underlying disorder in the abdominal cavity is required. For patients with pulmonary parenchymal disease, initial therapeutics may include: empiric trial with furosemide if there is evidence of heart failure; judicious fluid therapy if there is no evidence of heart failure; airway humidification; nebulization; coupage; antimicrobials; and/or antiinflammatory drugs. For animals with pleural cavity disease, thoracocentesis can be helpful therapeutically. For patients with PTE, oxygen supplementation is usually the main means of stabilization; once a diagnosis of the condition is made, anticoagulants and/or thrombolytics can be considered. Finally, patients with a look-alike syndrome will generally not be oxygen-responsive (since the disease is not primarily of the respiratory system) and a search for nonrespiratory diseases can be made.

CONCLUSION

Having a scheme to classify the causes of respiratory distress can help in the approach to patients presenting in an emergency situation. Identification of breathing patterns (inspiratory distress, expiratory distress, paradoxical breathing, and mixed inspiratory and expiratory distress) assists in localizing the site of respiratory disease. After stabilizing the patient, appropriate diagnostics and therapeutics can be targeted to focus on the location of the respiratory disease.

SECTION V
Toxicology

CHAPTER 144

Intoxication versus Acute, Nontoxicologic Illness: Differentiating the Two

Safdar A. Khan

CASE HISTORY

A complete and thorough case history is essential for differentiating a poisoning situation from a naturally occurring disease in an acutely ill animal. Obtaining a clear recent history may sometimes be quite challenging, especially in situations where the pet was unsupervised before the initiation of clinical signs.[1] History questions must include animal signalment (breed, sex, and age) and weight, previous medical history, vaccination history, and any medications the pet is taking. Initial information about any other animals present in the household, timeline of clinical signs, types of clinical signs reported by the owner, number of affected animals, pet's environment (indoor vs. outdoor), location (urban vs. rural), time of the year (summer vs. winter), recent renovations/ updates (construction material; lead in older farms/houses), availability of human medications in the pet's environment (antidepressants, pain killers, stimulants, nutritional supplements), presence or recent use of chemicals (insecticides, herbicides, rodenticides) in the house/yard, and information about indoor/outdoor plants may help provide clues to the clinician to narrow down the search for a possible cause for the pet's illness.

STABILIZING THE PATIENT

Before obtaining a complete case history, the first goal should be to stabilize the patient and preserve life of the acutely ill animal irrespective of the cause. Relying too much on specific antidotal treatment may be dangerous. A majority of clinical cases on presentation are treated supportively as only a very few specific antidotes are available or needed for treating specific poisonings. Therefore, on presentation, make sure the animal has a patent airway and adequate ventilation. Support and maintain cardiac functions. Monitor heart rate, rhythm, and blood pressure, and treat cardiac arrhythmias and blood pressure changes as needed. Hydration status, fluids, electrolytes, and acid-base balance should be checked and corrected accordingly. Treat central nervous system abnormalities (excitation, depression, seizures) as required, and maintain body temperature within the normal range (treat hypothermia or hyperthermia). After stabilizing the vital functions, obtain a history; then, provide other necessary treatment such as decontamination (administration of activated charcoal, bathing, dilution), supportive care, and carrying out other diagnostics (complete blood count, chemistries, radiographs, ultrasound) as needed.

TOXICOLOGIC VERSUS NONTOXICOLOGIC

Table 144-1 outlines some important toxicologic versus nontoxicologic rule-outs based on clinical abnormalities one must consider in an acutely ill animal. Where necessary, with each rule-out, along with major clinical abnormality, a brief description of other clinical signs is also provided. An acutely ill animal with sudden onset of clinical effects may often have multiple major clinical signs/abnormalities present. The purpose here is to provide an initial guideline for considering toxicologic versus nontoxicologic rule-out. Once a reasonable etiology has been narrowed down or established, the reader is encouraged to review a more detailed discussion on management of the particular poisoning or disease listed in this reference (see Table 144-1).

REFERENCES

The reference list can be found on the companion Expert Consult Web site at *www.expertconsult.com*.

Table • 144-1

Toxicologic versus Nontoxicologic Rule-Outs

MAJOR CLINICAL ABNORMALITY	TOXICOLOGIC RULE-OUTS	NONTOXICOLOGIC RULE-OUTS
CNS abnormalities (excitation and seizures)	• Strychnine (rapid onset, rigidity, hyperesthesia, wooden-horse–like stance) • Metaldehyde (hyperthermia, tremors, shaking) • Amphetamines or cocaine (ingestion in dogs: sympathomimetic effects and hyperthermia) • Tremorgenic mycotoxins (penitrem A, roquefortine) from eating moldy foods (GI signs, hyperthermia, and tremors) • Cold medications: pseudoephedrine, ephedrine, some antihistamines (sympathomimetic effects, hyperthermia) • Organophosphate or carbamate pesticides (cholinergic crisis; SLUD signs) • Pyrethrin/pyrethroid–type pesticides (especially permethrin in cats: tremors, shaking, ataxia, seizures, GI signs) • Organochlorine pesticides (tremors, shaking, ataxia, seizures) • Chocolate: caffeine, theobromine, methylxanthines (polydipsia, polyuria, GI and CV effects) • Zinc phosphide: mole or gopher baits (GI signs, shaking, pulmonary edema) • Bromethalin toxicosis: rat or mouse bait (paresis, weakness, ataxia, twitching) • Lead (GI signs, nucleated RBCs, basophilic stippling, anemia) • Metronidazole (toxicosis in dogs with repeated use: nystagmus, ataxia, weakness, paresis, seizures) • Nicotine: tobacco or cigarettes (ingestion in dogs: spontaneous vomiting, shaking, CV effects) • Tricyclic antidepressant toxicosis: amitriptyline, clomipramine, imipramine, nortriptyline (agitation, nervousness, ataxia, CV effects)	• Trauma/head trauma (outdoor animal, external or internal wounds/injuries) • Meningitis (fever, hyperesthesia, neck stiffness and pain) • Hydrocephalus (large, rounded head; ventrolateral deviation of eyes; seizures • Intracranial neoplasia (primary or secondary brain tumor: older animals) • Congenital portosystemic shunts (more common in certain breeds, <6 months of age, small liver) • Rabies (acute behavior changes, excitation, paralysis) • Canine distemper (young dogs: fever, respiratory, GI and CNS signs) • Hypocalcemia or hypercalcemia (hypocalcemic tetany, CV effects, CNS, renal effects from hypercalcemia) • Hypoglycemia (disorientation, ataxia, seizures, serum glucose <60 mg/dL) • Idiopathic epilepsy (dogs 1-5 years of age: blood work normal) • Polycythemia vera (primary or secondary, PCV 65%-81%, brick red mucous membrane) • Uremia (secondary to ARF or CRF) • Endotoxemia/septic shock (hemorrhagic GI signs, progressive weakness, abdominal pain)
CNS abnormalities (CNS depression and seizures)	• Ivermectin, moxidectin and other avermectin toxicosis (ataxia, weakness, depression, tremors, seizures, blindness) • Marijuana ingestion (ataxia, hypothermia, urinary incontinence) • Benzodiazepines ingestion: alprazolam, clonazepam, diazepam, lorazepam (hyporeflexia, ataxia, CNS excitation: paradoxical reaction) • Barbiturate overdose: short acting or long acting (coma, hypothermia, weakness, ataxia) • Ethylene glycol; see Acute Renal Failure (ataxia, drunkenness, disorientation, GI signs) • Methanol or ethanol ingestion (GI, signs, ataxia, weakness, depression) • Propylene glycol: antifreeze (depression, ataxia, GI signs) • Baclofen or other centrally acting muscle relaxant (ingestion in dogs: vocalization, ataxia, disorientation, coma, hypothermia) • Amitraz insecticide (depression, ataxia, CV effects, paralytic ileus)	• Thiamine deficiency in cats (cats fed mainly fish diet) • Coonhound paralysis (ascending flaccid paralysis; raccoon exposure within 2 weeks) • Feline infectious peritonitis: dry form (iritis; fever, weight loss, ataxia, seizures) • Feline leukemia (lymphadenopathy, nonregenerative anemia) • Feline panleukopenia (fever, GI signs, ataxia, neutropenia)

Table • 144-1

Toxicologic versus Nontoxicologic Rule-Outs—cont'd

MAJOR CLINICAL ABNORMALITY	TOXICOLOGIC RULE-OUTS	NONTOXICOLOGIC RULE-OUTS
Muscle weakness, paresis, paralysis	• Black widow spider bite (cats: swelling, pain) • 2,4-D and other phenoxy herbicides (in dogs: ataxia, weakness, GI signs) • Metronidazole, *see* Seizures (in dogs: nystagmus, ataxia, weakness, seizures) • Bromethalin rodenticide; see Seizures (paresis, CNS depression/excitation, twitching, seizures) • Coral snake envenomation (cats: local swelling, pain, puncture wound) • Macadamia nuts (ingestion in dogs: weakness, ataxia) • Concentrated tea tree oil exposure: *Melaleuca* oil (both cats and dogs: weakness, ataxia, CNS depression)	• Coonhound paralysis (muscle pain, ascending flaccid paralysis; raccoon exposure within 2 weeks) • Botulism (ascending paresis and paralysis) • Tick paralysis (flaccid ascending paralysis) • Aortic thromboembolism (cold extremities, weakness) • Profound anemia (measure PCV) • Severe hypokalemia • Hyponatremia • Severe hypovolemia • Marked hypo- or hyperthermia • Degenerative spinal cord diseases
Acute blindness	• Lead; see Seizures (GI signs, behavior changes, nucleated RBCs, basophilic stippling) • Ivermectin, moxidectin, and other avermectin toxicosis; see Seizures (ataxia, weakness, seizures, blindness reversible) • Salt poisoning (in dogs: excessive sodium chloride ingestion, polydipsia, GI signs, tremors, ataxia, seizures, serum sodium >160 mEq/L)	• Retinal detachment or hemorrhage • Glaucoma • Trauma (penetrating injury of head, face) • Acute cataract • Optic neuritis • Optic nerve disorders (optic chiasm, optic radiation, occipital cortex) • Sudden acquired retinal degeneration
Acute renal failure	• Ethylene glycol toxicosis (ataxia, drunkenness, GI signs, azotemia) • Easter lily (*Lilium longiflorum*), tiger lilies (*Lilium tigrinum, Lilium lancifolium*), rubrum or Japanese show lilies (*Lilium speciosum*), day lilies (*Hemerocallis* sp.) (reported in cats, initially GI signs, azotemia in generally 24-72 hours after ingestion) • Cholecalciferol rodenticide and other vitamin D_3 analogue: calcipotriene, calcitriol; see Hypercalcemia (initial GI signs, hypercalcemia, hyperphosphatemia, CV, and CNS effects, azotemia) • Grapes and raisins (ingestion in dogs: initial GI signs, then azotemia in >24 hours, possible pancreatitis) • NSAIDs: ibuprofen, naproxen, nabumetone, piroxicam, carprofen, diclofenac, ketoprofen, indomethacin, ketorolac, oxaprozin, etodolac, flurbiprofen, sulindac (initially GI signs, azotemia in 24-74 hours after ingestion in acute cases) • Zinc toxicosis; see Hemolysis (GI signs, pancreatitis, hemoglobinuria, anemia, renal failure) • Melamine and cyanuric acid contamination (outbreak in the United States in 2007 from contaminated dog and cat food: crystalluria, azotemia, GI signs)	• Renal infiltration (with lymphoma) • Renal thromboembolism • Infectious (pyelonephritis, leptospirosis, Rocky Mountain spotted fever, borreliosis, feline infectious peritonitis: cats) • Urinary tract obstruction • Renal lymphomas (more in cats than dogs) • Chronic renal failure (end stage) • Ischemic renal failure (hypotension, trauma, shock, congestive heart failure, anaphylaxis) • Neoplasia (adenocarcinoma in dogs; lymphosarcoma in cats) • Amyloidosis (immune mediated) • Hypercalcemia (due to any cause) • Transfusion reactions • Myoglobinuria/hemoglobinuria (due to any cause)

Continued

Table • 144-1

Toxicologic versus Nontoxicologic Rule-Outs—cont'd

MAJOR CLINICAL ABNORMALITY	TOXICOLOGIC RULE-OUTS	NONTOXICOLOGIC RULE-OUTS
Acute hepatic damage	• Carprofen and other NSAID-induced hepatopathies in dogs (within a few days after initiating therapy, GI signs, increased ALT) • Corticosteroids (steroid hepatopathy, long-term use) • Phenobarbital (chronic use) • Mushrooms: amanita type (delayed onset, 12 hours, GI signs, acute hepatic damage in 1-3 days) • Blue-green algae: *Microcystis* sp. (acute onset, GI signs, shock) • Iron: multivitamin ingestion (GI signs, shock, acute liver damage in 1-2 days) • Copper (copper storage disease; certain breeds can accumulate copper over a period of times) • Sago palm or cycad palm: *Cycas* sp. (ingestion: GI signs, liver damage in 1-3 days, seizures) • Acetaminophen toxicosis (methemoglobinemia within a few hours, GI signs, increased liver enzymes in 1-3 days) • Aflatoxicosis (dogs: mostly from contaminated dog food, several outbreaks reported in the United States) • Xylitol; *see* Hypoglycemia (ingestion in dogs: hypoglycemia within 12 hours, seizures, acute hepatic damage and coagulopathy in 1-3 days)	• Hepatic lipidosis (cats: period of stress, anorexia, obese animals) • Hepatic neoplasia (primary or metastatic, acute or gradual) • Infectious hepatitis (leptospirosis, infectious canine hepatitis, canine herpes virus, cholangiohepatitis, liver abscess, histoplasmosis, coccidiomycosis, babesiosis, toxoplasmosis, some rickettsial diseases, feline infectious peritonitis) • Acute pancreatitis (systemic) • Septicemia/endotoxemia (vomiting, diarrhea, hypothermia, collapse) • Heatstroke (high ambient temperature) • Shock (weak pulse, poor capillary refill time, progressive weakness) • Chronic passive congestion (secondary to cardiac problems)
Presence of acute oral lesions/ulcers	• Acid ingestion (corrosive lesions on lips, gums, tongue, salivation, vomiting, fever) • Alkali ingestion (same as with acid, esophageal perforation more likely) • Cationic detergents: present in several disinfectants (oral burns, salivation, vomiting, fever) • Alkaline battery (ingestion: oral burns, salivation, vomiting) • Potpourri ingestion (oral burns, salivation, vomiting, tongue protrusion, fever) • Bleaches: sodium or calcium hypochlorite (bleachlike smell, salivation, vomiting, wheezing, gagging) • Ingestion of phenolic compounds (especially in cats: oral ulcers/lesion may be present, Heinz body anemia and hemolysis may be seen)	• Uremic stomatitis (azotemia, GI signs) • Periodontal disease (associated with dental calculus; gingival lesions) • Trauma (presence of foreign body, grass, stick, bone, porcupine quills) • Electrical cord chewing (systemic signs such as dyspnea, pulmonary edema) • Systemic lupus erythematosus and other autoimmune diseases (oral lesions and other systemic and cutaneous signs present) • Infectious (feline calicivirus infection, FeLV, feline immunodeficiency virus, feline herpes virus, nocardiasis, ulcerative necrotizing stomatitis, fusobacterium)

Table • 144-1

Toxicologic versus Nontoxicologic Rule-Outs—cont'd

MAJOR CLINICAL ABNORMALITY	TOXICOLOGIC RULE-OUTS	NONTOXICOLOGIC RULE-OUTS
Acute methemoglobinemia, Heinz body anemia, hemolysis or blood loss (anemia)	• Acetaminophen (chocolate brown color mucous membrane within hours, dyspnea) • Local anesthetic toxicosis: lidocaine, benzocaine, tetracaine and dibucaine (methemoglobinemia, CV and CNS effects) • Phenazopyridine and other azo dyes toxicosis (methemoglobinemia, hemoglobinuria) • Naphthalene mothball ingestion (moth ball–like odor in the breath, hemolysis) • Onions and garlic toxicosis (hemolysis in 2-3 days, anemia, coffee-color urine) • Zinc toxicosis (metallic object in the GI tract, gastritis, pancreatitis, hemolysis, hemoglobinuria) • Iron (mostly see GI signs, hepatic damage, or shock) • Anticoagulants rodenticides: brodifacoum, bromadiolone, chlorophacinone, difethialone, diphacinone, pindone, warfarin (hemorrhaging, increased PT or aPTT, dyspnea, weakness) • Copper (certain breeds of dogs can accumulate copper in the liver) • Rattlesnake envenomation (swelling, pain, hemoglobinuria)	• Trauma (overt blood loss) • Immune-mediated hemolytic anemia • Thrombocytopenia (drug induced, infectious, or immune mediated) • Chronic renal failure (smaller kidneys, azotemia) • Infectious (ehrlichiosis, FeLV, hookworms, *Mycoplasma hemofelis*, babesiosis) • Severe liver diseases (deficiency of clotting factor can result in bleeding disorders) • Disseminated intravascular coagulation (secondary to underlying cause such as shock, neoplasia, septicemia, viral infections, pancreatitis) • Inherited bleeding disorders (von Willebrand disease, factor X deficiency, factor XI deficiency) • Epistaxis (primary or secondary, trauma, infectious, nasal polyps, malignant neoplasm)
Cardiac abnormalities	• Foxglove: *Digitalis* sp. (plant ingestion: GI signs and cardiac arrhythmias) • Lily of the valley: *Convallaria majalis* (plant ingestion GI signs and cardiac arrhythmias) • Oleander: *Nerium oleander* (GI signs and cardiac arrhythmias) • Bufo toads: *Bufo* sp. (GI signs collapse, seizures, and cardiac arrhythmias) • Azalea and other *Rhododendron* plant (GI signs and possible cardiac arrhythmias) • Antidepressant toxicosis (CNS signs, anticholinergic effects)	• Automobile trauma (evidence of other injuries) • Gastric dilation and volvulus (abdominal distension, dyspnea, shock) • Severe anemia (due to any cause of anemia) • Severe hypokalemia (due to any cause) • Acidosis (due to any cause) • Hypoxia (due to any cause) • Primary heart disease (cardiomyopathy, valvular heart disease, congenital heart problems, heartworm infestation: heart murmur, cardiomegaly, or evidence of congestive heart failure
Pulmonary edema	• Paraquat herbicide (rare; progressive dyspnea, panting, delayed onset after exposure) • Petroleum distillates: kerosene, gasoline and other hydrocarbons (hydrocarbon-smell in the breath, salivation, vomiting, CNS depression, diarrhea, aspiration) • Zinc phosphide (GI and CNS signs, pulmonary edema) • Smoke inhalation (dyspnea, collapse, panting, shock) • Organophosphate or carbamate pesticides (cholinergic crisis, SLUD signs) • Some organic arsenicals (mainly injectable, melarsamine)	• Cardiogenic (multiple causes of left ventricular failure) • Noncardiogenic (seizures, head trauma, electrical shock) • Hepatic disease (secondary to any cause of hepatic disease) • Renal disease (any cause of renal disease) • Drowning and near drowning • Shock (immune mediated, anaphylactic, trauma, transfusion reactions) • Neoplasia (primary or secondary)

Continued

Table • 144-1

Toxicologic versus Nontoxicologic Rule-Outs—cont'd

MAJOR CLINICAL ABNORMALITY	TOXICOLOGIC RULE-OUTS	NONTOXICOLOGIC RULE-OUTS
Gastrointestinal signs (vomiting, diarrhea, abdominal pain, drooling)	• Arsenical herbicides (initial stages: vomiting, abdominal pain, watery diarrhea) • Iron toxicosis (multivitamin ingestion in dogs: initial GI signs within hours) • Castor beans: *Ricinus communis* (initial GI signs within several hours) • Garbage poisoning (vomiting, diarrhea, dehydration, abdominal pain) • Chocolate toxicosis (initial stages: polydipsia, polyuria, vomiting, hyperactivity, tachycardia) • Fertilizer ingestion (NPK: vomiting, diarrhea, polydipsia) • Insoluble calcium oxalate containing plants: elephant's ear (*Caladium* sp.), dumb cane (*Dieffenbachia* sp.), philodendron (*Philodendron* sp.), peace lily (*Spathiphyllum* sp.) (vomiting, diarrhea, oral swelling, salivation) • Endotoxins and enterotoxins: staphylococcal, clostridial, *Escherichia coli, Salmonella* (severe GI signs, progressive lethargy, dehydration, hypothermia) • Zinc oxide (diaper rash ointment ingestion in dogs; mild to severe gastritis) • Zinc phosphide (GI and CNS signs, pulmonary edema; liver and kidney damage possible) • NSAID toxicosis (initial stages: GI signs with or without blood)	• Infectious (feline panleukopenia, canine distemper, canine parvovirus, canine coronavirus, infectious canine hepatitis, leptospirosis, salmonellosis) • Internal parasites (hookworms) • Dietary discretion (recent change in diet) • Foreign body (plastic, wood, metal, bones, partial or complete obstruction) • Gastric dilation, volvulus, intussusceptions (abdominal distension, pain, dyspnea, shock) • Liver diseases (secondary to liver disease) • Kidney diseases (secondary to renal disease, post–renal obstruction, uremia) • Metabolic disorders (diabetic ketoacidosis, hypoadrenocorticism) • Sudden change in the environment (traveling, weather change, boarding, moving) • Inflammatory bowel disease (generally immune mediated)
Hypernatremia (measured serum sodium >160 in dogs and >165 in cats)	• Paint ball ingestion (dogs: history of paintball ingestion, polydipsia, vomiting, diarrhea, ataxia) • Salt toxicosis (history of inducing emesis with sodium chloride, ingestion of excessive amounts of salt-containing objects [play dough] and foods) • Activated charcoal administration (can occur sporadically in some dogs possibly due to fluid-shift) • Sea water ingestion (history of visit to a beach, lack of access to fresh water, swimming)	• Due to pure water loss (nephrogenic diabetes insipidus, heatstroke, fever, burns, no access to water) • Due to hypotonic water loss (severe diarrhea, vomiting, diabetes mellitus, renal failure, hypoadrenocorticism)
Hypoglycemia	• Ingestion of xylitol-containing products (ingestion of sugar-free gum, bakery products, hypoglycemia within 12 hours) • Ingestion of oral diabetic/hypoglycemic agents (sulfonylureas)	• Insulinoma • Acute hepatic disease • Functional hypoglycemia (idiopathic in neonates, severe exercise) • Internal parasitism • Adrenocortical insufficiency • Endotoxemia

2,4-D, Dichlorophenoxyacetic acid; *ALT*, alanine aminotransferase; *aPTT*, activated partial thromboplastin time; *ARF*, acute renal failure; *CNS*, central nervous system; *CRF*, chronic renal failure; *CV*, cardiovascular; *FeLV*, feline leukemia virus; *GI*, gastrointestinal; *NPK*, nitrogen, phosphorous, potassium; *NSAID*, nonsteroidal antiinflammatory drug; *PCV*, packed cell volume; *PT*, prothrombin time; *RBC*, red blood cell; *SLUD*, salivation, lacrimation, urination, defecation.

CHAPTER 145

Food Safety and Toxicities

William Burkholder
Randall Lovell
Daniel G. McChesney

FOOD-RELATED ILLNESS

All animals have generally eaten or refused food within a day of their owner or caretaker noting the animal to be ill. Diagnosing whether this illness is due to something the animal ate can be difficult. For a definitive diagnosis one needs to be able to: (1) relate clinical and laboratory findings to a specific compound or class of compounds, (2) detect the compound or a metabolite of the compound in the animal, and (3) detect the compound in the food the animal has eaten at a concentration sufficient to produce the clinical signs. Although conceptually straightforward, meeting these criteria can be challenging.

For discussion of this topic we will define a food-related illness as any illness directly related to consuming a food containing an unsafe concentration of a substance. The substance could be a naturally occurring toxicant (e.g., aflatoxin or deoxynivalenol); result from microbial contamination of the food (e.g., *Salmonella* spp., *Clostridium* spp.); be intentionally added (e.g., melamine and cyanuric acid); be a contaminate of an ingredient (e.g., copper sulfate contaminated with polychlorinated biphenyls or ball clay with dioxins); or could be an ingredient present in the wrong concentration, (e.g., selenium or fat-soluble vitamins). An unsafe concentration could also be an insufficient amount of a required nutrient needed to support the animal's daily requirement (e.g., taurine, thiamine).

DIAGNOSING A FOOD-RELATED ILLNESS REQUIRES AN ADEQUATE DIETARY HISTORY AND A SAMPLE OF THE SUSPECTED FOOD

In 2007, reports of food-induced renal toxicosis resulted in one of the largest pet food recalls in history. Work done by veterinary schools, the United States Food and Drug Administration (FDA) and the pet food industry eventually showed that wheat gluten and rice protein concentrate, which were contaminated with melamine and cyanuric acid, were incorporated into many pet foods. This resulted in the formation of melamine cyanurate crystals in the kidneys of affected animals and caused numerous illnesses and deaths. The FDA received over 18,000 calls from consumers during these recalls.

A few weeks into the melamine cyanuric acid–related recalls, which lasted more than 8 weeks, the FDA worked with the Association of American Veterinary Laboratory Diagnosticians (AAVLD) to develop criteria for reporting cases along with required documentation. The FDA and the pet food industry estimated that the products involved represented slightly less then 1% of the all the pet food available. Even though the potential exposure theoretically involved more than 1 million animals and several veterinary internet sites reported thousands of dog and cat deaths associated with the contaminated pet food, very few of the reports received by FDA met the three criteria for definitively diagnosing a food-related illness.

The information that was most often lacking was an adequate dietary history and an unopened sample, or in most cases, any sample of the food(s) the animal had consumed. An adequate dietary history involves collecting information to answer what food(s) the animal ate, how much, and how often. Many times reports focus only on one food, excluding consideration of other foods or products the animal also received during the same time period.

The clinical manifestations of a food-related illness are often very similar to a variety of other diseases, especially those with clinical signs referable to the gastrointestinal tract, kidneys, and liver. For example, malignant neoplasias, cholecalciferol-analog rodenticides, and foods overformulated with vitamin D can all cause hypercalcemia and renal failure from metastatic calcification. Thus, a dog or cat presenting with signs of renal failure and hypercalcemia would need to have these differentials considered along with others before diagnosing the cause of the renal failure. In addition to clinical and laboratory findings, a dietary history and at least the preservation of a sample of suspected food(s) for possible testing along with the label(s) for explicit lot and manufacturing site identification become essential, especially if one wants to definitively diagnose a food-related illness. A contaminate in the food may not turn out to be the cause, but without an accurate dietary history and sample of the food it is difficult to either prove or eliminate.

OBTAIN ALL AVAILABLE CLINICAL, LABORATORY, AND PATHOLOGIC DATA

Because food-related illnesses rarely present with pathognomonic signs, a minimum data base (MDB) is often necessary. This MDB includes a thorough history, of which the dietary history is a part, a physical examination, and various clinical pathology (hematology, biochemical, urinalysis) assessments. This MDB helps to exclude more common as well as uncommon etiologies for any case suspected of being directly caused by food. Correlating MDB findings with possible causes can aid in limiting the candidate "toxicants" for additional tests as well as being useful in directing treatments.

Unfortunately, treatment is not always successful. If the patient dies, a necropsy with histologic evaluation of major organ systems is often needed for narrowing the differentials, particularly in food-related cases.

IDENTIFY COMPOUNDS OR CLASSES OF COMPOUNDS THAT HAVE BEEN REPORTED TO CAUSE CLINICAL, LABORATORY AND PATHOLOGIC FINDINGS CONSISTENT WITH THE INFORMATION AVAILABLE

Listing the primary clinical, laboratory, and pathologic findings for all potential contaminants is not possible. However, dogs and cats seem to be sensitive to certain potential con-

Table • 145-1

Toxicants Frequently Associated with Food

AGENT	COMMON SOURCE	ASSOCIATED FINDINGS
Aflatoxins	Corn, peanuts	Anorexia, icterus, ascites, hemorrhage, pale yellow-to-orange liver, edematous gallbladder, hepatic fibrosis[1-3]
Deoxynivalenol	Grains	Anorexia, weight loss, vomiting[4,5]
Tremorgenic mycotoxins (e.g., penitrem A, roquefortine, verruculogen)	Moldy food	Fine muscle tremors, ataxia, seizures, prostration, polyuria, polydypsia[6-8]
Theobromine/caffeine	Chocolate	Restlessness, hyperactivity, tachycardia, tachypnea, diuresis, vomiting, diarrhea, tremors, seizures[9-11]
Undetermined	Grapes/raisins	Acute renal failure[12-14]
Enterotoxin-producing bacteria (Salmonella, Escherichia, Clostridium, Staphylococcus, Streptococcus)	Garbage, spoiled	Vomiting, diarrhea, abdominal pain and distention, gastrointestinal statis[15-17]
Vitamin D	Food additive	Anorexia, lethargy, vomiting, diarrhea, hypercalcemia, soft tissue mineralization, renal failure[18-21]
Sulfur-containing compounds	Allium spp. fed in excessive amounts (garlic, onions)	Hemolytic anemia, Heinz body formation, eccentrocytosis, methemoglobinemia[22-26]

taminants and have recurring exposure to others in their food (e.g., mycotoxins, vitamin D, minerals). In addition, potential failures in processing the food (no or insufficient heating, inadequate low-acid canning procedures) can lead to microbial contamination. Table 145-1 lists the primary clinical, laboratory, and pathologic findings for several of the more common causes of food-related illnesses observed in dogs and cats.

TEST THE FOOD TO CONFIRM THE PRESENCE OF THE SUSPECTED COMPOUND AND TO CONFIRM THE DIAGNOSIS

If common and usual causes of illness have been ruled out and a food-related cause has not been eliminated as a possible cause of the illness or death, consideration should be given for contacting a regional or state veterinary diagnostic laboratory and/or the Center for Veterinary Medicine of the FDA. Food matrices present many unique chemical challenges when attempting to analyze for a contaminate. Laboratory tests that work in blood, urine, or tissue may not work at all in a food matrix. When conducting tests for the suspected compound, it is vital the laboratory use a method that has been validated in the food matrix being tested and that a full complement of standards are available. The results from the diagnostic workup already performed will be extremely valuable for a diagnostic laboratory to determine appropriate tests to run on the food(s).

REFERENCES

The reference list can be found on the companion Expert Consult Web site at *www.expertconsult.com*.

CHAPTER 146

Venomous Bites and Stings

Patrick M. Burns

The following monograph is a discussion of the indigenous venomous creatures of the United States; however, there is an increasing number of exotic venomous animals kept by herpetologists.[1] A snake identification guide is essential for any veterinarian in a snake-endemic area.[2] Expeditious transportation of the bite victim to the nearest veterinary facility followed by aggressive specific therapy are the cornerstone to a successful outcome.

CROTALIDS (PIT VIPERS)

Pit vipers cause approximately 150,000 veterinary emergency room visitations annually in the United States, most of which are in the southern half of the mainland.[3] The three genera of crotalids in the United States are *Crotalus* (rattlesnakes) (Figure 146-1, Web Figure 146-1), *Sistrurus* (pygmy rattlesnakes and massasauga) (Figure 146-2), and *Agkistrodon*

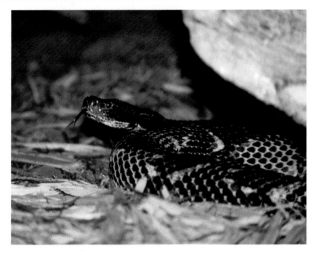

Figure 146-1 *Crotalus horridus*, timber rattlesnake.

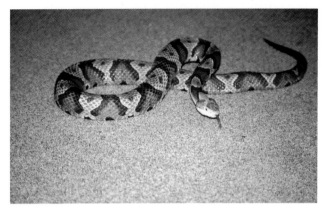

Figure 146-4 *Agkistrodon contortrix*, copperhead.

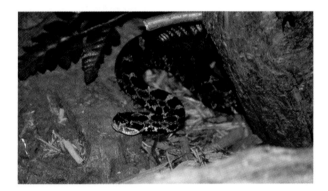

Figure 146-2 *Sistrurus catenatus*, eastern massasauga.

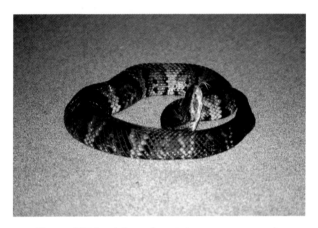

Figure 146-5 *Agkistrodon piscivorus*, cottonmouth.

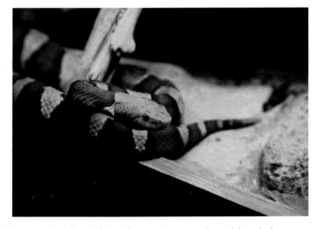

Figure 146-3 *Agkistrodon contortrix*, broad-banded copper snake.

(copperheads, cottonmouth water moccasins) (Figures 146-3, 146-4, and 146-5).

Crotalus catalinensis is the only rattlesnake that does not have a keratinized rattle on the end of the tail.

Pit vipers have characteristic retractable rostral maxillary fangs. They can control the amount of venom delivered with each bite, and the first, defensive bite often is "dry." This is, however, based upon a nonprovoked attack. Bites to the torso tend to develop more severe clinical signs, and bites are more serious during the spring and summer months due to larger venom production.

Crotalid venom is a mixture of enzymatic and nonenzymatic proteins.[3,4] Disintegrins, hyaluronidases, and collagenases are all enzymes that break down cellular adhesions to the extracellular matrix enabling the local penetration of toxins into the systemic circulation. Crotalid venom causes a disseminated intravascular coagulopathy-like syndrome characterized by defibrination. D-dimer levels are usually not elevated in the early stages of the envenomation.[4,5] Different toxins found among the various species affect the clotting cascade through different mechanisms and result in impaired platelet function, thrombocytopenia, activation of clotting factors, fibrinolysis, and vasculitis. Some crotalid envenomations induce neurologic signs only, such as convulsions and alterations in mentation.[3]

Clinical signs include localized pain, salivation, weakness, fasciculations, hypotension, alteration in respiratory pattern, regional lymphadenopathy, mucosal bleeding, ecchymoses, obtundation, and convulsions. The onset of these clinical signs may take several hours to occur. The severity of the local reaction does not correlate with the severity of the systemic signs.

Hematologic changes suggestive of envenomation include hemoconcentration followed by anemia, stress leukogram, spherocytosis, and echinocytosis. The erythrocyte membrane damage is likely due to the presence of phospholipase A_2 in the venom.[5] The coagulation panel may show prolongation of

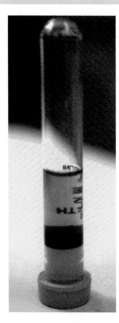

Figure 146-6   Disintegrated clot formation due to defibrination following snake envenomation.

the prothrombin time, activated clotting time, and partial thromboplastin time, with a reduction in fibrinogen and an increase in fibrin degradation products. The clot is characteristically unstable and will disintegrate over time (Figure 146-6).

Rhabdomyolysis may also be seen, especially with envenomation by Mojave, canebrake, and tiger rattlesnakes. Urinalysis can reveal proteinuria, hemoglobinuria, and myoglobinuria. Electrocardiographic abnormalities occur in more severely affected victims.

First aid should be aimed at keeping the patient calm, positioning the bite site below the level of the heart, and rapid transportation. Intravenous fluids are necessary to counteract the hypotension and pigmentary nephrosis. Diphenhydramine 1 to 2 mg/kg slow IV will provide mild sedation and may theoretically reduce the severity of any anaphylactic/anaphylactoid reactions. An equine-derived polyvalent antivenom (Antivenin Crotalidae Polyvalent, Fort Dodge Laboratories, Fort Dodge, Iowa) produced from the venom of *C. atrox* (western diamondback rattlesnake), *C. adamenteus* (eastern diamondback rattlesnake), *C. terrificus* (South American rattlesnake), and *Brothrops atrox* (fer-de-lance) is available. Slow IV infusion of the antivenom initially will help reduce the severity of any allergic reactions (urticaria, nausea, vomiting, or diarrhea) that may occur against the equine proteins in the antivenom. Epinephrine and prednisolone sodium succinate may be required in cases of severe envenomation and when reactions to the antivenom have occurred. Ideally the dose of the antivenom should be sufficient to neutralize the amount of venom received by the patient. This may require multiple vials. Local injection of antivenom is ineffective and not recommended.

A purified Fab-type antivenom (Crotalidae polyvalent immune Fab Ovine, Protherics, Inc., Brentwood, Tenn.) has been approved for use in humans. The antivenom is created against the following venoms: *C. atrox* (western diamondback rattlesnake), *C. adamanteus* (eastern diamondback rattlesnake), *C. scutulatus scutulatus* (Mojave rattlesnake), and *Agkistrodon piscivorus* (cottonmouth or water moccasin). The ovine antivenom has a number of advantages, including lower antigenicity, higher affinity, better tissue penetration, lower

chance of activating complement, and a theoretic lower chance of serum sickness. Apart from the higher cost, the main disadvantage is the potential need for repeat dosing due to the faster renal clearance of the antivenom. Delayed administration of the ovine antivenom up to 52 hours postenvenomation has been reported to be successful in human case reports; however, early administration is associated with a reduction in morbidity and mortality.[6]

The antivenom reverses the coagulopathy, electrocardiographic findings, and to a lesser degree neurologic changes. Tissue necrosis cannot be reversed by antivenom; however, the extent of the damage is limited. The practitioner should monitor the hemolysis and coagulation profile in order to judge the amount of venom required. Administration of blood products to reverse the coagulopathy without neutralization of the venom may result in further fibrinolysis and worsen clinical signs.[4] Fasciotomy is associated with an increased morbidity and has been shown to have little benefit in the vast majority of the cases.[7,8] Broad-spectrum antibiotics and opioid analgesics are indicated in patients with severe envenomation. A snakebite severity score has been formulated and may be helpful in monitoring a patient's therapeutic response.[3]

An anticrotalid venom vaccine was released in 2004 in the state of California for the protection against all North American crotalids except the Mojave rattlesnake. The vaccine induces an IgG response that will neutralize the venom. Obviously the protection against any venom is the amount of circulating IgG at the time of the envenomation, which will wane over time. It is possible for a vaccinated animal to still require antivenom therapy and should therefore be brought to veterinarian attention. This vaccination as yet has not undergone any laboratory or clinical scrutiny.[3]

ELAPIDS (CORAL SNAKES)

Most elapids are found in the southern and southeastern United States (i.e., *Micrurus fulvius tenere* [Texas coral snake]; *M. fulvius fulvius* [eastern coral snake]; *M. fulvius barbouri* [South Florida coral snake]; and *Micruroides euryxanthus* [Sonoran coral snake]). The incidence of elapid envenomation is extremely low compared with crotalids, and the percentage of dry bites is high because these snakes must "chew" on their victims to inject venom. Another difference between the elapids and crotalids is the lack of proteolytic enzymes in elapid venom (and therefore the lack of a local reaction). The neurotoxic venom of elapids affects the nervous system mainly by means of a nondepolarizing postsynaptic neuromuscular blocking activity, similar to the effect of curare. Some reports have mentioned an intravascular hemolysis, which is speculated to be mediated by phospholipase A_2.

The clinical onset of symptoms commonly is delayed 10 to 18 hours. In the dog, emesis, salivation, agitation, and central depression, followed by quadriplegia, hyporeflexia, intravascular hemolysis and, finally, respiratory paralysis, are seen. Cats show a loss of cutaneous nociception and hypothermia but not hemolytic anemia. Hematologic studies in dogs reveal erythrocyte membrane damage, such as burr cells and spherocytes similar to crotalid envenomation.

Application of a compression bandage, where possible, has been shown to be helpful.[9] North American coral snake antivenin (NACSA, Wyeth, Madison, N.J.) ceased production in 2006; however, another antivenom (Coralmyn, Bioclon, Mexico) has been shown to be effective against *Micrurus* species.[10] However, this antivenom is not effective against the Sonoran coral snake.

The same precautious should be used as mentioned above for the administration of this antivenom. Clinical signs and changes to the coagulation profile may be used to monitor response to antivenom therapy. In severe cases of envenomation, respiratory support by means of artificial ventilation may be required for several days. Broad-spectrum antibiotics are recommended for local wound infections. Treatment of Sonoran coral snake envenomation is supportive at this stage. Tick paralysis, botulism, polyradiculoneuritis, myasthenia gravis, and certain drugs can have clinical signs similar to those of elapid envenomation.

Latrodectus spp. (WIDOW SPIDERS)

The widow spiders belong to the genus *Latrodectus*. *Latrodectus mactans* (black widow), *L. variolus*, *L. bishopi* (red widow), *L. hesperus* (western black widow), and *L. geometricus* (brown widow) are the five species found in all the U.S. states except Alaska. *L. mactans* is the most common species. Females have an hourglass, reddish marking on the ventral abdomen. The cat seems more susceptible to latrodectism, as compared to dogs. Alpha-latrotoxin induces neurotransmitter release (acetylcholine, norepinephrine, dopamine, glutamate, and enkephalin) from nerve terminals causing depletion and subsequent blockade.[11,12] Approximately 10% of bites are "dry." Venom toxicity may also vary with the seasons, with a maximal effect during autumn and at its least in spring.[12]

Onset of clinical signs is usually within 8 hours of envenomation. Bites are characterized by no local reaction or minimal erythema. On the rare instance a small bite mark may be visible. Envenomation induces extremely painful states; hyperesthesia, muscle fasciculations, and muscle cramping of the torso are characteristic clinical signs. The motor signs may give way to a flaccid paralysis within 24 hours of the bite. Respiratory compromise, hypertension, tachycardia, and seizures may also occur. Cats also show vocalization, salivation, agitation, muscle cramping, and ataxia leading to paralysis. Death is usually due to cardiopulmonary collapse.

The diagnosis is based on the clinical signs and historical exposure to the spider habitat. Occasionally cats may vomit up a spider. A stress leukogram with hyperglycemia is often seen. The muscle cramping may lead to a rise in creatine phosphokinase. Urinalysis may reveal concentrated urine, casts, and an elevated albumin level. The reduction in urine output occurs secondary to dehydration and urinary retention.

The main treatment modality consists of administration of an equine-derived antivenom (Lyovac antivenin, Merck, Sharp & Dohme). This may be given slowly intravenously over 30 minutes to minimize the risk of anaphylaxis (~ 0.54% in humans).[12] Premedication with diphenhydramine may be helpful. One vial is usually enough, but at times a second is required. Relief of clinical signs is usually seen within 30 minutes. Correction of hypertension may be indicated following antivenom administration, particular in patients with preexisting cardiovascular disease. Intravenous fluids to correct dehydration and oliguria should be administered only after the hypertension has been corrected. Pulmonary edema has also been seen with latrodectism. Calcium administration is no longer recommended to treat muscle cramps. Opioids, diazepam, and cardiopulmonary support are all indicated, especially if no antivenom is available.[13]

LOXOSCELIDAE (RECLUSE OR BROWN SPIDERS)

Recluse spiders are members of the family Loxoscelidae, genus *Loxosceles*. They are also known as *violin spiders* due to a marking on the dorsum of the cephalothorax. Five species (*L. reclusa*, *L. refuscens*, *L. arizonica*, *L. unicolor*, and *L. laeta*) found in the south-central United States are capable of causing necrotic arachnidism. Two forms of loxoscelism (envenomation by recluse or brown spiders), cutaneous and viscerocutaneous, have been described. The cutaneous form, which is more common, starts with a bull's-eye lesion at the bite site. A pale center, caused by localized thrombosis, is surrounded by an area of erythema. Within 24 to 72 hours, a hemorrhagic bulla with an underlying eschar develops in the center. The eschar eventually sloughs, leaving an ulcer that may take months to heal. The severity of these lesions depends on the response of the immune system to the toxin.

The viscerocutaneous form involves the development of a Coombs'-negative hemolytic anemia that may last for 7 days, thrombocytopenia, and disseminated intravascular coagulopathy. The extent of the cutaneous lesion and the severity of the systemic signs do not appear to be correlated. A single bite can be lethal but in most cases results in dermonecrosis and prolonged wound healing (2 to 3 months). The bite itself is painless. Renal failure from the hemolytic anemia is the major cause of death from *Loxosceles* envenomation.

The exact mechanism of loxoscelism is unknown; however, it is likely the result both of the toxin and the immune response to the toxin. An immune-mediated vasculitis, hemolysis, and platelet abnormalities all play a part in the mechanism. Sphingomyelinase D is the major toxin. The venom causes rapid coagulation and thrombosis of the capillaries. Depletion of clotting factors VIII, IX, XI, and XII also occurs, with resultant prolongation of the activated partial thromboplastin time.

No definitive test for *Loxosceles* envenomation exists. The diagnosis is based on the history and clinical signs and on laboratory findings of a Coombs'-negative hemolytic anemia, hemoglobinemia, hemoglobinuria, and a prolonged activated partial thromboplastin time.[14] Hemolysis usually is seen only in the early stages and is followed by the cutaneous lesions. Systemic signs may be used to monitor the response to therapy. Other diagnostic possibilities include necrotizing fasciitis, mycobacterial infection, a burn wound, or a decubital ulcer.

Antivenin has had disappointing results when given after the lesions became obvious. Dapsone (1 mg/kg given orally for 14 days) has shown some efficacy in reducing the size of the cutaneous lesions. Dapsone inhibits chemotaxis, thereby minimizing the vasculitis caused by polymorphonuclear cells. Corticosteroids and surgery have not been shown to be efficacious in these cases. Viscerocutaneous symptoms may require intravenous fluids or blood products, and systemic antibiotics and analgesics may be necessary. Any analgesic that interferes with renal function should be avoided.

TICK PARALYSIS

Dermacentor andersoni, *D. variabilis*, and *Haemaphysalis cinnabarina* are found in the western United States and British Columbia; and *D. variabilis* and *Ixodes scapularis* are found in the central and eastern United States and in southern portions of Canada. However, tick paralysis does not occur at all locations, which suggests a variation in the potency of the toxin. This is also true for the transmission of tick-borne diseases. Tick paralysis is more likely to occur in the spring and summer months. Sporadic cases of tick paralysis are seen in livestock and wildlife.

Holocyclotoxin, a presynaptic neurotoxin at the neuromuscular junction, is secreted in the saliva of *Ixodes holocyclus*. It is similar to the toxin isolated from *D. andersoni*. The toxin inhibits the release of acetylcholine. Compound muscle action potentials are reduced to a greater degree than compound nerve action potentials, which suggest a neuromuscular transmission defect when using electrophysiologic diagnostics. The *Dermacentor* toxin can cause mortality, if left untreated, by means of a progressive, ascending paralysis that results in cardiorespiratory failure. Local effects of paralysis may be noted before the generalized form is seen. Recent studies on *I. holocyclus* toxins have shown a direct effect on the K⁺ channels of the heart,[15] causing a reduction in the fractional shortening and a prolongation of the QT interval as well as signs of acute left ventricular heart failure.[16] Aspiration pneumonia secondary to megaesophagus is not uncommon in severely affected animals.

Ascending flaccid paralysis, dysphonia, or localized signs of paralysis usually first appear 5 to 9 days after tick attachment. Pain perception is normal in these animals. The diagnosis is based on the clinical signs and a history of exposure to ticks. Most ticks are found around the head, neck, and forelegs, and clipping of the patient sometimes is necessary to find them.[17] Recovery from the paralysis usually occurs spontaneously within 3 days or more after removal of the tick. Treatment is supportive during this time, which in severe cases may mean artificial ventilation for respiratory failure. Fipronil sprays are a good alternative to organophosphates for eliminating other ticks. The main differential diagnoses for tick paralysis are polyradiculoneuritis, polyneuropathy, snake envenomation, fenthion poisoning, and botulism.

HYMENOPTERAN STINGS (INSECT BITES)

The bites and stings of some winged insects and fire ants (*Solenopsis* sp.) have the potential to cause serious toxic or allergic effects. Toxic reactions are dose dependent unless hypersensitivity to the toxin is a factor. The venoms of this group have three broad components: low–molecular weight toxins, peptides, and high–molecular weight toxins. Low–molecular weight toxins consist of histamine, dopamine, noradrenaline, amino acids, epinephrine, and acetylcholine and are involved only in the local reaction. Peptides (melittin, apamin, kinins, hemolysin, mast cell degranulating factors, and chemotactic factors) cause cytolysis and can act as neurotoxins, inducing hyperexcitability. High–molecular weight toxins consist of phospholipase A and B, hyaluronidase, and proteases and cause allergic reactions. Phospholipase A₂ and melittin can act synergistically to cause intravascular hemolysis.[18] Dialkydpiperidine is the main cytotoxic alkaloid found in fire ants. The lethal dose of Hymenoptera stings is approximately 20 stings/kg.[18]

Allergies are mediated by immunoglobulin E (IgE) and usually occur after a period of sensitization. The common bee (*Apis mellifera*) has the greatest propensity to cause an allergic reaction. Reactions to hymenopteran stings can include localized angioedema, urticaria, emesis, diarrhea, hematochezia, hemolysis, renal failure, respiratory distress, and death. Disseminated intravascular coagulopathy is possible in severe envenomation cases or allergic reactions. The most significant stings occur around the head and neck. Delayed immunologic reactions such as malaise, serum sickness, rashes, arthritides, and lymphadenopathies may be observed within a few weeks of the insect stings.

The diagnosis of hymenopteran stings is based on historical evidence of contact with stinging insects and clinical signs. Treatment consists of administration of corticosteroids and antihistamines and supportive care. In severe cases, prednisolone sodium succinate may be administered intravenously; however, most cases respond to dexamethasone sodium phosphate given intravenously or intramuscularly. Severe cases may require supportive care with oxygen therapy, intravenous fluids, gut protectants, positive inotropes, and vasopressors. Acute renal failure may require intensive fluid therapy with

attention to electrolyte imbalances and urine output. Patients with airway obstruction or bronchial constriction may require a tracheostomy or the use of bronchodilators.

HELODERMATIDAE LIZARD (GILA MONSTER)

The genus *Heloderma* includes two species of lizard that are venomous to humans (*H. suspectum* and *H. horridum*) (Figures 146-7 and 146-8). The venom of the helodermatids is a

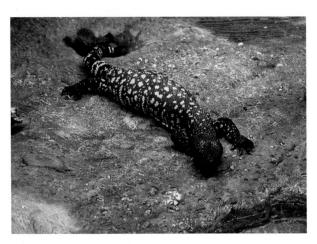

Figure 146-7 *Heloderma horridum*, beaded lizard.

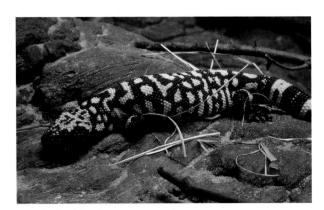

Figure 146-8 *Heloderma suspectum*, Gila monster.

Table • **146-1**

Toxins of the Gila Monster

TOXIN	ACTION
Gilatoxin	Acts as a neurotoxic protein
Helothermine	Reduces body temperature
Hyaluronidase	Damages local tissue, allowing toxins to spread
Phospholipase A₂	Causes release of histamine, serotonin, acetylcholine, kinins, and other slow-release substances
Helodermatine	Causes vasodilatation, increased permeability and edema
Arginine hydrolase	Causes release of bradykinin
Helospectin and helodermin	Have activity similar to that of vasoactive intestinal peptides

mixture of proteins and peptides (Table 146-1). The intravenous LD_{50} of the crude toxin is 0.4 to 2.7 mg/kg in mice; the toxic dose in dogs and cats is unknown.

Bite wounds typically are obvious and commonly are found around the face or forelegs. Clinical signs include salivation, lacrimation, emesis, tachypnea, respiratory distress, tachycardia, hypotension, and shock. Coagulopathies have not been reported, although a coagulation profile and minimum data base are indicated to help rule out snake envenomation. Treatment is symptomatic and may include intravenous fluids, respiratory support, debriding of the wound, and administration of broad-spectrum antibiotics and analgesics.

REFERENCES

The reference list can be found on the companion Expert Consult Web site at *www.expertconsult.com.*

CHAPTER 147

Plant Toxicities

Lynn Rolland Hovda

Animal exposures to plants and fresh flowers continue to be a common call to poison centers. Dogs, especially puppies and younger dogs, and cats make up the majority of the calls.[1] Ingestion generally occurs secondary to curiosity, boredom, or playfulness, although exposures by unknowledgeable owners still occur. Holiday plants and flower arrangements are frequently a source of problems as they are something new and different in the animal's environment. Many pet owners know little about the toxicities associated with their plants or the fact that some plants are far more harmful to a particular species than others.

One of the most common problems facing veterinarians is whether or not a plant exposure is responsible for clinical signs present in a pet. This is often frustrating because most ingestions are not witnessed and many pet owners do not know what plants are found in their house, garden, or yard or what flowers are present in an arrangement. Owners may report that they came home to find their houseplants uprooted or destroyed and their pet ill. Identification of the plant is difficult as many plants found in and around the house have several common names and the owner rarely knows the scientific name. Several reliable sources of plant identification aid the veterinarian, as does some baseline knowledge of toxic plants indigenous to the local area. Local nurseries, extension agents, and botanists are especially useful in plant identification.

Accurate identification and a thorough history are essential as ingestion of some plants can result in serious, life-threatening effects and others only in mild gastrointestinal problems. Very few antidotes are available for plant poisoning. Treatment generally consists of symptomatic and supportive care. Unless contraindicated, emesis or gastric lavage followed by activated charcoal with a cathartic should be performed. Identification of the specific plant, the quantity and parts ingested, the time of ingestion, and the age and breed of animal all are necessary for formulating a treatment plan. Examination of stomach contents (seeds, bulbs, flowers) may confirm ingestion, assist in plant identification, guide therapy, and offer a prognosis.

PLANTS KNOWN TO CAUSE SERIOUS SYSTEMIC EFFECTS

Lily (*Lilium* spp. and *Hemerocallis* spp.)
Easter lily toxicosis was first reported in cats 15 years ago and the list of suspect species has grown each year. It is believed that all parts of the Easter lily (*Lilium longiflorum*) (Web Figure 147-1), tiger lily (*L. tigrinum*), Japanese showy lily (*L. lancifolimu*) (Web Figure 147-2), rubrum lily (*L. speciosum* var. *rubrum*), stargazer lily (*L. auratum*), and some species of day lily (*Hemerocallis* spp.) (Web Figure 147-3) are toxic to cats.[2] A recent experimental study demonstrated that aqueous extracts of flowers and leaves of the Easter lily are the most nephrotoxic and pancreotoxic.[3] Ingestion of as little as 1 to 2 flower petals or leaves is associated with the onset of clinical signs. The toxin remains unidentified. Dogs, rabbits, and rats appear to be unaffected by the toxin.

Clinical signs generally occur within 3 to 12 hours with a reported range of 2 hours to 5 days. Early signs include vomiting, depression, and anorexia, followed in 1 to 3 days by acute renal failure. Laboratory work shows an increase in blood urea nitrogen (BUN), creatinine, potassium, and phosphorous. Epithelial casts have been found in the urine as early as 12 to 18 hours after ingestion. Proteinuria and glucosuria are common. Seizures unrelated to toxemia and pancreatic degeneration without a significant elevation in serum amylase have been reported. Early intervention is necessary for survival. Treatment includes early emesis, aggressive gastrointestinal (GI) decontamination with activated charcoal and a cathartic, and IV fluid diuresis for at least 48 hours. Peritoneal dialysis or hemodialysis may be helpful in anuric cats.[4] Prognosis is poor if treatment is delayed past 18 to 24 hours or anuria is present. Renal tubular epithelial cell necrosis precedes death.

Oleander (*Nerium oleander*), Lily of the Valley (*Convallaria majallis*), Kalanchoe (*Kalanchoe* spp.)
Common plants with cardiac glycoside activity include the common oleander (*Nerium oleander*) (Web Figure 147-4), lily

of the valley *(Convalleria majalis)*, and kalanchoe *(Kalanchoe spp)* (Web Figure 147-5). Five different types of cardiac glycosides (oleandrin, nerine, and several glucosides) have been identified in common oleander. The seeds, stems, leaves, and flowers of fresh and dried plants are toxic. Lily of the valley contains at least 15 toxins, with convallatoxin, convallarin, and convallamarin the most common. All parts of the plant contain cardiac glycosides with the highest concentration in the roots. The brightly red colored fruit is less toxic. Kalanchoe contains bufadienolides, with most poisonings occurring during the plant's flowering season.[5] The mechanism of action for all cardiac glycosides occurs at the cellular membrane level. Inhibition of the sodium-potassium ATPase pump causes slowed electrical conductivity with decreased active transport of sodium and an efflux of potassium.

The onset of signs varies depending on the species of plant. Signs associated with oleander ingestion occur as early as 45 minutes and may last for 4 to 5 days. Animals consuming lily of the valley or kalanchoe may show signs within a few hours of ingestion. Signs associated with cardiac glycoside–containing plants are generally related to either the cardiovascular system or GI tract, although kalanchoe also has a neurologic component. Vomiting and abdominal pain begin several hours before deterioration in myocardial function. Marked bradycardia with first-, second-, or third-degree atrioventricular (AV) block, ventricular arrhythmias, asystole, and sudden death can occur. Hyperkalemia is usually prominent, although scattered reports of hypokalemia exist. Sap from oleander plants has caused contact dermatitis and blistering of the nose and footpads. Diagnosis depends on physical identification of the plant. Digoxin assays have been successfully used in human beings for the identification of oleander.[6] Serum digoxin levels might be useful as a screening tool, but the correlation between the level and degree of toxicity is generally poor.

Treatment varies from case to case but early emesis and repeat doses of activated charcoal are essential as is correction of serum potassium abnormalities. An ECG is recommended for at least 24 hours to monitor abnormalities. Further treatment is symptomatic and includes addressing cardiovascular problems with drugs such as atropine, beta blockers, lidocaine or mexiletine, implantation of a temporary pacemaker, and digoxin-specific antibody fragments (Digibind, Glaxo Wellcome).[7] Fructose-1,6-diphosphate was used in one experimental study.[8] Prognosis is generally poor unless intervention is early and aggressive. An extremely bitter taste and spontaneous vomiting may help limit the number of deaths from oleander.

Azalea *(Rhododendron* spp.)

Azaleas *(Rhododendron* spp.) (Web Figure 147-6) are associated with severe toxicity and death. All parts of the plant, including the showy flowers and nectar, are toxic (Web Figure 147-7). The toxic agents are grayanotoxin glycosides. It appears that grayanotoxins (rhodotoxin, andromedotoxin, or acetylandromedol) act by binding to closed sodium channels. Slower opening and increased sodium permeabilities cause a decreased resting membrane potential in Purkinje fibers. Clinical signs include bradycardia or tachycardia, arrhythmias, severe weakness, hypotension, dyspnea, and respiratory failure.[9] GI signs unrelated to grayanotoxins include salivation, vocalization, vomiting, and diarrhea.

Treatment includes early induction of emesis followed by activated charcoal with a cathartic. An ECG should be used to monitor heart rate and rhythm; blood pressure should be monitored closely. The aggressive use of intravenous fluids and dopamine may be needed to support the cardiovascular system. Sodium channel–blocking drugs such quinidine and procainamide and atropine may be helpful in treating the cardiovascular abnormalities.

Sago Palm *(Cycas* spp.)

Cycad palms or sago palms *(Cycas* and *Macrozamia* spp.) are subtropical to tropical houseplants known to cause liver toxicity in dogs. All plant parts are toxic, with the seeds containing the greatest concentration. Ingestion of one or two seeds can result in death in a normal-size dog. Several important toxins have been identified: (1) cycasin and methylazomethanol, which are hydrolyzed by bacterial enzymes in the GI tract to methylazoxymethanol (MAM), the toxin responsible for liver necrosis and GI effects; (2) β-N-methylamino-L-alanine (BMAA), which causes neurologic effects; and (3) an unidentified high–molecular weight toxin associated with neurologic effects.[10]

The onset of action is variable, with signs occurring from an hour to several days. The most commonly reported signs are vomiting and diarrhea (with or without blood) followed by lethargy, depression, liver failure, and death. Neurologic signs include weakness, ataxia, seizures, and coma. Laboratory work shows a marked increase in liver enzymes (alanine transferase and alkaline phosphatase) and conjugated bilirubin. Coagulopathies may be present. Treatment includes early emesis, multiple-dose activated charcoal, control of GI and neurologic signs, and supportive care with special emphasis on the liver and secondary effects of acute liver failure. Blood transfusions and vitamin K_1 may be needed to provide clotting factors until the liver is capable of manufacturing its own.

Jequirity Bean *(Abrus precatorius)*, Castor Bean *(Ricinus communis)*

Abrus precatorius, the jequirity bean, is still used in Latin American to make necklaces and jewelry purchased by unsuspecting tourists. The plant is also cultivated in the subtropical portions of Florida and the Hawaiian Islands. Abrin, the toxin, is a toxalbumin similar to botulinum, cholera, and diphtheria. The castor bean plant *(Ricinus communis)* has similar toxic principals. Castor bean plants are widely used as an ornamental shrub throughout North America. Ricin, the toxalbumin, is concentrated in the seeds and ricine, an alkaloid, is present in leaves and seeds. Abrin and ricin are among the most deadly poisons in the world but must be released from their seed shell to be absorbed. Dogs are most often poisoned by chewing on the hard outer shell and ingesting the contents.[11] One well-chewed seed can be lethal to a normal-sized dog. Castor bean cake used as a fertilizer is another potential source of toxicity to dogs.[12] Once absorbed, abrin and ricin enter cells and inhibit protein synthesis resulting in cell death.

Signs of toxicity generally occur within 6 hours of ingestion and include severe abdominal pain, vomiting, watery diarrhea (with or without blood), depression, seizures, and cerebral edema. Laboratory analysis shows elevations in liver enzymes, BUN, creatinine, WBC count, and serum albumin and globulin.[13] Early induction of emesis followed by activated charcoal is indicated. Further treatment is symptomatic and supportive. Prognosis for recovery is poor once clinical signs develop.

Autumn Crocus *(Colchicum autumanale)*, Glory Lily *(Gloriosa* spp.)

Autumn crocus *(Colchicum autumnale)* and glory lily *(Gloriosa* spp.) contain colchicine, a toxic alkaloid that concentrates in the flowers, seeds, and corms (autumn crocus) and tubers (glory lily). Colchicine causes cell death by inhibiting normal cell division. Clinical signs include anorexia, vomiting and diarrhea (with or without blood), hypersalivation, abdominal pain progressing to depression, weakness, ataxia, and collapse. Signs progress further to include several organ systems and finally, multiple organ system collapse. Anemia or leukopenia may be present. Treatment is early decontamination and symptomatic and supportive care. The successful use of colchicine-specific Fab fragments has been reported in human beings. Filgastrim (Neupogen, Amgen) may be helpful in cases with myelosuppression.[14] Prognosis is poor if multiple organ systems are affected.

Yew (*Taxus* spp.)

The yew (*Taxus* spp.) is a common ornamental shrub found in the United States and Canada (Web Figure 147-8). Common species include the Japanese yew *(T. cuspidata)*, English yew *(T. baccata)*, Florida yew *(T. floridana)*, and ground hemlock *(T. canadensis)*. Bark, leaves, and seeds are toxic but not the fleshy part of the bright-red fruit (aril) (Web Figure 147-9). Taxine, a cardiotoxic alkaloid, causes conduction disturbances by direct effect on cardiac muscle ion channels.[15] Dogs and other pets are often exposed when shrub trimmings or sticks are used for toys or thrown into their pens. A little as 1 ounce of leaves is deadly to a normal-size dog. Caged birds may be poisoned by bark or other shrub pieces placed in their cages.

Clinical signs occur rapidly. In dogs, bradycardia or tachycardia, vomiting, diarrhea, mydriasis, weakness, muscle tremors, and seizures have been reported. Sudden death without signs may occur. Clinical signs in birds include crop regurgitation, ruffled feathers, dyspnea, weakness, ataxia, and sudden death. Early emesis is indicated in asymptomatic animals followed by activated charcoal. Further treatment is supportive and symptomatic. An ECG should be used to monitor heart rate and rhythm. Atropine may be helpful for bradycardia and IV lidocaine for arrhythmias. Prognosis is poor, and once clinical signs have occurred, further treatment is of limited value.

Yesterday, Today, and Tomorrow (*Brunfelsia* spp.)

Reports of toxicity in the United States and Australia associated with the ornamental garden shrub "yesterday, today, and tomorrow" (*Brunfelsia* spp.) are increasing. All parts of the plant are toxic, especially the juicy fruit portion. The plant contains many potential toxins with brunfelsamidine and hopeanine likely the most important. Both toxins are associated with central nervous system (CNS) effects; brunfelsamidine with excitation and hopeanine with depression. Toxicity may be specific only to the dog, rat, and mice.[16]

Depending on the particular species and amount consumed, signs can occur within minutes or up to 10 to 12 hours postingestion. Clinical signs are often similar to strychnine poisoning. Early signs include salivation, gagging, vomiting, retching, and agitation followed by nystagmus, decreased motor activity, muscle tremors, extensor rigidity, and seizures.[17]

Treatment in an asymptomatic animal is early emesis followed by activated charcoal with cathartic. Emesis should be undertaken with care as it may stimulate seizure activity. Further treatment, which may encompass several days, is primarily aimed at preventing and controlling seizures. A calm, dark isolation area with no external stimuli should be provided. Diazepam, barbiturates, or short-acting anesthetic agents are all choices for seizure control. Prognosis is good with early and aggressive care.

PLANTS WITH LESS SERIOUS SYSTEMIC EFFECTS

Oxalate-Containing Plants

Oxalate-containing plants (Araceae family) are the most frequently reported household plant exposure in cats and dogs. Plants in this family contain insoluble oxalate crystals in the leaves and stems. Plants in other families such as rhubarb (*Rheum* spp., Polygonaceae family) and the shamrock plant (*Oxallis* spp., Oxalidaceae family) contain soluble oxalate crystals.

Insoluble Crystals Common household plants in the Araceae family containing insoluble oxalate crystals include dumbcane (*Dieffenbachia* spp.) (Web Figure 147-10), philodendron (*Philodendron* spp.), peace lily (*Spathiphyllum* spp.) (Web Figure 147-11), calla lily (*Zantedeschia* spp.), and pathos (*Epiprennum* spp.) (Web Figure 147-12). There are hundreds of other less common species of plants in this family as well. Crystals or raphides are concentrated in the stem or leaf in a specialized cell known as an *idioblast*. Chewing on the plant releases the needle-sharp raphide crystals and other as yet unidentified enzymes. Clinically, stomatitis and glossitis, ocular, or systemic manifestations generally occur. Death from asphyxiation was reported in one dog who chewed the thick stem of a tall *Dieffenbachia picta* plant.[18]

Stomatitis and glossitis Irritation to the mucous membranes of the mouth and throat by embedded raphide crystals causes immediate and intense pain, local swelling, and profuse salivation. These may be accompanied by head shaking, loss of vocalization, and airway compromise. Treatment is symptomatic. The mouth should be thoroughly examined and any remaining plant pieces removed. Animals with swelling, erosions, or labored breathing should be monitored closely for glottal and epiglottal edema. Cool fluids, ice chips, and analgesics increase comfort until signs resolve. Most typically, it takes 30 to 90 minutes for this to occur, but signs can be prolonged for hours in animals with edema and airway compromise. An endotracheal tube or tracheal tube may be necessary in these animals.

Ocular Eye exposures, although rare in animals, cause severe burning pain and swelling. Left untreated, conjunctivitis, abrasions, and corneal ulcers develop. Treatment includes a 10- to 15-minute eye irrigation followed by a thorough eye examination with fluorescein dye staining or slit lamp examination. Ophthalmic protectant medications are used as indicated.

Systemic Systemic effects occur primarily in cats exposed to *Philodendron* spp. Signs are referable to the renal system and CNS and include hyperexcitability, tetany, and seizures. Treatment is symptomatic and supportive.

Soluble Crystals Rhubarb (*Rheum* spp., Polygonaceae family) (Web Figure 147-13), shamrocks (*Oxallis* spp., Oxalidaceae family) (Web Figure 147-14), and a few others contain soluble oxalate crystals. For rhubarb, the crystals are concentrated in the leaf while the stalk is edible. All parts of the shamrock plant contain soluble oxalates. When rhubarb leaves or shamrock plant material are ingested, soluble oxalates can be absorbed and bind to circulating calcium ions. Signs include diffuse GI tract irritation and infrequently systemic hypocalcemia. Oral calcium-containing products such as milk, yogurt, or antacids are used to bind oxalates in the GI tract. If systemic signs are noted, IV calcium gluconate or borogluconate should be administered to reverse the hypocalcemia. Calcium administration may have no effect on oxalate nephrosis, and acute renal failure may develop. It is likely the very bitter taste of the shamrock plant may limit exposure.

ORNAMENTAL HOLIDAY PLANTS

Ornamental holiday plants include holly (*Ilex* spp.) (Web Figures 147-15 and 147-16), poinsettia *(Euphorbia pulcherrima)* (Figure 147-1), and mistletoe *(Phoradendron flavescens)*. Well over 300 species of holly are found in the United States alone, making actual plant identification difficult. The toxin remains unidentified but may be ilicin (ilexanthin and ilex

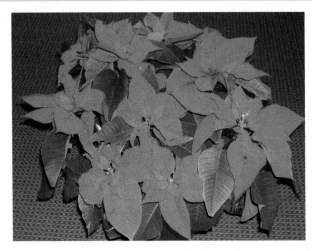

Figure 147-1 Poinsettia plant *(Euphorbia pulcherrima)*, which receives a lot of bad press but associated only with minor signs.

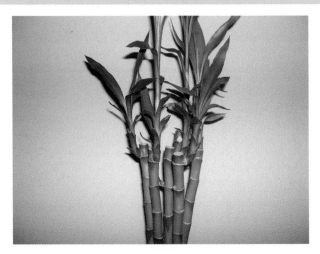

Figure 147-2 Lucky bamboo plant *(Dracaena sanderiana)*. This plant has become popular in homes and offices worldwide.

acids), a saponin causing GI effects. Poinsettias produce only mild toxicity.[19] The unidentified toxin in the latex sap, thought to be a diterpenoid ester, rarely causes more than mucous membrane irritation or contact dermatitis. Clinical signs include salivation, mild GI irritation, and occasional diarrhea. Conjunctival irritation and corneal ulcers can occur if the sap is rubbed into the eyes.[20] Mistletoe has the potential for more serious effects, although few animal case reports exist. The toxin is a phytotoxin or toxalbumin that can cause severe gastroenteritis with prolonged emesis. Signs occur up to 18 to 24 hours after ingestion of leaves, berries, or tea made from berries. Treatment associated with any of these plants is symptomatic and supportive. Demulcents and antacids are often of great benefit.

BULBS

Several varieties of poisonous plants grow from bulbs, tubers, or corms. Included are amaryllis *(Amaryllis* spp.); jonquil, narcissus, and daffodil *(Narcissus* spp.) (Web Figures 147-17 and 147-18); tulip *(Tulipa* spp.) (Web Figure 147-19); and iris *(Iris* spp.) (Web Figures 147-20 and 147-21). The toxic principal for most of them is unknown but at least several are thought to contain active alkaloids. Ingestion of the bulb has been associated with mild to severe gastroenteritis, tremors, and seizures. Hypothermia and cardiac effects were noted in a cat ingesting dried daffodil stems.[21] The iris *(Iris* spp.) plant is a special case as it contains specific irritant resins in the rhizomes. In addition to GI problems, damage to the liver and pancreas may occur. Treatment is symptomatic and supportive.

CHINABERRY TREE

The chinaberry tree *(Melia azedarach)* can be found throughout temperate regions of North America. All parts of the tree are toxic, although dogs are generally poisoned by eating fruit fallen from trees. Toxicity has been reported in rabbits, guinea pigs, rats, and other species. Many potential toxins have been isolated, with meliatoxins found in highest concentration in the fruit. Clinical signs usually occur within 1 to 2 hours after ingestion. Vomiting and diarrhea (with or without blood) are the most common signs, along with anorexia, severe abdominal pain, hypersalivation, and straining to defecate.[22] Neurologic effects are similar to nicotine, and signs include

depression, ataxia, seizures, and coma. Other reported signs include hyperthermia or hypothermia, tachycardia or bradycardia, mydriasis or miosis, and muscle rigidity. Death generally occurs from respiratory depression and arrest. Treatment is symptomatic and supportive.

Dracaena spp.

Many of the plants in this species are common indoor plants found in offices and homes throughout the United States. Popular species include the Janet Craig *(D. deremensis)* (Web Figure 147-22), lucky bamboo *(D. sanderiana)* (Figure 147-2), and corn plant *(D. fragrans)*. Easy access makes consumption likely in curious housebound dogs and cats. The toxic agent is unknown although it may be a saponin or glycoside. Signs are primarily related to the GI tract and include anorexia, salivation, vomiting (with or without blood). Other signs include depression, ataxia and weakness. Cats have developed mydriasis, difficult breathing, and tachycardia in addition to the other signs.[23] Treatment is symptomatic and supportive.

IVY

English ivy *(Hedera helix)* (Web Figure 147-23), a common houseplant and ground cover, contains hederagenin, a saponin associated primarily with GI irritation. Other compounds in the plant have been associated with contact dermatitis in human beings with a history of extensive exposure. Other *Hedera* spp. of ivy with suspected toxicity include Persian ivy *(H. colchica)*, Irish ivy or Atlantic ivy *(H. hibernica)*, and Nepal ivy *(H. nepalensis)*. Ingestion of leaves and berries causes profuse salivation, abdominal pain, vomiting, and diarrhea. Treatment is symptomatic and supportive.

NETTLE

Nettle toxicity (family Urticaceae) is seen primarily in hunting or field dogs. Some species of nettles contain hairs that break off when an animal rubs against them, allowing injection of the contents into the animal. The toxic agents are histamine, acetylcholine, serotonin, and formic acid. Clinical signs are variable and depend on which toxin predominates. Muscle weakness is the most common sign but may be accompanied by salivation, vomiting, pawing at the mouth, tremors, dyspnea, and a slow, irregular heartbeat. Atropine in large doses, antihistamines, and sedation are useful. Generally, animals respond to treatment in less than 24 hours.

SOLANINE-CONTAINING PLANTS

Solanine-containing plants are members of the Solanaceae family. Included are the tomato *(S. lycopersicon)*, potato *(S. tuberosum)*, eggplant *(S. melongena)*, bittersweet *(S. dulcamara)*, deadly or black nightshade *(S. nigrum)*, and Jerusalem cherry *(S. pseudocapsicum)*. The primary toxin is solanine. Some plants also produce tropane belladonna (deadly nightshade) or solanocapsine (Jerusalem cherry). Solanine is poorly absorbed orally, and most members of this family act only as GI irritants. Systemic absorption only occurs when substantial GI mucosa damage exists. Systemically, solanine causes CNS depression and cardiac arrhythmias. Deadly nightshade may cause a mixed picture, depending on which toxin is prevalent. Solanine usually predominates, but anticholinergic signs occasionally occur, and physostigmine may be indicated. Solanocapsine affects cardiac muscle, causing decreased heart rate and conductive changes. Treatment is symptomatic and supportive.

It is interesting to note that very few plants account for the most serious, life-threatening ingestions and yet the greatest number of calls to poison control centers involve plants with the potential for less serious outcomes. The early signs for the majority of all plant ingestions, life threatening or not, are nonspecific, making scientific and precise plant identification essential for quick diagnosis and treatment. Pet owners should be advised to accurately identify those plants with serious outcomes and remove them from their homes or at the very least, make them inaccessible to their pets. Other plants with less serious outcomes should be identified and access limited. Fresh flower arrangements, especially those containing lilies, in households with cats should be placed in an inaccessible area. If these steps can be accomplished, the number of animals with poor outcomes related to plant exposures will be limited.

REFERENCES

The reference list can be found on the companion Expert Consult Web site at *www.expertconsult.com*.

CHAPTER 148

Topical Toxins

Ahna G. Brutlag

Given the curious nature of cats and dogs, exposure to potential toxins is likely. This chapter will cover "topical toxins," encompassing those products both *applied* topically to cats and dogs, as well as those topical preparations accidentally *ingested* by cats or dogs such as common over-the-counter and prescription creams, ointments, and transdermal patches. Animals may be exposed to "topical toxins" through deliberate application by well-intentioned owners or, as is more common, by chewing into the containers of topical preparations. Outcome severity depends largely on the product and the dose ingested or absorbed. This chapter is organized based on the severity of the expected outcome—minor, moderate, or severe. A minor outcome reflects mild and self-limiting symptoms requiring little to no medical treatment. A moderate outcome reflects symptoms of a systemic nature that often require medical treatment but are typically not life-threatening. A severe outcome reflects a toxicity that, if left untreated, would likely result in permanent organ damage or death.

MINOR OUTCOMES

Zinc Oxide Ointment
Topical zinc oxide is found in diaper rash creams (such as Desitin) and other "skin protection" type products. Concentrations vary from 5% to 40%. In acute ingestions, elemental zinc toxicity is highly unlikely. Most animals will vomit following ingestion (thereby self-decontaminating).[1] Symptomatic and supportive care may be warranted if vomiting or

diarrhea becomes severe. To date, there is only one case report of a dog developing elemental zinc toxicity after ingestion of topical zinc oxide cream.[2] This dog was hospitalized following removal of a rectal mass. In an effort to alleviate discomfort, zinc oxide cream was frequently applied to the rectal area and the dog continually licked it off. It is estimated that he chronically ingested ¾ of a pound of 40% zinc oxide ointment over a 4-day period (approximately 4000 mg of Zn/kg total). By the fourth day, the dog developed clinical signs of zinc toxicity along with elevated serum and urine zinc levels. The dog recovered after whole blood transfusions and aggressive supportive care.

Corticosteroid Ointments and Solutions
Topical steroid ointments and ophthalmic preparations are common, containing up to 1% hydrocortisone, betamethasone, or triamcinolone. Toxicity is unlikely following oral exposure to these products.[1] Some animals may experience mild vomiting or diarrhea, most likely as a result of the petroleum-based carrier. A few dogs have developed self-limiting polyuria/polydipsia secondary to systemic absorption. Most often, no medical intervention is needed.

Antibiotic Ointments
Topical antibiotic ointments, such as Neosporin and Polysporin are commonly found in homes. Such products often contain a mixture of neomycin sulfate, bacitracin, and polymyxin sulfate. Acute ingestion may result in vomiting, diarrhea, and abdominal pain, with signs at least partially due to the petroleum-based carriers of these ointments. However, if

large amounts are ingested, the antibiotic portion of the ointment may alter normal gastrointestinal (GI) flora, thereby contributing to the GI signs. Treatment is symptomatic and supportive.

Anaphylactic reactions in cats to ophthalmic antibiotic compounds containing neomycin and polymyxin (both with and without bacitracin) have occurred.[3] In some of these cats, these antibiotic compounds were used to lubricate eyes during routine surgical procedures. While the incidence of anaphylaxis to these compounds is rare, it is recommended to use only pure ocular lubricants in situations where antibiotic therapy is not necessary.

MODERATE OUTCOMES

Tea Tree (Melaleuca) Oil

Tea tree oil (otherwise known as melaleuca oil) is an extract of the leaves of the Australian tea tree (Melaleuca alternifolia). It is similar in composition and toxicity to eucalyptus oil. This oil has proven antibacterial and antifungal properties and is a component of many face washes, shampoos, lotions, and ointments. It is also touted as an insect repellant and antiparasitic compound. The internet has multiple websites claiming this oil to be "completely safe and nontoxic" for pets and advocating its use as a parasiticide. Unfortunately, the propagation of such misinformation may be contributing to its common use and subsequent toxicity in dogs and cats, (i.e., topical application of 100% oil for parasite control).[4,5] It is unlikely that exposure to the diluted amount of oil found in shampoos and sprays would lead to toxicity.

Due to its highly lipophilic nature, the oil is rapidly absorbed from both the skin and GI tract.[5] Common clinical signs of toxicity include weakness, ataxia, muscle tremors, central nervous system (CNS) depression, and hypothermia.[4,5] The time period between dermal application and onset of clinical signs is 2 to 8 hours and resolution typically occurs within 1 to 2 days. While the toxic dose is not established, cases of toxicity following dermal administration of less than 10 mL of 100% oil on both dogs and cats have been reported to Pet Poison Helpline.[6] A separate case report described three cats, each of whom developed toxicity following dermal application of approximately 20 mL of 100% tea tree oil.[4] Additional case reports from the human literature describe children developing toxicity with symptoms ranging from confusion, disorientation, and ataxia to Glasgow Coma Scores of 5T (no verbal response, eye opening or response to painful stimuli) following the ingestion of 10 mL of tea tree oil.[7-9]

An antidote is not available and treatment consists mainly of decontamination and supportive care. Bathing the animal with a degreasing soap such as liquid hand dishwashing soap or benzyl peroxide shampoo will aid in the removal of the oil from the skin. The administration of activated charcoal may be an effective method of GI decontamination if there is risk of significant ingestion. There is evidence suggesting enterohepatic recirculation of structurally similar oils. Thus, multiple doses of activated charcoal may be beneficial.[5] Supportive care and baseline diagnostics should include the administration of IV fluids to maintain hydration, monitoring body temperature and providing thermal support, and monitoring vital signs, hepatic enzymes, and serum electrolytes.

The toxic components in tea tree oil are thought to be mainly cyclic hydrocarbons and terpene alcohols similar to those found in eucalyptus and pine oil.[7] Terpenes are primarily metabolized in the liver via phase I and II biotransformation. The terpene metabolites are primarily excreted in urine within 2 to 3 days of exposure. Since cats have limited ability to adequately perform glucuronidation, they may be at higher risk of toxicity than dogs. Cases of cats developing elevated liver enzymes following exposure to concentrated tea tree oil have been reported.[4]

Nicotine Transdermal Patches

Nicotine transdermal patches, used by people for smoking cessation therapy, may contain substantial amounts of nicotine. These patches are available both as over-the-counter and prescription products. When an animal chews on a patch and compromises the rate-controlling membrane, the majority of nicotine may be quickly released, leading to rapid onset of clinical signs. Individual patches contain anywhere from 7 to 114 mg of nicotine.[10] Use caution when interpreting the dose contents of patches as the total amount contained within the patch will likely be greater than the amount designed for release. For example, the Habitrol (Novartis Consumer Health, Inc.) patch, designed to release 21 mg of nicotine over 24 hours, actually contains a total of 52.5 mg of nicotine in each patch. Therefore, even used patches may contain significant amounts of remnant nicotine and pose a toxicity risk.

Historical studies have suggested that the oral LD$_{50}$ of nicotine for dogs was 9 to 12 mg/kg.[11,12] However, it seems likely that dogs can tolerate higher doses than these without fatality. Lethal dose data has not been reported in cats. It is interesting to compare studies in which transdermal patches were held to the buccal surface of dogs as opposed to ingested. In the dogs with buccal exposure (dosed at 11.5 mg/kg or less), nicotine was rapidly absorbed and peak plasma levels were recorded in less than 5 minutes of exposure.[13] Dogs ingesting patches (both intact and destroyed, dosed up to 13.4 mg/kg) developed peak plasma levels 60 to 120 minutes later.[14] Dogs with buccal exposure exhibited systemic toxic effects of toxicity within 1 to 2 minutes. Those signs were more severe than those seen in the group that ingested the patches. Dogs with buccal exposure developed severe, rapid-onset hypertension (systolic readings up to 400 mm Hg), marked sinus tachycardia, and ventricular arrhythmias.[13] Dogs that ingested the patches had few notable clinical effects other than vomiting, although cardiac parameters were not directly monitored.[14]

The amount of nicotine released following ingestion of transdermal patches may vary depending on the degree of damage done to the patch prior to ingestion and the composition of the patch. Experimentally, one patch recovered from the vomitus of a dog 15 minutes after ingestion had already released half its nicotine content.[14] Patches not vomited have a GI transit time of 25 to 57 hours.[14]

Signs of nicotine toxicity encompass multiple organ systems. Soon after ingestion, salivation and vomition may be observed. Nicotine acts as both a central nervous stimulant and a depressant. Therefore, in cases of severe toxicity, initial GI irritation may be followed by systemic signs: hypertension, tachycardia, tachypnea, hyperexcitability, mydriasis, tremors, and/or seizures. Delayed onset signs include neurologic depression, respiratory depression, ataxia, seizures, and death. Signs of central nervous depression would not be expected unless precipitated by central nervous stimulation. Therefore, if the animal did not ingest enough nicotine to cause stimulatory signs, it would be unlikely to develop delayed depressive signs.

Due to the rapid release of nicotine from altered or destroyed patches, treatment is usually focused on clinical signs rather than on patch removal. However, limited data exist on the rate of nicotine release in the GI tract from patches with *intact* rate-controlling membranes. Therefore, if a patch remains intact when ingested and is not removed, the release of nicotine could be slow (many hours versus 1 to 2 hours). This warrants removal via emesis, gastric lavage, or endoscopy. Alternatively, if the patch has passed into the intestines, surgical removal or multidose activated charcoal with cathartics may be warranted. Induction of emesis, unless instituted immediately postingestion by the pet owner, is best done under direct supervision of a veterinarian because of the possibility for neurologic changes.

Treatment is symptomatic and supportive as no antidote for nicotine toxicity is available. Heart rate and blood pressure should be monitored closely and treated if significantly abnormal. Beta-blockers may be used for tachycardia. Severe CNS stimulation or seizures may be treated with diazepam, barbiturates, or phenothiazines. Intravenous fluid administration may increase the rate of nicotine excretion. Antacids are not recommended as they may increase nicotine absorption from the stomach.[10]

MAJOR OUTCOMES

Fentanyl Transdermal Patches

Fentanyl is a synthetic opioid analgesic that binds to mu receptors.[15] It is 50 to 100 times more potent than morphine.[16] The transdermal patch is designed to release a constant amount of drug over a fixed time period. As with many transdermal patches, once the internal structure or patch matrix is disturbed (i.e., chewed on), a large amount of drug may be quickly released. Fentanyl patches contain significantly more fentanyl than is designed to be released during therapeutic transdermal absorption. For example, Duragesic 50 (Ortho-McNeil-Janssen Pharmaceuticals, Inc.) patches are designed to release 50 *micro*grams of fentanyl per hour for a duration of 72 hours. However, this same patch holds a total of 5 *milli*grams of drug. Studies have determined that fentanyl patches retain anywhere from 24% to 84% of their original drug following 3 days of wear in people.[17] Therefore, even a "spent" or used patch could still contain a significant amount of fentanyl and pose a lethal risk if ingested.

Transdermal fentanyl patches have been used in human medicine as an analgesic for nearly 20 years. Over the past decade, these patches have gained notoriety in veterinary medicine, and the incidence of patch ingestion by dogs and cats has risen precipitously. Because of the imminent danger associated with patch ingestion, it is highly recommended to not only secure a pet's patches extraordinarily well but to use Elizabethan collars whenever possible. Because children may accidentally chew on or ingest patches, clientele must be well educated about associated risks and proper disposal. There are multiple case reports of children developing severe or fatal toxicosis after chewing on or consuming fentanyl patches.[18-20] Fentanyl transdermal patches also have high potential for abuse by clients.[21-23]

Inadvertent overdose of an animal via transdermal administration is theoretically possible but the risk of causing serious toxicity is rather unlikely. Factors such as dermal blood flow, cutaneous vasoactivity, skin damage, environmental exposure, and hydration status all contribute to the rate of transdermal fentanyl absorption. Unintentional overdose from transdermal fentanyl patches may occur if cutaneous blood flow to the patch application site were significantly increased secondary to using heating pads or warmed surgical tables. However, the most common scenario in which a transdermal patch could lead to an overdose of fentanyl is from a cat or dog chewing on and/or ingesting a patch.

Species differences between cats and dogs with respect to fentanyl pharmacokinetics are marked. The time to first detectable plasma concentrations in cats is significantly shorter than in dogs (3 to 6 hours and 13 to 16 hours, respectively).[24,25] Also, the time needed to reach maximum plasma concentration in cats is less than in dogs. However, half-life is longer in cats than dogs (4 to 6 hours versus 2 to 4 hours). Additionally, signs of toxicity may vary between the species

as well. Dogs tend to exhibit more classic opioid effects, such as sedation and CNS depression, decrease of cardiac and respiratory rates, miosis, and hypothermia. Cats are more likely to exhibit paradoxical central nervous stimulation and mydriasis.

Decontamination of pets that have ingested a fentanyl patch needs to be managed with care. Unless the ingestion of the patch is less than 10 minutes prior to the induction of emesis, emesis is not recommended due to the potentially rapid onset of CNS changes. If the induction of emesis is not possible given the pet's neurologic status, the patch may be removed endoscopically or surgically. Because these patches are designed to release small amounts of fentanyl over a period of days, patch removal is important. Though the half-life of the drug is relatively short, signs of toxicity may theoretically continue for hours to days if the patch is not removed. Once removed, signs of toxicity should begin to resolve within 2 to 6 hours. Though not routine, systemic fentanyl levels may be measured in serum and urine.

In addition to decontamination, naloxone may be administered for the reversal of respiratory and CNS depression. Due to the short half-life of naloxone, it often needs to be redosed every 30 to 60 minutes until clinical signs resolve. The route of naloxone administration will determine the onset of action and the duration of effect. Consider giving the first dose IV for the most rapid onset and subsequent doses IM or SQ for more prolonged duration of effect. Seizures may be treated with diazepam. Additional treatments include IV fluids to support the cardiovascular system, thermal support, and mechanical ventilation, if necessary. Death following opioid toxicity is most often due to severe respiratory depression.[26]

SALICYLATES (ASPIRIN, OIL OF WINTERGREEN, ETC.)

Salicylates are a commonly used group of analgesics that also contain antipyretic and antiinflammatory properties. Salicylates also belong to a class of agents known as keratolytics and are therefore used, in humans, for the topical treatment of acne, psoriasis, ichthyoses, dandruff, corns, calluses, and certain warts. Acetylsalicylic acid (ASA), better known as aspirin, is commonly found in many over-the-counter and prescription analgesic ointments or liniments. Nonaspirin salicylates, such as salicylic acid, are found in over-the-counter topical acne control creams, lotions, sunscreens, and facial masks and pads, as well as "medicated" face washes and make-up (foundations and concealers). Brand name examples of such products include Clearasil, Noxzema, and Neutrogena' which may contain 1% to 5% salicylate. Methyl salicylate is found in concentrations up to 30% in over-the-counter and prescription liniments such as Bengay or HEET. It is also the active ingredient in oil of wintergreen.

In order to estimate the toxicity of certain nonaspirin salicylates, they are converted to an aspirin or acetylsalicylic acid equivalent. For example, 1 mL of oil of wintergreen, which is 98% methyl salicylate, is equivalent to 1400 mg of aspirin. To put this in perspective, 1 teaspoon (5 mL) of oil of wintergreen is equivalent to 21.5 adult aspirin (325 mg) tablets!

The therapeutic range and half-life of salicylates varies greatly between cats and dogs. For example, the therapeutic dose of aspirin in dogs is 0.5 to 25 mg/kg PO every 8 to 12 hours.[15] In contrast, the therapeutic dose for cats is 0.5 to 25 mg/kg PO every 2 to 3 days.[15] The large difference in dosing frequency is due to the decreased rate of salicylic acid elimination in cats. Salicylic acid is primarily metabolized via phase II conjugation with glucuronic acid. Because cats have a limited glucuronide pathway, they cannot metabolize and excrete salicylic acid as do dogs or humans. The half-life of oral ASA is dose-dependent. Half-lives range from 8 to 12 hours in dogs to 22 to 45 hours in cats.[27] In addition to oral dosing, topical dosing of salicylates has been studied in dogs. These studies have demonstrated drug penetration into deep tissues, synovial fluid, and the systemic circulation.[28] However, overdoses from topical exposure would not be expected unless large quantities were used chronically.

The range of salicylate toxicity between cats and dogs also varies greatly. Overall, cats are more susceptible to toxicosis. Though no outward clinical signs were noted in cats dosed orally with 25 mg/kg of ASA every 48 hours, pinpoint gastric erosions were noted 8 hours following a single IV dose of 20 mg/kg of ASA and death was seen in cats given 100 mg/kg ASA daily for 7 days.[27,29,30] Caution is warranted when any cat receives more than 30 mg/kg ASA or the equivalent. This is especially applicable in kittens, geriatric cats, or any cat with renal or hepatic disease. In dogs, chronic doses of ASA at 15 to 35 mg/kg dosed BID-TID led to submucosal gastric hemorrhages and erosions within 5 to 6 days.[31-33] Acutely, salicylates have a wider margin of safety in healthy dogs. Most healthy dogs will be able to tolerate acute oral doses of ASA less than 75 to 100 mg/kg without significant complication and can be managed at home. However, induction of emesis is indicated. These dogs should be observed closely by the owners for any signs of GI distress over the following 1 to 4 days and treatment quickly implemented should signs appear. Dogs acutely ingesting between 100 to 300 mg/kg of ASA should be evaluated by a veterinarian and supportive therapy instituted. Doses over 300 mg/kg of ASA warrant full and aggressive treatment. Ingestions of 400 to 500 mg/kg of ASA or greater carry a poor prognosis.[34]

Clinical signs of toxicity range from mild GI distress to death. GI irritation is the most common side effect of salicylate exposure. Vomiting, gastric erosion and ulceration, and GI hemorrhage are common results of overdose. Additionally, depression, hyperthermia, collapse, extreme weakness, tremors, seizures, bone marrow suppression, and cerebral edema have been documented. In severe cases, respiratory alkalosis may be noted soon after exposure, followed by significant metabolic acidosis with an increased anion gap. Finally, due to platelet inhibition and reduced production of prostaglandin, adverse coagulation and renal effects may be noted. In cats receiving an excessively high dose, salicylate-associated hepatitis has been reported.[35]

Treatment will vary from simple decontamination to aggressive life-support measures for survival. Emesis or gastric lavage may be indicated, followed by activated charcoal. A course of GI protectants including antacids, sulcralfate and misoprostil may be indicated for as long as 10 to 14 days.[33] If ulcerations are present, antibiotic treatment, analgesia, and blood transfusions may be needed. Baseline chemistry values, complete blood counts, and arterial or venous blood gases are recommended with treatments employed as indicated. Additional supportive care such as IV fluids, frequent monitoring of body temperature, and thermal support may be warranted. Seizures may be treated with diazepam.

5-Fluorouracil (5-FU)

Fluorouracil, also referred to as 5-FU, is an antineoplastic agent that has been used in both humans and animals since the mid-1900s. 5-FU is a fluorinated pyrimidine antimetabolite that substitutes for the uracil nucleotide. Ultimately, it interferes with the synthesis and processing of DNA and RNA, respectively. The ultimate result is programmed cell death. In healthy animals, the hematopoietic and epithelial cells (specifically the intestinal crypt cells) are most profoundly affected as they are the most rapidly dividing. In the United States, 5-FU is FDA approved for the topical treatment of human actinic keratosis and superficial basal cell carcinomas. Topical preparations are also used off-label for an array of other human dermal neoplastic conditions. Common topical preparations include a 0.5% to 5% topical cream and 1% to 5% topical solutions. Brand names of the drug include Efudex (2% and 5% solution and 5% cream from Valeant Pharmaceuticals International), Carac (0.5% cream from Sanofi Aventis), and Fluoroplex (1% cream and 1% solution from Allergan Pharmaceuticals).

Topical preparations are not often used in veterinary medicine due to the risk of inadvertent ingestion by animals and risk of toxicity to the owner from drug handling. A parenteral formulation has been administered to animals via IV, intraperitoneal, and intratumoral routes (the later for the treatment of equine sarcoids).[36,37] 5-FU is not FDA approved for veterinary use. Topical 5-FU creams have, historically, been used for treatment of feline cutaneous tumors such as squamous cell carcinomas. However, this practice is no longer recommended as both severe toxicity and death have been reported following "routine" use in cats.

Currently, the most common exposure of cats and dogs to 5-FU is via accidental oral exposure after chewing into a tube of the product. These preparations have an extremely narrow margin of safety and ingestion should be considered a medical emergency. Cats are extrermely sensitive to the effects of 5-FU, and even a few licks of the product may cause life-threatening toxicity. In dogs, the minimum reported toxic dose following oral exposure is 6 mg/kg followed by a minimum reported lethal dose of 20 mg/kg.[38,39] To put this in perspective, a 50-pound (22.7-kg) dog would only need to consume approximately 500 mg of 5-FU or roughly ¼ of the contents of a 40-g tube of Efudex 5% cream to achieve the minimum reported lethal dose. To date, the largest survived ingestion in a dog is 46 mg/kg of 5-FU.[40] The onset of clinical signs is rapid, typically beginning within 1 to 5 hours after ingestion.[38,40,41] Because of the rapid onset of toxicity, the induction of emesis by the pet owner is not often recommended. Thorough gastric lavage would be the preferred method of decontamination due to the miniscule toxic dose (if the ingestion was recent). Activated charcoal is recommended following gastric emptying. The most common signs of toxicity include rapid-onset vomiting, tremors, and seizures. The tremors and seizures are typically poorly responsive to diazepam. Additional manifestations of 5-FU toxicity include weakness, anorexia, abdominal pain, mucositis, diarrhea, GI erosions and ulceration, cerebellar ataxia, dose-dependent myelosuppression, cardiovascular collapse, myocardial ischemia, and death.[38-41] Treatment of toxicity must be aggressive. If seizures are not responsive to diazepam, other sedatives such as barbiturates, propofol, or gas anesthetics may be used if necessary. IV fluids, blood or plasma transfusions, thermal support, GI protectants, analgesics, and broad spectrum antibiotics may all be warranted. Laboratory evaluation should include frequent monitoring of chemistry profiles, complete blood counts, and coagulation profiles. Typically, clinical signs of myelosuppression take 2 to 3 weeks to resolve.[40]

References

The reference list can be found on the companion Expert Consult Web site at *www.expertconsult.com*.

CHAPTER **149**

Human Prescription and Street Drugs

Lynn Rolland Hovda

DRUGS OF ABUSE: PRESCRIPTION DRUGS AND ILLICIT DRUGS

Many animals are exposed each day to a variety of prescription drugs with a high potential for abuse. Some are also exposed to illicit street drugs. Dogs are the most commonly reported animals, but cats and ferrets as well as smaller pocket pets and birds also succumb to poisoning.

They may accidentally ingest drugs, contaminated baked goods, or illicit plants; be intentionally poisoned by having smoke blown into their faces; used as "pack mules" or "drug mules" to smuggle bags of heroin or cocaine, or be deliberately and maliciously drugged.[1] Police dogs and working search and rescue dogs are at a higher risk for exposure simply due to their occupation.[2]

PRESCRIPTION DRUGS

Amphetamines/Amphetamine-Like Compounds
One of the most common poisonings reported each year to the Pet Poison Helpline (PPH) is the ingestion of an amphetamine or amphetamine-like drug. Human prescription drugs in this group include dextroamphetamine and methylphenidate. Most of them are legally prescribed for children and some adults with ADHD/ADD or for treatment of narcolepsy. Sadly, these same medications, often referred to as "uppers," "speed" or "dexies," are widely sold on the street and in college dormitories as central nervous system (CNS) stimulants and diet aids.

Absorption is rapid and clinical signs often occur in 20 to 30 minutes after ingestion. Sustained-release products, including skin patches, are designed for slower onset and longer duration and the onset of clinical signs in these cases depends on whether the product was chewed or swallowed whole. Signs are generally related to CNS stimulation and include increased activity levels, irritability, twitches and tremors, and seizures. Other reported signs include hyperthermia, vocalization, tachycardia, premature ventricular contractions, changes in blood pressure, salivation, and mydriasis.[3]

Treatment is primarily symptomatic and supportive. Emesis is not recommended due to the rapid development of clinical signs. Gastric lavage followed by activated charcoal with a cathartic may be useful in early cases. Depending on the amount consumed, skin patches may need to be surgically or endoscopically removed. Temperature should be controlled with cooling measures including ice packs, cool towels, or a cooling blanket. The animal should be kept as calm as possible with little external stimuli. Chlorpromazine (10 to 18 mg/kg IV) has been successfully used in a number of cases to decrease seizures, hyperthermia, and heart rate.[4]

Sedative/Hypnotics
Barbiturates, especially phenobarbital, were at one time widely abused and animal overdoses were common. For the most part, they have been replaced with benzodiazepines and the newer, nonbenzodiazepine short-acting sleep aids.

Common benzodiazepine drugs include clonazepam, diazepam, estazolam, flurazepam, lorazepam, and temazepam. The onset and degree of signs vary with each drug and amount ingested. CNS signs predominate and include yawning, weaving, ataxia, inability to rise, and coma. More serious ingestions result in respiratory depression and cardiovascular instability.

Treatment for most ingestions is supportive; deaths are rare. Severe intoxications may benefit from the use of flumazenil (0.01 to 0.02 mg/kg IV), a benzodiazepine receptor antagonist. The short half-life of flumazenil may necessitate retreatment.[5] Animal exposures to nonbenzodiazepine sleep aids such as eszopidone, zalepon, and zolpiderm have skyrocketed in the past few years. The onset and duration or action depends on the drug ingested. Signs associated with CNS depression generally predominate, although several dogs and cats have shown behavioral changes associated with stimulation (excitement, agitation, hallucinations).[6] Treatment is symptomatic and supportive.

Opioids
The opioid group includes many legal and illegal synthetic drugs. Morphine and codeine are derived from the poppy plant *(Papaver somniferum)*. Oxymorphone and hydromorphone are legal prescription derivatives of morphine; heroin is an illegal derivative. Common synthetic opioids include buprenorphine, butorphanol, fentanyl, hydrocodone, meperidine, methadone, oxycodone, and propoxyphene. Oxycodone, hydrocodone, and fentanyl are perhaps the most commonly abused drugs in this group. Animals are often exposed through accidental ingestion.

Fentanyl is a special case because the number of dogs ingesting new or used fentanyl patches is large, as are those dogs that greedily eat fentanyl lollipops meant for human use. Absorption and onset of clinical signs depend on the specific opioid, formulation, and route of exposure; signs vary depending on species and age as well as the opioid. Dogs show early excitation with ataxia and increased respirations, vomiting, diarrhea, and urination followed by CNS depression, respiratory depression, hypothermia, hypotension, and death. Cats are at the opposite end of the spectrum and present with early excitation, aggressive behavior, hyperthermia, and absence of vomiting.

Treatment includes early decontamination, cooling measures for hyperthermia, symptomatic and supportive care, and naloxone (0.01 to 0.02 mg/kg IV, repeated as needed).[7] Ingested fentanyl patches often require surgical or endoscopic removal. Mechanical ventilation is needed for severe respiratory depression.

Ketamine
Ketamine, an analog of phencyclidine, is still widely used in veterinary medicine and less so in human medicine due to the dysphoric and dissociative effects. Stolen or otherwise illegally obtained ketamine is popular on the streets and referred to as "special k," "green jet," and "cat valium." Pets are exposed when they drink ketamine-spiked party punch, eat baked

goods or marijuana laced with ketamine, or inhale contaminated marijuana smoke.

The onset of action depends on the species, route of absorption, and other coingestants. Oral absorption may be limited. Commonly reported signs described in dogs and cats include opisthotonus, mydriasis, a blank stare, and zombielike state. Other noted effects include ataxia, agitation, rigidity, hallucinations, seizures, and death.

Animals should be kept in a quiet, dark room with little physical restraint. Diazepam is effective for control of excitation, hyperactivity, and seizures; phenothiazines are contraindicated.[8]

STREET DRUGS

Marijuana

Marijuana (Cannabis sativa), referred to as "grass," "Mary Jane," "pot," and "weed," is the most common street drug ingestion reported to the PPH. Pets are accidentally exposed by eating home-grown plants, marijuana cigarettes, or contaminated baked goods. They are also deliberately poisoned or intentionally exposed by people blowing smoke into their face to see what happens. Fortunately, marijuana has a wide margin of safety and death is rarely reported.

The onset of action varies depending on the route with signs beginning at 6 to 12 minutes after inhaling smoke and 30 to 60 minutes after ingestion. The majority of clinical signs in dogs are related to the CNS and include depression, disorientation, glassy eyes, mydriasis, recumbency, and behavioral changes.[9] A commonly described change in cats is "snatching at flies" when there are none. Other less common signs include gastrointestinal (GI) irritation, stupor, and seizures.

Treatment is primarily symptomatic and supportive and a full recovery is expected with appropriate therapy. Animals with smoke inhalation or mild intoxication often require only several hours of close monitoring for changes in body temperature, respiratory rate, and heart rate and rhythm. Asymptomatic dogs ingesting large amounts of plants and baked goods may benefit from early emesis; those with CNS depression should have gastric lavage followed by activated charcoal with a cathartic. Pets with severe CNS depression need to be closely monitored and abnormal behaviors treated with diazepam or another benzodiazepine.

Cocaine

Cocaine, an alkaloid obtained from Erythroxylon coca, is the most widely abused human street drug and second only to marijuana in animal abuse potential. Cocaine hydrochloride, the powdered form, is referred to as "coke," "nose candy," and "white girl." Cocaine can further be processed into the free alkaloid referred to as "crack," "crank," "ice," and "crystal." Both forms are highly toxic to animals, whether they inhale smoke, snort some lying around, or ingest a baggie full of cocaine that then ruptures in the GI tract.

Cocaine is rapidly absorbed across all mucosal surfaces including the nose, mouth, GI tract, and respiratory alveoli. The onset of clinically signs occurs within a few minutes and signs vary tremendously depending on route, tolerance, and adulterants. Early signs are related to CNS stimulation and include excitement, hyperesthesia, twitches, and seizures. Hyperthermia secondary to cocaine-induced heat production is life threatening.[10] Other associated signs include tachycardia, hypertension, arrhythmias, mydriasis, respiratory arrest, and death.

Emesis is not recommended due to rapid absorption and potential for seizures. Gastric lavage may be effective but caution needs to be taken in police dogs or "pack dogs" so the baggies do not rupture. Body temperature must be monitored closely and early and aggressive cooling measures undertaken. Diazepam, barbiturates, and chlorpromazine have all been used successfully to provide sedation, control seizures, and assist with hyperthermia. Diazepam alone may be effective in reversing tachycardia and hypertension. Sodium bicarbonate should be administered early to prevent arrhythmias associated with Na-K channel inhibition. Propranolol and other beta blockers may be effective in treating arrhythmias, but their use is controversial and should be reserved for life-threatening situations. Mechanical ventilation is often necessary in dogs with severe respiratory depression.

Heroin

This illegal synthetic opioid is generally injected but is sometimes smoked or snorted. Dogs are most often poisoned when used as "drug or pack mules" for the illegal movement of heroin. Heroin-filled baggies are either fed to them or surgically implanted in their peritoneal cavity. Extreme care needs to be taken when these products are removed so they are not ruptured. Death from infection is a distinct possibility as aseptic technique is not employed when these products are implanted.

Club Drugs

Club drugs or designer drugs are synthetic drugs that have become popular in the past 10 years. Common club drugs include GHB (gamma hydroxybutanoic acid), flunitrazepam, and designer amphetamines such as MDMA (methylenedioxymethamphetamine), 4MA, MDEA, and others. GHB and flunitrazepam are often referred to as the "date rape" drugs. There are few reports of animal ingestions but doubtless they are occurring.

GHB is a synthetic derivative of GABA that normally occurs in the body. Street names for GHB include "liquid x," "liquid ecstasy," and "scoop." Effects occur within 15 to 30 minutes after ingestion and usually last only several hours, although have persisted for over 8 hours in human beings.[11] Clinical signs are related to CNS depression and include lethargy, hypotonia, tremors, loss of consciousness, and respiratory depression. Emesis is contraindicated due to rapid onset of signs. The short duration of action limits treatment.

Flunitrazepam, a prescription benzodiazepine drug, is available in most countries but not in the United States. The blue-colored tablets are referred to as "rophies," "Mexican valium," and "rope." Clinical signs in human beings occur 20 to 30 minutes after ingestion and last up to 12 hours. The most commonly reported signs include confusion, sedation, amnesia, muscle relaxation, and hallucinations.[12] Flumazenil, a benzodiazepine antagonist, has been used successfully in human beings. The short half-life of flumazenil may necessitate retreatment.

MDMA, or "Ecstasy," is also called "lover's speed," "roll," and "disco biscuits." Structurally similar to amphetamine, it differs dramatically from GHB and flunitrazepam because it is a CNS stimulant. In dogs effects occur as early as 45 minutes and persist for up to 8 hours.[13] Signs are dose dependent and include hyperactivity, mydriasis, hyperthermia, seizures, and death. Treatment is similar to amphetamine drugs.

Hallucinogens

Lysergic acid diethylamide (LSD) is a powerful, synthetic hallucinogen. Street names include "purple acid," "cubes," and "dots." Little information exists regarding canine overdoses but it is expected that dogs mimic human beings. LSD is rapidly absorbed after oral ingestion with signs occurring within 90 minutes and persisting for up to 12 hours. Clinical signs are related primarily to abnormal mentation and include hallucinations, euphoria, disorientation, and incoordination. Cats exposed to LSD have developed bizarre postures, yawning, head twitching, body shaking, compulsive scratching, and abnormal movements.[14] Treatment is symptomatic and includes keeping the animal in a dark, quiet room, minimizing stimulation, and providing adequate sedation. Diazepam has been recommended for use in animal cases. Haloperidol has been used successfully in human beings and may be helpful in animals. Other less common hallucinogens found on the street pose a potential threat to animals.

Phenylcyclidine, a synthetic drug similar to ketamine, is referred to as "angel dust," "rocket fuel," and "love boat." While not strictly drugs, the seeds of the morning glory plant *(Ipomoea violacea)* and jimsonweed *(Datura stramonium)*; mescaline, the active ingredient in peyote; psilocybin, or "magic mushrooms"; salivia *(Salivia divornum)*; and nutmeg *(Myristica fragrans)* are all well-known hallucinogens.

The incidence of drug abuse, either by prescription or illicit drugs, is likely underreported in veterinary medicine. It is often difficult for a veterinarian to obtain an accurate history either because the owner does not know what happened or is reluctant to admit what occurred. Close attention to detail, astute questioning, and utilization of blood and urine drug screens may help with the diagnosis.

REFERENCES

The reference list can be found on the companion Expert Consult Web site at *www.expertconsult.com.*

CHAPTER 150

Chemical Toxicities

Ahna G. Brutlag

Given the common occurrence of animals inadvertently exposed to household chemicals, the number of serious outcomes is extremely rare. Most household chemicals have a very wide margin of safety and are merely minor dermal or gastrointestinal (GI) irritants. However, there are select categories of products that do pose a significant risk of toxicity to small animals.

Whenever an animal is exposed to a potential toxin, there are multiple resources available from which to obtain medical advice. The product manufacturer may be associated with a poison control center and be able to offer quality risk assessment and medical information. Additionally, one may contact an animal poison control center such as Pet Poison Helpline (800-213-6680) or the ASPCA Animal Poison Control Center (888-426-4435). Both are staffed 24/7 with experienced veterinarians board-certified in veterinary toxicology.

Another immediate information resource is the product label. The label is designed to convey product safety information to the consumer. In turn, this may be helpful to veterinarians trying to interpret the risk of toxicity to a pet. However, it is imperative to note that most of the animal testing that was done in order to establish a product's relative toxicity was on rodents or rabbits, not cats or dogs. As is well accepted, there can be significant interspecies differences with respect to chemical metabolism and sensitivity. Therefore, when in doubt, seeking out professional consultation from an animal poison control center is always recommended.

In order to interpret product labels, it is necessary to understand the specific signal words that correspond to acute toxicity of the finished product. These words, in order of increasing toxicity, are: CAUTION, WARNING, and DANGER.[1] The signal word is typically determined by the result of acute toxicity studies. For each exposure route, a *Toxicity Category* is determined (Table 150-1). The signal word is then assigned based on the most severe Toxicity Category or by the presence of certain inert agents (Table 150-2).

For example, any product containing a concentration of methanol at 4% or greater is automatically given the signal word DANGER. This is due to the risk of blindness in humans following methanol toxicity. Additionally, the word POISON and the skull and crossbones symbol are required for products classified as Toxicity Category I in acute oral, dermal, or inhalation toxicity studies.[1]

SOLVENTS AND ALCOHOLS

Acetone
Acetone, a commonly used solvent, is found in nail polish removers, wart removers, face washes, glues, paint strippers, and rubber cements. It is a clear, colorless, highly flammable liquid with a characteristic odor. Systemic toxicity is most common following oral ingestion but dermal absorption or inhalation exposure is possible. Overall, small exposures to acetone are unlikely to result in serious effects. Acetone has a relatively low order of toxicity with the lowest oral canine lethal dose being approximately 8 mL/kg. However, 2 to 3 mL/kg may produce clinical toxicosis.[2]

The most commonly reported acetone exposure to the Pet Poison Helpline is from dogs ingesting cotton balls with an acetone-based nail polish remover. To date, none of these exposures have lead to confirmed (or even suspected) acetone toxicity.[3] The more likely result of these exposures is a potential mild gastroenteritis or a bowel obstruction from the cotton balls.

Clinical signs of toxicity and treatment are discussed in the Isopropanol and Ethanol section.

Isopropanol and Ethanol
Isopropanol (isopropyl alcohol) and ethanol (ethyl alcohol) are common solvents and disinfectants that are found in glass/multisurface/all-purpose cleaners, antiseptics, personal care products, perfumes/colognes, foods, and alcoholic beverages (ethanol only). The term "rubbing alcohol" often refers to

Table • 150-1

Assignment of Toxicity Categories Based on Acute Toxicity Data[1]

STUDY	TOXICITY CATEGORY I	TOXICITY CATEGORY II	TOXICITY CATEGORY III	TOXICITY CATEGORY IV
Acute oral	≤50 mg/kg	>50 through 500 mg/kg	>500 through 5000 mg/kg	>5000 mg/kg
Acute dermal	≤200 mg/kg	>200 through 2000 mg/kg	>2000 through 5000 mg/kg	>5000 mg/kg
Acute inhalation (4-hour exposure)	≤0.05 mg/L	>0.05 through 0.5 mg/L	>0.5 through 2 mg/L	>2 mg/L
Primary eye irritation	Corrosive (irreversible destruction of ocular tissue) or corneal involvement or irritation persisting for more than 21 days	Corneal involvement or other eye irritation clearing in 8-21 days	Corneal involvement or other eye irritation clearing in 7 days or less	Minimal effects clearing in less than 24 hours
Primary skin irritation	Corrosive (tissue destruction into the dermis and/or scarring)	Severe irritation at 72 hours (severe erythema or edema)	Moderate irritation at 72 hours (moderate erythema)	Mild or slight irritation at 72 hours (no irritation or slight erythema)

Table • 150-2

Toxicity Category with Corresponding Signal Word[1]

TOXICITY CATEGORY	SIGNAL WORD
Toxicity Category I	DANGER
Toxicity Category II	WARNING
Toxicity Category III	CAUTION
Toxicity Category IV	None Required

70% isopropyl alcohol but can be used to describe concentrated ethyl alcohols as well.

Glass and multisurface/all-purpose cleaners may contain roughly 1% to 10% ethanol or isopropyl alcohol and/or trace (<1%) amounts of ethylene glycol. As a general class, these cleaners have a wide margin of safety and small exposures are unlikely to be problematic. The most likely effect from a small ingestion of these products would be mild, self-limiting vomiting. In the author's experience, animals ingesting the paper toweling or rags that were used for cleaning with these products are more at risk for a GI obstruction secondary to the foreign material ingested than a true alcohol poisoning. Additionally, the amount of ethylene glycol contained within these products is so miniscule that, unless massive amounts were ingested, the risk of ethylene glycol toxicity is highly unlikely and will not be discussed in this chapter. However, large ingestions of undiluted product may pose a greater risk for isopropanol or ethanol toxicity. Isopropyl alcohol is approximately twice as toxic as ethyl alcohol and roughly 80% of it is metabolized to acetone.[4] As little as 0.5 mL/kg of 70% isopropyl alcohol may cause adverse effects.[2]

Clinical signs from acetone and alcohol toxicity are similar. Due to rapid systemic absorption, the onset of clinical signs is typically within 30 minutes to a few hours. Animals will often present with vomiting, central nervous system (CNS) depression, ataxia, and respiratory depression or be comatose. Animals with oral exposures may have an acetone or alcohol odor to their breath. Also, elevated levels of urinary ketones may help to confirm acetone exposure. Additional laboratory findings secondary to acetone toxicity include hyperglycemia, ketonemia, and acidosis (similar to diabetic ketoacidosis).[2] Lab values from alcohol toxicity may reveal hypoglycemia, acidosis, and an elevated anion gap. Blood ethanol and isopropanol levels may be quickly obtained by most human hospitals for confirmation of exposure and to gauge prognosis. However, this is not routinely done in veterinary medicine.

Treatment of toxicity may include decontamination. However, the induction of emesis must occur quickly following ingestion due to the risk of CNS depression. Because of the rapid onset of clinical signs, emesis is not often recommended. Activated charcoal is of little value due to its limited ability to bind to acetone or alcohols. Therefore, treatment is primarily focused on supportive care with attention to acid-base status, blood glucose levels, and vital signs. Mechanical ventilation may be required. Hemodialysis is effective in removing isopropanol and acetone from the systemic circulation. Additionally, 4-methylpyrazole (4-MP) will prevent the metabolism of isopropanol to acetone.[4] The reported half-life of acetone in humans is 19 to 31 hours.[5] Therefore, a prolonged duration of treatment may be necessary.

ACIDS AND ALKALIS

While many household chemicals are weak acids or bases that cause only mild GI irritation, some are quite strong and have the potential to cause corrosive injury. As a general rule, corrosive injury is possible if the pH of the agent is below 2 or greater than 12.[6] However, some texts warn against esophageal injuries by substances with a pH of 10 or greater.[2] Additionally, as is discussed elsewhere in this chapter, product pH is not the sole determinant of corrosivity. Even substances with a neutral pH can exhibit corrosive behavior and cause massive tissue damage. Examples of this category include quaternary ammonium or cationic surfactants that have a neutral pH and concentrated phenolic compounds.[6,7]

Common products containing potentially corrosive acids include toilet bowl cleaners, rust or calcium/rust/lime-removing compounds, swimming pool additives and cleaners, automotive batteries, and gun barrel cleaning fluids (Table 150-3). These products often contain hydrochloric, sulfuric,

Table • 150-3

Examples of Potentially Corrosive Household Products[8-13]

PRODUCT CATEGORIES	BRAND NAMES	ACTIVE INGREDIENT(S)	% ACTIVE INGREDIENT(S)	pH OF ACTIVE INGREDIENT(S)
Toilet bowl cleaners	Professional Lysol Disinfectant Toilet Bowl Cleaner	Hydrochloric acid	9.5%	<1
	Clorox Disinfecting Toilet Bowl Cleaner with Bleach	Sodium hypochlorite Sodium hydroxide	1%-5% 0.1%-1%	13
Calcium/lime/rust removers	Easy-Off BAM Power Cleaner/ Grime and Lime Remover	Sulfamic acid	5%-10%	0.8
Drain cleaners and maintainers	Drano Clog Remover Liquid	Sodium hypochlorite Sodium hydroxide Sodium silicate	3%-7% 1%-5% 1%-5%	11.5-13.4
	Red Devil Drain Maintainer	Sodium hydroxide	100%	14
Oven cleaners	Professional Easy-Off Oven and Grill Cleaner	Sodium hydroxide	4%-6%	13.3

nitric, or phosphoric acid (or sodium bisulfate, which forms sulfuric acid in water). Additionally, aqueous solutions of free halogens such as chlorine, bromine, or iodine can also be corrosive. Ingestion of strong acids typically causes immediate and intense pain, which usually deters the animal from consuming large amounts. Following exposure to these products, animals may have evidence of corrosive lesions in the oral cavity and on the lips, be salivating excessively from pain and/or nausea, and develop vomiting, dysphagia, and refusal of food or water. If enough of an acidic compound was ingested to lead to corrosive esophageal injury, it is typical to see evidence of injury in the oral cavity. Rarely, with corrosive acid ingestions, would the oral cavity remain normal yet there would be significant esophageal damage.

Alkaline agents, on the other hand, have a different mechanism of action and, therefore, a different clinical presentation than acidic products. While acidic compounds tend to cause more superficial and localized injury (due to surface protein coagulation), alkaline compounds may lead to liquefactive necrosis causing deeper, more penetrating tissue damage. Therefore, full-thickness esophageal ulceration and the possibility of esophageal stricture are more likely to occur with ingestion of strong alkaline products. Despite tissue damage, alkaline agents can have a local anesthetic effect on tissue, and the onset of severe pain may be delayed for several hours. Additionally, the site of corrosive injury may be more localized to the lower esophagus than the oral cavity. Therefore, if an animal presents following a recent ingestion of a corrosive alkaline product but is not exhibiting significant pain and has a normal oral exam, there is still a strong possibility that esophageal injury is present.

Common alkaline-containing products include drain cleaners, toilet bowl cleaners (though less common than acids), dry cell batteries, and oven cleaners (see Table 150-3). These products often contain lye formulations such as sodium or potassium hydroxide, or sodium or potassium carbonate. They may also contain ammonium hydroxide and potassium permanganate. The physical characteristics of the product are an important factor in determining subsequent tissue damage. Thick, viscous products such as "cling" toilet bowl cleaners have a greater ability to coat larger surface areas than thin, less viscous liquids. Therefore, ingestions of more viscous products pose a greater risk of circumferential esophageal lesions. Powders or crystalline products may cause pinpoint areas of corrosive injury where they maintain contact with mucosal surfaces.

Baseline treatment for corrosive injury to the GI tract from strong acids and alkalis begins with dilution of the ingested product. This is best accomplished by rinsing the oral cavity with copious amounts of water or encouraging the animal to drink water or other neutral fluids. Adding tuna juice or chicken broth to water may entice animals to drink. Animals already exhibiting signs of GI pain are rarely willing to consume fluids orally. Inducing emesis is contraindicated following ingestion of corrosive material due to the potential for further esophageal damage. Likewise, activated charcoal is rarely recommended given the incidence of vomiting post-administration coupled with the poor binding capacity of charcoal to many of these compounds. Finally, an attempt to "neutralize" the ingested agent with a chemical of the opposite pH is seldom recommended due to the risk of an unintended thermal/chemical reaction. Any attempt at neutralization should only occur under the guidance of a knowledgeable toxicologist.

Determining the extent of the corrosive injury is very important. If esophageal or gastric ulceration is suspected, radiographs should be performed to evaluate the presence of free air (pneumoperitoneum, pneumomediastinum, and pneumothorax). Careful endoscopic examination of the upper GI tract should also be performed to evaluate the extent of injury. In order to prevent perforation, do not pass the endoscope beyond the first ulceration. Once esophageal or gastric ulceration has been confirmed, treatment is focused on administering GI protectants (namely sucralfate), maintaining hydration and nutrition (the use of a gastric feeding tube may be warranted), managing pain, and preventing systemic infection from bacterial translocation. Additionally, the possibility of esophageal stricture must be taken into account and monitored for.

BLEACHES

Bleach is a common household product to which animals are often inadvertently exposed. Most exposures occur through ingestion of dilute bleach and water solutions left out by the owner during cleaning. Chlorine bleaches are the most common household bleaches and often contain 3% to 6% sodium hypochlorite.[2,6] These products may also contain up to 0.5% sodium hydroxide (lye) to provide chemical stability along with small amounts of cationic surfactants to increase viscosity.[6] Nonchlorine bleaches ("color safe" bleaches) may contain sodium peroxide, sodium perborate, or enzymatic detergents. Additional, and potentially more problematic, are the "ultra" or "advanced" household bleach formulations. These products may contain 5% to 10% sodium hypochlorite and 0.5% to 2% sodium hydroxide.[6]

Overall, most companion animal exposures to household bleaches do not result in significant toxicity. Nonchlorine bleaches have a low order of toxicity causing mild gastritis and emesis. Household strength chlorine bleach is typically considered a mild to moderate GI irritant. Ultra bleaches have the highest risk of corrosive injury associated with them.

The clinical signs associated with bleach intoxication depend on the route of exposure. If ingested, vomiting, salivation, irritation of the oropharynx, transient anorexia, and abdominal pain are common. Corrosive injury to the oropharyngeal, esophageal, and gastric mucosa has been reported following ingestion of household-strength chlorine bleaches but the incidence rate is very low.[2] Likewise, systemic effects from household-strength chlorine bleaches are also rare. If they occur, they are likely secondary to localized tissue damage. However, intentional ingestions of massive amounts of bleach (greater than 5 mL/kg) in human beings have led to hyperchloremic acidosis and hypernatremia.[6] Thankfully, it is highly unlikely that an animal would consume this significant an amount of bleach.

When chlorine bleach is mixed with strong acids or ammonia, the combination may produce chlorine or chloramines gas, respectively. These gasses may be strong ocular and respiratory irritants. A common scenario under which this occurs is the mixing of an acidic drain cleaner with bleach. Clients may even report that they saw a green cloud of gas being released from the mixture.

Pulmonary irritation evidenced by coughing, gagging, retching, or dyspnea may also occur following inhalation of product fumes or powdered bleaches. Ocular irritation, lacrimation, blepharospasm, and/or corneal damage may occur secondary to direct ocular exposure or with exposure to chlorine and chloramines gasses. Additionally, dermal exposure may cause bleached patches of fur and irritated skin.

Treatment is largely symptomatic and supportive. If ingested, emesis, gastric lavage, or activated charcoal are not routinely recommended due to the potential for corrosive injury. Dilution with water is recommended instead.[14] GI protectants and antiemetics may be necessary. If corrosive injury occurs, aggressive management is required (refer to the Acids and Bases section for treatment advice). Following dermal exposure, bathe the animal well taking care to remove all bleach products (the fur may trap the bleach close to the skin). Following recent ocular exposure, flush the eye for 20 to 30 minutes with water or isotonic saline. Perform a thorough ophthalmic exam looking for evidence of corneal abrasion or ulceration. Animals with respiratory irritation should be moved to fresh air and provided oxygen if necessary.

SOAPS, DETERGENTS, GENERAL CLEANERS, FABRIC SOFTENERS

Products that fall into this category are among the most common chemicals companion animals are exposed to. For the most part, these products have a wide margin of safety and minimal risk of toxicity. Product examples include bar and hand soap, shampoos, liquid and powdered dishwashing products, laundry soaps and detergents, fabric softeners, and general or "all purpose" spray and foaming cleaners.

Soaps
The term *soap* typically refers to commercial hand, bar, body, and liquid dishwashing soaps. These products are comprised of nonionic, anionic, or amphoteric surfactants.[6] Ingestion of these products poses a low risk for toxicity with the exception of some homemade hand or laundry soaps, which may contain a larger amount of free alkali and pose a corrosive hazard.[2] Otherwise, soaps act as GI irritants that may lead to vomiting and/or diarrhea. Treatment for ingestion of these products is symptomatic and supportive. Emesis may be considered in large ingestions (providing the material is not corrosive). Common nonionic surfactants include alkyl ethoxylate, alkyl phenoxy polyethoxy ethanol, and polyethylene glycol stearate.[2]

Laundry and Automatic Dishwashing Detergents
Laundry detergents and automatic dishwashing detergents often contain anionic surfactants such as alkyl sodium sulfates, alkyl sodium sulfonates, dioctyl sodium sulfosuccinate, sodium lauryl sulfate, tetrapropylene benzene sulfonates, and linear alkyl benzene sulfonates.[2] Typically, intact skin provides an adequate barrier to anionic surfactants; however, they are well absorbed from the GI tract, where they may cause significant irritation. They are then metabolized in the liver with the metabolites being excreted in the urine. Intravascular hemolysis has been reported secondary to large ingestions.[2]

These detergents may also contain alkaline "builders" such as phosphates, sodium carbonate, sodium silicate, and sodium metasilicate. Builders are added to products in order to enhance the efficacy of cleaning in hard water, emulsify grease and oil, and maintain alkalinity.[6] Corrosive injury may occur from products containing concentrations of 0.5% sodium metasilicate, 15% sodium carbonate, and 20% sodium silicate or greater.[6] By law, products that may be corrosive are required to list this warning on their labels (see Tables 150-1 and 150-2).

Like soaps, most laundry detergents are merely GI irritants. However, some may contain large enough concentrations of builders to be considered corrosive. Ocular exposure to laundry detergents is most likely to result in a self-limiting conjunctivitis, while powdered detergents carry a risk for abrasive injury. Inhalation of a powdered product can be irritating to the mucosa of the nasal cavities and oropharynx, but significant harm is unlikely. Aspiration of vomitus containing such products may lead to a chemical pneumonitis.

Automatic dishwasher detergents are more alkaline than most laundry detergents due to the higher concentration of builders (possibly 70% to 80%).[6] Even small ingestions are likely to lead to GI irritation while larger ingestions may result in corrosive injury to the GI tract. Unless the pH of the product is known (this can often be obtained by calling the manufacturer or the medical information number listed on the label), emesis is not recommended. Treatment following ingestion includes irrigation of the mouth, encouraging the animal to consume fluids in effort to dilute the ingested product, and symptomatic and supportive care. Due to the risk of corrosive injury, ocular exposure warrants copious flushing of the eye for 20 to 30 minutes followed by a slit lamp exam with fluorescein staining.

Liquid Fabric Softeners and Disinfectants
Fabric softeners and disinfectant cleaners (sanitizers) may contain cationic surfactants, the most toxic of the surfactant groups. There are three main chemical groups of cationic surfactants: (1) quaternary ammonium compounds (benzalkonium and benzethonium chlorides); (2) pyridinium compounds (cetylpyridinium, cetrimonium); and (3) quinolinium compounds (dequalinium chloride).[15]

Overall, fabric softeners contain significantly less cationic surfactant than disinfectants. Concentrations below 7.5% are considered dermal, mucosal, and GI irritants and exposures pose risks similar to the previously mentioned surfactants.

However, ocular exposures to a 2% solution may be caustic to the cornea.[6] Concentrations above 7.5% may be corrosive to any tissue.

Cationic surfactants are rapidly absorbed from the GI tract and may lead to systemic toxicity. Isopropanol and ethanol, which are commonly added to cationic detergent solutions, significantly enhance GI absorption.[2] Clinical signs of toxicity include salivation, restlessness, vomiting with possible hematemesis, hypotension, muscle weakness, fasciculations, CNS depression, respiratory depression, circulatory collapse, seizures, and coma.[2,6,14] Death from shock or circulatory failure may occur as rapidly as 1 to 2 hours post significant ingestion.[16] Human deaths have been reported following ingestions of 100 to 400 mg/kg of benzalkonium chloride.[17]

Dryer and Fabric Softener Sheets

Dryer sheets or fabric softener sheets pose little risk of toxicity. While unused sheets may contain surfactants or other mild GI irritants, systemic toxicity is not an expected sequela following ingestion or oral exposure. The biggest risk to small animals is for a GI obstruction or a linear foreign body from the fibrous nature of the sheet.

REFERENCES

The reference list can be found on the companion Expert Consult Web site at *www.expertconsult.com*.

SECTION VI
Blood Pressure

CHAPTER 151

Pathophysiology of Systemic Hypertension and Blood Pressure Assessment

Rebecca L. Stepien

Systemic hypertension (HT) refers to the persistent elevation of systemic blood pressure (BP). Systemic hypertension is an increasingly recognized source of morbidity and, in some cases, mortality in human and veterinary patients.[1-7] Overt and sometimes devastating damage caused by HT is typically noted in the eyes,[5,8] central nervous system,[9,10] heart,[7,11-13] and kidneys.[2,6,14] Injury related to HT in these organ systems is often collectively termed *target organ damage* (TOD). TOD is often clinically obvious, especially in the ocular or nervous systems. In some cases, however, TOD can be insidious, resulting in undetected progressive deterioration of damaged organs (e.g., accelerated deterioration of renal function[6,9]).

Systemic HT is typically subclassified as primary ("essential") HT or secondary HT. Some veterinarians have attempted to distinguish essential, or primary, HT from idiopathic HT (i.e., systemic HT in the absence of overt, clinically apparent causal disease). Use of the term *idiopathic* acknowledges that there may be a causal disease (e.g., renal disease) that is responsible for HT but that the causal disease is in a preclinical phase.[15] In cases where the underlying disease is rare (e.g., pheochromocytoma), discovery of the cause of the HT is dependent on thorough diagnostic testing. In most dogs and cats, HT is a complication of a systemic disease rather than being primary.

The pathophysiologic mechanisms involved in the development and sustenance of human and veterinary HT remain unclear and may, at least in part, vary by causative disease. Mean arterial pressure is affected by both cardiac output and systemic vascular resistance. Both of the latter parameters are in turn affected by other physiologic factors (Figure 151-1).

Abnormalities in any of the contributing factors may alter mean arterial pressure. In the presence of normal renal function, increased BP leads to natriuresis and lowering of systemic BP. Regardless of the mechanism for the initial increase (e.g., catecholamine excess, alterations in renin-angiotensin-aldosterone axis activity), some abnormality in renal sodium handling that prevents appropriate response to HT is implicated in patients with HT.

PATHOPHYSIOLOGY OF TARGET ORGAN DAMAGE

Overview
Although damage to vascular beds causes widely varied clinical findings based on the system affected, TOD appears to be mediated by similar processes in the eye,[8] kidney,[3] and brain.[10] In dogs and cats, early cardiac changes induced by HT appear to be adaptive rather than pathologic, although this not the case in people with chronic HT.

Arterial blood flow is maintained at relatively constant levels in the brain, kidneys, and eyes through a process of vascular autoregulation. When systemic BP increases, small resistance vessels constrict, restricting flow in the vascular bed. When systemic BP falls, vessels dilate to maintain flow. Hypertensive damage in these organs occurs when these autoregulatory mechanisms fail. When resistance vessel constriction is inadequate, small vessels overdistend, breaking down endothelial tight junctions and allowing protein and plasma leakage into interstitial tissue. This leakage, augmented when high pressure is transmitted to the capillary bed, leads to tissue edema. If vascular resistance vessel constriction is excessive, ischemia of local tissues may result. Depending on the organ involved, focal hemorrhage and necrosis may also occur. Lastly, arteriolar hyalinosis and arteriosclerosis may develop, decreasing vascular distensibility (Figure 151-2).

Typical clinical manifestations of ocular, central nervous system, renal and cardiovascular TOD are found in Chapter 104.

Ophthalmologic Changes
Ophthalmologic changes secondary to HT are better described in cats than dogs and include intraocular hemorrhage (i.e., hyphema) and fundic changes. Three manifestations of fundic changes are possible and are termed hypertensive retinopathy, hypertensive choroidopathy, and hypertensive optic neuropathy,[5,8] respectively.

Hypertensive Retinopathy Abnormalities in vascular autoregulation allow high pressure to be transmitted to the

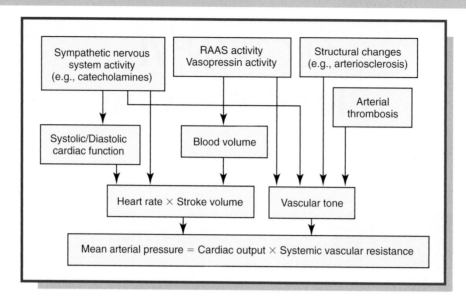

Figure 151-1 Physiologic contributors to systemic blood pressure regulation. Mean arterial pressure represents systemic blood pressure in this diagram. *RAAS*, Renin-angiotensin-aldosterone system.

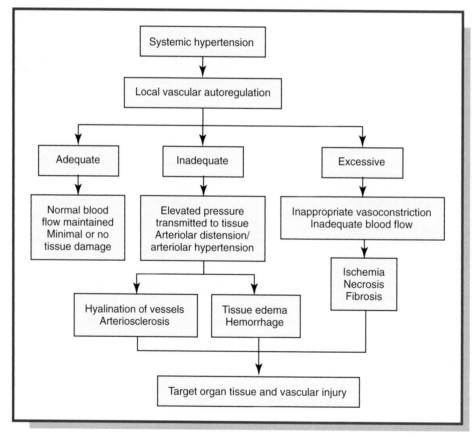

Figure 151-2 Common pathway of target organ damage due to systemic hypertension.

retinal arterioles, causing vascular distention and damaging endothelial cell junctions. Subsequently, gaps in the endothelial layer of the vessels allows breakdown of the blood-retinal barrier, retinal edema, and aggregation of focal intraretinal periarteriolar infiltrates. If terminal vessels are occluded, areas of retinal ischemia may develop. Lastly, retinal hemorrhage may develop later in the course of retinal changes.

Hypertensive Choroidopathy Leakage of vasoactive substances (e.g., angiotensin II) from the choriocapillaris

results in vasoconstriction and ischemia, which are followed by focal necrosis of the choriocapillaris and the retinal pigment epithelium. Exudation from the choriocapillaris into the subretinal space results in first bullous, then generalized, retinal detachment.

Hypertensive Optic Neuropathy As vasoconstrictive substances are released from damaged vascular beds, the blood supply to the optic nerve head is compromised. Chronic optic nerve head ischemia initially causes optic nerve edema, but eventually leads to loss of function and optic nerve atrophy.

Neurologic Changes

Similar to the eye, the autoregulatory system in the central nervous system maintains blood flow to the brain at optimal levels despite variability in relatively normal systemic BPs. When BP is far outside of the regulatory range, however, the autoregulatory system is less successful, and failure of adaptive vasoconstriction may result in cerebral edema, vascular hyalinosis, vascular sclerosis, or focal hemorrhage.[10] Inadequate vasodilation may result in areas of ischemia.

Renal Changes

In the kidneys, HT can lead to leakage of plasma proteins due to failure of autoregulation. Glomerular HT results in absolute protein loss through glomerular capillaries (i.e., proteinuria) as well as glomerulosclerosis. Proteinuria has been implicated as a cause of progressive renal tubulointerstitial damage and fibrosis. Proteinuria may contribute to progression of renal disease independent of BP.[16,17] The interaction of glomerular HT and subsequent proteinuria worsens renal function and provides a feedback loop for worsening HT. In addition to proteinuria, glomerular ischemia occurring though autoregulatory malfunction contributes to interstitial inflammation, fibrosis, and progression of renal damage.

Cardiovascular Changes

Left ventricular hypertrophy develops in patients with chronic HT as result of myocardial adaptation to increased afterload. Reductions in diastolic function may occur prior to overt cardiac hypertrophy in dogs.[18] Once hypertrophy occurs, the myocardium is more sensitive to adrenergic stimulation, has decreased coronary reserve, and is more susceptible to ischemic injury. In cats, LV diastolic functional changes were similar to those seen with hypertrophic cardiomyopathy.[19] Morphologic cardiac changes in hypertensive cats are heterogeneous and usually involve thickening of the left ventricular free wall, interventricular septum, or both. Additionally, some hypertensive cats exhibit left ventricular dilation, left atrial dilation, or abnormalities in systolic function indices.[11,13] Congestive heart failure secondary to hypertensive cardiac changes appears to occur rarely in dogs and cats, but they may exhibit increased sensitivity to fluid administration.

BLOOD PRESSURE ASSESSMENT

Assessing diagnostic BP values in dogs and cats has been comprehensively reviewed.[20] BP values obtained during diagnostic evaluation are assessed in conjunction with other clinical findings (e.g., evidence of retinal detachment, a history of polyuria and polydipsia), because these associated findings may point to the cause of the HT or indicate HT-associated end-organ damage. A single high BP value should never be used to diagnose systemic HT in the absence of other clinical information. BP measurements that exceed published normal ranges are not always indicative of disease. Patient distress[21] or physical manipulations, such as fluid administration, may elevate BP acutely. The degree of clinical concern associated with elevated BP should be proportional to the degree HT combined with the clinical signs and condition of the dog or cat.

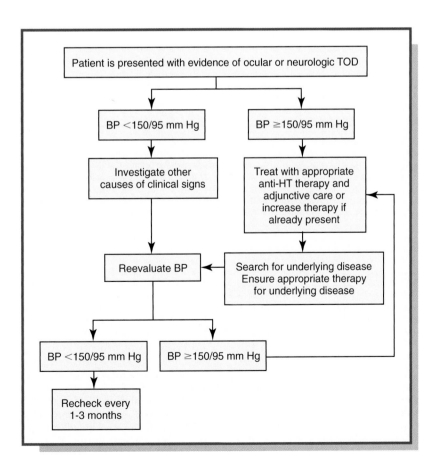

Figure 151-3 Recommendations for patients presented *with* evidence of ocular or neurologic target organ damage. *anti-HT,* Antihypertensive; *BP,* blood pressure; *TOD,* target organ damage.

Table • 151-1

Recommended Approach to Assessment of Abnormal Blood Pressure Values Based on Presence of Evidence of Target Organ Damage

PATIENT STATUS	BLOOD PRESSURE (mm Hg)	RISK OF TARGET ORGAN DAMAGE	RECOMMENDED ACTION
Overt evidence of ocular or neurologic target organ damage is present	≥150/95	Increased risk of BP as cause of clinical signs escalates with increasing BP	1. Treat with anti-HT or increase level of anti-HT 2. Supportive care as needed 3. When BP is controlled, investigate for causative disease
	<150/95	Questionable: other causes of clinical signs may be present	1. Recheck BP immediately to confirm 2. Investigate other causes of clinical signs (e.g., coagulopathy) 3. If no other cause for clinical signs identified, monitor BP over time
Patients at risk* for HT *without* overt evidence of ocular or neurologic target organ damage	≥180/120 160-179/100-120 150-159/95-100	High Moderate Low	1. Confirm with second measurement occasion within 7 days 2. If confirmed ≥160/100 mm Hg, consider anti-HT 3. Institute optimal therapy of underlying disease
	<150/95	Minimal	Remeasure in 3-6 months if at-risk disease is confirmed
Low risk or clinically healthy patient	≥150/95	Questionable	Likely to be artifactual in young, healthy animals 1. Recheck BP at another measurement occasion 2. Acclimate animal to measurement situation before second measurement 3. Screen carefully for evidence of underlying disease or target organ damage†
	<150/95	Minimal	Considered normal in animal without risk factors* or evidence of target organ damage

anti-HT, Antihypertensive medication; *BP,* blood pressure.
The clinical course of action should be tailored to the individual patient's circumstances. Recommendations may change as more clinical information becomes available. The normal BP range for healthy sight hounds may be higher than for other breeds.[28]
*Patients considered at risk for hypertension are those that have a disease condition or clinical signs of a disease known to be associated with hypertension in that species.
†Recommended screening tests for target organ damage include thorough physical examination (including funduscopic examination, cardiac auscultation, and neurologic examination), serum biochemistry, urinalysis (dogs and cats), and resting thyroxine concentration (cats).

DEFINITION OF NORMAL VALUES

Normal ranges for BP in dogs[22-28] and cats[29-33] are often expressed as a range within 2 standard deviations of the mean value for a normal population; animals with BP values outside this range are considered abnormal. The drawbacks to this approach to diagnosis of HT include inadvertent inclusion of normal animals with a BP value outside the "95% range" (leading to unnecessary diagnostic testing or therapy) or exclusion of HT as a diagnosis in an affected animal with mild or moderately elevated values (increasing the risk of end-organ damage). In addition, a dichotomous "normal" versus "too high" diagnostic result cannot take into account the differing risk of end-organ damage with increasing BP values.

Another approach to the diagnosis of HT is based on establishing diagnostic "cutoff" values at the level usually asso-ciated with clinically detectable disease. Clinical information regarding the BP typically associated with ophthalmologic,[5,34,35] neurologic,[10,36] and renal[6,9,14,37] abnormalities in spontaneous canine and feline HT is available, but there is no information about threshold BP values for end-organ damage in this group of patients. Furthermore, the "trigger point" at which elevated BP results in clinical signs likely differs from patient to patient and may be affected by the rapidity with which the HT develops.[20]

Previous high-end reference BP values for dogs varied between 160 and 180 mm Hg and between 160 and 200 mm Hg in cats. However, progression of renal damage in dogs is already enhanced with systolic BP values in this range and clinical studies have documented end-organ damage at systolic BP values as low as 170 mm Hg.[5,14] Accordingly, current recommendations consider a systolic BP greater than or equal to 160 mm Hg (as measured by oscillometric or Doppler ultrasonographic methods) worthy of further diagnostic concern in both dogs and cats,[20,38] although the use of antihypertensive medications may not be warranted if BP elevations are mild and causative situations can be remedied. The prevalence and importance of diastolic HT in dogs and cats are not well defined; therefore, most recommendations for BP assessment relate to systolic BP measurement.

APPROACH TO PATIENT GROUPS

Overview

HT detection goals in cats and dogs are to alleviate clinical signs, prevent future clinical signs, and prevent or delay subclinical deterioration of organ function. Clinical signs of "early" or mild HT in dogs and cats may appear to the owner or veterinarian as evidence of aging. Because the first overt clinical sign of HT in dogs and cats may be catastrophic (e.g., retinal detachment), detection of BP elevations below the level likely to produce clinical signs is preferable. Except for pets with overt clinical signs, detection of HT is a preventive measure.

BP assessment is a diagnostic test indicated in dogs and cats likely to have HT and as part of preventive medical care in those "at risk." Although acceptable BP ranges and measurement indications may change as data accumulate, persistent elevation of BP is a clinical finding that leads to further clinical investigation and may lead to consideration of therapy based on the presence of clinical signs and presence of causative disease.

Apparently Healthy Patients

The prevalence of HT in apparently healthy dogs is low.[28] Oscillometric and Doppler ultrasonographic test methods are moderately sensitive and specific at systolic BP cutoff values

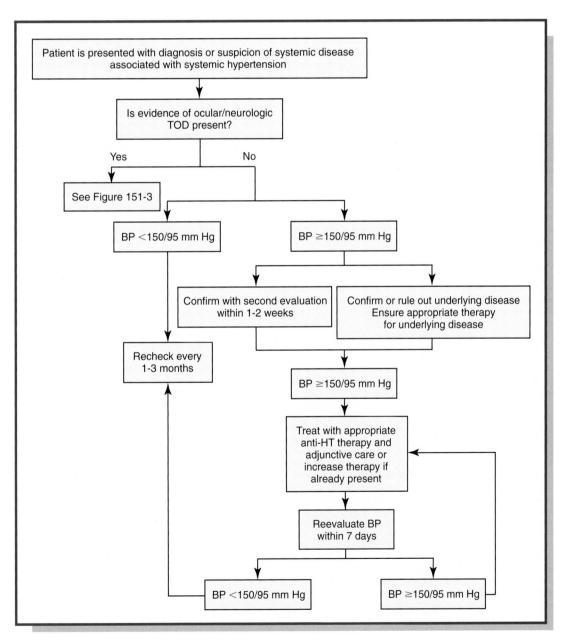

Figure 151-4 Recommendations for patients presented with *no* evidence of ocular or neurologic target organ damage. *anti-HT*, Antihypertensive; *BP*, blood pressure; *TOD*, target organ damage.

of ~160 mm Hg.[39] These test characteristics result in a low positive predictive value for abnormal test results in healthy dogs. Therefore, based on current information, routine screening of BP in this population is not recommended. The prevalence of HT in the healthy feline population is also low,[29] but the prevalence of renal disease and hyperthyroidism (both diseases commonly associated with feline HT) in older cats is high enough to prompt consideration of routine screening of cats over the age of 10 years.[5,20]

Patients with Clinical Signs of Ocular or Neurologic TOD

HT has been documented in association with overt clinical abnormalities of the ocular, neurologic, cardiovascular, and renal systems.* Effective therapy of HT in dogs or cats with any of these conditions typically eases, if not resolves, clinical signs.[5,40] Animals with HT, clinical signs of HT, and/or TOD should receive antihypertensive therapy (Figure 151-3, Table 151-1).

A detailed evaluation for known causes of HT in the species in question follows acute antihypertensive therapy. In

---

*References 5, 6, 9, 10, 12, 14, 34-37.

---

some cases, gaining control of the underlying disease (e.g., pheochromocytoma, hyperadrenocorticism) may result in lowering or normalization of BP.

Patients at Risk for Hypertension without Evidence of Ocular or Neurologic TOD

Patients considered at risk for HT are those with no clinical signs of HT that have a disease condition or clinical signs of a disease known to be associated with HT in that species.[30,41-43] Little reliable information is available on the effect of the duration of BP elevation and the extent of TOD in spontaneous canine and feline HT. With the exception of acute, extreme BP elevations, chronic BP elevations are more damaging than short-term elevations to target organ vascular beds. Therefore, early detection of elevated BP in dogs and cats at risk is aimed at detecting and managing any treatable underlying conditions and at attempting to maintain BP within a range less likely to lead to TOD (Figure 151-4; see Table 151-1).

REFERENCES

The reference list can be found on the companion Expert Consult Web site at *www.expertconsult.com*.

CHAPTER 152

Treatment of Hypertension

Anthony P. Carr

Hypertension in pets is a commonly recognized complication of a variety of diseases such as renal disease, hyperthyroidism, and hyperadrenocorticism. In older cats hypertension may also occur without a disease being present known to cause hypertension, best termed *idiopathic hypertension*. Once a definitive diagnosis of hypertension is made, treatment may be indicated in the hope of minimizing target organ damage (TOD) to eyes, kidneys, the heart and central nervous system. In some cases, successfully treating the initiating disease may resolve the elevation in high blood pressure; however, in many cases this is not adequate and antihypertensives are needed.

Hypertension can have a variety of deleterious consequences.[1] The risk of TOD increases with increasing blood pressure (Table 152-1).[2] Elevations in blood pressure can result in autoregulatory vasoconstriction in those vascular beds that have this capability. If this is sustained for a period of time, medial hypertrophy, ischemia, infarcts, and hemorrhage can occur. Organs that are commonly damaged in this manner include the eye (retinal detachments) and brain. In most instances hypertension is caused by an increase in systemic vascular resistance. This means that the heart has to pump blood into these narrower spaces. This translates into increased afterload, which can lead to cardiac compensatory changes such as left ventricular hypertrophy. Generally the healthy kidney is not susceptible to damage by increased blood pressure in small animal patients; however, the ability to autoregulate against elevated blood pressures is lost with renal insufficiency. With the loss of autoregulation systemic

pressure is transmitted to the glomerulus leading to renal injury. Loss of autoregulation has been demonstrated in dogs with reduced renal mass.[3] Loss of autoregulation also means that lower blood pressures are more poorly tolerated and can lead to loss of renal function and potentially acute renal failure.

Unfortunately, there is no cookbook approach to the treatment of hypertension as many factors need to be considered before treatment is initiated. Each patient's unique clinical situation will also influence which medications are preferred if treatment is initiated. When medical treatment is started, the treatment plan needs to take into consideration how fast blood pressure needs to be decreased and what the target

Table • 152-1

Classification of Hypertension on the Basis of Risk for Target Organ Damage

RISK CATEGORIES	SYSTOLIC PRESSURE (mm Hg)	DIASTOLIC PRESSURE (mm Hg)	RISK FOR TARGET ORGAN DAMAGE
I	<150	<95	Minimal
II	150-159	95-99	Mild
III	160-179	100-119	Moderate
IV	≥180	≥120	Severe

Table • 152-2

Medications Commonly Used to Treat Hypertension in Cats and Dogs

MEDICATION	CAT DOSAGE	DOG DOSAGE
Enalapril	0.25-0.5 mg/kg PO q12-24h	Same
Benazapril	0.25-0.5 mg/kg PO q24h	Same
Ramipril	0.125 mg/kg PO q24h	0.125-0.25 mg/kg PO q24h
Amlodipine	0.625-1.25 mg/cat/day PO (0.13-0.3 mg/kg q24h)	0.1-0.4 mg/kg PO q24h
Atenolol	2 mg/kg PO q12-24h (6.25-12.5 mg/cat PO q12-24h)	0.25-1.0 mg/kg PO q12-24h
Acepromazine	0.05-0.1 mg/kg SC, IV	Same
Hydralazine	2.5-5 mg/cat PO q12-24h	0.5-3.0 mg/kg PO q12h
Phenoxybenzamine	0.25-0.5 mg/kg PO q12h	0.25-1.5 mg/kg PO q8-12h
Prazosin	None	0.5-2.0 mg/dog PO q8-12h

blood pressure is. As an example, with suspected hypertensive encephalopathy or choroidopathy/retinopathy, more rapid reduction in blood pressure is needed than in a patient where TOD is not evident. Concurrent diseases may also significantly influence which medications are chosen. For example, an ACE inhibitor would be an ideal agent to use in an animal with hypertension and concurrent proteinuria or cardiac disease. If any medications are being used that could elevate blood pressure (e.g., corticosteroids, phenylpropanolamine), these should be discontinued or the dose reduced to the lowest possible.

It is uncertain if blood pressure control improves survival in pets as it does in humans. In a study of 141 cats, blood pressure control was not associated with survival. In these cats, proteinuria was the only variable that influenced outcome.[4] This study did not, however, assess diastolic blood pressure or pulse pressures, factors that influence outcome in humans. In addition, the overall treatment goal was to lower blood pressure below 160 mm Hg. In humans, however, it has been shown that more aggressive blood pressure control is associated with improved outcomes in patients with chronic renal disease, especially if proteinuria is present.[5] Although the current veterinary literature does not provide information on ideal therapies, there is little doubt that successfully treating hypertension will prevent or minimize TOD. Table 152-2 lists medications that have been suggested for the treatment of hypertension. Given the paucity of veterinary literature, some treatment recommendations have to be extrapolated from literature on human hypertensives.

ANGIOTENSIN-CONVERTING ENZYME INHIBITORS

Angiotensin-converting enzyme inhibitors (ACEIs) are commonly used antihypertensives in humans and pets. They also have many other beneficial effects that make them desirable medications to use in hypertensive patients, especially those with concurrent cardiac or renal abnormalities. ACEIs exert their effect by blocking the conversion of angiotensin I to angiotensin II (ANGII) by the angiotension-converting enzyme. ANGII can raise blood pressure by being a potent vasoconstrictor, decreasing antidiuretic hormone secretion, and increasing aldosterone secretion.

The blockade of ANGII by ACEIs has significant effects on the kidney that make ACEIs particularly well suited for treating hypertension in patients with renal impairment. The ACEIs (as well as angiotensin receptor blockers) lower intraglomerular pressure independent of the effects on systemic blood pressure by preferentially dilating the efferent arterioles. ACEIs also have been shown to reduce endothelial dysfunction, including on the renal vascular bed.[6] ACEIs also reduce proteinuria, stimulation of cytokines that lead to fibrosis, inflammatory cell recruitment, and compensatory hypertrophy.[7]

The use of ACEIs in hypertension can have adverse side effects. Because the ACEIs preferentially dilate the postglomerular (efferent) arteriole, glomerular filtration rate (GFR) can actually decrease as intraglomerular pressure drops. This is advantageous long term because the drop in intraglomerular pressure minimizes damage to the glomerulus and slows progression of renal disease. An increase in blood urea nitrogen and creatinine is not unexpected when ACEIs are used; however, it generally should not exceed a 10% to 20% rise. Acute renal failure can potentially develop, although it is rare and usually only seen with concurrent volume contraction (diuretic use, other sources of fluid loss) or if other medications are given that might be nephrotoxic (nonsteroidal antiinflammatory drugs, aminoglycosides). Given the potential for negative effects on kidney function, frequent monitoring of renal parameters and electrolytes is indicated when antihypertensives are used.

Generally blood pressure reduction achieved with an ACE inhibitor is modest at best. Poor response to ACEIs (benazapril or enalapril) as sole agents to control spontaneous hypertension have been reported in cats, with only 6 of 16 hypertensive cats being controlled adequately initially. After 6 months only 2 of 16 were still controlled.[8] In cats with induced renal insufficiency, benazepril caused a significant drop in blood pressure when compared to placebo. This decrease was approximately in the range of 10 mm Hg for systolic blood pressure.[9,10] There was no indication that dosages greater than 0.5 to 1.0 mg/kg/day were more efficacious at reducing blood pressure.[9] In dogs with induced renal insufficiency, enalapril at 0.5 mg/kg q12h resulted in a reduction in blood pressure similar in magnitude to that in cats.[11]

Ramipril is an ACEI that has been licensed for use in animals in Europe for some time. There are no peer-reviewed studies that have looked at its effect on hypertension; however, published data do suggest that it may be a more potent antihypertensive than other ACEIs. Twelve hypertensive cats treated with 0.125 mg/kg of ramipril daily resulted in good blood pressure control in all cats for up to 6 months. The antihypertensive effect was seen within 1 hour of administration. On average, blood pressure declined approximately 40 mm Hg.[12] In another study of cats with hypertrophic cardiac changes, blood pressure decreased around 40 mm Hg in those cats that were hypertensive (systolic blood pressure >180 mm Hg), whereas in normotensive cats no decrease was seen. Not all hypertensive cats responded to therapy.[13] Adverse side effects were not reported.

There is evidence from experimental studies and human data that suggest that ACEIs should be used when calcium channel blockers (CCBs) are used to control blood pressure. The main concern with CCBs is their effect on the renal vasculature. CCBs dilate the afferent arteriole, resulting in increased intraglomerular pressure. Increased renal damage has been documented in animal models of hypertension and renal disease.[14] In humans with proteinuric renal disease, CCBs as a sole agent were associated with increased proteinuria unless mean arterial pressure was dramatically lowered. This was not seen if an ACEI was given concurrently.[15] Similar results have been seen in diabetic nephropathy.[16] In healthy dogs the use of amlodipine resulted in a threefold increase in renin-angiotensin-aldosterone activity. This effect was blunted by the concurrent administration of enalapril.[17] The two drugs did work synergistically to decrease blood pressure. Given the evidence available, it would seem reasonable to start an ACEI when a CCB is used, though there is no specific data in pets to support this recommendation.

CALCIUM CHANNEL BLOCKERS

The management of hypertension in pets, especially cats, was problematic until the use of amlodipine was described. Amlodipine decreases calcium influx into both cardiac and vascular smooth muscle leading to vasodilation. Unlike other CCBs, amlodipine is not cardiodepressive and does not lead to a decreased heart rate. Amlodipine has a long duration of effect, so often once-daily dosing is adequate for blood pressure control. Blood pressure appears to decrease gradually as adverse side effects from a rapid drop in blood pressure (weakness, syncope, organ failure) are rarely reported.

Amlodipine (0.625 mg/kg/day) in one study of nine hypertensive cats was shown to reduce systolic blood pressure by approximately 40 mm Hg. This study also suggested that heavier cats required 1.25 mg/cat/day to achieve good blood pressure control.[18] A study in 30 cats with hypertension showed a similar magnitude decrease in blood pressure, which persisted for a prolonged period of time.[19] In cats with surgically induced renal insufficiency, the efficacy of amlodipine in keeping blood pressure under control was similar.[20] Systolic blood pressure was approximately 30 mm Hg and diastolic blood pressure 20 mm Hg lower in the group of cats given the medication. This substantial lowering also translated into clinical benefits for the cats treated. Only 1 of 10 cats treated had retinal lesions, whereas 7 of 10 untreated cats had ocular changes. Hypertension was severe enough in the untreated group that 2 cats succumbed to neurologic complications. Use of transdermal amlodipine also results in a decrease in blood pressure, though not as marked as with the same dose given orally.[21] Given the difficulty in administering oral medications to some cats, the transdermal route may be a viable option in some cats, though there may be more need for dose adjustments to achieve blood pressure control goals. To date there is no published data on the use of amlodipine in hypertensive dogs, though from personal experience it does appear effective and well tolerated.

ADRENERGIC BLOCKING AGENTS

Both alpha and beta blockers can be used to control blood pressure. Beta blockers have several effects that lead to a decrease in blood pressure, including decreasing heart rate and contractility; alpha$_1$-receptor blockers work by causing vasodilation. There are few reports of the use of these agents in veterinary patients.

Beta blockers are often used to help control hypertension in uncontrolled hyperthyroid cats. Atenolol is a good choice for a beta blocker as it often can be given once daily. Propranolol could also be used but requires TID administration, which will often negatively affect owner compliance. In hyperthyroid cats, not only is blood pressure reduced, but the medication may also be protective against arrhythmias and

other undesirable cardiac side effects of hyperthyroidism. If blood pressure control is inadequate, amlodipine can be added in as well. Beta blockers are contraindicated if the cause of hypertension is a pheochromocytoma.

Alpha$_1$-receptor blockers have been used on occasion to control hypertension. Phenoxybenzamine and prazosin are agents that belong to this group of medications. They can be considered when acceptable blood pressure control is not achieved with other medications. In patients with a pheochromocytoma, phenoxybenzamine is considered the drug of choice.

OTHER ANTIHYPERTENSIVE MEDICATIONS

Diuretics
Diuretics are commonly used in humans to treat hypertension and have been found to be efficacious. Information regarding the benefits of diuretics in hypertensive animals is lacking. Generally these medications are not used, the exception being cases where volume reduction may be of benefit (patients with edema or effusions).

Other Drug Therapy
Certain phenothiazine derivatives can decrease blood pressure. Both acepromazine and chlorpromazine are known to have this effect. The effect is related to alpha-adrenergic blockade. Hydralazine will also reliably decrease blood pressure in dogs and cats. Blood pressure can drop rapidly and to a great degree, so initial dosages should be low and titrated upward under close blood pressure control. Nitroprusside can be used in dogs with severe hypertension. It is administered as a constant rate infusion; continuous blood pressure and electrocardiogram monitoring is a necessity to avoid severe adverse side effects relating to hypotension.

ADJUNCTIVE THERAPY

Dietary manipulations are a consideration in treating certain hypertensive patients. Both sodium and potassium play a role in blood pressure control, at least in humans. Reducing the amount of salt consumed by humans can help to normalize blood pressure or at least make medications more efficacious. Whether salt reduction has a beneficial role in the treatment of hypertensive pets has not been investigated. Increased salt content does not appear to cause increases in blood pressure in healthy cats[22,23] or cats with experimentally reduced renal function.[22] In fact, reduced sodium diets (8.6 mg NaCl/g of food on dry matter basis) were associated with reduced GFR, activation of the renin-angiotensin-aldosterone system, and inappropriate kaliuresis. Generally moderate salt reduction can be considered in hypertensive patients especially if using a diet designed to help treat a concurrent disorder such as renal disease. It is of course important that the pet will continue to eat with the dietary change. Potassium also appears to play a role in blood pressure regulation based on epidemiologic data that shows that large potassium intake is associated with lower blood pressures.[24] The exact mechanism by which this occurs is unclear. Generally potassium supplementation is not indicated when an ACEI is being used.

Obesity is associated with hypertension in humans and dogs. Dogs have been frequently used as models of obesity-associated hypertension. In these models dogs are made obese in relatively short periods of time leading to increases in arterial blood pressure of approximately 15 to 20 mm Hg.[25,26] With weight loss, blood pressure normalizes.[25] Spontaneous obesity has also been associated with higher blood pressures in dogs.[27] Weight loss in spontaneously obese dogs leads to a modest decrease in blood pressure (unpublished data). The mechanisms by which increased body weight leads to increased blood pressure are complex, and many theories have been advanced to explain this phenomenon.[28] In an obese patient with hypertension, a weight loss regimen should be recommended as an adjunctive therapy that has many benefits besides lowering blood pressure.

MONITORING THERAPY

Since blood pressure can fluctuate it is important to monitor blood pressure frequently when antihypertensive medications are being used. It is of course also important to monitor blood pressure of normotensive patients with diseases known to cause hypertension in order to be able to intervene as soon as possible. Many of the medications used can adversely affect the kidney, so routine monitoring of renal parameters and electrolytes is recommended. These parameters should also be checked shortly after increasing drug dosages. In general, checking lab work 1 week after starting or increasing medications is indicated. Exact goals for blood pressure control have not been established, but maintaining blood pressure below 160 mm Hg systolic and 100 mm Hg diastolic is reasonable. Lower values would be ideal if the patient tolerates it.

REFERENCES

The reference list can be found on the companion Expert Consult Web site at *www.expertconsult.com*.

CHAPTER **153**

Hypotension

Lori S. Waddell

Blood pressure is measured as systolic, diastolic, and mean arterial pressures. Systolic and diastolic pressure correspond to the phases of the cardiac cycle. Mean arterial pressure (MAP) is calculated from the equation

$$MAP = Diastolic + [(Systolic - Diastolic) \div 3]$$

and is the most important value when considering perfusion of the organs and tissues. *Hypotension* is defined as a systolic arterial blood pressure of less than 80 mm Hg and/or a mean pressure of less than 60 mm Hg in either dogs or cats.

Causes of hypotension include decreased preload to the heart, decreased vascular tone, and cardiac dysfunction. Untreated hypotension can lead to shock from inadequate tissue perfusion and oxygen delivery to the tissues. Treatment of hypotension should consist of identifying and correcting the underlying problem. Recognition and treatment of hypotension are essential to prevent the development of refractory shock, organ failure, and death (Figure 153-1).

Blood pressure provides a measurement of tissue perfusion. The two are not equivalent, but blood pressure monitoring is the simplest means of obtaining an objective parameter. Subjective measures of tissue perfusion are obtained by physical examination; they include pulse quality, mucous membrane color, capillary refill time, and heart rate and rhythm. Combined with blood pressure monitoring, these parameters provide the basis for a more accurate assessment of tissue perfusion. A normal blood pressure does not necessarily mean that the tissues are adequately perfused, as blood pressure may be maintained with severe peripheral vasoconstriction and/or increased cardiac output.

CLINICAL MANIFESTATIONS

The clinical signs associated with hypotension depend on the severity and cause of the condition. In dogs, hypotension is usually associated with tachycardia, bounding to weak pulses, pale mucous membranes, slow capillary refill time, mental dullness, and weakness. If the underlying cause is sepsis, the mucous membranes may be injected or red with a rapid capillary refill time. Cardiac causes of hypotension can alter the clinical picture, with arrhythmias, weak, irregular pulses, and even severe bradycardia possible. Hypotensive cats also usually have tachycardia, poor pulse quality, pale mucous membranes, slow capillary refill time, mental dullness, and weakness. However, unlike dogs, cats with sepsis or systemic inflammatory response syndrome (SIRS) often have bradycardia rather than tachycardia and rarely have injected mucous membranes. In both species, hypotension is often associated with decreased urine output, hyperventilation, hypothermia, and cold extremities.

Inability to palpate pulses peripherally can be useful in assessing blood pressure. When metatarsal pulses are palpable, the systolic blood pressure is above 70 to 80 mm Hg. Although measurement of blood pressure confirms the presence of hypotension, the diagnosis can be made on physical examination findings alone.

PATHOGENESIS

Systemic blood pressure (BP) is dependent on cardiac output (CO) and systemic vascular resistance (SVR) (Figure 153-2):

$$BP = CO \times SVR$$

Cardiac output is determined by heart rate, contractility, preload, and afterload. The three main causes of hypotension are decreased preload, decreased cardiac function, and decreased vascular tone (Box 153-1). These may occur individually or in combination.

Systemic blood pressure is maintained via neural, hormonal, and local mechanisms. Smooth muscle in blood vessel walls is innervated by fibers from the sympathetic nervous system. Activation of this system results in vasoconstriction

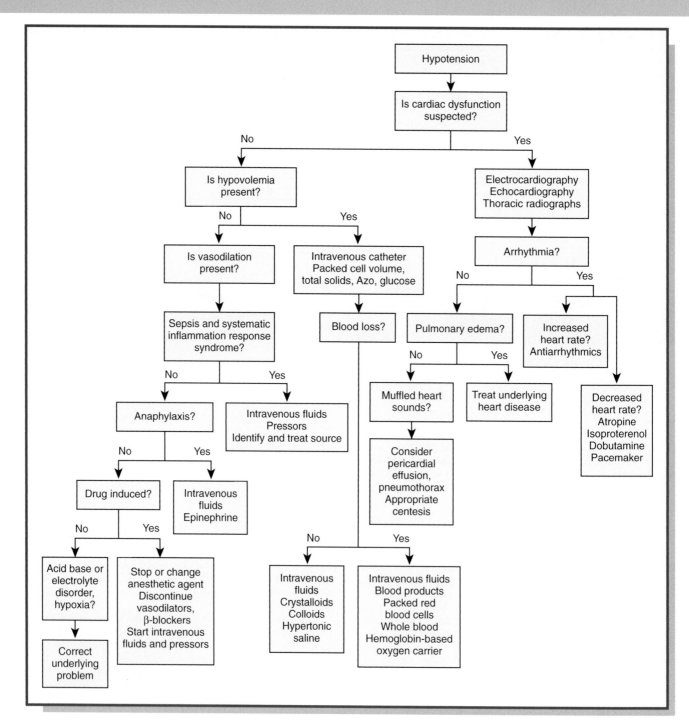

Figure 153-1 Algorithm for differential diagnoses and treatment of hypotension.

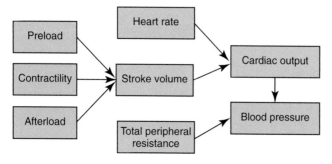

Figure 153-2 Cardiovascular parameters and their relationship to systemic blood pressure.

of vessels in tissue beds with the exception of skeletal muscle, where it causes vasodilation. Sympathetic innervation of cardiac muscle causes increased heart rate and contractility. Sympathetic stimulation occurs when the vasomotor center, located in the medulla oblongata, is activated. Hypovolemia and hypotension can lead to activation of the vasomotor center due to the baroreceptors in the carotid sinuses and aortic body sensing a lack of stretch, and the stretch receptors in the atria and pulmonary artery sensing a lack of distension and atrial filling. The vasomotor center is also activated by local hypoxia or hypercapnia causing stimulation of the chemoreceptors in the carotid sinus and aortic bodies, although this mechanism is less important than the baroreceptor reflex.

Box • 153-1

Causes of Hypotension

Decreased Preload
Hypovolemia
Hemorrhage
Trauma
Gastrointestinal losses
Polyuria
Hypoadrenocorticism
Effusions or third spacing of fluid
Burns
Heatstroke
Decreased Venous Return
Pericardial tamponade
Restrictive pericarditis
Severe pneumothorax
Positive pressure ventilation
Gastric dilatation and volvulus
Heartworm disease (caval syndrome)

Decreased Cardiac Function
Cardiomyopathy
Valvular disease
Bradyarrhythmias
Tachyarrhythmias
Electrolyte abnormalities
Acid-base disturbances
Severe hypoxia
Sepsis/systemic inflammatory response syndrome (SIRS)

Decreased Vascular Tone
Sepsis/SIRS
Anaphylaxis
Neurogenic
Drug induced (anesthetic agent, vasodilators [e.g., beta
    blockers, calcium channel blockers])
Electrolyte abnormalities
Acid-base disturbances
Severe hypoxia

---

from the gastrointestinal tract, impaired hepatic function, and activation of the coagulation cascade.

In addition to the mechanisms listed above, there are several other important effectors of blood pressure and vascular tone. Activation of the arachidonic acid cascade leads to production of prostacyclin and thromboxane A_2. Prostacyclin causes vasodilation, but thromboxane A_2 causes vasoconstriction. Nitric oxide (NO), produced by endothelial cells via nitric oxide synthase, is an important regulator of vascular tone, resulting in vasodilation. There are two types of nitric oxide synthase, the constitutive form and the inducible form. In sepsis and SIRS, there is a tremendous increase in NO production from inducible NO synthase, which is activated by a variety of inflammatory mediators including interleukin-1 (IL-1), IL-2, IL-6, and tumor necrosis factor. This overproduction of NO, coupled with depletion of vasopressin, downregulation of catecholamine receptors, and disruption of vascular smooth muscle calcium metabolism can result in vasoplegia, severe hypotension, and refractory shock.

Hypovolemia results in decreased cardiac output secondary to decreased venous return to the heart. This, in turn, results in decreased preload. Moderate to severe hypovolemia must be present to affect blood pressure due to the normal compensatory actions that occur, including increased heart rate to maintain cardiac output and increased peripheral vascular resistance secondary to vasoconstriction. The compensatory mechanisms maintain adequate blood pressure until more than 20% to 25% of the intravascular volume has been depleted. Hypovolemia can occur with blood loss or increased fluid losses secondary to vomiting, diarrhea, polyuria, or third spacing of fluid.

Restriction of cardiac filling can also result in decreased preload, decreased cardiac output, and hypotension. Pericardial effusion with tamponade and restrictive pericarditis can result in hypotension by this mechanism. Severe pneumothorax and positive pressure ventilation can also reduce venous return to the heart. Hypertrophic cardiomyopathy in cats reduces left ventricular volume, thereby reducing preload and cardiac output.

Bradyarrhythmias can affect blood pressure by reducing cardiac output, especially when the heart rate is extremely slow. Although pulses may be normal or strong in a dog or cat with bradyarrhythmia, overall cardiac output can be drastically reduced by the infrequency of systole. The resulting low cardiac output may be severe enough to cause syncopal episodes secondary to hypotension and decreased perfusion of the brain. Tachyarrhythmias can result in hypotension by reducing preload to the heart. At extremely rapid heart rates, filling of the heart is limited by the relatively short time for diastole. This can result in reduced cardiac output despite an increased heart rate. Also, coronary perfusion occurs during diastole, so at rapid rates, cardiac perfusion is significantly decreased and can eventually result in decreased contractility and decreased cardiac output.

Decreased cardiac output can also occur due to primary cardiac disorders. Dilated cardiomyopathy is characterized by reduced stroke volume and reduced cardiac output caused by decreased contractility. Valvular incompetence, resulting in regurgitant flow, can also lead to decreased stroke volume. Other causes of decreased cardiac contractility include myocarditis, myocardial infarction, myocardial depression secondary to sepsis, SIRS, anesthetic drugs, beta blockers and calcium channel blockers, and acid-base and electrolyte abnormalities.

Decreased systemic vascular resistance can also cause hypotension. Common causes of vasodilatation are sepsis/ SIRS; anaphylaxis; anesthesia; use of vasodilators, including beta blockers and calcium channel blockers; electrolyte abnormalities; and acid-base disturbances. Many of these mecha-

Hypotension also causes release of antidiuretic hormone (ADH) and adrenocorticotropic hormone (ACTH) from the pituitary, as well as release of catecholamines (norepinephrine and epinephrine) and cortisol from the adrenal glands. Increased concentrations of these hormones stimulates an increase in heart rate, vasoconstriction, and water retention by the kidneys. Simultaneously, the macula densa in the glomeruli are affected, and the renin-angiotensin-aldosterone system is activated, resulting in sodium retention by the kidneys and further vasoconstriction. These mechanisms serve to increase blood volume by means of sodium and water retention and to preferentially perfuse the brain and heart while decreasing perfusion to the skin, muscles, and abdominal organs, including the kidneys. Recognition and treatment of hypotension are essential to prevent the development of refractory shock and organ failure. Acute renal failure is one of the most common consequences of hypotension, but others include decreased coronary artery perfusion due to the increased heart rate, increased risk of bacterial translocation

nisms also affect cardiac contractility, resulting in hypotension mediated by decreased cardiac output and vasodilatation simultaneously.

MEASUREMENT OF BLOOD PRESSURE

Blood pressure monitoring can be divided into two main types, noninvasive and invasive methods. Noninvasive methods are most commonly used, and in dogs and cats usually consist of either an oscillometric system (Cardell Monitor, Sharn Veterinary, Tampa, Fla.; or Dinamap, Critikon, Tampa, Fla.) or Doppler methods (Parks Electronics, Aloha, Ore.). Invasive blood pressure monitoring is performed by direct arterial pressure measurement via placement of an arterial catheter and connection to a pressure transducer. Direct pressure monitoring is considered the gold standard of blood pressure monitoring.

TREATMENT

It is essential that initial treatment of hypotension always be aimed at correction of the underlying physiologic problem: decreased preload, cardiac dysfunction, or peripheral vasodilatation. Differentiation of cardiac and noncardiac causes of hypotension is a critical first step (see Figure 153-1). If the animal is hypovolemic, intravenous fluids and/or blood products should be administered until euvolemia has been attained. If hypovolemia is severe enough to cause hypotension, a shock bolus should be given. The standard doses of isotonic crystalloids are 60 to 90 mL/kg for dogs and 45 to 60 mL/kg for cats. If colloids are indicated in place of crystalloids, approximately one fourth of the crystalloid dose should be given. Hypertonic saline (5% to 7.5%) is a rapid intravascular volume expander and can be used when immediate resuscitation is needed. The dose for hypertonic saline is 5 mL/kg given over 5 to 10 minutes for dogs and 3 to 4 mL/kg given over the same time period for cats. After administration of hypertonic saline, it is essential to follow with one third to one half of a shock bolus of isotonic crystalloids to provide continued intravascular volume expansion and to replenish the interstitial space. If hypovolemia occurs secondary to blood loss, blood products, such as whole blood or packed red blood cells, or a hemoglobin-based oxygen-carrying solution may need to be administered to provide adequate oxygen-carrying capacity.

If the volume status is unknown or if there are concerns about overloading the animal with intravenous fluids, a central venous catheter can be placed for central venous pressure (CVP) monitoring. A low CVP (less than 0 cm H_2O) indicates hypovolemia due to fluid loss or vasodilatation secondary to decreased peripheral resistance. A high CVP (greater than 10 cm H_2O) indicates volume overload, right-sided heart failure, or increased pulmonary vascular resistance (afterload). If the significance of a low to normal CVP reading is questionable, a small test bolus of fluids can be given. A rapid bolus of 10 to 15 mL/kg of crystalloid or 3 to 5 mL/kg of colloid is

used. It is important to remember that the vascular bed is a compliant system, able to accommodate changes in volume with minimal changes in pressure. If the animal has a low CVP due to hypovolemia, the CVP will show either no change or a transient rise toward normal followed by a rapid decrease. The MAP also increases transiently. A bolus given to a dog or cat that is euvolemic usually causes a small increase in the CVP of 2 to 4 cm H_2O with a return to baseline within 15 minutes. A large increase (greater than 4 cm H_2O) followed by a slow return to baseline (longer than 30 minutes) is seen with hypervolemia or reduced cardiac compliance.

If the animal remains hypotensive once euvolemia has been achieved, the use of pressors should be considered. Commonly used pressors for treating vasodilation include dopamine, epinephrine, norepinephrine, and phenylephrine, administered for their alpha agonist effects, as constant-rate infusions. Only phenylephrine is a pure alpha agonist; the others have varying degrees of beta effects in addition to their alpha effects. Vasopressin can also be used in cases with vasodilatory shock. These drugs need to be titrated to effect, requiring frequent blood pressure monitoring. They should never be used in place of adequate volume expansion, because most patients with hypovolemic shock already have compensatory vasoconstriction.

Cardiac causes of hypotension must be addressed on a case-by-case basis. If tachyarrhythmias are the cause, antiarrhythmic therapy should be administered. Bradyarrhythmias may respond to medical therapy or may require placement of a pacemaker. Obstruction of cardiac filling by pericardial effusion or severe pneumothorax should be addressed by appropriate centesis. Positive inotropes such as dobutamine, a beta agonist, should be administered as a constant rate infusion when decreased cardiac contractility is suspected.

DIAGNOSTIC PLAN

Diagnosis of the underlying cause of the hypotension must often wait until after therapy has been initiated due to the critical nature of hypotension. History and physical examination abnormalities can often help in the determination of a tentative diagnosis, allowing therapy to be started. Initial diagnostics in an unstable hypotensive dog or cat should include packed cell volume, total solids, blood glucose, and an estimate of the blood urea nitrogen level (Azostix, Bayer Corporation, Elkhart, Ind.). Electrolytes, acid-base status, and lactate can also be helpful. Depending on the clinical signs, an electrocardiogram (ECG), abdominal and thoracic radiographs, abdominal ultrasonography, echocardiography, CVP and pulse oximetry determinations, and arterial blood gas analysis can be useful. A complete blood count, serum chemistry profile, and urinalysis should also be performed. If indicated by a suspicion of Addison's disease, an ACTH stimulation test should be completed. If sepsis is suspected, blood and urine cultures should be done unless the source of sepsis can be directly cultured.

SECTION VII
Therapeutic Considerations in Medicine and Disease

CHAPTER 154

Antibacterial Drug Therapy

Mark G. Papich

Antibiotic therapy has made many advances that have given veterinary medicine a large number of effective drugs and provided pharmacokinetic and pharmacodynamic information to guide dosing. Improved techniques for bacterial identification and susceptibility testing have helped to provide guidelines for the most appropriate drug selection. Despite these advances, treatment of infections in small animals continues to meet challenges with bacterial drug resistance, inability to maintain good compliance, and insufficient drugs to meet many of the needs of veterinary medicine. However, new drugs have become available, or are in development, that attempt to address the problems of drug availability and improved owner compliance. Although there are drugs available in veterinary medicine to treat the most common infections encountered in small animals, we are faced with using human-label drugs to meet other needs. Antibacterial drug therapy is more challenging when the infection is refractory, resistant, or is associated with another complicating factor. Susceptibility of the most common isolates has been documented well enough to make sound judgments and empirical antimicrobial drug choices. However, when the patient has a refractory and/or resistant infection, or is seriously ill with an infection, other strategies and drugs may be necessary. Throughout this chapter, several antibiotics are discussed. Complete dosage regimens and details about individual drugs are found in other sources written by this author.[1,2] You are encouraged to consult those references for more detail.

For the veterinary drugs, published data, approved labels, and freedom of information (FOI) summaries provide evidence for efficacy and guidelines for therapy. When specific information is not available through well-conducted clinical trials or inadequate veterinary clinical studies to support a recommended use and dose, dosing guidelines for these drugs have been based on extrapolation from human medicine, studies in laboratory animals, pharmacokinetic-pharmacodynamic (PK-PD) data, and susceptibility information.

BACTERIAL SUSCEPTIBILITY TESTING

Most of the time, bacteria isolated from infections in small animals include: *Staphylococcus pseudintermedius*, (formerly called *S. intermedius*), *Escherichia coli*, *Klebsiella pneumoniae*, *Pasteurella multocida*, beta-hemolytic streptococci, *Pseudomonas aeruginosa*, *Proteus mirabilis* (and occasionally indole-positive *Proteus*), *Enterobacter* spp. and *Enterococcus* spp.

Usually Susceptible Bacteria

If the bacteria are accurately identified, antibiotic selection is simplified because the susceptibility pattern of many organisms is predictable. For example, if the bacterium is likely to be *Pasteurella*, *Streptococcus*, or *Actinomyces*, susceptibility is expected to penicillin, ampicillin, amoxicillin, or amoxicillin-clavulanic acid (Clavamox). Cephalosporins (cephems) also will be active against these organisms, as well as other commonly used antibiotics such as tetracyclines or trimethoprim-sulfonamides.

Staphylococcus isolated from small animals is most likely to be *S. pseudintermedius* rather than *S. aureus* in dogs. Bacteria previously identified as *Staphylococcus intermedius* are most likely *S. pseudintermedius* and any future studies and papers will likely use the new terminology.[3] Occasionally other species of *Staphylococcus*—both coagulase-positive and coagulase-negative—are identified, including *S. aureus*. The typical wild-type strains of these staphylococci usually have a predictable susceptibility to antibiotics such as amoxicillin combined with a β-lactamase inhibitor (clavulanate; Clavamox), or β-lactamase–resistant first-generation cephalosporin such as cephalexin or cefadroxil, or the third-generation cephalosporins cefovecin (Convenia) and cefpodoxime (Simplicef). *Staphylococcus* also is susceptible to oxacillin and dicloxacillin but these are not used as commonly in small animal medicine. Reports of studies on *S. pseudintermedius* have shown that, despite frequent use of the above-mentioned drugs in small animals, the incidence of resistance has not increased.[4-6] Most staphylococci are also sensitive to fluoroquinolones, lincosamides (clindamycin, lincomycin), chloramphenicol, trimethoprim-sulfonamides, or erythromycin, but resistance can occur if the animals have been previously treated with these drugs.

Other bacteria also have been associated with predictable susceptibility. If the bacterium is an anaerobe (for example, *Clostridium*, *Fusobacterium*, *Prevotella*, *Actinomyces*, or *Porphyromonas*) predictable results can be attained by administering a penicillin, chloramphenicol, metronidazole, clindamycin, amoxicillin-clavulanic acid, or one of the second-generation

589

cephalosporins (cephamycins) such as cefotetan or cefoxitin. Metronidazole is consistently highly active against anaerobes including *B. fragilis*. The activity of first-generation cephalosporins, trimethoprim-sulfonamides/ormetoprim-sulfonamides, or fluoroquinolones for an anaerobic infection is unpredictable. If the anaerobe is from the *B. fragilis* group, resistance may be more of a problem because they produce a β-lactamase that may inactivate first-generation cephalosporins, penicillins, and ampicillin/amoxicillin. Some of these *Bacteroides* may also be resistant to clindamycin.[7]

Problem, or Resistant Bacteria

Staphylococcus   Despite the favorable rates of susceptibility listed above for *Staphylococcus*, in the last several years there has been an increase in the reports of emergence of methicillin-resistant *Staphylococcus* in companion animals.[8,9] Reports of these resistant isolates are becoming more frequent, just as methicillin-resistant *Staphylococcus aureus* (MRSA) in human hospitals and in the community has reached alarming rates. The relationship between human strains of methicillin-resistant staphylococci and the veterinary strains is an area of ongoing interest and debate.[10]

Staphylococcal resistance can be caused by altered penicillin-binding proteins (PBP2a), the resistance carried by the gene *mecA*. These are known as *methicillin-resistant staphylococci* (MRS).[8,9,11,12] If it is *S. aureus* the term *methicillin-resistant S. aureus* (MRSA) is used. Other *Staphylococcus* species also have been identified among veterinary isolates, such as coagulase-negative *Staphylococcus*. Oxacillin is now used more common than methicillin as a surrogate test for this type of resistance, and resistance to oxacillin is equivalent to methicillin resistance. If staphylococci are resistant to oxacillin or methicillin, they should be considered resistant to all other β-lactams, including cephalosporins and amoxicillin-clavulanate (e.g., Clavamox), regardless of the susceptibility test result. Adding a β-lactamase inhibitor will not overcome methicillin resistance. Unfortunately, these bacteria often carry coresistance to many other non–β-lactam drugs, including clindamycin, fluoroquinolones, macrolides, tetracyclines, and trimethoprim-sulfonamides. Use of fluoroquinolones and cephalosporins has been linked to emergence of resistance of methicillin-resistant staphylococci.[13] Because susceptibility to non–β-lactam antibiotics is unpredictable, a susceptibility test is needed to identify which drug to use for these infections. Clindamycin, chloramphenicol, rifampin, and trimethoprim-sulfonamides are drugs to consider for these infections if a susceptibility test can confirm activity. However, in some cases, the drug choices have been limited to some human-labeled drugs such as the glycopeptide vancomycin (Vancocin) or the oxazolidinone linezolid (Zyvox). Vancomycin can only be administered by intravenous infusion. Linezolid is the first in the class of oxazolidinones to be used in medicine, and it is used in people to treat resistant gram-positive infections caused by enterococci and streptococci.

Gram-Negative Bacteria   The most common resistant gram-negative bacteria in veterinary small animal medicine are the gram-negative bacilli, especially the enteric isolates. The most common resistant gram-negative bacilli that we encounter in small animal medicine is *Escherichia coli*. In some hospitals, there have been outbreaks of *Klebsiella pneumoniae*, *Enterobacter*, and indole-positive *Proteus*, but *E. coli* remains the most common. Another important gram-negative bacterium that is encountered in small animals is *Pseudomonas aeruginosa*. It is a nonfermenting, nonenteric bacterium but is inherently resistant to many antibiotics because they fail to penetrate the organism's outer membrane and produce β-lactamase.

A review of the recent literature on the susceptibility of *Escherichia coli* to veterinary drugs indicates that less than half of the isolates are susceptible to first-generation cephalosporins and aminopenicillins (ampicillin/amoxicillin).[14-16] In many studies the susceptibility was less than 30%. Recent studies also show an increase in resistance to fluoroquinolones among veterinary gram-negative isolates—as high as 20% to 23%. Based on these data as well as other studies, for initial therapy do not rely on ampicillin, amoxicillin, first-generation cephalosporins, or tetracyclines.

Wild-type strains of *E. coli* are ordinarily susceptible to third-generation cephalosporins, carbapenems, fluoroquinolones, and aminoglycosides. Many are also susceptible to amoxicillin-clavulanate (Clavamox) or ampicillin-sulbactam (Unasyn) combinations. Drugs that are *not* expected to have good activity against the wild-type strains are first-generation cephalosporins, ampicillin/amoxicillin, or macrolides. When resistant bacteria are suspected, after a susceptibility report is available, one may find that the only drugs to which some gram-negative bacilli are sensitive are the extended-spectrum cephalosporins, penems (carbapenems), or amikacin. The injectable cephalosporins consistently most active against these resistant strains are cefotaxime and ceftazidime, although individual veterinary hospitals have utilized others in this group. These drugs are more expensive than oral drugs and can only be administered by injection. Although there are some oral third-generation cephalosporins (cefpodoxime proxetil: Simplicef), their activity is not as good against gram-negative bacilli as the injectable formulations mentioned above.

Most of the *Pseudomonas aeruginosa* isolated from veterinary patients are from skin and ear infections. *Pseudomonas aeruginosa* is inherently resistant to many drugs, but it may be susceptible to fluoroquinolones, aminoglycosides (gentamicin, amikacin, tobramycin), ceftazidime, carbapenems (imipenem or meropenem), or extended-spectrum penicillin such as ticarcillin or piperacillin.[17-19] Of the currently available fluoroquinolones, (human or veterinary drugs) ciprofloxacin is the most active against *Pseudomonas aeruginosa*, followed by (in decreasing order) marbofloxacin, enrofloxacin, difloxacin, and orbifloxacin.[20,21] However, it is not established whether the in vitro differences in susceptibility translate to clinical efficacy. When administering a fluoroquinolone to treat *Pseudomonas aeruginosa*, the high end of the dose range is suggested.

BACTERIAL SUSCEPTIBILITY TESTING

Bacterial susceptibility to drugs has traditionally been tested with the agar-disk-diffusion test (ADD), also known as the Kirby-Bauer test. With this test, paper disks impregnated with the drug are placed on an agar plate and the drug diffuses into the agar. Activity of the drug against the bacteria correlates with the zone of bacterial inhibition around the disk. The inoculation variables must be well controlled and the test must be performed according to strict procedural guidelines.[22,23] The precise incubation time (usually 18 to 24 hours), selection and preparation of the agar, and interfering compounds should be known. The ADD test results provide qualitative (that is, the test determines only resistant vs. sensitive) rather than quantitative information. If this test is performed using standardized procedures, it is valuable, even though it may sometimes overestimate the degree of susceptibility.

MIC Determination

It is becoming more common for laboratories to directly measure the minimum inhibitory concentration (MIC) of an organism with an antimicrobial dilution test. Guidelines for testing have been published and standards established by the

Clinical Laboratory Standards Institute (CLSI), formerly known as the National Committee for Clinical Laboratory Standards (NCCLS).[22,23]

The test is usually performed by inoculating the wells of a plate with the bacterial culture and serial dilutions of antibiotics are arranged across the rows. The MIC can be directly determined by observing the lowest concentration required to inhibit bacterial growth. In some laboratories other methods to measure the MIC are being used such as the E-test (epsilometer test; AB Biodisk). The E-test is a quantitative technique that measures the MIC by direct measurement of bacterial growth along a concentration gradient of the antibiotic contained in a test strip.

Whether by dilution or the E-test, resistance and susceptibility are determined by comparing the organism's MIC to the drug's breakpoint as established by the CLSI.[22] After a laboratory determines an MIC, it may use the CLSI "SIR" classification for breakpoints (S, susceptible; I, intermediate; or R, resistant). In everyday practice, if the MIC for the bacterial isolate falls in the *susceptible* category, there is a greater likelihood of successful treatment (cure) than if the isolate were classified as resistant. It does not ensure success; drug failure is still possible owing to other drug or patient factors (for example, drug interactions, weakened immune status, or severe illness that compromises the action of antibacterial drugs). If the MIC is in the *resistant* category, bacteriologic failure is more likely because of specific resistance mechanisms or inadequate drug concentrations in the patient. However, a patient with a competent immune system may sometimes eradicate an infection even when the isolate is resistant to the drug in the MIC test.

The *intermediate* category is intended as a buffer zone between susceptible and resistant strains. This category reflects the possibility of error when an isolate has an MIC that borders between susceptible and resistant. The intermediate category is not intended to mean "moderately susceptible." If the MIC value is in the intermediate category, therapy with this drug at the usual standard dosage is discouraged because there is a good likelihood that drug concentrations may be inadequate for a cure. However, successful therapy is possible when drug concentrates at certain sites—in urine, or as the result of topical therapy, for example—or at doses higher than the minimum effective dose listed on the label. For example, fluoroquinolone antimicrobials have been approved with a dose range that allows increases in doses when susceptibility testing identifies an organism in the *intermediate* range of susceptibility. In these cases higher drug concentrations may make a cure possible if the clinician is able to safely increase the dose above the minimum labeled dose. (For example, in the case of enrofloxacin in dogs, this would be equivalent to a dose of 10 to 20 mg/kg/day, rather than the minimum dose of 5 mg/kg/day.)

PENETRATION TO THE SITE OF INFECTION

For most tissues, antibiotic drug concentrations in the serum or plasma approximate the drug concentration in the extracellular space (interstitial fluid).[24-26] This is because there is no barrier that impedes drug diffusion from the vascular compartment to extracellular tissue fluid.[27] There is really no such thing as "good penetration" and "poor penetration" when referring to most drugs in most tissues. Pores (fenestrations) or microchannels in the endothelium of capillaries are large enough to allow drug molecules to pass through unless the drug is restricted by protein binding in the blood. Tissues lacking pores or channels may inhibit penetration of some drugs (discussed below).

Diffusion into Tissues

Diffusion of most antibiotics from plasma to tissues is limited by tissue blood flow, rather than drug lipid solubility. If adequate drug concentrations can be achieved in plasma, it is unlikely that a barrier in the tissue will prevent drug diffusion to the site of infection as long as the tissue has an adequate blood supply. Rapid equilibration occurs between the extracellular fluid in tissues and plasma drug concentrations because of the driving force of the concentration gradient and the high surface area of capillaries available for diffusion. Drug diffusion into an abscess or granulation tissue can be impaired because, in these conditions, drug penetration relies on simple diffusion and the site of infection lacks adequate blood supply. In an abscess, there may not be a physical barrier to diffusion—that is, there is no impenetrable membrane—but low drug concentrations are attained because drug concentrations are slow to accumulate in a cavitated lesion.

Barriers to Diffusion   In some tissues a lipid membrane (such as tight junctions on capillaries) presents a barrier to drug diffusion. In these tissues, a drug must be sufficiently lipid soluble or be actively carried across the membrane in order to reach effective concentrations in tissues. These tissues include the central nervous system, eye, and prostate. A functional membrane pump (p-glycoprotein) also contributes to the barrier. Only some drugs can diffuse into these tissues because of their high lipophilicity or because of trapping of charged species of the drug. For example, drugs that are weak bases (trimethoprim, macrolides, lincosamides) are lipophilic in the pH of the blood and readily diffuse into cells and across membranes. But if the tissue is relatively more acidic than the plasma (for example, the central nervous system, leukocytes, and prostate), the drugs become charged, less lipophilic, and "trapped" in the tissue. There also is a barrier between plasma and bronchial epithelium (blood-bronchus barrier). This limits drug concentrations of some drugs in the bronchial secretions and epithelial fluid of the airways. Lipophilic drugs may be more likely to diffuse through the blood-bronchus barrier and reach effective drug concentrations in bronchial secretions.

LOCAL FACTORS THAT AFFECT ANTIBIOTIC EFFECTIVENESS

Local tissue factors may decrease antimicrobial effectiveness. For example, pus and necrotic debris may bind and inactivate vancomycin or aminoglycoside antibiotics (gentamicin or amikacin), causing them to be ineffective. Cellular material also can decrease the activity of topical agents such as polymyxin B. Foreign material in a wound (such as surgical implants or plant material) can protect bacteria from antibiotics and phagocytosis by forming a biofilm (glycocalyx) at the site of infection.[28,29] Cellular debris and infected tissue can inhibit the action of trimethoprim-sulfonamide combinations through the secretion of thymidine and PABA, both known to be inhibitors of the action of these drugs. This may explain why trimethoprim-sulfonamide combinations have not been effective in some infected tissues, particularly anaerobic infections.[30] Cations can adversely affect the activity of antimicrobials at the site of infection. Fluoroquinolones and aminoglycosides are two important drug groups diminished in activity by cations such as Mg^{++}, Al^{+3}, Fe^{+3}, and Ca^{++}. (Cations such as magnesium, iron, and aluminum also can inhibit oral absorption of fluoroquinolones.)

An acidic environment of infected tissue may decrease the effectiveness of clindamycin, erythromycin, fluoroquinolones, and aminoglycosides. Penicillin and tetracycline activity is not affected as much by tissue pH, but hemoglobin at the site of infection will decrease the activity of these drugs. An anaerobic environment decreases the effectiveness of aminoglycosides because oxygen is necessary for drug penetration into bacteria.

As mentioned previously, an adequate blood flow is necessary to deliver an antibiotic to the site of infection. Effective antibacterial drug concentrations may not be attained in tissues that are poorly vascularized (e.g., extremities during shock, sequestered bone fragments, and endocardial valves).

PHARMACOKINETIC-PHARMACODYNAMIC (PK-PD) PRINCIPLES

To achieve a cure, the drug concentration in plasma, serum, or tissue fluid should be maintained above the MIC, or some multiple of the MIC, for at least a portion of the dose interval. Antibacterial dosage regimens are based on this assumption, but drugs vary with respect to the peak concentration and the time above the MIC that is needed for a clinical cure. PK-PD relationships of antibiotics attempt to explain how these factors can correlate with clinical outcome.[31,32] Shown in Figure 154-1 are some terms used to describe the shape of the plasma concentration versus time profile.

The C_{MAX} is simply the maximum plasma concentration attained during a dosing interval. The C_{MAX} is related to the MIC by the C_{MAX}:MIC ratio. The AUC is the total area-under-the-curve. The AUC for a 24-hour period is related to the MIC value by the AUC:MIC ratio. Also shown in Figure 154-1 is the relationship of time to MIC measured in hours (T > MIC).

Antibiotics have been classified as being either bactericidal or bacteriostatic, depending on their action on the bacteria. However, the distinction between bactericidal and bacteriostatic has become more blurred in recent years. Drugs traditionally considered bactericidal can be "static" if the concentrations are low. Alternatively, drugs traditionally considered "static" can be "cidal" against some bacteria and under optimal conditions. Rather than "bacterio-static" or "bactericidal," drugs are now more frequently grouped as either *concentration-dependent* or *time-dependent* in their action. If concentration-dependent, one should administer a high enough dose to maximize the C_{MAX}:MIC ratio or AUC:MIC ratio. If time-dependent, the drug should be administered frequently enough to maximize the T > MIC. For some of these drugs the AUC/MIC also predicts clinical success.

Examples of how these relationships affect drug regimens are described below.

Aminoglycosides

Aminoglycosides (e.g., gentamicin, or amikacin) are concentration-dependent bactericidal drugs, therefore the higher the drug concentration, the greater the bactericidal effect. An optimal bactericidal effect occurs if a high enough dose is administered to produce a peak plasma concentration of 8 to10 times the MIC. This can be accomplished by administering a single dose once daily. This regimen is at least as effective, and perhaps less nephrotoxic, than lower doses administered more frequently.[33] Our current regimens in small animals employ this strategy. The single daily dose is based on the drug's volume of distribution (calculated using the area method). A once-daily dose for gentamicin is 5 to 8 mg/kg for cats, and 10 to 14 mg/kg for dogs. An appropriate dose for amikacin is 10 to 15 mg/kg for cats and 15 to 30 mg/kg for dogs once daily. The efficacy of these regimens has not been tested for conditions encountered in veterinary medicine, but the relationships are supported by experimental evidence and clinical experience. These regimens assume some competency of the immune system. If the animal is immunocompromised, one may consider a more frequent interval for administration. In animals with decreased renal function, longer intervals may be considered.

Fluoroquinolones

For the fluoroquinolone antimicrobials, investigators have shown that either C_{MAX}:MIC ratio or the AUC:MIC ratio may predict clinical cure in studies of laboratory animals, and in a limited number human clinical studies.[32,34-36] The optimal value for these surrogate markers has not been determined for infections in dogs or cats, but values attained with clinically proven dosages agree with targets established in laboratory animals and people. These experiences have shown that a C_{MAX}:MIC of 8 to 10 or an AUC:MIC of greater than 100 to 125 has been associated with a cure. The study that associated an AUC:MIC of greater than 125 with a cure involved critically ill human patients, but for some clinical situations AUC:MIC ratios as low as 30 to 55 have been associated with a clinical cure.[35] This difference may also be organism specific. Gram-positive bacteria infection cures have been associated with AUC:MIC ratios of 35 to 50.

Because wild-type sensitive bacteria from small animals often have an MIC for fluoroquinolones in the range of 0.125 mg/mL, (± one dilution), the approved label doses of the currently available fluoroquinolones usually meets the goal of a C_{MAX}:MIC ratio or a AUC:MIC ratio in the range cited above.[37] To take advantage of the wide range of safe doses for fluoroquinolones, low doses have been administered to treat susceptible organisms with low MIC, such as *E. coli* or *Pasteurella*. But for bacteria with a higher MIC (for example, gram-positive cocci), a slightly larger dose can be used. To achieve the necessary peak concentration for a bacterium such as *Pseudomonas aeruginosa*, which usually has the highest MIC among susceptible bacteria, the highest dose within a safe range is recommended. Bacteria such as streptococci and anaerobes are more resistant, and even at high doses a sufficient peak concentration or AUC:MIC ratio will be difficult to achieve.

β-Lactam Antibiotics

β-lactam antibiotics such as penicillins, potentiated-aminopenicillins, and cephalosporins are slowly bactericidal. Their concentration should be kept above the MIC throughout as much of the dosing interval as possible (long T>MIC) for the optimal bactericidal effect.[38] The time above MIC should exceed at least 30% to 50% of the dosing interval.

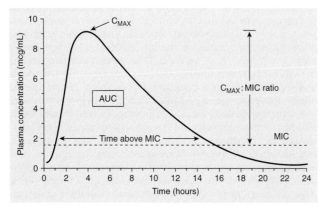

Figure 154-1 Plasma concentration versus time profile illustrating the principal pharmacokinetic-pharmacodynamic relationships for antimicrobial therapy. *AUC*, Area-under-the-curve; *MIC*, minimum inhibitory concentration.

Dosage regimens for the β-lactam antibiotics should consider these pharmacodynamic relationships. Therefore, for treating a gram-negative infection, especially a serious one, some regimens for penicillins and cephalosporins require administration 3 to 4 times per day. Some long-acting formulations have been developed to prolong plasma concentrations, and there are third-generation cephalosporins with long half-lives, and less frequent regimens have been used for some of these drugs (e.g., cefovecin, cefpodoxime proxetil, cefotaxime, and ceftiofur). (However, the long half-life for ceftriaxone in people does not occur in animals because of differences in drug protein binding.) Gram-positive organisms are more susceptible to the β-lactams than are gram-negative bacteria, and lower doses and longer intervals are possible when treating these bacteria. Additionally, because antibacterial effects occur at concentrations below the MIC (postantibiotic effect or PAE) for *Staphylococcus*, longer dose intervals may be possible for staphylococcal infections. For example, cephalexin or amoxicillin-clavulanate has been used successfully to treat staphylococcal infections when administered only once daily (although twice-daily administration is recommended to obtain maximum response). Cefpodoxime proxetil (Simplicef) is effective for once-daily administration, which is due to both high activity (low MIC values) and a longer half-life compared to other cephalosporins. Cefovecin (Convenia) has high protein binding in dogs and cats (approximately 99% or higher), and a half-life of 5 to 6 days. Because of this, cefovecin can be administered with a 14-day dosing interval and achieve cures for infections caused by susceptible bacteria in dogs and cats.

Other Time-Dependent Drugs

The drugs such as tetracyclines, macrolides (erythromycin and derivatives), sulfonamides, lincosamides (lincomycin and clindamycin), and chloramphenicol derivatives act in a time-dependent manner against most bacteria. Either time above MIC (T>MIC) or total drug exposure, measured as AUC/MIC, has been used to predict clinical success for these drugs.

The time-dependent activity is demonstrated by studies in which effectiveness is highest when the drug concentrations are maintained above the MIC throughout the dosing interval. Drugs in this group should be administered frequently to achieve this goal. However, a property of some is that they persist in tissues for a prolonged time, which allows infrequent dosing intervals. The macrolide derivative azithromycin (Zithromax) has shown tissue half-lives as long as 70 to 90 hours in cats and dogs, permitting infrequent dosing. Tissue concentrations of trimethoprim-sulfonamides persist long enough to allow once-daily dosing for many infections. Most published dosage regimens are designed to take the pharmacokinetic properties of these drugs into account.

EMPIRICAL TREATMENT BASED ON TISSUE SITE

Initiating antibiotic therapy often must be done before diagnostic microbiology information is available. Subsequently, treatment is often empirical—based on the clinician's best judgment and experience. To provide the patient with the best chance for a successful outcome, some knowledge is needed about the most likely pathogen, the susceptibility of the pathogen, and what drugs are the most practical for each type of infection. The drug choice should be based on the bacterial susceptibility, site of infection, and pharmacokinetic-pharmacodynamic properties of the drug.

Table 154-1 contains a list that includes some (but not all) possible choices for common infections encountered in veterinary medicine. In this list the "first choice" is a drug with a high likelihood of success, low expense, and few risks. If the

first choice has not been effective or if patient factors preclude using the first choice (e.g., allergy), the alternate choice should be considered.

Skin/Soft Tissue Infection

Many licensed small animal drugs are registered for skin infections. *Skin infections*, as listed in the product registration, do not always include pyoderma. However, many of these drugs, especially those registered more recently, are also active against the staphylococci that cause pyoderma. The drugs that have been shown to be effective for skin infections, based on the product's registration, available FOI data, or published studies, include: amoxicillin-clavulanate (Clavamox), cefadroxil (Cefa-Tabs, Cefa-Drops), cephalexin (generic), cefpodoxime proxetil (Simplicef), cefovecin (Convenia), clindamycin (Antirobe), trimethoprim-sulfadiazine (Tribrissen, Di-Trim), ormetoprim-sulfadimethoxine (Primor), and fluoroquinolones (enrofloxacin [Baytril], marbofloxacin [Zeniquin], orbifloxacin [Orbax], difloxacin [Dicural]). Treatment of more resistant infections was discussed earlier in this chapter.

Urinary Tract Infection

The most common bacteria encountered in canine urinary tract infections are *Escherichia coli*, and *Staphylococcus* spp. Other bacteria possible are *Streptococcus* spp., *Proteus mirabilis*, *Pseudomonas aeruginosa*, *Klebsiella*, *Enterobacter* spp., and *Enterococcus* spp. Primary urinary tract infections are rare in cats. However, infections may be more common in cats with other problems (for example, diabetes mellitus and chronic renal disease) and can be a complication of feline lower urinary tract disease. When infections occur, most are caused by staphylococci, streptococci, *E. coli*, *Proteus* spp., *Klebsiella* spp., *Enterobacter* spp., or *Pseudomonas* spp.

High antibiotic concentrations achieved in renal tubules and the urine after routine therapy. Therefore modest doses of antibiotics are often sufficient to cure lower urinary tract infections, even those that are caused by organisms identified on a susceptibility test as "intermediate" in sensitivity.[22,39] In animals that can concentrate their urine, urine concentrations of antibiotics are at least 100× the corresponding plasma concentrations because of the tubular concentration. When the infection is confined to the lower urinary tract, these high concentrations are an advantage.[40] Cures of urinary tract infections are possible, even when the antibiotic levels do not attain concentrations high enough for a systemic infection. However, clinicians should be aware that if the concentrating ability of the kidneys is compromised, antibiotic concentrations in the urine may be low. Patients may have dilute urine because of renal disease or treatment with corticosteroids, fluid therapy, or diuretics.

When the renal tissue is involved, high urine drug concentrations offer no advantage. Drug concentrations in renal tissue—which are equivalent to the renal lymph concentrations—are correlated to plasma drug concentrations, not the drug concentrations in the urine. Therefore, consideration must be given to drugs that attain high concentrations in the renal tissue and that can be administered at doses and intervals that are optimal to achieve the PK-PD relationships for a clinical cure.

The best empirical choices are drugs that are excreted by renal mechanisms in an active form and are broad spectrum to allow for the possibility of either gram-positive or gram-negative bacteria. Initial selection can be improved with a urinalysis, examination of urine sediment, a culture, and quantitation of the bacteria in the urine. Prior to culture results, empirical selection can be made with the following list of drugs (not necessarily in order of priority): amoxicillin, amoxicillin-clavulanate (Clavamox), first-generation cephalosporin, and trimethoprim-sulfonamide.

Table • 154-1

Empirical Antibacterial Drug Choices

INFECTION SITE	FIRST-CHOICE DRUGS	ALTERNATE-CHOICE DRUGS
Skin: pyoderma or other skin infection	Amoxicillin-clavulanate Cephalosporin*	Trimethoprim-sulfonamides Macrolide (erythromycin, azithromycin) Fluoroquinolone† Clindamycin Chloramphenicol
Urinary tract	Cephalosporin* Amoxicillin/Ampicillin Amoxicillin-clavulanate	Trimethoprim-sulfonamides, or ormetoprim-sulfadimethoxine Fluoroquinolone† Tetracycline‡
Respiratory tract	Amoxicillin-clavulanate Fluoroquinolone Cephalosporin*	Macrolide (erythromycin, azithromycin) Aminoglycosides (amikacin, gentamicin) Clindamycin Chloramphenicol Trimethoprim-sulfonamide (for some organisms) Extended-spectrum cephalosporin§ Carbapenems (for resistant infections)‖
Septicemia	Amoxicillin-clavulanate Cephalosporin* Fluoroquinolone†	Aminoglycoside (amikacin, gentamicin) Extended-spectrum cephalosporin§ Carbapenems (for resistant infections)‖
Bone and joint	Cephalosporins* Amoxicillin-clavulanate	Trimethoprim-sulfonamides Clindamycin Extended-spectrum cephalosporins§ Fluoroquinolones†

*Cephalosporins = cefazolin (injectable), cephalexin, cefpodoxime, or cefovecin.
†Fluoroquinolone = enrofloxacin, difloxacin, marbofloxacin, or orbifloxacin.
‡Tetracycline = oxytetracycline, tetracycline, doxycycline, or minocycline.
§Extended-spectrum cephalosporin = second- or third-generation drugs (e.g., cefotetan, cefotaxime, ceftazidime).
‖Carbapenems = imipenem or meropenem.

If a gram-negative bacilli is suspected as the cause of the infection and resistance to other drugs is a possibility, a fluoroquinolone cefovecin or cefpodoxime proxetil can also be considered.[14,41] If treatment has been refractory, some are resistant to fluoroquinolones. Treatment of resistant strains of *E. coli* and other bacteria was discussed previously in this chapter.

When treating urinary tract infections, rule out complicating factors such as cystic calculi, metabolic disorders such as diabetes mellitus or hyperadrenocorticism, and renal or prostate involvement. If the patient is an intact male dog, the prostate may be involved and a drug should be selected that will penetrate the prostate. Appropriate drugs are trimethoprim-sulfonamides or a fluoroquinolone.

Respiratory Infections

Upper and lower respiratory tract infections are common indications for empirical antibiotic therapy in animals. Upper respiratory infections are often self-limiting and will resolve without antibiotics However, many upper and lower respiratory infections are secondary, and the result of a more serious disease (e.g., megaesophagus), immunosuppression (e.g., cancer), or foreign body (nasal cavity infection).

Bacteria cultured from animals with respiratory tract infections include *Bordetella bronchiseptica, Streptococcus zooepidemicus, Escherichia coli, Pseudomonas aeruginosa, Klebsiella pneumoniae, Staphylococcus* spp., alpha- and beta-streptococci, and *Pasteurella multocida. Mycoplasma* may play a role in some infections, but its importance has been controversial. In cats, upper respiratory infections are most likely secondary to a viral infection, but organisms such as *Mycoplasma, Chlamy-dia, Pasteurella,* and *Bordetella bronchiseptica* may play a role.

Initial therapy for bacteria that cause respiratory infections may include: amoxicillin-clavulanate (Clavamox), cephalosporins, clindamycin (Antirobe), fluoroquinolones (enrofloxacin, marbofloxacin, orbifloxacin, or difloxacin), and chloramphenicol. For infections known to be caused by gram-positive bacteria or *Mycoplasma,* azithromycin can be considered. The choice of a first-generation cephalosporin versus a third- or fourth-generation cephalosporin depends on the possibility that the infection is caused by gram-negative bacteria with a high likelihood of resistance. If the infection is believed to be caused by a gram-negative bacteria (e.g., *E. coli, Klebsiella*) a third-generation cephalosporin, carbapenem (imipenem, meropenem), or aminoglycoside rather than a lower class should be considered.

In addition to the drugs listed, additional considerations are important in a patient with aspiration pneumonia or pyothorax that may be caused by anaerobic bacteria. In those cases consider metronidazole or clindamycin.

Because some of the organisms causing respiratory infections can become resistant, culture and sensitivity testing from respiratory secretions can be done from a transtracheal wash (TTW) or bronchoalveolar lavage (BAL). However, experienced clinicians realize that the results of a TTW or BAL may not always represent the bacterial pathogen causing disease deeper in the lung. Cultures from nasal secretions probably are not very representative of infection deeper in the airways. In situations in which sensitivity tests are not available, one study showed that most organisms cultured from the respiratory tract were sensitive to amikacin, enrofloxacin, a third-generation cephalosporin, and gentamicin. However, in vitro results may not always correlate with in vivo efficacy.

Treatment of infections of the airways is limited by penetration of the drug across the blood-bronchus barrier. Nonfenestrated capillaries of the alveoli may prevent drug diffusion from the plasma to epithelial lining fluid of alveoli.[42] This could potentially compromise treatment of pneumonia, but usually there is so much inflammation in the lungs of a patient with pneumonia that adequate drug concentrations leak into the epithelial lining fluid. Drugs such as macrolides (erythromycin, azithromycin), tetracyclines, and fluoroquinolones appear to achieve adequate concentrations in epithelial lining fluid.

Bordetella bronchiseptica presents a special case. *Bordetella* is a gram-negative nonfermentng bacilli (coccobacilli). Among its important virulence factors is the ability to adhere to the bronchial epithelium (ciliated epithelial cells) and produce exotoxins that inhibit neutrophil migration to the infection site. Infections are often mild and self-limiting and require no specific antibiotic treatment. When antibiotics are indicated, one should select a drug that achieves concentrations in bronchial secretions. Susceptibility tests are not standardized as well as they are for other organisms, and susceptibility results have varied. Drugs that often are active against *B. bronchiseptica* include aminoglycosides (gentamicin, tobramycin, and amikacin, some penicillins [ticarcillin], some of the extended-spectrum cephalosporins, chloramphenicol, and the tetracyclines). This organism is usually resistant to the macrolides (e.g., erythromycin, azithromycin). Despite their in vitro activity, aminoglycosides, cephalosporins, and penicillins may not achieve drug concentrations at the infection site and quinolones are not consistently active against this organism. Another treatment route that is considered is aerosolization of antibiotics (e.g., tobramycin).

Intracellular Infections, Flea- and Tick-Transmitted Infections

Since most bacterial infections are located extracellularly, it is sufficient for a cure to achieve adequate drug concentrations in the extracellular (interstitial) space rather than intracellular space. However, intracellular infections present another problem. Only lipid-soluble drugs are able to reach high concentrations in cells. Intracellular organisms such as *Brucella*, *Rhodococcus equi*, *Chlamydia*, *Rickettsia*, *Ehrlichia*, *Bartonella*, and *Mycobacteria* are examples of intracellular pathogens that may not respond to drugs that fail to penetrate cells. Staphylococci may, in some cases, become refractory to treatment because of intracellular survival.

Examples of drugs that accumulate in leukocytes, fibroblasts, macrophages, and other cells are fluoroquinolones (enrofloxacin, ciprofloxacin, difloxacin, marbofloxacin, and orbifloxacin), lincosamides (clindamycin, lincomycin), macrolides (erythromycin, clarithromycin), the azalides (azithromycin), and rifampin.[43] β-lactam antibiotics and aminoglycosides do not reach effective concentrations within cells.

Tetracyclines (e.g., doxycycline) and fluoroquinolones are often used to treat *Chlamydia*, *Ehrlichia*, *Bartonella*, *Mycoplasma hemofelis*, and *Rickettsia* infections because of their ability to kill intracellular organisms.

Sepsis and Fever

Often the only sign of a potential infection is fever. If there also is evidence that the patient is immunosuppressed, antibiotic therapy is justified. Immunosuppression may be attributed to neutropenia, corticosteroid administration, hyperadrenocorticism (Cushing's disease), or anticancer treatment. In these instances, it is not unusual to fail to identify a bacterial cause. Blood cultures are often recommended, but may be unrewarding, or the result of a blood culture may not be available for 2 to 3 days or longer. In these cases, one should select a drug protocol that gives maximum coverage with minimal risk of adverse effect.

Oral Drugs For patients that can be treated with oral drugs, a combination of a fluoroquinolone (enrofloxacin, difloxacin, marbofloxacin, orbifloxacin, or ciprofloxacin) plus a potentiated amoxicillin (Clavamox) or an oral cephalosporin (cephalexin, cefadroxil, or cefpodoxime proxetil) is a rational choice. This combination is safe and may be as efficacious as injectable drugs. However, if a patient is severely ill, do not rely on oral drug absorption alone and treatment should be initiated with an injectable regimen (see below). If oral therapy is used, the most common adverse effects from these combinations are those that affect the gastrointestinal system (nausea, vomiting, diarrhea).

Injectable Drugs If the patient is more critically ill, or if the infection becomes more life threatening, injectable drugs should be considered. In these cases, injectable enrofloxacin plus a cephalosporin (cefazolin), or potentiated ampicillin (Unasyn) is a rational choice, or, the combination of an aminoglycoside plus a cephalosporin or potentiated ampicillin. Although it is rare, if there is a possibility that the organism may be a *Pseudomonas*, ceftazidime and/or amikacin is recommended. If the organism has been refractory to therapy, resistance is possible because of infection caused by *Escherichia coli*, *Klebsiella*, or another gram-negative bacillus. In these situations, the administration of drugs with greatest activity should be considered. Rather than rely on *first line* drugs (listed above), these refractory cases should be treated with more active drugs. These include injectable drugs such as cefotaxime, ceftazidime, amikacin or possibly a carbapenem (imipenem-cilastatin, or meropenem).

REFERENCES

The reference list can be found on the companion Expert Consult Web site at *www.expertconsult.com*.

CHAPTER 155

Antifungal Drug Therapy

Dawn M. Boothe

Successful treatment of fungal disorders is facilitated by understanding the complexities of infection, particularly as they differ from bacterial infections. Pathogenic fungi generally are characterized by low invasiveness and virulence. Factors predisposing to infection include necrotic tissue, a moist environment, and an immunosuppressed host. Immunosuppression may benefit from the immunomodulatory actions exhibited by many antifungal drugs; newer therapies will likely include combinations of immunomodulatory drugs with antifungal drugs.[1] Successful therapy also is complicated by the generally fungistatic rather than fungicidal actions of drugs, particularly at concentrations achieved at infection sites. Barriers to drug penetration presented by the microbe include external coatings, encapsulating slime layers, or chitin of the cell wall. Host barriers, depending on the site and inflammatory response, may also limit tissue penetrability. Culture and susceptibility testing is not as helpful to antifungal as it is to antibacterial therapy, in part because acquired resistance is not common and techniques have not been well standardized. Testing focuses on resistance rather than susceptibility.[2] Inherent resistance by fungal organisms to antimicrobial drugs is common, limiting the spectrum of drugs. Target structure similarities between eukaryotic host and cell increases the risk of toxicity, often preventing dose increases that might otherwise enhance efficacy and decrease emerging resistance. Alternate delivery systems (e.g., lipid-based amphotericin B preparations) and combination therapy are two approaches by which therapeutic success might be enhanced.[3] The tendency to discontinue therapy as clinical signs resolve also contributes to therapeutic failure. In generally, antifungal therapy should extend well beyond clinical cure.

AMPHOTERICIN B

Amphotericin B remains one of the most effective antifungal drugs for treatment of systemic infections. It is a natural macrolide antibiotic secreted by *Streptomyces*. The complex molecule contains both lipid and water-soluble components. Amphotericin binds to cell membrane ergosterol, forming channels that alter K^+/H^+ exchange, increase loss of K^+, Mg^{2+}, and critical organic molecules, and disrupt cell metabolism (Figure 155-1).

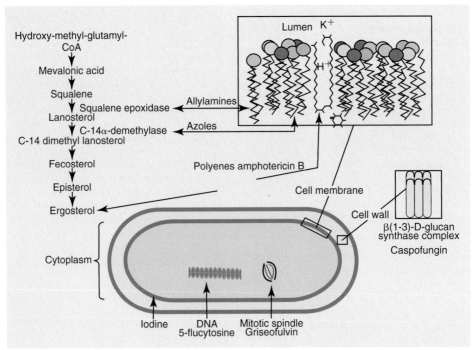

Figure 155-1 Mechanism of action of antifungal drugs. Most clinically relevant antifungals target cell wall ergosterol through different mechanisms. Amphotericin B binds to it, creating channels in the cell membrane. Azoles impair ergosterol synthesis by targeting lanosterol C-14α-demethylase while allylamines (e.g., terbinafine) inhibit squalene epoxidase. Drugs or drug classes that do not target ergosterol include 5-flucytosine, which impairs DNA synthesis upon its intracellular conversion to 5-fluouracil; griseofulvin, which impairs formation of the mitotic spindle; and caspofungin, an echinocandin that targets β-D-glucan synthesis in the fungal cell wall. Iodine may precipitate cellular proteins. (From Boothe DM: Small animal clinical pharmacology and therapeutics, in press.)

Although largely fungistatic, amphotericin B can be fungicidal at high concentrations. Amphotericin B appears to enhance both humoral and cell-mediated immunity as well as white blood cell (WBC) activity.[1] Its spectrum includes systemic dimorphic fungal infections (histoplasmosis, blastomycosis, cryptococcosis, and coccidioidomycosis) and disseminated sporotrichosis, phycomycosis (pythiosis, zygomycosis), aspergillosis, and candidiasis. Resistance is low. The disposition of amphotericin B has not been reported in dogs or cats and must be assumed from other species. It is not orally bioavailable, requiring parenteral (including local) administration. Binding to host cholesterol complicates kinetics. The half-life is long, with detectable drug in both bile and urine for up to 7 weeks in human patients. Based on other species, approximately 70% of drug in plasma can be anticipated to reach pleura, peritoneum, inflamed tissues, cerebrospinal fluid (CSF), and aqueous humor. Lipid-based amphotericin B preparations are preferentially distributed (in part by uptake by reticuloendothelial cells) to infection sites, thus decreasing exposure to kidneys and subsequent nephrotoxicity.[4] Preparations include a suspension of large lipid "ribbons" (ABLC: Abelcet), a colloidal preparation consisting of smaller cholesterol sulfate discs (ABCD: Amphotec), and a product comprised of even smaller liposomes (AmBisome).

Insoluble in water and unstable as a solution, amphotericin B rapidly decomposes with exposure to sunlight. It should be protected from light during storage but not necessarily during administration if it lasts less than 24 hours. Conventional (nonlipid) amphotericin B is prepared for injection as a lyophilized cake stabilized with the bile acid desoxycholate. A topical preparation (Fungizone) is also available in cream, lotion, and ointment forms. The injectable product should be reconstituted only with sterile water and diluted further only with 5% dextrose. When reconstituted according to label and refrigerated, it should remain stable for 1 week. Dilution with normal saline reduces strength by close to 45% within 2 hours. Reconstituted drug also can be divided and frozen. Amphotericin B should not be mixed with any other drug because of potential incompatibilities. Amphotericin B therapy is limited by renal toxicity, which is proportional to the total cumulative dose.[5] Intense renal arterial vasoconstriction occurs within 15 minutes of administration, may last 4 to 6 hours, and can be reduced by administration of sodium-containing fluids prior to treatment. However, fluid therapy may not be necessary for lipid-based products. Binding to distal renal tubular membrane cholesterol (see Figure 155-1) alters cell permeability, causing renal tubular acidosis, hypokalemia, and concentrating defects (polyuria/polydipsia). Potassium supplementation may be necessary. Administration as a "cocktail" containing 5% dextrose and mannitol (0.5 mg/kg) may decrease renal tubular swelling and increase renal blood flow. However, this approach is controversial and is based largely on anecdotal rather than evidential support.[5] Likewise, although sodium bicarbonate (1 to 2 mg/kg) theoretically may reduce tubular acidification, it should not be administered in the same fluid with amphotericin B. The risk of nephrotoxicity is substantially less for lipid-based preparations, and particularly liposomes. In humans, lipid preparations are indicated in lieu of conventional therapy in patients with renal insufficiency, hypomagnesia, hypokalemia, tubular acidosis, or polyuria.[5] Local deliveries that might decrease nephrotoxicity include subconjunctival (concentrations greater than 20 mg/mL are irritating), intravitreal, intrathecal (0.2 to 0.5 mg in either 5 mL of CSF or 10% dextrose two to three times per week), intranasal intraperitoneal, intravesicular (50 mg/mL infused into the bladder), or gastrointestinal. Subcutaneous administration (0.5 to 0.8 mg/kg diluted in 400 to 500 mL of fluid) may also be effective, including lipid-based preparations.[6] Catabolic drugs increase the risk of nephrotoxicity.[6] Examples include glucocorticosteroids, antineoplastic drugs, and antiprostaglandins (glucocorticoids and nonsteroidal antiinflammatory drugs). Amphotericin B also is associated with acute anaphylactoid reactions, most commonly manifested as vomiting, fever, and chills. Less common are thrombophlebitis and cardiac arrhythmias. Anaphylactoid reactions are probably more common with lipid preparations, with reactions least severe for the liposomal preparation (AmBisome).

Amphotericin B dosing is complicated, variable, and largely anecdotal, with no single dosing regimen fitting all patients. Various protocols are intended to minimize toxicity. The safest is probably IV administration (0.25 to 1.0 mg/kg) through a catheter over 4 to 6 hours diluted with 300 to 1000 mL of 5% dextrose or constant rate infusion.[7] However, rapid intravenous (IV) administration of the dose diluted in 10 to 60 mL, with simultaneous or subsequent supplemental saline-based fluids (in a different catheter) may also be safe, particularly for lipid-based products. The suggested frequency ranges from daily (lower doses) to alternate days (higher doses). Dosing continues to a cumulative dose of 4 to 12 mg/kg in dogs, or 4 to 6 mg/kg in cats. The higher dose is targeted whenever possible, but particularly for blastomycosis and coccidioidomycosis. For lipid-based preparations, daily and cumulative doses may be as high as 15 to 30 mg/kg (12 to 24 mg/kg potentially for cats), particularly for the liposomal product. Urine sediment may be the most sensitive indicator of nephrotoxicity. However, increased serum urea nitrogen indicates the need to discontinue therapy for 24 to 48 hours. Anaphylaxis might be reduced by pretreatment with antihistamines and short-acting glucocorticosteroids and pretreatment with a small test dose (0.1 mg/kg for cats or 0.25 mg/kg for dogs diluted in 10 mL infused over 15 minutes).

Amphotericin B remains the most effective antifungal for major nondermatophyte fungal pathogens. Indications include systemic dimorphic fungal infections. Amphotericin B appears to act synergistically with 5-flucytosine against cryptococcosis, and tetracyclines against coccidioidomycosis and azoles.

AZOLE DERIVATIVES

Azole antifungals are synthetic and include the imidazoles (clotrimazole, econazole, enilconazole, miconazole and ketoconazole), which contain two nitrogen atoms, and the triazoles (itraconazole, fluconazole and voriconazole, a fluconazole derivative "second-generation" drug), which contain three. Azoles inhibit fungal cytochrome P450 enzyme sterol-14α-demethylase, thus blocking fungal ergosterol synthesis (see Figure 155-1).[8] A lag time to efficacy may occur, reflecting in part slow synthetic activities. Cell membrane permeability increases and toxic 14-methylsterols accumulate. Effects are generally fungistatic, although selected drugs act fungicidal (econazole, clotrimazole), particularly if they also target other intracellular processes. Azoles are characterized by potentially beneficial immunomodulatory effects.[1]

Azoles are broad-spectrum antifungals, targeting dermatophytes, yeasts, dimorphic fungi, and selected opportunistic organisms, including some *Phycomycetes*. The general order of efficacy, from least to best, is ketoconazole, fluconazole, itraconazole, with voriconazole being best for *Aspergillosis*, followed by itraconazole. However, activity of voriconazole toward dimorphic fungi is only fair to good.[9] Clotrimazole and miconazole are used topically to treat dermatophytes, yeast, or nasal aspergillosis. Resistance to the azoles is not common, with the exception of fluconazole and *Candida*.

Oral absorption of the azoles varies with the animal, drug, preparation, gastric pH, and presence of other drugs. Absorption of itraconazole (tablet, not solution) and ketoconazole is enhanced by gastric acidity, and may be deceased with antisecretory drugs. Oral bioavailability of itraconazole capsules approximates 20% in dogs and even less in cats, whereas the solution is approximately 50% bioavailable. Fluconazole is completely absorbed in cats. Many azoles act as substrates for P-glycoprotein drug efflux transporters, which will decrease absorption. Distribution to tissues varies, being in order from best to worst, fluconazole, itraconazole and ketoconazole. Fluconazole and itraconazole can achieve effective CSF concentrations for some organisms. Azoles are generally highly bound to proteins. In the skin, binding may contribute to concentrations that exceed plasma by threefold to tenfold. Drug appears to be slowly released into the skin over a 2- to 4-week period after therapy is discontinued. Fluconazole is principally (70%) renally excreted while other azoles are extensively metabolized by hepatic cytochrome P450 enzymes. Metabolism may be dose dependent, declining at higher doses and longer half-life. The decline may also reflect (self)-inhibition of drug-metabolizing enzymes. The half-life of the azoles varies being shortest for ketoconazole (1.4 hours in dogs), longer for fluconazole (25 hours in cats), and longest for itraconazole (51 hours in dogs and 40 to 70 hours in cats). Long half-lives prolong time to steady-state, contributing to a lag time to efficacy.

Ketoconazole, itraconazole, and fluconazole are available for oral administration. Azoles are not water soluble. Fluconazole and itraconazole are available as IV preparations, although solubilizing agents may contribute to adverse reactions with injections. Cats tolerate a single 5 mg/kg IV dose of itraconazole or a slow IV drip of fluconazole. Ketoconazole, clotrimazole and miconazole are available as topical preparations. Clotrimazole and enilconazole have been used to treat nasal aspergillosis. Enilconazole is available in the United States as a 13.8% poultry dip (use 1:50 in water) and, in Canada, as a 10% solution approved for use in dogs and horses.

Because the azoles interfere with ergosterol synthesis, rather than binding to it, host toxicities typical of amphotericin B do not occur. Gastrointestinal side effects (nausea, vomiting, diarrhea) might be reduced by administration with food. Hepatotoxicity has been reported for ketoconazole, itraconazole, and fluconazole, with the risk increased at higher doses. Drug eruptions consistent with erythema multiforme and idiopathic vasculitis have been reported with itraconazole; and thrombocytopenia and hypokalemia with fluconazole. In humans, voriconazole is associated with diverse ocular side effects that warrant review prior to use in dogs or cats.[9] Drug interactions are common for all azoles and may cause serious adverse events. The most clinically relevant are those involving inhibition of cytochrome P450 drug-metabolizing enzymes (CYP). As a class, all azoles inhibit CYP3A4, a major enzyme with broad substrate specificity. For the remaining isoenzymes, ketoconazole inhibits the most, followed by fluconazole and voriconazole, with itraconazole inhibiting the fewest isoenzymes. Interactions involving P-glycoprotein may occur and extra caution should be taken when used in breeds predisposed to P-glycoprotein deletion deficiencies (e.g., working breeds). Finally, the azoles are also subject to the influence of other drugs that induce or inhibit drug-metabolizing enzymes.[9] In addition to drug-metabolizing enzymes, ketoconazole inhibits lanosterol C-14α-demethylase (cholesterol synthesis) responsible for endogenous steroid metabolism. Ketoconazole is associated with a change (lighter) in hair color of some dogs, and decreases basal cortisol, testosterone, and progesterone but not aldosterone concentrations. ACTH cortisol response is also reduced. The azoles may interact synergistically with a number of antifungal agents. These include 5-flucytosine against Candida and Cryptococcus and amphotericin B against a variety of organisms. However, for the azoles, timing of amphotericin B and azole therapy is important because impaired ergosterol synthesis by azoles may decrease efficacy of amphotericin B.

Ketoconazole has been reported to be effective treatment of dermatophytosis, mucocutaneous candidiasis, blastomycosis, histoplasmosis, coccidioidomycosis, and cryptococcosis.[6] Higher doses are indicated for systemic cryptococcosis and coccidioidomycosis. However, ketoconazole should probably only be used in combination (e.g., amphotericin B), especially for treatment of canine blastomycosis. Ketoconazole also has proven effective for treatment of Malassezia dermatitis (topical or systemic) and candidiasis but has little efficacy (43%) against Aspergillosis spp. Itraconazole and fluconazole are more commonly used for treatment of susceptible systemic fungal infections. Itraconazole is indicated for treatment of systemic dimorphic fungal disease, sporotrichosis, aspergillosis (up to 70% effective), dermatophytosis, dermatophytic pseudomycetomas, phaeohyphomycosis, and cutaneous Alternaria. In general, efficacy of fluconazole is not as favorable as itraconazole, but has treated canine blastomycosis, cryptococcosis, and nasal aspergillosis successfully. Voriconazole is likely to have greatest efficacy for aspergillosis but has not yet been studied in dogs or cats.

GRISEOFULVIN

Griseofulvin is produced from a Penicillium. It binds, in an energy-dependent manner, to mitotic spindle microtubules, inhibiting cell mitosis and cytotransport. It may be fungistatic or fungicidal. Efficacy is limited to dermatophytes, including Microsporum trichophyton and epidermophyton.

Oral absorption varies with particle size and preparation. Oral bioavailability of the ultramicrosize (particle size 2.7 μm; e.g., Fulvicin, Gris-Peg) is at least 50% greater than that of the microsize; the latter is best administered with a fatty diet. Although griseofulvin penetrates the stratum corneum, effective concentrations in hair, skin, and nails occur only following 4 to 6 weeks of systemic administration, the time necessary for deposition in keratin precursor cells. Griseofulvin undergoes hepatic metabolism; the half-life reportedly is 24 hours in the dog, allowing once-daily administration. Side effects include nausea, vomiting, and diarrhea, which might be minimized by administration of the dose in divided increments with a meal. Hepatotoxicity has been reported. Idiosyncratic toxicity occurs in cats independent of dose and duration. Clinical signs include gastrointestinal, neurologic, or bone marrow disease. Signs may or may not be reversible, depending on the severity. Cats with feline immunodeficiency disorders may be more likely to develop neutropenia. Selected breeds (Persians, Siamese, and Abyssinians) may be more commonly affected. At very high doses, the drug is teratogenic and carcinogenic in animals and should not be used in the first two trimesters of pregnancy. It a potent inducer of microsomal enzymes. Use with a shampoo (miconazole or chlorhexidine) enhances efficacy. Because of accumulation in keratin, griseofulvin is the drug of choice for nail infections.

5-Flucytosine

5-Flucytosine (FLU; 5-fluorocytosine), must be converted intracellularly by susceptible fungal cells to 5-flurouracil, where it interferes with fungal DNA synthesis. Its use is limited to resistance, particularly in rapidly growing organisms (e.g., Candida, Cryptococcosus) and as such, it is used only in combination with other antifungal drugs. Its spectrum is limited to Cryptococcus, Candidiasis and some cladosporiosis, aspergillosis, chromomycosis, and sporotrichosis. As a water-soluble drug, oral absorption of FLU is rapid and close to complete. Protein binding is minimal, facilitating CSF concentrations that approximate up to 90% of that in plasma concentrations. Its half-life is 3 to 6 hours. It is renally cleared; doses should be modified as needed based on serum creatinine. Bone marrow and gastrointestinal toxicity and alopecic dermatitis (in dogs) may occur.

ALLYLAMINES

The allylamines (e.g., terbinafine and naftifine) and the much older thiocarbamates (e.g., tolnaftate) competitively inhibit squalene epoxidase, depleting ergosterol. They are fungicidal. Efficacy toward dermatophytes and superficial pathogens is better than griseofulvin, in part because they are avidly taken up in the epidermis. Increasing evidence suggests efficacy toward other organisms, including systemic infections, *Sporothrix schenckii*, and *Aspergillus* when used in combination with other antifungal drugs. Activity is poor toward *Candida*. Terbinafine is available in oral and topical preparations. A dose of 20 to 40 mg/kg once daily in cats appears to be well tolerated and effective toward *M. canis*.[10]

IODIDES

The antifungal mechanism of iodides is not known. They are rapidly and completely absorbed orally, distributed to extracellular fluid, and concentrated in the thyroid gland. Available as 20% Na and K^+ salts, they are given PO or IV. Indications include cutaneous or lymphocutaneous forms of sporotrichosis. Iodide toxicity is more common in cats and is manifested as sweating, tachycardia, dry, scaly coat, diarrhea, and polyuria/polydipsia. Cardiomyopathy has been reported in cats.

ECHINOCANDINS

Echinocandins are the first new antifungal drugs to be developed in the last 15 years, with caspofungin as the first of the drugs to be approved in the United States.[11] They are synthetic modifications of lipoproteins secreted by fungal organisms, including *Aspergillus*. Echinocandins inhibit synthesis of β-D-glucan (the major glucan in the cell wall of *Aspergillus*). Disruption of the fungal cell wall results in rapid fungicidal effects for some organisms.[11] Their spectrum of activity is limited, but includes *Candida* sp. and its approved target, *Aspergillus* sp. The large molecular weight of the echinocandins limits use to IV administration due to poor oral absorption. Drug does not distribute well into the urine or central nervous system. Use in dogs and cats has not been described.

REFERENCES

The reference list can be found on the companion Expert Consult Web site at *www.expertconsult.com.*

CHAPTER **156**

Over-the-Counter Human Medications

Butch KuKanich

Over-the-counter (OTC) human medications are readily available, affordable, and generally perceived as "safe" by clients, but serious adverse effects, including death, can occur even with appropriate dosages. The wide variety of OTC medications under the same brand name may be confusing to clients and can result in serious adverse effects if client communication is not specific. For example, the veterinarian may recommend for a client to administer ½ tablet of the brand name Benadryl (diphenhydramine 25 mg) to a cat, but the client may mistakenly think Benadryl Allergy & Cold (Diphenhydramine 12.5 mg, acetaminophen 325 mg, phenylephrine 5 mg) is the same medication. Acetaminophen toxicity would occur after a single dose of Benadryl Allergy & Cold as signs of acetaminophen toxicity can occur after a single dose as low as 20 mg/kg in cats.[1] Therefore it is important that recommendations for the use of OTC medications are specific and not open to interpretation.

ANALGESICS

Aspirin (acetylsalicylic acid, ASA) is available in plain, buffered, and enteric coated formulations. Enteric coated aspirin is more variably absorbed in dogs than other formulations and therefore not recommended for routine use.[2] Plain and buffered aspirin are more consistently absorbed; however, the buffering in buffered aspirin is insufficient to produce any gastric protectant effects. Aspirin is available in 81, 325, and 500 mg tablets; therefore, it is important that the correct tablet strength is administered. Dogs are typically administered aspirin 10 to 15 mg/kg q8-12h PO, which has been well tolerated in some dogs during chronic administration. The adverse effects of aspirin are similar to other nonsteroidal antiinflammatory drugs (NSAIDs), which can produce gastrointestinal (GI), renal, and hepatic toxicity as well as inhibition of platelet aggregation. The GI adverse effects of aspirin may be decreased by coadministration of omeprazole (1 mg/kg q24h PO) or misoprostol (2 to 5 µg/kg q12h PO). In cats, the low-dose aspirin (81 mg) is the preferred formula, typically administered as ½ tablet per cat every other day. Cats rapidly metabolize aspirin to salicylate, the active metabolite, but salicylate is slowly eliminated necessitating a prolonged dosing interval (10 mg/kg q48h PO). Aspirin should not be administered concurrently with other NSAIDs. The efficacy of aspirin as an antithrombotic in cats is poor. Methyl salicylate is also available OTC, of which the primary active component (salicylate) is the same as aspirin. Therefore, the same considerations for aspirin should be used for methyl salicylate, although it is not frequently used in veterinary medicine.

Acetaminophen appears to be well tolerated in dogs at clinically recommended doses (15 mg/kg q8h PO), but the efficacy is questionable due to its short half-life (~ 1.5 hours). Acetaminophen is contraindicated in cats and should never be administered.

Ibuprofen (Advil and others) and naproxen (Aleve and others) should not be administered to dogs or cats due to the high risk of adverse effects.

ANTIHISTAMINES (H1)

A wide variety of antihistamines are available in OTC formulations. Antihistamines have been used for a variety of indications including allergies, insect bites/stings, motion sickness, and sedation in animals.

Antihistamines are typically thought of as having minimal adverse effects, but many first-generation antihistamines (diphenhydramine, chlorpheniramine) also have anticholinergic effects that can produce varying degrees of urinary retention, increased intraocular pressure, xerostomia, and subsequent polyuria and polydipsia.[3]

Other adverse effects that have occurred with antihistamines include sedation, paradoxical excitement, nausea, anorexia, constipation, and diarrhea[3].

The efficacy of antihistamines remains questionable for many allergic conditions in animals.[4] The efficacy of chlorpheniramine, cetirizine, and clemastine for canine atopy is poor and may not produce a better response than a placebo.[4,5] Further studies on clemastine indicated the oral bioavailability in dogs is approximately 3%, supporting it is not effective.[6] The pharmacokinetics of cetirizine have not been reported in dogs; therefore, the optimal dose has not been determined. Cetirizine (1 mg/kg q24h PO) resulted in only 18% of atopic dogs showing clinical improvement. Cetirizine is an active metabolite of hydroxyzine, which inhibited histamine wheal/flare response for 18 to 24 hours after hydroxyzine administration.[7] Therefore, it remains unclear if the pharmacokinetics or dose of cetirizine resulted in the poor efficacy or if other factors are involved as hydroxyzine (2 to 2.5 mg/kg q8h PO) appears to provide better efficacy for the treatment of canine atopy (~ 66% improved) than cetirizine, although a head-to-head comparison has not been reported.[4] The pharmacokinetics of cetirizine in cats are favorable with 5 mg per cat (~ 1 mg/kg) maintaining targeted plasma drug concentrations for 24 hours.[8] Diphenhydramine (2.2 to 2.5 mg/kg q8h PO) was the only OTC antihistamine that appeared to produce a favorable response in atopic dogs with 65% of animals showing improved clinical signs.[4] However, it is unclear if the currently recommended dose and interval of diphenhydramine are optimal, as no pharmacokinetic studies have been reported in dogs or cats. The pharmacokinetics or efficacy of orally administered loratadine have not been described in dogs or cats; therefore, any dosing recommendations are anecdotal.

ANTIDIARRHEALS

Loperamide (Imodium and others) (0.1 mg/kg q8-12h PO) is a highly efficacious opioid antidiarrheal that increases nonpropulsive rhythmic contractions of the GI tract and decreases GI secretions. In most animals loperamide is well tolerated with minimal adverse effects. Typical opioid effects (e.g., sedation, bradycardia, dysphoria) are not observed in loperamide-treated animals unless the animal has decreased functional P-glycoprotein efflux pumps such as P-glycoprotein–deficient Collies (or other breeds), or potentially animals treated with ketoconazole.[9] P-glycoprotein–deficient dogs suffer from typical opioid adverse effects for up to 24 hours after administration of the clinically recommended dose, which can be reversed with an opioid antagonist such as naloxone.

Bismuth subsalicylate (Pepto-Bismol and others) is an antidiarrheal with an undetermined mechanism of action.

Salicylate is absorbed systemically after administration; therefore, bismuth subsalicylate should not be used to animals on NSAIDs. The liquid formula contains 8.7 mg salicylate per mL (regular strength) or 15.7 mg/mL (maximum strength), while the tablet contains 102 mg salicylate. Bismuth subsalicylate will cause the feces to turn dark to black independent of GI bleeding. Doses should be repeated cautiously in cats as they eliminate salicylate slowly.

LAXATIVES, CATHARTICS, AND ENEMAS

A variety of choices are available for the treatment or prevention of constipation or obstipation in dogs and cats. Lubricant laxatives containing petrolatum or mineral oil are widely available and are labeled for use in cats, but can also be used in dogs. Direct oral administration of mineral oil is best avoided due to the risk of aspiration and pneumonia. Lubricant laxatives coat the surface of the feces to both lubricate the feces and retain fluid. Stimulant laxatives are rapidly acting and may produce effects by direct irritation of the intestines or by inhibiting glucose absorption and sodium-potassium pump (Na$^+$/K$^+$ ATPase). Senna (Senokot and others) and bisacodyl (Correctol and others) are both available OTC, but the precise dosing and efficacy has not been described in dogs or cats. Bulk laxatives are hydrophilic colloids, which attract fluid and mechanically distend the bowel and stimulate motility. A variety of formulations such as psyllium fiber laxatives (Metamucil and others) and calcium polycarbophil (Fibercon) are available. Stool softeners such as docusate sodium (Colace and others) are anionic surfactants that lower the surface tension in the feces resulting in increased fluid and fat content in the feces. Osmotic cathartics such as polyethylene glycol solution (Miralax), magnesium sulfate (Phillips' Milk of Magnesia) and magnesium sulfate (Epsom salts) are available OTC. Osmotic cathartics contain nonabsorbed or poorly absorbed ingredients that increase fluid content in the bowel by creating osmotic gradients. Some magnesium from the magnesium cathartics can be absorbed systemically and should be avoided in animals with or prone to hypermagnesemia, such as animals in renal failure, and can decrease the absorption of some drugs such as ciprofloxacin. Other adverse effects of the laxatives and cathartics can include fluid and electrolyte loss and dehydration, abdominal cramping, gas, and diarrhea. Laxatives containing phenolphthalein are no longer available in the United States due to safety concerns. Phosphate enemas (Fleet Saline Enema) and others should be avoided in dogs and cats due to the potential for phosphate absorption and toxicity. Mineral oil enemas (Fleet Mineral Oil Enema and others) are available OTC without the toxic potential of phosphate (saline) enemas.

ANTIEMETICS

The most common OTC antiemetics are antihistamines, used for motion sickness, primarily in dogs. Diphenhydramine (Benadryl and others) is often recommended for the treatment of motion sickness in dogs due to its availability and safety. Dimenhydrinate (Dramamine and others) is an antiemetic that contains approximately 54% diphenhydramine and 46% 8-chlorotheophylline. Dimenhydrinate is rapidly converted to diphenhydramine after oral administration in dogs, which is primarily responsible for its antiemetic effects. The 8-chlorotheophylline component may decrease drowsiness associated with diphenhydramine. The antiemetic efficacy of dimenhydrinate (dogs, 4 to 8 mg/kg q8h PO; cats, 12.5 mg per cat) or diphenhydramine (2.2 to 4 mg/kg q8h PO) for motion sickness has not been evaluated in dogs or cats. The bioavailability of oral meclizine in dogs is 22% with a 5.5-hour half-life; however, its efficacy against motion sickness in dogs has not been reported.[10] In humans, meclizine is less effective than dimenhydrinate at controlling motion sickness.[11] The pharmacokinetics or efficacy of cyclizine has not been reported in dogs, but cyclizine is less effective than dimenhydrinate in humans.[11]

Bismuth subsalicylate has antiemetic effects, but the dose required is high. Bismuth subsalicylate produced antiemetic effects in ipecac-treated dogs with 44 mg/kg producing an effective dose in 50% of the dogs, whereas 175 mg/kg was an effective dose in 90% of dogs.[12] The currently recommended dose of bismuth subsalicylate in dogs 4.4 mg/kg (10 times less than the dose providing antiemetic effects). It is important to note that the antiemetic dose (44 mg/kg) provides 22 mg/kg of salicylate (aspirin active metabolite), which may exacerbate the underlying condition; therefore, the antiemetic dose (44 mg/kg) is not recommended for use in dogs or cats.

EMETICS

Hydrogen peroxide is the OTC emetic of choice (0.25 to 0.5 mL/kg repeated if needed once at 5 to 15 minutes). Syrup of ipecac is no longer routinely available OTC due to its poor efficacy in eliminating the toxin, not as an emetic. Other emetics such as large doses of salt are not recommended due to the potential for toxicity. Emesis should not be initiated if a caustic (i.e., acid or base) substance is suspected, the animal is depressed or becoming unconscious, a CNS stimulant has been ingested and seizures are possible, or the substance is petroleum based.

ANTITUSSIVES

The most common OTC antitussive drugs are a combination of dextromethorphan with a variety of other drugs, which may include acetaminophen, an antihistamine, pseudoephedrine, phenylephrine, or guaifenesin. The efficacy of dextromethorphan as an antitussive has been questioned recently with a study in children indicating it was no more effective than a placebo.[13] The bioavailability of dextromethorphan is variable in humans, but an active metabolite, dextrorphan, is produced in high concentrations, which may be responsible for some of the pharmacologic effect in humans.[14] The efficacy of oral dextromethorphan has not been studied in dogs or cats. Pharmacokinetic data in dogs indicate dextromethorphan has a poor and variable bioavailability and the active metabolite is not produced in measurable concentrations, which questions the efficacy of oral dextromethorphan in dogs.[15]

GASTRIC ACID REDUCERS

A variety of drugs are available OTC that will reduce the acidity (increase pH) within the stomach and proximal duodenum. Antacids bind with hydrochloric acid to produce neutral salts and water. Calcium carbonate (Tums and others) (100 mg/kg per day, divided and administered with meals) is widely available, but has a short duration of action. Aluminum hydroxide and magnesium carbonate (Gaviscon and others) (10 to 20 mg/kg q8h PO, based on aluminum hydroxide content) is also widely available, but is also a short-acting antacid. Both antacids will bind dietary phosphate and can be useful in conditions of hyperphosphatemia, such as renal failure. Calcium-containing drugs may result in hypercalcemia with chronic administration to animals with decreased renal function, whereas magnesium-containing drugs may result in hypermagnesemia.[16] Antacids may reduce the absorption of fluoroquinolones, tetracycline, ketoconazole, iron supplements (calcium antacids only), and captopril, which may result in decreased drug efficacy.[17]

Famotidine (Pepcid AC and others), ranitidine (Zantac 75 and others), and cimetidine (Tagamet HB and others) are histamine H_2 receptor antagonists available as OTC products that inhibit acid secretion. Famotidine is often the H_2 antagonist recommended due to its safety, apparent efficacy, lack of adverse effects, and cost-effectiveness. Famotidine has a large safety profile with doses as high as 2000 mg/kg q24h PO producing minimal adverse effects in dogs (Pepcid Product Monograph). Famotidine (1 mg/kg q24h PO) appears to be more effective than ranitidine and cimetidine in dogs at reducing acid secretion and was also effective in decreasing the severity, but not the occurrence, of gastritis in sled dogs.[18-20] Famotidine (0.5 mg/kg q24h PO) is also recommended for use in cats, but extensive studies on it effectiveness after oral administration are lacking. However, IV studies have demonstrated famotidine effectively decreased gastric acid production in cats.[21] Famotidine is available OTC as 10- and 20-mg tablets. Cimetidine inhibits some of the drug-metabolizing cytochrome P 450 (CYP) microsomal enzymes and therefore has a greater potential of drug-drug interactions compared to ranitidine and famotidine. Additionally, cimetidine needs to be administered two to three times daily and therefore is not routinely recommended. Although studies have demonstrated ranitidine has GI prokinetic effects, clinical benefits of the enhanced motility have not been demonstrated, and with the potential of ranitidine being less effective in dogs at acid suppression, it is not routinely recommended. The extent of absorption of ketoconazole and itraconazole can be significantly decreased when coadministered with an H_2 antagonist.

Omeprazole (Prilosec OTC and others) is a H^+/K^+ ATPase inhibitor, also known as a proton pump inhibitor (PPI). The proton pump inhibitors provide the most effective reduction of gastric acid secretion in humans, dogs, and cats.[19,22] Omeprazole (OTC) is available in 20-mg tablets that contain a special coating to delay the release of the drug until is leaves the stomach, as omeprazole is unstable in acid. Therefore, tablet cutting or crushing results in drug degradation in the stomach and a resultant decrease in drug absorption, by up to 50%, and efficacy compared to intact capsules/tablets.[23] However, with multiple doses, and subsequently decreased stomach acidity, the amount of drug absorption may increase. The recommended dosage is 1 mg/kg q24h PO for cats and dogs. A study on the efficacy of omeprazole in sled dogs resulted in a greater than expected number of treated dogs developing diarrhea.[24] Clinically important drug interactions can occur with any drug decreasing gastric acidity. The most clinically recognized interaction is the decreased absorption of the antifungal drugs ketoconazole and itraconazole that can occur with any acid suppression therapy.[25]

TOPICAL DRUG THERAPY

The efficacy of many topical treatments in animals has not been extensively investigated. Drawbacks to topical therapy include the animal ingesting the topical medication, which will decrease efficacy but typically will not pose a serious toxicologic problem. Ointments and creams will result in hair, dirt, carpet fibers, and other debris accumulating at the treatment site, which may result in delayed response or healing.

A variety of topical ointments and creams are available OTC. Hydrocortisone is a glucocorticoid applied topically for allergic skin disease. A variety of antibiotic ointments are available, which typically include neomycin, bacitracin, and polymyxin, that provide a broad antimicrobial spectrum including gram-positive and gram-negative bacteria such as *Pseudomonas* spp. Diphenhydramine is available as a topical preparation also and may provide some efficacy for localized allergic skin disease.

A large variety of topical antifungal products are available OTC, primarily marketed to treat athlete's foot or yeast infections in humans. Clotrimazole, miconazole, tolnaftate, terbinafine, and others can be used topically for the treatment of localized dermatophyte infections in animals.

Products containing a local anesthetic such as benzocaine are poorly effective and may result in toxicity in susceptible animals, primarily cats, and therefore should be avoided. The efficacy of zinc oxide for the treatment of irritated skin or as a sunscreen is probably poor in animals. The risk of toxicity from small amounts of topically applied zinc oxide is minimal, but zinc toxicity has been reported.[26] A variety of artificial tears, wetting solutions, saline flushes, and other ophthalmic

products are available OTC. Routine use of these products should be discouraged until a definitive diagnosis is been made as they may mask the signs of a serious ophthalmic condition.

CONCLUSIONS

A wide variety of OTC medications are available including high-efficacy medications that are readily available and cost-effective. However, some of the medications can produce severe and life-threatening adverse effects if not appropriately used. Clients should be encouraged to contact their veterinarian before using any OTC medication.

REFERENCES

The reference list can be found on the companion Expert Consult Web site at *www.expertconsult.com*.

CHAPTER 157

Glucocorticoid Therapy

Leah A. Cohn

Glucocorticoid agents are among the most commonly used veterinary drugs. They exert myriad effects on nearly every tissue in the body resulting in both desired and undesired consequences. Effects vary with potency and preparation of the glucocorticoid product, dose and route of administration, duration of glucocorticoid exposure, and individual factors. Most often, the desired action of therapeutically administered glucocorticoids is suppression of inflammation or of a damaging immunologic response. Other properties of glucocorticoids are utilized in the treatment of hormonal deficiency states, metabolic disorders, neoplasia, and paraneoplastic syndromes.

Unfortunately, even for disease states in which glucocorticoid therapy is proven to be beneficial, there is often little scientific evidence of what constitutes an optimal treatment protocol. Instead, veterinarians rely largely on anecdote and experience to design glucocorticoid treatment regimens. Because effects vary with dose and potency, the veterinarian must be familiar with the equivalent dose range of various drug preparations required to produce physiologic, antiinflammatory, immunosuppressive, or other effects. As a general rule, glucocorticoids should be used "to effect" rather than at an arbitrary dose in order to minimize exposure and adverse effects.

PHYSIOLOGY

Glucocorticoid drug preparations are derivatives of the endogenously produced adrenal hormone cortisol. Cortisol and other glucocorticoid compounds move passively into cells and then bind intracytoplasmic receptors. Receptor numbers vary

with tissue and cell type. Bound receptors translocate to the nucleus, where they modify gene transcription. Proteins are either up- or down-regulated by glucocorticoids, which leads to specific cellular actions. Together, these actions affect the function of nearly every tissue type and result in a wide variety of effects (Box 157-1).

Metabolic, antiinflammatory, and immunosuppressive effects of glucocorticoids are particularly relevant to their therapeutic use. Metabolic effects are primarily catabolic and include insulin antagonism, increased glycogen formation, and increased gluconeogenesis. Glucocorticoids inhibit liberation of arachidonic acid to diminish production of eicosanoid proinflammatory mediators, and they increase production of antiinflammatory proteins.

Many antiinflammatory effects of glucocorticoids overlap with immunosuppressive effects. The glucocorticoid-induced stress leukogram (mature neutrophilia, lymphopenia and eosinopenia, and variable monocytosis) results from altered membrane expression of cellular adhesion molecules. Although glucocorticoids are typically described as "immunosuppressive" and are used to good effect in the treatment of immune-mediated disease, their actions are not so simple as to suppress all immune function. In fact, glucocorticoids can prime the innate immune response and promote humoral immunity at the same time that they dampen inflammation and suppress cellular immunity.[1] Dogs and cats are considered steroid-resistant species in that glucocorticoids induce apoptosis of only neoplastic or activated lymphocytes and not of resting lymphocytes.[2]

The release of endogenous glucocorticoids is controlled by an endocrine feedback axis consisting of the hypothalamus, the pituitary gland, and the adrenal gland (HPA axis) (Web

Box • 157-1

Selected Physiologic Effects of Glucocorticoids

Metabolic Effects
Increase gluconeogenesis
Increase protein catabolism
Antagonize insulin
Mobilize free fatty acids
Redistribute adipose tissue

Dermal Effects
Thinning or atrophic skin
Atrophic hair follicles

Cardiovascular Effects
Optimize catecholamine receptor numbers
Positive inotropic effects
Vasoconstriction

Gastrointestinal and Hepatic Effects
Induce alkaline phosphatase enzyme (dogs)
Decrease calcium and iron absorption
Promote hepatic fat and glycogen deposition
Alter mucin structure
Increase secretion of digestive hormones

Renal Effects
Increase glomerular filtration rate
Inhibit renal tubules' response to antidiuretic hormone
Promote water, sodium, and chloride retention
Promote potassium and calcium excretion
Proteinuria

Neurologic and Muscular Effects
Euphoria or behavioral change
Increase numbers or sensitivity of adrenergic receptors

Muscular atrophy
Muscular weakness

Endocrine Effects
Decreased adrenocorticotropic hormone production
Suppressed thyroid-stimulating hormone and T3/T4 concentrations

Hematopoietic Effects
Increase circulating mature neutrophils
Decrease circulating lymphocytes, lymphocyte sequestration, lymphoid tissue involution
Apoptosis of activated and neoplastic lymphocytes
Decrease circulating eosinophils
Increase circulating monocytes
Increase circulating red blood cells
Increase circulating platelets

Inflammatory and Immunologic Effects
Decreased eicosanoid (prostaglandin and leukotriene) formation
Inhibit mononuclear phagocytosis and chemotaxis
Decrease or increase cytokine production
Depress cell-mediated immunity
Diminish humoral immunity (secondary effect)

Miscellaneous Effects
Stimulate appetite
Inhibit fibroblast proliferation and collagen synthesis
Accelerate bone reabsorption
Stabilize lysosomal membranes
Antioxidant

Figure 157-1). The hypothalamus produces corticotropin-releasing hormone (CRH), which stimulates production of adrenocorticotropic hormone (ACTH) from the anterior pituitary gland. In turn, ACTH causes production and release of cortisol from the zona fasciculata and zona reticularis of the adrenal cortex. Cortisol then inhibits release of CRH and ACTH and dampens further glucocorticoid production. Pharmacologic derivatives of cortisol exert a similar negative feedback, but degree of suppression varies with glucocorticoid potency.

PHARMACOLOGY

Numerous modifications of the 17-carbon atom steroid nucleus have been developed to enhance or diminish particular glucocorticoid drug properties (e.g., mineralocorticoid or glucocorticoid potency, receptor binding strength). Intense efforts are currently underway to identify glucocorticoid receptor ligands that might retain desired actions while minimizing adverse events, but resulting drugs are not yet available commercially.[3] The majority of glucocorticoid in plasma is bound to proteins, but binding affinity varies with the particular product. Corticosteroid-binding globulin, and to a lesser extent other proteins including albumin, hold glucocorticoid unavailable for diffusion into the cell. Only glucocorticoid in excess of this binding capacity enters the cell and exerts a biologic effect.

Modifications of the basic glucocorticoid hormones have resulted in the development of numerous drug products available for either systemic or topical administration. The potency of these products is expressed as it relates to cortisol (Table 157-1). Importantly, the same metabolic effect can be attained by any of these glucocorticoid products when administered in a metabolically active form at equipotent dosages. The biologic half-life of systemically administered glucocorticoids is disparate from the plasma half-life. Because the biologic effects are largely due to alterations in genetic regulation of protein production, biologic effects are delayed and prolonged in comparison with plasma drug concentration. Glucocorticoid drugs are often divided into three groups based on duration of HPA suppression. Short-acting glucocorticoids typically suppress the HPA less than 12 hours; long-acting glucocorticoids more than 48 hours; and intermediate-acting products fall somewhere between.

Many glucocorticoid products are esterified in such a way as to alter water solubility of the compound and therefore affect rate of absorption of injectable preparations. Sodium

Table • 157-1

Comparison of Various Glucocorticoid Base Compounds

	RELATIVE ANTIINFLAMMATORY POTENCY	EQUIVALENT PHARMACOLOGIC DOSE (mg)	RELATIVE MINERALO-CORTICOID POTENCY	PLASMA HALF-LIFE DOGS/PEOPLE (HOURS)	BIOLOGIC HALF-LIFE IN PEOPLE (HOURS)
Short-Acting Glucocorticoids					
Hydrocortisone	1	20	2	1/1.5	8-12
Cortisone	0.8	25	2	?/1.5	8-12
Intermediate-Acting Glucocorticoids					
Prednisone	4	5	1	?/1	12-36
Prednisolone	4	5	1	1-3/2-3	12-36
Methyl-Prednisolone	5	4	0	1.5/3	12-36
Triamcinolone	5	4	0	?/4 or more	24-48
Long-Acting Glucocorticoids					
Dexamethasone	30	0.75	0	2/5 or more	35-54
Betamethasone	30	0.6	0	?/5 or more	>48

phosphate, hemisuccinate, and sodium succinate esters are the most water soluble and allow for rapid absorption and action. The duration of action of these esterified compounds is equivalent to that of the base glucocorticoid. Acetate and diacetate esters are poorly water soluble, whereas pivalate, diproprionate, hexacetate, and acetonide are least soluble. Slow absorption from the site of injection prolongs the duration of action of any glucocorticoid base with which these esters are combined. For example, although the biologic duration of methylprednisolone is 12 to 36 hours, the duration of the repositol formulation methylprednisolone acetate is 3 to 6 weeks.

Certain synthetic glucocorticoid compounds require conversion to an active metabolite. An example is prednisone, which requires hepatic conversion to prednisolone for activity; prednisone would therefore not be suitable for topical application. In the dog, hepatic conversion is rapid and thorough, allowing prednisone and prednisolone to be used interchangeably at equivalent dosages. In cats, however, prednisolone is preferred over prednisone. While it is unclear whether decreased gastrointestinal (GI) absorption or decreased hepatic conversion is to blame, pharmacokinetics of prednisone are inferior to those of prednisolone.[4] Cats are also unique in that they have fewer, less sensitive, cellular glucocorticoid receptors than dogs.[5] It has been suggested that cats may require twice the dose of glucocorticoid as dogs to achieve a similar effect, but the use of less available prednisone (vs. prednisolone) may have contributed somewhat to this clinical impression. Fortunately, cats seem to tolerate glucocorticoids with fewer "dog-common" adverse reactions, although when complications of glucocorticoid use arise in the cat, they can be serious (e.g., diabetes mellitus, congestive heart failure).[6,7]

CLINICAL UTILITY

Although glucocorticoids are used primarily for the treatment of disease, they are also used for disease diagnosis. Glucocorticoid (i.e., dexamethasone) is administered as a means to suppress the HPA axis for the diagnosis of hyperadrenocorticism (Web Box 157-1).

Glucocorticoids are used over a range of dosages to treat a wide variety of diseases; evidence supporting these usages varies from irrefutable (e.g., hypoadrenocorticism) to unsubstantiated (e.g., hemorrhagic shock). Even when good evidence exists to support the use of glucocorticoids to treat a given disease, there are few studies supporting a particular glucocorticoid formulation, dose strength, frequency, or duration of therapy.

Equipotent amounts of any metabolically active glucocorticoid exert a similar effect, which means that a higher dose of a less potent glucocorticoid can achieve the same effect as a lower dose of a more potent product. Physiologic actions of glucocorticoids occur at a much lower dose than do antiinflammatory effects, which, in turn, occur at a lower dose than do immunosuppressive effects. When choosing an initial treatment protocol, the veterinarian must begin by identifying a goal of glucocorticoid therapy (physiologic replacement, suppression of inflammation, suppression of immunity, or some other action). Additional variables relate to the patient (e.g., species, concurrent disease), the disease process (e.g., chronic or acute, localized or systemic), and available glucocorticoid products (e.g., solubility, duration of action, route of administration). Commonly used systemic veterinary glucocorticoid formulations and considerations for clinical utility are provided in Web Box 157-2, while Web Box 157-3 provides discussion regarding altering ongoing glucocorticoid regimens.

When glucocorticoid therapy is required in only a localized area (e.g., ocular inflammation), treatment can be administered topically, thus minimizing effects of glucocorticoids on other tissues. Systemic therapy using parenteral or oral products is best suited to situations in which several body systems and/or tissues are targeted for therapy (e.g., anaphylaxis, systemic lupus erythematosus). Realistically, glucocorticoids are often administered systemically even when only a single tissue is targeted.

Physiologic Replacement Therapy

Hypoadrenocorticism is the failure of the adrenal gland to produce enough corticosteroid hormones. Commonly, both mineralocorticoid and glucocorticoid deficiency exists, but isolated glucocorticoid deficiency can occur (atypical hypoadrenocorticism). Administration of prednisone or methyl-prednisolone, which are detected along with endogenous cortisol during assay, should be avoided prior to completion of diagnostic ACTH stimulation testing. If a delay in testing is unavoidable, dexamethasone may be administered (0.1 to 0.2 mg/kg) without altering diagnostic test results. Life-long hormonal replacement is the basis of continued therapy (see Chapter 294). Although some corticosteroid drugs (e.g., fludrocortisone) possess glucocorticoid and mineralocorticoid activity, separate mineralocorticoid (i.e., desoxycorticoste-rone pivalate) and glucocorticoid therapy are used more commonly. Glucocorticoid replacement is essential for animals with either typical or atypical hypoadrenocorticism. The glucocorticoid should be administered systemically at a physiologic dose. Predniso(lo)ne 0.2 to 0.3 mg/kg q24h is used most often; methylprednisolone tablets (0.1 to 0.2 mg/kg q24h) or hydrocortisone tablets (0.4 to 0.8 mg/kg q12h) may be used alternatively. During times of stress (e.g., boarding, illness) the amount of glucocorticoid administered should be temporarily increased (typically doubled) to meet increased physiologic demands.

Antiinflammatory Therapy

Glucocorticoids are used most often for their excellent antiinflammatory properties. Prior to initiating glucocorticoid therapy, attempts should be made to identify and eliminate the underlying cause of inflammation. Frequently, an underlying cause either cannot be found or cannot be entirely eliminated. Antiinflammatory therapy can be of benefit in such cases, and glucocorticoids are often the most effective such therapy.

It is particularly important to rule out infectious causes of inflammation, especially fungal infection, prior to beginning glucocorticoid therapy. Because of the suppressive effects of glucocorticoids on cell-mediated immunity, these drugs are relatively contraindicated during infection. Glucocorticoids often lead to a temporary clinical improvement in animals with inflammation secondary to infection, but failure to control infection can lead to worsening of disease or even death. Because glucocorticoids reduce fever, stimulate appetite, and can induce feelings of euphoria and suppress clinical evidence of inflammation, it can be difficult to detect worsened infection until later than would be ideal. There are exceptions to every rule, and glucocorticoids are actually indicated for the treatment of some infectious diseases.[8,9] Typically, they are combined with antimicrobial therapy to reduce inflammatory (e.g., *Pseudomonas* or *Malassezia* otitis) or immunologic (e.g., red cell destruction due to *Mycoplasma haemofelis*) consequences of infection.[10-12]

Specific treatment decisions regarding antiinflammatory therapy with glucocorticoids are based on a number of factors, including desired rapidity of action and expected duration of therapy. Rarely, a rapid onset of action is required, such as when respiratory inflammation compromises the animal's ability to breathe; injectable phosphate or succinate preparations are most useful in these situations. In most cases, antiinflammatory therapy will be required for days, weeks, or months. Intermediate-acting steroid preparations allow dosage to be titrated to effect and thereby minimized for chronic administration. The most often used antiinflammatory glucocorticoid is predniso(lo)ne at an initial dosage of 0.5 to 1.0 mg/kg/day for dogs or prednisolone 1 to 2 mg/kg/day for cats. Because the biologic half-life is 24 to 36 hours, there is little obvious advantage to division of the daily dosage. Once initial inflammation is suppressed, steroid dose is reduced to the lowest necessary level. Treatment with repositol products (e.g., methylprednisolone acetate) is not advisable in dogs even when long-term therapy is anticipated. Repositol therapy severely suppresses the HPA axis, prevents accurate dose

titration or early drug withdrawal, and is associated with more pronounced side effects. Additionally, such therapy can interfere with accurate diagnostic testing (e.g., allergen skin testing, endocrine testing) for long periods of time. Repositol therapy may be used to treat allergic or inflammatory skin conditions in cats (e.g., feline eosinophilic granuloma, indolent ulcer) when the owners are unwilling or unable to administer oral medications, but adverse reactions (e.g., congestive heart failure, iatrogenic hyperadrenocorticism, insulin resistance) may occasionally result.[7,13-16]

Regional inhibition of inflammation can often be accomplished via local application of glucocorticoids. Glucocorticoid products are available in a variety of formulations designed specifically for local application, and injectable preparations can be used to achieve a local effect. Because the intended actions are local rather than systemic, the products should include only metabolically active glucocorticoids (e.g., prednisolone rather than prednisone). Although local application minimizes unwanted effects, absorption does occur and can lead to systemic effects and suppression of the HPA axis.[17,18]

The eyes, skin, respiratory and GI tracts, and joints are the sites most often treated via local glucocorticoid application. Topical suspensions (e.g., 1.0% prednisolone acetate), solutions (e.g., 0.1% dexamethasone phosphate), or ointments (e.g., 0.05% dexamethasone phosphate) are indicated for controlling inflammatory disease of external structures, such as noninfectious conjunctivitis or uveitis. Therapy is typically titrated to effect by adjusting frequency of application (every 1 to 8 hours). Subconjunctival injections of glucocorticoids may reduce the need for frequent instillation of eye drops.[19] Contraindications to ocular glucocorticoid use include corneal ulceration or ocular infection. Ulcers can be exacerbated by glucocorticoids, and in the presence of infection, stromal melting may occur.[19] Because of its frequent association with infection, feline conjunctivitis is a relative contraindication to ophthalmic glucocorticoid use.

Dermatologic inflammation is often treated via systemic glucocorticoid administration, but topical products can augment or replace systemic glucocorticoids. Glucocorticoids should not be used to treat dermatologic disorders until serious attempts are made to diagnose a cause of the dermatopathy. They should only be used after efforts to eliminate or control precipitating and predisposing factors such as ectoparasites and food allergy. Alternatives to glucocorticoids should be considered when available (e.g., hyposensitization for atopy). When systemic steroids are used for atopy or other inflammatory skin conditions, they should be used sparingly; topical therapy may spare excessive tissue exposure. Glucocorticoids in the form of 1% hydrocortisone (the metabolically active form of cortisone) are available in shampoos, conditioners, lotions, creams, ointments, and otic medications. These products are particularly useful in reduction of pruritus associated with atopy when used in conjunction with other therapies such as antihistamine medications. Stronger glucocorticoid preparations, including triamcinolone acetonide (e.g., Panalog), betamethasone valerate (e.g., Gentocin Spray, Otomax), and fluocinolone acetonide (e.g., Synotic), are effective in reducing erythema, swelling, and pruritus. However, systemic absorption makes these products inappropriate for extended daily use, particularly when dermal barriers are no longer intact.

Glucocorticoids are frequently used to treat chronic respiratory inflammatory diseases such as feline reactive airway disease (e.g., asthma) and chronic bronchitis. Topical application of glucocorticoids to the airway epithelium may reduce inflammation while minimizing systemic glucocorticoid effects.[20-22] This can be particularly useful when systemic glucocorticoids are contraindicated, such as in the treatment of cats with asthma and concurrent diabetes mellitus, congestive heart failure, or active infection. Because the respiratory epithelium offers a vast absorptive area, minimization of systemic actions caused by inhaled glucocorticoids depends on the use of a product with limited systemic availability. Glucocorticoids like fluticasone and flunisolide have potent local activity but undergo rapid hepatic first-pass metabolism, thereby greatly diminishing systemic availability of active drug. Glucocorticoids can be delivered topically either via nebulization or a metered dose inhaler (MDI); more detail on inhalant glucocorticoid therapy is available at the associated website (Web Figures 157-2 and 157-3, Web Table 157-1, and Web Box 157-4).

Some dogs and cats with allergic or idiopathic rhinitis respond well to intranasal glucocorticoids. Such therapy should be delayed until neoplastic and infectious diseases have been ruled out. Nasal sprays are available, but two drops of ophthalmic 1% prednisolone acetate instilled in each nostril two to three times daily can be used successfully. Alternatively, aerosols delivered by nebulization or MDI can be used to target the nasal passages.

A number of inflammatory GI diseases are treated with either systemic (typically prednis[ol]one) or topical glucocorticoids. Topical therapy of GI disease is limited to the mouth, rectum, and colon. Although dogs with refractory colitis have been successfully treated with glucocorticoid suppositories and rectal foams, owners may find this treatment distasteful. Successful intralesional injection of oral eosinophilic granuloma with glucocorticoids has been described in cats.[23] Although not truly topical, there are glucocorticoid preparations designed specifically to act on the GI epithelium while minimizing systemic activity. Budesonide can be compounded from a powder form, or purchased as capsules containing budesonide-coated microgranules (Enterocort EC), which do not dissolve until reaching the distal small intestine. Although GI absorption of budesonide occurs, extensive first-pass hepatic metabolism to less active metabolites minimizes systemic drug availability. Although oral budesonide will suppress the HPA axis, other adverse effects typically attributed to glucocorticoid therapy have thus far not been noted in either healthy dogs treated with the coated product or dogs with inflammatory bowel disease treated with a compounded powder form of budesonide.[24,25] Budesonide may be especially useful for the treatment of inflammatory bowel disease in pets demonstrating adverse effects related to long-term systemic glucocorticoid administration.

Orthopedic pain and inflammation may be relieved by local injection of glucocorticoids, although such injections should never be considered curative. Although injections can bring about a rapid return to function, they are also associated with potentially devastating complications (e.g., cartilage damage and impaired healing of osteochondral defects, accelerated osteoarthritis, and joint sepsis).[26,27] Intraarticular glucocorticoid injections are used less often in small animals than in either horses or people.[28-30] Perhaps the best use of local glucocorticoid therapy in small animal orthopedic medicine is in the treatment of bicipital tenosynovitis in dogs. Typically, 1 mg/kg of repositol methylprednisolone acetate is injected directly into the tendon and tendon sheath.[31] Injection is followed with several weeks' strict rest prior to slow return to activity.

Immunosuppressive Therapy

Suppression of damaging immunologic responses in dogs and cats is most often achieved by the administration of systemic glucocorticoids at a dosage higher than that required to suppress inflammation. The beneficial role of glucocorticoids in the treatment of autoimmune disease is well documented. Additionally, glucocorticoids are used to suppress harmful immunologic reactions associated with diseases like feline infectious peritonitis or rejection of transplanted organs.[32,33] The use of an intermediate-acting glucocorticoid (e.g., prednis[ol]one or methylprednisolone) results in less HPA suppression and fewer adverse effects than would the use of long-acting glucocorticoid formulations and is, therefore, most appropriate for chronic immunosuppression. The initial dose of predniso(lo)ne required for immune suppression is purported to be 2 to 4 mg/kg/day for dogs or 2 to 8 mg/kg/day prednisolone for cats. Generally speaking, larger dogs should be treated with the lower end of the dose range. Despite predniso(lo)ne's biologic half-life of 24 to 36 hours, dividing this high dose and administering the drug twice daily may lessen GI irritation. At such high dosages, adverse effects of glucocorticoids are quite common. The addition of alternative immunosuppressive agents (e.g., azathioprine or cyclosporine) may have a steroid-sparing effect, thus allowing control of the disease at a lower glucocorticoid dose and facilitating a more rapid dose reduction. Ideally, once immune-mediated disease is controlled, the use of glucocorticoids can be slowly tapered until discontinued altogether. Some clinicians recommend initiating immunosuppressive therapy with dexamethasone rather than prednisone, but evidence for an advantage of one drug over the other at equipotent dosages is lacking.[34] Dexamethasone injection may be preferred when oral drug administration is difficult (e.g., due to vomiting or inability to swallow) but treatment should be switched to an intermediate-acting glucocorticoid when feasible (see Web Box 157-4 for information on switching between glucocorticoid formulations).

Antineoplastic Therapy

Glucocorticoids are useful in the treatment of several neoplastic and paraneoplastic conditions. Benefits can be attributed to direct tumoricidal effects, antiinflammatory and/or immunosuppressive properties, and to metabolic properties of glucocorticoids. Commonly, glucocorticoids are used in conjunction with other chemotherapeutic agents in the treatment of lymphoma.[35] Although glucocorticoids sometimes induce remission of lymphoma when used alone (predniso[lo]ne 2 mg/kg/day), rapid development of multidrug resistance leads to brief remission and decreases the chance that other, more aggressive chemotherapy protocols will be successful.[36] Because glucocorticoids induce apoptosis of neoplastic lymphocytes, the use of these drugs prior to diagnosis may interfere with the ability to cytologically or histologically confirm lymphoma. Other cancer types that may respond directly to glucocorticoids include multiple myeloma, certain leukemias, and mast cell tumors.[37-39]

Some paraneoplastic syndromes and some complications from neoplasia may respond to glucocorticoid therapy even when glucocorticoids are not directly tumoricidal. Glucocorticoids are antagonistic to insulin and are therefore used to increase plasma glucose concentrations in animals with insulinoma (predniso[lo]ne 0.5 mg/kg/day).[40] Hypercalcemia of malignancy may respond to systemic glucocorticoid therapy as well (predniso[lo]one 1 to 2 mg/kg/day).[41] In addition to direct effects on lymphoid neoplasia, they inhibit bone resorption, inhibit intestinal calcium absorption, and promote calciuresis. Edema and inflammation associated with many types of neoplasia are frequently treated with systemic glucocorticoid therapy on either a short- (e.g., during perioperative period surrounding tumor manipulation) or long-term basis (e.g., as palliative therapy for brain tumor).[42]

Miscellaneous Therapeutic Uses

In certain disease processes, glucocorticoids are used for short periods (often a single dose) in dosages much higher than those required to initiate immunosuppressive therapy. At such dosages glucocorticoids exert actions in addition to those mediated by gene transcription; these actions are somewhat nebulous but include antioxidant properties, membrane stabilization, and hemodynamic effects. Because a rapid onset of action is required, injectable succinate and phosphate esters are most appropriate. Animals with recent spinal cord injuries (<8 hours from time of insult) benefit from treatment with methylprednisolone sodium succinate (15 to 40 mg/kg IV).[43,44] Repeated boluses of 15 mg/kg may be administered 2 and 6 hours later, followed by either boluses of 7.5 mg/kg every 6 hours for 24 hours or by a 24-hour continuous rate infusion of 2.5 mg/kg/hr. A similar benefit has not been demonstrated for treatment of traumatic brain injury (human guidelines suggest avoiding glucocorticoids).[45]

Many veterinarians utilize short-term high-dose glucocorticoid therapy for treatment of conditions in which massive cytokine release is anticipated (e.g., gastric dilatation volvulus, snakebite envenomation). A beneficial role for glucocorticoids in most such situations has been neither confirmed nor denied. Serious complications from intensive short-term glucocorticoid treatment are rare, but they do occur.[46] Therefore it is difficult to recommend high-dose glucocorticoid therapy in the absence of proven benefit for these types of conditions.

High-dose glucocorticoid treatment for shock has fallen repeatedly in and out of favor. Anaphylactic shock is the only type for which routine treatment still involves the administration of high-dose glucocorticoids, although anaphylactic reactions to intravenous glucocorticoid administration itself have been reported.[47,48] Decades ago, high-dose glucocorticoids were used to treat hemorrhagic shock because of their ability to increase blood pressure; instead, treatment should focus on volume, colloid, and hemoglobin replacement. Although experimental studies in the 1970s seemed to suggest that high doses of short-acting glucocorticoids decreased morbidity from septic shock, clinical trials in people failed to support these claims. While high-dose steroid therapy in sepsis is not indicated, lower doses designed to counter relative adrenal insufficiency (RAI) may improve survival in humans.[49] Baseline cortisol may be within the reference range during RAI, but adrenal response to stress is inadequate and therefore contributes to the pathophysiology associated with critical illness.[50] Although relative adrenal insufficiency has been documented in septic dogs, it remains to be determined if low-dose glucocorticoid supplementation improves survival.[51]

ADVERSE EFFECTS

Adverse reactions associated with glucocorticoids are numerous and range from the merely bothersome to the life threatening (Box 157-2). Conditions exacerbated by glucocorticoid effects (e.g., infection, diabetes mellitus) are relative contraindications to their use. Generally speaking, the more potent the product, higher the dosage, and more prolonged the administration, the more serious are the adverse effects. The most common side effects of glucocorticoid use are polyuria, polydipsia, and polyphagia. Iatrogenic hyperadrenocorticism, distinguishable from pituitary- or adrenal-dependent hyperadrenocorticism only through clinical history and suppression of response to exogenous ACTH, can occur during prolonged glucocorticoid administration. Rapid withdrawal of exogenous glucocorticoids in an animal with suppression of the HPA axis can leave the adrenal gland unable to produce requisite levels of glucocorticoids, creating a state of adrenocortical insufficiency that can have life-threatening consequences. Rapid cessation of chronic (>2 weeks) therapy may result in a constellation of clinical signs including depression, decreased appetite, and vomiting.

Box • 157-2

Adverse Effects of Glucocorticoid Administration

Abortion
Alopecia
Calcinosis cutis
Colonic perforation
Comedones
Delayed wound healing
Diabetes mellitus
Gastrointestinal ulceration
Growth suppression
Hypercoagulable state
Hyperlipidemia
Iatrogenic hyperadrenocorticism
Immunosuppression (secondary infection, worsened infection, recrudescence of latent infection)
Insomnia, agitation, behavioral changes
Insulin resistance
Ligament and tendon rupture
Muscle atrophy
Muscle wasting
Myotonia/myopathy
Obesity
Osteoporosis
Panting
Polyphagia
Polyuria/polydipsia
Proteinuria
Psychosis/behavioral change
Seizure threshold lowered
Skin thinning
Vacuolar hepatopathy

Glucocorticoid administration can impact therapy with other pharmaceutical agents. For example, animals receiving immunosuppressive dosages of glucocorticoids should not be given modified live vaccines due to the risk of vaccine-induced disease.[52] Certain pharmaceuticals alter metabolism or clearance of the glucocorticoids, which results in either increased or decreased biologic glucocorticoid effects at a given steroid dose. Glucocorticoids can impact the effectiveness or toxicity of coadministered pharmaceuticals (Web Table 157-2). Additionally, intravenous administration of dexamethasone in a polyethylene glycol vehicle (e.g., Azium) may result in hemolysis, hypotension, and collapse.

GLUCOCORTICOID REDUCTION PROTOCOLS

Glucocorticoids should be used at the lowest dose possible to achieve the desired effect. When administered for more than 2 weeks, the dosage should be reduced slowly. This principle fits nicely with the ideal of adjusting the glucocorticoid dose "to effect," particularly in those cases requiring prolonged therapy (e.g., autoimmune disease).

Once clinical evidence suggests that the condition being addressed is controlled (e.g., red cell count normalized when treating immune-mediated hemolytic anemia [IMHA], diarrhea resolved when treating inflammatory bowel disease), the dosage of glucocorticoids should be tapered. There is no single ideal way to conduct this tapering, but certain principles apply. First, the clinical condition should be monitored closely. Worsening soon after a dose reduction suggests that the taper is too rapid. Second, the severity of the condition holds implications as to the rapidity of the taper. Glucocorticoids used to treat life-threatening disease (e.g., IMHA) should be tapered more slowly than glucocorticoids used to treat other conditions. Third, consolidated dosing with prolonged dosing intervals might spare HPA suppression while maintaining much of the desirable biologic drug effect. For example, if administering 5 mg prednisone twice daily, it may be better to first switch to 10 mg once a day rather than simply decreasing the twice daily dose. The daily dose can then be decreased incrementally. Dose interval is then changed to an every-other-day (EOD) basis, usually when the daily

dose nears a minimal antiinflammatory range (0.5 mg/kg for dogs). Initially, veterinarians may choose to increase the dose given on treatment days so that the total 2-day dose remains unchanged or only slightly decreased. Eventually, the glucocorticoid dose is lowered until it is discontinued altogether. Theoretically, EOD (or even every third day) dosing allows the HPA axis to recover from suppression during the "off steroid" day.[53,54] This type of EOD dosing scheme depends on the biologic duration of the steroid preparation and is thus only serviceable using intermediate-acting glucocorticoids.

REFERENCES

The reference list can be found on the companion Expert Consult Web site at *www.expertconsult.com*.

CHAPTER 158

Nonsteroidal Anti-Inflammatory Analgesics

Karol A. Mathews

Nonsteroidal antiinflammatory analgesics (NSAIAs) are a group of pharmaceutical agents that possess both analgesic and antiinflammatory properties. The NSAIAs are frequently used in human and veterinary medicine to relieve mild, moderate, and severe pain. The efficacy of many NSAIAs can be superior or equal to the pure mu agonist opioids (oxymorphone, morphine, hydromorphone, meperidine) and butorphanol or buprenorphine in managing soft tissue and orthopedic postoperative pain.[1-15] When used in combination with opioids, NSAIAs appear to confer synergism and may require reduced dosing of the opioid in mild to moderate, but not in severe, pain states. The NSAIAs concentrate in inflamed joints and tissues, likely contributing to duration of effect which varies between 12 to 24 hours.[16] The duration and efficacy of the NSAIAs makes them ideal for treating acute[1-15] and chronic pain[17-28] in veterinary patients; however, due to their potential for harmful adverse effects, patient and NSAIA selection must be considered prior to administration. Many veterinary publications review the clinical use of the NSAIAs in great depth with extensive citations of original studies,[29-39] and a critical review of published studies,[29] which is beyond the scope of this chapter; however, the reader is encouraged to read these.

PHARMACOLOGY

Cyclooxygenase enzymes oxidize arachidonic acid to various eicosanoids and related compounds, or prostanoids[40] (Figure 158-1). Nonsteroidal antiinflammatory analgesics are, with varying differences, inhibitors of cyclooxygenase enzyme 1 (COX-1), COX-2, or both, or COX-3, resulting in reduced prostaglandin (PG) synthesis. In addition to the peripheral action, a significant part of the NSAIAs' antinociceptive effect is exerted at the spinal cord and supraspinal levels.[41-47] This action, in addition to pain relief, may account for the observed overall well-being and improved appetite of patients receiving

injectable NSAIAs for relief of acute pain (personal observations). COX-1 can be induced in inflammatory states and is increased approximately twofold or threefold in tissue injury, and may also generate PGs at sites of inflammation (e.g., joints), it is present within the central nervous system, and active in transmission of pain, especially visceral nociception. COX-1 is also a constitutive enzyme, present in tissues, that ultimately converts arachidonic acid into prostanoids (thromboxanes, prostacyclin, and prostaglandins (PGE_2, PGF_2, and PGD_2) which are involved in many homeostatic functions.[46]

Cyclooxygenase 2 is also inducible and synthesized by macrophages and inflammatory cells, potentially increasing by twentyfold over baseline, especially in injured tissue and inflammatory conditions such as osteoarthritis.[42] The increased cyclooxygenase levels increase prostanoid production, where these compounds serve as mediators of inflammation and amplifiers of nociceptive input and transmission in both the peripheral and central nervous systems.[42] By this mechanism, COX-2 is responsible for a significant amount of pain and hyperalgesia experienced after tissue injury. As COX-2 appears to play an important role in nociceptive transmission, medications that prevent COX-2 activity and spare the constitutive COX-1 functions should be effective, with potentially fewer adverse effects, in the management of pain. Based on these findings emphasis is placed on COX-1 versus COX-2 activity of NSAIAs, with respect to safety and efficacy; however, it is important to note that COX-2 also has important constitutive functions,[47,48] and the notion of a "good versus bad COX" is misleading. The discovery of COX-3, characterized as generated from COX-1, is expressed in the brain and brain microvasculature in dogs and has been proposed to be a target of the analgesic/antipyretics acetaminophen and dipyrone.[46,49,50]

Currently, the presence of COX-3 appears to be restricted to dogs. Both acetaminophen and dipyrone have minimal effect on COX-1 and COX-2[46] and are frequently used to

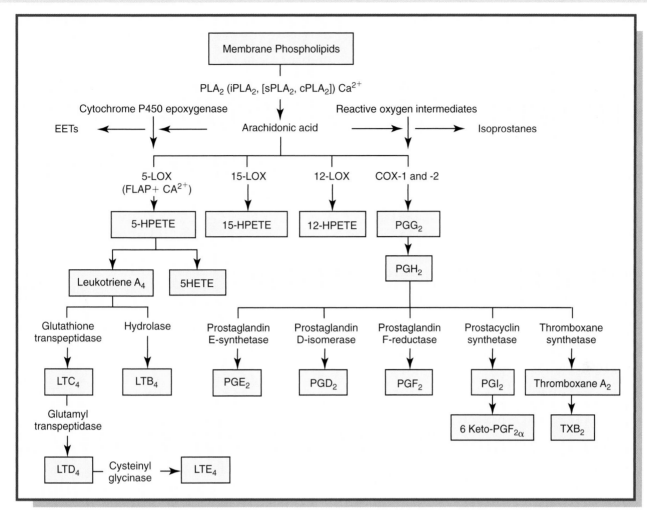

Figure 158-1 The arachidonic cascade. *COX*, Cyclooxygenase; *EETs*, epoxy-eicosatrienoic acids; *FLAP*, 5-lipooxygenase-activating protein; *HETE*, hydroxyeicosatetraenoic acid; *HPETE*, hydroperoxyeicosatetraenoic acid; *LOX*, lipooxygenase; *LT*, leukotriene; *PG*, prostaglandin; *PLA₂*, phospholipase A₂; *TXB₂*, thromboxane B₂.

reduce fever in animals with little gastrointestinal or renal adverse effects. Acetaminophen is toxic to cats. The COX-3 isoenzyme is more sensitive to NSAIAs that are analgesic and antipyretic but have low antiinflammatory activity, which again emphasizes the different niche for NSAIA therapy in managing pain of differing etiology. As the COX-3 isoenzyme genetic profile is derived from the COX-1 gene, this suggests that the COX-1 gene plays an integral role in pain and/or fever depending on the physiologic context.[44] New insights as to the role of various prostanoids continue to be discovered. Unlike other PGs, the J series of PGs (cyclopentenone PGs), formed by progressive nonenzymatic dehydration of PGD₂, has no known membrane receptor.[51] The COX-2–derived PGs also have an antiinflammatory role.[51] The PGJ₂ interact with nuclear receptors that comprise the peroxisome proliferator–activating receptor (PPAR) family, especially PPAR-γ. Activation of PPAR-γ can transrepress the activation of many transcription factors including nuclear factor κ-β (NF-κβ), an important promoter for inflammatory mediators. PPAR-γ is found in macrophages, dendritic cells, and B and T lymphocytes with potential roles in regulating inflammation and immunomodulation.[50,51]

Prostaglandins, especially COX-1 derived, are ubiquitous throughout the body and regulate many functions such as vascular and bronchial smooth muscle tone and fluid balance, just to name a few. Prostaglandins exert a negative feedback effect on cyclic adenosine monophosphate (c-AMP) with potential perturbations in many physiologic functions. As an example, renal water reabsorption depends on the action of antidiuretic hormone (ADH), which is mediated by c-AMP; inhibition of prostaglandin synthesis may lead to increased levels of c-AMP with a potential for enhanced ADH activity. Urine volume may be decreased through this mechanism but without renal injury.[46,52,53] In the inhibition of COX-2 activity when managing pain, the COX-2 enzyme has some important constitutive functions; there is a protective role for COX-2 in maintenance of gastrointestinal integrity and ulcer healing.[54] In addition, there is constitutive activity associated with nerve, brain, ovarian, and uterine function and bone metabolism.[52,55] COX-2 has constitutive functions in the kidney, which differ from those of COX-1. COX-2 is important in nephron maturation.[53,56] The canine kidney is not fully mature until 3 weeks after birth, nor optimally functional until 6 weeks after birth[56]; continual administration of a NSAIA during this time, or to the bitch prior to birth, may cause a permanent nephropathy. Most important is the dual role of the PGs as inflammatory and antiinflammatory mediators, where COX-2–derived PGs also function in resolution of inflammation.[47,50]

On the other hand, COX metabolites have been implicated in functional and structural alterations in glomerular and tubulointerstitial inflammatory disease. Administration of

COX-2 selective inhibitors decreased proteinuria and inhibited development of glomerular sclerosis in rats with reduced functioning renal mass.[53] Because COX-2 expression is also increased in glomerulonephritides such as lupus nephritis, it is possible that COX-2 inhibitors may also alter the natural history of glomerular inflammatory lesions.[53] COX-2–derived metabolite production is regulated and localized to the structures in the kidney that play an essential role in renal blood flow associated with renin activity and fluid-electrolyte homeostasis.[31,53,57] COX-2 is glucocorticoid sensitive, in that it is reduced following administration of glucocorticoids, which may partially explain the antiinflammatory and analgesic effects of this class of medications. Of interest, in addition to the COX-2 role in inflammation, aberrantly up-regulated COX-2 expression is increasingly implicated in the pathogenesis of Alzheimer's disease and possibly other neurologic conditions and a number of epithelial cell carcinomas, including colon, esophagus, breast, and skin.[58,59] The COX-2 inhibitors are being researched as potential anticarcinogenic agents. A potential role for NSAID use in the future may be as an adjunct to traditional therapies in the treatment of these neoplastic conditions in dogs and cats. A good review of the "Coxibs" is available; the background and pharmacology of the coxibs are reviewed elsewhere.[47,58,60]

Most NSAIAs that inhibit COX have been shown to result in diversion of arachidonate to the 5-lipooxygenase (5-LOX) pathway (see Figure 158-1). This results in an excessive production of leukotrienes (LT), which have been implicated in many pathologic states, including hyperalgesia and the creation of NSAIA-induced ulcers.[46,61,62] Leukotrienes are the products of 5-LOX cascade, where arachidonic acid is converted by a two-step mechanism into the conjugated triene epoxide leukotriene (LTA_4), the most biologically important intermediate LT.[47,62-64] LTA_4 is subsequently metabolized to LTB_4 and LTC_4. An LTD_4 is also recognized. Cells known to express 5-lipooxygenase include circulating polymorphonuclear leukocytes (PMNs), monocytes, basophils, eosinophils, tissue macrophages, and mast cells. These cells release LTA_4 and participate in transcellular biosynthesis of either LTC_4 or LTB_4.[65] As with the prostenoids, it is impossible to list all the activities of the LTs as these are also dependent on organ involvement. An in-depth discussion of dual inhibitors is available elsewhere.[39,47,66,68]

Associated with the use of NSAIAs is the risk of perturbation of the constitutive functions of COX-1 and COX-2 resulting in potential organ dysfunction. Depending on the NSAID selected, primary plug formation of platelets, modulation of vascular tone of all organs (the kidney and gastric mucosa being of specific importance), cytoprotective functions on the gastric mucosa, healing of intestinal mucosa, smooth muscle contraction, and regulation of body temperature will all be affected.[46,52] However, in this regard not all NSAIAs are created equal, as the COX-1, COX-2, and COX-3 enzymes variably control these functions. Some NSAIAs inhibit both COX-1 and COX-2 (aspirin, phenylbutazone, ketoprofen [Anafen, Merial], ketorolac [Toradol, Hoffman-LaRoche], flunixin meglumine [Flunixin, Schering-Plough]); while others may preferentially inhibit COX-2 and be a weak inhibitor of COX-1(meloxicam [Metacam, Boehringer-Ingelheim], carprofen [Rimadyl, Pfizer], etodolac [Etogesic, Fort Dodge], vedaprofen [Quadrisol-5, Intervet], tolfenamic acid [Tolfedine, Vetoquinol]); others selectively inhibit COX-2 (Deracoxib [Deramaxx, Novartis], firocoxib [Previcox, Merial]); while others, such as acetaminophen and dipyrone, may weakly inhibit both COX-1 and COX-2 but have greater inhibition of COX-3. Tepoxalin (Zubrin, Schering-Plough) is a dual COX/lipoxygenase (LOX) inhibitor and is reported to reduce COX-1, COX-2, and 5-LOX to some degree in dogs.[69] Licofelone, a new true dual inhibitor being evaluated in people and dogs, may have greater gastrointestinal safety than other NSAIAs.[70]

Throughout the remainder of this chapter, the generic names for the veterinary approved NSAIAs will be used. However, where the generic formulation also includes a human product, the human product will be stated, specifically meloxicam (Metacam the veterinary product, Mobicox the human product).

ADVERSE EFFECTS

All NSAIAs require accurate dosing to avoid potential adverse effects, especially when used long-term. Some patients may be receiving other medications and NSAIA interaction with these must be considered.[71] Based on the many important physiologic functions the prostanoids perform, one can appreciate the potential perturbation of normal homeostatic functions with administration of NSAIAs. The recommended dosages for the various NSAIAs rarely compromise these functions; however, should a patient be in a prostaglandin-dependent state, administration of NSAIAs frequently results in adverse effects (see Contraindications below). However, even in normal states the NSAIAs may result in gastrointestinal, renal, or hepatic abnormalities, or rarely a coagulopathy (predominately COX-1 NSAIAs) in the genetically predetermined individual. In humans, the COX-2–specific inhibitors appear to have fewer gastrointestinal adverse effects than those with COX-1 inhibition; however, long-term use in some people has resulted in gastrointestinal problems similar to those experienced with the COX-1 inhibitors, thereby identifying individuals intolerant to NSAIAs. While the incidence of gastrointestinal signs may be reduced with COX-2–specific targeted NSAIAs, adverse effects may also occur in dogs. Cyclooxygenase-2 expression has been identified in the duodenum of dogs, which increased significantly following 3 days of aspirin 10 mg/kg q12h when compared with effects of carprofen and deracoxib at recommended dosing.[72] Lesions were not observed by endoscopic examination. Up-regulation of COX-2 has been identified in the duodenum in response to mucosal erosion/injury performing an integral role in the daily healing process. Rarely, duodenal ulceration has been identified in dogs receiving appropriate dosing of deracoxib; therefore, it cannot be assumed that COX-2 specific inhibitors will be a "safe" treatment for all dogs with chronic administration. Duodenal ulceration/perforation has been reported in dogs prescribed deracoxib,[73] and similarly with meloxicam,[74] mostly associated with concurrent corticosteroid use and the higher than currently recommended dosages. This highlights the importance of contraindications (see below) for NSAIA administration. In addition, some reports of meloxicam toxicity have been associated with the use of Mobicox, the human formulation.[74] Mobicox 7.5 mg, 15-mg tablets can only accurately be dosed (0.1 mg/kg q24h) for a 75 kg to 150 kg, lean-weight dog. Splitting of the tablets results in inaccurate estimates of dose with potential for overdose. Unequal dispersion of drug within compounded products may also result in inaccurate dosing. When given per os, NSAIAs must be given with food to protect the gastric mucosa from high localized concentrations of the drug increasing the potential for gastric erosion. However, potential for gastritis/gastric erosion exists with all NSAIAs regardless of route of administration. It is necessary to advise owners on the importance of discontinuing the NSAIA immediately if inappetence or vomiting occurs as this may be the first sign of NSAIA intolerance, or occult inflammatory gastrointestinal pathology unmasked by the NSAIA.[74] Depending on severity of signs and presence of blood, gastric erosions/ulcers may exist requiring urgent assessment and appropriate therapeutic and supportive therapy. Serum creatinine should be measured to rule out renal injury as a cause of symptoms. If identified early, NSAIA-induced renal insufficiency is usually temporary and reversible with drug withdrawal and administration of IV fluids. An elevation in alanine aminotransferase (ALT) can potentially occur with all NSAIAs, and is usually reversible with NSAIA withdrawal. However, rare, acute hepatotoxicity after NSAIA administration has been recognized in dogs.[75] Recent package insert modification for firocoxib in Europe stipulates assessing for subclinical renal and hepatic disease prior to use, which is advisable prior to administration of any NSAIA. An adverse effect of administration of etodolac is keratoconjunctivitis sicca (KCS).[76] The incidence of KCS development is unknown and has not been reported with administration of other NSAIAs. The mean duration of etodolac administration prior to the development of KCS was approximately 8 to 9 months. Most dogs that developed KCS did not respond to treatment.

For specific details on reported adverse effects associated with NSAIA administration in dogs and cats refer to published reviews on this topic.[29-39]

GENERAL CONSIDERATIONS

As a group, NSAIAs are not reversible; it is, therefore, imperative that the general health of the patient be considered prior to prescribing NSAIAs. Where the large animal formulations of a NSAIA exists, it is not advised to dilute or estimate a dose for a cat or dog as a very small volume may easily result in serious overdose. Dosing should be calculated based on the ideal weight of a patient. Anecdotal incidents of single, accidental, large overdoses have been observed with no long-term adverse effects; however, short-term, gastric protection and intravenous (IV) fluids to support renal function is advised with high overdose. Relative overdose resulting in acute renal failure has also been observed in obese patients when dosed on true weight rather than ideal weight. Cats and dogs are more susceptible than people to the adverse effects of NSAIA administration; therefore, the reported safety of any NSAIA approved for the human patient should not be assumed to be so in the veterinary patient and should not be prescribed. Cats are even more of a concern than dogs as the potential for toxicity with certain NSAIAs is greater than for other species due to their limited ability to glucuronidate NSAIAs resulting in a prolonged duration of effect.[38] Carprofen, for example, has double the mean half-life in cats (20 hours with a range 9 to 49 hours), when compared to dogs.[77] Therefore, the potential for drug accumulation with daily administration is a major concern. Duration of efficacy is also difficult to predict due to half-life variability. Single dosing of carprofen has been reported for use in cats following ovariohysterectomy[11] and onychectomy.[37] Ketoprofen shows less variability in metabolism in cats and is approved for repeated dosing in this species. Meloxicam also shows less variability in metabolism and appears to be metabolized by the oxidative enzymes, and therefore daily dosing is possible in cats.[37,38] Meloxicam is approved for use in cats in many countries. A single dose of 0.3mg/kg is approved in the United States; however, it is the opinion of this author and others[38] that a dose of 0.1 or 0.2 mg/kg IV, SC, PO, depending on degree of surgical pain or lower for chronic pain, is effective allowing repeated daily dosing (see Osteoarthritis below). Tolfenamic acid is also approved for cats in several countries, but for only 4 consecutive days. NSAIAs should be restricted to animals older than 6 weeks of age, or may be older depending on the specific product directions. (Firocoxib [Previcox, Merial], for example, requires dogs to be 7 months of age or older.)

INDICATIONS FOR NSAIA ADMINISTRATION

The indications proposed here assume there are no contraindications (below) to their use. Table 158-1 lists recommended dosages.

Postoperative Pain

Patients undergoing orthopedic and selected soft tissue surgical procedures benefit from NSAIA administration, especially where extensive inflammation or soft tissue trauma is present. Opioid administration is beneficial immediately after most surgical procedures, due to the sedative and analgesic effects, to ensure a smooth recovery. Injectable NSAIAs can be coadministered with an opioid initially and subsequently used alone as the repeat analgesic following orthopedic and selected soft tissue surgery. The initial dose of NSAIAs depends on the expected severity of pain. Assuming a difficult fracture repair would require the recommended loading dose, then a laparotomy without complications could be successfully treated with half this dose. The administration of NSAIAs prior to surgical procedures is controversial due to their potential for harm. Some studies investigating preoperative administration of NSAIAs in veterinary patients did not specifically screen for adverse reactions.[31,32] Studies specifically assessing efficacy and safety of NSAIAs given preoperatively, where intraoperative fluid therapy was administered and patient monitoring conducted, noted rare adverse reactions with some of the NSAIAs.[31,32] Preanesthetic administration of meloxicam or carprofen to dogs receiving a painful stimulus for 45 minutes, without "intraoperative fluid administration, showed no significant difference in glomerular filtration rate when compared to saline.[78] Plasma levels of NSAIAs are effectively reached within 1 hour after oral administration, which must be considered when administered preoperatively for postoperative analgesia. A study evaluating the safety and efficacy of administration of meloxicam or carprofen prior to orthopedic or soft tissue surgery, where intraoperative fluids were administered, in both cats (meloxicam) and dogs (meloxicam or carprofen), demonstrated no ill effects.[9] In this study the NSAIA did provide very good to excellent analgesia, for longer than 24 hours, in ~70% of animals that underwent orthopedic procedures. The remaining patients required a much lower dose of the rescue opioid than expected to manage moderate to severe postoperative pain.[9] Meloxicam (Metacam) is approved for preoperative administration at 0.2 mg/kg to be continued q24h at 0.1 mg/kg as needed. Carprofen (Rimadyl) 4.4 mg/kg is also approved for preoperative administration to be continued q24h, or divided q12h. Deracoxib (Deramaxx) is approved for preoperative and postoperative use at 3 mg/kg once daily for 7 days; however, as with all NSAIAs, a reduction in dosing is suggested as soon as the postoperative pain diminishes, which may be 1 to 3 days, to avoid potential gastrointestinal lesions. The benefit of preoperative use of NSAIAs is the potential for a preemptive effect and the presence of analgesia upon recovery. Analgesia during the recovery period is essential. A cautionary note with presurgical administration of NSAIAs (especially COX-1 inhibitors) for oral procedures, including dentistry, is warranted. COX-1 inhibition reduces formation of thromboxane A_2, a platelet-activating and vasoconstricting eicosanoid; this in combination with the fibrinolytic activators present in the oral cavity and saliva, predisposes to hemorrhage. It is recommended that NSAIA administration be delayed until surgical bleeding is no longer a risk. Where NSAIAs are administered postoperatively, opioids should be administered concurrently as 45 minutes are required for therapeutic effect of the NSAIA. Another potential approach for longer procedures is to administer the NSAIA upon near completion of the surgical procedure, 30 to 45 minutes prior to extubation in the

Table • 158-1

Nonsteroidal Analgesic Dosing Regimen per Body Weight*

DRUG	INDICATION	SPECIES, DOSE, ROUTE	FREQUENCY
Ketoprofen	Surgical pain	**Dogs** ≤2.0 mg/kg, IV, SC, IM, PO	Once postoperative
		Cats ≤2.0 mg/kg, SC	Once postoperative
		Dogs and cats ≤1.0 mg/kg	Repeat q24h
	Chronic pain	**Dogs and cats** ≤2.0 mg/kg, PO	Once
		≤1.0 mg/kg	Repeat q24h
Meloxicam	Surgical pain	**Dogs** ≤0.2 mg/kg IV, SC	Once
		≤0.1 mg/kg IV, SC, PO	Repeat q 24h
	Chronic pain	**Dogs** ≤0.2 mg/kg PO	Once
		≤0.1 mg/kg PO	Repeat q 24h
	Surgical pain	**Cats** ≤0.2 mg/kg SC, PO	Once
		≤0.05 mg/kg SC, PO lean weight	Daily × 2-3 days
	Chronic pain	**Cats** ≤0.05 mg/kg SC, PO lean weight. Titrate reduction to comfort ~0.025 mg/kg ASAP.	Once daily Daily or 3-5 × weekly
Carprofen	Surgical pain	**Dogs** ≤4.0 mg/kg, IV, SC	Once upon induction
		≤2.2 mg/kg PO	Repeat q12-24h PRN
		Cats ≤2.0 mg/kg SC lean weight	Once upon induction
	Chronic pain	**Dogs** ≤2.2 mg/kg PO	q12-24h
Etodolac	Chronic pain	**Dogs** ≤10-15 mg/kg PO	Once daily
Deracoxib	Perioperative pain	**Dogs** 3.0 mg/kg PO	Once daily × ≤7 days
	Chronic pain	**Dogs** 1-2 mg/kg PO	Once daily
Firocoxib	Chronic pain	**Dogs** 5 mg/kg PO	Once daily
Tepoxalin	Chronic pain	**Dogs** 10 mg/kg PO	Once daily
Tolfenamic acid	Acute and chronic pain	**Cats and dogs** ≤4 mg/kg SC, PO	Once daily for 3 days. 4 days off. Repeat the cycle.
Flunixin	Pyrexia	**Dogs and cats** 0.25 mg/kg SC	Once
Meglumine	Ophthalmological procedures	**Dogs and cats** 0.25-1.0 mg/kg SC	q12-24h PRN for 1 or 2 treatments
Ketorolac	Surgical pain	**Dogs** 0.3-0.5 mg/kg IV, IM	q8-12h for 1-2 treatments
		Cats 0.25 mg/kg IM	Once only
	Panosteitis	**Dogs** 10 mg/**DOG** ≥30 kg, PO	Once daily for 2-3 days
		5 mg/**DOG** >20 kg <30 kg, PO	
Piroxicam	Inflammation of the lower urinary tract	**Dogs** 0.3 mg/kg, PO	q24h for 2 treatments, then q48h
Acetaminophen	Acute or chronic pain	**Dogs only** 15 mg/kg PO	q8h
Aspirin	Acute or chronic pain	**Dogs** 10 mg/kg PO	q12h

PRN, As required.
*See text for details on the contraindications for use.

stable patient. Ketoprofen is an excellent analgesic but is an inhibitor of both COX-1 and COX-2; therefore, unwanted side effects are a potential problem requiring careful patient selection. It is this author's opinion that ketoprofen be reserved for postoperative use, where hemostasis is guaranteed, to reduce the potential for hemorrhage. Flunixin meglumine is used as an antiinflammatory agent in selected ophthalmologic surgical procedures; however, the potential for side effects is of major concern[31] and potentially safer NSAIAs may be as effective

The four injectable formulations of NSAIAs available have been administered to cats and there appeared to be little difference in the efficacy of the NSAIAs, carprofen, ketoprofen, meloxicam, and tolfenamic acid for the treatment of acute surgical pain.[11] In the United States the injectable formulation of meloxicam is approved for a single preoperative dose at 0.3 mg/kg subcutaneously; however, it is this author's opinion (and others') that this dose is high, and many veterinarians

use lower doses (0.1-0.2 mg/kg, reducing to 0.05mg/kg) with good effect.[38] Carprofen, meloxicam and ketoprofen are now widely used in cats.[8-15]

Inflammatory Conditions

For relief of pain due to meningitis, soft tissue inflammation, polyarthritis, cystitis, otitis, severe inflammatory dermatologic diseases or injury (e.g., degloving, animal bites), NSAIAs appear to be more efficacious than opioids. As many of these patients may be more prone to NSAIA toxicity, careful patient selection and management is advised. Combination opioids and low-dose NSAIAs are also effective in these conditions. An exception may be necrotizing fasciitis, where NSAIAs are reported to increase morbidity and mortality.[79] However, this may be due to masking, through analgesia, of the critical nature of the problem and delaying surgical management rather than the NSAIA having a specific effect on morbidity.

Miscellaneous Conditions

Other indications for the use of NSAIAs are panosteitis, hypertrophic osteodystrophy (HOD), cancer pain (especially of bone), radiation-induced stomatitis in cats, and dental pain[32] (refer to surgical indications above). Ketoprofen or ketorolac (below) is suggested for the management of refractory pain associated with hypertrophic osteodystrophy and panosteitis. The HOD of Weimeraners is poorly responsive to NSAIA therapy and is better treated with high-dose, short-term, corticosteroids, provided infectious disease has been ruled out and clinical signs are consistent with HOD alone.[32]

Osteoarthritis

The NSAIAs certainly improve the quality of life for many dogs and cats with chronic pain due to osteoarthritis. The currently recommended NSAIAs for managing osteoarthritis variably target COX-1 and 2, or specifically COX-2, while sparing the constitutive functions of COX-1. However, as previously mentioned, adverse effects may still occur. Where long-term studies assessing efficacy and adverse effects of NSAIA treatment for osteoarthritis in dogs exist (carprofen, meloxicam, etodolac), adverse effects appear to be minimal; they are predominantly associated with the gastrointestinal tract.[17-25,31-36]

Carprofen was the first of the newer NSAIAs to be approved for canine use and there are several clinical trials evaluating efficacy and safety of this product. Following evaluation of five clinical trials designed to assess the use of carprofen to alleviate the clinical signs associated with osteoarthritis in dogs, Aragon et al concluded there was a moderate level of comfort that the substance and disease relationship is scientifically valid.[29,36] Clinical trials published since this report also support the efficacy of this NSAIA for the treatment of osteoarthritis.[80] Authors of a recent review of treatment for osteoarthritis comment that the strength-of-evidence ranking will likely increase from moderate to high as the number of clinical trials supporting carprofen use for the treatment of osteoarthritis increases.[36]

Etodolac is also one of the earlier approved veterinary NSAIAs. Although evaluation of the efficacy of etodolac was not the primary emphasis of one study, it appeared to be effective for the treatment of osteoarthritis with diarrhea occurring in some dogs.[18] Based on one randomized, etodolac/placebo-controlled study, Aragon et al concluded there was a moderate level of comfort that the substance and disease relationship is scientifically valid.[29,36]

Meloxicam (Metacam) has been evaluated in four clinical trials in dogs affected with osteoarthritis.[19,21-23] In all studies meloxicam was demonstrated to be effective for alleviating lameness. Aragon et al evaluated these four clinical trials and concluded there was a high level of comfort that the substance and disease relationship is scientifically valid.[29,36] Meloxicam has been reported to cause gastrointestinal ulceration; however, the majority of these cases were associated with inappropriate administration including the use of Mobicox.[74]

Deracoxib is reported to be effective for alleviating lameness associated with osteoarthritis in dogs.[20] As no independent clinical trials of deracoxib use are published, Aragon et al were not able to evaluate the clinical evidence regarding deracoxib for the treatment of osteoarthritis.[29,36] Deracoxib has been reported to cause gastrointestinal ulceration; however, the majority of these cases were associated with inappropriate administration.[73]

Tepoxalin, a dual COX/lipoxygenase inhibitor, is approved for management of osteoarthritic pain in dogs and is reported to reduce COX-1, COX-2, and 5-LOX to some degree in this species.[66-68] Tepoxalin has not been evaluated in clinical trials to date; therefore, safety and efficacy in treatment for osteoarthritis in dogs is not known.

Fircoxib is the most recently approved NSAID for administration to dogs and clinical trials have demonstrated its efficacy for treatment of osteoarthritis in this species.[24,25] While these studies were not evaluated by Aragon et al, employing the same criteria as the above-cited studies, others have concluded there is a moderate level of comfort that the substance and disease relationship is scientifically valid for firocoxib.[36]

As many patients with osteoarthritis are geriatric, a rapid reduction, with titration to achieving a comfortable state, is advised to reduce potential toxicity. For example, after titration to effect, administering meloxicam on every second or third day, with half the label-recommended dose, proved efficacious in some dogs during a 12-month period.[19] If a particular NSAIA appears ineffective in managing pain, prescribing a different NSAIA may be effective due to individual variation in response to the different analgesics. However, caution is advised when switching from one NSAIA to another as COX-2 dysregulation within the duodenal mucosa may predispose to ulceration. Currently it is difficult to predict in the individual patient what is a "safe" time to wait prior to starting a different NSAIA. In a recent study where the COX-2 inhibitor firocoxib was administered to dogs after a wash-out period from 1 to 7 days (most commonly >2 days) following discontinuation of another NSAIA, there was no increased risk when compared to a longer washout period.[81] The study examined only administration of firocoxib after another NSAID; therefore, the results cannot be extrapolated to other NSAIDs. Aspirin was not included in this study, which is important to note as aspirin up-regulates COX-2 and acts synergistically with 5-lipooxygenase to produce aspirin-triggered lipoxin, a mucosal protectant within the duodenum.[82] In another study where dogs were administered injectable carprofen followed by oral deracoxib within 24 hours, there was no evidence of NSAIA treatment–related lesions in the gastrointestinal tract.[83] Again, based on the individual intolerance and susceptibility to adverse effects of the NSAIAs, veterinarians and owners must be aware of the potential for gastrointestinal pathology when switching from one NSAIA to another, especially where intolerance to one is the reason for change, and not efficacy.

Osteoarthritis is being diagnosed more frequently in cats and NSAIAs appear to be effective in managing this disease in this species. Clarke and Bennett[26] reported a marked improvement in normal daily activities in 61% of cats, a moderate improvement in 14%, and a slight improvement in 25% within 4 weeks after initiating treatment with oral meloxicam. Ninety-six percent of cats readily accepted meloxicam either orally or in their food. In another study, there was no difference in response to treatment between meloxicam and ketoprofen in cats with chronic musculoskeletal disease, but meloxicam was definitely more palatable.[27] The approved dosing regimen in Australia and Europe for chronic use for meloxicam (Metacam 0.5 mg/mL) is 0.05 mg/kg once daily; however, many cats improve on lower doses (= 0.025 mg/kg) or on every-other-day dosing regimens. It is recommended that following an initial period of 0.05 mg/kg, the daily dose should be lowered to below 0.025 mg/kg as soon as possible to identify those cats that are managed with lower dosages.[38] As with dogs, the lowest effective dose should be used. This cautious approach will protect from potential adverse effects in those who may be susceptible. The kidney, being the more common affected organ in cats, warrants periodic monitoring of renal function. Occasional gastrointestinal effects may also be exhibited. As with dogs, discontinuation of any NSAIA is required should any behavioral changes occur or signs associated with gastrointestinal or renal pathology.

Where the adverse effects of an NSAIA are a concern, in both cats and dogs reducing the dose and adding an opioid may be equally as effective for chronic severe pain. Other options are also available.[36] However, for many geriatric animals with renal insufficiency and increased ALT, NSAIAs may be the only effective class of analgesic; for these animals the quality of life is of major importance. In this situation, a COX-1–sparing/COX-2–preferential NSAIA, at the lowest dose possible, may be suggested. Anecdotal reports indicate that worsening of renal function may not occur in some cats and dogs. Client understanding of potential worsening of renal function and ALT, however, is necessary prior to treatment. Water must be available at all times, and dietary indiscretions and stressful situations must be avoided. During NSAIA therapy all patients should be monitored for a nonspecific change in demeanor (potential first sign of intolerance), vomiting, increased water consumption, and hematochezia or melena. If this occurs, owners should be instructed to stop the medication and consult their veterinarian. Intermittent monitoring of creatinine and ALT is recommended when NSAIAs are prescribed chronically.

PYREXIA

Most veterinary–approved NSAIAs, aspirin, and acetaminophen are effective antipyretics. The antipyretic effect is obtained with a lower-than-analgesic dose. Dipyrone is an excellent antipyretic and is available as tablets and solution for injection. Dipyrone should be given intravenously to avoid the irritation when given intramuscularly. The analgesia produced is not adequate for moderate to severe postoperative pain. Gastric ulceration or nephrotoxicity is not a concern in the short term even in critically ill patients.

CONTRAINDICATIONS FOR THE USE OF NSAIAs

There are many potential interactions between NSAIAs and other medications, many of which are contraindicated during NSAIA use.[71] Nonsteroidal antiinflammatory analgesics should not be administered to patients with acute renal insufficiency, hepatic insufficiency, dehydration, hypotension, conditions associated with low "effective circulating volume" (e.g., congestive heart failure, ascites), coagulopathies (e.g., factor deficiencies, thrombocytopenia, von Willebrand disease), concurrent use of any other NSAIAs or corticosteroids, evidence of gastric erosion (vomiting with or without the presence of "coffee ground" material, melena), spinal injury (including herniated intervertebral disc as most of these patients receive corticosteroids with medical or surgical management). NSAIAs should never be administered to patients in shock, trauma cases upon presentation, or where hemorrhage is evident (e.g., epistaxis, hemangiosarcoma, head trauma). Patients with severe or poorly controlled asthma, or other moderate to severe pulmonary disease, may deteriorate with COX-1–inhibiting NSAIAs, especially aspirin. The administration of NSAIAs in head trauma, pulmonary diseases, or thrombocytopenia may prove to be safe with further study of the COX-2–preferential/COX-1–sparing NSAIAs. NSAIAs may have adverse effects on the reproductive tract and fetus as they may block prostaglandin activity resulting in cessation of labor, premature closure of the ductus arteriosus in the fetus and disruption of fetal circulation.[52] As COX-2 induction is necessary for ovulation and subsequent implantation of the embryo,[52] NSAIAs should be avoided in breeding females during this stage of the reproductive cycle.

Topically applied nonsteroidal antiinflammatory analgesics were significantly more effective than placebo in many human clinical trials involving acute and chronic painful conditions.[32] Topical NSAIAs were not associated with the gastrointestinal adverse effects seen with the same drugs taken

orally.[32] At the time of writing, there are no published studies investigating the use of topical NSAIAs in the veterinary literature for small animals.

NSAIAs NOT APPROVED FOR USE IN VETERINARY PATIENTS (OFF-LABEL USE)

Ketorolac (parenteral formulation and tablets) is comparable to oxymorphone in efficacy and to ketoprofen in duration and efficacy in managing postlaparotomy and orthopedic pain in dogs.[32] Only 1 to 2 doses should be administered. Ketorolac is included for the benefit of those working in the human research setting where the availability of ketorolac is more likely than other NSAIAs. Ketorolac has been used successfully for treatment of severe panosteitis in dogs when all other therapies had failed. Ketorolac given with food for 2 to 3 days in hydrated dogs cured approximately 99%; in the other 1%, signs recurred within a few days to months (unpublished observations). Misoprostol should be coadministered.

Aspirin is available in tablet form. It is most commonly used as an analgesic for osteoarthritic pain in dogs. It is formulated in combination with opioids, codeine or oxycodone for a synergistic effect for the treatment of moderate pain. However, dosing must be based on the aspirin dose rather than the opioid. It is also used as an antipyretic and anticoagulant in dogs and cats.

Acetaminophen is available in tablet form. It may be used as an antipyretic or as an analgesic. It is formulated in combination with opioids, acetaminophen and codeine, or acetaminophen and oxycodone. However, dosing must be based on the acetaminophen dose rather than the opioid . Acetaminophen should not be administered to cats.

Piroxicam (capsule formulation) is valuable for its antiinflammatory effects on the lower urinary tract in dogs with transitional cell carcinoma or cystitis and urethritis. Gastroprotectants are recommended.[84]

NSAIAs OF THE FUTURE

An extended duration of action NSAIA, Trocoxil (mavacoxib, Pfizer), in 6-mg, 20-mg, 30-mg, 75-mg, and 95-mg chewable tablets for dogs, is currently in the final stages of approval in Europe. The labeling is dosing of Trocoxil chewable tablets at 2 mg/kg of bodyweight. The initial treatment should be repeated 14 days later; thereafter the dosing interval is 1 month. A treatment cycle with Trocoxil should not exceed 7 consecutive doses (6.5 months). Trocoxil has an extended effect of duration (up to 2 months after administration of the second dose and following doses). Adverse reactions could occur at any point during this period.

A major concern with such a formulation is the perturbation in PG activity for up to 2 months after administration of a single tablet. Unforeseen situations will jeopardize the health of dogs taking this medication, as will inadvertent consumption by dogs and children, which does occur with many medications.

CONCLUSION

Over several years, many studies have reported the safety and efficacy of NSAIAs in various clinical settings; similar studies investigating the use of the recently approved COX-2–specific and dual cyclooxygenase/lipoxygenase inhibitors, with well-designed prospective large clinical trials and laboratory studies, are anticipated and should further determine the safety and efficacy of these NSAIAs in both the acute and chronic pain management settings. The NSAIAs are very effective analgesics in both the acute and chronic clinical settings. Millions of dogs and cats worldwide benefit from these analgesics on a daily basis. Due diligence on behalf of the veterinarian will reduce the potential for harm.

REFERENCES

The reference list can be found on the companion Expert Consult Web site at *www.expertconsult.com*.

CHAPTER **159**

Antioxidants, Nutraceuticals, and Dietary Supplements

John E. Bauer

Modern veterinary nutrition and food processing techniques have provided complete and balanced food formulations for companion animals that deliver consistent "functional food" ingredients in a convenient package. Recent pet food recalls and food safety concerns notwithstanding, advances in nutrition continue to be made by animal nutritionists and pet food manufacturers. As additional regulatory environments emerge, these advances will provide nutritional benefits beyond our present day understanding of optimal nutrition. Moving in parallel to these improvements, interest among pet owners regarding the benefits of dietary supplements and nutraceuticals also continues to emerge. Thus, pet owners are not only interested in dietary supplements, functional foods, and beverages for themselves but also wish to provide optimized nutrition for their animal companions. Thus it is no surprise that functional ingredients, treats, supplements, and even beverages are now readily available for dogs and cats. However, in spite of the considerable interest in nutraceuticals and dietary supplements, knowledge about their efficacy, modes of action, and safety is often lacking. Where data do exist, much of it may be proprietary and unpublished, or the published studies focus on humans or animals other than companion animals. With the myriad products and supplements currently available, veterinarians are often asked by clients to comment on nutraceuticals and often find themselves recommending some of them for pet health management. Thus it is important to obtain a better understanding of nutraceuticals, supplements, and functional food ingredients. This review, while not exhaustive, will primarily focus on studies that have appeared in the peer-reviewed scientific literature specifically in dogs and cats so that recommendations may be made from this perspective.

REGULATORY ASPECTS

Legal definitions for the term *nutraceutical* do not exist. The word was originally coined to refer to any substance that can be administered orally (as are foods) to promote good health and that is not a drug.[1] The Food and Drug Administration (FDA) defines a *food* as a substance that provides nutrition, taste, or aroma.[2] By comparison a *drug* is a substance that is either a food or nonfood substance used to treat, cure, mitigate, or prevent disease.[2] Drugs, by law, must undergo an approval process that substantiate their safety and efficacy. Therefore an important distinction between a food and a drug exists. In the midst of these definitions, nutraceuticals have found a place for themselves somewhere between foods and drugs. One well-known example of such a substance is fish oil, available in gel capsules from several manufacturers. These and other such substances are in use today in veterinary practice.

Presently, the term *nutraceutical* is used to describe a nutritional component that includes a food, plant, or other naturally occurring material, which may be purified or concentrated, that is used for the improvement of health by preventing or ameliorating a disease. Companies marketing nutraceuticals cannot advertise specific medical claims for their products. In the United States , however, a new product may be eligible for regulatory status as a dietary supplement (i.e., nutraceutical) under the Dietary Supplement Health and Education Act (DSHEA) passed by the U.S. Congress in 1994. The act established a new regulatory body for dietary supplements under the U.S. Federal Drug Administration. Unlike food, dietary supplements have been allowed to use a "nutrition support statement" relating to "structure-function" claims for the material in question.[3] A disclaimer that the supplement has not been evaluated by the FDA must be included on the product label. In addition, a statement that the "... product is not intended to diagnose, treat, cure, or prevent any disease" is also required. Of course, this act facilitated the availability of various nutritional products and supplements for human beings because it considered dietary supplements as a separate food category. It also opened the possibility of certain types of claims (i.e., structure/function claims) to be made without having any scientific evidence submitted to the FDA prior to marketing. However, DSHEA applied only to human foods. Discussion of animal dietary supplements was left out of the deliberations.

With respect to animal foods, responsibility for enforcing all aspects of the Food, Drug and Cosmetic Act that may apply to foods and drugs for animal use rests with The Center for Veterinary Medicine (CVM) of the FDA. This group is involved in reviewing food and feed additives. For reasons beyond the scope of this chapter, the CVM has essentially assigned "low regulatory significance" to most nutraceuticals. As a result, individual states were left to rule on market access to these substances.[4]

GENERAL GUIDELINES FOR DIETARY SUPPLEMENT SELECTION

Four important types of information should be considered when selecting a particular dietary supplement in companion animals, especially if long-term usage is envisioned.[5] The less that is known about a particular substance's information profile, the more cautiously one should proceed regarding dosage, indications, and patient monitoring. These four categories of information, which can be easily recalled using the acronym PETS and can be used to assist discussions with clients about a particular supplement, are briefly summarized below:

- Product Quality (P): The product quality of a substance should be documented and accessible.
- Efficacy (E): Efficacy of any therapy is established by scientific testing. Demonstrating efficacy of a nutraceutical substance requires rigorous and often expensive testing, depending on the extent to which claims for a product are being made and the regulatory environment surrounding that substance. Manufacturers should be asked to supply supportive documentation of efficacy.
- Tolerance (T): Tolerance for any nutraceutical must exist for it to be effective. It must be acceptable by the animal and to the pet owner.
- Safety (S): Safety is paramount and must be known before using a dietary supplement. Historical data on usage of certain substances may provide practical information regarding safety. Using a particular supplement in the absence of any published safety data in the target species is particularly risky and caution is advised.

ANTIOXIDANT NUTRACEUTICALS OF CURRENT INTEREST

Antioxidants and Free Radical Damage

Free radicals are molecular fragments that have at least one unpaired electron. This characteristic makes them highly reactive in biologic and other systems. Free radical reactions are ubiquitous in the animal body. They are associated with oxidation-reduction reactions, energy metabolism, biosynthesis, cell signaling, and body defense and detoxification mechanisms. Their reactivity can be beneficial due to oxidative burst reactions and other mechanisms that characterize neutrophil and other inflammatory cell functions that phagocytose and destroy bacterial invaders. However, when such free radicals are present in excess, oxidative metabolic damage and destruction of normal cell membranes and cell function occurs. Because not all of the molecular species that cause oxidative injury are free radicals (e.g., hydrogen peroxide), a more appropriate term is *reactive oxygen species* (ROS). The ROS are capable of reacting with all biologic molecules, including nucleic acids, proteins, carbohydrates, and lipids. Antioxidant mechanisms to quench these reactions are thus needed to normalize the effects of overabundant destructive cell processes.

Because of the potential adverse effects of ROS, cell systems utilize numerous defensive mechanisms. These systems include: direct interaction with reducing agents (e.g., vitamin C, glutathione); free radical scavenging (vitamin E, vitamin C, carotenoids, superoxide dismutase); reduction of hydroperoxides (e.g., glutathione peroxidase, catalase); removal of transition metals by protein binding (e.g., ferritin, ceruloplasmin, and other chelators); preventing reactive oxygen from reaching specific sites; and even repair of oxidative damage.[6]

The in vivo generation of free radicals and their related oxidative damage can be a consequence of stress, various diseases, aging, trauma, environmental stressors such as cigarette smoke or air pollution, infectious organisms, and other factors. As a by-product of oxidative metabolism, the generation of free radicals can probably not be halted entirely but only kept in check. Because free radicals arising from metabolism or environmental sources interact continuously in biologic systems, the oxidants and antioxidants are in a continual utilization and replenishment cycle that must be balanced to minimize cellular and tissue damage.

One of the most well-studied systems of biologic oxidative processes has been the effect of free radicals on lipid peroxidation in both cell-free and biologic systems. The well-known mechanism of lipid peroxidation consists of three stages: initiation, progression, and termination.[7,8] Initiation of lipid peroxidation occurs by way of the abstraction of a hydrogen atom from a methylene group such as exists on an unsaturated fatty acid by a free radical species. The resulting molecule is now a free radical that can react very rapidly with molecular oxygen to form a peroxy radical. The peroxy radical then abstracts another hydrogen atom from another unsaturated fatty acid to form another free radical species. Because a new free radical is formed, a chain reaction is created resulting in many free radicals being formed from one event. This chain reaction can be terminated when the chain-propagating species reacts with an antioxidant molecule to form non–free radical products. In the meantime, left to propagate, many highly reactive free radical species are formed. In their wake lies the numerous molecular markers of tissue destruction such as lipofuscin pigments, iosprostanes, carbonyl and nitrotyrosine protein derivatives, and DNA fragments. Antioxidants thus have the potential to terminate these chain reactions prior to their generating a large degree of cellular damage and hence provide cells the opportunity to complete their individual life cycles.

Dietary antioxidants that appear to fulfill a similar role in the animal body include the various tocopherols (vitamin E), vitamin C, and beta-carotene. Vitamin C is water soluble while the other two are lipid soluble. Among these free radical scavengers, vitamin E is the most well known and often promoted as a diet supplement or food ingredient. Vitamin E is absorbed from the intestines into the lymph system on lipoproteins then transported to the liver for utilization or storage. Compared to other fat-soluble vitamins (A, D, and K), vitamin E is not as efficiently stored.

Vitamin E

Vitamin E is the major lipid-soluble antioxidant present in plasma, erythrocytes, and tissues. The term *vitamin E* actually refers to a group of fat-soluble compounds known as the tocopherols. Its function as a scavenger of free radicals serves to prevent free radical or oxidative damage to polyunsaturated fatty acids in membranes, thiol-rich proteins of membranes, and nucleic acids. Support for an antioxidant role of vitamin E in vivo comes from observations that synthetic antioxidants can either prevent or alleviate certain clinical signs of vitamin E deficiency diseases. Vitamin E is located in the interior of the cell membrane near the polyunsaturated fatty acids. As such, should lipid peroxidation occur, vitamin E can terminate the process by becoming oxidized to a free radical, sparing any adjacent peroxidation. Vitamin C (ascorbic acid) then combines with the E radical forming a poorly reactive, water-soluble, vitamin C radical, regenerating vitamin E in the process. Vitamin C is the most abundant water-soluble antioxidant and it can directly scavenge ROS or regenerate vitamin E. Vitamin C can be synthesized by both dogs and cats, and hence is not considered a dietary essential. Nonetheless in response to stress, dietary supplementation may be beneficial.[9,10] Vitamin C may also help prevent oxidative damage induced by onion powder or propylene glycol ingestion in cats.[11]

Numerous studies have established vitamin E as an essential nutrient particularly with respect to maintenance of cell membrane integrity.[12,13] Beneficial effects on the canine immune system have also been reported.[14-17] One study reported that large doses improved some parameters of canine immune function. However, the control group in this study was deficient in vitamin E. Thus, it is unclear whether the effects seen were beyond a normal nutritional effect. Also it is unclear whether amounts above those normally required in the diet would be of additional benefit.[18] Other studies have shown in dogs that a prolonged dietary deficiency of vitamin E will cause oxidative damage and degeneration of the retina of the eye, and lead to reduced visual acuity.[19-21]

Beta-Carotene

Beta-carotene is a member of a class of substances called carotenoids that are principal pigments responsible for the red, orange, yellow, and green colors of fruits and vegetables. Beta-carotene along with alpha-carotene, lycopene, lutein, zeaxanthin, and beta-cryptoxanthin are the principal dietary carotenoids. Three of these carotenoids, alpha-carotene, beta-carotene, and beta-cryptoxanthin, can serve as dietary precursors of retinol (all-*trans* retinol, vitamin A). Collectively, these carotenoids are called provitamin A carotenoids or provitamin A. Dietary carotenoids that are not converted into retinol (lutein, zeaxanthin, lycopene) are referred to as *nonprovitamin A carotenoids*. Beta-carotene has been found to have antioxidant activity in vitro. It has been demonstrated to quench singlet oxygen, scavenge peroxyl radicals, and inhibit lipid peroxidation. The mechanism of beta-carotene's antioxidant activity is not clearly understood. Whether beta-carotene has significant antioxidant activity in vivo is unclear. In dogs beta-carotene can be converted to vitamin A (retinol) while cats cannot make this conversion. However, retinol *per se* appears to have low antioxidant activity. Therefore, possible in vivo antioxidant activity of beta-carotene is unlikely to be a consequence of its conversion to retinol.

Antioxidant Combinations

Vitamin E and other supplementary antioxidants are readily available as commercially manufactured over-the-counter products. However, their use as individual dietary supplements is not widespread in veterinary practice. Instead, combinations of antioxidants are often incorporated into present-day pet foods or as supplements containing one or more of these substances. Various combinations fed to dogs or cats have been reported to improve vitamin E status, benefit the adverse effects of exercise on immune function, decrease lipid peroxidation, and improve cognitive function.[22-25] One such combination included vitamin E, vitamin C, α-lipoic acid, L-carnitine, and fruit- and vegetable-based ingredients containing flavonoids and carotenoids in a pet food and noted that some age-dependent cognitive deficits of dogs were improved.[25] To the extent that oxidative stress is involved in the aging process, such an approach may have benefit. Another report of the use of a multiple combination of vitamins E, C, and beta-carotene resulted in increased serum vitamin E concentrations and suppressed a serum biomarker of lipid peroxidation (i.e., total serum alkenyls) in dogs and cats.[24] Also diet supplementation of sled dogs with beta-carotene, lutein, and vitamin E "normalized" adverse effects of exercise on immune status.[22]

Other studies in cats have also looked at potential protective effects of antioxidants in the feline Heinz body model. One bioflavonoid blend was offered before administration of acetaminophen and was found to provide some protection against Heinz body formation but did not prevent methemoglobinemia.[26] When cats were pretreated with vitamin E, vitamin C, or N-acetylcysteine, no beneficial effect on Heinz body formation induced with onion powder was seen. However, administration of N-acetylcysteine was associated with higher relative amounts of reduced glutathione concentrations in whole blood.[11] When propylene glycol was used to induce Heinz body formation, N-acetylcysteine again showed a significant beneficial effect.

OTHER NUTRACEUTICALS OF INTEREST

Chondroprotective Agents

Improvements in pet food quality and feeding practices combined with better veterinary care have resulted in increased longevity of companion animals. However, as with human beings, increased life expectancy has increased the risks for the development of chronic, progressive diseases such as osteoarthritis, obesity, renal failure, and their complications. With increased age, the genetically influenced degenerative diseases such as intervertebral disk disease, hip dysplasia, cognitive disorders, and familial disorders may also become exacerbated. In addition to specialty foods containing substances with purported benefits, dietary supplements to promote healthy joint function are also available. Dietary supplements include glucosamine, chondroitin sulfate, green-lipped mussel, methylsulfonyl methane, and trace minerals such as zinc, copper, and manganese. Many products use combinations of some but not all of these materials. Although it is often difficult to scientifically prove that one particular substance is efficacious when combined with others, there is growing evidence that some of these products have a beneficial effect on joint health. Some mention will be made of combination products that are available. However, to the extent possible, the discussion focuses on effects of single agents such as glucosamine and other compounds.

Glucosamine is an amino sugar and chondroitin sulfate is a sulfated *glycosaminoglycan* (GAG); both are naturally produced in the body. The GAGs are present in joints, tendons, ligaments, skin, and blood vessels. They are long-chain molecules that can hold water and allow the joint capsule to adapt to changes in pressure and therefore absorb shock induced by mechanical stress. Destruction of cartilage is characterized by destruction of the GAGs and loss of this property of the joint capsule. Theoretically, it is expected that provision of supplemental glucosamine to joint tissues will stimulate new GAG production. Data demonstrate that both substances can be absorbed via the gastrointestinal tract in dogs after oral ingestion and are taken up by articular cartilage.[27,28]

Combinations of chondroprotective agents are available. One proprietary product combines glucosamine with chondroitin sulfate and manganese ascorbate. It has been evaluated in several cell culture and animal studies in dogs and other species.[29-32] Survey data of practicing veterinarians indicate relief of pain as well as improved mobility with this type of combination product.[30]

Other substances may also benefit joint health including methylsulfonylmethane (MSM) and green-lipped mussel extracts. Purported benefits of MSM relate to it as a bioavailable source of sulfur, which is a component of several structural compounds found in joints.[33] However, the use of MSM in dogs or cats remains to be fully evaluated. Studies using green-lipped mussel extract, a mixture of glucosaminoglycans and omega-3 fatty acids and possibly other compounds, have been inconsistent in dogs exhibiting chronic lameness, with one study showing efficacy at a higher dose than another study[34,35] Additional proprietary combinations have also been evaluated.[36,37] In these cases, potential benefits of glucosamine may be further enhanced by the addition of other known collagen-matrix components or even antiinflammatory agents.

A biochemical basis for the use of glucosamine in treatment of chronic inflammatory disease has also been shown in the rat model of lipopolysaccharide-induced inflammation. Here it was found that glucosamine inhibits inducible nitric oxide synthesis. Excess nitric oxide mediates the pathogenesis of osteoarthritis.[38] Recently, in human osteoarthritis patients, the long-term effects of glucosamine sulphate have been evaluated using a randomized, placebo-controlled clinical trial (1500 mg orally).[39] Symptom-modifying and structure-modifying effects were found, which suggests the compound could mitigate osteoarthritis. Regarding the safety of this compound, no significant differences in adverse events compared with placebo were found.[39]

Long-term safety studies of the chondroprotective agents in dogs or cats have not been reported. However, some clinical benefit regarding osteoarthritis signs has been observed when the two materials have been fed in combination.[29-31]

Polyunsaturated Fatty Acids

Omega-6 fatty acids (e.g., linoleic acid) may be clinically useful to improve dry, flaky haircoat in which inflammation is not a part. Incorporation of linoleic acid into the lipid ceramide layer of the epidermis imparts a water barrier and provides precursors for physiologically important eicosanoid synthesis to help maintain cell membrane integrity.[40,41] Where inflammation is also present, marine-based eicosapentaenoic acid (an omega-3 fatty acid) may also provide relief of certain skin conditions. Plant-derived 18 carbon omega-3 fatty acids, such as alpha-linolenic acid, may also play a supportive role in the inflammatory response. However, their limited conversion to active long-chain derivatives and favored use as substrate for energy requires substantially greater dietary amounts to achieve such an effect compared with supplying the already-formed long-chain active fatty acids found in fish and marine sources.[42,43] Thus, the 18 carbon, omega-3 fatty acids

are not as potent a source for the above desired effects as are the 20/22 carbon types.

Long-chain omega-3 fatty acids, especially docosahexaenoic acid from marine source, are noted for their preferential role in neurologic development. A recent study showed improvements in retinal function and electroretinographic parameters in puppies from dams who had been fed high marine-based omega-3s during gestation, lactation/suckling, and weaning.[44] It should be noted that products that contain both 18 and 20/22 carbons omega-3 acids should have their labels carefully scrutinized as to the source, types, and amounts of the various fatty acids present. The dosage needed will be different, depending on the intended use of the product and whether vegetable or marine sources are included. High omega-3 fatty acid intake may have adverse effects on immune responses depending on the type and amounts of both omega-6 and omega-3 types.[45] The recommended safe upper limit for marine-based omega-3 fatty acids in dogs has recently been set at 0.37 g/(kg body wt)$^{0.75}$ by the National Research Council.[46]

REFERENCES

The reference list can be found on the companion Expert Consult Web site at *www.expertconsult.com*.

CHAPTER 160

Compounding Drugs

Ron Johnson

One of the greatest challenges to veterinarians can be the availability of appropriate drug dosage forms that enable easier dosing of small dogs and cats and improve owner compliance. Although advances have been made with new drugs and dosage forms approved for veterinary medicine, clearly there is an unmet need with drug formulation options and dosages. As such, drugs approved in one animal species are frequently used in another species, including human-approved drugs. Compounded drugs can alleviate some of the drug-related issues facing veterinary medicine provided compounding is approached in a rational manner. There is little doubt that compounded drug formulations can offer effective and safe delivery options to veterinary patients. Support for this comes from the large number of pharmacies offering compounded drug products for veterinary patients and the increasing number of peer-reviewed journal articles that involve compounded veterinary products. Ultimately, practitioners must ensure that the administration of compounded drugs to animals is justifiable, not driven by economics, and both safe and efficacious.

VETERINARY COMPOUNDED DRUGS: REGULATIONS

The compounding of veterinary drugs has continued to receive increasing regulatory attention. The Food and Drug Administration Center for Veterinary Medicine (FDA-CVM) provides regulatory surveillance and enforcement of drug compounding for veterinarian medicine under the authority of the Animal Medicinal Drug Use Clarification Act (AMDUCA) of 1994, which amended the Food, Drug and Cosmetic Act (FDCA).[1,2] The FDCA, an act of Congress, empowers the FDA-CVM with its regulatory role. The rules (administrative laws) that apply to the FDCA and AMDUCA are codified (arranged) in the Code of Federal Regulations (CFR) and published in the Federal Register by the executive agencies and departments of the Federal Government. The FDA-CVM will at times publish compliance policy guidelines (CPG) in order to facilitate interpretation of the regulations found in the CFR. These guidelines are not law (i.e., they are not legally binding); rather they represent current thinking by the FDA-CVM that may guide its regulatory actions, and can be subject to change over time.

The FDA-CVM does not currently define compounding; however, in an earlier guidance document, the FDA defined compounding as "any manipulation of the product to produce a drug dosage form other than that manipulation that is provided for in the directions for use on the labeling of the approved drug product."[2] This form of compounding will result in extra-label use of the approved drug product. Importantly, AMDUCA legitimizes compounding from approved animal and human drug dosage forms provided certain criteria are met.[1,2] The FDA-CVM also recognizes the need, in limited situations, to compound veterinary products from unapproved drugs and occasionally from bulk products (active ingredient in the unfinished form), provided again certain conditions are met. Compliance Policy Guideline 608.400:

"Compounding of drugs for use in animals," was written by the agency to outline guidelines for compounding from approved animal and human dosage form drugs, and unapproved drugs and bulk drugs that ordinarily will not merit regulatory action even though they are technically in violation of AMDUCA.[2,3]

Recent FDA concerns regarding compounding have focused on pharmacies generating large amounts of unapproved drugs for animal use that are largely copies of FDA-approved drugs. These practices constitute attempts to bypass the drug approval process and can be construed as illegal manufacturing disguised as compounding. The purpose of compounding by a veterinarian or pharmacist (under the order of a licensed practitioner) is to prepare an individualized drug treatment and not manufacture products for resale.[4,5] Position statements by the American Veterinary Medical Association (AVMA) on compounding for veterinary patients largely support the FDA-CVM.[2,6] The AVMA and other organizations such as the American College of Veterinary Clinical Pharmacology and the American Academy of Pharmacology and Therapeutics along with published literature in reputable journals represent valuable sources of information on compounding for animals that may assist the veterinarian with the complex and often confusing regulatory environment surrounding veterinary compounding.

UNDERSTANDING RISKS VERSUS BENEFITS WITH COMPOUNDED DRUGS

Pharmaceutical Issues

Compounding by medical professionals and pharmacists is not equivalent to the formulation of commercially manufactured products by reputable pharmaceutical firms. Drug formulation requires an understanding of the physical and chemical characteristics of the active pharmaceutical ingredient, along with the other agents (e.g., vehicles, excipients) used to produce the administered dosage form, in order to maintain the administered drug's effectiveness and safety profile. To this end, a compounded drug must possess adequate purity, potency, and demonstrate stability (shelf life) to maintain acceptable bioavailability (extent of systemic drug absorption) of the active pharmaceutical ingredient, but not produce toxicity or an ineffective preparation. However, for the vast majority of drugs compounded by veterinarians and most pharmacists, there is a lack of adequate pharmaceutical and clinical testing to ensure quality. Because drug pharmacokinetics, safety, and efficacy have not been determined for most compounded products, and are not likely to be, it is important for veterinarians to establish objective parameters to indicate whether a compounded product is efficacious, subtherapeutic, or toxic.[4] Objective parameters can include hematologic or clinical chemistry changes, serum drug levels when drug monitoring is available, and clinical signs and clinical end-points.

The mixing or combining of drugs or the addition of diluents (e.g., lactated Ringer's solution), vehicles (e.g., propylene glycol, dimethylsulfoxide), or flavoring agents to a drug may produce a chemical or physical interaction that may result in an inactive or toxic compound. Perhaps the most common cause of loss of active drug in a compounded preparation is from alterations in product pH as can occur when protective tablet coatings are disrupted, liquids are added to the product, or vehicles are altered.[7,8] Other evidences of active drug loss and instability of compounded formulations includes color changes (oxidation), separation of product phases or signs of cloudiness or precipitation in liquid dosage forms, or cracking, swelling or release of odors in solid dosage forms.[7] Manipula-

tions of the dosage form can also result in contamination of a sterile product meant for injection or affect drug bioavailability through alterations in drug-release rates. In general, the more extensive the manipulation of a drug preparation from its original formulation, the greater the chance that drug efficacy will be compromised.

While compounding from the finished formulation of an approved drug is recommended whenever possible, there are circumstances in small animal practice that warrant compounding from bulk ingredients. Approved drugs may not be available commercially due to backorder or withdrawal from the human market (e.g., cisapride for the treatment of gastrointestinal disorders in cats).[6] In other cases, there has never been an approved drug formulation containing the required ingredient (e.g., potassium bromide for seizure control).[6] Finally, approved drug formulations may be unacceptable for veterinary compounding for various reasons. When bulk substances are used to compound veterinary products, it is critical that the ingredient source be known and that all components of the compounded product meet either United States Pharmacopeia (USP) or National Formulary (NF) standards or another high-quality source such as analytical reagent or certified American Chemical Society, or have been inspected by the FDA.[9]

Transdermal Delivery of Drugs in Organogels

Transdermal administration of drugs for animals has the potential to be effective, safe, and can certainly enhance compliance. Absorption of drug via the transdermal route is primarily passive. As such, ideal molecules for this route of delivery are low molecular weight (<400 Daltons), lipophilic, and soluble in both water and oil.[10,11] Attention in veterinary medicine has focused on transdermal delivery of various drugs in organogels formulated for pulsed (single dose) therapy versus continuous release reservoirs (e.g., fentanyl patch (Duragesic).[12]

The growing list of drugs available in transdermal organogel formulations from compounding pharmacists includes antimicrobials, anticonvulsants, hormones, antineoplastics, prokinetic drugs, analgesics, and antiinflammatory agents. The vast majority of these compounded products are prepared in a pluronic lecithin organogel (PLO) vehicle. Lecithin is an emulsifying agent that forms a viscous gel when combined with water. Pluronic is a surfactant that enhances the formation of drug-containing micelles in a gel matrix. Together, these carriers can dissolve and deliver either hydrophilic or lipophilic molecules, making them convenient for delivery of a variety of chemical agents. The transdermal route of drug delivery provides for several advantages, including owner compliance, patient tolerance, ease of administration, and, most importantly, the ability to avoid first-pass hepatic metabolism.[10,11] However, the skin is also capable of metabolizing drugs.

Scientific reports of transdermal organogel compounded drug use in small animals, largely limited to cats, have been disappointing. Based on studies conducted in cats administered drugs compounded in PLO, overall systemic bioavailability is low (10% to 20%) compared to levels attained following oral dosing.[12,13] While doses of drugs administered transdermally should probably be increased compared to oral dosage recommendations, individual variation in attained drug levels and potential for drug accumulation following multiple dosing makes prediction of systemic drug levels challenging in the absence of drug monitoring or supporting scientific data. Interestingly, while methimazole administered transdermally in PLO was shown to be poorly absorbed in healthy cats, a separate repeat dose study conducted in hyperthyroid cats was able to demonstrate some clinical efficacy, suggesting transdermal methimazole may be an option in some cases.[14,15] Clinicians must assess both benefit and risk with this mode of drug delivery.

COMPOUNDING BY THE VETERINARIAN AND PHARMACIST: ROLES AND RESPONSIBILITIES

Compounding should be conducted in accordance with good pharmacy and compounding practices, relevant scientific literature, and applicable state laws. Pharmacy facilities used for compounding should have adequate room and equipment, be maintained in a clean and sanitary condition according to standard operating procedures in order to be effective, and prevent contaminations and errors. The USP 31-NF 26 contains a general chapter <1075> that addresses components of good compounding practices. These include responsibilities of the compounder, compounding facilities and equipment, recommendations for minimal training, and requirements for product packaging, labeling, and record keeping.[8] Importantly, there is now recognition of a separate veterinary compounding category by the USP-NF. The FDA Center for Drug Evaluation and Research has put forth a concept paper that evaluates drug products for human use that demonstrate difficulty when compounded because of reasons of safety or effectiveness.[16] The goal of the paper is to identify drugs that are demonstrably difficult to compound based on several evaluating factors that are also pertinent to compounding for veterinary use. Among these evaluating factors, training, facilities and equipment, and testing and quality assurance provides the clearest argument for separating compounding by qualified pharmacists versus the veterinarian, when other than minor manipulations to the product are required.[5,16] Products found notoriously difficult to compound and that should be avoided include sterile products, sustained-release products, and most transdermal delivery systems.[16] In contrast, candidates most suited for compounding includes drugs with a wide therapeutic index, drugs for which therapeutic drug monitoring or quantitative end-point measurements are possible, and drugs for which clinical data regarding their use in the intended species and condition are available.

Whenever possible, drug-specific stability data and literature should be consulted prior to compounding. The stability of a compounded preparation is critical to the determination of an expiry or beyond-use date, after which the compounded product should not be used. Good compounding practice requires all compounded products to be labeled with a beyond-use date. When a manufactured product is used as the active ingredient source for compounding nonsterile preparations, the manufactured product expiration date cannot be used to directly extrapolate a beyond-use date for the compounded product. In the absence of stability data applicable to a particular drug and specific compounded preparation, the conservative maximum beyond-use or expiry dates recommendations outlined in Box 160-1, which have been adopted

---

Box • 160-1

Guidelines for Maximum Expiry Dates for Nonsterile Compounded Drug Products

1. For solid dosage formulations and nonaqueous liquids where the manufactured drug product is the active ingredient source, the beyond-use date should not exceed 25% of the time remaining until the manufactured product's expiration (or 6 months, whichever is earlier). Where a USP or NF substance is the source of the active ingredient, the beyond-use date should be no later than 6 months.

2. For water-containing formulations prepared from active ingredients in solid form such as bulk drug (active ingredient in the unfinished form), capsules, or tablets, the beyond-use date should not exceed 14 days from preparation when the compounded product is cold-stored.

3. For other formulations, the beyond-use date should not exceed the duration of therapy (or 30 days, whichever is earlier) unless supportive stability data for the compounded preparation exists.

NF, National Formulary; *USP*, United States Pharmacopeia.

Box • 160-2

General Recommendations for Compounding Drugs for Companion Animal Use

1. The use of compounded drugs should be based on rational therapy originating from a veterinarian and not a pharmacist.
2. Compounding drugs in order to provide appropriate medical therapy may be necessary when: (i) a legitimate medical need exists such as suffering or death resulting from a lack of treating the affected animal, (ii) an appropriate dosage regimen does not exist for the species, size, age, or medical problem of the intended animal, or (iii) there is no marketed approved animal or human drug available, whether employed in a labeled or extralabeled manner, to treat the condition, or there is reason to believe the approved drugs will not be efficacious or safe in the intended animal.[2]
3. Compounding must be conducted within the limits of a legitimate pharmacy or veterinary practice.[2]
   Legitimate Pharmacist: A person dispensing pharmaceuticals based on a valid prescription while holding a valid license and conforming to state pharmacy laws.
   Legitimate Veterinarian: A person prescribing or dispensing pharmaceuticals based on a valid V-C-P-R while holding a valid license and conforming to state laws.
4. Seek the advice or assistance of pharmacists dedicated to reputable compounding.
5. Compounded drugs dispensed by a veterinarian (or pharmacist) must contain adequate labeling information to ensure safe and acceptable product use, and patient records must be kept.[2,9]
6. Veterinarians dispensing compounded products to be administered by the owner should do so in the confines of informed consent.
7. Compounded products should be sold to the individual client and not to other veterinarians or pharmacists for resale.[4,5]
8. The veterinarian should establish objective parameters that will indicate whether the compounded product is efficacious, subtherapeutic, or toxic.[4]
9. Report any suspected adverse events associated with the use of compounded veterinary products.

V-C-P-R, Veterinarian-Client-Patient Relationship.

from Chapter <795> of USP 31-NF 26, may serve as suggested general guidelines for nonsterile compounded drug products that are packaged in tight, light-resistant containers and usually stored at room temperature.[9]

Compounded products for use in veterinary medicine must be prepared in conjunction with a valid Veterinarian-Client-Patient Relationship (V-C-P-R), and can be compounded either by the veterinarian directly or by a licensed pharmacist under the order of the veterinarian. Other general recommendations for compounding drugs for companion animal use are outlined in Box 160-2.

The lack of FDA-approved animal products at an appropriate concentration, or formulated in a usable dosage form, or available in the required combination are some of the reasons for employing compounded drugs in animals. Also, palatability concerns with various oral preparations have prompted the use of flavoring agents to enhance preparation acceptability. Several pharmacists advocate cheese and fish flavoring with oral medications for cats, while dogs appear to prefer peanut butter, beef, and liver-flavored products.[17] Requests to pharmacists from veterinarians for compounded prescriptions often related to reformulation of human-labeled drugs for use in companion animals, particularly tablets and capsules.[5] Requests for the mixing of multiple drugs in a single product and formulation of novel systems for drug delivery such as transdermal organogels are also increasing. An earlier survey lists potassium bromide, metronidazole suspension, diethylstilbestrol capsules, methimazole liquid and prednisone liquid for oral administration, and protamine zinc insulin among the most commonly compounded veterinary products.[17] Perusal of Web sites for pharmacies offering compounding for veterinary patients supports these products as still being popular amongst veterinarians.

Most pharmacists will compound drugs for veterinarians; however, *substantial care must be exercised when choosing a compounding pharmacist.* Pharmacists with advanced training in compounding can provide valuable expertise and should be sought when the decision to use a compounded drug is made by a veterinarian. With the need for compounding on the rise, many pharmacists have become members of societies dedicated to reputable compounding including the International Academy of Compounding Pharmacists and the Professional Compounding Center of America, as well as veterinary pharmacy specific societies such as the Society of Veterinary Pharmacists and the American College of Veterinary Pharmacists. While encouraging, this underscores the lack of adequate standardized training in the science and practice of compounding by pharmacy schools, and certainly veterinary schools. Clearly, if veterinarians will continue to compound products for their patients, then greater attention must be given to the education of future veterinarians in academic programs, and of practicing veterinarians through continuing education on rational compounding of drugs.

REFERENCES

The reference list can be found on the companion Expert Consult Web site at *www.expertconsult.com.*

CHAPTER 161

Adverse Drug Reactions

Jill E. Maddison
Stephen W. Page

Any harmful and undesirable phenomenon occurring during treatment of a human or animal patient is termed an *adverse event* (AE). When drug treatment is associated with an AE it is termed an *adverse drug reaction* (ADR). An ADR can be defined as "an unintended or unexpected effect on animals, human beings or the environment, including injury, sensitivity reactions or lack of efficacy associated with the clinical use of a veterinary medicine (which includes pharmaceutical, biological and pesticide products)." An algorithm describing the logical process of classification of untoward observations is presented in Figure 161-1.

The study of ADRs, especially during postmarketing surveillance, is now termed *pharmacovigilance,* the science and activities relating to the detection, assessment, understanding and prevention of adverse drug reactions.

All drugs have the potential to result in an ADR. However, because it is frequently difficult to substantiate the cause of an adverse event, it is common to refer to an ADR as a suspected ADR until a clearer picture of etiology emerges. ADRs present a continuum of clinical significance, but of greatest concern are serious ADRs described as adverse drug reactions that are fatal, life threatening, disabling, or incapacitating or which result in permanent or prolonged adverse clinical signs. Figure 161-1 provides an overview of the rational approach to investigating AEs and ADRs.

In veterinary medicine, ADRs that are most frequently reported in dogs and cats involve vaccines, antimicrobial drugs, nonsteroidal antiinflammatory drugs (NSAIDs), ectoparasiticides, anthelmintics and anesthetic agents. These are also among the most commonly used therapeutic or prophylactic agents, thus the higher incidence of these ADRs may reflect usage patterns with the contribution of increased ADR potential more difficult to assess unless associated with an uncommon and unexpected sign (such as blindness in cats).

ADRs can result in additional treatment costs, ongoing disability, mortality, and the client's loss of trust in and diminished satisfaction with the veterinarian. To maintain the highest standards of care and to ensure that ADRs are not needlessly replicated, it is critical that suspected ADRs be fully investigated whenever possible.

CLASSIFICATION

The A to F mnemonic classification of suspected ADRs[1] highlights that ADRs may not only be related to or independent of dose but may also occur over an extended (even intergenerational) time period. Type A (augmented) ADRs are expected but exaggerated pharmacologic or toxic responses to a drug. This may be an exaggeration of the intended

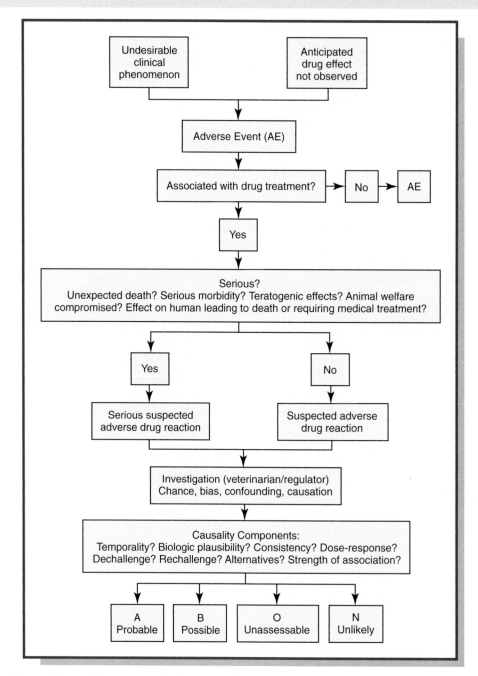

Figure 161-1 • Adverse event classification and a rational approach to investigating adverse events and adverse drug reactions.

response to the drug, a secondary response affecting an organ other than the target organ but predictable based on the pharmacology of the drug, or a toxic response. Most ADRs of this type are attributable to differences in drug disposition that result in higher drug concentrations at the site of action. This may occur as a result, for example, of increased drug absorption, organ failure, reduced protein binding (more likely due to decreased plasma protein than to displacement by another drug), hepatic enzyme induction or inhibition, decreased or absent transport protein function, or inappropriate dosage of a non–lipid soluble drug in an obese dog. They are usually dose-dependent and preventable if sufficient drug and patient information is available.

A second class of ADRs are Type B (bizarre) reactions. These are unexpected or aberrant responses that are unrelated to the drug's pharmacologic effect. They are not dose-dependent and are usually unpredictable and idiosyncratic.

Type B ADRs include allergic reactions, direct toxic effects on organs that are associated with actions unrelated to any desired therapeutic effect (the mechanisms for which may be complex and obscure), and aberrant responses in different species.

There are four further categories of ADR that are less commonly encountered in veterinary practice but nevertheless do occur and should be recognized in order to improve ADR detection and to prevent or minimize recurrences. Type C (chronic) ADRs occur only during prolonged treatment programs, as for example the induction of iatrogenic hyperadrenocorticism with chronic use of prednisolone or other corticosteroid. Type D (delayed) ADRs may be manifested some time after treatment. Second cancers developing in patients treated with alkylating agents such as cyclophosphamide are an example. Another example are clear-cell vaginal adenocarcinomas in daughters of women (inappropriately) administered diethylstilboestrol for maintenance of pregnancy

Table • 161-1

Most Common Signs Reported Related to Adverse Drug Events

DOG: TOP 10 SIGNS*	%	CAT: TOP 10 SIGNS*	%
Ineffectiveness	11%	Ineffectiveness	10%
Vomiting	9%	Death	6%
Anorexia	8%	Ataxia	5%
Depression/lethargy	8%	Vomiting	5%
Diarrhea	7%	Anesthetic recovery prolonged	4%
Death	5%		
Convulsion(s)	4%	Anorexia	4%
Alkaline phosphatase high	3%	Convulsion(s)	4%
		Depression/lethargy	4%
Trembling	3%	Fever	4%
ALT high	3%	Retina abnormal	3%

ALT, Alanine amino transferase.
*% of mentions in top 10 signs of products with at least 500 adverse drug reaction reports on the Center for Veterinary Medicine cumulative database (1987 to 2008).

in the 1950s and 1960s. Type E (end of treatment) ADRs occur when particular drug treatment is terminated suddenly. Examples include withdrawal seizures on terminating anticonvulsant therapy and adrenocortical insufficiency subsequent to cessation of chronic administration of glucocorticoids. Type F (failure of treatment) ADRs are the most commonly encountered ADR (Table 161-1) and can be particularly informative if thoroughly investigated.

There can be a multitude of reasons for treatment failure, and a direct drug-related cause is unusual.

INCIDENCE

The incidence of ADRs in veterinary medicine is difficult to accurately evaluate. Retrospective reviews of a large set of U.S. veterinary medical records recently revealed rates of 38.2 and 51.6 vaccine-associated adverse events per 10,000 dogs or cats vaccinated respectively.[2,3] In human medicine it has been estimated that 3% to 5% of all hospitalized patients are admitted because of an ADR. Some studies give a wide variety of estimates from 1.5% to 35% of patients developing an ADR while hospitalized. The answer to the question "How often do ADRs occur" is "It depends—on how intensively one searches, on what one means by an ADR, and on the group of patients in whom one looks."[4,5]

DIFFICULTIES IN DIAGNOSIS

One of the great challenges in determining the incidence of ADRs is the difficulty in accurate identification of ADRs. Appropriate diagnosis of an ADR is heavily dependent on the expertise of the attending clinician and the quality of the information available. Even experienced clinicians have difficulty in determining causality, and experts have been shown to agree less than 50% of the time when assigning causality to an ADR. Standardized causality algorithms are now routinely used by regulatory agencies but no method is free of individual judgment and inter-rater reliability can be low.[6]

The clinical signs of an ADR are almost always nonspecific and rarely if ever pathognomonic for an ADR. In human medicine the most common symptoms of ADRs (e.g., nausea/

vomiting, diarrhoea, abdominal pain, rash, pruritus, drowsiness, headache) are also reported in 80% of healthy patients on no medication.[7] A similar situation may also exist in veterinary medicine. An examination of the U.S. Center for Veterinary Medicine Freedom of Information summaries for seven NSAIDs reveals that concurrent placebo-treated dogs display similar incidences of the most commonly encountered adverse signs: vomiting, diarrhoea/soft stool, and inappetence. In addition, lethargy, dermatitis, pyrexia, abdominal pain, and even death were reported in the placebo group.

Placebo administration in humans causes an increase in the percentage of patients with symptoms and the number of symptoms per patient. Although a true placebo effect presumably does not exist in animals, veterinarians are reliant on the observations of owners who may be subject to various conscious or subconscious factors that may influence their interpretation of their pet's behavior.

Other factors that contribute to difficulties in determining whether a true ADR has occurred include multiple medications, underlying pathology, and the assumption that it is the active principle of a medication that is responsible for the ADR. Many reactions are due to excipients and some may be due to degradation products formed during storage (e.g., tetra ethyl pyrophosphates in some organophosphate preparations).

Even though all new drugs are extensively evaluated before release onto the market, evaluation before registration cannot ensure the safety of a drug. Premarketing clinical trials are usually too small, conducted for too short a period of time, and conducted in a select and nonrepresentative population to detect rare or delayed ADRs. If clinical signs caused by a drug reaction also occur in untreated populations (see Table 161-1), then additional patients would need to be observed before the reaction can be attributed to the drug. In addition, it is difficult to include in trials all groups of animals including different breeds, the aged, the young, diseased animals, and others that may have a higher risk of developing an ADR. Hence, postmarketing surveillance or pharmacovigilance of drug ADRs is very important in ensuring drug safety, detecting unusual and uncommon ADRs, and identifying individuals or populations at higher risk.

IDENTIFICATION

Any drug has the potential to affect a dog or cat adversely. The justification for using a drug includes a favorable balance of anticipated benefits to potential risks. In life-threatening situations, use of a drug with a narrow therapeutic ratio may be warranted, whereas the use of a drug with a narrow therapeutic ratio to treat trivial problems is more difficult to justify.

The likelihood, frequency, and severity of ADRs are dependent on the interaction of drug, animal, disease, and client factors. Table 161-2 provides information that should allow the risk of ADRs to be reduced in animals with compromised renal or hepatic function. Tables 161-3 and 161-4 identify drugs not recommended for use in cats and drugs where the toxicity profile is different in cats compared to dogs.

Assessment of causality of an ADR can also pose a significant challenge. Figure 161-1 summarizes the major steps in the process of attributing cause. These steps are explained in greater detail elsewhere.[8-10]

FACTORS THAT INFLUENCE TYPE A ADRs

The potential for a Type A ADR is higher in animals with organ dysfunction (see Table 161-2), particularly renal,

Table • **161-2**

Examples of Drugs That Should Be Avoided or Used with Caution in Patients with Hepatic or Renal Disease

DRUG CLASS	AVOID(*)/HEPATOTOXIC([†]) OR USE WITH CAUTION IN LIVER DISEASE	AVOID(*)/NEPHROTOXIC([†]) OR USE WITH CAUTION IN RENAL DISEASE
Antimicrobial drugs	Chloramphenicol	Aminoglycosides*[†]
	Chlortetracyclines*	Amphotericin*[†]
	Erythromycin estolate*	Fluoroquinolones
	Flucytosine	Lincomycin
	Griseofulvin	Naficillin
	Ketoconazole	Nalidixic acid
	Lincosamides	Nitrofurantoin
	Macrolides	Polymyxins[†]
	Metronidazole	Sulphonamide-trimethoprim
	Sulphonamide-trimethoprim*[†]	Sulphonamides
	Sulphonamides	Tetracycline (except doxycycline)
	Tetracyclines	
Anesthetics (general/local)/sedatives/ anticonvulsants	Barbiturates*[†]	Acepromazine
	Chlorpromazine	Chlorpromazine
	Diazepam[†]	Ketamine
	Halogenated anesthetics	Methoxyflurane*[†]
	Ketamine	Procainamide
	Lignocaine	
	Propofol	
Cardiac drugs	β-blockers	Angiotensin-converting enzyme inhibitors*[†]
	Lignocaine	Cardiac glycosides
	Quinidine	Procainamide
Diuretics		Spironolactone
		Thiazides
Antiinflammatories/analgesics	Butorphanol	Nonsteroidal antiinflammatories*[†]
	Corticosteroids	Pethidine
	Meclofenamic acid	Polysulphated glycosaminoglycan
	Phenylbutazone	
	Polysulphated glycosaminoglycan	
Cytotoxic drugs	Doxorubicin	Cisplatin*[†]
		Doxorubicin*[†]
		Fluorouracil
		Methotrexate*[†]
Miscellaneous	Doxapram	Allopurinol
	Heparin	Doxapram
	Suxamethonium	Gallamine
		Piperazine

hepatic, or cardiac dysfunction; in extremely young or old animals; in animals being given a number of drugs concurrently (potentially including all nonprescribed medications); in species for which safe use of the drug or class of drugs has not been established (see Tables 161-3 and 161-4 in relation to cats); and in obese or cachectic pets. Some factors result in qualitative differences in the effects of the drug and may preclude its safe use. Other factors may produce a quantitative change in the usual effects of the drug that can be offset by appropriate adjustment in dosage regimen. In general, type A ADRs should be preventable if the above factors are considered and dosage regimens are altered appropriately. The reader is referred to other sources for a more complete discussion of these factors.[8,11]

PHARMACOGENETIC DIFFERENCES

Pharmacogenetics refers to the effect of genetic and genomic differences between individuals on drug pharmacologic behavior. Genetic variability in the proteins responsible for drug transport, biotransformation (the enzymes of phase I and II processes), and receptors is heritable and determined by specific changes in the nucleotide sequences of specific genes. Genes in which particular nucleotide differences are present in at least 1% of the population are termed *polymorphic*. Heritable differences in a number of important hepatic enzymes have been well known in humans for decades. Application of pharmacogenetics to dogs is more recent and even fewer studies have been completed in cats. For example, there is a

Table • 161-3

Drugs Not Recommended for Use in Cats

Acetaminophen (paracetamol)	• Methemoglobinemia and Heinz body anemia
Apomorphine	• Significant central nervous system depression
Azathioprine	• Bone marrow suppression
Benzocaine	• Methemoglobinemia
	• Laryngeal edema
Cisplatin	• Fatal, acute pulmonary edema
Propylthiouracil	• Lethargy
	• Weakness
	• Anorexia
	• Bleeding diathesis
Phenytoin	• Sedation
	• Ataxia
	• Anorexia
	• Dermal atrophy
Scopolamine	• Tendency to cause behavioral changes
Sodium phosphate enemas	• Depression
	• Ataxia
	• Vomiting
	• Bloody diarrhea
Permethrin (high-concentration products)	• Hyperesthesia, generalized tremors, muscle fasciculations, hyperthermia, seizures, death

fourteenfold difference in activity of CYP2B11 (which metabolizes propofol) amongst mixed breed dogs. Other important pharmacogenetic differences affect N-acetyltransferase (involved in sulphonamide metabolism), thiopurine S-methyltrasnferase (involved in azathioprine metabolism), and P-glycoprotein (ABCB1) (mutations can result in increased substrate availability leading, for example, to ivermectin and vincristine toxicity).[12,13]

TYPE B ADVERSE DRUG REACTIONS (HYPERSENSITIVITY)

Type B ADRs are unrelated to dose, are difficult to predict, and, therefore, difficult to avoid. The major example of idiosyncratic ADRs or Type B ADRs are allergic or hypersensitivity reactions. Drug hypersensitivity reactions are more common in pets with a prior history of allergic reactions to the drug or atopic patients but they can occur in any individual.

Penicillin-induced hypersensitivity is the most well-characterized drug-induced hypersensitivity in small animals. Other drugs that have been reported to cause allergic reactions include sulphonamides, doxorubicin, penicillamine, dipyrone and quinidine. In humans, allergic drug reactions account for approximately 5% to 10% of ADRs.

Any component of a drug preparation may induce a hypersensitivity reaction and microbiologic contamination may also stimulate a hypersensitivity reaction. Relatively few drugs are responsible for inducing allergic drug reactions as most drugs are not capable of forming covalent bonds with proteins, a requisite step to render a molecule immunogenic. The drug/drug metabolite-protein complex must have multiple antigenic-combining sites to stimulate a drug-specific immune response and to elicit an allergic reaction. For those drugs that

Table • 161-4

Drugs That Are Therapeutically Useful in Cats but That May Have Different Toxicity/Activity Profiles Than in Dogs

Aspirin	• Hyperpnea
	• Hypersensitivity
	• Hyperthermia
Chloramphenicol	• Anemia
Digoxin	• Vomiting
	• Anorexia
	• Bradycardia
	• Arrhythmias
Doxorubicin	• Renal failure
Enrofloxacin	• Blindness
Furosemide	• Dehydration
	• Hypokalemia
Griseofulvin	• Leukopenia and thrombocytopenia
	• Nonreversible ataxia
Ketoconazole	• Dry haircoat
	• Weight loss
Lidocaine	• Myocardial and CNS depression
Megestrol acetate	• Mammary hypertrophy and neoplasia
	• Cystic endometritis
	• Diabetes mellitus
Methimazole	• Anorexia
	• Vomiting
	• Self-induced facial excoriation
	• Bleeding diathesis
	• Hepatopathy
	• Serious hematologic side effects
Metronidazole	• Disorientation
	• Ataxia
	• Seizures
	• Blindness
Opioids	• Inconsistent sedation
Morphine derivatives (excluding meperidine [pethidine], butorphanol and buprenorphine)	• Increased risk of excitation
Organophosphates	• Acute toxicity: hypersalivation, vomiting, diarrhea, muscle tremors
	• Chronic or delayed toxicity: paresis or paralysis that may or may not be reversible
Potassium bromide	• Greater prevalence of adverse effects in cats compared to dogs
	• Respiratory adverse effects reported: asthma (may be fatal), coughing of sufficient severity to lead to euthanasia or discontinuation of medication
Tetracyclines	• Hepatic lipidosis
	• Increased ALT activity
	• Ptyalism
	• Anorexia
Thiacetarsemide	• Drug fever
	• Respiratory distress
	• Fulminant pulmonary edema

ALT, Alaninie amino transferase; *CNS*, central nervous system.

are capable of inducing an immunologic response, it is generally the metabolites of the drug that are chemically reactive and that easily form covalent bonds with macromolecules.

Cross reactivity to other apparently unrelated drugs can occur if the particular portion of the drug molecule that is acting as the hapten also occurs in pharmacologically disparate groups of drugs. For example, the sulphamyl group is present in sulphonamide antimicrobial drugs as well as in furosemide/thiazide diuretics, the sulphonyl-urea group of oral hypoglycemic agents (e.g., glipizide and some coxibs). Thus an animal that has a reaction to a sulphonamide may also react to these seemingly unrelated drugs

Drug hypersensitivity may manifest in different ways. Acute anaphylaxis is associated with IgE and mast cell degranulation. It is characterized by one or more of the following clinical signs: hypotension, bronchospasm, angioedema, urticaria, erythema, pruritus, pharyngeal and/or laryngeal edema, vomiting, and colic. The main shock or target organ for anaphylactic reactions varies between species (e.g., hepatic veins are the main target in dogs and the bronchi, bronchioles and pulmonary vein in cats). Drug- or vaccine-induced anaphylaxis will generally be apparent within minutes to hours of drug administration, but can be delayed.

A systemic allergic reaction may also occur associated with drug use related to deposition of immune complexes in tissues and activation of complement. Clinical signs include nephritis, lymphadenopathy, neuropathy, vasculitis, arthritis, urticaria, and fever. Various hematologic perturbations may occur related to drug-induced antibody production resulting in hemolytic anemia, thrombocytopenia, and rarely agranulocytosis. Cutaneous reactions may also occur related to development of immune complex deposition or delayed hypersensitivity. Prior exposure to the drug is not essential as hypersensitivity may develop over the course of repeated drug administrations. In humans, 5 to 7 days is required for drug-drug hypersensitivity to develop in a patient previously unexposed to the drug.

Allergic drug reactions should be managed by withdrawing the drug and treating with corticosteroids if needed. Adrenaline and fluid therapy may be needed for acute anaphylactic reactions.

PSEUDOALLERGIC DRUG REACTIONS

Drug reactions may occur that resemble drug allergies but do not have an immunologic basis. These reactions are often termed *anaphylactoid reactions* and do not require prior exposure to the drug. They occur most frequently when a drug is given rapidly intravenously. Anaphylactoid reactions may be due to nonspecific release of mediators of hypersensitivity or can be due to the direct effects of the drug on tissues.

References

The reference list can be found on the companion Expert Consult Web site at *www.expertconsult.com.*

SECTION **VIII**
Dietary Considerations of Systemic Problems

CHAPTER **162**

Probiotics

Mary H. Bowles

Use of probiotics has been gaining popularity as a form of complementary or alternative medicine and is gradually becoming part of mainstream medical therapy and disease prevention. Probiotics have been defined by the World Health Organization as "live microorganisms, which when administered in adequate amounts, confer a health benefit on the host."[1] Within a few days of birth, the gastrointestinal (GI) tract (especially the colon) of animals and people develops a diverse population of microorganisms from the environment.[2-4] A portion of this population, notably *Lactobacillus*, *Bifidobacteria*, and *Enterococcus* bacteria, have the capability of providing protection against infectious agents and other potentially harmful substances. These bacteria also enhance beneficial immunologic responses.[4]

Following oral administration, probiotics are theorized to exert their beneficial effects by inhibition of pathogenic intestinal microorganisms through competition for nutrients and receptor sites, immunomodulation mechanisms, enhancement of gut digestion and pH balance, and alteration of host microorganism metabolic activity.[5,6] Probiotics should not be confused with *prebiotics*, defined as nonliving, nondigestible food ingredients such as oligosaccharides that beneficially affect the host by selectively stimulating growth of and/or activating the metabolism of a limited number of health-promoting bacteria in the intestinal tract.[7] When a probiotic is combined with a prebiotic for the purpose of producing a synergistic effect, the mixture is referred to as a *synbiotic*.[8]

FERMENTED DAIRY PRODUCTS

Fermented dairy products have been recognized for many years as a source of probiotics. In some cases, specific probiotic agents are actually added to such products to fortify the potential beneficial effects. However, in order for a probiotic to be safe and effective in the intestinal tract, the following conditions must be met: live microorganisms must be stable in product storage; present in large numbers; able to survive passage through the acidic gastric environment; nonresistant to antibiotics; and nonpathogenic, nontoxic, and incapable of absorption into the bloodstream following consumption.[9,10] Potential for beneficial effect also depends upon the interaction of the specific genus, species, and strain of the microorganism administered with the particular host species being treated.[9] Yogurt has long been advocated as a palatable, effective probiotic dairy product. Because pasteurized yogurt results in a product with heat-killed bacteria, nonpasteurized yogurt with live cultures is the logical choice for probiotic effect. Nonfortified yogurt generally contains *Lactobacillus bulgaricus* and *Streptococcus thermophilus*, organisms with questionable probiotic activity. Fortified yogurt frequently has added *Lactobacillus acidophilus* and *Bifidobacterium* species, enhancing the potential probiotic benefit.[11]

Although fermented dairy products and other products designed as human probiotic supplements may be beneficial to dogs and cats, relatively few controlled studies document their usefulness in promoting health or in preventing and treating disease. Controlled feline and canine studies supporting efficacy are also lacking in regard to products designed as pet foods or veterinary supplements with putatively probiotic or synbiotic ingredients. Probiotics are considered food supplements and are not subject to the same regulations applied to drugs. The results of two published studies reflect this lack of regulation, indicating that commercial probiotic supplements, especially veterinary products, are often poor in quality and that pet foods with probiotic additives frequently have inaccuracies related to probiotic content on the label.[9,12]

A variety of human health benefits have been attributed to the consumption of probiotic and synbiotic supplements (Box 162-1). Research efforts have indicated that some of these same benefits would occur in animals. Improved immune response, including increased fecal and blood levels of IgA, has been demonstrated in dogs and cats fed probiotics.[4,13,14] Control of pathogenic organisms through decreased numbers of fecal *Clostridia* and reduction in plasma endotoxins were observed in cats fed probiotics.[4,15] Similarly, fecal *Clostridia* species counts decreased in dogs fed a daily probiotic.[16]

POTENTIAL USE OF PROBIOTICS IN DOGS AND CATS

Probiotics appear to have the most potential for use in dogs and cats as nutritional aids in the treatment and prevention of diarrhea (Box 162-2). Reestablishing microbial flora after or during antibiotic administration has been one of the recognized benefits attributed to probiotics. When antibiotics are administered either as a specific treatment or prophylactically to prevent systemic infection, the functions of the normal microbial flora of the GI tract are altered. This disruption of

627

Box • 162-1

Human Health Benefits Attributed to Probiotics and Synbiotics

Gastrointestinal and Hepatic
Restoration of bacterial GI balance following administration of NSAIDs, glucocorticoids, antibiotics
Reduction of pathogenic bacterial intestinal overgrowth and fecal shedding of potentially pathogenic organisms such as *Salmonella, Campylobacter, Clostridia, Escherichia coli*
Prevention and treatment of traveler's (stress) diarrhea
Prevention and treatment of food allergies
Treatment of inflammatory bowel disease
Prevention of bacterial translocation from the intestine
Treatment of infection with *Helicobacter pylori*
Treatment of irritable bowel syndrome
Prevention and treatment of viral diarrhea in infants
Prevention and treatment of hepatic encephalopathy
Enhancement of mucosal immune system
Improvement in digestion of lactose
Modulation of mineral absorption
Reduction in oxalate absorption

Respiratory
Treatment of respiratory infection and allergies

Urogenital
Prevention and treatment of vaginal infections
Prevention and treatment of urinary tract infections
Reduction in formation of oxalate-associated uroliths

Dermatologic
Treatment of skin infections
Treatment of atopy

Miscellaneous
Positive effect on blood lipid levels and cholesterol
Production of anticarcinogenic effects
Reduction of blood pressure
Reduction in dental disease
Reduction in body fat and weight gain
Enhancement of cellular immunity and systemic immune responses
Reduction in inflammation associated with arthritis
Enhancement of growth
Enhancement of coagulation factor production
Promotion of antioxidant activity
Reduction in mutagenicity

From Laflamme DP: Bugs and guts: probiotics and the gastrointestinal tract. Research Report VET 11(1):2-5, 2007; Probiotics: considerations for human health. National Dairy Council Digest Archives, 2008. http://www.nationaldairycouncil.org/National DairyCouncil/Health/Digest. Center SA: Metabolic, antioxidant, nutraceutical, probiotic, and herbal therapies relating to the management of hepatobiliary disorders. Vet Clin North Am Small Anim Pract 34(1):67-172, 2004; Getting to know "friendly bacteria." CAM at the NIH: Focus on Complementary and Alternative Medicine 13(2): 2006. Available at: http://nccam.nih.gov/news/newsletter/2006_summer/bacteria.htm. Accessed May 20, 2009.
GI, Gastrointestinal; *NSAIDs*, nonsteroidal antiinflammatory drugs.

Box • 162-2

Causes of Canine and Feline Diarrhea Potentially Responsive to Probiotic Administration*

Medication-induced diarrhea
  Antibiotics
  NSAIDs
  Glucocorticoids
Stress-related diarrhea
  Boarding
  Travel
  Weaning
  Shelter or colony populations
  Working dogs
  Environmental changes
Viral, bacterial, or protozoal GI infections
Inflammatory bowel disease
Dietary change or indiscretion
Food intolerance or allergy
  Lactose intolerance
Maldigestion or malabsorption disorders
Small intestinal bacterial overgrowth
Spontaneous (idiopathic) diarrhea

From Laflamme DP, Bugs and guts: probiotics and the gastrointestinal tract. Research Report VET 11(1):2-5, 2007; Reynolds A, Simpson KW, et al: Probiotics: enhancing gastrointestinal health—a roundtable discussion. VET 1226 PVD Probiotics Roundtable: 2007. Available at: http://www.purinavets.com.
GI, Gastrointestinal; *NSAIDs*, nonsteroidal antiinflammatory drugs.
*Probiotic administration not recommended in patients less than 3 weeks of age or patients that are severely debilitated, immunosuppressed, or in acute phases of canine parvovirus or feline panleukopenia infection.

function suppresses protective mechanisms related to immune responses, toxin control, and containment of potentially pathogenic microorganisms.[4] The end result can lead to the development of diarrhea and/or other clinical signs of illness in the antibiotic-treated patient.

Multiple placebo-controlled human studies in adults and children have demonstrated efficacy in treating and reducing antibiotic-associated diarrhea using probiotics.[18-20] Many of these human studies support the concurrent administration of probiotics when administering antibiotics to reduce the incidence of diarrhea resulting from therapy, including antibiotic therapy for *Helicobacter pylori*.[21]

Feline and canine diarrhea unrelated to the administration of antibiotics may benefit from probiotic administration as well. The previously cited studies indicating reduction in *Clostridial* species counts in dogs and cats fed probiotics suggest that bacteria-related diarrhea may improve with probiotic therapy. Kittens fed a probiotic from weaning to 1 year of age had a markedly reduced incidence and duration of diarrhea episodes when compared with a control group of kittens.[4] A study indicating protection from *Giardia*-related GI signs and decreased duration of fecal shedding in gerbils suggested that probiotics have potential for management of recurrent *Giardia*-associated illness in dogs.[22] Bacterial species commonly used in probiotic preparations have been shown to reduce inflammation in mice serving as animal models for human inflammatory bowel disease.[23] Some evidence also exists that immunomodulating mechanisms and other potentially protective interactions with intestinal microflora may result from the use of probiotics in cats and dogs with inflammatory bowel disease.[24] Studies in rats and humans have indicated that probiotics and synbiotics may be helpful in the presence of liver disease to prevent bacterial translocation from gut to liver and to act prophylactically or therapeutically in those at risk for developing clinical signs from hepatic encephalopathy.[25] Although it has been suggested that feeding prebiotics and probiotics may be beneficial in dogs with lactose intolerance, food allergy, or small intestinal bacterial overgrowth, the proposed benefits have yet to be supported by controlled studies.

Probiotics and prebiotics have the potential to bring about positive effects in organ systems other than the GI tract. Preliminary evidence exists which indicates that urinary tract disorders may also derive benefit from probiotic administration. A study involving evaluation of in vitro oxalate degradation by canine and feline lactic acid bacteria and various prebiotics suggests that these agents could decrease levels of intestinal oxalate, reducing intestinal oxalate absorption.[26] Reduction in oxalate absorption could then result in decreased renal oxalate excretion, ultimately decreasing the potential for oxalate urolith formation. One synbiotic (Azodyl, Vetoquinol) has been marketed as a veterinary product to reduce azotemia and signs of uremia in cats and dogs with renal failure through intestinal metabolism of nitrogenous waste products. The manufacturer states that this synbiotic consists of the bacterial species Enterococcus thermophilus, Lactobacillus acidophilus, and Bifidobacterium longum. The prebiotic component consists of oligosaccharides that stimulate growth of colonic bifidobacteria. Evidence of efficacy of this synbiotic preparation in cats and dogs has been limited, but a canine, placebo-controlled study is currently being conducted.

Many probiotic preparations have been marketed for use as human or veterinary supplements. Most do not have published, well-designed studies to support manufacturer claims. When considering the administration of a probiotic or synbiotic as part of a treatment or prevention plan, it is best to select preparations from well-established companies. The manufacturer should disclose the number of live, microbial colony-forming units (CFU) available per unit weight as well as the specific genus, species, and, ideally, strain of each organism. The optimum guaranteed concentration of live microorganisms has not been established, but information presently available suggests numbers should be in the range of 1×10^8 to 1×10^{12} CFU/g of product to have the best chance of colonization of the GI tract and resulting efficacy.[17,27,28] Current information suggests that a minimum oral daily dose of 1×10^8 CFU/g should be administered for therapeutic effect.[27] Duration of administration depends upon the nature of the disorder being treated, ranging from a few days for acute diarrhea to several months for chronic disorders such as inflammatory bowel disease. The microorganisms administered are only transient residents of the GI tract. Consequently, when probiotics are indicated, they must be administered on a continuing basis to achieve the desired effect.[4] When given to maintain GI health in conjunction with antibiotic therapy, the probiotic should be administered for several days to weeks following discontinuation of antibiotic administration. If given concurrently with an antibiotic, the probiotic should be administered at a different time of day.

The specific microorganisms used as probiotics presently are usually not of canine or feline origin and vary with the manufacturer. Microorganisms most likely to be useful in a probiotic preparation administered to cats or dogs are the lactic acid bacteria Lactobacillus, Bifidobacterium, and Enterococcus bacterial species as well as the yeast Saccharomyces boulardii.[4,29] Lactobacillus acidophilus strain DSM13241 and Enterococcus faecium strain SF68 are two bacterial strains with information available indicating ability to survive in the GI

tract and provide immunomodulating efficacy.[27,28] Probiotics with lactic acid bacteria or Oxalobacter spp. have potential for use in the prevention of oxalate urolith formation.[26,30] Evidence in humans suggests that L. rhamnosus GG and Bifidobacterium Bb12 may be beneficial in reducing clinical signs related to allergies.[31] In addition, L. rhamnosus GG may provide protection against urogenital infection.[17] Fortified yogurt (e.g., Activia-Dannon—Bifidobacterium animalis DN 173010) has been shown to stabilize human intestinal transit, aiding in the production of more regular bowel movements.[32] Recently a veterinary probiotic supplement featuring a canine origin strain of B. animalis has become available (Prostora Max, IAMS). This supplement is currently being marketed in a chewable tablet form for enhancement of GI health in the dog.

STABILITY IN STORAGE AND HANDLING

Stability in storage and handling is an important issue in administering probiotics, considering that the cornerstone of their use is tied to the product containing live organisms. Particular attention should be paid to the manufacturer's recommendations concerning storage, administration, and shelf life. In general, products that are freeze-dried, microencapsulated, or contained in capsules, sachets, or, in some cases, tablets are more likely to deliver viable organisms when administered.[17,27,33] Such products include Azodyl (Vetoquinol—Enterococcus thermophilus, Lactobacillus acidophilus, Bifidbacterium longum), Fortiflora (Purina Veterinary Diets—Enterococcus faecium strain SF68), Prostora Max (IAMS—canine origin B. animalis), and Culturelle (Amerifit Brands—Lactobacillus rhamnosus strain GG). Fortified yogurt can be used as a probiotic, but variation in viability and concentrations of microorganisms is a limiting factor for its use.[23,27]

SAFETY AND POTENTIAL ADVERSE REACTIONS

Safety and potential adverse reactions must also be addressed when using probiotics. Food and Drug Administration designation of the chosen supplement's microorganisms as Generally Recognized As Safe (GRAS) is desirable. In general, probiotics should be used in dogs and cats older than 3 weeks of age that are not markedly debilitated with disease, immunosuppressed, or afflicted with severe clinical signs of intestinal infections such as canine parvovirus or feline panleukopenia.[25,27] In these situations the pet would be put at risk for opportunistic and, possibly, systemic infection developing from the probiotic microorganism itself.

CONCLUSION

Efficacy of probiotics in cats and dogs will undoubtedly become better defined as controlled studies with specific microbial strains in a canine or feline host are conducted. Host specificity of the various probiotic microbial strains is an important factor in determining efficacy of these microorganisms in maintaining health and preventing or treating disease. Currently, a microbial strain of B. animalis is the only probiotic of canine origin available, but Lactobacillus species have been isolated from the canine intestinal tract. The continued development of canine and feline origin probiotics offers the potential of expanding the role of probiotics as therapeutic and prophylactic aids in veterinary medicine.[34]

REFERENCES

The reference list can be found on the companion Expert Consult Web site at www.expertconsult.com.

CHAPTER 163

Nutritional Genomics

Dottie P. Laflamme
Steven S. Hannah

The recently completed sequencing of the human, feline, and canine genomes has ushered in the postgenomic era of medicine and nutrition, where new technologies are causing a shift in biomedical research and practice. Genomic sequencing efforts, coupled with advances in biotechnologies, have enhanced the ability to identify genes associated with disease and allowed the measurement of gene transcripts (mRNA), proteins, and metabolites associated with health and disease. Application of these technologies facilitates the ability to study the interactions between nutrients and gene expression, referred to as *nutritional genomics* (Figure 163-1).[1]

These approaches have already had an impact on human and veterinary clinical practice, and will continue to do so at an ever-increasing rate in the future. Therefore, it is important that veterinarians have an understanding of the mechanisms and applications of nutritional genomics.

WHAT IS NUTRITIONAL GENOMICS?

All cells in a body carry the same DNA. Yet, not all cells in the body express the same genes, allowing for different cells types. Controlled expression of genes is what allows the development of a phenotype, whether on a cellular level or a whole animal level. And expression of genes can be altered in response to environmental changes, including those caused by diet, drugs, or disease. The recognition that gene expression is important in a wide range of diseases and health conditions, and not just in inherited diseases, has contributed to the rapidly developing fields of functional and nutritional genomics. Genomics is defined variably, but generally refers to the study of the functions, interactions, and dynamics of all the genes in a cell or organism. This differentiates it somewhat from genetics, where the inheritance patterns of individual genes or traits are studied.

Nutritional genomics, or *nutrigenomics*, is the study of the interaction between dietary factors and gene expression. From one view, it reflects attempts to identify anomalies in genes (e.g., hereditary conditions) that might benefit from nutritional modification. This approach, best referred to as *nutritional genetics*, focuses on the genotypic variation of individuals and the subsequent phenotypic response to diet. This science also leads to the concepts of "personalized nutrition" or "tailored nutrition," as it focuses on the special needs of an individual or select group of individuals. Examples of this include

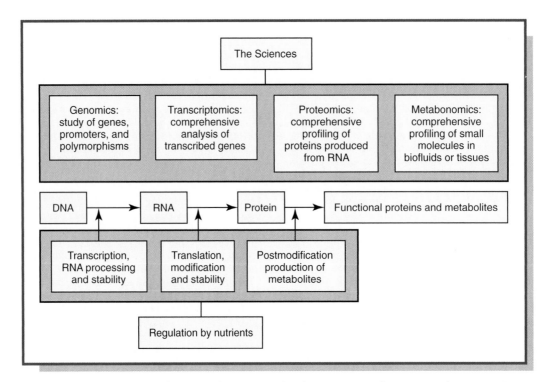

Figure 163-1 Science of nutritional genomic technologies. An animal's genetic makeup (DNA) cannot be changed, but its phenotype (expression of DNA) can be influenced by diet. This chart shows the steps from DNA to metabolites in the living organism, and the focus of each component of the sciences of molecular nutrition or functional genomics. (Adapted from Elliott R, Ong J: Nutritional genomics. Brit Med J 324:1438, 2002.)

inborn errors of metabolism such as phenylketonuria in humans, heritable diet-responsive hypercholesterolemia, or copper storage disease toxicosis in dogs. Taurine-responsive dilated cardiomyopathy in cats is another example of an interaction between genetics and nutritional need. The genetic basis for this problem suggests a heritable limitation on taurine absorption, metabolism, or excretion that can be overcome with additional intakes of taurine.[2]

On the other side of the nutritional genomics coin is the study of how diet can affect the global genome. Simply changing from a high-fat diet to a low-fat diet alters the expression of genes involved in metabolism, lipogenesis, and gluconeogenesis.[3] Understanding that nutritional modification can alter the expression of genes in such a way as to promote health or fight disease, this science focuses on improving nutritional health in the population at large. One example of this global effect is the up-regulation of genes encoding for antioxidant enzymes, resulting in reduced oxidative stress as well as reduced blood pressure, in animals fed soy isoflavones.[4] Another example is the role of dietary protein on protein turnover and protection of lean body mass. A classic study in dogs showed that total transcription rates (cellular RNA content) were more sensitive to inadequate protein intake, compared to the standard measure of nitrogen balance.[5] Clinically relevant was the demonstration that older dogs required 50% more protein to achieve a similar level of protein turnover compared to young dogs. Much more recently, the mechanisms by which specific amino acids in protein modify gene expression and protein turnover have been confirmed, as discussed later.[6]

Yet another application of nutritional genomics is to explore changes in gene expression associated with disease states, and attempt to correct these using dietary modification. One example of this includes the use of eicosapentaenoic acid (EPA) to reduce expression of inflammatory cytokines and chondrodestructive matrix metalloproteinases in canine osteoarthritis. Another example is the use of retinoic acid (vitamin A) to promote leukocyte maturation in the treatment of acute promyelocytic leukemia.[7]

HOW IS GENE EXPRESSION CONTROLLED?

Canines and felines, like all multicellular organisms with many cell types, must control gene expression so as to provide different cell lineages needed to develop various tissues and organs. For example, neurons and hepatocytes contain identical DNA, yet these cells are quite different because different subsets of genes within the DNA are expressed in each cell respectively. Differentiation of the tissues and organs occurs primarily during embryonic development, with different sets of genes being switched on and off. As one can imagine, a tremendous amount of regulation is required to ensure proper development of these tissues and organs. Regulation of gene expression within a differentiated, or mature, cell also occurs and is now recognized as a major regulatory point by which organisms adapt and survive in an ever-changing environment.

The expression of genes is controlled at multiple levels, including transcription (from DNA to RNA), translation (from RNA to protein), and posttranslational (modifications to activate or alter the function of a protein). Dietary molecules can affect the expression of genes, and it appears that about 80% of the direct effects of nutrients on gene expression occur at the level of transcription.[8]

A primary mechanism controlling gene expression is through the binding of specific transcription factors to sites on the DNA. Cells monitor their local environments for changes in extracellular conditions, usually via binding of extracellular molecules to cell-surface receptors. These extracellular molecules include signals from other organs of the body (e.g., hormones, cytokines, chemokines), threats to the cell (e.g., antigens, pathogens), substrates and products of metabolism (e.g., amino acids, organic acids, fatty acids), as well as various factors and cofactors needed for metabolism and other physiologic processes (e.g., vitamins, minerals, trace elements). Each of these classes of extracellular molecules represents signals to specific cell types.

The binding of signaling molecules to surface receptors initiates various mechanisms to transfer the information into the cell, triggering the appropriate cellular response. Often these mechanisms involve the process of signal transduction, a cascade of biochemical reactions resulting in the production or activation of a transcription factor that enters the nucleus and binds to DNA. Binding of the transcription factor to specific sites on the DNA modulates the expression of the target gene via a conformational change in the DNA that promotes or inhibits transcription.

Some genes produce factors (proteins) that can modify transcription of other genes. One such group of proteins is the nuclear receptor family. Nuclear receptors regulate the expression of genes involved in numerous physiologic functions, such as metabolism, reproduction, and development. The endocrine receptors that mediate the actions of steroids and thyroid hormones are perhaps the best known of these. Many other nuclear receptors have been discovered and their targets identified. One example is the family of peroxisome proliferator-activated receptors (PPAR α, γ, δ), which are activated by polyunsaturated fatty acids and eicosanoids, as well as other factors.[9] PPARγ is a regulator and promoter of adipogenesis, but also plays important roles in cellular differentiation, insulin sensitization, atherosclerosis, and cancer.[9] These nuclear receptors themselves can be regulated by dietary and pharmaceutical means. Dietary fat promotes an increase in fatty acid oxidation in the liver via a PPARα pathway, while PPARγ responds to increased dietary fat by up-regulating fat storage in adipose tissue.[3] The antidiabetic thiazolidinedione compounds (e.g., rosiglitazone) work by activating PPARγ, causing an up-regulation of genes involved in insulin sensitization.[7] Retinoic acid (vitamin A), used at pharmacologic doses, activates nuclear receptors to trigger the maturation of immature leukemic white blood cells in acute promyelocytic leukemia, supporting a cure rate reported to be near 90%.[7]

Nutrient modulation of gene expression is certainly not limited to effects on transcription. The translation step itself is regulated by a diverse array of mechanisms, including some involving macronutrients such as amino acids. A well-characterized example of amino acid–induced regulation involves a protein kinase referred to as the *mammalian target of rapamycin* (mTOR). The branched-chain amino acids, particularly leucine, work through the mTOR pathway to stimulate protein synthesis in skeletal muscle. In addition, leucine up-regulates other mediators of translation, facilitating the ribosomal binding of mRNA and initiation of translation into protein.[6] Leucine may also enhance insulin sensitivity in muscle, stimulating yet another pathway for protein synthesis.[10] In vivo, these effects of leucine result in an increase in muscle protein synthesis.

APPLICATION OF NUTRIGENOMICS TO VETERINARY PRACTICE

The advances in research technologies and bioinformatics have created the ability to study the impact of nutrition on phenotype in fine detail, identifying nutrient-gene interactions and nutrient-responsive biologic pathways. This should allow rapid advances in nutritional management of diseases, as well as improvements in nutrition to promote overall health. These same technologies are currently in use by pharmaceutical companies, and should result in more effective and safer drugs as well.

What can a veterinary clinician expect from companion animal nutrigenomics? Consider a scenario in which a dog's examination includes gathering genetic information identifying the dog's predisposition to various health issues. From this information, the veterinarian can provide a dietary regimen specifically targeting these risks to minimize the likelihood of onset (e.g., altering the expression of genes through diet so as to alter the disease phenotype). This example would represent the "nutritional genetics" application of nutrigenomics. In another scenario, a veterinarian might diagnose osteoarthritis in a dog and prescribe a diet that significantly reduces the pain and progression of the disease. It is likely that the development of that diet included research on how specific dietary components impacted not only specific metabolic enzymes and structural proteins but also the transcription of genes involved in arthritis. So while the veterinarian may not recognize the "genomic" contribution to the diet, indeed the field of nutritional genomics proved critical to the development of that diet.

Some current areas of application of nutritional genomics to veterinary nutrition are in the fields of obesity, diabetes, cardiology, oncology, and osteoarthritis. Recent studies in obesity confirmed that overfeeding high-fat diets leads to overexpression of numerous genes resulting in a decrease in insulin sensitivity, as well as increased expression of genes involved in inflammation, matrix formation, angiogenesis, and endothelial dysfunction.[11-13] Likewise, expression of GLUT-4

glucose transporter is significantly reduced in obese cats, contributing to insulin resistance is these animals.[14] Changes with weight loss included up-regulation of genes supporting insulin function.[15,16] However, hundreds of genes remain altered in animals following weight loss, including some associated with appetite regulation and adipogenesis, which may contribute to increased risk for weight rebound.[16] In addition to obesity itself, dietary composition can impact gene expression: isocalorically fed high-carbohydrate diets and high-fat diets induced very different changes in gene expression, and high-fat diets were associated with higher fasting blood glucose concentrations.[16] This may have implications for how obese-prone pets should be fed.

SUMMARY

Some nutrigenomic research already has led to commercial and clinical applications, such as diets for the nutritional management of canine osteoarthritis. Nutrigenomic research currently is underway in various fields such as obesity, diabetes, cardiology, oncology, and osteoarthritis. It is anticipated that other studies will result in improved knowledge about disease pathology and better treatment options, including dietary, for numerous conditions in the coming years.

REFERENCES

The reference list can be found on the companion Expert Consult Web site at *www.expertconsult.com.*

CHAPTER 164

Nutritional Assessment

Kathryn E. Michel

The purpose of nutritionally assessing a patient is to allow the clinician to answer the question, "Is intervention for this patient necessary?" and to aid the clinician in selecting the most appropriate nutritional intervention for that patient. The process involves evaluating both subjective and objective information regarding the patient and its dietary practices. In addition to aiding in the selection of a suitable diet and feeding management for the patient, it will also help the clinician to anticipate potential problems or complications and to devise strategies to avoid or monitor such developments.

TAKING A DIET HISTORY

The more information that is available about the patient's diet and feeding management, the better the clinician will be able to assess the adequacy of nutrient intake, the suitability of feeding practices, and the urgency for nutritional intervention. At the core of a dietary history is the careful gathering of information that will give an accurate picture of the foods that

the patient consumes. Ideally the person who is most responsible for feeding the patient should be questioned; however, it is important to find out who else resides in the household or has regular contact with the patient, including other pets. The patient's caregiver should be questioned about all foods that the patient receives (Box 164-1) and asked whether the information reflects what is typical for this pet, whether changes have occurred, and if so when they happened.

In addition to particulars about the patient's diet, the history should also include information regarding appetite, documented or perceived changes in bodyweight or condition, level of physical activity, and occurrence of any gastrointestinal (GI) signs. Again, the patient's caregiver should be queried as to whether the information reflects what is typical for this pet or whether (and if so when) changes have occurred. Although it is often the case that a pet owner cannot precisely recount an exact weight change, he or she may have an impression of the period of time over which the change occurred. Rapid weight loss and deterioration in body condition, particularly if associated with muscle wasting, suggests a greater degree of metabolic derangement or reduction in

Box • 164-1

Information to Be Included in a Diet History

- Commercial pet foods (brand and daily portion; dry foods should be weighed or measured with an 8-oz measuring cup; canned foods should be measured by can size and portion used)
- Commercial treats (brand, size, and frequency of use)
- Table foods or scraps (detailed information about type of food, portion size, and frequency of use)
- Treats for chewing (e.g., rawhide, pig's ears; size and frequency of use)
- Dietary supplements (brand and daily portion)
- Foods used for medication of the patient (type of food, portion size, and frequency of use)
- Pet's access to garbage
- Pet's ability to scavenge or roam

food intake (or both) and greater potential for significant malnutrition than a more gradual loss of weight.

PATIENT ASSESSMENT

Evaluation of body condition is the chief consideration in the assessment of the animal. Although some sophisticated techniques are currently being used in human patients or in a research setting (e.g., multiple-frequency bioelectrical impedance, dual-energy radiographic absorptiometry [DEXA], neutron activation), they have either not been sufficiently validated in companion animals or do not lend themselves to a clinical setting because of logistic considerations or expense. Body condition scoring, although subjective, is simple to learn, requires no special equipment, and has been shown to be repeatable and consistent among multiple observers.[1] The body condition scoring systems that have been published for companion animals are principally based on characterization of body silhouette and palpation of body fat (see Chapter 1). These systems are useful, particularly for identification of patients that have an overweight body condition; however, they may misclassify some malnourished patients. It is important to recognize that catabolism of lean body tissue can occur very rapidly and may account for a disproportionate amount of the body mass lost in sick patients. Although the purpose of adipose tissue is to serve as an energy reserve, no analogous reserve of endogenous protein exists. Because all endogenous protein is serving some function, continuous catabolism will eventually have deleterious consequences for the patient. Therefore, the process of body condition assessment should include not only the standard evaluation of body silhouette and evaluation of adipose tissue as assessment of energy reserves but also a separate evaluation of muscle mass as a subjective means of assessing lean tissue status. This can be accomplished by palpation of skeletal muscle over the axial skeleton and other bony prominences.

Other aspects of the physical examination of a patient that should be taken into consideration include haircoat quality and skin condition, evidence of peripheral edema or ascites (which may indicate hypoproteinemia), and clinical signs that may indicate specific micronutrient deficiencies such as neck ventriflexion or tetany.

SPECIAL CONSIDERATIONS REGARDING ASSISTED FEEDING

No definitive tests are available for establishing a patient's nutritional status. However, based on the information gathered from the patient's medical and dietary history and physical examination (as described previously), the clinician should be able to classify broadly the patient as being well nourished, mildly malnourished, or severely malnourished. The decision whether to intervene with some form of nutritional support for a patient has to balance the anticipated benefits with the potential risks and costs of the proposed intervention. Therefore, the intent of nutritional assessment should not simply be to diagnose inadequate food intake or malnutrition, but rather to identify patients that are at risk of a poor outcome as a result of their compromised nutritional status. Investigations of human patients have found increased risk of morbidity and mortality associated with various objective markers of nutritional status including hypoalbuminemia, lymphopenia, and attenuated delayed hypersensitivity reactivity. Other investigators have found that clinical assessment of patients based on a carefully performed history and physical examination, as described previously, has predictive value similar to that of objective markers of nutritional status such as serum albumin concentration.[2] Furthermore, investigations of the effect of nutritional support on improving clinical outcome suggest that the most significantly malnourished patients are the most likely to show benefit from nutritional support.[3]

There has been only limited investigation of the prognostic value of nutritional assessment in veterinary patients. Admission serum albumin concentration has been shown to correlate with risk of poor clinical outcome in critically ill dogs, and elevation of serum creatine kinase activity has been found to be associated with anorexia in feline patients.[4,5] To date there have not been any investigations of the prognostic value of subjective nutritional assessment or the impact of nutritional support on clinical outcome in companion animals; however, it is not unreasonable to expect results similar to those found in human patients. Therefore, it is recommended that patients assessed to be significantly malnourished on presentation or that are at risk of becoming significantly malnourished in the course of their illness due to decreased food intake, malassimilation of diet, or metabolic derangement, should be considered candidates for assisted feeding.

MONITORING NUTRITIONAL INTERVENTIONS

Once a dietary recommendation has been made, the patient should be reassessed after an appropriate interval of time. The actual timing of reassessment depends on the severity of the patient's illness and the type of nutritional intervention it has received. One should determine whether the prescribed recommendations are being followed if problems with diet acceptance or tolerance are seen, if the desired outcomes have been achieved, or if any adverse events associated with the diet or feeding management have occurred. A thorough nutritional assessment at the outset will often identify potential problems or complications and thereby determine what parameters should be monitored in the patient. At the least, bodyweight and condition should be reassessed regularly to ascertain that the patient is maintaining, gaining, or losing weight appropriately.

REFERENCES

The reference list can be found on the companion Expert Consult Web site at *www.expertconsult.com*.

CHAPTER 165

Body Composition of the Dog and Cat

Denise A. Elliott

Understanding body composition is essential for studying changes that occur with physiologic processes such as health, growth, aging and disease. Knowledge of body composition can be advantageous in the field of exercise physiology and athletic performance, where an optimal fat-to–lean tissue ratio may maximize performance. Objective quantification of body composition can also be used to assess nutritional status, to better understand and treat pathophysiologic processes associated with disease, and to monitor the effects of interventional therapies. A major clinical application of body composition analysis is to evaluate malnutrition. Obesity is the most prevalent form of malnutrition, affecting 25% to 30% of dogs and cats.[1,2] The ability to accurately measure body composition facilitates understanding of the causes and effects of obesity as well as short- and long-term responses to weight-reduction programs. Assessment of body composition is also crucial in the management of hospitalized dogs and cats at significant risk of protein-calorie malnutrition with depletion of the fat-free mass and associated body cell mass.[3] Alterations of body composition associated with critical illness can contribute to increased morbidity and mortality. Therefore, precise methods for the early assessment of body composition in critically ill animals are particularly important as medical and dietary interventions may be able to prevent or improve nutritional status and outcome in these patients.

Numerous methods exist for the assessment of body composition (Box 165-1). The most accurate way to establish the chemical composition of the body is by a direct method—chemical analysis of a cadaver. Although considered the "gold standard" criterion for the assessment of body composition, it is clear that this technique is not applicable for clinical evaluation of body composition or for monitoring serial changes in body composition. Indirect techniques including densitometry, total body potassium, computed tomography (CT) scans, magnetic resonance imaging (MRI) scans, total body electrical conductivity, and neutron activation analysis are not readily available. The remainder of this discussion will focus on clinically applicable methods.

The techniques to assess body composition are derived by subdividing the body into two or more physiologically distinct components (Figure 165-1). The traditional two-compartment model divides body weight into the fat mass (FM) and the fat-free mass (FFM).[4] Assessment of body composition in the form of FM and FFM provides valuable information about the physical and metabolic status of an individual. The FM can be considered to represent a calorie or energy storage depot. Conversely, the FFM may reflect the actual health of an animal. It is a heterogeneous entity consisting predominantly of total body water, minerals, glycogen, and protein. The FFM contains the body cell mass (BCM), which is the metabolically active part of the body responsible for determining most of the resting energy expenditure.[5] The BCM encompasses those lean tissues most likely to be affected by nutrition or disease over relatively short periods. Furthermore, the FFM is generally accepted as an index of protein nutrition, and therefore changes in FFM over time are assumed to represent alterations in protein balance.

The two-compartment model is dependent upon assumptions regarding the character of the FFM and the FM. The composition of the FFM is assumed to be relatively constant with a density of 1.1 g/mL at 37° C, a water content of 72% to 74%, and a potassium content of 50 to 70 mmol/kg. In addition, the major constituents of the FFM are presumed to be present in fixed ratios. In comparison, the FM is relatively homogenous in composition, anhydrous and potassium free with a density of 0.900 g/mL at 37° C.

BODY WEIGHT

Body weight is the simplest technique to assess body composition, and it should be included in the examination of every dog and cat. It not only provides a rough measure of total body energy stores but, in general, changes in weight parallel energy and protein balance. In the healthy animal, body weight varies little from day to day. Since there may be wide variation between scales, it is important to use the same scale for an individual animal each time it is examined. It is also important to use scales adapted for the size of the patient. Smaller scales are required for cats and toy breed dogs versus

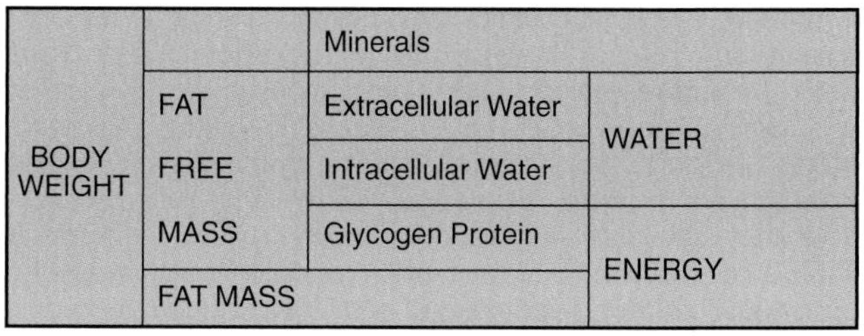

Box • 165-1

Techniques Available to Assess Body Composition

Clinically relevant	Research techniques
Body weight	Densitometry
Body condition score	Computed tomography
Cachexia score	Magnetic resonance imaging
Morphometric measurements	Total body electrical
Dilution techniques	conductivity
Bioelectrical impedance	Total body potassium
analysis	Neutron activation analysis
Dual energy x-ray	Cadaver analysis
absorptiometry	

Figure 165-1 Composition of the body based on the two compartmental model of body composition.

those utilized for large dogs. Scales should be routinely calibrated using standard known weights.

The problem with knowing body weight is that, by itself, it has little meaning. Knowledge that a Labrador Retriever weighs 70 pounds means little; the dog could be overweight, underweight, or in ideal body condition. Therefore, body weight should not be used in isolation. Body weight can be falsely altered by dehydration or fluid accumulation. In addition, body weight does not give an estimate of individual body compartments. For example, an overweight dog with heart failure may still have a loss of lean body mass that will not be detected by measurement of body weight.

BODY CONDITION SCORE

The body condition score (BCS) provides a quick subjective assessment of an animal's overall body condition. The two most commonly used scoring systems in small animal practice are a 5-point system, where a BCS of 3 is considered ideal, or a 9-point system where a BCS of 5 is considered ideal (Figure 165-2).[6,7]

The BCS in conjunction with body weight provides the clinician with a more complete perspective on body condition (see Chapter 1). It should be recorded in the medical record at every visit. Limitations of BCS include subjectivity inherent in scoring and interobserver variation. Finally, like body weight, BCS gives an overall assessment of body condition; it cannot differentiate between body compartments and does not provide any precise quantitative information concerning alteration in FFM relative to FM.

CACHEXIA SCORE

In many critically ill patients, weight loss is disproportional such that there is substantially greater loss of the metabolically active FFM compared to FM. This condition has been termed *cachexia*. In humans, skeletal muscle mass can be predicted by the circumference of the midarm muscle, the midarm muscle area, or the creatinine-height index. To the author's knowledge, such techniques have not yet been reported for cats or dogs. Initial loss of lean body mass can be subtle and is usually first noted in the epaxial, gluteal, scapular, or temporal muscles. Utilizing a subjective cachexia scoring system will facilitate the identification of those patients either with cachexia or at risk of impending cachexia (Table 165-1).[8]

MORPHOMETRIC MEASUREMENTS

Height and circumferential measurements of the abdomen, hip, thigh, and upper arm are commonly used to estimate percent body fat in humans. Pelvic circumference and distance from hock to stifle have been shown to predict body fat in dogs.[9] Circumferential measurements have also been developed to estimate the percent body fat in cats.[10] The Feline Body Mass Index (FBMI) is determined by measuring the rib cage circumference at the level of the ninth cranial rib (Figure 165-3, *A*) and the leg index measurement (LIM), which is the distance from the patella to the calcaneal tuber (Figure 165-3, *B*).

The percent body fat can be calculated as:

$$(1.54 \times \text{ribcage circumference}) - (1.58 \times \text{leg index measurement}) - 8.67$$

DILUTION TECHNIQUES

Total Body Water (TBW)

Dilution techniques rely on the principal of $C_1V_1 = C_2V_2$: that is, the volume of a biologic fluid can be calculated following the administration and equilibration of a known concentration of tracer. The tracer administered should be nontoxic, nonmetabolizable, easy to administer, and have the same distribution volume as the fluid under investigation. The TBW method relies on the assumption that fat has a negligible water content and the FFM has a fairly constant and known water content (mean 73.2%; range 0.70% to 0.76%).[11] FFM can be calculated as TBW/0.732, and since BW = Fat + FFM, an estimation of body composition can be made. The potential concern with this technique to determine body composition is the assumption of the hydration factor of the fat-free mass, which may change with age, sex, species, breed or disease.[12]

Isotopes of hydrogen (deuterium [D_2O] and tritium [^3H_2O]), urea, alcohol, N-acetyl-4-aminopyrine, and H_2O^{18} distribute in the TBW compartment and have been employed to quantify TBW. The most common method is dilution of the stable isotopes D_2O or H_2O^{18}. While these techniques have been successfully completed in dogs and cats and are appropriate for noninvasive studies, they do require expensive analytical equipment.[13-16] Deuterium and tritium undergo some exchange with nonaqueous H^+ and hence can overestimate TBW by 3% to 5%. H_2O^{18} provides the most accurate measure of TBW, although ^{18}O will exchange with labile oxygen atoms and hence can overestimate TBW by 0% to 1%.

Extracellular Fluid (ECF)

ECF is an important physiologic component of TBW that can be altered in illness. ECF can be measured by use of compounds including inulin, $^{35}S_2O^{3-}$, $^{35}SO_4^{2-}$, $^{34}SO_4^{2-}$, SCN^-, $^{36}Cl^-$, Br^-, and $^{82}Br^-$, which distribute within the extracellular space. However, some ECF markers may not distribute uniformly in the subcompartments of the ECF (plasma, interstitium, lymph, connective tissue), some markers penetrate cells to an extent that they cannot be precisely determined, or they may bind to some degree to endogenous components. Bromide is the most useful, safe, and widely used tracer for determination of ECW volume.[17] Simultaneous measurement of ECF and TBW enables the estimation of intracellular water (ICW) (i.e., ICW = TBW – ECW). ICW most closely approximates the BCM.

BIOELECTRICAL IMPEDANCE ANALYSIS (BIA)

Bioelectrical impedance analysis is an electrical method of assessing body composition that has the potential of estimating TBW, ECW, ICW, BCM, FFM, and FM. The composition of the body is calculated by measuring the nature of the conductance of an applied electrical current in the patient. Body fluids and electrolytes are responsible for conductance while cell membranes produce capacitance. Since adipose tissue is less hydrated than lean body tissues, more adipose tissue results in a smaller conducting volume or path for current and larger impedance to current passage. The FFM contains virtually all the water in the body, and thus if bioelectrical impedance is measured, a value for FFM can be determined.

A BIA test is performed by placing four small electrodes on the body, in a classic wrist/ankle configuration. The current is introduced from the distal electrodes. As it travels through the body, it experiences a slight delay due to cells, prior to detection by the proximal electrodes. Low frequencies (e.g., 5 kHz) pass primarily through the ECW because of high cell membrane capacitance. In contrast, at higher frequencies the

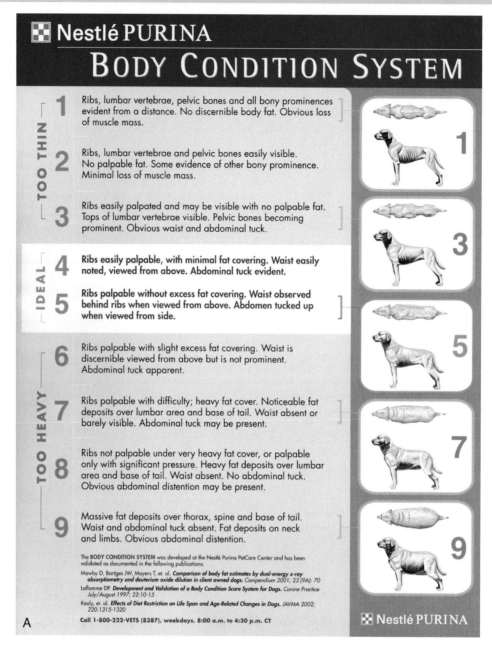

Figure 165-2 **A,** Nine-point body condition scoring system for dogs.

Table • 165-1

Subjective Cachexia Scoring System

CACHEXIA SCORE	DESCRIPTION
0	Good muscle tone, no evidence of muscle wasting
1	Early, mild muscle wasting, particularly noted in the hindquarters and lumbar region
2	Moderate muscle wasting evident in all muscle groups
3	Marked muscle wasting, with atrophy in all muscle groups
4	Severe muscle wasting

Data from Freeman LM: Nutritional modulation of cardiac disease. Waltham Focus 10(2):19-24, 2002.

effects of cell membrane capacitance are diminished, so the current flows through both the ICF and ECF environments, or TBW.

BIA may be affected by hydration status, consumption of food and water, skin and air temperature, recent physical activity, conductance of the examination table, patient age, size, shape, and posture, in addition to electrode positioning. Reliable BIA requires standardization and control of these variables. BIA requires further evaluation and validation in disease states, especially those associated with major disturbances in water distribution and states such as sepsis, which may alter cell membrane capacitance. It has been shown to be a safe, noninvasive, rapid, portable, and reproducible method to estimate body composition in healthy dogs and cats.[18-20] Calculation of ECF-ICF takes approximately 1 minute; hence BIA provides instantaneous quantitative information of body composition.

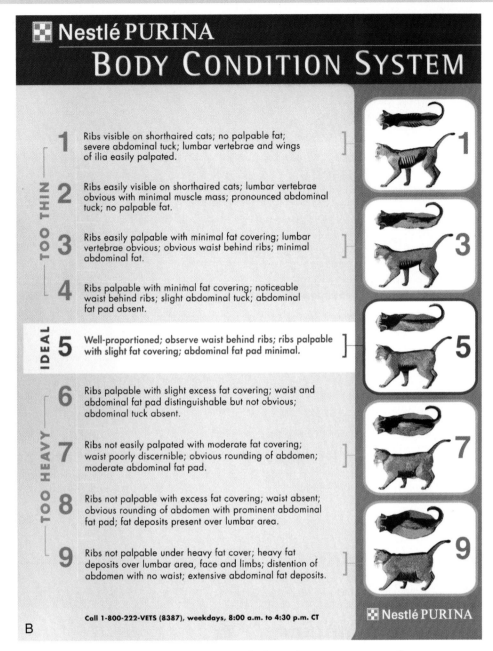

Figure 165-2, cont'd B, Nine-point body condition scoring system for cats.

DUAL-ENERGY X-RAY ABSORPTIOMETRY (DEXA)

DEXA is a technique originally developed for precise measurement of bone mineral content (BMC). However, it is now also used to measure both body fat and nonbone lean tissue. DEXA uses photons of two different energy levels (70 and 140 kVp) to distinguish the type and amount of tissue scanned. The x-ray source is positioned underneath the table supporting the patient, with the detector housed in an arm above. During a scan the source and detector move together over the patient. The detector measures the amount of x-rays that pass through the subject. The photons of the two different energy levels are impeded differently by bone mineral, lipid, and lean tissue. Algorithms are used to calculate BMC, FM, and lean body mass.

DEXA is safe, requires only 5 to 10 minutes for a whole-body scan, and radiation exposure is low. It does, however, require that the patient lie absolutely still, which necessitates a short-acting general anesthetic. Similar to other body composition techniques, DEXA relies on the assumption that lean body mass is uniformly hydrated at 0.73 mL water/g. The accuracy and precision of DEXA have been determined by comparison with cadaver analysis of cats and dogs.[16,21-25]

SUMMARY

Numerous methods exist for the assessment of body composition. The ideal body composition method should be accurate, safe, inexpensive, rapid, reliable, highly reproducible, and

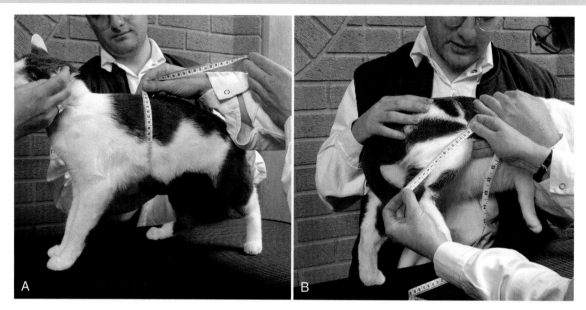

Figure 165-3 A, Measurement of the rib cage circumference at the level of the ninth rib. **B,** Measurement of the lower leg index measurement (LIM) from the middle of the patella to the calcaneus.

easy to operate. Although no such single method yet exists, the techniques of body weight, body condition score, cachexia score, and morphometric measurements fulfill several of these criteria. Some form of assessment should be included in the physical examination of every patient. Knowledge of body composition and how it changes in relation to health and disease can clarify the pathophysiologic adaptations occurring in a variety of clinical conditions. Body composition data are also used to monitor the effects of nutritional intervention and other therapeutic regimens.

REFERENCES

The reference list can be found on the companion Expert Consult Web site at *www.expertconsult.com.*

CHAPTER 166

Immunology and Nutrition

Nick Cave

The interactions between nutrition and immunity are complex and incompletely understood. Both pathogens and immune responses affect nutritional requirements and metabolism, and nutrients directly affect both the immune response and pathogens (Figure 166-1). Food also contains numerous antigens that normally stimulate harmless immune responses (oral tolerance), but can elicit harmful hypersensitivities. The nature of oral tolerance to dietary antigens is illustrated in Web Figures 166-1 and 166-2.

Nutrition can affect immunity by (1) enhancing or exaggerating, (2) suppressing or limiting, and (3) changing the nature of the response. There are multiple points during an immune response that nutrition can modulate (Figure 166-2).

Any effect can be either good or bad depending upon the specific disease and patient. It may be beneficial to enhance immunity to infection or neoplasia, or to attenuate immunity in hypersensitivities or in systemic inflammatory response

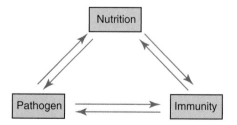

Figure 166-1 The interactions between nutrition, immunity, and pathogens are complex and multidirectional.

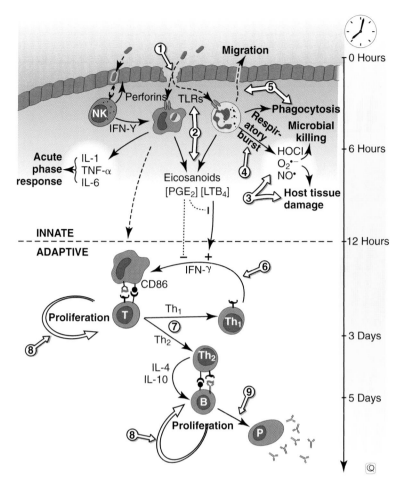

Figure 166-2 Schematic to show the multiple points within innate and acquired immune responses that can be modulated by nutrition. *1*, Epithelial integrity: vitamin A, protein-energy malnutrition. *2*, Toll-like receptor *(TLR)* signaling and eicosanoid production: polyunsaturated fatty acids (PUFA). *3*, Free-radical damage: antioxidants, protein-energy malnutrition. *4*, Respiratory burst: antioxidants, arginine, glutamine, genistein, carotenoids, taurine, obesity. *5*, Neutrophil migration and phagocytosis: glutamine, genistein, iron, taurine. *6*, Th$_1$ mediated responses: lutein, genistein, leptin. *7*, Th$_1$/Th$_2$ development: leptin, vitamin E, PUFA. *8*, Lymphocyte proliferation: lutein, genistein, Cu, Zn, B-vitamins, glutamine, glucose, antioxidants, PUFA. *9*, Immunoglobulin production: lutein, vitamin A, iron.

syndromes (SIRS). However, immunosuppression can lead to prolonged morbidity or even overwhelming sepsis, and enhancement of immunity may lead to increased self-damage in states already characterized by excessive or poorly regulated immune activation (e.g. SIRS, hypersensitivities). Clearly then, one diet cannot meet the needs of all.

NUTRITIONAL REQUIREMENTS FOR IMMUNITY

Nutrition can affect developing leucocytes at any time from fetal development to geriatric immunosenescence, the effects being greatest during development.[1]

Fuel and Cell Division
Glucose and glutamine are essential fuels for activated macrophages, neutrophils, and lymphocytes although both are only partially oxidized.[2] The incomplete oxidation is consistent with the need for leukocytes to operate in areas of low oxygen availability (e.g., ischemic tissue, or unvascularized spaces). Glucose and glutamine are also used for DNA synthesis during proliferation. Although fatty acids and ketones can be used by leukocytes, activation and proliferation does not increase their usage.[2,3] Low plasma glutamine makes lymphocytes more sensitive to apoptosis and leads to immunosupresion.[4] Glutamine supplementation enhances macrophage phagocytosis, increases circulating T-cell numbers, and normalizes lymphocyte function in severe sepsis.[5-8] Predictably, glutamine supplementation of TPN solutions has been shown to reduce morbidity in human sepsis.[5]

Antioxidants
Dietary antioxidants protect host cells and leukocytes against damage from free radicals produced by the activated leukocytes. Intracellular antioxidants in neutrophils and macrophages include taurine, glutathione, ascorbate, tocopherol, and carotenoids. Supplementation of glutamine can increase superoxide production by neutrophils by increasing glutathione production. The carotenoids β-carotene and lutein are incorporated into lymphocyte and neutrophil membranes protecting the lipid membranes from free-radical damage.[9-11] Plasma antioxidants (taurine, ascorbate, tocopherol, glutathione, and carotenoids), also limit free radical damage to the vascular endothelium and other tissues. Antioxidant deficiencies can impair lymphocyte proliferation and reduce numbers of circulating cells, while dietary enrichment can increase cell activity and antibody production.[12-15]

EFFECTS OF MALNUTRITION ON IMMUNITY

Malnutrition and starvation lead to physical and functional defects in epithelial barriers, atrophy of lymphoid organs, decreased circulating lymphocyte numbers and proliferation, reduced neutrophil chemotaxis, and reduced hepatic acute-phase protein production (Table 166-1).

During periods of weight loss, suppressed leptin secretion contributes to the immunosuppressive state, which can be corrected with either leptin administration or recovery of body fat mass.[16] Malnutrition during development can alter microbial colonization of mucosal surfaces, impair responses

Table • 166-1

The Effects of Specific Nutrient Deficiencies on Immunity

NUTRITIONAL DEFICIENCY	IMMUNOLOGIC DEFECTS	CLINICAL MANIFESTATION
Zinc	Thymic atrophy, lymphopenia, altered T-lymphocyte differentiation, reduced Th1 cytokine production, decreased antibody production	Diarrhea, increased susceptibility to infection from skin commensals
Copper	Lymphopenia, reduced lymphocyte proliferation, increased viral virulence	Neutropenia, anemia
Selenium	Impaired oxidant defense, increased viral virulence	Increased susceptibility to infection, increased organ oxidative damage
Iron	Decreased humoral responses, decreased phagocytosis and respiratory burst, reduced T-lymphocyte proliferation	Anemia, increased susceptibility to infection
Vitamin E	Increased IgE, increased PGE_2 production	Increased atopic disease signs? increased organ oxidative damage
Vitamin A	Mucosal barrier defects (squamous metaplasia), Lymphopenia, depressed antibody production, decreased Th2 responses, depressed neutrophil and macrophage maturation	General increased susceptibility to infection—especially respiratory infections, diarrhea
Protein	Impaired cell-mediated responses, decreased cytokine production,	General increased susceptibility to infection
Protein-energy malnutrition	Thymic atrophy, reduced lymphoid tissue mass (lymph nodes), decreased circulating T lymphocytes and B lymphocytes, Impaired cell-mediated responses, decreased cytokine production, reduced neutrophil migration	General increased susceptibility to infection from exogenous and endogenous sources, increased morbidity and mortality, diarrhea (villous blunting, chronic enteritis)

IgE, Immunoglobulin E; *PGE₂,* prostaglandin E₂.

to commensals and pathogens, increase susceptibility to infection, and decrease ability to resolve infection once established. Such defects may alter an animal's immunophenotype for life. The net result is an increased susceptibility to infection from both endogenous sources such as skin and intestinal commensals, and exogenous sources such as nosocomially derived organisms.[12,17]

Obesity

Obesity alters immune responses, which are normalized following weight reduction.[18-20] Reduced NK cell function, altered CD8:CD4 ratios, and reduced neutrophil respiratory burst have been described in obese dogs, humans, and rodents.[21] Simultaneously, obesity leads to increased circulating inflammatory cytokine concentrations and increased acute-phase protein production.[22] The cytokines are produced from activated macrophages within excessive adipose and from adipocytes themselves. The subclinical low-grade inflammation contributes to peripheral insulin resistance. In contrast, maintenance of a lean body condition reduces age-associated immunosenescence.[23]

EFFECTS OF IMMUNE RESPONSES ON NUTRITION

Immune responses to infection or neoplasia, or as the result of immune-mediated disease, affect the patient's nutritional status (Table 166-2). Almost always, food intake is reduced partly, or completely, which is mediated in part by interleukin-1 (IL-1), IL-6, and tumor necrosis factor-α (TNF-α) acting on central and peripheral nerves.[24] The universal finding

of anorexia in inflammatory disease across species suggests that it might be beneficial. Excessive force feeding of anorexic septic mice increases mortality, or the time to recovery in those that survive.[25] Systemic immune activation exaggerates postprandial insulin secretion, but most cells (especially the liver) resist glucose uptake. This resistance preserves blood glucose for glucose-dependent tissues. Increases in cortisol induce marked fat and muscle catabolism, increasing free fatty acid and amino acid delivery to the liver. Hepatic glucose production continues even after feeding, due to the insulin resistance, and hyperglycemia results.[26,27] Intracellular insulin signaling is dysregulated by IL-1, IL-6, and TNF-α (Figure 166-3).

In addition, although there is a relative insulin resistance, cellular glucose concentrations increase in neurons, endothelium, alveoli, vascular smooth muscle, and renal tubule cells. The net result is protein glycosylation and altered metabolism, ultimately resulting in acute renal failure, accelerated removal of erythrocytes, neuropathies, and immunosuppression. Prevention of hyperglycemia in severe inflammatory disease reduces morbidity and mortality.[28]

Recommendations for Feeding in Severe Inflammatory Diseases

Feeding excessive carbohydrate exacerbates the hyperglycemia and increases morbidity, while feeding excessive fat may lead to hepatic lipidosis and dysfunction. The general recommendations for feeding in severe inflammatory diseases are: (1) Feed no more than resting energy requirements (RER), (2) reduce food intake if hyperglycemia or hyperlipidemia occur, (3) feed a high-protein, high-fat diet unless contraindicated, and (4) feed enterally if possible.

Table • 166-2

The Effects of Immune Responses on Nutrition

EFFECT	MECHANISMS	SEQUELAE OR EXAMPLES
Depressed food intake	IL-1, IL-6, TNF-α: CNS and peripheral effects	Weight loss, loss of lean body mass, loss of fat mass, nutrient deficiency
Impaired nutrient absorption	Villous atrophy, enteritis	Decreased fat-soluble vitamin absorption, vitamin B_{12} deficiency
Increased loss	Enteritis, increased glomerular permeability	Hypoproteinemia, vitamin A deficiency
Increased requirements	Fever, leukocyte replication, tissue repair	Glutamine, tocopherol, folic acid, vitamin A, energy?
Altered metabolism and systemic transport	Altered insulin receptor signaling, fat and muscle catabolism	Insulin resistance and hyperglycemia, hyperlipidemia, decreased serum glutamine

CNS, Central nervous system; IL, interleukin; TNF, tumor necrosis factor.

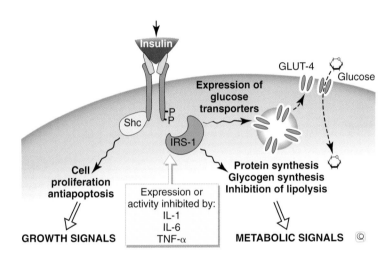

Figure 166-3   In systemic inflammatory states, peripheral and hepatic insulin resistance is induced by cytokine inhibition of the insulin-receptor substrate-1 (IRS-1), which prevents glucose transporter (GLUT-4). However, signaling via other pathways from the insulin receptor still occurs. The persistent hyperinsulinemia in response to the hyperglycemia leads to exaggerated signaling and cellular dysfunction. IL, Interleukin; TNF-α, tumor necrosis factor-alpha.

NUTRITIONAL MODULATION OF IMMUNITY

Nutrients capable of modulating immunity are legion, of which only a few are discussed here.

Polyunsaturated Fatty Acids

Dietary polyunsaturated fatty acids (PUFA) can modulate immunity via several mechanisms (Figure 166-4).[29-35] The dietary content of PUFA determines the proportions of the n-6 and n-3 PUFA incorporated into leukocyte cell membrane phospholipids. The n-3 PUFA eicosapentaenoic acid (EPA) competes with the n-6 arachidonate (AA) as a substrate for cyclooxygenase (COX) and lipoxygenase (LOX) after cleavage from the cell membrane, and the dietary proportions of n-6 and n-3 PUFA determine if the prostaglandins, thromboxanes, leukotrienes, and platelet-activating factor (eicosanoids) are produced from EPA or AA. EPA is a less efficient substrate for COX, resulting in reduced prostaglandin production. Eicosanoids produced from EPA range from antagonistic to equipotent to those derived from AA, and the overall effect on immunity is not explained simply by the reduced efficacy of EPA-derived eicosanoids. The effects and mechanisms of modulation of eicosanoids by dietary lipid are complex, although there is some value to the generalization that diets enriched in n-3 PUFA will reduce inflammation relative to diets enriched in n-6 PUFA.

PUFA also directly affect gene transcription through the peroxisome proliferator-activated receptors (PPARs), a family of cytosolic proteins that, once bound to an appropriate ligand, diffuse into the nucleus and promote or inhibit gene transcription. PPARs are expressed by macrophages, lymphocytes, and dendritic and endothelial cells.[36] Activation of PPARs by EPA leads to reduced TNF-α, IL-6, and IL-1 production by macrophages, and reduced IL-2 production by lymphocytes.[36-38]

Incorporation of EPA in place of AA in phospholipid membranes of lymphocytes affects the function of the lipid rafts within which T-cell receptors (TCR) are localized. This decreases signal transduction through the TCR, reducing T-cell activation.[35] Lastly, both EPA and docosahexaenoic acid (DHA) antagonize the interaction between gramnegative LPS and toll-like receptors, reducing the production of COX, TNF-α, IL-1, IL-6, and IL-8, and improving morbidity in severe sepsis.[32,39,40]

Predicting the effect of PUFA within a diet has to take into account (a) the total fat content, (b) the relative proportions of 18-carbon and 20-carbon n-3 and n-6 PUFA, (c) the absolute amounts of all individual n-3 and n-6 PUFA, (d) the previous dietary history of the animal, and (e) the duration of exposure to the diet in question. Describing the fat content of a diet by a simple ratio of n-6 to n-3 PUFA provides very limited and potentially misleading information. In addition,

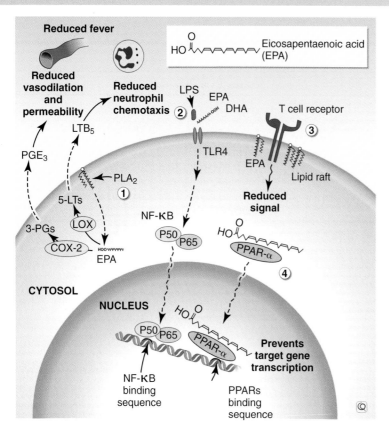

Figure 166-4 Dietary polyunsaturated fatty acids (PUFA) can modulate immune responses through several mechanisms. *1*, Incorporation of the 20 carbon PUFA EPA instead of AA gives rise to eicosanoids with differing biological actions. *2*, The n-3 PUFAs EPA and DHA can directly inhibit signaling through TLR4 by bacterial lipopolysaccharide (LPS). *3*, Incorporation of the 20 carbon PUFA EPA instead of AA into phospholipids changes the physical properties of membrane lipid rafts and leads to decreased signaling through the T-cell receptor. *4*, EPA binds to the cytosolic protein PPAR-γ, which then diffuses to the nucleus, where it binds to specific sequences and can inhibit gene transcription of inflammatory cytokines such as those induced by TLR signaling.

supplementation of a diet with a source of n-3 PUFA (e.g., marine fish oil) will have varying effects depending on the diet and patient. Most commercial diets are highly concentrated in n-6 PUFA, and the addition of a small amount of n-3 PUFA will achieve little.

Where information on specific dietary fatty acid concentrations is not available, a ratio of total n-6 to n-3 of less than 5 may be effective for reducing pruritus in atopic dermatitis, whereas a ratio less than 3.5:1 may be needed for more serious inflammatory diseases, and ratios as low as 1.3:1 may be optimal.[41-44] The exact amount of fish oil required to be added depends on the basal diet.

Genistein, Carotenoids, and Arginine

The isoflavone genistein is principally found in soy, clover, and alfalfa.[45] Genistein can interact with estrogen receptors, can inhibit numerous cell-cycling cascades by inhibiting tyrosine kinases, and can inhibit cellular proliferation by inhibiting DNA topoisomerase II. These effects can reduce leukocyte signaling, lymphocyte activation and proliferation, neutrophil activation and respiratory burst, macrophage phagocytosis, and humoral and delayed-type hypersensitivity responses (DTH).[46-54] Soy-based diets may contain sufficient genistein to affect mucosal, or even systemic, immunity.[55-57] Dietary carotenoids, including β-carotene and lutein, are incorporated into organelle membranes of neutrophils and lymphocytes acting as antioxidants.[9,58] Dietary lutein significantly increases DTH and humoral immunity in cats.[10] The availability of free

arginine limits the production of nitric oxide (•NO) after induction of iNOS in an activated phagocyte. An increase in available arginine increases •NO production in response to an inflammatory stimulus.[59] In immunity, •NO has many functions, which range from protective to pathogenic.[60-63] Overall it appears that supplemental arginine, either parenterally or orally administered, enhances the depressed immune response of individuals suffering from trauma, surgery, malnutrition, or infection, presumably by increasing leukocyte •NO production.[64] Although such an effect may be beneficial in some patients, it may also be detrimental, especially in SIRS.[64,65] Supplementation with arginine, beyond that provided by a conventional protein source, may be beneficial, while in other critically ill patients with SIRS, sepsis, or organ failure, it may be detrimental.[64] Diseases in which dietary-induced immunosuppression may be beneficial include chronic inflammatory diseases such as IBD, osteoarthritis, and atopic dermatitis. It is less clear in which states enhancement of immunity is beneficial, and in SIRS, it can be detrimental. Until more information is available in critically ill patients, nutritional support should focus primarily on preventing nutritional deficiencies and avoiding overfeeding and hyperglycemia.

References

The reference list can be found on the companion Expert Consult Web site at *www.expertconsult.com.*

CHAPTER **167**

Obesity

Patrick Nguyen
Marianne Diez

DEFINITION

Obesity is a pathologic condition characterized by excessive fat deposition leading to harmful consequences for health. Quantitatively, obesity is described as being 15% overweight as compared to optimal weight for the young adult animal after the end of growth and before the beginning of developing excessive fat stores. This body weight is used as a benchmark in both the initial and follow-up evaluations of the animal. In some cases the optimal body weight is unknown as the animal has always been overweight, even during the growth phase. This is especially true following early spaying.

The easiest way to assess and quantify overweight and obesity is probably morphometry and especially the combination between body weight and body index. Body index is a semiquantitative subjective evaluation method combining the evaluation of visible characteristics and palpation of specific regions of the body. This evaluation is conducted in accordance with simple criteria: the size and location of major adipose deposits, the visible and invisible skeletal structure, and the silhouette of the animal.

Several types of index have been proposed:

- 5 grades: 1 = gaunt; 2 = slim; 3 = optimal;
  4 = overweight; 5 = obese.[1]
- 9 grades: 1 to 4 = emaciated to slim; 5 = optimal; 6 to 9 increasingly overweight[2,3] (Figure 167-1).

Dogs presenting with an average index corresponding to an optimal weight have a fat mass of around 15%. When a 9-grade body index is used, every grade in the index represents a 9% increase in fat mass.[4] These systems can be easily applied by the clinician. Although it does not apply exclusively to the diagnosis of obesity, it helps with active prevention. It is important to weigh the animal during each routine consultation and to determine the body index.

Other tools are available to determine body fat content: ultrasound measurements, dual energy x-ray absorptiometry, dilution of heavy isotopes, and bioelectrical impedance. They are certainly more applicable to research settings than to clinical situations (Table 167-1).

HOW IS OBESITY A DISEASE?

Veterinarians should pay attention to obesity and do their best to inform and convince pet owners that in companion animals obesity is a disease by itself; obesity increases the risk for several chronic diseases; and above all obesity is a life-shortening factor that strongly penalizes the quality of life. These deleterious consequences arise from two mechanisms: metabolic and physical-mechanical. Metabolic changes are associated with excess fat and are linked to production of metabolic products, hormones and adipokines, with local, peripheral, and central effects. A physical-mechanical stress is related to the mass and weight (e.g., increased body mass, blood volume, heart work load). These two mechanisms do not act independently.

Obesity and Low-Grade Inflammation

Obesity is characterized by a chronic, systemic low-grade inflammatory state. Adipocytes and adipose tissue macrophages secrete proteins, termed cytokines (adipokines), that act in an autocrine, paracrine, or endocrine fashion to control various metabolic functions.[5] It has been suggested that inflammation in obesity is mainly an adaptive response to hypoxia in clusters of adipocytes within the expanding adipose mass.[6] Under normal weight conditions, cytokines contribute to homeostasis of glucose and lipid metabolism, but their dysregulated production in the obese state promotes insulin resistance (IR), inflammation, as well as atherosclerotic events.[7]

More than 50 adipokines have been identified and extensively reviewed.[8,9] **Tumor necrosis factor alpha** (TNF-α) has paracrine effects on adipose cells, and leads to IR in skeletal muscle[10]. It induces lipolysis, and down-regulates insulin receptor substrate-1 and the insulin-sensitive glucose transporter-4. **Interleukin 6** (IL-6) directly impairs insulin signaling in hepatocytes and adipocytes. TNF-α potently induces IL-6 mRNA expression and secretion in adipocytes. Plasma **leptin** concentrations are highly correlated with body mass index, and leptin influences food intake through a direct effect on the hypothalamus. In obese humans and animals, hyperleptinemia leads to tissue resistance to both leptin and insulin. Moreover, leptin modulates TNF-α production and macrophage activation. **Adiponectin** enhances insulin sensitivity in muscle and liver by enhancing insulin signaling.[11] Adiponectin also has antiinflammatory properties: it is able to suppress TNF-α–induced inflammatory changes. There is a negative correlation between adiponectin levels and adipose tissue (especially visceral), and plasma levels of adiponectin are down-regulated during obesity.[12] Plasma **C-reactive protein** (CRP) levels are strongly associated with obesity and IR,[13] and there is an inverse relationship between CRP and adiponectin in both plasma and adipose tissue.[14] **Apelin** and **visfatin** must also be mentioned since they are up-regulated in the obese state and both exert primarily beneficial effects.[15] Visfatin binds to the insulin receptor at a site distinct from insulin, reduces glucose release from liver, and stimulates glucose utilization in peripheral tissues.

Dog adipose tissue expresses a wide range of adipokine genes, similar to rodents and humans.[16] It has also been shown, at a transcriptional and plasma level, that genes involved in canine insulin resistance/sensitivity are influenced by IR in the same way as in man (overexpression of leptin mRNA; underexpression of adiponectin, GLUT-4, LPL, PPAR and UCP mRNAs).[17,18] Less information is available in cats but it is not different from other species.[19,20]

Obesity, Insulin Resistance, and Type 2 Diabetes Mellitus

Obesity leads to profound and proportional changes in the metabolism of glucose and the secretion of insulin.[21,22]

Adipocytes are cells highly responsive to insulin, which strongly regulates their biology,[23] and adipokines play a major

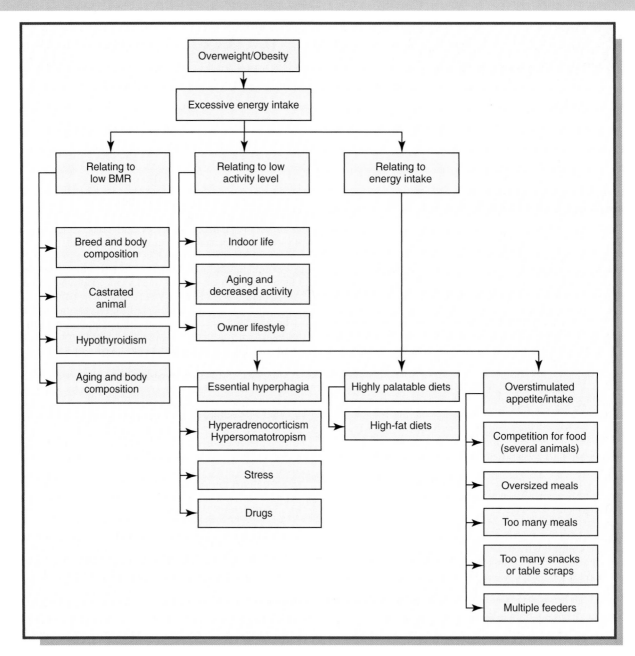

Figure 167-1 Algorithm for identifying causes for obesity. *BMR*, Basal metabolic rate.

role in obesity-related IR.[24] Leptin, TNF-α, IL-6, and resistin levels increase in obesity, whereas adiponectin levels decrease.

When obesity is induced by feeding with a high-fat diet, IR gradually develops in relation to an increase in adiposity.[25-27] and an increase in the production of adipocyte cytokines.[17,28-33] The omental adipose bed is a highly IR depot, and an increased fatty acid flux to the liver may account for hepatic IR.[34] In a long-term study, glucose disposal efficiency and insulin response were associated with increased quality and length of life in nonoverweight dogs.[35] Decreased gene expression of insulin-signaling genes in insulin-sensitive tissues has also been shown in obese cats.[36]

Obesity, Insulin Resistance, Dyslipidemia, Coronary Heart Disease

Dyslipidemia   Obesity, mainly with central fat, is associated with a dyslipidemia. Plasma triacylglycerol (TAG) and cholesterol are higher in obese dogs.[26,37,38] Studies identify the lipoprotein metabolism and the reverse cholesterol transport

(RCT) in healthy and IR dogs.[39,40] The anomalies observed in lipoprotein profiles in IR obese dogs were identical to those seen in IR man.[39,41] IR is associated with an increase in plasma VLDL, and a lower LDL-apo B100, due to reduced production, despite the higher catabolism. The LPL gene is underexpressed in IR dogs,[18] and the lipolysis is thus decreased.[41] In obese cats similar lipoprotein changes have been shown (increased plasma NEFA and TAG, and increased TAG and cholesterol in all lipoproteins, higher plasma VLDL, and lower HDL concentration).[42] However obesity is not associated with high risk for developing coronary artery disease because of their low-atherogenic RCT (mainly driven by HDL).[43,44]

Cardiac Failure   The connection between obesity and cardiovascular diseases (CVD) is not simple,[45] and there are at least three pathophysiologic mechanisms to explain the adverse effects of obesity on left ventricular function[46]: increase in ventricular preload due to increased plasma

Table • 167-1

Abbreviations

ABBREVIATION	MEANING
apoB100	apolipoprotein B100
BMR	basal metabolic rate
CAT	catechin
CLA	conjugated linoleic acid
CRP	C-reactive protein
CVD	cardiovascular disease
DAG	diacylglycerol
DNL	de novo lipogenesis
GFR	glomerular filtration rate
GLUT4	glucose transporter 4
HCA	hydroxycitric acid
HDL	high-density lipoprotein
HT	hypertension
IGF-1	insulin-like growth factor-1
IL	interleukin
IR	insulin resistance
LDL	low-density lipoprotein
LPL	lipoprotein lipase
ME	metabolizable energy
MTP	microsomal triglyceride transfer protein
MTPI	MTP inhibitor
NEFA	nonesterified fatty acid
OA	osteoarthritis
PCR	protein-to-calorie ratio
PPAR	peroxisome proliferator–activated receptor
RCT	reverse cholesterol transport
TAG	triacylglycerol
TDF	total dietary fiber
TGF-β	transforming growth factor beta
THL	tetrahydrolipostatin
TNF-α	tumor necrosis factor alpha
UCP	uncoupling protein
VLDL	very low-density lipoprotein

volume; increase in left ventricular afterload due to hypertension; and systolic and diastolic dysfunction due to changes in the myocardial genome and eventually coronary artery disease. Adipocytokines are responsible for hemodynamic and hormonal changes that profoundly modify gene expression of the myocardium, favoring myocyte hypertrophy and interstitial fibrosis.[47]

In cardiac failure secondary to obesity-related cardiomyopathy, loss of weight can lead to an improved functional status, a reduction of left ventricular remodeling, and an increase of the ejection fraction. Nevertheless these effects would depend on the duration and severity of obesity.[48,49]

In dogs the frequency of CVD increases with obesity.[50] Especially cardiac and vascular hypertrophy have been observed in obese dogs.[51]

Hypertension (HT) Two hemodynamic disturbances are commonly seen in obesity-associated HT: (1) increased intravascular volume and cardiac output, and (2) increased peripheral vascular resistance related to endothelial dysfunction, IR, hyperleptinemia, sympathetic nervous system stimulation, and adipokines (IL-6, TNF-α, etc.).[52] The increase in intravascular volume may result from a renal disturbance causing volume expansion due to activation of the sympathetic nervous system and renin-angiotensin aldosterone

system. Obesity, especially visceral obesity, is also responsible for physical compression of the kidneys. There may be a gradual loss of kidney function that exacerbates HT and makes blood pressure more and more difficult to control.[53] Moreover hyperleptinemia contributes to increased sympathetic activity and arterial pressure in obesity.[54]

Blood pressure is higher in overweight dogs,[55] but there are conflicting data and opinions about the origin and the mechanisms of HT in obese IR dogs, especially regarding the links between HT, hyperinsulinemia, cytokines, and the sympathetic nervous system.[56-59]

Obesity and Osteoarthritis

Weight control influences the degenerative joint disease process by reducing the stress on the joint.[60] However, the osteoarthritis (OA) prevalence in non–weight-bearing joints would suggest an alteration of the cartilage and bone metabolism, occurring independently of weight bearing. In vivo studies have shown increased concentrations of inflammatory cytokines and mediators in the joint in mechanically induced models of osteoarthritis.

In a long-term study, there was at all ages a greater frequency and severity of OA in ad libitum–fed compared to limit-fed fed dogs. Multifocal OA was mainly responsible for a shorter lifespan in dogs initially fed ad libitum.[61-63]

Obesity-Related Kidney Disease

Obesity leads to both structural and functional changes: glomerulomegaly, focal segmental glomerulosclerosis, increased glomerular filtration rate, renal blood flow, and renal hypertrophy. IR and hyperinsulinemia are associated with decreased endothelial production of nitric oxide and increased oxidative stress.[64,65] Leptin would trigger a paracrine interaction, in which glomerular endothelial cells secrete TGF-β, to which sensitized mesangial cells may respond, contributing to the glomerulosclerosis.[66] Apart from leptin, angiotensin II, when increased levels are combined with hyperinsulinemia, is related to glomerular hypertension and mesangial cell hypertrophy.[67]

Several changes may be the precursors of more severe glomerular injury associated with prolonged obesity: greater kidney weight, higher plasma renin activity, insulin concentration, arterial pressure, GFR, and renal plasma flow, expanded Bowman's capsule, increased mesangial matrix, and thickened glomerular and tubular membranes.[68] However, there is no evidence that chronic hyperinsulinemia and IR could cause hypertension in obese dogs.[69] On the contrary, several studies in dogs and humans suggested that the vasodilator action of insulin would tend to reduce blood pressure.[70]

Obesity and Cancer

An association between obesity, cytokines (e.g., leptin, adiponectin, IGF-1, TNF-α) and many types of cancers has been recognized.[71,72] Insulin-like growth factor-1 (IGF-1) stimulates anabolic metabolism, cell proliferation, and cell differentiation, and can inhibit apoptosis.[73] It is associated with diverse types of cancer (breast, ovarian, colorectal, lung, prostate, and bladder).[74] Leptin act as a mitogen and an angiogenic factor, and many types of cancer cells can respond to leptin as a mitogen/survival factor.[75,76] Adiponectin is inversely associated with endometrial[77] and breast[78] cancer risk. Although TNF-α has been used as a cytotoxic agent, recent preclinical cancer models have supported a link between chronic, low level TNF-α exposure and the acquisition of a promalignant phenotype.[79] The role of TNF-α remains controversial.

In the canine species, obesity at 1 year of age and 1 year before diagnosis of mammary nodules was found to be related to prevalence of mammary tumors,[80,81] but these observations contradict previous as well as more recent studies.[82,83]

Miscellaneous

- An epidemiologic study also shows that obesity increases the risk of acute hemorrhagic pancreatitis.[84]
- Obese animals or animals fed a diet with a high fat content are less resistant to infection than animals fed a balanced diet.[85-87]
- The hypothesis that there is a correlation between obesity and some forms of urinary incontinence, primarily in neutered bitches, has been suggested.[88]
- Obesity has been shown to be a factor linked with the onset of clinical signs of tracheal collapse.[89]
- Overweight dogs would also be more likely to develop urinary calcium oxalate calculi.[90]
- The risks associated with anesthesia are greater in obese dogs, but vary depending on the type of anesthetic used.[91]
- In bitches undergoing ovariectomy, the surgical time was significantly—on average 30%— longer among obese bitches.[92]

PATHOPHYSIOLOGY

In simple terms, obesity is the consequence of energy imbalance where intake exceeds expenditure for a variable period of time, which leads to a positive balance. There are a huge number of factors that can cause this situation, and the interaction between these factors rather than the action of any one of them is felt to be responsible for obesity.

Frequency

In the most recent studies, the frequency of obesity in dogs and cats presented at consultation varies from 20% to 45%, showing that obesity is a major medical problem in the companion animal population.[1,93-97]

In a recent study, when owners were asked to indicate body condition of their pets, 32.3% indicated a score of 4 or 5 (overweight or obese), but only 3 out of these 356 owners considered this to be a health problem.[98] In a study published just a decade ago (1999), veterinarians routinely did not recognize obese dogs and cats as having a health problem, even when body condition scores were available. In that study, veterinarians reported that only 2.0% of dogs and 1.8% of cats were obese, when, in fact, 28.3% of dogs and 27.5% of cats were assigned a body condition score that corresponded with overweight or obese.[99]

Risk Factors

- Breed: Breed may be a risk factor for obesity in the canine species and can be responsible for differences in basal metabolic rate (BMR; basal energy expenditure/kg $BW^{0.75}$) or in body composition (lean body mass is stronger determinant of BMR than body weight).
- Genetic factors: Genetic factors leading to obesity have been suggested in dogs but are still poorly understood.
- Age: The frequency of obesity increases with the age of the dog[95] but the frequency of obesity declines in dogs age over 12 years of age.[94]
- Sex: Females are more predisposed to obesity than males, due to a lesser lean body weight. Indeed in dogs of the same breed of comparable weight, the males are generally a little less fat than the females and so their expenditure is greater (on the order of 10%).[100]
- Neutering: Gonadectomy doubles the frequency of obesity in males and female dogs,[95] due to decreased BMR, increased food intake, and reduced activity. A 30% reduction in daily energy intake compared with intake before neutering has been shown to be necessary to maintain Beagle bitches at their ideal weight in the weeks following an ovariohysterectomy.[33]
- Endocrine diseases: Obesity may be associated with certain endocrine diseases, such as diabetes mellitus[21,22,101-104] and hypothyroidism.[103,105-108] According to the authors, at least 40% of bitches suffering from these conditions are obese. Obesity may also be secondary to hyperadrenocorticism.[109]
- Medications: Some medications may lead to hyperphagia and weight gain, particularly antiepileptics and glucocorticoids.
- Sedentary lifestyle and lack of exercise: Lack of exercise is a primary factor in the development of obesity because of a reduced total energy expenditure and BMR, and a decrease in lean body mass (and another secondary decrease in BMR). Dogs living in an apartment would be 1.35 time more prone to be obese than dogs living outdoors (31% versus 23%),[95] even if an open space or a confined environment are not the only determinant of spontaneous activity.
- Dietary pattern: The following dietary habits have been identified to contribute to obesity: dietary intake that does not take account of the energy requirements, and a fortiori ad libitum feeding; highly palatable food; treats or snacks not accounted for in the energy allocation.[95,110]
- High-fat diets: In humans the fat intake is the main determination in the development of obesity.[111] Indeed high-fat diets have a lower satiating power than high-protein low-fat diets.[112] High-fat diets also successfully induce obesity in dogs[26,113] and cats.[114] Altering the nutrient composition of a diet by only an 8% increase in fat content resulted in a significant increase in the deposition of abdominal fat in bitches.[27]
- Homemade diets, type of commercial food (wet versus dry), and not dividing an adequate daily diet into several meals has a particular influence on the frequency of obesity.[95,110]
- Social aspect of the food: The place of food in the relationship between the human and the dog plays a major role in the development of obesity: giving treats as signs of affection, interpretation of bulimia as a sign of good health, using foods as a palliative treatment to prevent unmonitored animals from becoming bored or destroying things.

Energy Balance

The Principles of Energy Balance   The fundamental principal of energy balance is:

$$\text{Changes in energy stores} = \text{energy intake} - \text{energy expenditure}$$

A positive energy balance is the consequence of energy intake exceeding expenditure, and, conversely, the balance is negative when expenditure exceeds intake. In normal conditions the energy balance oscillates meal after meal, day after day, week after week, without changing body weight and energy reserves in the long term. Many physiologic mechanisms play a role in adapting intake to expenditure and expenditure to intake so as to maintain a stable body weight in the long term. When the energy balance is positive, energy expenditure increases (increase activity of "futile" cycles such as continuous synthesis and hydrolysis with no net effect except the release of heat at the expense of ATP; increase activity of uncoupling proteins and futile cycle of proton pumping and proton leak across the mitochondrial inner membrane in dissipating energy) and, conversely, when the balance is negative, the energy expenditure decreases, which contributes to the resistance to weight loss.

Overestimation of Energy Expenditure and Requirement The second element in the equation is energy expenditure, which is split into three parts:
- Basal metabolic rate (BMR)
- Postprandial thermogenesis (production of heat subsequent to the meal)
- Physical activity

In sedentary human adults, these three parts represent respectively 60%, 10%, and 30% of energy expenditure. In dogs, the basal metabolic rate also represents 55% to 70% of the total expenditure,[115] but differences have been observed between breeds. For example Labradors have a lower basal metabolism rate than Great Danes or Spaniels. Lean body mass accounts for 90% to 95% of BMR versus 5% to 10% for fat mass. The BMR declines with age in dogs.[116] It is recommended to reduce the energy intake by 10% to 15% from age 7, while adjusting the diet depending on the physical condition of the individual. However, a low-calorie diet is not always justified for all old dogs.

The main factors of variation of energy expenditure have been reviewed in the Risk Factors section. The estimation of the energy requirement is not easy in dogs. There is a large quantity of data, but it is fragmented and difficult to generalize. Monitoring weight and knowing what the animal needs to consume to maintain a constant weight are the most important pieces of energy-requirement–based information for any given individual.

The situation is simpler in cats because of less variation in body weight. The average daily requirement differ mainly according to body composition; 100 kcal/kg $BW^{0.67}$ in lean cats; 130 kcal/kg $BW^{0.4}$ in overweight cats.[115] There are obviously also differences depending on activity but they would mainly be included in the fact the cats are lean or fat.

Dysregulation of Food Intake

Wild animals are generally active and even in an environment with plenty of food it is extremely rare for adult animals to be obese. The biologic mechanisms regulating body weight appear to be efficient in combating underconsumption. In domesticated animals, the lower environmental pressure would require the mechanisms that manage overconsumption to be even more efficient, and dysregulation of these mechanisms may account for pathophysiology of obesity.

Leptin acts as an energy balance modulation signal, both centrally (on the hypothalamus) and peripherally (e.g., liver, pancreas). It plays a key role in the regulation of food consumption. It also increases energy expenditure, at least in healthy individuals. Leptin is produced in proportion to the quantity of fat cells, and leptinemia increases in dogs during periods of weight gain.[17,32,33] However, there is an attenuated response to leptin in the obese state caused by reduced transport of leptin across the blood-brain barrier as well as a reduction in the ability of leptin to initiate cellular activation within the brain (leptin resistance).[117] Studies in rodents have shown that feeding animals a high-fat diet decreases leptin receptor levels within the hypothalamus and, consistent with this, leptin transport is reduced.[118]

Regarding **sex steroids** females are more sensitive to the appetite-inhibiting effects of leptin than males. Estrogen enhances the response to leptin, augmenting the satiety effect, and also increases transport of leptin into the brain.[119] In contrast, very little is known regarding the effects of testosterone on leptin sensitivity.

Ghrelin (growth hormone–releasing hormone) stimulates food intake in humans and rodents. Plasma ghrelin is lower in obese dogs than it is in healthy animals.[33,120] In contrast to ghrelin, **obestatin** has been initially reported to elicit anorexigenic effects in mice and rats, inhibit jejunal contraction, and decrease bodyweight gain.[121] It has been suggested that an imbalance of ghrelin and obestatin levels and a changed preprandial ghrelin–to-obestatin ratio may have a role in the pathophysiology of obesity.[122]

Adiponectin acts in synergy with leptin.[11] Its expression is reduced by half in obese dogs compared with healthy dogs.[18] Adiponectin is an important peripheral hormone related to insulin sensitivity, but whether or not it acts within the brain is not clear yet.[117]

Of course not all mechanisms are dysregulated. **TNF-α,** which is a proinflammatory molecule that participates in anorexia and cancer cachexia, has been found in particularly high quantities in the adipose tissue of obese animals and patients. The expression and the concentrations of TNF-α are positively correlated to the degree of obesity and the resistance to insulin[123] in dogs.[17] High TNF-α levels can limit the development of obesity (effect on both food intake and insulin sensitivity). It produces a potent anorexigenic effect in the hypothalamus, where it modulates insulin and leptin signaling and action.[124]

Many factors are therefore involved in the development of obesity, whether they are factors regulating food intake or energy expenditure.

Quality of Dietary Intake

For dogs and cats, the calculation of the energy provided (metabolizable energy ME) by a food is based on its chemical composition.

Fats are the nutrients that contain the most energy. The overconsumption of fatty food is accordingly an essential factor in the genesis of obesity. Indeed fat is often added to food to increase palatability. It also increases the energy density of the diet.

Food composition has great impact on satiety signals following food intake. Carbohydrates elicit strong satiety signals, particularly by stimulating insulin and amylin secretion. Complex and redundant pathways are involved in protein- and amino acid–induced satiety,[125] including the release of anorexigenic gut hormones. By contrast, fat has little effect on satiety and even disturbs satiety signals.

Moreover, when the net energy value is considered, the efficiency of protein utilization for energy is lower than that of fats or carbohydrates. Average efficiency of those nutrients would be 94%, 98%, and 77% respectively in simple-stomached animals.[126] That means that 100 kcal ME from carbohydrates, fats, or protein are not finally equal but would represent 94, 98, or 77 kcal net energy. Metabolizable energy overestimates net energy value of high-protein diets and underestimates that of high-fat diets.

A simple modification of food chemical composition—without modifying the apparent (metabolizable) total energy intake—can lead to changes in body composition and basal metabolic rate either by modifying satiety or true energy value or both.[27,127]

It therefore appears that the energy requirements of dogs are often incorrectly estimated and, accordingly, in many situations energy intake can be excessive. It is up to the clinician to determine whether the obesity is primary or secondary so as to establish the subsequent treatment. Figure 167-1 identifies the different components that may account for the development of obesity. Their knowledge would ensure a better and complete weight-reduction program.

NUTRITIONAL TREATMENT

Level of Energy Restriction

Two nutritional techniques can theoretically be used to reduce the body weight.

- Complete nutritional privation is applicable and effective provided the animal does not present with concomitant pathologies.[128-130] However, this method is not recommended for ethical reasons and because it does not involve the owner in long-term dietary modifications.
- The restriction of energy intake is therefore the only truly valid option, based on the information on the food habits.

The level of energy allocation depends mainly on the degree of weight excess, the actual energy intake, and the projected duration of weight loss. Because females and castrated animals commonly have a lower percentage of lean body mass and consequently a lower basal energy expenditure, they must be given less energy (approximately 15%) than males and intact animals.[33,131]

The first step consists of defining the ideal weight; the second of defining a target weight; the third is setting the energy restriction level. The diet is generally calculated to provide 40%—a very severe restriction[129]—to 60%[132] of the energy needed to maintain the target weight.

A very severe restriction might limit the duration of the diet but is not recommended because

- it may lead to a significant feeling of hunger in the animal, generating more activity after meals,[133] resulting in a lack of compliance;
- the loss of lean mass can be exaggerated by a sudden loss of weight, as it has been shown in humans[134];
- the rebound risk is more important following a more severe energy restriction,[135] due to a more reduced basal energy expenditure;
- severe caloric restriction may be counterproductive by inducing a decrease in activity,[28] and this exacerbates muscle mass loss.

A very severe energy restriction must therefore be reserved for the most severe cases of obesity, especially when there is a medical indication for rapid loss.

Various experimental and clinical trials have shown that a reasonable objective is to maintain a loss of 1% to 2% of the initial (obese) weight per week, or 4% to 8% per month. For a weight loss of 1.5% per week, approximately 4 months are needed to lower the body score by 2 points. Tables 167-2 and 167-3 shows the energy allocation based on parameters to be taken into account in dogs and cats respectively.

Table • 167-2

Energy Allocation and Protein-to-Calorie Ratio of Diets Given to Reduce Body Weight in Obese Dogs

DOG [Maintenance: 130 kcal EM/kg IBW$^{0.75}$; PCR: 45-55 g protein/Mcal ME]

Excess body weight	20%-30%		30%-40%		45% and more	
Body fat percentage	25%-35%		35%-50%		More than 50%	
Body condition score	7		8		9	
Daily energy allowance (kcal ME/kg TBW$^{0.75}$)	Male Entire	Female Spayed	Male Entire	Female Spayed	Male Entire	Female Spayed
Targeted ΔBW: −6% IBW/mo (approx. −1.5%/wk)	85	80	75	65	60	55
Probable duration of weight loss	12-18 weeks		18-24 weeks		25 weeks and more	
Recommended PCR	**≥70-85**		**≥85-105**		**≥105-120**	
Targeted ΔBW: ×7.5% IBW/mo (approx. −2.0%/wk)	80	75	65	60	55	50
Probable duration of weight loss	9-13 weeks		13-17 weeks		17 weeks and more	
Recommended PCR	**≥75-95**		**≥95-115**		**≥110-135**	

IBW, Ideal body weight; TBW, target body weight; PCR, protein-to-calorie ratio.

Table • 167-3

Energy Allocation and Protein-to-Calorie Ratio of Diets Given to Reduce Body Weight in Obese Cats

CAT [Maintenance: 100 kcal EM/kg IBW$^{0.67}$; PCR: 65 g protein/Mcal ME]

Excess body weight	20%-30%	30%-40%	45% and more
Body fat percentage	25%-35%	35%-50%	More than 50%
Body condition score	7	8	9
Daily energy allowance (kcal ME/kg TBW)	30	25	20
Probable duration of weight loss	9-13 weeks	13-17 weeks	17 weeks and more
Recommended PCR	**≥110**	**≥130**	**≥165**

IBW, Ideal body weight; TBW, target body weight; PCR, protein to calorie ratio

Modification in Nutrient Content

To achieve energy restriction by simply reducing the quantity of the food typically consumed must be absolutely avoided. This would lead to multiple deficiencies in essential nutrients as well as disturbed behavior.[28] The selection of a food specially adapted for weight loss is therefore imperative, and allows the dog to receive a sufficient food, while limiting energy intake.

Low-Calorie Diets The simplest way to reduce the energy concentration of a commercial food is to reduce the fat content and increase the dietary fiber content.

The volume of the ration must not be too small, and the food should have a sufficient satiating power. Several options are more or less controversial: increasing air content of kibbles to lower their density (and then increasing the volume of the ration), or increasing the hydration level of canned foods. Changing the size, texture, and shape of the kibble can increase the ingestion time and satiating power.

In the case of wet food, very high hydration (over 80% water) also helps maintain a relatively large volume. However, the impact on satiation is dubious, as the water is evacuated from the stomach in 20 to 30 minutes depending on the size of the particles. The addition of viscous dietary fiber that binds water can slow gastric emptying.[136]

Low-Calorie Diets: Low-Fat and High-Fiber The **fat content** of low-calorie foods is generally reduced to less than 25% of energy (25 to 30 g fat per Mcal ME). The most recent recommendations for maintenance are at least 14 and 22.5 g/Mcal in dogs and cats respectively to ensure provision of essential fatty acids and transport of fat-soluble vitamins.[115]

Fiber can be advantageous for the nutritional management of obesity in dogs. It is a bulking agent that reduces the energy density of a food with only a minor decrease in the volume of the food allowed. Its effect on the feeling of satiation remains controversial.[137-139] Soluble fiber slows down gastric emptying and induces slower absorption of nutrients in dogs[136] while insoluble fiber accelerates dietary transit.[140,141] A high-fiber diet reduced the energy intake and adiposity in dogs.[142,143] Adding short-chain oligosaccharides to the diet of obese dogs increased insulin sensitivity and modulated the transcription of genes involved in energy and fatty acid metabolism.[144]

Fiber also presents some inconveniences, which vary depending on the nature of the fiber and the rate of incorporation. It can adversely affect palatability,[145] and causes a reduction in the digestibility of certain nutrients like proteins and minerals. It increases the quantity of feces and the frequency of defecation, and may lead to gastrointestinal problems, such as flatulence and diarrhea.

Low-Calorie Diets and Essential Nutrients The content of all essential nutrients in low-calorie diets is extremely important. First of all the protein-to-calorie ratio (PCR) must be increased according to the energy restriction level so that, whatever the energy allowance, the protein intake is at least that required for the maintenance of target body weight (and lean body mass). The PCR should, for example, be 95 to 115 g protein/Mcal ME in dogs if the energy restriction is 50% and up to165 g protein/Mcal ME in cats given a very restricted diet. The same reasoning is obviously valid for all essential nutrients (including fatty acids); however, the protein level is more often taken into consideration because high-protein diets have been used successfully for many years and have demonstrated many benefits.

High protein levels are recommended in low-calorie diets for several reasons linked to amino acids requirement. They are also recommended for their impact on energy yield and satiety.

- Utilization of metabolizable energy from protein (amino acids) has a lower yield in terms of net energy intake than carbohydrates and fatty acids, due to the cost of synthesis of elimination forms of nitrogen (mainly urea).
- Many studies conducted on humans have shown that proteins have a higher satiating power compared to carbohydrates and fats[146] since, as amino acids, they are absorbed slowly. And because they mainly use gluconeogenesis, they induce little insulin secretion and delay appearance of hypoglycemia, which contributes to the feeling of hunger. The satiating power may, however, differ from one protein to another because of difference in the speed of digestion.

An increased protein-to-calorie ratio had positive effect on body composition by minimizing muscle wasting, maintaining lean tissue mass, and facilitating the loss of fat.[147,148] These effects have also been observed in dogs with diets having a PCR as high as 150 to 160 g protein per Mcal ME.[131,149] In cats fed a diet with a PCR of 105 or 133, the loss of lean tissue was reduced by approximately 50% in cats fed the diet with the highest PCR.[150] Moreover a higher protein intake resulted in a 50% lower bodyweight regain in human studies.[151] The quality of the protein is obviously also important since the requirement concerns essential amino acids.

Moreover it must be noted (even if this looks unrealistic) that the PCR should (in all diets, not only low-calorie diets) be expressed as g-digestible protein per Mcal ME, and even as g-available amino acids per Mcal ME.

Low-Calorie Homemade Diets Obese dogs can be fed homemade diets. However, the conditions described above must be respected. Low-fat ingredients should be selected (lean meat), as well as high-fiber sources of starch (complete cereals), vegetables, dietary fiber supplements in purified form (bran, soy fiber). The diet must be carefully formulated to ensure it is complete and balanced. Compared with a maintenance diet, the PCR must be higher as well as the concentration of other essential nutrients and the dietary fibre percentage. PCR must be adjusted to calorie restriction, between 88 and 135 g protein/Mcal ME in dogs, and between 100 and 165 in cats. By using dietary fibre supplements it is possible to increase the concentration to 25 to 30 g TDF/Mcal ME.

Examples of such homemade diets are shown in Table 167-4. In all cases an appropriate mineral and vitamin complement must be added in adequate quantity.

Special and Nutraceutical Ingredients

Lipase Inhibitors

- **Saponins:** In mice fed for 9 weeks either chikusetsusaponins (1% to 3%) isolated from *Panax japonicus*[152] or an extract of *Kochia scoparia* fruit[153] or ginseng saponins,[154] the expected increase in BW and adipose tissue was suppressed, following a high-fat diet. As fecal TAG levels increased, antiobesity effects of these saponins might be partly mediated by inhibiting lipase activity.
- **Chitosan:** Chitosan (acetylated chitin from the exoskeletons of crustaceans) would work as a "fat blocker" rather than an inhibitor of fat digestion. Mice given a high-fat diet with chitosan had less BW gain and fatty liver, and higher fecal fat excretion than control mice given high-fat diets.[155] Nevertheless, in two clinical trials, chitosan supplementation did not result in any reduction in BW in the doses used.[156,157]

Green Tea Catechins, Thermogenic Ingredients Green tea catechins (CATs) may play a role in the control of body composition via sympathetic activation of thermogenesis, fat oxidation, or both,[158,159] especially by inhibiting catechol-O-

Table • 167-4

Examples of Energy-Restriction Homemade Diets for Obese Dogs and Cats

OBESITY 1 (COD1)	per 1000 kcal ME
Turkey, breast without skin	575 g
Rice, cooked	120 g
Lentils, cooked	165 g
Wheat bran	40 g
Rapeseed oil	8 g

Nutrients Provided per 1000 kcal ME

Protein (PCR)	160 g
Protein calories	64%
Fat	16 g
Fat calories	15%
Fiber	26 g
Available carbohydrates	56 g
Calcium	220 mg
Phosphorus	2090 mg
Sodium	270 mg
Potassium	2920 mg
Magnesium	320 mg

OBESITY 4 (COD4)	per 1000 kcal ME
Haddock	560 g
Rice, cooked	265 g
Carrots (boiled, drained)	65 g
Wheat bran	50 g
Rapeseed oil	20 g

Nutrients Provided per 1000 kcal ME

Protein (PCR)	115 g
Protein calories	46%
Fat	26 g
Fat calories	24%
Fiber	25 g
Available carbohydrates	81 g
Calcium	160 mg
Phosphorus	1670 mg
Sodium	680 mg
Potassium	2570 mg
Magnesium	410 mg

OBESITY 2 (COD2)	per 1000 kcal ME
Haddock	750 g
Rice, cooked	135 g
Carrots (boiled, drained)	100 g
Wheat bran	45 g
Rapeseed oil	20 g

Nutrients Provided per 1000 kcal ME

Protein (PCR)	145 g
Protein calories	58%
Fat	27 g
Fat calories	24%
Fiber	23 g
Available carbohydrates	47 g
Calcium	200 mg
Phosphorus	1910 mg
Sodium	910 mg
Potassium	3090 mg
Magnesium	420 mg

OBESITY 5 (COD5)	per 1000 kcal ME
Turkey breast without skin	305 g
Rice, cooked	325 g
Lentils, cooked	55 g
Wheat bran	60 g
Rapeseed oil	20 g

Nutrients Provided per 1000 kcal ME

Protein (PCR)	95 g
Protein calories	38%
Fat	27 g
Fat calories	24%
Fiber	31 g
Available carbohydrates	102 g
Calcium	140 mg
Phosphorus	1600 mg
Sodium	150 mg
Potassium	2080 mg
Magnesium	380 mg

OBESITY 3 (COD3)	per 1000 kcal ME
Turkey breast without skin	430 g
Rice, cooked	270 g
Lentils, cooked	175 g
Wheat bran	45 g
Rapeseed oil	5 g

Nutrients Provided per 1000 kcal ME

Protein (PCR)	130 g
Protein calories	52%
Fat	13 g
Fat calories	11%
Fiber	30 g
Available carbohydrates	98 g
Calcium	190 mg
Phosphorus	1870 mg
Sodium	200 mg
Potassium	2580 mg
Magnesium	330 mg

OBESITY 6 (COD6)	per 1000 kcal ME
Beef, minced meat, 10% fat	305 g
Rice, cooked	260 g
French beans (canned)	300 g
Wheat bran	40 g
Rapeseed oil	10 g

Nutrients Provided per 1000 kcal ME

Protein (PCR)	75 g
Protein calories	30%
Fat	44 g
Fat calories	40%
Fiber	24 g
Available carbohydrates	80 g
Calcium	160 mg
Phosphorus	1190 mg
Sodium	940 mg
Potassium	2100 mg
Magnesium	340 mg

ME, Metabolizable energy; *PCR*, protein-to-calorie ratio.

methyl transferase enzyme, which degrades norepinephrine.[160] CATs also induce peroxisomal proliferation through the transactivation of PPARα.[161] In dogs nutritional doses of green tea extract improve insulin sensitivity and lipid profile and alter the expression of genes regulated by either PPARγ or PPARα that are involved in glucose and lipid homeostasis.[162]

Factors Affecting Metabolism and Nutrient Partitioning

- **Diacylglycerols** (DAGs): Synthetic diacylglycerols (DAGs) that directly reach the liver through the portal vein increase β-oxidation, enhance BW loss, suppress body fat accumulation, and lower postprandial plasma TAG levels. The increased FA oxidation might increase satiety.[163] Overweight DAG-fed dogs showed a BW and body fat reduction while the TAG-fed dogs maintained their obese BW.[164]
- **L-carnitine**: L-carnitine facilitates the transportation of long-chain fatty acids in the mitochondria, where they are subjected to β-oxidation. Addition of carnitine improved the lipid metabolism in obese rats.[165] In companion animals it would at least have a protective effect against fasting ketosis during obesity induction in cats.[166]
- **Conjugated linoleic acids** (CLA): The trans 10, cis 12 CLA (t10,c12-CLA) isomer has antiobesity properties and improves body composition because it decreases energy intake and increases FA oxidation in both muscle and adipose tissue, and increases energy expenditure.[167] CLA increases levels of mRNAs encoding lipid metabolizing and mitochondrial UCPs and stimulated both PPARγ and PPARα.[168] CLA reduced body fat in mice, rats, and chickens but produced less significant or inconsistent effects on BW and composition in pigs and humans,[169] and in cats (using a 0.4% CLA mixture[170]) and dogs,[143] and even in some rodent studies. The reasons for the inconsistency of CLA benefit in different species are many (e.g., doses used, variable dilution of t-10,c-12 in CLA isomer mixtures, diet composition, species-related differences in peroxisome proliferation[171]). Interestingly extract of bitter gourd activated PPAR α and γ, and decreased adiposity in rats.[172] It contains 9c,11t,13t-CLA, which has been identified as a PPARα activator.[173]
- *Garcinia cambogia* (hydroxycitric acid): *Garcinia cambogia* (brindle berry) contains hydroxycitric acid (HCA), which might limit de novo lipogenesis (DNL). HCA also inhibits serotonin uptake, and may be beneficial in controlling appetite.[174,175] However, a few clinical studies have shown controversial findings, even though a significant reduction in DNL has been shown in humans.[176] On the contrary no effect of *G. cambogia* was shown on fat-free mass or on energy expenditure in normal cats (0.3% of *Garcinia* extract).[170]
- **Ginseng saponins:** Due to their similarity with steroid hormones, ginsenosides would similarly bind to the nuclear receptors and alter gene expression. They would have PPARα modulatory[177] and hypolipidemic effects.[178]
- **Chromium:** As a dietary supplement chromium-picolinate increases lean body mass and decreases body fat. Its effectiveness is nevertheless controversial, even though it is supported by animal studies.[179,180]
- **Pyruvate:** Pyruvate would manipulate fat metabolism by increasing fat oxidation and decreasing carbohydrate oxidation. Two controlled trials in overweight patients reported reduction of fat mass and percentage body fat.[181]
- **Hydroxy-methylbutyrate:** Beta-hydroxy-β-methylbutyrate is a metabolite of leucine that has shown anticatabolic actions through inhibiting protein breakdown, resulting in larger gains in lean body mass and muscle strength.[182,183]

Pharmaceutical Aids

There are some drugs that can assist in obesity management. None of those that centrally act on food intake regulation will be discussed here because there are no clinical data regarding eventual benefits in dogs or cats. The intestinal lipase inhibitor, tetrahydrolipostatin (THL), and inhibitors of the microsomal triglyceride transfer protein (MTPI), dirlotapide and mitratapide, will be discussed below.

Tetrahydrolipostatin, a Lipase Inhibitor **Tetrahydrolipostatin** (THL; orlistat) is a lipase inhibitor that reduces fat absorption by around 30%.[184] In humans 120 mg three times a day is prescribed with meals. Clinical trials supporting the claim that THL helps reduce BW in obese patients include 2-year studies. At 12 months, patients adhering to a hypocaloric diet and receiving THL lost more BW than those receiving placebo (10.3 vs. 6.1 kg[185] and 8.8 vs. 5.8 kg,[186] respectively). At 24 months, BW regain (35%) in patients who continued to receive THL was less than in those who received placebo (63.4%). The major adverse effects with orlistat are gastrointestinal (e.g., oily stools). Psyllium would be helpful in controlling these GI side effects,[187] and coprescription of fat-soluble vitamins is recommended.

Dirlotapide and Mitratapide, Inhibitors of MTP Microsomal triglyceride transfer protein (MTP) plays an important role in the assembly of both VLDL (in the hepatocyte) and chylomicrons (in the enterocyte). MTP inhibitors (MTPIs) prevent atherosclerosis as they improve dyslipidemia. Indeed, they reduced both cholesterol and TAG levels in animals (rodents, rabbits, dogs) in clinical studies.[187-191] In rabbits, implitapide decreased plasma cholesterol and TAG by 70% and 45%, and VLDL secretion rate by 80%.[190] MTPI administration increased hepatic and intestinal TAG levels by 2.0-fold and 2.3-fold in mice fed a standard diet, whereas the increases reached 3.5-fold and 4.7-fold in animals receiving a high-fat diet.[188,190,192] Two compounds (mitratapide, dirlotapide) with antiobesity indication in dogs have been recently marketed, which are safe and have minimal side effects. They have selectivity for intestinal MTP compared with hepatic MTP and do not induce liver steatosis (as implitapide did in rabbits). These drugs must not be used in cats: indeed they are not intended for feline (no development or clinical trials have been conducted or published), possibly because cats are more prone to liver lipidosis than dogs.

Dirlotapide[193] is licensed for continuous use in the management of overweight and obese dogs for periods of up to 12 months. The dose must be regularly adjusted to the observed results. Significant weight reduction has been achieved in treated dogs, resulting primarily from a decrease in food intake and appetite, which has not been explained yet. There was also a significant effect on digestibility coefficients.[194-197] Although mitratapide is in principle a similar drug, the method of dosing is different: it is used short term and in conjunction with dietary management and behavioral modification. There are no published data supporting the efficiency of this drug.

Both drugs can easily be administered by the owner. Generally they are well tolerated, but side effects can occur, including occasional and transient gastrointestinal troubles, most notably vomiting. They are usually well tolerated after the first few weeks of administration. Owners must be forewarned that this may occur. Shortly after the drug is discontinued, appetite returns: feeding and behavioral strategies must be continued in order to avoid rebound in body weight to occur.

These drugs can be useful in the short or medium term, but other strategies are essential to ensure long-term success of a body weight loss programs. Whatever place any pharmacologic treatment will have, it should not be forgotten that in a global approach (behavioral and dietary) of obese dogs, medication should never be used alone as it does not change the owner and animal behavior.

Rationing in Practice

Dietary History   A discussion with the owner will be a source of direct and indirect information and input for the estimating the present ingested energy and avoiding pitfalls. The following information may prove useful:
- Regular food: brand, type, energy value
- Daily quantity
- Feeding method: ad libitum versus limited quantity
- Identification of the person who feeds the dog and other people involved
- Distribution of treats, leftovers, etc.
- Number of animals in the home and the obese animal's potential access to food.

In the case of extremely obese animals it is essential to ensure that the quantity of energy that will be prescribed is lower than that typically consumed by the animal. In the extreme obesity phase, energy expenditure, requirement, and intake can be very low.

Clinical Examination   The first aim of the clinical examination, and supplementary tests, is to check whether the state of obesity is secondary to an endocrine disease.

The second aim is determination of ideal weight and eventually appropriate target weight to determine the energy allocation. Target weight must be fixed with the agreement of the owner.

The length of the diet can be calculated on the basis of these data. Owners must nevertheless be forewarned that, depending on the quality of the dietary history, an adjustment could be necessary after 4 to 6 weeks according to the observed results. During this period the animal could not lose any weight or, in the worst situation, could even gain.

Selection of Food   Commercial foods for treating obesity in dogs and cats must have a low energy density, and be complete, balanced, and palatable. Especially essential nutrient content must be increased according to the intended level of energy restriction (see PCR in Tables 167-1 and 167-2).

Homemade diets can also be used taking into account the same conditions.

Energy and Food Allocation   The selection of the level of restriction and the type of food depends to a large degree on the initial situation. The aim is to produce a sustainable modification in the food that results in a sustainable reduction in body weight over the long term.

In most cases a severe restriction is not necessary if the animal is moderately obese and does not present clinical signs. A moderate restriction and a relatively slow loss of weight can certainly be contemplated in these cases. On the other hand, a much more radical approach will be necessary when the animal is severely obese and presents with surgical indication (such as a dog with a torn cruciate ligament). The surgeon may refuse to intervene before the animal has lost a significant amount of weight. Such a pathologic history generally results in the owner being highly compliant when the motivation is high enough to allow for a severe restriction.

Additional Advice   In addition to nutritional aspect of obesity management, the clinician can further enhance results by taking some of the following actions:
- Use clear, data-based messages that are much more persuasive than vague approaches
- Provide behavioral support
- Monitor the animal during the diet (establishing a weight loss curve, scheduling checkups)
- Prescribe reasonable physical exercise
- Monitor the animal postdiet to avoid a rebound effect that is generally observed in the absence of strict measures (providing the owner with advice on the selection of a maintenance food and the adequate quantity).

REFERENCES

The reference list can be found on the companion Expert Consult Web site at *www.expertconsult.com*.

CHAPTER 168

The Unique Nutritional Needs of the Cat

Debra L. Zoran

Cats are unique, often mysterious, creatures that once were known to us only in the shadows of farms, alleys, and remote places. Now, cats have surpassed dogs as the most common pet in Western society, and although they have become members of the family in ways similar to our canine companions, their role is entirely different. These new members of our extended family have come to fill a niche that only they can fill, but with our fascination and fawning over these wonderful creatures comes the realization that they are not small dogs. Their diseases are different, even as they are familiar in name, their behavior and social structure is undeniably feline and especially difficult for social humans to understand, and finally, possibly most importantly, their nutritional needs and metabolism reflect their feral background as true, obligate carnivores. Cats are truly wild animals that have decided to come live with us. As a result, it behooves us to recognize and understand normal feline metabolism and nutrition, particularly if we have any hope of being able to manage them during illness or prolonged anorexia, where their normal increased need for protein for energy and metabolism competes with the need for protein for repair, immune function, and the increased metabolic demands of illness. It is essential to recognize that although cats can and do use carbohydrate (CHO) as a source of metabolic energy, they have limited ability to spare protein utilization by using CHO, and they are better adapted for utilization of protein and fat in their diet, especially in times of illness. Despite these very specific and unique requirements, normal healthy cats can and have adapted well to the commercial diets that are universally available to them. These diets are typically formulated using a mixture of animal- and plant-derived nutrients, presented most commonly in dry kibble form that requires CHO for the expansion and cooking process. However, if the maxim: "let thy food be thy medicine" is true, the question remains: Should we as their caregivers (now that they are indoors and rely on us in many cases entirely for their nutrition) be providing diets that, while complete and balanced, do not mirror the natural diet for a cat? Or, alternatively, should our goal be to aim for optimal nutrition, not just formulated to meet basic needs, but to maximize health and prevent disease based on the unique nutritional profile of the cat? There is increasing evidence to suggest that many of the disorders and diseases of our indoor cats are either directly or indirectly related to their nutrition—and this is a completely fixable problem. This chapter will review the important and significant differences in feline nutrition, provide a framework for understanding the role of nutrients in feline nutrition, and discuss the feeding behavior in cats. All of this with one goal in mind: to help us better understand the unique nutritional needs of cats so that we can provide optimal nutrition for their health and longevity.

NUTRIENTS: THE IMPORTANCE OF PROTEIN AND AMINO ACIDS IN CATS

The natural diet of cats in the wild is based on consumption of small mammals, birds, and insects (i.e., meat-based) containing little CHO; thus, they are metabolically adapted to utilize protein and fat preferentially as energy sources in addition to having specific requirements for amino acids and fatty acids that come from these sources.[1] Thus, having a diet that primarily consists of protein and fat, cats are mandated to use protein for energy and maintenance of blood glucose levels even when sources of protein in the diet are limiting.[1-3] The requirement of cats to use protein for energy illustrates a significant difference in protein utilization between cats and omnivores, such as dogs, who utilize CHO or fat preferentially for energy when protein is limiting. For example, while the protein requirement of kittens is 1.5 times that of other species, adult cats require 2 to 3 times more protein in their diet than omnivores.[3-6] The greater requirement for dietary protein in adult cats is due to both an increased need for protein (nitrogen) and higher requirement for specific amino acids.[1] There are many possible explanations for the increased need for protein in feline diets, but the fact that cats depend on protein for energy, as well as for classic structural and synthetic purposes, is a major reason. Most omnivores, when fed a diet with low or modest protein levels, conserve amino acids by reducing the activities of aminotransferases and other enzymes involved in protein catabolism.[7] However, in a classic study by Rogers and coworkers, cats were fed both low (170 g/kg BW)– and high (700 g/kg BW)–protein diets to determine if they responded to low-protein conditions similarly to omnivorous species.[2] In cats fed either low or high levels of dietary protein, there was little adaptation in the activities of their aminotransferases or urea cycle enzymes.[2] Another study suggested that cats have a limited ability to adjust protein utilization to the level of protein in their diets; however, the primary finding was that protein oxidation increased in cats fed high-protein diets.[8] Protein oxidation in cats fed moderate protein diets did not decrease (low-protein diets were not evaluated).[8] Most recently, another group of researchers found that cats on low-protein diets had a net loss of protein (due to loss of muscle mass); however, the duration of the study was very short so the long-term effects were not evaluated.[9] Nevertheless, these experiments demonstrate that cats, as obligate carnivores, continually use proteins (i.e., dispensable nitrogen in the form of gluconeogenic amino acids) for production of energy and for other metabolic pathways (e.g., urea cycle) even in the face of low protein availability, and they seek to maximize protein uptake in times of low availability. Thus, while normal cats need increased dietary protein compared to other species to maintain their daily requirements for nitrogen, amino acids, and energy; sick, injured, or anorectic cats are in a particularly crucial situation. In this setting, cats now have the need for added protein for repair or to mount an immune response in addition to their unique nutritional needs. As a result, without appropriate nutritional support or intervention, they may develop protein malnutrition quickly. This essential need for protein is one of the main driving forces in the need for aggressive nutritional support of sick cats.

In addition to their increased need for dispensable protein, cats also have well-known needs for increased amounts of specific amino acids in their diet: taurine, arginine, methionine, and cysteine.[1,5] The natural diet of the feline contains an abundance of each of these specific amino acids (plus the 11 essential amino acids) (Table 168-1). The likely reason that the synthetic pathways for these amino acids are not present in cats is that they are redundant in an animal that would normally consume diets containing these amino acids in abundance. Further, even though cats do not have the ability to synthesize these amino acids, they are not conserved; in fact, the utilization of these amino acids (taurine, arginine, methionine and cysteine) is higher than in dogs or other species.

The most well-known essential amino acid in cats is taurine, a sulfur-containing beta amino acid that is essential for normal vision, cardiac muscle function, and for proper functioning of the nervous, reproductive, and immune systems.[5] Taurine is essential because cats cannot synthesize adequate quantities from the normal precursors, methionine or cysteine, as most other animal species are able to do. The enzymes required for synthesis of taurine (i.e., cysteine dioxygenase and cysteine sulfinic acid decarboxylase) are only minimally active in cats,[10,11] likely because cats consuming meat-based diets that contain large amounts of this amino acid did not need to have the metabolic machinery to make it. Further complicating matters, cats conjugate bile acids with taurine—not glycine, as do dogs and other species. This obligate use of the amino acid in bile results in a significant increased use of taurine and greater need for taurine in the feline diet.[10,11] Further, the requirement for taurine in cats is influenced by several common dietary factors, including the source of the protein in the diet, commercial processing, and presence of fiber in the diet.[12,13] For example, in pet foods formulated with plant source proteins or with added dietary insoluble fiber, taurine must be supplemented liberally to meet the taurine requirement. The reasons for these adjustments are: (1) taurine is only present in animal-source proteins, (2) insoluble dietary fibers reduce taurine absorption (among other amino acids), and (3) commercial heat processing reduces taurine bioavailability—a problem first discovered when Pion and coworkers noted that cats consuming commercially available taurine "replete" diets were still taurine deficient and developed the dilated form of cardiomyopathy.[14] This discovery in the late 1980s led to the supplementation of feline diets with additional taurine and resulted in a major decline in the incidence of dilated cardiomyopathy in cats, but

Table • 168-1

Essential and Nonessential Amino Acids in Cats[5]

AMINO ACID (AA)	ESSENTIALITY	GLUCONEOGENIC (G) OR KETOGENIC (K) OR BOTH	NOTES AND SOURCES
Arginine	Essential	G	Essential for urea cycle function and formation of nitric oxide and polyamines; cats synthesize less because they lack enzymes for synthesis of ornithine and citrulline; high concentrations in muscle proteins
Glutamine	Conditionally essential	G	Purine and pyrimidine nucleotide synthesis, important energy source for enterocytes, precursor to citrulline (and thus arginine in dogs), abundant in potatoes, synthesized from glutamate
Histidine	Essential	G	Formation of histamine; high levels in hemoglobin
Isoleucine	Essential	BOTH	Branched chain AA
Leucine	Essential	K	Branched chain AA
Lysine	Essential	K	Precursor for carnitine synthesis; can be easily lost with heat processing
Methionine	Essential	G	Sulfur-containing AA, converted to cysteine; important in polyamine synthesis (SAMe), carnitine synthesis, and as a methyl donor; may be limiting in cats
Phenylalanine	Essential	BOTH	Aromatic AA; degraded in liver to form tyrosine; may be limiting in cats
Taurine	Essential in cats		Conjugation of bile acids (cats only use taurine); essential for vision, reproduction, and muscle function (especially heart); synthesized from methionine and cysteine in dogs
Threonine	Essential	G	Energy source; muscle protein
Tryptophan	Essential	BOTH	Neurotransmitter
Tyrosine	Conditionally essential (source of methionine)	BOTH	Neurotransmitter; important in melatonin and dopamine metabolism; important in thyroid hormone synthesis; increased requirements in cats for hair color (black)
Aspartate	Nonessential	G	Neurotransmitter; purine and pyrimidine nucleotide synthesis; synthesized from glutamate and oxaloacetate
Cysteine	Nonessential	G	Important in synthesis of methionine, SAMe, and taurine (in dogs)
			Sulfur-containing AA; synthesized from serine
Glutamate	Nonessential	G	Neurotransmitter; precursor to alanine and glutamine synthesis in muscle; synthesized from branched chain AA
Glycine	Nonessential	G	Formation of creatine; purine and pyrimidine synthesis; synthesized from serine or choline
Proline	Nonessential	G	May be conditionally essential in cats, as they lack biosynthetic enzyme; synthesized from glutamate
Serine	Nonessential	G	Synthesis from glycolytic intermediates or pyruvate
Valine	Nonessential	G	Branched chain AA

SAMe, S-adenosylmethionine.

it also clearly illustrated that what was considered adequate based on feeding trials might not always be optimal or reflect the long-term effects of nutrient deficiencies that may cause subtle or no external signs initially. This is partly because prolonged deficiency of taurine (i.e., months or years) is required before significant signs of deficiency appear in most cats. The most common signs of deficiency are blindness (central retinal degeneration), reproductive failure or neonatal loss, and development of dilated cardiomyopathy.[5,14] Diagnosis of taurine deficiency in cats is confirmed by measurement of whole blood taurine concentrations, with normal concentrations of taurine in cats being greater than 300 nmol/mL and concentrations lower than 160 nmol/mL being consistent with deficiency.[5]

Arginine is an essential amino acid in dogs and cats, but, unlike dogs, cats are unable to synthesize enough ornithine or citrulline for conversion to arginine; thus arginine (an amino acid from meat sources only) must be present in their diet.[15,16] In addition, cats continually utilize large amounts of arginine in the urea cycle because there is minimal down-regulation of the cycle during fasting or in cats consuming low-protein diets.[1,2] Cats and kittens fed a diet devoid of arginine show clinical signs of hyperammonemia (ranging from salivation, neurologic abnormalities, hyperesthesia, emesis, and tetany, to coma and death) within hours.[15,16] Fortunately, arginine and citrulline are abundant in animal tissues, and thus arginine deficiency is rare in cats consuming appropriate foods. However, in cats fed diets with plant-origin protein sources, arginine must be supplemented to avoid a deficiency. This is also why cats with hepatic lipidosis should be given as much meat source protein (arginine) as they can tolerate (e.g., 35% to 50% of calories), as protein is essential to correction of the metabolic derangements and liver abnormalities occurring in idiopathic hepatic lipidosis.[17]

The requirement for methionine and cysteine in the feline diet is also much higher than for omnivores, including dogs.[5,18] A major reason for this is that both methionine and cysteine in cats are gluconeogenic amino acids that are catabolized to pyruvate and then subsequently oxidized for energy via the Cori cycle. Methionine and cysteine have many uses, but are primarily converted to taurine (in dogs), homocysteine, and s-adenosylmethionine (SAMe) and its metabolites (e.g., glutathione), which are important free radical scavengers and antioxidants.[5,18-21] In addition to the above pathways utilizing cysteine, the requirement for this amino acid is high in cats for production of hair and felinine, a sulfur-containing amino acid found in the urine of cats.[22] The highest concentrations of felinine are found in intact male cats (95 mg excreted/24 hr), with significantly lower concentrations in neutered males (29 mg/24 hr), intact females (19 mg/24 hr), and spayed females (13 mg/24 hr).[22] Thus, the dietary requirements for cysteine in intact male cats is significantly higher than in neutered males or female cats. Felinine function is largely unknown, but may be important in territorial marking, and the large rates of felinine excretion in male cats create another protein "sink."[22] Both methionine and cysteine are present in large quantities in animal tissues, so deficiency is uncommon in cats consuming an appropriate diet, but may occur in anorectic cats or in those fed diets with plant-origin proteins or human enteral formulations deficient in amino acids required by cats. Methionine or cysteine deficiencies are often initially seen clinically as poor growth in kittens, or crusting dermatoses and poor haircoat in adult cats.[5]

Tyrosine is considered to be a conditionally essential amino acid for cats and has an important role in the synthesis and homeostasis of melanin, present in black hair and skin pigment.[23] Tyrosine is synthesized from phenylalanine, an amino acid present in many proteins, but may not be high enough in feline diets to support tyrosine and subsequent melanin synthesis. As a result, tyrosine deficiency is most commonly observed in black cats whose hair becomes reddish/brown.[24] This effect can be reversed in cats fed diets containing increased concentrations of tyrosine, which includes diets high in animal-source proteins. Tyrosine is an excellent example of a nonessential amino acid that may become deficient in cats because utilization (of tyrosine for production of hair or its precursor, phenylalanine) for nonessential (degradative) functions is increased. The key point is that meat-source proteins provide these essential nutrients naturally, while diets formulated with proteins of other sources must be liberally supplemented to meet the need for these nutrients, and this supplemented diet may not provide optimal nutrition.

Carnitine is an amino group containing vitamin-like substance that is increasingly considered to be conditionally essential. However, until very recently, carnitine was not an approved by the American Association of Feed Control Officials (AAFCO) as a supplement in pet foods; thus, pet foods could not be fortified with carnitine, and to supply carnitine diets had to contain high carnitine ingredients. One major role for carnitine is transport of fatty acyl CoAs from the mitochondrial cytosol into the nucleus, thus making them available for beta oxidation.[25,26] Cats are able to synthesize carnitine from lysine and methionine—their major dietary source being meat and dairy proteins.[5] In cats, carnitine synthesis occurs in the kidney (in dogs and other species it occurs in the liver) and requires several B vitamins and iron; thus, synthesis may

be limited in anorectic, sick cats.[5,26] In humans, carnitine deficiency, either relative or absolute, causes hepatic lipid accumulation and liver dysfunction.[27] A similar connection is suggested in cats with idiopathic hepatic lipidosis (IHL), with current evidence suggesting carnitine supplementation hastens recovery and improves survival in affected cats.[28] Carnitine also increases lean muscle mass and enhances weight loss in obese cats.[29] While further investigation is necessary to better understand the role of carnitine in feline diets, supplementation of diets with carnitine (or its precursors) (250 to 500 mg carnitine/cat/day) is recommended for both obese cats and those with IHL.[29]

It is well known that cats have unique requirements for protein and amino acids in their daily diets, and that they use protein for energy through gluconeogenesis in a constant and continuous way. What was not clear until recently was the role of protein in metabolism, including glucose and lipid metabolism, and other aspects of intermediary metabolism, and its potentially important role in prevention of one of the most common nutritional disorders of cats: obesity. The role of protein in feline metabolism, both in the obese and lean state, was studied and several key findings have been reported: dietary protein levels are important in maintaining normal feline metabolic rates, in improving fat metabolism and turnover, and in preserving muscle mass.[30-32] In particular, Hoenig and coworkers showed in both obese and lean cats that diets high in protein (>45% metabolizable energy) resulted in greater heat production in lean cats (a measure of resting energy rate), improved fat metabolism and insulin sensitivity, improved fat loss during weight loss, preserved muscle mass (lean tissue) during weight loss (an essential factor in healthy weight loss), and improved glucose tolerance.[30-32] Conversely, in the obese or lean cats fed moderate protein but high-CHO diets, energy metabolism was lower during weight loss. Obese cats lost both lean and fat tissue, but lean tissue was lost at a higher rate, and high-CHO diets resulted in abnormal glucose tolerance tests.[30-32] These studies further illustrate the need for high levels of protein in feline diets to help maintain normal energy metabolism, but more importantly, in obese cats during weight loss, the requirement for high protein levels is even more acute to help normalize insulin sensitivity and fat metabolism and prevent loss of lean body mass.

NUTRIENTS: THE DIFFERENCES BETWEEN CARBOHYDRATE AND FAT METABOLISM

While it is clear that cats have a greater need for protein in their diet than dogs or other omnivores, it is also important to recognize that they are adapted to a low CHO and high fat intake. In wild felids consuming their natural diet of mice, their diet contains, on a dry matter basis, approximately 55% protein, 35% fat, and 10% CHO.[5] This lack of dietary CHO is not harmful because cats have a persistently high activity of gluconeogenic enzymes, which allows them to maintain their blood glucose by converting protein into energy.[33-35] Further illustrating these metabolic differences, cats have no salivary amylase, the enzyme responsible for initiating CHO digestion,[36] very low activities of intestinal and pancreatic amylase, and reduced activities of intestinal disaccharidases—the enzymes that break down CHO in the small intestine.[37] These specific differences do not mean cats cannot utilize starch—in fact they utilize simple sugars and some starches very efficiently—it simply underscores their development as carnivores and the expected low levels of grain in their normal diet. However, these digestive differences may mean that high levels of CHO in feline diets may have untoward effects. For example, high levels of CHO in cat diets decrease protein digestibility due to a combination of factors including increased passage rate and alterations in intestinal microflora.[38] Increased CHO in cat diets also causes a reduction in fecal pH, which is due to incomplete CHO fermentation in the small bowel resulting in increased microbial fermentation in the colon and increased production of organic acids.[38] Increased CHO present in the lumen also appears to lead to both different numbers and species of bacteria—changing the intestinal microbial flora in cats to an entirely different population than what would be expected if they were consuming a normal feline diet.[39]

Cats also have several distinct features that influence CHO metabolism and contribute to a unique feline pattern of glucose utilization. In most animals, both hepatic hexokinase (a constitutive enzyme) and glucokinase (an inducible enzyme) are active and responsible for phosphorylation of glucose for storage or oxidation. Cats differ in that they have minimally functioning glucokinase activity, and the activity is not adaptive (i.e., activity cannot be up-regulated when the diet contains large amounts of CHO).[34,40,41] In recent studies, this lack of adaptability to high glucose loads after a high-CHO meal has been illustrated in cats, where it may take anywhere from 8 to 10 hours for the blood glucose levels in a cat to return to normal, preprandial levels.[42,43] This observation is reinforced by other studies showing the increased time required for cats to eliminate glucose after an intravenous or oral glucose tolerance test, especially in overweight cats.[44,45] Chronic increases in blood sugar (even very small increases outside the normal range) result in persistent hypersecretion of insulin and can eventually lead to development of glucose intolerance and a prediabetic state, especially in obese cats. It is also important to note that different dietary CHO sources may have different effects on glucose and insulin secretion, so that not only the amount, but the type of CHO can affect glucose responses.[43,45] In addition to the above observations, cats also have minimally functioning hepatic glycogen synthetase (the enzyme responsible for converting glucose to glycogen for storage in the liver).[5] Again, the likely reason for low hepatic glucokinase and glycogen synthetase activity in cats is their evolutionary program to use gluconeogenic amino acids and fat in their diet for energy. Importantly, because carnivores utilize gluconeogenic protein catabolism to provide energy; additional starch in the diet that is not stored as glycogen or utilized for energy from exercise or other energy expenditure will be stored as fat. Hoenig and coworkers also reported that cats fed high-CHO diets had greater disappearance of fatty acids from their blood, which can only be explained by fat oxidation or lipid deposition—especially into muscle tissue and liver.[31] Using indirect calorimetry, the greater disappearance of nonesterified fatty acids was associated with increased fat production—not oxidation—a clear indication that cats consuming high-CHO diets that do not expend that CHO energy consumed via exercise have increased fat deposition.[31] This is a particularly keen issue in sedentary, indoor cats that often consume free-choice, CHO-based dry food—making it very easy to consume more calories than they burn, increasing their risk of obesity and also creating an increased postprandial CHO load that can lead to development of hyperinsulinemia and glucose intolerance. Finally, in addition to the differences in CHO handling illustrated previously, the feline liver also does not contain fructokinase, an enzyme necessary for metabolism of simple sugars. The lack of this enzyme was demonstrated in a study where cats consuming diets high in simple sugars became hyperglycemic and fructosuric.[46] Most cats are not attracted to foods with a sweet taste (as are dogs and people), but prefer foods with flavors from animal products (e.g., fats, meats). However, the reason cats are so willing to consume dry,

CHO-based diets is due to the fact that this biscuit is coated with digest (fat and protein) prior to packaging—thus making it quite appealing to the feline palate.

In the carnivorous diet, fat normally provides most of the fuel for energy, but is also very important in increasing the palatability and acceptance of food.[25,47] Meat-based diets, which also contain animal fat, supply the feline essential fatty acids: linoleic, linolenic, arachidonic acid, and some eicosotrienoic acid.[48] Most species can convert linoleic acid to arachidonic acid, the primary precursor for the 2-series prostaglandins, leukotrienes, and thromboxanes, and alpha-linolenic acid to eicosapentaenoic and docosahexaenoic acids, through desaturation and elongation pathways. Cats lack adequate hepatic delta 6–desaturase activity, and other hepatic desaturases as well, all of which are required for synthesis of arachidonic acid and eicosapentaenoate (EPA) and docosahexaenoate (DHA).[48,49] As with many other nutrients, cats evolved without the enzymatic machinery to synthesize derivatives of arachidonic acid or other long chain omega-3 polyunsaturated fatty acids because the end products were plentiful in the normal feline diet (if animal tissues containing fat were consumed). A deficiency of arachidonic acid and other essential fatty acids can lead to a number of skin and coat changes, poor vision and neurologic function, and reduced ability to respond to infection through prostaglandins and leukotrienes.

The need for fat in the feline diet to enhance palatability and provide essential fatty acids is well understood, but the role fat in diet as an energy source that is linked to the development of obesity also cannot be overlooked. Because of the increasing incidence of obesity in the feline population, multiple studies have attempted to answer the question relating fat intake of the typical feline diet to obesity. Clearly, obesity is a multifactorial problem, but several key aspects of feline metabolism revealed in these studies are worth consideration. First, neutered, indoor/inactive cats consuming diets higher in fat are able to increase their oxidation of fat—a response that is very unlike that of other species. This may help explain why cats have for long periods consumed diets higher in fat that other species without development of obesity.[50] However, also true in neutered cats, hormonal changes occur in their appetite, hormonal balance, and energy requirements that greatly increase their risk of obesity.[51-53] In particular, neutered cats with unrestricted access to food have increased intake and will gain weight rapidly after neutering. As a result, caloric intake and particularly fat intake (which represents the highest calorie component of diets) have received increased scrutiny as the source of increased calories contributing to obesity in young, neutered cats.[54,55] However, it may an oversimplification to blame only the fat content of the diet, when the metabolism of other nutrients in cats has such a profound effect on overall metabolism: protein increasing fat oxidation, CHO increasing fat deposition. Thus, adding high fat availability creates a readily available energy source that will likely be stored. Clearly, there is no debate that the effects of neutering on feline metabolism, hormonal balance, and appetite greatly increase the risk of development of obesity in young cats. But, it must also be abundantly clear that energy intake in these animals must be reduced following neutering by at least 25% to 30% or excess calories (whether they are of protein, CHO or fat) will be stored as fat.[51,56] This is the key first step in the process of prevention of obesity (and many other ills) in young cats, and it must start with a change in the way we feed cats: a reduction in free-choice feeding, calculation of more accurate caloric needs so that those that choose to feed dry foods can feed more correct amounts, and finally, choosing to feed cats foods that mirror their metabolic machinery to more optimally meet their nutritional needs.

FELINE NUTRITION ESSENTIALS: VITAMINS AND MINERALS

Not surprisingly, the vitamin needs of cats are also unique as compared to dogs those of and other omnivores. Cats require increased amounts of many of dietary water-soluble B vitamins, including thiamine, niacin, pyridoxine (B_6), and, under certain circumstances, cobalamin (B_{12}).[1,5] Pyridoxine is especially important because it is an essential cofactor in all transaminase reactions, which are constantly active in cats.[5] Cats can synthesize niacin, but their dietary requirement is four times higher than that of dogs because they have a much higher rate of catabolism of the vitamin precursors.[57] Thiamine deficiency can occur in both anorectic cats and in cats consuming diets high in thiaminase (high in seafoods) and is clinically evident as severe muscle weakness. Because most water-soluble B vitamins are not stored (the exception is cobalamin, which is stored to a small degree in the liver), a continually available dietary source is required to prevent deficiency. In anorectic or ill cats, daily supplementation with a multi–B complex vitamin solution (thiamine 5 to 30 mg/cat/day, riboflavin 2.5 to 5 mg/kg, or 0.5 to 1 mL multi–B complex/cat/day) will help prevent deficiency.[58] Deficiency is rare in cats consuming appropriate diets, as each of these B vitamins is present in high concentrations in animal tissues and is added to commercial cat diets.[5] Cobalamin deficiency is particularly common in cats with gastrointestinal (GI) diseases, as a complex series of events must occur for proper digestion of this vitamin in the ileum. Thus, any cat with anorexia, weight loss, chronic diarrhea, or vomiting should be evaluated for evidence of cobalamin deficiency as replacement therapy is essential to correction of the clinical signs.[59] However, it is important to recognize that cobalamin deficiency can also occur in any ill cat not consuming enough cobalamin (either due to anorexia or other causes), including cats with pancreatitis and liver diseases, and as such, evaluation and replacement of cobalamin levels in any sick cat is reasonable.[60]

Of the fat-soluble vitamins A, D, E, and K, cats have special needs for A and D. Vitamin A occurs naturally only in animal tissue and must be provided as the biologic form in feline diets because cats cannot convert beta-carotene (which is plentiful in plants) to retinol (the active form of the vitamin) because the intestinal enzyme is absent.[61] Vitamin A has a number of vital roles in physiology and clinical health, including maintenance of vision, bone and muscle growth, reproduction, and healthy epithelial tissue.[5] Vitamin A deficiency is rare in cats fed a commercial cat food and occurs slowly in a deficient diet, because the vitamin is stored in the liver. In fact, deficiencies are rare and only occur in cats with severe liver failure or GI disease resulting in fat malabsorption. Caution is strongly advised in supplementation of vitamin A, as toxicity can easily occur, resulting in hepatotoxicity or steatitis.[5,61] Recommended doses of vitamin A supplementation in cats with a deficiency are 625 to 800 IU/kg BW/day orally.[58]

Like vitamin A, cats also require a dietary source for vitamin D (e.g., calcitriol). Cats are unable to meet their metabolic needs for vitamin D via dermal photosynthesis because they lack the 7-dehydrocholesterol required for its synthesis.[62] Vitamin D is present in high amounts in animal liver and fat, so cats normally meet their needs for this vitamin via eating these foods. The primary functions of vitamin D are calcium and phosphorus homeostasis and enhancing the intestinal absorption, retention, and bone deposition of calcium. As with vitamin A, deficiency of calcitriol is rare and occurs slowly and is called rickets due to the skeletal changes that occur as a result of calcium/phosphorus imbalances. Nevertheless, supplementation should be approached cautiously and only in cats with severe hypocalcemia, as excesses of vitamin D cause significant hypercalcemia. The recommended oral doses of vitamin D_3 (calcitriol) supplementation in cats are 0.25 μg/kg BW every other day.[58] Calcitriol therapy should be monitored by measuring serum ionized calcium levels, a more accurate measure of available calcium and one that rapidly reflects potential overdoses.

Vitamin E is a generic descriptor for the biologic activity of alpha tocopherol. There are four naturally occurring tocopherol compounds, which are designated as alpha, beta, gamma, and delta.[63] Alpha tocopherol is the relevant compound for physiologic use in nutrition. Vitamin E is the major lipid-soluble antioxidant present in plasma, red blood cells, and tissues, where it functions as a free radical scavenger that decreases oxidative damage to fatty acids in cell membranes.[63] Vitamin E deficiency is not common in cats, but because of the nature of their diet (greater need for antioxidants due to higher fat metabolism), they are more susceptible than dogs. Signs of deficiency are anorexia, hyperesthesia, and nodular adipose tissue (due to steatitis).[64] In general, supplementation of cats should not occur unless hypovitaminosis E has been documented, as excess vitamin E supplementation can cause antagonism to the functions of both vitamins D and K.[58] Typical doses of vitamin E in cats are 100 to 400 U/cat orally once daily.[58]

Like vitamin E, vitamin K is a generic descriptor—in this case for menadione (2 methyl-1,4 naphthoquinone) and its derivatives that exhibit antihemorrhagic activity.[65] The naturally occurring compound is present in plants and is frequently called vitamin K_1 or phylloquinone. The unique function of vitamin K is to facilitate activation (carboxylation) of the glutamic acid residues in proteins that are vitamin K dependent: a tall order in cats that use protein carboxylation for many things, including (1) clotting proteins, (2) skeletal proteins, and (3) other proteins throughout the body.[65] Vitamin K is often not supplemented in commercially available pet food because most cats are able to meet their needs from the dietary ingredients and by intestinal synthesis of the vitamin from bacteria. However, in cats fed diets high in tuna or salmon, vitamin K deficiency can occur, so diets containing these ingredients must be supplemented with menadione.[66] The main situations where cats may require vitamin K supplementation are associated with consumption of anticoagulant rodenticides or in cats with severe liver disease.[67] However, because cats have a high need for vitamin K and often have subclinical deficiency with any form of severe liver disease or even severe inflammatory bowel disease (IBD) supplementation should be given to all cats with hepatic lipidosis, severe cholangitis, or severe IBD that results in decreased absorption of lipids.[67] The recommended dose of vitamin K_1 is variable, depending on the degree of hemorrhage or disease, but ranges from 1 to 5 mg/kg/day orally or SC.[58] Vitamin K_3 is not recommended for clinical use due to its poor absorption.

WATER

Water is an essential nutrient with innumerable functions in the body, but is often not considered in discussion of diet and dietary requirements. The water needs of cats reflect their early status as desert-dwelling animals and their development as strict carnivores that obtain most of their water requirements from prey and their need to concentrate their urine intensely to reduce water loss. Domestic cats have retained that ability to concentrate their urine, but have increased risks of other problems (e.g., urinary calculi) due to their diet. Cats have a less sensitive response to thirst and dehydration than dogs or other omnivores, and they adjust their water intake to the dry matter content of their diet (not the moisture content).[68] The composition of the food also affects water intake, as foods with a higher protein level result in an increased water intake and foods with a high CHO content result in a decreased water intake.[69,70] For example, cats consuming dry foods that are high CHO and low protein will consume approximately 50% less water (both in the diet and by drinking) as compared to cats eating canned foods.[5] Thus, in cats with a tendency to produce uroliths, feeding canned foods with an appropriate mineral profile and added water increases water intake and urine volume and decreases the concentration of urolith-forming minerals present in the urine. In older cats that are less able to produce concentrated urine, increasing water consumption becomes even more important to avoid dehydration and prevent risk of constipation and development of prerenal azotemia. As with their food preferences, cats will not consume water that is overly cold, contaminated with food, hair, or other particulates, or has particular odors or tastes (city water vs. bottled water). Some cats have a preference for aerated water (found in drinking fountains), while others prefer it still, and most will not drink from a water contained that is too close to the litter box. The key is to offer multiple options to the cats to best determine their individual preference.

FELINE FEEDING BEHAVIOR AND PREFERENCES

Food and taste preferences in cats are learned behaviors that are imprinted at a very early age—initially by interactions with the queen and then in the first weeks and months after weaning.[71] It is striking that feline dietary preference is not at all innate—it is a learned behavior that is acquired through social influences after birth and weaning.[72] In fact, kittens will choose to eat what their mothers eat, even if it is an "unusual" food for cats.[73] Kittens learn to imitate their mother's eating behavior down to the smallest detail—and there is a clear correlation between the mother's diet and that of the kittens. This period of development occurs primarily early in the weaning process and will be determined by 6 to 8 weeks of age. In addition to taste preferences, cats develop preferences for foods based on shape, mouth feel, and other physical characteristics.[72] Once taste and texture preferences are established in cats, they are particularly difficult to change. These preferences can also become "hard-wired" into the cat, so that later in life, the cat does not recognize as food those offerings that do not have the appropriate flavor, taste, shape, or physical characteristics. Some have called cats finicky, because they refuse to eat new or unusual foods, but in reality, they are cautious, careful eaters—an evolutionary blueprint for protecting them from eating foods that were new, spoiled, tainted, or potentially harmful. These behavioral characteristics are essential to understand, since many cats, as they age or develop diseases, will require foods of a new type (canned vs. dry) or possibly different flavor or physical characteristic. If the cat has not been introduced to these early in life (e.g., canned foods being introduced to a dry food–eating cat), they will, in many cases, refuse to eat them unless they have had previous exposure. This is not because they are finicky, but because they have not developed the preference. However, there is also a well-known phenomenon in cats, termed *neophilia*, that describes the tendency in cats that have been exposed to diverse diets to try a novel diet over a familiar one—almost as if they were "bored" with the old food.[72] The intensity of this behavior is directly related to the palatability of the new food. If the new food is as palatable as, or more palatable than, the old food, the cat will likely try the new food, and may be willing to continue to eat it, but the effect is typically short-lived (1 to 3 days) if the new food is less palatable or not preferred.[73,74]

Cats are extremely sensitive to external stimuli associated with their food: the odor (or aroma), the form (shape), texture (dry vs. canned, soft, moist), and palatability.[73,74] These different features are essential to determining preferences and regulating food intake in cats. Food odor is key for cats and is one of the major criteria for cats in food selection. Olfaction is the key factor to trigger good acceptance; anosmia or inability to breathe through the nose and perceive odors will result in food aversion or anorexia. The next key feature is the shape of the food, which again is primarily a learned behavior preference. There also appear to be breed preferences based on mouth size, as trials with Persians showed different preferences compared to domestic shorthair cats.[72] Texture is a common preference condition in cats, again owing to learned behaviors at a young age. For example, cats used to a certain texture or kibble shape may refuse a food of a different or new shape.

Finally, it is important to note that it is both fat and protein that are the primary determinants of taste preference in feline diets—rancid fat is a sure turnoff, as are protein sources (beef, chicken, fish, etc.) that are not preferred. This is also an important consideration for cats given a choice to eat dry versus canned foods—dry food is coated with digest (a fat and protein coating to enhance palatability) while canned food presents itself primarily as its protein flavor. Fat and crunch preferences are often very profound. Finally, practitioners can tell you that there is a high likelihood of cast needing a specific (usually canned) diet to meet a particular nutritional need at some point in their lifetime, such as when they have lower urinary tract disease, diabetes, obesity, renal disease, or GI disease. If they have not been introduced to canned food as kittens and fed some portion of their diet as canned, they will often refuse it. This unfortunate fact of feline feeding behavior complicates both the medical and nutritional management of their disease, and potentially reduces their quality (and quantity?) of life. Thus, a key concept is that it is a good idea to feed cats both canned and dry food early in life so they learn that both are food. This approach is beneficial not only to ensure that the cat will eat a particular food later in life, but also to provide the added water that they need in their diets. In addition, feeding canned food provides portion control that is necessary for indoor, neutered cats that have a lower resting energy metabolism, and with proper diet selection, a high-protein–low-CHO profile can be chosen to improve their metabolic status and meet their unique nutritional needs.

FELINE NUTRITION: WHAT IS AN APPROPRIATE AMOUNT OF FOOD?

Obesity is the most common nutritional and endocrine disorder in cats in the United States, with a reported incidence from 25% to 40%, depending on the study type and sources.[75] There are a large number of factors that contribute to this problem, including neuter status, sex, age, activity (indoor vs. outdoor), and feeding style (meal feeding vs. free choice). Both male and female neutered animals require significantly fewer (25% to 30%) calories for maintenance than intact animals—a fact that has been repeatedly proven in several recent studies evaluating the effect of neutering on intake, body fat mass, weight gain, and metabolism.[52-55] In a very recent study of ovariohysterectomized female cats who were allowed free access to a dry cat food, their fat mass increased from 18% to 33% in just 4 months—a staggering increase in body fat.[76] It is clear that specific guidelines for feeding cats a reduced amount of food are necessary, but all current maintenance energy equations (e.g., $90[BW_{kg}]^{0.75}$) and those recommendations present on the bags of food, are based upon *intact*, young, active animals. Using this equation to calculate a caloric intake for a typical 4- to 5-kg cat would mean that the cat should eat 300 kcal/day, which is clearly too much. Reducing this number by 30% to account for the decreased intake required of a neutered cat would reduce their intake to 200 to 210 kcal/day. In an ongoing study not yet published, Bauer and coworkers have shown that female cats require 60 to 70(BW)$^{0.67}$ (or approximately 200 kcal/day) to maintain a body condition score of 5/9.[77] Further studies are needed in male cats to determine their ideal energy intake, as evidence suggests that they may need even fewer calories to maintain ideal body condition. However, the key point is this: most neutered, indoor cats should receive about 200 kcal/day, preferably in meals, and many neutered males may require 10% to 20% less than this calculated amount to prevent obesity and maintain a lean body condition. Some active, thin cats that effectively self-regulate their food intake may be fed free choice; however, this method is still not recommended, as owners are less able to observe whether their cat is eating less or has even stopped eating if there are multiple cats in the household.

In summary, while a simple change in diet will not solve all of the ills of our feline patients, it is reasonable to believe that their lives are influenced by the foods we feed them. History has shown us this is true with respect to the many positive advances that have come in nutritional management of many diseases. While we may not agree on the cause, there are few that would question that nutrition plays a key role in the development of obesity, diabetes mellitus, hepatic lipidosis, and likely such complex diseases as IBD, cholangitis, and pancreatitis in cats. Although these problems are clearly very complex and multifactorial—having ties to genetic and environmental influences as well as to the nutritional factors outlined in this review—it is nevertheless to their peril that we ignore the unique nutritional needs of the cat—a true carnivore.

REFERENCES

The reference list can be found on the companion Expert Consult Web site at *www.expertconsult.com*.

CHAPTER 169

Dental Nutrition

Philippe Hennet

The first primitive mammals that appeared 250 million years ago already possessed two mandibles connected ventrorostrally by a symphysis and articulated to the skull by a temporomandibular articulation.[1] Evolutionary selection of mammals about 55 million years ago led to the apparition of all modern orders, including carnivores. Carnivores share a distinct anatomic character, the presence of a pair of carnassial teeth, which are the fourth premolar teeth of the maxilla and the first molar teeth of the mandible (Web Figures 169-1 and 169-2). In carnivore specialization, the temporomandibular articulation is located in the extension of the occlusal plane. It consists of a transversally oriented, hemicylindrical mandibular fossa, bordered ventrally by a powerful retroarticular process into which the head of the condylar process fits. This tight relationship between the condylar process and the mandibular fossa permits a hinge movement of the mandible with little lateral displacement, essential for achieving the crushing motion of carnassial teeth (Web Figures 169-3 and 169-4).[2] Due to the strong retroarticular process, high pressure can be placed unilaterally on the temporomandibular joint (TMJ) during carnassial crushing without risk of damage to the opposite TMJ.

Though zoologically classified as carnivores, dogs long have had an omnivore-carnivore or facultative omnivore diet.[3] Cats have a more specific carnivore diet, which is reflected in their dentition. Compared to dogs, cats have grinding/crushing molar teeth with an occlusal surface. Felids are characterized by a reduction in the number of teeth (evolutionary loss of premolars at the front of the row and of molars at the end of the row) and by a better adaptation to the cutting/crushing of preys through the use of teeth, especially carnassial teeth, longitudinally aligned as scissors blades (secodonte dentition).[4] Wild carnivores catch preys with their canine teeth, kill them through deep injuries induced by canine teeth and through crushing of caudal teeth, and tear and cut pieces of meat with their incisors with the help of strong muscular action of the neck. A big piece of meat can be subsequently cut, torn, and crushed through the action of carnassial teeth, while the animal can hold its prey with the forepaws. Felids and canids, opposite to humans, do not chew their food into very small pieces in order to mix it with salivary enzymes as a first stage of digestion (insalivation). They coat large pieces of meat with a mucus-rich saliva and swallow.

Though the original eating behavior of carnivores has mostly been lost in domestic animals, dental disease is not specific to modern carnivores. Wild canid and felid carnivores have been shown to have dental disease. In a study comparing periodontal disease among domestic cats and feral cats in Australia, it was found that domestic cats accumulated more calculus than feral cats but there was no statistical difference in the prevalence of periodontal disease between the two groups.[5] In another study on feral cats living on an Antarctic island, calculus was infrequently observed (9% of cats) but moderate to advanced tooth loss were reported in 62% of the cats.[6]

PERIODONTAL DISEASE, THE SINGLE MOST IMPORTANT DISEASE IN THE MOUTH OF DOGS AND CATS

In a large epidemiologic survey of more than 30,000 dogs and 15,000 cats examined in veterinary practices in the United States, it was reported that dental calculus and gingivitis were the most commonly diagnosed disorders.[7] Dental plaque accumulation, and its subsequent mineralization into calculus, leads to gingivitis, which, if not treated, may lead to periodontitis. Periodontitis is the most severe stage of periodontal diseases. It is characterized by alveolar bone destruction, tooth mobility, and tooth loss. Another study reported that ~60% of dogs had periodontal disease and 34% had missing teeth.[8] In another study of 115 dogs, 75% of dogs aged 2 to 8 years had radiographic signs of periodontitis.[9] Small-breed dogs are more severely affected. In a study of 769 dogs, dogs weighing less than 8 kg showed more severe disease.[10] In a study on 123 Poodles, 90% less than 4 years of age and all dogs older than 4 years had periodontitis involving at least one tooth.[11] In cats, 96% of 109 healthy colony cats had gingivitis and 92% (31% of teeth) had bone loss on radiographic examination.[12]

DENTAL PLAQUE AS THE CAUSE OF PERIODONTAL DISEASE

Periodontal disease is a local disease process initiated by dental plaque accumulation on tooth surface, as well as under the gingiva, which becomes infected. Periodontal lesions are the result of bacterial activity and host responses (release of cytokines and enzymes by granulocytes). Teeth, once erupted, are naturally bathed in the biologic fluid of the oral cavity, which contains more than 400 species of bacteria. Salivary glycoproteins, polypeptides and lipids form an acellular film on tooth surfaces, called the dental pellicle. Specific bacteria with adhesive properties, mainly gram-positive aerobes, colonize this dental pellicle. After adhesion of these initial (pioneer) bacteria, the biomass grows by division and multiplication. Further, colonization by other bacteria takes place. These bacteria attach to the pioneer bacteria (coaggregation). This "biofilm" (dental plaque) contains a diverse flora of bacteria embedded in a matrix of microbial and host origin polymers. Due to the complex organization of biofilm bacteria and subsequent phenotypic modifications compared to bacteria in cultures, chemical compounds have little effect in their destruction and mechanical disorganization of dental plaque is essential.

Inorganic substances from saliva are deposited into bacterial dental plaque and form calculus (commonly called *tartar*). Some species of bacteria act as catalysts of mineralization. Calculus can be located supragingivally and subgingivally. Blood and tissue exudates may be important for subgingival calculus formation. Calculus surface is rough and is colonized by dental plaque. In order to remove plaque, calculus has to be removed. Calculus may be clinically detectable on teeth as early as 2 weeks after thorough tooth cleaning. Calculus itself is not a primary cause of periodontal disease, but is always covered by plaque. Because of its rough surface, calculus favors plaque adhesion and accumulation. Therefore, calculus removal must be a component of treatment.

INFLUENCE OF DIET COMPOSITION

Though feeding a protein-deficient diet has been reported to induce degenerative changes of periodontal tissue, such deficiencies are unlikely with any commercially available pet food.[13] The addition of carbohydrate to a soft food was not associated with more plaque accumulation or more severe gingivitis in dogs.[14] Though data are limited, alteration of protein and carbohydrate content within AAFCO (Association of American Feed Control Officials) allowances is not considered to play a role in development of periodontal disease.

Feeding a low-calcium–high-phosphorus food may lead to secondary nutritional hyperparathyroidism and subsequent alveolar bone resorption, but in the absence of dental plaque, dogs are not more susceptible to periodontal disease.[15] Similar

to what is known about protein and carbohydrate content of diet, Ca-P ratio is strictly monitored in all commercial diets and the type of diet associated with those experimentally induced is not realistic. No specific influence of dietary vitamin content on development of periodontal disease in dogs or cats has been shown.

INFLUENCE OF DIET CONSISTENCY ("HARD" VERSUS "SOFT" DIETS)

In 1965, Egelberg et al showed that Beagle dogs fed a meal consisting of raw bovine trachea, esophagus, and muscles supplemented with vitamins, calcium, and iron showed less plaque accumulation and gingivitis compared to a control group fed the same diet that had been minced.[16] This report led to the incorrect belief that hard food was more beneficial than soft food in preventing periodontal disease. What was shown in Egelberg's study was that a diet requiring strong masticatory activity was beneficial. The original diet was not "hard" but rather made of large fibrous/cartilaginous pieces. A multicentric epidemiologic study conducted on a population of 1350 dogs showed that no significant difference could be observed between dogs fed soft versus those fed hard pelleted food. However, dogs offered a chewing device regularly showed less calculus accumulation, less gingivitis, and less alveolar bone resorption.[17] A study investigating commercial food reported that some canned and dry foods were less effective than a canned "reference" in reducing calculus accumulation.[18] A similar beneficial effect of hard food has been reported in cats.[19]

PERIODONTAL DISEASE CONTROL THROUGH DIETARY MEANS

Brushing Teeth
Dental daily tooth-brushing by owners is recognized as the best method for preventing dental plaque accumulation and subsequent periodontal disease development. However, most pet owners do not brush their pets' teeth due to lack of time, pet compliance, and practicality. Logically, pet food companies have investigated methods of promoting periodontal health that do not require direct action by owners. Since the early 1990s, pet food development has attempted to prevent plaque and calculus accumulation as a means of limiting periodontal disease progression.[18] The effect on calculus, plaque, and gingival inflammation of specific dental-oriented diets and chews or dietary bones has been investigated in many studies in dogs[20-25] but less in cats.[26,27]

Effect on Calculus Accumulation
Calculus, per se, is not the primary cause of periodontal disease. Living bacteria are required to produce periodontal disease. Calculus provides a rough tooth surface that enhances adhesion and retention of bacteria. Contrary to dental plaque, calculus can be readily identified by dog's owners. Prevention of calculus accumulation is therefore important for owners even though, in the absence of preventing plaque accumulation, it has minimal biologic significance. Control of calculus accumulation can be readily achieved through enhancement of the chewing activity and through the inhibition of calculus mineralization.[25,28,29] It has been shown that feeding dogs a commercial extruded dry food that simply has a 50% increase in kibble diameter results in 42% less calculus accumulation.[25] Coating food or biscuit with a calculus formation inhibitor (sodium hexametaphosphate or sodium tripolyphosphate) has been shown to further reduce calculus deposit on tooth

surface by 50% to 60%.[25,29] It has been shown that kibble size had no effect on maxillary incisor, canine, and third premolar teeth. However, kibble size had a significant effect on mandibular teeth, maxillary fourth premolars, and first molars.[25] Some teeth that did not show a reduction in calculus accumulation when kibble size was increased showed a reduction in calculus when the kibble was coated with a calculus mineralization inhibitor. This adjunct effect was due to the release of the chemical agent into the saliva.[25]

Effect on Plaque Accumulation

Inhibition of calculus formation without concomitant inhibition of dental plaque formation has limited value, as plaque is the etiological factor. The Veterinary Oral Health Council (VOHC), regulated by the American Veterinary Dental College (AVDC), scientifically evaluates studies on plaque/calculus retardation in dogs and cats. They award a "seal of acceptance" following review of data.[30] Since the mid-nineties, many studies on dental-oriented diets or chews have been performed using VOHC protocol guidelines. Fourteen percent to 39% reductions in plaque have been reported in publications utilizing various product (Web Figures 169-5 and 169-6).[20-25] Recently concerns have been raised regarding the validity of the methodology and, subsequently, pertinence of the results.[31-33] The index system that has been used in most of the older studies is no longer accepted by the VOHC.[30] It is accepted that short duration trials may be indicative of longer-term clinical relevance.[30] Screening the plaque retarding effect of a compound with mechanical or chemical activity can be performed over a brief time period (a few days) when studying the fast regrowth phase of dental plaque on tooth surface that have been thoroughly cleaned and polished (known as the "clean tooth model").[18,32] But it has yet to be shown that long term effects in real life situations can be predicted based on short trial experiments. When a specific diet or dental chew is inhibiting 25% of plaque accumulation, 75% remains. This large amount of dental plaque accumulating on the tooth surface, especially in critical areas such as along the gingiva, create favorable conditions for further plaque accumulation and plaque maturation. It might be questioned whether slight reductions in plaque accumulation have clinical value.

Effect on Gingivitis (Periodontal Disease Development)

Beyond the preventive effect of nutrition on the development the primary (dental plaque) or accessory (dental calculus) causes of periodontal disease, the preventive effect of the diet on the disease process itself needs to be investigated. Early studies demonstrated that soft sticky diets enhanced development of plaque accumulation and gingivitis.[13,16] However, the effect of dental-oriented diets and chews on gingivitis development is less known. Methodology again is critical in the assessment of periodontal disease indices. Gingivitis assessment, which is used to monitor periodontal disease development, is based on subjective "noninvasive" (redness, swelling) and objective "invasive" criteria (bleeding on probing).[32] However, standardized conditions (animals with nonpigmented or evenly pigmented gingiva to assess noninvasive criteria, use of standardized probing technique and of a pressure-control probe to assess the invasive criteria) are rarely met in most studies and therefore results obtained might be questionable.

While tooth brushing is still the gold standard in dental hygiene, lack of practicality in dogs and, more particularly, in cats dramatically limits its implementation. Therefore, it is legitimate to investigate other means of improving dental health in pets. Attempts to recreate a mechanical dental function when feeding dogs and cats may be essential as they have teeth that have been selected through evolutionary process to cut and crush food. However, how much of dental hygiene can really be achieved through this means is still unknown. Studying plaque inhibition and prevention of periodontal disease is a difficult task. Many studies have been performed, but many more will need to be performed in order to identify the optimal effect. Long-term studies are needed in order to evaluate the effect on periodontal health beyond the results that studies on plaque accumulation and gingivitis development can give.

REFERENCES

The reference list can be found on the companion Expert Consult Web site at *www.expertconsult.com*.

CHAPTER **170**

Nutrition of Healthy Dogs and Cats in Various Adult Stages

Andrea J. Fascetti
James G. Morris
Quinton R. Rogers

Although both dogs and cats are classified as carnivores, their nutrient requirements are not identical. The metabolism and nutritional needs of dogs approach those of omnivores, whereas the metabolism of cats is consistent with that of a strict meat-eating mammal.[1-3]

Dogs have the capability to use plant sources for synthesizing taurine, arachidonic acid, and vitamin A from their metabolic precursors present in plants, cysteine, linoleic acid, and beta-carotene, respectively. Cats, by contrast, either have diminished enzyme activities for synthesizing these nutrients (taurine and arachidonic acid) from their metabolic precursors, or they do not possess the enzyme. Cats must therefore obtain these nutrients from their diet. Both dogs and cats possess some similar metabolic characteristics such as an obligation to conjugate bile acids with taurine and an inability to synthesize vitamin D. However, the cat digests uncooked starch somewhat better than the dog, so not all evidence is fully consistent with the cat being a strict carnivore and the dog simply being an omnivore.

FOOD INTAKE AND PALATABILITY

The diet of feral cats is based largely on small mammals, birds, lizards, and insects. When domesticated cats are fed free choice, they eat 10 to 20 meals per day (12 mice per day provide the energy requirement of a normal cat) about equally divided between the light and dark period. Significant breed differences are seen in the feeding behavior of dogs: Beagles have feeding patterns similar to cats, whereas Basenjis and Poodles eat only during the daylight hours. The number of meals can vary widely from 5 to 20. Adult dogs adapt to one meal a day, and cats at maintenance can adapt to a similar regimen. During gestation and lactation, however, performance is enhanced by feeding several times a day or by feeding free choice. During the latter part of gestation and lactation, bitches should be offered food at least twice a day and preferably fed free choice.

Both cats and dogs prefer meat-based canned products rather than dry expanded diets, in part owing to the higher moisture content of canned products and in part because blood and fluids contain positive palatability factors. Texture is important; cats and dogs both prefer soft, moist foods to dry, powdery foods. Dogs respond positively to protein, peptides, certain free amino acids, sugar, and mononucleotides, together with certain electrolytes. The response of cats is neutral to protein and sugar, positive to peptides and certain free amino acids, and negative to mononucleotides. Good-quality animal fats enhance palatability for both cats and dogs. Medium chain triglycerides are strongly aversive to cats but not to dogs. Both dogs and cats respond positively to fresh meat extracts, whereas cats but not dogs generally show strong negative palatability to oxidized or rancid fats and breakdown products of trinucleotides or mononucleotides. In summary, cats are more sensitive to adulteration, oxidation, and rancidity in foods than are dogs. Cooked meat extracts (broth) are the most palatable natural ingredients to use to enhance the palatability of unpalatable foods for both dogs and cats.

Food intake of cats and dogs fed diets of low or high palatability is quite well controlled. The level at which the animal controls its weight is complex and depends on factors such as genetics (breed and strain), life stage, physical activity, food availability, food palatability, and whether the animal is neutered. Both dogs and cats maintain their weight and stay healthy if their diet is complete and balanced, even if the diet has poor palatability. Highly palatable, high-fat diets increase the risk for obesity. Nevertheless, dogs and cats control their food intake, albeit at a higher level of body weight, even when fed highly palatable high-fat diets. It is always easier to prevent obesity by selecting or manipulating the aforementioned factors before obesity occurs rather than to try to limit food intake to effect weight loss.

In most species, including cats and dogs, emetics (e.g., lithium chloride, apomorphine) induce an aversion to the taste of the food just previously eaten. This behavior is called a *learned taste aversion*. In cats there appears to be a neural disassociation between the neural response to the nutrient deficiency and feeding behavior. For those deficiencies and excesses that have been examined (protein deficiency and excess, individual essential amino acid deficiency and excess, sodium deficiency), no learned taste aversions have been demonstrated, despite the fact that food intake may have been depressed.[3,4] It is notable that even though cats do not appear to develop learned aversions to simple nutrient deficiencies or excesses, it has been shown that cats do avoid diets that cause hyperammonemia[5] or metabolic acidosis.[6] Thus palatability may override nutrient metabolic effects in cats, whereas nutrient metabolic effects (caused by nutrient deficiencies and

excesses) override palatability effects in herbivores and omnivores (Figure 170-1).

In herbivores and omnivores, food intake is depressed, and strong avoidance of a particular diet is exhibited when animals are fed diets with various nutrient deficiencies or excesses (e.g., deficiencies of thiamine, sodium, phosphate, protein, specific essential amino acids).

GENERAL FEEDING RECOMMENDATIONS

Practitioners should advise clients to choose a commercial diet that has passed an Association of American Feed Control Officials (AAFCO) animal protocol test for the particular life stage of the cat or dog. This ensures that the diet has undergone an animal feeding test. An AAFCO nutrient profile label means only that a diet meets a calculated nutrient profile. In most cases it is safest to feed a diet that has passed an AAFCO all-stages protocol. The exception would be if a particular dog or cat has a medical problem; then a specific therapeutic diet should be fed.

In selecting an appropriate therapeutic diet, one should always select a diet that has been tested for the intended purpose. Alternatively, one might recommend that a clinical nutritionist be consulted for advice or to formulate an appropriate balanced homemade diet. It is prudent to check whether a commercial diet (regular or therapeutic) has been properly tested in animals for the intended purpose. It is reasonable to feed a diet that has large, built-in safety factors in nutritional requirements, but there is no reason to pay for extra nutrients if they have not been shown to be of extra benefit to the cat or dog.

When a diet is complete, balanced, tested, and shown to be fully adequate in animals, there is no reason to feed a diet containing even more of one or more of the essential nutrients. Nevertheless, a paucity of information is available on specific nutrient requirements in adult life stages, including maintenance. There has been considerable research on the nutrient requirements for dogs and cats for growth, because it is the easiest life stage for which to determine requirements. The requirements for growth have been used to formulate requirements during pregnancy. Additional information from epidemiologic evidence and from other species has been used to formulate requirements for maintenance.

MEETING ENERGY NEEDS

About 80% of the food eaten by mature cats and dogs is used to provide their energy needs. The requirements for protein, minerals, and vitamins can be met in the remaining dry matter. Therefore, meeting energy needs is the first consideration in feeding cats and dogs. Energy, unlike individual amino acids, vitamins, and minerals, is not supplied by any single nutrient but is provided by the oxidation of substrates, primarily fats, carbohydrates, and proteins. The energy needs of dogs or cats may be supplied by diets with varying ratios of these three nutrients. The only avenue an animal has for disposal of excess energy is by oxidation to produce adenosine triphosphate or to store the excess energy in the form of adipose tissue. Mature dogs and cats that are in energy balance convert all the available or metabolizable energy (ME) from food into exercise and heat. To calculate the amount of food required by dogs or cats, the ME value of the food should be known.

The energy requirements of mature, nonpregnant cats and dogs are not constant but decrease on a unit-bodyweight basis with age, which is related to the reduction in general activity

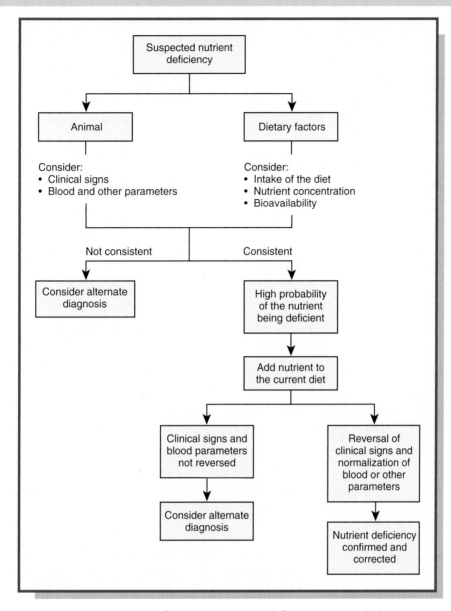

Figure 170-1 Algorithm for solving a nutrient deficiency in an adult dog or cat.

with age. As indicated, many individual cats and dogs adjust their energy intake from food to balance their energy needs. However, in some adults, this balance is not maintained, leading either to bodyweight loss, resulting in catabolism of body energy stores, or to obesity and bodyweight gain owing to excessive energy intake.

The maintenance energy requirements of adult cats and dogs may be estimated from formulas relating ME requirements to body weight. Because mature dogs have about a fiftyfold range in body weight, and because ME requirements per unit of body weight decrease with body weight, formulas generally include some power function of body weight (e.g., body weight raised to three-fourths power). A common linear formula used for dogs is ME = 39 W + 358, and an exponent formula is ME = 132 W$^{3/4}$, where W is body weight in kilograms and ME is kilocalories per day.[7]

The first equation approximates the relationship for small dogs such as Beagles but overpredicts energy requirements for large breeds. Because the bodyweight range of adult cats is much less than that of adult dogs, a power function is not recommended in normal weight, active cats. The formula currently recommended is ME = 70 W for active, lean cats with a body condition score of 5 or lower on a 9-point scale. For overweight cats (body condition score >5), the use of the exponent 0.4 may be justified to account for actual body mass (ME = 130 W$^{0.4}$).[7]

Although these formulas are useful starting points, they are not absolute requirements because considerable individual animal variation exists. It has been shown that a large variation exists in the prediction interval of maintenance energy requirement.[8] However, when enteral or parenteral nutritional support is necessary, a requirement estimate must be made. Similarly, when a weight reduction program is undertaken, an estimate of maintenance energy requirements is desirable, especially if a thorough diet history is not available. All adult cats and dogs that are voluntarily consuming food should be fed relative to their body condition and not by a formula. If an adult dog or cat is fed free choice and becomes obese, either the amount of food offered or the energy density (available caloric density) of the food should be reduced. When an adult cat or dog is not maintaining body weight, either more food or a more palatable food should be fed to increase intake, or a diet of a higher caloric density should be fed (or both should be done).

Pregnancy causes a demand for energy greater than normal adult maintenance requirements. Different responses to pregnancy occur in the ingestive behavior of bitches versus queens, even though the length of gestation is similar. Queens increase food intake soon after conception and have an almost linear increase in body energy stores with duration of gestation. In contrast, bitches normally do not increase food and energy intake until the latter stages of pregnancy. Queens and bitches in normal body condition may be given food free choice during pregnancy to allow for the increase in body tissue that will be mobilized during lactation and by fetal energy demands. Whereas the latter stages of pregnancy increase energy requirements by about a third, lactation places a huge demand on the bitch and queen and can result in energy intakes three to four times above maintenance. Depending on the number of kittens or pups, queens or bitches sustain a loss of body weight during lactation. This tissue loss should be largely the tissue gained during the prepartum period; with a good diet and normal litter size the weaning body weight of the mother should not be less than the body weight at conception.

PROTEINS AND AMINO ACIDS

Proteins are added to diets to provide essential amino acids and nitrogen. Nitrogen requirements are usually expressed as the crude protein requirement, because crude protein is defined as the quantity of nitrogen times 6.25. Nitrogen is used for the biosynthesis of dispensable amino acids, heme, purines, pyrimidines, and so forth. Both essential and dispensable amino acids are necessary at the cellular level for protein synthesis. Several amino acids are precursors for hormones and neurotransmitters. If the amino acid and crude protein requirements are known for each life stage, the clinical nutritionist can formulate a diet using amino acid composition tables for particular proteins and ensure that both essential amino acid and nitrogen requirements are met. However, a weakness of diet formulation using nutrient composition tables is that the bioavailabilities of amino acids and nitrogen from food sources are usually not known, or the effect of processing on the particular food (or food combinations) is not known. The most accurate way to tell if the diet is adequate in protein is to evaluate plasma amino acid concentrations during the absorptive state after feeding a particular diet. Amino acid patterns can be used not only to verify that essential amino acid requirements have been met but also to diagnose various nutritional problems (e.g., protein-energy malnutrition, essential amino acid deficiency) and metabolic problems (e.g., liver or kidney disease).

Carnivores have no problem meeting their protein or amino acid requirements if they eat other animals, because the body composition of various animals is quite similar and is high in good-quality protein. Nutritional problems arise only if a client attempts to feed a carnivore a vegetarian diet or a diet that has poor-quality ingredients (e.g., by-products that are high in collagen, such as skin and bone) or products that have been excessively processed. Quality control of ingredients in pet foods can be a concern, because large quantities of animal by-products do not always have a constant composition; thus these by-products may have variable digestibilities and bioavailabilities for nitrogen and amino acids. Specific amino acid deficiencies or excesses can cause a variety of problems, such as cataracts, dermatitis, hair loss or reddening of black hair or both, irritability, neurologic deficits, hyperammonemia, fatty liver, low glutathione, and emesis.

The most recent edition of the National Research Council's Nutrient Requirements of Dogs and Cats contains nutrient recommendations in terms of at least one of the following categories: minimal requirements, adequate intake, recommended allowances, and safe upper limits.[7] Recommendations from the AAFCO are in part based on this information.[9] Most cat and dog foods are formulated to meet or exceed these recommendations. Major pet food companies have competent nutritionists who take digestibility and bioavailability values into account in formulating diets, and most of the major diets have been tested. Therefore, veterinarians should be confident in recommending any pet food that has passed the AAFCO feeding protocol for the life stage in question. The bottom line is simple for adult dogs and cats: feed a commercial diet for the appropriate life stage from a reputable company. The only other safe course is consultation with a small animal nutritionist to attempt to evaluate a diet or to formulate a homemade diet. The latter is not recommended unless absolutely necessary because of the difficulty in predicting bioavailability of ingredient nutrients and the difficulty in getting good compliance in making and feeding such a diet.

MINERALS AND VITAMINS

Adult cats and dogs require the same minerals and vitamins that are essential to growing kittens and puppies. Although the requirements for growing kittens and puppies are fairly well defined, those for adults are not known with the same precision. The dietary concentration for growth satisfies adult requirements, even though the food intake of adults on a unit-bodyweight basis is less than that during growth. The function and clinical role of minerals and vitamins have been reviewed.[10,11]

Minerals

The published mineral requirements for cats and dogs have recently been reviewed and updated by the National Research Council.[7] Applying these values to practical diets requires bioavailability values to be taken into account. Although these have not been determined in cats and dogs, values originating in other simple-stomached species give useful approximations. The bioavailability of calcium, phosphorus, and magnesium from plant sources is considerably less than that from mineral salts or bone and should be discounted by 50%. In contrast, sodium, potassium, and chloride are readily exchangeable, and no adjustments are necessary concerning their source.

Bioavailability of trace elements, especially as they pertain to cats and dogs, is not known, but observations indicate that the availability of zinc and copper in diets containing high proportions of plant products is compromised. Zinc deficiency is common in dogs fed some of the lower-quality dry diets containing a high proportion of plant products. Clinical signs of copper deficiency have been reported in newborn kittens from queens given diets containing copper oxide as a supplementary source of copper. Reproductive performance of the queens was also reduced. The requirements for many of the major minerals (e.g., calcium, potassium, sodium) increase greatly in lactation. However, because food intake is also increased about twofold, the percentage in the diet need not change. Diagnosis of mineral deficiencies should be based on specific clinical signs, blood, plasma, or tissue concentrations for the species, as well as on reversal of clinical signs after supplementation with the specific mineral while the cat or dog is maintained on the same diet.

Vitamins

For the fat-soluble vitamins A, D, and E, the requirements are similar for adult cats and dogs. Cats, unlike dogs, are unable to use beta-carotene as a precursor for retinol, so they depend on preformed vitamin A in the diet. Neither cats nor dogs are capable of synthesizing vitamin D from ultraviolet (UV) light.[7,11,12] Although vitamins A and D are regarded as the most toxic of all the vitamins when given in excess, adult cats can tolerate large excesses (50 times requirement) of these two vitamins with no discernible deleterious effects. In normal cats and dogs, in contrast to most other animals, large concentrations of retinyl esters occur in plasma. Requirements for vitamin E are a function of the total polyunsaturated fatty acids (PUFAs) in the diet. Because cats frequently consume diets high in PUFAs, the requirement to prevent steatitis in cats is higher than that for dogs that are subjected to lower dietary inputs of PUFAs. Both cats and dogs have a metabolic requirement for vitamin K. Intestinal synthesis appears to be adequate to supply this need in dogs. When cats are fed some high-fish diets, they have a prolongation of clotting time and require supplemental vitamin K.

In contrast to the fat-soluble vitamins, the requirements for the water-soluble vitamins for cats versus dogs are different. Cats have a higher requirement than dogs for thiamine (vitamin B_1) and are exposed to dietary ingredients that often contain both thiaminases (e.g., raw fish) and to canned diets that have sustained extensive processing, causing loss of thiamine. As thiamine stores are rapidly exhausted, thiamine deficiency can readily occur in cats given deficient diets. Cats, unlike dogs, are unable to use tryptophan as a precursor for niacin synthesis, so niacin is an absolute essential dietary nutrient for cats. Niacin is normally obtained from foods by hydrolysis of nicotinamide adenosyl dinucleotide (NAD) and nicotinamide phosphodinucleotide (NADP) in the gut. Meats contain high levels of these nucleotides and thus are a principal source of this vitamin.

The published vitamin requirements[7] for growing kittens and puppies appear to satisfy the requirements of mature cats and dogs. However, in applying these values, it is necessary to take into consideration the bioavailability of the vitamin and its stability in the product. The bioavailability of the fat-soluble vitamins is high in the absence of most fat malabsorption syndromes, whereas the bioavailability of most of the B vitamins in natural products is variable and can be quite low.

TAURINE

Taurine, a beta-sulfur amino acid, occurs in all animal cells and is virtually the sole conjugate of the bile acids in cats and dogs. Taurine is synthesized de novo by dogs and cats from the sulfur amino acids cysteine and methionine. Although cat diets contain a higher level of sulfur amino acids than do dog diets, the rate of taurine synthesis by cats is low; cats given a low-taurine diet are readily depleted of this amino acid. This very low rate of taurine synthesis in cats is a consequence of low activities of two enzymes in the pathway of synthesis. Taurine depletion is associated with a wide range of clinical conditions, including feline central retinal degeneration, reversible dilated cardiomyopathy, reproductive failure in queens, and developmental defects and growth retardation in kittens. The amount of dietary taurine required for cats to maintain adequate blood concentrations varies twofold with the type of diet. For expanded (dry) diets, 1000 mg taurine/kg diet containing 4 kcal metabolizable energy/g is adequate.[7] Canned diets, which promote higher intestinal degradation of taurine exposed in the enterohepatic circulation, minimally require 1700 mg/kg diet containing 4 kcal metabolizable energy/g dry matter to maintain blood concentrations in the normal range.[7]

Until recently, diet-associated taurine deficiency in dogs has not been recognized. However, low blood taurine concentrations and dilated cardiomyopathy (DCM) have been identified in dogs that do not have a genetic predilection to this disease. A common finding among the cases was the consumption of commercial dry diets containing lamb meal, rice, or both as the primary ingredients. Cardiac parameters and blood taurine concentrations improved with treatment and taurine supplementation. Dogs that survived longer than 1 year were able to be removed from all cardiac medications except taurine, suggesting that these were not typical cases of DCM. Suggested mechanisms for taurine deficiency in these dogs were considered to be (1) insufficient synthesis of taurine, (2) extraordinary loss of taurine or its precursors in urine, (3) extraordinary gastrointestinal (GI) loss of taurine in bile acid conjugates (as found in cats), or (4) a reduction in protein digestibility. Based on clinical findings, blood taurine concentrations, and common diet histories, it appears that the consumption of diets with inadequate or unavailable sulfur amino acid (taurine precursors) results in taurine deficiency and low blood taurine concentrations in these dogs. The low plasma taurine concentrations can lead to the development of abnormal cardiac function and DCM.

ESSENTIAL FATTY ACIDS

The diets of healthy dogs and cats, like those of other animals, must contain PUFAs. Because these fatty acids cannot be synthesized de novo by animals, they are designated as essential fatty acids (EFAs). Dogs require two EFAs in the diet: linoleic acid C18:2 n-6 and linolenic acid C18:3 n-3. The letter followed by the number (e.g., n-6 or ω-6, n-3 or ω-3) refers to the location of the first double bond in the fatty acid from the methyl (or omega) end of the fatty acid. Animals cannot insert double bonds further than 9 carbons from the carboxyl end of a fatty acid. In addition to linoleic and linolenic acids, cats under certain conditions may require arachidonic acid, a member of the n-6 family of fatty acids in the diet. The activity of the hepatic delta-6–desaturase enzyme required in one of the pathways for the synthesis of arachidonic acid from linoleic acid is low in cats. This limited activity appears to be sufficient for growth and reproduction in male cats (where the testis also has delta-6–desaturate activity) but may be inadequate for sustained reproduction in queens. Other fatty acids, particularly those of the n-3 series, may also limit reproduction in queens.

Fatty acids function as precursors of eicosanoids, which include prostaglandin, leukotrienes, and thromboxanes. These extremely active biologic compounds have both paracrine and endocrine activity. As a group, the eicosanoids of the n-6 series tend to be involved in a more proinflammatory role, whereas those of the n-3 have an antiinflammatory or only a mildly inflammatory role.

Of the EFAs, the quantitative requirement of cats and dogs is greatest for linoleic acid. A deficiency of linoleic acid results in hyperkeratosis of skin, fatty degeneration of the liver, and degeneration of the testis. In addition, increased water loss through the skin occurs. Cats and dogs require about 1% to 2% of the calories as linoleic acid to prevent clinical signs of deficiency, though higher levels of total fat in the diet may result in better coat condition. The n-3 fatty acid, linolenic acid, occurs in high concentration in some plant oils, and higher homologues of this fatty acid occur in animal fats, particularly marine oils such as herring and tuna. In cats, the production of these higher n-3 homologues also appears to be limited, which may contribute to the poor reproductive performance of queens given some vegetable fat diets.

Clinical signs of arachidonate deficiency in cats are associated with eicosanoid dysfunction and include defective reproduction in queens and changes in blood platelet aggregation.

The requirement of cats for arachidonic acid has not been defined but appears to be of the order of 200 mg/kg dry matter. Arachidonate in natural diets comes from animal tissue membranes. Recently a fungal source of arachidonate has become commercially available, so it is possible to add this fatty acid to diets for cats without the inclusion of animal fat.

OTHER NUTRIENTS AND NUTRACEUTICALS

Choline is often included among the "essential" vitamins because it supplies labile methyl groups. Methionine and betaine can also supply methyl groups. A lack of total methyl groups in the diet leads to fatty liver because of an inability to mobilize hepatic fat.

Ascorbate, or vitamin C, is synthesized de novo by dogs and cats from glucose, and no substantiated evidence exists (except anecdotal reports in liver disease) to indicate that dogs or cats benefit from the addition of ascorbate to the diet. In contrast, some breeds of dogs have a limited capacity to syn-thesize adequate carnitine and benefit from its supplementation. Synthetic antioxidants are frequently added to human and animal diets to prevent lipid peroxidation during storage. Substantial evidence contraindicates the consumption of lipid peroxides. It is debatable whether these synthetic antioxidants are deleterious when used at the recommended concentrations in the diet. Natural antioxidants such as alpha-tocopherol, though less effective than the synthetic antioxidants, can also be used. A number of human foods such as onions and chocolate cause adverse effects in cats and dogs, respectively; thus some human foods should not be fed to cats and dogs indiscriminately. Food faddism in human nutrition has resulted in malnutrition, toxicities, and deficiencies. These same practices occur in dog and cat nutrition and should be avoided.

REFERENCES

The reference list can be found on the companion Expert Consult Web site at *www.expertconsult.com.*

CHAPTER 171

Neonatal and Pediatric Nutrition

Johnny D. Hoskins

The nutritional requirements, feeding, and care of puppies and kittens from birth to early adulthood are substantially different during their different stages of growth. The growth phase is a critical time in the life of a puppy or kitten; some will fail to grow to the size determined by their hereditary factors unless they consume appropriate food of adequate quality.

FEEDING THE PUPPY

Healthy puppies, during the first 2 to 3 weeks of life, should only eat and sleep. Nursing should be vigorous and active, with each puppy receiving sufficient milk from its mother. If the mother is healthy and well nourished, the puppy's nutritional needs for its first 3 to 4 weeks of life should be provided completely by her. Indications that the puppy is not receiving sufficient milk are constant crying, extreme inactivity, or failure to achieve weight gains in accordance with the general guidelines that a puppy should gain 1 to 2 g/day/lb (2 to 4 g/day/kg) of anticipated adult weight (or at least 10% gain per day).[1] For example, if the adult dog is expected to weigh 30 lb, as a puppy it should gain 30 to 60 g/day during its first 5 months of life.

The transition from mother's milk to solid food should be a gradual process beginning at about 3 weeks of age (4 weeks of age for toy breeds); however, if necessary, supplemental feeding may be started as soon as the puppy fails to show sufficient weight gain. During the changeover to solid food, the puppy can be offered a thick, gruel-like mixture of good-quality puppy food designed for growth and water (one part dry food blended with three parts water, or two parts canned food blended with one part water). To get the puppy eating, the gruel is placed in a shallow food dish, the puppy is encour-aged to lap the gruel by touching its lips to the food, or the feeder can put a finger in the gruel and then into the puppy's mouth. It can also be force-fed using a commercial dosing syringe. Once the puppy accepts the gruel, the amount of water is gradually reduced until it is omitted.

By 6 weeks of age, the puppy should be receiving at least 25% of its requirements from the weaning diet. The puppy may be permanently separated from the mother as soon as it learns to eat readily and drink satisfactorily. Most puppies are completely weaned at 7 to 8 weeks of age, depending some-what on size and breed. Early weaning and separation from littermates, prior to 6 weeks of age, however, can cause mal-nutrition or numerous behavioral problems later in life. Because of this, complete weaning should not be attempted until puppies are at least 6 weeks old and close human contact has been established.

Feeding the weaned puppy should always be directed to attaining the appropriate growth rate for the breed.[1] Instead of making food available to the puppy at all times (free-choice feeding), time-limited meal feeding is recommended. At each feeding, the puppy should be given 15 to 20 minutes to eat all that it wants; then the remaining food should be removed. From the time of weaning to 4 to 6 months of age (9 months for giant breeds), puppies are best fed at least three times a day at regular intervals. Thereafter, puppies should be fed twice a day on a regular schedule.

Some large and giant breeds of dogs (those over 30 kg body weight at maturity) have the genetic capacity to grow rapidly and will do so if provided with a food that meets or exceeds their nutrient and energy needs. However, a rapid growth rate is not compatible with normal skeletal growth and may result in certain types of developmental bone disease.[2,3] Beginning at weaning and continuing until they reach maturity, large and giant breeds of dogs should be fed for a moderate growth rate.

This can be accomplished by limiting food intake or, even better, by feeding a growth-formulated puppy food for large and giant breeds. If osteochondrosis or hypertrophic osteodystrophy occurs, nutritional management should be aimed at reducing caloric intake by decreasing the amount of food that is fed or feeding a growth-formulated puppy food for large and giant breeds.

FEEDING THE KITTEN

Healthy kittens, during their first 4 weeks of life, should nurse vigorously and actively. If the mother is healthy and well nourished, the nutritional needs of the kittens during this time should be filled completely by her. Each kitten should receive sufficient milk from its mother. Kittens not receiving sufficient milk cry constantly, are restless or extremely inactive, or fail to achieve the expected weight gain of 10 to 15 g/day.[1]

Kittens should be encouraged to begin eating solid food at 4 weeks of age. At this time, the kitten can be offered a thick, gruel-like mixture of good-quality kitten food designed for growth and milk or water (one part dry food blended with three parts milk, or two parts canned food blended with one part milk). The gruel is fed to kittens from a shallow bowl or force-fed by using a commercial dosing syringe. The feeder can encourage the kitten to eat the gruel by smearing some of the gruel on the kitten's lips, being careful not to get any in the nose, or placing a finger in the gruel and then into the kitten's mouth. This usually encourages the kitten to eat from a bowl at an early age. Once the kitten is eating the gruel well, the amount of milk or water in the gruel is gradually reduced until the kitten is consuming only solid food. The kitten may be permanently separated from the mother as soon as it learns to eat readily and drink satisfactorily. Most kittens are completely weaned at 6 to 8 weeks of age. Early weaning and separation from littermates before 6 weeks of age can result in behavioral problems such as slowness to learn and more suspicious, cautious, and aggressive actions.[4]

Food given to weaned kittens should be specifically formulated for growth. Feeding between 3 to 3.5 oz of dry food per day or 8 to 10 oz of canned food per day usually meets the growth requirements of most kittens. Because the kitten's eating habits are still in the formative stage after weaning, it is important that easily digested, high-quality, calorically dense food is provided. Cow's or goat's milk is often fed to kittens after weaning and is a good food, provided that it does not cause diarrhea. Milk should never be given in place of fresh water.

Kittens should be fed all the food they will consume. Excessive caloric intake and excessively rapid growth rate are seldom problems in growing kittens. Most kittens are not voracious. When food is always available, they nibble at it frequently. Kittens fed unlimited amounts of food (free-choice feeding), regardless of the form of food (dry or canned), eat every few hours. Free-choice feeding, or at least three-times-a-day feeding, is preferred during growth.

At 12 weeks of age the kitten's energy needs are three times greater than those of an adult cat, or more than 200 kcal/kg of bodyweight. As kittens mature past 6 months of age, their growth rate slows and their food needs decrease. Their energy needs are still greater than adult cats, or approximately 90 kcal/kg of bodyweight.

REARING NURSING PUPPIES AND KITTENS

Newborn puppies and kittens are unable to effectively control their body temperature.[5] During their first 4 weeks of life, they gradually progress from being largely poikilothermic to being homeothermic. That is, for the first week of life their body temperature is directly related to the environmental temperature, and a steady ambient temperature of 30° to 32° C (86° to 90° F) is needed. Over the next 3 weeks, the ambient temperature can be gradually lowered to 24° C (75° F). Humidity should be maintained at 55% to 60%. It is equally important that sudden changes of environmental conditions be avoided.

The most obvious alternative to a mother rearing her own young is for another nursing mother to act as a foster mother. If a foster mother is not available, it is necessary to hand-feed the puppies or kittens a replacement food that is a prototype of nutritive substance formulated to meet the optimum requirements of the puppy or kitten. Mother's milk is the ideal food. Various modifications of homemade and commercially prepared formulas simulating mother's milk have been used with good success.[5-7] Commercially prepared formulas are preferred, because they closely compare to mother's milk. These formulas generally provide 1 to 1.24 kcal of metabolizable energy per milliliter of formula. The caloric needs for most nursing-age puppies and kittens are 22 to 26 kcal per 100 g of body weight. Therefore the average puppy or kitten should daily receive approximately 13 mL of formula per 100 g of body weight during the first week of life, 17 mL of formula per 100 g of body weight during the second week, 20 mL of formula per 100 g of body weight during the third week, and 22 mL of formula per 100 g of bodyweight during the fourth week. These amounts of formula should be given in equal portions three or four times daily. For the first 3 weeks of life, the formula should be warmed before each feeding to about 100° F (37.8° C) or to a temperature near the animal's body temperature.

After each feeding, the abdomen should be enlarged but not overdistended. When a formula is used, less than the prescribed amount should be given per feeding for the first feedings. The amount should then be gradually increased to the recommended feeding amount by the second or third day. The amount of formula should then be increased accordingly as the puppy or kitten gains weight and a favorable response to feeding occurs. Puppies should gain 1 to 2 g/day/lb (2 to 4 g/day/kg) of anticipated adult weight for the first 5 months of their lives. At birth the kitten should weigh 80 to 140 g (most weighing around 100 to 120 g) and gain 50 to 100 g weekly.[1]

When preparing formula, the clinician should always follow the manufacturer's directions for its proper preparation and keep all feeding equipment scrupulously clean. A good way of handling prepared formula is to prepare only a 48-hour supply at a time and divide this into portions required for each feeding. Once formula is prepared, it is best stored in the refrigerator at 4° C.

The easiest and safest way of feeding prepared formula to nursing-age puppies and kittens is by nipple bottle, dosing syringe, or by tube.[1] Nipple bottles made especially for feeding orphan puppies or kittens or bottles equipped with preemie infant nipples are preferred. When feeding with a nipple bottle, the clinician or other staff member should hold it so that the puppy or kitten does not ingest air. The hole in the nipple should be such that when the bottle is inverted, milk slowly oozes from the nipple. It may be necessary to enlarge the nipple hole with a hot needle to get milk to ooze from the bottle when inverted. When feeding, a drop of milk should be squeezed onto the tip of the nipple and the nipple should be inserted into the animal's mouth. Milk should never be squeezed out of the bottle while the nipple is in the animal's mouth; doing so may result in laryngotracheal aspiration of the milk into the lungs. In addition, prepared formula should never be fed to a puppy or kitten that is chilled or that does not have a strong sucking reflex. Only when the sucking reflex is present should feeding with nipple bottle be attempted.

Tube feeding is the fastest way to feed orphaned puppies or kittens. Most owners can do it easily with a little training. The following may be used: a 5-French (F) infant feeding tube for puppies or kittens weighing less than 300 g, an 8- to 10-F infant feeding tube for puppies or kittens weighing over 300 g, or an appropriately sized, soft, male urethral catheter. Once weekly, the feeding tube should be clearly marked to indicate the depth of insertion to ensure gastric delivery (i.e., the distance from the last rib to the tip of the nose can be measured and marked off on the feeding tube as a guide). The animal should never be fed into the distal esophagus. When feeding, a syringe should be filled with warm, prepared formula and fit it to the feeding tube. The clinician or staff member should be sure to expel any air in the tube or syringe. The animal's mouth should be opened slightly and, with the animal's head held in the normal nursing position, the feeding tube should be gently passed to the marked area. If an obstruction is felt or coughing occurs before reaching the mark, the tube should be assumed to be in the trachea. If this does not happen, the prepared formula should be slowly administered over a 2-minute period to allow sufficient time for slow filling of the stomach. Regurgitation of formula rarely occurs, but if it does, the feeding tube should be withdrawn and feeding interrupted until the next scheduled meal.

A vital aspect of tending orphaned puppies and kittens is to simulate, after feeding, the mother's tongue action on the anogenital area, which provokes reflex micturition and defecation. Application of this stimulus has to be taken over by the person tending the puppies or kittens. The clinician can achieve the necessary result by swabbing the anogenital area with moistened cotton or dry, soft tissue paper to manually stimulate the elimination reflex. It is sometimes possible to effect the same response simply by running a forefinger along the abdominal wall. This stimulation should be regularly provided after each feeding using nipple bottle or tube. After they reach about 3 weeks of age, puppies and kittens are usually able to relieve themselves without simulated stimulation.

Most puppies and kittens benefit from gentle handling before feeding to allow for some exercise and to promote muscular and circulatory development. In addition, at least once a week the orphaned puppy or kitten should be washed gently with a soft moistened cloth for general cleansing of the skin, simulating the cleansing licks of the mother's tongue.

REFERENCES

The reference list can be found on the companion Expert Consult Web site at *www.expertconsult.com*.

CHAPTER 172

Nutrition-Related Skeletal Disorders

Todd L. Towell

Nutrition-related skeletal disorders include conditions related to imbalances of key nutrients (calcium, phosphorous, and vitamin D) and a spectrum of developmental orthopedic diseases. Nutritional imbalances can affect dogs and cats of any age but are most detrimental in growing animals. Developmental orthopedic disease (DOD) includes a diverse group of musculoskeletal disorders that occur in growing animals, most commonly fast-growing large- and giant-breed dogs whose adult weight will exceed 25 kg. Understanding the role of nutrition in the pathophysiology of these diseases facilitates prevention, diagnosis, and treatment.

NUTRITIONAL SECONDARY HYPERPARATHYROIDISM

Although more than 99% of total body calcium (Ca) is stored in the skeleton, it is the extracellular fluid (plasma) calcium concentration ($[Ca^{2+}]$) that is critical for a multitude of cellular, contractive, and enzymatic processes. As a result, plasma $[Ca^{2+}]$ is tightly controlled by a complex homeostatic mechanism involving fluxes of calcium between the extracellular fluid and kidney, bone, and gut. Three major hormones: parathyroid hormone (PTH), calcitonin, and 1,25-dihydroxyvitamin D ($1,25[OH]_2D_3$) regulate the influx (gastrointestinal [GI] absorption and bone resorption) and efflux (GI and renal loss and skeletal mineralization of the less labile bone pool), of calcium.[1] Increased plasma $[Ca^{2+}]$ inhibits PTH and stimulates calcitonin secretion resulting in Ca transport to cell

organelles, storage of Ca in the labile Ca pool of bone, and increased glomerular Ca excretion.[2] Nutritional secondary hyperparathyroidism occurs when chronic insufficient Ca intake or absorption stimulates PTH secretion. Parathyroid hormone activates osteoclasts (mobilizing calcium from bone), increases renal tubular reabsorption of calcium (conserving free calcium), increases urinary phosphate excretion (lowering serum phosphate level), and increases conversion of vitamin D to its active dihydroxy form in the kidneys (augmenting GI calcium absorption)[3,4] (Figure 172-1).

If increased Ca absorption in the intestine is insufficient to meet daily requirements, Ca will be resorbed at the endosteal surface of the diaphyses and in the areas of cancellous bone. In addition to chronic inadequate Ca intake, excessive phosphorus (P) intake coupled with inadequate calcium intake may result in nutritional secondary hyperparathyroidism. The excess phosphorus reduces the ionized calcium concentration in serum via mass action equilibrium, resulting in hypersecretion of PTH. Excessive osteoclasia and pathologic fractures of growing bone are sequelae to long-term hyperparathyroidism. Mineralization of osteoid and cartilage will be undisturbed.[5,6]

CLINICAL AND RADIOLOGIC EXAMINATION

Although animals of any age can be affected, most animals with nutritional secondary hyperparathyroidism are young individuals eating foods deficient in Ca. For example, animals

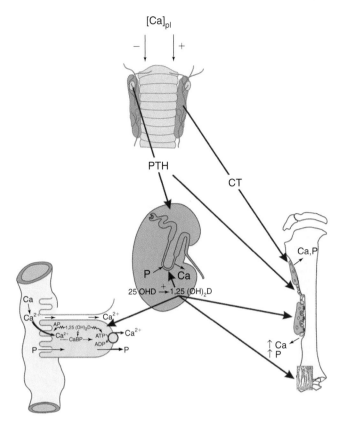

Figure 172-1 Calcium homeostasis regulated by calciotropic hormones. An increase (+) of plasma calcium ($[Ca]_{pl}$) concentration $[Ca]_{pl}$ stimulates secretion of calcitonin (CT) from the thyroid glands. This enhances renal excretion and inhibits bone resorption of calcium, which in the long term will disturb skeletal remodeling and endochondral ossification. A decrease (−) of $[Ca]_{pl}$ stimulates parathyroid hormone (PTH) secretion from the parathyroid glands causing (1) shrinkage of osteoblasts, allowing osteoclasts to resorb bone, and (2) increased reabsorption of Ca and excretion of phosphorus (P) and increased formation of $1,25(OH)_2vitD$ in the kidney. As a result of the latter, active absorption of Ca and P is increased, renal Ca and P reabsorption is increased, and mineralization of newly formed osteoid and cartilage is stimulated.

fed improperly formulated homemade foods or all-meat diets may receive insufficient calcium and/or excessive phosphorus. Commercial foods may result in Ca deficiency if the source of Ca has poor bioavailability, especially in young large-breed dogs. Clinical signs may include reluctance to move and play, lameness, uncoordinated gait, sternal recumbency, loose teeth, and painful mastication. Pathologic fractures can occur in any affected animal but are most common in the femur of young (<6 months) male dogs (Figure 172-2).[7]

Blood calcium concentrations are generally within normal limits although such values can, uncommonly, be increased. Increases in serum PTH and calcitriol ($1,25[OH]_2vitD_3$) concentrations can be detected [4,6] (see Figure 172-1). Radiographs may reveal thin cortices, wide medullary cavities, folding (green stick) fractures, normal height of growth plates with relatively white metaphyseal borders, as well as compression fractures of cancellous bone of epiphyses and vertebrae.[5,6]

DIFFERENTIAL DIAGNOSIS

Rule-outs for radiographic abnormalities and pathologic fractures include nutritional secondary hyperparathyroidism and inborn errors of metabolism that include osteogenesis imperfecta, mucopolysaccharidosis, and other rare diseases (see Figure 172-2). Hyperparathyroidism may be primary or secondary (nutritional or renal). Chronic Ca deficiency may be complicated by vitamin D deficiency if all-meat diets are the sole food source.

THERAPY

Correction of the diet includes utilizing a commercially available, complete and balanced dog or cat food. The absolute amount of calcium in the food is more important than the calcium-phosphorus ratio in young growing dogs.[8,9] Foods should provide 0.8% to 1.2% dry matter (DM) calcium and the calcium-phosphorus ratio should be kept within physiologic limits (1.1:1 to 2:1). It is preferred to have the ratio 1.2:1.[10] Improved mineralization of the skeleton should be evident in 3 to 4 weeks.[4] During this time it is important to prevent pathologic fractures, especially of the vertebrae. Supplementing Ca as Ca carbonate or Ca lactate (and not Ca phosphate or bone meal) at 50 mg Ca/kg bodyweight may accelerate osteoid mineralization. Corrective osteotomies can be planned, if necessary, after the skeleton is normally mineralized. Even pets with compression fractures of the spinal cord may have a full recovery.

RICKETS

Since dogs and cats are not capable of synthesizing vitamin D (vitD), they require a source of this essential vitamin (hormone) in their food.[2,5] Vitamin D is absorbed in the small intestine by bile salt–dependent passive diffusion. It is then transported to the liver, where it is hydroxylated into 25-OHvitD.[2] A second hydroxylation takes place in the kidney, either to $24,25(OH)_2vitD$ or to $1,25(OH)_2vitD$ (calcitriol).[2] Calcitriol is the metabolite that stimulates active intestinal and renal absorption of Ca and P. Both metabolites (Ca and P) are necessary for osteoid and cartilage mineralization.[2] Rickets is characterized by defective mineralization of newly formed bone and cartilage as well as metaphyseal thickening.[5,11] *Rickets* is the term used to describe hypovitaminosis D in young animals; in adults it is referred to as *osteomalacia*. Hypovitaminosis D arises most commonly from inadequate intake or endogenous production of vitD, but rickets lesions can also occur secondary to decreased phosphorous intake or an increased and abnormal calcium-to-phosphorus ratio.[12-14] Additionally, rickets can occur despite normal vitD intake if intake of calcium is excessive at an early age (~3 weeks of life). This causes hypercalcemia, secondary hypoparathyroidism, and tertiary decreased calcitriol formation.[6,13]

CLINICAL AND RADIOLOGIC EXAMINATION

A thorough dietary history is critical. Since commercial pet foods contain 2 to 10 times the Association of American Feed Control Officials (AAFCO) minimum recommended amounts of vitamin D, rickets is generally only seen in animals fed improperly formulated homemade foods such as unsupplemented strict vegetarian foods or animals with biliary atresia or inborn errors of vitD₃ metabolism.[15-19] Radiographs dem-

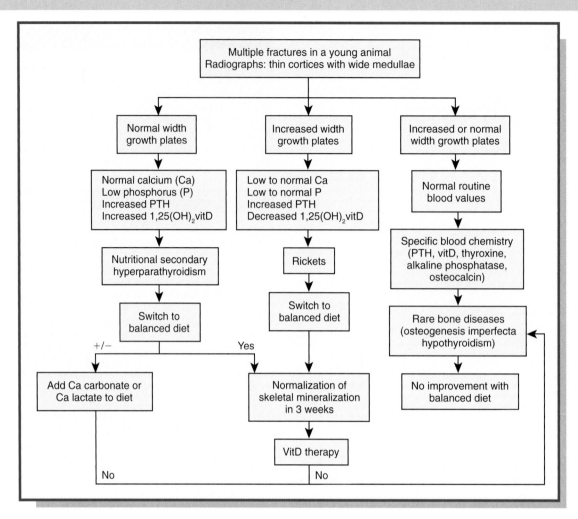

Figure 172-2 An algorithm for multiple pathologic fractures in young dogs and cats. *PTH,* Parathyroid hormone; *vitD,* vitamin D.

onstrate thin long bone cortices and extremely thickened growth plates. Increased growth plate width is not associated with low-calcium/high-phosphorous foods but is a strong indicator of rickets. Despite hyperparathyroidism, plasma $[Ca^{2+}]$ and phosphorus can be normal or low-normal. Diagnosis of vitD deficiency can be made by measuring circulating levels of vitD metabolites. In rickets levels of $1,25(OH)_2$vitD will be decreased, whereas in nutritional or renal secondary hypoparathyroidism $1,25(OH)_2$vitD will be increased.[2,15]

TREATMENT

Transition to a nutritionally balanced commercial dog or cat food is generally sufficient to resolve rickets. Mineralization of bone cortices, callus, and growth plates will occur within 3 weeks. If the dog or cat fails to respond to a balanced diet, vitD therapy can be recommended.

DEVELOPMENTAL ORTHOPEDIC DISEASE

The pathogenesis of DOD in the dog is multifactorial, involving genetic susceptibility, environmental influences, and nutrition. DOD is a common cause of secondary osteoarthritis and degenerative joint disease (DJD) in dogs. Osteoarthritis is the most commonly diagnosed nontraumatic orthopedic condition in dogs, with an estimated 20% incidence in adults.[20,21] Canine hip dysplasia and osteochondrosis make up the overwhelming majority of DOD with a nutrition-related etiology. Specific risk factors for DOD in young dogs include: (1) large or giant breeds (genetics) (>25 kg adult weight), (2) free-choice feeding (management), particularly of high-energy foods (nutrition), and (3) excessive intake of calcium and vitamin D from food, treats, and supplements (nutrition).[22-30] The key nutritional factors that contribute to DOD are excesses of calcium and energy.[24] Excess calcium intake results in disturbed endochondral ossification, retained cartilaginous cores, and delayed skeletal maturation.[5] Excess energy promotes both rapid growth and obesity.

CANINE HIP DYSPLASIA

Canine hip dysplasia (CHD) is a polygenic disease with complex inheritance. As such, environmental factors such as nutrition and lifestyle have a profound influence on both its incidence and its severity.[31] Excessive energy intake appears to be paramount to the phenotypic expression of CHD in growing and adult dogs. One long-term study of dogs genetically predisposed to CHD documented that prevalence and severity of osteoarthritis/DJD (the phenotypic expression of CHD) is greater in dogs with body condition scores (BCSs) above normal.[32] Over their lifespan, the median age of radiographic evidence of CHD/osteoarthritis was significantly lower (6 years) in overweight versus normal weight dogs (12 years).[31] Additionally, the mean age at which 50% of the dogs required long-term treatment for clinical signs attributable to osteoarthritis was significantly earlier (10.3 years, p<0.01) in the overweight dogs as compared to the dogs with normal BCSs (13.3 years).[33]

CLINICAL AND RADIOLOGIC EXAMINATION

The diagnosis of CHD/DJD is based on both clinical examination and pelvic radiography. Physical examination should include neurologic assessment as well as a thorough orthopedic examination. Joints, muscles, tendons, ligaments, and long bones should be palpated for evidence of swelling, heat or pain. Joints should be assessed for crepitus, range of motion, collateral stress, abduction, and adduction abnormalities (instability). Muscle atrophy, hypertrophy, or asymmetry should be noted, as this may be indicative of the most clinically affected joint. However, early diagnosis is challenging since most dogs with CHD/DJD do not exhibit clinical signs early in life or, necessarily, at any time. Although epidemiologic data are not available, based on clinical experience one study estimated that fewer than 5% of dogs with radiographic evidence of DJD (i.e., phenotypic expression of CHD) will have clinical signs such as pain, lameness, and gait alterations.[34]

Three categories of radiographic methods are currently used to diagnose CHD: (1) evaluation of hip capsule laxity, (2) evaluation of osseous conformation and evidence of osteoarthritis, and (3) evaluation of functional subluxation.[35] The traditional standard for the assessment of CHD in the United States, as adopted by Orthopedic Foundation for Animals (OFA), is subjective radiographic evaluation of ventrodorsal extended-hip radiographs at 2 years of age. In subjective hip scoring systems, a diagnosis of CHD is typically made if there is radiographic evidence of hip subluxation (joint laxity), DJD, or both. Radiographic evidence of DJD includes one or more of the following: femoral periarticular osteophyte formation, subchondral sclerosis of the craniodorsal acetabulum, osteophytes on the cranial, or caudal acetabular margin or joint remodeling from chronic wear.[36] Unfortunately, subtle arthritic changes defy detection by conventional radiographic methods, and not all dogs genetically predisposed to CHD/DJD express these changes by 2 years of age. As a result, conventional hip-extended radiography tends to underestimate the presence of CHD/DJD. In a lifelong study of Labrador Retrievers, 55% of the dogs graded normal by OFA-type scoring became dysplastic by the end of life.[35] This high rate of false-negative diagnosis explains the lack of progress in reducing the frequency and severity of CHD by selective breeding based on OFA certification. Evaluation of hip joint laxity by calculating a distraction index (DI) shows promise as an early, reliable indicator of genotypic susceptibility and phenotypic expression of clinical signs.[36-38]

OSTEOCHONDROSIS

Osteochondrosis (OC) is common in young, rapidly growing, warm-blooded, domesticated species and man. In all species, the etiology is considered multifactorial. In dogs, risk factors for OC include age, gender, breed, rapid growth, and nutrient excesses (primarily calcium and energy).[24,25,27,28] All large- and giant-breed dogs are at increased risk for OC. However, Great Dane, Labrador Retriever, Newfoundland, and Rottweiler breeds are at greatest risk.[27] Osteochondrosis is a disruption in endochondral ossification that results in a focal lesion but is considered a systemic disease.[39,40] Osteochondrosis occurs in the physis and/or epiphysis of growth cartilage, most commonly in the shoulder, stifle, hock and elbow. Acute inflammatory joint disease (or DJD) may ensue when the cartilage surface is disrupted and subchondral bone is exposed to synovial fluid. Inflammatory mediators and cartilage fragments are released into the joint (osteochondritis dissecans), which perpetuates the cycle of DJD.[41]

CLINICAL AND RADIOLOGIC EXAMINATION

Clinical signs of OC include pain and lameness. Clinical signs observed are related to severity and location of disease. When OC affects physeal cartilage, it may cause growth abnormalities in long bones such as angular limb deformities. In dogs with OC, palpation and extension of shoulder, elbow, stifle, and tibiotarsal joints may demonstrate pain and/or swelling. Circulating concentrations of Ca, P, calcitonin, and calcitriol have usually been within normal limits. Survey radiographs are generally sufficient for diagnosis. However, other imaging techniques, including arthroscopy, may provided earlier evidence of lesions.[42] The radiographic appearance of OC varies with the area of involvement.

DEVELOPMENTAL ORTHOPEDIC DISEASE TREATMENT

To help prevent DOD in a large- to giant-breed puppy (>25 kg adult weight), it is best to feed a commercial food specific for their unique nutrient requirements. The recommended intake of most nutrients in fast-growing, large- and giant-breed puppies is similar to that of other breeds. However, it is important to note that the recommendations are more stringent for energy density, dietary fat, calcium, and the calcium-phosphorus ratio (energy density = 3.5 to 4.1 kcal/g, fat = 8.5% to 17% DM, calcium = 0.8% to 1.2% DM, Ca:Phos from 1.1 to 2:1 with lower end of range [1.2:1] preferred). Several commercial foods specifically formulated for fast-growing, large- and giant-breed puppies are available. Select a food that is most similar to the key nutritional factor benchmarks. To prevent imbalances and excesses, the addition of vitamin or mineral supplements to balanced foods is not recommended. This is particularly true for calcium, phosphorus, vitamin D, and vitamin A. If a nutritionally adequate growth food is being fed, supplementation is contraindicated. The large- to giant-breed puppy should be fed to maintain a BCS between 2/5 and 3/5 (~4/9). Dietary deficiencies are of minimal concern in this age of commercial foods specifically prepared for young, growing dogs; the major potential for harm results from excess consumption of energy and calcium. A balanced food fed at an appropriate quantity will help to optimize the conditions of skeletal development and decrease the risk of DOD.

Although prevention is preferred, if DOD is manifested a multifaceted therapeutic approach is warranted (Figure 172-3). When appropriate, surgical correction of underlying conditions should be considered. Once DJD/osteoarthritis is diagnosed, the cornerstone of multifaceted therapy is therapeutic nutrition. Nutritional treatment of DOD/osteoarthritis should initially focus on weight reduction if the BCS is greater than 3/5. Foods designed for dogs with osteoarthritis should supply age-appropriate nutrition and specific nutrients that may help reduce inflammation and pain, slow the degradative

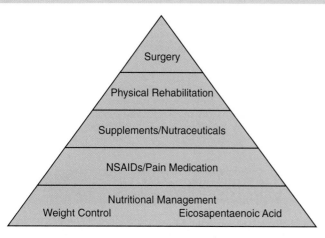

Figure 172-3 Multimodal approach to management of osteoarthritis secondary to developmental orthopedic disease. *NSAIDs,* Nonsteroidal antiinflammatory drugs.

process, complement prescribed medications, and provide tangible improvement in symptoms of osteoarthritis. Clinical studies indicate that nutritional management using a therapeutic food supplemented with n-3 fatty acids helped reduce the clinical signs of osteoarthritis in dogs as noted by pet owners, clinical orthopedic examination, and gait analysis of ground reaction forces.[43-45] Based on these studies, a food designed to aid in the management of osteoarthritis in dogs should provide levels of total omega-3 fatty acids between 3.5% to 4.5% (DM) and specifically 0.4% to 1.1% (DM) eicosapentaenoic acid. The n-6 to n-3 fatty acid ratio should be less than 1:1. Dogs consuming the therapeutic food should receive an average of 50 to 100 mg EPA/kg BW/day.

REFERENCES

The reference list can be found on the companion Expert Consult Web site at *www.expertconsult.com.*

CHAPTER 173

Adverse Reactions to Foods: Allergies versus Intolerance

Philip Roudebush

An adverse reaction to food is a clinically abnormal response to an ingested food or food additive. In general, the pathogenic mechanisms that cause adverse food reactions include ingestion of the inciting agent followed by interaction of the agent with a biologic amplification system that leads to inflammation and clinical signs.

In view of the number of diverse foods that are routinely ingested by animals, it is not surprising that adverse reactions develop to dietary substances. The fact that food-related reactions appear relatively infrequently is testimony to the effectiveness of the gastrointestinal (GI) mucosal barrier and oral tolerance. Adverse reactions to food have been blamed for a variety of clinical syndromes in cats and dogs, usually involving the skin and GI tract.

TERMINOLOGY

Adverse reactions to food comprise a variety of subclassifications based on pathomechanisms. The following terms and definitions are recommended by the American Academy of Allergy, Asthma and Immunology (Figure 173-1).[1-3] *Food allergy (food hypersensitivity)* is an adverse reaction to a food or food additive with a proven immunologic basis. *Food anaphylaxis* is an acute food allergy with systemic consequences, such as respiratory distress, vascular collapse, and urticaria. *Food intolerance* is a nonimmunologic, abnormal physiologic response to a food or food additive. Food intolerance can be further classified as food idiosyncrasy, food poisoning, and pharmacologic reactions to food. *Food idiosyncrasy* is an abnormal response that resembles food allergy but that does not involve immune mechanisms. A direct nonimmunologic action on the host of food or a toxin in food is termed *food poisoning.* Adverse reactions due to a druglike or pharmaco-

logic effect of a food substance on the host are called *pharmacologic reactions to food.* When adverse reactions result from such behaviors as gluttony, pica, or ingestion of indigestible materials, the term *dietary indiscretion* is used. Traditionally, the term *food allergy* has been used to describe all adverse reactions to food in dogs and cats, including reactions that were actually food intolerance.

FOOD ALLERGENS

The specific food allergens that cause problems in animals have been poorly documented. In general, the major food allergens that have been identified in human beings are water-soluble glycoproteins that have molecular weights ranging from 10,000 to 70,000 daltons and that are stable when treated with heat, acid, or proteases.[4,5] Other physiochemical properties that account for their unique allergenicity are poorly understood.[6]

Fifteen different studies, representing a total of 278 dogs, have described cutaneous lesions associated with adverse reactions to specific foods or ingredients.[7] These studies reported findings from a wide geographic area, including the United States, United Kingdom, France, Australia, and Japan. Adverse reactions to beef, dairy products, and wheat accounted for two thirds of reported cases in dogs. Adverse reactions to chicken, chicken eggs, lamb, or soy accounted for approximately 25% of reported canine cases. Adverse reactions to corn, pork, rice, or fish ingredients are rarely reported in dogs. Allergens identified in serum from food-allergic dogs include chicken serum albumin (chicken), bovine IgG (cow's milk, beef), muscle phosphoglucomutase (beef, lamb), ovine IgG (lamb), and Gly proteins 50 and 75 kD (soy).[8-10]

In cats, 10 different studies, representing a total of 56 animals, have described cutaneous lesions or gastroenteric signs associated with adverse reactions to specific foods or ingredients.[7] These studies have also reported findings from a wide geographic area, including the United States, United Kingdom, France, New Zealand, and Japan. Adverse reactions to beef, dairy products, and fish accounted for more than 80% of reported cases. No specific allergens have been identified in food allergic cats.

Human allergy reference books often have phylogenetic tables of animal and vegetable foods so that food-allergic individuals can avoid other closely related foods. Cross-reactivity among food allergens has been only briefly investigated in pet animals.[10,11]

FOOD INTOLERANCE

Nonimmunologic, abnormal physiologic reactions to food include food intolerance and dietary indiscretion (see Figure 173-1). Like the term *food allergy*, the term *food intolerance* has been applied inappropriately to any and all adverse reactions to food. Food intolerance mimics food allergy except that it can occur with the first exposure to a food or food additive, because nonimmunologic mechanisms are involved. The incidence of food intolerance versus food allergy in animals is unknown.

Idiosyncratic adverse reactions to food additives often occur in human beings. Although food additives are frequently cited as the cause of problems in dogs and cats, few data confirm this perception. Propylene glycol and onion ingredients have been documented to cause hematologic abnormalities in cats.[12,13]

Another cause of food intolerance is pharmacologic reactions to substances found in food. Vasoactive or biogenic amines such as histamine cause clinical signs when present in excessive levels in food. Adverse reactions to histamine in scombroid fish (e.g., mackerel, tuna) have been observed in cats and dogs.[14] Vasoactive or biogenic amines may not be present in levels high enough to cause clinical signs, but they may lower the threshold levels for allergens in individual dogs and cats.

The diarrhea, bloating, and abdominal discomfort that occur when animals with lactose intolerance ingest milk are relatively common metabolic adverse reactions in dogs and cats. Osmotic diarrhea often occurs when excessive levels of lactose are consumed. Puppies, kittens, or adult animals may develop diarrhea when given cow's or goat's milk because these milk sources contain more lactose than either bitch's or queen's milk.

Intolerance to disaccharides commonly occurs secondary to enteritis or rapid food changes. Loss of intestinal brush border disaccharidase activity contributes to the diarrhea associated with enteritis. Inadequate intestinal disaccharidase activity is another factor responsible for diarrhea subsequent to rapid food changes. Several days are required for intestinal disaccharidase enzyme activity to adapt to changes in food carbohydrate sources.

CLINICAL FEATURES

Dermatologic Responses in Dogs

Reports of adverse food reactions in dogs with cutaneous disease did not document a gender predisposition, and ages ranged from 4 months to 14 years. However, up to one third of canine cases may occur in dogs less than 1 year old. Because many adverse food reactions occur in young dogs, the index of suspicion for food allergy may rise above that for atopic dermatitis when intense pruritus occurs in dogs less than 6 months old. Most investigators have not found a breed predilection, whereas others have found that Cocker Spaniels, Springer Spaniels, Labrador Retrievers, Collies, Miniature Schnauzers, Chinese Shar-Peis, West Highland White Terriers, Wheaten Terriers, Boxers, Dachshunds, Dalmatians, Lhasa Apsos, German Shepherds, and Golden Retrievers are at increased risk.

Adverse food reactions in dogs typically occur as nonseasonal pruritic dermatitis, often accompanied by GI signs. The pruritus varies in severity. Lesion distribution is often indistinguishable from that seen with atopic dermatitis; the feet, face, axillae, perineal region, inguinal region, rump, and ears are often affected. Many dogs with adverse food reactions have lesions only in the region of the ears. This finding suggests that adverse food reactions should always be suspected in dogs with pruritic, bilateral otitis externa, even if it is accompanied by secondary bacterial or yeast infections.

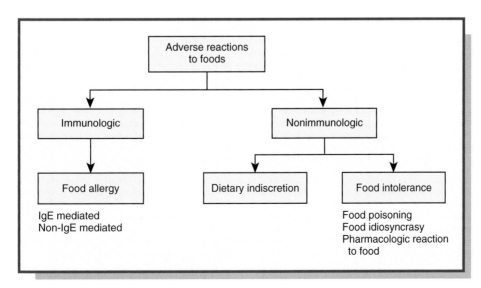

Figure 173-1 Classification of adverse reactions to food. *IgE*, Immunoglobulin E.

Adverse food reactions often mimic other common canine skin disorders, including pyoderma, pruritic seborrheic dermatoses, folliculitis, and ectoparasitism. Twenty percent to 30% or more of dogs with suspected adverse food reactions may have concurrent allergic disease, such as flea allergy or atopic dermatitis.

Food anaphylaxis is an acute reaction to food or food additives with systemic consequences. The most common clinical manifestation in dogs occurs in localized form and is referred to as *angioedema* or *facioconjunctival edema*. Angioedema is typically manifested by large, edematous swellings of the lips, face, eyelids, ears, conjunctivae, and/or tongue, with or without pruritus. Most veterinary practitioners attribute angioedema solely to insect envenomation (biting or stinging insects); however, a number of other common causes are food, drugs, vaccines, infections, atopy, and blood transfusions. Urticarial reactions (hives) are characterized by localized or generalized wheals, which may or may not be pruritic. They usually occur within minutes of allergen exposure and generally subside after 1 to 2 hours.

Dermatologic Responses in Cats

Gender predisposition has not been documented in adverse food reactions in cats, and ages have ranged from 6 months to 12 years. Siamese and Siamese-cross cats may be at increased risk, because they have accounted for nearly one third of cases.

Dermatologic signs include several different clinical reaction patterns, such as (1) severe, generalized pruritus without lesions; (2) miliary dermatitis; (3) pruritus with self-trauma centered around the head, neck, and ears; (4) traumatic alopecia; (5) moist dermatitis; and (6) scaling dermatoses. Angioedema, urticaria, and conjunctivitis occur commonly in cats with adverse food reactions. Adverse reactions to food may also cause self-inflicted alopecia (psychogenic alopecia, or neurodermatitis), eosinophilic plaques, and indolent ulcers of the lips in some cats. Concurrent flea allergy or atopic dermatitis may occur in up to one third of cats with suspected adverse food reactions.

Moderate to marked peripheral lymphadenomegaly and absolute eosinophilia are commonly found in cats with dermatologic manifestations of food allergy.

Gastrointestinal Responses in Dogs and Cats

Gender predilections have not been established for GI disease resulting from adverse reactions to foods. Similarly, there are no well-documented breed predispositions to GI food allergy, but Chinese Shar-Peis and German Shepherd Dogs are commonly affected. Gluten-sensitive enteropathy has been well documented in Irish Setters. A wide age range of patients can be affected, including dogs and cats as young as weaning age.

Every level of the GI tract can be damaged by food allergies. In cats and dogs, clinical signs usually relate to gastric and small bowel dysfunction, but colitis can also occur. Vomiting and diarrhea are prominent features. The diarrhea can be profuse and watery, mucoid, or hemorrhagic. Intermittent abdominal pain is occasionally observed. Concurrent cutaneous signs may be seen. GI disturbances such as soft feces, excessive flatus, intermittent diarrhea, and frequent defecation (three or more times per day) occur in up to half of dogs and cats with cutaneous manifestations of food sensitivity.

The role of food allergy in canine and feline inflammatory bowel disease is unknown. Hypersensitivity to food is probably involved in the pathogenesis of this syndrome; at least some affected animals could be more appropriately diagnosed as suffering from food protein–induced enterocolitis.

Irritable bowel syndrome is a disease of dogs characterized by chronic recurrent abdominal pain and large bowel diarrhea. Feeding changes often alleviate the signs of irritable bowel disease, implying that food allergy or food intolerance plays a role in this syndrome.

DIAGNOSIS

Dietary elimination trials are the main diagnostic method used in dogs and cats with suspected adverse food reactions (Figure 173-2). At the present time, intradermal skin testing, radioallergosorbent tests (RASTs), and enzyme-linked immunosorbent assays (ELISAs) for food allergy are considered unreliable in animals.[15,16]

The ideal elimination food should (1) include a protein hydrolysate or reduced number of novel, highly digestible protein sources; (2) avoid protein excesses; (3) avoid additives and vasoactive amines; and (4) be nutritionally adequate for the animal's life stage and condition.[17] Excess protein levels should be avoided so as to reduce the amount of potential allergens to which the dermatologic patient is exposed. However, a higher protein level may be necessary to counteract protein losses from the GI tract or impaired absorption in patients with hypoproteinemia and weight loss associated with severe GI disease. Although elimination trials are performed only for several weeks to months, the food used in the trial should be nutritionally complete and balanced for the intended species, age, and lifestyle of the animal. Elimination trials are often performed with young animals, in which nutritionally inadequate foods are more likely to result in nutritional disease.

Homemade Elimination Foods

Homemade foods are often recommended as the initial test food for dogs and cats with suspected food allergy. Homemade test foods usually include a single protein source or a combination of a single protein source and a single carbohydrate source. However, many homemade foods fail to meet nutritional requirements because they are made from a minimum of ingredients.[17,18] In general, homemade foods lack a source of calcium, essential fatty acids, certain vitamins, and other micronutrients and contain excessive levels of protein, which are contraindicated in animals with food allergy. Feeding nutritionally inadequate homemade foods for more than 3 weeks may result in nutritional disease, especially in young animals.

Commercial Elimination Foods

A variety of foods with limited and different protein sources are manufactured by several companies. These commercial products are attractive because they are convenient and nutritionally complete and balanced for either cats or dogs. The newest concept for managing animals with suspected adverse food reactions is use of commercial foods containing hydrolyzed protein ingredients. Veterinary therapeutic foods containing protein hydrolysates offer several hypothetical advantages over traditional commercial or homemade elimination foods. Protein hydrolysates of appropriate molecular weight (less than 10,000 daltons) do not elicit an immunologically mediated response and may be regarded as truly "hypoallergenic" ingredients.[8] Novel or unique protein sources are less important with protein hydrolysates. Protein hydrolysates have been used for many years in human infant formulas and for human patients with various GI diseases.

Few commercial foods have been adequately tested in dogs and cats with known adverse food reactions; only a few commercial foods have undergone the scrutiny of clinical trials using patients with dermatologic or GI disease. In published clinical trials, two thirds to three fourths of patients with suspected adverse food reactions showed significant improvement in clinical signs when fed appropriate commercial foods.

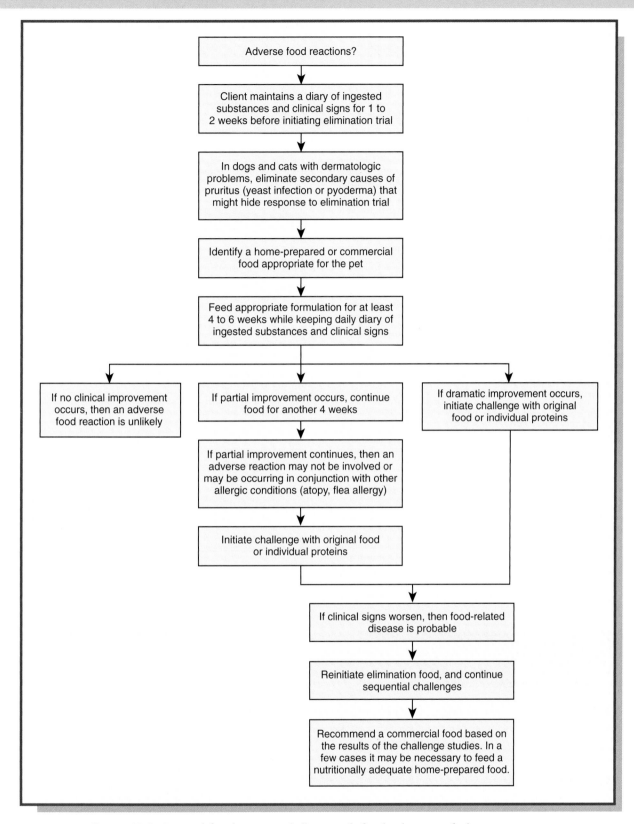

Figure 173-2 Protocol for elimination-challenge trials for the diagnosis of adverse reactions to food. (From Roudebush P, Guilford WG, Jackson HA: Adverse reactions to food. In Hand MS, Thatcher CD, Remillard RL, et al, editors: Small animal clinical nutrition, ed 5, Topeka, Kan, 2010, Mark Morris Institute.)

Performing an Elimination Trial in Patients with Dermatologic Disease

Before an elimination trial is initiated, the client should feed the animal its usual food for several days. During this time, the client should record the type and amount of food ingested, any other ingested food items (e.g., table scraps, treats, and snacks), and the occurrence and character of adverse reactions. The patient is then fed a controlled elimination food for 4 to 12 weeks. During the elimination trial, no other substances should be ingested, including treats, flavored vitamin supplements, chewable medications, fatty acid supplements, or chew toys. To improve compliance, canine and feline treats are now available containing hydrolyzed protein sources, which are less likely to influence results of an elimination trial. The client should document daily the type and amount of food ingested and the occurrence and character of adverse reactions. A daily food diary helps document progression of clinical signs during the elimination trial and whether a strict elimination trial was performed in the home environment. Examples of food diaries can be found in other publications.[17]

A tentative diagnosis of an adverse food reaction in dermatologic patients is made if the level of pruritus markedly decreases. This improvement may be gradual and may take 4 to 12 weeks to become evident. A diagnosis of an adverse food reaction is confirmed if clinical signs reappear 10 to 14 days after the animal's former food and other ingested substances are offered as a challenge.

Elimination trials are often difficult to interpret because of concurrent allergic skin disease. Patients with other allergic diseases may only partially respond to an elimination trial. Flea-allergy and atopic dermatitis are the most common canine and feline allergies and should be eliminated through other diagnostic testing.

Performing an Elimination Trial in Patients with Gastrointestinal Disease

Elimination-challenge trial designs for patients with GI food disease are similar to those for patients with dermatologic problems (see Figure 173-2). However, shorter elimination periods (2 to 4 weeks) are usually satisfactory. In chronic relapsing conditions, the elimination period chosen must be greater than the usual symptom-free period of the patient to allow reliable assessment of how food sensitivity contributes to the patient's signs.

As with skin disease, the degree of clinical improvement during the elimination trial will be 100% only if food allergy or food intolerance is the sole cause of the patient's problems. For instance, resolution of allergies acquired as a result of GI disease will not eliminate the clinical signs due to the primary GI disease process. Recrudescence of GI signs after challenge of a food-sensitive patient with the responsible allergen usually occurs within the first 3 days but may take as long as 7 days, particularly if the responsible allergen was removed from the food for longer than 1 month.

TREATMENT

For most food allergies, avoiding the offending foods is the most effective treatment. How selective or meticulous an avoidance diet must be depends on the individual animal's sensitivity. Some dogs and cats may suffer adverse reactions to even trace amounts of an offending food, whereas others may have a higher tolerance level. Concurrent allergies influence the threshold level of clinical signs in some animals. Symptomatic therapy in pruritic animals can also include corticosteroids and antihistamines. Corticosteroids, along with dietary change, are often used in animals with inflammatory bowel disease.

Both homemade and commercial foods can be used for long-term maintenance of patients with suspected food allergy. It is very important that any homemade recipe for long-term maintenance ensures a nutritionally adequate ration. An attempt should always be made to find an acceptable commercial food that will increase owner compliance with the dietary change and ensure a nutritionally adequate ration.

REFERENCES

The reference list can be found on the companion Expert Consult Web site at *www.expertconsult.com.*

CHAPTER 174

Nutritional Management of Gastrointestinal Conditions

Debra L. Zoran

GENERAL GUIDELINES

The gastrointestinal (GI) tract is a complex tubular system primarily responsible for accepting and digesting food, absorbing nutrients and water, and expelling wastes from the body in the form of feces. A proper diet and normally functioning GI tract are integral to the delivery of nutrients, prevention of malnutrition, repair of damaged intestinal epithelium, restoration of normal luminal bacterial populations, promotion of normal GI motility, and maintenance of normal immune function (e.g., both tolerance of and protection from pathogens).[1] Dietary characteristics, such as the amount of food, its form, the frequency of feeding, and the composition of the diet, also have important effects on GI function and may be used to help ameliorate signs of disease. Both nutrients and nonnutritional components of a diet support normal GI function, but they also may cause or influence the development of GI pathology (e.g., antibiotic-responsive diarrhea [ARD], inflammatory bowel disease [IBD], and dietary intolerance or sensitivity/allergy). In chronic or severe GI disturbances, such as protein-losing enteropathies (PLE), diet may have a profound effect on intestinal recovery and successful management of the disease.

Traditionally, nutritional management of acute, nonspecific GI disease has included institution of a short-term period of fasting, or by altering food intake with the general intent to "rest" the gut. This approach is believed to be beneficial by allowing healing as well as slowing gastric and peristaltic contractions.[2] For many acute, non–life-threatening GI disturbances, withholding of food and water for 24 to 48 hours, along with correction of fluid and electrolyte deficits, may be quite effective. If vomiting is a significant problem, this period of nothing per os (NPO) may be essential to allow antiemetic therapy the opportunity to be effective.[3] However, prolonged fasting or "rest" of the GI tract should be avoided, as it can contribute to delayed recovery of intestinal function, development of malnutrition, or lead to problems that occur from a lack of enteral nutrition (e.g., ileus, bacterial disruption, bacterial translocation, villous blunting).[4]

For example, in puppies with parvoviral enteritis, the long-held belief was that nutritional support should either be given parenterally, or withheld, until the vomiting and diarrhea were controlled. However, it has now been shown that puppies given early enteral nutrition—even in tiny amounts—had significant benefit in resolution of clinical signs, weight gain, and reduced evidence of gut permeability. This was assessed by sugar permeability, an indicator of reducing bacterial translocation risk.[4] Thus, the current recommendation for all dogs (and cats) with acute gastroenteritis, is to maximize the period of fasting to12 to 36 hours, or the shortest period necessary to achieve control of vomiting. Then, one should gradually introduce a liquid or highly digestible intestinal diet (i.e., minimal fat and easily digested protein and carbohydrate [CHO] sources). When indicated, a gradual reintroduction of the original diet or a more appropriate diet for long-term management can be given.

In previously healthy animals, short-term fasting for 2 to 3 days is not expected to be harmful nutritionally, systemically, or to the GI tract. However, in injured or sick animals there is a shift in metabolism toward a catabolic state (Table 174-1).[5]

Thus, in sick animals or those with nutritional compromise that are fasted longer than 3 to 4 days, the increased catabolic state leads to a deficiency of protein and calories. In turn, these animals are predisposed to immune system dysfunction, reduced availability of antioxidants and free radical scavengers, reduced energy for vital cellular functions, lack of precursors for repair of injured or diseased tissue, and, ultimately, loss of lean body mass.[5,6] Prolonged fasting also deprives the GI epithelium of its primary metabolic fuel source, glutamine,

which is present in chyme and is necessary not only for replacement of the GI mucosal cells lost in normal turnover (every 3 to 5 days) but also for repair of mucosal injury and normal immune function.[7]

A good general rule of thumb for induction of nutritional support is the "3- to 5-day rule": By day 3 of anorexia, planning should begin for implementation of nutritional support, and by day 5 the plan should be implemented. Once the determination is made that nutritional support is needed, the next step is to determine how to provide that nutrition. Again, the rule of thumb is: if the gut works, use it, and use as much of the GI tract that is functional—in other words, provide nutrition as normally as is feasible. There are a wide variety of options available for providing enteral nutrition, including oral force-feeding, nasoesophageal tube feeding, esophageal (E) tube feeding, gastrostomy (G) tube feeding, or jejunostomy (J) tube feeding. Each of these different feeding methods has pros and cons that may influence choice (Table 174-2).

Interested readers are referred to several recent reviews on clinical considerations for placing feeding tubes and technical information needed to perform the procedures.[8] One key is that the feeding method selected should be able to provide all of the protein and energy needs without significantly increasing morbidity or stress to the animal or to the caregiver. For example, while the benefit of force-feeding a cat is avoiding placement of a feeding tube, the negative is that in most cats it is difficult, if not impossible, to attain their caloric needs. Further, in some cats, force-feeding results in significant stress to both cat and caregivers. Force-feeding may also result in development of food aversion—to the foods being force-fed.

Alternatively, nasoesophageal tubes are generally not good for large animals because the volume of liquid nutrition that must be administered to meet their caloric needs makes this approach impractical. These and other issues, including anesthesia, diet choices, and management of feeding tubes are reviewed elsewhere. In dogs or cats that are vomiting, or unable to eat enterally, alternative approaches to nutritional support, such as parenteral nutrition, may have to be considered.[6] But in most pets with GI disease, enteral nutrition, delivered in an appropriate amount, form, and frequency, is the best way to provide the necessary nutrition for the gut and for the whole animal.

Selection of a diet in managing dogs or cats with GI disease should be based on several factors: (1) the specific GI disease (if it can be determined), (2) the area of the GI tract affected, (3) any prior diets used in the management of the disease (a dietary history is essential to success in many dietary therapy chosen), and (4) understanding any other health issues that may influence the diet choice (e.g., kidney disease). There are several specific characteristics to be considered when selecting a diet for management of GI disease, including the type and amount of protein, CHO, fat, fiber, and their digestibility. The first, and possibly most important, consideration in choosing a diet to feed an animal with GI disease is nutrient digestibility. If the animal is fed a diet novel in both protein and CHO but the nutrients are not highly digestible, the malassimilation of those ingredients due to poor digestibility could contribute to worsening of the clinical signs (e.g., osmotic diarrhea, malodorous feces) and, potentially, the disease itself (e.g., overgrowth of bacterial pathogens). Typical commercially available maintenance pet foods have protein and CHO digestibilities ranging from 70% to 85% on a dry matter (DM) basis.[9,10] Less known specialty brands or pet foods available from bulk sellers may consist of ingredients with highly variable quality and digestibility. Sometimes this information is not available on the food label. Thus, if such foods are to be fed to pets with GI disease, further investigation to determine the digestibility of the food may be needed.

Table • 174-1

Energy Metabolism in Starvation

	STARVATION	HYPERMETABOLISM
Energy expenditure	Decreased	Increased
Mediator activation	+	+++
Fuel sources	Glucose/fat	Protein/fat
Gluconeogenesis	+	+++
Protein synthesis	Decreased	Greatly decreased
Catabolism	Not occurring	+++
Amino acid oxidation	+/−	+++
Ureagenesis	+/−	++
Ketosis	+/−	+
Responsiveness	+++	+
Rate of malnutrition	+	+++

Table • 174-2

Feeding Methods and Tube Feeding

ENTERAL FEEDING METHOD	POSITIVES	NEGATIVES
Oral/force-feeding	No tube placement, easy if patient accepts food	Difficult to meet caloric needs in hard-to-feed cats, may increase stress or food aversion in cats
Nasoesophageal tube	Tube placement requires only local anesthetic (in nose)	Can only use liquid diets in tube,
		Only tolerated for short-term in most
	Allows excellent short-term feeding method for cats with normal gastrointestinal tract, but not interested in eating	Must ensure that tube is in esophagus, not trachea, to avoid aspiration
		Should not use in vomiting patients
Esophageal tube	Allows long-term feeding of canned gruel diets	Requires short-term general anesthesia to place tube
	Relatively quick and easy to place with practice	Must wrap neck to protect tube from accidental removal
	Does not require special equipment to place tube	Site infection can occur
	Can be removed at any time after placement	
Gastrostomy tube	Allows feeding of canned or gruel diets	Requires general anesthesia to place tube
	Well tolerated for very long-term feeding with minimal patient discomfort	Requires special equipment to place tube
		Must not be removed after placement for 10-14 days to allow seal to form around stoma
		Leakage around tube or poor tube seating can result in peritonitis
Jejunostomy tube	Enteral feeding method of choice for pets with pancreatitis or gastric outflow disturbances	Requires general anesthesia to place tube
	Allows feeding when vomiting is severe	Surgical procedure, laparoscopy or special endoscopic expertise required to place
	Tube can be removed at any time after placement	Can use only liquid diets

Pet foods formulated for dietary therapy of GI disease (e.g., highly digestible or low-residue enteric diets) should have CHO and protein digestibilities of at least 88% DM.[9,11] Such diets should also have low to moderate levels of fat (~15% DM in cats and between 6% and 15% DM in dogs), be lactose free, and have reduced amounts of dietary fiber or other poorly digestible CHO. There are many different, highly digestible therapeutic diets available. Each formula is unique and therefore can elicit a different individual response. For example, each diet is likely to have different protein or CHO sources and varying levels and types of fat (e.g., some add omega-3 fatty acids), and some are formulated with ingredients designed to enhance GI health, such as the prebiotic fructo-oligosaccharides (FOS). Although the benefits of these individual additives have not been proven in large clinical trials, feeding highly digestible diets to pets with both acute and chronic GI diseases is widely accepted as beneficial.

ROLE OF CONSISTENCY, FREQUENCY, AND MEAL SIZE

The amount of food fed should be calculated based on the energy needs of the individual animal and the ability of the GI tract to assimilate different foods. Although there is ongoing discussion among nutritionists regarding the best method for determining energy requirements of well or sick animals, the goal should be to meet the animal's daily resting (or basal) energy requirements (RER).[12] One generally accepted equation for determining resting energy requirements in dogs and cats is $70 (BW_{kg})^{0.75}$ (dogs) and $60 (BW_{kg})^{0.67}$ (cats).

Once energy requirements have been determined, meal size, frequency, and consistency should be considered. In most

animals with GI disease, small meals (e.g., less than one third of stomach capacity) are recommended several times each day (three to six meals). This approach reduces gastric distention and reduces risk of vomiting. This also increases the mixing and digestion of the food present in the stomach. The feline stomach has a smaller capacity (approximately 60 mL/kg) and is less distensible than the stomach of a dog (capacity is nearly 80 to 90 mL/kg), which has greater capacity due to its distensibility.[13] Feeding small meals reduces gastric acid secretion and may reduce nausea and gastroesophageal reflux.[1,9]

In general, liquid diets empty faster from the stomach than canned foods, and canned foods faster than dry.[9] Thus, many animals with GI disease may benefit from small meals of a liquid or canned form. Liquid diets have primarily been used in specialized circumstances (e.g., for nasoesophageal or jejunostomy tube feeding) or with certain GI conditions (e.g., esophageal stricture, selected cases of megaesophagus, or gastric outflow disturbances) to reduce the risk of regurgitation or vomiting. However, one key is to remember that if liquid diets are fed too quickly or in large volumes, diarrhea may occur due to rapid emptying of the stomach, which will overwhelm the capacity of the small intestine. One good use of liquid diets is to substitute them for water (either for syringe or tube feeding) to reduce the caloric dilution.

DIET COMPOSITION

A variety of nutritional and nonnutritional diseases affect the GI tract and their treatment may be enhanced by appropriate diet selection. Numerous therapeutic diets are available for GI disease therapy, including some that are highly digestible, have novel antigen, are hypoallergenic, contain hydrolyzed protein, or include increased fiber content. Each of these dietary components may be used in management of GI disturbances; however, selection of the most appropriate diet requires an understanding of the differences in the nutrient composition of these formulations. Furthermore, under some circumstances, specific diets (e.g., homemade or elemental) are required for successful dietary management of severe GI disease.

PROTEIN

There are many diseases of the small intestine that result in impaired digestion (e.g., EPI) or absorption (e.g., IBD, ARD, PLE) of protein. The effects of protein malassimilation on the GI tract are often less clinically obvious than those involving fat or CHO, but they are no less important. Protein in the GI tract increases lower esophageal sphincter pressure and can be a potent stimulus for secretion of hormones, including gastrin and pancreatic hormones. Protein in the GI tract also increases both gastric emptying and intestinal transit.[1,9] Protein malassimilation can lead to protein malnutrition, which can further impair GI function, repair of mucosal injury, and the mucosal immune response.[14] In addition, intact protein reaching the distal small intestine and colon increases bacterial ammonia production, alters bacterial numbers, and can alter the bacterial species present. Change in the bacterial flora can lead to production of abnormal fecal consistency, odor, and flatus. More importantly, change in flora may contribute to development of bacterial enteritis, colitis, or colonic hypersensitivity.[15] Feeding highly digestible diets is essential in the initial approach to the dietary management of any kitten or young cat with diarrhea as both protein quality and high digestibility are critical. Cats have a shorter GI tract than dogs and greater need for protein.[13]

Protein-losing enteropathies (PLEs) are a group of potentially severe intestinal diseases that occur as primary enteropathies (e.g., lymphangiectasia) or familial enteropathies (e.g., Soft-Coated Wheaten Terriers, Basenjis, Irish Setters). PLEs also include enteropathies occurring secondary to infectious, neoplastic, or inflammatory processes that infiltrate the GI mucosa and result in protein loss either as a result of maldigestion, malabsorption, or leakage across damaged mucosa.[16-18] In addition to protein loss, secondary PLEs also result in loss of mucosal function, motility disturbances, and other gut functions.[16,18] Protein loss may also occur from a lack of available or functional enzymes, such as occurs with exocrine pancreatic insufficiency (EPI). Regardless of cause, nutritional therapy is essential in managing PLE. In mild forms of PLE, feeding a highly digestible, low-fat diet, in addition to specific therapy for the primary disease, may be sufficient. In dogs with severe intestinal disease, such as lymphangiectasia, significant hypoalbuminemia (serum albumin less than 1.5 g/dL) and severe inability to digest and absorb fat may occur. Disease progression can result in subsequent development of GI mucosal edema and further nutrient malassimilation.[18,19] In these animals, ultra–low-fat diets (fat concentrations less than 3 g/100 kcal or less than 10% DM) to prevent further steatorrhea and hydrolyzed protein or elemental diets that provide amino acids instead of intact protein may be necessary to achieve successful dietary control.[16]

In animals with the most severe forms of PLE, a combination of parenteral and enteral nutrition may be needed to replace proteins whose loss results in systemic decreases in oncotic pressure. Appropriate nutrition may also help resolve gut edema and correct protein-calorie malnutrition.[16,19] Once serum albumin concentrations are stable at greater than 1.75 g/dL, highly digestible, low-fat diets containing intact protein may be tolerated. However, some dogs with PLE may require feeding of ultra–low-fat homemade diets (e.g., nonfat turkey breast, nonfat cottage cheese, egg whites, rice, and cooked potatoes). Some dogs benefit from combinations of hydrolyzed, ultra–low-fat (less than 10% fat DM), or elemental diets, indefinitely.[16] The elemental diet lowest in fat (~5%) that has been used successfully is Vivonex TEN (Abbott). This is a human product and not balanced for dogs. However, it can be used as a short-term supplemental diet. Vivonex should not be used in cats without supplementation of several important amino acids and additional protein.

Adverse reactions to food are generally classified as immunologic (immune-mediated) or nonimmunologic. The immunologic causes of adverse reactions to food are true food allergies or food sensitivities. They can be IgE or non-IgE mediated and are most commonly caused by a dietary protein.[20] Immunologic reactions to food are usually associated with dermatologic and/or GI disease in dogs and cats. One could guess that the condition is both readily diagnosed and common, based on the number of exclusion diets available on the pet food market. In reality, neither is true. There is general agreement that other causes of diarrhea and pruritus are more common and that many GI disturbances appear to respond to dietary manipulation. The incidence of food allergy as a cause of GI or dermatologic signs is reported to be between 7% and 19% of all dogs.[3,18,21,22] Thus, other common causes of GI signs or pruritus should be ruled out before initiating a diet elimination trial, especially since such trials are difficult in households with more than one pet. Food trials should be completed before invasive tests or procedures are considered.

Nonimmunologic adverse reactions to food include both food intolerance and dietary indiscretion. Food intolerances usually cause only GI upset but, occasionally, dermatologic signs such as pruritus can be observed. This combination of signs can make diagnosis confusing. Food intolerance may be caused by metabolic (e.g., lactose intolerance), pharmacologic (e.g., intolerance of food additives), or idiosyncratic (any food substance, additive, preservative, etc., that results in an adverse reaction in the GI tract).[20,23] In several studies in cats with diarrhea, 35% to 50% improved after changing their diet to one that was highly digestible. This suggests that dietary intolerance is a major factor in development of diarrhea in cats.[3,23] Food poisoning can also be a form of food intolerance. Most animals with food intolerance will respond well (in a period of 2 to 3 weeks) to a diet that does not contain the offending agent(s). This may or may not require feeding an exclusion/novel antigen or hydrolyzed diet. Regardless, dogs and cats respond well to such diets because they are devoid of offending agents.

Ideally, diets used to treat adverse food reactions should contain: (1) a reduced number of novel protein sources or a protein hydrolysate (no intact proteins, molecular weights <10,000 daltons), (2) highly digestible protein, (3) no food additives or vasoactive substances (e.g., preservatives, antimicrobials, humectants, coloring agents, flavors, flavor enhancers, emulsifying agents, stabilizers, and thickeners), and (4) adequate nutrition for the animal's lifestage.[24] The above recommendations can be achieved with a commercial novel antigen or hydrolyzed diet or by preparing a homemade elimination diet. For the purposes of a dietary trial, a homemade elimination diet (using a single, novel protein source and a single, highly digestible CHO source) may be reasonable and effective. However, for long-term feeding, homemade diets must be balanced or risk nutritional deficiencies. This is particularly important in cats because of their specific and unique nutritional requirements. Trials for dietary sensitivity should last a minimum of 8 to 12 weeks. Trials for dietary intolerance can be much shorter, and, in general, a positive response will be seen within 2 weeks if the diet is appropriate. One key is recognizing that a single dietary trial with a therapeutic, elimination, or hydrolyzed diet may not be sufficient to rule out an adverse reaction to a food (either food allergy or intolerance). This is a frustrating reality. One must recognize that even a trial with hydrolyzed diets is not 100% effective for ruling out allergy. Multiple diet trials may be needed to identify the most appropriate diet. This information should allow clinicians to appropriately communicate with clients.

FATS AND FATTY ACIDS

In general, dietary fat is more digestible than CHO or protein—average digestibility of fat in commercial foods is higher than 85% and can be as high as 95% in premium diets.[9] Therefore, fat malabsorption is unusual. However, because digestion and absorption of fat is a complex process requiring multiple steps, malassimilation of fat in animals with GI disease is common. Thus, the amount of fat present in the diet is important and in treating dogs and cats with GI disease. In commercial therapeutic highly digestible diets formulated for GI disease, a reduced amount of fat, ranging from 4% to 15% DM, is present. In hypoallergenic diets, there is variability in fat content but, in general, higher amounts of fat are present. The wide variation in dietary fat content can influence response to treatment, especially in severe enteropathies. The major roles of fat in diets for companion animals are to provide energy, building blocks for cells (lipoproteins and cholesterol), and essential fatty acids. Dietary fat is also important in pet food as a palatability enhancer—which can create a problem with diet acceptance in some of the low-fat, highly digestible diets.

Like protein, fat also has some direct effects on the GI tract, including slowing gastric emptying in dogs and humans but not in cats.[1,3,25] In contrast to the effects of protein, increased levels of dietary fat decrease the tone of the lower esophageal sphincter and may lead to increased risk of gastroesophageal reflux or vomiting.[25] Thus, low-fat, highly digestible diets improve gastric emptying in dogs and may reduce vomiting. In animals with GI disease, undigested fat or fatty acids that reach the distal ileum or colon may increase bacterial fermentation (especially nonbeneficial species), resulting in formation of proinflammatory and prosecretory hydroxy fatty acids. This can cause osmotic diarrhea.[15,17] Nevertheless, complete absence of dietary fat is also undesirable and may lead to a deficiency of essential fatty acids.

There has also been focus on adding antiinflammatory omega-3 fatty acids (fish oils) to diets used for GI disease therapy. In humans with ulcerative colitis, addition of fish oils to diets resulted in less inflammatory mediators, improved mucosal function and fluidity, and reduced need for antiinflammatory drugs to maintain disease control.[26] The clinical benefit of fish oils in treating canine inflammatory skin disease is well recognized; however, studies specifically assessing a reduction of intestinal inflammation in dogs and cats fed omega-3 fatty acids are less well documented.[27] Nevertheless, adding omega-3 fatty acids to therapeutic diets should not be harmful and may be beneficial. Therefore, some highly digestible diets are formulated to contain added omega-3 fatty acids and fewer omega-6 (proinflammatory) fatty acids.

CARBOHYDRATES/DIETARY FIBER

There are no requirements for dietary CHO for dogs or cats. They are present in pet foods to provide a readily available energy source, to reduce fat or protein content of food, and to make the diets more economical to produce. The CHOs present in pet foods are primarily plant starches, such as rice, potato, corn, wheat, and barley.[25] These vary in digestibility, glycemic index (ability to increase blood sugar rapidly), and glycemic load (ability to increase total glucose over time). In diets for dogs with GI disease, the overall quantity of CHO is less important than its digestibility. This may not be true in cats, recognized as obligate carnivores with less ability to digest and metabolize dietary CHO.[28] In cats with IBD, CHO malabsorption was detected by the presence of increased breath hydrogen, but not related to overt changes in clinical signs.[29]

CHO digestibility is determined by its source and whether it has been cooked; for example, rice and wheat are generally highly digestible, whereas uncooked corn or potato starch is less digestible.[25] CHO malassimilation can cause osmotic diarrhea, increased intestinal gas (flatus), loss of water and electrolytes, enhanced fermentation of bacteria in both the small intestine and the colon, and overgrowth of pathogenic bacteria. Further, CHO malassimilation contributes to acidification of the colonic luminal environment, which promotes formation of hydroxy fatty acids and other potentially toxic intermediates.[9,25] White rice is the CHO of choice for most dogs (and is the most commonly used CHO in therapeutic diets), because it is gluten free (some dogs, especially Irish Setters and Soft-Coated Wheaten Terriers, are sensitive to gluten or may develop sensitivity to gluten, which is present in wheat, oats, and barley), highly digestible, and nonantigenic.[2,3,9,18] Other gluten-free CHO sources include potato, corn, and tapioca. Potato and tapioca are less digestible than white rice and corn may be antigenic to animals prone to food sensitivities. The glycemic index and glycemic load of starches present in pet foods are generally not important for managing GI disease in dogs or cats; however, they may be important in cats due to their reduced ability to handle a glucose load, or in animals with cancer or pancreatic or liver disease.

Another class of CHOs present in some diets are the beta-linked polysaccharides (i.e., those not readily broken down by mammalian amylases), which include the dietary fibers.[25] Dietary fibers are a large, complex group of CHOs that include starch and nonstarch polysaccharides found in plants; they are readily digested by bacterial enzymes but less well digested by mammalian enyzmes[25]. Traditionally, fibers were classified as soluble (highly fermentable) or insoluble (poorly fermented or nonfermentable) based on their digestion by amylase; however, a physiologically relevant classification, based on their activity in the GI tract, is currently recommended (Table 174-3).

Fibers are soluble if they form gels in solution (thus attracting water), delay gastric emptying, slow intestinal transit, inhibit absorption of cholesterol and some other nutrients, are poor bulking agents, are highly fermentable in the colon (i.e., increase the numbers of bacteria and increase short chain fatty acids [SCFAs], especially butyrate, an essential colonic fuel source), acidify luminal contents, and stimulate colonic cellular proliferation.[1,25,30] Examples of soluble fibers include FOS, pectins, psyllium, oats, barley, guar gum, fruits, and some legumes.[25]

Insoluble fibers do not form gels, have no effect on gastric emptying, increase or "normalize" intestinal transit, have no effect on nutrient absorption, are good bulking agents (i.e., dilute colonic content and thus bind noxious agents in the colon), are fermented less and therefore produce fewer SCFAs, and increase fecal weight.[1,30] Typical examples of insoluble fibers are cellulose, wheat and rye fibers (most cereal fibers), and the woody parts of plants (e.g., lignins).[25] In general, diets containing dietary fibers are used primarily in diseases of the colon, with soluble fibers being used to promote colon health in colitis or other infectious or inflammatory

Table • 174-3

Comparison of Fermentable and Nonfermentable Fiber Effects on the Gastrointestinal Tract

EFFECT	SOLUBLE (FERMENTABLE) FIBER (e.g., BEET PULP, GUAR GUM)	INSOLUBLE (NONFERMENTABLE) FIBER (e.g., CELLULOSE, METHYLCELLULOSE)
Transit time	No effect on transit in colon, slows transit of ingesta in small intestine	Normalizes transit in the colon by increasing segmentation (mixing) and improving propulsion, appears to increase speed of transit in small bowel
Fecal bulk	Decreased—stool smaller and softer	Increased—stool larger, drier
Bacteria/fermentation	Increases (more fermentation, may support beneficial bacteria such as lactobacilli or bifidobacteria)	Fermentation occurs, but to a very minor extent—minimal change in fecal flora
Water binding	High water binding, forms thick gels, increases fecal water, feces is wetter and smaller	Water absorption is efficient—feces can become quite dry if it is not expelled quickly or the pet is dehydrated

diseases of the colon, and insoluble fibers being used to normalize motility (e.g., hair or irritant colitis), act as an adsorptive agent (e.g., colitis due to toxins or bacterial colitis), or in animals prone to constipation that need the propulsive effects of a bulking agent. It should be noted that insoluble fibers acting as bulking agents should not be used in dehydrated animals or in cats with decreased colonic function (obstipation/megacolon).

FOS are kestose or nystose sugars present in a variety of fruits, vegetables, and grains that behave in the GI tract like soluble fibers. These sugars have generated considerable interest in both human and veterinary medicine, because they are preferentially fermented by beneficial bacterial species (e.g., *Lactobacillus* and *Bifidobacteria* spp.) and prevent the growth of pathogenic species.[31,32] In studies of humans with IBD or colitis, adding FOS to the diet greatly improved the response to therapy, clinical disease was reduced, and relapses were fewer.[33] Only a few studies in dogs (and even fewer in cats) have evaluated the role of FOS in the dietary therapy of GI disease. However, preliminary evidence supports the finding in humans that FOS increases the numbers of beneficial bacteria in the colon of both dogs and cats[31] and may prove beneficial in controlling bacterial overgrowth, ARD, or other inflammatory diseases believed to have a bacterial origin (e.g., IBD).

NUTRITIONAL DEFICIENCIES RESULTING FROM GASTROINTESTINAL DISEASE

Nutritional deficiencies may occur as a consequence of GI disease. Protein and calorie malnutrition is the most common nutritional deficiency in severe or chronic GI disease. Not surprisingly, deficiencies of electrolytes (e.g., sodium, potassium, chloride, and bicarbonate) and divalent cations (e.g., magnesium, zinc, and calcium) are also common and

should be corrected.[34] A variety of vitamin deficiencies may occur as a result of severe intestinal disease, but deficiencies of B vitamins, especially cobalamin, folate, and of some of the fat-soluble vitamins (E and K), are the most common and clinically important micronutrient deficiencies recognized in dogs and cats.[1,3,34,35] Little is known about deficiencies of microminerals; however, it is reasonable to assume that levels of copper, selenium, zinc, and others may be affected and deficiencies thus corrected by nutritional support.

Cobalamin (vitamin B_{12}) is an essential cofactor in many body energy reactions, cellular growth and repair processes, and in liver glutathione (antioxidant) metabolism.[34] Many dogs and cats with severe intestinal disease have cobalamin deficiency—which until corrected can be associated with persistent diarrhea or poor response to therapy. Measurement of cobalamin levels is particularly important in any cat with anorexia or GI disease because of their higher need for all B vitamins, and cobalamin in particular, so deficiency can occur quite quickly. Deficiency is corrected by replacement with injectable cyanocobalamin at a dose of 25 μg/kg once/week SC for 4 to 6 weeks in dogs, or 250 μg/cat/wk SC for 4 weeks, then once monthly thereafter, as needed to maintain normal serum levels. Some dogs and cats may require lifelong therapy to control their signs, and in those patients it is possible they will require lifelong B_{12} injections as well. Remember, it may take as long as 3 to 4 weeks, once starting appropriate therapy, to see any response, so it is important to be patient and to recheck values to be sure normal levels have been achieved.

References

The reference list can be found on the companion Expert Consult Web site at *www.expertconsult.com*.

CHAPTER 175

Nutritional Management of Hepatic Conditions

Craig G. Ruaux

Among the myriad roles of the liver in metabolic homeostasis, extraction of assimilated nutrients and potentially toxic compounds from the portal circulation is particularly critical. Because the source of both the assimilated nutrients and many potentially toxic compounds is either directly from the diet or from alteration of dietary components by the intestinal microbiota, dietary modification has obvious potential for benefit in animals with hepatic disease.

Nutritional interventions in pets with hepatic disease should be aimed towards optimizing the ability of the liver to heal and regenerate, including provision of sufficient metabolic energy to meet the needs of the patient, considering the disease state of the animal. In most cases, protection of animals from hepatic encephalopathy is not as important as the provision of adequate dietary energy intake and preservation of body mass though adequate caloric intake and provision of adequate protein intake.

METABOLIC ENERGY AND PROTEIN REQUIREMENTS IN CHRONIC HEPATIC DISEASE

Animals with hepatic disease are typically in a catabolic state. While little work has been published regarding energy requirements of hepatic disease in companion animals, studies in human beings suggest that inflammatory/necroinflammatory diseases such as chronic active or acute hepatitis are associated with up to a twofold increase in resting metabolic energy requirements.[1] Even within human medical practice, there is a lack of consensus regarding metabolic energy demands of patients with liver disease. Human clinical nutritionists who specialize in gastrointestinal disease assign a higher disease stress factor for decompensated liver disease than those who do not specialize in these cases.[2]

In animals with acute hepatic inflammatory disease or chronic active hepatitis, protein requirements to maintain a positive nitrogen balance may be substantially higher than in normal dogs.[3] Dietary protein restriction in this group of patients may actually slow recovery. A sizable proportion of this increased metabolic energy and protein requirement is due to increased protein turnover. In the absence of adequate dietary intake, common in animals with liver disease, protein-calorie malnutrition can develop. Protein-calorie malnutrition is associated with loss of lean body mass, blunted immune responsiveness, decreased hepatic albumin synthesis with a resultant loss of plasma oncotic pressure, and increased risk of dehiscence of surgical wounds.[4]

Hepatic disease is often accompanied by conditions that predispose animals to malassimilation. Cholestasis, for instance, is associated with decreased ability to digest and absorb fat due to reduced intestinal availability of bile acids. Cats with cholangitis/cholangiohepatitis often have other diseases of the gastrointestinal tract, such as pancreatic disease or inflammatory bowel disease (IBD), that may further compromise nutrient absorption through decreased digestive enzyme activity or mucosal dysfunction, respectively.

Patients with liver disease often experience significant nausea and anorexia. As hepatic functional mass declines, less glycogen storage capacity is available within the liver, necessitating the use of lean muscle glycogen stores and protein as substrates for gluconeogenesis to maintain blood glucose concentrations. Together, reduced voluntary intake due to nausea/anorexia and increased muscle protein mobilization to provide substrates for gluconeogenesis lead to rapid weight loss in animals with hepatic disease. Muscle tissue is also a storage site for a large proportion of the total body pool of ammonia, which is a major encephalopathic toxin. Failure to meet the animal's metabolic energy requirements and maintain a positive nitrogen balance through provision of adequate dietary protein and fat can thus promote the development of hepatic encephalopathy through release of muscle ammonia stores. Given the difficulty of detecting hepatic encephalopathy in more mildly affected animals, many clinicians will prescribe protein-restricted diets early in the course of liver disease. This may actually worsen the clinical state if low-protein diets with decreased palatability lead to insufficient caloric intake. The first aim of nutritional support for most animals with hepatic disease should be to ensure adequate caloric intake to meet metabolic energy requirements.[5] Normal canine maintenance diets utilizing high-quality, readily digestible protein sources are indicated in most dogs with liver disease, unless overt hepatic encephalopathy is present.

Provision of adequate calories via dietary fat and carbohydrate is sparing for lean muscle protein, and allows the use of ingested amino acids for synthesis and repair of muscle mass. While the actual metabolic energy requirements of animals with hepatic disease are not well defined, clinical experience suggests that most of these patients require at least the same dietary metabolic energy input as healthy, active animals. Unfortunately, many diets utilized to protect animals from hepatic encephalopathy have reduced palatability, particularly in animals with nausea due to liver disease, making the provision of adequate caloric intake from these diets difficult.

In cats, the provision of adequate protein intake is even more important to maintain lean body mass. As obligate carnivores, cats have a minimal dietary protein requirement two to three times greater than dogs and other omnivores.[6] Several amino acids (e.g., taurine, arginine, methionine and cysteine) are either essential in cats or become conditionally essential in disease states featuring decreased voluntary intake. Bile acids in the cat are exclusively conjugated to taurine.[7] As bile acids are lost in feces or deconjugated by intestinal bacterial activity, there is a constant demand for additional taurine, which must be met either from dietary intake or mobilization of muscle protein.[8] Total body taurine deficiency can thus develop rapidly in cats with hepatic disease. The importance of adequate protein and essential amino acid input in cats is discussed further in the section describing hepatic lipidosis.

Representative major nutrient compositions of diets from several manufacturers that are either directly labeled for use in animals with hepatic disease or recommended by the manufacturer for use in liver disease, are summarized in Table 175-1.

Table • 175-1

Major Nutrient Compositions of Representative Veterinary Prescription Diets with a Labeled Indication for Use in Hepatic Disease or Hepatic Encephalopathy

DIET	PROTEIN (%DM)	PROTEIN g/100 kcal ME	FAT (%DM)	CARBOHYDRATE (%DM)	MANUFACTURER RECOMMENDED INDICATIONS
Canine					
Hills l/d, dry	17.6	3.7	24.1	50.7	Liver disease, hepatic
Hills l/d, canned	17.6	3.9	24.2	49.3	encephalopathy, copper storage
Purina NF Kidney Function, dry	15.9	3.6	15.7	62.8	Renal failure, hypertension, early
Purina NF Kidney Function, canned	16.5	3.6	27.4	50.4	CHF, hepatic disease with encephalopathy
Purina EN GastroENteric Formula, dry	26.9	7.6	12.6	53.4	Hepatic disease not associated with
Purina EN GastroENteric Formula, canned	30.52	7.6	13.8	48.9	encephalopathy, enteritis, pancreatitis, IBD
Royal Canin HEPATIC LS 14	14.0	4.0	14.0	51.4*	Hepatic insufficiency, hepatic disease, hepatic encephalopathy, portosystemic shunts, disorders of copper metabolism
Feline					
Hills l/d, dry	31.8	7.1	23.2	37.4	Liver disease, hepatic lipidosis,
Hills l/d, canned	31.6	6.7	23.2	38.0	hepatic encephalopathy
Purina NF Kidney Function, dry	28.5	7.2	12.8	50.6	Renal failure, hypertension, early
Purina NF Kidney Function, canned	31.1	6.0	29.5	30.6	CHF, hepatic disease with encephalopathy
Purina EN GastroENteric Formula, dry	56.2	12.9	18.4	16.7	Enteritis, diarrhea, gastritis, hepatic lipidosis
Royal Canin HYPOALLERGENIC HP 23	23.5	6.2	18.0	3.6.*	IBD, dietary intolerance, pancreatic insufficiency, elimination diet trials, hepatic disease
Royal Canin RENAL LP, dry	21.0	5.4	42.6	9.5*	Chronic renal failure, hepatic encephalopathy

Values are rounded to one significant figure. Data and indications obtained from respective company websites or printed materials as of October 2008.
CHF, Congestive heart failure; *DM*, dry matter; *IBD*, inflammatory bowel disease; *ME*, metabolizable energy.
*Royal Canin quotes carbohydrate content of their diets as % as fed rather than on a dry matter basis.

Many diets recommended for use in liver disease feature reduced protein content. While reduced protein content may be protective against hepatic encephalopathy, the use of these diets in animals with nonencephalopathic disease carries the risk of inducing protein-calorie malnutrition. The majority of liver diseases encountered in companion animals do not carry a risk of encephalopathy except in end-stage (Table 175-2); thus the use of "liver" diets with markedly reduced protein content is not recommended for all animals with liver disease.

Diets with mildly reduced protein content utilizing a high-digestibility protein (such as the renal and hypoallergenic diets listed in Table 175-1) are a preferred choice in most companion animals with liver disease.

NUTRACEUTICALS IN HEPATIC DISEASE

A reasonable definition of the term *nutraceutical* would be a food, food-derived compound, or dietary supplement that is given with the intent to modulate disease or provide health benefits. Many nutraceutical compounds have been suggested as supplements in human beings and animals with hepatic disease[9]; however within the veterinary literature only two

compounds/products, s-adenosylmethionine (SAMe) and silymarin, have received meaningful attention.

SAMe is a compound derived from the essential amino acid methionine and ATP. SAMe is an important donor of methylpropyl, sulfhydrylpropyl, and aminopropyl groups in many reactions occurring within the hepatocyte. These reactions are involved in many of the liver's essential metabolic processes, including detoxification of drugs and xenobiotics via transulfuration and transmethylation pathways.[10] Adequate availability of SAMe is also critical to the synthesis and reduction of glutathione (GSH), which is one of the most important early protection mechanisms within the cell against oxidant stress.[10-12] Oxidative stress, with subsequent mitochondrial dysfunction and activation of cell death pathways, is a major cause of hepatocyte death in many disease processes.[13]

SAMe, presented as a stable 1,4-butanedisulfonate salt in enteric-coated tablets (Denosyl SD4, Nutramax Laboratories, Edgewood, Md.), has been assessed prospectively in healthy, untreated cats and in healthy dogs receiving chronic prednisolone therapy.[10,14] In both dogs and cats increases in hepatic GSH, with an increase in the ratio of reduced to oxidized GSH, were noted. In the dog study, however, no significant

Table • 175-2

Common Canine and Feline Liver Diseases

CANINE	FELINE
Vacuolar Hepatopathy	
Glucocorticoid induced	Glucocorticoid induced
Diabetes mellitus	Diabetes mellitus
Chronic illnesses	Chronic illnesses (pancreatitis, IBD)
(pancreatitis,	Hepatic lipidosis syndrome
inflammatory bowel	**Very severe cases may have**
desease [IBD])	**encephalopathy**
Infiltrative Diseases	
Acute hepatitis	Cholangiohepatitis
Chronic active hepatitis	Lymphosarcoma
Lymphosarcoma	
Biliary Tree Diseases	
Major bile duct obstruction	Major bile duct obstruction
Biliary mucocele	Cholangitis
	Neoplasia (biliary carcinoma)
Primary or Metastatic Neoplasia	
Metastases of	Hepatocellular carcinoma (rare)
hemangiosarcoma	
Massive hepatocellular	
carcinoma	
Other	
Primary portal vein	**Cirrhosis**
hypoplasia/microvascular	
dysplasia	
Cirrhosis	**Portosystemic vascular anomalies**
Portosystemic vascular	
anomalies	
Juvenile fibrosis	
disorders (rare)	

Modified from Center SA: Nutritional support for dogs and cats with hepatobiliary disease. J Nutr 128:2733S-2746S, 1998. Conditions associated with risk of hepatic encephalopathy are in bold type. Note that the majority of "liver disease" diagnoses in companion animals are not associated with hepatic encephalopathy, except in an end-stage state.

effect was seen on clinicopathologic or histologic manifestations of glucocorticoid-induced vacuolar hepatopathy.[14] Successful therapeutic use of SAMe has been reported in a dog with acetaminophen toxicity, severe Heinz-body anemia, and markedly increased aspartate aminotransferase activity.[15]

Cats are particularly susceptible to acetaminophen-induced hepatotoxicity, and SAMe appears to be a rational therapeutic selection for this condition. Unfortunately, controlled studies of the effect of SAMe therapy on a model of acetaminophen hepatotoxicity in the cat showed little to no effect, with most changes failing to reach statistical significance.[11] There are no well controlled clinical studies assessing the efficacy of SAMe as a therapy for chronic liver disease in dogs or cats.

Silymarin, a mixture of flavonolignans extracted from the milk thistle (Silybum marianum L.), has been shown to have potent antioxidant efficacy in several models of oxidant-mediated liver disease.[16] There is substantial recent interest in the use of silymarin in many diseases that feature oxidant-mediated pathology, including alcoholic liver disease and

human viral hepatitis.[17,18] Studies in companion animals are lacking, although the oral bioavailability of a silybin-phosphatidylcholine complex has been described.[19] Metaanalysis of clinical trials using silymarin in human beings reveal little evidence for clinical benefit except in Amanita phalloides mushroom poisoning. This is likely a reflection of poor study design of many of these trials.[20]

There is a strong theoretical underpinning for the use of many of the active ingredients in nutraceutical preparations in some hepatic disease conditions.[21] Unfortunately, if applying a strict "evidence-based" approach to medical decision making, there is no convincing evidence of benefit from these compounds in management of chronic hepatic disease in dogs and cats. Overall, accurate diagnosis of the primary liver disease and implementation of therapy directed towards this diagnosis are recommended in preference to empirical therapy with nutraceutical compounds at this time.

COPPER-RESTRICTED DIETS

Hepatic copper accumulation is a feature of several diseases in dogs. Copper (Cu) accumulation hepatopathy is well recognized as an autosomal recessive disorder in the Bedlington Terrier. In these dogs a genetic defect in the COMMD1 gene has been identified.[22] In several other breeds, including the Doberman Pinscher, Cocker Spaniel, West Highland White Terrier, Skye Terrier, and Labrador Retriever,[23,24] there is evidence of excessive Cu accumulation in some liver diseases. Because Cu can accumulate with cholestasis as well as primary hepatocellular disease, the significance of Cu accumulation as a primary pathologic event is less clear in these dogs; however, preliminary evidence from Labrador Retrievers in the Netherlands suggests that chelation therapy and reduced Cu diets are associated with improvement in chronic inflammatory liver disease and reduced disease progression.[25]

Animals with hepatic Cu accumulation sufficient to cause overt hepatopathy are best treated with specific therapy using chelating drugs such as d-penicillamine, at least until hepatic Cu content is reduced below toxic levels. Dietary Cu restriction can be useful in the maintenance phase of management for dogs with these diseases. Typical maintenance canine diets will contain a minimum of 7.3 ppm Cu, while Cu-restricted diets may contain as little as 3 ppm Cu on a dry matter basis.

Additional dietary manipulations to decrease hepatic Cu accumulation include supplementation with ascorbic acid and elemental zinc (Zn). Zn supplementation increases the intestinal expression of metallothionein, an avid metal binding protein within the enterocytes. Metallothionein has a higher affinity for Cu than Zn. Administration of Zn between meals leads to increased metallothionein expression in the enterocytes, Cu in the diet is then bound with high affinity within the mature enterocyte and lost in the feces as the enterocyte is shed.[26] Zinc is given at a loading dose of 100 mg elemental Zn per os twice weekly for 3 weeks, followed by a maintenance dose of 50 mg elemental Zn per os twice weekly. Vomiting and nausea may both occur as side effects of Zn therapy; administration of the Zn with a small amount of food may reduce these side-effects. Ascorbic acid supplementation increases urinary excretion of both Cu and Zn, as well as increasing the intestinal synthesis of metallothionein.

VITAMIN AND MINERAL SUPPLEMENTATION

Animals with liver disease often have vitamin and/or mineral deficiencies. Several factors, including reduced voluntary intake, fat malabsorption, reduced gastrointestinal mucosal function, and loss of reserve stores in hepatic tissue can all contribute to the development of vitamin and mineral deficiencies.

Water-soluble vitamins such as folic acid, thiamine, cobalamin, niacin and riboflavin are often critical cofactors in enzymatic pathways carried out in hepatic cells. In cats with hepatic lipidosis, deficiencies of these vitamins are common.[27] Most water-soluble vitamins do not have substantial body stores and daily replacement from dietary sources is necessary. Administration of multivitamin supplements is cost-effective, simple, and should be included in any nutritional support plan for patients with liver disease.

In the cat, cobalamin malabsorption due to small intestinal disease is commonly documented in association with liver disease.[28] Cobalamin malabsorption due to intestinal disease cannot be overcome by increased dietary supplementation with this vitamin; parenteral therapy is necessary.[29] A dose range previously described for use in cats with cobalamin deficiency due to intestinal disease is 250 µg/cat injected subcutaneously, once a week for 6 weeks, once every 2 weeks for 6 weeks, then once a month thereafter.[29] The concentration of cobalamin in standard injectable multivitamin preparations is insufficient to supply this amount of cobalamin in a reasonable injection volume; the use of pure preparations of cobalamin in addition to multivitamin products is recommended in dogs and cats with documented cobalamin deficiency.

In animals with more severe, long standing liver disease, fat malabsorption and subsequent deficiencies of fat-soluble vitamins can occur. Significant elevations in the plasma concentration of proteins induced by vitamin K antagonism (PIVKA) have been documented both in cats with hepatic lipidosis and cats with cholangiohepatitis associated with IBD.[30] Vitamin E deficiency reduces cellular defenses against oxidant-mediated damage, potentially playing a role in copper-associated hepatoxicity.[31,32] Empirically, regular provision of vitamin E, A, and D supplementation by intramuscular injection at 3- to 4-month intervals is recommended in companion animals with longstanding liver disease, particularly if this is complicated by the presence of steatorrhea. Cats with hepatic lipidosis should be screened for vitamin K deficiency, particularly if there is any evidence of bleeding tendencies. If detected (ideally via PIVKA assay), subcutaneous vitamin K administration at 1 to 5 mg/kg/day for 2 to 3 days is indicated.

Carnitine and choline are essential cofactors for hepatic cellular fatty acid transport. Carnitine is essential within the mitochondria for beta-oxidation of long chain fatty acids. Choline is essential for the synthesis of phosphatidyl choline, necessary for export of very low–density lipoproteins (VLDL) from hepatocytes. Carnitine and choline supplementation are both potentially important in the management of feline hepatic lipidosis, discussed below.

NUTRITIONAL INTERVENTION IN HEPATIC ENCEPHALOPATHY

Hepatic encephalopathy (HE) results from loss of hepatic detoxification function and subsequent accumulation of encephalotoxins within the systemic circulation and central nervous system (CNS). These encephalotoxins may be directly toxic to neurons (e.g., ammonia) or may act as "false" neurotransmitters, interfering with CNS function.[33] In human patients, HE is graded via a variety of physiologic and neurologic scoring systems, most of which refer back to the West Haven Criteria.[33] Under this scoring system, HE is scored from 0 (no encephalopathy) to 4 (hepatic coma) (Table 175-3).[34]

Subtle neurologic impairments, equivalent to inattention or mild tremor, are difficult to detect in small animals; therefore most animals with a diagnosis of HE will fall within the West Haven Criteria scores 2 to 4. Most animals with liver disease, however, do not meet these criteria. According to a recent consensus statement of the European Society of Parenteral and Enteral Nutrition, protein restriction is not indicated in human patients with an HE score of 0 to 2, as negative protein balance and resultant malnutrition are negative prognostic factors.[1] Protein restriction is indicated in human patients with West Haven Criteria scores of 3 or 4. Such scores are a strong negative prognostic factor, with most dying within 1 year.[1] Assuming a similar relationship in animals with a diagnosis of liver disease, most of whom do not fall within scores 2 to 4 of the West Haven Criteria, aggressive protein restriction may be counterproductive, even in mildly encephalopathic patients.

Recommendations for dietary protein content in diets fed to animals with severe HE vary. Most dogs can be managed with diets containing 3 to 4 g of protein per 100 kcal of diet, while cats require at least 6 to 7 g/100 kcal. Note that the recommendation is for protein proportion within the diet, not for protein intake/kg of animal. Several commercially available diets are formulated to meet these recommendations (see Table 175-1).

The amino acid makeup of the diet used in patients with HE is another area of interest and controversy. It has been suggested that aromatic amino acid (AAA)–rich diets are likely to potentiate HE, the AAAs potentially acting as substrates for the production of encephalotoxins.[3] The molar ratio of AAA to branched chain amino acids (BCAAs) in plasma has been shown to be increased in animals with HE.[3] BCAAs are important substrates for gluconeogenesis; thus the presence of protein/calorie malnutrition will lead to depletion of these amino acids in the plasma. While these changes in the AAA:BCAA are well documented in veterinary and

Table • 175-3

West Haven Criteria of Altered Mental Status in Hepatic Encephalopathy Patients

STAGE	CONSCIOUSNESS	INTELLECT AND BEHAVIOR	NEUROLOGIC FINDINGS
0	Normal	Normal	Normal
1	Mild lack of awareness	Shortened attention span; impaired addition or subtraction	Mild ataxia or tremor
2	Lethargic	Disoriented, inappropriate behavior	Obvious ataxia, "head pressing" in small animals
3	Somnolent but rousable	Gross disorientation, bizarre behavior	Muscular rigidity, clonus, hyperreflexia
4	Coma	Coma	Decerebrate posture

Modified from Hassanein TI, Hilsabeck RC, Perry W: Introduction to the Hepatic Encephalopathy Scoring Algorithm (HESA). Dig Dis Sci 53:529-538, 2008.

human patients, their significance as a direct cause of HE rather than as a epiphenomenon is unclear. Experimental studies using dogs with surgically created portosystemic vascular anomalies found more pronounced HE and higher blood ammonia concentrations in the dogs receiving a low–AAA:BCAA diet; however, the dogs receiving this diet ate more than those receiving a high–AAA:BCAA diet, resulting in greater total protein intake.[35] Based on metaanalyses of studies in human beings with HE, BCAA supplementation is recommended in patients who develop HE scores of 3 or 4 during enteral nutrition.[1] The situation is less clear with lower grade HE human patients and by extension most veterinary patients. In most cases BCAA supplementation is unlikely to lead to a net negative benefit unless voluntary intake is reduced. Most veterinary prescription diets specifically labeled for hepatic disease are formulated to achieve a higher BCAA content and derive a significant proportion of metabolizable energy from fats and carbohydrates.

Feeding of several small meals throughout the day is often of benefit for animals with overt HE, reducing the total ammonia load following each meal. Other strategies used to control HE in small animals include antibacterial therapy with neomycin or metronidazole and the use of enteric lactulose therapy (oral or via enema) to reduce ammonia production and absorption, respectively, from the gastrointestinal tract.

HEPATIC LIPIDOSIS IN CATS

Appropriate nutritional management is absolutely central to successful resolution of hepatic lipidosis (HL) in cats.[36] While the underlying pathology of hepatic lipid accumulation in cats is not entirely clear, there is consensus that reduced caloric intake and protein-calorie malnutrition are important predisposing factors. Obese cats are commonly felt to be at increased risk[27,37,38]: however, this is not exclusively a disease of the overweight cat. It has been stated that more than 95% of cats have an underlying illness that predisposes the cat to enter a catabolic state.[27] Successful management in the medium to long term will require addressing the underlying disease process to allow a return to more normal appetite. In the short term, diligent attention to restoration of a positive caloric balance is necessary. Often this must be achieved in order to make the cat sufficiently stable to allow a rational diagnostic workup for underlying disease.

The feline liver has relatively small glycogen stores; thus the cat becomes dependent upon systemic lipolysis and hepatic metabolism of triglycerides relatively rapidly with the onset of starvation or anorexia. The underlying biochemical defect leading to hepatic accumulation of these lipids is not clear. Both carnitine/choline deficiency and arginine deficiency have been suggested. Cats with HL fed arginine-deficient diets, even if fed in quantities necessary to supply adequate caloric intake, can rapidly develop severe HE as the urea cycle is compromised.[27] Choline and carnitine are both important in mitochondrial fatty acid transport and packaging of fatty acids into VLDLs for export from the hepatocyte; thus deficiency of these trace elements may contribute to fat accumulation. Arginine, choline, and carnitine supplementation are commonly recommended in the nutritional management of cats with HL. If the diet used for initial feeding is deficient in arginine, as is the case with most human formulations, this amino acid should be supplemented at dose of 250 mg/100 kcal of diet delivered. The author empirically supplements HL cats with arginine, carnitine, and taurine regardless of the enteral nutrition formula used. Oral admin-

istration of L-carnitine, 250 to 500 mg/day, and taurine, 250 to 500 mg/day are also recommended.[27,36,37]

Most cats with HL are severely anorectic. Assisted feeding should be implemented as soon as feasible in these patients. Oral forced alimentation is not recommended; cats will rapidly develop food aversion, while the stress of handling and syringe feeding can precipitate rhabdomyolysis in hypokalemic and hypophosphatemic cats, as can occur with refeeding syndrome (see below). Medical agents for appetite stimulation in cats are variably effective, often ineffective in HL cats, and may require hepatic detoxification. Early placement of a feeding tube, at the minimum an esophagostomy tube, should be considered the standard of care. With critically ill cats, where even a short anesthetic procedure to place an esophagostomy tube is felt to carry excessively high risk, initial feeding with a nasoesophageal tube (5 to 8 F) can be attempted. However, these tubes are more prone to clogging and failure due to vomiting, regurgitation, or removal by the patient. Nasoesophageal tubes require placement and maintenance of an Elizabethan collar as many cats do not tolerate them. The small lumen of the tube limits diet choice to liquefied formulations. Placement of an esophagostomy tube allows use of larger bore tubes (10 to 14 F) that make feeding easier and open up the possibility of blenderized diets. Percutaneous endoscopically placed gastrostomy (PEG) tubes are larger still (up to 20 F), and allow greater movement of the head and neck of the cat (as these areas are not bandaged), which appears to reduce morbidity in some cats by allowing self-grooming. Clinicians experienced in this technique can place a tube in a 10- to 15-minute procedure. If a large bore PEG tube can be placed, assisted feeding by owners becomes more feasible in the home environment. As some cats require assisted feeding for weeks to months, this can be an important aspect of successful home care. Given that many cats show vitamin K deficiency and elevated PIVKA with HL,[30] administration of subcutaneous vitamin K for 1 to 2 days before either esophagostomy or PEG tube placement is recommended. Surgical placement of gastrostomy tubes via celiotomy in cats with HL is associated with high risk for postoperative morbidity and an unacceptable risk of stomach displacement.[27]

During initial reinstitution of feeding, dramatic and potentially life-threatening electrolyte derangements can occur, particularly in serum potassium (K^+) and phosphate (PO_4^{3-}). These are both predominantly intracellular ions, but during periods of extended malnutrition both K+ and PO_4^{3-} move into the extracellular space to maintain cellular membrane potentials. With refeeding and renewed insulin activity, there is a rapid shift of both ions back into the intracellular fluid; this shift can be fast enough to result in both rhabdomyolysis and hemolysis in some severely affected cats. These changes should be anticipated, and in severely affected cats parenteral administration of PO_4^{3-} and K^+ should begin preemptively. K^+ replacement can be dosed using routine sliding dose scales, while PO_4^{3-} is commonly administered intravenously at 0.01 to 0.03 mmol/kg/hr. PO_4^{3-} is commonly available with K^+ as a cation; care should be taken to ensure that the total K^+ input dose not exceed 0.5 mEq/kg/hr. Oral administration of K^+ as the gluconate salt is also recommended. Twice daily measurement of serum electrolytes, including magnesium, is recommended. Electrolyte abnormalities should be anticipated during the first few days of therapy, and should be addressed as early as possible though judicious fluid supplementation.

Many cats with HL have water-soluble vitamin deficiencies. These are commonly supplemented by admixing multivitamin preparations into IV fluids at a dose of 1 to 2 mL/1L bag, and the bag and lines should be protected from light. Cobalamin deficiency is also common, and can be addressed with subcutaneous cobalamin injections. Thiamine deficiency is particularly insidious. Both thiamine and K⁺ deficiencies can result in obtundation, weakness, and neck ventroflexion. These signs may be misinterpreted as HE, and these abnormalities should be screened for and corrected before instituting low-protein diets for presumed encephalopathy. While very severe cases of HL in cats can result in HE and necessitate the use of low-protein diets for a short period, HE is not a feature of most cases of HL, and use of low-protein diets may be associated with an adverse outcome.[39]

REFERENCES

The reference list can be found on the companion Expert Consult Web site at *www.expertconsult.com*.

CHAPTER 176

Nutritional Management of Endocrine Disease

Sean J. Delaney
Sally C. Perea

Several commonly encountered endocrinopathies have nutritional strategies that can be useful as an aid in therapy. These endocrinopathies include diabetes mellitus, hyperadrenocorticism, and hypothyroidism. Although of unknown etiology, one strategy for the nutritional management of feline idiopathic hypercalcemia is included (Figure 176-1).

DIABETES MELLITUS

The nutritional management of diabetes mellitus focuses on improving glycemic control. This means attempting to minimize the rapid absorption of glucose from dietary carbohydrates.

Using Fiber to Minimize the Rapid Absorption of Glucose

The absorption rate of glucose from digested dietary carbohydrate within the intestinal tract may be decreased by dietary fiber. There are two types of dietary fiber—soluble and insoluble. Soluble fiber absorbs water and is responsible for the gelling effect associated with ingredients like pectin, derived from fruit. Insoluble fiber does not form gels, primarily adds bulk, and is usually derived from woody plant material. Both fiber types have been shown to be effective at improving glycemic control, presumably by blunting the absorption of glucose.[1-6] It appears that mixed soluble and insoluble fiber sources may be most effective in decreasing carbohydrate absorption.[6] However, fiber, especially soluble fiber, may have unwanted effects. Specifically, increased levels of dietary soluble fiber can adversely affect the absorption of minerals[7] and can cause loose stools.[1,6] These issues are not typically of concern in therapeutic foods formulated with soluble fiber, but are a concern when supplemental soluble fiber is added to pet food exclusively and aggressively. Although the impact on mineral absorption is not predictable, the effect on stool firmness can be assessed by titration. Generally, supplemental fiber recommendations are:
- If a mixed source of fiber is desired, psyllium (e.g., Metamucil) can be added to the diet in amounts of 1 to 3 tablespoons per day.
- If a source of soluble fiber is needed, 2 to 4 teaspoons of guar gum (e.g., Benefiber) can be added to the diet each day. *This dose is lower than the recommended amounts for mixed or insoluble sources due to a concern about soluble fiber's effect on stool quality, not because soluble fiber is more "potent" for managing diabetics.*
- If a source of insoluble fiber is needed, 1 to 3 tablespoons of coarse wheat bran can be added to the diet each day.

Initially the lowest dose should be used and then titrated to increased amounts as long as poor stool quality remains acceptable. Care should be taken when selecting supplemental fiber products, as they potentially could contain the toxic artificial sweetener, xylitol. If the mixed fiber source, canned pumpkin, is used, one should recognize that it is actually quite low in fiber (0.4 g/tbsp compared to 9 g/tbsp for psyllium). Further, canned pumpkin pie filling should not be used since it contains a great deal of sugar. Most, if not all, concentrated fiber sources need to be mixed with canned food. For insoluble fiber this is mainly due to poor palatability. When a mixed fiber or soluble supplement is used, it generally needs to be mixed with canned food to enable it to be safely consumed and increase palatability. Safe consumption is a concern as many forms of soluble fiber can rapidly gel and, at least in humans, can represent a choking hazard (a warning of this choking hazard can often be found on human fiber supplements).

A convenient alternative to fiber supplementation is use of high-fiber therapeutic foods (Table 176-1). Most of these products rely heavily on insoluble fiber, and several have been shown to be effective in the management of diabetes mellitus.[2-5] Generally it is recommended that transitioning to a high-fiber food be done carefully in a newly diagnosed diabetic. Insulin therapy is quite challenging for most clients and the potential for an adverse experience is higher when diet is changed at the same time. Specifically, a concern among many nutritionists is that the high-fiber food may not be as palatable to the pet and that the client might not recognize poor appetite or anorexia prior to a scheduled insulin injection. This combination, however, can lead to an insulin overdose. Such a hypoglycemic episode early in treatment may frighten the client and reduce their resolve for treating their diabetic pet. Therefore, it is recommended that the transition to a new high-fiber food be delayed for a few weeks or that clear instructions be given to the client on the need to slowly transition to the new food.

Using a Low-Carbohydrate Food to Minimize the Absorption of Glucose

Another approach to the nutritional management of diabetes mellitus is the use of lower carbohydrate foods. Altering car-

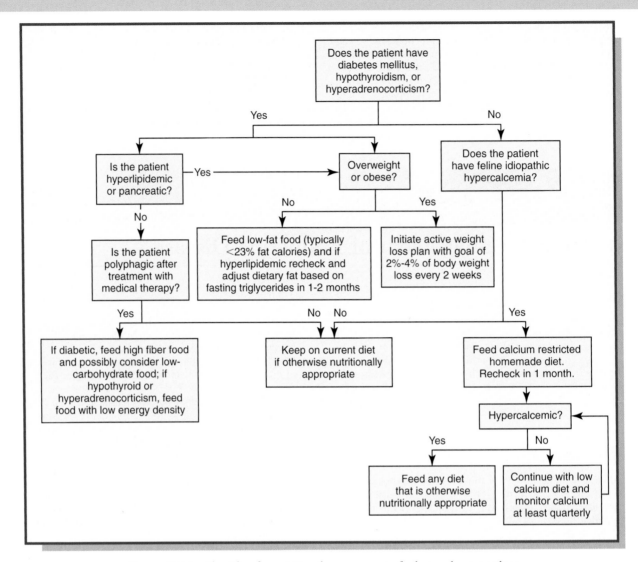

Figure 176-1 Algorithm for nutritional management of select endocrinopathies.

bohydrate amount and/or source has been a strategy in the management of people with diabetes mellitus for more than a century. For pets, a "lower carbohydrate" diet is a relatively new concept and has come to mean a food that has about 20% of its calories supplied by carbohydrate (Table 176-2). The premise behind this approach is that peaks in glucose absorption will be blunted as less carbohydrate is consumed. Exogenous insulin should be more effective if peaks and valleys in blood glucose concentration are avoided. This, in turn, should result in longer periods of circulating glucose concentrations closer to normal, which, in turn, may translate into better glycemic control.

Low-carbohydrate foods can decrease the dose of insulin needed. The clinical significance of this mainly is that the need for exogenous insulin may dissipate in cats with "type 2" disease. For cats with "type 1" disease and for almost all dogs, their dose of insulin might significantly decrease when switching from a higher carbohydrate food to a low-carbohydrate food.[8] The magnitude of this change may be muted if the higher carbohydrate food was also high in fiber. Therefore, it is recommended to ensure that food be made available at all times when transitioning a pet to a low-carbohydrate food, that a blood glucose curve be performed soon after the transition, and that the client is educated on how to recognize and respond to a hypoglycemic event.

Low-Carbohydrate Foods and Dietary Fat Intolerance

Unfortunately, by their very nature, low-carbohydrate foods are generally higher in fat and protein. Since some diabetics may concurrently be fat intolerant,[9,10] one must be cautious when using a low-carbohydrate and higher fat food for the management of diabetes. If concurrent or historical pancreatitis is suspected, it might be better to manage a diabetic dog or cat with a high-fiber food as these tend to also be lower in fat. In addition to pancreatitis, hypertriglyceridemia may also be a concurrent concern in some diabetics. In part this may be related to the endocrinopathy and may resolve with insulin therapy. Therefore, it might be preferable to start with a lower fat and higher fiber approach if the pet is hypertriglyceridemic. Then if the hypertriglyceridemia resolves based on fasting triglyceride measurements, one can slowly transition to a low-carbohydrate food with close blood monitoring. Alternatively, it might be best to avoid a low-carbohydrate food that is higher in fat in all dogs and cats with a history of hypertriglyceridemia.

Using Foods with a Low Glycemic Index to Minimize the Absorption of Glucose

The avoidance of foods with a high glycemic index (GI) is a concept popular for people with diabetes. GIs are based on

Table • 176-1

High-Fiber Veterinary Therapeutic Foods

	% CARB ME BASIS	g CRUDE FIBER/mcal
Canine Foods		
Hill's Prescription Diets		
r/d dry	41.6%	41.0
r/d dry with Chicken	40.6%	42.0
r/d canned	45.9%	71.0
w/d dry	55.0%	54.0
w/d dry with Chicken	55.0%	55.0
w/d canned	52.0%	35.0
Iams Veterinary Formulas		
Restricted-Calorie dry*	57.0%	6.54
Restricted-Calorie canned*	32.0%	8.14
Purina Veterinary Diets		
DCO Dual Fiber Control dry	46.3%	20.8
OM Overweight Management dry	47.6%	34.4
OM Overweight Management canned	25.2%	77.7
Royal Canin Veterinary Diets		
Calorie Control CC High Fiber dry	37.5%	55.98
Calorie Control CC High Fiber canned	45.1%	24.49
Diabetic HF 18 dry	51.4%	36.52
Feline Foods		
Hill's Prescription Diets		
r/d dry	36.0%	41.0
r/d dry with Chicken	34.5%	41.0
r/d canned	36.5%	55.0
r/d canned with Liver and Chicken	34.2%	50.0
w/d dry	37.0%	22.0
w/d dry with Chicken	36.0%	22.0
w/d canned	26.0%	27.0
w/d canned with Chicken	25.0%	31.0
Iams Veterinary Formulas		
Restricted-Calorie dry*	42.0%	6.76
Restricted-Calorie canned*	21.0%	3.81
Purina Veterinary Diets		
OM Overweight Management dry	23.3%	17.6
OM Overweight Management canned	22.4%	26.0
Royal Canin Veterinary Diets		
Calorie Control CC High Fiber dry	37.2%	43.0
Calorie Control CC High Fiber canned	27.6%	18.7
Diabetic HF 18 dry*	24.6%	13.4

ME, Metabolizable energy.
*These foods utilize low glycemic index ingredients (such as barley) as part of the primary strategy for the management of diabetes mellitus (relying less on total crude fiber content).

Table • 176-2

Low-Carbohydrate Veterinary Therapeutic Foods

	% PROTEIN ME BASIS	% FAT ME BASIS	% CARB ME BASIS
Feline Foods			
Hill's Prescription Diets			
m/d dry	43.0%	44.0%	13.0%
m/d canned	46.0%	41.0%	13.0%
Purina Veterinary Diets			
DM Dietetic Management dry	49.7%	37.4%	12.9%
DM Dietetic Management canned	46.3%	47.1%	6.6%
Royal Canin Veterinary Diets			
Calorie Control CC High Protein canned	45.4%	46.5%	8.1%
Canine Foods			
Royal Canin Veterinary Diets			
Calorie Control CC High Protein canned	42.6%	53.1%	4.2%

ME, Metabolizable energy.

effect on the types of starch and sugars present in the food, one can generally predict a food's GI based on the food's relative fiber and carbohydrate content. Therefore, in pet foods it is suggested that a greater focus be put on total dietary fiber and carbohydrate contents rather than on the GI of the individual ingredients.

Weight Management in the Diabetic Patient

Many diabetic dogs and cats are overweight or obese. In cats, weight loss may aid in reverting a cat from insulin dependence to no longer requiring insulin.[8] As obesity can also shorten lifespan,[12] it is recommended that controlled weight loss be attempted in all diabetic pets. Unfortunately, the better managed a diabetic patient, the more challenging weight loss becomes. This is because poor diabetic control contributes to weight loss while insulin, being anabolic, contributes to weight gain. Therefore, it is important to distinguish weight loss due to poor glycemic control from weight loss due to an effective weight loss plan. Fortunately, many foods appropriate for active weight loss are higher in fiber and/or lower in carbohydrate, and thus consistent with the nutritional management of a diabetic. If weight loss is initiated, close monitoring of glycemic control with blood glucose curves and of weight loss rate are recommended. In general dogs and cats should not lose more than 2% to 4% of body weight between biweekly weigh-ins.

Exercise is an important part of any weight loss plan. Given the high likelihood that diabetic dogs will develop cataracts and not undergo corrective surgery, newly diagnosed, overweight, diabetic dogs should be immediately put on an exercise regimen of daily leash walking. Then as their vision deteriorates, the pet will already be adapted to trusting the client and used to going on walks even when blind, thereby enabling exercise to be part of concurrent or future weight loss plans.

healthy test subjects' blood glucose response after eating test doses of foods rich in carbohydrates. A higher GI value indicates that the food causes a greater increase in blood glucose. Although no standardized in vivo test for pets has been established, this concept has garnered a small level of interest in veterinary medicine.[11] However, if one reviews the assembled lists on GI, it becomes apparent that GI in large part seems to correlate with both fiber and carbohydrate content. For example, a legume that is rich in fiber and low in carbohydrate has a lower GI than polished rice. Although there is some

HYPERADRENOCORTICISM AND HYPOTHYROIDISM

The nutritional management of hyperadrenocorticism and hypothyroidism centers around the management of polyphagia, a slow metabolism, and/or hyperlipidemia. Polyphagic patients are inherently prone to obesity. To combat weight gain, "lite" over-the-counter foods can be helpful. These foods have legally defined limits on how many calories they can contain. Such foods also have a larger volume, which can potentially assist with satiety. It should be noted that some products carry comparative titles, such as "reduced" or "lower" calories. These products do not have specific limits and, as such, care should be used during selection to ensure that they are actually as low in caloric content as desired. Increasing meal frequency and using low-calorie treats may also be helpful while managing polyphagic patients. For dogs with hyperadrenocorticism, successful treatment should eliminate all clinical signs, including polyphagia. Further, successfully treated dogs regain muscle strength and are more capable of exercise. Therefore, dietary modifications may be unnecessary following treatment unless obesity already exists. For hypothyroid dogs, thyroid hormone supplementation should increase muscle strength, ability to exercise, and metabolic rate to normal levels. These effects should greatly assist with weight management.

For pets with secondary hyperlipidemia, treatment of the causative endocrinopathy may resolve the dyslipidemia. For those pets whose medical treatment alone does not or cannot resolve their obesity, hunger, or hyperlipidemia, dietary therapy is an important facet of the overall management. For overweight or obese pets, a weight loss plan should be created around a food designed for active weight loss. If the dog or cat is concurrently hyperlipidemic, then use of a low-fat weight loss food is critical (Table 176-3). If the patient is merely hyperlipidemic, a low-fat food that is not designed for active weight loss can also be used (Table 176-4).

As with any dietary intervention, monitoring is a key to successful long-term management. For overweight or obese patients this typically means biweekly weigh-ins with adjustment in calories fed depending on response. Generally a weight loss rate between 1% to 4% of body weight every 2 weeks is the goal. For hyperlipidemic patients, a fasting triglyceride measurement 1 to 2 months after initiation of a low-fat diet is helpful in determining if further fat restriction is needed. Clinical experience suggests that all hyperlipidemic patients can be treated with dietary therapy alone (assuming that the responsible endocrinopathy is well managed). However, it should be noted that fat content of the diet may need to supply less than 15% of the calories. For such a requirement, a homemade diet must be prepared since no severely fat-restricted (<15% fat calories) commercial food options exist.

FELINE IDIOPATHIC HYPERCALCEMIA

No underlying endocrinopathy has been identified as a cause for feline idiopathic hypercalcemia. Experience with calcium-restricted dietary therapy has been occasionally successful. Since no over-the-counter or therapeutic commercial food is calcium restricted, such dietary approaches to therapy require the use of homemade diets. It is unclear if some other aspect of a home-cooked diet may be responsible for the limited success that has been documented or whether the response has been coincidental. It does appear that hypercalcemia can be transient in some cats (unpublished data). If a dietary trial is desired, it is recommended to restrict calcium to 0.6 g per megacalorie (~40% of commonly recommended adult main-

Table • 176-3

Lower-Fat Veterinary Therapeutic Foods Appropriate for Weight Loss

	% PROTEIN ME BASIS	% FAT ME BASIS	% CARB ME BASIS
Canine Foods			
Hill's Prescription Diets			
r/d dry	36.9%	21.5%	41.6%
r/d dry with Chicken	37.0%	22.4%	40.6%
Iams Veterinary Formulas			
Restricted-Calorie dry	24.0%	19.0%	57.0%
Purina Veterinary Diets			
OM Overweight Management dry	33.5%	18.9%	47.6%
OM Overweight Management canned	51.2%	23.6%	25.2%
Feline Foods			
Hill's Prescription Diets			
r/d dry	39.6%	24.4%	36.0%
r/d canned with Liver and Chicken	41.3%	24.5%	34.2%
Purina Veterinary Diets			
OM Overweight Management dry	56.2%	20.5%	23.3%
Royal Canin Veterinary Diets			
Calorie Control CC High Protein dry	44.4%	23.4%	32.1%

ME, Metabolizable energy.

Table • 176-4

Low-Fat Veterinary Therapeutic Foods (Not for Weight Loss)

	% PROTEIN ME BASIS	% FAT ME BASIS	% CARB ME BASIS
Canine Foods			
Hill's Prescription Diets			
w/d dry	21.0%	24.0%	55.0%
w/d dry with Chicken	21.0%	24.0%	55.0%
Iams Veterinary Formulas			
Optimum Weight Control dry	29.0%	21.0%	50.0%
Royal Canin Veterinary Diets			
Digestive Low Fat LF dry	24.8%	15.2%	60.0%
Digestive Low Fat LF canned	31.6%	15.3%	53.1%
Feline Foods			
Hill's Prescription Diets			
w/d dry	39.0%	24.0%	37.0%
w/d dry with Chicken	40.0%	24.0%	36.0%

ME, Metabolizable energy.

tenance levels) or less. At the same time, fish oil or organ meats should be avoided as these ingredients can be quite high in vitamin D. If dietary restriction is ineffective, the cat may be nonresponsive to calcium restriction and dietary therapy may be unnecessary.

REFERENCES

The reference list can be found on the companion Expert Consult Web site at *www.expertconsult.com*.

CHAPTER 177

Nutritional Modulation of Heart Disease

Lisa M. Freeman
John E. Rush

The goal of nutrition is no longer just to prevent deficiencies. It is now known that modification of diet can be an important part of medical therapy for heart disease. In the 1960s, the main nutritional recommendations for dogs with congestive heart failure (CHF) were to feed a low-sodium diet (for all stages of heart disease), to feed a restricted protein diet, and to provide supplemental B vitamins.[1] Few changes to these recommendations were made until the 1980s, when the question of how early to institute sodium restriction was raised and one of the first mentions of cardiac cachexia appeared in veterinary medicine.[2] It was also in the late 1980s that the discovery of the relationship between taurine deficiency and feline dilated cardiomyopathy (DCM) was published.[3] Now, research is beginning to show that nutrition may be able to modulate heart disease, either by slowing the progression, minimizing the number of medications required, improving quality of life or, in rare cases, actually curing the disease. There is potential for the use of diet as an important adjunct to medical therapy for animals with heart disease.

The main goals of diet therapy for heart disease are to maintain optimal body weight, to avoid nutritional deficiencies and excesses, and to take advantage of the potential benefits of pharmacologic doses of certain nutrients.

OPTIMAL WEIGHT MAINTENANCE

A key goal for the optimal management of heart disease is to maintain optimal bodyweight, because both weight loss and obesity can adversely affect health.

Cachexia

Cardiac cachexia is the muscle wasting commonly seen in patients with CHF. In one study of dogs with DCM, more than 50% of patients had some degree of cachexia.[4] The weight loss that occurs in animals with CHF is unlike that seen in a healthy dog or cat that loses weight. In a healthy animal receiving insufficient calories to meet requirements, metabolic adaptations allow fat to be used as the primary fuel source, thus preserving lean body mass. Conversely, the primary fuel source in animals with an acute or chronic disease, including heart disease, is amino acids from muscle; therefore, these animals quickly catabolize muscle and lean body mass. Thus the distinguishing feature of cachexia is a loss of lean body mass, which has direct and deleterious effects on strength, immune function, and survival.[5] Cachexia is often mistakenly viewed as an end-stage syndrome manifested by an emaciated dog or cat. In fact, cachexia is a progressive

process of muscle loss that can be very subtle initially and can even occur in an obese animal. Recognizing the process of cachexia at an early stage provides better opportunities to manage it effectively.

The loss of lean body mass in cardiac cachexia is a multi-factorial process caused by anorexia, increased energy requirements, and metabolic alterations.[5] The anorexia may be secondary to fatigue or dyspnea or may be due to medication toxicity or feeding of an unpalatable diet.[5] Anorexia is present in 34% to 75% of dogs and cats with clinically significant heart disease.[4,6-8] However, increased production of inflammatory cytokines, such as tumor necrosis factor (TNF) and interleukin-1 (IL-1), is the primary mediator of cachexia.[5] These inflammatory cytokines directly cause anorexia, increase energy requirements, and increase the catabolism of lean body mass. TNF and IL-1 also cause cardiac myocyte hypertrophy and fibrosis and have negative inotropic effects.

Cardiac cachexia is typically recognized only after CHF has developed. It is more common in dogs than in cats and is most often seen in DCM or right-sided heart failure. Loss of lean body mass is most readily evident in the epaxial, gluteal, scapular, or temporal muscles. A number of cachexia scores have been proposed but the authors use a 0 to 4 scheme (where 0 = no muscle wasting, 1 = mild, 2 = moderate, 3 = marked, and 4 = severe).[4] Nutritional considerations for cardiac cachexia should include management of anorexia, if present. Nutritional modulation of cytokine production also may be helpful. One method of decreasing the production and effects of cytokines is omega-3 (n-3) polyunsaturated fatty acid (PUFA) supplementation (see below). Supplementation of fish oil, which is high in n-3 fatty acids, can decrease cytokine production in dogs with CHF and improve cachexia.[4] In some but not all dogs with CHF-induced anorexia, fish oil supplementation can improve food intake.[4] In addition, n-3 fatty acid intake has been associated with longer survival in dogs with heart failure.[8]

Obesity

Overweight (i.e., over ideal body weight) and obesity (i.e., more than 20% over ideal body weight) are common in the pet population, and can have detrimental effects on health. Therefore, maintaining an optimal bodyweight and body condition score should be a goal for dogs and cats with asymptomatic cardiac disease. The effects of obesity are less clear in heart failure. Obesity is common even in animals with heart failure, with 41% of dogs in one study being overweight or obese at the time of diagnosis of heart failure.[8] Obesity is a known risk factor for heart disease in people. However, several recent studies have shown that in people with heart failure, obesity actually is associated with a longer survival time; this is called the "obesity paradox."[9-13] Results of one study of dogs with heart failure showed that dogs that gained or maintained weight had a longer survival time than those that lost weight.[8] This supports the concept that weight loss is very detrimental in heart failure and careful attention to body weight, muscle loss, and appetite are of critical importance in animals with cardiac disease. While these findings may call into question the merits of weight loss once CHF is present, if an animal is obese (>7/9 body condition score) and obesity is negatively impacting quality of life, a careful weight loss program is indicated. Owners often find that severely obese dogs and cats with cardiopulmonary disease that successfully lose weight appear less dyspneic and more active. All animals with heart failure, even those that are overweight or obese, should be carefully monitored for unintentional weight loss. In addition, it is important to be aware that cachexia (i.e., muscle loss) can occur even in obese animals, so monitoring of muscle mass is important.

MODULATION OF SPECIFIC NUTRIENTS

Nutritional deficiencies once were a common cause of cardiac disease in people and probably animals. In cats, taurine deficiency was a common cause of heart disease until as recently as the late 1980s. Identifiable nutritional deficiencies are now uncommon in dogs and cats (unless owners are feeding homemade, vegetarian, or otherwise nutritionally unbalanced diets) but still could play a role in the etiology of some heart diseases. Nutritional deficiencies also may develop secondary to the disease or its treatment. A new area of nutritional research is that of nutritional pharmacology, the concept that supplementation of certain nutrients may provide benefits above and beyond their known nutritional effects. Therefore modulation of various nutrients by reducing or increasing their intake (either by a small amount or to pharmacologic levels) may be recommended for animals with heart disease.

Protein and Taurine

Protein   In the 1960s, authors recommended a restricted protein intake for dogs with CHF to prevent "metabolic stress" on the kidneys and liver.[1] There is no evidence that protein restriction is necessary for dogs and cats with CHF and, in fact, it probably is deleterious, because these patients are predisposed to loss of lean body mass. Many of the diets designed for dogs with cardiac disease are low in protein (3.3 to 4.2 g/100 kcal), and protein-restricted diets designed for renal disease are recommended by some authors for animals with heart disease. Unless severe renal dysfunction is present (i.e., serum creatinine >2.5 to 3.0 g/dL), high-quality protein should be fed to meet canine (5.1 g/100 kcal) and feline (6.5 g/100 kcal) minimum levels according to Association of American Feed Control Officials (AAFCO).[14]

Taurine   Taurine is an amino acid found in high levels in the myocardium. Despite knowledge of the role of taurine deficiency in feline DCM, a small number of cats still develop DCM.[3] Most current cases of feline DCM do not involve taurine deficiency but it should be suspected in all cases of this disorder. A dietary history should be elicited from owners to determine whether the cat has been fed a poor-quality, homemade, vegetarian, or otherwise unbalanced diets. Plasma and whole blood taurine should be measured, and treatment with taurine (125 to 250 mg PO q12h) should begin concurrently with medical therapy. If the taurine concentration is

found to be normal, taurine supplementation can be discontinued.

Unlike cats, dogs are thought to be able to synthesize adequate amounts of taurine, which is not considered a requirement in canine diets. Most dogs with DCM do not have taurine deficiency, but low taurine concentrations have been found in some dogs with the disorder.[15-18] The most common breeds in which DCM has been reported to be associated with taurine deficiency are the American Cocker Spaniel, Golden Retriever, Labrador Retriever, Portuguese Water Dog, Saint Bernard, English Setter, and Newfoundlands.[15-21]

Diet appears to play some role in the development of taurine deficiency in dogs as very low protein, lamb and rice, and some high-fiber diets have been associated with taurine deficiency, but the exact role of diet remains unknown.[15,17-26] Taurine deficiency also may be the result of increased renal or fecal loss of taurine, higher requirements, or other metabolic defects present in certain breeds.

While some dogs with DCM have low circulating taurine concentrations, not all of these respond to taurine supplementation. One small prospective study showed that Cocker Spaniels supplemented with taurine and carnitine had clinical and echocardiographic improvements.[27] It is not known whether the response would be similar with either taurine or carnitine alone. A retrospective study of 12 dogs with taurine deficiency and DCM documented improved cardiac contractility after taurine supplementation.[18] In a study of Portuguese Water Dog puppies, plasma taurine was low in all puppies tested, and DCM was diagnosed in eight of nine puppies.[21] Taurine supplementation was instituted in six of the puppies, which significantly increased circulating taurine concentrations and cardiac function.[21] Finally, in a study of Beagles fed a low-taurine, very low protein diet for 48 months, one dog developed DCM but showed significant improvement in cardiac contractility after supplementation of taurine.[22]

Dogs with DCM and taurine deficiency that do respond to taurine supplementation generally do not have as dramatic a response as do taurine-deficient cats with DCM. Nonetheless, measurement of plasma and whole blood taurine concentrations is warranted in certain breeds of dogs with DCM such as the Cocker Spaniel, Newfoundland, or Golden Retriever, or in breeds that are not typically associated with the development of DCM (e.g., Border Collie, Dachshund). Taurine concentrations also should be measured in dogs with DCM eating lamb meal and rice-based diets, very low protein, vegetarian, or high-fiber diets. Taurine analysis is not recommended in typical breeds that develop DCM (e.g., Doberman Pinschers, Boxers). Supplementation with taurine (250 to 1000 mg PO q8-12h) is recommended in dogs with documented taurine deficiency, although the exact dose required for repletion is not known. Some of the potential benefits of taurine in dogs with DCM may be due to its positive inotropic effects or role in calcium regulation in the myocardium.

The AAFCO minimum for taurine for adult cats is 25 mg/100 kcal for dry food and 50 mg/100 kcal for canned foods.[14] Because taurine is a nonessential nutrient in dogs (i.e., it is not thought to be required in the diet), no minimum level has been established for commercial dog foods. The dietary taurine content of commercial dog foods varies widely (less than 5 to over 50 mg taurine/100 kcal). To achieve a dose of 500 mg q12h for a 40 kg dog (although this has not been determined to be the *optimal* dose of taurine for a dog with DCM), a diet would have to contain approximately 50 mg/100 kcal of taurine.

Fat

Fat provides calories and increases the palatability of pet foods but it also can significantly affect immunologic, inflammatory, and hemodynamic parameters. The n-3 fatty acids, eicosapentaenoic acid (EPA) and docosahexaenoic acid (DHA), are long chain fatty acids in which the first double bond is at the position of the third carbon from the methyl end (vs. the n-6 PUFA, linoleic, γ-linolenic, and arachidonic, in which the first double bond is at the sixth carbon). This minor chemical difference conveys different structural and functional characteristics to the fatty acid. Plasma membranes normally contain very low concentrations of n-3 fatty acids, but levels can be increased by a food or supplement enriched in n-3 fatty acids. Dogs with CHF have been shown to have plasma fatty acid abnormalities, including decreased concentrations of EPA and DHA compared to normal dogs.[4] In one study of dogs with DCM and CHF, fish oil supplementation normalized these plasma fatty acid abnormalities.[4]

Another potential benefit of n-3 fatty acid supplementation is that breakdown products of the n-3 fatty acids (series 3 and 5 eicosanoids) are, in general, less potent inflammatory mediators than eicosanoids derived from n-6 fatty acids (series 2 and 4 eicosanoids). This decreases the production of cytokines and other inflammatory mediators, which may reduce cachexia.[4] Finally, n-3 fatty acids have antiarrhythmic effects in a variety of species including Boxers with ventricular arrhythmias.[28] The authors currently recommend a dose of 40 mg/kg EPA and 25 mg/kg DHA for dogs and cats with anorexia or cachexia. This dose also can be used as an adjunct to medical therapy for arrhythmias. With the exception of a few specially designed therapeutic diets, commercial diets do not achieve this level of n-3 fatty acids, so supplementation is usually necessary. The amount of EPA and DHA in individual fish oil supplements varies widely, so it is important to know the exact amount in brand of supplement recommended. The most common formulation of fish oil, however, is 1-g capsules that contain approximately 180 mg EPA and 120 mg DHA and can be purchased over the counter at most human pharmacies or health food stores. At this concentration, fish oil can be administered at a dose of one capsule per 10 pounds of bodyweight to achieve the authors' recommended EPA and DHA dosage. Fish oil supplements should contain vitamin E as an antioxidant, but other nutrients should not be included to avoid toxicities. Cod liver oil and flax seed oil should not be used as sources of n-3 fatty acids.

Minerals

Sodium Studies in the 1960s showed that very–low-sodium diets could help to control fluid accumulation in dogs with CHF.[1] Authors in the 1960s and 1970s recommended changing animals to a severely sodium restricted diet when a heart murmur was first detected, even before clinical signs were present. More recently, questions have been raised about severe sodium restriction in asymptomatic cardiac disease due to activation of the renin-angiotensin-aldosterone system.[29,30] One study of dogs with asymptomatic chronic valvular disease (CVD) showed that a low-sodium diet resulted in increased aldosterone concentrations and heart rate, with no improvement in cardiac size or function.[30] Because of lack of documented benefits and potential adverse effects of severe sodium restriction in asymptomatic disease, the authors recommend only mild sodium restriction (<100 mg/100 kcal) in asymptomatic heart disease (International Small Animal Cardiac Health Council [ISACHC] Stages 1a and 1b). However, this is an opportune time to begin educating the owner about the animal's overall dietary patterns—the pet food, treats, table food, and how medications are administered—as it is generally much easier to institute dietary modifications at this stage, before the animal develops clinical signs of CHF. Most owners are unaware of the sodium content of pet foods and human

Table • 177-1

*Examples of Low-Sodium Treats**

	kcal/ TREAT	SODIUM PRODUCT (mg/TREAT)
Dog Treats		
Purina Veterinary Diets Lite Snackers	15	11
Iams Original Formula Biscuits (small)	22	10
Hill's Prescription Diet Canine Treats	13	5
Stewart Fiber Formula Dog Biscuits (medium)	25	5
Baby carrots	4	4
Apple (raw, 1 slice) or orange (1 section)	10	0
Cat Treats		
Purina Whisker Lickin's Brand Crunchy Cat Treats Tartar Control	2	2
Stewart Fiber Formula Cat Treats	1	1

Treats to Avoid

Baby food; pickled foods; bread; pizza; condiments (e.g., ketchup, soy sauce); lunch meats and cold cuts (e.g., ham, corned beef, salami, sausages, bacon, hot dogs); most cheeses, including "squirtable" cheeses (unless specifically labeled as low sodium); processed foods (e.g., potato mixes, rice mixes, macaroni and cheese); canned vegetables (unless labeled as no salt added); snack foods (e.g., potato chips, packaged popcorn, crackers); soups (unless homemade without salt); and most other pet treats.

*Even low-sodium treats, if fed in large quantities, can provide a large dose of sodium (this especially can be a problem in cats or small dogs).

foods and need very specific instructions regarding appropriate foods and acceptable low-salt treats (Table 177-1).

When CHF first arises, additional sodium restriction is recommended (<80 mg sodium/100 kcal). This can be achieved with a therapeutic diet designed for animals with early heart disease or with certain other therapeutic diets (which may be designed for other disease) or even some over-the-counter diets. The content of sodium and other nutrients, such as protein, can be found by consulting manufacturers' product guides or by calling the companies. Be cautious with canine senior diets, which often are reduced in protein (which is not recommended for animals with heart failure). Similarly, diets designed for animals with renal disease are not recommended because of the protein restriction (unless severe renal dysfunction is present). As CHF becomes more severe, more sodium restriction (i.e., <50 mg/100 kcal) may allow lower dosages of diuretics to be used to control clinical signs. To achieve this degree of sodium restriction, commercial therapeutic diets should be selected (e.g., Royal Canin Veterinary Diet Canine Early Cardiac EC 22, Purina Veterinary Diets JM Joint Mobility, or Hill's Prescription Diet j/d; note that all three contain relatively high levels of n-3 fatty acids). Avoid diets that are restricted in protein unless indicated for significant renal dysfunction. The one commercially available cardiac diet for cats (Purina Veterinary Diets CV Cardiovascular Feline Formula) meets feline nutritional requirements but also provides a palatable, high-protein option for canned food in dogs with CHF requiring severe sodium restriction.

Potassium   Hypokalemia causes muscle weakness, predisposes patients to digitalis toxicity, and potentiates arrhythmogenesis. In addition, Class I antiarrhythmic drugs (e.g., mexiletine, quinidine) are relatively ineffective in the face of hypokalemia. Hypokalemia can be precipitated by the use of loop diuretics (e.g., furosemide), thiazide diuretics (e.g., hydrochlorothiazide), or inadequate dietary intake (often associated with anorexia). In the past, when the mainstays of therapy were diuretics and digoxin, hypokalemia was recognized to be a significant problem in people and dogs with CHF.

Now, angiotensin-converting enzyme (ACE) inhibitor therapy has gained widespread use in the management of dogs with CHF, and this class of drug results in renal potassium sparing. Angiotensin-converting enzyme inhibitors cause increased serum potassium and some animals develop hyperkalemia. Spironolactone, now used in some dogs with cardiac disease, is an aldosterone antagonist and a potassium-sparing diuretic. Whereas animals receiving ACE inhibitors or spironolactone can develop hyperkalemia, it is not a very common occurrence unless they are eating a diet that contains high levels of potassium.

Commercial diets vary widely in potassium concentrations. Commercial reduced-sodium diets range from 143 to 270 mg potassium/100 kcal, with an AAFCO minimum of 170 mg/100 kcal for dogs and 150 mg/100 kcal for cats. If hyperkalemia is present in an animal with cardiac disease, a diet with a lower potassium content should be selected. Conversely, if an animal is hypokalemic, a diet higher in potassium or oral potassium supplementation may be indicated.

Magnesium   Magnesium plays an important role in normal cardiac function. Alterations in magnesium homeostasis can occur in people and dogs and can have deleterious effects in a variety of cardiovascular conditions including hypertension, coronary artery disease, CHF, and cardiac arrhythmias. Some cardiac drugs, including digoxin and loop diuretics, are associated with magnesium depletion. Therefore, animals with heart failure receiving these medications have the potential to develop hypomagnesemia. Hypomagnesemia can increase the risk of arrhythmias, decrease cardiac contractility, cause muscle weakness, contribute to renal potassium loss, and can potentiate the adverse effects of certain cardiac medications.

Hypomagnesemia has not been a consistent finding in studies of animals with heart disease, but this may be because serum magnesium concentrations are a poor indicator of total body stores.[31,32] Therefore, normal serum magnesium does not necessarily mean there are adequate total body stores. We recommend routine measurements of serum magnesium, especially in animals with arrhythmias or those on large doses of diuretics.

Like potassium, magnesium concentrations vary widely in commercial pet foods. Commercial reduced-sodium diets for dogs can contain between 10 and 40 mg magnesium/100 kcal (AAFCO minimum of 11 mg/100 kcal for dogs and 10 mg/100 kcal for cats). A diet high in magnesium would be indicated for an animal with a low serum magnesium concentration. In some animals with low serum magnesium concentrations, diet adjustment alone will not correct the problem and oral supplementation will be required.

Vitamins

B Vitamins   Thiamine deficiency is known to be a cause of cardiomyopathy in people, but there has been little investigation into the role of B vitamins as a cause of heart disease in dogs and cats. Anorexia and urinary loss of water-soluble vitamins can contribute to low B vitamin concentrations in patients with heart failure. In one recent study of human CHF patients, for example, 33% were thiamine deficient.[33] As with other nutrients such as potassium, B vitamin deficiencies may have been much more common when furosemide was the primary means of therapy for patients with CHF. Research suggests that vitamins B_6, B_{12}, and folate may be significantly lower in cats with cardiomyopathy than in healthy controls, an effect that appeared to be unrelated to diet or furosemide use.[34,35] Animals with cardiac disease (at least those receiving diuretics) may have higher B vitamin requirements. Most commercial cardiac diets contain increased levels of water-soluble vitamins to offset urinary losses.

Other Nutrients

Carnitine   L-carnitine is concentrated in skeletal and cardiac muscle and is critical for fatty acid metabolism and energy production. Carnitine deficiency is associated with primary myocardial disease in a number of species, including a family of Boxer dogs.[36] Anecdotal reports exist regarding the efficacy of carnitine in canine DCM, but no blinded prospective studies have been done so a causative role has not been established. Even if carnitine deficiency is not the inciting cause of DCM, L-carnitine supplementation could be beneficial by improving myocardial energy production. In human DCM patients, most studies of L-carnitine have not been well controlled. However, one randomized, double-blind, placebo-controlled study showed improved 3-year survival in human DCM patients receiving 2 g/day L-carnitine.[37] In dogs, it is not yet clear whether the carnitine deficiency seen in some dogs with DCM is the cause of the disease or merely secondary to the development of CHF. A study of rapid pacing–induced heart failure in dogs showed that myocardial concentrations decreased in normal dogs after the onset of CHF.[38] There are few side effects of L-carnitine supplementation but high cost is a deterrent for some owners. We currently offer the option of L-carnitine supplementation (50 to100 mg/kg PO q8h) to owners of dogs with DCM.

Antioxidants   Much attention has been given to antioxidants for their potential role in the prevention and treatment of human cardiac diseases. Reactive oxygen species are a by-product of oxygen metabolism for which the body normally compensates through the production of endogenous antioxidants. An imbalance between oxidant production and antioxidant protection, however, could increase the risk for heart disease. Antioxidants are produced endogenously but also can be supplied exogenously. The major antioxidants include enzymatic antioxidants (e.g., superoxide dismutase, catalase, glutathione peroxidase) and oxidant quenchers (e.g., vitamin C, vitamin E, glutathione, and beta-carotene). Most of the research in human cardiology has been in coronary artery disease. but in dogs with CHF due to either DCM or CVD, there is an imbalance between increased oxidant production and reduced antioxidant protection, particularly as the disease becomes more severe.[39,40] Supplemental antioxidants are now included in many commercial veterinary diets, including at least one cardiac diet, and can increase circulating antioxidant concentrations and reduce oxidation.[30] However, potential clinical benefits of antioxidant supplementation require additional study.

Coenzyme Q10   Coenzyme Q10, like carnitine, is a cofactor in a number of energy-producing reactions but is also an antioxidant. Although coenzyme Q10 supplementation has anecdotally been reported to be beneficial, controlled prospective studies are necessary to accurately judge the efficacy of this product. One study of experimentally induced CHF in dogs showed that serum coenzyme Q10 levels were not reduced and that coenzyme Q10 supplementation increased serum, but not myocardial, concentrations.[41] Most human studies of coenzyme Q10 supplementation have not been well controlled and results are conflicting. The current recommended dose in dogs is 30 mg PO BID, although up to 90 mg PO BID has been recommended for large dogs. Possible reasons for the purported benefits of supplementation include correction of a deficiency, improved myocardial metabolic efficiency, or increased antioxidant protection.

PRACTICAL ASPECTS OF FEEDING THE PATIENT WITH HEART DISEASE

There is not a single "best" diet for managing heart disease. It is important to match the nutritional needs of an individual patient to the diet or diets that best suit those needs. Patients with heart disease vary in terms of their clinical signs, laboratory parameters, and food preferences, and these all affect diet selection. For example, animals with asymptomatic heart disease require less severe sodium restriction than animals with CHF. Dogs with cardiac cachexia require a calorically dense diet while an overweight dog should be fed a calorically restricted diet. Concurrent diseases also influence diet choice and, in one study, were present in approximately 61% of dogs and 56% of cats with heart disease, respectively.[7,42] For example, a cat with hypertrophic cardiomyopathy and a history of struvite urolithiasis would need a diet that is sodium restricted but also one that has nutritional modification to reduce the risk of struvite urolith formation. Finally, laboratory results, such as the presence of hypokalemia or hyperkalemia, also can alter diet selection.

Based on these and other patient parameters, diets can be matched to the individual patient. There currently are a number of commercial veterinary diets available that are specifically designed for animals with cardiac disease. Specific characteristics of these foods vary, but they are moderately to severely sodium restricted, generally contain increased levels of B vitamins, and vary in their protein content. Some cardiac diets also may include increased levels of taurine, carnitine, antioxidants, or n-3 fatty acids. Above all, the diet must be palatable enough that the animal will willingly eat it. The authors typically determine several diets that would be appropriate for an individual animal. These diets are offered as choices for the owner and the pet. Having dietary choices is particularly beneficial for more severely affected patients, in which a cyclical or selective loss of appetite is common. All diet recommendations should also include discussion of treats, table food, and foods used for medication administration.

As mentioned earlier, anorexia is a common problem in animals with heart failure and can contribute to the syndrome of cachexia. Another important problem with anorexia is that it may affect survival by influencing an owner's decision to euthanize the pet. In one study of owners of dogs euthanized for CHF, anorexia was one of the most common contributing factors to the euthanasia decision.[6] Anorexia becomes more common as the cardiac disease becomes more advanced. Recommendations for managing anorexia are listed in Box 177-1.

Finally, a note of caution: In animals with an acute episode of CHF, avoid changing the diet until the patient is stabilized. Once the animal is home and stabilized on medications, a gradual change to a new diet can be made. Forced dietary

---

Box • 177-1

Keys to Managing Anorexia in Patients with Cardiac Disease

- Assess the patient for optimal medical control of heart failure.
- Assess the patient for side effects of medications (e.g., digoxin toxicity or azotemia).
- Feed more frequent but smaller meals.
- Warm the food to body temperature (for cats). Try different temperatures of food for dogs.
- Gradually introduce a more palatable diet (e.g., switch from a dry food to a canned food, change to a different brand, or have a nutritionist formulate a balanced homemade diet).
- Use flavor enhancers, such as cooked meat or fish or low-sodium tuna juice for cats, and cooked meat or sweeteners (e.g., yogurt, maple syrup, or honey) for dogs.
- Administer fish oil supplements if the diet does not contain high concentrations of omega-3 fatty acids.

Box • 177-2

Methods for Administering Medication to Dogs and Cats

1. Teach the owner to pill the animal without using foods.
2. Use a Pet Piller or Pet Pill Gun (Jorgensen Laboratories, Loveland, Colo.).
3. Use a compounded, flavored liquid medication instead of a pill (remember that compounding may alter the pharmacokinetics of a drug).
   Caution: Always determine the sodium content of a compounded product.
4. Insert medications into appropriate foods, such as the following:
   - Fruit (e.g., banana, orange, melon)
   - Low-sodium cheese
   - Low-sodium canned pet food
   - Peanut butter (labeled as "no salt added")
   - Home-cooked meat (without salt); not lunch meats

---

changes when the animal is sick or starting new medications may induce food aversions.

In many cases, the desired nutrient modifications can be achieved through diet alone. However, supplementation of certain nutrients may be desirable if they are either not in a particular diet or not at high enough levels to achieve the desired effect. It is important to be aware that dietary supplements currently do not require proof of safety, efficacy, or quality control to be marketed. Therefore, veterinarians should consider recommending specific brands of dietary supplements that bear the logo of the United States Pharmacopeia Dietary Supplement Verification Program (DSVP), which tests human dietary supplements for ingredients, concentrations, dissolvability, and contaminants. Another good resource is Consumerlab.com, which performs independent testing of dietary supplements (primarily human supplements but also some pet products).

In addition to finding a diet that has the desired nutritional properties and palatability, it also is important to devise an overall dietary plan that meets the owner's expectations. This includes finding a diet that the owner perceives the pet to enjoy, providing acceptable treats, and devising a satisfactory method for administering medications. In one study, over 90% of dogs with heart disease received treats and these treats are often high in sodium.[42] Fewer cats (33%) receive regular treats but this additional source of nutrients also should be addressed with cat owners.[7] In addition, the majority of people administering medications to their dogs use foods as a way to administer the medication (Box 177-2).[42]

Only 34% of cat owners use foods to administer medications but because of the difficulty of this activity in cats, special care should be taken to ensure that the cat owner can be successful and adherent in medication administration.[7] Including information regarding all sources of food from pet food, treats, table food, and medication administration in the overall diet plan is important to achieve success with nutritional modification.

REFERENCES

The reference list can be found on the companion Expert Consult Web site at *www.expertconsult.com.*

CHAPTER 178

Nutritional Management of the Lower Urinary Tract Conditions

Denise A. Elliott

Lower urinary tract disease (LUTD) refers to a heterogeneous group of disorders characterized by clinical signs that can include hematuria, dysuria, stranguria, pollakiuria, inappropriate urination (periuria or signs of irritative voiding outside of the litter-box), and partial or complete urethral obstruction. LUTD is not a single disease; rather it is simply a term indicating mucosal irritation of the urinary tract that may be caused by the presence of infectious agents, congenital abnormalities, tumors, urethral plugs, uroliths, or crystals. In many cases of feline LUTD, no specific cause of the disorder can be found, and these cats are considered to have "idiopathic" disease. Investigation of LUTD involves a rational approach to ascertain the precise etiology so that an appropriate treatment plan can be formulated. Nutrition has a fundamental role in the management of urolithiasis and idiopathic cystitis.

UROLITHIASIS

Uroliths are polycrystalline concretions composed primarily of minerals and smaller quantities of matrix. Urinary crystals form when urine is supersaturated with respect to a specific mineral or mineral compound. Precipitation is a result of increasing supersaturation. The initial phase, or nucleation, of urolith formation involves the formation of a crystal nidus. This phase is dependent on supersaturation of urine with calculogenic crystalloids and is influenced by the extent of renal excretion of the crystalloid, the urine pH, urine temperature, the presence or absence of various inhibitory factors, and the presence of promoters of crystallization (e.g., dead cells, cellular debris, protein, bacteria, or other crystals). Crystal growth depends on the ability of the nidus to remain within the urinary tract, the duration of supersaturation of the urine, and the physical ultrastructure of the crystal. The actual rate of growth of the urolith depends on numerous factors including mineral composition and risk factors such as infection.

Urine supersaturation is the driving force for the formation of crystals within the urinary tract. More than 40 years ago, researchers began exploring ways of evaluating urine parameters and predicting risk of urolithiasis. This led to a research methodology called *Relative Supersaturation (RSS) ratio*, a technique first introduced in human medicine in the 1960s by Dr. W.G. Robertson.[1] The measurement of the RSS predicts the crystallization potential of that urine. This technique has become the gold standard for urine evaluation in humans,[2] and the technique has been validated for use in dog and cat urine.[3-5]

In order to study urine parameters using RSS, it is necessary to obtain complete urine collections over a 48-hour period. The urine is analyzed for the concentration of 10 solutes (calcium, magnesium, sodium, potassium, ammonium, phosphate, citrate, sulfate, oxalate, and uric acid) and pH.[4] The number of interactive complexes that could occur between these ions, together with each salt activity coefficient, are calculated and the activity product determined. The activity product indicates likelihood of urolith formation. The activity product is divided by the thermodynamic solubility product of the crystal and the resultant RSS ratio is produced. The thermodynamic solubility product is the activity product at which a urolith will remain static and not grow or dissolve.

Each crystal type has a unique RSS. RSS can be used to define three different zones of urine saturation: undersaturated, metastable, or oversaturated. The higher the RSS, the greater the risk of crystal formation.[4] A RSS of less than 1 indicates urine under saturation and that crystals will not form. In a complex media such as urine, it is possible to have a RSS higher than 1 without spontaneous precipitation of crystals.[5] This is due to electrical fields (ionic strength) induced by the numerous ions in solution and presence of crystallization inhibitors. Both prevent free mineral fractions (e.g., calcium and oxalate) to interact and form crystals. This level of supersaturation is qualified as *metastable supersaturation*. At this level of saturation, calcium oxalate crystals will not spontaneously form, but might occur in the presence of a nucleus. In the zone of metastable supersaturation, crystals, and thus uroliths, will not dissolve. At higher urine mineral concentration, crystals form spontaneously within minutes to hours. This is the labile supersaturation zone. The limit between metastable and labile supersaturation is called the *formation product*. Kinetic precipitation studies in urine have shown that the RSS for the formation product for struvite is 2.5 and for calcium oxalate is 12. The advent and validation of RSS technology to evaluate dog and cat urine has allowed researchers to explore the influence of nutritional alterations on the risk of LUTD.

GENERAL MANAGEMENT OF UROLITHIASIS

General strategies include increasing water consumption to lower the supersaturation of the urine, adjusting and controlling urinary relative supersaturation, reducing ingestion or absorption of calculus components, and preventing urinary tract infection. For some uroliths, one can attempt to adjust and control urine pH or utilize drugs to block formation of calculi or to form soluble complexes with the mineral components of the urolith.

Stimulate Diuresis

The unifying feature of the management of all mineral types is to stimulate diuresis by increasing water intake and thereby lower the urinary saturation of mineral components. In addition to lowering urinary mineral concentration, the risk of calculus formation can be reduced because higher urine volume and increased frequency of urination increases the elimination of crystalloids before they can aggregate into larger particles. Water consumption should be increased such that the urine specific gravity is maintained at or below 1.020 to 1.025. Small dog breeds (Miniature Schnauzers) produce less urine, urinate less frequently, and have more concentrated urine than large breed dogs (Labrador Retrievers).[6] This may be important in the pathophysiology of stone formation in high-risk small breed dogs.

To stimulate diuresis, drinking must be encouraged. An increase in water turnover can be achieved by feeding diets that contain 80% to 85% moisture (canned, pouch, tray), by increasing feeding frequency (increasing number of meals per day), by increasing the sodium chloride (NaCl) content of the diet, by adding water to the diet, and by providing novel and unique methods of water presentation. Practical methods to encourage water intake include providing water bowls in multiple sites, ensuring water is fresh at all times (water fountains, frequent water changes), using different "varieties" of water (e.g., tap, distilled, bottled), using different formats of bowl (e.g., ceramic, glass, stainless steel), and, especially for cats, utilizing large-diameter water bowls to ensure that the cats' sensitive whiskers do not touch the edge of the bowl.

Cats that were fed two identical diets except for moisture content tended to consume less water, urinate less frequently, produce less urine, and produce more concentrated urine on the lower moisture diet.[7] The water intake of a cat is significantly influenced by the number of meals per day. Kirschvink et al reported that that water intake increased from 72 mL/cat/day to 95 mL/cat/day by feeding three meals rather than one meal per day.[8] Therefore, for a given energy level, water intake can be increased significantly by adding to the meal frequency. Diet digestibility also influences the absolute amount of water available to dilute urine. Less digestible diets have been associated with increased fecal water loss. The increased loss of water into the feces decreases the amount of water absorbed and subsequently excreted in the urine.

A comparison was made on the composition of canine urine after feeding a dry diet (7% moisture) or one supplemented with water (73% moisture).[9] Increasing the moisture content of the diet was associated with significant reductions in urine specific gravity, urinary oxalate concentrations, and calcium oxalate RSS. This suggests that feeding a high-moisture diet to high-risk breeds may reduce the risk of urolithiasis.

Increased dietary sodium content has been shown to increase water intake, increase urine volume, and decrease urinary supersaturation in cats and dogs.[9-17] Healthy cats fed 1.1 g Na/1000 kcal had a mean urine volume of 11 ± 5 mL/kg/day, which increased significantly to 20 ± 7 mL/kg/day when the dietary sodium intake was increased to 2.5 g Na/1000 kcal.[10] Historically, there has been controversy about the use of NaCl to stimulate thirst and diuresis because of the theoretical effect that salt would have on urinary calcium excretion and on blood pressure. However, recent studies have refuted these concerns and support the use of moderate increases in sodium to help maintain urinary tract health. The effect of sodium on increasing calcium excretion may be countered by the positive effect that excess sodium has on urine dilution and volume.

A sodium intake of 1.04% dry matter basis (DMB) was associated with an increase in 24-hour calcium excretion and urine output.[11] However, as urinary output increased by 100%, the sodium intake did not alter urine calcium concentration but did decrease oxalate concentrations when compared with a sodium intake of 0.30% to 0.39% DMB. Due to the significant effect of sodium on urine volume, increasing dietary NaCl does not increase the urinary calcium oxalate RSS and therefore does not increase the risk for calcium oxalate urolith formation. Further, epidemiologic studies demonstrate that dogs consuming diets with a salt content of 1.43 to 3.70 g/1000 kcal have a decreased risk of calcium oxalate urolith formation when compared with dogs eating diets containing 0.48 to 0.77 g/1000 kcal.[18]

The effect of the dietary sodium content of 23 commercially available extruded diets was evaluated with respect to water intake and urine composition in 55 healthy adult cats.[12] Cats fed diets containing moderate dietary sodium content had significantly higher water intake and urine volume, significantly lower urine specific gravity, and lower calcium oxalate RSS values compared to cats fed lower sodium diets. Urinary calcium concentration did not differ significantly between cats fed the moderate and lower sodium diets. The results of this study indicate that dietary sodium concentrations up to 4 g/1000 kcal did not increase the urine calcium concentrations in cats, but did, however, increase water turnover and urine volume compared to cat fed diets with sodium content less than 1.75 g/1000 kcal. The effect of dietary sodium content on water intake, urine volume, urine specific gravity, mineral excretion, relative supersaturation and activity product ratios of calcium oxalate and struvite were evaluated in 9 healthy cats.[13] Increasing sodium content from 0.4% to 1.2% DMB was associated with a significant increase in urine volume but no increase in calcium excretion. The effect of 11 extruded diets with sodium contents ranging from 0.44% to 1.56% DMB were compared to urinary parameters in healthy cats.[14] A significant linear correlation was found between dietary sodium and calcium oxalate RSS, demonstrating that increasing dietary sodium content significantly decreases calcium oxalate RSS in cats by increasing urine volume. Increased moisture intake has also been shown to reduce calcium oxalate RSS in urolith-forming cats.[15] The effect of feeding 0.2 g Na/100 kcal versus 0.3 g Na/100 kcal to 15 dogs (7 Labrador Retrievers, 8 Miniature Schnauzers) for 36 days was studied. Increasing dietary sodium content was associated with significantly increased water intake and urine production, significantly decreased urinary concentrations of oxalate, and significantly decreased RSS for calcium oxalate.[16] Collectively, results of these studies suggest that the addition of sodium to dry diets may reduce the risk of urolithiasis.

Effect of Dietary Sodium on Blood Pressure and Renal Function

The long-term risks of increased (1.75 to 3.25 g/1000 kcal) dietary NaCl intake on the health of dogs and cats is controversial. However, recent studies have reported that the levels of dietary NaCl that will stimulate diuresis do not appear to affect blood pressure in healthy pets or canine and feline models of renal failure.[19-23] Moreover, an epidemiologic study concluded that feeding cats higher levels of Na, among other nutrients, reduced their odds of suffering from chronic renal failure.[24] Short-term feeding of high-sodium foods (0.46% vs. 1.02% Na DMB) to young, healthy cats for 14 days was associated with a significantly increased water intake and decreased urine specific gravity. Blood pressure measurements remained within the reference range throughout the study in all 10 cats.[19] The effect of dietary sodium concentration (0.22% vs. 1.3%) on renal function in adult cats indicated no differences in plasma creatinine, blood urea nitrogen, or glomerular filtration rate (GFR) (assessed by exogenous plasma creatinine clearance).[20] These data suggest that extremes of dietary salt have no short-term effect on renal function in healthy cats. Feeding diets containing 0.18% versus 1.3% sodium (DMB) for 4 weeks in eight partially nephrectomized dogs caused no significant differences in GFR.[21,22]

The effect of salt intake on blood pressure in cats with induced azotemia similar in degree to IRIS Stages II and III in cats was evaluated.[23] Salt intake had no effect on blood pressure. Further, the lowest level of salt intake was associated with the lowest values for GFR, hypokalemia, kaliuresis, and activation of the renin-angiotensin-aldosterone system. The results of this study suggest that, similar to healthy cats and dogs and dogs with induced renal disease, cats with induced renal disease are not salt-sensitive.

Adjusting Urine pH

Adjusting urine pH via dietary manipulation or medical means can be an effective adjunct in the management of some, but not all, uroliths. Urine acidification markedly increases struvite solubility and is essential in the medical dissolution of these uroliths.[25] In contrast, urine alkalinization is important in increasing the solubility urate and cystine uroliths. Calcium oxalate uroliths appear at any urine pH and medical dissolution is not possible.[26] Alkalinization above 7.5 is not recommended as this may contribute to calcium phosphate urolithiasis.

UROLITHIASIS

Struvite Uroliths

Struvite uroliths form when the urine becomes supersaturated with magnesium, ammonium, and phosphorus. Diets containing 0.15% to 1.0% magnesium (DMB) are associated with formation of struvite uroliths. The "form" of magnesium also influences the formation of struvite uroliths. For example, cats fed 0.45% magnesium chloride did not form struvite uroliths, whereas cats that were fed 0.45% magnesium oxide did.[27] The difference in struvite formation susceptibility was due to magnesium oxide promoting formation of alkaline urine, whereas the chloride salt promoted protective acidic urine.

Excess dietary protein provides additional urea that is converted to ammonia and excess glutamine that can be converted to ammonium. Supersaturation of the urine with magnesium, ammonium, and phosphorus can occur with intravascular volume depletion and water conservation. Hypokalemia increases the risk of struvite urolithiasis by promoting intracellular acidosis, which stimulates urinary excretion of ammonium. Alkaline urine increases the proportion of trivalent phosphate (PO_4^{3-}) as the reaction of HPO_4^{2-} is shifted to the right (i.e., $HPO_4^{2-} \rightarrow H^+ + PO_4^{3-}$). Struvite uroliths can also occur secondary to the presence of urease-producing bacteria *(Staphylococcus, Proteus, Ureaplasma)*. The bacteria hydrolyze urea from dietary protein to ammonium and bicarbonate. In dogs, more than 60% of struvite uroliths are associated with a concurrent bacterial infection caused by urease-producing organisms. However, the majority (90%) of urine samples from cats with struvite uroliths are sterile.

Pure sterile struvite uroliths can be easily dissolved by the administration of a digestible diet that is high in moisture and with reduced quantities of protein, magnesium, and phosphate. The diet should promote the formation of an acidic urine (6.0 to 6.3), with a relative supersaturation less than 1. The diet should contain adequate quantities of sodium to promote water intake and the formation of dilute urine. The mean time to achieve dissolution is 1 to 4 months.[28-31] It is recommended that dissolution therapy should continue for 1 month after radiographic documentation of struvite dissolution. At that time, the dissolution diet should be altered to one designed to prevent the recurrence of struvite urolithiasis. Concurrent antimicrobial therapy is indicated for those cats and dogs with a clearly documented infection. If the urolith does not dissolve, then owner compliance with the dietary recommendations should be reevaluated. It is more likely, however, that a different mineral type or a complex mineral type may be involved with the urolith and further medical evaluation is indicated. Indeed, 76% of canine struvite stones are of a mixed composition.

The basis of preventing struvite formation is to reduce the urinary concentrations of magnesium, ammonium, and trivalent phosphate. For dogs with struvite urolithiasis secondary to urease-producing bacteria, specific preventive nutritional therapy may not be required. For the remainder, nutritional recommendations include a modified protein, magnesium, and phosphate diet that promotes the formation of dilute acidic urine with a relative supersaturation value less than 2.5. The diet should be highly digestible, have high water content, and contain adequate concentrations of taurine and potassium since urinary acidification can increase taurine and potassium excretion.

Calcium Oxalate Uroliths

Risk factors for the formation of calcium oxalate uroliths include excess dietary intake of calcium, oxalate, vitamin D, or vitamin C. Further, diseases that promote hypercalcemia or the intestinal hyperabsorption of calcium are risk factors. Diets designed to minimize struvite urolithiasis through urine acidification may have increased the occurrence of calcium oxalate urolithiasis in cats.[18] Metabolic acidosis promotes skeletal mobilization of carbonate and phosphorus to buffer hydrogen ions. Simultaneous mobilization of calcium coupled with inhibition of renal tubular reabsorption of calcium results in hypercalciuria. Cats fed diets formulated to produce a urine pH between 5.99 and 6.15 were three times as likely to develop calcium oxalate uroliths as cats with urine of a higher pH.[18] However, many cats are fed acidifying diets, yet few appear to develop hypercalcemia, metabolic acidosis, or calcium oxalate urolithiasis. Therefore, additional factors such as gastrointestinal hyperabsorption or increased renal excretion of calcium and/or oxalate may be important in susceptible cats.

Studies in both cats and dogs have reported that those fed diets low in moisture and low in protein had an increased risk of calcium oxalate urolithiasis.[18,32,33] Cats and dogs that consume high-protein diets are reported to have increased water consumption, urine volume, and urinary phosphorus excretion, while calcium excretion is not increased. Dietary factors associated with a decreased risk of calcium oxalate include increased dietary intake of water, protein, calcium, phosphate, magnesium, sodium, potassium, and chloride.

Excessive dietary oxalate (e.g., asparagus, broccoli, spinach, rhubarb, rice cakes) will increase renal clearance of oxalate and risk of urolithiasis in humans. These high-risk foods are not traditionally fed to dogs or cats. Furthermore, these ingredients are not typically used in the production of commercial dog and cat foods. Hyperoxaluria has been reported in related cats with a deficiency of hepatic D-glycerate dehydrogenase.[34] This enzyme is responsible for the metabolism of oxalic acid precursors.

In humans, calcium oxalate stones have also been associated with excessive consumption of vitamin C. Vitamin C is metabolized to oxalic acid and excreted in urine. The effect of dietary vitamin C supplement on urinary oxalate concentration has been studied in 48 healthy adult American Domestic Short Hair cats.[35] Cats were fed a nutritionally complete and balanced dry control food for 2 weeks before they were fed for 4 weeks a diet containing 40 mg/kg, 78 mg/kg, 106 mg/kg, or 193 mg/kg of vitamin C, respectively. Vitamin C supplementation up to 193 mg/kg did not affect urinary oxalate concentration in the healthy cats.

Experimentally induced vitamin B_6 deficiency resulting in increased urinary oxalate concentrations and oxalate nephrocalcinosis has been reported in kittens.[36] Pyridoxine increases the transamination of glyoxylate to glycine. Therefore, pyridoxine deficiency increases the endogenous production and subsequent excretion of oxalate. However, a naturally occurring form of this syndrome has not yet been reported. Furthermore, supplementation with vitamin B_6 does not decrease urinary oxalic acid excretion compared with a diet containing adequate levels of vitamin B_6.[37]

Magnesium has been reported as a calcium oxalate crystallization inhibitor in rats and people. Both dietary magnesium restriction and magnesium supplementation have been associated with increased risk of calcium oxalate urolithiasis in cats. Magnesium reduces calcium oxalate supersaturation by combining with oxalate. In humans, dietary supplementation with excess magnesium has been associated with increased urinary calcium excretion. Hence, to minimize calcium oxalate urolithiasis, diets should neither be severely restricted nor supplemented with magnesium. Hypophosphatemia will stimulate the production of vitamin D and augment intestinal calcium absorption and urinary excretion of calcium. Diets low in phosphate have been reported to increase the risk of calcium oxalate urolithiasis in cats.

Most dogs and cats with calcium oxalate uroliths have recurrences.[38,39] Crystallization of calcium oxalate, the first step in the formation of uroliths, cannot occur unless the urine is supersaturated with these crystalloids. Therefore, diets promoting production of urine undersaturated with calcium oxalate should prevent reoccurrence. While the degree of urinary saturation provides the driving force for crystallization, inhibitors and promoters of this process, and subsequently of crystal growth or agglomeration, may also be important.

Nutritional recommendations include a diet that is high in moisture with reduced quantities of calcium, oxalate, vitamin C, and vitamin D. The diet should not be restricted in phosphate, magnesium, or pyridoxine, and should produce urine with an RSS value lower than 12. Excessive dietary calcium and dietary oxalate should be avoided. However, absolute restriction of dietary calcium should be avoided unless intestinal hyperabsorption of calcium is documented. A reduction in dietary calcium should be accompanied with a concurrent reduction in oxalate, as reducing consumption of only one of these constituents will increase the availability of the other constituent for intestinal absorption.

Administration of potassium citrate has been recommended as a component of managing calcium oxalate disease in cats and dogs. The mechanism of action was postulated to be twofold: alkalinization of the urine to reduce the solubility of calcium oxalate crystals and to increase the urinary concentration of citrate to bind oxalate. Oral potassium citrate (doses ranging from 0 mg/kg/day to 150 mg/kg/day) in 12 healthy adult dogs did not cause any significant difference in urine volume, urine specific gravity, or urine citrate concentrations.[40] There was a dose-dependent effect on urine pH. Potassium citrate did not alter the RSS for calcium oxalate. However, there was a significant effect of potassium citrate on increasing the risk of struvite disease. Therefore, not only is there no benefit of potassium citrate for calcium oxalate disease, supplementation may increase the risk of struvite disease.

In nine confirmed stone-forming Miniature Schnauzers, the mean urinary RSS was in the supersaturated zone at 13.7. After 1 month of feeding a diet specifically designed for the management of calcium oxalate urolithiasis, the mean urinary RSS value for calcium oxalate was significantly decreased to 4.26, placing it in the metastable zone.[41] A significantly lower level of saturation was maintained throughout a period of 12 months, when compared with the prestudy urine RSS values. Spontaneous homogenous crystallization will not occur at this level of supersaturation; therefore, feeding this diet would be expected to reduce the reoccurrence of stone formation in these dogs.

Calcium Phosphate Uroliths

Risk factors for the formation of calcium phosphate uroliths (hydroxyapatite, carbonate apatite, brushite) include hypercalciuria, hyperphosphaturia, alkaline urine, and decreased urine volume. Pure calcium phosphate uroliths are usually associated with a metabolic disorder such as primary hyperparathyroidism or idiopathic hypercalcemia. If a pet is hypercalcemic, a complete medical workup is indicated to identify and treat the underlying cause. Prevention of calcium phosphate urolithiasis involves increasing the water intake to obtain a urine specific gravity of 1.020 to 1.025 and adjusting the relative supersaturation of the urine for calcium phosphate. Nutritional recommendations include a diet that is high in moisture with reduced quantities of protein, calcium, sodium, and vitamin D. The diet should not be restricted or contain excess phosphate.

Urate Uroliths

Risk factors for the development of urate urolithiasis (ammonium urate, sodium urate, potassium urate, calcium urate, uric acid) include hyperuricosuria (secondary to hepatic failure, portosystemic anomalies, excess dietary purines, increased nucleic acid breakdown from lymphoma, diffuse tissue destruction), hyperammonuria (excess dietary protein, metabolic acidosis, aciduria, hypokalemia, urinary tract infection from urease-producing bacteria), aciduria, and decreased urine volume. A genetic defect in uric acid metabolism resulting in increased serum and urinary concentrations of urate is the most common etiology for canine urate disease.[42]

Dissolution of urate uroliths can be achieved in dogs within 14 weeks by raising the urinary pH and lowering the urine concentrations of uric acid and ammonium.[43] There have not been any published reports on dissolution protocols for feline urate urolithiasis. The urinary excretion of purines should be reduced by providing a low-purine diet. Historically this has been achieved by utilizing an extremely protein-restricted diet and by avoiding protein sources that are high in dietary purines (such as organ meats and fish). However, it has recently been reported that severe protein restriction is not mandatory to decrease purine urinary excretion.[44] Rather, purine restriction can be achieved via appropriate selection of protein sources. Potassium citrate or sodium bicarbonate should be administered to promote the formation of alkaline urine (pH 7.0 to 7.5). Urinary alkalinization alters the ratio of ammonium to ammonia. Allopurinol, an inhibitor of xanthine oxidase, can be used to lower urinary urate excretion in dogs. The safety and efficacy of allopurinol has not been reported in cats. Xanthine oxidase is the enzyme that converts xanthine and hypoxanthine to uric acid. As a direct result of inhibition of xanthine oxidase by allopurinol, the excretion of hypoxanthine and xanthine increases. To reduce the risk of xanthine urolithiasis, allopurinol must be administered in conjunction with a low-purine diet, and the dose adjusted to maintain 24-hour urinary excretion of uric acid below 300 mg/kg.[45] Prevention following dissolution or surgical removal is necessary due to the high risk of urolith reoccurrence. The ideal preventive diet should not be severely protein restricted, yet be extremely low in purine concentration and promote the formation of dilute, alkaline urine.

Cystine Uroliths

Cystine stones are due to an inherited defect of proximal renal tubular reabsorption of several basic amino acids especially cystine.[46,47] Lysine, arginine, and ornithine are also found in abnormal amounts in the urine of cystinuric pets.[48] To facilitate cystine dissolution, a low-purine, taurine, carnitine, and potassium citrate supplemented diet has been recommended.[49] The aim of preventive therapy is to reduce the concentration of cystine in the urine and to increase the solubility of cystine in urine. Reducing dietary protein intake will reduce the intake and subsequent urinary excretion of cystine. Furthermore, utilizing protein sources that are limited in methionine (e.g., soybean protein) will reduce the urinary excretion of cysteine as methionine is a precursor of cystine. The solubility of cystine is highly dependent on urinary pH. Therefore, the urine should be alkalinized to achieve a fasting pH between 7.5 and 8.0, at which level cystine is markedly more soluble. Alkalinization can be achieved with the addition of potassium citrate. In addition, water consumption should be encouraged to lower urine specific gravity and increase the frequency of urination. Thiol-containing drugs bind cystine to form disulfide complexes, which are more soluble in urine than cystine. 2-MPG (mercaptopropionyl-glycine) is the most commonly used drug, at 20 mg/kg BID. D-penicillamine has been used, but its use is associated with undesirable side effects.

MISCELLANEOUS UROLITHS

Xanthine uroliths have been sporadically reported in dogs.[50,51] The majority of xanthine stones develop secondary to allopurinol therapy for urate urolithiasis or leishmaniasis. There have not been any reports of effective dissolution protocols. Management requires a low-purine diet in conjunction with lowering of the allopurinol dose.

Silica stones have been reported in dogs with pica or dogs consuming diets high in silicates (corn gluten, soybean hulls).[52] Prevention requires a high-quality, highly digestible diet.

Potassium magnesium pyrophosphate uroliths have been reported in Persian cats.[53] The etiology is unknown, and specific management beyond stimulation of diuresis is unknown at this time. Similarly, dried, solidified blood clots have been reported in cats.[54]

IDIOPATHIC DISEASE

In approximately 50% of cats with feline lower urinary tract disease, the etiology of hematuria, pollakiuria, stranguria, and inappropriate urination remains unknown.[55,56] These cats are classified as having idiopathic or interstitial cystitis. The diagnosis of feline interstitial cystitis requires documentation of signs of chronic irritative voiding (dysuria, hematuria, pollakiuria, inappropriate urination), sterile and cytologically negative urine, and cystoscopic observation of submucosal petechial hemorrhages.[57] It is not yet known if feline interstitial cystitis is a specific disease or merely a pathologic response of the bladder to several different diseases.

Abnormalities in the local, sensory, central, and efferent nervous systems have been suggested to be involved in the pathophysiology of feline interstitial cystitis.[57] It has been postulated that stressors in a sensitive cats' environment precipitate clinical signs. Stress activates the efferent sympathetic nervous system, which stimulates the dorsal root ganglia. The dorsal root ganglia cause the peripheral release of neuropeptides and inflammatory mediators responsible for inflammation and pain. Therefore, one of the cornerstones of therapy is to identify and relieve stressors in the cat's environment. Stress is, however, difficult to quantitate. Potential sources include environmental aspects such as changes in weather, activity, litter-box placement, litter type, diet, owner work schedule, and the addition or removal of people or animals. Stress can be managed by providing the cat with hiding places and something that allows the cat to express predatory behavior, such as climbing posts and toys that can be chased and caught.[58]

Diet plays a role in the pathophysiology and treatment of interstitial cystitis. An abrupt change in diet has been associated with the recurrence of clinical signs. Therefore, it is reasonable to limit the frequency of diet changes in sensitive cats. Recurrence of clinical signs has also been associated with feeding dry formulation. In a prospective study, the recurrence of clinical signs was evaluated in 54 cats fed either a moist or dry diet.[59] Cats were evaluated for 12 months or until signs recurred. Recurrence of clinical signs occurred in 39% of cats receiving the dry formulation versus 11% of cats receiving the moist formulation. The exact nature of the beneficial effect of the canned diet was not elucidated. The renal solute load and urine pH were not different between the two groups of cats. However, the urine specific gravity of the cats receiving the moist diet was significantly lower than that of the dry formulation group (1.032 vs. 1.052, respectively). The results of these findings suggest that feeding a moist diet protected nearly 90% of cats from recurrence of clinical signs for up to 1 year. The reduction in clinical signs associated with increased water intake may be a result of a reduction in urinary solute concentration, urine osmolality, and/or increased urine volume.

CONCLUSION

Nutrition has a fundamental role in the management of urolithiasis and feline idiopathic cystitis. Clearly, urine dilution, achieved by promoting water intake, is the most important universal dietary strategy that is essential to all forms of urolithiasis and idiopathic cystitis. Additional therapeutic endeavors include reducing urinary mineral saturation, and for some types of uroliths, manipulating urinary pH or administering drugs that affect the metabolic pathways of the components of the calculus, administering agents that increase the solubility of the mineral complexes, and eliminating or preventing bacterial infection.

REFERENCES

The reference list can be found on the companion Expert Consult Web site at *www.expertconsult.com*.

CHAPTER 179

Parenteral Nutritional Support

Daniel L. Chan

OVERVIEW

Metabolic responses to illness or injury place critically ill animals at high risk for malnutrition and its deleterious effects. These problems include alterations in energy metabolism, compromised immune function, decreased wound healing, and probably a negative impact on overall survival.[1-3] Whereas healthy animals lose primarily fat when they do not receive adequate calories (simple starvation), sick or traumatized patients catabolize lean body mass when they are not provided with sufficient calories (stressed starvation). Inadequate calorie intake is a common problem in critically ill animals due to anorexia, an inability to eat or tolerate feedings (e.g., vomiting), or decreased absorptive capabilities.[1,4]

Because malnutrition may occur quickly, it is important to provide nutritional support by either enteral or parenteral means if oral intake is not adequate. The goals of nutritional support are either to prevent development of malnutrition or to treat malnutrition. Although unproven in dogs and cats, it is logical to assume that treatment or prevention of malnutrition decreases morbidity and mortality.[1,2,5-7] Whenever possible, oral nutritional support (enteral) should be used because it is safest, most convenient, most physiologically sound, and least expensive. Although enteral nutrition is preferred in critically ill animals, parenteral nutrition (PN) is an established method of providing nutritional support to patients whose gastrointestinal tracts cannot tolerate enteral feedings.[3,5,6,8,9]

Although the use of parenteral nutritional support has become more common, there remains a perception that this is technically difficult, associated with complications, and limited to university hospitals and referral centers. In reality, parenteral nutritional support can be adopted in many practices. Further, complications can be significantly reduced with proper management techniques. The goals of this chapter are to outline the identification process of dogs and cats most likely to benefit from PN, to review the process of formulating, implementing, and monitoring parenteral nutritional support, and to discuss how PN can be incorporated into various practice situations.

NUTRITIONAL ASSESSMENT

The first step in the consideration of nutritional support is appropriate patient assessment. Assessing nutritional status via objective measurements of body composition (e.g., anthropometry, bioelectrical impedance, dual energy x-ray absorptiometry, or serum indicators of malnutrition) is rarely employed in clinical veterinary medicine. Therefore subjective clinical assessment remains paramount in the identification of malnourished animals that require nutritional support as well as those imminently at risk for malnutrition. Indicators of malnutrition include weight loss, poor haircoat, muscle wasting, signs of inadequate wound healing, hypoalbuminemia, lymphopenia, and coagulopathies. However, these abnormalities are not specific to malnutrition and do not occur early in the process. In addition, fluid shifts may mask weight loss in critically ill patients. Given these limitations, it is crucial to identify early risk factors that may predispose pets to malnutrition (e.g., anorexia of greater than 3 days duration), serious underlying disease (e.g., trauma, sepsis, peritonitis, pancreatitis, gastrointestinal surgery), or significant protein losses (e.g., protracted vomiting, diarrhea, protein-losing nephropathies, draining wounds, or burns).

Nutritional assessment should also identify factors that can affect the nutritional plan, such as the identification of specific electrolyte abnormalities; hyperglycemia, hypertriglyceridemia, or hyperammonemia; or comorbid illnesses, such as renal or hepatic disease. Such findings require adjustments to be made to the formulation of PN and in some cases prompt changing the nutritional plan. Appropriate laboratory analyses (e.g., serum biochemical profile, urinalysis) should be performed in all dogs and cats to assess these parameters.

GOALS OF NUTRITIONAL SUPPORT

The goals of nutritional support are to provide for the animal's ongoing needs, prevent or correct deficiencies or imbalances, minimize metabolic derangements, and prevent further catabolism of lean body tissues. Restoration of optimal body condition should not necessarily be the goal of nutritional support in the acute stages of diseases. In severely malnourished dogs and cats, nutritional support is directed towards preservation of lean body tissue and organ function, rather than complete reversal of malnutrition, which is accomplished when the patient becomes convalescent. The necessity for instituting nutritional support is dictated by individual needs and not necessarily by the specific disease. The ultimate goal of nutritional support is to provide the necessary nutrients and calories until the dog or cat voluntarily consumes an adequate amount of food in its own environment.

THE NUTRITIONAL PLAN

One key to successful nutritional management of critically ill animals lies in the proper diagnosis and treatment of their underlying disease. While an attempt is made to diagnose and treat that underlying illness, a crucial care factor is selection of an appropriate route for nutritional support (Figure 179-1).

Providing nutrition via a functional digestive system is always preferred. Therefore, particular care should be taken to determine whether enteral feedings would be tolerated. Even if only small amounts of enteral nutrition would be tolerated, this route of feeding should be pursued and supplemented with PN as necessary. Based on the nutritional assessment, anticipated duration of support, and appropriate route of delivery (i.e., enteral or parenteral), a nutritional plan can be formulated.

The first steps of instituting nutritional support include reestablishing proper hydration status, correction of electrolyte or acid-base disturbances, and achieving hemodynamic stability. Commencing nutritional support before such abnormalities are addressed can increase complication risk and, in some cases, further compromise the animal. Implementation of the nutritional plan should be gradual, with a goal of reaching the target level of nutrient delivery in 48 to 72 hours being appropriate.

CALCULATING NUTRITIONAL REQUIREMENTS

Ideally, the provision of nutritional support should provide ample substrates for gluconeogenesis, protein synthesis, and energy necessary to maintain homeostasis. The clinician must ensure that enough calories are being provided to sustain critical physiologic processes (e.g., immune function, wound repair, cell division and cell growth). Therefore calculating the animal's total energy expenditure is necessary. However, as clinically available direct measurements of energy expenditure in dogs and cats are still in the developmental phase, use of mathematical formulas are the only practical means of estimating energy requirements. The resting energy requirement (RER) is defined as the number of calories required per day for maintaining homeostasis at rest in a thermoneutral environment while the animal is in a postabsorptive state.[10] While there are several formulas proposed to calculate the RER, a widely used allometric formula can be applied to both dogs and cats, regardless of bodyweight. For animals weighing between 2 and 30 kg, there is also a linear formula that provides reasonable estimation of the RER:

$$RER = 70 \times (\text{current body weight in kg})^{0.75}$$

or for animals weighing between 2 and 30 kg:

$$RER = (30 \times \text{current body weight in kg}) + 70$$

Despite the convention of multiplying the RER by an illness factor between 1.0 and 2.0 to account for increases in metabolism associated with different diseases and injuries, less emphasis is now being placed on such subjective and extrapolated factors.[4] The current recommendation is to use more conservative energy estimates (i.e., start with the animal's RER) to avoid overfeeding. Overfeeding can result in metabolic and gastrointestinal complications, hepatic dysfunction, and increased carbon dioxide production.[9] One study demonstrated that use of "illness factors" in calculating energy requirements for cats was strongly associated with the development of hyperglycemia.[11]

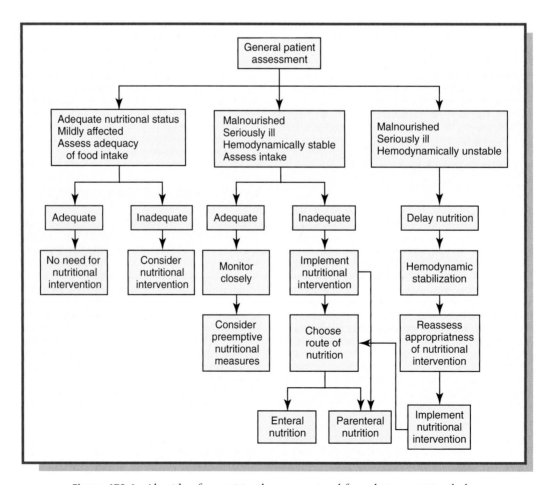

Figure 179-1 Algorithm for nutritional assessment and formulating nutritional plan.

As the preservation of lean body mass is a primary goal of nutritional support, close monitoring of bodyweight, fluid distribution, response or tolerance to feedings, and changes in the underlying condition should dictate whether to increase the number of calories provided in the nutritional plan. Typically, if an animal continues to lose weight on nutritional support, the number of calories provided should be increased by 25% and the plan should be reassessed in a few days. Additional adjustments to the nutritional plan might also include the addition or restriction of electrolytes such as magnesium and potassium as dictated by serial biochemical profiles.

NUTRITIONAL SUPPORT

A major advantage of enteral over parenteral nutrition is superior maintenance of intestinal structure and function. The presence of nutrients within the intestinal lumen elicits trophic effects that mediate mucosal cell proliferation. It has also been proposed that a lack of enteral nutrition contributes to the impairment of mucosal barrier function, which allows for the translocation of intestinal bacteria or endotoxins leading to sepsis and a systemic inflammatory response.

However, in animals unable to tolerate enteral feedings, such as those that are vomiting, regurgitating, or unable to protect their airway, PN should be considered. Inability to tolerate enteral feedings is the only major indication for parenteral nutritional support. Although obtaining enteral access in critically ill animals can be difficult, every effort must be made to ensure that a functional gastrointestinal tract is not bypassed. A more extensive review of enteral nutrition is provided elsewhere (see Chapter 85).

PARENTERAL NUTRITION

PN has sometimes been characterized as a technique fraught with complications. In reality, many of the complications attributed to PN in the past might have had more to do with overfeeding or "hyperalimentation," rather than with the route of feeding itself. Although metabolic complications can be associated with PN, these complications are generally mild, have minimal consequences, and rarely require discontinuation of nutritional support. Septic complications associated with PN can be dramatically minimized with careful attention to aseptic technique in the compounding of PN, placement of dedicated PN catheters, and careful monitoring of the catheter site.

Types of Parenteral Nutrition

The most commonly used term for PN is "total" parenteral nutrition (TPN). However, there is some controversy regarding use of the term *total* because it is recognized that most veterinary preparations of PN are not complete and do not meet all of the nutrient requirements of dogs and cats. Given that the different types of PN can be defined in a number of ways, it may be simpler to categorize the different types of PN in terms of calories provided, that is, when PN is formulated to meet 100% of an animal's energy requirements, it is referred to as *total parenteral nutrition*. PN formulated to provide only a portion of the energy requirements, typically 40% to 70%, is termed *partial parenteral nutrition* (PPN). The lower osmolarity of PPN solutions, as compared to TPN solutions, is achieved by diluting the solution (ideally to less than 800 mOsm/L), which decreases the caloric and protein density but makes it suitable for administration via peripheral veins. For this reason, PPN may also be referred to as *peripheral parenteral nutrition*. The lower osmolarity is achieved in part, by utilizing 5% dextrose instead of 50% dextrose in the preparation of PPN and sometimes by the addition of isotonic and sometimes hypotonic crystalloids. As such, PPN is intended for short-term use (less than 5 days) and should be limited to dogs and cats that are not debilitated. PPN is also sometimes used as interim nutritional support until TPN can be formulated, or it is used when specific contraindications to the placement of jugular catheters exist, such as increased intracranial pressure or coagulopathies.

COMPONENTS OF PARENTERAL NUTRITION

PN is formulated as a mixture of a carbohydrate (dextrose), amino acids, and, usually, fat (lipid) (Web Figure 179-1). Carbohydrate, in the form of dextrose (typically 5% or 50%), may have benefits in addition to acting as a fuel substrate. These potential benefits include stimulation of insulin secretion, reduction of muscle protein catabolism, and inhibition of hepatic glucose output, which may spare muscle protein from being catabolized for gluconeogenesis. However, administration of dextrose or supplementation of maintenance fluids with dextrose as the sole source of calories, in most cases, does not amount to adequate nutritional support and should be discouraged. For example, a 5% dextrose infusion provides only 170 kcal per liter of solution, and would provide less than 25% of the RER for a dog or cat at maintenance fluid rates. Dextrose infusions are more appropriate for the treatment of hypoglycemia rather than for nutritional support.

Crystalline amino acid solutions are an essential component of PN. The importance of supplying amino acids relates to maintenance of positive nitrogen balance and repletion of lean body tissue. This may be vital as critically ill dogs and cats begin to recover from illness. Supplementation of amino acids may support protein synthesis and spare tissue proteins from being catabolized via gluconeogenesis.[9] The most commonly used amino acid solution (Travasol, Clintec Nutrition, Deerfield, Ill.) contain most of the essential amino acids for dogs and cats. The exception is taurine. However, as PN is typically not used for more than 10 days, the lack of taurine does not become a problem in most circumstances.

Amino acid solutions are available in different concentrations from 4% to 10%, but the most commonly used is 8.5%. Amino acid solutions are also available with and without electrolytes. Animals with normal serum electrolyte concentrations typically receive amino acid solutions with electrolytes, whereas those with electrolyte disturbances may benefit from amino acid solutions without electrolytes. Special formulations of amino acid solutions containing higher concentrations of the branched chain amino acids are available, although at much greater expense. Although these solutions were originally thought to be useful in the management of highly catabolic metabolic diseases or when hepatic encephalopathy was present, studies have not confirmed a clear benefit in overall survival.[12]

Lipid emulsions are the calorically dense component of PN and a source of essential fatty acids. Lipid emulsions are isotonic and are available in 10% to 20% solutions (Intralipid, Clintec Nutrition, Deerfield, Ill.). These commercially available lipid emulsions are made primarily of soybean and safflower oils. They predominantly provide long chain polyunsaturated fatty acids that include linoleic, oleic, palmitic, and stearic acids. These solutions are emulsified with egg yolk phospholipids and their tonicity is adjusted with glycerol. The emulsified fat particles are comparable in size to chylomicrons and are removed from the circulation via the action of peripheral lipoprotein lipase. A common misconception exists with respect to the use of lipid-containing PN for animals that have pancreatitis. Although hypertriglyceridemia may be a risk factor for pancreatitis, infusions of lipids have not been shown to increase pancreatic secretion or worsen pancreatitis. Such therapies are, therefore, considered safe[13] except when the serum triglyceride concentration is increased. This would indicate a clear failure of triglyceride clearance. According to the most recent guidelines provided by the American Society of Parenteral and Enteral Nutrition, humans with serum triglycerides exceeding 400 mg/dL should have the lipid proportion in PN markedly reduced or eliminated altogether.[14] Although specific data regarding the maximal safe level of lipid administration in dogs and cats are not available, it would seem prudent to maintain normal serum triglyceride concentrations.

Another concern regarding use of lipids in PN is its purported immunosuppressive effect. This may develop via impairment of the reticuloendothelial system, particularly when PN solutions containing a high percentage of lipid are used.[9] Despite in vitro evidence supporting the notion that lipid infusions can also suppress neutrophil and lymphocyte function, studies have not yet correlated lipid use and increased rates of infectious complications.

Daily vitamin recommendations for dogs and cats receiving PN are extrapolated from established oral nutritional requirements.[9] Multivitamin preparations intended for IV administration provide a convenient and practical means for vitamin supplementation.

It is recommended to add 0.2 mL/kg of a multivitamin preparation (M.V.I.-12 NeoSan Pharmaceuticals Inc., Wilmington, N.C.) to each PN bag at the time of compounding, up to 10 mL/day. This provides most of the water- and fat-soluble vitamins except for vitamin K. In certain situations (e.g., longstanding malnutrition, malabsorptive disorders), 0.5 mg/kg of vitamin K can be administered SQ, once weekly. Some research suggests that the addition of D-alpha-tocopherol (vitamin E) could reduce the amount of peroxidation in PN solutions.[14] Trace metals (4 Trace Elements, Abbott Laboratories, North Chicago, Ill.) can also be added to the PN solution at a dose of 0.1 mL/kg (up to 5 mL/day) in order to provide zinc, manganese, copper, and chromium. Although vitamins are commonly added to PN solutions, trace metals are usually only added when PN is to be administered for more than 5 days or when food has not been consumed for a prolonged period.

Addition of other parenteral medications to PN admixtures is possible; however, their compatibility must first be verified. Drugs that are known to be compatible and sometimes added to PN include heparin, insulin, potassium chloride, and metoclopramide. While the addition of insulin to PN is often required in people receiving PN, the hyperglycemia seen in dogs and cats receiving PN does not usually require insulin administration. However, diabetic pets require adjustments to their insulin regimen. Although there is a described veterinary protocol for the addition of insulin directly to PN, it is often easiest to manage diabetics receiving PN with SQ injections of insulin.[9]

PARENTERAL NUTRITION COMPOUNDING

Based on the nutritional assessment and plan, PN can be formulated according to the worksheets found in Boxes 179-1 and 179-2. For TPN (see Box 179-1), the first step is the calculation of the patient's RER. Protein requirements (grams of protein required per day) are then calculated, taking into consideration factors such as excessive protein loss, severe hepatic disease, or significant renal disease. Although some recommendations meet all energy requirements with only

dextrose and lipids, the protocol listed accounts for energy also provided from amino acids in the calculations and subtracts the calories provided by amino acids from the daily RER to estimate the total nonprotein calories required. Nonprotein calories are then usually provided as a 50:50 mixture of lipids and dextrose. This 50:50 ratio can be adjusted in cases of persistent hyperglycemia or hypertriglyceridemia (e.g., a higher proportion of calories would be given from lipid in an animal with hyperglycemia). The calories provided from each component (amino acids, lipids, and dextrose) are then divided by their respective caloric densities, and the exact amounts of each component are added to the PN bags in an aseptic fashion. The amount of TPN delivered will often provide less than the daily fluid requirement, and additional fluid can either be added to the PN bag at the time of compounding or be provided as a separate infusion.

For formulation of PPN, Box 179-2 provides a step-by-step protocol in which animals of various size can receive 70% of their RER and approximately meet their daily maintenance fluid requirement. In extremely small animals (≤3 kg), the amount of PPN will exceed the maintenance fluid requirement and increase the risk for fluid overload, so volume adjustments are necessary. Also, in animals requiring conservative fluid administration (e.g., congestive heart failure), these calculations for PPN may provide excessive fluid volumes. This formulation has been designed so that the proportion of each PN component is dependent on animal weight such that a smaller animal (between 3 to 5 kg) will receive proportionally more calories from lipids, compared to a large dog (greater than 30 kg), which would receive more calories in the form of carbohydrates. This allows the resulting formulation to approximate the daily fluid requirement.

Ideally, compounding of PN should be done aseptically under a laminar flow hood using a semiautomated, closed-system, PN compounder (e.g., Automix Compounder, Clintec Nutrition, Deerfield, Ill.; Web Figure 179-2).

If an automated compounder is not available, manual compounding can be done under a laminar flow hood with strict adherence to aseptic technique using a 3-in-1 bag (All-In-One EVA container, Clintec Nutrition, Deerfield, Ill.). New regulations implemented by the United States Pharmacopeia in 2004 require strict adherence to sterile compounding of PN solutions.[15] Given these ideal conditions, it is often easier and more cost-effective to have a local human hospital or a human home health care company compound PN solutions. A few specialized veterinary centers can also compound PN for use in general practice. Alternatively, commercial ready-to-use preparations of glucose or glycerol and amino acids are available for IV use (Table 179-1).

While these ready-to-use preparations are convenient, they provide only 30% to 50% of caloric requirements when administered at maintenance fluid rates and as a result should only be used for interim nutritional support or to supplement low-dose enteral feedings.

PARENTERAL NUTRITION ADMINISTRATION

The administration of any PN requires a dedicated, aseptically placed catheter, used solely for PN administration. Most critically ill dogs and cats that receive PN require placement of a new or additional catheter, because PN should not be administered through previously existing catheters placed for reasons other than PN. Long catheters composed of silicone, polyurethane, or tetrafluoroethylene are recommended for use with any type of PN to reduce the risk of thrombophlebitis.[3,4] Multilumen catheters are often recommended for TPN administration. Multilumen catheters can remain in place for long time periods. Such catheters can be used for blood

Box • 179-1

Total Parenteral Nutrition (TPN) Calculations

1. Calculate resting energy requirement (RER)

   RER = 70 × (current bodyweight in kg)$^{0.75}$

   or for animals weighing between 2 and 30 kg:

   RER = (30 × current body weight in kg) + 70   RER = _____ kcal/day

2. Protein requirements

	Canine (g/100 kcal)	Feline (g/100 kcal)
*Standard	4	6
*Reduced (hepatic/renal disease)	2-3	3-4
*Increased (excessive protein losses)	6	6

   (RER ÷ 100) × _____ g/100 kcal = _____ g protein required/day
   $\underset{\text{protein req}}{}$

3. Volume of nutrient solutions required

   a. 8.5% amino acid solution = 0.085 g protein/mL

   _____ g protein required/day ÷ 0.085 g/mL   = _____ mL/day of amino acids

   b. Nonprotein calories: The calories supplied by protein (4 kcal/g) are subtracted from the RER to get total nonprotein calories needed.

   _____ g protein req/day × 4 kcal/g   = _____ kcal provided by protein

   RER – kcal provided by protein   = _____ total nonprotein kcal/day required

   c. Nonprotein calories are usually provided as a 50:50 mixture of lipid and dextrose

   *20% lipid solution = 2 kcal/mL

   To supply 50% of nonprotein calories

   _____ lipid kcal required ÷ 2 kcal/mL   = _____ mL of lipid

   *50% of dextrose solution = 1.7 kcal/mL

   To supply 50% of nonprotein calories

   _____ dextrose kcal required ÷ 1.7 kcal/mL   = _____ mL of dextrose

4. Total daily requirements

   _____ mL of 8.5% amino acid solution

   _____ mL of 20% lipid

   _____ mL of 50% dextrose

   _____ total mL of TPN solution to be administered over 24 hrs

*Using a common 8.5% amino acid solution containing potassium (i.e., Travasol), TPN made according to this worksheet will provide potassium at higher than maintenance levels. Therefore, you may not need to supplement potassium in any other fluids your patient is receiving. TPN for animals that are hyperkalemic should be formulated using amino acid solutions without electrolytes. Rates of other IV fluids being concurrently administered should be adjusted accordingly.

sampling, administration of additional fluids, and IV medication administration, and they negate the need for separate catheters placed at other sites.[5,16]

Although placement of multilumen catheters does require more technical skill than conventional jugular catheters, they can be valuable in the treatment of any critically ill animal. The high osmolarity of TPN solutions (often ~1200 mOsm/L) requires administration through a central venous (jugular) catheter, while PPN solutions can be administered through either a jugular or peripheral venous catheter. The concern with administering fluids high in osmolarity has been risk of thrombophlebitis, although this side effect has not been demonstrated in dogs or cats.

Because of the various metabolic derangements associated with critical illness, TPN should be instituted gradually over 48 hours. It is recommended that TPN be started at 50% of the RER on day 1 and then increased to the targeted amount by the second day. In this manner, serum electrolyte, glucose, acid-base status, total fluid requirements, and other parameters can be monitored as TPN is administered. In most cases, PPN can be started without gradual increase. It is also impor-

tant to adjust the rates of other fluids being concurrently administered. For both TPN and PPN, the animal's catheter and infusion lines must be handled aseptically at all times to reduce the risk of PN-related infection (Web Figure 179-3).

PN should be delivered as continuous rate infusions over 24 hours via fluid infusion pumps. Inadvertent delivery of massive amounts of PN can result if administration is not properly regulated. Cyclic administration of PN (i.e., alternating PN with other parenteral fluids every 12 hours) has also been described. However, this practice is not recommended as it circumvents maintenance of a closed-system for PN administration and can increase the rate of complications. Once a bag of PN is set up for administration, it should not be disconnected even for walks or diagnostic procedures. The drip regulator can be decreased to an extremely slow rate and can accompany the animal if it needs to be moved. Administration of PN through an in-line filter (Air Eliminating Filter, Clintec Nutrition Division, Deerfield, Ill.) is also recommended and is attached at the time of setup. This set-up process is performed daily with each new bag of PN. Each bag should only hold one day's worth of PN, and the accompany-

Box • 179-2

Partial Parenteral Nutrition (PPN) Calculations

1. Calculate resting energy requirement (RER)

    RER = 70 × (current bodyweight in kg)$^{0.75}$
    or for animals weighing between 2 and 30 kg:
    RER = (30 × current bodyweight in kg) + 70   RER = ____kcal/day

2. Calculate the partial energy requirement (PER)

    Plan to supply 70% of the animal's RER with PPN: PER = RER × 0.70 = ____kcal/day

3. Proportion of nutrient requirements according to bodyweight:
    (Note: For animals ≤3 kg, the formulation will exceed maintenance fluid requirements)
    a. Cats and Dogs 3-5 kg:
       PER × 0.20 = ____kcal/day carbohydrate required
       PER × 0.20 = ____kcal/day protein required
       PER × 0.60 = ____kcal/day lipid required
    b. Cats and Dogs 6-10 kg:
       PER × 0.25 = ____kcal/day carbohydrate required
       PER × 0.25 = ____kcal/day protein required
       PER × 0.50 = ____kcal/day lipid required
    c. Dogs 11-30 kg:
       PER × 0.33 = ____kcal/day carbohydrate required
       PER × 0.33 = ____kcal/day protein required
       PER × 0.33 = ____kcal/day lipids required
    d. Dogs >30 kg:
       PER × 0.50 = ____kcal/day carbohydrate required
       PER × 0.25 = ____kcal/day protein required
       PER × 0.25 = ____kcal/day lipid required

4. Volumes of nutrient solutions required:
    a. 5% dextrose solution = 0.17 kcal/mL

       ____kcal carbohydrate required/day ÷ 0.17 kcal/mL   = ____ mL/day dextrose
    b. 8.5% amino acid solution = 0.34 kcal/mL

       ____kcal protein required/day ÷ 0.34 kcal/mL   = ____ mL/day amino acids
    c. 20% lipid solution = 2 kcal/mL

       ____kcal lipid required/day ÷ 2 kcal/mL   = ____ mL/day lipid
                                                  = ____ total mL of PPN to be administered over 24 hrs

Note: This formulation provides approximately a maintenance fluid rate. Commonly used 8.5% amino acid solutions (i.e., Travasol) with electrolytes contain potassium. For animals ≤35 kg, the PPN solution made according to this worksheet will provide approximately maintenance levels of potassium. For animals >35 kg, the potassium contained in the PPN solution will be lower than maintenance levels. Rates of other iv fluids being concurrently administered should be adjusted accordingly.

Table • 179-1

Commercially Available Alternatives for Partial Parenteral Nutrition (PPN)

PRODUCT NAME	FEATURES	MANUFACTURER
Clinimix	2.75% amino acids, 5% dextrose	Clintec Nutrition, Deerfield, Ill.
Quickmix	2.75% amino acids, 5% dextrose	Clintec Nutrition, Deerfield, Ill.
ProcalAmine	3% amino acids, 3% glycerol	B. Braun, McGraw Inc., Irvine, Calif.
Vamin 9 Glucose	5.9% amino acids, 10% dextrose	Fresenius Kabi, Bad Homburg, Germany

ing fluid administration sets and in-line filter are changed at the same time using aseptic technique. Discontinuation of PN should be done when the animal resumes consuming an adequate amount of calories of at least 50% of RER. Whereas TPN should be gradually discontinued over a 6- to 12-hour period, PPN can be discontinued abruptly.

COMPLICATIONS

As with any therapy intended for critically ill animals, complications can occur. Complications associated with PN can include mechanical complications of the catheter and lines, thrombophlebitis, metabolic abnormalities, and sepsis. Mechanical complications such as inadvertent catheter removal, catheter occlusion, and line disconnection or breakage are probably not inherently related to PN and are likely no more common than in any dog or cat with an IV catheter. Metabolic complications are much more likely to be related to PN and include hyperglycemia, hypertriglyceridemia, hyperbilirubinemia, increased alkaline phosphatase activity, azotemia, electrolyte shifts, and hyperammonemia.[2,5,11,16,17] The more commonly encountered complications, namely hyperglycemia and hypertriglyceridemia, are usually transient and can be effectively managed without serious consequences. However, one study did demonstrate higher mortality rates in cats receiving TPN that developed hyperglycemia within the first 24 hours of TPN support.[17] Decreasing the infusion rate for 12 to 24 hours is often effective, although in some instances reformulation of PN is required. Animals with biochemical changes subsequent to initiation of PN should have more frequent laboratory parameter evaluations.

Septic complications, including catheter-site infection with and without systemic sepsis, have been reported in dogs and cats receiving PN. This complication is uncommon, ranging from 3% to 12% in dogs and cats receiving PN.[5,16,17] Septic complications can be minimized by strict adherence to established protocols and careful attention to early signs of problems relating to catheter care. Any catheter suspected of causing fever, increase in white blood cell count, or other sign compatible with infection should be removed and cultured.

One of the proposed advantages of PPN over TPN is lower risk of complication. This concept has been supported by a study documenting lower rates of complications in dogs and cats receiving PPN, compared to previously reported complication rates associated with TPN in dogs.[5,16] Although direct comparisons between the two patient populations cannot be made, there were approximately 0.17 complications per day of PPN administration in dogs and cats, versus 0.53 complication per day of TPN administration in dogs[5,16] and between 0.30 and 0.62 complications per day of TPN in cats.[11,17] Reasons for these differences could be attributed to differences in severity of illness between these animal populations. Hypocaloric nutritional support may actually confer some benefit, including lower complication rates, in certain patient populations.[18]

MONITORING

Given the potential for complications, monitoring of dogs and cats receiving PN is a vital part of nutritional support. This monitoring should be similar to that already in place for any critically ill animal. Careful monitoring of the catheter site is recommended to detect problems early (e.g., signs of inflammation or malposition) and should be done on a daily basis. Catheters should be evaluated for patency and bandages changed daily. At a minimum, body weight, body temperature, respiratory rate, catheter site, and serum glucose should be evaluated daily. All blood tubes should be inspected for visible lipemia. Monitoring of other parameters (e.g., electrolytes, acid-base status, complete blood count, biochemical profile) may also be indicated. Persistent hyperglycemia, hypertriglyceridemia, or signs of encephalopathy should prompt reevaluation and may necessitate decreasing rate of infusion or reformulation of PN and serial evaluation of blood work.

SUMMARY

With the growing recognition that nutritional support is an integral part of the therapeutic regimen of many critically ill animals, it is becoming increasingly important for veterinarians to be able to incorporate parenteral nutritional support in their practice or to refer these cases to facilities capable of providing such therapy when necessary. Proper identification of dogs and cats most likely to benefit from PN and the ability to formulate, administer, and monitor PN are key factors in ensuring the successful incorporation of parenteral nutritional support in their care.

References

The reference list can be found on the companion Expert Consult Web site at *www.expertconsult.com*.

CHAPTER 180

Nutritional Management of Renal Conditions

Joseph W. Bartges

Chronic renal failure is a common disease of older dogs and cats that occurs occasionally in younger animals, is typically irreversible, stable for some period of time, but ultimately progresses. Studies on dogs[1] and cats[2-5] with naturally occurring chronic renal failure have demonstrated that dietary modification can slow progression of disease, provide longer survival times, and improve quality of life.

TWO-STEP PROCESS OF DOGS AND CATS WITH RENAL DISEASE

The first step in nutritional problem solving is the assessment phase, involving assessment of the patient, diet, and feeding method. The second phase is initiation of nutritional management, assessment of response, and alteration of management, if necessary.[6]

Assessment Phase

Assess the Patient Dogs and cats with chronic renal failure may appear healthy or may have signs of chronic disease such as poor haircoat, weight loss, and muscle wasting. Additionally, signs of uremia may be present including gastrointestinal ulcers and uremic halitosis. The International Renal Interest Society (http://iris-kidney.com) has developed a staging system for dogs and cats with chronic renal failure (see Chapter 311).[7] Staging is based on degree of azotemia, whether proteinuria is present, and whether systemic arterial hypertension is present.

Pets with chronic renal failure may exhibit some degree of anorexia. Causes of anorexia and nausea include retention of uremic toxins, dehydration, biochemical alterations (azotemia, metabolic acidosis, electrolyte imbalances, and mineral imbalances), anemia, renal secondary hyperparathyroidism, and uremic gastroenteritis.[8] Gastric ulcers occur less commonly in dogs and cats than in people; however, many dogs and cats with chronic renal disease have gastric pathology including vascular changes and edema[9] and probable gastric hyperacidity associated with hypergastrinemia from decreased renal excretion.[10]

Assess the Diet

Energy Body weight and body condition is variable in dogs and cats with chronic renal failure. Patients that are obese may be prone to systemic arterial hypertension,[11] while those that are underweight or cachectic may be prone to complications such as intolerance of medications, secondary infections, and poor quality of life. Decreased energy intake from inappetence or advanced renal failure may lead to poor body condition.

Fatty acids Average fat content of adult dog and cat foods is approximately 12% (dry matter basis) containing predominantly n-6 polyunsaturated fatty acids, unless fish oil is added. Cytokines derived from membrane-bound n-6 fatty acids include prostaglandins, thromboxanes, and leukotrienes of the 2- and 4-series. These cytokines are typically proinflammatory and vasoactive. In people with chronic renal failure and dogs with induced chronic renal failure, intrarenal free radical production and antioxidant depletion occurs, which may promote disease progression.[12-14]

Antioxidants Chronic renal failure is a prooxidant state occurring early in the course of the disease and progressing in severity.[14,15] Modification of oxidative stress may have benefit in managing chronic renal failure.[16]

Water-soluble vitamins Theoretically, water-soluble vitamins are lost at an increased rate with renal failure due to the polyuric state.

Electrolytes Hypokalemia and whole body potassium depletion is uncommon in dogs but occurs in 20% to 30% of cats with chronic renal failure. Hyperkalemia was reported in 13% of 186 cats with chronic renal failure.[17] Consequences of hypokalemia include weakness due to polymyopathy and progression of renal failure.[18] Amlodipine may promote hypokalemia in some cats with chronic renal failure,[19] and enalapril and benazepril may promote hyperkalemia.

Serum sodium concentrations are typically normal in pets with chronic renal failure. The role of dietary sodium in systemic arterial hypertension and chronic renal failure is controversial. High salt intake has not been associated with systemic arterial hypertension in dogs or cats; however, these studies were on healthy animals, animals with induced disease, or of short duration.[19,20] In a longer term study of cats that were healthy, were obese, older, or that had renal insufficiency, high dietary salt increased water intake and urine output in all cats except those with renal insufficiency.[21] High salt intake was not associated with increased blood pressure in any group; however, it was associated with increased serum concentrations of urea nitrogen, creatinine, and phosphorous in all, with the greatest increase in those with renal insufficiency.

Acid-base balance Metabolic acidosis occurs commonly in dogs and cats with chronic renal failure. Retention of metabolic acids, lactic acid production, electrolyte imbalances, and consumption of dietary acids are responsible. As renal function declines, capacity to excrete hydrogen and reabsorb bicarbonate is reduced and metabolic acidosis occurs. Metabolic acidosis may exacerbate hypokalemia, increase muscle catabolism and loss of lean mass, disrupt intracellular metabolism, and promote osteodystrophy. Cats appear to adapt to chronic renal failure, and metabolic acidosis does not appear to occur until later in the course of the disease.[22]

Moisture Due to the polyuric nature of chronic renal failure, dehydration may occur, especially in cats. Canned formulated diets contain 70% to 80% moisture and dry formulated diets contain 10% to 12% moisture; therefore, dehydration is more likely to occur in animals consuming a dry formulated diet.

Protein Azotemia is by definition an increase in nitrogenous compounds in blood, the majority of which are derived from dietary protein or catabolism of endogenous protein. The rationale for formulating a diet that contains reduced quantity of highly biologically available protein and adequate nonprotein calories is based on the premise that controlled reduction of nonessential protein results in decreased production of nitrogenous compounds. This may aid in amelioration of clinical signs associated with renal azotemia. Whether reduction of dietary protein alters progression of renal failure is less certain.[23-31]

Minerals Renal secondary hyperparathyroidism occurs commonly in dogs and cats with chronic renal failure.[1,32] Relative and absolute deficiency of calcitriol (vitamin D_3) has been hypothesized to play a pivotal role in development of renal secondary hyperparathyroidism,[33] but phosphorous retention also appears to play a role. Hyperphosphatemia due to phosphorous retention occurs early in chronic renal failure, playing a role in renal secondary hyperparathyroidism and progression of renal failure.[25,26,34,35]

Assess the Feeding Method
The most important aspect of nutritional management of chronic renal failure is appetite and whether food intake is adequate. Question owners as to the volume of food provided, how frequently it is provided, and how much of the meal is consumed by their pet. Determine whether the pet has a preference for a certain form of diet.

Initiation and Monitoring Phase

Selection of Diet
Several available diets are formulated and marketed for feeding dogs and cats with chronic renal failure. These diets are similar, although differences in ingredients and nutritional composition exist. Additionally, homemade diets can be formulated by certified veterinary nutritionists (Box 180-1).

Energy Sufficient energy must be provided to maintain body condition and bodyweight and to minimize endogenous protein catabolism, which can result in malnutrition and exacerbation of azotemia and uremia. Caloric requirements for dogs and cats with chronic renal failure are unknown, but are believed to be similar to those of healthy dogs and cats. Daily resting caloric requirements can be estimated using one of two formulas:

$$\text{Linear:} \ (30 \times BW_{kg}) + 70$$

$$\text{Exponential:} \ 70 \times BW_{kg}^{0.75}$$

Resting caloric requirement is then multiplied by a factor, usually 1.0 to 1.6, to arrive at the estimated daily maintenance caloric requirement.[36] This is only an estimate and individual

Box • 180-1

Veterinary Nutrition Centers and On-Line Sites That Can Formulate Complete and Balanced Homemade Diets for Use in Chronic Renal Failure in Dogs and Cats

Angell Memorial: telephone consults (617) 522-7282

Balance IT: http://www.balanceit.com/

Michigan State University: telephone consults
  (517) 432-7782; diet analysis (517) 353-9312

Ohio State University: telephone consults (614) 292-1221 or
  (614) 292-3551

Tufts University: telephone consults (508) 839-5395
  extension 84,696; VetFax 800-829-5690

University of Tennessee: telephone consults (865) 974-8387

University of California, Davis: telephone consults (530)
  752-1387 (veterinarians); (530) 752-1393 (clients)

variability can be significant; therefore, serially monitor body weight, body condition, and appetite, adjusting intake as needed. As chronic renal failure progresses, dogs and cats may exhibit partial or complete anorexia with associated weight loss. Consuming diets that are more calorically dense than maintenance adult foods promotes adequate energy intake with less volume intake resulting in less gastric distention and nausea. Because dietary fat is more calorically dense than dietary protein and carbohydrates, these diets are typically higher in fat when compared with maintenance adult foods. Available diets formulated for renal failure contain 12% to 30% crude fat (dry matter basis). Nausea and anorexia associated with chronic renal failure may also occur because of hypergastrinemia and gastric hyperacidity.[9] Administration of histamine-2-receptor antagonists or other antacids may be beneficial.

Fatty acids   In people, chronic renal failure is associated with increased free radical production and antioxidant depletion that may promote progression of disease. Dogs fed diets containing 15% fat with fish oil had a more sustained glomerular filtration rate (GFR) when compared with dogs fed beef tallow or safflower oil.[37] This benefit has not been demonstrated in cats.

Antioxidants   Cats fed a therapeutic diet formulated for managing chronic renal failure that was supplemented with vitamin E (742 mg/kg), vitamin C (84 mg/kg) and beta-carotene (2.1 mg/kg) had a significant reduction in oxidative DNA damage.[38] In an unpublished study of 6- to 8-year-old Beagles using the remnant kidney model, dogs were divided into four dietary groups: high n-3 fatty acids, high n-3 fatty acids plus antioxidant supplementation, high n-6 fatty acids, and high n-6 fatty acids plus antioxidant supplementation.[13] Specific antioxidants were vitamin E, carotenoids, and lutein (amounts not specified), and dietary total (n-6 + n-3) polyunsaturated fatty acid content was approximately 2.5% (dry matter basis). Results demonstrated independent and additive protective effects of antioxidant therapy and n-3 fatty acids. GFR rate of decline was slowed by n-3 fatty acids and by addition of antioxidants; effects were additive and were associated with reduced magnitude of proteinuria, glomerulosclerosis, and interstitial fibrosis.

Water-soluble vitamins   Although B vitamin deficiency has not been demonstrated with chronic renal failure, many diets formulated for managing chronic renal failure contain higher amounts of B vitamins when compared with adult maintenance diets. B vitamin supplementation may also stimulate appetite.

Electrolytes   Diets formulated for chronic renal failure are typically higher in potassium content than adult maintenance foods; potassium citrate is often used in order to provide a source of potassium as well as alkalinization. The goal is to maintain serum potassium concentrations in the middle to upper half of the laboratory reference range. If necessary, potassium can be supplemented orally as gluconate or citrate salts. Potassium chloride is not recommended because of poor palatability and acidifying nature. Potassium gluconate is administered orally at 2 to 6 mEq/cat/day and potassium citrate is administered at 40 to 75 mEq/kg/day depending on the body weight and severity of hypokalemia. Routine low-dose potassium supplementation has been recommended for cats with chronic renal failure; however, a recent clinical study failed to show that supplementation with 4 mEq/day of potassium gluconate improved muscle potassium stores when compared with sodium gluconate.[39] In this study, median muscle potassium content did increase in the potassium-supplemented group to a level approaching potassium content of normal cat muscle, and no significant adverse events were reported. Based on current data, no recommendation can be made for or against low-dose potassium supplementation.

Whether dietary sodium content should be restricted with chronic renal failure is controversial. In one study, high dietary sodium intake in cats with naturally occurring chronic renal failure was associated with worsening azotemia[21]; however, in another study of induced chronic renal failure in cats, sodium restriction was associated with hypokalemia.[19] Thus, salt supplementation and salt restriction must be done cautiously and patients should be monitored. Increased dietary sodium may increase urinary calcium excretion and can contribute to ongoing renal damage in cats with marginal renal function and to possible development of calcium oxalate urolithiasis.

Acid-base balance   Treatment options for managing metabolic acidosis associated with chronic renal failure include dietary modification and alkalinization therapy. Dietary protein is a major source of organic acids; therefore, reduction of dietary protein decreases metabolic acidosis. Most diets formulated for renal failure are reduced in dietary protein and contain potassium citrate, an alkalinizing compound. Oral sodium bicarbonate may be used for additional alkalinization therapy. Because the effects of gastric acid on oral sodium bicarbonate are unpredictable, dose should be individualized; initial starting dosage is 8 to 12 mg/kg PO q8-12h. Many dogs and cats will not willingly accept oral sodium bicarbonate administration. Potassium citrate is another alkalinizing agent that has an additional advantage of providing potassium to cats prone to or affected with hypokalemia. Starting dosage is 40 to 80 mg/kg PO q8-12h.

Moisture   Voluntary water intake may be insufficient to maintain hydration, especially in cats. Feeding a canned formulated diet, which contain 70% to 80% water, may provide adequate fluid intake. In patients that cannot maintain hydration by voluntary consumption of water, additional fluids may be administered SQ or by a feeding tube. Lactated Ringer's solution is used most commonly for SQ fluid administration; use of glucose-containing solutions is discouraged because of risk of infection. Typically, cats and small dogs receive 75 to 150 mL SQ q24-72h. Amount administered and frequency of administration should be based on response to fluid administration. Nasogastric, esophagostomy, or gastrostomy feeding tubes may be placed in order to facilitate fluid administration in animals that do not tolerate SQ administration of fluids. Warm tap water may be administered via feeding tube.

Protein Dietary protein requirement for dogs and cats with chronic renal failure is unknown. Diets formulated for managing dogs with renal failure typically contain 13% to 18% protein (dry matter basis) and diets formulated for managing cats with renal failure typically contain 25% to 32% protein (dry matter basis). Another means to decrease blood concentrations of nitrogen-containing compounds (blood urea nitrogen and creatinine) is to facilitate excretion of nitrogen through the gastrointestinal tract. This can be accomplished by providing probiotics or soluble fiber. New supplements, including fiberlike polysaccharides derived from chitin and bacterial productions, are available as phosphate binders and agents that reduce azotemia. Limited data exist as to efficacy, and maximal effect occurs when combined with nutritional therapy.[40-44]

Minerals Dietary phosphorous restriction decreases the degree of hyperphosphatemia and hyperparathyroidism and slows progression of chronic renal failure in dogs and cats.[3,25,26,34,45] Dietary phosphorous content for management of chronic renal failure should be 0.2% to 0.5% (dry matter basis) while maintaining a Ca:P ratio of 1.1-1.3:1.0. In stage I and II renal failure, feeding a phosphorous-restricted diet may decrease parathyroid hormone concentrations to normal.[35,45]

Clinical studies of dietary modification in dogs and cats with chronic renal failure Several studies have demonstrated longer survival times and better quality of life in dogs and cats with chronic renal failure fed accordingly.[1-4] Most of these studies showed at least a twofold increase in survival in dogs and cats fed a "renal failure" diet. Diets were most effective with stage II renal failure. Efficacy with stage I renal failure has not been demonstrated.

Selection of Feeding Method Most dogs and cats with chronic renal failure are fed orally and some require administration of appetite stimulants such as mirtazapine; however, nutritional support can be provided using feeding tubes.[46] The formulation of the diet, dry versus canned, may be modified to stimulate adequate nutritional intake as well as moisture intake. Feeding canned diets increases moisture intake and may help prevent dehydration from occurring due to polyuria of chronic renal failure. It may also be necessary to modify feeding frequency if animals are unable or unwilling to consume large meals. Some dogs and cats require feeding smaller amounts, three or four times daily.

Monitoring Patient Response Chronic renal failure is a progressive disease; therefore, serial monitoring is important. Monitoring of nutritional management of chronic renal failure involves body condition score, body weight, appetite, quality of life, and biochemical parameters. Frequency of monitoring should be individualized to the patient and to the stage of chronic renal failure. Most animals should be monitored every 4 to 6 months in stage I or II renal failure and more frequently in stage III and IV, or if renal failure is unstable or progressing rapidly.

REFERENCES

The reference list can be found on the companion Expert Consult Web site at *www.expertconsult.com*.

CHAPTER 181

Dietary and Medical Considerations in Hyperlipidemia

Denise A. Elliott
Patricia A. Schenck

Hyperlipidemia is a consequence of elevated plasma concentrations of triglyceride and/or cholesterol and is due to a disturbance in plasma lipoprotein metabolism. In the fasted state, hyperlipidemia is an abnormality caused by accelerated production or delayed degradation of lipoproteins. The lipoproteins function to transport insoluble triglyceride and cholesterol through the blood. The major classes of lipoproteins differ in their lipid content, apoprotein content, size, density, and electrophoretic mobility.[1]

Lipoproteins are categorized according to their density as chylomicrons, very–low-density lipoprotein (VLDL), low-density lipoprotein (LDL), and the high-density lipoprotein (HDL). The system is dynamic; one class produces another during its metabolism (Figure 181-1). The chylomicron and VLDL are involved primarily in triglyceride metabolism, whereas HDL and LDL are involved primarily in cholesterol metabolism.

PATHOPHYSIOLOGY

After digestion and absorption, cholesterol and triglyceride are packaged into chylomicron particles by enterocytes. Chylomicrons are secreted into mesenteric lymph, through which they ultimately reach the systemic circulation. Endothelial lipoprotein lipase (LPL) hydrolyzes the triglyceride core of chylomicrons to free fatty acids and glycerol. The free fatty acids diffuse into adjacent tissues and are either resynthesized into triglyceride and stored (adipocyte) or used for energy (myocyte). Depletion of the triglyceride component of the chylomicron alters the surface so that the chylomicron is converted into a chylomicron remnant; the remnant is then recognized and removed from the circulation by specific hepatic receptors. Chylomicrons are usually present in plasma 30 minutes to 2 hours after a fat-containing meal, and hydrolysis is normally complete within 6 to 10 hours of eating.

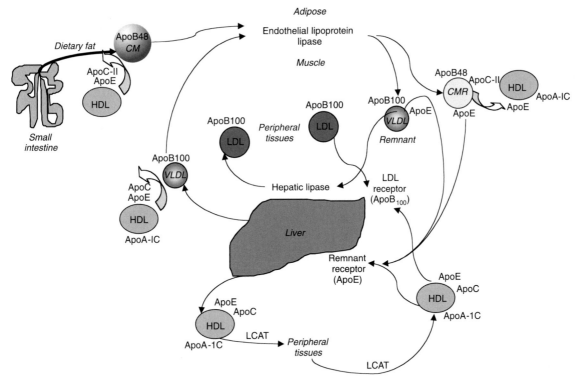

Figure 181-1 Schematic representation of lipid metabolism. *CM,* Chylomicron; *CMR,* chylomicron remnant; *HDL,* high-density lipoprotein; *LCAT,* lecithin:cholesterol acyl transferase; *LDL,* low-density lipoprotein; *VLDL,* very–low-density lipoprotein.

Excess free fatty acids in the liver that are not directly oxidized for energy are transformed by the hepatocyte into triglyceride, packaged into VLDL particles, and secreted into blood. Endothelial LPL then removes and hydrolyzes the triglyceride portion of the VLDL into free fatty acids and glycerol. Removal of the triglyceride core converts the VLDL to a LDL particle. The LDL particle is a cholesterol- and phospholipid-rich entity that functions to transport cholesterol to tissues, where it may be used for membrane synthesis or steroid hormone production. Ultimately, LDL particles bind to LDL receptors, and are removed by the liver.

The liver also secretes nascent HDL particles into the circulation. HDLs are rich in proteins with lower amounts of lipid. HDL transfers ApoC and ApoE to chylomicron and VLDL particles. Excess tissue cholesterol is transferred to HDL particles as plasma lecithin:cholesterol acyl transferase (LCAT) esterifies cholesterol to hydrophobic cholesteryl esters. HDLs scavenge excess unesterified cholesterol from cells and other lipoproteins and return it to the liver for excretion into bile. This process is often referred to as *reverse cholesterol transport.* In humans, a second enzyme (cholesteryl ester transfer protein [CETP]) can function to transfer HDL cholesteryl esters to chylomicrons and VLDL and LDL particles in exchange for triglyceride. However, dogs and cats have very low levels of CETP; thus there is little transfer of cholesterol ester to LDL,[2,3] and most cholesterol is contained within HDLs rather than LDLs.

Hypertriglyceridemia can develop secondary to increased chylomicron production (excessive dietary intake of lipid), ineffective clearance of the chylomicron particle, increased VLDL production (excessive dietary intake of lipids and/or carbohydrate, excessive endogenous production, or mobilization of lipids), and ineffective clearance of the VLDL particle (Box 181-1). Likewise, hypercholesterolemia (see Box 181-1)

Box • **181-1**

Pathophysiologic Mechanisms Contributing to Hypertriglyceridemia and Hypercholesterolemia

Hypertriglyceridemia	*Hypercholesterolemia*
Increased chylomicron production	Increased production of VLDL
Excessive dietary lipid intake	
Reduced chylomicron clearance	Reduced clearance of LDL
Increased VLDL production	
Excess dietary lipid intake	Reduced clearance of HDL
Excess dietary carbohydrate intake	
Excess endogenous free fatty acid production	
Excess mobilization of free fatty acids	
Reduced VLDL clearance	

HDL, High-density lipoprotein; *LDL,* low-density lipoprotein; *VLDL,* very–low-density lipoprotein.

can arise from increased production of the LDL precursor (VLDL), or reduced clearance of the LDL or HDL particle.

CLASSIFICATION

Postprandial hyperlipidemia is the most common cause of hyperlipidemia in the dog and cat. This is a normal physiologic manifestation caused by the production of triglyceride-rich chylomicrons and usually resolves within 2 to 10 hours. In contrast, pathologic abnormalities (Box 181-2) in plasma lipids and lipoproteins may be of genetic or familial origin (primary) or arise as a consequence of disease (secondary). Primary hyperlipoproteinemias have been reported in several breeds of dogs including the Shetland Sheepdog, Beagle, Miniature Poodle, Cocker Spaniel, and the English Cocker Spaniel.[4] Idiopathic hyperlipidemia of the Miniature Schnauzer is the most commonly recognized canine hyperlipoproteinemia. Although all mechanisms and genetics have not been fully elucidated, it is characterized by excessive VLDL particles with or without concurrent hyperchylomicronemia, mild hypercholesterolemia, and a significant reduction in LPL activity.[4-7] Feline familial hyperlipidemia is characterized as a fasting hyperchylomicronemia with a slight increase in VLDL and is due to production of an inactive LPL.[8-12] Idiopathic hyperchylomicronemia has also been observed in dogs and is characterized by hypertriglyceridemia, hyperchylomicronemia, and normal serum cholesterol concentrations.[12] Idiopathic hypercholesterolemia due to an increase in HDL_1 has been observed in Briards[13] and in other breeds.

Diseases associated with secondary hyperlipidemia include endocrine disorders (hypothyroidism, diabetes mellitus, hyperadrenocorticism), nephrotic syndrome, cholestasis, pancreatitis, and drug-induced.[1,14] A summary of the lipoprotein changes associated with disease is presented in Table 181-1. With treatment of the underlying disease, many of the lipid abnormalities are reversed. Hypothyroidism is the most common cause of hypercholesterolemia in the dog.[15] There is a decrease in lipid degradation; lipid synthesis also decreases, but to a lesser degree. Decreased LPL activity impairs the removal of triglyceride-rich lipoproteins, and thyroid hormone deficiency reduces the biliary excretion of cholesterol. The resultant increase in intrahepatic cholesterol down-regulates the hepatic LDL receptor, increasing the level of circulating LDL and HDL.[1] Naturally occurring atherosclerosis has been associated with hypothyroidism in the dog.[16]

In diabetes mellitus, insulin deficiency reduces the production of LPL, with subsequent decreased clearance of triglyceride-rich lipoproteins. Furthermore, hormone-sensitive lipase is activated, causing the release of large quantities of free fatty acids into the blood; these free fatty acids are converted by the liver into triglycerides, packaged into VLDL, and secreted back into the circulation. Thus the hypertriglyceridemia seen with diabetes mellitus is attributed to both a reduction of LPL and increased production and decreased clearance of VLDL particles. Insulin deficiency increases the synthesis of cholesterol in the liver. The increased intrahepatic cholesterol concentration down-regulates the hepatocyte LDL receptor and consequently reduces the clearance of circulating LDL and HDL particles.

The mechanism of hypertriglyceridemia associated with hyperadrenocorticism is probably due to stimulation of hormone-sensitive lipase with release of free fatty acids into the circulation. Similar to diabetes mellitus, excess free fatty acids are converted into VLDL particles. In addition, glucocorticoids inhibit LPL activity, thereby reducing the clearance of triglyceride-rich lipoproteins.

Box • 181-2

Primary and Secondary Causes of Hyperlipidemia in the Dog and Cat

Primary Disorders	Idiopathic hyperlipoproteinemia (Miniature Schnauzers, Briards, Beagles)
	Idiopathic hypercholesterolemia (Briards)
	Inherited hyperchylomicronemia of cats
	Idiopathic hyperchylomicronemia
	Primary hypercholesterolemia
Secondary Disorders	Postprandial
	High-fat diets
	Pancreatitis
	Hypothyroidism
	Cholestasis
	Diabetes mellitus
	Nephrotic syndrome
	Hyperadrenocorticism
	Obesity

Table • 181-1

Expected Lipoprotein Changes in Hyperlipidemias

CONDITION	CHOLESTEROL	TRIGLYCERIDE	CHYLOMICRON	LDL/VLDL	HDL₂	HDL₁	LPL*
Idiopathic hyperlipoproteinemia	↑	↑↑	±	↑		±	↓
Idiopathic hypercholesterolemia	↑	N	N	N	N	↑	N
Idiopathic hyperchylomicronemia	↑	↑↑	↑↑				↓†
Hypothyroidism	↑	↑		↑↑		↑	
Hyperadrenocorticism	↑	↑		↑			
Diabetes mellitus	↑	↑		↑↑		↑	↓‡
Nephrotic syndrome	Early ↑	Later ↑	±	↑↑			↓
Cholestasis	↑			↑		↓	
Pancreatitis	↑	↑		↑	↓	±	↓
High-fat diets	↑			↑		↑	
Ultra–high-fat diets	↑	↑		↑		↑	
Obesity	±		±	↑			↓

HDL_1, high-density lipoprotein-1; HDL_2, high-density lipoprotein-2; *LDL*, low-density lipoprotein; *LPL*, lipoprotein lipase; *N*, normal; *VLDL*, very–low-density lipoprotein.
*Lipoprotein lipase activity.
†Presumptive decrease based on literature reports and human findings.
‡Presumptive decrease based on human findings.

CLINICAL FEATURES

Waxing and waning vomiting, diarrhea, and/or abdominal discomfort are the most common clinical presentations associated with hypertriglyceridemia. Severe hypertriglyceridemia (>1000 mg/dL) has been associated with pancreatitis, lipemia retinalis, seizures, cutaneous xanthomas, peripheral nerve paralysis, and behavioral changes.[11,17-23] Cutaneous xanthomas, which represent lipid-laden macrophages and foam cells, are the most common manifestation of hypertriglyceridemia in the cat.[21] Severe hypercholesterolemia has been associated with arcus lipoides corneae, lipemia retinalis, and atherosclerosis.

DIAGNOSIS

If a dog or cat has hyperlipidemia after a 10- to 12-hour fast, the length of fasting should be verified. Secondary causes of hyperlipidemia should be ruled out first; primary hyperlipidemia is considered when fasting hyperlipidemia occurs and all causes of secondary hyperlipidemia have been ruled out (Figure 181-2). Every attempt should be made to determine if the hyperlipidemia is primary or secondary, as hyperlipemia secondary to an underlying disorder will typically resolve or improve with correction of the metabolic disturbance. Therefore, each dog or cat requires a full history, physical examination, complete blood count, serum biochemistry panel, and urinalysis. Additional diagnostic tests such as thyroxine concentrations, bile acids, abdominal ultrasound, and evaluation of adrenal function may be indicated.

Serum turbidity can provide an estimation of the triglyceride content. Clear serum usually has a triglyceride concentration of <200 mg/dL. Serum appears hazy when triglyceride concentration is about 300 mg/dL and has the appearance of skim milk at a triglyceride concentration around 1000 mg/dL.[1] Patients with pure hypercholesterolemia do not exhibit hyperlipidemia. Samples to confirm hypertriglyceridemia should be obtained after a 12- to 18-hour fast (Figure 181-3). A serum sample rather than whole blood or plasma should be submitted for assessment, and the sample can be refrigerated or frozen for several days without affecting test results. During assessment of the sample for hypertriglyceridemia, the laboratory should not clear the sample prior to determination of the triglyceride concentration. Clearing hyperlipidemic samples by centrifugation removes chylomicrons, which artificially lowers the triglyceride concentration.

The refrigeration test (Figure 181-4) can help delineate if the hyperlipidemia is predominantly due to excess chylomicrons or VLDLs.[23] When a hyperlipidemic sample is refrigerated overnight (about 12 hours), chylomicrons will float and form a cream layer. If the infranatant remains cloudy, then VLDLs are present in excess. Formation of a cream layer over a cloudy serum layer suggests both excess chylomicrons and VLDL particles.

Lipoprotein electrophoresis can be utilized to distinguish the lipoproteins in serum.[24] Electrophoresis separates lipopro-

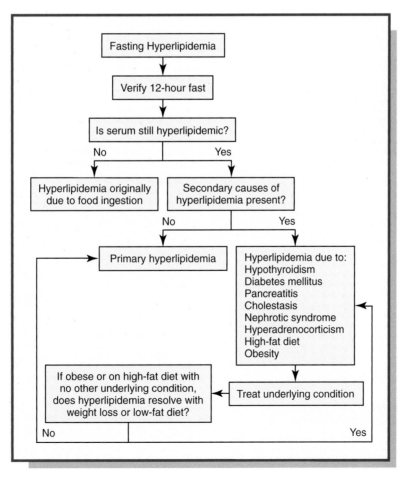

Figure 181-2 Algorithm to determine the cause of hyperlipoproteinemia. (From Encyclopedia of canine clinical nutrition, Royal Canin.)

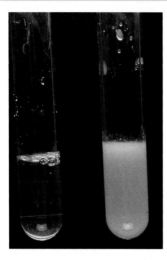

Figure 181-3 The appearance of normal *(left tube)* and hyperlipidemic serum *(right tube)*. Normal serum should be clear, with no evidence of turbidity. Fasting serum that is turbid indicates the presence of excess lipid in the serum *(right tube)*.

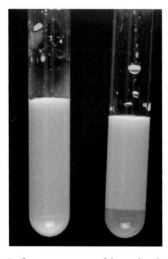

Figure 181-4 Refrigeration test of hyperlipidemic serum. On the left is a fasting hyperlipidemic serum sample from a dog. Following a refrigeration test, a lactescent layer ("cream layer") appears on the top of the serum. This layer is due to increased chylomicron particles present in the serum sample. Note that the serum below the top lactescent layer is also turbid, indicating the presence of other excess lipoproteins.

teins based on their charge and mobility on agarose gel, and provides a semiquantitative determination of lipoproteins present. Serum that has not been frozen should be used for electrophoresis, and the results should be interpreted by someone knowledgeable of canine or feline lipoproteins (not a human laboratory). Lipoprotein electrophoresis is most useful for monitoring effectiveness of treatment.

MANAGEMENT

A recommendation to treat primary hyperlipidemia involves a lifelong commitment. If the hyperlipidemia is secondary to another disease process, treatment of the underlying disease will typically decrease or eliminate the hyperlipidemia. In general, serum triglyceride >500 mg/dL or cholesterol

>750 mg/dL should be treated. A realistic goal of therapy is to reduce the triglyceride concentrations to less than 400 mg/dL. While dogs and cats are resistant to the development of atherosclerosis, naturally occurring atherosclerosis has been reported in dogs with diabetes mellitus and hypothyroidism.[16,25-27] Persistent hyperlipidemia may lead to pancreatitis, diabetes mellitus, and can contribute to progressive renal injury.[28-30]

A switch to a low-fat diet with moderate protein content is the initial therapy. The low-fat diet should contain less than 20% fat on a metabolizable energy (ME) basis for dogs, and less than 25% fat on a ME basis for cats. The diet must be chosen based on ME; the percent fat as stated on the diet label does not represent the amount of fat being consumed on an ME basis. Treats should be restricted to 5% or less of the daily caloric intake and changed to low-fat commercial varieties. If the pet is overweight, caloric restriction is indicated and beneficial as it decreases the production of VLDL from excess dietary energy. Fructooligosaccharides and beet pulp in the diet are also beneficial as this blend has been shown to decrease the triglyceride and cholesterol concentrations in dogs.[31] An increase in soluble fiber can decrease serum cholesterol by about 10% due to an interference with bile acid reabsorption.

The presence of hyperlipidemia should be reevaluated after 6 to 8 weeks of feeding the low-fat diet. If hyperlipidemia is still present, the dietary history (especially the feeding of treats) should be carefully reviewed. A diet lower in fat can be chosen; however, a low-fat diet alone may not result in resolution of hyperlipidemia in some animals.[32] If hyperlipidemia is still present, fish oil (1 g/10 lb or 1 g/4.55 kg body weight daily) can be added to the treatment regimen. Fish oils are rich in omega-3 fatty acids, and are effective at lowering serum triglyceride and cholesterol in many patients. Fish oil supplementation may act by decreasing the production of VLDL, stimulating the activity of LPL, decreasing the intestinal absorption of lipid, and increasing the secretion of cholesterol into bile.[33-35]

A combination of a low-fat diet with fish oil therapy has been effective in resolving the hyperlipidemia in the majority of animal patients.[1] No long-term studies to ensure safety of lipid-lowering agents have been performed in dogs or cats; however, in other species, the addition of dietary fish oils has been relatively safe. Since fish oils are a dietary supplement, they are easily obtained and relatively inexpensive.

Treatment using pharmaceutical lipid-lowering agents has been attempted with variable results.[36] All of these pharmaceuticals have toxic effects, are not approved for use in animals, and should be used with caution. Until further studies evaluate the dose, effect, and toxicity, drug therapy should only be attempted in those animals that have severe hypertriglyceridemia that cannot be ameliorated by a low-fat diet and fish oil therapy.

Gemfibrozil (a fibric acid derivative) can lower serum triglyceride in humans by as much as 40%, and its use has been used in the dog (200 mg/day) and cat (10 mg/kg BW q12h). Reported adverse effects include abdominal pain, vomiting, diarrhea, and abnormal liver function tests. Niacin (100 mg/day, dog) may lower serum triglyceride concentrations, but adverse effects are frequent and include vomiting, diarrhea, erythema, pruritus, and abnormalities in liver function tests.[32] The statins (lovastatin, simvastatin, pravastatin, fluvastatin, cerivastatin, atorvastatin) primarily suppress cholesterol by 20% to 40% in humans, but can also decrease triglyceride by 10% to 15%. Adverse effects include lethargy, diarrhea, muscle pain, and hepatotoxicity. Lovastatin (10 to 20 mg PO once daily) may be tried in dogs with persistent severe hypercholesterolemia that does not respond to diet and fish oil therapy. Lovastatin should not be used in patients with hepatic disease. Probucol has been used in humans as a cholesterol-lowering agent, but should be avoided as it often causes cardiac arrhythmias. Bile acid sequestrates such as cholestyramine (1 to 2 g PO BID) are effective at lowering serum cholesterol but have been associated with constipation. Cholestyramine also interferes with the absorption of other oral medications, and may increase serum triglyceride concentration.

CONCLUSION

To establish a diagnosis of primary hyperlipidemia, postprandial and secondary causes must be ruled out by a complete medical and diagnostic evaluation. Treatment of the underlying secondary causes that contribute to the disease results in resolution of the hyperlipidemia. A low-fat diet, possibly with the addition of fish oil, is the cornerstone for management of the patient with primary hyperlipidemia.

REFERENCES

The reference list can be found on the companion Expert Consult Web site at *www.expertconsult.com.*

CHAPTER 182

The Principles and Implementation of Enteral Nutrition

Stanley L. Marks

Nutritional support is aimed at minimizing development of malnutrition in animals at risk, while maintaining or enhancing immunologic and intestinal barrier function. The goal of nutritional support is to provide a formula of fuels and nutrients in proportions that can be utilized by animals with maximal efficiency. Choosing the proper enteral access technique requires knowledge of the limitations and benefits of techniques available for obtaining enteral access. The reader is encouraged to read Chapter 85 for a thorough review of the techniques and complications associated with placement of these devices.

RATIONALE FOR ENTERAL NUTRITIONAL SUPPORT

Enteral feeding is indicated for animals unable to ingest adequate amounts of calories but that have sufficient gastrointestinal function to allow digestion and absorption of feeding solutions delivered into the gastrointestinal tract via an enteral feeding device. The rationale for prescribing enteral nutrition rather than parenteral nutrition (PN) is based on the superior maintenance of intestinal structure and function, safety of administration, and reduced cost of enteral alimentation. The average daily cost of total parenteral nutrition (TPN) for maintaining the caloric requirements of a 20-kg dog is approximately 5 to 30 times greater (excluding catheter costs) than the cost of a commercial liquid enteral formula, and 60 times greater than the cost of a commercial intestinal canned diet. The most important stimulus for mucosal cell proliferation is the direct presence of nutrients in the intestinal lumen. Bowel rest due to starvation or administration of TPN leads to villous atrophy, increased intestinal permeability, and a reduction in intestinal disaccharidase activities.[1,2] Prolonged fasting in the stressed, critically ill animal can lead to intestinal barrier failure and increased permeability to bacteria and endotoxins. However, enteral nutrition may result in underfeeding, perceived intolerance, aspiration, access-related complications, and diarrhea.

PATIENT SELECTION FOR NUTRITIONAL SUPPORT

Efforts to assess nutritional status and attempts to decide whether nutritional support is required on the basis of a single biochemical measurement or bodyweight determination are simplistic and of limited value. Objective methods of assessing nutritional status such as body composition measurement (anthropometry, bioelectrical impedance measurements, dual energy x-ray absorptiometry) are still in their infancy in clinical veterinary medicine, with the result that a subjective global assessment of an animal's nutritional status needs to be performed. This technique is based on easily collected historical information (changes in oral intake, degree of weight loss, presence of vomiting or diarrhea) and changes found on physical examination (muscle wasting, body condition, and presence of edema or ascites).

Although body weight is routinely determined in sick animals, it is important to appreciate its limitations. The appearance of the animal cannot be equated with its state of nourishment because body weight does not differentiate between fat, lean tissue, and extracellular water. The animal's serum albumin concentration and total lymphocyte count are insensitive determinants of nutritional status. The large number of disease processes that influence these parameters are unrelated to malnutrition. Nutritional support should be considered for animals that demonstrate recent unintentional weight loss that exceeds 10% of optimal body weight or for those whose oral intake has been or will be interrupted for more than 5 days. Animals with increased nutrient losses from chronic diarrhea or vomiting, wounds, renal disease, or burns should also be considered for nutritional support.

Numerous methods exist for quantifying body composition and body fat mass in companion animals. In a clinical setting, the most widely accepted and practical method of body condition evaluation is scoring using visual assessment and palpation. This method affords a reproducible and useful assessment of nutritional status. The body condition score (BCS) is not affected by fluid shifts that can readily impact body weight, facilitating the improved assessment of nutritional status in the hospital or intensive care environment. The most widely accepted system is the nine-integer scale system, which has previously been shown to correlate well with body fat mass determined by dual energy x-ray absorptiometry (DXA).[3] Body condition scoring schemes do not incorporate the loss of lean body tissue, although the recent implementation of a muscle condition score could further enhance the assessment of nutritional status.[4]

CALCULATION OF NUTRITIONAL REQUIREMENTS

Nutritional support provides substrates for gluconeogenesis and protein synthesis and provides the energy needed to meet additional demands of host defense, wound repair, cell division, and growth. The anticipated duration of nutritional support should be determined and factored into the nutritional support plan. In addition, the most optimal route of nutritional support should be determined (enteral vs. parenteral) based on the underlying disease process, the integrity of the gastrointestinal tract, and the pet's clinical signs (e.g., intractable vomiting, diarrhea, dysphagia). Appetite stimulants are usually of little to no benefit in the management of hospitalized critically ill patients, and are best reserved for animals that are recovering sufficiently or are at home.

The provision of nutritional support should provide sufficient substrates for gluconeogenesis, protein synthesis, and energy to sustain vital physiologic processes such as immune function, wound repair, and cell division. Energy expenditure has been determined using indirect calorimetry in research populations of dogs; however, utilization of mathematical formulas remains the most efficient, cost-effective, and practical means of estimating a patient's energy requirement. An estimate of an animal's resting energy requirement (RER) is needed to determine the minimum amount of food necessary to sustain critical physiologic processes. The RER is the animal's energy requirement at rest in a thermoneutral environment and in a postabsorptive state. A linear formula can be applied to determine the RER of dogs and cats weighing between 2 and 45 kg, or alternatively, an allometric formula preferred by the author can be applied to dogs and cats of all weights.

Allometric formula: $\text{RER (kcal/day)} = 70 \, (\text{BW in kg})^{0.75}$

Linear formula: $\text{RER (kcal/day)} = 30 \, (\text{BW in kg}) + 70$

Until recently, many clinicians multiplied the RER by an "illness factor" between 1.1 to 2 to account for the increased metabolism associated with different disease states and injuries. Veterinary nutritionists discourage the implementation of this extrapolated and subjective practice, and advocate a more cautious approach to minimize the likelihood of overfeeding and its associated complications. Nutritional support in hospitalized patients should initially deliver sufficient calories and protein to meet the patient's RER at its current weight, adjusted for body condition. This is a rational and safe estimate that decreases likelihood of metabolic complications such as refeeding syndrome. Close observation of changes in body weight, physical examination findings (decreased subcutaneous fat stores, muscle wasting, and presence of edema or ascites), and ongoing losses (diarrhea, vomiting, exudative wounds) will help determine whether to increase or decrease the patient's caloric intake. Weight changes often reflect fluid dynamics in the early period following injury.

DIET SELECTION

Type of feeding formula depends on the selected route of feeding, the functional status of the gastrointestinal tract, and the animal's nutrient requirements. Other factors, such as cost, availability, and ease of use, may also be important. Animals fed via nasoesophageal or jejunostomy feeding tubes are limited to receiving liquid enteral formulas that have a caloric density of approximately 1 to 1.3 kcal per mL. When selecting a liquid formula for feeding, veterinary professionals should pay particular attention to the amount of protein in the formula, the type of protein (intact proteins, peptides, and amino acids), and the quality of the protein. Whole egg has the highest biologic value, followed by cow's milk, lactalbumin, beef, soy, and casein. Most human liquid formulas contain less than 20% protein calories, precluding their use for the long-term (longer than 2 weeks) feeding of cats. The lower protein formulas should be supplemented with protein modules such as Promod (Ross Laboratories, Columbus, Ohio), Casec (Mead-Johnson, Evansville, Ind.) or Promagic (Animal Nutrition Laboratories, Burlington, N.J.) at 15 to 30 g casein or whey powder per 8–fl-oz can. Almost all human liquid enteral formulas lack taurine, an essential amino acid in cats, which necessitates its supplementation (250 mg taurine per 8–fl-oz can) in this species. High-protein commercial human liquid formulations contain between 21% to 42% protein calories and include Impact (Novartis Nutrition, Minneapolis, Minn.), Immun-Aid (McGaw, Inc., Irvine, Calif.), Alitraq (Ross Laboratories, Columbus, Ohio), Promote (Ross Laboratories, Columbus, Ohio), and Traumacal (Mead-Johnson, Evansville, Ind.).

Polymeric solutions contain macronutrients in the form of isolates of intact protein (casein, lactalbumin, whey, egg white), triglycerides, and carbohydrate polymers. The carbohydrates are usually glucose polymers in the form of starch and its hydrolysates. Fats are of vegetable origin. The osmolality varies between 300 and 450 mOsm/kg in solutions with a caloric density of 1 kcal/mL; however, the osmolality may reach 650 mOsm/kg in solutions with a greater caloric density. Monomeric solutions contain protein as peptides or amino acids, fat as long chain triglycerides (LCT), or a mixture of LCT and medium chain triglycerides (MCT), and carbohydrates as partially hydrolyzed starch maltodextrins and glucose oligosaccharides. These solutions require less digestion and their absorption is more efficient than that of regular foods or polymeric solutions; however, the partially digested macronutrients contribute to the higher osmolality, which is between 400 and 700 mOsm/kg.

Commercial blenderized pet food diets are recommended for feeding via esophagostomy or gastrostomy tubes. In select cases, the feeding of a liquid enteral formulation may be indicated (nasoesophageal or jejunostomy tube feeding). There are a number of complete and balanced veterinary enteral formulations (Table 182-1) that contain adequate amounts of protein, taurine, and micronutrients, which precludes the need for supplementation in most situations.

Feeding should be delayed for 12 to 24 hours after placement of a gastrostomy tube, to allow return of gastric motility and formation of a fibrin seal. In contrast, feeding can be instituted immediately after esophagostomy tube placement, once the animal has fully recovered from anesthesia. Diet can be administered as bolus feedings or continuous infusion when a gastrostomy tube is used for feeding. Improved weight gain and decreased gastroesophageal reflux have been reported in humans given continuous feedings,[5] although similar studies are lacking in the veterinary literature. If continuous feeding is employed, it should be interrupted every 8 hours to determine the residual volume by application of suction to the

Table • 182-1

Macronutrient Composition of Selected Veterinary Enteral Formulations

PRODUCT	PROTEIN TYPE	CALORIC DENSITY (kcal/mL)	NUTRIENTS (% OF TOTAL kcal)		
			PROTEIN	FAT	CARBOHYDRATE
Prescription diet a/d Canine/Feline (Hill's)	Pork liver, poultry liver, chicken, corn flour, pork protein isolate	1.1	33	55	12
Maximum-Calorie Canine & Feline (Iams)	Chicken, chicken by-product meal	2.1	29	68	3
CliniCare Canine/Feline liquid diet (Abbott)	Sodium caseinate, whey protein	1.0	30	45	25
Clinicare RF Feline liquid diet (Abbott)	Sodium caseinate, whey protein	1.0	22	57	21
CV Cardiovascular Feline Formula (Purina)	Liver, beef, corn, fish	1.37	32.6	49.8	17.7
Veterinary Diet Feline and Canine RS (Royal Canin)	Chicken liver, chicken, casein	1.0	38.9	54.8	6.3

feeding tube. If the residual volume is more than twice the volume infused in 1 hour, feeding should be discontinued for 2 hours and the rate of infusion decreased by 25% to prevent vomiting. Treatment with metoclopramide (1 to 2 mg/kg/24 hour as a continuous infusion) may be used to enhance gastric emptying and prevent vomiting.[6]

With bolus feeding, the required daily volume of food should be divided into four to six meals. Dogs and cats are usually fed approximately 25% of their caloric requirement on the first day of feeding, with a gradual increase of 25% of the caloric requirement per day. Most animals are able to reach their energy requirement by the fourth or fifth day of feeding. The food should be warmed to room temperature and fed slowly through the tube to prevent vomiting. Flushing of the tube with 15 to 20 mL of lukewarm water helps prevent clogging. Before each feeding, aspirate the tube with an empty syringe to check for residual food left in the stomach from the previous feeding. If more than half of the last feeding is removed from the stomach, the feeding should be skipped and residual volume rechecked at the next feeding.

Jejunal feeding can be started within 6 hours of tube placement if peristalsis is present. Continuous feeding should be used with jejunostomy feeding to avoid abdominal cramping and diarrhea associated with bolus feeding via this route. Continuous infusion is recommended at an initial flow rate of 1 mL/kg/hr and increased gradually over 48 hours until the total daily volume can be given over a 12- to 18-hour period.[7]

REFERENCES

The reference list can be found on the companion Expert Consult Web site at *www.expertconsult.com*.

CHAPTER 183

Home-Prepared and Raw Diets

Sally C. Perea
Sean J. Delaney

Although a majority of pet owners in the United States feed complete and balanced commercial pet foods,[1] there is a growing interest in home-prepared and raw food diets. A recent survey of pet owners in the United States and Australia reported that noncommercial foods (table scraps, leftovers, or homemade foods) were fed as part of the main diet in 30.6% of dogs and 13.1% of cats. These noncommercial foods comprised at least one quarter of the diet in 17.4% of dogs and 6.2% of cats. Fewer than 3% of pet owners in this survey reported feeding exclusively home-prepared diets, but approximately 7% of dogs received at least half their diet as home-prepared foods. Ninety-three percent of the dogs and 100% of the cats fed at least half of their daily diet from home-prepared foods were given raw bones or meat as part of their primary diet.[1]

The motivation to feed home-prepared or raw food diets varies. Some proponents of home-prepared or raw food diets cite benefits such as control over ingredients selected, avoidance of artificial preservatives, preservation of natural enzymes, and incorporation of phytonutrients.[1] Other reported motives include a desire to pamper the pet, provide a more wholesome or nutritious diet, provide a medical benefit, improve dental health, or provide a diet that more closely resembles that of wild canids or felids.[1]

Because commercial foods are consistent, complete, and balanced formulations, they are generally preferred over home-prepared foods, which are subject to recipe deviations and inconsistencies. Commercial foods that have undergone Association of American Feed Control Officials (AAFCO) feeding tests also have the advantage of demonstrating performance of the food within a species, and bioavailability of the nutrients. However, there are some indications for home-prepared foods, such as when a commercial food is not available to meet the patient's needs. A common example of this is when a pet has multiple disease conditions that require multiple nutrient modifications that are not available in one commercial food.

NUTRITIONAL ADEQUACY

One of the primary concerns with feeding home-prepared foods is appropriate nutritional balance and adequacy. Of 54 pet owners feeding their pet at least half of the diet from homemade foods in the survey mentioned above, only 16 reported use of a recipe designed for pets. Of these recipes, 8 were from a veterinarian, 3 were obtained from the Internet, and 5 were from other sources.[1] Although the nutritional adequacy of these diets was not evaluated, it raises concerns regarding potential misinformation available to the public regarding home-prepared diets for dogs and cats. Even more concerning is the large portion of owners who fed home-prepared foods that were not designed for pets.

Nutritional inadequacy and/or improper balance are problems that can affect both home-cooked and raw food diets. One study evaluating the nutritional adequacy of homemade pet diets from six published resources (49 maintenance and 36 growth diets) found that 86% of the diets had inadequate levels of various minerals, 62% had inadequate levels of various vitamins, and 55% had an inadequate protein or essential amino acid level.[2] Another study evaluating the nutritional adequacy of five raw diets (two commercially prepared and three home prepared) found that all of the diets had levels of essential nutrients below minimum recommended AAFCO levels.[3] In addition to a variety of nutrient deficiencies, all three of the home-prepared raw diets had improperly balanced calcium-to-phosphorus ratios, two had excessive levels of vitamin D, and one had excessive levels of vitamin E.[3]

In addition to deficiencies in nutrient profiles, clinical nutrient deficiencies secondary to unbalanced home-prepared foods have been reported.[4-6] Inadequate calcium and improper calcium-to-phosphorus ratio is one of the most common problems reported in both dogs and cats fed unbalanced home-prepared foods.[4,5] Calcium deficiency, with or without concurrent vitamin D deficiency, may cause nutritional secondary hyperparathyroidism. Young growing animals will commonly develop long bone abnormalities, while adult animals have been reported to develop bone resorption of the mandible and maxilla, resulting in a rubber jaw syndrome.[4,5] One report of a 6-year-old dog maintained on an unbalanced home-prepared diet for the management of lymphocytic-plasmacytic enterocolitis documented nutritional secondary hyperparathyroidism, low serum 25-hydroxycholecalciferol concentration, and clinical and computed tomography findings consistent with rubber jaw syndrome.[5] This dog had been on the unbalanced diet for 18 months. As with most nutritional deficiencies, underlying calcium deficiency is not commonly recognized until calcium stores are significantly depleted. Thus, pets on unbalanced diets may not display obvious clinical signs of underlying nutritional insufficiency. Similarly, many nutrient deficiencies, such as calcium, are not readily apparent on routine blood work because serum concentrations are tightly regulated despite severe dietary deficiency.

METHODS FOR EVALUATING NUTRITIONAL ADEQUACY OF HOME-PREPARED FOODS

Chemical nutrient analysis is the ideal method to assess nutrient composition of a home-prepared food. Unfortunately, this is cost prohibitive; therefore, most diets are evaluated based on computer evaluations. Nutrient profiles of individual ingredients can be obtained from nutrient databases, such as the USDA Nutrient Database (Table 183-1).

The nutrient profiles of individual ingredients can vary widely based on cooking method and other factors, such as the cut of meat, portion of the plant fed, and season in which the plant was grown. Therefore, a detailed diet history is the first and most important step in evaluating nutritional adequacy. Once a complete diet history is collected, the pet's daily diet can be evaluated with the use of formulation software or self-developed spreadsheets. The nutrient content of the diet can then be compared to the established nutrient requirement for the appropriate species and life stage of the pet.

While detailed evaluations should be conducted to carefully assess the nutritional adequacy and balance of a diet, there are simple items that can be evaluated quickly to assess general completeness (Figure 183-1). The first question to answer is the amount of unbalanced foods provided in the daily diet. Although feeding a diet comprised of primarily home-cooked foods will raise flags of concern, there are many pet owners who feed a lower percentage of unbalanced foods that may still be compromising the nutritional adequacy and balance of the diet. The rule of thumb is that unbalanced foods and treats should provide no more than 10% of the total daily caloric intake. When unbalanced foods are added to a complete and balanced diet, nutrient dilution occurs and essential nutrients may fall below minimum requirements. In addition, additions of unbalanced foods can also cause nutrient imbalances. For example, meats are high in phosphorus, and when added to a complete and balanced diet may result in unbalanced calcium-to-phosphorus ratios. Other foods used as treats may provide high levels of some nutrient that can reach above safe upper limits. An example of this is feeding liver as a treat. Because liver can be high in some vitamins and minerals, such as vitamin A, daily feeding can cause total dietary levels to reach unsafe amounts.

If unbalanced foods do provide more than 10% of the total daily caloric intake, an assessment should be made to determine the presence of the major categories of essential nutrients in the diet. The first step is to identify an adequate source of protein and essential amino acids, such as meat, or potentially a vegetarian protein, such as soy protein for dogs. In generally, the protein source should make up a minimum of one third of the diet by volume (higher amounts may be required for some vegetarian sources such as legumes). While dogs can generally perform well on vegetarian protein sources, providing the appropriate protein and amino acid levels with vegetarian ingredients is more challenging in cats. One reason for this is that vegetarian protein sources are generally limiting in essential sulfur-containing amino acids, such as methionine. Vegetarian protein sources also lack arachidonic acid, which is an essential dietary fatty acid for cats, but not for dogs. Arachidonic acid (20:4 n-6) is found primarily in animal fats and is therefore difficult to provide in vegetarian diets. However, a recent study in cats demonstrated that feeding high amounts of borage oil, a source of γ-linolenic acid (GLA), results in arachidonic acid enrichment of red blood cells, suggesting that diets containing high amounts of GLA may be a suitable substitute for preformed arachidonic acid.[7]

In addition to a source of arachidonic acid for cats, both dogs and cats require a source of linoleic acid (18:2 n-6). Linoleic acid is an essential fatty acid for dogs and cats and plays an important role in skin and coat health.[8] Animal fats often provide some linoleic acid, but most diets require an additional source to meet the pet's requirement. Vegetable oils such as corn oil, canola oil, safflower oil, and soybean oil can serve as dietary sources of linoleic acid. Of the readily

Table • 183-1

Nutrition Resources

NAME	WEB SITE	TELEPHONE
Institutions with Clinical Nutrition Faculty and Residents Available for Consultation		
University of California, Davis	www.vetmed.ucdavis.edu/vmth/small_animal/nutrition/default.cfm	530-752-1387
University of Missouri	www.vmth.missouri.edu	573-882-7821
University of Tennessee	www.vet.utk.edu/clinical/sacs/nutrition.php	865-974-8387
Tufts Cummings School of Veterinary Medicine	www.tufts.edu/vet	508-839-5395, x84696
Virginia Tech	www.vetmed.vt.edu/vth/nutrition.asp	540-231-4621
Home-Cooked Diet Formulations for Veterinarians Only		
Veterinary Nutritional Consultations	www.petdiets.com	800-649-2043 508-429-2043
Balance IT Vet Express*	www.balanceit.com	888-346-6362
University of California, Davis	www.vmth.ucdavis.edu/vmth/services/nutrition/nutrition.html	530-752-1387
The UCVMC-SD Clinical Nutrition Program	www.ucvmc-sd.vetmed.ucdavis.edu/nutrition.cfm	858-875-7505
Home-Cooked Diet Formulations Accessible by Clients Directly		
Veterinary Nutritional Consultations	www.petdiets.com	800-649-2043 508-429-2043
Balance IT for Pet Lovers*	www.balanceit.com	888-346-6362
Veterinary Nutrition Organizations		
American College of Veterinary Nutrition	www.acvn.org, specialty college	
American Academy of Veterinary Nutrition	www.aavn.org	
Human Foods Nutrient Content Information		
USDA Nutrient Database	www.nal.usda.gov/fnic/foodcomp/search/	

*Balance IT is owned by the authors.

available vegetable oils, corn oil has the highest concentration of linoleic acid; therefore, less corn oil is required to meet the minimum requirement and, accordingly, is frequently used by veterinary nutritionists.

Many pet owners like to cook with olive oil and may substitute recommended vegetable oils with olive oil. Olive oil has a high content of monounsaturated fatty acids (MUFA). Studies in people have shown that MUFAs can help protect against heart disease by controlling low-density lipoprotein (LDL) cholesterol levels ("bad" cholesterol), while raising high-density lipoprotein (HDL) cholesterol levels ("good" cholesterol).[9] Therefore, olive oil is often recommended as part of a healthy diet for humans. However, dogs and cats do not maintain LDLs in circulation as humans do, which prevents oxidation and formation of atherosclerotic plaques.[10] Thus, the same health benefits that are promoted for humans do not carry over to dogs and cats. In addition, olive oil has low levels of linoleic acid, requiring four to five times the amount of olive oil (compared to corn oil) to meet the minimum requirement. Because this can significantly increase the fat content of the diet, olive oil is generally avoided or used in combination with another dietary source of linoleic acid.

Although alpha-linolenic acid (18:3 n-3) has not previously been considered an essential fatty acid for dogs and cats,

more recent studies suggest that providing alpha-linolenic acid in the diet provides some benefits for optimal health, especially in growing and reproducing animals.[8] Similarly, docosahexaenoic acid (DHA) is now known to be essential for optimal brain and retinal development in puppies.[11,12] The fatty acid content of commonly supplemented oils and fats are summarized in Table 183-2. Although alpha-linolenic acid is commonly provided by terrestrial vegetable oil sources such as canola or flax seed oils, algal or fish oil sources must be used to supply long-chain omega-3 fatty acids such as eicosapentaenoic acid (EPA) and DHA in the diet.

After assessing any home-cooked diet for essential protein, amino acid, and fatty acid needs, one should identify the source of essential vitamins and minerals. Although many foods will contribute to the vitamin and mineral content of a diet, a supplemental form is generally required to ensure that recommended allowances are met. Table 183-3 outlines the National Research Council recommended levels of nutrient in a 1000-kcal diet for a dog and compares them to the levels provided in some commonly available supplements.

Depending on the supplements used, additional sources may be required to meet all essential needs. For example, a human One-A-Day Maximum multivitamin/multimineral tablet will provide enough of most of the needed vitamins and trace minerals. However, additional supplementation with

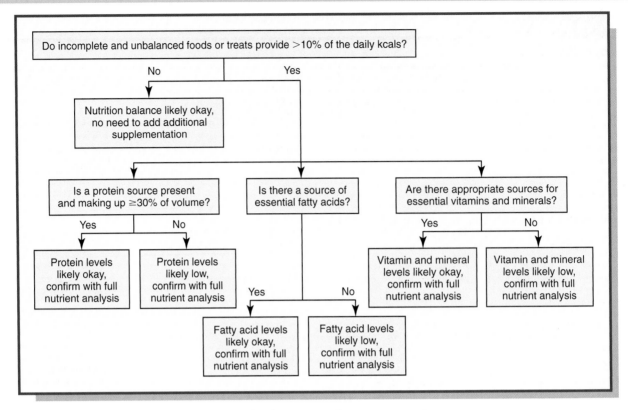

Figure 183-1   Quick assessment for nutrient completeness.

Table • 183-2

Fatty Acid Contribution of Commonly Supplemented Oil and Fat Sources

| INGREDIENT (QUANTITY) [USDA #]* | SATURATED FAT (g) | TOTAL MUFA (g) | TOTAL PUFA (g) | OMEGA-3 FATTY ACIDS | | OMEGA-6 FATTY ACIDS | | |
				LA 18:2† (g)	AA 20:4† (g)	ALA 18:3† (g)	EPA 20:05 (g)	DHA 22:05 (g)
Corn oil (1 tsp–4.5 g) [04518]	0.583	1.241	2.46	2.395	0	0.052	0	0
Canola oil (1 tsp–4.5 g) [04582]	0.331	2.847	1.332	0.855	0	0.411	0	0
Safflower oil (1 tsp–4.5 g) [04511]	0.279	3.359	0.646	0.646	0	0	0	0
Olive oil (1 tsp–4.5 g) [04053]	0.621	3.283	0.474	0.439	0	0.034	0	0
Flaxseed oil (1 tsp–4.5 g) [42231]	0.426	0.916	2.992	0.576	0	2.416	0	0
Salmon oil (1 tsp–4.5 g) [04593]	0.894	1.307	1.815	0.069	0.03	0.048	0.586	0.135
Butter, unsalted (1 tsp–4.7 g) [01145]	2.431	0.995	0.144	0.129	0	0.015	0	0
Chicken fat (1 tsp–4.2 g) [04542]	1.27	1.907	0.892	0.832	0.004	0.043	0	0

AA, Arachidonic acid; *ALA*, alpha-linolenic acid; *DHA*, docosahexaenoic acid; *EPA*, eicosapentaenoic acid; *LA*, linoleic acid; *MUFA*, monounsaturated fatty acids; *PUFA*, polyunsaturated fatty acids.
*Fatty acid compositions acquired from the USDA National Nutrient Database.
†Some values approximated from undifferentiated values when n-3 or n-6 differentiation was not reported by the USDA.

calcium, phosphorus, potassium, chloride, iodine, choline, and taurine (for cats) is commonly needed to meet minimum requirements. More recently all-in-one veterinary supplements (Balance IT) have become available to make supplementation easier.

For those multivitamin and multimineral supplements that fall short of necessary levels, calcium can be provided in a calcium-only supplement (such as calcium carbonate or calcium citrate), or a calcium and phosphorus supplement (such as dibasic or tribasic calcium phosphate or bone meal). Commonly, both a calcium-only and a calcium and phosphorus supplement should be used in combination to create an appropriate calcium-to-phosphorus balance. Bone meal is a readily available calcium and phosphorus supplement;

Table • 183-3

Comparison of National Research Council (NRC) Nutrient Requirements and Nutrition Composition of Common Multivitamin/Multimineral Supplements for Dogs*

NUTRIENT	NRC ADULT DOG REQUIREMENT AMOUNT PER 1000 kcal	ONE-A-DAY MAXIMUM MULTIVITAMIN/ MULTIMINERAL PER TABLET	BALANCE IT CANINE PER SCOOP (4.4 g)	PET-TABS PLUS FOR DOGS PER TABLET	RX ESSENTIALS FOR DOGS PER TSP (5 g)	THORNE CANINE BASIC NUTRIENTS PER CAPSULE
Vitamins						
Vitamin A (IU)	1263.3	2500.0	467.4	1500	500	500
Vitamin D (IU)	136	400	46.8	150	75	75
Vitamin E (IU)	17.8	30	19.77	15	15	50
Thiamine (mg)	0.56	1.5	0.114	0.24	5	10
Riboflavin (mg)	1.3	1.7	0.260	0.65	5	7
Pantothenic acid (mg)	3.75	10	0.773	0.68	5	10
Niacin (mg)	4.25	20	1.073	3.4	3	13
Pyridoxine (mg)	0.375	2	0.027	0.24	5	7
Folic acid (mcg)	67.5	400	0.0179	50	0.005	0.01
Vitamin B_{12} (mcg)	9	6	2.5	0.7	0.003	0.01
Choline (mg)	422	0	107.84	40	0	5
Minerals						
Calcium (g)	1	0.162	0.561	0.071	0.075	0.05
Phosphorus (g)	0.75	0.109	0.351	0.071	0	0.025
Potassium (g)	1	0.08	0.444	0.011	0.0004	0.0001
Sodium (g)	0.2	0	0.045	0.0028	0	0
Chloride (g)	0.3	0	0.073	0.0028	0	0
Magnesium (g)	0.15	0.1	0.035	0.0043	0.005	0.0005
Iron (mg)	7.5	18	7.239	3	0.25	0.25
Copper (mg)	1.5	2	0.666	0.1	0.005	0.01
Manganese (mg)	1.2	3.5	0.458	0.25	1	0
Zinc (mg)	15	15	10.69	1.4	1.5	0.5
Iodine (mg)	0.22	0.15	0.148	0	unknown	0.01
Selenium (mg)	0.088	0.02	0.016	0	0.005	0.01

*This table serves only as an informational tool to evaluate supplement completeness. The appropriate amount of supplement needed to balance a home-prepared diet must be determined by first calculating the nutrient contribution of foodstuffs, followed by evaluation of minimum allowances, safe upper limits, and appropriate balance of all nutrients.

however, it has fallen out of favor with many veterinary nutritionists due to concerns of lead contamination. In the United States, the only commercially available non–bone meal calcium and phosphorus supplement available is tribasic calcium phosphate (available under the brand name Posture). When using this and other calcium supplements, care should be taken to account for any additional vitamin D added. This is especially true when used in combination with other vitamin and mineral supplements that already provide needed vitamin D levels.

Salts can be used in home-cooked diets to provide additional sodium, chloride, potassium, and iodide. There are three basic salt supplements that are readily available for this use. The first is standard iodized salt, which provides sodium, chloride, and iodine. The second is salt substitute (such as Morton Salt Substitute), which is a potassium chloride mixture, but provides no iodine. And the third is lite salt (such as Morton Lite Salt) that provides a 50:50 mixture of iodized salt and salt substitute.

Another nutrient that may require additional supplementation is choline. Choline serves as a component of choline phospholipids and as a methyl donor for methylation reactions in the body. Other methyl donors, such as methionine, can serve as choline equivalents in the diet. Therefore, methionine levels in the diet above the dietary requirement can serve to meet a portion of the choline requirement. However, because methionine can be a limiting amino acid, especially in reduced-protein diets, additional choline supplementation is generally required. Finally, depending on the limiting nutrient in the multivitamin/multimineral supplement, additional sources may be required. Examples of this are vitamin B_{12} and zinc, which are common limiting nutrients when using One-A-Day Maximum in home-cooked diet formulations. Because simply adding higher quantities of the One-A-Day can push other nutrients toward safe upper limits, an additional vitamin B_{12} or zinc supplement may be needed.

ADDITIONAL CONCERNS WITH RAW FOOD FEEDING

In addition to nutritional inadequacy, additional risks that may come with feeding of raw food include pathogenic bacterial infection, environmental contamination, and potential gastrointestinal obstruction by bones. Contamination with pathogenic bacteria in raw pet foods has been well documented.[13-15] Although the number of pets developing illness when feeding raw food is unknown, clinical cases have been well documented and reported in the scientific literature. One report described salmonellosis in two cats from the same household fed a raw beef–based diet.[16] The first cat from this household was a 14-year-old, intact male exotic shorthair cat that died. Clinical signs prior to death included weight loss, soft stools, and at least 1 week of anorexia. Tissue cultures taken from the lung, liver, spleen, and kidney at necropsy were shown to be positive for *Salmonella typhimurium*. Unfortunately, samples from this cat's diet were not available for culture. The second cat, a 10-week-old, intact male exotic shorthair kitten, was examined 9 months later. The kitten was moribund on presentation, and euthanasia was performed at the owner's request. Necropsy revealed suppurative pneumonia and enteritis with villous blunting and erosion. Tissue cultures and subtyping revealed *Bordetella bronchiseptica* in the lung and *Salmonella newport* in both lung and small intestine samples. Samples of the raw ground beef fed to this kitten where subsequently shown to be positive for *S. newport*, confirming the raw meat as the source of infection.

Many of the studies on raw food feeding practices have been conducted in Greyhound racing and breeding facilities, where feeding of raw meat is common. One investigation of an outbreak of diarrheal disease and death of young puppies at a Greyhound breeding facility revealed *Salmonella enterica* infections that where traced back to raw beef fed to the animals.[17] Necropsies of deceased puppies revealed *S. enterica* septicemia, enteritis, and colitis. Multiple samples where collected from the facility, and *S. enterica* was recovered from 88 of 133 total samples taken. Of 61 fecal samples, 57 (93%) where found to be positive. Seventy-five percent of raw meat samples being fed at the facility were also positive. Other positive samples where collected from the soil, food bowls, water buckets, the kitchen sink, cleaning tools, floor surfaces, and flies. Serotyping of the 88 samples positive for *S. enterica* revealed 94.3% *newport*, 3.4% *typhimurium*, 1.1% *anatum*, and 1.1% *uganda*. Samples with serotype Newport were identified in multiple samples of the raw meat, confirming the raw meat as the primary source of the infection.

Pets not developing clinical illness when fed contaminated raw meat products still introduce a risk to humans and other pets in the environment through shedding of organisms in the feces.[18,19] Children, seniors, immunosuppressed, and immunocompromised individuals are at the greatest risk through environmental contamination. In response to public health concerns, the FDA prepared a set of guidelines for pet owners on the proper handling of raw pet foods to help minimize the risk of cross-contamination of pathogens.[20] From this guideline, "The FDA does not advocate a raw meat, poultry or seafood diet for pets, but is stepping up its efforts to minimize the risk such foods pose to animal and human health because we understand that some people prefer to feed these types of diets to their pets." This educational approach is also one that should be implemented by veterinarians when discussing raw pet foods with clients. After discussing these risks with owners, alternative feeding options that will improve safety can be offered. There are many commercially available cooked pet foods that offer caloric distributions similar to those of raw foods and incorporate similar feeding philosophies such as avoidance of grains, the use of vegetables, the addition of probiotics, and the use of natural preservatives and ingredients. For pet owners who prefer home-made preparations, a complete and balanced home-cooked diet can be suggested as an alternative.

INDICATIONS FOR HOME-COOKED DIETS

When available, a complete and balanced commercial pet food is preferred to preparing a home-cooked diet. The major advantages of home-cooked diets are that the ingredients and nutrients selected can be tailored specifically to the pet's needs. This can become important for patients that have multiple disease conditions that require multiple nutritional approaches not available in a single commercial food.

When selecting the appropriate nutritional management for any patient, the clinician should ask a series of questions: (1) What is the appropriate caloric distribution of macronutrients in this patient's diet? (2) Are there any micronutrients that should be modified to meet this pet's needs? (3) Are there specific ingredients or dietary antigens that must be avoided? and (4) Are there any commercial foods that meet the needs identified in questions 1 to 3?

To address the first question, the clinician should consider if any modifications to dietary protein, fat, or carbohydrate levels are indicated. If the clinician concludes that more than one of these macronutrients must be reduced or restricted, the commercial food options may be limited. For example, a patient with a history of renal disease and pancreatitis will require both protein and fat restriction. However, most commercially available foods designed for the management of renal disease are moderate to high in fat. The second and third questions consider what micronutrients in the diet should be modified and if any ingredient must be avoided. Again, if multiple disease conditions are present, the required nutrient modifications may not be available in one diet. For example, a cat with a history of struvite urolithiasis and food allergies may not tolerate the ingredients provided by commercially available foods designed for the management of struvite urolithiasis, but foods designed for the management of food allergies may not provide appropriate levels of phosphorus and magnesium to address the struvite urolithiasis.

After determining the nutritional modifications that are required for the patient, commercial foods should be explored for potential options. There may be cases where exploring the options can reveal a commercial food that addresses all of the patient's needs. For the example of concurrent renal disease and pancreatitis, currently available foods designed for the management of renal disease should be evaluated for varying fat levels. The questions should then be asked, "What is this patient's fat tolerance?" and "Are there any commercial foods that can meet his needs?" The level of fat restriction required will vary from patient to patient and is generally related to the level of dietary fat that initially contributed to the pancreatitis episode. If the patient was on a high-fat food when pancreatitis developed, the pet may be able to tolerate a moderate fat level provided by a commercially available food designed for the management of renal disease. However, if the patient is sensitive to fat and cannot tolerate moderate fat levels, most, if not all, commercially available options will be eliminated, and home cooking may be the only viable option to address both conditions.

If the choice is made to treat with a home-cooked diet, the next step is to acquire an appropriate and nutritionally balanced home-cooked diet formulation. An individual consultation with a board-certified veterinary nutritionist will often provide the most guidance and individual tailoring of a diet to meet the patient's needs (see Table 183-1). Other veterinary software programs and published recipes are also options available to veterinarians looking for more standardized dietary formulations or recommendations (see Table 183-1). Formal consultations and the use of nutrition software are generally preferred to published recipes, as they provide more up-to-date nutritional strategies and can be formulated for the individual pet's specific caloric and nutrient requirements. Most important, one should acquire a diet that is complete and balanced for long-term feeding and that has been developed by a qualified board-certified veterinary nutritionist. As with all veterinary therapeutic diets, regular rechecks and monitoring of the patient are essential to ensure that the dietary therapy is meeting the patient's needs. Most veterinary nutritionists encourage feedback on how the home-cooked diet formulation is working for the patient and can provide reformulations and adjustments to the diet as needed.

REFERENCES

The reference list can be found on the companion Expert Consult Web site at *www.expertconsult.com*.

SECTION IX
Hematology and Immunology

CHAPTER 184

Problem-Oriented Differential Diagnosis of Autoimmune Skin Diseases

Karen A. Moriello

Immune-mediated skin diseases are uncommon in clinical veterinary practice; they accounted for fewer than 1.5% of all skin diseases seen in a university referral dermatology service (Figure 184-1). Nonetheless, they are problematic to veterinarians because they can appear similar to other skin diseases that are more common. Immune-mediated skin diseases are divided into two major categories: primary autoimmune diseases, in which the disease is the result of attack against self-antigens, and secondary immune-mediated diseases, in which the disease is the result of an attack against a foreign antigen. Common foreign antigens that cause tissue damage include drugs, bacteria, and viruses. This chapter provides an overview of the more common autoimmune skin diseases and highlights key features that may narrow the list of differential diagnoses or may answer the question, "Should I be thinking of an autoimmune skin disease?"

CLINICAL CLUES IN THE HISTORY AND PHYSICAL EXAMINATION FINDINGS

Two common conditions are encountered in pets with autoimmune skin diseases (ASDs). One is the "textbook presentation" of the disease, which includes an acute onset of severe lesions. These patients are rarely problematic with regard to diagnosis, because suspicion is high from the onset. The clinician suspects something serious and an aggressive diagnostic evaluation usually results in a diagnosis. In the other situation, the disease manifests itself in a less obvious way, waxes and wanes, partially responds to treatment for a different disease, is a mild form of the ASD, or occurs concurrently with another chronic skin disease (e.g., atopic patients that develop pemphigus). The following points should raise suspicion of a possible immune-mediated skin disease:

Historical Clues
- Any severe skin disease with an acute or rapid onset
- Reports that the lesions wax and wane, especially in relatively short cycles of 7 to 10 days
- Intermittent episodes of depression, fever, and anorexia, especially if they coincide with the development of lesions

- Lack of response to seemingly appropriate therapy. For example:
  - A routine case of otitis externa that does not respond to therapy, with evidence emerging of primary lesions on the inner pinnae
  - Dogs or cats that continue to develop pustular lesions despite appropriate antibiotic therapy, especially if therapy has continued for longer than 3 weeks
  - Continued development of oral lesions on gums after appropriate dental therapy
- Difficulty eating or drinking (an early historical finding in dogs with oral ulcers)

Suspicious Physical Examination Findings
- Pruritus (variable in ASD, and its presence does not rule out ASD; evidence of pruritus may come from the history or may be obvious on examination [e.g., excoriations, observed self-trauma])
- Symmetry of skin lesions or marked regionality (e.g., lesions limited to nose)
- Skin disease (mild or moderate) with concurrent signs of systemic illness (fever, anorexia)
- Large numbers of easily found, intact primary lesions all in the same stage, especially pustules, vesicles, or bullae
  - Intact or recently ruptured pustules on the inner pinnae
  - Intact pustules near the mammae of cats
  - Intact, flaccid pustules spanning several hair follicles, often yellow-green in color
- Thick, adherent crusting on the body
  - Crusting only on the face and/or footpads
  - Crusting that includes the face, footpads, and body
- A strong, offensive odor, with exudation and serum accumulation on the trunk, causing matting of the haircoat, especially if oily seborrhea is not present
- Ulcerations or erosions. For example:
  - Oral ulceration and/or erosions, drooling, with or without halitosis
  - Mucocutaneous ulcerations and/or erosions, matting of the haircoat in these areas, and odor (often prominent findings)

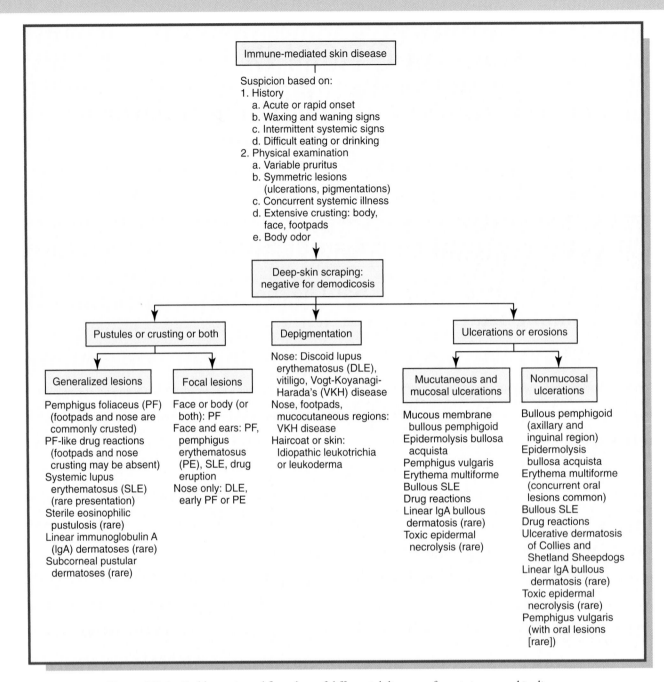

Figure 184-1   Problem-oriented flow chart of differential diagnoses for autoimmune skin diseases based on common presentations.

• Ulcerations and erosions in the axillary and/or inguinal region
• Depigmentation of the nose or mucocutaneous junctions
• Acute development of erythroderma with or without edema

PROBLEM-ORIENTED APPROACH TO DIFFERENTIAL DIAGNOSIS

The dermatologic problems most commonly associated with ASD are pustular eruptions, crusting and scaling, mucocutaneous ulcerations, nonmucocutaneous ulcerations, depigmentation, erythroderma, and miscellaneous problems such as noninflammatory focal alopecia or lesions localized to one site

(e.g., nose). Box 184-1 presents a problem-oriented list of differential diagnoses for ASDs. Because of the variation in clinical signs, some diseases fit into several categories. Box 184-2 provides a summary of the key diagnostic findings for skin biopsy and immunologic tests in various ASDs that help confirm the diagnosis. Skin scrapings and dermatophyte cultures should be negative in ASD. However, mite infestations and/or dermatophytosis can develop secondary to immunosuppressive disorders and occasionally occur concurrently. Adult-onset demodicosis can precede the development of an ASD. In a "classic" ASD case, bacterial cultures of intact pustules should be reported as "no growth" or "scant" growth. If heavy growth of bacteria is found, this may indicate that the pustular disease is bacterial in origin, that bacteria have colonized skin lesions caused by the ASD, or that staphylo-

Box • 184-1

Differential Diagnosis of Autoimmune Skin Diseases

Generalized Pustular Eruptions and/or Crusting Dermatoses (Involving the Body, Head, Face, or Feet)

- Pemphigus foliaceus (PF) (footpad and nose commonly are crusted)
- Superficial pustular drug reactions (nasal and footpad crusting may be absent)
- Paraneoplastic pemphigus
- Lupus erythematosus, exfoliative cutaneous lupus erythematosus of German Short Haired Pointers
- Sterile eosinophilic pustulosis (rare disease)
- Linear IgA pustular dermatosis (rare disease)
- Subcorneal pustular dermatosis (rare disease)
- Sterile pustular erythroderma of Miniature Schnauzers

Focal Pustular Eruptions and/or Focal Crusting

- Face and/or footpads: PF
- Face and ears only: PF (early), pemphigus erythematosus (PE), drug eruptions, lupus erythematosus
- Nasal only: lupus erythematosus, PE (early), PE

  NOTE: Pustules are quite transient, and many of the generalized pustular diseases also present as generalized, malodorous, crusting dermatoses. The major differential diagnoses here are bacterial pyoderma, dermatophytosis/superficial pustular dermatophytosis, severe seborrhea, hepatocutaneous disorder, and zinc deficiency. Bacterial pyoderma rarely affects the head, and dermatophytosis is a nonsymmetric skin disease. Most cases occur in young animals (dermatophytosis) or sled dogs (zinc deficiency). Severe, oily seborrhea may also appear as a crusting dermatosis and can mimic PF if nasal and digital hyperkeratosis is present; the major differentiating factor is that primary seborrhea starts out at a young age. Zinc-responsive skin diseases may present as widespread or focal crusting dermatoses and can mimic PF. Some diseases are breed related (e.g., sterile pustular erythroderma of Miniature Schnauzers).

Mucocutaneous and Mucosal Ulcerations

- Pemphigus vulgaris (PV) (may also have oral ulcerations)
- Mucous membrane pemphigoid
- Epidermolysis bullosa acquisita
- Erythema multiforme (EM) (target lesions, cutaneous ulcerations also may be present)
- Bullous systemic lupus erythematosus
- Drug reactions
- Paraneoplastic pemphigus
- Linear IgA bullous dermatosis (rare)
- Toxic epidermal necrolysis (TEN) (rare)

  Note: The primary lesions in these diseases are vesicles and bullae, which are quite transient and rupture, leaving erosions

and ulceration. The adjacent haircoat becomes matted and odorous. The major differential diagnoses of concern are candidiasis, ulcerative mucocutaneous bacterial pyoderma, and cutaneous lymphoma.

Nonmucosal Ulcerations (Axillae, Inguina, Pinnae, or Other Haired Areas)

- Bullous pemphigoid
- Epidermolysis bullosa acquisita
- Linear IgA bullous dermatosis
- Bullous systemic lupus erythematosus
- Vesicular cutaneous lupus erythematosus of Shetland Sheepdogs and Collies
- Erythema multiforme
- Toxic epidermal necrolysis
- Drug eruptions
- Pemphigus vulgaris (with concurrent mucocutaneous lesions)

  NOTE: The primary lesions are vesicles and/or bullae, which are quite transient. These patients commonly present with fever, pain, a matted haircoat, and exudation. The major differential diagnoses of concern are deep bacterial pyoderma, deep pyoderma caused by demodicosis, and cutaneous deep and intermediate mycoses.

Depigmenting Skin Diseases

- Nasal only: Discoid lupus erythematosus, vitiligo-like syndrome, uveodermatologic syndrome, early PF or PE
- Nose, footpads, lips, eyelids, and mucocutaneous regions: Uveodermatologic syndrome (these animals have concurrent uveitis)
- Haircoat or skin: Idiopathic leukotrichia or leukoderma

Miscellaneous

- Focal alopecia: Alopecia areata, rabies vaccine, focal vasculitis
- Widespread noninflammatory alopecia: Alopecia areata, pseudopelade
- Erythematous target lesions: Erythema multiforme
- Nodular ulcerative lesions: Nodular panniculitis, canine pyoderma gangrenosum
- Purpura, hemorrhage, "punched out" lesions: Vasculitis, erythema multiforme
- Ear margin necrosis, pineal erosions: Vasculitis, proliferative necrotizing otitis of kittens, cryoglobulinemia and cryofibrinogenemia, proliferative thrombovascular necrosis of the pinnae
- Dependent edema with erythema: Vasculitis
- Sloughing nails: Lupoid onychitis
- Nasal lesions: PF, PE, lupus, mucous membrane pemphigoid

---

coccal bacteria from the clinician's fingers contaminated the culture. In some cases skin biopsies are diagnostic, and in other cases a trial of antibiotic therapy or a review of previous therapies may answer the question. Cytologic specimens may also show concurrent *Malassezia* overgrowth. It is important to rule out candidiasis in dogs and cats with mucocutaneous

or ulcerative dermatoses. This is best done by fungal culture at a reference laboratory (a swab is submitted) and by cytologic examination of exudate (unfixed, unstained slides of debris scraped from the lesion margins are submitted).

Cytologic examination of the contents of an intact pustule may be extremely valuable for making a diagnosis. This diag-

Box • 184-2

Key Diagnostic Findings in Common Autoimmune Skin Diseases

Skin Biopsy
- *Pemphigus vulgaris:* Suprabasilar acantholysis with cleft and vesicle formation; basal cells attachment to basement membrane resembles a row of tombstones.
- *Pemphigus foliaceus:* Intragranular or subcorneal pustules with acantholysis.
- *Pemphigus erythematosus:* Intragranular or subcorneal pustules with acantholysis with a lichenoid reaction.
- *Bullous pemphigoid, epidermolysis bullosa acquisita, linear IgA bullous dermatosis, mucous membrane pemphigoid,* and *bullous systemic lupus erythematosus:* Subepidermal cleft and vesicle formation, no acantholysis, and possible lichenoid reaction.
- *Systemic* or *discoid lupus erythematosus (DLE) (the histologic findings for both systemic and discoid lupus erythematosus are identical, except that pigmentary incontinence may be more prominent in DLE):* Hydropic and/or lichenoid interface dermatitis of the epidermis and possibly of the outer root sheath of the hair follicles, apoptosis of basal cells and, less commonly, subepidermal vesicles.
- *Erythema multiforme (EM) (the histologic findings with EM vary greatly; a key finding is apoptosis of keratinocytes throughout the epidermis):* Interface dermatitis with prominent single cell apoptosis of keratinocytes throughout the epidermis and outer root sheath of the epidermis.
- *Toxic epidermal necrolysis:* Hydropic degeneration of basal cells, full-thickness coagulation necrosis of the epidermis, and minimal dermal inflammation.

- *Uveodermatologic syndrome:* Lichenoid interface dermatitis with large histiocytes, as well as prominent pigmentary incontinence; hydropic degeneration of epidermal basal cells is rare.

Antinuclear Antibody Testing
- *Pemphigus erythematosus:* Weak positive titer may be seen.
- *Systemic lupus erythematosus:* Strong positive titer.

Direct Immunofluorescence Testing
- *Pemphigus complex:* Positive intercellular fluorescence.
- *Pemphigus erythematosus:* Positive intercellular and basement membrane fluorescence.
- *Bullous pemphigoid (50% to 90% of cases), epidermolysis bullosa acquisita, linear IgA dermatosis, mucous membrane pemphigoid, systemic or cutaneous lupus erythematosus (50% to 90% of cases):* Positive basement membrane fluorescence.

  NOTE: Direct immunofluorescence testing usually is negative in the other autoimmune skin diseases; however, this is not always the case, and nonspecific staining may be seen.

Indirect Immunofluorescence Testing
- Indirect immunofluorescence testing using a salt split-skin as a substrate is a relatively new method of differentiating the autoimmune subepidermal bullous diseases.

---

nostic test may be helpful for corroborating a diagnosis of pemphigus foliaceus (PF). Intact pustules are rare in cats, and if found, especially on the inner pinnae and near the mammae, are almost always caused by PF. In dogs, it is rare to easily find large numbers of intact pustules. The pustules of pemphigus are large, flaccid, and filled with a copious amount of pus. The specimen should be stained and examined for acanthocytes, which are round, deeply basophilic epidermal cells often present as rafts (i.e., numerous cells adhered together). In dogs these cells tend to be found in PF and in cases of severe bacterial pyoderma. Cytologic specimens should be carefully examined for eosinophils. In dogs, eosinophils can be seen in pustular specimens from PF. A finding of eosinophils should prompt the clinician to consider other differential diagnoses, such as allergic disease (small numbers of eosinophils), sterile eosinophilic pustulosis (almost pure fields of eosinophils), or parasitic diseases (variable). In cats, a finding of large numbers of eosinophils requires some thought on the part of the clinician, because many allergic skin diseases of cats can mimic ASDs.

CHAPTER 185

Immune-Mediated Diseases and Therapies

Oliver A. Garden

THE SPECTRUM OF IMMUNE-MEDIATED DISEASE

Immune-mediated diseases of the dog and cat are many and varied, accounting for a large number of clinical cases presented to veterinarians each year.[1-6] The spectrum of immune-mediated disease is wide, ranging from disorders involving specific organs to those involving multiple body systems (Figure 185-1).[1,4,7,8]

A cardinal feature of the non–organ specific diseases is the anatomically dispersed nature of the antigens to which the immune system responds, often involving the systemic deposition of immune complexes leading to vasculitis[9,10]; in contrast, the organ-specific diseases are characterized by immune

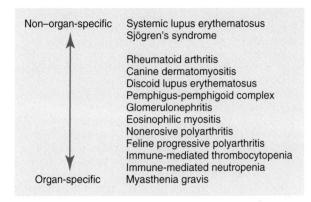

Figure 185-1 The spectrum of immune-mediated disease in dogs and cats. Examples of immune-mediated diseases of various etiologies are shown, lying along a spectrum from those showing no organ specificity to those showing discrete sites of immunological assault.

reactions to specific tissue antigens.[11] The conventional classification of immune-mediated diseases into primary (idiopathic) or secondary etiologies further helps to rationalize their diagnosis and therapy, since elimination of identifiable underlying factors such as drug usage, neoplasia, or infection is necessary for the effective treatment of diseases in which they play a role[3] (Web Figure 185-1). However, the ever-expanding spectrum of infectious agents—many of which have immunopathologic sequelae—raises the possibility that several of the currently labeled "idiopathic" diseases may in due course be associated with specific underlying pathogens as knowledge in this area grows.[12-17] Indeed, there is increasing recognition of the possibility of coinfection of individual patients with multiple pathogens.[18-21]

A proportion of immune-mediated diseases are truly autoimmune, involving inappropriate immune responses to self-antigens.[11,22-24] This chapter focuses on the diagnosis and clinical management of common autoimmune diseases. The reader is urged to refer to the electronic version of the chapter for additional information and learning resources; specific textbooks devoted to veterinary immunology and immune-mediated disease also exist.[5,25,26]

ETIOLOGY, PATHOGENIC MECHANISMS, AND THE ROLE OF INFECTION

Both humoral and cellular mechanisms of tissue damage have been identified in human and veterinary autoimmune diseases, involving one or more of the four basic Coombs' and Gel immune responses (Web Figure 185-2).[27-29] Key to the development of such immunopathogenic responses is a loss of self-tolerance, defined as a state of nonresponsiveness or of nonpathogenic responsiveness to self-antigens.[11,24] Such tolerance operates within both the primary lymphoid organs ("central tolerance"), in which various mechanisms censor the release of potentially autoreactive T cells from the thymus or autoreactive B cells from the bone marrow, and the peripheral lymphoid organs ("peripheral tolerance"), in which cells managing to escape the central censorship mechanisms are nevertheless controlled by processes such as deletion by apoptosis, functional inactivation by anergy, and suppression by regulatory T cells (Tregs).[30-34] Indeed, autoimmunity itself is a natural phenomenon and may have roles in neuroregeneration[35-37] and the removal of senescent red blood cells[38,39]; only when it is associated with a lack of regulation and the development of progressive inflammation does it become pathogenic, forming the basis of autoimmune disease.[22,23,40,41]

Loss of self-tolerance may occur in various ways, all of which may foster the development of autoaggressive immune responses.[41,42]

> For more information on this topic, please visit the companion Expert CONSULT Web site at www.expertconsult.com.

Autoimmune disease is multifactorial, involving genetic, environmental, and hormonal influences.[1,4,6,97,98] Inherited factors include genes encoding major histocompatibility complex (MHC) molecules or single nucleotide polymorphisms of regulatory proteins, while environmental influences include viral infection and exposure to xenobiotic agents.[23,42,99,100] Vaccination has also been linked to various immune-mediated and inflammatory sequelae in both human[101-104] and veterinary patients, the latter including systemic lupus erythematosus (SLE),[105] immune-mediated hemolytic anemia (IMHA),[106] polyarthritis,[107] steroid-responsive meningitis,[108] focal cutaneous vasculitis,[109] and necrotizing granulomatous panniculitis[110] in dogs (but not thyroiditis in laboratory Beagles[111]); transient caliciviral-induced lameness in kittens[112]; and necrotizing granulomatous panniculitis in cats[110] (Web Figure 185-3). A number of potential mechanisms—including nonspecific immune activation by adjuvants or microbial superantigens, exposure to cross-reactive tissue proteins incorporated into vaccines, and molecular mimicry between vaccinal microbes and autoantigens—have been proposed, but they currently remain largely unsubstantiated.[104,113] Rabies and feline leukemia virus (FeLV) vaccines have also been associated with the development of sarcomas in cats.[114-117]

The specificity of the autoimmune response elicited by factors compromising peripheral tolerance is determined in part by the genetic background of the patient, as can be shown by the variable clinical manifestations arising from the depletion of Tregs in various murine strains, ranging from limited, organ-specific inflammation to severe, polysystemic disease.[118,119]

> For more information on this topic, please visit the companion Expert CONSULT Web site at www.expertconsult.com.

Hormonal influences are important in the pathogenesis of human autoimmune disease, in which women are overrepresented in the majority of conditions—for example myasthenia gravis (MG) and SLE, which are respectively three and nine times more prevalent in women than men.[144] The impact of gender in canine and feline patients is less clearly defined, confounded by the influence of neutering and differing results between studies. For example, some studies of canine IMHA have documented greater prevalence of disease in females than males regardless of reproductive status[121,127,128,145]—though whether animals were neutered was not always recorded[126]—while others have found (i) greater prevalence in neutered than intact females, which in turn showed greater prevalence than males,[124,125,146] or (ii) no difference between males and females, particularly when the effect of gender was corrected for breed and age.[122,123,147] By comparison, feline IMHA is generally thought to be more prevalent in males than females.[148-150]

> For more information on this topic, please visit the companion Expert CONSULT Web site at www.expertconsult.com.

DIAGNOSIS OF IMMUNE-MEDIATED DISEASE

Signalment, History, and Physical Examination
Diagnosis of immune-mediated disease requires:
- Recognition of the signalment and evaluation of the history and physical examination
- Careful analysis of laboratory tests, imaging, and biopsy results

- When available, fulfillment of diagnostic criteria or algorithms—for example, those used to facilitate the diagnosis of SLE

In general, canine IMHA, immune-mediated thrombocytopenia (ITP), and SLE are overrepresented in middle-aged animals—with a mean or median age at presentation of five to seven years in various studies*—though dogs of any age may be affected; by comparison, canine patients with idiopathic immune-mediated polyarthritis show an average age at presentation of between 3[172] and 5[173-176] years, while those with masticatory muscle myositis are on average 3 years old at presentation[195]—though, again, cases can present at any age. Cats tend to show a more variable age of presentation on average—5 to 7 years in some studies,[129,196] but younger than 5 years[148,149,178,197] or older than 7 years[178,198] in others. As discussed above and online, gender influences are less apparent in canine and feline than human patients. Immune-mediated disease may be characterized by periods of remission and exacerbation, with overall deterioration with time, or acute exacerbation that necessitates immediate medical attention to avoid life-threatening sequelae.[3,4] Historical features of the polysystemic immune-mediated diseases may include lameness with or without muscle pain; mucocutaneous lesions; lethargy and dyspnea; weight loss with inappetence; polyuria and polydipsia; and even seizures and behavioral changes[3,168,193,194]; those with organ-specific disease show more specific signs referable to the affected organ.[3] Physical findings may include swollen, painful joints and muscles; cutaneous erythema, macules, papules, pustules, seborrhea, erosion or ulceration, pyoderma, depigmentation, alopecia, nasal dermatitis, and purpura; pallor and petechiae of the mucous membranes; cardiac arrhythmias; and lymphadenomegaly and splenomegaly[3,168,193,194] (Web Figure 185-6). Individual cases may show one or a number of these signs (Figure 185-2), but joint, skin and hematologic abnormalities are often prominent in SLE.[3,168,193,194]

Diagnostic Tests

Possible diagnostic tests for immune-mediated disease include a complete blood cell count (CBC), serum biochemical profile, urinalysis, coagulation profile, radiography, arthrocentesis, immunological tests, and biopsies[199]; the problem list of each presenting case—and whether organ-specific or polysystemic disease is suspected—will dictate which tests are applied. Generally, diagnostic tests should be carried out before administration of blood products.

CBC/Coagulation Profile   Abnormalities that may be encountered in immune-mediated disease include:
- Anemia: This may be regenerative with macrocytosis when caused by immune-mediated hemolysis, or nonregenerative when caused by infection, uremia, chronic bleeding, or immune-mediated assault of erythroid precursors.[200] Spherocytes, red blood cells (RBCs) that have suffered damage to the plasma membrane or partial phagocytosis—with decreased surface area–to-volume ratio, assumption of a spherical shape, and loss of central pallor—are often associated with immune-mediated disease, being observed in ~90% dogs with IMHA[201] (Web Figure 185-7); however, alternative differential diagnoses may include severe hypophosphatemia,[202,203] microangiopathic injury referable to disseminated intravascular coagulation, vasculitis, and other causes such as splenic torsion[204] (Web Figure185-8), Heinz body hemolytic anemia,[205] congenital red cell enzymopathies such as pyruvate kinase (PK) deficiency,[206] zinc toxicosis,[207] and coral snake envenomation.[208] Since feline erythrocytes

lack obvious central pallor, spherocytes are much more difficult to discern in this species.[205] Congenital enzymopathies should be considered in the differential diagnosis of regenerative anemia, since the clinicopathologic manifestations may be deceptively similar to IMHA in some cases.[206,209-214]
- Thrombocytopenia: This may be caused by antiplatelet antibodies, which not only compromise the function of platelets[215,216] but also promote their elimination by the reticuloendothelial system (RES).[217] One study observed that a proportion of ITP cases were characterized by an initial microthrombocytosis—thought to be specific for ITP—followed by a regenerative macrothrombocytosis[218]; however, a more recent paper was unable to differentiate the various causes of thrombocytopenia on the basis of platelet volume.[219] In the cat, platelets are a similar size to RBCs, prompting caution in the interpretation of automated counts from machines based on aperture impedance flow cytometry, which attempt to differentiate the two cell types by size[220]; similar considerations apply to Cavalier King Charles Spaniels, which show autosomal recessive macrothrombocytopaenia.[221,222] Evaluation of a blood smear is an important part of the CBC in both species, but particularly so in these contexts.[200,205,223]
- Neutropenia: This may be an idiosyncratic manifestation of drug toxicity—for example, associated with anticonvulsant administration[224]; part of polysystemic immune-mediated disease—for example, SLE[166,167,169]; and, rarely, idiopathic.[225-232] Antineutrophil antibodies have been demonstrated in human SLE,[233] but not to the author's knowledge in the canine or feline disease.
- Lymphocytosis: Though rare in dogs with IMHA, lymphocytosis may be observed in up to ~50% of cats with IMHA, thought to reflect chronic antigenic stimulation of the cells; these patients may also be hyperglobulinemic for the same reason, without any evidence of alternative causes such as feline infectious peritonitis and neoplasia.[129,149] Lymphocytosis has been described in other feline hemolytic anemias, including pyruvate kinase deficiency and increased osmotic fragility in Abyssinian and Somali cats, which may similarly be associated with hyperglobulinemia.[234]

For more information on this topic, please visit the companion Expert CONSULT Web site at www.expertconsult.com.

- Coagulation abnormalities: Pulmonary thromboembolism (PTE)[241] is a significant cause of mortality in IMHA,[125,241-245] prompting consideration of Virchow's triad of contributing factors—vascular stasis, hypercoagulability and endothelial damage.[246] Stasis alone does not appear to be sufficient to induce coagulation unless it is combined with endothelial damage and, or hypercoagulability.[247] The pathogenesis of thromboembolism in IMHA is thought to be multifactorial,[248] including:
  - Hypercoagulability—potential causes include (i) disseminated intravascular coagulation (DIC)[125,243] secondary to tissue factor activation by anti–red cell antibodies, lysed RBCs, and inflammatory mediators[249]; (ii) platelet activation[250]; (iii) corticosteroid administration[251]; and (iv) loss of antithrombin (AT) and hypoalbuminemia—with increased platelet aggregability—if there is concurrent glomerulonephritis (GN)[252,253] and protein-losing nephropathy (PLN).[254-258] Current evidence suggests that antiphospholipid antibodies do not play a major role in thromboembolism of canine IMHA,[243] in contrast to their significance in human IMHA and SLE; however, a lupuslike "anticoagulant," which prolonged the activated partial thromboplastin time (APTT) but paradoxically predisposed to thromboembolism in vivo, has been

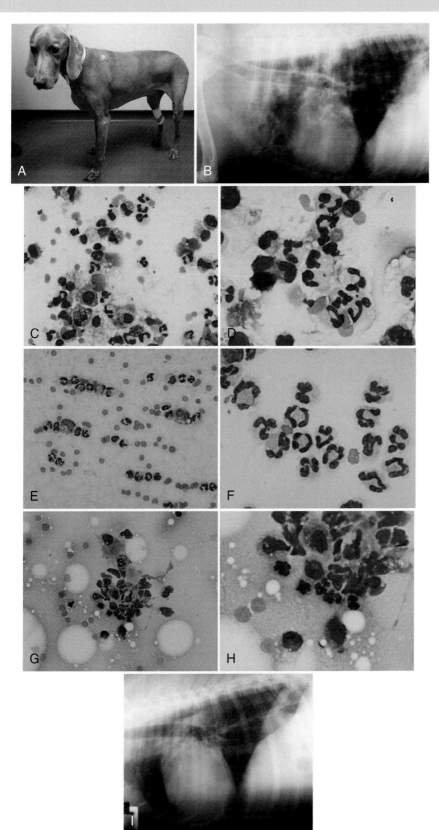

Figure 185-2 Polysystemic immune-mediated disease in a Weimaraner. **A,** A 9-year-old, neutered male Weimaraner dog presented with a 1-week history of dyspnea and lameness. Physical examination revealed pyrexia, pain, and effusion of multiple joints and numerous subcutaneous nodules on the ventral neck, sternum, and lateral thoracic regions. Thoracic radiographs revealed a patchy, peripheral interstitial pattern and a cranioventral alveolar pattern, for which principal differential diagnoses included angiostrongylosis (lungworm infestation), bacterial bronchopneumonia, eosinophilic or other immune-mediated bronchopneumopathy, and lymphoma. Inflated left and right lateral, and ventrodorsal, views were taken under general anesthesia. **B,** Left lateral view. **C** and **D,** A fecal Baermann test was negative and bronchoalveolar lavage (BAL) revealed neutrophilic inflammation and increased mucin. **E** and **F,** Bacterial, mycoplasmal, and fungal cultures of the BAL were all negative. Synovial aspirates revealed nonseptic neutrophilic inflammation, shown on both the direct smears—which illustrate typical "windrowing"—and the cytocentrifuged preparations. **G** and **H,** Aspirates of the subcutaneous nodules revealed mixed, neutrophilic, and histiocytic inflammation on a background of pink matrix with associated lipid, consistent with panniculitis; bacterial (including mycobacterial) and fungal cultures of nodular aspirates were negative. Bacterial cultures of urine and blood were also negative. Following a lack of response to initial broad-spectrum, bactericidal antibiotics while awaiting culture results, immunosuppressive doses of prednisolone were administered, leading to a resolution of all clinical signs within 48 hours. Repeated thoracic radiographs performed 3 days after starting immunosuppressive therapy revealed near-complete resolution of the original lesions. **I,** Conscious left lateral view, which may be compared to **B.** A serum antinuclear antibody titer in this patient was negative. (Patient managed by Dr. Isuru Gajanayake; images of the BAL, synovial fluid, and nodular aspirates reproduced with permission from Dr. Balazs Szladovits; all other images reproduced with permission from Dr. Oliver Garden.)

documented in the dog.[259] Hypercoagulability presents a challenge to measure in clinical practice, but the recent validation of thromboelastography (TEG) (Haemoscope Corporation, Niles, Ill.) as a technique to assess global clotting function in dogs goes some way towards addressing this deficit[260-266] (Figure 185-3). However, samples need to be run within 1 to 2 hours of collection and the availability of TEG machines is currently limited; nevertheless, when available, this methodology yields information on both coagulation and fibrinolysis.[241,254] Though validated for use in dogs, clinical utility of TEG in cats is not yet established, though reference ranges for TEG parameters in cats have recently been defined.[267,268]

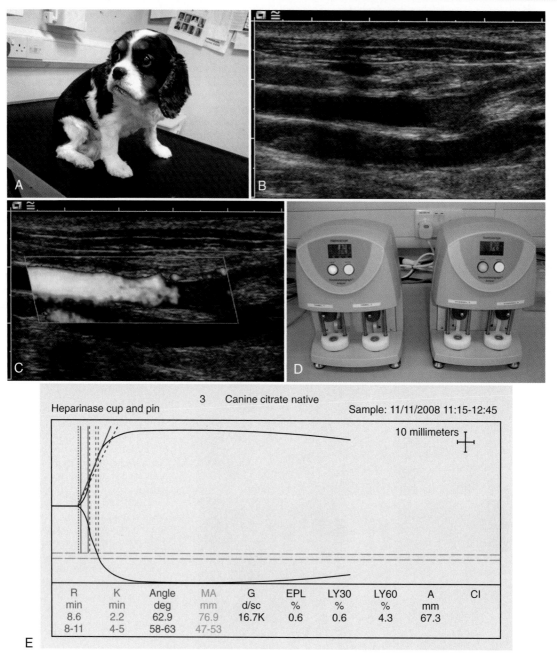

Figure 185-3 For legend, see opposite page

- Endothelial injury mediated by inflammatory mediators and hypoxia[248]; in contrast to human IMHA, antiendothelial antibodies are unlikely to play a major role in the canine disease.[269]
- Vascular stasis—thromboemboli tend to inhibit blood flow, exacerbating the ongoing process[248]; furthermore, vasodilatory responses may be blunted by the binding of nitric oxide by even trace amounts of free hemoglobin.[270]
- Thromboembolism appears to be an uncommon sequela of feline primary IMHA, which is less prevalent as a disease in this species than in the dog[129,149,271,272]; indeed, cats appear to suffer generally lower mortality in primary IMHA (20% to 25%)[129,149] than dogs (30% to 70%).*

*References 121-123, 125, 126, 128, 145, 191, 192, 273, 274.

Serum Biochemical Profile Abnormalities may include:
- Increased concentrations of blood urea nitrogen (BUN), creatinine, and inorganic phosphate, which may be referable to dehydration or chronic glomerular lesions.
- Hypoalbuminemia and hypercholesterolemia, which may be referable to PLN caused by GN[275-280]; mild hypoalbuminemia may also be secondary to a negative acute phase response in the course of severe inflammatory disease.[281]
- Hyperbilirubinemia, which may occur as a consequence of hemolysis or hepatobiliary causes, including impairment of (i) bilirubin uptake by hepatocytes, (ii) cytosolic transport, (iii) storage, (iv) conjugation and (v) canalicular egress—secondary to hypoxic, thromboembolic, and/or hepatic endothelial cell damage.[128] Increased serum bilirubin concentrations—often higher than 10 mg/ dL—have been associated with a negative prognosis in many,[121-123,125,128,282] but not all,[124,192] studies of canine

Figure 185-3 Aortic thrombosis in a Cavalier King Charles Spaniel with protein-losing nephropathy. **A,** An 11-year-old, neutered female Cavalier King Charles Spaniel presented with an acute history of collapse and paresis of the pelvic limbs, associated with pain and marked attenuation of the femoral pulses. A diagnostic workup revealed the presence of a hyperechoic structure within the abdominal aorta, consistent with a thrombus. **B** and **C,** Ultrasound images of the caudal abdominal aorta (cranial to left of image): **B** reveals the hyperechoic structure within the abdominal aorta, located cranial to the origin of the external iliac arteries; **C,** Application of power Doppler, demonstrating the absence of color and thus blood flow at this level. Thromboelastography (TEG) was performed, confirming significant hypercoagulability. Urinalysis revealed marked proteinuria—likely to be of glomerular origin (noninflammatory sediment; bacterial culture negative)—thereby providing a mechanistic explanation for the hypercoagulability. **D,** The two TEG machines at the Royal Veterinary College, UK. **E,** TEG tracing of patient on presentation: the low-normal reaction time *(R)*, decreased clot formation time *(K)*, high-normal angle *(Angle)*, and increased maximal amplitude *(MA)* confirm the hypercoagulable nature of this sample. This patient was successfully treated with low-dose aspirin, dalteparin and benazepril—monitored with serial measurements of systolic blood pressure by Doppler technique, serum biochemical profiles, routine urinalyses, urine protein: creatinine ratios, abdominal ultrasound examinations, and TEG assays—with return of femoral pulses and locomotor function of the pelvic limbs, despite sonographically-documented persistence of a residual thrombus in the distal aorta; the patient has remained ambulatory and bright, with no other clinical signs in the 7 months since initial presentation. A comprehensive search for underlying infection or neoplasia was unremarkable, suggesting a working diagnosis of "idiopathic" glomerulonephritis—though renal biopsies were not obtained in this case. (Patient managed by Dr. Silke Schmitz; ultrasound images reproduced with permission from Dr. Livia Benigni; TEG tracings courtesy Dr. Robert Goggs and Daniel Chan, reproduced with permission from Dr. Oliver Garden.)

IMHA; other factors predicting a negative outcome on survival have included a lack of robust reticulocytosis (corrected reticulocyte count <3%),[122] packed cell volume (PCV) below15%,[122] leukocytosis (>28 × 10³/μL) with a neutrophilic left shift and toxic change,[121,124,128,191] red cell macrocytosis,[192] thrombocytopenia,[121,128] prolongation of the prothrombin time (PT),[124] increased serum alkaline phosphatase[123] and creatine kinase (CK)[128] activity, hypoalbuminemia,[128] hypokalemia,[128] and increased serum BUN concentration.[121]

- Hyperglobulinemia, which may develop with B cell activation in immune-mediated disease—for example, polyclonal B cell activation and expansion in SLE.[166,167,169,283-285]
- Increased serum CK activity, which may occur as a consequence of polymyositis and/or myocarditis, especially during the acute phase of disease.[286] If the inflammation is localized to a particular muscle or group of muscles—for example in MMM—serum CK activity may show only a mild increase and then return to normal as the disease becomes chronic.[195] Alternative causes of increased serum CK activity include marked hemolysis and hyperbilirubinemia; traumatic venipuncture, surgery and intramuscular injections; and noninflammatory etiologies such as prolonged recumbency, heat stroke, and intense physical activity.[287] Furthermore, young animals and small dogs have inherently higher serum CK activity[287] and significant muscle necrosis may also increase serum ALT activity.[288]

Urinalysis   Abnormalities may include:
- Proteinuria, which is gauged by measurement of a urine protein (mg/dL): creatinine (mg/dL = μmol/L × 88.4⁻¹; Up:c) ratio following either suspicion for excessive urinary protein loss on the basis of routine tests, including dipstick evaluation and—if performed—a sulfosalicylic acid (SSA) turbidimetric assay, or proactive screening in high-risk animals.[289] While the upper limit of normality was historically considered to be 1.0 in both dogs and cats, more recent studies have suggested that normal Up:c ratios are typically 0.2 to 0.3 or less; indeed, the

upper limit in dogs is now considered to be 0.5 and for cats, 0.4.[290] Up:c ratios that exceed these values should raise concern for glomerular or tubulointerstitial renal disease, if prerenal and postrenal causes of proteinuria have been ruled out; furthermore, values greater than 2.0 are generally suggestive of glomerular lesions.[291] Though rarely required in the context of immune-mediated disease, sensitive semiquantitative point-of-care tests that measure urine albumin are now available, offering the ability to detect concentrations of albumin that are greater than normal but less than the limit of detection of conventional dipsticks (e.g., ≤30 mg/dL; microalbuminuria); these tests have found greatest utility in the early diagnosis of chronic idiopathic renal disease.[290]

- If a urinary tract infection (UTI) can be ruled out, the discovery of a Up:c ratio of ≥2.0 should prompt consideration of potential antigenic triggers for GN, including occult infection with a variety of organisms examined on the basis of geographical prevalence—for example, *Dirofilaria immitis, Angiostrongylus vasorum, Ehrlichia* spp., *Borrelia burgdorferi, Rickettsia rickettsii, Bartonella* spp., *Leishmania infantum, Babesia* spp., and *Leptospira interrogans.* Only when such infections have been ruled out can "idiopathic" GN be diagnosed.[292]
- Hematuria, pyuria, erythrocyte casts: In the absence of an active UTI, such findings could be consistent with severe GN; infectious agents should again be considered as a source of antigen.[293]

Serum Protein Electrophoresis

For more information on this topic, please visit the companion Expert CONSULT Web site at www.expertconsult.com.

Specific Immunologic Tests

Direct antiglobulin (Coombs') test   In the absence of an alternative explanation such as blood loss, the presence of anemia—especially if regenerative—should prompt in-saline agglutination testing as an initial diagnostic step: a drop of blood drawn from an EDTA tube is mixed with two to four drops of 0.9% saline solution on a slide, before microscopic examination for agglutinating clumps of RBCs (Web Figure 185-10). These are distinguishable from rouleaux, which look like stacks of coins and are generally dispersed by saline dilution.[128,205,301-303] This test is thought to be the consequence of IgM or large quantities of IgG autoantibody coating the RBCs[302,303] and typically yields a positive result in 35% to 78% of cases[123,125,128,146]—though one study noted that only 4 of 42 (9.5%) patients demonstrated persistent autoagglutination following the washing of patient RBCs in 0.9% saline,[122] a more rigorous variant of the "bedside" test.[302,303] Both autoagglutination without prior washing[128] and persistent autoagglutination with washing[122] have been associated with severe disease and higher rates of mortality in canine patients. Data in the cat are more sparse, one report documenting autoagglutination in 10% of cases[304] and a second describing macroscopic agglutination in 100% cases, but persistent agglutination postwashing in only 21%.[149] Autoagglutination is compatible with IMHA and would usually preclude subsequent immunodiagnostic testing, which is reliant on agglutination as a readout. The osmotic fragility test, based on the decreased ability of RBCs coated with antibodies to withstand osmotic challenge, may also help to make a diagnosis of IMHA,[121,149,305] but in practice is only occasionally performed (Web Box 185-1). Both the in-saline agglutination and osmotic fragility tests need to be interpreted carefully, and lack of autoagglutination does not rule out a diagnosis of IMHA. The direct antiglobulin test (DAT), or Coombs' test—which detects antibodies associated with the surface of RBCs—should be carried out if immune-mediated anemia is suspected and autoagglutination cannot be demonstrated. The primary reagent in this test is polyvalent rabbit antidog or anticat immunoglobulin G (IgG), IgM, and complement factor (C) 3 antiserum, but a full test also uses a panel of monospecific antisera.[146,150,304,306-311] The test should ideally be performed in duplicate at both 37° C and 4° C; a recent study suggested that the sensitivity of the test could be optimized by inclusion of the incubation step at 4° C, which identified 10 of 65 cases that yielded negative results at 37° C.[312] A positive response is detected by agglutination of patient RBCs and an end-point dilution of the antiserum reagent is determined. Results are either reported as a reciprocal titer or a "positive/negative" result, depending on the house style of the clinical pathology laboratory; while some studies have suggested that the magnitude of the titer may have diagnostic significance, becoming negative with remission,[126,311] others have been unable to show such a correlation and indeed have suggested that in a minority of patients a positive titer may persist during remission.[146,307]

The sensitivity of the direct Coombs' test in the dog has varied from 33% to 96% in different studies,* though as a rule of thumb is generally thought to be positive in approximately two thirds of cases; its specificity—when examined—has generally exceeded 90%,[306,308,310] though one study documented weak positive titers in 19 of 38 dogs that did not meet additional criteria for IMHA.[146] Surface IgG—with or without IgM and/or C3—is the most common finding in Coombs' tests employing monospecific antisera, accounting for 42% to 95% of positive results; IgM—with or without IgG and/or C3—is less commonly observed, being present in 1.5% to 52% of cases; while C3—with or without IgG and/or IgM—accounts for 5.3% to 87% of positive results.† One study documented a high prevalence of C3 alone in minimally anemic dogs, often with underlying disorders,[306] while a more recent study suggested that dogs with specific reactivity at 4° C—rather than 37° C—were more likely to be suffering from secondary IMHA.[312] Data in the cat are sparse, reflecting the paucity of

documented cases: a recent study suggested that IgG autoantibodies are more common than those of IgM isotype; furthermore, none of the cats in this series demonstrated Igs against C3.[149] However, an earlier study suggested that the direct Coombs' test lacked specificity in the cat, with 8 of 20 nonanemic, control cats yielding weak positive titers.[304] The predominant cause of false-negative results is thought to be the limited analytical sensitivity of the assay, which is unable to detect low surface densities of Igs or C3 on RBCs, which may nevertheless be of pathogenic significance.[310,314-316] This shortcoming has prompted the development of the direct enzyme-linked antiglobulin test (DELAT), which is based on the elaboration of a color product by an enzyme conjugated to the antiserum reagent in the style of an enzyme-linked immunosorbent assay (ELISA) test.[314-316] Though the DELAT has performed well in a number of studies, it is not widely available in practice. Still greater sensitivity has been achieved by the development of flow cytometric assays,[313,317] though availability is limited to those diagnostic laboratories offering flow cytometry as a specific expertise. Immunosuppressive therapy generally does not influence Coombs' test results until substantial increases in PCV are achieved, usually after 1 to 2 weeks after the inception of therapy.[126]

The most common cause of false positives in the Coombs' test is prior blood transfusion. Incompatible RBCs can react with preexisting alloantibodies or stimulate the production of new antibodies: both are detectable in the Coombs' test, even in the absence of clinical evidence of transfusion incompatibility.[307] Positive results are also occasionally obtained in association with overt infection or neoplasia, even in the absence of anemia, thought to be of questionable pathogenic significance[306]; if there is attendant anemia, the positive Coombs' test results may signal secondary IMHA.[306,312] Both Coombs' and ANA-positive results have been induced experimentally in cats using the drug propylthiouracil.[90,318] Finally, the low-level auto-Ig involved in the clearance of senescent RBCs in health[38,39] is thought to be below the sensitivity of the Coombs' test and is thus not a cause of false positive results.

Antinuclear antibodies   Serum ANAs are a hallmark of human, canine, and feline SLE.[171,319-324] Indirect immunofluorescence or—less commonly—immunoperoxidase tests are used to detect ANAs, in which the antibodies bind to nuclei of a substrate tissue and are visualized with a fluoresceinated or enzyme-linked polyvalent secondary antibody[150,321,325] (Web Figure 185-11). Substrate tissues have included rat liver, vero (monkey kidney), and human epithelial (HEp-2) cells, though canine studies have suggested that HEp-2 cells are superior to rat liver, yielding fewer low-level positive titers in healthy animals.[326] Patient serum is generally screened at a dilution of 1 in 10 to 1 in 40—depending on the individual laboratory—and, if positive, an end-point dilution is determined; titers in excess of 1 in 100 to 1 in 160 are considered to be significant.[150,322,323,327] Various positive-staining patterns are recognized in human patients, including homogeneous, peripheral, speckled, and nucleolar.[328,329] Of these, the two commonest in canine SLE are the speckled pattern with no staining of chromosomes in mitotic cells and the homogeneous pattern, with positive chromosomal staining in mitotic cells[326,330-332]—though a recent study has suggested that most of the patients with speckled patterns of reactivity represent "SLE-related disease" rather than SLE, since their predominant clinical signs were limited to the musculoskeletal system.[325] Documented feline patients, though fewer in number, have similarly shown homogeneous and speckled ANA patterns.[150,171] Specificities of ANAs differ between human and canine SLE; thus, anti-DNA antibodies occur in the majority of human SLE patients,[333] in contrast to canine patients, in which these antibodies are rare and antihistone

*References 121, 123-126, 128, 145, 310, 313.
†References 121, 122, 145, 306, 310, 312.

antibodies are the most common.[319,330-332,334-338] In human patients, anti-DNA antibodies are thought to play a role in the pathogenesis of lupus nephritis[339]; antihistone antibodies may play a similar role in canine lupus, binding to cationic histones that have planted onto the negatively charged glomerular basement membrane.[336] The fine specificity of ANAs in cats is currently unknown.[150]

ANA testing is indicated when SLE is suspected on the basis of compatible clinicopathologic markers.[327] The results of the ANA test must be interpreted with caution: positive ANA results have been recorded in various canine diseases other than SLE, including rheumatoid arthritis,[321] "idiopathic" immune-mediated polyarthritis,[321] atopic dermatitis,[340] symmetrical lupoid onychodystrophy, and black hair follicular dysplasia of Gordon Setters,[341] animals with seroreactivity to *Bartonella vinsonii* subsp. *berkhoffii*, *Ehrlichia canis* and *Leishmania infantum*, hepatozoonosis,[332] autoimmune thyroiditis,[342] bacterial endocarditis,[343] and neoplasia, pemphigus erythematosus, pemphigus vulgaris, and dirofilariasis.[169] Similarly, up to 20% of normal dogs[323] and 10% of normal cats[150] may show low titers of ANAs, though high titers have occasionally been observed in healthy German Shepherd Dogs[338] and other breeds when rat liver was used as the test substrate.[326] Positive results have also been documented in feline IMHA,[150] ITP,[150] nonerosive and erosive polyarthritis,[150] aural hematoma,[344] plasma cell pododermatitis,[345] hyperthyroidism,[346] cholangitis,[4] and transiently in FeLV infection.[4] Occasional canine cases—typically less than 10%—fulfill many of the criteria for SLE and yet show negative ANA test results.[167,169,335,347,348] Possible explanations cited in the literature include a prozone phenomenon, shortcomings of the nuclear substrate for anticytoplasmic antibodies, improper fixation of the substrate, immunosuppressive treatment, binding of antibodies by circulating immune complexes and deposition in tissues, renal loss of antibodies, use of monovalent rather than polyvalent fluoresceinated conjugates, and genuine lack of production.[349-351] Though there is little information in the veterinary literature to explain this phenomenon, an early study examining antibodies against extractable nuclear antigens (ENAs) demonstrated the potential fallibility of the ANA test by noting that two of the six canine lupus patients were ENA-positive but ANA-negative.[335] Surprisingly few studies have examined ANA titers in animals undergoing remission of disease: while the magnitude of the titer correlated with severity of disease and decreased with remission in both dogs[168] and cats[171] in two studies, other authors have documented discordant, high titers in asymptomatic patients.[352]

Rheumatoid factor

For more information on this topic, please visit the companion Expert CONSULT Web site at www.expertconsult.com.

Antiplatelet antibodies

For more information on this topic, please visit the companion Expert CONSULT Web site at www.expertconsult.com.

Antineutrophil antibodies

For more information on this topic, please visit the companion Expert CONSULT Web site at www.expertconsult.com.

Thyroxine (3,5,3',5'-tetraiodothyronine; T4), 3,4,3'-triiodothyronine (T3), and thyroglobulin autoantibodies

For more information on this topic, please visit the companion Expert CONSULT Web site at www.expertconsult.com.

Acetylcholine receptor autoantibodies Of the immune-mediated neuromuscular disorders, acquired MG is the most common in both dogs and cats.[389,390] A high relative risk has been identified in the Akita, Scottish Terrier, German Short-Haired Pointer, and Chihuahua[391,392]—and in the Abyssinian and related Somali cat breeds.[393] The disease may present in various forms,[394] including (i) focal, in which the weakness localizes to the esophageal and pharyngeal musculature; (ii) generalized, in which the weakness shows a more global distribution; (iii) acute fulminating, in which the weakness shows a generalized distribution, but is acute in onset and severe in nature; and (iv) paraneoplastic, in which neoplasia underlies the disease. The molecular lesion underlying all of these forms of MG is an autoimmune response against acetylcholine receptors (AChRs) at the neuromuscular (NM) junction.[395] Acquired MG may be associated with hypothyroidism,[396] hypoadrenocorticism, other autoimmune disorders, thymoma, thymic cysts, cholangiocellular carcinoma, osteogenic sarcoma, anal sac adenocarcinoma, and dysautonomia.[390,397-400] The onset or exacerbation of MG may be associated with bacterial or viral infection, and estrous cycles, gestation, or whelping may initiate or exacerbate MG in female dogs, prompting the recommendation to neuter these animals when they are clinically stable.[390,399] The disease in cats is much less common than in dogs[401] and is more often associated with a cranial mediastinal mass—19% of feline versus 3.4% of canine patients in comparative case series[391,393] (Web Figure 185-12). The gold standard for the diagnosis of acquired MG in both dogs and cats is the documentation of autoantibodies against muscle-type nicotinic AChRs by a species-specific immunoprecipitation radioimmunoassay, involving the precipitation of serum IgG and IgM antibodies binding to solubilized AChR complexed with a high-affinity peptide antagonist[125]—labeled α-bungarotoxin. The γ-emission of the precipitate allows the amount of AChR bound to Ig to be quantified.[390,399,402] This test shows excellent sensitivity and specificity: while false positives are extremely rare, some 2% of dogs with "generalized MG" on the basis of clinical signs, edrophonium challenge (Tensilon) testing, and fatigable repetitive nerve stimulation may be seronegative.[399] Possible causes of seronegative MG include:[399] (i) antibodies directed against non-AChR endplate antigens, or against the α-bungarotoxin–binding site; (ii) antibodies bound to the endplate without detectable serum Ig (antigen excess); (iii) antibodies directed against antigens that may be lost during the AChR extraction procedure; and (iv) observation of the disease in its early stages, when the patient may still be seronegative. AChR autoantibody titers should be measured every 6 to 8 weeks with treatment, since they may return to the normal range with clinical remission of the disease.[390] Indeed, spontaneous remission of canine MG is also known to occur from a few weeks to 1 year following the initial diagnosis,[179,403,404] though the mechanistic basis for this phenomenon remains unclear.

2M myofiber autoantibodies Masticatory muscle myositis is an idiopathic immune-mediated disease of the 2M myofibers of the muscles of mastication—the temporalis, masseter, rostral digastricus, and pteyroids—directed specifically at myosin.[286,405,406] Cavalier King Charles Spaniels, Samoyeds, Dobermans, Rottweilers, and German Shepherd Dogs are overrepresented.[195] Clinical signs may include swelling and/or eventual atrophy of the muscles of mastication; jaw pain and trismus; and exophthalmos followed ultimately by enophthalmos, owing to swelling and then atrophy of the pterygoid muscles in the respective acute and chronic phases of the disease.[195,406] Demonstration of autoantibodies against 2M myofibers of the temporalis muscle in an immunocytochemical assay—using a staphylococcal protein-A horseradish peroxidase conjugate—is diagnostic, showing high sensitivity (85% to 90%) and specificity (100%).[405] More recently, an ELISA for 2M autoantibodies has largely replaced the immunohistochemical test, showing similarly impressive sensitivity and specificity.[195]

Radiography and Arthrocentesis   Nonseptic, suppurative joint lesions are a common manifestation of polysystemic autoimmune disease[166,167,169,358] and are the hallmark feature of immune-mediated polyarthritis.[172,174-177,407,408] Generally, there is a nonerosive pauciarthropathy (involvement of up to five joints) or polyarthropathy (involvement of six joints or more), with soft tissue swelling and occasional development of small osteophytes and erosions; rare canine cases have been documented with prominent erosive lesions but polysystemic signs of anemia and leukopenia suggestive of SLE, consistent with the occasional overlap of usually distinct autoimmune phenotypes.[283] Arthrocentesis of up to four to six joints should be considered if shifting lameness is a feature of the history or multiple joint effusions are detected during the physical examination: carpal, tarsal and stifle joint spaces are commonly sampled[409,410] (Web Figure 185-13). Scrupulous sterile technique is essential! Synovial fluid analysis is diagnostic of nonseptic, inflammatory arthritis, with over 5000 WBC/mm^3 (reference range 250 to 3000/mm^3), 15% to 95% well-preserved neutrophils (normal <6%), low viscosity, and poor mucin clot formation; a protein content of 2.5 to 5.0 g/dL (reference range 2.0 to 2.5 g/dL) is typical.[409-411]

Cerebrospinal Fluid Analysis

For more information on this topic, please visit the companion Expert CONSULT Web site at www.expertconsult.com.

Biopsies   Biopsies may be useful in the further characterization of both organ-specific and polysystemic immune-mediated diseases, though care must be taken to procure suitable samples. Mucocutaneous lesions should be sampled across the interface with normal tissue and may demonstrate leukocytoclastic vasculitis, interface dermatitis, or stomatitis.[169,428-436] However, such lesions are not specific for any one disease, illustrating the importance of interpreting the biopsy results in the context of the entire clinicopathologic database. Muscle biopsies also merit special mention.[437] Biopsies should be collected from sites distant to those evaluated by electromyography (EMG) to avoid needle-induced artifact. If biopsies are being taken from the temporalis muscle, the opposite muscle to that evaluated by EMG is sampled; furthermore, care must be taken to sample the temporalis and not the overlying frontalis muscle, since the latter is not involved in masticatory muscle myositis and may yield false-negative results.[195]

Immune deposits in lesional tissue may be demonstrated by immunoperoxidase or immunofluorescence methods.[436,438,439] The immunoperoxidase method allows retrospective staining of formalin-fixed, paraffin-embedded tissue used for conventional light microscopy, while immunofluorescence techniques are better suited to frozen sections or cold, ethanol-fixed tissues;[438] however, immunofluorescent methodologies have recently been developed for use in formalin-fixed, paraffin-embedded human specimens,[440] thus paving the way for the application of these techniques in the investigation of immune-mediated disease in veterinary patients. SLE is characterized by the deposition of immunoglobulins and/or complement within the basement membrane zone and occasionally the intercellular spaces of the epithelium, and within walls of small dermal blood vessels.[169] Localization of immune deposits within the basement membrane has given rise to the name *lupus band test*, suggesting specificity of this pattern of staining for SLE and discoid lupus erythematosus (DLE)[169,430] (Web Figure 185-14). This is in fact not the case, since bullous pemphigoid, DLE, and cutaneous drug eruption also give rise to similar basement membrane staining.[169] Furthermore, IgM deposition within the basement membrane of the footpads and nose should be regarded as incidental, since healthy dogs possess interface IgM at these locations.[441-443]

Renal biopsies may be informative in cases with glomerular proteinuria.[444,445] Though there has traditionally been a reluctance among practitioners to obtain biopsies of the kidneys, increasing recognition of both their diagnostic value in appropriate patients[445,446] and the relatively low rate of complications associated with their procurement when performed with due diligence[447] has encouraged the submission of these biopsies in recent years. A pathologist with appropriate expertise should be identified before the collection of samples. Renal biopsies should ideally be submitted in: (i) formalin for routine light microscopy; (ii) 4% w/v formalin with 1% w/v glutaraldehyde in sodium phosphate buffer for electron microscopy; and (iii) ammonium sulphate-N-ethylmaleimide fixative (i.e., Michel's solution) for immunofluorescence staining.[445,446,448] (Snap-freezing is another option for immunofluorescence staining, but is less convenient in the clinic.[447]) Biopsies may reveal membranous or membranoproliferative GN in both SLE-like diseases and various infections with immune-mediated sequelae; sclerosis and hyalinization of glomeruli may occur, with development of chronic renal failure.[166,167] Glomerular immune complex deposition may be demonstrated with immunostaining techniques to identify immunoglobulin or complement[277,449-451] (see Web Figure 185-14). Bacterial culture of urine should be performed as a matter of routine prior to renal biopsy, both to rule out the possibility of a UTI and pyelonephritis and to avoid the possibility of abdominal dissemination of bacteria.

Emerging Diagnostic Modalities: Flow Cytometry

For more information on this topic, please visit the companion Expert CONSULT Web site at www.expertconsult.com.

Diagnostic Schemes and Predictive Algorithms: SLE

For more information on this topic, please visit the companion Expert CONSULT Web site at www.expertconsult.com.

THERAPEUTIC OPTIONS

Overview: The Cell Cycle, Immunosuppression, and Supportive Therapies

Treatment of both organ-specific and polysystemic immune-mediated disease in the dog and cat relies on halting ongoing immune-mediated damage, while satisfying the nutritional, nursing, and—when applicable—analgesic requirements of the patient. Currently, nonspecific immunosuppression is central to the treatment of most "idiopathic" immune-mediated diseases and is achieved by the administration of corticosteroids with or without adjunctive agents.* For example, prednisolone or prednisone is usually administered to patients with polysystemic immune-mediated disease, with the option of adding azathioprine or other cytotoxic agents as appropriate.† The vinca alkaloids, notably vincristine, have been used for the treatment of ITP,[152,156,158,483,484] and a number of novel agents have now been evaluated in preclinical or small clinical studies with the promise of more potent and targeted immunosuppression for the future.[477,485-494]

---

*References 149, 158, 174, 176, 195, 198, 364, 369, 390, 471-480.
†References 166, 167, 169-171, 472, 479, 481, 482.

Discussion of the various classes of immunosuppressive drugs necessitates an understanding of the cell cycle, which is briefly reviewed here.[495] The beginning of the cycle is marked by phase M, or mitosis, which is followed by a G1 phase (gap 1) characterized by RNA and protein synthesis of varying duration from tissue to tissue, sometimes extending up to days or weeks. From G1, cells may enter a resting, nonproliferating state (G0) in which they may remain for long periods of time—or from which they may return quickly to G1, to proceed with cell division. A period of DNA synthesis (S phase) follows G1 and generally lasts about 2 hours. This is succeeded by G2 (gap 2), another period of RNA and protein synthesis that generally lasts about 6 to 8 hours. The immunosuppressive drugs described in the following paragraphs generally all inhibit proliferating immune cells, though their mechanisms of action and cell phase specificity vary widely. Owing to their potentially severe side effects and—in some cases—high cost, they are employed only when a definitive diagnosis has been reached. The following section summarizes key information of relevance to the clinical use of immunosuppressive drugs in the treatment of small animal immune-mediated disease, with an important caveat: in many cases, objective evidence of the benefit of these drugs—beyond that of corticosteroids alone—is lacking. Further work in this area of small animal medicine, in the form of blinded, controlled, prospective clinical trials, is clearly warranted, especially in the case of those drugs that are either expensive or associated with severe side effects in a proportion of patients.

Various supportive treatment measures should be considered alongside immunosuppression, including:
• Gastrointestinal cytoprotection

For more information on this topic, please visit the companion Expert CONSULT Web site at www.expertconsult.com.

• Whole blood, or packed red cell, transfusions

For more information on this topic, please visit the companion Expert CONSULT Web site at www.expertconsult.com.

• Thromboprophylaxis

For more information on this topic, please visit the companion Expert CONSULT Web site at www.expertconsult.com.

• Danazol

For more information on this topic, please visit the companion Expert CONSULT Web site at www.expertconsult.com.

• Erythropoietin-α

For more information on this topic, please visit the companion Expert CONSULT Web site at www.expertconsult.com.

• Antihypertensive drugs

For more information on this topic, please visit the companion Expert CONSULT Web site at www.expertconsult.com.

• Diet

For more information on this topic, please visit the companion Expert CONSULT Web site at www.expertconsult.com.

• Topical skin products, avoidance of excessive sunlight

For more information on this topic, please visit the companion Expert CONSULT Web site at www.expertconsult.com.

• Splenectomy

For more information on this topic, please visit the companion Expert CONSULT Web site at www.expertconsult.com.

• Therapeutic plasmapheresis

For more information on this topic, please visit the companion Expert CONSULT Web site at www.expertconsult.com.

Specific Immunosuppressive and Immunomodulating Agents

Corticosteroids Corticosteroids form the mainstay of immunosuppressive therapy, showing both genomic and nongenomic effects.[613] The genomic effects are mediated by binding to a cytoplasmic receptor, of which at least three isoforms are recognized in different tissues.[614-617] Following dissociation from plasma-binding proteins such as transcortin and albumin, corticosteroids either passively diffuse into the cell or engage with a plasma membrane receptor, which has been described in monocytes, B cells, and neutrophils; this membrane receptor is thought to mediate some of the nongenomic effects of these drugs.[618-620] A conformational change of the cytoplasmic receptor occurs following binding of the corticosteroid, which releases the heat shock and immunophilin proteins that associate with the receptor in the resting state.[614,615] This activation event unmasks the DNA-binding domain of the receptor, which is then able to associate with specific DNA sequences called *glucocorticoid responsive elements* (GREs) following translocation to the nucleus. The rate of transcription of nearby genes is either increased (positive GRE) or decreased (negative GRE), thereby inducing or inhibiting the translated proteins.[621-624] An example of a protein undergoing positive regulation is Iκβ, an inhibitory factor that associates with the transcription factor NFκβ, thereby preventing the up-regulation of several genes that do not themselves have GREs. The receptor and corticosteroid are eventually metabolized by the liver and other target tissues, with renal excretion of inactive metabolites; the cellular half-life of the activated complex is approximately 10 hours.[622]

Despite being the mainstay of immunosuppressive therapy, corticosteroids are associated with various systemic side-effects, particularly if required for long periods[474,625]; often they may be more optimally combined with other immunosuppressive agents, thus allowing a "dose-sparing" effect in the longer term (Box 185-1). Local therapy may also be appropriate for the treatment of certain immune-mediated diseases, such as inflammatory bowel disease (IBD)[626] and asthma,[627-629] in an endeavor to minimize systemic toxicity. Budesonide is a nonhalogenated glucocorticoid that has been used in aerosol form since the early 1980s to treat human asthma and allergic rhinitis[630]; indeed, the dog was used as an animal model in early evaluation of the efficacy and mechanisms of action of inhaled budesonide.[631,632] More recently, it has been used to treat human IBD.[633,634] After absorption across a mucosal surface, budesonide undergoes extensive (~90%) first-pass hepatic metabolism by the cytochrome P-450 system, yielding metabolites—primarily 16-α-hydroxyprednisolone and 6-β-hydroxybudesonide, which undergo renal excretion—with one-tenth to one-hundredth the activity of the parent molecule.[635] Budesonide has a concentrated local effect, because it is reversibly converted to lipophilic esters upon uptake into the cell; gradual hydrolysis of these esters releases active budesonide with time, thus prolonging its local effects.[636,637] Budesonide has been administered to dogs with IBD—with variable results[626,638]—when systemic effects of corticosteroids have been particularly undesirable, for example in patients with diabetes mellitus (DM) or those being treated for hyperadrenocorticism. Studies in both dogs with IBD[639] and healthy Beagles[640] have demonstrated that budesonide suppresses the hypothalamo-pituitary-adrenal (HPA) axis, despite showing none of the other clinicopathologic manifestations of systemic corticosteroids when administered for up to

---

Box • 185-1

Potential Adverse Effects of Corticosteroids

Central Nervous System
Polyphagia
Euphoria/restlessness

Musculoskeletal System
Osteopenia
Myopathy
Decreased intestinal calcium absorption

Gastrointestinal tract
Ulceration
Pancreatitis
Colonic perforation, especially perioperative spinal cases
    treated with dexamethasone

Fluid and Electrolyte Balance
Retention of sodium and water
Inhibition of action of antidiuretic hormone (ADH) on renal
    collecting tubules (nephrogenic diabetes insipidus) and an
    increase in glomerular filtration rate
Central diabetes insipidus: inhibition of release of ADH from
    neurohypophysis

Metabolic
Hyperlipidemia
Lipolysis
Protein catabolism
Glucocorticoid hepatopathy (dogs): multifocal or diffuse
    hepatic vacuoles containing glycogen

Endocrine
Hypothalamo-pituitary-adrenal axis suppression
Diabetogenic
Decreased synthesis of thyroid hormone

Immune System
Decreased bacterial killing
Increased risk of infection
Recurrent urinary tract infection (UTI): all animals receiving
long-term glucocorticoids should have periodic urine cultures
to rule out occult UTI

---

a month. Fluticasone propionate is an androstane glucocorticoid used in the treatment of childhood and adult asthma when administered by the inhaled route[641-643]; in humans, it has approximately twentyfold higher affinity for the glucocorticoid receptor than that of dexamethasone.[644,645] Like budesonide, fluticasone undergoes extensive first-pass hepatic metabolism by the cytochrome P-450 system, yielding an inactive metabolite (17β-carboxylic acid) that undergoes biliary excretion.[644,645] Fluticasone has been used in the treatment of chronic bronchitis and eosinophilic bronchopneumopathy in dogs[646] and chronic bronchitis and asthma in cats.[647,648] A recent study in healthy dogs revealed that fluticasone—like budesonide—suppresses the HPA axis, though less so than oral prednisone.[649] In the future, blinded, controlled, prospective clinical trials are required to substantiate the clinical efficacy of both budesonide and fluticasone in dogs and cats.

Relative immunosuppressive potency and duration of action of the orally administered corticosteroids varies, but prednisolone and prednisone are generally used as first-line drugs (Table 185-1). Therapeutic actions of corticosteroids in immune-mediated disease are thought to include[474,616,621,650-652]:

- Decreased egress of inflammatory cells from the bloodstream into peripheral tissues
- Decreased elaboration of inflammatory mediators, including prostaglandins and leukotrienes
- Suppression of macrophage and neutrophil bactericidal functions
- Decreased macrophage Fc receptor expression, with less effective phagocytosis
- Decreased antigen presentation to Th cells, with decreased T cell help for B cells
- Decreased effector cell function, including that of natural killer (NK) cells
- Inhibition of the passage of immune complexes through basement membranes
- Inhibition of the amplification pathways of the complement cascade

Antimetabolites   The antimetabolites impair cell function either by interfering directly with the action of an enzyme or by causing the synthesis of an aberrant molecule that fails to function properly within the cell.[653] These drugs are "phase-specific," interfering with the S phase of the cell cycle.[472,473] Three groups are recognized, based on their mechanisms of action. They include the purine analogs (azathioprine, 6-mercaptopurine), the antifolates (methotrexate), and the pyrimidine analogs (5-fluorouracil, cytosine arabinoside), of which azathioprine is the drug most often used to treat immune-mediated disease.[473,654]

The most commonly used of the thiopurines is azathioprine, which is converted to the active metabolite 6-mercaptopurine by the liver.[473,654] Further hepatic metabolism to the active compounds 6-thioinosinic and 6-thioguanylic acids then occurs, followed by xanthine oxidase–catalyzed breakdown to thiouric acid, a metabolite that undergoes renal excretion.[655] Coadministration of the xanthine oxidase inhibi-

---

Table • 185-1

Relative Immunosuppressive Potency of the Corticosteroids

DRUG	IMMUNOSUPPRESSIVE POTENCY	IMMUNOSUPPRESSIVE DOSE (MG/KG/DAY)	DURATION OF ACTION
Predniso(lo)ne	1	2.0-4.0	12-36 hrs
Methylprednisolone	1.25	2.0-4.0	12-36 hrs
Dexamethasone	7-10	0.2-0.5	>48 hrs
Betamethasone	7-10	0.2-0.5	>48 hrs

tor allopurinol increases the intracellular concentrations of the active metabolites of azathioprine, prompting the recommendation in human medicine to administer azathioprine at one fourth to one third the usual dose if the patient is also receiving allopurinol[656,657]; similar hazards presumably also exist in veterinary patients. The purine analogs compete with endogenous adenine and guanine, resulting in the formation of nonfunctional nucleic acid strands that prevent cellular proliferation; immunosuppression results from reduced DNA and RNA synthesis, with inhibition of coenzyme formation and mitosis.[473,655] Both humoral and cell-mediated immunity are inhibited; the effects on T cells are profound and include the inhibition of inflammatory gene expression,[658] induction of their apoptosis following activation,[659] and suppression of their conjugate formation with antigen-presenting cells.[660] Azathioprine may also reduce the elaboration of proinflammatory cytokines by monocytes and macrophages.[661,662] While the immunosuppressive effect of azathioprine may theoretically take several weeks to become apparent, inhibition of lymphocyte blastogenesis in vitro was demonstrated in one study after only 1 week of therapy[663]; though the in vitro system can never entirely recapitulate the behavior of the drug in vivo, these results accord with the author's impression that the clinical effect of azathioprine may be observed within the first 2 weeks of therapy when combined with corticosteroids.

Azathioprine has been used in the management of lymphocytic and granulocytic leukemias and various immune-mediated diseases, often being administered alongside a corticosteroid, thus capitalizing on its "steroid-sparing" effect.[472,473,654] Several studies have suggested that azathioprine confers a beneficial impact on clinical signs and survival in canine IMHA,[121,123,124,128] while a fifth revealed a potential benefit that failed to reach statistical significance—perhaps because of underpowering of the study.[273] Though this evidence has all been derived from retrospective clinical studies, which immediately undermines the confidence with which predictions can be made,[664-666] it is nevertheless the best evidence that we currently have available and provides a rationale for the coadministration of azathioprine with a corticosteroid in the management of canine IMHA, unless there is a specific contraindication against the use of this drug. Azathioprine is generally well tolerated in the dog, but gives rise to profound and often irreversible myelosuppression if used above the safe dose of 0.3 mg/kg PO every 48 hours in the cat[667]; since accurate dosing is difficult to achieve with 50-mg tablets and the therapeutic window of this drug is particularly narrow in cats, its use in this species is **not** recommended. Potential toxic manifestations of this drug in the dog include neutropenia, thrombocytopenia, anemia, acute pancreatitis, nonspecific gastrointestinal signs (vomiting and diarrhea), and hepatopathy.[473,654] Neuromuscular blockade is a potential additional adverse effect in the cat.[654]

Methotrexate

For more information on this topic, please visit the companion Expert CONSULT Web site at www.expertconsult.com.

Cytosine arabinoside (cytarabine)

For more information on this topic, please visit the companion Expert CONSULT Web site at www.expertconsult.com.

Mitotic Inhibitors: Vinca Alkaloids The vinca alkaloids were originally extracted from the common periwinkle plant, *Vinca rosea*, purported to have hypoglycemic properties by common folklore. Despite ultimately demonstrating only minimal hypoglycemic effects, crude extracts from this plant were found to have cytotoxic properties.[696,697] Vincristine and vinblastine are the two most common vinca alkaloids employed in modern veterinary practice[697,698]; vinorelbine, a semisynthetic derivative of vinblastine, was recently evaluated in the treatment of dogs with cutaneous mast cell tumors, but yielded disappointing results with significant toxicity,[699] despite encouraging earlier data.[700] Vincristine and vinblastine have similar chemical structures, based on a common multi-ringed complex with a formyl (vincristine) or methyl (vinblastine) side chain attached to a catharanthine ring.[697] Both drugs bind to tubulin, a dimeric protein resident in the soluble fraction of the cytoplasm, blocking its polymerization and leading to arrest of the cell cycle in metaphase.[701] Vinca alkaloids also lead to the breakdown of preformed microtubules, which function in the maintenance of cellular structure and the provision of a conduit for secretions and the movement of neurotransmitters along axons.[696,701] Interference with these functions may be responsible for both the increased release of platelets from megakaryocytes and the neurotoxic side effects of these drugs.[696,702] While vincristine is considered to be phase-specific, acting during mitosis, vinblastine also blocks the cellular use of glutamic acid, thereby inhibiting purine synthesis and the S phase of the cell cycle.[696,697]

The principal indication for the vinca alkaloids is in the treatment of lymphoma and lymphoid leukemias, usually as a component of a combination protocol,[698,703] but vincristine has also been administered to dogs with hemangiosarcomas,[704] and vinblastine is used in the chemotherapy of mast cell tumors.[705,706] Vincristine is also the drug of choice for the treatment of canine transmissible venereal tumor[707] and vinblastine—less often associated with neurotoxicity—may be considered as an alternative to vincristine if a peripheral neuropathy has developed in the course of treatment.[708,709-713] Vincristine has also been used in the therapy of ITP, either being administered intravenously as a bolus injection[152,156,364,369,484] or used to load platelets prior to a transfusion of platelet-rich plasma (PRP).[483] Loading the platelets with the vinca alkaloid in this manner targets toxic amounts of the drug to the reticuloendothelial system, thereby helping to eliminate the principal sink of platelets in ITP. Vincristine binds more avidly to platelets than vinblastine, so may be preferable for this mode of therapy. A method for loading platelets in vivo has also been described, involving dilution of vincristine in isotonic saline solution and slow infusion over 4 to 8 hours; both the solution and giving set need to be covered with aluminum foil to prevent degradation of the drug by ultraviolet light.[714] Both of the vinca alkaloids must be given intravenously, since they act as severe irritants in the extravascular tissues, leading to pain, necrosis, and even tissue sloughing.[696,715] If extravasation occurs, the injection should be stopped immediately, the area infused with hyaluronidase (150 U through the patent catheter or needle),[716] and heat applied to the area for 15 to 30 minutes 4 times daily for 48 hours, in an effort to disperse the drug and minimize tissue irritation; cold packs should not be applied, since they tend to exacerbate tissue ulceration in the case of vinca alkaloids.[717] Topical application of 90% dimethylsulphoxide may also be carried out several times daily for 72 hours, for its antiinflammatory, free radical–scavenging, and analgesic properties.[718]

Vincristine is generally not myelosuppressive in the dog, though it may occasionally induce significant neutropenia in the cat.[719] Inappetence, nausea, vomiting and constipation may be observed with both vincristine and vinblastine in the dog and cat.[697,714] Vinblastine has myelosuppressive activity in both species, the nadir for neutrophil counts usually occurring within 4 to 9 days of administration; recovery after withdrawal of the drug usually takes from 7 to 14 days.[720] One of the more debilitating side effects of long-term treatment with vincristine and, rarely, vinblastine is the development of an iatrogenic sensory and motor neuropathy, seen most often in cats.[709-712] Neuronal degeneration with axonal swelling may occur, with secondary demyelination of peripheral nerves; if therapy is not immediately stopped, severe, generalized motor weakness may develop.[710,711,713] Signs of the neuropathy generally abate in the months following cessation of therapy, though some of the lesions may be irreversible. Pulmonary edema has also recently been documented in a cat with chronic lymphocytic leukemia given vincristine as part of a combination chemotherapy protocol.[721] Finally, the syndrome of inappropriate ADH release (SIADH) has been recorded in human patients receiving vincristine,[696] though this side effect appears to be rare in the dog and cat.[697,714] The vinca alkaloids are eliminated primarily by biliary excretion of the parent drug, alongside some urinary excretion of the parent drug and metabolites.[722] The enzyme responsible for metabolizing vinca alkaloids in dogs and cats has not been identified, but biliary excretion in other species is dependent on the drug transporter P-glycoprotein, which is present on biliary canalicular and renal tubular epithelial cells.[723] A recent study documented a greater prevalence of hematologic toxicities—thrombocytopenia and neutropenia—in dogs with the ABCB1-1Δ (formerly MDR-1) mutation, which encodes functionally inactive P-glycoprotein; thus, accumulation of the drug was thought to occur as a consequence of its compromised excretion.[724,725] A pharmacogenetic approach to vincristine therapy was therefore recommended, involving the submission of a polymerase chain reaction (PCR) test for the mutation in any patient falling within one of the herding breeds—which show increased prevalence of the mutation[726,727]—before therapy commences: if the patient was homozygous or heterozygous for the mutation, vincristine would be administered at a reduced dose—though the appropriate dose reduction has not yet been established and currently remains empirical.[725]

Calcineurin Inhibitors The calcineurin inhibitors, ciclosporin and tacrolimus (formerly FK506), function by binding to specific intracellular receptors called *immunophilins*: ciclosporin binds to cyclophilin, while tacrolimus binds to the FK506-binding protein.[728-730] The heterodimeric complex thus formed then associates with and inhibits the calcineurin-calmodulin complex, a calcium-dependent serine-threonine phosphatase that results in the dephosphorylation of regulatory proteins. Following translocation to the nucleus, the dephosphorylated regulatory proteins act as subunits of transcription factors such as NF-AT (nuclear factor of activated T cells), which promotes transcription of the interleukin (IL)-2 gene.[729-733] The calcineurin inhibitors thus suppress transcription of key cytokines involved in the innate and adaptive arms of the immune response, including IL-2, a T cell growth factor, and interferon-α, a monocyte and macrophage activation factor[729-735]; blockade of the transition from cell phase G_0 to G_1 thus occurs. Ciclosporin also inhibits the proliferation of canine keratinocytes and their synthesis of prostaglandin E_2 following exposure to lipopolysaccharide, mechanisms that may contribute to its antiinflammatory and immunosuppressive action in the treatment of canine allergic skin disease.[736] In addition, both ciclosporin and tacrolimus stimulate the activation of latent transforming growth factor-β via the generation of reactive oxygen intermediates, contributing to the excessive deposition of extracellular matrix that underlies the nephrotoxicity of these agents in humans.[737] Various studies have suggested that the calcineurin inhibitors also inhibit the number and/or function of Tregs, which would work against attempts to correct the abnormal immune responses underlying autoimmune disease,[738-742] but this observation remains controversial.[743-745] Tacrolimus is 10 to 100 times more potent than ciclosporin[746-748] but has a low therapeutic index and is associated with severe side effects in dogs, including inappetence, vasculitis, hepatotoxicity, and intestinal intussusception.[731,749-751] Therefore, its systemic use in small animals cannot currently be recommended. However,

topical tacrolimus has found utility in the management of canine atopic dermatitis,[485,752] perianal fistulae, DLE, pemphigus erythematosus, pemphigus foliaceus, alopecia areata, and vitiligo, but usually only as an adjunctive or secondary treatment[753-755]; furthermore, ocular tacrolimus has shown promise in the management of canine keratoconjunctivitis sicca,[756] but the skin product (Protopic; Astellas Pharma) should **not** be placed in the eye since it contains propylene carbonate, an ocular irritant.[753] As a topical therapy, tacrolimus is associated with minimal toxicity, showing neither atrophogenic nor adverse systemic effects[485,753,754]; however, care should be taken to prevent the patient from inadvertently ingesting the drug by licking the area to which it has been applied.

Cyclosporine A, now known simply as *ciclosporin*, is a cyclic polypeptide metabolite extracted from the fungus *Tolypocladium inflatum Gams*.[757] The drug is lipophilic and hydrophobic, and must be solubilized before administration.[758] The intravenous preparation (Sandimmune Injection; Novartis) is an ethanol-polyoxyethylated castor oil mixture (Cremophor EL) that must be diluted in 0.9% sodium chloride or 5% dextrose in water prior to administration,[759] while the oral preparation (Neoral) and the veterinary-licensed product Atopica; Novartis) is a microemulsion formulation[760-763]; the older, soft gelatin–capsulated oral preparation (Sandimmune; Novartis) shows poor bioavailability and is not recommended.[764,765] Ciclosporin has a large volume of distribution, most accumulating in red blood cells and leukocytes; remaining circulating drug is bound to plasma lipoproteins.[766,767] Metabolism is primarily hepatic, with predominantly biliary excretion; only a small percentage of metabolites undergo renal excretion.[766,767] While the presence of food decreased the bioavailability of the micoremulsified preparation of ciclosporin by 22% in dogs,[768] it appeared to make no difference to clinical response in the treatment of canine atopic dermatitis[769]; thus, the usual recommendation to administer the drug 2 hours before or after feeding may be redundant in some clinical scenarios.

The need for therapeutic drug monitoring of ciclosporin is controversial. Recent studies of canine patients with both atopic dermatitis[768,770] and perianal fistulae[771,772] suggest that the reliable bioavailability of the microemulsified preparation and the lack of correlation between blood concentrations and clinical response argue against routine monitoring of blood ciclosporin concentrations for these disorders. The side effects are dose-related and clearly discernible, one of the most serious in human patients—nephrotoxicity—not being encountered in small animals at the commonly recommended doses of the drug.[485,766,767,773] However, the author would recommend the measurement of whole blood ciclosporin concentrations in the context of hematologic or other systemic immune-mediated diseases—or when a clinical response to a regular dose of ciclosporin has not been observed in a dermatologic application, to exclude the possibility of poor drug absorption in the individual patient. A third scenario in which drug monitoring may be helpful is to monitor dogs with a known ABCB1-1Δ mutation and thus defective P-glycoprotein function, in which systemic accumulation of the ciclosporin may occur as a consequence of decreased biliary and renal excretion—as both ciclosporin and tacrolimus are known to be P-glycoprotein substrates.[727] Decreased lymphocyte efflux of ciclosporin may also occur,[774] adding to the potential for toxicity, though to the author's knowledge this possibility has not so far been explored in small animals and appears to be complicated in humans owing to the large number of polymorphisms and their differential effects on P-glycoprotein function.[775] Whole blood or plasma levels of ciclosporin can be determined by high-pressure liquid chromatography (HPLC), fluorescence polarization immunoassay, and specific monoclonal antibody radioimmunoassay: trough ciclosporin concentration is measured just prior to administration of the next dose.[776] While an optimal blood concentration has not been objectively determined for any of the systemic immune-mediated disorders in small animals, authors have variously suggested maintenance of a trough concentration of at least 200 ng/mL,[777,778] or targeting a trough concentration of 400 to 500 ng/mL,[776,779] in both the dog and cat—based on extrapolation from the human literature, anecdotal evidence, and experience gained in the setting of allotransplantation. Measurements are begun 48 hours after the start of therapy, repeating at 1, 2, and 4 weeks, and ideally continuing every 1 to 3 months thereafter in an endeavor to ensure maintenance of immunosuppressive effect without inadvertent overdosing.[780] In order to reduce the cost of therapy—especially in large dogs—ketoconazole may be administered with the ciclosporin: the ketoconazole inhibits the hepatic microsomal cytochrome P-450 isoenzyme 3A12 involved in the metabolism of ciclosporin, thus reducing the dose by as much as 60%.[766,776,781-786] Side effects of dual therapy have not been noted, though chronic administration of ketoconazole to dogs may induce the formation of cataracts.[787] The administration of fluconazole alongside ciclosporin would tend to have the same effect, increasing blood concentrations of ciclosporin and prompting the recommendation to monitor blood levels and—if necessary—to reduce the dose of ciclosporin commensurately in this situation.[788]

Ciclosporin tends not to be nephrotoxic or hepatotoxic in dogs and cats at the doses recommended in the veterinary literature—in contrast to the susceptibility of human patients to such toxicities—and is generally well tolerated in these species.[766,770,789,790] However, it may nevertheless cause inappetence and predispose to opportunistic bacterial and fungal infections in both cats and dogs at routine doses[766,791-793]; recrudescence of dormant infections—for example, toxoplasmosis[794]—may occasionally also be observed. Long-term ciclosporin therapy may also increase the probability of neoplasia—in particular lymphoma[795,796]—especially with concurrent prednisone or prednisolone therapy. Other side effects noted in dogs have included vomiting, diarrhea, weight loss, gingival hyperplasia, papillomatosis, involuntary shaking, inhibition of insulin release, and peripheral insulin resistance—all signs that tend to abate with a reduction in dose.[731,766,776,777,797] Finally, hirsutism may be observed in both dogs and cats.[766,770,797,798]

Ciclosporin has been used successfully in small animal patients in the context of renal transplantation[776,799] and various immune-mediated disorders, including keratoconjunctivitis sicca (KCS; topical therapy),[800-802] perianal fistulae,[771,772,781-783,803] pemphigus,[767,804] atopic dermatitis,* sebaceous adenitis,[807,808] alopecia areata,[808] pure red cell aplasia,[809] vesicular cutaneous LE,[810] MG,[811] meningoencephalomyelitis of unknown etiology (MUE),[812-815] and steroid-refractory IBD.[816] However, a prospective, placebo-controlled clinical trial found that the drug offered no advantage over standard care in the management of idiopathic GN,[817] and reports of the therapeutic potential of ciclosporin in the treatment of IMHA remain mixed, some suggesting that it shows efficacy[818,819] and others failing to substantiate any clinical benefit in this setting.[273,820] Finally, ciclosporin has also been used in the treatment of canine[157,819] and feline[164] ITP, but its clinical benefit in this disease remains unsubstantiated.

Rapamycin

For more information on this topic, please visit the companion Expert CONSULT Web site at www.expertconsult.com.

Novel Antimetabolites
Leflunomide

For more information on this topic, please visit the companion Expert CONSULT Web site at www.expertconsult.com.

Mycophenolate mofetil

For more information on this topic, please visit the companion Expert CONSULT Web site at www.expertconsult.com.

Alkylating Agents These drugs possess alkyl radicals (R-CH_2-CH_3^+) that react covalently with DNA, causing breaks in the molecule and cross-linking of the twin strands, actions that interfere with DNA replication and RNA transcription.[473,879] These agents thereby inhibit protein synthesis in resting cells, prevent mitosis, and kill dividing cells.[473,879] This group includes cyclophosphamide, ifosfamide, chlorambucil, melphalan, mechlorethamine, nitrosoureas (carmustine and lomustine), procarbazine, and dacarbazine, though only chlorambucil is in current use as an immunosuppressive drug in small animals. Various studies have demonstrated the neutral or negative impact of cyclophosphamide on the outcome of IMHA,[124,126,128,273] and the author does **not** therefore recommend the use of this drug for small animal immune-mediated disease. Indeed, a number of recent studies have demonstrated that Tregs show a differential sensitivity to the lymphotoxic effects of cyclophosphamide, which is thought to underlie its ability to accelerate the expression of type 1 DM in NOD mice,[880,881] and combination therapy with corticosteroids may even amplify cyclophosphamide-induced effects on Treg number and function.[882] This potentiating effect on the immune response at low doses is thought to be the basis of metronomic therapy for neoplasia.[883-886]

Chlorambucil is a cell cycle–nonspecific alkylating agent that shows high oral bioavailability and is highly plasma protein–bound; it is a noncytotoxic prodrug that is rapidly metabolized in the liver to phenylacetic acid mustard, the principal active metabolite.[473,887-889] Further metabolism to inactive compounds that are excreted in the urine and feces occurs.[890,891] Chlorambucil is the slowest acting and least toxic of all the alkylating agents commonly used in veterinary medicine[473]; myelosuppression—which is dose-related—is generally not observed until the drug has been administered for at least a month, and is usually reversible within a 2-week period if noted sufficiently early.[888,892,893] Additional side effects may include inappetence, vomiting and diarrhea, referable to gastrointestinal toxicity,[893] generalized myoclonus,[894] and grand mal seizures,[895] which have been observed in cats receiving high-dose pulse therapy. Chlorambucil is generally administered without food, which interferes with its passive absorption.[896,897] It is used in combination chemotherapy protocols for chronic lymphocytic leukemia, low-grade lymphoma, intermediate to high-grade lymphoma (maintenance protocols), mast cell tumors, multiple myeloma, and to replace cyclophosphamide in cases of sterile hemorrhagic cystitis.[893,895,898-900] It has also found utility as an adjunctive immunosuppressive agent in the treatment of canine and feline pemphigus foliaceus,[804,901] feline eosinophilic granuloma complex, and a variety of immune-mediated diseases in cats (e.g., IMHA, ITP, and IBD) when used in combination with corticosteroids.[893] Corticosteroids and chlorambucil may also benefit patients with membranous GN, which results from the deposition of immune complexes—most often containing IgG—onto the subepithelial aspect of the glomerular basement membrane.[902] In common with many of the alternative immunosuppressive drugs in the dog and cat, objective evidence for the efficacy of chlorambucil in this and other potential indications is currently lacking; further work is required in this area.

---

*References 485, 768, 789, 790, 805, 806.

Intravenous Immunoglobulin Human intravenous immunoglobulin (hIVIG) is a purified preparation of polyspecific IgG derived from the pooled plasma of healthy blood donors, used in human medicine to provide passive immunity in patients with primary or secondary immunodeficiency syndromes and in the treatment of a number of immune-mediated disorders, including chronic inflammatory demyelinating polyneuropathy and multifocal motor neuropathy; ITP, IMHA, autoimmune neutropenia and pure red cell aplasia; acute, decompensating MG; Guillain-Barré syndrome; Kawasaki disease; and dermatomyositis.[903-905] Indeed, hIVIG has been used in the treatment of almost 100 human diseases, though it has been approved by the Food and Drug Administration for only 6.[904,906,907] Plasma used for the preparation of hIVIG is typically derived from 3000 to 100,000 healthy blood donors screened for antibodies to human immunodeficiency virus, hepatitis B and hepatitis C, following multiple fractionation and processing steps to reduce its infectious risk and to harvest the therapeutic component.[903] Each preparation contains antibodies from across the spectrum of the normal human IgG repertoire, including antibodies to external antigens—for example, from food, intestinal bacteria, pathogens—and autoreactive and antiidiotypic antibodies (an *idiotype* is an antigenic determinant of the variable region of an antibody: antiidiotypic antibodies are those with specificity for other antibodies); hIVIG also contains traces of IgA, IgM, Th2 cytokines and cytokine antagonists.[903,908] While the mechanisms of action of hIVIG have not all been fully elucidated, they are thought to include:[908-911] (i) blockade of Fcγ receptors on monocytes and macrophages, thus inhibiting antibody-dependent cellular cytotoxicity; (ii) saturation of the neonatal Fc receptors (FcRn) present on endothelial cells, thus rendering the FcRn unable to bind to—and protect from degradation—autoAbs within lysosomes; (iii) neutralization of autoAbs by idiotypic Abs in IVIG; (iv) inhibition of the interaction of autoreactive T cells with antigen-presenting cells, by virtue of soluble CD4, CD8, and MHC molecules, and anti–T cell receptor Abs, present in the IVIG product, all of which block key molecular interactions in the immunologic synapse; (v) simultaneous ligation of B cell–inhibitory FcγRIIB and the B cell receptor idiotype, with resultant inhibition of B cell activation and induction of anergy and, or apoptosis—thus helping to ameliorate autoantibody production; (vi) immune deviation from Th1 to Th2, by virtue of the presence of Th2 cytokines and both Abs and antagonists of Th1 cytokines within the IVIG product; (vii) inhibition of the differentiation and function of dendritic cells, in part by enhancing the production of IL-10; (viii) prevention of the generation of the membrane attack complex (C5b-9), by scavenging active complement components and diverting them away from cellular targets; and (ix) inhibition of leukocyte recruitment to inflamed tissues, by direct inhibition of selectin and integrin function.[912] Most of these mechanisms remain unsubstantiated in small animals, but binding of hIVIG to canine lymphocytes and monocytes has been demonstrated, the latter Fc-mediated.[913] Furthermore, the ability of hIVIG to inhibit phagocytosis of antibody-coated canine RBCs was confirmed using a mononuclear cell phagocytic assay.[913]

hIVIG has been employed alongside conventional immunosuppressive therapy in various immune-mediated diseases of dogs, including: (i) nonregenerative anemia, in which reticulocytosis was observed within 1 to 4 days of administration in five of five dogs, two of which required a further infusion by 52 days after initial treatment, which elicited a similar, but blunted response[914]; (ii) IMHA, in which hIVIG appeared to elicit an increase in PCV of at least 4% within 3 to 4 days in 10 of 13 dogs,[915] an increase in hemoglobin concentration of at least 2 g/dL within 14 days in 8 to 10 dogs[916] and a potential beneficial effect in 9 dogs, which showed similar mortality to 13 patients not receiving hIVIG despite suffering from more severe disease[917]; (iii) severe ITP, in which 4 of 5 dogs showed an apparent response to treatment, the mean platelet count increasing from 2500/μL to 50,600/μL 24 hours after infusion;[918] (iv) concurrent IMHA and ITP (Evans' syndrome) in a diabetic Miniature Schnauzer immunosuppressed only with leflunomide and hIVIG, the platelet count increasing from 2000/μL to 116,000/μL within 24 hours of the infusion[856]; and (v) various immune-mediated skin diseases, including severe pemphigus foliaceus,[919] Stevens-Johnson syndrome[920] and other suspected cutaneous drug reactions,[921] and epidermolysis bullosa acquisita[922]—all of which experienced an improvement in clinical signs after hIVIG infusion. Experience of hIVIG in the treatment of feline immune-mediated disease is limited: to the author's knowledge, only a single case report of its use in the treatment of severe erythema multiforme in a domestic shorthair cat has been published, suggesting a beneficial response.[923] In the same publication, the authors allude to a case of toxic epidermal necrolysis in a dog that was also treated with hIVIG. Several authors have hypothesized that hIVIG may allow a temporary cessation of erythrolysis in IMHA, thus allowing additional time for other forms of treatment to become effective.[924] Indeed, the short half-life of hIVIG in dogs (7 to 9 days[916]) suggests that its benefits may be limited to the short term, supported by its apparent inability to improve long-term survival of canine patients with IMHA in one study.[916] However, the possibility of a longer term impact on cells of the immune system—perhaps extending beyond the physical presence of hIVIG itself—cannot be excluded and may explain its association with long-term clinical remission in dogs with nonregenerative anemia.[914] One of the potentially beneficial effects of hIVIG in the treatment of immune-mediated skin disease is the blockade of *Fas* receptors expressed by diseased keratinocytes,[925] though there is no proof of this mechanism operating in small animals. Despite these initially encouraging reports of the use of hIVIG in a number of canine immune-mediated diseases, a recent blinded, placebo-controlled, randomized clinical trial of hIVIG in dogs with IMHA failed to demonstrate any improvement in initial clinical response or shortening of the period of hospitalization—though the authors conceded that their study was underpowered when examined posthoc.[282]

hIVIG has been administered at doses varying from 0.5 to 1.5 g/kg in the form of a solution diluted in 0.9% saline or sterile water—according to the individual product—infused over 4 to 12 hours[924]; prophylactic diphenhydramine was also administered immediately prior to the infusion in several studies, owing to the potential for a hypersensitivity response.[282,856,915,916,918-924] Side effects of hIVIG treatment in canine patients appear to be uncommon, resonating with the low prevalence of severe side effects in human patients.[926] Pilot studies documented mild, transient thrombocytopenia in healthy dogs given hIVIG[916]; furthermore, the potential for allospecific hypersensitivity reactions exists with repeated administration, though multiple doses were administered over a 31-week period in a dog with pemphigus foliaceus without adverse effects.[919] An increased tendency for thromboembolism has been documented in human patients,[926] but a recent prospective clinical study of hIVIG in canine IMHA documented only mild and transient side effects, with no evidence of increased PTE in the treated animals.[282] A drawback to the widespread use of hIVIG therapy is its high cost and inconsistent availability to veterinarians, owing to constant demand for the product in human medicine.[904] Further, controlled clinical studies are required in the future to define with more certainty the therapeutic benefits and potential side effects of hIVIG in dogs and cats.

Levamisole

For more information on this topic, please visit the companion Expert CONSULT Web site at www.expertconsult.com.

Practical guidelines for therapy

For more information on this topic, please visit the companion Expert CONSULT Web site at www.expertconsult.com.

Problems and solutions in therapy of immune-mediated disease

For more information on this topic, please visit the companion Expert CONSULT Web site at www.expertconsult.com.

REFERENCES

The reference list can be found on the companion Expert Consult Web site at *www.expertconsult.com*.

CHAPTER 186

Immune-Mediated and Infective Arthritis

David Bennett

Immune-mediated and infective arthritis form the two main categories of inflammatory arthropathy (Figure 186-1) and are characterized by an elevated white cell count in the synovial fluid, mainly comprising neutrophils. Synovial fluid analysis is mandatory for diagnosis of these conditions, and it distinguishes them from the more common degenerative arthropathies (see Chapter 187).[1] Infective arthritis is defined as an inflammatory arthropathy caused by an infective agent that can be cultured from the affected joint or joints; however, it is not always possible to culture the organism, and it is important to assume infection where only a single joint is affected with an inflammatory type of arthritis. Bacteria are the most common cause of infective arthritis. The use of the polymerase chain reaction (PCR) to detect microbial RNA and DNA may, in the future, challenge our present understanding of joint infections[2]; it can certainly help in detecting the presence of microbial agents that cannot be cultured; however, its extreme sensitivity must be recognized. A recent study, for example, reported bacterial DNA in 37% of stifle joints of dogs with cranial cruciate ligament failure but without sepsis and thus the pathogenetic significance is unclear.[2]

Immune-mediated arthritis is defined as an inflammatory disease where microbial organisms cannot be cultured from the joints and where the immune system plays an important role in its pathogenesis, in the form of immune complex formation, and autoimmunity. The failure to culture microorganisms does not rule out their involvement, but unlike the true infective arthropathies, there are no living organisms within the articular cavity. Unlike bacterial infective arthritis, they are generally polyarthropathies, although some of the more uncommon infections can involve multiple joints. Although the etiology of immune-mediated arthritis is unknown, certain microbial infections have been implicated. Immune complex formation in response to microbial infection, either locally in the joint or systemically with subsequent deposition into the joint is a favored hypothesis.[3] Transportation of microbial antigens to joints, with a subsequent immune response, is another possibility. Canine distemper viral antigens and antibodies have been identified in the immune complexes from the synovia of dogs with immune-mediated arthritis[4]; macrophages containing distemper antigens have also been demonstrated in the synovial membrane.[5] The theory of molecular mimicry has also been proposed, where antibodies against certain bacteria or viruses may cross-react with cartilage components. Some researchers think that polyclonal B-cell activation, as may occur in a persistent or serious infection, may lead to the emergence of autoantibodies against joint "self-antigens," which can result in joint pathology. For example, autoantibodies against heat shock proteins may stimulate immune complex formation in joints or may even cross-react with cartilage epitopes.[6] Similarly antiglobulins (rheumatoid factors) can be involved in immune complex formation. Potential antigens may also originate from nonmicrobial sources, such as tumor antigens, drug antigens/haptens, and dietary antigens. Once the joint inflammation has been established, by whatever mechanism, various autoantigens, such as altered collagen, are produced. These autoantigens will also stimulate an immune response, thereby helping to perpetuate the inflammation.[7,8]

It is likely that certain individuals are genetically predisposed to immune-mediated arthritis, particularly through genetic variations in the immune response. Certain of the histocompatibility antigens, in particular the DLA-DRB1 alleles (DRB1 002, 009, and 018), have been associated with immune-mediated arthritis in the dog; furthermore, it appears that a conserved amino acid motif in the third hypervariable region in some DRB1 alleles of both humans and dogs is associated with immune-based arthritis in both species.[9]

Lameness is an important clinical feature in both infective and immune-based arthritis, although many immune-mediated polyarthropathies present as cases of "pyrexia of unknown origin." Lameness may be an obvious limp, although generalized stiffness is most often seen with the immune-mediated polyarthropathies. Bacterial infections generally have an acute onset, although a more chronic, insidious onset is possible, the so-called "low-grade" infections. The joint is usually swollen and painful on manipulation, and heat may be detectable. Only about one third of infective arthropathies have systemic signs, as compared to two thirds of the immune-mediated cases. The immune-mediated arthropathies tend to have a sudden onset, with multiple joints swollen and painful in a bilaterally symmetric fashion. In some cases obvious joint swelling and pain may not be apparent, but multiple arthrocenteses and fluid analyses confirm the diagnosis. Multiple synovial fluid analyses should be performed in all cases of "pyrexia of unknown origin"; immune-mediated polyarthritis is the single most common diagnosis of such cases in a referral practice.[10] Local lymphadenopathy is common with both the

WWW. To view a video on this topic, go to **www.expertconsult.com.**

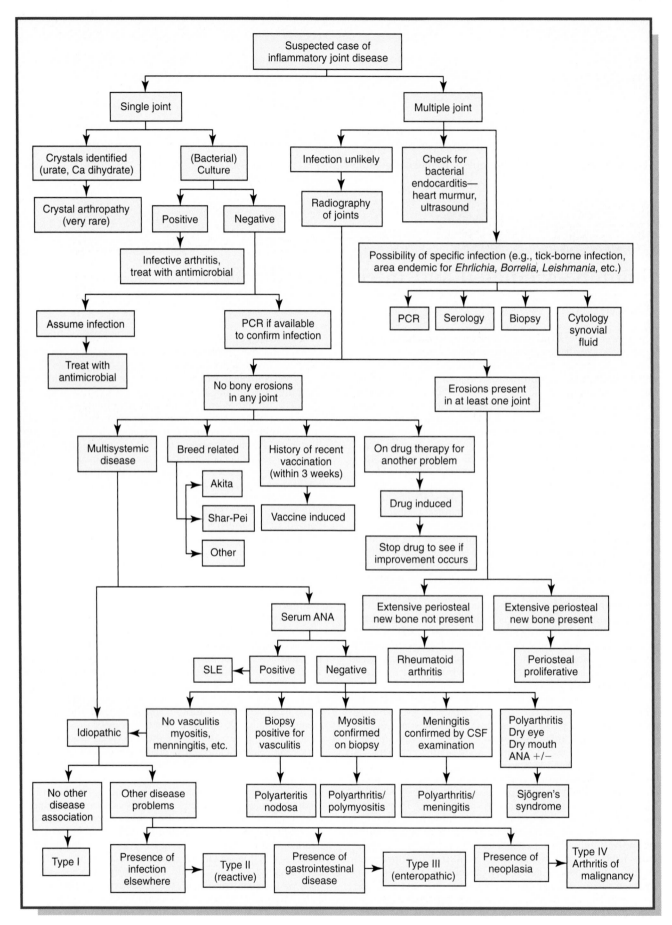

Figure 186-1 Algorithm showing how to identify a specific type of inflammatory arthropathy. The initial identification is made on synovial fluid examination—a fluid containing a high neutrophil count. *ANA*, Antinuclear antibody; *CSF*, cerebrospinal fluid; *PCR*, polymerase chain reaction; *SLE*, systemic lupus erythematosus.

infective and the immune-mediated arthropathies. Diseases of other body systems are common with the immune-mediated arthropathies, although these can occur with certain infections as well.

BACTERIAL INFECTIVE ARTHRITIS (SEPTIC ARTHRITIS, SUPPURATIVE ARTHRITIS)

Beta-hemolytic streptococci of Lancefield group G, *Staphylococci*, hemolytic *Escherichia coli*, *Pasteurella* sp., and *Erysipelothrix* sp. are the bacteria most commonly isolated from septic joints.[11-13] Less commonly isolated organisms include *Corynebacterium*, *Salmonella*, *Brucella*, and *Pseudomonas* spp. and anaerobic organisms. In some cases a mixed infection may be present, involving both aerobic and anaerobic bacteria. Infection can be introduced by direct penetration of a joint, iatrogenic infection after open joint surgery, or through road accident injuries. Most joint infections in cats are associated with bite wounds incurred in fights. In most dogs, infection occurs by the hematogenous route, and the source of infection is often unknown. Preexisting joint disease such as osteoarthritis and/or prior surgical intervention predisposes the joint to opportunistic infection as a result of seeding of organisms in the compromised synovial tissues.[12] Trauma can also predispose a joint to subsequent infection and lameness; an initial mild injury may resolve, but the lameness returns a few days later after hematogenous localization of infection to the joint.[11] Bacterial infections may also spread to joints from infected foci in neighboring soft tissues or bone. Most cases involve only a single joint, but two joints may be affected at the same time, or a second joint may be affected some time after the first (Web Figure 186-1).

Involvement of more than two joints most often occurs secondary to a severe systemic bacterial infection, such as bacterial endocarditis[14] or omphalophlebitis, that has a significant bacteremic component. Confusingly, bacterial endocarditis can result in a true infective arthritis or in an immune-mediated arthritis. These dogs often have lesions of other body systems, and a cardiac murmur is generally present. Ultrasonography may show the vegetative endocarditic lesion.

Bacterial infective arthritis affects dogs of all ages. The larger breeds are most often affected, and the male to female ratio is 2:1. The elbow and stifle joints are most often affected although any joint can be involved. The radiographic features vary with the type of infection and its duration. The earliest radiographic change is soft tissue swelling (Web Figure 186-2). A marked periosteal reaction often develops in the later stages, and calcification of the joint capsule may be seen. Subchondral bone erosions may appear as discrete radiolucencies or as more extensive bone destruction (Figure 186-2). Patchy sclerosis of subchondral bone is often seen. Some infected joints show an overall loss of bone density (see Figure 186-2). Leukocytosis, as a result of neutrophilia and a left shift, is an inconsistent finding.

The diagnosis of bacterial infective arthritis is confirmed by culture of the organism from synovial fluid or synovial membrane (or both); however, negative cultures are common. Both aerobic and anaerobic cultures should be made and it is important to place the sample immediately into culture medium if anaerobes are to be isolated. Blood cultures are sometimes worthwhile if the animal is pyrexic. Bacterial sensitivity testing should be performed on positive cultures to aid therapeutic planning.

The mainstay of therapy is a prolonged course of systemic antibiotics, which should be initiated in all suspect cases pending confirmatory laboratory results. A broad-spectrum bactericidal antibiotic is used. Clavulanate-potentiated amoxicillin, fluoroquinolones and cephalosporins are all useful. The

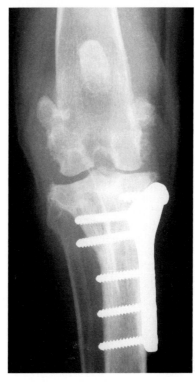

Figure 186-2 Craniocaudal radiograph of an infected stifle joint showing advanced pathology. Bony destruction is obvious, as shown by an increased intercondylar notch and bony loss at the articular margins of the femur and tibia. Overall loss of bone density of the distal femur also is present. There is evidence of previous surgery, specifically a tibial plateau leveling osteotomy for cranial cruciate ligament failure.

antibiotic should be changed only if indicated by subsequent antibiotic sensitivity tests. Metronidazole is sometimes used in combination with other antibiotics to improve activity against anaerobes. Local gentamicin beads or sponges can be used with resistant gram-negative aerobes such as *Pseudomonas*.[15] Systemic antibiotic therapy is continued for at least 4 to 6 weeks, or for 2 weeks after complete resolution of clinical signs. Joint lavage and drainage are particularly indicated if the clinical signs are severe or if the patient is an immature animal with open growth plates. Rest of the joint, by means of strict confinement and, where appropriate, support bandaging, is important in the early stages. Analgesics are generally necessary, and the nonsteroidal antiinflammatory drugs (NSAIDs) are ideal for this. During the recovery phase, controlled exercise, such as passive flexion and extension or gentle lead walks, should be initiated to maintain range of movement in the joint. The level of exercise can be gradually increased after the first 4 weeks.

LYME ARTHRITIS

Lyme disease is a tick-borne, multisystemic illness that affects humans and a number of domestic animals. It is caused by infection with the spirochete *Borrelia burgdorferi*, which is primarily transmitted by ticks of the *Ixodes* genus.[16-18] A European study reported *B. burgdorferi* sensu stricto as the species most likely to be found in joints.[19] Dogs often present with an acute lameness associated with a monoarthritis or pauciarthritis that may be migratory. True polyarthritis is rare, although an immune-mediated polyarthritis has been reported with Lyme disease. Episodes of lameness typically last only a few days, although repeat episodes may occur. Other manifestations include neurologic and cardiac signs and general malaise. Radiographs of affected joints may be normal or may show only soft tissue swelling in the joints.

A diagnosis of Lyme disease is difficult to establish with certainty. *B. burgdorferi* is notoriously difficult to culture from clinical cases although PCR can be used. Serologic testing is of value, although subclinical and asymptomatic infections can occur. Approximately 20% of normal dogs with a history of a tick bite are seropositive for *B. burgdorferi*; therefore, the mere presence of a positive serum anti-*Borrelia* antibody test in a lame dog is insufficient to establish a diagnosis of Lyme disease.[17]

Lyme disease is treated with antibiotics, such as tetracycline, penicillin derivatives, and erythromycin. A response normally is seen within 7 days of the start of treatment, but antibiotic therapy should be continued for at least 2 weeks after resolution of all clinical signs. Most cases have an excellent prognosis, particularly if diagnosed and treated promptly.

Cats undoubtedly are exposed to *B. burgdorferi*, in that 4.2% to 15% of normal cats are seropositive for the organism, but little evidence of clinical disease exists in this species.[20-22] The reason for this is unclear, but the cat's immune response does differ from the dog's in that felines shown an early response to OspA and B antigens.[21]

BACTERIAL L-FORMS AND ARTHRITIS

L-form bacteria are cell wall–deficient bacteria, and these organisms have been associated with pyogenic subcutaneous abscesses and arthritis in cats. The infection spreads locally and hematogenously to involve other joints and subcutaneous sites. The infection is resistant to many antibiotics but is susceptible to tetracyclines.

MYCOPLASMAL ARTHRITIS

Mycoplasmal infection of joints may arise as a result of the spread of organisms from localized sites of active or latent infection in the mucous membranes of the airways, conjunctivae, or urogenital tract. This is most likely to occur in debilitated or immunodepressed animals. *Mycoplasma gatae* and *Mycoplasma felis* have been associated with polyarthritis and tenosynovitis in cats. Infection with *Mycoplasma spumans* is associated with a polyarthritis syndrome of young Greyhounds[23,24]; it is essentially a nonsuppurative polysynovitis, usually associated with severe destruction of articular cartilage. The organisms may be seen in a synovial fluid smear stained with Wright, Leishman, or Giemsa stain. Mycoplasmal arthritis can be treated with tylosin, gentamicin, or erythromycin.

FUNGAL ARTHRITIS

Fungal arthritis is very rare. It usually occurs as an extension of fungal osteomyelitis but may also present as a primary granulomatous synovitis. Fungal infections of joints have involved a range of organisms, including *Coccidioides immitis, Blastomyces dermatitidis, Filobasidiella (Cryptococcus) neoformans, Sporotrichum schenckii,* and *Aspergillus terreus.* The organisms may be seen in synovial fluid smears or cultured from the joint.

RICKETTSIAL ARTHRITIS

Polyarthritis increasingly is recognized in association with rickettsial infections in dogs. *Rickettsia rickettsii,* the causative organism in Rocky Mountain spotted fever (RMSF), is transmitted by ticks of the *Dermacentor* genus and is endemic in wooded areas of the central United States and the eastern seaboard. RMSF is a severe disease associated with rapid dissemination of *R. rickettsii* from the site of the tick bite to many organs in the body, resulting in widespread vasculitis. Polyarthritis is one possible clinical sign.

Canine ehrlichiosis (*Ehrlichia canis* infection transmitted by the tick *Rhipicephalus sanguineus*) may present as a polyarthritis in certain geographically restricted areas, including Missouri and Tennessee. Cats are thought to suffer infection by rickettsiae of the *Ehrlichia* genus, but case reports are lacking.

PROTOZOAL ARTHRITIS

Leishmaniasis is a chronic systemic disease caused by the protozoan parasite *Leishmania donovani* (United States) and *infantum* (Europe). *Leishmania* is transmitted by insect vectors, mainly sandflies, and is endemic in areas such as the Mediterranean, Africa, Asia, and South America. The dog is the main reservoir host in many areas. In addition to polyarthritis, signs such as fever, malaise, weight loss, dermatopathy, lymphadenopathy, and hepatosplenomegaly may occur in the dog.[25] The disease has a long latent period and may appear in nonendemic areas despite prolonged quarantine procedures. The synovitis is usually associated with an infiltrate of large numbers of macrophages filled with *Leishmania* bodies. An immune-mediated polyarthritis may also be seen in association with the infection. Cats can become infected, but clinical disease is rare.

Toxoplasma gondii infection is well known in the cat and does occur rarely in the dog; lameness can be a feature, but joint involvement is poorly documented. *Neospora caninum* infection can cause a polymyositis as well as neurologic disease; only experimental infection in the cat has been reported.

Infection with *Hepatozoon canis* can cause polyarthritis and polymyositis in both the dog and the cat. Infection occurs by ingestion of the vector tick *(R. sanguineus)*, which contains the organism in its digestive tract.

Infection with *Babesia* spp. most often causes severe anemia, although polyarthritis and polymyositis have very rarely been described. *B. canis* and *B. gibsoni* affect the dog, and *B. felis, B. cati, B. herpailuri,* and *B. pantherae* affect the cat. Babesioses are tick-borne diseases carried by ixodid ticks, and concurrent infection with other protozoal organisms can occur.

VIRAL ARTHRITIS

Calicivirus can produce a true infective arthritis in the cat, most often under cattery conditions, and certain strains are more likely to be involved. Experimental studies have shown that calicivirus can infect joints and cause synovitis, and that live virus can be recovered from these joints.[26,27]

IMMUNE-MEDIATED ARTHRITIDES

The immune-based arthropathies are divided into two broad categories, erosive and nonerosive,[28-33] based on whether bony destructive changes are present on the radiographs. The diseases that cause bony destruction generally have a poorer prognosis. Within each of these categories there are further classifications into different syndromes and types, in an attempt to help diagnosis and treatment, but there is overlap between them. A radiographic survey of several joints should always be made.

Erosive Immune-Based Arthritides

Rheumatoid Arthritis Rheumatoid arthritis (Figure 186-3 and Web Figure 186-3) can affect any breed or cross-

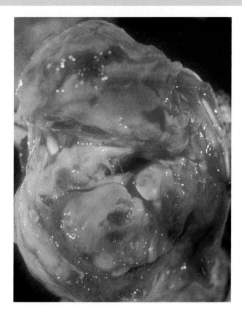

Figure 186-3 Gross appearance of the carpus of a dog with rheumatoid arthritis. Two obvious areas of cartilage and bone loss can be seen, and the resultant ulcers have been replaced with granulation tissue. The synovium is thickened and discolored. Multiple, symmetric joint involvement was apparent in this dog.

breed of dog and also the cat.[28,34,35] Animals are usually adult, although the exact age of onset varies (an average age of 5 to 6 years is reported).[28] The classic radiologic feature of rheumatoid arthritis is the presence of subchondral bone destruction, visualized as an irregularity of the articular surface or as "punched out" erosions (Web Figure 186-4). Advanced cases may show extensive bone destruction with gross joint deformity (Web Figure 186-5).

A more generalized loss of mineralization of the epiphysis can be another feature, and soft tissue swelling around or synovial effusion within the joint may be present. Calcification of the soft tissues around the joint may be seen. In some early cases, radiographic evidence of bone destruction may be absent; such evidence generally appears within 6 months if the disease persists.

Rheumatoid arthritis is commonly but not invariably associated with the presence of circulating autoantibodies against immunoglobulin G, collectively known as rheumatoid factor.[36] However, rheumatoid factor is not specific for this disease and cannot be relied upon as a diagnostic test. It occurs in the other immune-mediated arthropathies and in other disease states, particularly those of a chronic nature, in which antigen-antibody interaction occurs.[36]

Periosteal Proliferative Polyarthritis Periosteal proliferative polyarthritis is more common in the cat compared to the dog.[34] It affects mainly the hocks and carpi, and the characteristic feature is marked periosteal new bone formation, often extending beyond the confines of the joint (Web Figure 186-6). Also, one or more joints show localized bony erosions. Bony destruction and proliferation can also occur at the attachment of ligaments and tendons, lesions known as enthesiopathies. Cats of any age can be affected, although the disease is said to be common in young adults. Male castrated cats appear to be affected more often.

Nonerosive Immune-Based Arthritis

Systemic Lupus Erythematosus Systemic lupus erythematosus (SLE) is a multisystemic disease characterized by simultaneous or sequential development of autoimmune hemolytic anemia, immune-mediated thrombocytopenia, leukopenia, glomerulonephritis, dermatitis, polymyositis, pleuritis, central nervous system (CNS) disease, and symmetric polyarthritis.[30] SLE occurs in both dogs and cats, and because the clinical signs are so variable, diagnosis of the disease can be difficult.

The pathogenesis of SLE involves two main components, autoimmunity and immune complex hypersensitivity. Antibodies against red blood cells, platelets, and leukocytes are important in the development of hemolytic anemia, thrombocytopenia, and leukopenia; the deposition of immune complexes (possibly nuclear antigen and antinuclear antibody) in the kidneys (glomeruli), joints (synovial blood vessels), and skin (dermal/epidermal junction), and possibly in other organs, explains the inflammatory changes in these tissues. Joint radiographs may show no obvious abnormalities, although occasionally soft tissue swelling or synovial effusion is present.

SLE is characterized by the presence of circulating antinuclear antibody (ANA), a group of autoantibodies targeted against nuclear material.[37] Although ANA is found in various chronic disease states, a diagnosis of SLE according to some scientists cannot be justified unless the ANA test result is positive at a reasonably high titer. However, many veterinarians believe that the ANA test is completely nonspecific and, therefore, a test that should not be utilized in veterinary medicine, although tests that detect specific nuclear antigen antibodies might be more reliable.

Polyarthritis/Polymyositis Syndrome In polyarthritis/polymyositis syndrome, polyarthritis is complicated by polymyositis. This syndrome is most often seen in Spaniel breeds.[31] The dogs test negative for ANA; therefore, the disease cannot be categorized as SLE. These dogs present with marked stiffness and poor exercise tolerance, and they often adopt a crouched stance. Widespread muscle atrophy is usually apparent, although in the early stages, muscle swelling and pain may be seen. Muscle atrophy can be associated with fibrosis and contracture, resulting in reduced joint motion; this may be seen in the limb joints and also in the temporomandibular joints, leaving the dog unable to open its mouth.

The muscle enzymes creatine kinase and aldolase are often increased, but not in all cases. Electromyography may show focal areas of spontaneous activity in affected muscles. The myositis is confirmed by multiple muscle biopsy examination (at least six different muscles should be biopsied), although the inflammatory change can be patchy and may be absent from some muscles (myositis should be seen in at least two of the biopsy samples).

Polyarthritis/Meningitis Syndrome Polyarthritis/meningitis syndrome has been seen in several breeds, including the Weimaraner, Newfoundland, German Short-Haired Pointer, Boxer, Corgi, Nova Scotia Duck Tolling Retriever, and Bernese Mountain Dog. It also is reported in the cat. These animals present with pyrexia, stiffness, and neck pain and in some cases with nervous signs. Cerebrospinal fluid shows increased protein, white cell, and creatine kinase levels, indicating an inflammatory lesion of the CNS.

Sjögren's Syndrome In humans, Sjögren's syndrome was originally described as a syndrome comprising keratoconjunctivitis sicca ("dry eye"), xerostomia ("dry mouth"), and a polyarthritis, which may be an erosive (rheumatoid) arthritis or a nonerosive arthritis. Dry eye in the dog has been reported with SLE and lymphocytic thyroiditis.[1] Sialadenitis with rheumatoid arthritis has also been documented.[1]

Familial Shar-Pei Fever Dogs with familial Shar-Pei fever present with episodes of fever (105° to 107° F) and with swelling of one or both hock joints and occasionally other joints.[38,39] It is an autosomal recessive disease characterized by increased production of interleukin-6. In some cases the inflammation appears to be periarticular rather than within the joint itself and in these cases the synovial fluid cytology may be normal. Enthesiopathies are also seen and these animals appear to be susceptible to other problems such as immune-mediated renal disease and thromboembolism. The age of onset of signs is variable (young puppies or adult dogs); the period between attacks is variable and an attack may be "triggered" by a stress situation that, if identified, might be avoidable, thus reducing the incidence of attacks. In some affected dogs, amyloid deposits occur in several organs, but renal amyloidosis and hepatic amyloidosis are the conditions most significant to the prognosis. Amyloidosis, when it occurs, will eventually result in renal or hepatic failure, which may occur any time between 1.5 and 6 years of age; 25% of cases will develop renal failure. Some authorities believe that Shar-Pei fever and amyloidosis are separate hereditary diseases in this breed which may coexist in an individual animal. It is true that not all cases of Shar-Pei fever develop amyloidosis and not all cases of amyloidosis ever have episodes of lameness and fever. At present, there is no specific laboratory test for confirming the diagnosis of the disease or for screening its presence in clinically normal animals. All dogs with Shar-Pei fever should have a urinanalysis every 3 months and routine blood examinations every 6 to 12 months.

Polyarthritis of the Adolescent Akita Polyarthritis of adolescent Akitas affects dogs less than 1 year of age.[40] Meningitis may also be present, as may other organ involvement. These dogs have an unfavorable prognosis, because the response to antiinflammatory and immunomodulatory drugs is poor.

Polyarteritis Nodosa Polyarteritis nodosa is an inflammatory condition of the small arteries, often of a granulomatous nature, that can be diagnosed only by histologic examination of biopsy or autopsy material. Polyarthritis, polymyositis, and meningitis can occur. The attacks are often cyclical, although persistent signs can occur

Drug-Induced Arthritis Drug-induced vasculitides are basically hypersensitivity reactions involving the deposition of drug antibody complexes around blood vessels in different areas of the body. The drug may act directly as an antigen or may combine with host proteins as haptens to form neoantigens. Polyarthritis is only one feature of these disease syndromes; fever, lymphadenopathy, and macular-papular or bullous-type hemorrhagic rashes are common. Thrombocytopenia, hemolytic anemia, polymyositis, retinitis, and glomerulonephritis are also reported. The most commonly incriminated drugs are antibiotics, particularly sulfa drugs, lincomycin, erythromycin, cephalosporins, and penicillins. The Doberman Pinscher appears particularly susceptible to sulphadiazine-trimethoprim.[41] The diagnosis is made on the basis of worsening clinical signs while the animal is undergoing drug therapy and very rapid improvement (2 to 7 days) after the drug is stopped. To become sensitized the animal usually has to have encountered the drug previously or have been undergoing long-term therapy.

Vaccination Reactions Occasionally an immune-based polyarthritis can develop after vaccine inoculations. It is most likely to occur after the first injection of a primary vaccination course, particularly in kittens.[42] The polyarthritis is generally seen 5 to 7 days after the first inoculation, and the lameness is usually only transient, lasting for 24 to 48 hours. The calicivirus component appears to cause the condition, and calicivirus antigens have been identified in synovial macrophages of vaccinated (F9 strain) and naturally infected (A4 strain)

cats.[26] The presence of these antigens has been associated with an active synovitis. Persistent polyarthritis in the dog has been reported after recent vaccination,[43] and canine distemper virus may be the component involved.

Idiopathic Polyarthritis Idiopathic polyarthritis includes all those cases of inflammatory arthropathy that cannot be classified into the other groups. It is still the most common type of polyarthritis in both the dog and the cat.[32,44]

The idiopathic group can be divided into four subcategories[1,32]:
- Type I: Uncomplicated idiopathic arthritis; this is the most common subgroup.
- Type II: Idiopathic arthritis associated with infections remote from the joints (reactive arthritis). The infections commonly occur in the respiratory tract, tonsils, conjunctiva (e.g., *Chlamydophila* in the cat), urinary tract, uterine tract, skin (including anal furunculosis) and oral cavity.[32]
- Type III: Idiopathic arthritis associated with gastrointestinal disease (enteropathic arthritis). The gastroenteritis is usually characterized by vomiting and/or diarrhea. Sometimes blood is present in the feces. Cases of intestinal bacterial overgrowth and malabsorption have been complicated by polyarthritis, and very occasionally the intestinal disease is an ulcerative colitis.[32]
- Type IV: Idiopathic arthritis associated with neoplasia remote from the joints (arthritis of malignancy). The neoplastic lesion may not be apparent by clinical assessment; some are recorded only during a *postmortem* examination. Neoplasias have included squamous cell carcinoma, heart base tumor, leiomyoma, and mammary adenocardinoma.[32] In the cat, myeloproliferative disease is the most common association,[34] and cats with a nonerosive polyarthritis that do not respond well to therapy should always have a bone marrow examination and should be tested for feline leukemia virus (FeLV) and feline immunodeficiency virus (FIV).

The age of onset can vary from a few months to 11 years; many animals are young adults (1 to 3 years) when first presented, especially in type I cases. The pathology is generally an acute/subacute synovitis (Web Figures 186-7 and 186-8). Soft tissue swelling and/or synovial effusion may be apparent on radiography (Web Figure 186-9), although often no abnormality is visible.

Disease of other body systems is not uncommon. A detailed clinical examination, and extensive blood and urine analyses, should be carried out.

TREATMENT

The treatment and prognosis vary with the different types of polyarthritis. Repeated synovial fluid analysis is the most sensitive method of monitoring the effectiveness of treatment. A fall in the total cell count and a reduction in the proportion of polymorphs are good prognostic signs. The erosive arthropathies and animals with multiple-system disease tend to have a poorer prognosis. In a recent study of idiopathic type I cases, the most common type of polyarthritis, 56% of affected dogs made a complete recovery following immunosuppressive therapy. Continuous antiinflammatory medication was required in 18% of cases, relapses were treated successfully in 13%, and 15% of dogs died or were euthanatized as a result of the disease.[44]

The initial treatment in most cases is to attempt immunosuppression with high doses of corticosteroids. These are given orally for 2 weeks (prednisolone, 2 to 4 mg/kg) in a daily divided dose, and the dosage then is gradually reduced over the next 4 to 8 weeks. Generally a marked response occurs within a few days, but it is important that therapy be maintained to help prevent relapses. Repeat arthrocenteses and synovial fluid analyses of joints initially sampled for diagnostic purposes are performed at 2 weeks; if the white cell count has fallen below 4000/mm³ and most of the cells are mononuclear, the prognosis is reasonably good. A simple method of evaluating joint fluid is to make slides using the same protocol as with peripheral blood. The slide can be stained in-hospital using common modified Wright's solutions. Once stained, the slide can be examined microscopically under "high" magnification and the average number of neutrophils per high power field multiplied by 1000. Normal joints contain fewer than 3 to 5 white blood cells per high power field and most such cells are mononuclear. A greater number than 3 to 5 neutrophils per high power field is absolutely abnormal. This is a simple, reliable, and cost-effective means of diagnosing and then monitoring therapeutic response in dogs with idiopathic polyarthritis.

If the polymorph counts remain increased despite high-dose steroid therapy, it should be continued for a longer period. Relapses are always possible; therefore, the prognosis overall is guarded.

If relapses occur or if the response to prednisolone therapy is poor, a combination of prednisolone and cytotoxic drugs can be tried. The cytotoxic drug of choice is cyclophosphamide, given orally at a dosage of 1.5 mg/kg (for dogs over 30 kg), 2 mg/kg (for dogs 15 to 30 kg), or 2.5 mg/kg (for dogs under 15 kg). The drug is given on 4 consecutive days of each week or as close to this regimen as possible, allowing for the fact that, because of health and safety issues, tablets should not be divided. In addition, oral prednisolone is given each day at an antiinflammatory dosage (0.25 to 0.5 mg/kg) to help control pain by reducing the articular inflammatory load. This treatment is continued for 2 to 4 months, even though clinical remission may occur much earlier. Cyclophosphamide should not be used for longer than 4 months because of bladder toxicity problems. The urine can be tested weekly for blood, but the drug does not need to be stopped unless overt blood is visible.

Once cytotoxic therapy has been instigated, blood counts should be monitored every 7 to 14 days. If the white cell count falls below 6000/mm³ or the platelet count below 125,000/mm³, the dosage should be reduced by one fourth; if the white cell count falls below 4000/mm³ or the platelet count below 100,000/mm³, the drug should be discontinued for 2 weeks and then recommenced at half the original dosage.

In dogs (but not in cats), azathioprine can be used as an alternative to cyclophosphamide, at a daily oral dosage of approximately 2 mg/kg every other day, together with low-dose prednisolone given every other day (alternating with the azathioprine). Bone marrow suppression is more likely with azathioprine.

If the response to cytotoxic drugs and prednisolone is still poor or if relapses occur, a combination of a cytotoxic drug, low-dose prednisolone, and levamisole can be tried. Levamisole may act as an immunomodulatory drug (i.e., it may suppress helper T cells). It is administered as a liquid oral preparation at a dosage of 5 to 7 mg/kg every other day up to a maximum of 150 mg daily.

Whatever the therapeutic regimen used, the intention is to stop therapy after 3 to 6 months. Generally the cytotoxic drug and levamisole are stopped first, and the steroid is continued at an ever-decreasing dosage.

Gold injections (sodium aurothiomalate or aurothioglucose) have been used in cases of rheumatoid arthritis with some success. It is important to administer a small test dose before full treatment is begun to check for any adverse sensitivity to the drug, and the animal must be checked regularly during treatment for toxic side effects. The dose ranges from 5 to 40 mg, given by intramuscular injection at weekly intervals for 6 weeks. Generally, low-dose prednisolone also is given. Auranofin (Ridaura), an oral preparation of gold, is also available. Auranofin, which is given at a dosage 0.05 to 2 mg/kg administered twice daily, is less toxic than the injectable gold preparation, but diarrhea is a common side effect.

A combination of oral methotrexate and leflunomide has been used in the cat to treat rheumatoid arthritis[35] and can be tried in other forms of immune-mediated arthritis and in the dog although, to date, the author has little experience with these drugs. The methotrexate dose is given once weekly; on the day it is given, the dose is 7.5 mg divided into three separate and equal doses of 2.5 mg each. The leflunomide dose is 10 mg daily and is given by oral administration. When significant improvement has occurred, the doses are reduced to 2.5 mg of methotrexate once weekly and 10 mg of leflunomide twice weekly.

Constant corticosteroid therapy sometimes is necessary to keep an animal in clinical remission, and this is perhaps acceptable if only a small dose is required. A few patients spontaneously recover within a day or two without any treatment. NSAIDs can be used in mild cases or while laboratory results are awaited.

Treatment of idiopathic arthritis types II, III, and IV is directed primarily against the infective, alimentary, or neoplastic lesion, although corticosteroid therapy may be necessary. Colchicine treatment has been used in attempts to control the amyloidosis seen in some cases of Shar-Pei fever, but its effectiveness has not been proved although there is some anecdotal evidence that it reduces the episodes of fever and lameness. Acute episodes of fever and lameness can be treated with aspirin or other NSAIDs.

It is important to provide supportive therapy, when appropriate, for animals undergoing therapy for immune-mediated arthritis. Rest, avoidance of stress environments, and good nutrition are essential. Patients receiving immunosuppressive therapy should be checked regularly for secondary infections, and owners should be warned to avoid potential disease environments. Because of the possible involvement of canine distemper virus in immune-mediated arthritis, dogs that have suffered immune-mediated polyarthritis should be screened for distemper antibody levels when a booster inoculation is due; if the levels are consistent with protection, the booster should exclude the distemper component.

REFERENCES

The reference list can be found on the companion Expert Consult Web site at *www.expertconsult.com*.

CHAPTER 187

Canine and Feline Osteoarthritis

David Bennett

Osteoarthritis (OA) is a common and complex, progressive disease. In pathologic terms, OA has been defined as "an inherently noninflammatory disorder of movable (synovial) joints characterized by deterioration of articular cartilage and by the formation of new bone at the joint surfaces and margins." From the etiopathogenesis perspective, it has been defined as "a complex of interactive degradative and repair processes in cartilage, bone and synovium, with secondary components of inflammation" and clinically, it may be defined as "a slowly evolving articular disease characterized by the gradual development of joint pain, stiffness, and limitation of motion." OA is the most common arthropathy of dogs and cats (Figure 187-1).

CANINE

ETIOPATHOGENESIS

The inevitable progression of OA can largely be attributed to enzymatic degradation of the articular cartilage. The initiation of OA is not well understood, but several theories have been extended to explain how different stimuli may give rise to a progressive, degenerative disorder. These hypotheses can broadly be divided into those that propose abnormal stresses acting on normal cartilage and those that propose a consequence of normal stresses acting on abnormal cartilage. OA arising from abnormal stresses acting on normal cartilage or as a consequence of other recognizable joint disease such as infection, immune-mediated inflammation, osteochondrosis, hip dysplasia, elbow dysplasia, and cruciate disease is often termed *secondary osteoarthritis*. Secondary OA is the most common form of the disease in dogs. The term *primary osteoarthritis* describes an important subset of OA in which there is believed to be a fundamental defect in the biomaterial properties of the articular cartilage. Normal loading then leads to progressive degradation of the cartilage matrix. Prevalence of primary OA increases with increasing age, but genetic factors may modify the age at onset and the progression of the disease.

Heritability has also been recognized as an important factor in some underlying diseases, such as hip dysplasia and elbow dysplasia, which lead to secondary OA. There is significant variation in the severity and rate of progression of the disease between individual animals with the same inciting cause, and this may be due to environmental (e.g., amount of exercise, body weight) and/or genetic influences. Once established, both primary and secondary OA progress along a "final common pathway" of anatomic and biochemical changes in the joint. In a minority of cases, OA presents as a more aggressive disease in which subchondral bone erosions are a feature. The term *erosive osteoarthritis* is used to describe this particularly severe clinical presentation.

PATHOLOGY

The earliest gross anatomic changes in OA cartilage include localized areas of softening associated with disruption or fibrillation of the surface cartilage matrix. *Flaking* is said to occur when this disruption is superficial and fragmentation is tangential to the cartilage surface. Deeper disruption of the cartilage matrix gives rise to fragments oriented perpendicular to the cartilage surface, and this phenomenon is termed *fissuring*. The fissuring progresses to loss of cartilage and culminates in full-thickness cartilage loss, exposure of subchondral bone, and eburnation (Web Figures 187-1 and 187-2). Full thickness loss of cartilage can take 3 to 5 years in the cranial cruciate ligament-deficient stifle joint of the dog.[1]

In some cases, changes in the subchondral bone may precede the cartilage pathology. The proposed theory is that stiffening of the subchondral bone may result in an increased load on the cartilage.[2,3] The formation of osteophytes at the articular margins is an important feature of OA and is part of the remodeling process by which the joint alters its shape in an attempt to create a more functional articulation (Web Figures 187-3 through 187-5).[4] New bone deposition can also occur at the attachments of ligaments and tendons (enthesiophytes). Soft tissue thickening and synovial effusion are common and there may be calcification of articular and periarticular soft tissues.

Although OA is classed as a degenerative disorder, it has an important inflammatory component. A moderate to marked synovitis is seen in approximately 50% of surgical specimens from dogs with OA. The synovitis is characterized by hyperplasia and hypertrophy of synovial lining cells, villous proliferation, and a mild infiltration of lymphocytes, plasma cells, and mononuclear phagocytes.

Molecular Events in Osteoarthritis

Throughout life there is a constant turnover of cartilage matrix, which is under the control of the matrix metalloproteinases (MMPs) and their inhibitors (the inhibitors of the matrix metalloproteinases or TIMPs). In OA the activity of the MMPs and the aggrecanases is increased substantially, homeostasis is lost, and there is a net loss of cartilage matrix. The increased enzymatic activity is driven by release of inflammatory cytokines such as interleukin (IL)-1, tumor necrosis factor-α, and IL-6, which stimulate the release of MMPs and aggrecanases from synovial cells and chondrocytes themselves (Web Figures 187-6 and 187-7).[5]

Cytokines, released from synoviocytes and chondrocytes, are also involved in prostaglandin and nitric oxide release. Interestingly as OA becomes more chronic, fewer TIMPs and cytokine inhibitors are produced and more cytokine receptors are expressed on articular cells, all contributing to progression and perpetuation of the disease.

 To view a video on this topic, go to **www.expertconsult.com**.

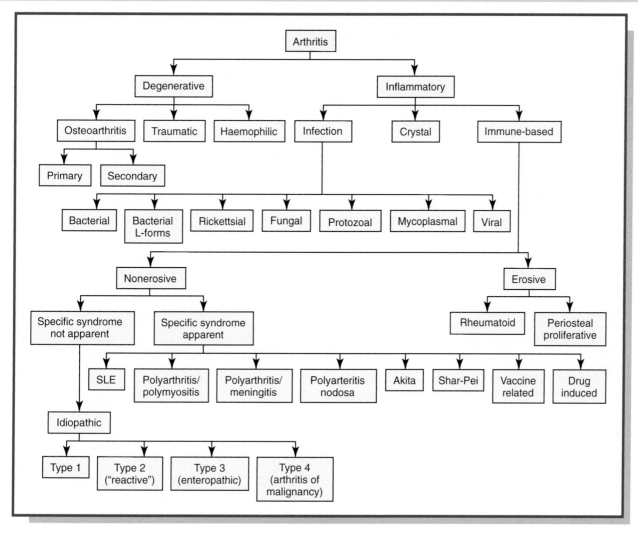

Figure 187-1   Algorithm showing the classification of arthritis in the dog and cat. *SLE*, Systemic lupus erythematosus.

DIAGNOSIS

History and Clinical Signs   OA in dogs most commonly presents as lameness, which may have a sudden or insidious onset. Acute presentations of OA are commonly associated with episodes of minor trauma or excessive exercise superimposed on preexisting disease. However, acute episodes of lameness may be the result of infection localizing to the osteoarthritic joint.[6] If this is suspected (particularly if the lameness has not improved after a couple of days of rest and analgesia), a synovial fluid sample should be taken for cytology and culture. In secondary OA, clinical signs referable to the underlying disease may precede the onset of clinical OA by many months or years. It is important to remember that the disease may have progressed considerably before becoming clinically apparent and that there will be considerable preexisting structural damage to the joint. Often the earliest sign noted by the owner is a loss of normal performance, although it is generally the onset of lameness that prompts the owner to seek veterinary advice.

Stiffness after rest is a cardinal sign of joint disease and is frequently present in OA before the onset of the overt lameness. The stiffness usually lasts only a few minutes after rising from a period of rest, in contrast to the prolonged or continu-

ous stiffness seen in inflammatory joint diseases. This clinical sign may be exacerbated by obesity, long periods of exercise, and cold or damp conditions. Only in advanced cases of OA is stiffness a problem for prolonged periods of time, and this is invariably accompanied by obvious lameness. In some animals there may be behavioral effects of constant joint discomfort, including increased nervousness, aggression, depression and loss of appetite.

The clinical signs of OA are limited to the musculoskeletal system. In secondary OA, there may be clinical signs referable to the primary disease, such as a drawer sign in rupture of the cranial cruciate ligament. Osteoarthritic joints are usually swollen and painful on palpation. The swelling occurs as a consequence of periarticular new bone formation, joint capsule fibrosis, and synovial effusion. The range of movement of the joint may be reduced, and pain is particularly evident when the joint is manipulated to the limits of extension and flexion. Crepitus is an inconsistent finding, most commonly present with chronic disease. Heat and redness are usually not detected in OA joints unless there is superimposed trauma or infection.

Diagnostic Imaging   Radiography remains the primary diagnostic imaging modality for suspected cases of OA. Radiographic changes in osteoarthritic joints may be seen in both soft and mineralized tissues (Web Figures 187-8 through

187-10), although radiographic signs may be absent in pathologically affected joints.

It is also true that radiographic changes may not necessarily be associated with clinical disease. The earliest radiographic sign of OA is usually increased periarticular soft tissue opacity and/or synovial effusion. This feature is difficult to evaluate in some joints. It is readily seen, for example, on a mediolateral view of the stifle joint, where it manifests as an apparent reduction in the size of the infrapatellar fat pad and a soft tissue swelling visualized caudal to the femorotibial articulation (see Web Figure 187-8).

New bone, in the form of periarticular osteophytes, becomes radiologically apparent within 2-3 weeks of the onset of OA although histologically these can be defined after 2 to 3 days.[4] Osteophytes are most readily identified on films, where they can be seen protruding from the surface of the bone, although they are also appreciated as an area of sclerosis along the articular margin (see Web Figures 187-8 and 187-10). It is important to remember that due to the remodeling process, osteophytes can become less obvious with time.[7] Osteophyte formation itself is likely to be genetically influenced since, for example, some breeds produce more osteophytes than others given the same degree of hip laxity.[8] The joint space (cartilage thickness) will increase in the early stages of the disease (within the first year after rupture of the cranial cruciate ligament) due to increased hydration and matrix formation; in the later stages the joint space decreases as cartilage is lost.[9,10] In dogs joint space changes are difficult to evaluate because of the difficulty in achieving weight-bearing views. Subchondral cyst formation, commonly seen in man, is rare in the dog.

Bony trabeculae in the subchondral area may thicken (subchondral sclerosis), and this is an important feature of radiographic OA (see Web Figures 187-8 through 187-10). It is seen as an increased radiopacity of the subchondral bone. However, subchondral sclerosis as seen radiographically may be explained by true subchondral trabecular thickening by superimposed osteophytes around the margins of the joint, by mineralized plaques within the joint capsule overlying the bone, or by mineralized free bodies within the joint cavity, again superimposed on the bone. The interpretation of sclerosis is not obvious. One study involving boarded radiologists suggested agreement in identifying sclerosis was uncommon.[7] In severe cases of OA, there may be wearing away, or attrition, of subchondral bone, particularly at weight-bearing surfaces.

Calcification of both intraarticular and periarticular soft tissues may occur in chronic OA. Intraarticular calcification usually occurs in the joint capsule. Initially there is cartilaginous metaplasia followed by endochondral ossification, leading to the formation of synovial osteochondromas. Mineralized free bodies may also be seen radiographically. Free bodies most likely form within the synovium and become detached during joint motion. They consist of fibrous tissue, calcified cartilage, and bone; they derive nutrition from the synovial fluid and can increase in size. In secondary OA, radiologic changes typical of the primary disease may be superimposed on the changes typical of OA (see Web Figure 187-10). In advanced cases, the changes may be so extensive that the original cause of the disease is difficult, or impossible, to establish from the radiographs.

There are many other imaging modalities used in the evaluation of OA. Computed tomography can provide detailed information on the bony changes associated with OA and is particularly relevant for the elbow joint, where it can be used to identify underlying causes such as coronoid disease.[11] Arthroscopy is generally not necessary purely for diagnosis, although it can be used to inspect and grade the severity of articular cartilage pathology; the saline irrigation that accompanies arthroscopy may assist in relieving clinical signs by flushing mediators of inflammation from the articular cavity. Scintigraphy has been used to image OA joints but is of limited clinical value. Ultrasonography has also been applied to OA joints, mainly to screen for underlying causes or complications such as meniscal damage. Magnetic resonance imaging (MRI) is now the gold standard for assessing loss of cartilage from human OA joints. MR scans are being used in dogs, although a high-quality scanner is needed because of their thinner articular cartilage. There are different methods of assessing cartilage loss, including estimating cartilage volume, thickness mapping, and delayed gadolinium-enhanced MRI (dGEMRI) of cartilage.

Laboratory Findings Despite much research, no diagnostically reliable serum or hematologic markers of OA exist. Analysis of synovial fluid from osteoarthritic joints reveals cytologic and biochemical changes consistent with degenerative joint disease: low white cell counts, principally macrophages and lymphocytes (Table 187-1).

TREATMENT AND MANAGEMENT OPTIONS

Client education and support is essential when treating dogs with OA. The nature of the disease should be explained to the owner, particularly the inability to cure. The condition is

Table • 187-1

Diagnostic Characteristics of Synovial Fluid

	NORMAL JOINT	OSTEOARTHRITIS	IMMUNE–MEDIATED ARTHRITIS	BACTERIAL INFECTIVE ARTHRITIS
Color	Clear/pale yellow	Yellow	Yellow (+/–blood tinged)	Yellow (+/– blood tinged)
Clarity	Transparent	Transparent	Transparent or opaque	Opaque
Viscosity	Very high	High	Low/very low	Very low
Mucin clot	Good	Good/fair	Fair/poor	Poor
Spontaneous clot	None	+/–	Often	Often
White cells (/mm³)	<1000	100-11,000; avg 1500	>5000; avg 30,000	>5000; avg 45,000
Neutrophils	<5%	<10%	10%-95%; avg 65%	>90%
Mononuclear cells	>95%	>90%	5%-90%	<10%
Protein (g/dL)	2.0-2.5	2.0-3.0	2.5-5.0	>4.0
Glucose (% of serum value)	>90	N/A	N/A	<50

"managed" and it is progressive. Client-based questionnaires can help owners to assess the progress of their pets.[12,13] It is essential to establish therapeutic goals that are acceptable to the animal, the owner, and the clinician. The ultimate aims of therapy will be influenced by several factors, including the severity of the clinical problem, the type of dog and its usage, the requirements of the owner, the age and size of the dog, concurrent disease or drug therapy that may interfere with the use of antiinflammatory drugs, and any financial constraints.

General and Supportive Measures and Lifestyle Changes

Obesity Animals are considered obese if their body weight exceeds their ideal weight by 20% or more. Many osteoarthritic dogs are obese. In addition to assessing animals by measuring bodyweight, body condition scoring should also be used. Many obese dogs with clinical OA become free of signs once they have achieved their ideal body weight or be able to manage with lower doses of analgesic/antiinflammatory drugs.[14] There are now several different reducing diets available, and obesity clinics can be effectively run by nursing staffs. There are also drugs available that alter the dogs' metabolism to encourage weight loss; these are the MTP (microsomal triglyceride transfer protein) inhibitors. Dirlotapide and mitratapide are examples—they reduce lipid absorption and release hormones that signal satiety to the brain.

Exercise Exercise is also a key factor in OA management.[15] Inactivity can lead to soft tissue complications of muscle weakness and joint stiffness that compound the clinical problems associated with arthritis. Overexercise, on the other hand, can precipitate or exacerbate clinical signs. In many cases, inability to exercise is equated with poor quality of life, and so restoration of the capability to exercise is a key target. Exercise can be used as a tool in management, acting to reverse or preclude problems by ensuring flexibility, muscular strength, joint mobility, and cardiovascular fitness. Of course exercise is more likely to precipitate problems in the obese patient. The type of exercise regimen to be used depends on the type of clinical problem exhibited by the dog. Exercise should be strictly controlled or prevented when the joints are extremely painful or when exercise itself produces pain. Different types of mobilization or exercise are appropriate depending on the clinical situation, stage of the disease and the interest and compliance of the owner.

Passive movement The aim is just to maintain mobility and flexibility until the clinical problem improves through, for example, the use of nonsteroidal antiinflammatory drugs (NSAIDs). This exercise requires no exertion by the pet since the joint is moved through a complete range of motion by the owner or therapist. Slow movement is performed, alternately flexing and extending each joint in turn, 10 to 15 times, and repeating this approximately 3 times daily.

Active assisted exercise Animals are encouraged to perform active assisted exercise to move both joints and muscles without pain or damage but they require some assistance with extreme movements as they lack strength. Assistance is usually provided in the form of slings or a towel, used to support some of the animal's bodyweight when walking or rising. Hydrotherapy is a method of assisted exercise that is assuming increasing popularity. In hydrotherapy, buoyancy is used to counter the effect of gravity and bodyweight. The actual amount of assistance derived from the water can be set by the degree of immersion of the animal, up to the point where the animal must swim. Swimming is an excellent form of mobilization and strengthening without the weight-bearing impact forces that can be so destructive and painful to diseased joints. Specialist hydrotherapy pools are increasing in number, and this offers the opportunity to use controlled swimming or hydrotherapy as a therapeutic aid in dogs with arthritis. Initially only short sessions of 1 to 3 minutes once or twice weekly are used and these can be gradually increased to 5 to 10 minutes two or three times weekly. Underwater tread mills are also being used to exercise arthritic patients—the amount of water is varied to provide varying degrees of assistance.

Active resisted exercise This is used to augment exercise programs by strengthening particular areas of the body in preparation for unassisted exercise. Examples include approximation, short-leash walking, wheel barrowing, dancing, pattern walking, rising/sitting, walking on inclines or stairs, and walking with weights.

Controlled voluntary movement This is the exercise enjoyed by the owner and dog together. Moderate exercise should be encouraged and may be defined as exercise within the capability of the dog that does not increase pain, lameness, or excessive stiffness, either during or following the exercise period. Moderate exercise requires that an acceptable exercise regimen be designed for each dog. Short-lead exercise can be used in the early stages and gradually increased over a period of time. Programs should consist of several short exercise periods that should, if possible, be spaced evenly throughout the day. Exercise patterns should be almost identical every day, with little variation at weekends, for example, when the client may have more time to spend with the dog.

Other Physical Therapies There are other physical therapies that can be used to improve joint and muscle function. These techniques can often involve specialist equipment and training and are usually carried out by a physical therapist or physiotherapist. These include superficial heat therapy, cryotherapy, ultrasound and diathermy, and electrotherapy.

Medical Treatment of Osteoarthritis

Drugs, particularly analgesics, are important in the management of OA, but they should be used judiciously and in combination with lifestyle adjustments. Many dogs with osteoarthritis have only transient or intermittent joint pain, and relatively few suffer severe, unrelenting pain requiring permanent full-dose analgesic therapy. However, most dogs with clinical OA require drug therapy at some stage. In an attempt to clarify nomenclature: *symptom-modifying OA drugs (SYMOAD)* is the name given to compounds that reduce pain, such as NSAIDs. Those agents that have the potential for structural modification (i.e., they reverse or slow the structural pathologic changes) are termed *structural modifying OA drugs (STMOAD)*. Most of these are potentially found in the nutraceutical group.

Nonsteroidal Anti-Inflammatory Drugs These are still the mainstay of drug treatment for OA and there is much evidence to support their effectiveness.[16] NSAIDs act predominantly by blocking the inflammatory effects of prostaglandins through inhibition of the breakdown of arachidonic acid by cyclooxygenase (COX); some NSAIDs also inhibit lipoxygenase, thus inhibiting leukotriene production. Research has shown that there are two principal forms of COX, an endogenous form, COX-1, and an inducible form, COX-2. The endogenous form is responsible for the production of protective prostaglandins that help to maintain the integrity of the gastric mucosa and vascular endothelium and to protect renal blood flow in times of circulatory crisis. COX-2 is produced as part of the inflammatory response, responsible for producing inflammatory prostaglandins such as PGE_2. It has thus been proposed that NSAIDs that preferentially or selectively inhibit COX-2 or are COX-1 sparing are preferable since they are associated with fewer side effects. However, COX-1 does play an important part in the inflammatory process and pain perception and COX-2 is important in resolving inflammation. Recently, splice variants of COX-1 have been identified including COX-3 and partial COX-1 proteins (PCOX-1a and COX-1b).[17]

Factors to consider when selecting a NSAID include safety, license for use in the species (particularly in long-term therapy), efficacy, ease of administration, and cost. There are several available (Table 187-2). The two most commonly used in the United Kingdom are meloxicam and carprofen. Carprofen appears to be only a weak inhibitor of COX and its exact mode of action is not certain. Meloxicam preferentially inhibits COX-2; it is easy to administer as a liquid, mixed with food. Tepoxalin (TN Zubrin), a pyrazole derivative, is a dual inhibitor of both COX and lipoxygenase. Although it is not a preferential inhibitor of COX-2, there is evidence that it is tissue selective in its inhibition of prostaglandin production. The elimination pathway for tepoxalin is almost exclusively via the feces; only about 1% is found in the urine. This may help explain why renal toxicity is rarely encountered; it is the only NSAID licensed for use in dogs with renal impairment. The coxibs are a relatively new subgroup of COX-1–sparing NSAIDs, and two are currently used in the dog—deracoxib and firocoxib. Both appear effective with a good safety margin.[18] They are as effective as other NSAIDs but appear to have fewer gastrointestinal side effects.[19] Paracetamol (acetaminophen) (in combination with codeine in the United Kingdom) is still sometimes used to treat OA in dogs.

When using NSAIDs it is advisable to always start with the recommended dose for a minimum of 3 to 4 weeks. If symp-

toms resolve the drug can then be stopped; if not, the drug should be continued for 2 or 3 more weeks. If improvement occurs, the dose should be continually reduced until an effective minimal dose is attained. If no improvement occurs, another NSAID or analgesic compound should be tried. NSAIDs can be used in combination with other agents and this may enable further lowering of the NSAID dose. If one particular NSAID appears ineffective or becomes ineffective with time, it is worth trying another. Also, if toxic signs are seen with one NSAID, this may not be the case when trying another. Alternatively, the same NSAID at a lower dose can sometimes result in side effects disappearing. If side effects do occur, it is important to stop therapy completely until signs of toxicity have been absent for at least 3 to 4 days. The coxibs should be considered for dogs susceptible to gastrointestinal upset. Alternatively, the use of NSAIDs together with gastric protectants (e.g., sucralfate), H_2 antagonists (e.g., ramitidine, cimetidine), or proton pump inhibitors (e.g. omeprazole) can minimize the gastrointestinal signs in susceptible animals. PGE agonists such as Misoprostol (a PGE analogue at a dose of 2 to 5 µg/kg twice or three times a day) can be used in severe cases.

All NSAIDs carry some risk of systemic side effects, particularly through damage to the gastrointestinal tract. Some NSAIDs cause a reduction in the glomerular filtration rate, which may be clinically significant in dogs with compensated renal failure. Carprofen has also been associated with hepatic toxicity in susceptible dogs.[20] Furthermore, excretion of NSAIDs may be reduced in dogs with clinical or subclinical renal, cardiac, or hepatic disease. Such animals require lower doses to achieve therapeutic serum drug concentrations without risk of toxicity. Hepatic and renal parameters should be checked in all dogs before prolonged administration of NSAID therapy. Care should be taken if the dog is receiving other drug therapies since there may be competition for plasma protein binding.

There is much discussion as to the effects of NSAIDs on articular cartilage. Some of the older NSAIDs have toxic effects on chondrocytes in culture. In contrast, carprofen has been shown to stimulate chondrocyte activity in culture[21] and to slow the progression of early OA in the experimental canine cruciate ligament model.[22] Meloxicam has also been shown to have stimulatory effects on proteoglycan production in cartilage.[23] The effect of the coxibs on cartilage is influenced by whether healthy or diseased cartilage is studied, but positive effects can occur.[19]

Corticosteroids Corticosteroids can be given systemically or locally by intraarticular injection. They are potent antiinflammatory drugs and are certainly symptom-modifying. Low-dose oral prednisolone is the most commonly used regimen; this may involve doses as low as 2 to 5 mg per day for a Labrador-sized dog. The side effects normally associated with corticosteroids are minimal with these low doses, although they will occur with continuous therapy. Intraarticular corticosteroids are regularly used by some clinicians. An experimental study in the dog using the cruciate sectioning model has shown beneficial effects of intraarticular corticosteroids, both methylprednisolone acetate and triamcinolone.[24] Overall the injected joints showed less cartilage erosion, less osteophyte production, less stromelysin activity, and less chondrocyte proliferation. This study did not investigate the effects of long-term therapy and was only concerned with relatively early OA. There are several disadvantages of intraarticular corticosteroids, particularly with repeated injections, which are not recommended. Corticosteroids are generally indicated in cases of OA where there is a significant inflammatory component (e.g., a relatively high neutrophil count in the synovia) or where NSAIDs are ineffective or causing unac-

Table • 187-2

Nonsteroidal Anti-Inflammatory Drugs Used in the Dog to Treat Osteoarthritis

DRUG	FORMULATION	LICENSED DOSE FOR DOGS IN UNITED KINGDOM
Carporfen	Tablets	4 mg/kg q24h
Deracoxib*	Tablets	1-2 mg/kg q24h
Etadolac*	Tablets	10-15 mg/kg q24h
Firocoxib	Palatable tablets	5 mg/kg q24h
Ketoprofen	Tablets	1 mg/kg q24h (for up to 5 days)
Meloxicam	Oral suspension	0.2 mg/kg on day 1; thereafter 0.1 mg/kg q24h
Paracetamol + codeine	Tablets	33 mg/kg q8h (for up to 5 days)
Phenylbutazone	Tablets	2-20 mg/kg q24h for 14 days, then review
Tolfenamic acid	Tablets	4 mg/kg q24h (for up to 3 days; may be repeated every 7 days)
Tepoxalin	Lyophilized tablets	10 mg/kg q24h
Vedaprofen	Gel	0.5 mg/kg q24h for 28 days, then review

*Not available in the United Kingdom.

ceptable side effects. Corticosteroids should never be used in combination with NSAIDs.

Pentosan Polysulphate Pentosan polysulphate (PPS) is a semisynthetic glycosaminoglycan prepared from beech wood shavings and is structurally similar to heparin.[25] It has been available as the sodium salt for several years and is given as a course of four weekly subcutaneous injections. A calcium salt (Na) is also available that can be given orally. Many actions have been attributed to PPS. Being structurally similar to heparin, the drug exhibits anticoagulant and fibrinolytic properties. Anecdotal evidence suggests that a clinical response may not be seen until the third or fourth injection, but may last for some considerable time after the cessation of treatment. Intraarticular NaPPS was used alone or in combination with insulin-like growth factor-1 to treat experimentally induced OA in the dog (cranial cruciate ligament transection model).[26] At 6 weeks postsurgery, the severity of articular cartilage histopathology was decreased in PPS-treated animals compared to untreated dogs but was greater than in unoperated control dogs. Moreover, the levels of active, but not total, neutral metalloproteinase were decreased in cartilage from dogs treated with PPS compared to untreated dogs with induced OA. A clinical study suggested that the sodium salt given SQ has symptom modifying properties in chronic canine OA.[27] However, another study using oral PPS failed to show evidence of symptom or structure modification in naturally occurring canine stifle OA secondary to cranial cruciate ligament deficiency.[28] Injectable polysulphated glycosaminoglycan (PGAG) is a similar preparation available for use in dogs in the United States but not in the United Kingdom.

Nutritional Supplementation

There has been an increased interest in the application of nutritional supplementation in the management of OA in small animals in recent years. The term *nutraceutical* is often used to cover those nutrients that are used in this way. A nutraceutical is defined as a substance produced in a purified or extracted form that is administered orally to provide or stimulate the production of raw materials required for normal bodily function. Two of the most commonly used are glucosamine and chondroitin sulphate, which can be regarded as matrix supplements and were originally introduced based on the assumption that they could prevent or reverse the degradation of articular cartilage by increasing availability of components required for proteoglycan matrix manufacture. They are now also thought to have antiinflammatory/analgesic effects. Essential fatty acids can also be regarded as nutraceuticals and are increasingly used in an attempt to reduce the inflammatory load in osteoarthritic joints.

Chondroitin Sulphate The form and source of chondroitin sulphate appears to influence its pharmokinetic profile.[29] Mammalian sources appear to be superior to marine sources and the molecular weight (ideally 5000 to 20,000 Daltons) and the degree of sulphation are important. Labeling with H^{3+} has demonstrated distribution to articular cartilage in dogs.[30] However, in another study 6 hours after oral administration of tritiated chondroitin sulphate to rats, the majority of radioactivity in articular cartilage was from oligosaccharides, monomer, and tritiated water, suggesting the chondroitin molecule itself is not incorporated.[31] In experimental animals, chondroitin has been demonstrated to have antiinflammatory effects. In particular, it was shown to reduce edema formation in a rat carrageenin model.[31]

Glucosamine Oral glucosamine sulphate is 90% absorbed and diffuses into the articular tissues.[32] In addition to the sulphate form, glucosamine is also available as the

hydrochloride and as N-acetylglucosamine; although many different claims are made, there appears to be little difference in the efficacy of the different forms. Evidence does, however, favor glucosamine sulphate as being more effective, with the suggestion that the sulphate molecule itself might be clinically important, a factor that might also be relevant to chondroitin.[33] An amide of palmitic acid and glucosamine (glupamid) is another formulation used and that has improved bioavailability and antiinflammatory properties.

There have been several studies of the efficacy of glucosamine in relief of pain and disability associated with OA. Most of these have been on humans. The results of studies have varied and there have been problems with study design and size of study groups. For example, one showed treatment with glucosamine to be as effective as ibuprofen[34] but another study showed no beneficial effect of glucosamine over placebo.[35] Metaanalyses suggest that there may indeed be symptom modification from use of glucosamine in human OA[36] but there is general agreement that there is a likely publication bias toward positive results and more studies are required to confirm therapeutic effects.[36-38] A randomized double-blind placebo-controlled trial investigated the effects of long-term glucosamine sulphate therapy in human knee OA. It involved 212 people who were randomly assigned 1500-mg sulphate oral glucosamine or placebo once daily for 3 years.[39] There was no significant mean joint-space narrowing in the 106 patients receiving glucosamine (–0.06 mm); there was significant loss (–0.31 mm) in those patients receiving placebo. This is the first reported evidence that nutraceuticals can have a definite structure-modifying effect in the treatment of human OA. A clinical study in Spain (the GUIDE study) also showed a positive effect of glucosamine.[33]

Glucosamine and Chondroitin in Combination Most nutraceutical preparations have glucosamine and chondroitin in combination. In a survey involving 3080 veterinary practitioners, 64% recommended the use of glucosamine/chondroitin to treat OA, with 83% of those reporting an improvement in symptoms within 4 weeks.[40] A recent study in 1583 people (the Glucosamine/Chondroitin Arthritis Intervention Trial [GAIT]) with symptomatic knee OA demonstrated that glucosamine, chondroitin, or the two in combination did not reduce pain compared to placebo.[41] However, the results suggested that the combination of glucosamine and chondroitin may be effective in a subgroup of patients with moderate-to-severe knee pain. The study did show a high placebo response (60.1%), which is unusual and difficult to explain. This initial publication reported the short-term results (24 weeks of therapy); the long-term results are awaited. A limited study by Moreau et al in dogs with clinical OA showed no beneficial effects with matrix supplements, in contrast to both carprofen and meloxicam.[42] A randomized double-blind positive-controlled trial showed that a chondroitin and glucosamine preparation improved 81% of dogs with OA by day 70, as far as pain, weight bearing, and overall assessment was concerned.[43] This compared to 94% of dogs receiving carprofen, although this group also showed improvement in lameness and joint motion. Interestingly, 67% of the glucosamine/chondroitin group showed continued improvement at day 98, after the medication had been withdrawn (compared to 65% in the carprofen group). In an experimental study in rabbits using sectioning of the cruciate ligaments and partial meniscectomy to induce arthritis, the administration of glucosamine/chondroitin significantly reduced cartilage damage.[44]

Which product to use? There are several preparations of glucosamine and chondroitin sulphate available on the market. Regulation of these products is confusing since in some countries the products are licensed whereas in others they are not.

Quality control can thus be lacking. One study indicated that 84% of products did not meet label claims.[45] If using these products, it is advisable to use those produced by reputable veterinary companies that can guarantee the quality of their products. Although cheaper versions may be available, they are best avoided.

The exact dose of glucosamine and chondroitin is unknown and serum concentrations that have been detected are often much less than the levels used in tissue culture systems to produce positive effects. They appear to be safe products; gastrointestinal signs are sometimes encountered and polydipsia/polyuria less so. An association between glucosamine and diabetes mellitus in humans or insulin resistance appears unfounded. However, if using these preparations in diabetic animals, it is advisable to decrease the monitoring intervals. Glucosamine is protein bound in the blood, and again care should be taken when used in combination with NSAIDs in case of competition between the two leading to toxicity. Polysulphated preparations (most of these are injectable) should perhaps not be used in combination with NSAIDs since the former have anticoagulant properties and would perpetuate any gastrointestinal bleeds initiated by the NSAID.

The manner in which the nutraceuticals should be used is also a matter of debate. They may be used on their own in clinically affected cases or in combination with NSAIDs, which is how the author most often uses them. There is an argument that they should be used in a prophylactic fashion to prevent or slow the progression of OA. Dogs with hip or elbow dysplasia or cruciate disease that will inevitably develop OA would be candidates. Other examples could be amputees, dogs having suffered joint trauma (e.g., a dislocated hip), or dogs having undergone joint surgery.

The majority of nutritional supplements contain other ingredients besides the glucosamine and chondroitin sulphate. These include methylsulphonylmethane, which may help in matrix formation, and the curcuminins, quercetin and vitamin C, which are antioxidants. Avocado/soya bean unsaponifiable extracts have been included as an antiinflammatory agent in one of the nutraceutical products. Micronutrients such as manganese and zinc, which are involved in enzymatic reactions within cartilage, are present in some products also.

Essential Fatty Acids The essential fatty acids (EFAs) are normal constituents of cell membranes and are involved in lipid transport. They are also precursors to the eicosanoid family of inflammatory mediators. There are two main types of fatty acid, the omega-3 and the omega-6, and both these compete for incorporation into phospholipids and as substrates for COX and lipoxygenase. A higher proportion of omega-6 fatty acids within cell membranes is believed to promote the production of the inflammatory prostaglandins, leukotrienes, and thromboxanes. Diets containing omega-3 fatty acids (e.g., fish oils) and certain of the omega-6 fatty acids may help to reduce the production of proinflammatory prostaglandins within arthritic joints Miller et al reported clinical improvement in dogs with arthritis which were receiving fatty acid therapy for skin disease.[46] In vitro studies have shown that the addition of omega-3 EFAs can prevent inflammatory and matrix degradative processes initiated by chondrocytes,[47,48] specifically down-regulating aggrecanase activity. There is a prescription diet specifically for the management of OA in the dog. This contains high levels of omega-3 fatty acids, particularly eicosapentaenoic acid, and has a reduced ratio of omega-6–to–omega-3 fatty acids. The diet also contains glucosamine and chondroitin as well as antioxidants and weight-reducing ingredients. There is also a reduced-calorie version of the diet that is particularly useful for dogs prone to increasing their bodyweight. There are several clinical trials that support the effectiveness of an EFA-based diet in reducing the clinical signs of chronic OA. Although the antiinflam-

matory properties of green-lipped mussel have been attributed to a variety of pharmacologically active components, the omega-3 EFAs are commonly cited as being the main factor. Green-lipped mussel extract has produced improvement in clinical OA in some studies.[49]

Viscosupplements

Synovial fluid viscosity is generally reduced whenever an arthropathy occurs, and this results in inefficient lubrication, which can exacerbate pain. There are several preparations of hyaluronic acid that can be injected intraarticularly to improve synovial fluid quality and are more often used in the horse. There is no licensed product for use in small animals, but nonlicensed products are used by some clinicians. The matrix supplement nutraceuticals have been shown to stimulate hyaluronic acid production and improve synovial fluid viscosity, and other agents such as PPS/PGAG may also improve synovial fluid viscosity.

Multimodal Drug Therapy

There is now a growing trend to use several drugs together to provide greater osteoarthritic pain relief.[50,51] This is based on the hypothesis that pain transmission involves multiple pathways, mechanisms, and transmitter systems and therefore it is unlikely that a single class of analgesic such as the commonly used NSAID, whatever the dose, will provide complete pain relief. The combination of two or more classes of analgesic is likely to be more effective, and since the analgesic effect from these drugs is often synergistic, smaller doses of the individual drugs can be used, which decreases the likelihood of side effects from any one drug. However, there is no published scientific evidence that multimodal drug therapy is of benefit over monomodal therapy in animals suffering from OA. Drugs used in addition to NSAIDs include opioids, N-methyl-D-aspartate (NMDA) receptor antagonists, tricyclic antidepressants, anticonvulsants and calcium channel blockers, and sodium channel blockers. The glucosamine/chondroitin preparations and the polysulphated glucosaminoglycans might also be included as adjunctive products since there is some evidence they have an antiinflammatory and analgesic effect. The use of adjunctive drug therapy is indicated for animals not responding to NSAIDs or in those cases where the initial improvement with NSAIDs has decreased and quality of life is becoming affected. The most commonly used individual drugs are amantadine, tramadol, gabapentin, and amitriptyline (Table 187-3).

Other Treatments

There are many other approaches to the control of chronic pain in animals that have been described and these include acupuncture, electroacupuncture, acupressure, transcutaneous nerve stimulation, laser therapy, and the implantation of gold beads. There is much anecdotal evidence to support their use but more detailed studies are required.

Surgical Treatment of Osteoarthritis

The surgical treatment of arthritic joints includes joint replacement (prostheses are now available for the hip, elbow, and stifle), excision arthroplasty, and arthrodesis. The reader is referred to surgical texts for more details. It is perhaps relevant to mention irrigation of an osteoarthritic joint with saline or lactated Ringer's solution, under general anesthesia. This simple procedure will often produce a clinical improvement that can last for several months. Generally, joint irrigation is combined with an arthroscopic examination of the diseased joint, which provides important information on the state of the articular cartilage. During an arthroscopic examination of the elbow, for example, approximately 1 to 2 liters of fluid will be flushed through the joint. Also, it is possible during arthroscopy to remove free bodies that might be contributing

Table • 187-3

Adjunctive Drugs Used in Canine Osteoarthritis Pain Management*

DRUG	CANINE DOSE	COMMENTS
Amantadine	3-5 mg/kg orally once daily	May take up to two weeks to see positive effects Side effects appear to be mild agitation in some dogs Marketed as 100-mg capsules Suggest one capsule for dogs weighing 20-37 kg, and two capsules for dogs weighing 37-65 kg
Amitriptyline	0.5-2 mg/kg orally once daily	Bitter taste Should not be used concurrently with tramadol
Gabapentin	5-10 mg/kg orally twice daily (up to 10 mg/kg three times daily)	Most common side effect appears to be sedation
Polysulfated glycosaminoglycans (Adequan)	5 mg/kg intramuscularly twice weekly for four weeks, then once a month	No noted side effects
Tramadol	4-5 mg/kg orally twice or three times daily	Side effects appear to be sedation and vomiting (likely opioidergic effects) Should not be used concurrently with amitriptyline

Modified from Lascelles BDX: Beyond NSAIDs for canine osteoarthritis patients; multimodal drug therapy. Proceedings BVOA Scientific Meeting, Austin Court, Birmingham, United Kingdom, April 11, 2007, pp 18-23.
*Many of these drugs have not been properly evaluated in the dog and should be used with care. Although they can be used on their own as a painkiller, they are intended to be used in combination with nonsteroidal antiinflammatory drugs.

to the clinical problem. The symptomatic response may be the result of flushing out mediators of inflammation, destructive enzymes, and general debris and also a reduction in synovial fluid volume, which causes joint distension and pain. Figure 187-2 summarizes the therapeutic approach to cases of OA in the dog.

FELINE

Traditionally, it has been assumed that OA in the cat is either rare or cats do not suffer clinical disease. The disease shows many differences and peculiarities when compared with its presentation in dogs and thus deserves to be considered separately. One of the main reasons that the disease has been ignored for so long is the assumption that lameness is the main clinical feature, but this is certainly not the case, and it is changes in lifestyle and behavior that give the clue to the cat being in chronic pain.[52,53] Pathologic changes within affected joints can be severe (Web Figures 187-11 and 187-12).

PREVALENCE

The radiographic prevalence of OA in the cat is significantly high. Clarke and colleagues examined 218 cats, which included animals of all ages (mean age 6.5 years), and found a prevalence of appendicular OA of 16.5%.[54] Hardie et al found a prevalence of 64% (90% if all types of degenerative disease were included), but they only examined cats older than 12 years of age (mean age 15.2 years).[55] Godfrey examined 292 cats with an average age of 9.5 years and found a prevalence of appendicular OA of 22%.[56] There are no reports of the clinical prevalence of feline OA, but it is likely to be high in the older cat.[52]

ETIOPATHOGENESIS

Unlike the dog, most cases of OA in the cat appear to be of a primary or idiopathic nature. Secondary OA in the cat

can be associated with previous trauma, and hip dysplasia can result in secondary hip OA; this accounts only for approximately 20% of hip OA, the rest being primary. Acromegaly is another cause of secondary OA.[57] Overall, 60% to 75% of cases of OA in the cat appear to be idiopathic.[52,54]

CLINICAL FEATURES

The most common features of OA in the cat are a reduced level of activity and a reduced ability to jump.[52,53,58,59] Since OA is more common in the older cat, these changes in lifestyle are most often explained as the effects of old age rather than as an indication of chronic pain. Owners are most likely to recognize the signs of OA in cats. Reduced activity levels include less time spent outdoors, less time spent playing/interacting with the owner, and less time hunting. The reduced ability to jump includes hesitation and refusal to jump or jumping only reduced heights. Other changes in behavioral patterns have also been associated with chronic pain in the cat, including seeking seclusion, vocalization on handling, aggression and/or resentment to handling, changes in urination/defecation, alterations in grooming, and changes in appetite.[52] Stiff gait and/or an obvious limp are sometimes reported by the owner although not necessarily confirmed at the time of clinical examination. Assessment of lameness in cats during a physical examination is not easy, for obvious reasons.

The elbow (59%) and hip (48%) joints were the most commonly affected with only 5.5% of shoulders, 7% of stifles and 9% of hocks showing clinical disease.[52] Bilateral involvement is very common and multiple joints may be affected. Unlike in the dog, periarticular joint thickening is often subtle and difficult to detect on palpation. Synovial effusion is not obvious in many cats and few show a reduced range of motion of affected joints. Crepitus is also exceedingly rare. Obviously, assessment of pain in the cat is difficult since many cats do not willingly accept palpation and manipulation of their joints even if disease-free.

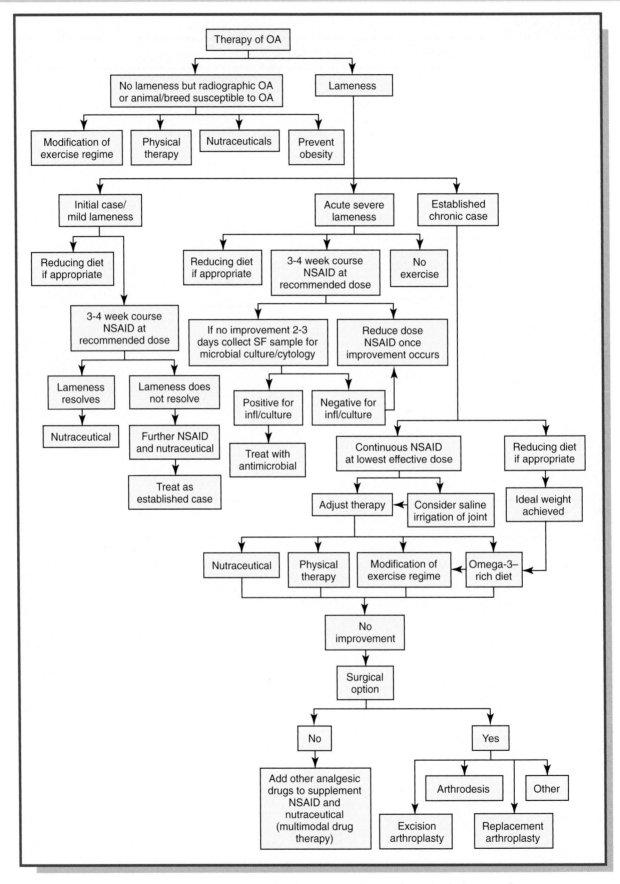

Figure 187-2 Algorithm illustrating the therapeutic selection for individual cases of canine osteoarthritis *(OA)*. *NSAID,* Nonsteroidal antiinflammatory drug; *SF,* Synovial fluid.

DIAGNOSTIC IMAGING

Radiography is the most commonly used modality for helping to diagnose feline OA. The radiographic features of feline versus canine OA can be different, with soft tissue mineralization and intraarticular mineralized bodies being considerably more common.[52,54] As in the dog, the presence of osteophytes is regarded as the key radiographic feature of OA, although these can sometimes be difficult to identify. Soft tissue thickening and synovial effusion are generally less apparent in feline OA.

Elbow Joint Although subjective, the presence of subchondral bone sclerosis beneath the ulnar notch is a key feature of elbow OA (Web Figures 187-13 through 187-15). Sclerosis is more easily assessed in the feline patient compared to the dog since there is less variation in the anatomy between different types and breeds of cat and thus it is easier for the clinician/radiologist to appreciate changes in bone density. Apparent subchondral bone sclerosis can be due to increased thickening of the bony trabeculae beneath the articular surface, by osteophyte formation at the articular margin, or by soft tissue mineralization/mineralized bodies superimposed on the bone. Most osteophyte formation appears to occur on the medial side of the joint, the distal humerus, and proximal ulna (see Web Figure 187-14). Bony reaction on the medial epicondyle (sometimes referred to as *medial epicondylitis*) is often present. It is important to remember the sesamoid bone in the supinator muscle of the feline elbow joint, which is present in all elbows but is radiographically visible in about 40% of normal joints.[60] However, the sesamoid does become more obvious in an osteoarthritic joint and is often increased in size. It is sometimes difficult to distinguish the sesamoid bone from soft tissue mineralization. More severe pathology appears to occur within the medial compartment of the joint (see Web Figure 187-12).

Hip Joint Although hip dysplasia is well documented in the cat, it only accounts for about 20% of cases of hip OA.[52] This of course is influenced by how hip dysplasia is presently defined. Keller et al reported a 6.6% prevalence of hip dysplasia in a hospital population of cats and demonstrated no statistical difference in the prevalence of hip dysplasia between domestic shorthair and pure-bred cats. There was no effect of sexual status.[61] The Maine Coon breed is reported as having a prevalence of 18%, and genetic influences are thought to be involved in feline hip dysplasia.[62] Increased joint laxity within the feline dysplastic hip has been demonstrated,[63] and more research is required into the relevance of feline hip laxity and arthritis. Clarke and Bennett recorded a Norberg angle for the dysplastic hip of 87.5 degrees compared with 99.2 degrees for the normal.[52] The normal Norberg angle is much less than that for a dog, indicating a shallower acetabulum. OA of the hip joint is characterized by osteophyte formation, particularly on the cranial effective acetabular rim and femoral neck, where it often appears as a sclerotic line (Web Figure 187-16).

There appears to be two distinct morphologic types of hip dysplasia in the cat, one typified purely by less than 50% coverage of the femoral head by the dorsal acetabulum and the other by an abnormally shaped femoral head, where there may also be poor acetabular coverage.

Stifle Joint OA of the stifle is characterized by osteophyte formation on the patella, around the trochlear margin (where, again, it will appear as a sclerotic line), and on the caudal edge of the tibia. Soft tissue mineralization is often seen. Remember the cat often only has one fabella (the lateral)

visible on the radiograph; the medial fabella is often insufficiently mineralized to be seen. It is common in the cat to see mineralization in the cranial pole of the medial meniscus, and this may represent degenerative calcification within the meniscus or possibly the presence of a meniscal sesamoid bone, the lunula[64] (Web Figure 187-17).

In most cases mineralization of the medial meniscus is an incidental finding of no clinical significance. Mineralization within the cranial cruciate ligament may occasionally be seen. Enthesiophyte formation at the attachment of the patellar ligament on the tibial tuberosity is another feature that may be seen. This may occur as part of stifle OA but is often seen as a solitary lesion, which appears to be of little clinical significance.

Shoulder Joint OA of the shoulder joint is characterized by osteophyte formation on the caudal rim of the glenoid and on the caudal edge of the humeral head (Web Figure 187-18).

There often appears to be a line of separation between the osteophyte and the edge of the glenoid, and this may represent a situation where the osteophyte has not become completely incorporated within the epiphysis, or it may not be a true osteophyte but an osteochondroma. It is sometimes possible to appreciate a reduced joint space on the caudal aspect of the joint. The clavicle is very obvious in the feline shoulder and should not be confused with a pathologic lesion. The cat also has a very prominent coracoid process of the glenoid and its appearance is influenced by the radiographic positioning; it is easily mistaken for new bone formation on a caudocranial or craniocaudal film.

Hock and Carpus OA of the hock is characterized by osteophyte formation and soft tissue mineralization, most of the pathology occurring within the lateral aspect of the joint. OA of the carpus is rare in the cat, although osteophyte formation on the distal radius and on the carpal bones may be seen.

TREATMENT

The general approach to treatment is similar to that of the dog, although there is only one NSAID licensed for use long term in the cat (meloxicam).

Supportive Measures Obesity can be a feature of cats with OA (approximately 14%), and such cats should be placed on a reducing diet until their target weights are achieved. However, losing weight in the feline patient is more of a challenge than in the canine. Modifying the cats' environment such as providing comfortable bedding, reducing the necessity for jumping, using shallow litter trays or ramps, and modifying the cat flap can all be considered. Physical therapy is again more of a challenge in the cat than it is in the dog, but there have been recent developments in this area for the feline arthritic patient, including the use of hydrotherapy pools.

Environmental Enrichment Cats are territorial animals and changes in their territorial environment can challenge their security leading to increased anxiety. It is likely that such an event in a cat suffering chronic pain can compound the problem. Thus, the owner should be encouraged to ensure that there have not been any recent changes in the cats' immediate environment that could be upsetting it and contributing to the problem. Ways of improving the immediate environment include providing places where cats can hide, such as cardboard boxes or igloo beds, and ensuring more than one access to and from their core territory (owner's house). Food bowls should be well placed, and there should be more than one distributed throughout the house, again to ensure that the cat feels secure but also to encourage exercise by movement throughout the house. Water bowls should be placed away from the food and more than one should be provided. Litter trays should be well placed and there should be at least one per cat and again easily accessible. The owner should be encouraged to play with the cat for at least three sessions per day and for several minutes at each session. Playing with the cat encourages exercise and mental stimulation. The owner should also be encouraged to hold and stroke the cat, particularly around the head, since this is known to release neurotransmitters that can improve the cats' mood and its ability to cope with chronic pain. Similarly, grooming several times a day and for several minutes each time will have a similar effect. Pheromonatherapy is another possible approach. There are products that contain feline pheromones (the F3 fraction of feline facial pheromone and the F4 fraction). These are provided as a spray that can be released into the environment or as a diffuser that plugs into the electrical socket.

NSAIDs Meloxicam is an effective NSAID for treating chronic pain in OA cats. The dose is 0.1 mg/kg orally on day 1 and then 0.05 mg/kg orally once daily. In the study by Clarke and Bennett, there was a marked improvement in over 60% of cases.[52] Meloxicam is easy to administer since it is mixed with the food and the palatability is excellent. Side effects are rare although occasional vomiting and diarrhea are reported. It is recommended to always give a full course of treatment for 3 to 4 weeks. If continuous therapy is required, the dose can be reduced based on clinical response. Meloxicam is thought to be metabolized by oxidative pathways and thus the relative low capacity for hepatic glucuronidation of exogenously administered drugs seen in the cat is not a problem. A molecular genetic basis for the latter has been identified; domestic cats have fewer hepatic UDP-glucuronosyltransferase (UGT) isoforms and may have mutations of UGT or pseudogenes.[65-67] Since it is mainly older cats that suffer OA, routine blood analyses are advisable to assess liver and kidney status. It is important to encourage adequate fluid intake in cats receiving NSAIDs, and thus feeding moist tinned or sachet food is important, particularly when on long-term therapy. Meloxicam is highly protein-bound in the blood and

	All of the time	Some of the time	None of the time
• My cat sleeps more and/or is less active			
• My cat goes out less			
• My cat is less willing to jump up or down			
• My cat will only jump up or down from lower heights			
• My cat shows signs of being stiff at times when he or she walks or runs			
• My cat is more reluctant to come and greet me or interact with me			
• My cat plays with other animals or toys less			
• My cat hunts less			
• My cat has a poor coat			
• Overall my cat is less agile			
• My cat shows signs of lameness or limping			
• My cat has more accidents outside the litter tray			
• My cat has difficulty getting in or out of the cat flap			
• My cat has difficulty going up or down stairs			
• My cat is grooming less			
• My cat is grooming more			
• My cat does not like to be groomed by me			
• My cat does not like being picked up			
• My cat does not like being stroked			
• My cat does not like strangers			
• My cat seems restless at home			
• My cat vocalizes a lot			
• My cat seems frightened by sudden noises			
• My cat is scratching (post/furniture) more			
• My cat is scratching (post/furniture) less			
• My cat has changed his/her toileting			
• My cat is spraying in the house			
• My cat has become more aggressive toward me			
• My cat has become more aggressive to other cats			
• My cat has become aggressive to visitors			

Figure 187-3 Owner-based mobility/lifestyle/behavioral questionnaire used to help identify clinical osteoarthritis in the cat.

thus care is always needed when it is given to a cat receiving other drugs, such as ACE inhibitors and diuretics, where there might be competition for protein binding. These cats should be particularly carefully monitored for possible side effects. Multimodal analgesic therapy is also being applied to the cat although this is very much in its infancy and side effects are more common than with the dog.

Nutritional Supplements As with the dog there is a prescription diet that is rich in EFAs and has been shown to have a positive effect in reducing the clinical features of OA in the cat. The EFAs required by the cat are different from those required by the dog; docosahexaenoic acid and alpha-linolenic acid are those most relevant to the feline species. The diet can be used together with meloxicam, in which case the moist form of the diet should be used. The nutraceuticals containing glucosamine and chondroitin are available for use in the cat, and although there are no published clinical trials, there is much anecdotal evidence that these preparations can reduce the pain and clinical features of feline OA. They are very safe agents to use in the cat and can be used on their own or together with NSAIDs. The oral administration of glucosamine and chondroitin has been associated with mild gastrointestinal upset in cats.

CONCLUSION

Although there is now an increasing awareness of feline OA, it is still a much underdiagnosed disease in general practice,

and many cats suffering chronic pain require therapy. Currently the feline population is an ageing one[68]; for example, in the last 10 years the percentage of cats in the United States over 6 years of age has increased from 24% to 47%, the percentage over 10 years has increased by 15%, and over 15 years has increased from 5% to 14%. The average age of cats in Europe has increased from 4.7 to 5.3 years over a similar period. Owners are key to making the diagnosis since they know if the animal's lifestyle has changed in any way, but they must be asked the right questions. It is recommended that the owners of all cats over 6 years of age should regularly complete a "mobility questionnaire" with the veterinary clinician or one of the nursing/technical staff. Figure 187-3 shows the questionnaire used by the author for this purpose. Making an accurate diagnosis can be difficult since the clinical examination can be a challenge and it is sometimes difficult to know whether a joint is truly thickened or painful. Radiography can help to confirm a diagnosis but this requires a general anesthetic or heavy sedation and many clinicians will be hesitant to anaesthetize an old cat because of the associated risks. Thus it is often the case that the diagnosis is made purely on the lifestyle and behavioral changes and the response to an initial course of analgesic therapy.

REFERENCES

The reference list can be found on the companion Expert Consult Web site at *www.expertconsult.com*.

CHAPTER 188

Immune-Mediated Hemolytic Anemia and Other Regenerative Anemias

Kelly Mitchell
Stephen Kruth

REGENERATIVE BONE MARROW RESPONSE

Anemia is defined as a reduction in the number of circulating red blood cells (RBCs), hematocrit, and hemoglobin, resulting in decreased oxygen-carrying capacity. A normal animal will regenerate the erythron by accelerating erythropoiesis via erythropoietin-mediated effects on erythroid progenitor cells. Under accelerated erythropoiesis, reticulocytes leave the marrow early, causing an increase in number of circulating reticulocytes. The most reliable indicator of regeneration is an increase in aggregate reticulocytes in peripheral blood. After erythropoietin stimulates the marrow, it usually takes 2 to 5 days before reticulocytes can be identified in circulation, with peak numbers occurring 4 to 7 days following stimulation. Following severe acute blood loss, healthy dogs can increase reticulocyte production sixfold to eightfold, and cats threefold to fivefold.

Reticulocytes can be identified by staining cytoplasmic RNA with new methylene blue or brilliant cresyl blue and enumerated by hand or automated cell counters. Dogs normally produce only aggregate reticulocytes. In cats, aggregate reticulocyte counts more accurately reflect the regenerative state than do punctate reticulocyte counts; clinical pathology

laboratories usually report aggregate reticulocyte numbers. Normal dogs usually have less than 1 reticulocyte/100 erythrocytes and normal cats less than 0.4 reticulocytes/100 erythrocytes; however, it is more useful to evaluate aggregate reticulocyte counts as absolute reticulocyte counts. Healthy dogs usually have less than 60,000 and cats less than 42,000 reticulocytes/μL; higher values are suggestive of accelerated erythropoiesis. Other findings consistent with a regenerative response include polychromatophilia, anisocytosis, macrocytic and/or hypochromic indices, Howell-Jolly bodies (nuclear remnants), increased red cell distribution width (RDW), and appropriate rubricytosis.[1,2] Regenerative anemias can be classified as those associated with hemolysis or those associated with acute or chronic blood loss. Rarely, cats with erythroid neoplasia have responsive anemias. The examination of the blood film may yield important information regarding the cause of the anemia, including hemoplasma, *Babesia* or *Cytauxzoon* organisms, spherocytes suggestive of immune mediated injury to erythrocytes, evidence of oxidative injury (Heinz bodies, eccentrocytes), or other changes in erythrocyte morphology (acanthocytes, schizocytes, keratocytes) that can be evidence of vasculitis, hemangiosarcoma, or intravascular coagulation. Bone marrow examination is rarely indicated in patients with regenerative anemias. An approach to the patient with regenerative anemia is presented in Figure 188-1. One of the most common causes of regenerative anemia of dogs is immune-mediated hemolytic anemia (IMHA).

IMMUNE-MEDIATED HEMOLYTIC ANEMIA

PATHOPHYSIOLOGY

Antibody-mediated RBC destruction is the hallmark of IMHA. Canine IMHA occurs most frequently (60% to 75% of cases) as an idiopathic disorder characterized by immune system dysregulation, antibody production against unaltered RBCs, and the absence of identifiable underlying disease.[3,4] Less frequently, infectious diseases, neoplasia, or drug administration alter RBC surface antigens such that autoreactive antibodies are produced and secondary IMHA occurs (Box 188-1). A causal relationship between development of IMHA and a possible predisposing factor can be difficult to prove and may more accurately reflect a temporal or coincidental association (e.g., hypothyroidism, bladder calculi, chronic renal failure[4]), parallel manifestations of the same disorder (e.g., multisystemic autoimmune disease[5,6]) or a nonimmunologic mechanism of hemolysis (e.g., envenomation[7]).

In the setting of primary IMHA, the exact mechanism(s) by which loss of immunologic tolerance toward unaltered erythrocyte self-antigen(s) occurs is unknown. Mechanisms implicated in the initiation of autoreactivity in human IMHA include regulatory T-lymphocyte dysfunction, defective development of peripheral or central tolerance, exposure of previously ignored or hidden self antigens and cross reactivity between self and foreign antigens.[8] Autoreactive T lymphocytes have been isolated from the peripheral blood of dogs with IMHA, suggesting loss of immunologic self-tolerance.[9-11] Erythrocyte glycophorins, RBC anion channel band 3,[12] and the cytoskeletal protein spectrin[11] have been implicated as autoantigens in canine IMHA. Autoreactivity to spectrin is expected in hemolytic disease as a consequence of exposure to hidden RBC antigens and may represent a mechanism for removal of senescent erythrocytes, having been identified in clinically normal dogs.[10,11]

Phagocytosis of opsonized RBC occurs following binding of the fragment crystallizable or constant fragment (Fc) of the immunoglobulin molecule to Fc receptors on cells of the mononuclear-phagocytic system.[6,13] Appropriate Fc receptors are expressed on blood monocytes and hepatic Kupffer cells; however, the primary site of extravascular erythrophagocytosis is the spleen.[6,13] The interaction of RBC-bound autoantibody with macrophages results in either complete phagocytosis or partial internalization of a portion of the RBC membrane, followed by resealing of the membrane and reentry of the remaining red cell into circulation as a spherocyte. In addition, antibody binding can initiate complement fixation and formation of a transmembrane pore (membrane attack complex) with resultant intravascular osmotic hemolysis.[13,14]

Antibodies of the IgG subclass, alone or in combination with IgM, are the most commonly identified erythrocyte-bound immunoprotein in canine IMHA.[4,15-18] Antibodies to only IgM or complement protein C3b were infrequently implicated as the autoreactive immunoprotein in older reports, but have not been identified using newer flow cytometric techniques.[17,19,20] IgG antibodies are relatively poor activators of the classical complement pathway and IgG-sensitized RBCs are generally eliminated through extravascular hemolysis.[21] IgM-sensitized RBCs are generally eliminated through a combination of intravascular hemolysis (due to IgM-mediated activation of the classical complement pathway) and extravascular phagocytosis.[21]

The most common complication and cause of death in canine IMHA is confirmed or suspected thromboembolic disease (TED), including pulmonary thromboembolism (PTE) and disseminated intravascular coagulation (DIC).[22,23] The relative incidence of postmortem-confirmed TED in dogs with IMHA has been reported to range from 10.6% to 80%.[4,23-27] In addition to PTE, necropsy evaluations of dogs with IMHA have revealed evidence of thromboembolism in the spleen, lungs, kidneys, liver, heart, pituitary gland, stomach, skin, and lymph nodes.[4,24,27] Three or more laboratory criteria of DIC (thrombocytopenia, prolonged prothrombin time, activated partial thromboplastin time, low antithrombin activity, low fibrinogen concentration, increased fibrinogen degradation product concentration, increased D-dimer concentration) are identified in 19% to 45% of dogs with IMHA.[4,23,26] Findings that have been associated with an increased risk of TED include severe thrombocytopenia, hypoalbuminemia, negative direct antiglobulin test (DAT), intravenous catheterization, and increased serum alkaline phosphatase (ALP) activity.[26] Although the exact etiology of TED has not been determined, vasculitis, antiphospholipid antibodies, liberation of RBC stroma, tissue factor production and release from leukocytes and indirect procoagulatory effects of free hemoglobin have been hypothesized to play a role.[23,26] Many of the suspected clinical risk factors for development of TED are unavoidable in treatment of the disease, including intravenous catheterization, administration of exogenous glucocorticoids or cytotoxic agents, and blood transfusion.[27]

Box • 188-1

Conditions That Are Reported to Underlie or Predispose to Canine Immune-Mediated Hemolytic Anemia

Infectious
Haemobartonellosis
Salmonellosis
Ancylostoma caninum infection[4,137]
Anaplasma phagocytophilum infection[138]
Trichuris vulpis infection[4]
Babesiosis

Neoplastic
Lymphoma[139]
Leukemia
Soft tissue sarcoma[140]
Bronchoalveolar carcinoma[4]
Mast cell tumor
Splenic hemangioma

Inflammatory
Pancreatitis[4]
Prostatitis/cystitis[4]
Systemic lupus erythematosus[141]

Drugs/Toxins
Levamisole
Carprofen[142]
Cephalosporin antibiotics
Griseofulvin
Recent vaccination[38]
Bee-sting envenom[7]

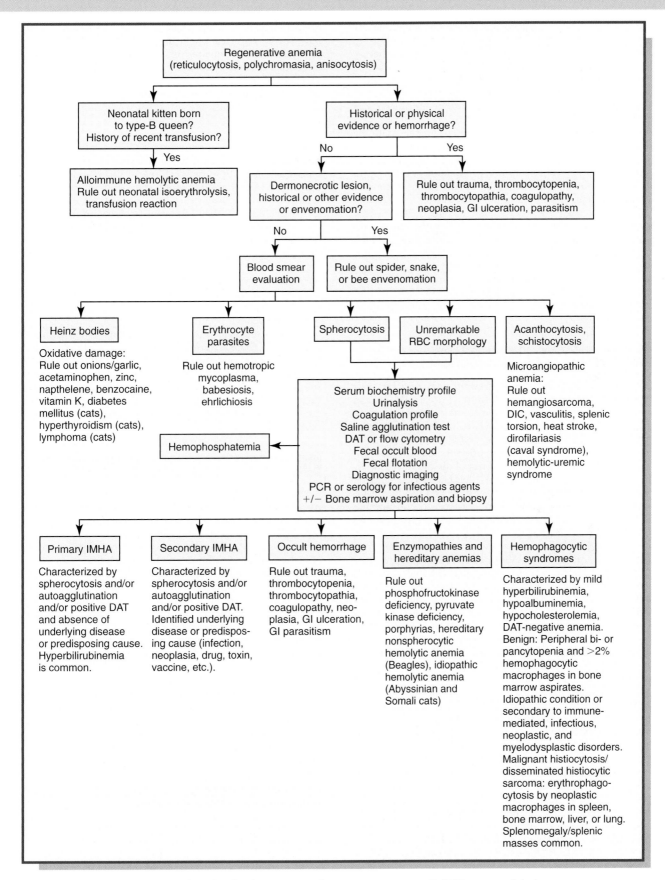

Figure 188-1 Algorithm for the patient with regenerative anemia. *DAT,* Direct antiglobulin test; *DIC,* disseminated intravascular coagulation; *GI,* gastrointestinal; *IMHA,* immune-mediated hemolytic anemia; *PCR,* polymerase chain reaction; *RBC,* red blood cell.

Increasing evidence suggests that a systemic inflammatory response coincides with the period of acute hemolysis in canine IMHA.[28] The occurrence of an acute inflammatory response is supported by the findings of moderate to marked leukocytosis[29] as well as by changes in the serum concentration of several acute phase proteins, including C-reactive protein, α-1 acid glycoprotein, ceruloplasmin, fibrinogen, von Willebrand factor antigen, and albumin.[23,26,30,31] Severe systemic inflammation promotes a hypercoagulable state by increasing tissue factor expression, increasing fibrinogen concentration, increasing platelet responsiveness and P-selectin expression, and by inhibiting the production or activity of anticoagulant molecules including antithrombin, thrombomodulin, protein C, and plasminogen activators.[28,32] The net result is an increase in procoagulant activity, a decrease in anticoagulant activity, and decreased fibrinolysis. The significant morbidity and mortality associated with canine IMHA despite apparently successful immunosuppression and appropriate supportive care suggests that the pathophysiology of this disease cannot be explained by autoimmunity and anemia alone. Rather, inflammatory processes and associated abnormalities in hemostasis could play a major role in the progression of this disease.

PATIENT PRESENTATION

Signalment, Seasonality of Presentation, and Possible Association with Recent Vaccination Primary IMHA can occur in any canine breed, although breed predispositions are well described. The American Cocker Spaniel (ACS) represents 11% to 33% of affected dogs* and is reported to be 3.3 to 12.2 times more likely than other breeds to develop IMHA,[3,4,33,34] without an increased risk of disease related mortality.[24,33] ACS who do not express dog erythrocyte antigen (DEA) 7 have been reported to be at increased risk for development of IMHA compared to an all-breed control population.[34] However, the proportion of DEA 7–positive dogs did not differ between ACS with or without IMHA,[34] suggesting the absence of DEA 7 may be a common feature of the breed regardless of disease status. Although differential representation of dog leukocyte antigen (DLA) class II haplotypes have been identified in dogs with IMHA compared to an all-breed control group, strong breed-associated DLA heterogeneity precluded identification of breed-specific associations between DLA haplotype and development of IMHA.[16] Attempts to identify genetic or familial risk factors for development of IMHA may be hampered by the inadvertent identification of breed rather than disease associated traits. Other breeds that have been reported to be at increased risk of development of IMHA include Miniature Schnauzer,[3,24] Collie,[3,4,16,34] English Springer Spaniel,[3,4,16] Poodle,[3] Bichon Frise, Miniature Pinscher, Finnish Spitz,[34] and Old English Sheepdog.

Although IMHA can occur in dogs of any age, it is most commonly a condition of young adult to middle-age dogs, occurring less frequently in dogs under 2 years of age[24] and more frequently in dogs in the age ranges of 2 to 4 years, 5 to 7 years,[3] or greater than 6 years.[24] Female dogs have been indentified to be at increased risk of IMHA.[15,22,24,26,33-37] The overrepresentation of female dogs and neutered dogs of either sex has been offered as evidence that androgens are protective against development of IMHA.[24,26] However, only one report identified sexually intact male dogs to be at decreased risk of disease[24] while others have been unable to demonstrate an association between sex or spay/neuter status[34] and development of IMHA. Importantly, sex may not be a significant factor after controlling for breed and age.[3]

*References 4, 15, 16, 22, 24, 26, 33.

Inconsistent seasonal trends in the month of diagnosis have been reported for canine IMHA.[4,24,35] Reasons for the potential seasonality of IMHA include undiagnosed infectious disease,[35] seasonality of routine health care (e.g., vaccination, parasite prophylaxis), and changes in microvascular autoagglutination due to appendicular hypothermia,[24] all of which would be subject to additional geographic variation.

A temporal association between vaccination and development of IMHA has been suggested.[38] While subsequent investigations have been unable to confirm such an association,[24,26,39] individual associations between recent vaccination and development of IMHA are frequently described within larger case series.[3,4,33] Mechanisms by which vaccination could induce IMHA include antibody formation against erythrocyte membrane–attached vaccine components, nonspecific immune stimulation, and macrophage activation or exacerbation of preexisting disease.[38] Given the suspected multifactorial etiology of the disease, the relationship between vaccination and development of IMHA may be causal in some patients and nothing more than a temporal association in others. There is no evidence that vaccination increases the incidence of IMHA within the general population of dogs.

While it seems intuitive to refrain from revaccinating dogs with IMHA, there are no evidence-based guidelines pertaining to revaccination of dogs with a history of IMHA. Suggestions include vaccinating only when there is significant risk of exposure or if required by law and administration of individual vaccines on a sequential schedule. The relative risks of attenuated, inactivated, and recombinant products for inducing relapse are unknown.

CLINICAL PRESENTATION

Clinical signs and physical exam findings vary with the severity and rapidity of onset of the anemia. Lethargy, depression, weakness and anorexia are the most common clinical complaints.[3,4,13,15,18] Collapse and tachypnea can occur with severe or acute anemia. Vomiting, diarrhea, polydipsia, and pica (usually soil) are less frequently reported.[15,18] Epistaxis, petechial hemorrhage, melena, or other bleeding tendencies may be the presenting clinical complaint in dogs with concurrent thrombocytopenia.[13,18] Dogs with intravascular hemolysis may present with hemoglobinuria, a shorter history of illness, and more severe clinical signs.[15,18]

Mucous membrane pallor is noted on physical examination in the majority (76% to 97%) of patients.[3,4,13,15,18] Other common physical exam findings attributable to anemia include tachycardia, tachypnea, hemic systolic heart murmur, and prolonged capillary refill time.[3,4,13,15] More specific indicators of extravascular hemolysis such as icterus, splenomegaly, and hepatomegaly are observed at presentation in 25% to 50% of cases.[3,4,15] Abdominal discomfort, lymphadenopathy, and hyperthermia are less common physical exam findings.[13,15,18]

DIAGNOSIS

Complete Blood Count, Serum Biochemical Profile, and Urine Analysis A moderate to marked regenerative anemia, spherocytosis, and autoagglutination are characteristic of IMHA. However, the absence of one or more of these findings on a complete blood count (CBC) does not exclude the diagnosis. Blood smear evaluation is essential for identification of spherocytosis and RBC parasites and helpful for estimation of the adequacy of the regenerative response, leukocyte and platelet numbers. Moderate to marked spherocytosis is identified upon initial evaluation in 52% to 95% of reported cases.*

Mean hematocrit (Hct) reported for dogs with IMHA at admission to hospital ranges from 13.0 to 21.0 L/L,[3,4,15,18,24,33] with greater than 80% of dogs in some reports presenting with Hct less than 20 L/L.[4,29] A regenerative anemia (corrected reticulocyte count >1% or absolute reticulocyte count >60 × 10^3 cells/μL) is present in the majority (42% to 85%) of dogs at initial diagnosis.[3,4,22-25,33] Dogs with anemia of acute onset may present before sufficient time has elapsed for development of a regenerative response, but should demonstrate adequate reticulocytosis within 3 to 5 days.[4] Persistent ineffective erythroid regeneration is suggestive of immune-mediated destruction of erythroid precursors, anemia of inflammatory disease, paraneoplastic syndrome, lack of erythropoietin (e.g., chronic renal insufficiency), or bone marrow disorders including myelophthisis, myelofibrosis and myeloproliferative disorders. Persistent nonregenerative anemia or leukopenia are indications for bone marrow aspiration and biopsy.

Moderate to marked leukocytosis is a common hematologic abnormality in dogs with IMHA,[29] reported in 66% to 98% of dogs at the time of diagnosis.[3,18,22,23,33] While tissue necrosis secondary to anemic hypoxia and thromboembolism is the suspected stimulus for the leukocytosis,[29] others have suggested that the typical absence of leukocytosis with other anemic disorders is evidence of a cytokine response to inflammation and necrosis which is unique to IMHA.[2]

Concurrent thrombocytopenia is identified in 25% to 70% of dogs with IMHA at the time of diagnosis† and is typically assumed to be due to concurrent immune-mediated platelet destruction (Evans' syndrome). Dogs with IMHA and concurrent thrombocytopenia should not be assumed to have concurrent immune-mediated thrombocytopenia (ITP) until evaluation for DIC has occurred. Failure to recognize DIC may explain why some reports[24,26] have identified an association between thrombocytopenia and increased mortality.

The most consistently reported serum biochemical abnormality in dogs with IMHA is hyperbilirubinemia. Serum total bilirubin concentration is increased in 60% to 86%[3,4,23,33] of dogs with IMHA and has been inconsistently linked with increased mortality. Although it is assumed that much of the hyperbilirubinemia is of prehepatic (hemolytic) origin, increased serum ALP (80% to 90% of dogs),[3,33] alanine aminotransferase (33% to 58% of dogs),[3,4,33] and aspartate aminotransferase (69% of dogs)[33] activities suggest hypoxia or drug-induced hepatocellular damage could contribute. Artifactual hypophosphatemia due to interference from hyperbilirubinemia and possibly hemoglobinemia has been described.[40] Decreased packed cell volume (PCV) with normal serum total protein concentration (total solids) is consistent with hemolysis. Intravascular hemolysis is suggested by the presence of hemoglobinuria and/or hemoglobinemia.

Saline Agglutination Test All dogs with suspected IMHA should be evaluated for the presence of RBC autoagglutination by means of a saline agglutination test. Briefly, one drop of EDTA-anticoagulated blood is combined with equal parts saline on a microscope slide. Persistence of RBC agglutination after saline dilution is suggestive of antibody-mediated clumping of cells.[40] However, microscopic evaluation of the saline-diluted RBCs is necessary to differentiate autoagglutination from rouleaux formation. If microscopic distinction between autoagglutination and rouleaux formation is not immediately obvious, further dilution of the patient sample

with saline (1 part blood to 2 to 3 parts saline) or comparison to a comparably diluted control blood sample can be performed.

Detection of Antierythrocyte Antibodies The direct antiglobulin test (DAT), or Coombs' test, detects erythrocyte-bound immunoglobulin or complement, the presence of which is strongly supportive of a diagnosis of immune-mediated hemolysis.[41] A positive slide agglutination test confirms the presence of erythrocyte-bound immunoglobulin and precludes performance of the DAT.

The DAT is performed via addition of species-specific antiserum containing antibody to one or more of IgG, IgM, or complement protein C3 to a suspension of washed patient erythrocytes.[17,42] Interaction between erythrocyte-bound immunoglobulin or complement and the antiserum results in grossly visible agglutination of erythrocytes.[13,42] Results are reported as the highest dilution of antiserum at which autoagglutination is observed.[17] Hemolytic conditions, other than IMHA, that have been associated with DAT-positive anemia include acute or delayed hemolytic transfusion reactions, infection with erythrocyte parasites, drug-induced hemolytic anemia, lymphoproliferative disorders, and neonatal isoerythrolysis.[21,42]

DAT-negative canine IMHA, characterized by clinical evidence of hemolysis, absence of identifiable underlying disease, and a negative DAT, is a common clinical occurrence, with a reported incidence of 23% to 63%.[3,24,26] Estimates are complicated by the lack of agreement with regards to the definition of a positive DAT titer. Factors that have been implicated in false-negative DAT results include low level of membrane-bound immunoglobulin or complement, low binding affinity or high dissociation constant of membrane-bound antibody, previous corticosteroid therapy, and technical error (e.g., improper antisera to antibody ratio, improper washing or dilution of cell preparations).[17,41,43]

The use of flow cytometry for detection of anti-RBC antibodies is more sensitive and specific than regenerative anemia with spherocytosis for diagnosis of canine IMHA and more sensitive than direct antiglobulin testing for detection of anti-RBC antibodies.[20] By flow cytometry, anti-RBC antibodies are detected in 17.7% and 8.3% of anemic and nonanemic dogs, respectively.[20] Among anemic dogs, anti-RBC antibodies are detected in 77%, 36%, and 4% of dogs with IMHA, thrombocytopenia, and neoplasia, respectively.[17,19,44]

Diagnostic Imaging Diagnostic imaging in patients with hemolytic anemia is indicated to detect underlying conditions that may mimic IMHA (e.g., gastrointestinal zinc foreign body) and to identify underling neoplasia or systemic illness.[35] Thoracic radiographs are generally unremarkable although a pronounced interstitial lung pattern, patchy alveolar opacities, and mild pleural effusion have been associated with the development of PTE.[45] Descriptions of abdominal ultrasound findings in dogs with IMHA are limited. Hepatomegaly,[6,14] splenomegaly,[5,14] and anechoic peritoneal effusion[3,14] were the most common ultrasound findings reported by Mason and colleagues.[22] Pleural and peritoneal effusions may occur as a consequence of thromboembolism or vasculitis while hepatomegaly and splenomegaly are assumed secondary to extravascular phagocytosis.

Ancillary Testing Indications for ancillary testing for blood-borne infectious agents, polysystemic autoimmune disease, or other systemic illness will depend on patient history (including travel), clinical signs, geography, seasonality, and results of the initial diagnostic evaluation.

In summary, diagnostic criteria for primary canine IMHA include anemia (characterized by spherocytosis, autoaggluti-

---

*References 3, 4, 18, 22-26, 33, 35, 38.
†References 3, 4, 18, 22, 23, 25, 26, 33.

nation and/or presence of anti-RBC antibodies [DAT or flow cytometry]), absence of identifiable underlying disease or predisposing cause, and negative or stable infectious disease titers, as indicated by the geographic region or travel history. Concurrent nonhematologic disease of presumed autoimmune etiology or positive antinuclear antibody titer should prompt consideration of a multisystemic autoimmune condition such as systemic lupus erythematosus (SLE).

THERAPY

Supportive Care and Transfusion Therapy Supportive care of the canine patient with IMHA will depend on the severity of clinical signs. Treatment of suspected or confirmed underlying disease and withdrawal of any nonessential or potentially causative drugs are essential. Antibiotic therapy is only indicated to address suspected or confirmed bacterial infection or as empirical therapy for geographically common (consider travel history) infectious diseases (e.g., *Mycoplasma* spp., *Babesia* spp.). Appropriate intravenous fluid support should not be withheld from anemic patients over concerns of further decline in Hct as vascular volume is essential to effective tissue perfusion. If concerns over the degree of anemia and associate clinical signs exist, a transfusion of packed RBCs should be administered rather than restriction of fluid therapy.

Most dogs with IMHA (44% to 90%) have anemia of sufficient severity to require a blood transfusion.* Transfusion therapy of human patients with IMHA is not associated with an increased risk of alloimmunization or aggravation of hemolysis[46] and is considered a life-saving measure.[47] Compared to dogs that were not transfused, transfusion of packed RBCs to dogs with IMHA has been reported to increase survival without appreciable hemolytic transfusion reactions.[33] Receipt of a blood transfusion and the number of transfusions received were recently identified as negative predictors of survival in dogs with IMHA;[18] however, whether this was related to disease severity or direct transfusion complications was not specified. Although widely discussed in the human medical literature, the clinical relevance of the time-dependent metabolic and biochemical changes that occur in stored blood (e.g., loss of 2,3-diphosphoglycerol [2,3-DPG]) has not been thoroughly evaluated in veterinary patients.[48,49] Until it can be determined whether the age of the transfused RBCs affects morbidity and mortality in canine IMHA, it is suggested that younger blood products be administered when possible.

Ideally, all patients requiring a RBC transfusion would receive a type and cross-match compatible blood product. As subjective interpretation of agglutination is the end point of both tests, interpretation of blood typing and cross matching can be hampered by persistent (i.e., despite saline washing) RBC autoagglutination. Dogs with no previous history of transfusion or dogs having received their first transfusion no more than 5 days prior can receive DEA 1.1-negative blood products, "universal donor" (DEA 1.1, 1.2, 3, 4, 5, and 7 negative) blood products, or commercial bovine hemoglobin solution.[50] A cross match must be attempted for all dogs with a history of blood product transfusion, as the presence of preformed alloantibodies increases the risk of acute hemolytic transfusion reaction. If persistent autoagglutination precludes interpretation of cross-match results, transfusion with universal donor blood or bovine hemoglobin solution may be required.

Immunosuppressive Therapy Administration of glucocorticoids at immunosuppressive doses is the foundation of

acute and chronic treatment of canine IMHA.[51,52] The specific mechanisms of effectiveness in IMHA remain speculative but are assumed to include rapid impairment of macrophage-mediated erythrophagocytosis, delayed (within 14 days[53]) decrease in immunoglobulin concentration, and altered T lymphocyte generation and function secondary to decreased interleukin (IL)-6 production.[13,52,54] The often slow or poor clinical response of intravascular hemolysis to glucocorticoid therapy could potentially be explained by the lack of immediate glucocorticoid effects on immunoglobulin and complement concentrations.

Prednisone (2 mg/kg/day) and dexamethasone (0.25 to 0.5 mg/kg/day) are the most frequently recommended glucocorticoid agents for initial treatment of canine IMHA.[13,50,54,55] There is no documented advantage to higher corticosteroid doses or of one glucocorticoid over another. Adverse side effects associated with corticosteroid administration are common and typically include polyuria, polydipsia, polyphagia, panting, steroid myopathy, gastric ulceration, vacuolar hepatopathy, iatrogenic hyperadrenocorticism, cutaneous atrophy, and alopecia.[50,54,56] Exogenous corticosteroid excess is a suspected clinical risk factor associated with TED in dogs,[57] a significant cause of morbidity and mortality in canine IMHA. Measures to minimize the side effects of glucocorticoid therapy—including determination of the minimum effective dose, extended dosing interval, shortened duration of therapy, intermittent or "pulse" therapy and dosing based on body surface area—have yet to be investigated in the management of canine IMHA.

Despite recommendations to reserve adjunctive immunosuppressive agents for dogs with severe disease (persistent autoagglutination, intravascular hemolysis, nonregenerative anemia) and dogs that fail to respond to initial glucocorticoid therapy,[13,50] the negative side effects of glucocorticoids and the poor prognosis associated with the acute hemolytic crisis have resulted in a trend towards combination immunosuppression in canine IMHA. Due to its association with increased survival time,[3,33] azathioprine has become the primary adjunctive immunosuppressive agent for canine patients with IMHA.[50] Azathioprine is a purine analogue antimetabolite, metabolized in the liver to 6-mercaptopurine and further converted to active cytotoxic thioguanine nucleotides.[13,58,59] The thioguanine nucleotides act as purine antagonists and induce immunosuppression by impairing RNA, DNA and protein synthesis, thereby inhibiting lymphocyte proliferation[60,61] without affecting absolute lymphocyte numbers or serum immunoglobulin concentration.[53,62] Canine lymphocyte blastogenic response is significantly inhibited following 7 days of azathioprine therapy at a dose of 2 mg/kg/day and returns to baseline within 1 week of treatment cessation.[62]

The recommended initial dose of azathioprine in canine IMHA is 2 mg/kg q24h.[3,13,24,51] There are no controlled clinical trials to support how long a daily dosing regimen should be maintained. Some authors recommend alternate day dosing once prednisone therapy has been tapered to every other day[13] while others recommend a transition to alternate day therapy within 4 to 7 days,[3,24] presumably believing this will minimize the risk of adverse effects.

Side effects of azathioprine therapy are infrequent but include acute pancreatitis,[63] bone marrow toxicosis,[63,64] hepatotoxicosis, and gastrointestinal illness.[13,50] Of the few described cases of azathioprine-associated bone marrow toxicosis in the dog,[58,63,64] all dogs received a similar azathioprine dose (2 to 2.2 mg/kg/day) for periods ranging from 3 to 16 weeks at the time bone marrow suppression was identified. Azathioprine-associated bone marrow toxicosis in the dog is not related to RBC thiopurine methyltransferase (TMPT) activity as has been demonstrated in human patients.[58,65]

---

*References 3, 4, 18, 23, 24, 26, 33.

Reports of the use of cyclosporine in management of canine IMHA are increasingly frequent in the veterinary literature. Cyclosporine binding of the intracellular protein cyclophilin and the resulting inhibition of calcineurin, prevent nuclear translocation of a family of proteins (nuclear factor of activated T cells) essential for transcription of the IL-2 gene.[66,67] The absence of IL-2 prevents further activation and proliferation of T lymphocytes and secondarily results in IL-4, interferon-γ, and granulocyte colony-stimulating factor suppression,[55,66,68] but does not affect peripheral lymphocyte count or serum immunoglobulin concentrations.[69]

To date, no prospective trials have reported on the efficacy of cyclosporine in dogs with IMHA, and its use is often reserved for patients with severe clinical presentations or dogs that fail to respond to standard prednisone and azathioprine therapy. In one retrospective evaluation, survival to discharge in dogs with IMHA who received cyclosporine was not significantly different than that of dogs who did not receive the drug.[51] In small preliminary investigations, cyclosporine was effective in normalization of the PCV in two of three dogs with refractory IMHA[70] and was an effective long-term treatment either alone (one dog) or in combination with prednisone (four dogs).[71] However, short-term (5 days) cyclosporine monotherapy did not resolve autoagglutination in six dogs with newly diagnosed IMHA.[71]

Monitoring of cyclosporine blood levels following organ transplantation was adopted as routine practice in human medicine due to large individual variability of drug blood levels.[66] While the pharmacokinetics of cyclosporine in the dog have been described,[68,72] the relationship between blood concentration and therapeutic efficacy has not been established for canine IMHA. The initial recommended dose of cyclosporine for management of canine IMHA is 5 to 10 mg/kg administered orally once or twice daily.[13,50,51] Monitoring of trough plasma concentrations every 2 to 4 weeks to maintain concentrations between 100 to 300 ng/mL has been suggested.[13]

Reported side effects of cyclosporine therapy in the dog include gastrointestinal illness (specifically vomiting), gingival hypertrophy, papilloma-like skin lesions, and hair loss.[66] Increased susceptibility to opportunistic infections and cancer are accepted complications of chronic immunosuppression in human solid organ transplant recipients.[73] Presumed infectious pneumonia and bacterial hepatitis due to *Clostridium piliforme*[23] have been reported as causes of death in dogs receiving immunosuppressive treatment for IMHA. In a preliminary study evaluating the effect of oral cyclosporine in dogs with refractory IMHA (three dogs) or ITP (four dogs), one dog died of sepsis and another of systemic aspergillosis soon after cyclosporine was added to their chronic immunosuppressive regimen.[70] In addition, a dog with multicentric lymphoma diagnosed on postmortem examination after 697 days of intermittent prednisolone and cyclophosphamide therapy for IMHA and ITP has been described.[15] The risk of immunosuppression-related infection and neoplasia in canine IMHA warrants consideration before long-term immunosuppression is recommended.

Leflunomide, mycophenolate mofetil, and liposomal-encapsulated clodronate are among the novel immunosuppressive and immunomodulating agents to be investigated in canine IMHA. Leflunomide and mycophenolate mofetil inhibit *de novo* pyrimidine and purine biosynthesis respectively, thereby inhibiting DNA synthesis, reducing the generation of effector lymphocytes, and decreasing antibody production.[50,74] Neither drug has been critically evaluated for use in autoimmune disease in veterinary medicine; however, mycophenolate mofetil was used successfully in treatment of warm-type IMHA in a small human trial[75-77] and in treatment of aplastic anemia in a single canine case report.[78] Lefluno-

mide therapy was initiated in five dogs with IMHA exhibiting poor responses to conventional therapy with an excellent response (return to normal Hct) documented in four dogs.[79] Despite reports of effectiveness in the human medical literature,[76] treatment of canine IMHA with human monoclonal anti-CD20 antibody (rituximab) is unlikely to be effective as the molecule does not appear to bind to or deplete canine B lymphocytes.[80] Short-term CD4 and CD8 monoclonal antibody therapy has been successfully used in combination with cyclosporine and azathioprine to induce tolerance to renal allografts in dogs.[81] The potential of CD4 and CD8 monoclonal antibodies to induce rapid immunosuppression in canine autoimmune hemolytic anemia remains to be investigated. When incorporated into liposomes, the drug clodronate is preferentially phagocytosed by macrophages leading to macrophage depletion via rapid apoptosis and decreased clearance of opsonized cells.[82] In a small preliminary study, liposomal clodronate infusion was well tolerated in dogs with severe IMHA and was associated with decreased RBC clearance in two of seven treated dogs.[82] Macrophage depletion is unlikely to be of benefit in anemia mediated by IgM or C3b, where complemented mediated destruction predominates.[82] In the absence of controlled clinical trials or more widespread use, the potential adverse effects of these agents are unknown. Anecdotally, gastrointestinal adverse reactions are common side effects of leflunomide and mycophenolate mofetil.

Thromboprophylaxis Development of thromboembolism is an important complication of canine IMHA; however, an ideal prophylactic anticoagulant has yet to be identified.[24] Randomized, prospective evaluation of anticoagulant therapy in canine IMHA is lacking. In a retrospective evaluation of 29 dogs with IMHA, treatment with unfractionated heparin was not associated with prolonged survival.[33] While the ability of low–molecular weight heparins to inhibit coagulation via neutralization of Factor Xa may prove efficacious in canine IMHA, variable pharmacokinetics in veterinary species[83] and increased cost currently limit their use.

The identification of hyperresponsive, activated platelets in dogs with IMHA[84] and improved short- and long-term survival in dogs with IMHA treated with aspirin (0.5 mg/kg/day)[24] provide pathophysiologic and circumstantial clinical justification for antiplatelet therapy in acute IMHA. Aspirin exerts its antiplatelet effects by inhibition of cyclooxygenase-mediated synthesis of thromboxane A_2, a powerful stimulant of platelet aggregation.[85,86] The recommended aspirin dose for prevention of thromboembolism in the dog (0.5 mg/kg/day) is presumably based on an unpublished pilot study of whole blood platelet aggregometry in clinically normal dogs.[24] Whether aspirin therapy effectively inhibits platelet aggregation in dogs with IMHA and whether this translates into decreased incidence of TED and increased survival is currently unknown.

Chronic Disease Management There are few evidence-based guidelines pertaining to chronic monitoring and management of canine IMHA. Serial CBC evaluations (specifically Hct, resolution of autoagglutination, and spherocytosis) are used as an indication of response to initial therapy, continued disease remission and as a guide for tapering immunosuppressive medications. With the inclusion of newer potentially myelosuppressive drugs in the treatment regimen and the increasing recognition of bone marrow disorders (e.g., myelofibrosis, bone marrow necrosis) occurring in association with IMHA, CBC evaluation is preferable to monitoring of PCV alone. However, transfusion therapy, frequent blood sampling, bone marrow disease, and persistent mild anemia in patients whose disease is otherwise in remission can make interpretation of serial CBCs difficult. At best, the CBC should be used as a marker of disease remission and acknowledged as a late marker of disease relapse. The ability of flow cytometry to quantify the percentage of RBCs with surface-bound immunoglobulin may prove useful for monitoring the effectiveness of immunosuppressive therapy.

Evaluation of the patient by means of a history, physical examination, and CBC should be performed once to twice weekly until resolution of anemia, then biweekly until tapering of immunosuppressive medications is initiated. Anecdotal guidelines suggest maintenance of an immunosuppressive glucocorticoid dose until the patient's Hct is stable or rising followed by a 25% to 50% dosage reduction every 2 to 4 weeks such that drug withdrawal occurs over a 3- to 6-month period.[13,50] A CBC should be performed prior to each dosage reduction to confirm ongoing hematologic remission. Despite recommendations for cautious and extended drug tapering, successful withdrawal of immunosuppressive therapy in canine IMHA has been reported to occur over as few as 6 to 13.2 weeks.[15,40] Current evidence suggests that under appropriate circumstances complete withdrawal of prednisolone and azathioprine can be achieved over a period of 3 months,[18] but there is no evidence to suggest more protracted drug tapering is mandatory or protective against disease relapse.

Relapse of clinical disease is perceived as a common complication of canine IMHA.[50] Collating dogs from multiple studies that were discharged from hospital and available for long-term follow up, 16.2% (25/154) of dogs experienced clinical disease relapse as immunosuppressive therapy was withdrawn or following cessation of therapy.[15,24,33,40,87] Therapy should be reinstituted at original immunosuppressive doses should hematologic evidence of IMHA return during drug tapering or following cessation of therapy. While a requirement for extended or even life-long therapy is recognized in a minority of patients,[18,50] there is no evidence to suggest that indefinite prednisone or azathioprine therapy at subimmunosuppressive doses is protective against disease relapse. In addition, while tapering (rather than abruptly discontinuing subimmunosuppressive glucocorticoid dosing regimens) theoretically permits recovery of the hypothalamic-pituitary axis, there is little evidence to justify tapering subtherapeutic doses of immunosuppressive agents such as azathioprine and cyclosporine.

PROGNOSIS

Published reports generally denote a guarded to poor prognosis for long-term survival. With few exceptions,[26] studies suggest 50% to 88% of dogs with IMHA will survive to discharge from hospital.* For patients who survive to hospital discharge, death or euthanasia due to ongoing IMHA or complications thereof occurs most frequently within the first 2 months.† The wide variation in median survival times reported for dogs with IMHA may be partially attributable to the high early mortality rate.

Several attempts have been made to correlate objective hematologic and biochemical markers with prognosis in dogs with IMHA.[13,50] Variables that have been associated with increased mortality in more than one report include hyperbilirubinemia/icterus,[4,24,26,29,38] autoagglutination,[4,24,38] increased band neutrophil count,[18,24] thrombocytopenia,[18,24,26] and hypoalbuminemia.[24,26] Furthermore, lower PCV, lower reticulocytes count,[4] marked leukocytosis,[33] hypokalemia, increased creatinine kinase (CK) concentration,[24] increased prothrombin time,[33] increased serum ALP activity,[3] increased plasma urea concentration, receiving a blood transfusion, and

number of transfusions[18] have all been associated with an increased risk of mortality in individual reports. With the exception of hyperbilirubinemia, prognostic indicators in canine IMHA are inconsistently reproducible between studies.[50]

Feline IMHA

Compared to dogs, primary IMHA occurs infrequently in cats. Nonimmunologic (e.g., toxicosis-related oxidative damage, inherited erythrocyte defects, hypophosphatemia) and immune-mediated hemolysis secondary to infection (e.g., feline leukemia virus [FeLV], *Mycoplasma hemofelis, Cytauxzoon felis*), drug reaction (e.g., methimazole, propylthiouracil), neoplasia (e.g., lymphoma), or other disease process (e.g., cholangiohepatitis[89]) occur more frequently than the idiopathic, autoimmune form of the disease. Primary IMHA is reported to occur predominantly in younger (≤ 6 years), male, domestic shorthair/mixed-breed cats.[13,90,91] Himalayans were overrepresented in a single, preliminary report.[90] The most frequently reported clinical signs and physical exam findings are lethargy, anorexia, pica, mucous membrane pallor, systolic heart murmur, and occasionally icterus.

Severe anemia at initial presentation (mean Hct of ≤ 12%)[89-91] is characteristic of feline primary IMHA. The small size and lack of central pallor of the normal feline erythrocyte generally precludes identification of spherocytes. Although the severity of the anemia along with the insidious and nonspecific nature of the clinical signs are suggestive of a chronic condition, the anemia is generally nonregenerative (≥58% of cats) at the time of initial evaluation[89,91] and may suggest immune-mediated destruction of erythroid precursors or pure red cell aplasia. Unlike the canine form of the disease, neutrophilic leukocytosis is uncommon (≤12%).[89-91] Lymphocytosis (31% to 52%) and thrombocytopenia (33% to 42%) have also been described.[89-91] Among 36 cats with nonregenerative primary IMHA, neutropenia and thrombocytopenia were common findings, occurring in 53% and 67% of cases, respectively.[91] In a recent study of cats with primary IMHA, serum biochemical abnormalities were generally limited to mild hyperbilirubinemia (68%), hyperglobulinemia (53%), hypoalbuminemia (21%), and mild to moderate increases in serum ALP (5%), alanine transferase (52%) and aspartate transferase activities (16%).[89]

Among 19 cats with primary IMHA, macroscopic slide agglutination of erythrocytes was identified in all cats.[89] Macroscopic agglutination in cats must be interpreted with caution given the propensity of feline erythrocytes for rouleaux formation. Autoagglutination should be confirmed by means of a saline agglutination test as described for dogs. Autoagglutination that persists despite saline washing and precludes performance of the DAT is described in 17% to 40% of feline patients.[89-91] In the absence of identifiable underlying disease and persistent autoagglutination, the DAT is useful in identifying primary feline IMHA.[89] Clinical evidence of intravascular hemolysis (i.e., hemoglobinemia, hemoglobinuria) has not been identified in feline primary IMHA despite IgM and C3b positive DAT results.[89-91] Bone marrow aspiration and biopsy are indicated if persistent ineffective erythroid regeneration or multiple cytopenias are identified.

The tendency for hemolytic anemia in cats to be of secondary immune-mediated origin necessitates exclusion of underlying disease by means of serologic testing for retroviruses (FeLV and feline immunodeficiency virus [FIV]), negative blood film examination and/or polymerase chain reaction (PCR) for hemotropic *Mycoplasma*, normal diagnostic imaging or cytologic/histologic exclusion of neoplasia. While radiographic or ultrasonographic evidence of splenomegaly and/or hepatomegaly may reflect extramedullary hematopoiesis or extravascular hemolysis,[89] enlargement of either organ should

---

*References 3, 4, 15, 22-26, 33, 51, 87, 88.
†References 3, 4, 15, 23, 24, 33, 38, 87.

prompt cytologic evaluation for neoplasia, namely lymphoma or mast cell disease.

Supportive care of the feline IMHA patient is generally as discussed for the canine patient, including the likely necessity for RBC product transfusion. Assuming accurate pretransfusion blood typing or cross matching, blood product transfusion is safe in cats with hemolytic anemia and does not carry an increased risk of transfusion reaction or acute mortality compared to other anemic conditions.[92,93] Multiple transfusions can be safely administered to cats with severe anemia.[94] Glucocorticoids (dexamethasone, prednisone, or prednisolone) are the initial recommended immunosuppressive agents. Initial prednisone or prednisolone doses of 2 to 4 mg/kg/day have been reported[89,90] An empirical course of doxycycline in case of hemotropic *Mycoplasma* infection can be considered in the absence of PCR testing. Although based on very limited descriptions, cyclosporine and/or cyclophosphamide/chlorambucil have been administered in addition to glucocorticoids in nonresponsive or poorly responsive cases.[90,91]

Primary feline IMHA is associated with a lower overall mortality rate (24% to 32%) than the canine form of the disease possibly due to a lower incidence of thromboembolic complications.[89,90] Recent retrospective reports suggest persistent or relapsed anemia necessitates protracted (possibly life-long) glucocorticoid therapy and/or alternate immunosuppressive regimens in up to 50% of cases.[90,91] Relapse of clinical disease following cessation of therapy is reported in 16% to 19% of cats with primary IMHA.[89,90]

OTHER HEMOLYTIC ANEMIAS

Alloimmune Hemolysis: Transfusion Reactions

Acute hemolytic transfusion reactions can develop when a dog or cat having preexisting antibodies to erythrocyte antigens undergoes transfusion with erythrocytes displaying those antigens. Binding of alloantigens (antigens occurring in a genetically different individual of the same species) by preformed alloantibodies leads to complement activation and intravascular hemolysis of the transfused erythrocytes.

In dogs, alloantibodies are produced during pregnancy, parturition, or after blood transfusion. Blood typing helps to identify potentially antigenic glycoproteins or glycolipids that are components of the erythrocyte membrane. Although 12 or more DEAs have been identified, DEA 1.1, 1.2, and 7 are the most likely to induce alloantibody formation. However, transfusion reactions due to DEA 4 and the *Dal* blood types have been reported.[95,96] Dogs do not have naturally occurring alloantibodies; thus initial exposure will not likely cause an acute transfusion reaction. However, once alloantibodies have been formed subsequent to exposure to alloantigens, only a small quantity of alloantigen is required to cause a transfusion reaction; there are enough erythrocytes and erythrocyte membrane fragments in fresh-frozen plasma to cause clinically significant acute reactions.

Feline erythrocyte antigens are termed *type-A*, *type-B*, or *type-AB*. The erythrocyte antigen *Mik* has also been recently described in domestic shorthair cats.[97] The incidence of these blood types varies among cat breeds and geographic locations, with type A consistently being the most prevalent blood type. Type-B cats have been most commonly identified in Australia, Turkey, Japan, and Europe.[98-100] Breeds with increased prevalence of type-B blood include Abyssinian, Birman, Japanese Bobtail, Persian, Himalayan, Somali, Sphinx, Cornish Rex, British Shorthair, and Devon Rex; prevalence of blood types within breeds is influenced by geographic location.[101,102] Type-AB cats are rare, and they do not produce alloantibodies.

In cats, alloantibodies occur naturally; however, the epitopes that induce these antibodies have not been identified. A severe reaction may occur on the *initial* exposure to blood, without prior sensitization by previous transfusion or pregnancy. The naturally occurring anti-B antibodies of type-A cats are weak agglutinins and hemolysins; if type-B blood is transfused into a type-A cat, the erythrocyte half-life falls to 2.1 days. Clinical signs associated with this mismatch are usually mild, and may include listlessness, tachycardia, tachypnea, hemoglobinemia, and hemoglobinuria. Anti-A alloantibodies present in type-B cats appear to be strong hemolysins and agglutinins and can induce severe acute hemolytic transfusion reactions. If type-A blood is transfused into a type-B cat, the erythrocyte half-life falls to minutes to hours, and potentially fatal systemic anaphylaxis and hemolysis can follow. Clinical signs may include hypoventilation, apnea, vomiting, diarrhea, vocalization, arrhythmias, hemoglobinemia, and hemoglobinuria. Shock, systemic inflammatory response syndrome, multiorgan dysfunction syndrome, and DIC may ensue.

Blood typing and major cross matching reduce the possibility of a hemolytic transfusion reaction.[93] It is not necessary to blood type or cross match a dog before the first transfusion. Sensitization occurs within 3 to 5 days of initial transfusion, and subsequent transfusion should be preceded by typing and major cross match. For cats, blood typing and major cross match should precede all transfusions.[102,103]

Alloimmune Hemolysis: Neonatal Isoerythrolysis

Neonatal isoerythrolysis is most commonly recognized in kittens, and occurs when type-A or type-AB kittens ingest colostrum containing anti-A alloantibodies from a type-B queen. Ingested alloantibodies are absorbed across the intestine, enter the blood, and attach to the neonate's paternally derived erythrocyte surface antigens. The opsonized erythrocytes are then lysed by macrophages or complement.

Kittens at risk are healthy at birth and nurse normally. Clinical signs develop hours to days following ingestion of colostrum, and variably include sudden death, weakness, failure to thrive, reluctance to nurse, dyspnea, hemoglobinuria, jaundice, and necrosis of the tail tip secondary to thromboembolism. A moderately regenerative anemia may be present, a Coombs' test on the neonate will be positive and a cross match between the queen's serum and neonate's erythrocytes will be positive. Anti-B alloantibodies of type-A queens have weak activity and are not usually associated with clinical signs. Type-AB cats do not produce alloantibodies. Neonatal isoerythrolysis is preventable if queens and toms of breeds with a high prevalence of type-B blood are blood typed prior to breeding.

In dogs, neonatal isoerythrolysis is rare, occurring when a DEA 1.1–negative bitch develops anti-DEA 1.1 antibodies after being transfused with DEA 1.1–positive blood, and then passes those antibodies to DEA 1.1–positive puppies. Affected puppies become pale within 1 to 2 days after birth; deaths may occur within the first 72 hours.

Infection-Associated Hemolysis

Acute infection with one or more hemotrophic *Mycoplasma* species ("hemoplasmas") can be associated with acute hemolytic anemia. In cats, the most important organism appears to be *Mycoplasma haemofelis*, while "*Candidatus* M. haemominutum" and "*Candidatus* M. turicensis" do not appear to cause anemia as uncomplicated infections in otherwise healthy cats. Cats may be infected with multiple hemoplasma species, or be coinfected with FeLV or FIV. Clinical signs associated with acute infections in cats include lethargy, anorexia, fever, anemia, and occasionally icterus and splenomegaly. In dogs, *M. haemocanis* and "*Candidatus* M. haematoparvum" appear to cause anemia only in splenectomized or immunosuppressed dogs. Fleas in cats and *Rhipicephalus sanguineus* in dogs appear to be important arthropod reservoirs and vectors.

Hemoplasmas reside on the surface of RBCs and may induce antibodies that react with either the parasite or erythrocyte antigens that are exposed as a consequence of infection. The mechanism(s) responsible for the pathogenicity of hemoplasmas has not been completely defined; however, it appears that the host's immune response plays an important role in the development of acute hemolytic anemia.

Hemolysis is primarily extravascular and is usually associated with moderate to severe macrocytic hypochromic regenerative anemia. Infected dogs may have spherocytosis, autoagglutination, and a positive DAT. Hemoplasmas are sometimes identified on the blood film; however, this is an insensitive test for infection. Conventional or real-time quantitative PCR of the 16S rRNA gene are the diagnostic tests of choice. Doxycycline and fluoroquinolones appear to effectively control acute infections in cats; however, they do not consistently clear the organisms. Imidocarb dipropionate may be indicated in refractory cases; however, no clinical studies evaluating efficacy are currently available. Prednisolone (2 to 4 mg/kg/day) is often recommended to moderate the host immune response; however, many cats respond to antibiotics alone.[104-106]

Hemolytic anemia can be caused by infection with *Babesia canis*, *B. gibsonii*, and *B. conradae* infections in dogs. Parasitemia results in hemolysis and the development of a responsive anemia; infected dogs commonly have erythrocyte autoagglutination and positive DATs. While direct parasitic damage of erythrocytes contributes to the anemia, proteases produced by the parasite, immune-mediated responses, and oxidative injury all appear to contribute to the hemolytic process. Diagnosis is based upon identification of organisms in erythrocytes, immunodiagnostics, and PCR testing.[107-110]

Cytauxzoon felis, a tick-borne protozoon parasite affecting erythrocytes, causes acute hemolytic anemia; however, due to the acuteness of presentation, the anemia is not usually regenerative. Infections have been reported in cats from the south central and southeastern United States. The clinical disease course is rapid, with fever, lethargy, and anorexia, leukocytosis, hemolytic anemia, icterus, and elevated liver enzymes usually present. Definitive diagnosis is based on microscopic identification of parasites. Effective medical therapy has not been described; however, some cats have survived infection.

Erythrocyte Metabolic Defects

Oxidative Damage: Heinz Body and Eccentrocytic Hemolysis   When oxidative injury exceeds the reductive capacity of the erythrocyte, hemoglobin is converted to HgbFe^{3+}, which precipitates and aggregates as Heinz bodies on the inner surface of erythrocyte membranes. Erythrocytes with Heinz bodies are less deformable and more fragile than normal erythrocytes and are lysed in spleen. Additionally, there may be redistribution of band-3 proteins and formation of an antigen that is recognized by autologous antibodies, leading to secondary immune-mediated hemolysis. In Wright-stained films, Heinz bodies appear as slightly pale structures that create membrane defects or protrude from erythrocytes. Heinz bodies can visualized with new methylene blue stain as pale blue round structures associated with and sometimes protruding from erythrocyte membranes. In cats, Heinz bodies may be a normal finding due to inefficient splenic pitting of abnormal erythrocytes, and because feline hemoglobin has more sulfhydryl groups and is more prone to form more disulfide bridges than dogs. In addition, feline erythrocytes may have less reductive capacity than erythrocytes of other species. While Heinz bodies do occur in dogs, oxidative injury of canine erythrocytes can be more localized to the erythrocyte membrane and cytoskeleton, leading to the formation of "eccentrocytes" (erythrocytes that have their hemoglobin shifted to one side of the cell).[111-113] Chemicals associated with erythrocyte oxidative injury in to dogs include acetaminophen, benzocaine, n-propyl disulfide (onions, chives, garlic, leek, shallot, and related plants of the genus *Allium*), vitamins K$_1$ and K$_3$ (or possibly vitamin K antagonists rather than vitamin K), thiols in skunk musk, and zinc (ingestion of zinc toys, pennies, pet carrier fasteners, zippers, zinc oxide).[114-117] Common chemicals associated with erythrocyte oxidative injury in cats include acetaminophen, benzocaine, and n-propyl disulfide.

The diagnosis of Heinz body anemia is based on the findings of regenerative anemia, evidence of hemolysis, demonstration of Heinz bodies on erythrocytes, and history of exposure to an oxidant. It should be noted that zinc toxicity is usually associated with hemolytic anemia; however, Heinz bodies are present in only one third of affected dogs, that eccentrocytosis and mild spherocytosis can be present, and that a DAT can be positive. Management of Heinz body hemolytic anemia includes supportive care (including transfusion therapy if required), removal of zinc objects and possibly s-adenosyl-l-methionine (SAMe).[118]

Hereditary Hemolytic Anemias   In humans, hereditary erythrocyte disorders are classified into those affecting heme/hemoglobin, erythrocyte membranes, or erythrocyte enzymes. Membrane disorders and erthroenzymopathies have been documented in dogs and cats; however, hemoglobinopathies have not been recognized in dogs/cats. These disorders are rare, and all have autosomal recessive inheritance, except for one form of feline porphyria, which appears to have autosomal dominant inheritance. The relatively more common hereditary erythrocyte abnormalities that cause anemia are described here. Further information can be found in Chapter 270 of the previous edition of this text.[2]

Hereditary Hemolytic Anemias: Membrane Defects
Stomatocytosis   Stomatocytes are bowl-shaped macrocytes that have well demarcated slitlike pallor and increased fragility that is caused by the lack of a cytoskeletal protein. Affected individuals can have mild regenerative anemia. Hereditary stomatocytosis is reported in Alaskan Malamutes, Drentse Patrijshonds, and Miniature Schnauzers. The phenotype of affected Alaskan Malamutes includes chrondysplastic dwarfism; Drentse Patrijshonds have hypertrophic gastritis, hepatic bile duct proliferation, and abnormalities of the central nervous system. Affected Schnauzers have an otherwise normal phenotype.[119]

Increased osmotic fragility   Anemia caused by markedly increased osmotic fragility of erythrocytes, possibly caused by an inherited membrane defect, has been described in Somali, Abyssinian, Siamese, and Domestic Shorthair cats. Affected cats have recurrent anemia, splenomegaly, weight loss, lymphocytosis, and hyperglobulinemia. Some of these cats may respond to prednisolone therapy.[2]

Hereditary Hemolytic Anemias: Erythroenzymopathies   Phosphofructokinase (PFK) deficiency is reported in field trial English Springer Spaniels in the United States, Great Britain, and Denmark, as well as in an ACS and mixed-breed dogs. PFK is a rate-controlling enzyme of glycolysis. This disorder is caused by a mis-sense mutation of the muscle-type PFK gene, resulting in truncation and rapid degradation of the unstable protein. Homozygous affected dogs have persistent compensated hemolytic anemia. Signs during crisis include lethargy, anorexia, fever, icterus, hemolytic anemia, hemoglobinemia, and hemoglobinuria/hyperbilirubinuria. Signs of an exertional myopathy also occur, including exercise intolerance, muscle cramps, and mildly increased CK activity. Between crises, there may be persistent hyperbilirubinemia and reticulocytosis despite a normal Hct. Exercise, hyperventilation, excessive barking, or high ambient temperature can cause mild respiratory alkalemia. Affected erythrocytes are extremely "alkaline fragile" due to reduced adenosine triphosphate (ATP) production and decreased 2,3-DPG concentrations, which leads to unstable erythrocyte membranes and hemolysis. PCR testing accurately discriminates between normal, carrier, and affected dogs. Affected dogs should not be encouraged to exercise, and carriers and affected dogs should not be bred.

Pyruvate kinase (PK) deficiency has been described in English Springer Spaniels in the United States, Great Britain, and Denmark, as well as an ACS and mixed breed-dogs and Abyssinian, Somali, and Domestic Shorthair cats. Homozygous affected dogs usually show signs in first few weeks of life, which include decreased exercise tolerance, tachycardia, heart murmurs, pale mucous membranes, and splenomegaly.

Erythrocyte R-type PK catalyzes the last ATP generation step of glycolysis; erythrocytes in homozygous affected dogs completely lack R-PK activity and express a fetal or leukocyte M_2-PK that is not functional in erythrocytes. Without PK activity, erythrocytes become ATP-deficient, membranes become defective, and hemolysis occurs. Prolonged hemolytic anemia in dogs results in excessive absorption of iron from the intestine, leading to iron overload. Iron overload causes progressive marrow (myelofibrosis, osteosclerosis) and hepatic injury (hemosiderosis, hemochromatosis, fibrosis, failure). Affected dogs usually die between 1 and 5 years of age.

These animals have moderate anemia, moderate to extreme reticulocytosis, mild to moderate icterus, and decreased erythrocyte PK (R-type) activity. PCR testing is available for Basenji, Beagle, Dachshund, Toy Eskimo, West Highland White Terrier, and Cairn breeds. PK enzyme testing with isozyme characterization is required to diagnose PK deficiency in other breeds.

Total erythrocyte PK activity is reduced in cats with PK deficiency, with no M_2 activity as in dogs. The feline disorder may be asymptomatic, or cause chronic anemia or intermittent macrocytic hemolytic anemia and mild splenomegaly, but no osteosclerosis. Clinical signs are generally observed before 3 years of age. The genetic defect is a splicing defect in the R-PK gene, causing a 13-base pair deletion. A molecular screening test is available. Because PK deficiency can be asymptomatic in cats, testing of Abyssinian and Somali cats used for breeding is recommended. Mean osmotic fragility of erythrocytes from cats with PK deficiency is usually within the reference range, differentiating this disorder from the osmotic fragility syndrome described in Abyssinian and Somali cats. Prednisone and splenectomy appear to ameliorate the clinical signs of intermittent anemia in cats with PK deficiency.[2,120,121]

Porphyrias are a group of hereditary disorders in which heme precursors accumulate in cells and body fluids because of deficient enzyme activity in the heme synthetic pathway. Cats with erythropoietic porphyria have hemolytic anemia and discolored (red, orange, or brown) teeth that fluoresce when irradiated with near-ultraviolet light. Porphyria in domestic shorthair cats is characterized by only a mild anemia, while porphyria in Siamese cats is can be associated with severe macrocytic, hypochromic anemia with poikilocytosis, Howell-Jolly bodies, and nucleated RBCs. Photosensitization, which has been described for other species, has not been seen in cats.

Hypophosphatemia Severe hypophosphatemia has been reported to cause extravascular hemolysis and Heinz body formation in dog and cats receiving insulin, hepatic lipidosis, enteral and parenteral hyperalimentation, and oral administration of phosphate binders. Decreased ATP production, depletion of DPG, and reduced glutathione lead to increased erythrocyte fragility and susceptibility to oxidative injury and hemolysis. Management includes aggressive oral and parenteral phosphate supplementation.[2]

Microangiopathic Anemias

Fragmentation of normal red cells can occur from mechanical trauma as they circulate though vasculature containing fibrin strands or abnormal rheologic forces. These microangiopathic hemolytic anemias are characterized by reticulocytosis and changes in erythrocyte morphology. Fragmented erythrocytes can appear as schistocytes (often triangular) or keratocytes (helmet-shaped). Microangiopathic anemias have been associated with DIC, vasculitis, hemangiosarcoma and other splenic disorders, hemolytic uremia syndrome, valvular heart disease, hepatic disease, glomerulonephritis, myelofibrosis, chronic doxorubicin toxicosis, heartworm caval syndrome, increased red cell fragility associated with severe iron deficiency, and potentially intravenous catheters.[2,122,123]

The diagnosis of microangiopathic anemia is based upon finding mild to moderate anemia, no to moderate reticulocytosis, schistocytosis, and often thrombocytopenia and other evidence of a consumptive coagulopathy. Regardless of the degree of anemia, the finding of schistocytosis should prompt the clinician to search for disorders associated with abnormal microvasculature.

Envenomation

Hemolytic anemia has been reported to occur in dogs following envenomation by brown recluse spider (*Loxosceles recluse*),[124] Eastern Diamondback rattlesnake (*Crotalus adamanteus*),[125] Eastern Coral snake (*Micrurus fulvius*),[126] and Red-Bellied Black snake (*Pseudechis porphyriacus*).[127] Phospholipase A and sphingomyelinase D are the components of venom suspected to have direct hemolytic effects.[124,126,127] Geography, seasonality, history and identification of dermonecrotic lesions, coagulopathy, cardiac arrhythmias, renal and/or neurologic dysfunction may help to distinguish brown recluse spider or snake envenomation from other more common causes of hemolysis. Spherocytic hemolytic anemia and neurologic dysfunction have been infrequently reported to occur in dogs following bee sting envenomation.[7] Components of bee venom suspected to have direct hemolytic properties include hyaluronidase, melitin, and phospholipase A.[7,128] Prolonged hemolysis and successful treatment with glucocorticoid immunosuppression[7] suggest development of an immunologic response against previously hidden erythrocyte antigens or altered erythrocyte membranes.

Histiocytic Disorders

The hemophagocytic form of malignant histiocytosis/disseminated histiocytic sarcoma is characterized by invasion of phagocytic, neoplastic histiocytes arising from spleen and bone marrow macrophages with subsequent intravascular invasion and spread to the liver and lungs.[129] Bernese Mountain Dogs, Rottweilers, and Golden, Labrador, and Flat-Coated Retrievers are most commonly affected.[129-131] The common features of regenerative anemia, thrombocytopenia, and splenomegaly can result in an initial misdiagnosis of IMHA/ITP. Normal or slightly increased serum bilirubin concentration, hypoalbuminemia, hypocholesterolemia, and DAT-negative anemia are features of hemophagocytic histiocytic sarcoma that may help differentiate hemophagocytic histiocytic sarcoma from IMHA.[129,131] Diagnosis requires cytologic or histologic demonstration of erythrophagocytosis by neoplastic macrophages in spleen, bone marrow, liver, or lung.[129] The disease is rapidly progressive and carries a grave prognosis for recovery.

Hemophagocytic histiocytic sarcoma should not be confused with hemophagocytic syndrome, a nonneoplastic proliferative disorder of macrophages characterized by peripheral bicytopenia or pancytopenia and more than 2% hemophagocytic macrophages in bone marrow aspirates.[132-134] Hemophagocytic syndrome is differentiated from malignant histiocytic conditions by the lower percentage of histiocytic cells in bone marrow specimens, absence of cytomorphologic features of malignancy, and smaller macrophage size as determined by flow cytometric scatter plots.[132,135] Hemophagocytic syndrome occurs as an idiopathic condition or in association with immune-mediated, infectious, neoplastic, and myelodysplastic disorders.[132] Tibetan Terriers may be overrepresented.[132] Although based on a limited number of cases, canine hemophagocytic syndrome generally carries a grave prognosis for recovery, with the possible exception of disease associated with a treatable infectious condition.[132,134]

Blood Loss Anemia

Bleeding from wounds—into the gastrointestinal or urinary tracts, or into the pleural, pericardial, or peritoneal cavities or subcutaneous tissues—may lead to acute or chronic anemia. Hemorrhage may be induced by trauma, ulceration, neoplasia, acquired or congenital factor deficiencies, von Willebrand disease, or thrombocytopenia/thrombocytopathia. Chronic iron-deficiency anemia has been associated with inflammatory bowel disease.[136] Heavy hookworm, tick, or flea burdens may cause anemia, as can bleeding blood donors or frequent phlebotomy for diagnostic purposes.

During the first few hours following blood loss, fluid shifts from the extravascular space, causing anemia and hypoproteinemia, with proportionate decreases in albumin and globulin concentrations. Otherwise normal animals should respond with evidence of accelerated erythropoiesis in 3 to 4 days. If hemoperitoneum or hemothorax is present, the animal may autotransfuse, with resorption of approximately 80% of erythrocytes within 1 to 2 weeks.[2]

The diagnosis of blood loss anemia is based upon history (including administration of nonsteroidal antiinflammatory drugs; pica is suggestive of iron deficiency), physical examination (including rectal examination for melena), and the findings of anemia, hypoproteinemia (if losses are external), and reticulocytosis (if there has been sufficient time for the marrow to accelerate erythropoiesis and the animal has not developed severe iron deficiency anemia). Hct and plasma protein concentrations may not change until fluid shifts occur (hours to days); thus the Hct may significantly underestimate the magnitude of acute blood loss. Urinalysis, testing for fecal occult blood, fecal examination for hookworms, and ultrasonographic examination of the abdomen, pleural, and pericardial spaces may be indicated. Management of acute blood loss anemia includes volume resuscitation, prevention of further hemorrhage, transfusion with appropriate blood products, and management of the underlying cause. When hemorrhage has been controlled, resolution of the anemia should occur within 1 to 2 weeks.

Chronic Blood Loss and Iron Deficiency

Iron is absorbed in the proximal small intestine and stored in spleen, liver, and bone marrow as ferritin (soluble and mobile) and hemosiderin (insoluble). Iron is transported in plasma by transferrin, which is normally 20% to 60% saturated with iron. If external hemorrhage becomes chronic, iron deficiency may develop. Young animals are at greatest risk due to relatively small iron stores and large iron requirements during growth.

Depending upon the magnitude of iron loss, the anemia may be regenerative or nonregenerative and may be characterized by microcytic normochromic to microcytic hypochromic indices. Marked anisocytosis may be present, and the RDW is increased. A pronounced reticulocytosis is usually found. Thrombocytosis is a common finding in iron deficiency anemia. Other typical findings include mild to moderate hypoproteinemia, hypoferremia (may be normal or slightly elevated if the sample is hemolyzed, or if there was a recent transfusion), low transferrin saturation, decreased serum ferritin concentration (may be elevated in inflammatory conditions), normal to slightly elevated iron binding capacity, and depleted iron storage sites. Characteristic bone marrow findings include mild to moderate erythroid hyperplasia with nuclear distortion with no stainable iron (note that cats normally store little iron).

Animals with severe iron deficiency are reported to have impaired intestinal absorption of iron, thus management is initiated with one injection of iron dextran (10 to 20 mg/kg IM). Supplementation is continued with oral ferrous sulfate (11 mg/kg PO daily with food); weeks to months of supplementation are usually required to correct the deficiency state. Whole blood or PRBC transfusions could put the animal at risk for volume overload, and should be used judiciously.[2]

REFERENCES

The reference list can be found on the companion Expert Consult Web site at *www.expertconsult.com*.

CHAPTER 189

Immune-Mediated Thrombocytopenia, von Willebrand Disease, and Platelet Disorders

Marjory B. Brooks
James L. Catalfamo

PRIMARY HEMOSTASIS

Platelets play a critical role in the initiation, regulation, and localization of hemostasis. The term *primary hemostasis* refers to the interactions among platelets, von Willebrand factor (VWF), and the vessel wall that culminate in the formation of a platelet plug (Figure 189-1). These reactions begin with platelet contact with the damaged vessel and VWF-mediated adhesion; proceed through platelet activation, degranulation, and aggregation; and conclude with the devel-

does not differentiate patients with primary IMT from those with secondary IMT, and nonspecific antibody binding may complicate interpretation of test results. Microthrombocytosis (MPV less than 5.5 fL) has been described as a feature of primary and secondary IMT and is seen early in the disease course. In a case review, severe thrombocytopenia (less than 20,000/μL) and microthrombocytosis were found almost exclusively in dogs with IMT; however, only half of the IMT patients had these abnormalities.[16] Accurate MPV determination is affected by the anticoagulant used; platelets stored in ethylenediamine tetraacetic acid (EDTA) rather than citrate may have artifactual increases in MPV.

Thrombocytosis

Mild to moderate increases in the platelet count ("reactive" thrombocytosis) are seen in association with chronic blood loss, neoplasia, systemic inflammatory disease, and hypercortisolism.[17] High platelet counts may occur after splenectomy. A persistent and markedly high platelet count (greater than 900,000/μL) is suggestive of primary bone marrow disease (e.g., myelodysplasia, essential thrombocythemia) and is an indication for bone marrow examination. The clinical features of essential thrombocythemia in human beings and dogs include splenomegaly and hemorrhage caused by platelet dysfunction.[18]

Platelet Function Tests

The buccal mucosa bleeding time (BMBT) is an in vivo screening test of primary hemostasis (Figure 189-6). If thrombocytopenia has been ruled out, a long BMBT is compatible with either platelet dysfunction or VWF deficiency.[19] Platelet dysfunction is definitively diagnosed using more comprehensive tests of platelet structure and activation response (Table 189-3). To ensure platelet viability, functional assays are best performed within 2 to 3 hours of sample collection. The PFA 100 (Dade Behring, Newark, Del.) can be used to measure platelet adhesion and aggregation with small volumes of whole blood (less than 2 mL) under conditions that simulate blood flow.[20,21] More specific assessment of platelet function is performed by monitoring agonist-induced responses of shape change, aggregation, and release of dense granule contents (Figure 189-7).[22]

Flow cytometry is used to assess platelet function by means of detection of membrane glycoproteins (required for adhesion and aggregation) and activation markers, such as P-selectin, fibrinogen, and surface PS.[23] These markers are evidence of effective alpha granule release and procoagulant activity (Figure 189-8).

Detailed evaluations of platelet function, physiology, and ultrastructure are usually reserved for characterization of hereditary thrombopathias.

SPECIFIC PLATELET DISORDERS

Thrombocytopenia

Thrombocytopenia is the most common acquired hemostatic defect of dogs and cats.[10] Many different pathogens cause thrombocytopenia (Table 189-4), often through combined marrow suppression and an increased rate of peripheral loss.

Arthropod-borne agents are increasingly identified as the cause of cytopenias in dogs and cats.[8,24] Infectious agents usually cause systemic signs, producing physical examination findings and complete blood count (CBC) abnormalities beyond those of thrombocytopenia alone. Although dogs and

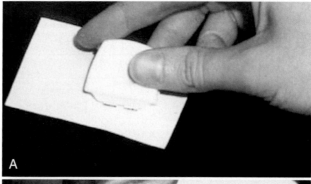

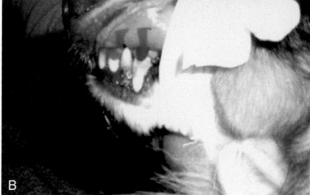

Figure 189-6 Buccal mucosal bleeding time. **A,** Template device (Simplate II; Organon Teknika, Durham, N.C.) with spring-loaded blades that make incisions of uniform depth and length when the device is triggered. **B,** Incised buccal bleeding time wounds in a Shetland Sheepdog affected with type 3 von Willebrand disease. After incision, shed blood is collected by gently blotting below the wounds with gauze or filter paper. The time from incision to cessation of blood flow is the buccal bleeding time.

cats with infectious thrombocytopenias may initially respond to steroid administration, sustained platelet response and disease resolution require specific treatment. It therefore is important to rule out infectious thrombocytopenia (through serology, cytology, or PCR) before an immunosuppressive steroid regimen is begun.

Mild to moderate thrombocytopenia is seen in association with many tumor types, with more severe depression likely in hematopoietic neoplasia such as multiple myeloma, lymphoma, and leukemia.[5] DIC is a common cause of thrombocytopenia in hemangiosarcoma, and tests to define a DIC process (see Table 189-2) should be performed in any cancer patient with a falling or low platelet count. In addition to tumor-mediated thrombocytopenia, cancer patients are at risk of developing thrombocytopenia arising from cytotoxic drug therapy.

A thorough drug history is indicated for any patient with thrombocytopenia, because numerous drugs have been reported to impair platelet production, induce secondary immune destruction, and/or cause platelet dysfunction (Table 189-5).[25] Establishing the causality of drug-induced thrombocytopenia is difficult, but ancillary diagnostics can help define possible underlying mechanisms. The findings of pancytopenia and megakaryocytic hypoplasia indicate bone marrow suppression, and the presence of platelet-bound antibody is compatible with an immune-mediated process.

Idiopathic, or primary, IMT is an autoimmune disease, usually mediated by IgG directed against platelet membrane

Table • 189-3

Platelet Function Assays

TESTS	SPECIFIC ASSESSMENTS
Dilute whole blood	GPII$_b$III$_a$-mediated clot retraction
Platelet aggregation studies	Aggregation response to specific agonists: adenosine diphosphate (ADP), collagen, arachidonate, epinephrine, platelet-activating factor
Platelet secretion studies	Secretion of dense granule contents: ADP, adenosine triphosphate (ATP), serotonin
Flow cytometry	Detection of constitutive membrane antigens: GPIIbIIIa (CD61 = GPIIIa); GPIb (CD42b = GP1bα)
	Detection of activation markers: P-selectin (CD62p), phosphatidylserine (annexin-V), fibrinogen binding site (CAP1), platelet-bound fibrinogen (antifibrinogen antibody)
	Platelet calcium entry and release: Fluo-3
Spectrofluorimetry	Platelet calcium entry and release: Fura-2AM
Electron microscopy	Platelet ultrastructure: shape change, cytoskeleton, intracellular organelles (granules, dense bodies, lysosomes), dense tubular system

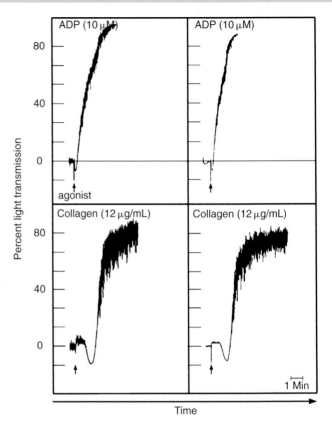

Figure 189-7 Platelet aggregation profiles of platelet-rich plasma obtained from two healthy dogs. Platelet activation was initiated by the addition *(arrow)* of adenosine diphosphate *(ADP)* *(top panels)* or collagen *(bottom panels)*. Aggregate formation is evidenced by an increase in light transmission. ADP induces a rapid aggregation response. In contrast, collagen stimulation is followed by a lag phase before aggregation ensues.

GPII$_b$III$_a$. The disease is uncommon in cats, but in case reviews of canine thrombocytopenia, primary IMT accounts for approximately 5% to 15% of patients, with overrepresentation of females and certain breeds (Cocker Spaniels, Poodles, and Old English Sheepdogs).[4,11] The diagnosis of primary IMT is generally based on combined clinical and laboratory criteria: exclusion of other underlying disease processes, the presence of severe thrombocytopenia (less than 50,000/μL), normal to increased megakaryopoiesis, microthrombocytosis, platelet-bound antibodies, and response to immunosuppressive therapy.

Breed-specific, clinically asymptomatic thrombocytopenias occur in dogs. Healthy Greyhounds have a platelet count somewhat lower than that of other breeds, with a mean platelet count of approximately 150,000/μL.[26] Cavalier King Charles Spaniels have a hereditary macrothrombocytopenia associated with a beta-tubulin defect. Affected dogs have platelet counts ranging from 25,000/μL to 100,000/μL.[27]

Acquired Platelet Dysfunction

Many common drugs and disease syndromes impair platelet function, but the clinical significance is highly variable.[28] A mild to moderate bleeding tendency may complicate management of disease syndromes such as anemia, liver failure, uremia, DIC, and paraproteinemia. The pathogenesis of platelet dysfunction in these disorders is complex and multifactorial and includes intrinsic alterations in platelet metabolism and extrinsic changes in blood viscosity. Many drugs demonstrate in vitro platelet inhibition (see Table 189-5) by a variety of different mechanisms. The antiplatelet effects of aspirin are

caused by a well-characterized, irreversible inactivation of intraplatelet cyclooxygenase (COX).[29] Other nonsteroidal antiinflammatory drugs (NSAIDs) cause transient COX inhibition, and newer NSAIDs that selectively inhibit the COX-2 isoform are predicted to have fewer antiplatelet effects. Although drugs with potential antiplatelet effects may not cause spontaneous or severe bleeding, they should be given cautiously, if at all, to thrombocytopenic patients, patients undergoing surgery, or patients with signs of abnormal hemostasis.

Hereditary Platelet Dysfunction

Hereditary platelet function defects (thrombopathias) are rare but likely are underdiagnosed because of logistic difficulties in performing platelet function studies. Diseases are broadly grouped as defects of membrane glycoproteins, storage granules, signal transduction, or procoagulant activity.[20] Breed-specific defects within these functional classifications have been identified in dogs and cats (Table 189-6).

Defects in the GPII$_b$III$_a$ complex, referred to as thrombasthenic thrombasthenia, have been identified in Otter Hounds and Great Pyrenees as the result of two distinct GPIIb mutations.[30,31] It is likely that the platelet function defects found in unrelated breeds are caused by unique mutations.

von Willebrand Disease

VWD is the most common canine hereditary hemostatic defect.[32] The clinical signs of VWD overlap with those of

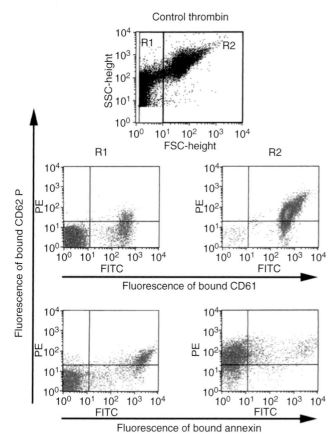

Control thrombin

Figure 189-8 Flow cytometry analyses of canine platelet response to thrombin stimulation. The dot plot at top displays activated platelets in region R2. Region R1 contains platelet membrane-derived microparticles, debris, and machine noise. The four composite cytograms display the fluorescence intensity of labeled probes bound to the events in R1 or R2. The activated platelets (R2) display high-intensity labeling with CD61 and CD62P probes, denoting the presence of the membrane integrin GPIIIa and externalization of alpha granule constituent P-selectin, respectively. Most thrombin-activated platelets, however, are not labeled with the annexin probe, indicating low surface phosphatidylserine. In contrast, platelet membrane-derived particles (R1) display both P-selectin and phosphatidylserine. In all cytograms, events in the lower left quadrant represent nonspecific background fluorescence. *FITC*, Fluorescein isothiocyanate; *FSC*, forward scatter; *PE*, phycoerythrin; *SSC*, side scatter.

other primary hemostatic defects, including mucosal hemorrhage, cutaneous bruising, and prolonged bleeding after injury. Petechiation, however, is not typical of VWD.

Disease Classification

Canine VWD is classified into one of three subtypes based on the clinical severity, plasma VWF concentration (VWF:Ag), and VWF multimer composition.[33,34] In general, a single type of VWD predominates in each affected breed (Table 189-7). Type 1 VWD, the most common form, is typically a mild to moderate bleeding diathesis characterized by low plasma VWF:Ag and normal multimer distribution. Type 2 VWD is a moderate to severe bleeding diathesis with a variable reduction in VWF:Ag and a disproportionate loss of high–molecular weight (HMW) multimers. Type 3 VWD is a severe bleeding disorder caused by a total lack of VWF.

Table • 189-4

Pathogens That Cause Infectious Thrombocytopenia

TYPE OF AGENT	PATHOGEN
Viral agents	Canine: Distemper virus, herpesvirus, parvovirus, adenovirus
	Feline: Feline leukemia virus (FeLV), panleukopenia virus, feline immunodeficiency virus (FIV), feline infectious peritonitis (FIP) coronavirus
Arthropod-borne agents	*Ehrlichia* spp. (*E. canis, E. platys, E. ewingii*); also *Babesia, Haemobartonella, Rickettsia, Leishmania, Cytauxzoon, Borrelia,* and *Dirofilaria* spp.
Fungal and bacterial agents	Septicemia: Various agents *Histoplasma, Candida,* and *Leptospira* spp.

Diagnosis of von Willebrand Disease

The screening test findings compatible with VWD include a normal platelet count, normal coagulation panel, long BMBT, and long PFA closure time, with definitive diagnosis confirmed by the finding of low plasma VWF:Ag (see Figure 189-4). Comprehensive analyses for VWD subtype classification include quantitative, functional, and qualitative VWF assays (Table 189-8).

Inheritance and Expression

VWD is an autosomal trait; males and females experience the bleeding tendency and transmit the defect to offspring with equal frequency.[35] Expression of type 1 VWD is complex, with evidence for both incomplete dominant and recessive patterns.[36,37] Type 1 VWD is common in Doberman Pinschers, and in this breed clinical signs of VWD are typically seen in dogs with a VWF:Ag of 15% or lower.[38,39] Homozygosity for a splice-site mutation in the VWF gene and for certain VWF marker alleles is associated with a low plasma VWF.[40,41] The clinical severity of type 1 VWD for an individual dog (or human patient) cannot be explained fully by current molecular or biochemical tests. Risk of hemorrhage represents a continuum, with severe signs typically associated with relatively severe reduction in plasma VWF concentration (Figure 189-9). In contrast, type 2 and type 3 VWD in dogs appear to be simple recessive traits. Clinically affected dogs inherit a mutant VWF gene from each parent and express a bleeding tendency. The carrier parents are clinically normal, although their plasma VWF is typically low (less than 50% VWF:Ag). Mutations causative for type 3 VWD have been described in Scottish Terriers and Dutch Kooiker Dogs.[42,43] Mutation detection tests for these breeds and for less well-defined VWF mutations in other breeds are available commercially (vetGen, Ann Arbor, Mich.).

TREATMENT OF PLATELET DISORDERS AND VON WILLEBRAND DISEASE

Effective management of platelet disorders and VWD requires control of active sites of bleeding, stabilization of the patient to reverse signs of blood loss anemia and hypovolemia, and identification and correction of the primary disease that caused or exacerbated the hemostatic defect. Initial treatment modalities include both nontransfusion and transfusion

Table • 189-5

Drugs That Have Antiplatelet Effects

CATEGORY	DRUG	DISORDER/MODE OF ACTION
Antibiotics and antifungal drugs	Carbenicillin	Thrombopathia: Unknown action
	Cephalosporins	Thrombopathia: Membrane action*
	Chloramphenicol	Thrombocytopenia
	Penicillin	Thrombocytopenia
	Sulfonamides	Thrombocytopenia
Antiinflammatory drugs	Aspirin	Thrombopathia: Prostaglandin (PG) inhibition
	Ibuprofen	Thrombopathia: PG inhibition
	Naproxen	Thrombopathia: PG inhibition
	Phenylbutazone	Thrombocytopenia and thrombopathia: PG inhibition
Cardiac and respiratory drugs	Aminophylline	Thrombopathia: Phosphodiesterase inhibition
	Diltiazem	Thrombopathia: Calcium blocker
	Isoproterenol	Thrombopathia: Membrane action
	Procainamide	Thrombocytopenia
	Propranolol	Thrombopathia: Membrane action
	Verapamil	Thrombopathia: Membrane action, calcium blocker
Cytotoxic drugs	Azathioprine	Thrombocytopenia
	Chlorambucil	Thrombocytopenia
	Cyclophosphamide	Thrombocytopenia
	Doxorubicin	Thrombocytopenia
Miscellaneous	Dextran	Thrombopathia: Membrane action
	Estrogen	Thrombocytopenia
	Methimazole	Thrombocytopenia

*Membrane action is interaction or interference with membrane receptors.

Table • 189-6

Hereditary Platelet Function Defects

DEFECT	BREED	LABORATORY FINDINGS
Thrombasthenia	Otter Hound, Great Pyrenees	Absent or reduced GPII$_b$III$_a$ complex, abnormal adhesion, absent or severely reduced aggregation to all stimuli, abnormal clot retraction, distinct GPIIb mutations
Signal transduction	Basset Hound, Landseer	Abnormal cAMP metabolism, defective GPII$_b$III$_a$ activation, abnormal adhesion, aggregation only in response to thrombin, normal clot retraction
	Spitz	Abnormal adhesion, absent or trace aggregation in response to most stimuli, normal clot retraction, distinct CalDAG-GEF1 mutations
Storage pool	Persian cat	Chédiak-Higashi syndrome, low dense granule number, failure to secrete ADP and serotonin, abnormal aggregation, normal clot retraction
	American Cocker Spaniel	Normal dense granule number, abnormal ADP storage and secretion, abnormal ADP-induced aggregation, normal clot retraction
Signal transduction and storage pool	Collie	(Associated with cyclic neutropenia and stem cell defect), defective dense granule serotonin and ADP release, abnormal aggregation storage pool and to all stimuli but ADP
Undefined	Boxer	Abnormal aggregation to ADP and collagen, normal shape change, normal granule ATP/ADP content, normal fibrinogen and VWF binding
Procoagulant deficiency	German Shepherd Dog	Abnormal membrane phosphatidylserine exposure, abnormal microparticle release, abnormal prothrombinase activity, normal shape change, normal aggregation, normal clot retraction

ADP, Adenosine diphosphate; ATP, adenosine triphosphate; cAMP, cyclic adenosine monophosphate; VWF, von Willebrand factor.

Table • 189-7

Classification of Canine von Willebrand Disease

CLASSIFICATION	VWF PROTEIN	SEVERITY	REPORTED BREEDS
Type 1	Low concentration/all multimer forms present	Variable	Airedale, Akita, Dachshund, Bernese Mountain Dog, Coton de Tulear, Doberman Pinscher, German Shepherd Dog, Golden Retriever, Greyhound, Irish Wolfhound, Kerry Blue Terrier, Manchester Terrier, mixed breed dogs, Papillon, Pembroke Welsh Corgi, Schnauzer, Shetland Sheepdog
Type 2	Low concentration/disproportionate loss of high–molecular-weight multimers	Moderate to severe	German Shorthaired Pointer, German Wirehaired Pointer
Type 3	Absent	Severe	Chesapeake Bay Retriever, Dutch Kooiker, Scottish Terrier, Shetland Sheepdog Sporadic cases: Australian Shepherd, Border Collie, Cocker Spaniel, Eskimo Dog, Labrador Retriever, Maltese, Pit Bull, Rottweiler

Table • 189-8

von Willebrand Factor Analyses

TEST	PARAMETER MEASURED	TYPICAL RESULTS WITH VWD	NORMAL VALUES*
Buccal mucosal bleeding time (BMBT)	Primary hemostasis—vessel, platelet, VWF interaction	Type 1: 5 to >12 min Type 2: >12 min Type 3: >12 min	2-4 min
Platelet function analyzer (PFA 100) ADP/collagen closure time	VWF-dependent platelet adhesion and platelet aggregation	Type 1: 150-200 sec Type 2: >300 sec Type 3: >300 sec	47-119 sec
von Willebrand factor antigen (VWF:Ag)	VWF concentration	Type 1: 5%-20% Type 2: 1%-5% Type 3: <0.1%	>50%
Ristocetin and botrocetin cofactor activities (VWF:RCo; VWF:BCo)	VWF-dependent platelet agglutination	Type 1: Cofactor activity = VWF:Ag Type 2: Cofactor activity <VWF:Ag Type 3: Cofactor activity absent	>50%
Collagen binding capacity (VWF:CB)	Quantitative measure of VWF bound to collagen	Type 1: VWF:CB = VWF:Ag Type 2: VWF:CB < VWF:Ag Type 3: VWF:CB absent	>50%
VWF multimer composition (Western blot)	Distribution and size of VWF multimer forms	Type 1: All VWF multimers present Type 2: Low/absent HMW forms Type 3: no VWF	Complete size array

ADP, Adenosine diphosphate; *HMW,* high molecular weight; *VWD,* von Willebrand disease.
*Expected values for healthy dogs in authors' laboratory.

support. Although the BMBT is a useful screening test of primary hemostasis for diagnostic purposes, it is not an accurate predictor of disease severity or surgical hemostasis.

Nontransfusion Therapy

Most animals with thrombocytopenia or acquired platelet function defects are effectively treated through identification and correction of the underlying disease process. Drugs with antiplatelet effects, invasive surgery, and jugular catheterization should be avoided, and cage rest is indicated to minimize trauma in severely thrombocytopenic patients. Based on the geographic location, history, and initial workup, institution of appropriate therapy for infectious thrombocytopenia (e.g., doxycycline for *Ehrlichia, Rickettsia,* and *Haemobartonella* spp.) is indicated pending confirmatory test results.[8] Immunosuppressive doses of prednisone (2 mg/kg given every 12 to 24 hours) are administered if the diagnostic workup indicates that primary IMT is likely.[11] Primary IMT patients usually demonstrate resolution of petechiae and an increased platelet count within 2 to 5 days of starting therapy. Refractory primary IMT can be effectively treated with vincristine (0.02 mg/kg given intravenously every 7 days).[44] Immunosuppressive therapy for IMT can be considered successful if a stable platelet count (preferably at or above 100,000/μL) is

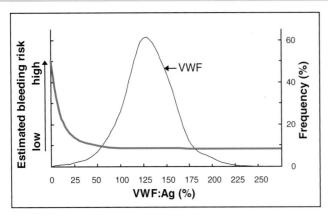

Figure 189-9 Graphic model representing the relationship between plasma von Willebrand factor *(VWF)* level (%) and potential risk for bleeding. The curve labeled VWF represents the frequency distribution of plasma VWF levels in a population of dogs. The red line estimates the risk for bleeding relative to VWF level. Bleeding risk is low when VWF level is >50% and increases sharply as patient plasma VWF levels go below 25%.

attained. Maintenance involves slow, gradual tapering of immunosuppressive therapy, with minimal exposure to unnecessary drugs, vaccination, or stress conditions to avoid relapse.

Desmopressin acetate (DDAVP; deamino 8 D-arginine vasopressin) is a synthetic vasopressin analog used in human medicine to treat a variety of hemostatic defects, including acquired platelet function defects and mild VWD.[45] Desmopressin (1 μg/kg given subcutaneously) has been reported to shorten the BMBT and the PFA-100 closure time and to provide surgical hemostasis when administered 30 minutes before surgery to Doberman Pinschers with type 1 VWD.[46,47] Desmopressin therapy could be considered for other mild to moderate acquired or hereditary platelet function defects. Close monitoring to determine the extent and duration of response is required, and transfusion should be available if the response to desmopressin is inadequate.

Transfusion Therapy

Transfusion with products to replace red cells (Table 189-9) is indicated for patients with acute blood loss and/or severe anemia that cannot be stabilized with fluid therapy alone. Transfusion solely to supply platelets (see Table 189-9) is rarely indicated or beneficial for thrombocytopenic patients or those with acquired platelet function defects. The survival of transfused platelets in IMT patients may be less than 1 day, which further limits their clinical utility. Platelet transfusions should be considered, however, in patients with persistent and uncontrolled bleeding or signs of central nervous system hemorrhage. Dogs and cats affected with severe hereditary thrombopathias may benefit from platelet transfusion as prophylaxis for surgery or if they develop severe spontaneous bleeding.[20,48]

Fresh whole blood, as platelet replacement, must be maintained at room temperature, collected in a citrate-based anticoagulant, and transfused as soon as possible after collection.[49] This product is best used for patients with active bleeding or when no other platelet product is available.

Platelet components are labor intensive to produce, because platelets require special processing and storage techniques to maintain viability. Platelet-rich plasma (PRP) is prepared by centrifugation of whole blood at low G force within 6 hours of collection.[49] The expected platelet yield is

Table • 189-9

Guidelines for Transfusion Therapy

PRODUCT	DOSE	INTERVAL BETWEEN REPEAT PRODUCT TRANSFUSIONS
Products for Red Cell Replacement		
Fresh whole blood	12-20 mL/kg	Every 24 hours (volume overload limits interval)
Packed red cells	6-12 mL/kg	Every 12-24 hours
Oxyglobin	10-30 mL/kg*	Once
Products for Platelet Replacement		
Fresh whole blood	12-20 mL/kg	Every 24 hours (volume overload limits interval)
Platelet-rich plasma	6-10 mL/kg†	Every 8-12 hours
Platelet concentrate	1 U/10-15 kg‡	Every 8-12 hours
Products for von Willebrand Factor Replacement		
Fresh whole blood	12-20 mL/kg	Every 24 hours (volume overload limits interval)
Fresh frozen plasma	10-12 mL/kg	Every 8-12 hours
Cryoprecipitate	1 U/10 kg§	Every 6-12 hours (as needed)

*Infusion guidelines for cats (off-label use): Infuse up to maximum dose of 10 mL/kg.
†Platelet count ≥ 0.5 to 1×10^9/mL.
‡Platelet count ≥ 5×10^9/mL.
§Unit defined as cryoprecipitate prepared from 200 mL of fresh frozen plasma.

approximately 80% of the platelets, in one-third volume, of the starting whole blood unit. In accordance with human blood banking standards, units of PRP, prepared from 450-mL units of whole blood, are expected to contain at least 50 billion platelets.[50] Low-volume platelet concentrates (PC) are prepared from PRP by a second centrifugation step. Platelet-rich plasma and PC must be maintained at room temperature from the time of collection until transfusion, with administration as soon as possible after collection, and maximum storage of 3 days. Preliminary studies of dimethylsulfoxide (DMSO) cryopreserved canine platelet concentrates have been published recently and a commercial product is available (Midwest Animal Blood Services, Stockbridge, Mich.). This product may widen the availability of platelet transfusion beyond referral centers capable of producing components in-house, however treatment trials have not yet confirmed efficacy. Strict attention to aseptic technique is critical during collection and transfusion of platelet products to prevent contamination or disease transmission. Transfusion to supply active VWF (see Table 189-9) is highly effective in controlling hemorrhage in VWD patients.[51] The best strategy is early, rapid transfusion to increase VWF to hemostatic levels and wound therapy to control hemorrhage from a single site. After initial transfusion, severely affected patients may require a second or third transfusion to sustain hemostasis for an additional 24 to 48 hours. Stabilization of the hematocrit and cessation of active hemorrhage indicate that hemostatic levels of VWF have been attained. Plasma components are the safest and most effective products for treating VWD. Plasma cryoprecipitate is prepared from fresh frozen plasma (FFP) and contains a fivefold to tenfold concentration of active VWF in approximately one-tenth volume of the starting plasma.[49] Cryoprecipitate is the best product for rapid replacement of VWF, but fresh frozen plasma is an acceptable alternative if cryoprecipitate is unavailable. The use of plasma components rather than whole blood prevents sensitization to red cell

antigens, eliminates the need for canine type-matched donors, and minimizes the risk of volume overload.

REFERENCES

The reference list can be found on the companion Expert Consult Web site at *www.expertconsult.com.*

CHAPTER 190

Systemic Lupus Erythematosus

Michael Stone

What is systemic lupus erythematosus (SLE)? A single definition is lacking. Veterinary patients with SLE classically demonstrate at least two separate manifestations of autoimmunity in addition to the presence of antinuclear antibody (ANA). However, some patients demonstrate clinical features of multisystemic autoimmunity yet lack serum ANA. This article will discuss the pathogenesis, clinical signs, diagnosis, and therapy of SLE.

PATHOGENESIS

Autoimmune disease may be defined as a clinical syndrome caused by the activation of T cells or B cells, or both, in the absence of an ongoing infection or other discernible cause. With SLE, immune system dysregulation leading to immune complex formation is postulated to induce tissue damage (type III hypersensitivity); however, direct antibody-mediated cytotoxicity (type II hypersensitivity) and cell-mediated autoimmunity (type IV hypersensitivity) also occur.

Effectors

1. Pathogenic antibodies: SLE patients produce antibodies directed against a broad range of nuclear, cytoplasmic, and cell membrane molecules. Autoantibodies may cause damage through the formation of immune complexes, opsonization of target cells, and interference with cellular physiology. Antibodies may penetrate living cells and bind to cytoplasmic or nuclear structures, alter cell function, and contribute to disease by mechanisms other than classic complement-mediated injury.[1]
2. Pathogenic immune complexes: Immune complexes, formed every time antibody meets antigen, are normally removed by the mononuclear phagocyte system. When there is continued production of autoantibody to a self-antigen, overload of the mononuclear phagocyte system may occur. Circulating immune complexes will deposit in walls of blood vessels where there is physiologic outflow of fluid, such as glomeruli, synovia, and choroid plexus. Some immune complexes are "tissue tropic" and prone to bind in tissues because of cationic charge or because the antibodies they contain are directed against tissue components. Trapped immune complexes activate complement, attracted neutrophils will release lysosomal enzymes, and tissue damage is caused.[2]
3. Autoreactive T cells: T cells may directly cause tissue damage in SLE. Dermatologic lesions, polymyositis, and

vasculitis have been associated with cytotoxic T cell–mediated damage.[3]

Genetics

In mice, more than 25 genes have been identified that can contribute to an autoimmune diathesis.[1] Most genes are associated with the major histocompatibility complex (MHC), encoding cytokines, antigen coreceptors, members of cytokine- or antigen-signaling cascades, costimulatory molecules, molecules involved in pathways that promote apoptosis or inhibit it, and molecules that clear antigen or antigen-antibody complexes. For example, a consequence of inheriting Fc receptors that weakly bind immunoglobulin may be the impaired ability to clear immune complexes, predisposing to the sequelae of circulating immune complexes. Protective genes exist that prevent the development of SLE even if multiple susceptibility genes are inherited. In dogs SLE is clearly inherited and experimental colonies of dogs with SLE have been established.[4-6] SLE in dogs has been associated with the allele dog leukocyte antigen (DLA) A7, along with a negative (or "protective") association with DLA A1 and B5.[7] Dogs with a specific allotype of the fourth component of complement may be predisposed to SLE[8] as well as dogs with decreased serum IgA.[9] SLE may occur more frequently in purebred cats, also suggesting genetic influence.[10]

Environmental Factors

The lower than expected rate of SLE concordance among identical human twins strongly suggests that an environmental trigger exists.[3] Exposure to UV light causes disease flares in up to 50% of humans with SLE and has been reported in both dogs[5,11] and cats.[12] The importance of gender is demonstrated by the fact that 90% of cases occur in women, particularly during their reproductive years. Such gender distribution has not been identified in either the dog or cat. Exposure in early life to infectious agents may suppress the development of allergic and autoimmune disorders.[13] It has been suggested the increase in allergy and autoimmune disease recognized in humans is related to decreased exposure to endotoxin during early development. Adequate stimulation may be important in the ontogeny of the normal immune system.[14]

Drugs

Certain drugs may induce SLE-like disease in humans[15] (Box 190-1). This disease is probably different from true SLE. The clinical manifestations of drug-induced lupus in humans are predominantly arthritis, serositis, fatigue, malaise, and low-

Box • 190-1

Causes of Drug-Induced Systemic Lupus Erythematosus in Humans

Allopurinol	Hydralazine	Penicillamine	Propylthiouracil
Captopril	Isoniazid	Penicillin	Quinidine
Chlorpromazine	Lithium	Phenothiazines	Streptomycin
Clonidine	Lovastatin	Phenylbutazone	Sulfasalazine
Danazol	Mesalazine	Piroxicam	Sulfonamides
Diphenylhydantoin	Minocycline	Primidone	Tetracycline
Griseofulvin	Salicylic acid	Procainamide	Valproate

Adapted from Mutasim DF, Adams BB: A practical guide for serologic evaluation of autoimmune connective tissue diseases. J Am Acad Derm 42:159, 2000.

grade fever; nephritis and central nervous system (CNS) diseases are rare. The manifestations disappear in most patients within a few weeks of discontinuation of the offending drug, never to reappear unless reexposure occurs.[3] Propylthiouracil has been associated with hemolytic anemia, thrombocytopenia, and development of ANA in cats.[16] Methimazole has been associated with development of ANA in cats, but clinical signs of SLE have not been reported.[17] Hydralazine has been associated with development of ANA in the dog.[18]

Infectious Agents

No infectious agents have been identified that cause SLE. However, it is possible that infectious agents and/or their antigenic products can worsen SLE in patients with the appropriate predisposing genes. Microbial antigens have the potential to initiate autoreactivity through molecular mimicry, polyclonal activation, or the release of previously sequestered antigens. The immunogenicity of autoantigens may be increased by inflammation in the target organ, explaining flares of immune-mediated disease induced by vaccination or infection. Molecular mimicry describes infection with an agent that has antigens immunologically similar to host antigens but sufficiently different to allow an immune response. As a result, tolerance to autoantigens breaks down and the pathogen-specific immune response cross-reacts with host tissues.[19] In cats the viruses feline leukemia virus (FeLV) and feline immunodeficiency virus (FIV) can induce disease similar to SLE, and serum ANA may occur in the early stages of FeLV infection.[20] Whether FeLV- or FIV-induced disease is truly similar to SLE is debated.[21] Feline ehrlichial disease has also been associated with positive ANA.[22]

In summary, the ability to manufacture pathogenic immunoglobulin and sustain its production depends upon inheriting an appropriate number of susceptibility genes, lack of protective genes, and an environmental stimulus that sets the whole process into action.

CLINICAL FINDINGS

The clinical signs reported in dogs and cats with SLE are summarized in Table 190-1. It must be noted that the process of deriving criteria from diagnosed cases is inherently circular, because criteria are based on diagnosed cases of SLE.

Nonerosive polyarthropathy is the most frequent primary complaint in dogs. The smaller joints (carpi, tarsi, elbows, stifles) are most frequently involved. Synovial fluid analysis reveals neutrophilic inflammation with greater than 10,000 cells/mm³. In cats articular symptoms are also common. Some cats may demonstrate joint swelling and abnormal synovial fluid yet lack signs of lameness.

Fever is frequently reported in both dogs and cats and may be either persistent or intermittent.

In humans, the kidney is commonly involved, with biopsy demonstrating involvement in almost all SLE patients.[23-25] Renal involvement may be benign and asymptomatic or relentlessly progressive and fatal. The earliest manifestation is proteinuria. In dogs, proteinuria and glomerular lesions are also frequent. Biopsy may reveal mesangial and/or endothelial hypertrophy, proliferative and/or membranous glomerulonephritis, and sclerotic changes. Proteinuria and/or glomerulonephritis are also commonly reported in the cat.

Cutaneous manifestations in dogs may include erythema, scaling, crusting, depigmentation, and alopecia. Lesions may develop in the skin, mucocutaneous junctions, and oral cavity. Preferential localization of lesions may occur in areas poorly protected by the haircoat and be exacerbated by exposure to sunlight. Biopsy reveals inflammatory infiltrates at the dermoepidermal junction and vacuolar change in the basal columnar cells. Immunofluorescence stains demonstrate immunoglobulin and complement deposits at the epidermal basement membrane. The cutaneous lesions in 25 reported cases in cats have included erythema, ulceration, crusts and depigmentation of the face, ears, and paws in 7, biopsies consistent with pemphigus foliaceus or plasmacytic pododermatitis in 4, ulcerative stomatitis in 3, and seborrheic dermatitis in 1 case.

Only rarely is anemia, leukopenia, or thrombocytopenia the presenting feature of human SLE without concomitant problems of the skin, joints, CNS, or cardiopulmonary systems. In dogs, although it is common to find anemia of chronic inflammation, Coombs-positive anemia is uncommon. Thrombocytopenia may be severe enough to cause bleeding, but the association with antiphospholipid syndrome and thromboembolic disease should also be considered. Leukopenia has been frequently reported. Complement concentrations were decreased in three of eight dogs with suspected SLE.[8] As in dogs, hemolytic anemia is uncommon in cats and thrombocytopenia rare. Complement levels were decreased in one studied cat.[10]

Thrombosis associated with the "lupus" anticoagulant was reported in one dog with SLE.[34] The "lupus" anticoagulant is an antibody directed against membrane phospholipids. The antibody causes in vitro prolongation of the activated partial thromboplastin time (thus the paradoxical name anticoagu-

Table • 190-1

Clinical Signs in Dogs and Cats with Suspected Systemic Lupus Erythematosus

CLINICAL SIGN	DOGS (INCIDENCE*)	DOGS (PERCENTAGE)	CATS (INCIDENCE*)	CATS (PERCENTAGE)
Nonerosive polyarthritis	236/302	78%	9/25	36%
Fever	186/275	68%	11/21	52%
Renal disorders	167/302	55%	10/25	40%
Dermatologic lesions	138/302	46%	15/25	60%
Lymphadenopathy/splenomegaly	66/175	38%		
Leukopenia	54/302	18%		
Hemolytic anemia	45/302	15%	6/25	24%
Thrombocytopenia	40/302	13%	2/25	8%
Myositis	16/275	6%		
Central nervous system disorders	16/302	5%	6/25	24%
Neuropathy	7/302	2%		

Summarized from references 10-12, 21, and 26-33.
*Number of patients affected/number of patients described.

lant). The antibody's effect in vivo, however, causes platelet activation and hypercoagulability.

Memory impairment, headache, epilepsy, and personality changes may accompany lupus in humans. Sole involvement of the CNS without other clinical or laboratory features of SLE is unusual. In animals, subtle behavioral disturbances may go unrecognized. In cats, reported CNS involvement has included racing around the house, twitching of the ears, tail, and hindlimbs, repeated licking of paws and tail base, generalized seizures, hyperesthesia along the dorsum, restless crying, disorientation, ataxia, loss of conscious proprioception, nystagmus, and ventroflexion of the neck.[10] Polymyositis was suspected in several dogs and cats. Polyneuritis, characterized by hyperesthesia of the nerve courses, has been reported in a dog.[11]

In humans, chest pain with or without pleural effusion is the most common sign of cardiopulmonary involvement. Fibrosis, pulmonary embolism, capillary leak, or serositis may affect the lungs. The heart valves, myocardium, or conducting system may be affected and pericardial effusion may develop. Neutrophilic myocarditis was demonstrated in four dogs with SLE.[28] Serositis of the pleura or pericardium was not observed in any of the cats. Subclinical lung changes were noted on thoracic radiographs of one cat.[10]

DIAGNOSIS

Criteria have been developed for the diagnosis of SLE in humans (Table 190-2), and these criteria may be modified to apply to veterinary patients (Table 190-3). Veterinary patients with SLE classically demonstrate at least two separate manifestations of autoimmunity along with positive ANA. Patients with three or more separate manifestations of autoimmunity may also be considered to have SLE despite the absence of detectable ANA. The most common syndrome recognized in the dog is immune-mediated polyarthritis, in combination with immune-mediated skin disease, glomerulonephritis, hemolytic anemia, or thrombocytopenia. Similar signs occur in the cat; however, neurologic signs may be more common.

Diagnostic testing of suspected SLE patients should include hematology, biochemistry, urinalysis, imaging, joint fluid cytology, histopathology of the skin and/or kidney, and serum ANA. Cats should be tested for FeLV and FIV. Infectious and neoplastic disease must be excluded through imaging, culture of urine, blood and/or joint fluid, serology for tick-borne and fungal disease, and therapeutic antibiotic trials. In tick-infested areas, a 3- to 7-day course of doxycycline should be considered prior to concluding the presence of immune-mediated disease.

Immunodiagnostic investigations may include Coombs' testing, platelet autoantibodies, rheumatoid factor, coagulation testing for antiphospholipid antibodies, serum immunoglobulin, complement, circulating immune complex concentrations, and endocrine autoantibodies (i.e., thyroglobulin). Immunohistologic investigation may include immunoperoxidase and immunofluorescence staining and electron microscopic evaluation.[40]

Biopsies may be supportive but are rarely diagnostic of SLE by themselves. When the skin is biopsied, care should be taken to avoid ulcers or erosions, since an intact epidermis is necessary to substantiate the diagnosis. Oral biopsy specimens are rarely beneficial, since ulcers, which are inherently not diagnostic, are common in this location. Erythematous areas adjacent to ulcers yield the most diagnostic results.[41]

The diagnosis of SLE in cats is less well defined. In some studies all cats with positive ANA test results were diagnosed with SLE, but whether these patients truly had SLE is debatable. Another unanswered question is how to categorize FeLV- or FIV-positive patients. Some reports include FeLV-positive cats while others exclude them.[10,21,29-31,42] Because of the possibility of ehrlichial disease, it has been recommended that all cats receive a course of doxycycline before the diagnosis of immune-mediated disease is made.[43]

SPECIFIC TESTING

LE Cell Test

Clotted blood is mashed to release free nuclei. The presence of circulating antibody directed against nucleoprotein will bind and opsonize the nuclear complex. A lupus erythematosus (LE) cell is recognized as a neutrophil that contains phagocytized nuclear material. Interpretation depends upon the experience and diligence of the technician performing the test, and false negative results are common.[26,27,44] Because of technical, sensitivity, and specificity problems, the LE cell test has been largely replaced by the more sensitive ANA test. LE cells may rarely be seen on smears of pericardial, pleural,

Table • 190-2

American College of Rheumatology Revised Criteria for the Classification of Systemic Lupus Erythematosus[35]

CRITERIA	DEFINITION
1. Malar rash	Fixed erythema, flat or raised over the malar eminences, tending to spare the nasolabial folds
2. Discoid rash	Erythematous raised patches with adherent keratotic scaling and follicular plugging; atrophic scarring may occur
3. Photosensitivity	Skin rash as a result of unusual reaction to sunlight
4. Oral ulcers	Oral or nasopharyngeal ulceration, usually painless
5. Arthritis	Nonerosive arthritis involving two or more peripheral joints
6. Serositis	a. Pleuritis—pleuritic pain or rub or evidence of pleural effusion, OR b. Pericarditis—pericardial effusion
7. Renal disorder	a. Persistent proteinuria, OR b. Cellular casts—may be red cell, hemoglobin, granular, tubular or mixed
8. Neurologic disorder	a. Seizures—in the absence of offending drugs or known metabolic derangements or electrolyte imbalance, OR b. Psychosis—in the absence of offending drugs or known metabolic derangements or electrolyte imbalance
9. Hematologic disorder	a. Hemolytic anemia—with reticulocytosis, OR b. Leukopenia—less than 4000/mm^3 on 2 or more occasions, OR c. Lymphopenia—less than 1500/mm^3 on 2 or more occasions, OR d. Thrombocytopenia—less than 100,000/mm^3 in the absence of offending drugs
10. Immunologic disorder	a. Anti-DNA: antibody to native DNA in abnormal titer, OR b. Anti-Sm: presence of antibody to Sm nuclear antigen, OR c. Positive finding of antiphospholipid antibodies based on 1) an abnormal serum level of IgG or IgM anticardiolipin antibodies, 2) a positive test result for lupus anticoagulant, or 3) a false-positive serologic test for syphilis
11. Antinuclear antibody (ANA)	An abnormal titer of ANA at any point in time and in the absence of drugs known to be associated with "drug-induced lupus"

From Tan EM: The 1982 revised criteria for the classification of systemic lupus erythematosus. Arthritis Rheum 25:1271,1982.
For the purposes of identifying patients in clinical studies, a person shall be said to have systemic lupus erythematosus if any 4 or more of the 11 criteria are present, serially or simultaneously, during any interval of observation.

Table • 190-3

Proposed Criteria for the Diagnosis of Systemic Lupus Erythematosus (SLE)

CRITERIA	DEFINITION
1. ANA	Abnormal titer of ANA in the absence of drugs, infectious, or neoplastic conditions known to be associated with their development
2. Cutaneous lesions	Depigmentation, erythema, erosions, ulcerations, crusts, and/or scaling with biopsy findings consistent with SLE
3. Oral ulcers	Oral or nasopharyngeal ulceration, usually painless
4. Arthritis	Nonerosive, nonseptic arthritis involving two or more peripheral joints
5. Renal disorders	Glomerulonephritis or persistent proteinuria in the absence of urinary tract infection
6. Anemia and/or thrombocytopenia	Hemolytic anemia and/or thrombocytopenia in the absence of offending drugs
7. Leukopenia	Low total white cell count
8. Polymyositis or myocarditis	Inflammatory disease of the skeletal or cardiac muscles
9. Serositis	Presence of a nonseptic inflammatory cavity effusion (abdominal, pleural or pericardial)
10. Neurologic disorders	Seizures or psychosis in the absence of known disorders
11. Antiphospholipid antibodies	Prolongation of activated partial thromboplastin time that fails to correct with a 1:1 mixture of patient and normal plasma, in the absence of heparin or fibrin degradation products

Adapted from references 28 and 36-39.
ANA, Antinuclear antibody.
A diagnosis of SLE is established if a patient manifests three or more criteria simultaneously or over any period of time.

peritoneal, joint, cerebrospinal, and blister fluid and when present are highly suggestive of SLE.

Antinuclear Antibodies

Antinuclear antibodies are a heterogeneous population of antibodies directed against various nuclear antigens. ANA may be detected using frozen sections of rat liver or cultured cell lines (e.g., Vero cells, HEp-2 human epithelial cells). There is no universally accepted protocol for ANA testing used by veterinary laboratories. The result of an ANA test is commonly reported as a serum titer and, sometimes, pattern of nuclear staining. The most commonly observed patterns are speckled or homogenous staining, but there is no clear association between patterns and the nature of clinical disease. A clinically significant titer must be distinguished from low ANA titers that may be present in up to 10% of normal animals and animals with any chronic inflammatory, infectious or neoplastic disease.[45,46]

In humans, substrates tend to remain comparable in their ability to detect common ANA but differ substantially in the quantitation of antibody titer.[47] In dogs, it has been suggested that multiple substrates be used to increase the sensitivity of the test.[48] Two canine studies found markedly different ANA results when rat liver and HEp2 cell substrate were compared[48,49]; however, results were well correlated in a third report.[50] Feline ANA test results were found to have a low coefficient of correlation when identical sera were sent to different laboratories.[51]

In conclusion, the most appropriate substrate, conjugate, and methodology for ANA testing remains undefined and each laboratory's value should be interpreted individually. ANA-negative SLE cases have been described in veterinary patients,[5,26-28] and a positive ANA should be neither required nor sufficient in itself to make a diagnosis of SLE. SLE should not be diagnosed or excluded based upon this single test result.

Autoantibodies

Suspicion of human SLE leads to testing for specific antibodies that provide diagnostic and prognostic information (Table 190-4). The following summarizes autoantibody studies that have been performed in veterinary patients (Table 190-5).

Antibodies to DNA Serum antibodies may recognize denatured (single-stranded) or native (double-stranded) DNA. Anti–single-stranded DNA has low diagnostic value in humans and has not been studied in veterinary medicine. Anti–double-stranded (native) DNA is highly specific for the diagnosis of human lupus, even though only 60% to 83% of patients are positive. Anti–double-stranded DNA has been found infrequently in dogs with SLE.

Extractable Nuclear Antigens Extractable nuclear antigens (ENA) are molecules extracted from the soluble fraction of cell nuclei (DNA and histone proteins are insoluble and therefore excluded). There have been more than 20 saline-extractable antigens identified, and the term *ENA* generically refers to this group of nuclear proteins. The binding of serum antibodies to commercially available tissue extracts is the basis for serologic testing. Important ENA include Sm, Ro, La, and ribonucleoprotein (RNP). In veterinary medicine, antibodies against ENA have not yet been shown to offer the diagnostic and prognostic significance they do in human patients.

Antihistone Antibodies Histones are a group of proteins that bind the DNA helical structure into supercoil formation. Histone antibodies are characteristic of drug-induced SLE in humans. Investigators at one university[11,53,54] detected antihistone antibodies in 61% to 72% of dogs with SLE. Antihistone antibodies have been detected in canine sera by other investigators; however there was no significant difference in concentration between ANA positive and negative sera,[49] and antihistone antibodies were detected in conditions other than

Table • 190-4

Autoantibody Associations in Human Systemic Lupus Erythematosus (SLE)

EPITOPE	COMMENTS
ds-DNA	Highly specific for the diagnosis of SLE
Sm	Associated with membranous nephropathy
RNP	Associated with Raynaud's phenomenon, pulmonary and muscle involvement
SS-A/Ro	Associated with cutaneous manifestations, sicca complex, neonatal lupus
SS-B/La	Associated with neonatal lupus
Phospholipid	Associated with thrombocytopenia, thrombosis, infertility

From Edworthy SM: Clinical manifestations of systemic lupus erythematosus. In: Kelley's textbook of rheumatology, ed 6, Philadelphia, 2001, Saunders, pp 1105-1119.
ds-DNA, Double-stranded DNA; *Sm, Ro, La*, extractable nuclear antigens named for the first two letters of the patient from which the antigen was first described (e.g., Sm = Smith); *RNP*, ribonucleoprotein; *SS-A*, Sjögren's syndrome A antigen (or its equivalent, Ro); *SS-B*, Sjögren's syndrome B antigen (or its equivalent, La).

Table • 190-5

Positive Autoantibody Results in Suspected Canine Systemic Lupus Erythematosus Patients

EPITOPE	INCIDENCE*	INCIDENCE (PERCENT)	REFERENCE
ds-DNA	6/38	16%	Costa, 1984[52]
	1/3		Bennett, 1987[44]
	1/47	2%	Brinet, 1988[53]
	2/100	2%	Monier, 1992[54]
	0/43		Monestier, 1995[55]
Sm	9/34	24%	Costa, 1984[52]
	2/30	7%	Hubert, 1988[5]
	12/75	16%	Fournel, 1992[11]
	0/20		White, 1993[56]
	1/64	2%	Henriksson, 1998[57]
RNP	4/38	10%	Costa, 1984[52]
	0/12		Monier, 1988[6]
	0/30		Hubert, 1988[5]
	6/75	8%	Fournel, 1992[11]
	0/20		White, 1993[56]
	5/64	8%	Henriksson, 1998[57]
SS-A/Ro	1/12		Monier, 1988[6]
	0/30		Hubert, 1988[5]
	3/75	4%	Fournel, 1992[11]
	0/20		White, 1993[56]
SS-B/La	0/30		Hubert, 1988[5]
	0/12		Monier, 1988[6]
	1/75	1%	Monier, 1992[54]
	0/20		White, 1993[56]
"Type 1" (antibody to a 43-kd nuclear antigen, also known as hnRNP G)	10/38	38%	Costa, 1984[52]
	15/75	20%	Fournel, 1992[11]
"Type 2"	5/38	13%	Costa, 1984[52]
	7/75	9%	Fournel, 1992[11]
Phospholipid	1/1		Stone, 1990[34]
	2/20	10%	Scott-Moncrieff, 2001[58]
	1/1 (feline)		Lusson, 1999[59]

*Number of positive patients /number of tested patients. See Table 190-4 for abbreviations.

canine SLE.[52] The use of antihistone antibodies as an indicator of drug-induced SLE in veterinary patients has not been reported.

Antiphospholipid Antibodies Antiphospholipid antibodies bind to cell-associated phospholipids, such as the cell membrane. The antibody interferes with the function of procoagulant phospholipids in clotting tests in vitro. Patients with the lupus anticoagulant have prolonged activated partial thromboplastin time that fails to correct with a 1:1 mixture of the patient's plasma and normal plasma. Their presence is associated in humans with thrombocytopenia, thrombosis, and fetal loss. Antiphospholipid antibodies were described in one dog with SLE,[34] 2 of 20 dogs with hemolytic anemia,[58] and one cat with SLE.[59]

MANAGEMENT

Sunlight should be avoided if photosensitization occurs. Most patients also require corticosteroid administration. Prednisone 1 to 2.2 mg/kg/day orally is initially started; lower doses may be effective in less severe cases. A combination of prednisone and immunosuppressants is recommended in more severe cases, especially those affecting the kidneys. Full doses are administered until the disease is in complete remission, defined as resolution of clinical signs as well as radiographic or laboratory changes that were initially present. After remission is attained the dose is tapered, generally in half, for approximately 4 weeks. Reevaluation is performed, and if signs of disease are absent (on physical and laboratory evaluation), the dose is again halved. Tapering is repeated monthly until the animal either relapses or stops medication. The recommended minimum duration of therapy is 6 months. If relapse occurs during taper, the dose should be increased to the most recently effective dose and held there for a few months. If the maintenance requirement is unacceptable because of side effects, an additional immunosuppressive agent is added.

Some cats do not respond to prednisone. Cats that do not completely respond to prednisone should be treated with an alternate steroid (prednisolone, methylprednisolone, triamcinolone, or dexamethasone) prior to instituting additional immunosuppressant therapies.

Combination immunosuppression therapy allows a lower dose of corticosteroid to be used. Azathioprine (Imuran) is the drug most frequently used in dogs. The dose is 2.2 mg/kg orally once daily until remission occurs, then the same dose is administered every other day. Prednisone and azathioprine are frequently used in combination. The drugs are administered together once daily and tapered after remission is attained. Tapering should be performed every 2 to 4 weeks, with the minimum duration of therapy being 6 months.

Azathioprine is not recommended for use in cats. Instead, chlorambucil may be administered along with corticosteroids for cats that require additional immunosuppression. Chlorambucil (Leukeran) is used in cats at 15 mg/m² orally (4 mg for most cats) once daily for 4 days, and repeated every 3 weeks. Alternatively 2 mg chlorambucil (total dose) may be administered every 2 to 3 days. Potential side effects include anorexia and bone marrow suppression. In cats, the dosage of chlorambucil should be tapered before the prednisone is tapered.

Alternative immunosuppressants may include cyclosporine (5 mg q12-24h IV or PO) or mycophenolate mofetil (10 to 20 mg/kg q12-24h IV or PO). Immunoglobulin G (0.5 to 1 g/kg IV q24h 1 to 4 days) may be useful of refractory cases.

Novel therapeutic approaches include prednisone (1 to 2 mg/kg daily) combined with levamisole (2 to 5 mg/kg, max 150 mg) every 48 hours.[11] The prednisone is tapered and discontinued after 2 months, while levamisole is given continuously for 4 months and then stopped. If there is relapse of disease, levamisole is readministered for a further 4-month period. Approximately 75% of dogs treated with such therapy were reported to attain remission. Side effects included agranulocytosis, excited behavior, and aggressiveness.[39]

In humans, an antimalarial drug such as hydroxychloroquine may provide additional relief. Antimalarial agents have multiple sun blocking, antiinflammatory, and immunosuppressive effects, although their mechanism of action is not completely understood.[60] Their use has not been reported in dogs or cats with SLE.

PROGNOSIS IN VETERINARY PATIENTS

The natural course of SLE in veterinary patients is not known. Patients may be well controlled and medications may be tapered; however, relapses should be anticipated. Routine evaluation should include hematology, biochemistry, urinalysis, and serum ANA every 1 to 3 months. The titer of ANA may correlate with clinical severity and fall with clinical improvement, but the antibody may persist at low titer during clinical remission. It has been suggested that therapy should be more aggressive when the clinical presentation includes renal disease.[10,39] Renal function should be monitored for life in all patients suspected of having SLE.

REFERENCES

The reference list can be found on the companion Expert Consult Web site at *www.expertconsult.com.*

CHAPTER 191

Nonregenerative Anemia

Anthony Abrams-Ogg

Anemia is a clinical problem and not a specific diagnosis, and may be caused by many diseases. Anemia is classified by pathophysiology as being due to hemolysis, hemorrhage, [erythroid] hypoplasia, or hemodilution (4 Hs); one or more may be involved in a case. Hemolytic and hemorrhagic anemias may be either regenerative (most frequent occurrence) or nonregenerative, while hypoplastic anemia is, by definition, nonregenerative. Anemia is also classified by duration as acute or chronic, but there is a spectrum in between the two. Acute anemias are caused by either hemo-

stomach, resulting in pernicious anemia.[117] Cobalamin deficiency results in elevated blood levels of methylmalonic acid and homocysteine. Folate and/or cobalamin deficiency affects other organs, in particular the gastrointestinal tract and nervous system, and associated signs as well as overall well-being may be affected without overt hematologic changes.

Naturally occurring dietary folate and cobalamin deficiency has not been reported in dogs, and dogs are resistant to experimental folate deficiency.[119] Serum folate declines in dogs during pregnancy, and supplementation has been associated with a reduction in congenital defects.[120,121] In cats, naturally occurring megaloblastic anemia responding to folate and cobalamin supplementation has been reported infrequently,[113,122,123] and megaloblastic anemia has occurred in experimental dietary folate deficiency.[114,124] The anemia is normocytic to macrocytic.

Serum levels of folate and/or cobalamin may be reduced in dogs and cats with various gastrointestinal, pancreatic and hepatic disorders (see Chapters 174, 270, and 282-283). Anemia or macrocytosis (in cats) may occur but are not common.[125-129] Bone marrow is typically not evaluated in these disorders.

Cobalamin deficiency resulting from a genetic disorder of intestinal malabsorption has been reported in Giant Schnauzers, Border Collies, Beagles, Australian Shepherd Dogs, and presumptively in one cat.[115,116,130-134] Intrinsic factor deficiency has not been identified in these cases. Signs and severity vary, but generally are associated with failure to thrive. Megaloblastic and other dysplastic changes are present in the bone marrow resulting in normocytic normochromic anemia, increased RDW, and megaloblasts in the peripheral blood. Intramedullary erythrophagocytosis has also been seen, consistent with destruction of dysplastic erythroid cells. Animals have had elevated levels of methylmalonic acid in the urine and/or serum. Dogs treated with parenteral cobalamin have had correction of anemia and have thrived; the one cat was not treated.

Chronic treatment with azathioprine in dogs and methotrexate in cats in the author's practice has been associated with macrocytosis in some cases. Poodles have an inherited disorder of megaloblastic dyshematopoiesis and macrocytosis but are not anemic.[135]

Starvation   Idiopathic bone marrow failure and serous atrophy causing pancytopenia was associated with prolonged anorexia in four cats; malnutrition may have been contributory.[136]

Development Dam Deep in the Bone Marrow

Nonregenerative Immune-Mediated Hemolytic Anemia   As discussed in Chapter 188, IMHA is classically characterized by peripheral destruction of red cells and a strong regenerative response. However, less commonly, an immunologic attack on erythropoiesis occurs "deeper" in the bone marrow instead of, or in addition to, the peripheral blood. This attack may occur at several levels and act as a "dam" in the bone marrow preventing normal maturation and resultant lack of a regenerative response.[7,25,26,136-143] While in dogs regenerative IMHA is more common than nonregenerative IMHA, this is not the case in cats.

At the first level, an attack on reticulocytes in the blood results in lack of reticulocytes on a hemogram but evidence of synchronous erythroid hyperplasia on bone marrow biopsy. At the next level, an attack on erythroid cells causes a maturation arrest. In some cases the expansion of immature erythroid cells behind the immunologic dam is so prominent that it may be mistaken for erythroid leukemia, similar to the previously discussed situation with early myeloid hyperplasia. In other cases of ineffective erythropoiesis, erythroid production tapers

into the later stages on bone marrow biopsy. In both scenarios erythroid dysplasia may be pronounced. If the immunologic attack occurs at the level of the earliest committed erythroid progenitor cells, then a bone marrow biopsy reveals attenuation or absence of all stages of erythropoiesis, and the diagnosis is erythroid hypoplasia or aplasia. If the immunologic attack occurs at the level of pluripotent hematopoietic progenitor cells, then a hemogram reveals pancytopenia and a bone marrow biopsy reveals trilineage hypoplasia or aplasia, often with replacement with adipocytes, and the diagnosis is "aplastic anemia." Historically, the term *aplastic anemia* has been used to denote trilineage bone marrow aplasia, while *pure red cell aplasia* has been used to identify the condition where only erythroid production is impaired. These are linguistically bad terms, but are conventional. Further permutations on this theme are possible. For example, cases of erythroid and megakaryocytic hypoplasia with normal neutrophil and monocyte production have been seen,[144] because platelets and red cells differentiate from each other after their common progenitor cells differentiate from the neutrophil-macrophage progenitor cells.

In most cases of immunologic attack in the bone marrow the anemia is normocytic normochromic. Serum iron and transferrin levels may be elevated.[138] There is no pathognomonic finding on bone marrow biopsy.[25,26,139,143] Bone marrow plasma cell hyperplasia or lymphocytosis support the diagnosis, but its absence does not rule it out, and caution must be exercised in diagnosing mild plasma cell hyperplasia against a background of reduced bone marrow cell density.[145] Immune-mediated erythroid hypoplasia and related disorders are presumptively diagnosed on the basis of ruling-out other causes of erythroid hypoplasia, supportive bone marrow biopsy findings, and on response to immunosuppression. Because immunosuppression is not always successful with immune-mediated diseases, lack of response does not rule-out the diagnosis. The diagnosis is also supported by concurrent typically immune-mediated disorders (e.g., polyarthritis), positive antinuclear antibody titer, positive Coombs' test, and spherocytes and, if thrombocytopenia is present, positive tests for antiplatelet and antimegakaryocyte antibody.

Feline immune-mediated dyserythropoiesis most commonly occurs in young cats and is more likely to explain a FeLV-negative nonregenerative anemia than is a false-negative FeLV test.[7,136,140,141] In addition, while the anemia in some cats has responded to prednisone therapy alone, many cases appear to require more intense immunosuppression. The author prefers to initiate treatment with prednisone, cyclophosphamide, or chlorambucil, and cyclosporine at standard doses. Because the role of hemotropic mycoplasma and ehrlichial infections in the pathogenesis of the disorder is not known, treatment with doxycycline or marbofloxacin is recommended.[7,146] Testing by polymerase chain reaction (PCR) at a laboratory with a proven track record in quality control may be considered. Over 70% of cats are expected to recover.

The signalment of dogs with immune-mediated dyserythropoiesis is typical of IMHA and other immune-mediated disorders, with middle-aged spayed female dogs at increased risk.[137,138,147] The tendency is to also treat dogs with a combination of immunosuppressive agents (see Chapter 188), although the benefit of doing so is not known. Over 70% of dogs are expected to recover, but the response may take weeks. The prognosis may be better in dogs with subacute-to-chronic disease than with typical peracute to acute IMHA because dogs without acute peripheral hemolysis and its associated systemic inflammatory response are at less risk for pulmonary thromboembolism and disseminated intravascular coagulation.

Serum EPO levels are anticipated to be elevated in immune-mediated nonregenerative anemia, therefore EPO therapy is usually not recommended.[7,141] However, rhEPO therapy has been beneficial in cases of immune-mediated aplastic anemia in humans despite elevated serum EPO levels.[148] Nonetheless, routine treatment with rhEPO is not recommended in dogs and cats where treatment may trigger another antierythroid immune response.

Feline Leukemia Virus Infection FeLV is not cytopathic but infection of erythroid cells alters or arrests their development, causing a normocytic normochromic anemia.[149] In some cases this may be by mechanisms similar to anemia of inflammatory disease.[149,150] Macrocytic anemia may occur with some subgroup A strains.[123,149,151] Subgroup C causes pure red cell aplasia and may also be responsible for aplastic anemia.[149,152] Cats infected with FeLV may also develop anemia secondary to hemotropic mycoplasma infections, hematopoietic and nonhematopoietic neoplasia, and possibly IMHA.[149,154] Endogenous EPO levels are elevated and in principle rhEPO therapy should not help, but there are anecdotal reports of benefit.[150,153] Treatment of FeLV infection is further discussed in Chapter 212.

Diversion of Hematopoietic Cells

Acute Myeloid (Myelogenous) Leukemia (AML) Myeloid leukemia refers to neoplasia arising from hematopoietic cells in the bone marrow, be they of erythropoietic, thrombopoietic, granulopoietic, monocytopoietic, mixed-lineage, or pluripotent stem cell origin, with or without overt peripheral blood involvement. The term *myeloid* in the context of leukemia is thus used to distinguish these leukemias from lymphoid leukemias, while in the context of normal hematopoiesis myeloid refers to granulocyte-monocyte lineage cells as distinct from erythroid cells. Hematopoiesis is diverted into production of malignant cells, with a resulting decrease in normal blood cell production. The malignant clone arises from a mutant stem cell with pluripotent properties, but it is not known if the mutation occurs in normal hematopoietic stem cells or in more differentiated cells that then acquire stem cell properties.[155] Any AML may cause anemia, but the most profound tend to be seen with leukemias arising from erythropoiesis, namely erythroleukemia and erythremic myelosis.[156-165] The classification and nomenclature of myeloid leukemias is an evolving process,[166,167] but generally *erythroleukemia* is a broader term referring to leukemia arising from a common erythrocyte and leukocyte precursor, while *erythremic myelosis* refers to leukemia strictly of erythropoietic origin. In AML arising from mixed-lineage or pluripotent cells, an animal is more likely to be presented for clinical signs due to neutropenia and thrombocytopenia, analogous to the situation with bone marrow destruction. In contrast, in erythremic myelosis, leukocyte and platelet production is more spared, and an animal is more likely to be presented for signs due to anemia. These rules are not absolute, in part because normal blood cell production is also affected by displacement and depression, and the malignant clone may change in character.[168,169]

Animals with AML are usually presented for inappetence and lethargy. The main physical examination finding in an animal with erythroid leukemia is pallor. Petechiation and ecchymoses may be present if there is thrombocytopenia, but they are more difficult to see compared to an animal with immune-mediated thrombocytopenia because of the anemia. Fever may be present, especially if the animal is neutropenic. Hepatomegaly and/or splenomegaly may occur from leukemic cell infiltration.[157,170] Lymph node infiltration may also occur, but lymphadenopathy is not typically as marked as with lymphoma.

A hemogram may reveal many combinations of leukemic cells and cytopenias. Abnormal erythroid cells may resemble any prereticulocyte stage of erythropoiesis. Marked nonregenerative anemia is typical, and it is important not to misdiagnose the presence of rubricytes and metarubricytes as a sign of regeneration. Bone marrow biopsy is needed for diagnosis if only anemia with or without other cytopenias is present. If leukemic cells are present in the blood, bone marrow biopsy is not strictly necessary but helps to further characterize the disorder. Bone marrow biopsy of an animal with erythremic myelosis will reveal marked erythroid hyperplasia with maturation arrest and erythrodysplasia.

Following on the previous discussion of immune-mediated dyserythropoiesis, it is difficult to distinguish malignant from nonmalignant causes of erythroid hyperplasia with dyserythropoiesis on the basis of morphology alone.[7] Indeed, in some models of erythroid leukemia the defect is an oncogene-based maturation arrest.[171] Bone marrow tissue culture, and cytogenetic and molecular studies of clonality, may potentially be used in an attempt to prove malignancy; however, such studies are not well developed and/or not readily available for dogs and cats.[139,172]

How then is acute erythroid leukemia, which carries a poor prognosis, distinguished from an immunohematologic disorder with morphologic mimicry, which carries a relatively good prognosis? First, in cats, a positive ELISA test for FeLV supports the diagnosis, as FeLV is a proven cause of AML.[172,173] Cases of ELISA-negative, PCR-positive cats have been reported from laboratories with stringent quality control, but unfortunately, in the author's experience poor laboratory PCR technique (as shown with PCR for FIV)[173a] is another explanation and confirmation of the result by another laboratory is advised. In dogs there is no equivalent cause to FeLV, accounting for the rarity of the diagnosis. The only risk factor for erythroleukemia in the dog is chronic irradiation.[174]

Second, more than 30% blast cells in the bone marrow has been suggested as a diagnostic criteria for AML in dogs and cats, based in part on this being a criteria to distinguish AML from MDS in humans.[167] The author respectfully disagrees. Three cats ultimately diagnosed with immune-mediated dyserythropoiesis were initially diagnosed with AML based on that criterion.[7] Nonetheless, the greater the percentage of blasts the greater the likelihood of AML.

Third, nonmalignant dyshematopoiesis may yield dysplastic cells in the peripheral blood, but the greater the presence of abnormal cells, the greater the likelihood of leukemia. However, in one dog in the author's practice ultimately diagnosed with immune-mediated or toxin-induced pancytopenia, 30% of peripheral blood nucleated cells were dysplastic. A complete remission was attained after 2 weeks of treatment with prednisone alone.

Fourth, if hepatomegaly, splenomegaly, or lymphadenomegaly are present, biopsy of these organs may reveal neoplastic cell infiltration. Organomegaly on its own is not sufficient evidence, as this may also occur due to lymphoid hyperplasia in immune-mediated blood disorders. Furthermore, in the latter case biopsy may also reveal extramedullary hematopoiesis, which may mimic neoplasia.

Fifth, the presence of disorders and positive test results characteristic of immune-mediated disorders supports immune-mediated dysmyelopoiesis, although these may have an underlying neoplasm.

Finally, AML appears to be uncommon in dogs and FeLV-negative AML is uncommon in cats. Because of the difficulty in confirming a diagnosis of erythroid leukemia, especially in the absence of peripheral blast cells, and the tendency to euthanize animals with AML, if there is ever a place for the clinician to stand by the old adages of "treat for the treatable" and "never let an animal die without the benefit of prednisone," it is here. Erythroid leukemia is treated with cytotoxic chemotherapy and specific protocols are discussed in

Chapter 324. Fortunately these protocols are also immuno-suppressive. Another approach to the treatment of various forms of AML is to promote differentiation of neoplastic cells stuck in maturation arrest, which thereby mature out of malignant behavior. Several agents have been used for this purpose including physiologic agents (rhEPO and other hematopoietic growth factors, vitamin D, retinoids, methylprednisolone), and nonphysiologic agents, including cytotoxic drugs, often given at lower than conventional doses.[175-178]

Myelodysplastic Syndrome (MDS) MDS is characterized by peripheral blood cytopenias, but normal to increased marrow cellularity with dysplastic changes, and a risk of progression to AML. As the name implies, it is a syndrome, not a single disease, and as with AML, classification and nomenclature are evolving.[166,167] The unifying concept is an abnormal clone of hematopoietic progenitor cells that may suppress, displace, and progressively replace normal hematopoietic tissue. The hematologic and clinical progression is highly variable. It is one more of the many hematologic disorders associated with FeLV infection in cats.[173,179]

Even more than with AML, MDS and immune-mediated dyshematopoiesis may mimic each other morphologically,[25,26,139,143,180-182] but the confusion has less immediate clinical impact as MDS does not prompt euthanasia as quickly as AML. There are also numerous other causes of myelodysplasia that mimic MDS as discussed elsewhere in this chapter, and workup should include investigation for infectious diseases, drugs, toxins, nutritional deficiencies, non-AML neoplasia, and inherited disorders. Myelodysplastic changes may also be normal in elderly humans.[183] Similar to AML, primary MDS appears to be uncommon in dogs, and a positive FeLV ELISA supports the diagnosis of MDS in cats. As with non-regenerative IMHA, positive ANA and Coombs' tests support immune-mediated myelodysplasia. Detection of more than 5% monoblasts identified by cytochemistry is another criterion proposed as strongly supportive of MDS in dogs.[139] It is unlikely that there are any other discriminatory clinical or laboratory features. Treatment of MDS has historically relied on supportive transfusions and later treatment of AML if it occurs. Early hematopoietic stem cell transplantation is being evaluated in humans,[184] but is not feasible for most dogs and cats. Differentiation therapy with rhEPO for a subtype of MDS characterized by erythroid predominance is beneficial in humans, even in the presence of elevated endogenous EPO.[185] This treatment was successful in a dog with this form of MDS, although treatment also included prednisone.[186] Immunosuppression and observation of response is the most practical course in many cases.

Displacement of Erythroid Tissue (Myelophthisis)

Erythroid cells may be crowded out by metastatic cancer cells,[187,188] nonmyeloid hematopoietic neoplasia (acute lymphoid leukemia, multiple myeloma, mast cell neoplasia), granulomatous inflammation (e.g., histoplasmosis), or myelofibrosis. In addition to physical displacement, neoplastic cells may depress erythropoiesis by molecular mechanisms.[189] As with other causes of generalized bone marrow injury, neutropenia and thrombocytopenia may be more responsible for clinical signs than anemia. Bone marrow biopsy is diagnostic, and usually nonmyeloid hematopoietic neoplasms do not pose the same diagnostic dilemmas as do AML and MDS.

Another mechanism of displacing hematopoietic cells is myelofibrosis. Myelofibrosis is a nonspecific finding: it may be idiopathic, the result of FeLV infection in cats, chronic inflammation in the bone marrow (including autoimmunity—it is a common finding in immune-mediated erythroid hypoplasia), secondary to a primary leukemia, or in some cases a primary tumor of bone marrow stromal cells.[138,143,149,190-195] Although

neutropenia or neutrophilia, and thrombocytopenia and thrombocytosis, may occur, leukocyte and platelet numbers are often normal, and moderate to severe nonregenerative anemia is the salient finding. The anemia is typically normocytic normochromic, but macrocytosis in one case series of dogs was observed and was associated with a better prognosis.[192] Idiopathic myelofibrosis is usually treated with standard immunosuppressive agents.

Osteopetrosis is a rare condition of young dogs that may cause nonregenerative anemia or pancytopenia secondary to thickening of the cortices and narrowing of the medullary cavity.[196,197] Osteopetrosis may be a feature of FeLV subgroup C–induced bone marrow failure.[149,198]

Depression by Disease ("Anemia of Chronic Disease")

Nonhematologic diseases depress the erythron at various levels and by various mechanisms. Diseases include infectious diseases, nonseptic inflammation, neoplasia, chronic liver diseases, chronic renal failure, and some endocrinopathies. Congestive heart failure is a common cause of anemia and pseudoanemia in humans, but does not appear to be in dogs and cats, although one small study identified lower Hct in dogs with severe heart failure.[199-201] Some mechanisms of anemia are shared by some of the disorders, but there are enough differences in mechanisms and in onset of anemia that render "anemia of chronic disease" too broad a term. It has been hypothesized that reduced activity associated with chronic illness results in fatty replacement of hematopoietic tissue and that this is a common mechanism that has been overlooked.[202]

Anemia of Inflammatory Disease (AID) and Cancer-Associated Anemia Anemia of inflammatory disease (AID) is caused by complex cytokine derangements that decrease EPO production, EPO function, iron metabolism, and red cell lifespan.[203-205] A key event is the sequestration of iron, which is considered to be an adaptive mechanism that renders the micronutrient unavailable to infecting microorganisms.[206,207] These mechanisms are present in acute inflammation, and Hb levels begin to decrease in several days, but actual anemia develops only in more chronic inflammation because of red cell lifespan. The anemia is usually mild to moderate, but may be severe, especially in cats, in part because of the shorter red cell lifespan.[208] The anemia is initially normocytic and normochromic, but may progress to microcytic and hypochromic in dogs. Serum iron should be low-normal to low, but in contrast to iron deficiency, AID is supported by documenting low-normal to decreased transferrin, and high-normal to elevated ferritin. Bone marrow biopsy should reveal normal to mildly depressed erythropoiesis with normal to increased iron in dogs.

Cancer-related anemia is common in humans and is widely considered to be common in animals, although this not extensively documented.[209] The mechanisms responsible for AID are considered responsible for cancer-related anemia not attributable to other causes, and the anemia is initially mild, normocytic, and normochromic. Iron sequestration has been shown in dogs with lymphoma and osteosarcoma.[210] Causes of cancer-related anemia are further discussed in Chapter 333.

Anemia at diagnosis and during therapy may be negative prognostic factors for various tumors in humans, and definitely have a negative impact on quality of life.[211-216] Tumor hypoxia is a well-recognized mechanism of resistance, and it is possible that anemia favors resistance to treatment and tumor progression.[217] Conversely, increasing iron load with transfusion or rhEPO treatment is potentially detrimental. Analogous to iron sequestration in AID being a protective mechanism against microbial proliferation, iron sequestration in paraneoplastic AID may be protective. Neoplastic cells have a higher iron requirement due to rapid proliferation, and iron chelators have anticancer properties.[218] An additional concern is that treatment with EPO may stimulate tumor progression, perhaps because some tumors express EPO receptors.[219] However, EPO may also have an anticancer effect in some tumors such as multiple myeloma.[220] Treatment with EPO increases the risk of venous thrombosis.[216] Correcting anemia improves quality of life, but the effect on tumor response, tumor progression, and overall patient survival is not clear.[216]

The current recommendation in veterinary medicine is to treat anemia in the oncology patient using the same transfusion triggers as with patients with nonneoplastic disorders. Some patients with advanced cancer and chronic anemia have been transfused in the author's practice at a higher trigger than with chronic anemia due to other causes, in an effort to improve quality of life. Response has been variable, consistent with the observation in humans that factors other than anemia contribute to fatigue.[221] Treatment with rhEPO has also anecdotally been used for this purpose in dogs and cats. It is not known if the risk for antibody formation is the same in this group of patients as in patients with chronic renal failure.

Feline Immunodeficiency Virus (FIV) Anemia was present in 36% of FIV-positive cats in one case series.[222] Some of the anemias seen with FIV are due to secondary diseases, including hemotropic mycoplasma infections and neoplasia, but anemia may occur without these.[149,223,224] The virus is not cytopathic and does not infect erythroid cells, and serum from FIV-positive cats does not depress erythropoiesis in tissue culture.[225] Recent studies have shown that, similar to HIV, FIV does infect megakaryocytes and bone marrow stromal cells, and the latter is likely involved with in depressing erythropoiesis through alterations in the marrow inductive microenvironment.[226] Another mechanism may be infection of T cells involved in regulating hematopoiesis.[227] Bone marrow findings include erythroid hyperplasia with megaloblastic dysplasia and ineffective erythropoiesis.[66,222] As in humans with HIV-associated anemia, rhEPO therapy is beneficial in ameliorating anemia, and FIV-positive cats are at low risk of anti-EPO antibody formation.[228]

Chronic Liver and Kidney Disease Anemia is common in liver disease and is multifactorial.[229] Mechanisms include AID, malnutrition, reduced red cell lifespan, and hemorrhage due to gastrointestinal ulceration, coagulopathy, and hepatic rupture. Excluding major hemorrhage, the anemia is usually mild to moderate normocytic normochromic and is not responsible for presentation to the clinic. Poikilocytosis is common, including target cells in dogs, probably due to abnormal lipids in the red cell membrane.[230]

Anemia in chronic renal failure may result in a mild to marked anemia due to EPO deficiency, decreased red cell lifespan, and uremic bleeding.[231,232] Treatment with rhEPO is discussed in Chapter 311. The benefits of EPO supplementation go beyond the correction of anemia and hopefully routine supplementation will become easier in the future.[23,233]

Endocrine Disorders Anemia in hypothyroidism is considered an adaptation to decreased oxygen demands due to decreased basal metabolic rate, and thus is a consequence, rather than cause, of lethargy. Thyroid hormone normally stimulates burst-forming units–erythroid and colony-forming units–erythroid directly and indirectly via EPO, and it also stimulates 2,3-DPG synthesis.[234,235] In two series of 66 and 50 dogs, 32% and 40% were anemic, respectively, while in a series of 7 dogs with severe hypothyroidism characterized by

altered mental status or myxedema, 57% were anemic, with the lowest value being 23%.[236-238] The prevalence and severity of decreased red cell mass may be underestimated by these figures, as plasma volume is also decreased in hypothyroidism.[234] Anemia is typically normocytic normochromic with normal red cell survival.

Dogs with both typical and glucocorticoid only–deficient hypoadrenocorticism often have low-normal to low Hct.[239-241] Glucocorticoids enhance erythropoiesis and this is part of a normal stress response.[242] The mechanisms are not completely known, but they include stimulation of glucocorticoid receptors on erythroid progenitor cells. Anemia is normocytic normochromic and is usually mild to moderate. With chronic hypoadrenocorticism the anemia may be severe. Acute gastrointestinal hemorrhage from ulceration may also contribute to anemia, and may also be a mechanism for hypoalbuminemia.[243,244] Anemia may be masked on presentation by dehydration. In one case series of dogs, 34% were anemic at presentation with a mean Hct of 39% (range 15% to 57%), while after 24 hours of fluid therapy 71% were anemic with mean Hct of 28% (range 8% to 40%).[245] Hypoadrenocorticism is less common in cats than dogs, and anemia is both less common and less severe.[255-257]

Critical Illness Anemia is common in critically ill patients because of repetitive blood sampling, surgery, gastrointestinal ulceration, AID, decreased red cell lifespan, and nutritional deficiencies.[258-260] Transfusion triggers are controversial. Because transfusion has been associated with worse outcomes in some situations, rhEPO is being used with increasing frequency in humans. The current recommendation in dogs and cats is to transfuse based on the same criteria as in anemia due to other causes.

Dilution (Pseudoanemia)

Fluid Therapy Fluid therapy with either crystalloids or colloids will decrease Hct. This is not usually a concern in anemic animals as red cell mass is not affected. Indeed, in anemic dehydrated animals there is likely to be improved tissue oxygenation because of improved circulation. The main concern is volume overload as previously discussed.

Pregnancy Plasma volume expansion occurs during pregnancy, probably due to systemic vasodilation and the resulting increase in vascular capacitance.[261] Erythropoiesis also increases during pregnancy, but the degree of plasma volume expansion is relatively greater than the increase in red cell mass; therefore, Hct decreases. (Albumin levels also decrease, although altered albumin metabolism is also involved.[262]) The volume expansion and erythroid hyperplasia are believed to be adaptive mechanisms to improve placental circulation, in part by lowering blood viscosity. Other benefits include a mechanism to counter the increased risk of thrombosis due to thrombocytosis and elevated fibrinogen, and a volume reserve to buffer hemorrhage during parturition. In dogs, the Hct slowly declines and is usually <40% by day 35 of gestation and <35% at term, and in one report the degree of drop in the Hct was positively correlated with the number of fetuses.[263-265] Reticulocytosis was not discussed. In a study of six cats, mean Hct 1 day after breeding was 36% and dropped to 28% at term.[266] A mild increase in aggregate and punctuate reticulocytes was reported. Consistent with other observations of the poorer tolerance of cats to volume expansion, congestive heart failure due to volume expansion has been reported in pregnancy.[267]

Drugs

Many drugs may cause an idiosyncratic nonregenerative anemia, either as an isolated finding or accompanied by other cytopenias. In some cases the mechanism is probably immunologic and in other cases toxic. Noncytotoxic drugs with a known or suspected risk for partial or complete bone marrow suppression in dogs include estrogens (previously discussed); phenylbutazone, meclofenamic acid, carprofen; captopril, quinidine; thiacetarsemide, albendazole, metronidazole, and phenobarbital.[268-274] Phenytoin may cause macrocytosis.[271] In cats griseofulvin may cause bone marrow failure (especially in FIV-positive cats), and antithyroid drugs may cause anemia and other cytopenias.[136,275] Cephalosporins and trimethoprim-sulfonamides at normal doses have been rarely associated with adverse hematologic reactions in both species.[276,277] Trimethoprim-sulfonamides at high doses has caused mild anemia from folate inhibition in normal dogs and delayed recovery in

dogs during bone marrow transplantation.[278,279] Chloramphenicol causes reversible erythroid suppression by inhibiting Hb synthesis in all species.[280-282] Unlike in humans, there is not a risk for idiosyncratic aplastic anemia in dogs and cats. Recombinant human EPO may result in immune-mediated pure red cell aplasia in both species with a risk of 20% to 25%.[23] Recombinant human interleukin-11, a thrombopoietic cytokine, causes dilutional pseudoanemia.[283]

REFERENCES

The reference list can be found on the companion Expert Consult Web site at *www.expertconsult.com.*

CHAPTER 192

Acquired Coagulopathies

Marilyn E. Dunn

A coagulopathy is any defect in the body's ability to clot. Defects in blood clotting can lead to either a state of hypocoagulability or hypercoagulability. This chapter will review common causes of hypocoagulability, hypercoagulability, and thrombosis in small animals.

VITAMIN K DEFICIENCY

Vitamin K deficiency is one the most commonly acquired coagulopathies in small animals. Deficiency most commonly results from ingestion of vitamin K antagonist rodenticides; however, decreased synthesis from the intestinal microflora along with decreased vitamin K absorption have also been reported.

Vitamin K is a fat-soluble vitamin found in 3 forms: vitamin K_1 (phylloquinone), vitamin K_2 (menaquinone), and synthetic vitamin K_3 (menadione). Vitamin K_1 is derived from green leafy plants and is absorbed through the lymphatics in the proximal small intestine. Vitamin K_2 is synthesized by bacterial microflora (*E. coli and Bacteroides* predominantly) in the ileum and colon. Vitamin K_3 is a synthetic form that must be metabolized to vitamin K_2 to be activated.[1]

Vitamin K plays an important role as a cofactor in the intrinsic, extrinsic and common pathways where it is essential in the activation of the vitamin K–dependent clotting factors II, VII, IX, and X and proteins C and S. Factors II, VII, IX, and X are produced in the liver as inactive precursors. These precursors contain gamma glutamyl amino acid groups that, in the presence of vitamin K, will undergo carboxylation, allowing calcium binding and thus clotting. The carboxylation reaction requires reduced vitamin K. However, during carboxylation, vitamin K becomes oxidized by the enzyme vitamin K epoxidase and becomes vitamin K epoxide. To allow continued factor activation, this vitamin K epoxide must be once again reduced by vitamin K epoxide reductase. Some anticoagulant rodenticides currently on the market

inhibit this process leading to the release of dysfunctional forms of the clotting factors II, VII, IX, and X into circulation[1,2] (Figure 192-1). Recently, the key protein, vitamin K epoxide reductase complex subunit 1 has been identified as the key protein of the vitamin K cycle and is an area of intense research. Inhibition of vitamin K epoxide reductase leads to rapid depletion of the vitamin K–dependent clotting factors. Because factors II, VII, IX, and X have very short half-lives in the dog (42, 6.2, 13.9, and 16.5 hours, respectively), a coagulopathy quickly develops.[1,2]

Ingestion of coumarin-based rodenticides is the most common cause of vitamin K–deficient coagulopathy in small

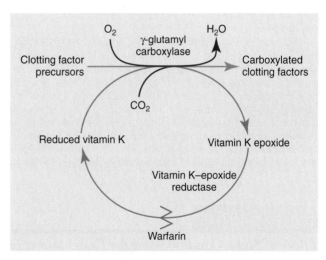

Figure 192-1 Vitamin K epoxidase cycle illustrating the carboxylation of clotting factors and the site of warfarin inhibition. (Courtesy Dr. Christian Bédard.)

 To view a video on this topic, go to **www.expertconsult.com.**

animals. Approximately 10% of calls to poison control centers involve dog or cat anticoagulant rodenticide poisoning. These are available as powders, pellets, and blocks. Warfarin was the first of the anticoagulant rodenticides developed; however, rats quickly developed resistance to warfarin leading to the development of the more potent second generation products with longer half-lives (bromadiolone, brodifacoum, and diphacinone). Once ingested, warfarin is transported to the liver and excreted through either urine or bile, where it may undergo enterohepatic recirculation.[1-3]

Dogs and cats consuming rodents intoxicated with anticoagulant rodenticides are unlikely to be affected. The amount of rodenticide ingested by the rodent or the residue concentration is believed to be so small that a large number of intoxicated rodents would have to be ingested to result in toxicosis. As an example, tissue residues in rodents fed a warfarin-based rodenticide was 2 ppm. Rodenticide typically contains 50 ppm. Toxicity in the dog occurs at doses of 1 mg/kg, and therefore a dog would have to consume 20 g of rodenticide or 500 g of rodents per kg.[3]

Diagnosis is usually based on appropriate history, clinical signs, and laboratory testing. Clinical signs associated with anticoagulant rodenticide toxicity develop 2 to 5 days following exposure. Based on a retrospective of 21 dogs, the most common presenting complaints and physical examination findings were dyspnea (57%), lethargy (48%), coughing/hemoptysis (30%), pallor (26%), epistaxis (17%), vomiting (17%), melena (17%), hematochezia (13%), lameness (13%), spontaneous subcutaneous hematoma (13%), ecchymoses (13%), hematoma at intramuscular injection sites (9%), hematuria (9%), gingival bleeding (9%), and collapse (9%).[4]

Following ingestion, the first test to show an abnormal result is the proteins induced by vitamin K absence (PIVKA) within 12 hours, followed by the prothrombin time (PT) within 36 to 72 hours, then the partial thromboplastin time (PTT). Animals presenting with clinical signs typically have a prolonged activated clotting time (ACT), PT, and PTT. Anemia (83%), thrombocytopenia (61%), hypoproteinemia (57%), and increased fibrin degradation products (FDP) (55%) were also reported in the previous study (Table 192-1).

PIVKA has been shown to have high sensitivity and specificity for rodenticide antocoagulants.[5,6] Measurement of rodenticide concentrations in serum, blood or tissue is necessary to confirm exposure, especially in cases having legal implications.

Following acute ingestion, emetics, adsorbents and cathartics should be given to minimize absorption. As the amount absorbed is often uncertain, therapy with vitamin K$_1$ can be initiated at a dose 2.5 to 5 mg/kg as a subcutaneous injection divided and given in several sites. Oral therapy can be followed up 6 to 12 hours later at a dose of 2.5 mg/kg once a day for a week. PT should be measured 48 hours after discontinuation of therapy. Therapy in a bleeding patient consists of restoring functional clotting factors. This can be done through plasma or blood transfusion and the administration of vitamin

K$_1$. As it may take up to 12 hours before functional clotting factors are present in circulation following initiation of vitamin K therapy, a transfusion may be necessary. Length of administration is based on the half-life of the ingested rodenticide. A 2- to 4-week therapy has been recommended for second generation rodenticides. A PT should be measured 48 hours following discontinuation of therapy, and if it is prolonged, therapy should be resumed for 2 more weeks. Vitamin K$_1$ should never be given intravenously as it has been associated with anaphylaxis. Vitamin K$_3$ should not be used as it has a delayed onset of activity and has been reported to cause Heinz body anemia.[1-3]

Although less common, vitamin K deficiency can also develop secondary to decreased synthesis by the intestinal microflora. This can result from chronic antibiotic therapy. Severe fat malabsorption such that can occur secondary to complete bile duct obstruction, exocrine pancreatic insufficiency, and lymphangiectasia can result in vitamin K deficiency. Therapy should be aimed at correcting the underlying disorder and parenteral vitamin K$_1$ administration.[1]

LIVER DISEASE

The liver plays a central role in coagulation homeostasis. Hemostatic abnormalities are common in liver disease and have been estimated to occur in 70% to 85% of human patients; however, clinical bleeding is much less common (<2%). The liver is the site of synthesis of all clotting proteins and their inhibitors (antithrombin, alpha$_2$-macroglobulin, alpha$_1$-antitrypsin, alpha$_1$-acid glycoprotein and proteins C and S) except for von Willebrand factor. Factor VIII is synthesized in the liver but also in nonhepatic sinusoidal endothelial cells. The liver is also the site of synthesis of fibrinolytic proteins (plasminogen, plasminogen activators and proactivators).[7-9]

Liver disease is typically associated with coagulopathies when liver reserve is poor. Liver failure results in multiple changes in the hemostatic system because of reduced synthesis of procoagulant and anticoagulant factors. Factor deficiency is attributed to decreased factor synthesis, abnormal factor synthesis, and excessive consumption. Clotting factor deficiencies have been correlated to the degree of hepatocellular necrosis and the concurrent decrease in albumin. In some instances, prolonged bleeding times may be documented before the decrease in albumin given the shorter half-lives of the clotting factors. Added to all these other anomalies is vitamin K deficiency which was previously discussed. During failure, the liver is unable to clear activated hemostatic proteins and inhibitor complexes from the circulation. Given these various anomalies, the global effect of liver failure on hemostasis is complex and may result in bleeding or thrombosis.

Sluggish blood flow through the portal vein secondary to hypertension can also lead to portal vein thrombosis.[7-9]

Table • 192-1

Effect of Some Conditions on the Coagulation Test Results

CONDITION	PLATELETS	PROTHROMBIN TIME	PARTIAL THROMBOPLASTIN TIME	FIBRIN DEGRADATION PRODUCTS
Liver disease	Normal to ↓	Normal to ↑	Normal to ↑	Normal to ↑
Disseminated intravascular coagulation	↓	↑	↑	↑
Rodenticide toxicity	Normal to ↓	↑	↑	Normal to ↑

In people with liver failure, the following abnormalities favoring bleeding have been reported: thrombocytopenia, impaired platelet function and vessel wall interaction, decreased levels of clotting factors II, V, VII, IX, X, XI, dysfibrinogenemia, and decreased alpha$_2$-antiplasmin. The following abnormalities favoring thrombosis have been reported: elevated levels of factor VIII and von Willebrand factor, decreased proteins C and S and antithrombin, and decreased levels of plasminogen. Thromboelastography in people with cholestatic liver disease show either a normo- or hypercoagulable tracing[7] (Box 192-1).

The liver is also responsible for the clearance of activated clotting proteins. The mononuclear phagocytic system clears these products such as FDP, prothrombinase, fibrin monomers, and tissue thromboplastin. Increased FDP have been observed in liver failure.[7-9]

Despite these abnormalities, spontaneous clinical bleeding in small animals due to liver failure is rare. It has been estimated that at least 80% of the functional capacity of the liver must be lost before observing hypoalbuminemia and decreased clotting factors. It is generally accepted that clinical bleeding will not occur until clotting factor levels decrease below 15%. The nature of the liver disease, its severity and rate of onset may also affect clotting status.[7]

Liver disease may also result increased fibrinolysis which can explain oozing and continued bleeding from surgical or venipuncture sites in some patients with liver failure.

In severe liver disease, prolongation of the PT, PTT, increased PIVKA, thrombocytopenia and increased FDP and D-dimer may be observed. Similar coagulation profiles can be found in patients with disseminated intravascular coagulation (DIC). There has been some controversy as to whether patients in liver failure may suffer from low grade DIC; however, autopsies in cirrhotic patients have not demonstrated microvascular thrombosis. Differential diagnosis based only on laboratory tests may be impossible.[1]

Typically, therapy for coagulopathies in liver disease is only undertaken in the bleeding patient or prior to invasive procedures such as surgery. Administration of vitamin K$_1$ may help improve vitamin K–dependent clotting factor synthesis. Administration of blood products (fresh frozen plasma, cryoprecipitate, platelet concentrates, recombinant factor VIIa) may be necessary in the actively bleeding patient or prior to more invasive procedures in hemostatically unstable patients.

Ideally, therapy should be aimed at treating or supporting the underlying liver disease.[1,7-10]

NEOPLASIA

Patients with neoplasia may present with bleeding or thrombosis from various causes. Hemostatic abnormalities reported in cancer patients can be caused by thrombocytopenia, thrombocytopathia, DIC, release of factors from tumor cells, tumor-induced organ dysfunction, microangiopathy, endothelial invasion by neoplastic cells, and the administration of various chemotherapeutic agents. The pathogenesis of DIC in cancer patients is multifactorial and results from systemic generation of thrombin and plasmin leading to fibrin polymerization and subsequent fibrinolysis. As this cycle continues, it results in depletion of clotting factors, platelets. and fibrinogen.

A number of case reports in veterinary medicine have documented alterations in hemostasis with various tumor types.

Tumors most commonly associated with DIC were hemangiosarcoma, inflammatory mammary tumors, thyroid carcinoma, primary lung tumors, and intraabdominal carcinomas. Other tumors associated with hemostatic abnormalities in small animals are multiple myeloma, mast cell tumors and lymphoma.[11-13]

A number of chemotherapeutic drugs have been found to interfere with hemostasis.[1]

Therapy should be targeted at the underlying neoplasia while hemostatically supporting the patient as needed.

DISSEMINATED INTRAVASCULAR COAGULATION

DIC, also known as *consumptive coagulopathy*, is a syndrome that can complicate many disease processes and lead to life-threatening hemorrhage. It is considered a secondary disease because an original insult predisposing to thrombosis must be present to initiate DIC. It can be defined as a pathologic activation of clotting factors leading to formation of disseminated microthrombi. Microthrombi consume clotting factors along with platelets, resulting in their depletion. Severe clotting factor depletion then leads to hemorrhage from venipuncture sites or digestive, respiratory, urinary, or reproductive tracts. Microthrombi result in poor tissue and organ perfusion, which may lead to multiple organ dysfunctions. Regardless of the underlying disease, once initiated, the pathophysiology of DIC is similar.[14] A critical mediator of DIC is the release of tissue factor, a transmembrane protein present on the surface of most cells. In health, tissue factor does not come into contact with the general circulation. However, in inflammation, tissue factor can be expressed on endothelial cells within the circulation and on some neoplastic cells. Tissue factor can also be released into circulation in response to proinflammatory cytokines (interleukin-1, tumor necrosis factor) and endotoxin. Once in circulation, tissue factor forms a complex with factor VIIa, a potent stimulus for thrombin formation. Excess circulating thrombin cleaves fibrinogen leaving behind multiple fibrin clots leading to microvascular and macrovascular thrombosis. Thrombin and fibrin production become exaggerated. DIC is a mixed coagulopathy as throughout its course, the patient may undergo phases of hypo- or hypercoagulability. Coagulation inhibitors are also consumed in this process. Decreased inhibitor levels lead to more clotting so that a feedback system occurs in which increased clotting leads to more clotting. Concurrently, thrombocytopenia due to entrapment in clots and excessive consumption also occur. Clotting factors are consumed in the development of

---

Box • 192-1

Hemostatic Changes in Liver Disease Which May Lead to Either Hemorrhage or Thrombosis

Lead to hemorrhage	Lead to thrombosis
Thrombocytopenia	Elevated factor VIII
Thrombocytopathia	Elevated von Willebrand factor
Impaired platelet/vessel wall interaction	Decreased levels of plasminogen
Decreased production of clotting factors II, V, VII, IX, X, XI	Decreased levels of antithrombin
Dysfibrinogenemia	Decreased levels of proteins C and S
Decreased alpha$_2$-antiplasmin	Decreased levels of plasminogen

multiple clots, which contributes to the bleeding seen with DIC.[1,14,15]

Simultaneously, excess circulating thrombin results in the conversion of plasminogen to plasmin, leading to fibrinolysis. Fibrinolysis results in excess amounts of FDPs, which have anticoagulant properties, possibly contributing to hemorrhage. Excess plasmin also activates the complement and kinin systems, leading to clinical signs such as shock, hypotension, and increased vascular permeability. The hypercoagulable state occurs early in the course of DIC and prolonged clotting times accompanied by bleeding usually occur later in its course.[1,14,15]

Diagnosis of DIC is based on clinical findings and laboratory testing; however, given its dynamic nature and considerable variation in coagulation profiles of affected dogs, establishing a diagnosis can be challenging. Any animal having experienced prolonged hypotension, systemic inflammatory response syndrome, disturbed blood flow to a major organ, or major tissue trauma is at high risk of developing DIC. Patients in acute fulminant DIC present with bleeding; however, in more chronic forms patients may only show signs related to the underlying disorder.[1]

No single laboratory test can be used to diagnose DIC. The diagnosis is usually established by documenting a known condition predisposing to DIC and a combination of the following laboratory findings: prolongation of coagulation times, thrombocytopenia, elevation of d-dimer or soluble fibrin, decrease in antithrombin, clinical or postmortem evidence of thrombosis. A recent study reported that thromboelastography was valuable in the assessment of 50 dogs presenting in DIC. The majority of these patients were found to have hypercoagulable tracings.[16] In this study, mortality was associated with high D-dimer, low antithrombin, and hypocoagulable thromboelastographic tracings as compared to survivors. A canine study indicated that a negative D-dimer test excludes DIC as a diagnosis with a confidence interval of 95%.[1,14,15]

Therapy is multifaceted and should be aimed at ensuring adequate tissue perfusion, eliminating the initiating cause, supporting target organs, replacing blood components, and initiating anticoagulant therapy. Blood component replacement can be provided by plasma transfusions, which can help replace clotting factors in order to rebalance coagulant and anticoagulant proteins. Fresh whole blood, platelet-rich plasma, or concentrates may be indicated in some patients. Antithrombin replacement has been attempted in people with no improvement in mortality seen. Activated protein C may reduce organ damage in human patients with sepsis and DIC but this has yet to be investigated in veterinary medicine.[1,13]

Heparin therapy for DIC is controversial. The efficacy of its administration in patients with low antithrombin levels is unclear. Heparin is a glycosaminoglycan that exerts its effects by binding to antithrombin and accelerating its interaction with activated factors IIa (thrombin), IXa, Xa, XIa, and XIIa. Thrombin and factor Xa are most responsive to inhibition by antithrombin. Thrombin inactivation requires formation of a ternary complex involving heparin, AT, and thrombin. Heparin is an indirect anticoagulant, exerting most of its effect through potentiation of AT activity. The drug is administered either intravenously or subcutaneously, as it is very poorly absorbed orally. Heparin has long been the mainstay of DIC therapy despite few reports documenting its true benefit. Increased morbidity has been reported in people in DIC who receive heparin while actively bleeding. Heparin does not eliminate existing thrombi but may prevent the formation of new thrombi. Empiric heparin therapy in veterinary medicine for DIC varies widely, encompassing a subcutaneous dosage range of 50 to 200 IU/kg q6-12h.[17]

Overall prognosis for DIC is poor and varies depending on the underlying disorder. DIC has also been referred to as "death is coming."

THROMBOSIS

Thrombosis is a major cause of mortality in people with heart disease, cancer, and stroke, which are the three most common causes of death in developed countries. Hereditary defects of coagulation inhibitors, referred to as *thrombophilias*, further increase the burden of thrombus formation in human populations. Aspirin, heparin, and warfarin have long been the mainstays of antithrombotic therapy in human medicine.

Although hereditary thrombophilias have not been identified in dogs or cats, thrombosis is recognized as a common complication of many acquired diseases, including cardiac, endocrine, inflammatory, and neoplastic disorders. Advances in our understanding of pathologic thrombus formation and recent pharmacokinetic studies of antithrombotic drugs in dogs and cats hold promise for the development of effective thromboprophylactic regimens in small animal practice.

Normal hemostasis is maintained through an intricate balance between endogenous anticoagulants and procoagulants. The net effect is preservation of blood flow in the systemic vasculature with localized coagulation at sites of vessel injury. Changes in this balance can tip the scales to either excessive bleeding or widespread thrombus formation (hypercoagulability). The concept of "Virchow's Triad" (endothelial damage, alterations in blood flow, and hypercoagulability) refers to underlying factors that act singly or together to promote thrombus formation in various disease states. The primary disorder influences the site of thrombus formation (arterial or venous vasculature), the composition of the occluding thrombus, and the approach to antithrombotic therapy.

Clinical signs of a thrombus can be variable and depend on the affected organ. Clinical signs result from compromised blood flow to the organ. Thrombi may obstruct flow locally or break off and lodge downstream, where the vessel caliber is smaller and there is slower flow. Acute pulmonary thromboembolism is associated with dyspnea. Renal arterial thromboembolism can be associated with acute renal failure.[17,18]

Diagnosis of hypercoagulability is a great challenge in veterinary medicine. Routine coagulation tests (PT, PTT) are designed to detect "hypocoagulability" and assays that measure consumption of anticoagulant proteins and fibrinogen are generally insensitive indicators of subclinical thrombosis. Nevertheless, low plasma AT activity and high FDP, D-dimer, and fibrinogen levels provide laboratory evidence of hypercoagulability. In human studies, platelet hyperaggregability and expression of platelet activation markers such as P-selectin have been observed in patients with thrombotic tendencies. Thromboelastography (TEG) is a technique that depicts global hemostasis, beginning with clot formation and ending with clot lysis. Characteristic changes in the TEG profile have been associated with hypercoagulability in people. Evaluation of platelet function and TEG may prove useful in future veterinary studies to detect hypercoagulability and to monitor antiplatelet and anticoagulant therapy.[17,18]

Actual detection of thromboemboli can be very difficult. A combination of Doppler ultrasonography, angiography, venography, and ventilation perfusion scans can aid in their identification; however, many cases of thromboembolism likely go undiagnosed in small animals.[1,18]

Treatment of thrombosis can be aimed at reducing thrombogenesis or dissolution of existing clots through the use of thrombolytic agents. Reducing thrombogenesis can be achieved with antiplatelet drugs or anticoagulants. Antiplatelet agents act through inhibition of platelet activation pathways or interference with membrane receptors. The three classes of antiplatelet drugs in current use include nonsteroidal antiinflammatory drugs (cyclooxygenase inhibitors), thienopyridines (ADP receptor antagonists), and GPIIb/IIIa blockers (fibrinogen receptor antagonists).[17]

Aspirin is the most common antiplatelet drug used in veterinary medicine. It acts through irreversible acetylation of the platelet cyclooxygenase active site leading to decreased thromboxane A_2 synthesis. The effects of aspirin are permanent and last for the lifespan of the platelet (7 to 10 days). In a retrospective study of IMHA in dogs, improved survival was attributed, in part, to low-dose (0.5 mg/kg PO) aspirin administration.[17,19]

Thienopyridines irreversibly inhibit the binding of ADP to specific platelet ADP receptors (P2Y12). ADP receptor blockade impairs platelet release reaction and ADP-mediated activation of GPIIb/IIIa, thereby reducing primary and secondary aggregation response. These drugs must be metabolized by hepatic cytochrome p450, with platelet inhibition occurring by 3 days after initiation of therapy. Clopidogrel, given to cats at dosages of 18.75 to 75 mg PO q24h was well tolerated and resulted in significant antiplatelet effects.[17,20]

Anticoagulants inhibit the generation of fibrin, but do not dissolve preexisting fibrin clots.

There are currently three anticoagulants in clinical use: warfarin, heparin, and low–molecular weight heparins.

Warfarin is a vitamin K antagonist that alters the synthesis of vitamin K–dependent clotting proteins (Factors II, VII, IX, X) and the anticoagulants, proteins C and S. Warfarin interferes with hepatic reductase activity leading to impaired post-translational carboxylation. Warfarin's anticoagulant activity is delayed (4 to 5 days) as the newly synthesized inactive clotting proteins gradually replace their functional counterparts. Warfarin is administered orally at an initial dose of 0.2 mg/kg PO q12h in dogs and 0.1 to 0.2 mg/kg PO q24h in cats. Close monitoring for dosage adjustment is essential because warfarin's anticoagulant effect is highly variable from one patient to another. Therapy is monitored based on PT, with a target prolongation to 1.5 times baseline. Due to the variability in PT reagent sensitivity, the World Health Organization has recommended that the PT be expressed as a ratio (International Normalized Ratio [INR]). The INR formula incorporates a factor (ISI) specific to each thromboplastin reagent, and is calculated as follows: INR = (patient PT/control PT)^{ISI}. An INR target range of 2 to 3 is considered optimal, without causing excessive bleeding, for most human thrombotic syndromes. INR or PT monitoring is recommended daily for the first week of warfarin therapy, twice weekly for 3 weeks, then once a week for 2 months, then every 2 months. Dose adjustments should be based on the total weekly dose. Despite close monitoring, bleeding complications commonly (20%) occur.[17]

Heparin has been the anticoagulant of choice for thromboprophylaxis and treatment of thrombosis in human and veterinary medicine. Despite its widespread use, heparin has a complex pharmacokinetic profile that produces an unpredictable anticoagulant effect. For treatment of thrombosis in people, UH is typically initiated with a bolus dose of 60 to 80 IU/kg, followed by infusion of 12 to 15 IU/kg/hr. Heparin therapy is then monitored by measurement of the PTT, with dosage adjustment to prolong values to 1.5 to 2.5 times the control value. Please consult the section on DIC for further dosing recommendations.[17]

Low–molecular weight heparins (LMWHs) are produced by depolymerization of heparin. Like heparin, LMWHs bind to AT and accelerate its inhibition of Factor Xa. LMWHs bind poorly to plasma proteins and cells and undergo first order renal clearance. The pharmacokinetics of two LMWHs and enoxaparin have been investigated in healthy dogs and cats, using anti-Xa activity to monitor anticoagulant effect. Dalteparin given to dogs at 150 U/kg q8h resulted in anti-Xa activity in the range 0.2 to 1.0 U/mL.

In contrast, the predicted dosages required to maintain anti-Xa activity at levels equal to or higher than 0.5 U/mL in cats were 150 IU/kg q4h for dalteparin and 1.5 mg/kg q6h for enoxaparin. LMWHs have the advantage of less intense monitoring and can be administered on an outpatient basis, thus facilitating thromboprophylaxis.[17]

Thrombolytic drugs are less commonly used and target the clot directly by accelerating fibrinolysis. These agents can be infused directly into the clotted vessel if given systemically. Tissue plasminogen activator, streptokinase, and urokinase have also been used with variable outcomes in veterinary patients.[18]

ACQUIRED ANTICOAGULANTS

Acquired anticoagulants or inhibitors of coagulation have been reported in humans, laboratory animals, and small animals. These circulating anticoagulants are primarily made up of immunoglobulins of the IgG class directed against one or many coagulation factors.

The presence of an inhibitor is suspected when coagulation test results do not fit the clinical image.

References

The reference list can be found on the companion Expert Consult Web site at *www.expertconsult.com*.

CHAPTER **193**

Leukocytes in Health and Disease

Marion L. Jackson

OVERVIEW OF LEUKOCYTE PRODUCTION AND KINETICS

In the dog and cat, peripheral blood leukocytes comprise granulocytes (neutrophils, eosinophils, and basophils), lymphocytes, and monocytes (Figure 193-1). Mast cells and plasma cells are not usually present in the circulation unless associated with certain inflammatory, immunologic, or neoplastic disorders. This chapter will focus on the five main leukocytes in situations of health and nonneoplastic disease; neutrophils will receive the greatest emphasis.

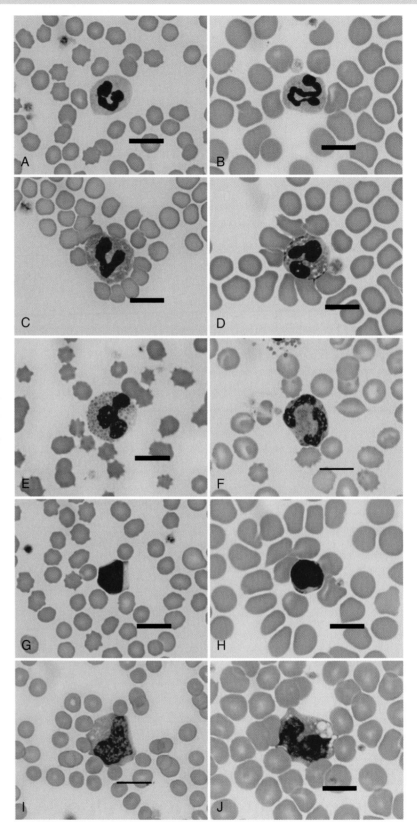

Figure 193-1 Feline and canine leukocytes. **A,** Feline neutrophil. **B,** Canine neutrophil **C,** Feline eosinophil. **D,** Canine eosinophil. **E,** Feline basophil. **F,** Canine basophil. **G,** Feline lymphocyte. **H,** Canine lymphocyte. **I,** Feline monocyte. **J,** Canine monocyte. Wright-Giemsa stain. Bar = 10 microns.

Peripheral blood leukocytes are formed in the bone marrow and occasionally in extramedullary sites, such as spleen and liver. The absolute number of leukocytes in the peripheral blood is relatively constant in health as production and loss maintain a steady state. Leukocytes respond when the body confronts invaders, tissue injury, inflammation, stress, or immunologic stimuli, and the response is often reflected in leukogram changes on the complete blood count (CBC). The leukogram includes the total white blood cell (WBC) count, the differential count (percent and absolute number) for each leukocyte type, grading of toxic change (if present) in neutrophils, and recording of any unusual leukocyte morphology.

Hemopoietic stem cells give rise to common myeloid progenitors and common lymphocyte progenitors in the bone marrow. These multilineage progenitors differentiate, through several steps, to unilineage committed progenitors under the influence of specific growth factors. These include: granulocyte colony-stimulating factor (G-CSF) for neutrophils; interleukin (IL)-5 for eosinophils; stem cell factor (SCF) for basophils; macrophage colony-stimulating factor (M-CSF) for monocytes; IL-7 and IL-2 for T lymphocytes; IL-15 for natural killer lymphocytes; and IL-4 for B lymphocytes.[1]

Granulopoiesis, the production of neutrophils, eosinophils, and basophils, takes about 6 days from hemopoietic stem cell to mature granulocyte in dogs and cats. One half of this time is spent in the proliferating/mitotic pool and the other half in the maturing/storage pool.[2,3] Studies suggest that the first cells entering the storage pool are the first to enter the peripheral circulation. Transit times can be markedly shortened with increased demand, particularly from infections.[4] Neutrophils live in the peripheral blood for about 12 hours and can survive in tissues for another 12 hours. Although the longevity of neutrophils in tissues is generally controlled by the rate of programmed cell death (apoptosis), inflammatory processes can have marked effects on survival times in tissues as well as transit times in bone marrow and peripheral blood. Senescent neutrophils are lost from mucosal surfaces, particularly in the gastrointestinal and respiratory tracts, or are phagocytosed by tissue macrophages.

Neutrophils exist in one of two compartments in the peripheral blood—the circulating pool or the marginating pool (Figure 193-2). Both compartments are freely interchangeable and about equal in size. Cells in the marginating pool travel close to the inner vessel wall and, mainly in small capillaries, roll slowly along the endothelial surface in preparation to migrate into a site of inflammation. Neutrophils in the marginating pool are also available to enter the circulating pool in response to epinephrine release or strenuous exercise. Venipuncture draws from the circulating leukocyte pool; therefore, leukogram findings represent the total number and specific leukocyte types in the circulating pool.

Neutrophils leave the circulation in a random manner, i.e., those that have just arrived from the bone marrow are as likely to exit as those that have been circulating for several hours.[4] Migration of neutrophils into sites of inflammation varies between the rich capillary bed in the lung and postcapillary venules. Physical trapping of neutrophils in small diameter capillaries is an important means of sequestering inflammatory cells, whereas, adhesion molecules are required to draw neutrophils to inflammatory sites in postcapillary venules. Inflammation normally follows a certain pattern: increased local blood flow; increased vascular permeability; and recruitment of leukocytes. Leukocytes in the marginating pool engage in low-affinity rolling interactions with the endothelium via selectins. However, with local production of inflammatory mediators, expression of complementary adhesion molecules is up-regulated on rolling leukocytes and endothelial cells.[5,6] Firm adhesion is mediated primarily by integrins, expressed on leukocyte surfaces, binding to their ligands on endothelial

cells.[7] Leukocytes then migrate between or through endothelial cells and across basement membranes toward the site of infection or injury.[8] Chemoattractants elaborated at the inflamed site are responsible for the unidirectional migration of leukocytes toward the damaged tissue. Neutrophils are usually first to arrive, followed by macrophages and lymphocytes; however, the pattern may change depending on the nature of the invader.

NEUTROPHILS AND THEIR DISORDERS

Neutrophil disorders include neutrophilia, neutropenia, and functional defects. Neutrophilia is usually a consequence of inflammation, infection, or necrosis. However, neoplastic processes (e.g., as a paraneoplastic event or primary neoplasia of neutrophils) and functional defects (e.g., canine leukocyte adhesion deficiency) can also result in neutrophilia. Changes in absolute neutrophil counts resulting from inflammation are discussed in the section Interpreting the Leukogram. In addition to acute, overwhelming inflammation, neutropenia can result from increased peripheral destruction (e.g., immune-mediated neutropenia or destruction by aberrant cell populations, usually neoplastic and non-neoplastic monocyte lineage cells)[9] or from decreased production related to bone marrow pathology (e.g., necrosis; certain viral infections, such as parvovirus and feline leukemia virus; drug reactions, such as phenobarbital[10]; toxicity, such as estrogen administration or abnormal endogenous production[11]; and myelophthisis [replacement of hemopoietic tissue in the bone marrow by abnormal tissue]).

EOSINOPHILS AND THEIR DISORDERS

Eosinophil production is influenced greatly by IL-5; as such, diseases characterized by T helper 2 (Th2) lymphocyte-mediated immune responses and excess IL-5 release may result in eosinophilia.[12] However, eosinophilia can occur in the absence of Th2 dominance, suggesting that other eosinophil mediators are responsible for eosinophil stimulation and recruitment with certain conditions. The lower reference limit for absolute canine and feline eosinophil numbers is 0 or near 0; therefore, eosinopenia is not recognized in these species and abnormalities detected on the leukogram are restricted to eosinophilia and morphologic changes. Given that the eosinophil is primarily a tissue-dwelling cell, considerable accumulation of eosinophils can occur within tissues without an accompanying eosinophilia, particularly if the process is well established and a "steady state" has been reached between bone marrow production of eosinophils and egress into the site. Eosinophilia can be associated with: allergic reactions; parasitic infections; inflammatory processes associated with release of eosinophilotropic factors; neoplasia (eosinophilic leukemia); paraneoplastic process (e.g., secondary to mast cell neoplasia or T lymphocyte neoplasia)[13]; hypoadrenocorticism; or idiopathic causes (e.g., idiopathic hypereosinophilic syndrome),[14] which can be difficult to distinguish from eosinophilic neoplasia. Morphologic changes can be seen in circulating eosinophils with increased demand, neoplasia, breed-related finding (e.g., Greyhound dogs),[15] and Pelger-Huët anomaly (discussed later).

BASOPHILS AND THEIR DISORDERS

Basopenia (or basophilopenia), like eosinopenia, is not appreciated given the lower limit of the reference interval for these cells in peripheral blood. Basophilia may accompany eosino-

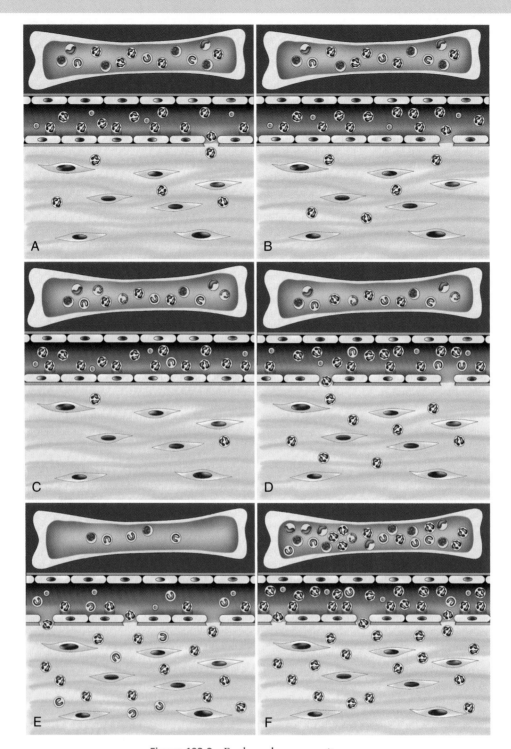

Figure 193-2   For legend, see opposite page

philia in allergic reactions and parasitic infections. Basophil numbers can also be increased with neoplasia (basophilic leukemia) or as a paraneoplastic event (e.g., mast cell tumor or other myeloproliferative disorder).

LYMPHOCYTES AND THEIR DISORDERS

Lymphopenia is one of the most common leukogram changes identified in veterinary medicine, probably because most CBCs are performed on sick animals and these animals are likely to be "stressed" and producing increased levels of endog-

enous corticosteroids. Return of lymphocyte numbers often parallels recovery in these animals, serving as a good prognostic sign. Additional causes of lymphopenia are: hereditary and acquired immunodeficiency diseases; acute viral and bacterial infections (not distinguishable from a stress response); immunosuppressive therapy and chemotherapy; and internal or external loss of lymph. Lymphocytosis should be interpreted relative to age of the animal, vaccination history, and whether the animal is clinically ill. Lymphocyte numbers that are within reference limits or increased in an ill dog suggest the possibility of a glucocorticoid deficiency. Fractious cats, or cats likely to have high levels of endogenous epinephrine for

Figure 193-2 Granulocyte kinetics. **A,** Health. About one half of the neutrophils in the peripheral blood are in the circulating pool and one half are in the marginating pool, loosely bound to endothelial receptors. **B,** Epinephrine response. Epinephrine release or administration results in decreased binding of neutrophils to endothelial receptors. The circulating neutrophil pool expands as a result of decreased neutrophil margination. **C,** Corticosteroid/stress response. Corticosteroid administration or increased endogenous production causes neutrophilia in three ways: release of neutrophils and sometimes bands from the storage marrow pool is increased; neutrophils move from the marginating pool to the circulating pool in the peripheral blood; and decreased migration of neutrophils into tissues occurs. **D,** Acute mild inflammation. Peripheral blood findings are highly variable depending on the nature of the inflammation. This figure demonstrates increased release of neutrophils and low numbers of bands from the marrow, as well as increased migration into tissues. Neutrophilia accompanied by a mild left shift would be expected on the leukogram. **E,** Acute, overwhelming inflammation. The tissue demand for neutrophils is high resulting in depletion of the storage pool in the bone marrow. Immature neutrophils, including bands and sometimes metamyelocytes and myelocytes, are also released into the peripheral blood resulting in a severe left shift. Absolute neutrophil numbers in peripheral blood may be within reference limits or below reference limits due to the marked egress into tissue sites. **F,** Chronic inflammation. Although there is high tissue demand for neutrophils, the bone marrow has had sufficient time to respond to the need. Neutrophil hyperplasia occurs in the bone marrow and moderate/marked neutrophilia, possibly accompanied by a mild/moderate left shift, would be expected on the leukogram. (Courtesy Dr. Juliane Deubner, Medical Illustrator, Western College of Veterinary Medicine, University of Saskatchewan.)

any reason, may have transient lymphocytosis that relates to circumstances around the time of venipuncture. A follow-up CBC when the cat is more relaxed can aid in differentiating epinephrine-induced lymphocytosis from other causes of lymphocytosis. Additional causes of lymphocytosis include chronic antigenic stimulation, recent vaccination, and neoplasia. Morphologic features sometimes aid in differentiating neoplastic and nonneoplastic lymphocyte disorders; however, there is considerable overlap between features of reactive/immunologically stimulated lymphocytes and neoplastic lymphocytes.

MONOCYTES AND THEIR DISORDERS

Similar to eosinophils and basophils, the lower reference limit for canine and feline monocyte numbers in peripheral blood is 0 or close to 0, so monocytopenia may be undetectable. Monocytosis can accompany a stress/corticosteroid response and can also be seen with inflammation. Monocytosis is expected with, but not restricted to, inflammatory processes requiring considerable phagocytic activity (e.g., immune-mediated hemolytic anemia or extensive necrosis); chronic situations; and those caused by foreign material or organisms that elicit granulomatous or pyogranulomatous inflammation. Monocytosis accompanied by cytopenias of other hemopoietic cell lines and aggressive phagocytosis of hemopoietic cells in peripheral blood, bone marrow, or other tissues could indicate monocyte neoplasia or hemophagocytic syndrome, a nonneoplastic proliferation of histiocytes.[16]

INTERPRETING THE LEUKOGRAM

Excitement can lead to epinephrine release and movement of neutrophils from the marginating pool to the circulating pool (see Figure 193-2). The net result of this shift is a relative increase in total WBC count attributable to an increase in the number of mature neutrophils. However, an epinephrine response does not necessarily produce an absolute neutrophilia since reference intervals have likely been established under similar circumstances.

Chronic or acute illness, pain, trauma, or other disturbance in homeostasis, may result in increased production of endogenous corticosteroids and a "stress" leukogram. The classic stress leukogram comprises neutrophilia, lymphopenia, and monocytosis. However, lymphopenia is the most consistent leukogram finding with stress, and is caused by altered movement of lymphocytes between the peripheral blood and lymph nodes, bone marrow, and other lymphocyte-rich tissues,[17,18] coupled with lymphocyte lysis over the longer term. Whether neutrophilia and monocytosis also accompany a stress lymphopenia, may be dependent on the degree of corticosteroid elevation, duration, species, and presence or absence of concurrent illness. Corticosteroids may affect neutrophil kinetics as follows: increased release from bone marrow; decreased margination in peripheral blood; and decreased migration into tissues (see Figure 193-2). Together, these result in neutrophilia, as noted on the CBC. Occasionally low numbers of band neutrophils are released from the bone marrow as well as mature neutrophils with stress. Administration of exogenous corticosteroids produces leukogram changes similar to the innate stress response, but may be more exaggerated and, therefore, more difficult to distinguish from an inflammatory leukogram. Additional clinical information and monitoring the leukogram over time are useful in differentiating these processes.

Exposure to lipopolysaccharide (LPS), a component of the cell wall of gram-negative bacteria, can result in endotoxemia. Endotoxemia causes widespread activation of inflammatory responses, sometimes leading to shock, organ failure, and suppression of wound healing processes.[19] Neutrophils have heightened oxidative burst potential, become hyperadhesive to endothelium, and are unable to migrate across vascular endothelium into tissues to counter-invading organisms. Results are generalized endothelial damage, neutropenia, and thrombocytopenia on CBC results, and indicators of organ failure on additional laboratory tests.

Inflammation produces myriad leukogram changes reflecting the severity, extent of tissue involvement, duration, and offending agent. A grass awn lodged between the digits causes pustule formation and considerable discomfort, but is unlikely to result in leukogram abnormalities. The same grass awn migrating through the lung parenchyma may cause extensive tissue damage and inflammation, marked systemic effects, and usually severe leukogram changes.

The duration of the inflammation usually cannot be determined based on leukogram changes alone. Exceptions are acute, overwhelming inflammation and severe chronic inflammation. Most of the leukograms that clinical pathologists and clinicians confront are neither of these; therefore, establishing a timeframe is not possible. Acute mild inflammation can result in neutrophilia with a mild left shift (see Figure 193-2); however, leukograms representing recovery from acute, overwhelming inflammation and chronic inflammation can be identical at certain points in the process. Anatomic pathologists are better able to assess duration of inflammatory processes because the tissues being examined are the focal point of the reaction. Sampling the peripheral blood provides a window into only one component of a dynamic process. It is helpful to embrace the concept of this dynamic situation and consider the bone marrow and tissue environments when interpreting leukogram changes.

Acute, overwhelming inflammation as might occur with septic peritonitis caused by bowel perforation, would be expected to quickly deplete the peripheral blood of its neutrophils and the bone marrow of its postmitotic pool of neutrophils and bands (see Figure 193-2). Although neutrophil production is accelerated as a result of increased demand, the bone marrow is unable to meet these needs in the short term. The rapid movement of neutrophils into an extensive site of inflammation can result in a WBC count that is within reference intervals (WRI) or decreased. The leukocyte differential count is particularly important in these situations as immature neutrophilic granulocytes may equal or surpass the number of mature neutrophils, a situation that alerts the clinician to the fact that the inflammation is acute and overwhelming, and the bone marrow is not yet responding adequately to the tissue damage or infection. This left shift (presence of immature neutrophilic granulocytes in the peripheral blood) can be called degenerative if the absolute number of mature neutrophils is within or below the reference interval and immature neutrophilic granulocytes (e.g., bands, metamyelocytes, myelocytes) equal or surpass the mature stages in number. Toxic change is often recognized within mature and immature neutrophil cytoplasms in this situation (Web Figure 193-1).

Toxic change results from accelerated granulopoiesis and is characterized by any of the following cytoplasmic changes: retention of primary, azurophilic granules; blue granularity due to ribosome retention; vacuolation; and Döhle bodies, which are deposits of rough endoplasmic reticulum. Although these features can occur in any combination, often the type of toxic change that is present is relatively consistent within that sample. Evaluation of canine and feline blood smears for toxic change in neutrophils provides useful clinical information and aids in prognostication.[20,21]

Severe inflammation of longer duration than the situation of acute bowel perforation described above may be characterized by a severe left shift. However, the total leukocyte count is often increased due to increased mature and immature neutrophilic granulocytes. Pyometra is an example of such a pathologic process. Although there is a severe left shift suggesting the bone marrow is not entirely capable of meeting the demands for neutrophils, bone marrow examination would reveal granulocytic hyperplasia. Also, when the focus of tissue demand, the uterus in this example, is removed, a marked rebound neutrophilia is often seen and several days may pass before neutrophils return to normal numbers and immature neutrophils disappear from the peripheral circulation.

Chronic inflammatory processes can produce variable leukogram changes reflecting the nature of the offending agent, the surface area involved, and the host response. Moderate to severe neutrophilia, with a mild or no left shift and moderate to marked monocytosis, are the classic findings with chronic inflammation (see Figure 193-2). However, a long-standing, well–walled-off abscess may produce subtle to no leukogram changes.

Monitoring the leukogram over time can be useful to assess the significance of abnormalities and to predict whether problems are ongoing or resolving. Bone marrow examination is indicated when there are unexplained and persistent leukogram changes. For example, neutropenia without a left shift or toxic change is not usually explained by an inflammatory process. Mild neutropenia could represent normal fluctuation in a clinically healthy animal. However, persistent moderate to severe neutropenia may signal bone marrow pathology.

LEUKOCYTE MORPHOLOGY OR FUNCTION ABNORMALITIES

Canine Leukocyte Adhesion Deficiency
Canine leukocyte adhesion deficiency (CLAD) is a rare hereditary disease affecting Irish Setter dogs, Irish Setter–cross dogs and Irish Red and White Setter dogs.[22,23] The disease is characterized by recurrent bacterial infections beginning shortly after birth, often including omphalophlebitis, gingivitis, and pyoderma. The marked leukocytosis seen on CBC is due to the inability of neutrophils to adhere to and transmigrate the vascular endothelium, migrate to infection sites in tissues, and phagocytose bacteria. The defect is caused by a missense mutation in the gene encoding β-2 integrin, the CD18 subunit of several heterodimeric leukocyte adhesion proteins. The single missense mutation in the ITGB2 gene encoding CD18, is a guanine to cytosine transversion at position 107 resulting in the replacement of cysteine with serine at residue 36 in the protein (C36S). Genetic testing supports a worldwide distribution of this mutation in Irish Setter dogs. As an autosomal recessive inherited disease, carrier dogs are not clinically affected whereas homozygotes for the mutation experience serious infections that significantly shorten their lives even with antibiotic therapy and other supportive care. Genetic testing involves polymerase chain reaction (PCR) amplification of the gene followed by restriction enzyme digestion. The mutation changes the restriction site allowing identification of carrier (heterozygous for the mutation) and affected (homozygous for the mutation) animals.[24] The disease has been successfully treated using a foamy virus vector expressing canine CD18.[25]

Chédiak-Higashi Syndrome
Chédiak-Higashi syndrome is a rare autosomal recessive condition reported in several species, including Blue Smoke Persian cats.[26] The syndrome is characterized by hypopigmentation of skin, eyes, and hair; superficial bleeding; and variable susceptibility to infections. Large peroxidase-positive cytoplasmic granules containing lysosomal enzymes are present in most nucleated cells, including neutrophils (Web Figure 193-2).

Chédiak-Higashi syndrome is considered to be a lysosomal storage disorder caused by mutation of the lysosomal trafficking gene (LYST).[27,28] Accumulation and lack of mobilization of lysosomal granule contents in melanocytes, neutrophils, natural killer lymphocytes, and platelets are responsible for cell dysfunction and corresponding clinical signs.

Cyclic Hemopoiesis
Cyclic hemopoiesis is a rare stem cell disorder with autosomal recessive inheritance in gray Collie dogs. Affected dogs experience cyclic fluctuations in production of all hemopoietic

cells and maturation arrest and apoptosis of developing marrow cells at the onset of neutropenia.[29] Neutrophil numbers decline every 10 to 12 days, followed by rebound. Increased susceptibility to infections correlates with episodes of neutropenia. Mutation of AP3B1, the gene encoding adaptor protein complex 3 β-subunit, is responsible for the disease in dogs, resulting in near undetectable levels of the protein. This protein is required for trafficking of neutrophil elastase into the primary granules of neutrophils.[30,31] Carrier and affected dogs can be detected with DNA-based testing and G-CSF is an effective long-term treatment.[31,32]

Neutrophil Anomaly of Birman Cats

An inherited anomaly of neutrophil granulation and staining has been identified in Birman cats as an autosomal recessive trait.[33] Affected cats are clinically healthy but their neutrophils contain reddish-purple cytoplasmic granules with Romanowsky stains (Web Figure 193-3), similar to primary granules of progranulocytes. Granules do not stain with alcian blue or toluidine blue dyes, ruling out accumulation of mucopolysaccharide. The anomaly is thought to represent alteration in the content of lysosomal granules resulting in increased affinity for acidic dyes. The trait was prevalent in a survey of Birman cats.

Pelger-Huët Anomaly

Pelger-Huët anomaly is an inherited disorder of leukocyte and megakaryocyte development that has been identified in many species, including dogs and cats.[34-36] The characteristic finding in neutrophils, eosinophils, and basophils is hyposegmentation of the nucleus, but chromatin is coarse and clumped and cytoplasmic features are normal (Web Figure 193-4).

Nuclei are bilobed, dumbbell-shaped, band-shaped, or round; female dogs lack Barr bodies or sex chromatin "drumsticks" in circulating granulocytes. The anomaly has been reported in several purebred and mixed breed dogs and had a 9.8% incidence in a study of Australian Shepherd dogs.[37] The disorder is probably inherited as an autosomal dominant trait with incomplete penetrance in the Australian Shepherd breed. Heterozygotes for the anomaly are clinically healthy and neutrophil function is normal. Homozygosity may be lethal in utero and there is one report of homozygous Pelger-Huët anomaly and chondrodysplasia in a stillborn kitten.[38] Six related Samoyed dogs were reported to have hematologic abnormalities with similarities to Pelger-Huët anomaly. Findings were hyposegmentation of eosinophils and scarcity of Barr bodies in female dogs. These dogs also had ocular and skeletal abnormalities leading to the possibility of a multifaceted hereditary disorder.[39] In human Pelger-Huët anomaly, mutations in the gene for lamin B receptor have been identified; this receptor targets heterochromatin and lamins to the nuclear membrane.[40] The genetic basis of the anomaly has not been determined in animals. Although not of clinical significance in heterozygotes, peripheral blood findings can initially be misinterpreted as a severe left shift suggestive of inflammation. The lack of cytoplasmic abnormalities (toxic change) in neutrophils and persistence of the abnormal nuclear features in the healthy animal help to distinguish between inflammation and Pelger-Huët anomaly. Transient hyposegmentation of leukocytes, sometimes referred to as pseudo-Pelger-Huët anomaly, may occur with inflammation, neoplasia, or drug therapy and can usually be differentiated from Pelger-Huët anomaly by monitoring of the CBC and identifying an underlying condition.

Neutrophil Function Defects

Neutrophil function defects have been reported in eight closely related Doberman Pinscher dogs.[41] Affected dogs experienced chronic rhinitis and pneumonia. Neutrophils were morphologically normal but had impaired bactericidal ability that may have been related to an inability to generate oxygen radicals normally upon stimulation. Neutrophil functional abnormalities have also been identified in Weimaraner dogs.[42,43] Affected dogs had a variety of clinical signs including fever, depression, pneumonia, stomatitis, osteomyelitis, vomiting, diarrhea, joint pain, conjunctivitis, and pyoderma. Although neutrophil function defects were not identified in one group of dogs,[42] abnormal neutrophil chemiluminescence was identified in another study.[43] The exact nature of these defects has not been further elucidated.

Lysosomal Storage Diseases

Naturally occurring lysosomal storage diseases are reported in animals, and although affected cats and dogs may appear healthy at birth, the progressive accumulation of nondegraded substrate in lysosomes can lead to skeletal abnormalities, growth retardation, organomegaly, and visual defects.[44,45] The presence of abnormal cytoplasmic granules or vacuoles in peripheral blood leukocytes is suggestive of one of many types of lysosomal storage diseases. These diseases include, but are not restricted to: glycoproteinoses (fucosidosis; mannosidosis); oligosaccharidoses; sphingolipidoses (GM_1 and GM_2 gangliosidosis, Gaucher disease, globoid cell leukodystrophy, Niemann-Pick disease); mucopolysaccharidosis (MPS I, II, III, VI, VII); and the proteinoses (ceroid lipofuscinosis).[45] The mucopolysaccharidoses are inherited lysosomal storage diseases caused by deficiency of one of several glycosaminoglycan (GAG)-degrading enzymes. Each disease has a characteristic phenotype and urinary GAG excretion profile.[46] Granules representing accumulated GAG in leukocytes appear as eosinophilic cytoplasmic deposits with Romanowsky stains (Web Figure 193-5) and stain metachromatically with toluidine blue and alcian blue. GM_1-gangliosidosis is caused by an enzyme defect leading to lysosomal accumulation of GM_1-ganglioside and other galactose-containing glycoconjugates.[47] Vacuolated lymphocytes can be seen in peripheral blood of dogs and cats with GM_1-gangliosidosis (Web Figure 193-6).

GM_2-gangliosidosis results in accumulation of GM_2-ganglioside and related glycolipids in lysosomes, especially in neurons.[48] Pink granules can be seen in neutrophils and lymphocytes of dogs and cats with GM_2-gangliosidosis (Web Figure 193-7).

Specific metabolic, enzymatic, or molecular evaluation is needed to diagnose these storage diseases. For those diseases with known mutations in the gene encoding the defective enzyme, DNA-based testing is available. Genetic studies indicate that most of these diseases are inherited as an autosomal recessive trait.[49]

Infectious Agents as Inclusions in Peripheral Blood Leukocytes

Thorough peripheral blood smear evaluation may provide an etiologic diagnosis when disease is caused by certain viral, bacterial, yeast, or parasitic organisms. Such examples include canine distemper virus inclusion bodies in neutrophils and erythrocytes; bacterial infections resulting in bacteremia or septicemia; *Anaplasma phagocytophilium* infection in dogs; *Histoplasma capsulatum* yeast infections; and *Hepatozoon americanum*, an apicomplexan parasite (Web Figure 193-8).

Miscellaneous Leukocytes and Leukocyte Morphology

In addition to peripheral blood leukocytes of normal morphology, the following may be encountered: hypersegmented neutrophils, from sample aging, corticosteroid influence, or administration of certain drugs; canine eosinophils devoid

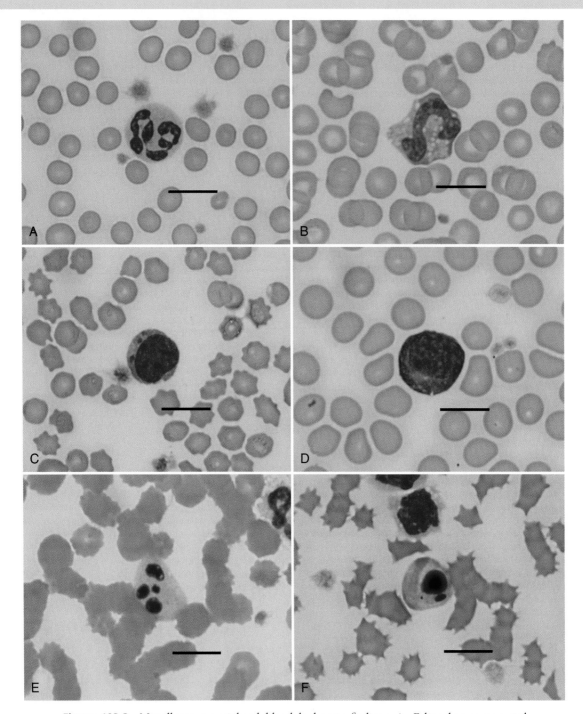

Figure 193-3 Miscellaneous peripheral blood leukocyte findings. **A,** Feline hypersegmented neutrophil. **B,** Eosinophil from a Greyhound dog. Note lack of granule staining. **C,** Feline large granular lymphocyte. **D,** Canine reactive lymphocyte. **E,** Canine apoptotic (pyknotic) cell—probably a neutrophil. **F,** Feline apoptotic (pyknotic) cell—probably a neutrophil. Wright-Giemsa stain. Bar = 10 microns.

of eosinophilic-staining granules commonly seen in Greyhound dogs; lymphocytes with large magenta cytoplasmic granules—large granular lymphocytes representing natural killer cells, cytotoxic T cells, or a neoplastic lymphocyte population; large, darkly staining lymphocytes indicating an immunologically stimulated state (reactive lymphocytes) or neoplasia; and cells undergoing apoptosis or pyknosis, which is usually due to aging of the sample prior to smear preparation (Figure 193-3).

See Figure 193-4, an algorithm depicting quantitative and qualitative peripheral blood leukocyte abnormalities.

REFERENCES

The reference list can be found on the companion Expert Consult Web site at *www.expertconsult.com.*

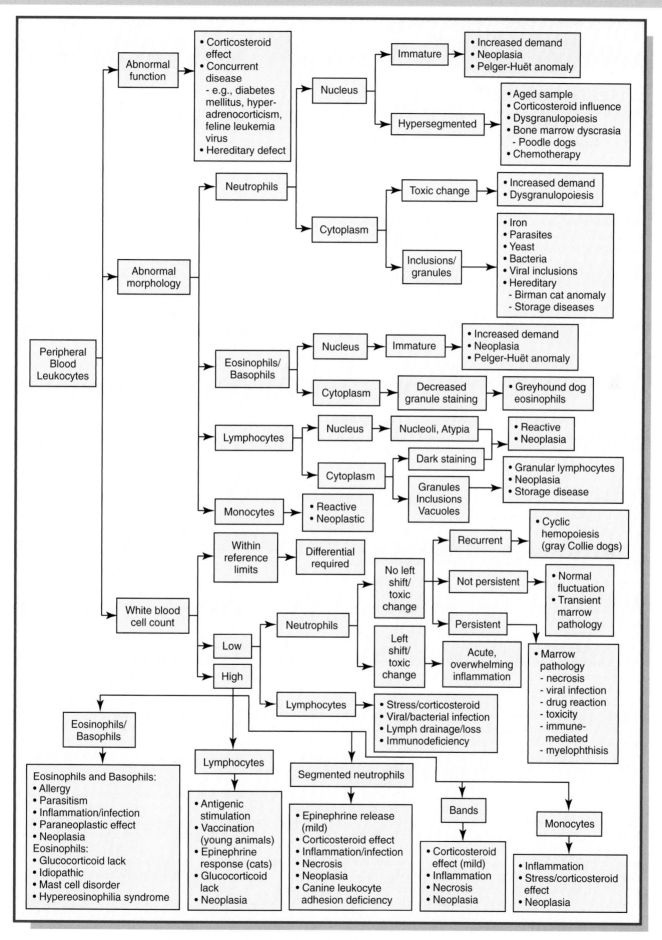

Figure 193-4 Algorithm of peripheral blood leukocyte abnormalities.

CHAPTER 194

Diseases of the Spleen

Helio Autran de Morais
David J. Argyle
Robert T. O'Brien

"Spleen is like the tongue of an ox [or] the sole of the foot; slightly bowed out on the left side, a little concave on the inner side, toward the stomach. It has an uneven surface and is a little rough with some tubercles ..."

"Similarly [according to] other physicians the spleen [is] the receptacle of melancholy as the gall bladder of gall; wherefore the spleen causes one to laugh."

William Harvey, Lectures on the Whole of Anatomy (1653)

For many years, the ability to laugh was for long considered a sign that the spleen was working well. Regarded as the repository of the most noxious substance of the body—black bile (in Greek: *melanos kholis*), the spleen prevented the onset of melancholia by containing the bodily fluid that produced this mental state. Understanding of the spleen has greatly improved over the last several centuries. However, clinical evaluation of this organ remains mostly morphologic, based on palpation, radiographs, and especially ultrasound examination, followed by cytology or histopathology. No biochemical tests have been designed to assess splenic function. Consequently, although splenomegaly is common in clinical practice, it is often hard to isolate the cause.

PREVALENCE

Prevalence of spleen disorders cannot be easily estimated in dogs and cats. Splenomegaly can be asymptomatic, and in the absence of splenomegaly, it is difficult to determine, on the basis of clinical signs, that the spleen is responsible for the animal's condition. Most prevalence studies in dogs and cats are based either on necropsy or biopsies. Necropsy-based studies overestimate diseases with poor prognosis or with no clinical relevance. Diseases that are treated by surgery are overestimated in prevalence studies based on biopsies, but are underestimated in prevalence studies based on necropsy data. This might explain the absence of hemangiosarcoma and the low ratio hemangiosarcoma/hematoma found in necropsy studies in dogs. Based on biopsies submitted to regional diagnostic laboratory from 1372 dogs[1] and 455 cats,[2] spleen samples from dogs represented 1.3% of all submissions to the laboratory, whereas spleen samples from cats represented 0.3%. However, these percentages do not represent true prevalence, because biopsies from all species were included in the total submission number.[1]

In two necropsy surveys, nonneoplastic diseases represented approximately 50% of feline splenic disorders.[2,3] Congestion, lymphoid hyperplasia, capsulitis, extramedullary hematopoiesis, and hyperplastic nodules accounted for more than 50% of the cats with nonneoplastic splenic disease. Unfortunately, those were pathologic descriptions with the underlying disease not apparent in many cases. In two retrospective studies that looked at prevalence of arrhythmias in

dogs with splenic masses,[4,5] hematomas were found in 17%[5] to 44%[4] of the cases. In a prospective study that looked at prevalence of arrhythmias in dogs undergoing splenectomy, 38% of the dogs had neoplasia and 32% had hematomas.[6] Nodular hyperplasia, immune-mediated disease unresponsive to medical therapy, and splenic torsion each accounted for 10% of the cases. Nodular hyperplasia, hematoma, extramedullary hematopoiesis, congestion, and lymphoid hyperplasia were the most common nonneoplastic lesions found in the spleen of dogs at necropsy or biopsies.[1,7-9] In a lifetime study of Beagles chronically exposed to radioactive radium and strontium, splenic abnormalities were present in 105 of the 865 dogs. Hyperplastic nodules with or without hematoma, and diffuse lymphoreticular hyperplasia accounted for 66% of the splenomegalies found in these dogs.

Thus, the ratio of nonneoplastic to neoplastic splenic disease in dogs varies among studies. Populations that included all cases of splenomegaly or masses,[1,8] show a higher than 50% prevalence of nonneoplastic diseases. A higher prevalence of tumors is found in populations submitted to splenectomy[6,9] and in dogs with splenic masses and arrhythmias.[4,5] Nonneoplastic masses, therefore, are as common as neoplastic masses in the spleen of dogs.

CLINICAL MANIFESTATIONS

Owner complaints for dogs and cats with splenic disorders are usually vague, and these signs may arise from the underlying disease. Common complaints include vomiting, anorexia, weakness, collapse, abdominal enlargement, and weight loss. Polyuria and polydipsia may occur; the mechanism is unclear, but it resolves after splenectomy. Clinical signs are usually related to abdominal distention from a mass, uniform splenomegaly or intraabdominal bleeding. Lethargy and collapse may occur due to hypovolemia, arrhythmias, or anemia.

Signs related to the underlying disorder may also be present (Box 194-1). Ventricular tachyarrhythmias appear to be highly prevalent in dogs with splenic masses (hematoma, hemangiosarcoma or leiomyosarcoma),[4-6] particularly if the mass has ruptured.[6] Dogs subjected to splenectomy, regardless of the reason, are also prone to arrhythmias during and after surgery.[6]

The most reliable clinical sign of splenic disease is palpable splenomegaly. However, not all splenomegalies are abnormal. Breed variations in spleen size exist, particularly in dogs. German Shepherds have larger spleens; in some other breeds (e.g., Miniature Schnauzer, Cocker Spaniel, Greyhounds) have the spleen located more caudally in the abdomen and may be perceived as enlarged under palpation.[10] It is important to remember that not all enlarged spleens are palpable.

The major laboratory abnormalities accompanying splenic disease are related to the underlying systemic illness. Changes in blood cell counts may be due to the primary disease or

Box • 194-1

Clinical Signs of Splenic Disease in Dogs and Cats

Abdominal distention
    Splenomegaly
    Splenic mass*
    Intraabdominal bleeding*
Arrhythmias
Nonspecific signs and signs of the underlying disorder
    Lethargy
    Weakness
    Collapse
    Anorexia
    Pu-Pd
    Diarrhea
    Pale mucous membranes
    Jaundice

*Signs suggestive of tumors.

caused by the abnormal spleen. Erythrocyte counts are usually normal or decreased, but can be increased in patients with splenomegaly associated with polycythemia vera.[11] Schistocytosis, which is highly indicative of a neoplastic splenic disorder, was observed in 23% of patients with splenic tumors, but only in 3% of dogs with nonneoplastic disease.[9] Granulocyte and platelet counts also can be decreased, normal, or increased.

Extramedullary hematopoiesis can occur in the spleen. Because the spleen maintains the ability for hematopoiesis but does not retain the normal inhibitory mechanisms present in the bone marrow, it releases young blood cells into the circulation.[12] Increases in nucleated red blood cells and immature white blood cells (leukoerythroblastic effect) may appear in the peripheral blood in patients with splenic disorders.

DIAGNOSTIC APPROACH

Splenomegaly can be detected by physical examination or by abdominal radiographs or ultrasound. Although splenomegaly can be identified during palpation, the severity of the enlargement cannot be reliably assessed in dogs with this technique alone. Differentiating between a splenic mass (localized splenomegaly with at least one large mass) and diffuse splenomegaly (uniform enlargement of the spleen) helps to narrow the number of potential diagnoses (Box 194-2). Fine needle aspiration of the spleen may provide the final diagnosis or characterize the type of inflammation present. A sequential approach to diagnose the origin of splenomegaly is shown in Figure 194-1.

Abdominal Radiography
Radiographically, the spleen is apparent in both the dog and cat. The dorsal extremity (head) is commonly seen on ventrodorsal projections in the cranial left abdomen caudal to the gastric fundus and cranial to the left kidney along the left body wall. On this projection, the splenic head is triangularly shaped. The body of the spleen may be directed transversely across the abdomen immediately caudal to the stomach, along the left body wall, or anywhere in between. In dogs, the ventral aspect (tail) is often seen along the ventral body wall immediately caudal to the liver in the lateral projection. Dis-

tension of the stomach may caudally displace the tail. The tail of the spleen is uncommonly seen in cats.

Generalized splenomegaly may increase splenic length. The spleen may also fold up from the ventral wall, extending to varying lengths up the right body wall or expand more caudally towards the urinary bladder. In the cat, visualization of the splenic tail along the ventral body wall supports a diagnosis of splenomegaly. Alternatively, with generalized enlargement or focal masses, the spleen produces a mass effect, displacing the intestines caudally. The spleen is a very common origin for masses in the midcranial and left cranial abdomen. Atypical splenic location, with changes in shape, may occur in dogs with splenic torsion. Concurrent peritoneal effusion is common. Lesions rarely cause changes in splenic radiopacity.

Abdominal Ultrasonography
Ultrasonography is a very effective tool for evaluation of the size, shape, and vascular supply of the spleen. There are no objective criteria for normal splenic size. As a rule, cats have much smaller spleens than dogs of similar size. Normal variations in dogs include capsular invagination (hyperechoic foci adjacent to splenic veins), a bent spleen, or a portion folded back upon itself. Generalized isoechoic enlargement may be a normal variation in German Shepherd and other dog breeds, and in some cats. Overall spleen length and evidence of intestinal displacement are the criteria used to assess for splenomegaly. A true decrease in splenic size (microsplenia) may occur with acute anemia due to contraction of the spleen. Ultrasonography is more sensitive than radiography for detecting alterations in the shape and outer margination of the spleen. Irregularities in shape and focal changes in echogenicity are the major criteria for characterization of splenic disease in dogs and cats.

Nodular disease is easily detected in the middle and tail regions of the spleen. Often the head of the spleen is within the rib cage, and masses in the dorsal extremity may require a rigorous examination with an intercostal approach. Benign masses may be hypoechoic, hyperechoic, or mixed echoic. Benign masses cannot be differentiated from malignant masses solely based on gray-scale ultrasonography. Extramedullary hematopoiesis and nodular hyperplasia (Figure 194-2), which are common regenerative lesions, are usually hypoechoic and are seen in the spleen of older dogs. These lesions are much less common in cats.

Certain lesions have a more characteristic sonographic appearance. Myelolipoma, a benign tumor seen in older dogs, is both very echogenic and attenuating. The result is a classic hyperechoic and indistinctly shadowing lesion (Figure 194-3). Unlike with mineralization, the attenuation is not complete, and the internal architecture of the lesion can be seen to varying depths.

The spleen has a high prevalence for vascular disease, because it is attached at only one pole and is prone to harbor diffuse neoplasia. Splenic torsion and diffuse tumor invasion may result in uniform diffuse hypoechogenicity or a more mixed "Swiss cheese" appearance (Figure 194-4). Doppler examination of the splenic veins is an important step to verify lack of venous return. As with portal vein flow, splenic venous flow is low velocity and essentially nonpulsatile. Power Doppler is especially valuable as this modality is more sensitive to very low velocity flow. Thrombosis may occur after mechanical torsion, tumor vascular invasion, or thromboembolic diseases. Regional infarctions are commonly seen in dogs with disseminated intravascular coagulation (DIC) and autoimmune conditions, such as immune-mediated hemolytic anemia and immune-mediated thrombocytopenia. Infarcted regions are usually peripheral, hypoechoic, and swollen (Figure 194-5). Necrosis may be seen with chronic severe

Box • 194-2

Causes of Splenomegaly in Dogs and Cats

Splenic mass (asymmetric or nonuniform splenomegaly)
  Nodular hyperplasia
    Lymphoid*
      Fibrohistiocytic (D)
  Hematoma*
  Malignant tumors*
    Hemangiosarcoma*
    Fibrosarcoma
    Leiomyosarcoma
    Histiocytic sarcoma
    Metastatic disease
  Benign tumors
    Hemangioma
    Myelolipoma
  Abscess
  Extramedullary hematopoiesis (C)
  Granuloma
Uniform (symmetric)
  Congestion
    Drugs*
    Portal hypertension*
    Right-sided congestive heart failure*
    Splenic torsion
Hyperplasia†
  Chronic infection*
  Inflammatory bowel disease
  Systemic lupus erythematosus
  Polycythemia vera
Extramedullary hematopoiesis†
  Chronic anemia*
  Immune-mediated hemolytic anemia*
  Immune-mediated thrombocytopenia*
Neoplasia
  Neoplastic infiltrative diseases
  Lymphoma*
  Leukemias*
    Multiple myeloma
    Primary erythrocytosis (polycythemia vera)
    Primary mast cell tumor (C)
    Metastatic mast cell tumor
    Disseminated malignant histiocytosis

Nonneoplastic infiltrative diseases
  Hypereosinophilic syndrome (C)
  Amyloidosis
Inflammatory‡
  Suppurative
    Sepsis*
    Bacterial endocarditis*
    Infectious canine hepatitis
    Toxoplasmosis
    Foreign body
    Penetrating wounds
    Tumors
Granulomatous
  Cryptococcosis
  Histoplasmosis (C)
  Mycobacteriosis
  Leishmaniasis
Pyogranulomatous
  Feline infectious peritonitis* (C)
  Blastomycosis
  Sporotrichosis
Eosinophilic
  Eosinophilic gastroenteritis
  Hypereosinophilic syndrome (C)
  Tumors
Lymphoplasmacytic
  Ehrlichiosis*
  Anaplasmosis*
  Hemotropic mycoplasmosis* (C)
  Lymphoplasmacytic enteritis*
  Pyometra
  Brucellosis
Necrotic tissue
  Torsion
  Necrotic center of neoplasms
  Infectious canine hepatitis (D)
  Anaerobic infection
  Tularemia
  Systemic calicivirosis (C)
  Salmonellosis

C, Cats. D, Dogs.
*More common diseases.
†The causes of extramedullary hematopoiesis and hyperplasia can overlap.
‡The typical inflammatory response for each organism; some degree of overlap exists.

vascular disease and result in formation of free gas in the spleen and free fluid in the peritoneum.

An additional ultrasound modality for evaluation of focal nodular and vascular diseases of the spleen is contrast harmonic ultrasound. Second generation ultrasound contrast agents are liposome encapsulated inert gas spheres that are injected intravenously and small enough (3 to 5 μm) to pass through the pulmonary circulation without embolization. Harmonic ultresound software technology allows detection of sound waves that are multiples of the transmitted frequency. Ultrasound contrast bubbles are very powerful generators of

harmonic frequencies, and, combined with tissue signal suppression, they create a novel method to image perfusion of organs. These contrast media, which can be used as blood pool agents, will cause infarcted regions to appear hypoechoic compared to the surrounding normally perfused spleen. Preliminary studies indicate that ultrasound contrast agents may help discriminate between malignant and benign masses by exploiting differences in blood supply. Hemangiosarcomas have very poor overall perfusion with distinct peripheral vessels. This perfusion pattern has been noted in hemangiosarcoma masses in the liver, lung, peritoneum, and the spleen. In the liver,

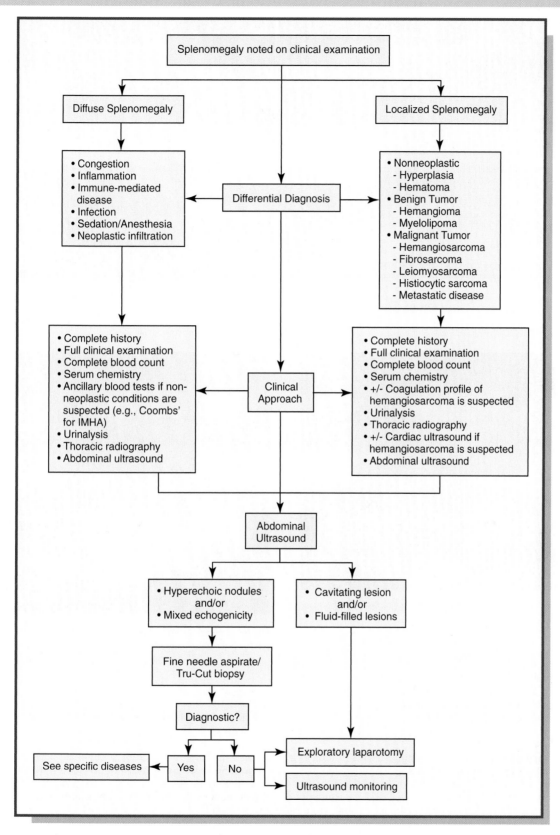

Figure 194-1 Diagnostic approach to a patient with splenomegaly. *IMHA,* Immune-mediated hemolytic anemia.

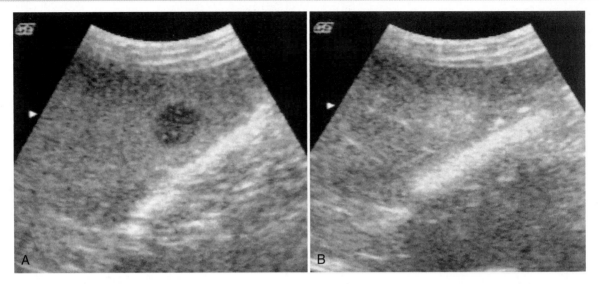

Figure 194-2 Nodular hyperplasia. Note the contrast enhancement pattern on precontrast (**A**) and postcontrast (**B**) images.

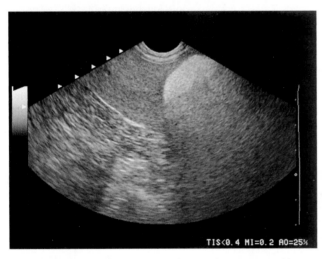

Figure 194-3 Myelolipoma. Note hyperechogenicity and hyperattenuation pattern.

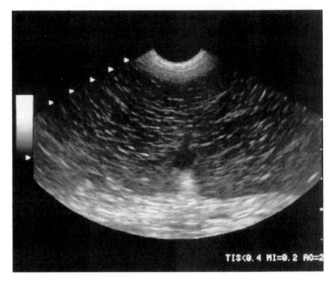

Figure 194-4 Splenic torsion. Note "Swiss cheese" echogenic pattern of splenic necrosis.

metastatic nodules have a more rapid wash-in and wash-out compared to normal liver or benign liver nodules. Benign nodular hyperplastic nodules in the spleen have good overall perfusion.

Fine Needle Aspiration

Although imaging of the spleen only rarely results in a diagnosis, an aspirate may provide a cytologic sample and the answer. Core biopsy is possible, but not usually necessary. Most diseases of the spleen exfoliate well and are suitably sampled with fine needle techniques. Splenic aspirates correctly identified the underlying problem in over 60% of cases in one study. Incorrect diagnosis occurred in 15% of the cases, and histopathology was required to distinguish between neoplastic and reactive conditions in 22% of the cases.[13] Of the fine needle techniques, the variation that seems to provide the most cells without undue hemodilution involves no negative pressure with the attached syringe and multiple thrusting motions with the needle. With the plunger already pulled

back in the barrel of the syringe prior to insertion of the needle, it thereafter is easy to expel the content of the needle by depressing the plunger. This technique works well for nodular hyperplasia and extramedullary hematopoiesis–benign nodules, metastatic carcinomas, and hematopoietic tumors. Solid sarcomas may not exfoliate well with aspiration techniques and a core sample may provide a better result. Cavitated lesions should only be sampled with the utmost care, if at all.

Fine needle aspiration appears to be safe even in presence of coagulopathies or thrombocytopenia.[14] As a general rule, all abnormal spleens that do not have cavitated lesions should be aspirated. Aspiration is not necessary in patients with splenic torsion whenever lack of adequate blood flow can be determined by Doppler ultrasonography, or in patients with myelolipoma if only lesions with the classic acoustic properties are present. Aspiration also may not be required for

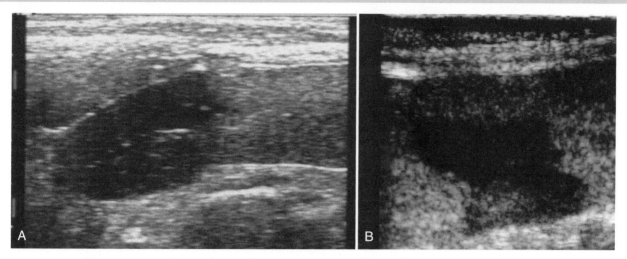

Figure 194-5 Infarcted spleen in two dogs. **A,** Note hypoechoic infarcted portion of spleen on gray-scale ultrasound image. **B,** On the contrast harmonic ultrasound image, the infarcted portion was not seen on gray-scale ultrasound but was hypoechoic compared to surrounding well-perfused, contrast-enhanced spleen.

patients with diffuse homogeneous splenomegaly and no clinical signs attributable to splenic disorders, and in patients with a known cause of congestion (e.g., tranquilizers, portal hypertension, right-sided heart failure), or for "classic" infarct lesions in asymptomatic patients.

Fine needle aspiration can provide the final diagnosis in neoplastic disorders or, when the organism can be identified, in infectious disease. Aspirates of normal spleen reveal small lymphocytes with occasional medium and large lymphocytes and rare neutrophils. A few macrophages and plasma cells may be present.[15] Precursors of all three cell lines may be seen in patients with extramedullary hematopoiesis, but erythroid cells are more common. In hyperplasia resulting from antigenic reaction, there is an increase in medium and large lymphocytes and in macrophages and plasma cells.[15] Patients with splenitis have an increase in inflammatory cells. Identification of the predominant cell type narrows the number of potential diagnosis. Inflammation can be further characterized based on the predominant cell type in suppurative, granulomatous, pyogranulomatous, eosinophilic, or lymphoplasmacytic. The most common causes for each type of inflammation are shown in Box 194-2.

Splenic Biopsies/Splenectomy

Spleen biopsies can be obtained in patients where the primary diagnosis of a mass is not obtained by fine needle aspiration. Care should be taken with impression smears made from spleen biopsies. Inadvertently making impressions of the capsular surface instead of parenchyma will reveal uniform sheets of loosely attached mesothelium that will be nondiagnostic.[15] Splenectomy should be considered in animals with cavitated masses without metastasis or necrosis.

Other Diagnostic Tests

In addition to image techniques and fine-needle aspiration, urinalysis, complete blood count, and biochemical profile are necessary in all patients with splenomegalic. Cats need be tested for infection with feline leukemia virus (FeLV) and feline immunodeficiency virus (FIV). Chest radiographs should be obtained in patients with splenic masses to rule out metastasis, and bone marrow examination may be indicated in patients with alterations in blood cell lines.

COMMON CAUSES OF SPLENOMEGALY IN DOGS AND CATS: NEOPLASTIC DISEASES

In both the dog and the cat, the spleen can be the site for both malignant and benign tumors as well as nonneoplastic disease. In dogs, around two thirds of splenic masses are diagnosed pathologically as neoplastic. Of these lesions, around one half to two thirds are diagnosed as hemangiosarcoma. In cats, around one half of splenic lesions submitted for pathologic examination are diagnosed as neoplastic. Tumors of the spleen usually present either as localized or diffuse splenomegaly and can be confused with nonneoplastic conditions. The actual clinical features of primary splenic tumors can be very vague, except in cases of splenic rupture and bleeding.

Malignant Tumors of the Canine Spleen

Hemangiosarcoma Hemangiosarcoma is a highly malignant tumor arising from the vascular endothelium. It is most common in the larger breeds of dog (especially German Shepherd), with the median age of affected dogs being 10 years. The most common primary site of hemangiosarcoma in the dog is the spleen, but it can also affect cutaneous sites. Around 25% of dogs with splenic hemangiosarcoma also have concurrent hemangiosarcoma affecting the right atrium.

The classical presentation of hemangiosarcoma in dogs is that of a solitary cavitated lesion that bleeds causing hemoperitoneum and sudden-onset hypovolemic collapse. Dogs often present with sudden-onset collapse, pallor, tachycardia and tachypnea, and distended abdomen. Abdominocentesis reveal frank hemorrhage. If possible, platelet count and clotting profile should be performed. Approximately 50% of dogs that present with abdominal bleeding are in DIC. Anemia and thrombocytopenia are common. Reticulocytosis and polychromasia may occur depending on when the bleed took place. A peripheral blood smear may reveal schistocytosis as red cells shear as they course through the tortuous lesion in the spleen.

DIAGNOSIS AND CLINICAL STAGING

Dogs with hemoperitoneum and concurrent hematologic changes such as schistocytosis and thrombocytopenia with concurrent anemia should carry a high suspicion for hemangiosarcoma. Clinical staging to determine the nature and extent of disease should include three-view thoracic radiography (right and left lateral views and dorsoventral), complete blood count and serum chemistry, coagulation profile, cardiac and abdominal ultrasound, and potentially exploratory laparotomy. The World Health Organization staging system for canine hemangiosarcoma is given in Box 194-3.[16] The only way to definitively diagnose hemangiosarcoma is by histopathology following splenectomy. Cytology is often unrewarding, and the gross appearance of the spleen is often a poor indicator of the underlying disease. Large hematomas or benign hemangiomas can have an identical "appearance" to hemangiosarcoma at surgery, and no decision on elective euthanasia can be taken at surgery unless there is evidence of gross metastatic disease. To achieve a good pathologic diagnosis, it is also important to submit the most appropriate samples to the pathologists. If your pathologist is not on site, then it will be difficult to submit a spleen in its entirety as it will not properly fix in formalin. In addition, multiple sites need to be sampled and fixed because the spleen will also contain multiple areas of hemorrhage and fibrosis that grossly may look like tumor. Large samples can be sliced like a loaf of bread to ensure even penetration of formalin.

TREATMENT

The treatment of choice for primary splenic hemangiosarcoma is splenectomy. Dogs that present in acute hypovolemic shock are not surgical candidates and should be stabilized before surgery is contemplated. Often dogs present following one major bleed, but if bleeding does not continue, these patients will autotransfuse and become better surgical candidates over the subsequent 24-hour period. It is noteworthy that around 20% of dogs can develop ventricular arrhythmias associated with splenic tumors. Dogs should be monitored electrocardiographically before and during surgery and in the immediate postoperative period. In some of these dogs arrhythmias can be difficult to control until the spleen has been surgically removed.

Splenectomy will relieve abdominal distension caused by the tumor and prevent any further bleeding. However, the role of surgery alone in improving survival is difficult to determine because of the rapid growth of metastasis. The most common cause of death in dogs is metastasis, and many chemotherapy protocols have been described as adjunctive therapies to improve survival. Survival times following surgery with or without chemotherapy are shown in Table 194-1. Overall the prognosis should be considered poor even with adjunctive chemotherapy. The most promising improvements in survival came from a study that combined both chemotherapy (doxorubicin and cyclophosphamide) and liposome-encapsulated muramyl tripeptides (LMTP). LMTP is a nonspecific biologic that enhances macrophage activation. In this study, the median survival time improved from 179 days (chemotherapy alone) to 273 days. At the time of writing, LMTP is no longer available.

Nonangiomatous, Nonlymphoid Sarcomas of the Spleen

Fibrosarcoma, leiomyosarcoma, myxosarcoma, osteosarcoma, liposarcoma, and undifferentiated sarcoma have all been described as primary splenic malignant tumors. Unlike hemangiosarcoma, the clinical signs associated with these tumors are usually vague and typically involve progressive anorexia and lethargy. In rare cases where the tumor has become large, it may result in splenic torsion.

The treatment of choice is surgery, with no large-scale clinical trials describing the benefits of adjunctive chemotherapy. As a group, a median survival time following splenectomy is reported to be around 4 months, but there is a large variation depending on tumor type. The mitotic index at histopathologic examination has prognostic implications. Tumors with a mitotic index less than 9 have a better prognosis that those with an index greater than 9.

Histiocytic Sarcoma   Canine histiocytic disorders represent a range of diseases that are a diagnostic and therapeutic challenge. This disease is most common in the Bernese Mountain Dog and Retriever breeds, but has been reported in a number of other breeds. The spleen can be a site for primary histiocytic sarcoma or a site of dissemination from malignant histiocytosis. Primary splenic histiocytic sarcoma has been associated with a hemophagocytic syndrome characterized by a Coombs'-negative anemia due to erythrophagia by malignant histiocytes. Whether primary or part of a secondary disease complex, histiocytic disease associated with the spleen carries a poor prognosis. Dogs will often die from disseminated disease even after splenectomy. Lomustine

---

Box • 194-3

The World Health Organization Staging System for Canine Hemangiosarcoma

T	Primary tumor
T0	No evidence of tumor
T1	Tumor confined to spleen
T2	Tumor confined to spleen but ruptured
N	Regional lymph nodes
N0	No regional lymph node involvement
N1	Regional lymph node involvement
N2	Distant lymph node involvement
M	Distant metastasis
M0	No evidence of distant metastasis
M1	Distant metastasis

From Wood CA, Moore AS, Gliatto JM, et al: Prognosis for dogs with stage I or II splenic hemangiosarcoma treated by splenectomy alone: 32 cases (1991-1993). J Am Anim Hosp Assoc 34:417-421, 1998.

Table • 194-1

Survival Times for Dogs Treated for Splenic Hemangiosarcoma

TREATMENT	MEDIAN SURVIVAL TIMES
Splenectomy alone (stage 1 or 2)	86 days
Splenectomy plus VAC*	164 days
Splenectomy plus AC*	179 days
Splenectomy plus doxorubicin	60 days if evidence of gross disease after splenectomy
	172 days if no evidence of further disease

Adapted from Murphy and Brearley, 2008.
AC, Doxorubicin, cyclophosphamide; VAC, vincristine, doxorubicin, cyclophosphamide (plus chlorambucil and methotrexate).
*Stage unknown.

(CCNU) or liposome-encapsulated doxorubicin have been suggested as adjunctive therapies but large-scale clinical studies are lacking.

Benign Tumors of the Canine Spleen

A number of benign tumors have been reported in the canine spleen. In general, these carry a good prognosis with long survival times following splenectomy.

Myelolipomas are tumors containing a mixture of adipose tissue and hematopoietic tissue. Lipomas are benign fat tumors that may affect the spleen. Hemangiomas are benign tumors arising from the vasculature. They can be distinguished from hemangiosarcoma only on histopathology. Splenectomy is considered curative.

Metastatic Tumors of the Canine Spleen

As well as being a site for primary neoplasia, the spleen is also a site for secondary tumor deposits or infiltrates. Notable among these are lymphoma, leukemias, multiple myeloma, primary erythrocytemia (polycythemia vera), high-grade metastatic mast cell tumors, and carcinomas. The management of secondary splenic tumors revolves around management of the underlying primary malignancy and usually involves systemic chemotherapy.

Malignant Tumors of the Feline Spleen

Mast Cell Tumor In cats, the spleen is a common site for primary mast cell tumor. Typically, these patients present with a history of dullness and lethargy, progressive anorexia, occasional vomiting (histamine release), and diffuse splenomegaly on clinical examination. Mastocytosis is observed on a complete blood count, whereas malignant mast cells can be seen in lymph nodes, liver, and bone marrow.

Diagnosis is usually made by ultrasound-directed fine needle aspirate of the spleen. The treatment of choice is splenectomy, with a mean survival time of around 12 to 18 months following surgery. However, this is a high-risk surgery because excessive handling of the spleen could lead to massive histamine and heparin release leading to shock and ultimately death. Presurgical therapy with antihistamines, careful surgical technique, and proper anesthetic monitoring are essential for success. Following surgery the mastocytosis usually clears without any chemical therapy. Adjunctive use of chemotherapy is controversial with no large-scale clinical studies proving their benefit.

Feline Splenic Hemangiosarcoma Compared to the canine disease, feline splenic hemangiosarcoma is rare. Cats with this condition will normally present with nonspecific clinical signs such as anorexia, weight loss, and vomiting. Very rarely will cats have hypovolemic shock and collapse. There is a paucity of feline cases reported in the literature although those that have been described have been associated with metastatic disease. A median survival of 20 weeks following surgery has been reported. There are no large-scale clinical studies showing the benefit of chemotherapy following surgery.

Other Malignant Tumors As with dogs, other primary sarcomas (e.g., fibrosarcoma) have been reported but are very rare. Treatment of choice is surgery, and there is no information on the use of adjuvant therapies.

Benign Tumors of the Feline Spleen

A number of benign tumors have been reported in the feline spleen. In general these carry a good prognosis with long survival times following splenectomy. These include hemangiomas, which are benign tumors arising from the vasculature. Splenectomy is considered curative.

Metastatic Tumors of the Feline Spleen

The feline spleen can be a site for both primary neoplasia and for secondary tumor deposits or infiltrates. Notable amongst these are lymphoma, leukemias, multiple myeloma (rare in cats), and carcinomatosis. The management of secondary splenic tumors revolves around management of the underlying primary malignancy, and usually involves systemic chemotherapy.

COMMON CAUSES OF SPLENOMEGALY IN DOGS AND CATS: NONNEOPLASTIC DISEASES

Generalized splenomegaly occurs not only with tumor infiltration, but also may be caused by congestion, splenic hyperplasia/extramedullary hematopoiesis, inflammation, or cellular infiltration. Splenic masses are usually due to neoplasia, hematoma, abscess, or nodular hyperplasia.

Congestion

Congestion is commonly seen as a consequence to sedation or anesthesia, portal hypertension, or splenic vein thrombosis. Administration of phenothiazine sedatives (e.g., acepromazine) or ultrashort acting barbiturates (e.g., thiopental) produces substantial splenomegaly. Splenomegaly can be severe, because up to 30% of the blood volume can be pooled in the spleen. Administration of propofol to dogs, however, did not produce statistically significant splenomegaly.[17]

Congestion can also be secondary to portal hypertension with hepatic disease and systemic venous hypertension in right-sided heart failure or intrathoracic caudal vena cava compression. Chronic congestion of the spleen may lead to splenic hyperplasia. No changes in echogenicity were subjectively noted in congested spleens, although significant increased attenuation and a trend towards increased backscatter (echogenicity) were noted.[17] Diffuse changes in splenic echogenicity in patients with a known cause of congestion, therefore, are likely due to another underlying condition.

Splenic pedicle torsion is a special cause of congestion in dogs. It usually develops in large, deep-chested dogs, especially the German Shepherd and Great Dane.[18] Males represented 79% of the cases in one study.[18] Acute torsion causes profound systemic signs with shock and abdominal discomfort, whereas chronic torsion is associated with vague signs including vomiting, anorexia, lethargy, and icterus. Radiographically, a decrease in abdominal detail, displacement of other abdominal organs, and loss of visualization of the body of the spleen in the left cranial of the abdomen are seen in the ventrodorsal view. In the lateral view, the spleen is enlarged, is abnormally positioned or shaped, and may have intrasplenic gas.[19] Ultrasonographically, the spleen is diffusely enlarged and abnormally located. It is usually hypoechoic with decreased flow through splenic veins. In one study, intravascular thrombi could be identified in 50% of the cases.[18] Supportive therapy should be instituted immediately in these patients and the spleen removed surgically. If appropriately treated, splenic torsion carries a favorable prognosis.[18]

Splenic Infarction

Infarcts can be observed in patients in hypercoagulable states associated with liver disease, renal disease, or hyperadrenocorticism.[20] It also can occur with preexisting uniform splenomegaly[20] or splenic torsion.[18] Splenic infarction is a sign of abnormal coagulation or blood flow, and the clinical signs are related to the underlying cause. Ultrasonographically, infarct regions are usually peripheral and have hypoechoic, swollen areas. After contrast injection, they appear hypoechoic when compared to the surrounding, normally perfused spleen.

Infarcted regions may resolve with appropriate therapy of the underlying disease.

Splenic Hyperplasia/Extramedullary Hematopoiesis

The splenomegaly seen with splenic hyperplasia and extra-medullary hematopoiesis reflects "work hypertrophy" resulting from removal of abnormal blood cells from circulation, increased activity of mononuclear phagocytic and lymphoid cells, and increased blood cell production. In immune-mediated hemolytic anemia and thrombocytopenia, the spleen serves as a site of antibody production and also as an important site of removal of antibody-sensitized cells. Chronic increased destruction of red blood cells in some non–immune-mediated hemolytic diseases also appears to cause hyperplas-tic splenomegaly in dogs and cats.[21] Chronic antigen stimulation by infectious agents (e.g., bacterial endocarditis), blood parasites, or immune-mediated disease can stimulate hyperplasia of mononuclear phagocytic and lymphoid cells.

In work hypertrophy, the spleen is uniformly enlarged and may be hypoechoic on ultrasonographic examination. Cyto-logically, small lymphocytes still predominate, but there is an increase in medium- and large-sized lymphocytes, and plasma cells are commonly observed.[15]

Extramedullary hematopoiesis (EMH) may accompany splenic hyperplasia in patients with concomitant anemia, thrombocytopenia, or leukopenia. It is a very common cyto-logic diagnosis in dogs with uniform splenomegaly[14] and may also occur with a variety of splenic neoplasms. EMH is also common in cats; it was diagnosed in 21% of cats in one study.[22] A nodular pattern is more common in cats with EMH. The presence of nucleated red blood cells in peripheral blood suggests EMH. Cytologically, precursors of all three cell lines may be observed in this condition.[15] A finding of hematopoi-etic precursors with large amount of vacuoles in the back-ground suggest the presence of a myelolipoma rather than EMH.[15]

Nodular Hyperplasia/Hematoma

Nodular hyperplasia is a nonneoplastic regional proliferation of components cells normally found in the parenchyma of the canine spleen.[23] Nodular hyperplastic lymphoid proliferation is the most common form in dogs, but it is not common cats.[1,2] A high percentage of splenic lesions in dogs have features of hematomas and nodular hyperplasia, which suggests that these disorders may be different stages of the same process. Lymphoid elements are usually observed with superimposed hematomas.[1] It has been suggested that marginal zoning dis-tortion caused by nodular hyperplasia disrupts regional splenic blood flow in and around the hyperplastic nodule, eventually leading to hematoma formation.[1] Cats have a "nonsinusal" type of spleen and a different architecture and blood flow pattern of the intermediate circulation bordering the white pulp.[2] Those differences could render the feline spleen less vulnerable to disrupted blood flow and hematoma formation.

Nodular hyperplastic lesions are usually hypoechoic on ultrasonographic examination. Splenic hematomas in dogs are associated with large splenic masses. A history of trauma is rare.[24] Most dogs with splenic hematoma are relatively healthy and do not have acute splenic rupture,[21] although they may develop hemoabdomen.[25] Large hyperplastic nodules and splenic hematoma cannot be differentiated from hemangiosa-rcoma grossly. Splenectomy is the treatment of choice for hematomas and hyperplastic nodules large enough to cause splenomegaly.[26]

A particular variation of hyperplastic nodule in dogs is the fibrohistiocytic nodule.[23] Nodular fibrohistiocytic prolifera-tion is characterized by a mixed population of histiocytoid or spindle cells intertwined with hematopoietic elements,

plasma cells, and lymphocytes. These nodules appear to form a continuum between lymphoid nodular hyperplasia and malignant splenic fibrous histiocytoma.[23] Histologically, the lymphoid:fibrohistiocytic ratio is the most important predic-tor of survival in these dogs. A higher proportion of lymphoid to fibrohistiocytic type cells was associated with increased long-term survival.[23]

Box • 194-4

Infectious Causes of Splenomegaly/Splenitis*

Viral Diseases
Feline immunodeficiency virus (C)
Feline infectious peritonitis (C)
Feline leukemia virus (C)
Infectious canine hepatitis (D)
Systemic calicivirosis (C)

Rickettsial and Mycoplasmal Diseases
Ehrlichiosis and anaplasmosis (canine and feline)
Hemotropic mycoplasmosis
Q fever (*Coxiella burnetii*)
Rocky Mountain spotted fever (*Rickettsia rickettsii*)

Bacterial
Bacteremia
Bartonellosis
Canine brucellosis
Endotoxemia
Florida borreliosis
Lyme borreliosis
Myeloidosis

Mycobacterial Infections
Nocardiosis
Plague
Salmonellosis
Tularemia

Fungal
Blastomycosis
Cryptococcosis
Histoplasmosis
Sporotrichosis
Opportunistic infections
Paecilomycosis
Monocillium indicum (D)
Systemic candidiasis

Protozoal
Babesiosis
Cytauxzoonosis (C)
Hepatozoonosis (*Hepatozoon canis*, D)
Leishmaniasis
Toxoplasmosis
Trypanosomiasis

C, Cats. D, Dogs.
*Infectious disease may affect the spleen directly or cause splenom-egaly by causing chronic anemia, chronic antigen stimulation or disturbances in blood flow (e.g., endotoxemia).

Inflammatory Splenomegaly

Inflammatory splenomegaly (splenitis) is a uniform splenomegaly usually secondary to infection. In addition to the inflammatory response associated with hyperplasia, patients with splenitis also have increases in other inflammatory cells. It is important to classify the splenitis according to the predominant cell type, because different etiologic agents are associated with different types of inflammation. Some overlap exists, and the same organism can cause a different inflammatory response in a different patient. For example, lymphoplasmacytic splenitis has been observed in patients with feline infectious peritonitis, histoplasmosis, and blastomycosis. Care must be taken in diagnosing suppurative splenitis in patients with peripheral neutrophilia or eosinophilic splenitis in patients with peripheral eosinophilia. The most common causes of splenitis according to the predominant inflammatory response are listed in Box 194-2. Infectious agents that can cause splenitis or lead to splenomegaly by chronic antigen stimulation, disturbances of blood flow, or by causing chronic anemia are listed in Box 194-4.

PATIENT WITH A SPLENIC NODULE

Splenic nodules without associated splenomegaly are a relatively common finding in older dogs undergoing abdominal ultrasound for unrelated reasons. Most splenic nodules in this age group are benign and might require no further action. Myelolipomas can be easily identified, whereas lymphoid hyperplasia, EMH, and splenic infarcts may be more difficult to differentiate from an early neoplastic lesion. Further diagnostics should be attempted in breeds with high risk for hemangiosarcoma, patients with systemic tumors likely to involve the spleen (e.g., lymphoma, hemangiosarcoma), hematologic abnormalities, fever, or other signs of systemic infectious disease.[27] Fine needle aspiration should be attempted in all splenic nodules. The main risk associated with the procedure is contamination of abdominal cavity with tumor cells in case

of hemangiosarcoma. Hemangiosarcoma is not likely to manifest itself as one or few small nodules, but it may be a risk in predisposed breeds. A more conservative approach involving repeating the ultrasonographic examination in 4 weeks has been suggested.[27] Any increase in size in the nodule over this period should then be pursued aggressively. It should be remembered that a change in diameter from 1.0 to 1.2 cm is associated with a doubling in volume for a spherical mass.[27]

GENERAL MANAGEMENT OF A PATIENT WITH SPLENIC DISEASE

Diffuse splenomegaly is usually managed medically. Most diseases that cause diffuse splenomegaly are systemic, and treatment should be directed at the underlying cause. Splenic torsion in dogs is the exception to the rule. A few tumors and myeloproliferative disease can also benefit from removal of the spleen. Splenectomy can also be considered in patients with immune-mediated anemia or thrombocytopenia refractory to therapy. It is important to demonstrate bone marrow hyperplasia in the cell line with decreased peripheral numbers before splenectomy is performed. Spleen removal is the treatment of choice for patients with splenic masses.

Removal of the spleen may predispose the patient to infections. Splenectomized humans are more likely to die of sepsis, but this predisposition has not yet been confirmed in dogs and cats. A few organisms that infect blood cells (e.g., as in babesiosis, hemotropic mycoplasmosis, and ehrlichiosis) are known to occur more in splenectomized patients. Ideally, dogs and cats should be tested before splenectomy and treated accordingly if infected.

References

The reference list can be found on the companion Expert Consult Web site at *www.expertconsult.com*.

CHAPTER 195

Skeletal Diseases

Kenneth A. Johnson

Animals with bone disease may have signs of lameness, deformity, or dysfunction that could be confused with, or complicated by, joint, muscle, or neurologic disorders.[1] Therefore a systematic approach is necessary in evaluating animals with these signs. The expertise of a radiologist and bone pathologist will often be invaluable in establishing a diagnosis. Traumatic injuries should also be considered in the differential diagnosis but are not discussed here, because excellent descriptions exist elsewhere. Some bone diseases that also affect joints are described in Chapter 186.

The precise cause of many bone diseases that affect dogs and cats is unknown. Furthermore, some conditions have multiple causes, such as the congenital, heritable, and metabolic disorders. This makes logical classification difficult. A causative system is used here for want of a better alternative.

BONE PATHOPHYSIOLOGY

Structural Organization of Bone

Bone is a living tissue with several important functions, including storage of calcium, phosphorus, and other minerals. Bones act as a series of levers that facilitate the action of muscles and joints in movement, and they provide support and protection for other body systems. In addition, bone marrow stroma provides an inductive environment for hematopoiesis and is a source of osteogenic precursor cells.[2,3] Bones are structurally composed of compact (cortical) and cancellous (trabecular) bone (Figure 195-1).[4] The microstructural units of cortical bone are osteons that, in cross-section, have concentric layers of collagen fibers and a central canal.

Trabeculae of cancellous bone have a three-dimensional lattice arrangement and large intertrabecular spaces containing hemopoietic or fatty marrow tissue. Long bones have

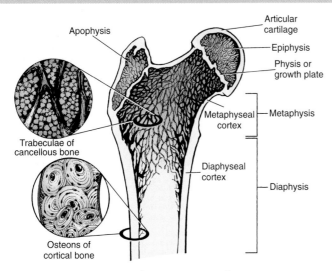

Figure 195-1 Regions and microstructure of an immature proximal femur.

several distinct regions: diaphysis, metaphysis, and epiphysis (see Figure 195-1). In growing animals, each epiphysis contains one or more ossification centers, is covered by hyaline cartilage on the articular surface, and is separated from the metaphysis by the physis or growth plate.[5,6] For reasons not well understood, many diseases have a predilection for certain regions of bone or even for particular bones.

Bone cells are derived from two separate cell systems: (1) the stromal fibroblastic (osteoblasts and osteocytes) and (2) hemopoietic (osteoclasts) systems.[2,3] During bone formation, osteoblasts synthesize collagenous matrix called *osteoid*, which is mineralized to become bone. Osteoblasts entrapped in newly forming bone become osteocytes. At sites of normal skeletal growth and remodeling, osteoblasts are derived from determined osteoblast precursor cells that reside in bone marrow stroma, endosteum, and periosteum. In injury or disease, inducible osteogenic precursor cells derived from other mesenchymal tissues, such as muscle and fibrous tissue, can be stimulated to differentiate to osteoblasts and form extraperiosteal ectopic bone. Osteoblasts can form several different types of bone.[4] Lamellar bone has collagen fibers in a parallel array and is found in osteons and mature trabecular bone. Formation of lamellar bone requires a preexisting matrix, such as calcified cartilage matrix (so-called endochondral ossification) or old bone that has been partially removed by osteoclastic resorption. Woven bone is characterized by random orientation of its collagen fibers. It can be deposited de novo, without preexisting bone or cartilage, and is formed when new bone is laid down rapidly in growth, fracture repair, and bone disease.[7] Normally it is remodeled to lamellar bone but may persist in rapidly growing osteogenic tumors.

Osteoclasts are large, multinucleate cells formed by fusion of circulating mononuclear cells. They are found on the surface of bone trabeculae and within remodeling osteons and are responsible for bone removal during growth, modeling, and remodeling of the skeleton. Osteoclasts erode mineralized bone first by solubilizing mineral, then digesting the protein.[3] This leaves concave pits in the bone surface, called Howship's lacunae. Formation and resorption of bone is regulated systemically by parathyroid hormone (PTH), calcitonin, and vitamin D (see Chapter 286). The principle action of PTH is to activate osteoclastic bone resorption and increase blood calcium concentration. Osteoblasts have PTH receptors, but osteoclasts do not. The increase in osteoclast number and activity induced by PTH is mediated by osteoblasts via a complex coupling mechanism involving several cytokines, including receptor activator of nuclear factor—kappa B (RANK) ligand, interleukins, and tumor necrosis factor (TNF).[2,3]

Bone Growth and Development

Growth of the axial and appendicular skeleton is primarily by endochondral ossification at the physes. Most physeal growth is longitudinal, but the zone of Ranvier and subperiosteal appositional growth contribute circumferential expansion as well. Physes have various zones that reflect chondrocytic structure and metabolic activity, but the transition between zones is gradual (Figure 195-2). Once formed, each chondrocyte remains in a fixed anatomic location throughout its life and there accomplishes all its functions.[8,9] The two most prominent stages involve proliferation and hypertrophy (including mineralization of matrix), prior to tissue resorption during vascularization. Most of the longitudinal growth of a physis is due to the tenfold increase in chondrocyte volume that is maximal in the hypertrophic zone. Defects in any part of the sequence, such as incomplete chondrocyte maturation, cause dwarfism or disordered bone growth (see Figure 195-2).

Modeling of Bone Modeling is the process that molds and sculpts the contours of expanding bones during growth. Within the metaphysis, the primary spongiosa is modeled to secondary spongiosa, which in turn is resorbed to form the marrow cavity of the shaft. Simultaneously, bone diameter decreases rapidly in the metaphyseal cutback zone as redundant bone is removed by subperiosteal osteoclastic resorption. In modeling, bone formation rates are frequently unequal to resorption rates, but unlike remodeling, bone formation is not dependent on resorption to precede it.[10] Modeling can correct the shape of malunited fractures, deformities, and bone subjected to altered loading, as predicted by Wolff's law. However, because the modeling process is closely coupled to growth, it is usually less effective after maturity.[10]

Normal and Pathologic Bone Remodeling

Remodeling is the process in which bone renews itself throughout life.[10] It always follows the sequence of activation → resorption → formation, and the packets of cells at a remodeling site are collectively called *bone multicellular units*.[10,11] Remodeling occurs in three bone envelopes: (1) the periosteal surface, (2) the endosteal-trabecular (cancellous bone) surface, and (3) the osteonal (intracortical) surface (Figures 195-3 and 195-4). In normal remodeling, bone formation equals resorption, whereas in bone disease a pathologic imbalance of resorption and formation often results in osteopenia of cortical and cancellous bone. Bones subjected to disease, trauma, or disuse exhibit a response termed the *regional acceleratory phenomenon*, in which the number of activated bone multicellular units increases suddenly.[10] This results in increased cortical porosity and trabecular thinning that reaches a peak at approximately 2 to 3 months; it may take up to 1 year to be reversed, during which time resorption sites are refilled with new bone.[12]

DIAGNOSIS OF BONE DISEASE

History and Signs

Initially, it is important to establish the age, breed, and sex of the patient because these factors may be associated with increased risk of a particular disease. Common complaints from owners are lameness, deformity, difficulty in rising, and reluctance to exercise. One must ascertain the duration and intensity (shifting, constant, intermittent, worsening) of the

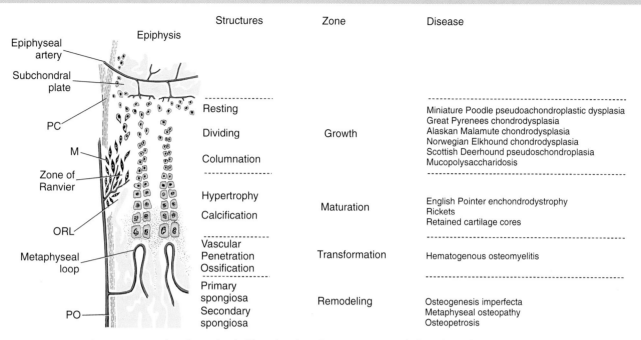

Structures	Zone	Disease
Epiphysis		
Resting		Miniature Poodle pseudoachondroplastic dysplasia
Dividing	Growth	Great Pyrenees chondrodysplasia
		Alaskan Malamute chondrodysplasia
Columnation		Norwegian Elkhound chondrodysplasia
		Scottish Deerhound pseudoschondroplasia
		Mucopolysaccharidosis
Hypertrophy		English Pointer enchondrodystrophy
Calcification	Maturation	Rickets
		Retained cartilage cores
Vascular Penetration	Transformation	Hematogenous osteomyelitis
Ossification		
Primary spongiosa	Remodeling	Osteogenesis imperfecta
Secondary spongiosa		Metaphyseal osteopathy
		Osteopetrosis

Labels on figure: Epiphyseal artery; Subchondral plate; PC; M; Zone of Ranvier; ORL; Metaphyseal loop; PO

Figure 195-2 The physis divided based on histologic structure and physiologic function (growth, maturation, transformation, and remodeling). Regions affected by some diseases of growth and remodeling are indicated. In the zone of Ranvier, undifferentiated mesenchymal cells *(M)* give rise to chondroblasts. The periosteum *(PO)* and perichondrium *(PC)* are continuous in this region. The metaphyseal cortex also extends into this region, becoming the osseous ring of Lacroix *(ORL)*, which acts as a peripheral restraint to the cell columns but does not impede latitudinal growth of the adjacent zone of Ranvier. (Adapted from Ogden JA: Skeletal injury in the child, ed 2, Philadelphia, 1990, Saunders, p 37.)

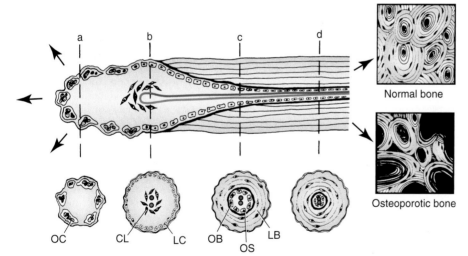

Labels: a, b, c, d; OC; CL; LC; OB; OS; LB; Normal bone; Osteoporotic bone

Figure 195-3 Remodeling osteon in cortical bone shown in longitudinal section. Components of this bone multicellular unit are shown in four transverse sections on the lower level. *a,* Cutter cone with osteoclasts *(OC)* resorbing bone. *b,* Capillary loop *(CL)* with undifferentiated lining cells *(LC)* in the quiescent zone between resorption and formation. *c,* Closing cone with centripetally advancing osteoblasts *(OB)*, separated by an osteoid seam *(OS)* from radially deposited new lamellar bone *(LB)*. *d,* Completed osteon (Haversian system).

problem, any known trauma, and any previous illness, medication, or surgery, as well as response to therapy. The owner should be asked whether exercise or rest exacerbates the problem, and whether swelling, drainage, or apparent pain had been noticed. Recognition of similar problems in related animals may indicate heritable disease. The type and quantity of foods, vitamins, and minerals fed should be determined.

Physical Examination
In conjunction with the normal physical examination, special attention is paid to lameness and gait abnormalities and to the musculoskeletal system (see Chapters 30, 263, and 264).[13,14] Visual appraisal might detect abnormalities in limb length and symmetry. The bony prominences and distal limb bones are palpated to detect pain, swelling, dyssymmetry, or crepitus. By comparison with the contralateral limb, muscle atrophy or altered range of joint motion may be identified. Each abnormality alone is rather nonspecific but aids in region localization. Before proceeding with sedation and radiography, further testing should be considered to exclude neurologic disease as a contributing factor (see Chapters 52 and 258).

Radiology
Radiology is the most useful method for routine noninvasive evaluation of skeletal lesions. To appreciate subtle lesions, radiographs must be excellent. Two or more views are always

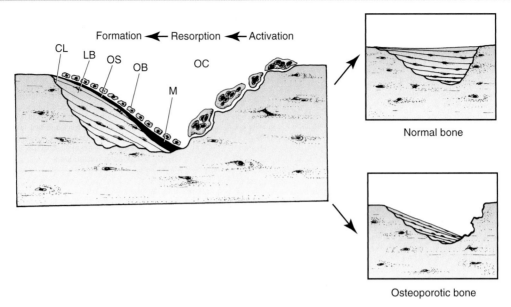

Figure 195-4 Trabecular bone remodeling with the components of bone multicellular unit: osteoclasts *(OC)*, nonmineralized matrix *(M)*, osteoblasts *(OB)*, osteoid seam *(OS)*, new lamellar bone *(LB)*, and cement line *(CL)* separating it from original bone. Normally, formation equals resorption, but in diseases causing osteoporosis, bone formation is inadequate or defective.

necessary, with the limb properly positioned. Comparison with radiographs of the contralateral limb or a radiographic atlas is useful to distinguish real bone lesions from anatomic and breed variations.[15]

Bone has a limited number of ways of responding to injury or disease. Lesions should be characterized according to changes in bone density, size, shape, or contour; the type of margination; the nature of any periosteal reaction; region of bone involved; and soft tissue changes.[16-18] The finding of a particular response, such as periosteal new bone, is not necessarily diagnostic of a specific disease (Box 195-1). Abnormalities could result from traumatic, neoplastic, infectious, idiopathic, or other processes. When considered in conjunction with signalment, history, and physical abnormalities, radiographic findings may lead to a diagnosis or a list of diagnostic alternatives. At this point it is valuable to consult descriptions of various bone diseases, to evaluate the possibilities, and to decide what further tests are indicated. Tests that are directed at confirming the most likely diagnosis, yet are least invasive and have low morbidity, are done first.

Nuclear Imaging

Scintigraphy is highly sensitive in detecting skeletal lesions, but it is not widely available and is generally not specific for cause.[19,20] After a radiopharmaceutical, usually [99m]technetium labeled methylene diphosphonate ([99m]TcMDP), is injected intravenously, it is incorporated into sites of new bone formation and remodeling and in regions of increased blood flow. The distribution of radionuclide in bone is detected with a gamma camera and is an indication of skeletal metabolic activity, complementing the structural information from radiographs. In cases of lameness in which physical examination and radiographs are unremarkable, scintigraphy may pinpoint a region of increased uptake in bone or a joint.[21] Further procedures such as computed tomography (CT), biopsy, culture, or surgical exploration would then be necessary to determine the cause of the "hotspot."

Tumor metastases in bone have a characteristic multifocal distribution, detectable by scintigraphy before they are seen on radiographs.[20] Although scintigraphy also detects primary bone tumors, it is seldom necessary for their diagnosis. Scintigraphy with [99m]TcMDP may help detect osteomyelitis before radiographic signs appear, but it is not specific for the disease.

Computed Tomography

High-resolution CT provides excellent cross-sectional images of lesions not found with radiographs. Its greatest application in the musculoskeletal system has been in evaluating the complex anatomy of skull, spine, and pelvis; in delineating boundaries of tumors involving soft tissues or bone; and in detecting early bone destruction.[22] For bone tumors this information allows more precise presurgical planning for en bloc resection of cranial and pelvic lesions and for limb salvage in appendicular lesions (Figure 195-5).[23-25]

Magnetic Resonance Imaging

Advantages of magnetic resonance imaging (MRI) are that high-resolution, serial, multiplanar images of skeletal soft tissues, such as ligament, tendon, menisci, and articular cartilage, can be obtained without the use of ionizing radiation. However, because this imaging modality relies on detection of changes in the orientation of mobile tissue protons within a strong magnetic field, the signal intensity of mineralized bone matrix is low. Adjacent soft tissues (periosteum, endosteum, fat, articular cartilage, and bone marrow) mainly define contours of bone. Subtle lesions of metaphyseal cancellous bone can be appreciated, as can displacement, compression, and invasion of soft tissue by expansile osseous lesions.[26] However, cortical bone lesions are better visualized using CT.

Chemistry

Estimation of blood calcium and inorganic phosphate concentrations and of alkaline phosphatase activity will be occasionally useful in diagnosing some bone diseases, but these variables are maintained within reference ranges in many skeletal diseases. Validated assays for canine PTH, PTH-related protein, and vitamin D metabolites are useful in hypercalcemic disorders (see Chapter 286).

Box • 195-1

Radiologic Signs of Some Common Bone Diseases

Bone Loss
1. Generalized and diffuse
   Primary hyperparathyroidism
   Renal secondary hyperparathyroidism
   Nutritional secondary hyperparathyroidism
   Disuse osteoporosis
2. Thin cortices
   Primary hyperparathyroidism
   Renal secondary hyperparathyroidism
   Nutritional secondary hyperparathyroidism
   Disuse osteoporosis
   Neoplasia
   Osteomyelitis
   Bone cyst
3. Focal
   Osteomyelitis
   Neoplasia
   Bone cyst
   Multifocal: myeloma, lymphosarcoma, metastases
4. Cystic
   Congenital bone cysts
   Aneurysmal bone cysts
   Subchondral bone cysts
   Central giant cell granuloma

Bone Production
1. Cortical
   Osteopetrosis
   Trauma
   Remodeling of deformity
   Fracture healing
2. Medullary
   Enostosis
   Myelosclerosis
   Osteomyelitis
   Sequestration
   Neoplasia
   Infarcts
   Fracture healing
3. Periosteal
   Hypervitaminosis A
   Mucopolysaccharidosis (MPS)
   Multiple cartilaginous exostoses
   Enostosis
   Metaphyseal osteopathy
   Craniomandibular osteopathy
   Secondary hypertrophic osteopathy
   Osteomyelitis
   Neoplasia
   Trauma

Adapted from Allan GS: Radiographic signs of diseases affecting bone. In Proceedings No. 87, Orthopaedic surgery in dogs and cats, Sydney, Australia, 1986, The University of Sydney Postgraduate Committee in Veterinary Science, p 247.

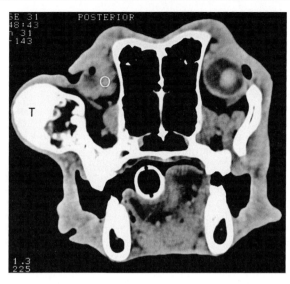

Figure 195-5 Computed tomography image of an osteoma *(T)* of the zygomatic arch that caused ocular *(O)* displacement.

Hematology
Alterations in circulating leukocyte numbers may be consistent with acute osteomyelitis, but the hemogram is usually unremarkable in chronic osteomyelitis and other bone diseases.

Biopsy and Histopathology
Histologic examination of a representative bone biopsy is the most reliable way to establish a diagnosis when radiographic signs are not highly characteristic of a particular disease. Biopsy may be necessary to distinguish between malignant and benign neoplasia, osteomyelitis, developmental lesions, and degenerative conditions. It also specifically identifies tumor type and grade, establishes the prognosis, and may dictate appropriate treatment. For various reasons, mistakes are frequent at this stage of the investigation. The most common pitfall is inappropriate sampling and submission of a biopsy that is reactive bone formed secondarily to the actual disease. Because processing of bone for histology can take 1 week or more, such an outcome can be frustrating and misleading.

Closed needle biopsies of medium-to-large, solid, solitary lesions of appendicular long bones are obtained using a 4-inch, 8- or 11-gauge Jamshidi bone biopsy needle (Sherwood Medical Co., St. Louis, Mo.) (see Chapter 99).[27] This method has less postsurgical morbidity (pain, hematoma, infection, tumor seeding, pathologic fracture) than incisional biopsy. The clinician should carefully evaluate the radiograph to ensure that the biopsy is obtained from the center of the lesion and that dense reactive bone is avoided. The skin puncture site and biopsy tract must be situated so that they can be subsequently excised if the lesion is surgically resected. Two or three cores of tissue are taken by redirecting the needle through the same skin opening. Needle orientation can be guided with image intensification or radiography. Jamshidi needle biopsy is not suitable for lesions of small bones or lesions with recent pathologic fractures because there may be significant hematoma in the latter. For cystic and fluid-filled lesions or those associated with extensive osteolysis and tumor necrosis, an open incisional wedge biopsy through a limited surgical approach might be necessary. Bone that appears abnormal can also be collected with a bone curette, taking care to avoid mutilating the specimen.

For investigation of diseases affecting growth and endochondral ossification, physeal biopsies can be obtained percutaneously from the greater tubercle of the humerus with a Jamshidi needle.[28] For suspected metabolic bone diseases, larger specimens of cancellous bone are collected with an 8-mm Michele trephine from the iliac crest or by excision of a segment of rib or distal ulnar diaphysis.[29]

The surgical borders of lesions excised en bloc are labeled with India ink for examination by the pathologist to ensure tumor-free margins.[30] Specimens can also be radiographed using nonscreen film or industrial film in a Faxitron cabinet system. Biopsies are fixed in neutral buffered formalin for 6 to 24 hours; they must not be frozen.[7] Large bone specimens should be cut into 5-mm slabs to ensure proper fixation.[7] If osteomyelitis is suspected, a portion of the biopsy should be separated for bacteriologic culture before the remainder is fixed in formalin. Bone specimens that cannot be cut with a scalpel are decalcified in 10% formic acid prior to embedding in paraffin. Rapid decalcification in strong acids or excessive decalcification will destroy cellular detail and render the biopsy nondiagnostic. Nondecalcified bone biopsies embedded in methylmethacrylate and sectioned with a sledge microtome are necessary for diagnosis of some metabolic bone diseases.[31] Histologic evaluation of bone is rather specialized and requires the expertise of a pathologist with special interest and training. Most pathologists will want to review the clinical data and radiographs as well before making a diagnosis.

Cytology

Cytologic examination of fluids and exudates obtained by sterile aspiration is valuable in early detection of acute osteomyelitis, before obvious radiographic changes occur in bone.

Microbiology

Isolation and identification of bacteria are helpful in confirming a diagnosis of osteomyelitis, and in vitro susceptibility testing aids in antimicrobial drug selection. Cultures of pus from externally draining tracts are less than 50% accurate in identifying the pathogens causing osteomyelitis because the tracts become colonized by skin organisms and gram-negative bacteria. It is preferable to culture fluid collected by sterile aspiration, or from pus, necrotic tissue, and sequestra collected during surgical débridement. Both aerobic and anaerobic culture are advisable because anaerobic bacteria are involved in up to 60% of bone infections in small animals.[32] Samples for aerobic culture should be collected into a sterile container, taken to the laboratory, and plated out on agar within 10 to 15 minutes. Specimens for anaerobic culture require special handling because a few minutes of exposure to air will kill sensitive anaerobes and prevent subsequent isolation. Fluid for anaerobic culture can be collected into a syringe if air is expelled and the needle capped with a rubber stopper.

When the anticipated delay in plating out samples exceeds 15 minutes, tissue samples and swabs are placed into a reduced Cary-Blair, solidified anaerobic holding media (Becton Dickinson, Franklin Lakes, N.J.) to exclude oxygen. Both aerobes and anaerobes may be isolated from such preparations because most aerobic bacteria are facultative anaerobes.

CONGENITAL BONE DISORDERS

Embryonic and postnatal skeletal development is complex and exquisitely susceptible to errors. Skeletal growth disorders that are apparent at birth or manifest later in young animals are of two main types: (1) generalized dysplasias and (2) localized malformations of individual bones. Some are caused by inherited defects and sporadic mutations, and some are due

to teratogens and unidentifiable embryopathies. In humans, more than 100 such disorders, mostly inherited, have been listed in the Paris Nomenclature for Constitutional Disorders of Bone.[33] This classification is based on specific clinical, genetic, radiologic, histologic, and biochemical features. Animal diseases are not sufficiently characterized to allow complete adoption of the Paris system,[34] although some general groupings are possible (Box 195-2). Generalized dysplasias are described later with developmental and genetic disorders or with joint diseases (see Chapter 186), whereas dysostoses are considered here.

Box • 195-2

Some Congenital Skeletal Disorders of Small Animals

Osteochondrodysplasias (Abnormalities of Cartilage, Bone Growth, and Development)
A. Defects of growth of tubular bone or spine
   Multiple epiphyseal dysplasias: Beagle
   Pseudoachondrodysplasia: Miniature Poodle
      Scottish Deerhound
   Chondrodysplasia: Alaskan Malamute
      Cocker Spaniel
      English Pointer
      Great Pyrenees
      Norwegian Elkhound
   Ocular-skeletal dysplasia: Labrador Retriever
      Samoyed
   Pelger-Huët anomaly: cats
   Scottish Fold osteochondrodysplasia: cats
B. Disorganized development of cartilage and fibrous
      components
   Multiple cartilaginous exostoses (osteochondromatosis)
   Enchondroma
   Fibrous dysplasia
C. Abnormalities of density, cortical diaphyseal structure,
      or metaphyseal molding
   Osteogenesis imperfecta
   Osteopetrosis

Primary Metabolic Abnormalities
Vitamin D–dependent rickets
Mucopolysaccharidosis (MPS)
Fucosidosis
GM gangliosidosis
Gaucher's disease

Dysostoses with Malformation of Individual Bones, Singly or in Combination
Hemimelia
Phocomelia
Amelia
Syndactyly
Polydactyly
Ectrodactyly
Segmental hemiatrophy

Adapted from Sharrard WJW: Pediatric orthopaedics and fractures, ed 3, London, 1993, Blackwell Scientific Publications.

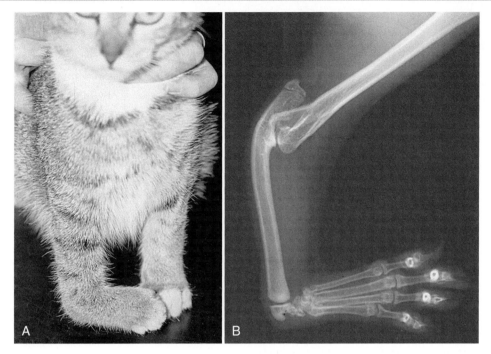

Figure 195-6 Kitten with radial agenesis. **A,** Radial agenesis and a 90-degree varus angulation of the metacarpus. **B,** The radius and radial carpal bone are absent. The proximal ulna is misshapen, the distal ulna thicker than normal, and the carpus malarticulated. (From Winterbotham EJ et al: Radial agenesis in a cat. J Small Anim Pract 26:393, 1985.)

Dysostoses include the malformations of individual bones either singly or in combination.[35] They can involve the craniofacial region, the axial bones, and extremities. Embryonic limb bud development commences with a projection of mesoderm covered by ectoderm. Three signaling centers within the limb bud that control and coordinate limb development are (1) the apical ectodermal ridge, (2) the zone of polarizing activity, and (3) the Wingless-type signaling center.[36] The apical ectodermal ridge is a thickened layer of ectoderm overlying the distal tip of the limb bud that acts as a signaling center guiding proximal to distal limb development. It also causes interdigital necrosis, thereby separating webbed digits, probably by the local expression of FGF genes.[37] The zone of polarizing activity exerts control via the signaling molecule sonic hedgehog protein, and the Wingless-type signaling center controls limb alignment with respect to dorsal orientation.[36] Subsequently, the individual bones form from cartilage anlages and the secondary centers of ossification.[5,37] Three mesodermal rays (ulnar, radial, and central) contribute to pectoral limb formation; disturbances of one or more rays or of the signaling centers will result in perturbations of the corresponding components of bone and associated soft tissue. For example, failure of the apical ectodermal ridge may produce syndactyly of the digits or result in a truncated limb similar to congenital amputation.[36] Except for a few heritable disorders that will be mentioned, most dysostoses in dogs and cats occur sporadically.

Hemimelia, Phocomelia, and Amelia

In these conditions the animal has a congenital absence of portions of the normal structures in an extremity. Hemimelia is either longitudinal (paraxial), with absence of the ulnar, radial, or central regions in the forelimb, or transverse, with the distal portion of the limb completely absent.

Radial agenesis is the most common paraxial hemimelia in cats and dogs. It is usually unilateral and sporadic. Bilateral radial agenesis might be an inherited autosomal recessive trait in Chihuahua dogs.[34] In radial agenesis, the radius is partially or completely absent, and the ulna is shorter, thickened, and curved (Figure 195-6). The radial carpal bone and first digit are often absent as well. Lack of a radial head support allows humeroulnar subluxation, and the range of elbow motion is reduced. The metacarpus deviates into varus, severely impairing limb function. One hypothesis is that radial agenesis and other hemimelias are a consequence of neural crest injury because limb bud embryopathies often have a segmental pattern that corresponds to the distribution of the segmental sensory nerves.[38] Treatment of radial agenesis by reconstructive surgery may be very successful in the restoration of limb function.[39] Another, less common paraxial hemimelia is tibial agenesis.[34]

Complete absence of a distal portion of a limb (congenital amputation) can be caused by transverse hemimelia, strangulation by constrictive bands, or in utero accidents.[40,41] The cause may be impossible to determine in young animals because postnatal trauma can also cause amputations.

In phocomelia, an intercalary segment of limb is missing. In severe cases the paw with rudimentary digits is attached to the trunk like a seal flipper. Proximal femoral focal deficiency is a phocomelia with a missing segment of femur. In man, this is usually a unilateral defect that is not inherited.[42] A young Dalmatian with proximal femoral focal deficiency had unilateral hindlimb shortening and muscle atrophy that became accentuated with further growth.[43] Radiographically, bone in the intertrochanteric, neck, and head regions of the femur was absent, and there was marked femoral shortening.

Amelia is complete absence of one or more limbs. Two kittens with bilateral hindlimb amelia have been reported.[34] Most animals affected by amelia probably die or are euthanized at birth.

Syndactyly

Two or more digits are fused in a bony or soft tissue union in syndactyly.[7,34] This is not clinically important in pets, and surgery is generally unwarranted unless the deformity causes lameness.[44] Congenital synostosis of adjacent metatarsal bones is a variation on digital fusion (Figure 195-7).

Polydactyly

Polydactyly is the presence of extra digits, usually on the medial side of the paw in dogs and cats. An inherited syndrome of skeletal defects exists, including polydactyly and syndactyly in Australian Shepherd dogs.[7] An X-linked gene was suspected. Polydactyly is an inherited autosomal dominant trait in cats.[34] Multiple hindlimb dewclaws in Great Pyrenees have similar inheritance.

In Saint Bernard dogs, dewclaws may be associated with anomalous tarsal bones. Some have a large curved bone that seems to be an extension of the central tarsal bone on the medial side of the proximal row of tarsal bones (Figure 195-8). These tarsal anomalies occur bilaterally, are not associated with clinical signs, and are probably inherited.

Ectrodactyly

Often called split hand or lobster claw deformity, ectrodactyly is caused by incomplete fusion of the three rays or absence of the central ray.[42] Classically, the third metacarpal bone and digit are absent, producing a deep cleft that divides the paw into radial and ulnar parts, but many variations occur. The third metacarpal bone may be present and hypoplastic, and neighboring digits and metacarpal bones may be absent or hypoplastic.[45-47] The cleft between metacarpal bones may terminate just below the carpus or extend proximally through the carpus, separating radius and ulna entirely (Figure 195-9).[45-47] Asynchronous radial and ulnar growth can contribute to the structural disorder at the carpus. Half of the affected dogs have concomitant congenital elbow luxation. It is usually an isolated deformity without breed predilection in dogs but may be inherited in cats.[7,34] Function can be improved by reconstructive surgery or arthrodesis.[45,48]

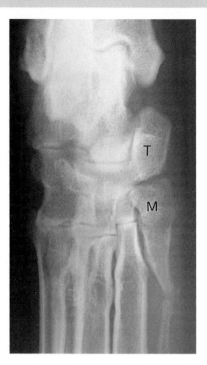

Figure 195-8 Vestigial first metatarsal bone *(M)* and an anomalous tarsal bone *(T)* extending medially from the central tarsal bone in a Saint Bernard.

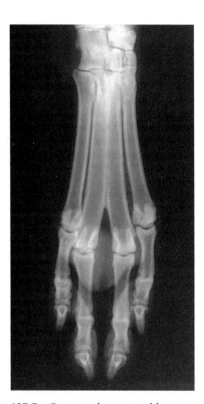

Figure 195-7 Congenital metatarsal bone synostosis.

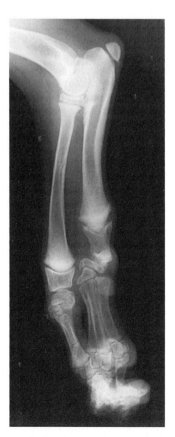

Figure 195-9 Forelimb of 12-week-old mixed-breed dog with ectrodactyly, including distal radial and ulnar separation.

Segmental Hemiatrophy

Hemiatrophy is a misnomer because the condition is actually limb hypoplasia rather than atrophy of a normal structure. The affected forelimb is noticeably shorter and slimmer, especially in the antebrachium and paw.[49] An affected Golden Retriever also had darker pigmentation of skin and hair of the abnormal limb and horny keratinization of pads and nails, but it had no pain or discomfort.[50] Radiographically the carpal bones were smaller, and the numbered carpal bones were misshapen. The metacarpal bones were 3 cm shorter than contralateral bones and half normal diameter. This is a sporadic deformity and probably not inherited. It must be distinguished from atrophy that follows long-term limb immobilization.[12] A similar type of distal hypoplasia of metacarpus and digits is seen in immature dogs, subsequent to accidental trauma or surgery to the antebrachium.[50] Ilizarov limb lengthening may be indicated if shortening impairs function.

DEVELOPMENTAL AND GENETIC BONE DISORDERS

Osteopetrosis

Defective osteoclastic resorption of bone is the principal feature of osteopetrosis. In growing bones, failure of normal bone modeling results in accumulation of primary spongiosa, so the diaphysis remains filled with bone and a marrow cavity does not form. Affected bones have a marbled, densely homogeneous radiographic appearance, but they are actually quite fragile. Many forms of osteopetrosis exist. Osteoclasts may be absent, be present in reduced numbers, or be defective in their ability to resorb bone.[7] The disorder is rare and not very well characterized in dogs and cats.[7,51] Idiopathic acquired osteopetrosis of adult cats was characterized by thickening of diaphyseal cortices and vertebral bodies.[51] Feline leukemia virus (FeLV) also produces medullary sclerosis and nonregenerative anemia in growing cats, probably through infection of hemopoietic precursor cells from which osteoclasts arise.[7]

Osteogenesis Imperfecta

Osteogenesis imperfecta comprises a group of heritable diseases characterized by osteopenia, excessive bone fragility, and increased susceptibility to fracture. Fractured bones form callus and heal, but unless stabilized adequately, malunion and deformities occur.[52-54] Radiographically there can be generalized osteopenia, thinning of diaphyseal cortices, and multiple fractures in various stages of union. The fundamental defect in humans and dogs is abnormal type I collagen production, mostly due to mutations of genes that normally code for procollagen synthesis.[52,53] The resulting type I collagen fibrils are thin and fail to mineralize. Osteogenesis imperfecta is rare in dogs and cats, and the mode of heritability and exact biochemical defects are unknown.[34,54,55] Animals may have multiple fractures, with minimal or no trauma. Some may also have dentinogenesis imperfecta (seen as pink teeth), stunted growth, and apparent weakness.[55] Two litters of rough-coated Dachshund puppies suffering from osteogenesis imperfecta showed signs of pain when handled, as well as brittle, translucent, and fractured teeth.[56] However, they were well proportioned without evidence of deformity or dwarfism. The diagnosis of osteogenesis imperfecta is made by analysis of type I collagen from cultured skin fibroblasts,[55] but the more common causes of osteopenia, including renal and nutrition secondary hyperparathyroidism, should be eliminated first.

Mucopolysaccharidosis

The mucopolysaccharidosis (MPS) disorders are rare genetic lysosomal storage diseases caused by specific defects in lysosomal enzymes that are involved in metabolism of glycosaminoglycans. Compounds normally degraded by these enzymes accumulate intracellularly, interfering with cellular function and producing characteristic clinical signs. Several MPS disorders have been recognized in cats (MPS I, VI, and VII) and dogs (MPS I, II, IIIA, IIIB, VI, and VII),[57] but the presence and severity of skeletal abnormalities produced by them are different.

MPS VI is caused by decreased arylsulfatase B activity and leads to intracellular accumulation and increased urinary excretion of dermatan sulfate. Feline MPS VI has been recognized mainly in Siamese cats, as an autosomal recessive disorder, but has also been described in domestic shorthaired (DSH) and long-haired cats, and a Siamese and DSH cross.[57-59] MPS VI has also been reported in dogs of several breeds.[57] Skeletal disease is the predominant abnormality. Clinical features become evident in affected cats from age 6 to 8 weeks and include small head and ears, flattened face, corneal clouding, pectus excavatum, growth retardation, skeletal deformity, and hindlimb paresis or paralysis from spinal cord compression by bone lesions. They have a crouching gait, and manipulation of joints and cervical spine causes pain. Radiographic features include epiphyseal dysplasia, thinning of long-bone cortices, generalized osteopenia, bilateral coxofemoral subluxation, secondary osteoarthritis, and vertebral fusion.[60] Diagnostic confirmation is provided by demonstration of excess dermatan sulfate in urine with the toluidine-blue (Berry) spot test, metachromatic granules in neutrophils, and reduced arylsulfatase B activity in leukocytes.[57] A PCR-based screening method allows detection of carrier cats.[58]

MPS I in DSH cats is an autosomal recessive disease due to decreased activity of alpha-L-iduronidase.[57,61] Clinical features are similar to MPS VI, but facial dysmorphism may not be as striking as in Siamese, and metachromatic granules are usually less distinct in leukocytes than in MPS VI and MPS VII.[62] Radiographic features are similar to MPS VI, except that epiphyseal dysplasia and dwarfism are absent. Neurologic abnormalities due to spinal cord compression by bone proliferation occur relatively later, after 2 years of age. Excretion of dermatan sulfate and heparin sulfate in urine is detectable using the toluidine-blue spot test.[61] MPS I has also been reported in dogs. Affected animals are dwarfed and have swollen painful joints, glossoptosis, corneal clouding, and progressive motor and visual deficits. Radiographic features include epiphyseal dysgenesis, periarticular bone proliferation, and enlargement of femoral diaphyses.[63]

MPS II was diagnosed in a 5-year-old male Labrador Retriever with coarse facial features, macrodactylia, generalized osteopenia, progressive neurologic deterioration, and a positive urine test for glycosaminoglycan.[64] Iduronate sulfatase activity was deficient in cultured dermal fibroblasts.

Canine MPS VII (beta-glucuronidase deficiency) has been described in dogs and cats.[58] Affected dogs appear normal at birth, but by age 2 to 3 months develop hindlimb paresis and have a disproportionately large head, flattened face, swollen lax joints, bowed limbs, dorsoventrally flattened rib cage, and corneal clouding.[65] Radiographic features include bilateral coxofemoral luxation, abnormally shaped carpal and tarsal bones, generalized epiphyseal dysplasia, cervical vertebral dysplasia, and platyspondylisis. Feline MPS VII is characterized by growth retardation, delayed dental eruption, corneal clouding, abdominal distension, and multiple skeletal abnormalities.[66-68] In both species, peripheral leukocytes contain metachromatic inclusions and urinary excretion of chondroitin sulfate is increased.[66,69] Genetic tests can distinguish phenotypically normal MPS VII carrier dogs and cats from homozygous normal animals.[66,70]

Several therapeutic strategies for MPS have been trialed with some success, including enzyme replacement therapy, heterologous bone marrow transplantation, and somatic cell gene transfer, but all require further development.[57,71]

Dwarfism

Various disorders causing small stature in dogs and cats listed in Box 195-3 are reviewed in other chapters. Considered here are skeletal dysplasias and some endocrinopathies (hyposomatotropism and hypothyroidism) that are more commonly associated with dwarfism in small animals.

Skeletal Dysplasias (Osteochondrodysplasias) Osteochondrodysplasias are disorders characterized by abnormalities in growth and development of cartilage, bone, or both (see Box 195-2). Disorders of this type have been reported in several breeds of dogs. Box 195-4 summarizes the better-characterized entities. Most have known or suspected genetic basis and autosomal recessive inheritance is common. They frequently cause disproportionate dwarfism, with discrepant development of axial and appendicular skeleton producing reduced limb length relative to the trunk (Figure 195-10).

Another type of genetic dwarfism occurs in achondroplastic dog breeds, such as Bulldog, Boston Terrier, Pekinese, Pug, and Shih Tzu. These animals have been bred selectively for achondroplasia and thus have shortened maxilla, depressed nasal bridge, flared metaphyses, and short bowed limbs as part of accepted breed standards.[34] Hypochondroplastic breeds, such as Basset Hound, Beagle, Dachshund, Dandie Dinmont Terrier, Scottish Terrier, Skye Terrier, and Welsh Corgi have similarly shaped legs as a breed characteristic, although their skulls are normal.[34] In humans, many of these skeletal diseases originate from various mutations in the FGFR3 gene; a similar mutation seems not to be involved in the Bulldog, Bassett Hound, or Dachshund.[87-89] These forms of dwarfism differ from the nonpathologic, mutant, proportionate reduction in stature in dogs that has led to the establishment through selective breeding of many miniature and toy breeds.

An osteochondrodysplasia with autosomal dominant inheritance has been described in Scottish Fold cats.[90,91] Along with the folded ears typical of this breed, affected individuals show signs of lameness; reluctance to jump; stiff and stilted gait; short, misshapen distal limbs; and short, thick, inflexible tail. Radiographic features include irregular size and shape of bones of tarsus, carpus, metatarsus, metacarpus, phalanges, and caudal vertebrae. In addition, these animals have narrowing of apparent joint spaces, new bone production around distal limbs joints, diffuse osteopenia, and formation of a plantar exostosis caudal to the calcaneus in advanced cases (Figure 195-11). However, the severity and rate of progression of changes are quite variable. Treatment is noncurative, but pentosan polysulfate, glycosaminoglycans, nonsteroidal antiinflammatory drugs (NSAIDs), or irradiation might be palliative.[90,92]

A chondrodysplasia in two unrelated kittens with shortened, bowed forelimbs was described.[77] Radiographic signs included long-bone bowing, metaphyseal flaring, and a gross enlargement of physeal cartilage that resembled rickets. Serum calcium, phosphorus, and 1,25-dihydroxyvitamin D_3 concentrations were normal, but PTH concentrations were below the reference range. Furthermore, treatment of the kittens with oral 1,25-dihydroxyvitamin D_3 for 3 months did not resolve the radiographic abnormalities or correct the stunted statue. The disorder is considered to be an (osteo) chondrodysplasia of unknown heritability rather than rickets.[93]

Pituitary Dwarfism hypopituitarism and consequent dwarfism, inherited in autosomal recessive fashion in German Shepherd and Karelian Bear dogs, have also been described in other dog breeds (Weimaraner, Spitz, Toy Doberman Pinscher) and cats.[94,95] A cystic, vestigial adenohypophysis is present in many affected German Shepherds, but some have a hypoplastic or a normal-appearing pituitary gland. The syndrome is dominated by effects of hyposomatotropism, but deficiency of other adenohypophyseal hormones can lead to degrees of accompanying secondary hypothyroidism, hypoadrenocorticism, and hypogonadism.[96] Affected animals are usually recognizable by the age of 2 or 3 months. They grow slowly but retain near-normal body proportions. The soft puppy-hair coat is retained initially, but symmetric alopecia and hyperpigmentation develop with age. Accompanying abnormalities include abnormal behavior (aggression, fear biting), delayed dental eruption, short mandible, cardiac disorders, cryptorchidism, megaesophagus, and testicular atrophy or estral abnormalities.

Radiographically, limb bones are shortened, with delayed closure of growth plates in some cases. Epiphyses may show disordered and incomplete calcification, suggesting hypothyroidism. Hormonal testing can be undertaken to confirm the diagnosis if necessary. Most pituitary dwarf animals can be expected to remain small for life. However, two unusual cases with typical clinical features at 10 weeks of age grew steadily and appeared normal when 1 year old.[97] Both had normal hormonal test results, indicating that growth hormone secretion ideally should be evaluated in suspected cases to clarify prognosis.

Replacement therapy with growth hormone (if available and economical) and thyroxine or glucocorticoid, if indicated, could be considered, but long-term prognosis is poor.[94] Another promising approach involves chronic progestin administration to induce growth hormone production from mammary ductular cells of affected dogs of either sex.[98]

Congenital Hypothyroidism Skeletal development is abnormal in congenital hypothyroidism, which is rare in dogs and cats. Although cases are usually encountered sporadically in various breeds, some familial occurrences are known: secondary hypothyroidism with autosomal recessive inheritance in Giant Schnauzers,[99] primary dyshormonogenesis with autosomal recessive inheritance in Abyssinian cats,[100] thyroid

---

Box • 195-3

Some Causes of Small Stature in Dogs and Cats

Nonendocrine
Malnutrition
Malassimilation
Portal systemic shunt (PSS)
Cardiovascular defects
Glycogen storage disease
Skeletal dysplasia
Mucopolysaccharidosis (MPS)
Hydrencephalus
Renal disease

Endocrine
Hyposomatotropism
Hypothyroidism
Hypoadrenocorticism
Hyperadrenocorticism
Diabetes mellitus

Modified from Feldman EC, Nelson RW: Canine and feline endocrinology and reproduction, ed 3, Philadelphia, 2004, Saunders.

Box • 195-4

Canine Osteochondrodysplasias: Clinical and Radiologic Signs, and Inheritance Pattern

Alaskan Malamute Chondrodysplasia[7,72]
Short limbs, bowed forelegs, carpal joints enlarged, paws deviated laterally; ulna growth plate thickened, irregular and flared; associated hemolytic anemia; autosomal recessive trait, complete penetrance, variable expression

Beagle Multiple Epiphyseal Dysplasia[7,72]
Short limbs, enlarged joints, kyphosis; stippled mineralization of epiphyses, especially femur and humerus, disappeared by 5 months; vertebrae short; dysplastic hips; osteoarthropathy in adults; autosomal recessive trait

Bull Terrier Osteochondrodysplasia[73]
Abnormal hind leg gait, femoral neck fractures; nonossified foci in femoral necks and metaphyses of long bones; some long bones distorted; dwarfing not noted; littermates affected but inheritance not known

English Pointer Enchondrodystrophy[7,74,75]
Short limbs, bowed forelegs, abnormal locomotion; wide irregular growth plates; possibly inferior prognathism; probable autosomal recessive trait

Great Pyrenees Chondrodysplasia[7,72,76]
Very short limbs, forelegs bowed with valgus deformity; body length reduced slightly; flared, flattened metaphyses; poorly developed epiphyses and cuboidal bones; vertebrae poorly ossified and irregular; autosomal recessive trait

Irish Setter Hypochondroplasia[77]
Mildly short limbs and spine, variable radius and ulna bowing and carpal valgus; growth plates, epiphyses and metaphyses radiographically normal; autosomal recessive trait

Labrador Retriever Ocular-Skeletal Dysplasia[7,78]
Short limbs, prominent elbows and carpi, paws deviated laterally, hind legs hyperextended; tubular bones short and wide, cortices thin, metaphyses flattened and flared, increased metaphyseal opacity; epiphyses and cuboidal bones large and misshapen; hip dysplasia, abnormal elbows; cataracts, retinal dysplasia and detachment; autosomal trait, recessive effect on skeleton, incompletely dominant on eye

Miniature Poodle Multiple Enchondromatosis[79,80]
Short bowed limbs, femoral neck fractures; lucent areas extending from growth plates into metaphyses and some diaphysis;

diaphyses distended and distorted; ribs and vertebrae also affected; sternum lacked bone; autosomal nondominant trait

Miniature Poodle Multiple Epiphyseal Dysplasia[72]
Similar to disorder in Beagle; inheritance unknown, but two of three affected were littermates

Miniature Poodle Pseudoachondroplasia[7,72]
Poor growth, abnormal gait; short, bent legs, enlarged joints; possible inferior prognathism; vertebrae short, limb bones short and thick with bulbous ends; stippled densities in epiphyses; ossification complete by 2 years of age, but limbs remained short and deformed; probable autosomal recessive trait

Newfoundland Osteochondrodysplasia[81,82]
Radiographically evident irregularities in the metaphysis and distal diaphysis of the radius and ulna, characterized by distinct opaque islands of trabeculae in longitudinal striations. May be a focal failure of conversion from primary to secondary spongiosa. Usually an incidental radiographic finding that is not associated with any clinical signs or gross deformity.

Norwegian Elkhound Chondrodysplasia[7,72]
Shortened body, disproportionally short limbs, especially forelegs, which may be bowed; metaphyses flared and flattened, with denser band; ventral vertebral bodies irregular, delayed union of vertebral end plates; may have glucosuria; autosomal recessive trait

Samoyed Ocular-Skeletal Dysplasia[7,83,84]
Short forelegs, varus deformity of elbows, valgus of carpi, premature closure of ulnar growth plates, bowed radii; domed forehead; cataracts, retinal detachment, hyaloid artery remnants eosinophilia; autosomal recessive trait

Scottish Deerhound Pseudoachondroplasia (Osteochondrodysplasia)[85,86]
Retarded growth, short bowed limbs, exercise intolerance, small head, short trunk, lax joints, kyphosis; vertebrae and long bones short, epiphyseal ossification irregular and delayed; later osteopenia, severe deformity; single autosomal recessive inheritance suspected

---

unresponsiveness to thyroid-stimulating hormone (TSH) with autosomal recessive inheritance in Japanese cats,[101] and thyroid unresponsiveness to TSH in related Scottish Deerhounds.[102]

Abnormalities may be detectable by the age of 1 or 2 months. Affected animals are disproportionate dwarfs, with short limbs and spine, blocklike trunks, and broad short skulls. The radiographic features are epiphyseal dysgenesis and delayed skeletal maturation (Figure 195-12). Nonskeletal findings include delayed dental eruption, macroglossia, leth-

argy, mental dullness, persistent puppy haircoat progressing to thinning and alopecia, mild nonregenerative anemia, and hypercholesterolemia. Thyroid gland enlargement can accompany congenital dyshormonogenesis[103] but is absent if a hypothalamic-pituitary defect is causing thyroid understimulation[104] or thyroids are unresponsive to TSH.

A low blood plasma thyroxine concentration is expected, but results of other thyroid tests will differ, depending on whether the defect is of thyroidal, pituitary, or hypothalamic origin. The plasma growth hormone response to provocative

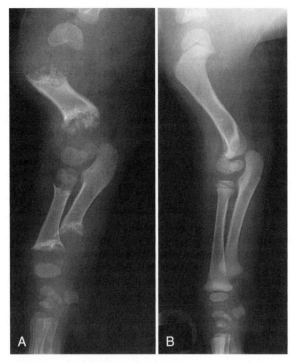

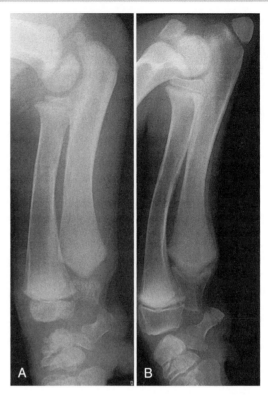

Figure 195-10 **A,** Radiograph of a 5-week-old Alaskan Malamute with chondrodysplasia. Physeal cartilage is widened, and adjacent metaphyseal bone roughened and irregular. **B,** Radiograph of a normal littermate of same age for comparison.

Figure 195-12 **A,** Forelimb of 15-week-old Great Dane with features of congenital hypothyroidism. Reader should note the disordered and irregular ossification of epiphyses (epiphyseal dysgenesis) in humerus, radius, and ulna; the absence of an olecranon apophysis; and delayed skeletal maturation. **B,** Normal Great Dane of similar age for comparison. (Courtesy R.B. Lavelle.)

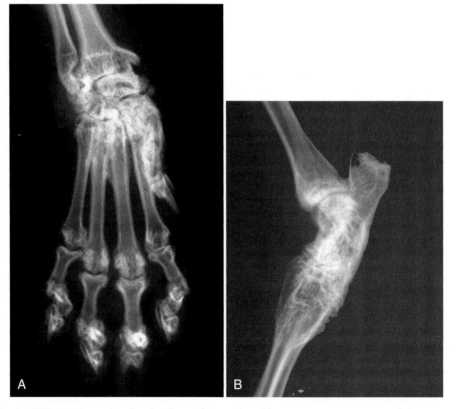

Figure 195-11 Osteochondro-dysplasia of Scottish Fold cats. **A,** Exostoses around the carpus. **B,** Exostoses and ankylosis of the tarsal joints. (Courtesy Veterinary Imaging Associates, Sydney, Australia.)

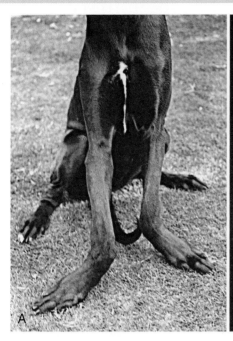
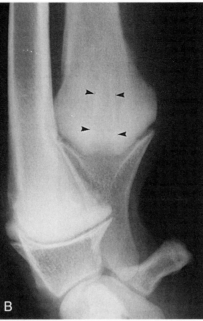

Figure 195-13 **A,** Seven-month-old Great Dane with bilateral forelimb deformities caused by retained cartilage cores in the distal ulnar physes. **B,** Radiograph demonstrating retained cartilage core *(arrowheads)* extending from distal ulnar physis into the metaphysis. (From Johnson KA: Retardation of endochondral ossification at the distal ulnar growth plate in dogs. Aust Vet J 57:474, 1987.)

stimuli may be suppressed (see Chapter 284).[98,104] Treatment with thyroxine can reverse many of the abnormalities but should commence early and continue for life.

Retained Cartilage Cores

In young large and giant breed dogs, cartilage cores sometimes form in the metaphysis of the distal ulna. Physeal hypertrophic chondrocytes fail to mature and mineralize adjacent matrix, and they accumulate in long columns in the primary spongiosa.[105] The cause of the disorder is unclear. In Great Dane pups, formation of cartilage cores in the distal ulnar and tibial metaphyses was associated with feeding diets containing three times the recommended content of calcium.[106]

Radiographically a central, radiolucent core of cartilage exists that is 5 to 10 mm wide and 2 to 6 cm long, extending from distal ulnar physis into metaphyseal bone (Figure 195-13). Lesions are usually bilateral. They may be a subclinical radiographic finding or be associated with varying degrees of growth retardation after 5 months of age. Retarded ulnar growth causes relative shortening of the ulna, valgus, and rotation of the paw, cranial bowing of the radius, and carpal and elbow subluxation (see Figure 195-13).

Craniomandibular Osteopathy

Craniomandibular osteopathy occurs mainly in young West Highland White, Scottish, Cairn, Boston, and other terriers, and occasionally in nonterrier breeds.[107] Autosomal recessive inheritance is known in West Highland White Terriers,[108] and a hereditary predisposition may exist in Scottish Terriers. However, the sporadic occurrence in unrelated breeds suggests other causative factors are also involved. Canine distemper virus (CDV) infection of bone has been mentioned as a possible cause,[107] although an epidemiologic study did not indicate a direct relationship.[109] The condition is usually recognized at 3 to 8 months of age, when affected pups develop mandibular swelling, drooling of saliva, prehension difficulties, pain on opening the mouth, or some combination of these signs. The clinical course may fluctuate, with periods of remission and exacerbation. Abnormal physical findings comprise firm, often painful, swelling of mandible, temporomandibular region, or both areas. Periods of pyrexia occur in some cases. Restricted jaw movements and atrophy of masticatory

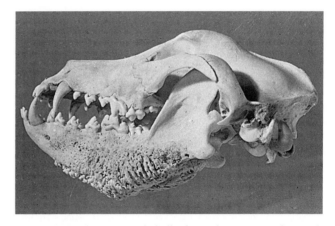

Figure 195-14 Macerated skull of a Doberman Pinscher with craniomandibular osteopathy. Reader should note extensive bone changes involving mandible. Tympanic bullae, petrous temporal bones, and temporomandibular joint regions were unaffected in this dog. (From Watson ADJ et al: Craniomandibular osteopathy in Doberman Pinschers. J Small Anim Pract 16:11, 1975.)

muscles may be obvious in severely affected dogs. Mandibular swelling without pain or eating difficulties occurs in some dogs, especially of larger breeds.

Radiographic changes are generally bilateral but often asymmetric, with irregular bony proliferation involving the mandible and tympanic bulla-petrous temporal bone areas in about 50% of cases. However, changes can be confined to the mandible (33% of cases) (Figure 195-14) or the tympanic bulla-petrous temporal region (13%). The calvarium and tentorium ossium are often thickened (Figure 195-15), and other skull bones are sometimes affected. Concurrent long bone lesions resembling later stages of metaphyseal osteopathy have been observed in a few terriers with craniomandibular osteopathy.

The diagnosis is straightforward in cases with typical clinical and radiographic features. Routine laboratory tests are unlikely to be helpful. Bone biopsy may be useful in atypical

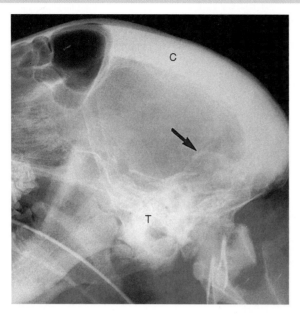

Figure 195-15 Skull of Scottish Terrier with craniomandibular osteopathy. The tympanic bulla-petrous bone area *(T)* shows dense sclerotic bone changes. Reader should note thickened calvarium *(C)* and tentorium osseum *(arrow)*.

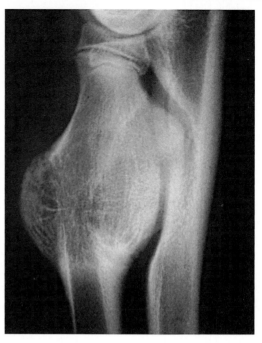

Figure 195-16 Radiograph demonstrating a solitary multiple cartilaginous exostosis-type lesion in the forelimb of a young dog. Reader should note the expansile lesion of the proximal radius, causing malalignment of the radius and attenuation of adjacent ulna. (Courtesy R.B. Lavelle.)

cases, such as dogs of rarely affected breeds with lesions confined to the mandible, especially if unilateral. The histopathology involves resorption of existing lamellae, proliferation of coarse trabecular bone beyond normal periosteal boundaries, replacement of marrow spaces by vascular fibrous stroma, and infiltration at the periphery of new bone by inflammatory cells. A mosaic pattern of irregular cement lines is present in the new primitive bone.[110]

Craniomandibular osteopathy is self-limiting. Abnormal bone proliferation eventually slows and becomes static at about 1 year of age. Lesions then tend to regress, although radiographic abnormalities or impaired prehension sometimes persist. Antiinflammatory drug treatment can reduce pain and discomfort, but the effect on lesions is unknown. The prognosis is guarded when extensive changes affect the tympanic-petrous temporal areas and adjacent mandible. Ankylosis and adhesions may then develop, permanently restricting jaw movements and eating.

Multiple Cartilaginous Exostoses

In rare instances these benign lesions (osteochondromatosis, multiple hereditary osteochondromata) occur in dogs and cats, as single or multiple exostoses.[111,112] The disorder may be inherited as an autosomal dominant trait in humans, horses, and dogs.[113,114] Protuberances consist of cancellous bone covered by a cap of hyaline cartilage and arise in the metaphyseal region of bones formed by endochondral ossification. With continued physeal growth and elongation of long bones, exostoses may be finally located in the diaphysis. Lesions develop and grow most rapidly in immature animals, becoming senescent at maturity. Malignant transformation of exostoses to chondrosarcoma occurs rarely in aged animals.[115,116]

The cause is unknown. One hypothesis is that congenital or acquired defects in the perichondrial ring allow an island of physeal cartilage to be pinched off and trapped in metaphyseal bone. This physeal cartilage continues to grow radially, giving rise to exostoses. However, this does not explain the similar lesions found occasionally in nonskeletal sites, such as tracheal cartilages.

Superficially located exostoses may be palpable. Signs may include paresis due to progressive spinal cord compression in young animals (see Chapter 262) or pain due to impingement of exostoses on adjacent tissues.[117] Radiographically, lesions are rounded to cauliflower-like in outline, with a smooth thin shell of cortical bone (Figure 195-16). They protrude above the bone contour and may extend into the medullary cavity. Internally, exostoses have well-defined bone trabeculae that are continuous with the medullary cavity, and diaphyseal cortex in the region is interrupted by the lesion. Adjacent bones such as ulna and metacarpals may be deformed by expanding exostoses (see Figure 195-16). Solitary exostoses are biopsied to allow differentiation from neoplastic lesions. Surgical excision of exostoses that are causing spinal cord compression or lameness is recommended (see Chapter 262).[117] All exostoses should be monitored for malignant transformation.

IDIOPATHIC BONE DISORDERS

Enostosis

Enostosis (panosteitis, eosinophilic panosteitis) is a relatively common disease causing lameness in medium-, large-, and giant-breed dogs.[118] Among breeds at greatest risk are Great Pyrenees, Basset Hound, Shar-Pei, Mastiff, Giant Schnauzer, and German Shepherd.[119] Two thirds of affected dogs are male. The age of onset is 6 to 18 months; older dogs are rarely affected. Lameness is acute in onset, not associated with trauma, and intermittent in one or more limbs. Each episode of lameness lasts 2 to 3 weeks but, with recurrent bouts, enostosis may persist for 2 to 9 months. Other signs in early stages include anorexia, lethargy, pyrexia, and weight loss. On physical examination, pain is detected on deep palpation of affected bones. Bones commonly affected are the ulna, humerus, radius, femur, and tibia. Ilium, metatarsal, and other bones are rarely affected. The disease begins in the medullary bone marrow, in the region of a nutrient foramen.

The cause is unknown: Genetic predisposition, hemophilia, bacterial infection, vascular abnormality, metabolic disease, allergy, hyperestrogenism, and endoparasitism have been proposed, but the evidence for most of these is scant.[118] Viral infection is considered a possible cause, based on clinical features of the disease, transmission experiments, and in situ hybridization demonstration of virus in bone cells of dogs infected with CDV.[118,120] A relationship between enostosis and ingestion of protein-and-energy-rich foods was suggested recently, and changes in protein or amino acid metabolism were reported in affected dogs.[121]

Three radiographic stages are recognizable.[118] The first stage, with medullary radiolucency due to bone marrow degeneration, is infrequently seen. Most often detected is the second stage (Figure 195-17). A granular, hazy increased radiopacity that begins in the region of the nutrient foramen may extend to fill the entire medullary cavity. Formation of new endosteal bone and a thin layer of smooth periosteal bone are secondary changes. In the final stage, most bones return to normal appearance, but some have residual thickening of medullary trabeculae and cortical deformity.

Histopathologically, lesions are characterized initially by replacement of normal marrow by fibrous tissue, followed by excessive remodeling of cortical and medullary bone in the affected areas, with endosteal new bone formation generally

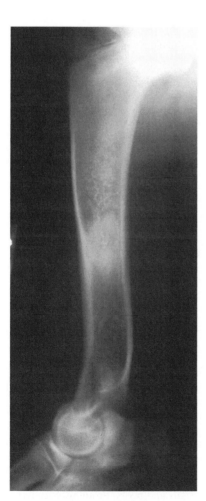

Figure 195-17 Radiograph of a forelimb of a young dog with enostosis, showing patchy intramedullary densities in the humeral diaphysis. (Courtesy Veterinary Imaging Associates, Sydney, Australia.)

more prominent.[118] Basenjis and West Highland White Terrier dogs with inherited pyruvate kinase (PK) deficiency can develop intramedullary osteosclerosis but, unlike enostosis, new trabecular bone formation is uniform throughout the medullary cavity.[122]

Enostosis can occur concurrently with developmental diseases such as ununited anconeal process and osteochondritis dissecans, and it may be difficult to determine which disease is causing lameness. Leukocytosis and eosinophilia occur inconsistently in affected dogs; serum chemistry is unremarkable. Enostosis is self-limiting, usually by age 18 months, but analgesic NSAIDS may help alleviate pain and lameness.

Metaphyseal Osteopathy

Metaphyseal osteopathy (hypertrophic osteodystrophy) is a disease of young, rapidly growing dogs of larger breeds. Breeds at particular risk include Great Dane, Weimaraner, Boxer, Irish Setter, German Shepherd, and Labrador and Golden Retrievers.[119] Signs usually begin at 3 to 4 months of age (range 2 to 8 months), with metaphyseal swelling and pain, accompanied by depression, inappetence, and variable pyrexia. Some cases recover within a few days, but others have one or more relapses during the following weeks before they finally recover. In a few instances, repeated relapses and consequent pain, cachexia, and debility necessitate euthanasia. Unexplained deaths have been observed rarely.

Radiographic changes occur especially in metaphyses of limb bones and are usually bilateral. Scapulae and ribs may also be affected. In the early stage, an irregular radiolucent zone is present in the metaphysis, separated from the normal-appearing growth plate by an opaque band (Figure 195-18, A). Surrounding soft tissue may be swollen. Later radiographs may show metaphyseal enlargement with irregular periosteal new bone formation, although not all affected dogs develop these changes (Figure 195-18, B). Once the disease is no longer active, bone changes undergo repair and remodeling, but some diaphyseal distortion and exostoses may remain (Figures 195-18, C, and 195-19).

Hematologic and biochemical tests contribute little to the diagnosis, although neutrophilia, monocytosis, and lymphocytopenia can occur during active disease, reflecting stress and inflammation. The principal histologic changes involve the primary spongiosa of metaphyses, with acute suppurative osteomyelitis, necrosis, trabecular microfractures, and defective bone formation. Trabecular resorption produces the radiolucent metaphyseal zone. The opaque band near the growth plate results from trabecular collapse and secondary bone formation. Periosteal thickening, with subperiosteal fibrosis and inflammation, periosteal new bone formation, extraperiosteal dystrophic calcification, or a combination of these abnormalities may be seen.[123]

The cause of metaphyseal osteopathy is unknown. Prior suggestions implicating hypovitaminosis C, overnutrition, or copper deficiency have not been substantiated. Attempts to identify a causative infectious agent or to transmit the disease have not been successful. However, CDV RNA has been detected within bone cells of dogs with metaphyseal osteopathy, suggesting a role for this virus in the etiopathogenesis.[124] Other circumstantial evidence supports this[123-125]: Metaphyseal osteopathy may be accompanied or preceded by respiratory or gastrointestinal (GI) signs; dental enamel hypoplasia, a sequel to distemper infection, was found in two dogs with metaphyseal osteopathy; three of seven dogs inoculated with blood from dogs with metaphyseal osteopathy developed distemper; and typical bone changes have developed in some pups 4 to 21 days after inoculation with live distemper virus vaccine. However, the osteosclerotic metaphyseal lesions found in a series of dogs clinically affected with distemper differed macroscopically, radiographically, and histologically

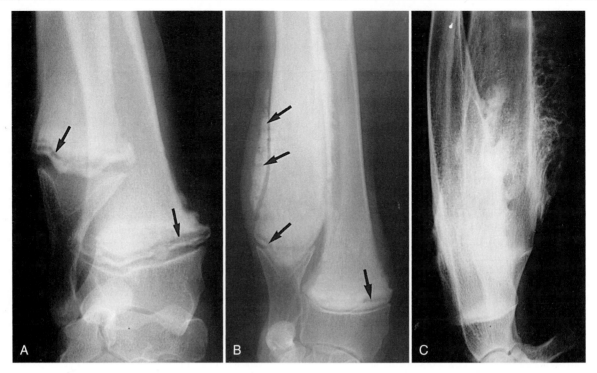

Figure 195-18 Radiographs of metaphyseal osteopathy. **A,** Early stage with irregular radiolucent zone *(arrows)* separated from the physis by a narrow radiopaque band. **B,** Later stage with radiolucent metaphyseal zones *(bottom two arrows)* adjacent to the physes still evident. Periosteal new bone and soft tissue mineralization *(top two arrows)* adjacent to the metaphyseal cortex. **C,** Inactive stage with residual diaphyseal deformity and spiculated periosteal exostoses.

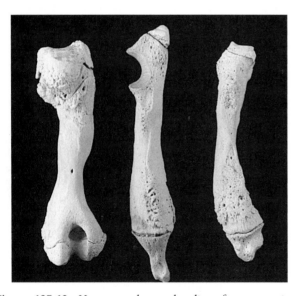

Figure 195-19 Humerus, ulna, and radius of a young giant-breed dog that suffered metaphyseal osteopathy. Reader should note the severe deformities and periosteal new bone.

from metaphyseal osteopathy.[126] Any relationship between distemper virus, metaphyseal osteopathy, and other hyperostotic bone diseases (craniomandibular osteopathy and enostosis) remains uncertain. An epidemiologic study concluded that, apart from the obvious age effect, risk factors for metaphyseal osteopathy, craniomandibular osteopathy, and CDV infection were dissimilar.[109] Metaphyseal osteopathy has been reported in related dogs of several breeds, including Weima-

raner littermates.[125-127] However, most cases are sporadic, affecting isolated pups in a litter.

No specific treatment exists for metaphyseal osteopathy. Dietary imbalances or excesses should be avoided and an antiinflammatory analgesic given as needed to reduce pain. Good nursing care may be required to avoid dehydration, undernutrition, and pressure sores.

Calvarial Hyperostosis

An unusual hyperostosis affecting frontal and parietal bones was reported in two unrelated Bullmastiffs.[123,128] From age 6 months there was progressive outward thickening of the calvarium (the cranial cavity was unaffected) with pyrexia, lymphadenopathy, and eosinophilia. The swelling stabilized at maturity, then regressed. The lesion was a subperiosteal hyperostosis with initial deposition of new woven bone followed by secondary osteonal remodeling. Similarities were noted with cases of craniomandibular osteopathy, inherited PK deficiency, and human infantile cortical hyperostosis.[122,129,130]

Multifocal Osteopathy

An idiopathic multifocal osteopathy was described in four young adult Scottish Terriers, of which at least three were genetically related (fourth pedigree unavailable).[131] The condition was characterized by multifocal absence of bone in skull, cervical spine, radius, ulna, and femur (Figure 195-20). Histopathologic findings in one case indicated osteoclastic osteolysis and replacement of bone by fibrous tissue. Associated clinical signs included reluctance to move, stiff and stilted gait, carpal valgus and laxity, drooling, and dysphagia.

Avascular Necrosis of the Femoral Head

Avascular (or aseptic) necrosis of the femoral head (Legg-Calve-Perthes disease) occurs in adolescent dogs. Miniature-

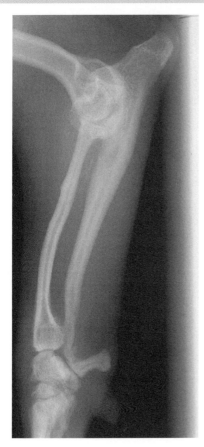

Figure 195-20 Radiograph of the antebrachium of a Scottish Terrier with multifocal osteopathy. Reader should note the marked attenuation in diameter of the radial diaphysis. (Courtesy C.W. Hay.)

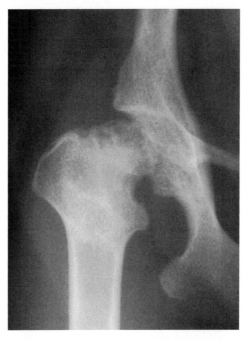

Figure 195-21 Later stage Legg-Calvé-Perthes disease. Reader should note the multifocal osteolysis of the femoral head, thickened femoral neck, and increase in width of joint space. (Courtesy Veterinary Imaging Associates, Sydney, Australia.)

and small-dog breeds are mostly affected, but Australian Shepherd dogs also have increased risk of developing this disorder.[119] Within the predisposed small breeds, about 2% of individuals are affected, without apparent sex predilection. Clinically affected individuals are commonly presented at 4 to 11 months of age with hind leg lameness, usually unilateral but sometimes bilateral (12% to 20% of cases). The onset of lameness is usually gradual, though there may sometimes be a history of trauma. The severity varies from a slight limp to complete non-weight-bearing lameness. Pain and reduced range of movement are found on palpating the affected joint. Crepitus, shortening (up to 2 cm) of the affected limb, and muscle atrophy may be evident at initial presentation.

The cause of this condition is unknown, but autosomal recessive inheritance has been suggested for West Highland White and Yorkshire Terriers, Toy and Miniature Poodles, and Pug dogs.[132] Early exposure to sex hormones, a consequence of precocious sexual maturity in small breeds, may be a factor. Another suggestion is that injury or infection and increased synovial fluid in the hip joint disrupt the blood supply to the femoral epiphysis while the growth plate is present. Continued weight bearing could then lead to collapse and remodeling of the femoral neck and head.

One of the earliest radiographic changes in this disorder is increased radio-opacity of the affected femoral head. Later changes include an apparent increase in joint space width, shortening and widening of the femoral neck, irregular opacity of femoral epiphyseal and metaphyseal regions, and flattening and irregularity of femoral articular cartilage (Figure 195-21). Secondary osteoarthrosis and acetabular osteophytes may also be evident.

Conservative treatment (short walks on a leash several times daily, swimming, analgesic drug as needed) produces satisfactory outcomes in 25% to 30% of affected dogs, whereas femoral head and neck excision, when performed correctly, gives good to excellent results in 67% to 85% of cases, though slight intermittent lameness may remain.[114,133] Excision arthroplasty is advisable if conservative treatment does not produce clinical improvement within 4 weeks.[133]

Secondary Hypertrophic Osteopathy

In secondary hypertrophic osteopathy (pulmonary hypertrophic osteoarthropathy), firm nonedematous swelling develops in all four limbs, usually in response to intrathoracic disease, most often neoplasia. Of 180 canine cases, 98% had intrathoracic disease, and 92% of these had either metastatic lung neoplasia or primary tumors of lung or thoracic esophagus.[134] A few dogs had pneumonitis, endocarditis, or dirofilariasis. Of four cases lacking intrathoracic disease, three had urinary rhabdomyosarcoma and one had hepatic carcinoma. Because of the association with neoplasia, secondary hypertrophic osteopathy occurs mostly in older animals. No breed or gender predilection exists in dogs. The disorder is rare in cats.

Signs related to limb changes often precede signs of thoracic disease, but they can begin simultaneously with or after thoracic signs. Affected animals are stiff and reluctant to move. Swelling occurs in all limbs, which are warm, firm, and may be painful. Thoracic disease may be manifested by cough, dyspnea, abnormal lung sounds, or cardiac displacement. Abnormal laboratory findings, if any, are related to the underlying intrathoracic disease.

Radiographic changes are characteristic: soft tissue swelling of distal extremities initially, then periosteal new bone formation as irregular nodules perpendicular to the cortex or smoother parallel deposits (Figure 195-22). Bone changes begin distally and may spread proximally to involve humerus and scapula, femur, and pelvis. Ribs and vertebrae are sometimes affected.

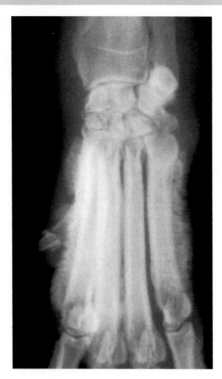

Figure 195-22 Radiograph of distal forelimb of a dog with secondary hypertrophic osteopathy. Periosteal new bone growth occurs, with nodular appearance affecting the metacarpals and digits. Adjacent soft tissues are thickened. (Courtesy Veterinary Imaging Associates, Sydney, Australia.)

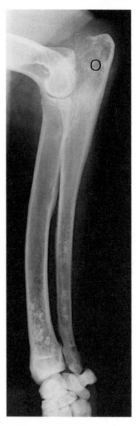

Figure 195-23 Radiograph demonstrating medullary bone infarction in an aged dog with osteosarcoma *(O)* of the olecranon. The multiple areas of medullary sclerosis in the radius and ulna are infarcts.

On histologic examination, the bones are surrounded by highly vascular, dense connective tissue containing numerous thick-walled arteries. The osteogenic layer of the periosteum is hyperplastic and overlies maturing and remodeling trabecular bone. The pathogenesis of secondary hypertrophic osteopathy involves increased blood flow to the distal extremities, then overgrowth of connective tissue and subsequent osteoneogenesis. This seems to involve a neural reflex originating in the thorax and affecting connective tissue and periosteum of the limbs. The efferent pathway apparently involves nerve fibers that leave the lung near the bronchi and join the vagus in the mediastinum. The nature of the efferent connection, whether neural or hormonal, is unknown. Regression of secondary hypertrophic osteopathy may follow (1) removal of the source of afferent impulses by excision of the lung lesion or (2) interruption of the afferent fibers by peribronchial dissection or vagotomy. There may be an alternate afferent pathway from parietal pleura along intercostal nerves because regression has sometimes followed thoracotomy and section of intercostal nerves or extensive resection of a neoplasm of the thoracic wall. The rare association with intraabdominal lesions is more obscure.

Treatment should be directed against the underlying thoracic disease, using appropriate medical or surgical methods. Successful resection of lung lesions by lobectomy or pneumonectomy can quickly remove pain, soft tissue swelling, and lameness. The bone abnormalities usually regress gradually over several months. Where complete removal of lung lesions is not possible, the skeletal signs may be ameliorated by removal of larger lesions even if multiple small lesions remain. Relief may also follow intrathoracic vagotomy on the same side as the lesion or on the worse affected side if metastases are bilateral.

Medullary Bone Infarction

Medullary bone infarcts do not cause clinical signs in dogs. They affect older dogs and are usually found in conjunction with osteosarcoma and, occasionally, skeletal fibrosarcoma or renal adenocarcinoma.[135,136] Bone infarcts are characterized radiographically by numerous, irregularly demarcated areas of increased radiopacity in the medullary cavities of one or more bones (Figure 195-23). The densities obliterate medullary cavities to varying degrees. Any bone may be affected, but infarcts are mainly found distal to elbow and stifle.[135]

The pathogenesis of the disorder is unknown and does not seem to be due to metastatic tumor cell dissemination. However, intramural collagen deposition causes occlusion of nutrient arteries, hypoxia and widespread necrosis of medullary soft tissues and bone, and new bone proliferation on endosteum and medullary trabeculae.[135] Common causes in humans are dysbaric conditions, fat embolization, hyperadrenocorticism, hyperviscosity, hemoglobinopathy, and anemia. Medullary bone infarcts should be differentiated from enostosis, bacterial and fungal osteomyelitis, and metastatic neoplasia.

Bone Cyst

Benign cystic bone lesions, either monostotic or polyostotic, are uncommon in dogs and cats. Young dogs of larger breeds are affected most often, with Doberman Pinschers and German Shepherds overrepresented.[114,137] Males are affected twice as often as females. The cause is unknown but may involve intramedullary metaphyseal hemorrhage, local disturbance of bone growth, or other factors.[134] Heritable factors might also be implicated because lesions occurred in three

Doberman Pinscher littermates and in three Old English Sheepdog littermates and both parents.[114]

Bone cysts may be subclinical until they are large or fracture with trauma. Pain, lameness, and local swelling may ensue. The lesions occur in metaphyses and adjacent diaphyses of long bones, sparing growth plates and epiphyses. The distal radius or ulna (or both) are affected most often. The cysts are lined by a thin membrane and contain fluid that may be blood tinged. Radiographically, the lesions are lytic and expansile, with thinned cortex and little or no periosteal reaction. There may be one or several chambers, partially divided by bony ridges or partitions (Figure 195-24).

Alternative diagnoses are atypical bone neoplasia, aneurysmal bone cyst, and fibrous dysplasia of bone. Fine needle aspiration biopsy and cytologic examination may be useful: only a benign bone cyst is likely to be fluid filled, although the other lesions may contain areas of cystic degeneration or hemorrhage. If uncertainty persists, surgical biopsy and histopathologic study are indicated. To stimulate healing of bone cysts, surgery has been advocated, using drainage, curettage, bone grafting, and external support to prevent fractures. Some untreated cysts heal spontaneously without surgery, although pathologic fracture of cystic bone is a risk.[138]

Aneurysmal Bone Cyst

Aneurysmal bone cyst is a nonneoplastic lesion that results in considerable local bone destruction. Although common in man, it is rare in dogs and cats. Lesions arise in ribs, pelvis, scapula, spine, and metaphyses of long bones in young adults and geriatric animals.[139,140] The cause is unknown, but tumors, developmental abnormalities, and trauma-induced hemorrhage causing venous obstruction or arteriovenous shunts in bone marrow have been suggested as initiating factors.[7] Localized partial disruption of medullary blood flow results in endosteal bone resorption and outward displacement of the periosteum. The periosteum forms successive layers of woven

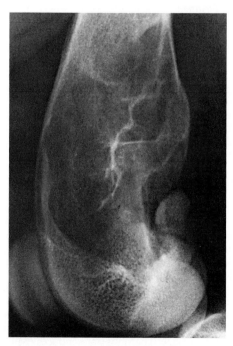

Figure 195-24 Bone cyst in distal femur of a young Doberman Pinscher. The lesion has expansile, lytic appearance, with thinning of overlying cortex. Bony ridges or partitions are evident internally.

bone that are resorbed as the lesion expands, producing the appearance of a ballooning aortic aneurysm.[7] Blood-tinged fluid and fibrovascular tissue fill the lesion, which has a honeycomb appearance with huge vascular channels. Radiographically, it appears as a large expansile cyst, with minimal internal trabecular septation, surrounded by thin rim of mineralized soft tissue or bone (Figure 195-25). A triangle of laminated periosteal new bone (Codman's triangle) forms at the junction between cyst and adjacent normal diaphyseal bone. Some have an underlying tumor (osteosarcoma, giant cell tumor) that complicates diagnosis. Signs may be suddenly exacerbated by neoplastic erosion of vessels and intralesional hemorrhage or by fracture.[140] Uncomplicated lesions have a good prognosis when treated by en bloc resection, amputation, or curettage.[141] Nonresectable lesions in man are irradiated to stop bleeding and lesional growth, but postirradiation sarcoma can ensue.

Subchondral Bone Cyst

Subchondral bone cysts are benign lesions in subchondral bone between growth plate and articular cartilage.[142] They are usually lined with synovium and occasionally communicate with the articular synovial membrane. Radiographs show a single or multilocular radiolucent defect with well-circumscribed borders. They are common in horses and pigs and usually a manifestation of osteochondrosis.[7] This association was also noted in a dog.[142]

Fibrous Dysplasia

Fibrous dysplasia is a rare fibro-osseous lesion of bone believed to be of developmental origin.[7] It affects mainly young or newborn animals and may be monostotic or polyostotic. The lesions are expansile and may cause problems of disfigurement or compression of adjacent structures or bone weakness and fracture (Figure 195-26). Monostotic lesions have been reported in the jaw or infraorbital bone of dog, and in mandible, maxilla, or distal ulna of cats.[143,144] Fibrous dysplasia, aneurysmal bone cysts, and benign bone cysts are distinct entities but have been confused in the veterinary literature.[145]

The lesions have marked homogenous radiopacity and are composed of firm, gray fibrous tissue that is gritty when cut. Histologically, they consist of fibrous connective tissue stroma containing spicules of woven bone replacing normal osseous tissue. Cavities of various size containing clear or bloody fluid may be scattered throughout.[7] Two feline lesions were resected, and both patients were free of recurrence 4 years later.[143]

Central Giant Cell Granuloma

This rare, nonneoplastic lesion affects the tooth-bearing regions of maxilla and mandible of young dogs.[146] Trauma-associated intraosseous hemorrhage seems to be an initiating factor. Radiographically the lesion is a rounded to ovoid, expansile, uniloculated radiolucency that is well demarcated from surrounding tissue by a thin rim of smooth nonreactive bone. Adjacent teeth may lose their laminae dura and be displaced, but tooth root resorption is rare. The center of the lesion consists of tan-colored soft tissue composed mainly of loose fibrovascular stroma containing pleomorphic mesenchymal cells and numerous large, irregular multinucleated giant cells. These cells arise from mesenchymal tissue; they are not osteoclasts and are not involved in bone resorption. The lesions resemble giant cell tumors histologically. The latter are potentially malignant tumors that cause extensive destruction at the ends of long bones. Because central giant cell granuloma is rare, diagnosis should be confirmed by biopsy. Treatment is by curettage or en bloc resection.[146]

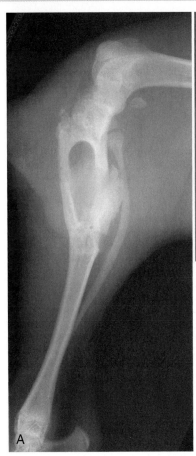

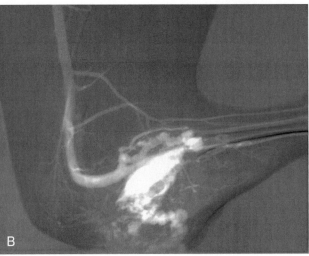

Figure 195-25 Aneurysmal bone cyst of the tibia in a 2-year-old Boxer dog that had sustained a tibial fracture as a puppy. **A,** Reader should note the angular deformity of the diaphyses of the tibia and fibular due to fracture malunion. A large cystic cavity in the proximal tibia is associated with a soft tissue mass cranial to the tibia. **B,** Arteriogram showing a dilated, tortuous arteriovenous fistula extending from the tibia into adjacent soft tissue. (Courtesy J.H. Marti.)

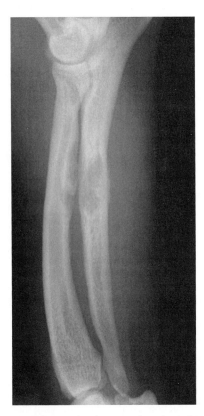

Figure 195-26 Fibrous dysplasia in the ulnar diaphysis, with secondary lysis and new bone formation in adjacent radial cortex. (Courtesy P.A. Manley.)

METABOLIC, NUTRITIONAL, AND ENDOCRINE BONE DISORDERS

The term *metabolic bone disease* is used here to encompass various conditions that cause generalized reduction in bone mass, or osteopenia. Osteopenia can be categorized into excessive bone resorption, or osteolysis, as occurs in hyperparathyroid states, and defective bone formation. The latter is further subdivided into insufficient formation of osteoid, or osteoporosis, and defective mineralization of osteoid, or rickets-osteomalacia.

Major causes of metabolic bone disease involve nutritional or hormonal processes (or both). The more important causes discussed here are nutritional secondary hyperparathyroidism, rickets, renal osteodystrophy, and hypervitaminosis A. Other metabolic bone diseases that rarely produce bone-related clinical signs are mentioned briefly.

Nutritional Secondary Hyperparathyroidism

Nutritional secondary hyperparathyroidism is a metabolic disorder in which bone production is normal but osteopenia results from excessive bone resorption. It is caused by diets providing excess phosphate, insufficient calcium, or both.[114] Affected animals have usually been fed mainly meat, organ tissue, or both. This provides adequate phosphate but insufficient calcium and Ca/P ratios of about 1:16 to 1:35,[147] which contrast with the recommended 1.2:1 for dogs and 1:1 for cats. Added cow's milk provides insufficient calcium to correct the imbalance. The imbalance induces hypocalcemia, which increases secretion of PTH. Increased parathyroid activity tends to normalize blood calcium and inorganic phosphate concentrations by promoting mineral resorption from bone, enhancing intestinal calcium absorption, and facilitating

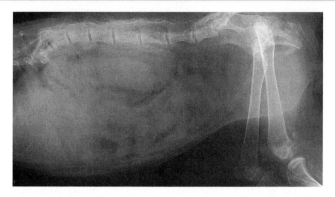

Figure 195-27 Abdomen of kitten with nutritional secondary hyperparathyroidism. Reader should note poor contrast in radiopacity between bones and soft tissues such as liver and kidneys. The cortices of long bones are thin, vertebrae are lucent, and the vertebral column is deformed in the thoracolumbar area.

renal phosphate excretion and calcium retention. However, continued ingestion of the defective diet sustains the hyperparathyroid state and causes progressive skeletal demineralization and consequent clinical signs.

Nutritional secondary hyperparathyroidism causes clinical disease in pups and kittens of all breeds, but it also occurs occasionally in adults. Signs in young animals are lameness, reluctance to stand or walk, and skeletal pain. Costochondral junctions and metaphyses may appear swollen, and pyrexia is sometimes present. Bone fractures can follow relatively mild trauma. Limb deformity may be evident. Paresis or paralysis may result from vertebral compression, and constipation may follow pelvic collapse. Effects are less dramatic in adults, but generalized osteopenia and skeletal pain are sometimes seen, and resorption of alveolar bone may cause loosening and loss of teeth.

Radiographically, decreased bone density and thin cortices are seen, with or without fracturing (Figure 195-27). Growth plates are normal, but metaphyses may be mushroom shaped. An area of relative radio-opacity occurs in the metaphyses adjacent to growth plates, representing the area of primary mineralization, and may be best appreciated in the distal radius and ulna (Figure 195-28).

Blood biochemical tests are of little value in confirming nutritional secondary hyperparathyroidism. The calcium concentration is usually within the reference range because of compensatory changes. Concentrations of inorganic phosphate and alkaline phosphatase may appear high but should be interpreted carefully because growing animals often have higher values than adults.

Affected animals should be confined for the first few weeks of treatment to reduce the risk of fractures and deformity. A good-quality, nutritionally complete commercial ration should be fed. For all but mildly affected cases, sufficient calcium carbonate should be added to produce a calcium/phosphorus ratio of 2:1. This is maintained for 2 to 3 months, after which the supplement is withdrawn. Oversupplementation with calcium should be avoided. For severely affected cases parenteral administration of calcium (e.g., 10 to 30 mL of 10% calcium gluconate solution by slow intravenous infusion daily for 3 days) may help reduce pain and lameness initially, but it does little to correct the calcium deficiency. An NSAID might be useful for short-term analgesia. The prognosis is generally good, unless skeletal deformity and disability are marked.

Rickets

Clinical cases of rickets are rare in dogs and cats. Rickets and its adult equivalent, osteomalacia, occur when insufficient

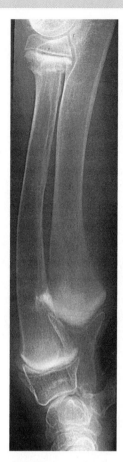

Figure 195-28 Foreleg of a pup with nutritional secondary hyperparathyroidism. Bone is abnormally radiolucent and cortices are thin. Growth plates are normal, but relatively radiopaque zones are present in the adjacent metaphyses (representing areas of primary mineralization of osteoid).

calcium, phosphorus, or both is available for mineralization of newly formed osteoid. The more likely causes of rickets in dogs and cats are hypovitaminosis D (dietary deficiency),[148] inborn error in vitamin D metabolism,[149] or low availability of minerals from the diet (inadequate concentration, impaired absorption). Dogs and cats do not synthesize cholecalciferol (previtamin D_3) in skin exposed to ultraviolet (UV) light and are mainly dependent on dietary intake.[150-152]

Affected animals may be lame and reluctant or unable to walk. Fractures or bending of long bones can occur. Enlargement of costochondral junctions and metaphyses may be evident. Other possible abnormalities are delayed dental eruption, weakness, listlessness, and neurologic signs (excitability, tremor, convulsion, and coma) from hypocalcemia. Potential blood test abnormalities include low calcium, low inorganic phosphate, increased alkaline phosphatase, increased PTH, and low 25-hydroxycholecalciferol (the storage form of vitamin D).[148,149,153]

Characteristic radiographic findings are axial and radial thickening of growth plates and cupping of adjacent metaphyses (Figures 195-29 and 195-30). The distal ulnar growth plates are consistently the most severely affected, and this finding reflects a failure of mineralization of cartilage that is being produced at the normal rate. Additional findings are osteopenia, thin cortices, and bowed diaphyses.

When dietary deficiency is suspected, therapy requires a regular diet with adequate and not excessive amounts of calcium, phosphorus, and vitamin D.[148,153] The regimen

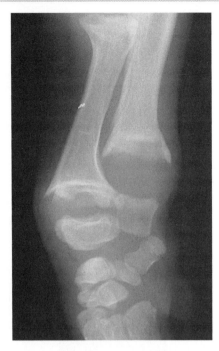

Figure 195-29 Foreleg of a 12-week-old Saint Bernard with rickets due to an inborn error in vitamin D metabolism. Enlarged physes and cupping of adjacent metaphyseal bone are features of rickets. (From Johnson KA et al: Vitamin D-dependent rickets in a Saint Bernard dog. J Small Anim Pract 29:657, 1988.)

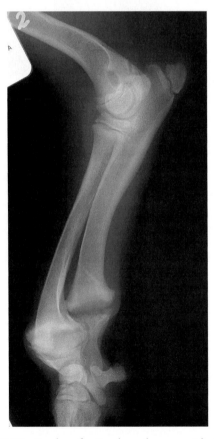

Figure 195-30 Foreleg of a Greyhound puppy with rickets due to dietary deficiency of vitamin D. Reader should note the axial and radial enlargement of the physes and cupping of the adjacent metaphyseal bone. (Courtesy R. Malik and Veterinary Imaging Associates, Sydney, Australia.)

described for nutritional secondary hyperparathyroidism would be appropriate. Treatment with dihydrotachysterol was effective in a dog in which an inborn error in vitamin D metabolism was suspected.[149]

Renal Osteodystrophy

Renal osteodystrophy is an osteopenic disorder that results from chronic renal failure (CRF). This complex abnormality involves both hyperparathyroidism (excessive bone resorption) and rickets-osteomalacia (impaired osteoid mineralization). Hyperparathyroidism results from impaired renal excretion of phosphate and consequent hyperphosphatemia. This lowers blood calcium concentration, increases parathyroid gland activity, and induces bone resorption. Although this tends to normalize blood calcium concentrations, the hyperparathyroid state is maintained by persisting hyperphosphatemia. Concurrently, synthesis of 1,25 dihydroxyvitamin D declines because of reduced functional renal mass. This and other metabolic derangements lead to severe depression of enteric calcium absorption, impaired mineralization of osteoid, and thus rickets-osteomalacia.

The syndrome is dominated by signs of renal failure and uremia. Bone disease is more likely to be recognized clinically in growing dogs or, rarely, cats with early-onset renal failure. Changes may be most evident in the head. The mandible and maxilla may be pliable and swollen, owing to bone resorption and fibrosis, and teeth may be malaligned, loose, or lost. Skeletal pain, fractures, and bowing of long bones can also occur. Osteopenia of the mandible and maxilla leads to enhanced radiographic contrast between teeth and bone, and teeth may appear almost unsupported by bony tissue.[154]

Treatment is directed against the underlying disease, if possible. Reduced phosphate intake, coupled with oral phosphate binder (aluminum hydroxide or carbonate) as needed, can help to control hyperphosphatemia. Once this is achieved, consideration can be given to administering calcium to improve calcium balance or administering calcitriol to control hyperparathyroidism (see Chapters 309 and 311).

Hypervitaminosis A

Prolonged intake of excessive vitamin A supplements or ingestion of mainly liver diets can cause osteopathy. The major finding in older cats is extensive, even confluent, exostoses and enthesophytes involving cervical and cranial thoracic vertebrae (Figure 195-31). Enthesophytes may also form around limb joints, especially shoulder or elbow, which may reflect increased sensitivity of tendon, ligament, and joint capsule attachments to the effects of tension.[134,155]

The lesions are painful in the early stages and may ankylose, causing neck stiffness and abnormal posture. Associated clinical signs are lethargy, depression, irritability, poor grooming, lameness, and gingivitis.[134] Experimental vitamin A toxicosis in young animals depressed chondrocyte and osteoblast activities, which produced thin bone cortices, retarded long-bone growth, and produced loose or lost teeth in kittens.[155,156] Puppies had joint pain, thin bone cortices, and retarded bone growth.[157]

Treatment necessitates avoiding the source of vitamin A. Mature cats will improve clinically, but rigidity from ankylosis will probably remain despite bone remodeling. Bone growth may be retarded permanently in young animals.[155]

Other Endocrine and Nutritional Bone Disorders

Primary Hyperparathyroidism With uncontrolled hyperplastic or neoplastic proliferation of parathyroid tissue, excessive secretion of PTH may cause increased bone remodeling and skeletal demineralization. This could lead to lameness, pain, fractures, vertebral collapse, loose or lost teeth, and pliable, possibly swollen jaw bones (Figure 195-32). However,

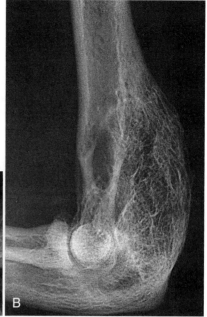

Figure 195-31 Cat with hypervitaminosis A. **A,** Confluent exostoses affect the dorsum of the spine from the second cervical to the fifth thoracic vertebrae. **B,** Exuberant exostoses of distal humerus and proximal ulna are ankylosing the elbow.

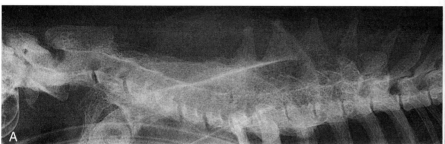

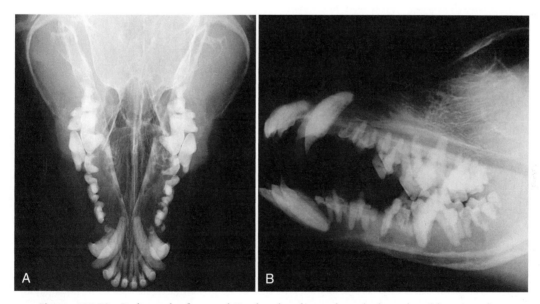

Figure 195-32 Radiograph of an aged Keeshond with parathyroid adenoma and hyperparathyroidism, with profound osteopenia of the skull and mandible. **A,** In the ventrodorsal view, osteolysis of the zygomatic arch, maxilla, facial bones, and mandible occurs. **B,** In the lateral view, loss of the lamina dura and mandibular cortex occurs, except for the thin ventral cortex.

the predominant findings usually relate to hypercalcemia[158] and include polydipsia (PD), polyuria (PU), listlessness, incontinence, weakness, inappetence, and urocystolithiasis (see Chapter 286).

Humoral Hypercalcemia of Malignancy With certain neoplasms, especially lymphosarcoma or adenocarcinoma of the anal sacs in dogs, widespread skeletal demineralization ensues through the humoral action of PTH-related protein.[158,159] Although skeletal dysfunction can occur as with primary hyperparathyroidism, findings are usually dominated by changes related to the underlying tumor and the effects of hypercalcemia (see Chapter 286).

Hyperadrenocorticism Chronic glucocorticosteroid excess due to iatrogenic excess or naturally occurring hyperadrenocorticism causes osteopenia. Retarded growth and delayed growth plate closure may occur in young dogs,[160] and spontaneous fractures and increased prevalence of intervertebral disk disease have been suggested.[161] Osteopenia in spontaneous canine hyperadrenocorticism is attributable primarily to decreased bone formation; bone resorption is apparently normal, although parathyroid hyperplasia is present in some cases (see Chapter 157).[161]

Hypogonadism Hypogonadism, whether a developmental defect or produced surgically, can delay growth plate closure.[7] In dogs, closure was delayed by neutering in both sexes, and the extended growth period resulted in longer radius and ulna in all males, as well as in bitches neutered at 7 weeks.[162] Gonadectomy in cats delayed distal radial physeal closure but did not affect bone length.[163] However, neutered male cats are predisposed to spontaneous, nontraumatic fractures of the femoral capital physis between the ages of 5 and 24 months.[164-166] Fractures are often bilateral. Radiographic signs include physeal fracture displacement and lysis of the metaphyseal bone, producing an "apple core" appearance. Histologic examination of specimens resected at surgery revealed that the articular cartilage and epiphyseal bone of the capital epiphysis had normal structure and viability, but the physeal cartilage was thickened and necrotic.[165] Normally this physis closes at 7 to 9 months of age in sexually intact cats. Delayed physeal closure after early gonadectomy apparently allows the persistence of cartilage that is unable to support normal weight-bearing activities.

Hepatic Osteodystrophy   Severe hepatic disease can produce rickets-osteomalacia due to malassimilation of fat and vitamin D (and secondarily of calcium) and impaired production of 25-hydroxyvitamin D.[167] Osteoporosis may also occur due to diminished hepatic protein synthesis.[167] Although well-recognized in human patients, hepatic osteodystrophy has yet to be characterized in dogs and cats.

Anticonvulsant Osteodystrophy   Prolonged high-dose anticonvulsant therapy with primidone, phenytoin, or phenobarbitone can cause osteodystrophy in human epileptics.[167] These drugs induce hepatic enzymes that enhance catabolism and excretion of vitamin D, resulting in calcium malabsorption, hypocalcemia, secondary hyperparathyroidism, and osteomalacia. Phenytoin also directly inhibits intestinal calcium transport and bone resorptive responses to PTH and vitamin D metabolites.[167] The significance of these changes to veterinary patients is unknown.

Hypovitaminosis A   Vitamin A is important for growth, maturation, and remodeling of bone. Hypovitaminosis A decreases osteoclastic activity and impedes bone remodeling, causing long bones to be deformed. Affected animals are usually lame. The condition is probably rare.[134,168]

Hypervitaminosis D   Skeletal demineralization follows massive intake of vitamin D, its active metabolites or analogs. Although osteopenia, bone deformation, and retarded growth are possible, the major clinical effects are related to hypercalcemia and soft tissue mineralization.[168] Correcting intakes of vitamin D, calcium, and phosphate should resolve the bone problems, but soft tissue damage may persist.

Zinc-Responsive Chondrodysplasia   This form of dwarfism occurs in Alaskan Malamutes and possibly other northern breeds.[168] Affected dogs have short, bowed legs; flared, irregular, thickened growth plates; and coarse, disorganized metaphyseal trabeculae. Hemolytic anemia with macrocytosis, hypochromia, and stomatocytosis are also present. Lifelong supplementation with zinc sulfate or gluconate was suggested.[168]

Copper Deficiency
Lameness and bone fragility can occur in dogs on copper-deficient diets.[7] Radiographic features are thickened growth plates and flared metaphyses, with osteopenia and epiphyseal slipping in severe cases. Histologically the animal has thickening of the zone of hypertrophic chondrocytes plus disorganization and collapse of the primary spongiosa.[169] The condition is rare.[7]

Lead Poisoning   Although skeletal signs are absent in plumbism, lead lines are seen radiographically in bones of some affected immature dogs. The lines are radiopaque bands in metaphyses adjacent to growth plates of long bones (Figure 195-33). They result from accumulation of thick mineralized trabeculae at these sites because of impaired osteoclastic activity. The presence of lead itself adds little to the radiopacity.

Overnutrition in Growing Dogs   Provision of balanced diets in quantities in excess of recommended daily intake or feeding diets that contain greater than the recommended content of protein, energy, minerals, or vitamins have been referred to as *overnutrition* or *overfeeding*. Experimental studies of young growing Great Danes found that feeding of an excessively supplemented diet was associated with development of wobbler syndrome, enostosis, osteochondrosis, and metaphyseal osteopathy.[170] Subsequently, it was found that diets with excessive protein content have no adverse effects on skeletal development.[171] However, Great Dane puppies fed a diet containing triple the recommended calcium requirement had elevated absorption and retention of calcium and disturbed endochondral ossification, and they developed osteochondrosis, retained cartilage cores, radius curvus syndrome, and had stunted growth.[106,172,173] Another study of Great Dane puppies fed diets with calcium/phosphorus ratios of 1.2:1, but with lower than recommended concentrations of calcium, found that bones had lower bone mineral content throughout the growth period.[174] Long-bone growth was also delayed until 6 months of age, but after this time bone growth caught up and was normal by 12 months of age, despite dietary deficiency in calcium.

Young Great Danes fed ad libitum with a balanced commercial diet initially had greater increases in body weight and height than littermates fed a restricted (two thirds of the

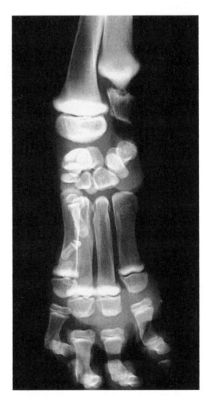

Figure 195-33 Radiograph of distal forelimb of a puppy with lead poisoning. Radiopaque bands are present in metaphyses adjacent to growth plates.

caloric intake) diet.[153] The restricted puppies later had a period of catch-up growth, and by age 7 months long bones were of identical length.[153] Restricted feeding (25% reduction in total intake) of a balanced diet limited the incidence and severity of osteoarthritis secondary to hip dysplasia in Labrador Retriever dogs.[175] Accordingly, overfeeding and oversupplemented diets should be avoided in growing pups. Ad libitum feeding is not recommended because it does not result in larger adult dogs, and it increases risk of orthopedic problems such as hip dysplasia.[153,175]

NEOPLASTIC BONE DISEASE[176]

Neoplasia of the skeletal system can be categorized into primary bone tumors, metastatic bone tumors, tumors of soft tissues extending into adjacent bone, and benign bone tumors.[176] These conditions are discussed elsewhere in this text. Nonneoplastic conditions of bone, such as cystic lesions and fibrous dysplasia, which may be confused with primary bone cancer, are important differentials. Bone cysts and fibrous dysplasia of bone are discussed earlier in this chapter.

BONE INFECTION

Bone infection (osteomyelitis) may be bacterial, fungal, or possibly viral (see Metaphyseal Osteopathy) in origin. Beta-lactamase–producing *Staphylococcus* cause approximately 50% of cases of bacterial osteomyelitis, often as monomicrobial infections.[32] Polymicrobial infections may have mixtures of *Streptococcus* and gram-negative bacteria (*Escherichia coli, Pseudomonas, Proteus,* and *Klebsiella*), and sometimes anaerobic bacteria. More common anaerobic isolates are *Actinomyces, Peptostreptococcus, Bacteroides,* and *Fusobacterium.*[177] Anaerobes are especially common in bite wound infections. *Nocardia, Brucella canis,* and tuberculosis cause osteomyelitis in rare instances.[176] Mycotic genera that cause osteomyelitis include *Coccidioides, Blastomyces, Histoplasma, Cryptococcus,* and *Aspergillus.* Fungal osteomyelitis is often a component of disseminated mycotic infections that occur in certain specific regions of the world. Diagnosis and treatment of deep mycoses are discussed in Chapters 217 to 220.

PATHOPHYSIOLOGY

Bacterial contamination of bone can occur with open fractures, surgery, bite wounds, foreign-body penetration, gunshot injury, extension from soft tissue, and hematogenous spread. However, bone is relatively resistant to infection unless the animal has concurrent soft tissue injury, bone necrosis, sequestration, fracture instability, implanted foreign material, altered host defenses, or some combination of these problems.[178] In chronic infections, avascular fragments of cortical bone (sequestra) are colonized by bacteria, surrounded by exudate, and may persist for long periods. New bone formed by periosteum (involucrum) incompletely encapsulates the focus of infection and sequestrum. Exudate draining from the bone follows sinus tracts that discharge through skin openings, generally in a more dependent location. Osteomyelitis is exacerbated by fracture and instability. Cortical bone at the fracture site is resorbed because of infection and interfragmentary motion, and this causes further widening of the fracture gap and additional instability.

Extraneous material (wood, soil, asphalt, and surgical implants) may incite a foreign-body response, interfere with local host defense mechanisms, and provide a nidus for infection.[178,179] Bacteria have unique mechanisms for bonding to surfaces of implanted foreign material. Initially the surfaces of implants become coated with matrix and serum proteins, ions, cellular debris, and carbohydrates (Figure 195-34).[180] Fibronectin, collagen, and fibrinogen are especially important in bacterial binding to biomaterial. Staphylococci and other gram-positive bacteria possess numerous cell membrane receptors for binding to fibronectin on implant surfaces.[180] Gram-negative bacteria are less effective at binding and have pili and fimbriae that specifically bind cellular proteins, matrix proteins, and glycolipids.[180] Bacteria also bind to exposed collagen matrix proteins (sialoprotein) and hydroxyapatite crystals of damaged bone.[180-182]

Once adherent, bacteria have two important mechanisms that ensure their persistence: (1) slime production and (2) phenotypic transformation.[182,183] Adherent staphylococci and some other bacteria produce a slime composed of extracel-

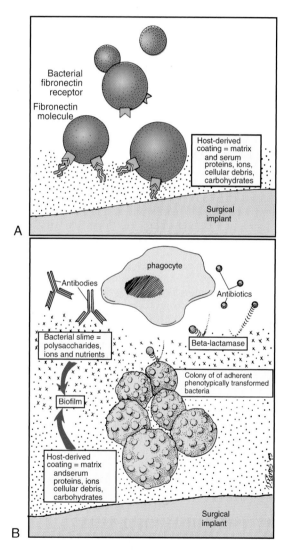

Figure 195-34 Mechanisms of bacterial persistence in chronic osteomyelitis. **A,** Foreign material such as surgical implants become coated with host-derived material containing fibronectin that binds with membrane receptors of contaminating bacteria. **B,** Adherent staphylococci and some other bacteria produce a slime that together with the host-derived material is called biofilm. Biofilm increases bacterial adhesion, protects bacteria from phagocytes and antibodies, and may also contain beta-lactamase. In addition, some adherent bacteria are phenotypically transformed to more virulent strains. (From Johnson KA: Osteomyelitis in dogs and cats. J Am Vet Med Assoc 205:1882, 1994.)

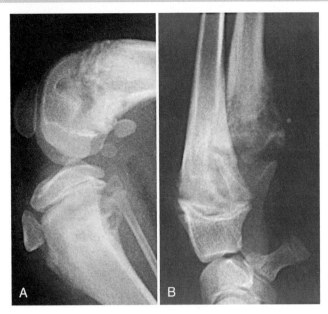

Figure 195-35 Polyostotic metaphyseal osteomyelitis in a Border Collie pup that had persistent neutropenia. **A,** Disruption of metaphyseal architecture of distal femur and proximal tibia, with irregular areas of radiolucency and sclerosis and some periosteal new bone adjacent. **B,** Similar changes are evident in distal humerus and proximal radius.

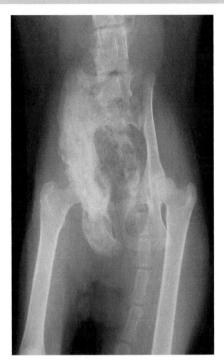

Figure 195-36 Pelvis of a cat with chronic osteomyelitis probably due to a bite wound from another cat. The hemipelvis is thickened by the formation of irregular, speculated new periosteal bone. (Courtesy Veterinary Imaging Associates, Sydney, Australia.)

lular polysaccharide, ions, and nutrients. Slime, together with host-derived material (matrix and serum proteins, ions, cellular debris, and carbohydrate), envelopes bacterial colonies and is called *biofilm* or *glycocalyx* (see Figure 195-34). Biofilm is a virulence factor because it increases bacterial adhesion, shields bacteria from phagocytes and antibodies, and modifies drug susceptibility.[180] Most antimicrobial drugs diffuse through biofilm, but biofilm may contain high concentrations of beta-lactamase, which protects some bacteria. In addition to providing physical protection, biofilm causes adherent bacteria to transform phenotypically to more virulent strains that are more resistant to antimicrobial drugs than when they are tested in vitro.[180]

The metaphyses of long bones are commonly affected in young animals with acute hematogenous osteomyelitis.[184] These regions may be especially vulnerable because capillary endothelium therein is discontinuous, allowing extravasation of erythrocytes and possibly bacteria.[178] When local defenses are compromised, osteomyelitis may ensue. This probably accounts for the development of metaphyseal osteomyelitis in Irish Setter pups with leukocyte adhesion protein deficiency and Border Collies with neutropenia due to impaired release of neutrophils from bone marrow (Figure 195-35).[185,186]

DIAGNOSIS

Acute osteomyelitis may produce signs of systemic illness including pyrexia, inappetence, dullness, and weight loss, together with neutrophilia and left shift. Heat, pain, and swelling in muscle and periosteum surrounding the infected bone may be evident. In chronic osteomyelitis, abscessation with single or multiple sinus tracts is a prominent sign. Lymphadenopathy, muscle atrophy, fibrosis, and contracture accompany chronic disease, but hematologic alterations are uncommon.

Radiographs are usually necessary for diagnosis (see Radiology). In acute osteomyelitis, soft tissue swelling (but no

osseous changes) occurs, except perhaps in young animals with acute metaphyseal osteomyelitis. In chronic osteomyelitis, periosteal new bone forms early and tends to be extensive, spiculated, and radially orientated (Figure 195-36). Bone resorption produces cortical thinning, medullary lysis, and rounding of fractured bone ends. In young animals, the diaphyseal cortex may be entirely resorbed and replaced by a shell of involucrum. The finding of sequestra is virtually diagnostic for osteomyelitis. Sequestra may be small and obscured by surrounding bone, but it should always be suspected in cases of persistent bone infection. Contrast radiography may help delineate sinuses and foreign bodies. A water-soluble contrast media (10 to 20 mL of Urografin, 76%) is injected slowly through a Foley catheter into each sinus. Incomplete delineation of sinuses is a problem. Isolation of bacteria from the site of suspected bone infections should be attempted to confirm the diagnosis and determine in vitro drug susceptibility. The diagnosis can usually be made from the history, physical examination, radiology, microbiology, or some combination of these factors.

TREATMENT

Contrary to long-held beliefs, most antimicrobial drugs penetrate bone well. However, osteomyelitis can be difficult to treat because of factors discussed under pathophysiology. Beta-lactam agents (penicillins, cephalosporins), tetracyclines, and aminoglycosides readily traverse the capillary membrane in normal and infected bone, and they are widely distributed in interstitial fluid.[187] Peak tissue concentrations of these drugs are reached 25 to 45 minutes after intravenous administration in normal and infected bone, and concentrations in bone closely reflect those in blood.[187] Therefore factors other than drug penetration (such as toxicity, administration routes, in vitro susceptibility, and cost) should dictate drug selection. Acute bacterial osteomyelitis may be cured by 4 to 6 weeks of antimicrobial drug therapy, provided bone necrosis is limited and no fracture occurs. However, in chronic osteomyelitis, drug treatment is futile without surgical intervention to remove sequestra and débride necrotic tissue.[178] Débrided wounds are left open to heal by secondary intention, protected with sterile dressings, and irrigated daily with sterile physiologic saline. Fractures must be stabilized and bone defects grafted with autologous cancellous bone. Treatment of chronic osteomyelitis is invariably prolonged and expensive and may be frustrated by episodes of recurrence. Treatment of recurrent osteomyelitis may necessitate a further search for sequestra, repeated débridement and drainage, reassessment of fracture stability, and reevaluation of microbiology and antimicrobial drug therapy.

REFERENCES

The reference list can be found on the companion Expert Consult Web site at *www.expertconsult.com*.

SECTION X
Infectious Disease

CHAPTER 196

Laboratory Diagnosis of Infectious Disease

Michael R. Lappin

There are two primary methods for diagnosing infectious diseases, detection of the organism or detection of antibodies against the organism. Infectious agents are detected in biological specimens most frequently by culture, cytology, fecal examination, histopathology, immunologic techniques, and nucleic acid amplification techniques. Polymerase chain reaction (PCR) assay and reverse transcriptase PCR (RT-PCR) assay are the most commonly used nucleic acid amplification techniques. Detection of the organism gives the most information supporting a clinical diagnosis of an infectious disease, but these assays are neither available nor optimal for all agents. Thus, antibody detection is still commonly used to aid in the diagnosis of some infectious diseases. In some clinical situations, the combination of organism detection and antibody detection assays is indicated.

When evaluating the results of infectious disease diagnostic tests, the *analytical sensitivity* defines the minimum detectable amount of the substance in question that can accurately be measured; the *analytical specificity* defines whether the substance detected cross-reacts with other substances. The *diagnostic sensitivity* is the proportion of positive test results from known infected animals; the *diagnostic specificity* is the proportion of negative test results from known uninfected animals. The *predictive value of a positive test* (PPV) is the probability that a test positive animal is diseased; the *predictive value of a negative test* (NPV) is the probability that a test negative animal is normal. The lower the prevalence of disease, the lower the PPV. Disease prevalence has little effect on negative predictive values.

Sensitivity, specificity, PPV, and NPV vary with each assay. Many of the infectious disease agents encountered in small animal practice colonize normal animals as well as induce disease in some individuals. For example, *Giardia* spp. antigen was detected in approximately 10% of normal dogs in a recent study.[1] Thus, when *Giardia* spp. antigen is detected in the feces of a dog or cat with diarrhea, the test result alone does not prove *Giardia* is the cause of the clinical signs (PPV <100%). Thus, veterinarians generally need to use a combination of findings to aid in the clinical diagnosis of an infectious disease:

- Appropriate signalment and history for the infectious agent suspected
- Clinical signs referable to the agent
- Detection of the agent (cytology, culture, antigen assay, PCR assay) or antibodies against the agent
- Exclusion of other causes of the clinical syndrome
- Response to an appropriate treatment

When these criteria are met, the suspected infectious agent might have been the cause of the clinical disease. However, it is always possible that the disease process resolved in spite of the therapy prescribed.

The following is a discussion of the some of the most common infectious disease organism detection and antibody detection techniques used in small animal practice. Also see the sections of the textbook for each infectious agent for more detailed information.

ORGANISM DETECTION

Culture

Culture can be used to document the presence of some bacteria, rickettsia, fungi, viruses, and protozoans in biologic specimens. However, some bacteria (e.g., hemoplasmas) have never been cultured, and many rickettsia, viruses, and protozoans are difficult to culture. Thus, PCR assays are now being used frequently to document these infections (see Nucleic Acid Amplification section). However, for many bacteria and fungi, culture is still the optimal way to document infection. For example, for most aerobic bacterial diseases, culture is superior to PCR assay because antimicrobial susceptibility testing can be used to determine optimal drug therapy.

In small animal practice, aerobic bacterial culture is used most frequently. To minimize organism death or overgrowth of normal flora, the material to be cultured should be collected without contamination, the material should be transported to the laboratory as quickly as possible in the most appropriate medium, and the most appropriate culture materials should be used. For routine aerobic bacterial culture, swabs containing transport medium should be used if a delay of greater than 3 hours is expected. If cultures are not to be started within 4 hours, the swabs should be refrigerated (or transported with cold packs) to inhibit bacterial growth; some bacteria will grow more rapidly than others, potentially masking fastidious organisms. Most aerobes will survive at 4° C (routine refrigeration temperature) in tissue or on media-containing swabs for 48 hours. Routine aerobic culture is generally successful on fluid samples (e.g., urine, airway washings) stored at 20° C for 1 to 2 hours, 4° C for 24 hours, or 4° C for 72 hours if placed in transport medium. See the bacterial endocarditis and *Bartonella* spp. sections of the textbook for a discussion of optimal blood culture techniques.

If feces are to be cultured for *Salmonella* spp. or *Campylobacter* spp., the laboratory should be provided approximately 2 to 3 g of fresh feces for optimal results. A transport medium should be used if a delay is expected. The laboratory should be noticed of the suspected pathogen so that appropriate culture media can be used. *Tritrichomonas foetus* and *Giardia* spp. can also be cultured from feces but these techniques are rarely performed because antigen assays (*Giardia* spp.) or PCR assays (both organisms) are now widely available (see Chapter 207).[1-4]

In certain situations, anaerobic, *Mycoplasma* spp., *Mycobacterium* spp., or fungal culture may also be indicated. Solid-phase transport media that will support the growth of most aerobes, anaerobes, *Mycoplasma* spp., *Mycobacterium* spp, and fungi for several days if refrigerated are available. Amies medium or modified Stuart bacterial transport medium are also often used to transport materials for *Mycoplasma* spp. culture. *Mycoplasma* and *Ureaplasma* cultures are most commonly performed on airway washings, synovial fluid, exudates from chronic draining tracts in cats, urine from animals with chronic urinary tract disease, and the vagina of animals with genital tract disease. *Mycobacterium* spp., *Mycoplasma* spp., *Bartonella* spp., and fungal culture may be indicated if pyogranulomatous inflammation is present. Most commercial laboratories do not provide *Mycoplasma* spp., *Mycobacterium* spp., anaerobic bacteria, or fungal antimicrobial susceptibility testing, so positive samples should be saved for transport to specialized laboratories as indicated.

In-house culture systems are available for cutaneous fungal agents. Materials from dogs or cats with suspected systemic fungal infection can be transported to the laboratory as described for bacteria, and the laboratory can be told specifically that fungal culture is needed. The mycelial phase of some systemic fungi like *Blastomyces dermatitidis* and *Histoplasma capsulatum* occurs in culture and can infect humans, so in-house culture for these agents is not recommended.

Viral agents can be isolated from tissues or secretions at some laboratories. However, for most routine viral infections of dogs and cats, PCR assays are now available (see Nucleic Acid Amplification section).

Cytology and Histopathology

Cytologic evaluation of exudates, bone marrow aspiration, blood smears, synovial fluid, gastric brushings, duodenal secretions, urine, prostatic washings, airway washings, fecal smears, tissue imprints, and aspiration biopsies is an inexpensive and extremely valuable tool for the documentation of current infections. For demonstration of most blood-borne infectious agents, thin smears are preferred. Cells in airway washings, prostatic washings, urine, aqueous humor, and cerebrospinal fluid (CSF) should be pelleted by centrifugation at $2000 \times g$ for 5 minutes before staining. Multiple slides should always be made. After being placed on the microscope slide, the material is air-dried at room temperature, fixed if indicated by the procedure used, and stained. Slides that are not stained immediately should be fixed by dipping in 100% methanol and air-dried. Cytologic specimens can be stained with routine stains; immunocytochemical techniques for certain pathogens are available (see Immunologic Techniques). Stains routinely used for the diagnosis of infectious diseases in small animal practice include Wright-Giemsa stain, Diff-Quik, Gram stain, and acid-fast stain.

One slide for cytologic evaluation is generally stained initially with Wright-Giemsa or Diff-Quik stains. If bacteria are seen (Table 196-1), Gram stain is applied to another slide to differentiate gram-positive and gram-negative agents that can be used to aid in the empiric selection of antibiotics.

Actinomyces (nonacid fast) and *Nocardia* (generally acid fast) can be differentiated by acid-fast staining characteristics. If pyogranulomatus inflammation is present, acid-fast staining is indicated to assess for *Mycobacterium* spp. within the cytoplasm of macrophages.

The hemoplasmas (see Table 196-1), some rickettsial agents (Table 196-2; *Ehrlichia* spp., *Anaplasma* spp.), and some protozoans (*Babesia* spp., *Cytauxzoon felis*) can be noted on cytologic examination of thin blood smears. However, organism numbers can fluctuate and so cytology can be falsely negative.

Wright-Giemsa stain is the best stain to use in practice for these organisms. Hemoplasmas can leave the surface of the red blood cell when the blood is placed into ethylenediaminetetraacetic acid (EDTA). Thus, making thin blood smears immediately with blood that has not been placed into anticoagulant may give optimal results (Figure 196-1). Collection of blood from an ear margin vessel for blood smear cytology may improve the likelihood of detecting *Ehrlichia* spp. or *Anaplasma* spp. morulae within white blood cells (Figure 196-2).

Fecal or rectal cytology should be performed on all dogs and cats with diarrhea. A small amount of fecal material should be collected from the surface of the feces or the wall

Table • 196-1

Characteristic Cytologic Morphology of Common Small Animal Bacteria

AGENT	MORPHOLOGIC CHARACTERISTICS
Actinomyces spp.	Gram-positive, acid fast–negative filamentous rod within sulfur granules
Anaerobes	Usually occur in mixed morphologic groups
Bacteroides fragilis	Thin, filamentous, gram-negative rods
Campylobacter spp.	Seagull-shaped spirochete in feces
Chlamydophila felis	Large, cytoplasmic inclusions in conjunctival cells or neutrophils
Clostridium spp.	Large, gram-positive rods
Clostridium perfringens	Large, spore-forming rods in feces
Hemoplasmas*	Rod- or ring-shaped on the surface of red blood cells
Helicobacter spp.	Tightly coiled spirochetes in gastric or duodenal brushings
Mycobacterium spp.	Intracytoplasmic acid fast rods in macrophages or neutrophils
Nocardia spp.	Gram-positive, acid fast–positive filamentous rod within sulfur granules
Leptospira spp.	Spirochetes in urine; dark-field microscopy required
Yersinia pestis	Bipolar rods in cervical lymph nodes or airway fluids

*Mycoplasma hemofelis, "*Candidatus* M. haemominutum," and "*Candidatus* M. turicensis" infect cats, and *M. haemocanis* and "*Candidatus* M. haematoparvum" infect dogs.

Table • 196-2

Characteristic Cytologic Morphology of Common Small Animal Rickettsial Agents

AGENT	MORPHOLOGIC CHARACTERISTICS
Ehrlichia canis	Clusters of gram-negative bacteria (morulae) in mononuclear cells
Ehrlichia chaffeensis	Clusters of gram-negative bacteria (morulae) in mononuclear cells
Ehrlichia ewingii	Clusters of gram-negative bacteria (morulae) in neutrophils
Anaplasma phagocytophilum	Clusters of gram-negative bacteria (morulae) in neutrophils and eosinophils
Anaplasma platys	Clusters of gram-negative bacteria (morulae) in platelets
Neorickettsia risticii	Clusters of gram-negative bacteria (morulae) in mononuclear cells

of the rectum by cotton swab, which is rolled on a microscope slide multiple times to give areas with varying smear thickness (Figure 196-3). After air drying, the slide is generally stained with Diff-Quik stain and examined for white blood cells and bacteria morphologically consistent with *Campylobacter* spp. (spirochetes; Figure 196-4) or *Clostridium perfringens* (spore-forming rods; Figure 196-5). It is also possible that *H. capsulatum* or *Prototheca* may be observed in the cytoplasm of mononuclear cells. Other stains can be applied to aid in identification of the enteric protozoans (see Chapter 207).

Arthrospores and conidia of dermatophytes can be identified cytologically. Hairs plucked from the periphery of a lesion are covered with 10% to 20% potassium hydroxide on a microscope slide to clear debris. The slide is then heated but not boiled, and it is examined for dermatophytes. All dogs or cats with chronic, draining skin lesions should have imprints of the lesions made and evaluated cytologically for the presence of fungal organisms (Table 196-3). This is very important if *Sporothrix schenckii* is on the differential list as this organism is capable of zoonotic transmission to people (Figure 196-6).[5]

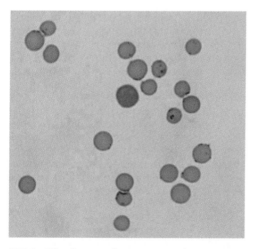

Figure 196-1 Blood smear from a cat with acute *Mycoplasma haemofelis*. Note the epicellular location of the organisms (1000×).

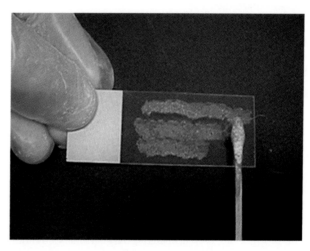

Figure 196-3 Preparation of a slide for rectal cytology. The cotton swab is rolled across the slide.

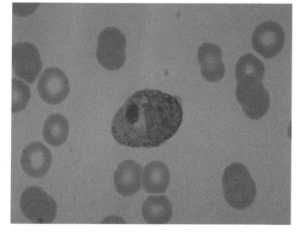

Figure 196-2 *Ehrlichia canis* morula in the cytoplasm of a circulating mononuclear cell (1000×). (Courtesy Dr. Ed Breitschwerdt, North Carolina State University.)

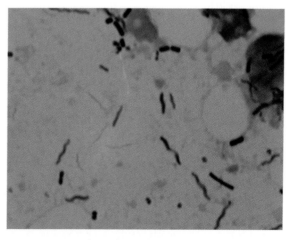

Figure 196-4 Fecal cytology showing several different spirochete bacteria (1000×).

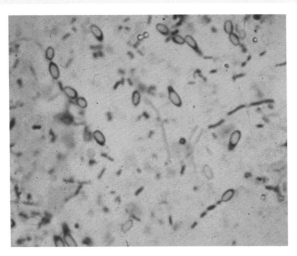

Figure 196-5   Fecal cytology showing spore-forming rods consistent with *Clostridium* spp. (1000×).

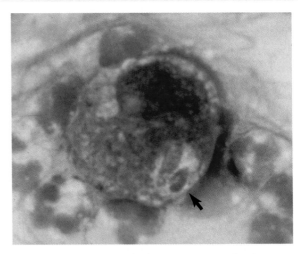

Figure 196-6   *Sporothrix schenkii (two organisms by the arrow)* in a macrophage from the draining tract of a cat (1000×).

Table • 196-3

Characteristic Cytologic Morphology of Small Animal Systemic Fungal Agents

AGENT	MORPHOLOGIC CHARACTERISTICS
Blastomyces dermatitidis	Extracellular yeast, 5 to 20 μm in diameter, thick, refractile double-contoured wall, broad-based bud, routine stains are adequate
Cryptococcus neoformans	Extracellular yeast, 3.5 to 7.0 μm in diameter, thick unstained capsule, thin-based bud, violet color with light red capsule with Gram stain, unstained capsule with India ink
Coccidioides immitis	Extracellular spherules (20 to 200 μm in diameter) containing endospores, deep red to purple double outer wall with bright red endospores with periodic acid–Schiff stain
Histoplasma capsulatum	Intracellular yeast in mononuclear phagocytes, 2 to 4 μm in diameter, basophilic center with lighter body with Wright's stain
Sporothrix schenckii	Intracellular yeast in mononuclear phagocytes, 2 to 3 μm × 3 to 6 μm in diameter, round, oval, or cigar-shaped

Canine distemper virus infection causes inclusions in circulating lymphocytes, neutrophils, and erythrocytes of some dogs. Rarely, feline infectious peritonitis virus results in intracytoplasmic inclusions in circulating neutrophils. Feline herpesvirus 1 (FHV-1) transiently results in intranuclear inclusion bodies in epithelial cells. However, cytology is commonly falsely negative for canine and feline viral diseases. Immunocytochemical or nucleic acid amplification techniques are generally more sensitive and specific than cytology for these agents.

Tissues collected from animals with suspected infectious diseases can be evaluated by several different techniques. Specimens for culture should be collected from the fresh samples and then tissues can be frozen, placed into 10% buffered formalin solution, or placed into glutaraldehyde-containing solutions. Routine histopathologic evaluation is performed on formalin-fixed tissues. Special stains can be used to maximize the identification of some infectious agents, and the clinician should alert the histopathology laboratory to the infectious agents suspected. Frozen specimens can be superior to formalin-fixed tissues for immunohistochemical staining and nucleic acid amplification techniques. Glutaraldehyde-containing fixatives are superior to other fixatives for electron microscopic examination of tissues.

Fecal Examination

Infectious agents are commonly associated with gastrointestinal disease. A number of fecal examination techniques, including direct saline smear, fecal or rectal cytology, fecal flotation, Baermann funnel technique, immunologic techniques, and nucleic acid amplification techniques are used to evaluate dogs and cats with vomiting or diarrhea (see Chapter 83). In addition, some fecal examination techniques can aid in the diagnosis of respiratory parasites as these agents are often swallowed and passed in feces (see Chapters 228 and 230).

Fecal flotation is indicated in dogs or cats with gastrointestinal signs of disease. Cysts, oocysts, and eggs in feces can be concentrated to increase the sensitivity of detection. Most eggs, oocysts, and cysts are easily identified after centrifugation in zinc sulfate solution or Sheather's sugar solution.[6] These procedures are superior to passive flotation techniques for identification of most parasites, in particular *Giardia* spp. If diarrhea is present, the fecal flotation is often combined with microscopic examination of fresh, liquid feces or a wet-mount examination for the presence of protozoal trophozoites (*Giardia* spp. [small bowel diarrhea], *T. foetus* [large bowel diarrhea], and *Pentatrichomonas hominis* [large bowel diarrhea]. A 2 mm × 2 mm × 2 mm quantity of fresh feces or mucus is mixed thoroughly with one drop of 0.9% NaCl or water, a coverslip is applied, and the slide is evaluated immediately for motile organisms by examining it under 100× magnification.

Immunologic Techniques

A number of immunologic techniques are used to identify infectious agents or their antigens in body fluids, feces, cells, or tissues. In general, polyclonal or monoclonal antibodies against the agent in question are used in a variety of different test methodologies, including direct fluorescent antibody assay with cells, tissue, or feces, immunohistochemistry with tissues, and agglutination assays and enzyme-linked immunosorbent assays (ELISAs) for antigen detection in serum, plasma, blood, or feces. Sensitivity, specificity, NPV, and PPV vary among assays but are generally high for most assays. Some assays require specialized equipment like fluorescent microscopes and so are only available at diagnostic laboratories. Other assays are available as point of care tests.

Currently available antigen assays for use with serum or plasma from dogs or cats include *Dirofilaria immitis*, *Cryptococcus neoformans*, *B. dermatitidis*, *H. capsulatum*, and feline leukemia virus. Parvovirus, *Cryptosporidium parvum*, and *Giardia* spp. antigen detection procedures are available for use with feces. Immunocytochemistry and immunohistochemistry techniques are available for the documentation of a variety of infectious diseases. These procedures are particularly valuable for the detection of viral diseases, detection of agents present in small numbers, and for differentiating among agents with similar morphologic features. In general, these techniques are more sensitive and specific than histopathologic techniques and are comparable to culture. See individual chapters for further discussion of these assays.

Nucleic Acid Amplification Techniques

The PCR reaction amplifies DNA. Very low DNA copy numbers can be amplified to detectable levels with this technique (Figure 196-7). By use of a reverse transcriptase step, RNA is converted to DNA; therefore, the technique can also be used to detect RNA (RT-PCR). Depending on the infectious agent in question, the techniques can be more sensitive than other available assays. In addition, PCR assay results can often be returned within 24 hours of sample submission, which is generally quicker than culture. However, the assays must always be shipped to a diagnostic laboratory as special equipment is required. If the organism in question is difficult to culture (e.g., *Ehrlichia* spp.) or cannot be cultured (e.g., hemoplasmas), PCR assays are of particular benefit for documenting infection.

Specificity of PCR assays can be very high, depending on the primers used in the reaction. For example, primers can be designed to detect one bacterial genus but not others. Primers can also be designed to identify only one species. For example, a PCR assay can be developed to detect all *Anaplasma* spp. or just one species such as *A. phagocytophilum*.

PCR assays are prone to false-positive results if sample contamination occurs during collection or at the laboratory performing the procedure. False-negative results can occur if the sample is handled inappropriately while being collected or transported. Some PCR assay results may also be affected by administration of antimicrobial drugs prior to sample collection. For example, hemoplasma or *Bartonella* spp. PCR results can be transiently negative during antibiotic treatment even though infection still persists. Acute infections generally have higher DNA (or RNA) copies in samples than chronic infections because in chronic infections, the immune response has attenuated the organism. Thus, the optimal sample for assessment by PCR assay is usually one collected during the acute phase of illness prior to antimicrobial treatment.

While many commercial laboratories are offering nucleic acid amplification assays, there is minimal to no standardization of assays. In addition, there may be little external quality control at some laboratories. For example, samples from cats with and without feline immunodeficiency virus (FIV) infection were sent to four different laboratories offering FIV PCR assay.[7] The laboratory with the best performance obtained the correct result on 90% of the samples; two of the laboratories obtained the correct result on <60% of the samples.

While PCR assays are very sensitive, the PPV of many assays can be very low. For example, because the technique detects DNA or RNA of both live and dead organisms, positive test results may be achieved even if the infection has been controlled. When the organism being tested for commonly infects the background population of healthy pets, interpretation of results for a single animal can be difficult. For example, feline calicivirus (FCV) is an important pathogen of cats. However, the organism is also commonly carried by healthy cats and modified live vaccine strains colonize cats.[8] Thus, although FCV RT-PCR is a sensitive way to document infection by FCV, the PPV of a FCV RT-PCR result is actually very low. In one study of cats with and without stomatitis, the PPV of FCV RT-PCR assays results from oral swabs was 0%.[9] Similar problems exist for FHV-1 PCR assay results.[10,11] In one study of cats with and without conjunctivitis, more FHV-1 positive tests were detected in the healthy control group than the group with conjunctivitis.[10]

Real-time PCR or fluorogenic PCR is a type of PCR assay that can be used to determine the amount of microbial DNA in a sample (Figure 196-8).[12-15] This technique can be used to monitor response to drug treatment.[13-15] It is possible that the DNA or RNA load in a sample will correlate to the presence of disease for some agents. However, that does not appear to be true for chronic FHV-1 conjunctivitis, *Mycoplasma haemofelis*, or "*Candidatus* M. haemominutum" infections.[12-14]

Based on these observations, it is very important that small animal practitioners carefully assess the predictive values of currently available PCR and the expertise and reliability of the laboratory that will be performing the assays. New PCR assays are being developed almost daily. See specific chapters for a discussion of the use of PCR for the detection of individual agents.

ANTIBODY DETECTION

Serum Antibodies

Once exposed to foreign antigens the immune system generates serum antibodies (humoral immune response). Complement fixation, hemagglutination inhibition, serum neutralization, agglutination assays, agar gel immunodiffusion,

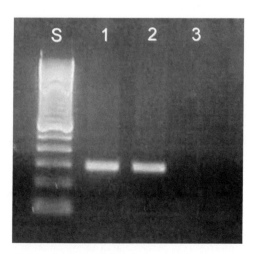

Figure 196-7 Conventional polymerase chain reaction assay example. *S*, Standards; *1*, positive amplicon; *2*, positive amplicon; *3*, negative sample.

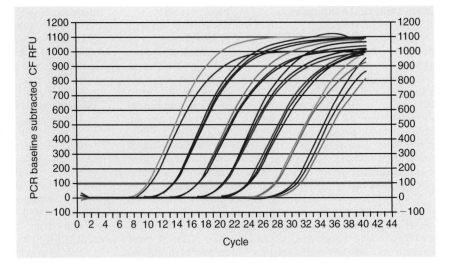

Figure 196-8   Example tracing from a fluorogenic real-time polymerase chain reaction *(PCR)* assay. *CF RFU,* Curve-fit relative fluorescence units.

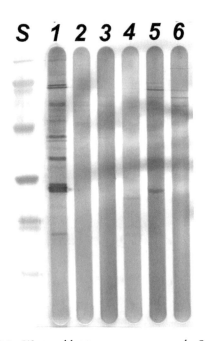

Figure 196-9   Western blot immunoassay example. *S,* Molecular mass standards; *1,* positive control; *2,* negative control; *3,* negative sample; *4,* positive sample; *5,* positive sample; *6,* negative sample.

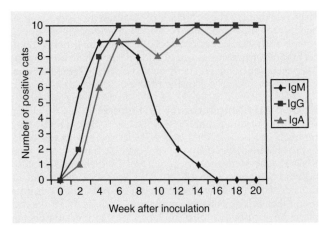

Figure 196-10   Hypothetical example of the serum IgM, IgG, IgA responses over time to an antigen.

indirect fluorescent antibody assay (IFA), ELISA, and Western blot immunoassay are commonly used to detect serum antibodies against infectious agents. Complement fixation, hemagglutination inhibition, serum neutralization, and agglutination assays generally detect all antibody classes in a serum sample. Specific antibodies most commonly assayed for include immunoglobulin M (IgM), immunoglobulin G (IgG), immunoglobulin A (IgA), and immunoglobulin E (IgE). ELISA, Western blot immunoassay, and IFA are the assay types that are usually adapted to detect specific IgM, IgG, or IgA responses. Western blot immunoassays have the potential advantage of allowing the determination of the different antigens recognized by the humoral immune responses (Figure 196-9).

Comparison of IgM, IgA, and IgG antibody responses against an infectious agent can be used to attempt to prove recent or active infection. In general, IgM is the first antibody

produced after antigenic exposure.[16] Antibody class shift to IgG occurs in days to weeks. Serum IgA responses often mirror those of IgG (Figure 196-10).

Timing of antibody testing is important. In general, serum antibody tests in puppies and kittens cannot be interpreted as specific responses until at least 8 to 12 weeks of age due to presence of antibodies from the dam passed to the puppy or kitten in colostrum. Most infectious agents can induce disease within 3 to 10 days after initial exposure; using many assays, serum IgG antibodies are usually not detected until at least 2 to 3 weeks after initial exposure. Based on these facts, false-negative serum antibody tests during acute disease are probably common in small animal practice. If specific serum antibody testing is negative initially in an animal with acute disease, repeat antibody testing should be performed in 2 to 3 weeks to assess for seroconversion. Documentation of increasing antibody titers is consistent with recent or active infection. Because of a slight potential for interassay variation, it is preferable to assess both the acute and convalescent sera in the same assay on the same day.

Many of the infectious agents encountered in small animal practice infect a large percentage of the population resulting in serum antibody production, but only induce disease in a small number of animals in the infected group. Notable examples include coronaviruses, *Bartonella henselae, Toxoplasma gondii*, and *Borrelia burgdorferi*.[16-18] For these examples, even though assays with good sensitivity and specificity for the detection of serum antibodies are available, the PPV for presence of disease is extremely low, since antibodies are commonly detected in nondiseased animals. Diagnostic utility of some serologic tests is also limited due to the presence of antibodies induced by vaccination. Examples include feline coronaviruses, some *Borrelia burgdorferi* assays, FHV-1, FIV, parvoviruses, calicivirus, and canine distemper virus.

Positive results in serum antibody tests should always be interpreted only as evidence of present or prior infection by the agent in question. Recent or active infection is suggested by the presence of IgM, an increasing antibody titer over 2 to 3 weeks, or seroconversion (negative antibody result on the first test, positive antibody result on convalescent testing). If detected, documentation of increasing antibody titers can suggest recent exposure to an antigen. However, the time period from the first positive result and maximal antibody titers can be very short. For example, some cats experimentally inoculated with *T. gondii* will go from the first detectable titer to the maximal titer within 1 to 2 weeks.[16]

Detection of recent infection based on antibody testing does not always prove disease due to the agent in question, especially if most infected animals are subclinical. *Borrelia burgdorferi*, *T. gondii*, and *B. henselae* are common examples. Conversely, failure to document recent or active infection based on serologic testing does not exclude a diagnosis of clinical disease. For example, many dogs with ehrlichiosis and dogs or cats with systemic fungal infections develop clinical signs of disease after serum antibody titers have reached their plateau.

Individual animals vary in their humoral responses against specific antigens. Some animals are high responders and produce large concentrations of specific antibody whereas others do not. Thus, the magnitude of an antibody titer does not definitely document that an antigenic exposure was recent, active, or associated with clinical disease. This is particularly true for the IgG class of antibody and for agents resulting in persistent infections. For example, many healthy

cats experimentally inoculated with *T. gondii* have IgG antibody titers >10,000 6 years after the last inoculation.[16] Since there are no antibody test results that alone prove the presence of disease, they must be combined with other clinical parameters.

Antibodies in Body Fluids

Some infectious agents induce disease of the eyes and central nervous system (CNS). Documentation of agent-specific antibodies in aqueous humor, vitreous humor, or CSF can be used to document the involvement of these tissues. Quantification of ocular and CSF antibodies is difficult to interpret if serum antibodies and inflammatory disease are present because serum antibodies leak into ocular fluids and CSF in the face of inflammation. Detection of local production of antibodies within the eye or CNS has been used to aid in the diagnosis of canine distemper virus infection (see Chapter 204), FHV-1 (see Chapter 214), feline bartonellosis (see Chapter 216) and feline toxoplasmosis (see Chapter 217). The following is a method to prove local antibody production by the eye or CNS.

$$\frac{\text{Aqueous humor or CSF}}{\text{specific antibody}} \times \frac{\text{Serum total antibody}}{\text{Aqueous humor or CSF}}$$
$$\frac{}{\text{Serum specific antibody}} \times \frac{}{\text{total antibody}}$$

If this ratio is greater than 1, it suggests that the antibody in the aqueous humor or CSF was produced locally. This formula has been used extensively in the evaluation of cats with uveitis. Approximately 60% of cats with uveitis in the United States have *T. gondii*–specific IgM, IgA, or IgG C values >1.[19] The technique was also used to help prove that FHV-1[20] and *B. henselae*[21] are causes of uveitis in cats.

References

The reference list can be found on the companion Expert Consult Web site at *www.expertconsult.com*.

CHAPTER 197

Companion Animal Vaccines and Vaccination*

Richard B. Ford

Vaccination guidelines for the cat were first published in 1998; the first iteration of canine vaccination guidelines followed in 2003. By the end of 2006, both sets of guidelines had been reviewed extensively and updated. Today, the complete text of both the American Animal Hospital Association (AAHA) Canine Vaccine Guidelines–revised[1] (available at: www.aahanet.org; search: Vaccine Guidelines) and the American Association of Feline Practitioners (AAFP) Feline Vaccine Guidelines[2] (available at: www.catvets.com; search: Information Briefs) are available to

the entire profession. However, the reader is reminded that since publication of vaccination guidelines, new vaccines have been licensed and updated information on existing vaccines has been published. AAHA and AAFP Vaccination Guidelines are updated, but at any point in time, they may not represent the most current information available.

Published vaccination guidelines for the dog and cat are recommendations only. They do not represent vaccination standards and are not intended to represent any form of universal vaccination protocol that veterinarians are expected to follow when selecting and using vaccines. It is still the responsibility of the individual practice/clinician to establish a vaccination protocol that addresses the risk of exposure and infection faced by the individual patient. Because

---

*Dedication: To Dr. James R. Richards (1948-2007), whose dedication and commitment to feline health has meant so much to so many!

veterinarians do have discretion in the selection and use of vaccines, canine and feline vaccination guidelines have been developed to facilitate development of a rational vaccination protocol.

The concept of core versus noncore vaccines is highlighted in both the AAHA Canine Vaccine Guidelines and the AAFP Feline Vaccine Guidelines. While core vaccines are recommended for administration to all dogs and all cats, it is the clinician who must ultimately make the decision as to which vaccines will be actually be administered and when. Rabies vaccination remains the only exception, wherein vaccination requirements are defined by State or local statute.

This chapter does not represent a summary of the AAHA or AAFP Vaccine Guidelines. Instead, it is intended to offer insight on developing a rational vaccination protocol based on information provided in the 2006 Vaccine Guidelines and the most current published information available.

VACCINE TECHNOLOGY

Today, there are over 25 vaccine types (e.g., killed, modified-live, recombinant) for the dog and approximately 16 for the cat. This is represented by over 160 proprietary (trade name) vaccines. Despite the unprecedented number of products on the market today, significant differences among vaccines for the same disease do exist. Comparative data on all vaccines are not available, yet over the past decade a number of studies have been published that demonstrate important differences among various vaccine types that should be taken into consideration when implementing a vaccination protocol. When selecting vaccines for administration to companion animal patients, veterinarians should consider known differences between the various vaccine types.

Inactivated Vaccines

Also called *noninfectious* or *killed* vaccines, inactivated viral and bacterial vaccines are licensed for used in both dogs and cats. While such products do offer an element of safety (i.e., they can not revert to virulence and are safe in immune suppressed and pregnant animals), they are generally less immunogenic, are associated with a slower onset of immunity (weeks), and shorter duration of immunity (months to years) compared to attenuated live vaccines, and are associated with a higher risk of local and systemic adverse reactions.[3] Killed vaccines primarily stimulate humoral immunity. Generally, a minimum of two initial doses of a killed vaccine are considered necessary to induce a protective immune response.

Most killed vaccines used in companion animals today contain adjuvant, a compound added to enhance the immunogenicity of noninfectious antigens. All killed viral and bacterial vaccines licensed for cats contain adjuvant. Adjuvant-induced inflammation has been implicated in metaplastic changes in mesenchymal cells (e.g., fibrocytes) leading to injection site sarcomas in (genetically predisposed?) cats.[3-7] The 2006 AAFP Feline Vaccine Guidelines recommend veterinarians avoid the use of inflammatory vaccines (e.g., those that contain adjuvant) when feasible.

Modified-Live (or Attenuated) Vaccine

Modified-live viral (and avirulent live bacterial) vaccines offer several advantages over killed vaccines. In contrast to killed vaccines, attenuated vaccines induce rapid onset (days) and prolonged (exceeding 5 years for most viral vaccines) immunity. Attenuated vaccines tend to induce both humoral immunity as well as a cell-mediated immune response. In contrast to killed vaccines, attenuated vaccines are able to induce a protective immune response when administered topically (e.g., intranasally). (Note: Only vaccines approved for mucosal administration should be administered topically.) The most significant disadvantage to modified-live vaccines is the fact that whole viral antigen, although attenuated, does replicate following administration. Replication of attenuated viral and bacterial vaccines can occur at sites distant from the point of inoculation. In some cases, mild to moderate clinical signs of disease can occur following inoculation, particularly when using vaccine approved for topical administration. Although rare, attenuated vaccines do have potential to revert to virulence.

Recombinant Vaccine

Recombinant vaccines (designated by an *r* preceding the antigen) are among the latest vaccine types to be introduced into veterinary medicine. Today, licensed recombinant vaccines are available for administration to a variety of species including dogs, cats, horses, and ferrets. Recombinant vaccine, also referred to as *genetically engineered vaccine*, fundamentally entails transferring selected segments of DNA or RNA from one virus or bacterium into another. The USDA recognizes three categories of recombinant vaccine: Category I: so-called "subunit" vaccines contain purified antigens derived from recombinant organisms (e.g., OspA in the rLyme vaccines); Category II: so-called "gene-deleted" vaccines (none are currently licensed for use in dogs or cats); and Category III: so-called "vectored" vaccine contain a benign virus that serves as a vector for delivering unique genes capable of expressing immunogenic proteins (e.g., rDistemper vaccine expressing the fusion protein and hemagglutinin).

Unlike killed and modified-live vaccines, recombinant categories I and III vaccines contain only the genetic material (e.g., DNA) that encodes for immunogenic protein. Since the pathogenic agent is not present in the vaccine, there is no opportunity for a category I or III recombinant vaccine to induce the disease it is intended to prevent. Recently published studies have demonstrated that the duration of immunity of the recombinant canine distemper virus vaccine is at least 3 years.[8] In addition, in a shelter-challenge model, the recombinant distemper vaccine was able to induce protective immunity in puppies despite the presence of maternal antibody. Use of a recombinant canine distemper virus vaccine in shelters facing high risk of distemper exposure should be considered.

DNA Vaccine

Sometimes dubbed the "third revolution" in vaccine development, DNA vaccines are unique in that the patient is inoculated with DNA only. In this case, the recombinant DNA expressing the desired antigen is directly injected into the patient, wherein immunogenic quantities of the desired antigen (protein) are directly produced by host cells. In 2007, the first DNA vaccine was licensed as a therapeutic vaccine specifically for the treatment, not prevention, of canine malignant melanoma.[9] This is a unique vaccine that has limited distribution and, at this writing, is only available to practicing oncologists and selected internists in the United States.

CORE VACCINES

The designation of certain vaccines as *core* is terminology used by the AAHA Canine Vaccine Task Force and the AAFP Feline Vaccine Advisory Panel to recommend which vaccines should be administered to all dogs and cats. Core vaccines recommended for the dog are: modified-live virus (MLV) or recombinant canine distemper virus (CDV), MLV canine parvovirus (CPV-2), MLV canine adenovirus-2 (CAV-2), and killed rabies vaccine (Table 197-1).

Table • 197-1

Core Canine Vaccines and Recommendations for Administration (Based on the 2006 Report of the American Animal Hospital Association Canine Vaccine Task Force)

CORE VACCINES	PRIMARY PUPPY SERIES (≤16 WEEKS)	PRIMARY ADULT SERIES (>16 WEEKS)	BOOSTER INTERVAL
Distemper Recombinant, or Modified-live	Administer one dose at 6-8 weeks of age, then every 3-4 weeks until 15-16 weeks of age	Administer two doses 3-4 weeks apart	Administer one dose 1 year following completion of the initial series, then every 3 years thereafter
Parvovirus Modified-live	Same as above	Same as above	Same as above
Adenovirus-2 Modified-live (SQ injection)	Same as above	Same as above	Same as above
Rabies Killed—1 year Killed—3 year (SQ injection)	Administer one dose (1-year rabies) at 12-16 weeks of age	Administer one dose (1-year rabies)	Administer one dose (3-year rabies) 1 year following administration of the first dose, then every 3 years thereafter

NOTE: Requirements for canine rabies vaccination are established by state and/or local statutes and may differ from the recommendations listed above.

Table • 197-2

Core Feline Vaccines and Recommendations for Administration (Based on the 2006 Report of the American Association of Feline Practitioners Feline Vaccine Advisory Group)

CORE VACCINES	PRIMARY KITTEN SERIES (≤16 WEEKS)	PRIMARY ADULT SERIES (>16 WEEKS)	BOOSTER INTERVAL
Parvovirus (panleukopenia)	Administer one dose as early as 6 weeks of age, then every 3-4 weeks until 16 weeks of age	Administer two doses, 3-4 weeks apart	Administer one dose 1 year following completion of the initial series, then every 3 years thereafter Note: Annual booster of cats against FHV-1 and FCV may be recommended in cats housed in high-risk environments
Herpesvirus-1 and Calicivirus Modified-live (nonadjuvanted), or Killed (adjuvanted) (SQ or intranasal administration)	Same as above	Same as above	Same as above
Rabies Recombinant (nonadjuvanted) (SQ injection)	Administer one dose at 12-16 weeks of age	Administer one dose	Annually
Rabies Killed—1 Year Killed—3 Year (adjuvanted) (SQ injection)	Administer one dose at 12-16 weeks of age	Administer one dose	Administer one dose 1 year following administration of the first dose, then every 3 years thereafter

NOTE: Requirements for feline rabies vaccination are established by state and/or local statutes and may differ from the recommendations listed above.
FCV, Feline calicivirus; *FHV-1,* feline herpesvirus-1.

Core vaccines for the cat are: panleukopenia (feline parvovirus [FPV]), herpesvirus-1 and calicivirus* (combined), and either recombinant or killed rabies vaccine (Table 197-2).

Vaccines are designated as core on the basis of the severity and prevalence of the infection, vaccine efficacy, safety, as well as the potential for the infection to be zoonotic (i.e.,

rabies). Vaccination intervals recommended for puppies and adults by the AAHA Canine Vaccine Task Force may vary from those published on the manufacturer's label.

Canine Initial Vaccination Series
Puppies should be inoculated at least three times between the sixth and sixteenth weeks of age with a MLV or recombinant CDV vaccine, a MLV CPV-2 vaccine, and a MLV (parenteral) CAV-2 vaccine. A 3- to 4-week interval is commonly recommended. Vaccines should not be administered at intervals of less than 2 weeks, regardless of antigen. Perhaps the

---

*Designation of feline calicivirus vaccine as "core" for cats does not include vaccines for the prevention of virulent systemic feline calicivirus (VS-FCV) infection.

most common recommendation for the initial vaccination in puppies is to administer a three-dose combination core vaccine series at 2 months, 3 months, and 4 months of age. Alternatively, some practices report inoculating puppies at 3-week intervals beginning as early as 6 weeks of age. This dictates administration of a four-dose initial vaccination series that should conclude not earlier than 14 to 16 weeks of age. Because of the risk for maternal antibody interference when using MLV vaccines, the AAHA Task Force recommends administering the final dose of the initial core vaccine series at 14 to 16 weeks of age. A single dose of killed (1-year) rabies vaccine is generally administered between 12 and 16 weeks of age. Rabies vaccination requirements are stipulated by state or local ordinance where applicable.

Although veterinarians do have discretion in the selection and use of a licensed vaccine, it is impractical to recommend vaccination against every disease for which a vaccine is available. Where risk of infection is considered to be particularly high, canine vaccines designated by the AAHA Task Force as *noncore* are appropriately recommended. For example, Lyme borreliosis vaccination is commonly designated as a "core" vaccine in practices located in areas of the United States geographically endemic for canine Lyme disease.

It is recommended that all dogs receive a single dose of the core vaccines 1 year following the last dose of the initial vaccination series (i.e., at 1 year and 4 months of age). Despite the absence of any studies documenting a maximum interval between initial vaccine doses in puppy and primary adult vaccination, it is reasonable to recommend that vaccination intervals exceeding 6 weeks should prompt 2 additional doses 3 to 4 weeks apart.

Canine Adult Vaccination

Practice recommendations for the administration of core vaccines to adult dogs vary significantly throughout the United States. The AAHA Canine Vaccine Task Force does recommend that, regardless of manufacturer, all MLV and recombinant CDV vaccines (there are no killed CDV vaccines), and all MLV parvovirus and adenovirus-2 vaccines be administered at 3-year intervals following the 1-year (post–initial series) booster inoculation. Durations of protective immunity are expected for at least 3 years postvaccination for the core canine vaccines listed by the AAHA Canine Vaccine Task Force.

For rabies vaccination in adult dogs, the AAHA Canine Vaccine Task Force follows the recommendations of the National Association of State Public Health Veterinarians as published annually in the Compendium of Animal Rabies Prevention and Control.[10] Unless otherwise stipulated by State or local ordinance, all adult dogs should be inoculated every 3 years with a licensed rabies vaccine.

Although optional, triennial revaccination with core vaccines, as recommended in the 2006 report of the AAHA Canine Vaccine Task Force, does represent a standard of care in veterinary medicine today. Annual vaccination is commonly practiced and also represents a standard of care in the United States. There is no legal or ethical requirement that dictates a veterinarian must only use a 3-year labeled vaccine in a triennial vaccination protocol.

Canine Adult Primary Vaccination

Dogs over 16 weeks of age when presented for initial vaccination are not expected to have interfering concentrations of passively acquired maternal antibody. Therefore, a single dose of a MLV (or a recombinant CDV) vaccine should provide a protective immune response. However, current recommendations and conventional practice is that initial vaccination of dogs over 16 weeks of age should include two doses of core vaccines, 3 to 4 weeks apart. Use of any killed viral or bacterial

vaccine requires two doses be administered, preferably 3 to 4 weeks apart.

Canine High Exposure Risk

Administration of core vaccines to dogs housed in shelters or other environments considered to pose a high risk of exposure to distemper virus, parvovirus, parainfluenza virus, or adenovirus justifies a different vaccination schedule than would be recommended for a household pet dog presented for routine vaccination. It is important that these vaccines be administered at the time of admission to the facility. Use of modified-live and recombinant core vaccines are recommended over killed vaccines. Any delay in administering vaccine could increase the risk of infection among unvaccinated dogs.

In the absence of a valid vaccination history, it is reasonable to assume that dogs admitted to a shelter have never been vaccinated or are overdue for vaccination. Therefore, all puppies should receive one inoculation of core vaccines at the time of admission, then an additional dose every 2 weeks until they are determined to be at least 16 weeks of age. Adult dogs should receive a single dose of core vaccines on admission and again 2 weeks later if still housed in the facility.

Administration of a 1-year rabies vaccination is generally indicated in dogs that are from 12 to 16 weeks of age. For adult dogs admitted to an animal shelter, administration of a 1-year rabies vaccine would typically only be recommended at the time of discharge from the facility. Specific regulations dictating rabies vaccination of shelter-housed dogs may apply depending on facility regulations, local, or State statutes.

Feline Initial Vaccination Series

All household pet cats should be vaccinated against panleukopenia (FPV), herpesvirus-1 (FHV-1), feline calicivirus (FCV), and rabies. Recommendations for administering the initial vaccination series to kitten vary slightly from the label recommendations provided by most manufacturers. Recent studies support extending the initial vaccination series beyond 12 weeks of age in an attempt to prevent interference by maternally derived antibody. The AAFP Feline Vaccine Advisory Panel recommends beginning as early as 6 weeks of age and every 3 to 4 weeks until 16 weeks of age. Implementing a three-dose protocol, similar to that recommended in puppies, is a reasonable inoculation schedule wherein one combination vaccine is administered at approximately 2, 3, and 4 months of age. In communities where feline rabies vaccination is required, veterinarians are expected to comply with local or state statutes. In locations that do not have rabies vaccination requirements for cats, it is recommended that veterinarians follow the recommendations outlined in the 2006 AAFP Feline Vaccine Guidelines: a single dose of a 1-year rabies vaccine at 12 to 16 weeks of age followed by a booster inoculation 1 year later.

AAFP Feline Vaccine Guidelines do not stipulate a preference for either MLV or killed core vaccines. However, in 1993, a causal link was established between both killed feline rabies and killed feline leukemia vaccination and risk for development of fibrosarcoma.[4] Although the precise mechanism whereby these vaccines lead to malignant changes has not been definitively established, the pathogenesis of vaccine-associated sarcoma (also called *injection-site sarcoma*) suggests an association between cancer and adjuvant-induced inflammation in genetically predisposed cats.[5-8] In the United States all killed viral and bacterial vaccines licensed for cats are adjuvanted. Attenuated-live (MLV) and recombinant feline vaccines do not contain adjuvant.

Current feline vaccine recommendations stipulate that veterinarians should avoid the use of inflammatory vaccines when feasible.[2]

Feline Adult Vaccination

Administration of core vaccines for FPV, FHV-1, and FCV is recommended every 3 years in adult cats receiving MLV or killed virus vaccine. Challenge studies have demonstrated durations of protective immunity lasting for at least 5 years.[11] Other than for rabies vaccination, booster inoculation intervals for adult cats is left to the discretion of the individual clinician. Rabies vaccination in adult cats is established by local or State statutes when applicable. Several states, however, do not require feline rabies vaccination. However, it is still recommended that all cats receive routine inoculations for rabies.

Feline High Exposure Risk

Vaccination of kittens and adult cats housed in high-risk environments are assumed to be at significant risk for exposure to viral respiratory infection as well as panleukopenia virus infection. Kittens should be inoculated with a combination MLV vaccine for FPV, FHV-1, and FCV at the time of admission to the facility. Vaccination should be considered in kittens as early as 4 to 6 weeks of age. Subsequent inoculations should be administered every 2 weeks until 16 weeks of age for cats that remain in the facility.

Adult cats (older than 16 weeks of age) should receive a single dose of a combination MLV vaccine at the time of admission and 2 weeks later if they remain in the facility. A single dose of a 1-year rabies vaccine is indicated in kittens at 12 to 16 weeks of age; adults cats should receive a single dose of a 1-year rabies vaccine at the time of discharge.

Shelter-housed cats are considered to have a higher risk for exposure to a virulent (systemic) strain of FCV than household pet cats. Confirmed infections in the United States and the United Kingdom, however, remain rare. In 2007, a combination feline calicivirus–virulent systemic feline calicivirus was licensed in the United States. Shelters interested in using this vaccine will need to consider price, infection risk and disease prevalence. At this writing, cross-protection against naturally occurring calicivirus infections has not been demonstrated. An Information Brief published on the AAFP Web site (www.catvets.com) offers additional insight regarding VS-FCV infection and vaccination.

NONCORE VACCINES

While vaccines for the most serious infectious diseases are indicated in all dogs and cats (core vaccines), other licensed vaccines are not. The AAHA Canine Vaccine Task Force and the AAFP Feline Vaccine Advisory Panel have recommended that certain vaccines are not necessary in all dogs and all cats. The decision to administer, or not to administer, a particular vaccine is determined by the individual clinician after reasonable assessment of risk. Risk for exposure and infection to those diseases for which licensed vaccines are available varies significantly depending on factors such as housing, geographic endemicity of pathogens, age, travel opportunities, and health status. Canine vaccines designated as noncore are indicated for protection against *Bordetella bronchiseptica*, parainfluenza virus, leptospirosis, and *Borrelia burgdorferi* (Lyme borreliosis) (Table 197-3).

Feline vaccines designated as noncore are indicated for protection against feline leukemia virus (FeLV), feline immunodeficiency virus (FIV), *Chlamydophila felis* (formerly, *Chlamydia psittaci*), and *Bordetella bronchiseptica* (Table 197-4).

Canine *Bordetella bronchiseptica* and Parainfluenza

Vaccination against *B. bronchiseptica* and parainfluenza virus has proven to be an important component of infectious tracheobronchitis (ITB) prevention, particularly in high-density environments, such as shelters, kennels, and rescue groups.[12] Canine vaccines are available for both topical (avirulent-live bacteria for intranasal use only) as well as parenteral (cellular antigen extract) administration. Most of the intranasal vaccines approved for use in dogs include MLV parainfluenza virus. Some products also contain MLV canine adenovirus-2.

A recently published challenge study documented the ability of topically administered vaccine to prevent postchallenge shedding of *B. bronchiseptica*; parenterally administered vaccine did not prevent shedding following challenge.[13] Regardless of the route of administration, most authors agree that vaccinated dogs experience substantially less coughing following challenge with *B. bronchiseptica*. Because a wide spectrum of pathogenic viruses and bacteria are associated with canine ITB, vaccination should not be expected to completely eliminate the risk of infection or the development of mild upper respiratory signs following exposure. Administering vaccine by the topical route can be less desirable for both patient and clinician. A single dose of intranasal vaccine has been demonstrated to induce a protective immune response within 72 hours.[14]

Although two initial doses of an intranasal vaccine, 3 to 4 weeks apart, are commonly recommended, a single dose can induce a protective immune response by 72 hours postvaccination. The durations of immunity following administration of a single dose, versus two doses, are not known. For puppies housed in a high-risk environment, the intranasal vaccine can be administered as early as 3 to 4 weeks of age. Booster inoculation using the intranasal vaccine is recommended at least 5 days prior to a known exposure risk (e.g., boarding).

Parenteral *B. bronchiseptica* vaccine requires two initial doses be administered 2 to 4 weeks apart with the first dose administered as early as 6 weeks of age. The onset of immunity following vaccination with the parenteral (cellular antigen extract) vaccine has not been published. A protective immune response is expected several days following administration of the second dose. Dogs that become aggressive during attempts to administer intranasal vaccine should be vaccinated by the parenteral route.

There are no published studies that compare the duration of immunity subsequent to parenteral versus intranasal vaccination. Intranasal vaccines have been demonstrated to prevent clinical signs following challenge for periods of 12 to 14 months postvaccination. The manufacturer recommends administration of the parenteral *B. bronchiseptica* vaccine annually, although independent studies demonstrating duration of immunity have not been published for this vaccine. Annual vaccination is appropriate for dogs with low to moderate risk of exposure. It is the author's recommendation that dogs having high risk of exposure (boarding, dog day-care) may benefit from vaccination every 6 months.

Leptospirosis

Leptospirosis vaccines are currently available for up to four serovars: *canicola*, *icterohaemorrhagiae*, *grippotyphosa*, and *pomona*. The decision to vaccinate individual dogs against leptospirosis is complicated by the fact that confirmed infections are relatively uncommon, reliable geographic prevalence data is limited, duration of immunity studies are difficult to perform, serovars other than those for which vaccine is available are believed to cause clinical illness in dogs (e.g., *L. bratislava*), and vaccines have a reputation for causing acute adverse reactions (e.g., facial edema and hives). Vaccination can prevent development of clinical signs following exposure. Although canine leptospirosis vaccines are capable of mitigating clinical signs, none of the current leptospirosis vaccines

Table • 197-3

Noncore Canine Vaccines and Recommendations for Administration (Based on the Report of the 2006 American Animal Hospital Association [AAHA] Canine Vaccine Task Force)

NONCORE (OPTIONAL) VACCINES	PRIMARY PUPPY SERIES (≤16 WEEKS)	PRIMARY ADULT SERIES (>16 WEEKS)	BOOSTER INTERVAL
Bordetella bronchiseptica + Parainfluenza Avirulent-live (intranasal administration ONLY)	A single dose is recommended by the manufacturers and may be given as early as 3-4 weeks of age Two doses, 2-4 weeks apart are recommended May be given as early as 3-4 weeks of age	A single dose	Annually; animals in a high risk/exposure environment may benefit from a booster if longer than 6 months since the previous dose
Bordetella bronchiseptica Antigen extract (SQ administration)	Administer two doses, 2-4 weeks apart beginning as early as 8 weeks of age	Administer two doses, 2-4 weeks apart	Annually; animals in a high-risk/exposure environment may benefit from a booster if longer than 6 months since the previous dose
Leptospirosis (serovars: canicola, icterohaemorrhagiae, pomona, grippotyphosa) Killed bacterin (SQ administration)	Administer two doses, 2-4 weeks apart beginning as early as 12 weeks of age (Vaccination of dogs less than 12 weeks of age is generally not recommended)	Administer two doses, 2-4 weeks apart	Annual booster is recommended for dogs with a defined risk of exposure. Vaccination is not recommended for all dogs. Exposure risk should be considered prior to recommending
Lyme borreliosis Recombinant, or Killed bacterin (SQ administration)	Administer two doses, 2-4 weeks apart beginning as early as 12 weeks of age	Administer two doses, 2-4 weeks apart	Annual booster is recommended for dogs with a defined risk of exposure. Vaccination is not recommended for all dogs
Crotalus atrox* (Western Diamondback Rattlesnake vaccine) Toxoid (SQ administration)	Recommendations vary depending on size of the dog and risk of exposure. See manufacturer's recommendations	Recommendations vary depending on size of the dog and risk of exposure. See manufacturer's recommendations	Not stipulated Duration of immunity studies has not been conducted
Porphyromonas spp.* Killed bacterin (SQ administration)	Administer two doses, 3 weeks apart beginning as early as 7 weeks of age (manufacturer recommendation)	Administer two doses, 3 weeks apart	Not stipulated Duration of immunity studies has not been conducted

*The AAHA Task Force has not categorized this vaccine as core or noncore.

will consistently or completely prevent infection and subsequent shedding of spirochetes.

Duration of immunity in dogs vaccinated against leptospirosis is difficult to assess and may vary significantly from dog to dog. Following initial vaccination, antibody titers are not sustained beyond a few months. Antibody titer does not consistently correlate with protective immunity. Annual vaccination is recommended in dogs considered to be at risk of exposure. Most authors support current recommendations that only dogs at high risk should be vaccinated, especially outdoor sporting breeds and hunting dogs. Administering vaccine to at-risk dogs is commonly recommended in the spring, since infections are generally diagnosed most often in the summer and fall months. Although dogs living rural areas are often targeted to be at greatest risk for exposure, infections have been documented in dogs living in strictly urban communities.

In addition to environmental factors, many clinicians do not recommend leptospirosis vaccination in dogs younger than 12 weeks of age or smaller than 12 pounds body weight. Miniature Dachshunds and Pugs may be at greater risk for developing acute hypersensitivity reactions subsequent to administration of a leptospirosis vaccine.[15] While there is only limited data supporting these recommendations, doing so is intended to minimize the consequence of hypersensitivity reactions should they occur. Dogs that do experience an acute postvaccination hypersensitivity reaction may recover spontaneously. Reactions deemed severe should be hospitalized and closely observed for respiratory distress and pulmonary edema. Treatment with corticosteroids may be indicated. Dogs with a history of having developed facial edema or hives following a previous leptospirosis vaccination are frequently treated with a single dose of diphenhydramine, 2 to 4 mg/kg, orally, 20 to 30 minutes prior to vaccination. Efficacy of diphenhydramine in preventing or mitigating postvaccination reactions is unknown. Veterinarians do report development of postvaccinal "hives" despite administration of diphenhydramine prior to vaccination. Postvaccination observation for

Table • 197-4

Noncore Feline Vaccines and Recommendations for Administration (Based on the 2006 Report of the American Association of Feline Practitioners [AAFP] Feline Vaccine Advisory Group)

NONCORE (OPTIONAL) VACCINES	PRIMARY KITTEN SERIES (≤16 WEEKS)	PRIMARY ADULT SERIES (>16 WEEKS)	BOOSTER INTERVAL
Feline Leukemia Recombinant (nonadjuvanted) (Transdermal administration ONLY)	Administer two doses, 3-4 weeks apart beginning as early as 8 weeks of age	Administer two doses, 3-4 weeks apart	Annual booster; booster vaccination is *not* recommended for all cats. Exposure risk should be considered prior to recommending
Feline Leukemia Killed (adjuvanted) (SQ administration)	Administer two doses, 3-4 weeks apart beginning as early as 8 weeks of age	Administer two doses, 3-4 weeks apart	Annual booster; booster vaccination is *not* recommended for all cats. Exposure risk should be considered prior to recommending
Chlamydophila felis Avirulent live (nonadjuvanted) (SQ administration)	Administer two doses, 3-4 weeks apart beginning as early as 9 weeks of age	Administer two doses, 3-4 weeks apart	Annual booster; booster vaccination is not recommended for all cats. Exposure risk should be considered prior to recommending
Chlamydophila felis Killed (adjuvanted) (SQ administration)	Administer two doses, 3-4 weeks apart beginning as early as 9 weeks of age	Administer two doses, 3-4 weeks apart	Annual booster; booster vaccination is *not* recommended for all cats. Exposure risk should be considered prior to recommending
Feline Immunodeficiency Virus (FIV) Killed (adjuvanted) (SQ administration)	Administration of three initial doses is required Beginning as early as 8 weeks of age, administer two additional doses 2-3 weeks apart	Administration of three initial doses is required. Each dose should be administered 2-3 weeks apart	Annual booster; vaccination is *not* recommended for all cats. Exposure risk should be considered Note: A single dose of FIV vaccine will cause a false-positive test result on all commercial FIV tests
Bordetella bronchiseptica Avirulent live (nonadjuvanted) (Intranasal ONLY)	Administer a single dose as early as 8 weeks of age	Administer a single dose	Annually, but only in cats with established risk of exposure
Virulent Systemic Calicivirus* Killed (adjuvanted) (SQ administration)	Administer two doses, 3-4 weeks apart beginning as early as 12 weeks of age	Administer two doses, 3-4 weeks apart	Duration of immunity is not known Annual booster is recommended by the manufacturer

*The AAFP Advisory Panel has not categorized this vaccine as core or noncore.

at least 30 minutes is indicated in any patient with a history of acute hypersensitivity reaction associated with vaccine.

Borrelia burgdorferi (Lyme Borreliosis)

Risk assessment for vaccinating dogs against Lyme borreliosis is generally based on geographic prevalence of infection risk. It is appropriate to recommend vaccination of dogs residing in the northeastern states, the upper Midwest, and coastal regions of northern California, Oregon, and Washington. In fact, veterinarians practicing in endemic areas of the United States may recommend vaccination against Lyme borreliosis as core. However, despite the well-published geoprevalence of Lyme disease in humans and dogs, there is growing evidence that exposure and clinical illness associated with infection occurs outside the traditional boundaries of geoprevalence. Some infections are likely to be associated with pet travel into endemic areas. Other cases seem to represent exposure to vector ticks in areas outside traditionally endemic areas.

Two types of Lyme borreliosis vaccines are licensed for use in dogs: inactivated (killed) whole spirochete vaccines and recombinant outer surface protein A (OspA) vaccines. All licensed vaccines, regardless of type, induce protection by their ability to induce antibody to the OspA protein. Uniquely, the interaction between the antibody and the antigen occurs in the tick, not in the dog. Ticks that feed on vaccinated dogs ingest OspA antibody. Because OspA is only expressed on spirochetes residing in the midgut of the tick, prevention of disease is the result of failure of the tick to transmit infectious spirochetes to the host.

The decision to vaccinate dogs against Lyme borreliosis has been controversial for several reasons.[16] Vaccine efficacy, vaccine-associated risks, and low disease prevalence have been used to argue against routine vaccination. Today, most authors agree that it is better to prevent infection than to attempt clearing spirochetes from infected dogs. Natural immunity following infection is negligible. Furthermore, antibiotic treatment of infected dogs is generally regarded as insufficient to fully clear the patient of spirochetes. Although published challenge studies are limited, there is reasonable evidence supporting the fact that vaccine can prevent infection. Concerns over the risk of vaccine-induced Lyme nephropathy appear not to be justified, as the majority of confirmed cases studied at Cornell University had no history of prior vaccination (RE Goldstein: personal communication). Vaccination has no role in the treatment of canine Lyme borreliosis.

Dogs selected for vaccination should receive at least two initial doses as early as 9 to 12 weeks of age. A second dose should be administered 2 to 4 weeks later. Annual booster inoculations are recommended in dogs considered to be at risk of exposure. It is strongly recommended to test dogs for *Borrelia burgdorferi* antibody prior to vaccination.

Feline Leukemia Virus

The consequences of FeLV infection are well known. In susceptible cats, infection can lead to persistent immune suppression, anemia, neoplasia, and death. However, vaccination against FeLV infection is recommended as noncore on the basis that the risk of exposure and infection varies significantly depending on the lifestyle and age of the cat. Healthy adult cats are known to be significantly more resistant to FeLV infection than kittens.[17] Therefore, the AAFP Feline Vaccine Advisory Panel highly recommends administration of FeLV vaccine to all kittens. Although adult cats are more resistant to FeLV infection than kittens, resistance is not absolute. Annual vaccination of adult cats is still indicated for those cats that are allowed to roam. Annual vaccination of strictly indoor adult cats should also be considered if housed with cats that do spend unsupervised time outside.

There are currently four licensed FeLV vaccines in the United States. Three are parenterally administered, killed-adjuvanted vaccines. A recombinant (nonadjuvanted) viral canarypox-vectored FeLV vaccine is available in the United States for transdermal (needle-free) administration only. A recombinant (nonadjuvanted) FeLV vaccine is available in Europe and the United Kingdom for parenteral injection. Regardless of the vaccine type, two initial doses are recommended 3 to 4 weeks apart; the initial dose can be administered as early as 8 weeks of age. Annual vaccination is recommended for cats considered to be at risk of exposure. Most studies support a 12-month duration of immunity; it is unlikely that vaccine-induced immunity persists longer. The AAFP Advisory Panel on Retrovirus Testing recommends all cats be tested and found to be negative for the presence of FeLV antigen prior to administering vaccine.[18] Although vaccination of FeLV-positive cats is not known to be harmful, there is no therapeutic benefit to be gained from doing so.

Feline Immunodeficiency Virus

In the United States, there is currently only one licensed feline immunodeficiency virus (FIV) vaccine. This product is a whole virus, dual subtype (clades A and D), killed-adjuvanted vaccine. Limited numbers of challenge studies involving the FIV vaccine provide conflicting results regarding the ability of the vaccine to protect cats against heterologous virus challenge. A single dose of vaccine will induce an antibody response capable of causing false-positive test results on all commercially available FIV tests for a period of at least 1 year. Additionally, FIV vaccine antibody can be passed from queen to kitten resulting in false-positive test results in kittens until approximately 12 weeks of age.[18,19]

Recommendations for FIV vaccination should be limited to those cats with known risk for exposure, especially through bite wounds from other cats. Three initial doses, 1.0 mL per dose, are recommended by the manufacturer. Annual revaccination is recommended in cats with sustained risk for exposure. It is recommended that all vaccinated cats be permanently identified (e.g., microchip) and that the owner be advised that future tests for FIV are likely to be "positive."

Chlamydophila felis (formerly Chlamydia psittaci)*

Chlamydophilosis is a bacterial infection affecting the conjunctiva and causing a persistent mild to serious mucoid to mucopurulent ocular discharge and possibly sneezing. Clinical signs are not diagnostic. Confirmation of infection generally requires culture or polymerase chain reaction (PCR) technology. Infection in the United States among the pet cat population is considered to be uncommon. Whole bacterial-adjuvanted and avirulent live-nonadjuvanted vaccines are currently available in the United States. Risk for exposure and infection is difficult to assess because the documented prevalence of disease is very low. Because bacteria from the upper respiratory tract can be transmitted directly to other cats, vaccination is generally limited to households where multiple cats reside, where the opportunity for cat-to-cat contact is high, and *C. felis* infection can be documented. *C. felis* vaccines may mitigate the severity of clinical signs associated with infection. They do not, however, consistently prevent infection or shedding of infectious bacteria.

Cats selected for vaccination against *C. felis* should receive two initial doses of vaccine as early as 9 weeks of age. A second dose is administered 3 to 4 weeks later. Cats determined to be at risk of exposure should be vaccinated annually as long as the risk of exposure continues.

Bordetella bronchiseptica

Several species of animals, and occasionally humans, are susceptible to infection by the gram-negative coccobacillus *Bordetella bronchiseptica*. In cats, as well as in dogs, it appears that these bacteria can exist as commensal organisms in the respiratory tract, but also as a pathogen capable of causing mild to serious respiratory infections involving both the upper and lower respiratory tract. The ability of *B. bronchiseptica* to vary its virulence pattern is likely attributable the presence of virulence genes that may, subject to yet unknown stimuli, become active resulting in the production of several proteins capable of causing significant cellular injury. Outbreaks have been reported within multiple-cat households, particularly among kittens. In the author's experience, *B. bronchiseptica* infection is particularly serious in kittens coinfected with FCV. Among cats housed in shelters and multiple cat households, the seroprevalance may be quite high. Seroprevalance, however, does not always correlate with infection or the ability to isolate bacteria.

The only *B. bronchiseptica* vaccine currently available for administration to cats is an avirulent live, nonadjuvanted vaccine approved for intranasal administration. There is no parenteral vaccine approved for use in cats. Initial inoculation requires only a single dose, administered as early as 8 weeks of age. The duration of immunity is not known to extend beyond 1 year. Therefore, cats considered to at risk for exposure can be revaccinated annually. Anecdotal reports from veterinarians suggest that clinical signs of nasal discharge and cough have been seen within a few days of vaccination in some cats, particularly in kittens. The duration of immunity subsequent to intranasal vaccination in cats has not been reported.

---

*Despite recent reclassification of *Chlamydia psittaci* to *Chlamydophila felis*, vaccine labels may not reflect this change.

MISCELLANEOUS VACCINES

Since publication of the AAHA and AAFP Vaccine Guidelines, additional vaccines have been licensed for use in dogs or cats: *Crotalus atrox* (canine), *Porphyromonas* spp. (canine), and virulent systemic calicivirus (feline). To date, there have been no independent studies published that evaluate the efficacy or duration of immunity associated with these products. It is this author's recommendation that the following vaccines are reasonably designated as noncore and should be administered at the discretion of the veterinarian only after careful consideration of the patient's risk for exposure.

Crotalus atrox Toxoid

The "rattlesnake vaccine" is a conditionally licensed vaccine recommended by the manufacture for administration to healthy dogs at risk for rattlesnake envenomation, particularly the Western Diamondback Rattlesnake. The vaccine is administered most often to dogs living in the southwestern United States. In most dogs two doses, 1 mL per dose given subcutaneously, are recommended at an interval of 4 weeks to complete the initial vaccination series. Annual boosters are recommended. The manufacturer does recommend administration of vaccine approximately 1 month prior to potential exposure (i.e., the beginning of rattlesnake "season"). It has been recommended that booster inoculations be administered at 4- to 6-month intervals in small dogs and dogs that are considered to be at high risk for encounters with rattlesnakes. The vaccine does not necessarily preclude the need to administer emergency treatment or the need to administer antivenin. Anecdotal reports from veterinarians with considerable field experience using the rattlesnake vaccine suggest that the vaccination does seem to mitigate the severity of envenomation and may actually increase survivability in dogs requiring extended transit times (hours) when seeking medical attention.

Postvaccination reactions have been observed as an injection site "lump." Veterinarians have reported removing sterile fluid from the injection site several days following inoculation. Firm, subcutaneous masses may persist for several days or weeks (granuloma?) postinoculation, but most seem to spontaneously resolve with time.

Table • 197-5

Vaccines Not Generally Recommended for Routine Administration to Dogs and Cats *

VACCINE	REASON
Killed CPV Inactivated canine parvovirus	Compared to MLV canine parvovirus vaccines, inactivated vaccines are generally regarded to be less immunogenic and have a shorter duration of immunity. Killed vaccines are susceptible to maternal antibody interference in puppies as old as 16-18 weeks of age.
Killed CAV-2 Inactivated canine adenovirus-2	Parenteral killed CAV-2 vaccines are considered to be less immunogenic than MLV CAV-2 vaccines administered parenterally.
MLV CAV-2 (topical) Modified live vaccine canine adenovirus-2 for intranasal administration	Some intranasal vaccines for *B. bronchiseptica* and parainfluenza also contain MLV CAV-2 for protection against hepatitis and infectious tracheobronchitis. However, all manufacturers currently provide a parenteral MLV CAV-2 vaccine combined with canine distemper and parvovirus. There is no advantage to administering CAV-2 vaccine by both the intranasal and parenteral routes.
MLV and Killed CAV-1 MLV and inactivated canine adenovirus-1	Risk of postvaccination adverse reactions, especially corneal edema ("blue-eye") and nephritis, in dogs is significant. MLV CAV-2 vaccines are significantly safer and provide cross-protection against CAV-1 (hepatitis).
MLV and Killed CCV MLV and inactivated canine coronavirus	Canine coronavirus infection causes mild to subclinical illness in young (usually less than 6 weeks of age) puppies that is self-limiting. Routine vaccination of dogs is not justified. Dual virus (CPV + CCV) challenge studies in dogs demonstrate that neither the MLV nor killed vaccine reduce severity of clinical illness. Duration of immunity studies are inconclusive since neither the CCV vaccinates nor control dogs develop clinical signs of illness following challenge.
Killed *Giardia* Inactivated canine and feline *Giardia lamblia*	Not recommended for administration to either dogs or cats on the grounds that data supporting the ability of the vaccine to prevent infection and clinical signs is lacking. The vaccine is *not* labeled for use in treatment of infected cats or dogs. Limited studies in infected dogs and cats do not support a therapeutic role for this vaccine. The product is adjuvanted.
FIP (topical) MLV feline infectious peritonitis vaccine for intranasal administration	Studies documenting the ability of the FIP vaccine to consistently provide a protective immune response in cats are lacking. The potential for the vaccine to provide protection has only been demonstrated in coronavirus-negative cats. However, (benign) coronavirus infection is common among healthy cats and kittens, especially in multiple cat households. Most authors agree that the virulent coronavirus biotype (the FIP virus) is not contagious from cat to cat; therefore, routine vaccination of household pet cats is not recommended. Also, vaccination of cats residing in multiple-cat households where FIP is known to exist is not recommended. Earlier concerns over the ability of this vaccine to induce a systemic humoral immune response and potentiate severe clinical consequences subsequent to infection ("antibody dependent enhancement" of disease) appear to be unfounded.

*Canine and feline vaccines included in this table are based on recommendations published in the 2006 American Animal Hospital Association Canine Vaccine Task Force and the 2006 American Association of Feline Practitioners Feline Vaccine Advisory Panel, respectively. All vaccines listed are licensed by the USDA and can be selected for administration at the discretion of the veterinarian.

Porphyromonas Vaccine

The *Porphyromonas* vaccine is a killed, adjuvanted bacterin. The vaccine contains three types of inactivated bacteria: *P. denticanis, P. gulae,* and *P. salivosa.* Initial vaccination entails subcutaneous administration of two doses (1 mL per dose), 3 weeks apart. Although the vaccine is recommended as a aid in the prevention of periodontitis in dogs, canine challenge studies are not available. At this time, the manufacturer has not stipulated revaccination intervals. Six- and 12-month intervals are reportedly being studied. The product does contain formaldehyde, which may explain the relatively high rate of postvaccination reactions. Three types of reactions are observed most commonly: injection site "lumps" (which may resolve spontaneously), pain at the injection site, and transient (days) lethargy. Assessment of the efficacy of this vaccine will be very difficult to establish because of the inability to perform a controlled challenge study.

Virulent Systemic Feline Calicivirus (VS-FCV) Vaccine

Highly prevalent in the general feline population, caliciviruses are well known for their ability to cause contagious upper disease in kittens and adult cats. Clinical signs characteristically include sneezing, nasal and ocular discharge, secondary bacterial rhinitis/conjunctivitis, fever, and gingivostomatitis. In contrast to feline herpesvirus-1, multiple strains of FCV have been identified and are known to vary somewhat in their ability to cause clinical illness. A small group of FCV strains have been recognized to cause acute, severe systemic disease. Designated *virulent systemic feline calicivirus* (VS-FCV) or *hemorrhagic calicivirus,* infected cats develop rapidly progressive signs associated with upper respiratory infection, systemic vasculitis, facial and/or limb edema, cutaneous ulceration, multiorgan failure, and disseminated intravascular coagulation with spontaneous bleeding and death. Adults cats, as well as kittens, can be affected regardless of prior vaccination against the more common calicivirus associated with upper respiratory disease. Over the past decade a small number of outbreaks, most often among shelter-housed cats, attributed to a highly pathogenic strain of calicivirus have been documented in both the United States and the United Kingdom.[2,20,21]

In 2007, a VS-FCV vaccine was licensed in the United States. Veterinarians considering the use of this product should review the AAFP Information Brief on VS-FCV and the shelter medicine website before recommending its use in household pet cats. (www.catvets.com and www.sheltermedicine.com). At this writing, there have been no independent studies documenting field efficacy of the vaccine or its duration of immunity. Although most documented cases have occurred among shelter-housed cats, risk for exposure is difficult to assess in household pet because VS-FCV strains arise from calicivirus mutations and the overall disease incidence appears to be very low. It is currently not known whether the strain of VS-FCV used in the vaccine will protect cats from challenge by a unique (heterologous) calicivirus strain as each outbreak strain documented appears to have been caused by a VS-FCV that is antigenically and genetically distinct.

VACCINES GENERALLY NOT RECOMMENDED

The AAHA Canine Vaccine Task Force and the AAFP Feline Vaccine Advisory Panel have recommended that some vaccines, although licensed by the USDA for administration to dogs and cats, are generally not recommended for routine use (Table 197-5). These recommendations are based on various criteria, including: the vaccine may be associated with serious adverse events (e.g., canine adenovirus-1), data supporting the ability of the vaccine to induce a sustained, protective immune response are lacking (e.g., feline infectious peritonitis, *Giardia,* canine coronavirus), or a superior (more immunogenic) product is available (e.g., inactivated parvovirus).

NOTE: each vaccine listed as "not recommended" is licensed by the USDA; veterinarians are not obligated to follow either the AAHA or AAFP Vaccine Guidelines in making decisions regarding the administration of any of these products.

NEW VACCINES

In 2009, two additional canine vaccines were licensed in the United States: canine influenza virus (CIV) and a bivalent Lyme borreliosis bacterin expressing borreliacidal antibodies to the outer surface proteins A (OspA) and C (OspC). At this writing, neither vaccine has been reviewed or categorized by the AHAA Canine Vaccine Task Force. It is the author's recommendation that these vaccines not be recommended for use in all dogs and that veterinarians should limit administration to dogs considered to have reasonable or known risk for exposure.

CIV infection has been identified in dogs in at least 30 states and the District of Columbia (see Chapter 230). Naturally occurring infections are highly contagious, but clinical disease is generally mild. Cough and lethargy are characteristic; clinical signs appear to resolve spontaneously (uncomplicated cases) within 2 weeks following onset. Severe respiratory disease and death is uncommon but has been reported. Kennel/shelter-housed dogs appear to be at greatest risk of exposure. Following infection, viral shedding is short-lived (7 to 8 days). The conditionally licensed CIV vaccine is a monovalent, killed (adjuvanted) product. The manufacturer recommends two initial doses 2 to 4 weeks apart in dogs as young as 6 weeks of age with annual revaccination. A single dose of vaccine is unlikely to induce a protective immune response. Field efficacy studies are not available. The vaccine is reported by the manufacturer to reduce severity of clinical signs caused by infection and to reduce the duration of virus shedding among infected dogs. The vaccine does not prevent infection or shedding following exposure (nonsterile immunity). It is the author's recommendation that administration be limited to use in dogs deemed to be at risk of frequent exposure to multiple dogs, especially those maintained in cluster housing environments. However, animal shelters that do not maintain dogs longer than 3 weeks are not likely to derive benefit from the use of this vaccine.

The most recent Lyme borreliosis vaccine, licensed for administration to dogs in the United States, is a killed (adjuvanted) bacterin that produces borreliacidal antibodies to both OspA and OspC. The vaccine contains both conventional *Borrelia burgdorferi* spirochetes and a unique (ospA and ospB-negative) spirochete strain expressing only OspC.[22] The manufacturer recommends administration of two initial doses, 2 to 4 weeks apart to dogs as young as 8 weeks of age. Revaccination is recommended annually. The vaccine is an aid to the prevention of subclinical arthritis in dogs at risk of exposure to *B. burgdorferi.* To date, no studies have been published that demonstrate enhanced efficacy of this bivalent vaccine over any other killed or recombinant vaccine that expresses OspA exclusively.

REFERENCES

The reference list can be found on the companion Expert Consult Web site at *www.expertconsult.com.*

BACTERIAL DISEASES

CHAPTER 198

Leptospirosis

Richard E. Goldstein

ETIOLOGY

Leptospirosis is a zoonotic disease of major worldwide significance that has been diagnosed in animals and humans. The disease is caused by the spirochetal bacterium of the genus *Leptospira*.[1] These are highly motile obligate aerobic spirochetes that share features of both gram-negative and gram-positive bacteria. Morphologically, they are thin, flexible, filamentous bacteria made up of fine spirals with hook-shaped ends. They are motile through writhing and flexing movements while rotating on their long axis.[1] Canine leptospirosis was first described in 1899. Prior to 1960, *L. interrogans* serovars icterohaemorrhagiae and canicola were believed to be responsible for most cases of canine leptospirosis. Infection was described as causing acute or subacute hepatic and renal failure and was typically thought to be characterized by acute hemorrhagic diathesis, icterus, or uremia.[2] Confusion may arise about the classification of leptospires because serogrouping used in the past overlaps with newer classifications based on genetic methodologies.

Another source of confusion is the subdivision to serogroups that each contain one or more similar serovars. Most of the commonly diagnosed canine pathogenic serovars are still classified (as before) as belonging to the *L. interrogans* species, although the common canine serovar grippotyphosa, for example, is typically classified as belonging to the *L. kirschneri* species.[1] Approximately 250 different serovars have been identified in the *Leptospira* complex.[3] Although the pathogenic importance of many serovars is unknown, 6 to 8 are thought to be pathogenic in the dog.[4-6] Each serovar has a primary host that maintains the organism and contributes to its dissemination in the environment. Although all mammals are susceptible to infection, clinical signs are expected to be most severe with non–host-adapted serovars.[7]

Historically *L. interrogans* serovars icterohaemorrhagiae and canicola were most common in dogs. These were the primary components in bivalent vaccines. After this vaccine came into widespread use, the incidence of "classic" lept-ospirosis in dogs appeared to have decreased,[8] although a cause and effect between the widespread use of the vaccine and the reduction of infection with these serovars has not been proven. In the past 20 years multiple reports of increased incidence of the disease in dogs have been published with few cases due to the "classic" serovars in North America (Table 198-1).

The most common serovars seen today in the United Sates are thought to be *L. kirschneri* serovar grippotyphosa, *L. interrogans* serovar pomona, and *L. interrogans* serovar bratislava.[6,7,9] The recent increased incidence of the diagnosis of the disease does appear to be real and not just an effect of increased testing.[9]

New vaccines have been marketed that include *Leptospira* serovars grippotyphosa and pomona. It is too soon to assess a potential serovar shift following use of newer vaccines. In recent years increasing incidence of *L. kirschneri* serovar autumnalis has also been documented as many commercial laboratories have added this serovar to their testing panel.[9,10] Little is known about this serovar in the dog in terms of experimental infection, but it may emerge as an important cause of renal and nonrenal leptospirosis. Table 198-1 includes many of the recent reviews assessing suspected serovar incidence in confirmed cases of leptospirosis in different regions of North America. Other serovars have been documented from different areas of the world. Serogroup Australis has been incriminated in a Canadian outbreak and has been documented as the cause of chronic canine hepatitis in France and leptospirosis in Italy. In Germany, the predominant serovars appear to be grippotyphosa, icterohemorrhagica, saxkoebing, canicola, and bratislava; a recent survey in Italy identified bratislava and grippotyphosa[7,8,11-16]

EPIDEMIOLOGY

The bacteria are maintained in the renal tubules of the reservoir host and excreted in the urine. Hosts are not typically ill and may be able to shed bacteria for their entire life. The dog

Table • 198-1

Recent Reviews Documenting the Most Common Serovars in Dogs with Leptospirosis from Different Areas of North America

FIRST AUTHOR (REGION)	JOURNAL	YEAR	NO. OF CASES	PREDOMINANT SEROVARS
Goldstein (New York)	JVIM	2006	55	Grippotyphosa, pomona
Ward (Indiana)	JAVMA	2004	90	Grippotyphosa
Prescott (Ontario)	Can Vet J	2002	31	Autumnalis, bratislava
Adin (California)	JAVMA	2000	36	Pomona, bratislava
Ribotta (Quebec)	Can Vet J	2000	19	Grippotyphosa, pomona

is not the reservoir host for any pathogenic serovars, excluding *L. interrogans* serovar canicola. The reservoir hosts for the other serovars include common rodents, skunks, raccoons, and deer. These animals can carry and excrete the bacteria in their urine for extended periods.[3] This may also be true for dogs as well, but most likely specifically for dogs infected with *L. interrogans* serovar canicola. It is less likely, yet still not completely known, whether such a carrier state exists in dogs infected with other serovars that have not adapted for persistence in the dog.

Leptospires can be transmitted directly between hosts in close contact through urine, venereal routes, placental transfer, bites, or ingestion of infected tissues as the organism penetrates mucosa or broken skin. Shedding by infected animals occurs, usually via urine. The exact duration of shedding and potential spread to other dogs or humans is uncertain and may depend on the serovar and be more common with canicola that the other serovars in dogs. Indirect transmission, which happens more often, occurs through exposure of susceptible animals or humans to a contaminated environment (e.g., soil, food, or bedding). Water contact is the most common means of spread, and habitats with stagnant or slow-moving warm water favor organism survival. *Leptospira* organisms invade the host through skin wounds or through intact mucous membranes from the water. Because optimal survival conditions include a neutral or slightly alkaline pH, the organism survives only transiently in undiluted acidic urine (pH 5.0 to 5.5), whereas dilute urine provides a suitable habitat. Ambient temperatures between 0° and 25° C favor survival; freezing markedly decreases survival. Rainfall, temperature, and pH requirements explain the apparent increased incidence of canine leptospirosis in late summer and early fall, in the southern, semitropical belt of the United States, and in similar climatic regions worldwide. Clustering of cases depends on environmental factors. Seasonality is clearly associated with rainfall,[6,17-19] and disease outbreaks often occur during or immediately after periods of flooding. This was most apparent in a large human outbreak in triatheletes in Illinois. People became infected after swimming in a lake a short time after strong rains and flooding.[20]

Once in a susceptible host, leptospires begin to multiply as early as 1 day after entering the vascular space.[21] Following the leptospiremic phase, which lasts a few days, they can invade a variety of organs, including the kidneys, liver, spleen, central nervous system (CNS), eyes, and genital tract. Leptospires damage organs by replicating and inducing cytokine production and inflammatory cell invasion. Initial replication mainly damages the kidneys and liver. The extent of damage to internal organs varies, depending on the virulence of the organism and host susceptibility.[22]

Recovery from infection depends on the production of specific antibodies. As serum antibodies increase, the organism is cleared. Renal colonization occurs in most infected animals that do not have adequate protection from prior exposure or vaccination. Without appropriate antibiotic treatment, the organism may persist in renal tubular epithelial cells, possibly shedding from the kidneys for weeks to months after clinical recovery. The prognosis is highly dependent on conservation of renal function.

PATHOGENESIS

Understanding the molecular basis for leptospiral virulence is crucial in the effort to produce more effective diagnostics, vaccines, and in appreciating the spectrum of clinical disease that result from infection. Identifying surface antigens that are expressed during active infection in vivo, in addition to their obvious potential for vaccines, may also facilitate distinction

between active infection, vaccination, or exposure. For example, *Leptospira* immunoglobulin–like protein A (LigA) contains domains homologous to proteins with attachment and invasion functions and is expressed in vivo but not in vitro.[3] *Leptospira* organisms penetrate abraded skin or mucous membranes and replicate rapidly in the bloodstream. The sequence of events after infection is amazingly variable and likely depends on:

- Virulence and numbers of bacteria. It has been shown that suspected *L. interrogans* serovar pomona infections induced significantly more severe kidney disease and had a worse outcome that infection suspected to be from other serovars.[7]
- Immune response. Previous exposure (naturally occurring or vaccinal) to the same serovar is likely to provide some degree of immunity, although immunity duration is unknown. There is some evidence to suggest that the immunity may last a few years. A study comparing different commercially available vaccines demonstrated only mild serologic responses to a series of two vaccinations but good immunity when challenged 1 year after the second vaccine.[23]
- After infection the following organs may be affected:
  - Kidneys: Renal colonization. Organisms persist and multiply in the renal tubular epithelial cells causing acute nephritis. If not fatal and not treated appropriately, this MAY lead (information is mostly experimental from *L. canicola*) to chronic interstitial nephritis and a persistent carrier state.
  - Liver: Liver damage. Centrilobular necrosis and subcellular damage, bile canaliculi, and duct occlusion may cause icterus. This is not seen as commonly as with *L. icterohaemorrhagiae*.
  - Endothelial damage and DIC: Tissue edema and disseminated intravascular coagulation (DIC) may occur rapidly and result in acute endothelial injury and hemorrhagic manifestations. *Leptospira* lipopolysaccharides stimulate neutrophil adherence and platelet activation, which may be involved in inflammatory and coagulatory abnormalities.
  - Other body systems may also be damaged during the acute phase of infection. Benign meningitis resulted when leptospires invaded the CNS; however, this is more common in humans. Uveitis occasionally is present in naturally occurring and experimentally induced canine leptospirosis. Abortion and infertility resulting from transplacental transmission of leptospires associated with serovar bataviae infection have been described. Pulmonary manifestations include labored respiration and coughing. Interstitial pneumonia has been documented in humans. Lung changes in dogs infected with leptospirosis are associated with pulmonary hemorrhage, most likely due to endothelial damage and vasculitis.[24] Secondary immune-mediated disease (e.g., polyarthritis, hemolytic anemia) have been suspected to occur, but the incidence of canine cases is unknown.

DIAGNOSIS

Establishment of a diagnosis is important because animals can serve as reservoirs and pose potential zoonotic risks. The diagnosis of leptospirosis in dogs is difficult for a few reasons. First, clinical signs can be vague and nonspecific. Clinicopathologic data is more indicative of the end-organ damage and is relatively nonspecific, requiring more targeted testing. Specific leptospirosis testing in practice is limited to serology, which lacks both sensitivity (negative results early in the disease process) and specificity (reacts positively with vaccinal antibodies) when a single test is preformed. Thus the index of suspicion must be broad, and veterinarians may have to submit repeated samples to obtain a definitive diagnosis.

SIGNALMENT AND HISTORY

It would be valuable to identify dogs likely to be infected with *Leptospira* organisms to narrow the need for specific and sometimes expensive testing. This knowledge may also help in deciding which dogs should be vaccinated. Geographic region and season should be taken into account, although large amounts of epidemiologic data by region are not always available.[25] Roaming dogs and those exposed to standing water contaminated by wildlife urine are candidates. Some studies suggest male dogs are more likely to develop the disease.[19,26] Anecdotally, though, it does appear that even small dogs in urban environments contract the disease, forcing the veterinary practitioner to maintain a wide index of suspicion and think broadly when dogs have appropriate clinical signs and when making vaccine decisions.

CLINICAL SIGNS

Clinical signs of leptospirosis in dogs can be nonspecific. Signs of hepatic and renal dysfunction and of coagulation defects usually predominate. Severity of clinical signs depends on age and immunocompetence of the host, environmental factors affecting the organisms, and the virulence and quantity of the acquired bacteria. Younger dogs (less than 6 months) are more severely affected and develop more signs of hepatic dysfunction. A majority of experimental leptospiral infections in dogs are subclinical. It is unknown what percentage of naïve, naturally infected dogs show obvious clinical signs. Peracute leptospiral infections may also exist. Experimentally these are characterized by massive leptospiremia, causing shock and often death with few premonitory signs. Signs found to be most common in dogs diagnosed with leptospirosis in New York State included lethargy, vomiting, anorexia, and polydipsia. Icterus and fever on initial presentation were found to be relatively uncommon and should not be relied on to determine which dogs should be tested for the disease.[7]

CLINICOPATHOLOGIC DATA

There is no single result on a serum chemistry profile, complete blood count, or urinalysis that would allow diagnosis of leptospirosis. Azotemia, increased serum liver enzyme activity, electrolyte disturbances, and mild increases in serum bilirubin concentrations are common. Coagulation parameters may be altered in severely affected animals. Leukocytosis and thrombocytopenia are relatively common. Since these findings are not common with other causes of acute kidney injury (possibly with the exception of pyelonephritis), a combination of such findings and azotemia suggests leptospirosis. Urinalysis often reveals decreased specific gravity, glucosuria, granular casts, and low-grade proteinuria, all markers of tubular injury.[7]

IMAGING

Characteristic changes have been described in the lungs on thoracic radiographs[24] and in the kidneys on abdominal ultrasound[27] in dogs with leptospirosis. These were not controlled studies, and it is unclear how often or how specific these findings are in dogs. Leptospiral infection can lead to similar clinical signs independent of the etiologic serovar,[7,15] at least with regard to the serovars commonly seen today in dogs in North America and in Europe. This makes the serovar identification of the organism much less important than a yes or no answer for the disease. Based on results of signalment, history, physical examination, and clinicopathologic data, the decision regarding specific testing for leptospirosis can be made. Figure 198-1 suggests a possible approach for diagnosing canine leptospirosis.

SPECIFIC TESTING

Detection of antibodies using the microscopic agglutination test (MAT) is the most common diagnostic method currently used in the United States for the diagnosis of canine leptospirosis.[28] Serial dilutions of the canine sera are mixed with cultured *Leptospira* organisms of different serovars representing different serogroups. The titer against a specific serogroup is defined as the highest dilution of the sera that caused 50% agglutination with the organisms representing that serogroup. The problem in interpretation of MAT or other antibody test results is the high prevalence of subclinical infections and the persistence of antibodies. In addition, leptospiral vaccines induce antibodies, therefore the presence of antibodies in itself does not necessarily reflect disease. However, a high MAT titer (≥800) to a nonvaccinal serovar and a negative or low (≤400) titers against vaccinal serovars, accompanied by clinical signs of leptospirosis, is typically considered highly suggestive of active infection.[28]

In a study of naïve puppies vaccinated against four serovars, the MAT titers were often highest to the nonvaccinal serovar auntumnalis.[29] Similarly, in infected dogs, crossreactive results may make identification of the infecting serovar difficult. High titers to a specific serovar may not definitely identify the causative serovar, because shared epitopes among organisms of related serovars frequently induce production of cross-reactive antibodies.[25] In a recent human study where urine cultures and MAT results were compared, the MAT accurately predicted serovar in only 46% of the cases.[30] Laboratory variation and differences in host-specific humoral immune responses sometime make correct assignment of antibody tests even more difficult. Fortunately for the veterinary practitioner, though, the infecting serovar is not crucial information to have as the disease appears to be similar and the treatment identical, regardless of serovar.[7,15] These data are important from an epidemiologic perspective.

Perhaps the most reliable diagnostic criterion widely available is a fourfold increase in MAT titers. Because antibody test results are often negative in the first week of illness, especially in young dogs (less than 6 months of age), a second serum sample should be obtained within 1 to 2 weeks. Negative initial antibody tests can be explained by the 7- to 9-day period required before MAT antibodies are detected. MAT titers become positive after about 1 week, peak at 3 to 4 weeks, and remain positive for months after both natural infection and vaccination.[28] Therefore, to confirm current infection versus previous infection or vaccination, a rising titer should be demonstrated. Antimicrobial therapy early in the course of the disease may decrease the magnitude of the titer rise. Lower levels of antibodies to leptospiral antigens used in the MAT may also indicate exposure to infection with nonleptospiral spirochetes (e.g., oral spirochetal infections). However, dogs exposed to ticks harboring *Borrelia burgdorferi* that developed high titers to that organism did not show significant increases in anti-*Leptospira* titers on the MAT. In contrast, leptospiral infections can affect antibody results for borreliosis.

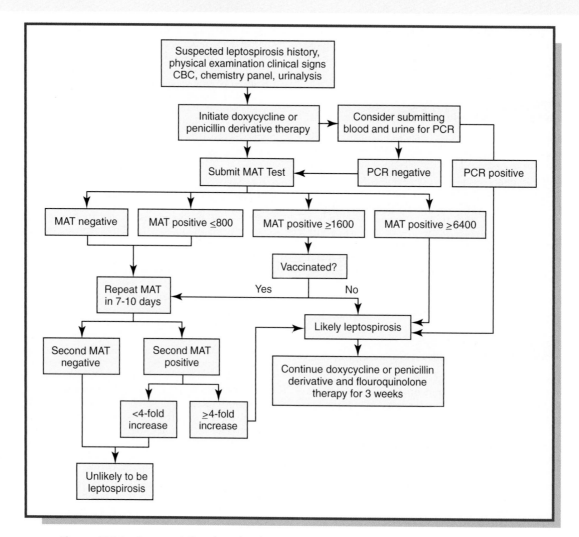

Figure 198-1 Suggested flowchart for the current diagnosis of canine leptospirosis using the microscopic agglutination test *(MAT)*. *, Recommended serovars for testing in North America include grippotyphosa, pomona, bratislava, canicola, icterohaemorrhagiae, and autumnalis; *CBC*, complete blood count; *PCR*, polymerase chain reaction.

In addition to the widely used MAT, a combined IgM/IgG ELISA[15,31,32] or immunofluorescent assay (IFA)[33] can be used to measure leptospiral antibodies. IgM antibodies increase within the first week of infection (before the MAT titer); the maximum IgM titer develops within 14 days and decreases thereafter. IgG antibody tests turn positive 2 to 3 weeks after infection and persist for months, with a maximum titer after 1 month.[28] A combined IgM/IgG test from a single sample is better suited to distinguishing natural infection from vaccine-induced immunity than is the MAT, because dogs that have been vaccinated and have received boosters demonstrate a high IgG titer but low or negative IgM antibodies. However, these combined tests cannot distinguish between different serovars.

The organisms can be directly identified using one of several techniques. Visualization of organisms in fresh urine can be accomplished using dark-field microscopy. Organisms may be seen in tissue sections or on air-dried smears using light microscopy. Organisms may be detected via culture or by detection of deoxyribonucleic acid (DNA) by polymerase chain reaction (PCR). However, such direct methods are reliable only with positive results. A negative result never excludes the presence of the infectious agent. Identification of leptospires in urine by dark-field microscopy[34] is frequently unre-

warding, and both positive and negative results should be followed by culture or antibody testing. Leptospires sometimes can be seen by light microscopy in tissue sections or on air-dried smears with Giemsa stain or silver impregnation. Immunofluorescence and immunohistochemical staining techniques have been adapted to identify *Leptospira* organisms in tissues imprints of liver and kidney and in body fluids such as blood or urine, and these techniques potentially can be used to identify animals shedding organisms in urine when culture is impossible or too time-consuming[35] (Figure 198-2).

Although culture of the organism from blood, urine, or cerebrospinal fluid (CSF) would be ideal, leptospires are difficult to culture and may take weeks to months to grow. They are fastidious, and sampling should always precede institution of antimicrobial therapy. Dogs are leptospiremic during the first week of infection, but the number of circulating organisms subsequently decreases as serum antibodies increase. Urine (sampled by cystocentesis to avoid overgrowth by normal flora) is the best fluid for culture. If animals are adequately hydrated, administration of a low dose of a diuretic such as furosemide (0.5 mg/kg) just before urine collection may facilitate recovery of organisms. Urine should be alkalinized to or above a pH 8.0 during transport. Special liquid, semisolid, or solid culture media should be used. Definitive

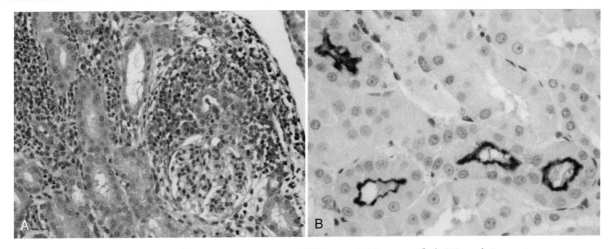

Figure 198-2 The above images represent H&E-stained, 20× magnified **(A)** and *Leptospira* immunohistochemistry–stained, 40× magnified **(B)** renal histopathology from dogs experimentally infected with *L. kirshneri* serovar grippotyphosa. Note the marked inflammatory response **(A)** and the dark brown–staining *Leptospira* organisms along the inner lining of the renal tubules **(B)**.

differentiation of the etiologic serovar can also be accomplished using culture.

PCR has been used to detect leptospires in blood, CSF, aqueous humor, and urine. Urine testing is recommended because concentration of leptospires is highest in urine, although such testing will be negative early in the disease process or following antibiotic therapy. In two studies comparing PCR, culture, and antibody testing in healthy and diseased animals, PCR was significantly more sensitive than the other methods in identifying shedders and diagnosing the disease.[36,37] Because culturing of urine is time-consuming and insensitive, the PCR approach may be most useful for direct detection of the organism, especially when testing for subclinical infection or chronic shedding. Quantitative PCR may be a commercially available option for the identification of organisms in blood in early infection and later in the urine.[38] Recent advances in PCR techniques have allowed not only diagnosis of leptospirosis but perhaps also identification of specific *Leptospira* serovars.[39] Future diagnostics will most likely include quantitative PCR of blood and urine as well as serologic testing, looking for specific antibodies produced only with natural infection. These tests will not be serovar-specific but should provide a reliable "yes" or "no" diagnosis early in the disease using a single blood sample and will not be influenced by vaccination.

IDENTIFICATION IN TISSUE

In the event that kidney tissue is obtained either via antemortem biopsy or postmortem, *Leptospira* organisms can be relatively easy to identify within tubules adjacent to the lining of the tubular cells via special stains (modified Steiner or silver), immunohistochemistry (see Figure 198-2), or via PCR. In addition to the presence of the organism, leptospirosis can be suspected based on the inflammatory injury to the kidney. The liver is another major parenchymatous organ damaged during leptospiremia. Profound hepatic dysfunction may occur without major histologic change because damage is subcellular. The degree of icterus in both canine and human leptospirosis usually corresponds to the severity of hepatic necrosis. Chronic active hepatitis and hepatic fibrosis may also occur as a chronic sequela to *Leptospira* infection in dogs. Presumably, initial hepatocellular injury and persistence of the organism in the liver result in altered hepatic circulation

and immunologic disturbances that perpetuate the chronic inflammatory response.

TREATMENT

Supportive therapy for animals with leptospirosis depends on the severity of the clinical signs and whether renal or hepatic dysfunction is present. Antimicrobial therapy is essential to terminate bacteremia and should be initiated quickly after leptospirosis is suspected and even prior to confirmation of the diagnosis. A study in humans revealed that if antibiotics were delayed by 4 days after presentation, there was no longer an advantage to their administration.[40] Treatment can be divided into two stages. The goal of the first stage is to immediately inhibit multiplication of the organism and rapidly reduce fatal complications of infection, such as hepatic and renal failure. Doxycycline or penicillin and its derivatives are the antibiotics of choice for terminating leptospiremia.

If oral drugs can be administered, use of doxycycline (5 mg/kg given every 12 hours) or amoxicillin (22 mg/kg every 12 hours) is recommended. Ampicillin (22 mg/kg given IV every 8 hours) or amoxicillin, if available for IV use (22 mg/kg given every 12 hours) are preferred for vomiting, uremic, or hepatically compromised animals. These drugs prevent shedding and transmission of organisms within 24 hours, and, therefore, also significantly decrease the risk of zoonotic transfer. They may not, however, clear renal infections or eliminate the carrier state and chronic shedding.

The goal of the second stage, therefore, is to eliminate the carrier state through administration of drugs such as tetracyclines, fluoroquinolones, or the newer erythromycin derivatives. Doxycycline (5 mg/kg given orally every 12 hours for 3 weeks) is the drug of choice, when tolerated. Doxycycline treatment should start as soon as oral therapy is possible and liver function is uncompromised. Doxycycline is usually given orally, although IV administration is also available. Oral administration, however, can cause gastrointestinal side effects. Doxycycline can be given regardless of the degree of renal dysfunction. The doxycycline dose does not need to be adjusted in animals with kidney disease because it is predominantly excreted in the feces. Therefore, in a dog suspected of being infected with leptospirosis, the common protocols include doxycycline alone for both stages in animals that can tolerate oral therapy or a penicillin derivative that is later either combined with a fluoroquinolone or switched to doxycycline after the diagnosis has been confirmed.

The extent of renal damage after treatment determines the overall prognosis for affected dogs. Aggressive fluid therapy should accompany antimicrobial treatment as is described for other causes of acute renal injury (see Chapter 309). Hemodialysis has been shown to be beneficial in dogs that develop anuria, oliguria, or are refractive to fluid therapy.[6] Some dogs have an apparent clinical recovery after treatment, whereas others develop persistent azotemia with an overall survival rate approaching 80%.[6,7]

PREVENTION

Inactivated bacterins against icterohaemorrhagiae and canicola infection have been widely used, and this strategy has reduced the prevalence of highly virulent forms of illness. However, these vaccines are not cross-protective against the serovars responsible for most of the current infections in dogs. Currently two bacterin-based vaccines that contain grippotyphosa and pomona strains, either as bivalent or quadrivalent products (Duramune LGP or Duramune LCI-GP, Fort Dodge Animal Health, Fort Dodge, Iowa, and Vanguard L4, Pfizer Animal Health, New York, N.Y.), are now marketed in the United States. These vaccines are recommended annually, following a two-injection initial series in a puppy or previously unvaccinated dog. Unfortunately, no data regarding the duration of immunity are published for the vaccines containing these new serovars. Good protection has been shown to persist for 1 year despite low MAT antibody titers at the time of challenge for other bacterin type of vaccines containing serovars canicola or icterohaemorrhagiae.[23] Debate has arisen over the necessity of routine vaccination in dogs. As inactivated bacterins, leptospiral vaccines have been thought to cause allergenic reactions, especially in certain breeds, and when combined with other adjuvanted agents. However, many manufacturers have improved and purified their leptospiral vaccines, producing safer multicomponent products. Such vaccines were not shown to be more reactive than other commonly used vaccines.[41] Icterohaemorrhagiae and canicola infections continue to occur in unvaccinated animals, which indicate that these agents have not been eradicated.

Wild animal reservoirs and subclinically affected domestic animals continue to harbor and shed organisms. Therefore, control of rodents in kennels, maintenance of environmental conditions to discourage bacterial survival, and isolation of infected animals are important steps in preventing the spread of disease. Complete control of shedding by wild animal reservoirs is impossible. For these reasons, vaccination of dogs is essential.

LEPTOSPIROSIS IN CATS

The prevalence of clinical illness is low in cats, despite the presence of leptospiral antibodies in the feline population and the exposure of cats to leptospires excreted by wildlife. Serovars canicola, grippotyphosa, and pomona have been isolated from cats. Outdoor cats have the highest antibody prevalence, and transmission from rodents is suspected. Cats may also be exposed to the urine of cohabiting dogs. Although cats develop antibodies after exposure, they appear to be less susceptible than dogs to both spontaneous and experimental infection. Clinical signs are usually mild or not apparent in feline leptospirosis, despite the presence of leptospiremia and leptospiruria and histologic evidence of renal and hepatic inflammation. The lack of clinical cases may be related partly to cats' aversion to water and partly to natural resistance to infection.

PUBLIC HEALTH CONSIDERATIONS

The majority of leptospiral infections in humans are identified among those involved in water-related activities, either through work or leisure activities. In some outbreaks, simultaneous exposure of humans and dogs occurs. Urine from infected dogs can cause disease in humans when it comes in contact with mucosal surfaces or a break in the epidermal barrier. Latex gloves are necessary when urine or urine-contaminated items are handled, and face masks and goggles should be worn when contaminated kennel areas are hosed down. Urine-contaminated areas should be cleaned with dry paper first (to avoid dilution of urine), then washed with detergent and treated with iodophor disinfectants, to which the organism is susceptible. Shedding dogs can be identified with urine PCR. All dogs known to be or suspected of shedding should be treated with doxycycline.

REFERENCES

The reference list can be found on the companion Expert Consult Web site at *www.expertconsult.com*.

BACTERIAL DISEASES

CHAPTER 199

Lyme Disease

Richard E. Goldstein

ETIOLOGY

Tick-borne spirochetoses are a group of diseases that affect humans and animals worldwide. They can be divided into the Lyme disease group (Lyme borreliosis), caused by *Borrelia burgdorferi* and transmitted by *Ixodes* ticks, and the relapsing fever group, which is transmitted by soft ticks. The Lyme disease group was recognized more recently and is now the most commonly diagnosed vector-borne disease in humans.[1] Like most spirochetes, *Borrelia* organisms are small, corkscrew-shaped, motile, microaerophilic bacteria of the order Spirochaetales that can move in connective tissue using their flagella. Borreliosis has been known in Europe since the early

1900s; Alan Steere of Yale University first described the disease and the connection to tick bites after a 1975 outbreak in Lyme, Connecticut (which led to the name *Lyme disease*). However, evidence suggests that this infection in indigenous wildlife and their tick vectors is a bit older. Studies have demonstrated that ear skin samples from museum specimens of white-footed mice collected near Dennis, Massachusetts, in 1894 contained *Borrelia* DNA.[2] *Borrelia* organisms also were detected in British ticks from 1897.[3] Lyme disease has now become prevalent in many areas of North America, Europe, and Asia and over the last 20 years has evolved into a major health concern in much of the United States and Europe in both humans and dogs.[1] Experimentally induced and naturally occurring Lyme borreliosis has been described in dogs, cats, and other domestic animals.[1] Antibody prevalence in dogs in endemic areas correlates with living in forested and urban areas and time spent outdoors.

At least six species of borreliosis have been found in dogs and humans. *B. burgdorferi sensu stricto* predominates in humans and dogs in the United States. It also is found in Europe but only in about 10% of isolates. *B. garinii* and *B. afzelii* are the most common species in Europe. In cats, the natural disease is poorly documented, although cats can be infected experimentally. Cats seem to be less susceptible to clinical signs than dogs, and dogs less susceptible than humans.

This chapter will address the most common clinical questions facing veterinarians practicing in Lyme-endemic regions around the world, or that are presented with dogs that travel to those regions. Such questions include:

- How is the disease transmitted? And what causes clinical disease in some dogs after infection?
- What are the common clinical signs of Lyme disease? How can one diagnose Lyme disease in dogs that have appropriate clinical signs? How should they be treated?
- Should we be monitoring nonclinical dogs for anti-*Borrelia* antibodies, and, if identified should they be treated?
- How can we prevent dogs from becoming infected in Lyme-endemic areas?
- Is Lyme disease truly associated with severe or fatal clinical disease in dogs such as cardiac arrhythmias, neurologic disease, and proteinuric kidney disease?

PATHOGENESIS

Unlike the related spirochete *Leptospira* spp., *Borrelia* organisms do not survive free living in the environment. They are host associated and are transmitted between vertebrate reservoir hosts and hematophagous arthropod vectors. The principal vectors of *B. burgdorferi sensu lato* are various species of hard ticks of the *Ixodes* complex. *I. ricinus* and *I. persulcatus* are the primary vectors in Europe and Asia, respectively. In the United States, the closely related black-legged ticks *I. scapularis* (Northeast, Midwest, and Southeast) and *I. pacificus* (West) are the main vectors. These small *Ixodes* ticks (less than 3 mm) generally feed on more than one host during their life cycle. *I. scapularis* is a three-host tick with a 2-year life cycle. Infected nymphs overwinter, and in the spring they transmit infection to reservoir hosts, which in turn infect feeding larvae. Larvae and nymphs feed primarily on rodents and small mammals (northern *I. scapularis*) and reptiles (southern *I. scapularis*), whereas adult ticks feed on deer or larger mammals. Humans and pets are usually infected by nymphs or adult ticks. Because reptiles are not competent reservoir hosts, the infection rate of southern *I. scapularis* ticks is much lower than that of northern *I. scapularis* ticks. Fur-

thermore, because the southern *I. scapularis* ticks do not always feed on mammals, the prevalence of *Borrelia* infection is relatively low in the southern regions.[1] Other ticks and insect vectors have been found to harbor *Borrelia* organisms but do not seem to maintain infection or to be important for transmission. Direct transmission of *Borrelia* spirochetes between reservoir hosts is extremely unlikely, as is transovarial transmission in ticks. Canine urine is also an unlikely source of spread. In a natural infection model, control dogs in direct contact with infected dogs for up to 1 year did not develop antibodies, and organisms could not be isolated from the urine of infected dogs. These studies also did not document any evidence of in utero spread.[4] However, *Borrelia* organisms can survive freezing and storage, which makes artificial insemination a potential source of infection.[5] Blood transfusions also offer another uncommon but potential source of infection.

Natural spirochete transmission requires 48 hours of tick attachment, during which time organisms multiply and cross gut epithelium into the hemolymph, disseminate to the salivary glands, and infect the host through tick saliva.[6] This process of translocation from being adhered to the tick gut epithelial lining to eventually migrating to the salivary glands and from there into the next host is actually triggered by the blood meal itself and is accompanied by major changes of the *Borrelia* surface proteins. Outer surface proteins (Osps) coat the *Borrelia* organisms at all times. In the gut of the tick the major Osp expressed on the *Borrelia* surface is OspA. As a reaction to the warm mammalian blood entering the gut of the tick, a shift in expression is triggered within the *Borrelia* so that OspA is down-regulated and OspC is up-regulated and becomes the predominant Osp.[7] Understanding this shift is crucial to the understanding of the diagnostic and prevention strategies for this disease. Once in the body, *Borrelia* spirochetes usually cause persistent infection.

Experimental evidence suggests that *Borrelia* organisms exist extracellularly and, in an undetermined way, can evade immune clearance. Organisms can persist and proliferate for extended periods (probably lifelong in most animals) in intercellular spaces. Most infected animals never develop clinical signs and in these animals, it is likely that *Borrelia* organisms persist but do not invade connective tissues. In some dogs, *Borrelia* organisms proliferate and migrate from the skin at the site of the tick bite through connective tissues, including joints, beginning in close proximity to the tick bite. Clinical illness in these dogs results from the host's inflammatory response to their presence. Despite treatment for months or years, *Borrelia* spirochetes can persist in the skin, connective tissues, joints, and nervous system and be detected by polymerase chain reaction (PCR) and occasionally culture of these tissues.

It is still not known why specific individuals develop clinical signs.[8] Pathogenicity does depend on the *Borrelia* species in humans, and *B. burgdorferi sensu stricto* seems to be more pathogenic in dogs than the species mainly found in Europe. Evidence suggests that about 5% to 10% of dogs with antibodies in endemic areas in the United States develop clinical disease within 2 to 5 months of infection[9]; the percentage is much lower in endemic areas in northern Europe. Experimental studies indicate that the number of infected feeding ticks is critical. Age and immune status of the animal also appear important. Treatment with high doses of glucocorticoids at the time of infection has been shown to increase likelihood of clinical signs. Development of immune complications, such as arthritis, is probably related to multiple host factors in addition to the virulence and inoculum of the *Borrelia*. Humans with certain haplotypes of the major histocompatibility complex may also be prone to more severe clinical manifestations of the disease.[10]

CLINICAL SIGNS

Experimental infections in dogs have used *B. burgdorferi sensu stricto* strains; therefore, the clinical condition caused by this organism is relatively well described. In experimentally infected dogs, overt clinical illness begins 2 to 5 months after tick exposure. Clinical signs include fever, inappetence, lethargy, lymphadenopathy, and episodic shifting limb lameness related to polyarthritis (Web Figure 199-1). Arthritis begins in the joint closest to the tick bite. Release of proinflammatory cytokines, especially interleukin-8 (IL-8), plays an important role in the pathogenesis of acute and possibly more chronic progressive arthritis in dogs.[11,12] The clinical signs that develop in natural infection or in infections caused by other *Borrelia* species have been less definitively characterized. Some questions remain regarding more serious, but less common syndromes associated with Lyme infection in dogs including: protein-losing glomerular disease (Lyme nephritis), cardiac disease (myocarditis), and neurologic disease.[13] Another question yet to be answered is whether some dogs develop the devastating chronic recurrent disease seen in some infected humans.

The lack or apparent lack of clinical signs in most dogs with active Lyme infection makes both the diagnosis and the study of this disease difficult. This is different than the human disease in which a large percent of people exhibit a characteristic rash around the area of the tick bite during or immediately after *Borrelia* transmission.[14] This rash is not typically seen in dogs and no specific hematologic or biochemical changes are associated with canine Lyme disease. In contrast to leptospirosis, leukocytosis is not seen, probably because *Borrelia* organisms rarely spread hematogenously. Dogs with renal manifestation may have proteinuria due to glomerulonephritis and sometimes secondary azotemia, hematuria, pyuria, and tubular casts. Synovial fluid analysis findings are typical for a suppurative polyarthritis, with leukocyte counts ranging from 2000 to 100,000 nucleated cells per microliter.

Cardiac arrhythmias secondary to myocarditis and myocarditis, similar to those reported in humans, have also been uncommonly reported in dogs.[1]

DIAGNOSING LYME DISEASE

Bacterial Culture

This is very difficult in the case of *Borrelia* due to the small number of infecting organisms and the complicated techniques required for culture success. Special media (e.g., modified Barbour-Stoenner-Kelley medium) are required, but even then culturing is insensitive.[15] Skin appears to be the most consistent tissue for premortem or postmortem culture when specimens are taken at or near the site of tick attachment.[16] Xenodiagnosis, in which uninfected ticks become infected after feeding on suspect infected hosts, has proved reliable in research laboratory settings but is too time-consuming and not useful for routine clinical diagnosis.

PCR can be highly specific but rarely clinically useful. The best materials for diagnosis are skin samples, which should be taken at a location closest to the tick bite. If the tick bite location is unknown, a sample should be taken close to the joint in which the first lameness or swelling was observed. If arthritis is not present, the sample should be taken from an area that is generally most exposed to ticks (usually the front part of the dog). PCR can also be performed using urine,[17] which is even less sensitive. Blood is not useful for PCR, because *Borrelia* organisms rarely spread hematogenously. Joint fluid,[18] synovia samples, or cerebrospinal fluid (CSF) samples are excellent PCR material if appropriate clinical signs are present. Inherently PCR cannot distinguish between live and dead organisms. Some studies have suggested that small DNA fragments of *Borrelia* may persist in synovial membranes after treatment,[16,19] and these fragments may induce positive PCR results. However, experimentally injected *Borrelia* DNA (without replicating *Borrelia*) was destroyed and was not detectable after 3 weeks. The sensitivity of PCR is high, but the sample must contain *B. burgdorferi* DNA. A negative PCR result, therefore, never excludes the presence of the organism elsewhere in the body.

Serology

Clinical signs in conjunction with serology are utilized in diagnosis. There are currently three types of serologic testing commercially available:

- *Nonspecific enzyme-linked immunosorbent assay (ELISA).* This is a sensitive test aimed at identifying any antibodies produced against *Borrelia* whole-cell antigens. It does NOT differentiate between antibodies produced in reaction to Lyme infection versus Lyme vaccination. Paired titers are not helpful in the diagnosis of Lyme disease because high antibody titers usually persist for long periods. Simultaneous measurement of IgG and IgM in a single specimen theoretically would provide more information in other diseases. However, in naturally *Borrelia*-infected dogs and humans, IgM persists for many months; therefore a positive IgM titer does not help confirm recent exposure or infection.[13,20,21] False-negative antibody test results are rare. Early antibody testing is usually negative because the immune response to *B. burgdorferi* develops gradually. Experimentally infected dogs have ELISA-positive results by 4 to 6 weeks after exposure. Titers were highest at 3 months after exposure. Titer increases almost always precede clinical lameness and fever in experimentally infected dogs[4]; therefore, a negative titer in an animal with clinical signs rules out Lyme disease with a high probability.
  - Since one can never be sure of infection status and, at times, of vaccination status, a positive nonspecific ELISA should ideally be followed up with an additional test that would confirm infection (i.e., Western blot[22] or a C6 antibody test[23]).
- *C6 antibody testing.* Recently the antigenic properties of a 26 amino acid–long invariable region located within the central domain of the VlsE molecule, the variable surface of *B. burgdorferi*, were investigated. This region, named IR (invariable region) 6, was determined to be antigenetically conserved among strains of the *B. burgdorferi sensu lato* complex and to be immunodominant in both human and canine hosts.[24] An in-house canine C6 ELISA using the IR6 sequence as a peptide (C6) biotinylated at the N-terminus, recently became available in the United States. The anti-C6 antibody response is highly specific for *B. burgdorferi* and is more sensitive than whole-cell ELISA tests in early infection, detecting antibodies as early as 3 weeks postexposure.[25] It also is more sensitive in detecting *Borrelia* infection in Europe than other commercial ELISA kits.[26] Dogs with leptospirosis, Rocky Mountain spotted fever, babesiosis, ehrlichiosis, and heartworm disease do not have antibodies to C6. Furthermore, C6 is not affected by the currently available Lyme vaccines.[27] C6 antibody levels also may correlate to *Borrelia* loads, dropping relatively quickly after antibiotic therapy,[28,29] whereas conventional whole-cell ELISA results stay at medium levels for a longer time period even following successful treatment.[16] It is still important to remember, though, that the C6 ELISA, although specific, only indicates infection by to *B. burgdorferi* and not clinical disease.

- There are currently two commercially available ELISA tests for canine anti-C6 antibodies. This peptide is expressed only during infection; therefore, both these tests are meant to be positive only in the event of natural exposure and negative in naive dogs or vaccinated dogs.[23,30] These tests include the in-house SNAP 3Dx or SNAP 4Dx tests and the quantitative C6 antibody test available through IDEXX Laboratories (Westbrook, Me.). Some logical uses of these tests:
  - The SNAP 3Dx and 4Dx are excellent for screening dogs for Lyme infection. This can be done as part of a screening program for nonclinical dogs or when Lyme disease is suspected. A positive result is indicative of active Lyme infection.[31] The SNAP 3Dx test also detects canine heartworm antigen, and antibodies against *Ehrlichia canis*. The SNAP 4Dx detects those as well as antibodies against *Anaplasma phagocytophilum* and *Anaplasma platys*.
  - The quantitative C6 antibody test also detects anti-C6 antibodies with results reported in titer units after comparing to a standard curve. While much remains to be learned, the quantitative C6 titer does drop nicely with therapy[29] and it has been shown that the titer correlated well with circulating anti-Lyme immune complexes.[32] More studies are warranted to characterize when and how exactly to use the results of this titer, but even today this quantitative titer may be a useful tool regarding treatment decisions of nonclinical dogs.

Western Blot

Western blot assays are able to detect a spectrum of antibodies, including a pattern of antibody reactivity after natural infection that differs from that produced by vaccination. After natural exposure to *B. burgdorferi*, antibodies develop to several proteins, including Osps. One of these outer surface proteins, OspC, appears to be expressed by *Borrelia* organisms in the host at warmer temperatures but is lost at lower temperatures in the tick or with in vitro cultivation. However, OspC is a prominent protein response to infection, and high amounts of anti-OspC antibodies are produced after natural infection. In contrast, the protein OspA is mainly expressed by *Borrelia* during the arthropod state (or if cultured in vitro). Therefore, reactivity to OspA but not OspC occurs in vaccinated dogs (because the vaccine strains are cultured in vitro) but is lacking in naturally infected dogs. This effect is even more prominent if recombinant vaccines containing OspA are used rather than whole *Borrelia*. Thus, the Western blot antibody pattern expressed by vaccinated dogs differs from that of naturally infected dogs.[33]

However, The Western blot is relatively expensive and labor-intensive and its interpretation requires significant expertise. As we have learned more about the SNAP 4Dx and quantitative C6 assays, they have superseded use of the Western blot as a confirmatory assay. Western blot is only recommended in dogs where the vaccinal antibody status is uniquely important to the veterinarian.

In humans, CSF antibody titers have been compared with serum antibody titers in an attempt to diagnose neuroborreliosis. Intrathecal production of specific antibodies to *B. burgdorferi* can be demonstrated if the ratio of CSF to serum *B. burgdorferi* antibodies is greater than the CSF to serum concentration of albumin, total IgG, or specific IgG against another infectious agent. An increased intrathecal antibody concentration was demonstrated in dogs with neurologic dysfunction. The results of such reports are difficult to assess

because the dogs were from endemic areas, and no supporting histopathology or culture findings were supplied.[1]

Interpreting the Results of Lyme Testing in a Dog with Clinical Signs

The challenge in diagnosing this disease is not the quality of available tests, since they are excellent. The problem is the large proportion of dogs in an endemic area that could be infected with *Borrelia*, the vast majority without clinical signs. Many dogs that are clinical for other diseases will test positive for Lyme serology. Thus a positive test alone does not diagnose the disease! The following is a practical approach to the diagnosis of the Lyme disease (Figure 199-1):

1. Are the clinical signs appropriate? These include acute monoarthritis or polyarthritis, lethargy, fever and pain. If not, consider other diseases.
2. Is the test used specific for *Borrelia* infection (SNAP 3Dx, SNAP 4Dx, or Western blot). If not, then one of these tests should be used to verify that a positive dog on a nonspecific ELISA is truly positive for *Borrelia* infection.

If the answers to the two previous questions are both yes, it may make sense to obtain a minimal data base of complete blood count, serum chemistries, and urinalysis including testing for proteinuria. The dog should be treated for presumptive Lyme disease and response to therapy monitored. The diagnosis should remain presumptive because there is no test that can prove that *Borrelia* is the agent causing the clinical signs. If a dog responds rapidly and does not redevelop clinical signs during or immediately following therapy, then a presumptive diagnosis of Lyme disease can remain, although in reality coinfection or other disorders such as immune-mediated polyarthritis as well as spontaneous remission have not been ruled out. If response to therapy is inadequate or there is a rapid reoccurrence of clinical signs, then additional diagnostics should be preformed, and Lyme disease becomes an unlikely diagnosis.

Screening Nonclinical Dogs for *Borellia* Infection

Relatively inexpensive and accurate tests for screening nonclinical dogs exist (SNAP 3Dx or SNAP 4Dx) and are readily available. However, this is not reason to use testing to routinely screen nonclinical dogs for *Borrelia* infection. There are pros and cons to screening of nonclinical dogs.[13] If the practitioner is treating all positive nonclinical dogs, then screening is necessary to identify those dogs. A detailed discussion regarding the evidence for and against treatment of nonclinical dogs will follow. However, even if practitioners are not treating nonclinical dogs, there are still many reasons to screen nonclinical dogs annually in Lyme-endemic areas:

1. To document infection rate in the area of a specific practice and for dogs with specific lifestyles. This is essential for decision making regarding prevention strategies of tick control and vaccination that can vary greatly from region to region.
2. To monitor for tick exposure and evaluate the efficacy of the preventive strategy (tick control ± vaccination) employed by the veterinarian and the dog owner.
3. To provide information regarding possible coinfections that can also be diagnosed using the same test (e.g., *Anaplasma phagocytophilum*).
4. To assist in possibly identifying early Lyme nephritis cases by following up a positive SNAP test with an assay for proteinuria.
5. To provide information regarding Lyme incidence that could be used for human health purposes by individual families of positive dogs or the human health authorities.

Potential reasons not to screen nonclinical dogs:

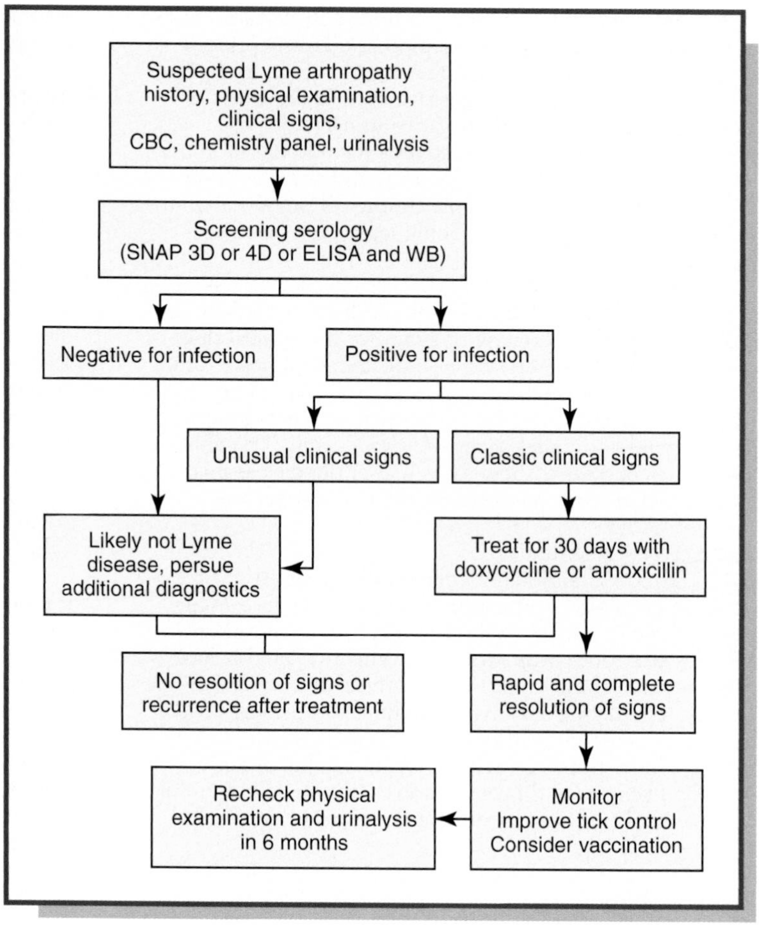

Figure 199-1 A possible flow chart for the diagnosis of Lyme disease in dogs with appropriate clinical signs in Lyme endemic regions. *CBC,* Complete blood count; *ELISA,* enzyme linked immunosorbent assay; *WB,* Western blot.

1. Most dogs are nonclinical anyway.
2. There is no definitive evidence that nonclinical dogs should be treated and screening these dogs could lead to overtreatment.
3. Despite the fact that the specificity of the SNAP test is high (>96%), the positive predictive value will be low in areas of very low Lyme prevalence.

It appears that the benefits of screening nonclinical dogs far outweigh potential risks. This is independent of whether positive nonclinical dogs should be treated, and does mandate that veterinarians understand the value of a positive SNAP test and the possibility of false positives, especially in nonendemic regions, and not overreact to a single positive test result.

TREATMENT

Because of the difficulty involved in obtaining an accurate diagnosis, antibiotics often are given empirically in an attempt to make a therapeutic diagnosis. Many reports exist of successful recovery after institution of antimicrobial therapy in dogs "diagnosed" with Lyme arthritis. However, clinical improvement after any therapeutic intervention should be viewed with caution, because of coinfections, and because acute limb and joint dysfunction is intermittent and often resolves after several days to weeks, regardless of whether antibiotics are given.[34] Doxycycline, the drug of choice, by itself has been shown to be chondroprotective in noninfectious arthritis in dogs[35] and thus may lead to improvement also in arthritis not related to Lyme disease.

The antibiotics that are most effective for treating *Borrelia* infection are the tetracyclines, ampicillin or amoxicillin, some third-generation IV cephalosporins, and erythromycin and its derivatives. Doxycycline (5 mg/kg given orally every 12 hours or 10 mg/kg given once daily for 30 days) is the first choice because it is a lipid-soluble and relatively low in cost. The other drugs are usually reserved for refractory or chronic infections. Improvement often occurs within 24 to 48 hours of initiating therapy. Greatest success is achieved in initial phases of clinical illness.

Many studies suggest that the organism is difficult to eliminate from animals with established infection and that relapses occur despite seemingly adequate treatment regimens.[34,36] While treatment should be continued for a minimum of 30 days, clearance of the organism is questionable. Relapse can occur, and PCR results can become positive after discontinuation of antimicrobials.[37,38] Also, inflammatory changes that occur in various tissues, such as the joints, may become self-perpetuating. Intraarticular persistence of *Borrelia* organisms may stimulate chronic immune and inflammatory processes. The current recommendations for treating chronic or recurrent borreliosis are to repeat the 30-day antibiotic treatment four or five times at 3-month intervals or every time there appears to be a reoccurrence of clinical disease.

Nonsteroidal antiinflammatory medications may be helpful for pain relief during episodes of recurrent arthritis. Immunosuppressive doses of glucocorticoids should be avoided, because immunosuppression may potentiate infection exacerbation.[37] Tick-exposed dogs that recovered from clinical signs of Lyme disease and then were treated with oral prednisolone for a 2-week period 16 months after original exposure again demonstrated lameness and polyarthritis.[34]

Treating Nonclinical Dogs

The question as to whether to treat nonclinical Lyme positive dogs has no definitive answer at this time. There is no definitive proof that treatment of a nonclinical dog lessens the chance of developing clinical signs down the road, of developing chronic disease, or of developing Lyme nephritis. Therefore, without such proof many experts do not recommend treatment of nonclinical, Lyme-positive dogs.[13] However, it appears that many practitioners in Lyme-endemic regions are routinely treating all or most Lyme positive nonclinical dogs identified on routine screening. The decision to treat may stem from owner pressure or from fear that clinical signs would be more likely to develop in an untreated dog. The rationale for not treating nonclinical dogs includes the following:

- There is no definitive proof that a treated nonclinical dog is less likely to develop clinical signs than a nontreated dog.
- The risks to the individual dog being treated include side effects of the antibiotic as well as the unnecessary expense for the owner.
- The more global effects of excessive antibiotic use on the development of resistant strains of bacteria.

Current literature suggests that there may be benefit for treating a subset of Lyme positive nonclinical dogs. The two tools suggested to assist in making decisions regarding the treatment of nonclinical dogs are proteinuria and the quantitative C6 assay.[13]

- Proteinuria (Figure 199-2). Microalbuminuria is not merely secondary to being Lyme-positive in nonclinical dogs.[39] It is thought to be likely, although unproven, that dogs suffering from early Lyme nephritis will develop proteinuria prior to azotemia and overt clinical signs. Therefore, screening nonclinical Lyme-positive dogs for proteinuria may be a method of identifying dogs with early Lyme nephritis. It is strongly recommended that all Lyme-positive dogs be tested for proteinuria, and all dogs with proteinuria be tested for Lyme, and if positive for both these dogs should be treated.[13]

- Quantitative C6 (see Figure 199-2). Studies have documented a decline in serum quantitative C6 concentrations following doxycycline treatment of Lyme positive clinical[32] and nonclinical dogs.[29,32] The quantitative C6 titers were shown to be more likely to drop if they initially were ≥30 ELISA units.[29] IDEXX Laboratories have recommended using the magnitude of the quantitative C6 titer in decision making regarding treating nonclinical dogs (see Figure 199-2). Obviously a decreasing titer does not in itself justify therapy. The theory behind this recommendation is that a decreasing titer may reflect decreasing antigen load and therefore may be seen as a sign of a success of therapy. This theory is supported to some degree by finding that Lyme-specific immune complexes also drop following doxycycline therapy and correlate well with the drop in quantitative C6 titers.[32]

PREVENTION

Tick control using residual insecticides or growth regulators is a supportive measure that must be used to reduce the prevalence of infection in dogs. The proper use of these agents will decrease the risk of Lyme infection and, coupled with fastidious grooming and avoidance of areas with an abundance of ticks, may suffice for Lyme prevention in areas of relatively low prevalence. It is unlikely that tick control products alone will prevent dogs from becoming infected in dense endemic regions. It is in these regions of the Northeast, Midwest, and Northern Pacific West Coast of the United States that Lyme vaccination should be considered as potential component of the Lyme prevention strategy.

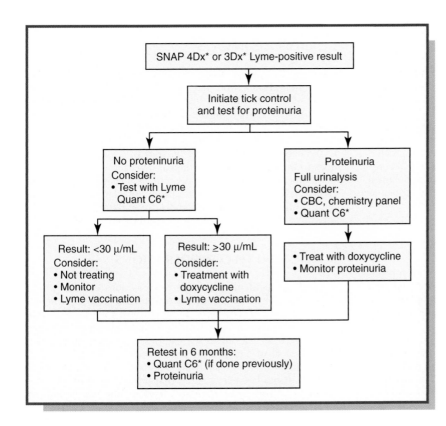

Figure 199-2 A flow chart demonstrating the possible use of proteinuria and the quantitative C6 assay as aids in decision making regarding the treatment of nonclinical Lyme-positive dogs in Lyme-endemic regions. *, IDEXX Laboratories, Westbrook, Me.; *CBC*, complete blood count.

In United States, whole-cell bacterins and recombinant protein OspA vaccines for dogs are commercially available. Both types of vaccine produce anti-OspA antibodies in well-vaccinated dogs. These antibodies have no effect in the dog but, when taken up by the tick during the blood meal, they bind to the OspA-coated *Borrelia* in the tick hindgut and are subsequently killed. Thus these vaccines prevent transmission from the tick versus priming the canine immune system to produce bactericidal antibodies in vivo as other vaccines commonly do. Cell culture–grown whole-cell bacterin vaccines contain OspA antigen as do the recombinant OspA–only vaccines. The concern of extraneous protein increasing the risk of vaccine reactions has precluded development of a whole-cell bacterin from consideration as a human vaccine. All human vaccines that have been sold in the United States were based on recombinant DNA production of Osp products, but even they are no longer on the market because of lack of sales. In Europe and other geographic areas, only whole-cell bacterins are available for dogs (and no vaccines are available for humans) because the multiplicity of infecting strains makes the development of a recombinant product that would protect against the different *Borrelia* species difficult. Multiplicity of infecting strains also makes questionable the protection induced by whole-cell vaccines (which are now on the market in Europe containing *B. burgdorferi sensu stricto* stains), because cross-protectivity between *B. burgdorferi* species cannot be demonstrated.

The advantage of recombinant protein OspA vaccines is that they induce antibodies only to OspA, the protein that is expressed in the tick and not in the dog. Vertebrate hosts infected by *Borrelia* organisms through tick bites rarely, if ever develop antibodies to OspA. OspA is expressed by *Borrelia* in unfed ticks but is changed to OspC during transmission from the vector due to the warm conditions during feeding on the vertebrate host. During feeding, antibodies against OspA that are present in the vertebrate's blood due to vaccination enter the tick and neutralize *Borrelia* before the organism enters the host. Antibodies to OspA from the host cause an arrest of growth and salivary gland invasion in the ticks.[40] Spirochetes then are either killed instantly by antibody-induced complement lysis or their mobility is reduced such that they cannot continue their migration to the salivary glands of the ticks.[41] In the vaccinated host, only OspA antibodies are present, and these cannot bind to *Borrelia* organisms expressing OspC. Thus the risk of the development of immune complex diseases is likely to be reduced compared with whole-cell *Borrelia* vaccines.[42]

Western blot or C6 ELISA testing must be performed to distinguish vaccine induced from natural exposure antibodies in a vaccinated dog. The vaccination of an already-infected animal does not clear current infection, and thus not recommended in a dog with clinical signs. Vaccination of nonclinical Lyme-positive dogs is necessary to prevent new infections as natural immunity is limited.

LYME NEPHRITIS

There is little existing proof of cause and effect or even proof that the disease exists. The syndrome was first defined in a case report in 1988[43] and a large retrospective histopathologic study performed at the University of Pennsylvania and published in 1997.[44]

This large histopathologic study really first characterized the devastating clinical syndrome that has become known as "Lyme nephritis." This study described a common pathologic lesion noted in 49 dogs within a 6-year period. The common finding in all of the dogs was a unique renal histopathologic

lesion including immune-mediated glomerulonephritis, diffuse tubular necrosis and regeneration, and lymphocytic-plasmacytic interstitial nephritis. Approximately 50% of the samples evaluated were obtained at necropsy and 50% were from biopsies of dogs alive at the time, but that died shortly thereafter. The clinical syndrome is one of severe proteinuric glomerular disease progressing to acute renal failure and death. All affected dogs had severe uremia and hypoalbuminemia. Twenty-one dogs were shown to have immune complex glomerulonephritis with IgG, IgM, and basement membrane complement (C3) deposition. All dogs evaluated with urinalyses were proteinuric. The main connection to Lyme disease in these dogs was that 18 of 18 dogs that were tested serologically for Lyme were positive. Thirteen also had a history of a recent lameness. Affected breeds included: Labrador Retrievers: 14/49 (29%); Golden Retrievers: 10/49 (20%); and 15 other breeds. Since publication, it has been learned that *Borrelia* organisms are not present in the kidneys of dogs that are Lyme-positive and die with clinical disease and histopathologic lesions that fit with Lyme nephritis. This has been shown using extremely sensitive molecular techniques of PCR, quantitative PCR, and fluorescent *in situ* hybridization.[45,46] It has, therefore, been suggested that if this syndrome is caused by *Borrelia* infection, then immune complex disease is the most likely pathologic mechanism.[13] We have demonstrated recently (unpublished data) that there are immune complexes present in the kidneys of the dogs that have died from this syndrome and that they include anti-*Borrelia* antibodies, the first real evidence for a cause and effect relationship between Lyme disease and "Lyme nephritis."

The timeframe of progression from Lyme infection, proteinuria, azotemia, and the development of Lyme nephritis is yet unknown. It appears reasonable to assume, though, that positive Lyme serology and proteinuria precede severe clinical disease. Therefore, it is strongly recommended to screen every Lyme-positive dog (whether clinical or not) for proteinuria and every proteinuric dog in Lyme-endemic regions for Bb antibodies (see Figure 199-2). Dogs positive for both should be considered clinical and treated aggressively.[13]

BORRELIOSIS IN CATS

Cats have been found to be antibody-positive for *Borrelia*, and experimental infection has been produced, but naturally acquired disease has not been documented. Approximately 13% of cats tested in the United States had antibodies; however, there was no difference in positive results from cats with or without lameness.[1] In the United Kingdom, 4% of tested cats had antibodies.[47] Cats may be more resistant than dogs to the development of clinical signs. However, when cats were inoculated experimentally with organisms directly from arthropods, they developed multiple limb lameness and had joint, pulmonary, lymphoid, and CNS inflammation at necropsy. Arthritis and meningitis predominated.

PUBLIC HEALTH CONSIDERATIONS

There is no evidence that infected pet dogs or cats pose a direct risk to humans except by introducing unfed tick stages into a household. The ticks do not survive long indoors and, if fed, tick stages do not reattach without molting. However, partly fed ticks can refeed and can pose a greater risk of infection because of the shorter required period of attachment. Direct horizontal spread from dogs and cats to humans is unlikely. It has been speculated that urine from infected dogs could be a source of human infection. *Borrelia* organisms, however, deteriorate quickly in urine, and there is no evidence that human infections have occurred after contact with infected dogs.[48] In addition, in a recent study in the Netherlands, no positive correlation was observed between antibody prevalence in hunters compared with their dogs.[49] Although Lyme disease is classified as an indirect zoonosis, dogs, cats, and humans are incidental hosts for a sylvan cycle that exists in nature. Lyme borreliosis in humans is usually associated with outdoor activities that result in exposure to tick vectors.

REFERENCES

The reference list can be found on the companion Expert Consult Web site at *www.expertconsult.com*.

CHAPTER 200

Mycobacterial Infections in Cats and Dogs

Danièlle A. Gunn-Moore

Mycobacteria are bacteria with a high mycolic acid content in their cell wall, which gives them many of their characteristic traits. These include being acid-fast with Ziehl Neelsen (ZN) and similar stains, being environmentally resistant, and having the ability to survive and multiply within mononuclear phagocytes, thereby inducing granulomatous to pyogranulomatous host responses.[56,138]

Several species of mycobacteria can cause disease in veterinary species, being either primary pathogens, or becoming pathogenic under certain circumstances. Traditionally, mycobacteria of veterinary importance have been divided into three groups: (1) obligate primary pathogens that require a mammalian host to perpetuate their life cycle, e.g., the tuberculosis complex group, and *M. lepraemurium*, (2) saprophytes that can become facultative pathogens causing local or disseminated disease and being further divided into fast-growing and slow-growing opportunistic (or atypical) nontuberculous mycobacteria (NTM), and (3) mycobacteria that are difficult to grow so their environmental niche cannot be determined; this latter group includes the organisms responsible for some cases of feline leprosy and for canine leproid granuloma syndrome.[25,77,109]

Tuberculosis can be caused by a number of different, but closely related, bacteria. Relevant members of the tuberculosis complex group include *Mycobacterium tuberculosis*, *M. bovis* (the "bovine bacillus"), and *M. microti* (the "vole bacillus"). *M. tuberculosis* causes over 90% of tuberculosis in man, but rarely infects other mammals, except for dogs.[132] *M. bovis* is the main cause of tuberculosis in cattle, and can also cause disease in dogs and cats. *M. microti* causes tuberculosis in voles[175] and cats.[63] *M. avium* causes tuberculosis in birds, and can also infect man, dogs, and cats.[164] Although *M. avium* is a member of the *M. avium–intracellulare* complex (MAC) and a slow-growing saprophyte, it is often considered with the tuberculosis complex as it can cause clinical disease indistinguishable from that caused by members of this group.

Other mycobacteria that can be potentially pathogenic in cats and dogs include *M. lepraemurium*, which causes leprosy in rats and is one of the causes of feline leprosy[100,109,148]; and opportunistic NTM, which are usually saprophytes, but can cause disease in cats and dogs. In cats these include the fast-growing *M. chelonae-abscessus* group (containing *M. chelonae* and *M. abscessus*), the *M. fortuitum* group (containing *fortuitum* and *M. peregrinum*), the *M. smegmatis* group, *M. phlei*, *M. thermoresistible*, *M, flavescens*, *M. mucogenicum*, *M. alvei*,

and *M. septicum*, and the slow-growing *M. genavense*, *M. terrae*, *M. xenopi*, *M. malmoense*, *M. ulcerans*, *M. szulgai*, and *M. simiae*.* This type of infection is seen less commonly in dogs, but it has been seen associated with the fast-growing *M. fortuitum*, *M. chelonei*, and *M. smegmatis*, and the slow-growing *M. genavense.*†

Mycobacterial taxonomy is notoriously complex, with divisions being made relating to whether the bacteria will grow using standard mycobacterial culture techniques and, if they do grow, on their speed of growth, culture characteristics, and biochemical properties. However, with the advent of molecular techniques the true genetic relationships are now being determined and this has complicated the picture even further.[166,90] It is therefore perhaps most sensible to consider the mycobacterial infections seen in cats and dogs by way of their clinical presentations, rather than focusing entirely of the taxonomic subgrouping of the bacteria involved. Mycobacterial syndromes seen in cats and dogs therefore include (1) tuberculosis (localized or disseminated cutaneous and/or internal granulomas); (2) feline leprosy and canine leproid granuloma syndrome (localized cutaneous nodules); and (3) NTM mycobacteriosis (subcutaneous or disseminated granulomatous inflammation). Unfortunately, the differentiation and classification of feline mycobacterial infections into feline cutaneous tuberculosis, feline leprosy, and NTM infections is arbitrary at best, particularly when infection with *M. avium* is placed in the tuberculosis group, and the differentiation between feline leprosy and NTM infections is often based simply on the ability to culture the causal organism, and not on any clinical or pathologic difference. Indeed, as molecular techniques develop it is likely that the number of mycobacteria found to infect cats and dogs will increase considerably, and the classification of the diseases they cause will have to be altered.

Mycobacterial infections are rare in both cats and dogs. However, more cases are seen in cats; the majority of which present as skin lesions. These are typically seen as cutaneous nodules, draining tracts, and/or ulceration. In some cases, the disease may become generalized secondary to skin inoculation, but only occasional cases present with primary systemic

---

*References 4, 11, 29, 37, 42, 71, 77, 78, 136, 180, 181, 183, 190, 191.
†References 45, 48, 61, 62, 92, 97, 109, 169, 185.

disease. Where systemic disease is seen, infection with a member of the tuberculosis group or a MAC organism is most likely,[7,63] although occasional cases have been seen with some NTM (e.g., *M. fortuitum*, *M. thermoresistible*, *M. visibilis*, *M. simiae* or *M. xenopi*).[4,28,104,190,191] In the latter cases, infection can usually be related to percutaneous injury, contamination via soil or the presence of devitalized tissue. These factors tend to be reflected in the distribution of the lesions.

It is difficult to determine the current prevalence of mycobacterial infections in cats and dogs. Data from the Veterinary Laboratories Agency (VLA) in United Kingdom reveal that of the 337 ZN-positive feline samples they received from 2005 to 2007,[91b,124,194] *M. microti* was identified in 19%, *M. bovis* in 12%, *M. avium* in 7%, *M. malmonoense* in 1%, unclassified mycobacterium in 4%, and the samples failed to culture in 55%. A positive culture was only gained in 45% of samples in part because the culture system used by the VLA is optimized for *M. bovis*. Therefore, many of the NTM would not have been identified by this system and even with optimized systems these organisms can be exceedingly difficult to grow. Unfortunately, there is currently no way to correlate these findings to the number of cats actually developing mycobacterial infections in the United Kingdom and there generally are even less data from other countries.

TUBERCULOSIS

CLINICAL BACKGROUND

Epidemiology and Etiopathogenesis

Historically, tuberculosis used to be common in cats and dogs, with prevalence levels in necropsy studies from Europe and other countries of 1% to 13% in cats and 0.1% to 13.5% in dogs.[154] In cats, over 95% of tuberculosis was historically caused by *M. bovis*,[49,136] with only a few cases of *M. tuberculosis*,[132] and occasional cases of either *M. avium*[39,73,88,157] or *M. microti*.[63,81,172] In dogs, *M. tuberculosis* caused approximately 75% of cases, with most of the rest being due to *M. bovis*,[49,101,132] and only occasional cases of *M. avium* infection.[164] Most cases of tuberculosis in cats and dogs were believed to result from ingestion of milk from tuberculous cattle or arose secondary to living in close proximity to *M. tuberculosis*–infected people.[101,132,154] Hence, with the reduction of tuberculosis from national herds, the pasteurization of milk, and the reduction of human tuberculosis, there has been a marked decline in the prevalence of disease seen in cats and dogs.[3,64,86,132,151]

Currently, tuberculosis in cats and dogs is recognized infrequently.[64] When it is diagnosed it is usually caused by infection with either *M. bovis* or, in the case of cats, *M. microti*. Of the recent cases of tuberculosis in cats in the United Kingdom (approximately 100 cases identified in the last 3 years), 61% were caused by *M. microti* and 39% by *M. bovis* or, if you include MAC organisms then 50% were caused by *M. microti*, 32% by *M. bovis* and 18% by MAC organisms.[124,194] Infection of cats with *M. tuberculosis* is exceedingly rare,[5] probably because they are naturally resistant to this bacterium.[151] Although dogs appear to be less resistant to *M. tuberculosis* than cats, this disease is now very rare in the developed world; only five cases of tuberculosis have been confirmed by the VLA in dogs from the United Kingdom in the past 20 years; all of which were due to *M. bovis*.[3,41] There have also been a handful of published case reports, most of which involved *M. bovis*,[5,9,34,41,160,149] although one case from France was caused by *M. microti*[31] and four cases resulted from *M. tuberculosis* infection; two originating from Africa, one from Spain, and one from the United States.[5,66,133,168]

For more information on this topic, please visit the companion Expert CONSULT Web site at www.expertconsult.com.

The *current epidemiology of tuberculosis in cats* is unclear. Two main theories currently exist; (1) indirect spread from cattle and/or badgers or (2) direct spread from wild rodents and other small mammals.

Direct infection from cattle or badger as been proposed as the specific strains (spoligotypes) of *M. bovis* identified in cats in the United Kingdom are typically the same as those seen in cattle and badgers from the same geographic location.[124] In addition, some of the owners of the infected cats have commented that badgers have visited their gardens or that a badger sett was located close to their property.[124] However, close contact is typically needed for the spread of *M. bovis* infection, which is something that rarely occurs between cats and cattle or badgers. Classically, cattle infected cats via contaminated milk, so the lesions developed within their alimentary tract. Currently, few cats develop this type of lesion, with the majority developing cutaneous lesions. It has been suggested that infection could occur following heavy environmental contamination,[14] for example, where extensive endemic *M. bovis* infection is present in local cattle, badger, or other species (e.g., deer). The risk of feline infection would therefore vary in each geographic area and be dependent on the likely close interaction between infected species, their environments, and domestic cats.

In cats, cutaneous lesions are typically seen affecting the "fight and bite sights" (i.e., the face and legs), which are the areas most likely to be bitten when playing with prey. In addition, some of the risk factors that have been identified in feline tuberculosis include being keen hunters, and regularly catching small rodents.[63] Studies have shown that in the United Kingdom wild field voles (*Microtus agrestis*), bank voles (*Clethrionomys glareolus*), and wood mice (*Apodemus sylvaticus*) can all be naturally infected with *M. microti*[20] and an even wider range of wild mammals can be infected with *M. bovis* (e.g., foxes, stoats, polecats, wild ferrets, common shrews, yellow-necked mice, wood mice, field voles, grey squirrels, moles, and rats), with the infection being seen most commonly in small animals that cats like to hunt (e.g., field and bank voles, common shrews [*Sorex araneus*] and wood mice).[32,33] In addition, the *M. bovis* spoligotypes that have been identified in these wild animals are typically the same as those seen in the cattle and badgers from the same region.[33] Therefore, the author believes that the most likely mechanism by which cats become infected is by hunting small wild rodents. While few people debate the likelihood that this is the most probable method by which cats are exposed to *M. microti* infection, this is not necessarily supported by the genotypic evidence.[186] Some authors suggest that there is currently no evidence for a significant self-maintaining reservoir of *M. bovis* in small wild mammals in the United Kingdom.[32,33] That said, whether a self-sustaining reservoir is needed is debatable, as new members of these spillover species are constantly being infected with *M. bovis* from cattle and badger.

All members of the tuberculosis complex pose potential *zoonotic risks*. However, there have been no recently reported cases of cats or dogs passing tuberculosis onto humans. By far the greatest risk of tuberculosis to humans is spending time with infected humans or, less frequently, handling infected cattle. *M. tuberculosis* and *M. bovis* can both cause *reverse zoonoses* and there have been a small number of cases where humans have infected their cats and dogs with *M. bovis*[43,69,132,149] or *M. tuberculosis*.[43,66] Dogs and cats are spillover hosts and as such are believed to present a low risk of further dissemination, either to humans or other animals.[49]

For more information on this topic, please visit the companion Expert CONSULT Web site at www.expertconsult.com.

Predisposition

Many cases of feline and canine tuberculosis may be subclinical in nature.[155] Infection usually occurs after protracted exposure (e.g., repeated exposure to infected small mammals, living on a farm housing tuberculous cattle, or living for prolonged periods with infected humans or poultry). Tuberculosis is therefore seen mainly in adult animals,[86] although younger animals may develop disease if exposed to very high levels of infection[83] or when MAC organisms are involved.[74,129] No gender predisposition is seen in dogs, but male cats appear to be overrepresented.[63] Little evidence of immunosuppression has been found and most cats tested for feline immunodeficiency virus (FIV) and feline leukemia virus (FeLV) have been negative.[63,15,7] However, MAC infections have been seen in a number of immunosuppressed cats, including occasional cases of FeLV infection,[99] concurrent toxoplasmosis,[15] or the administration of immunosuppressive drugs following renal transplantation.[60] Dogs are believed to be more susceptible to *M. tuberculosis* and *M. bovis* than cats, but relatively resistant to MAC infections.[70] Certain breeds appear to be predisposed to infection with MAC organisms, including Siamese[39,73,88] and Abyssinian breeds of cat,[7,150] and Bassett and Miniature Schnauzer breeds of dogs.[8,19,40,67,122,174] While the nature of this predisposition is unknown, similar inherited predispositions in humans have been found to result from defective interferon-gamma (IFN-γ)–mediated immunity.[2,140]

Clinical Signs

Depending on the route of infection, affected cats and dogs may present with systemic signs related to the alimentary and/or respiratory tracts or with localized disease affecting the skin (which may later develop pulmonary involvement).[86,151] Historically, cats most commonly developed alimentary lesions (secondary to being infected by drinking tuberculous milk) while dogs developed pulmonary lesions (secondary to inhaling infected droplets of their owner's sputum); in dogs the initial pulmonary lesions then tended to spread so the animals typically died with widely disseminated disease.[49,86] Currently, there are really too few cases in dogs to comment; but most appear to present with pulmonary and/or alimentary signs.[3,9,31,34,41,168] However, the most usual presentation for tuberculosis in cats is now the cutaneous form, with respiratory and alimentary forms being seen less frequently.[64] In cats, the primary complex is often incomplete, especially when the infection gains entry via the mouth or intestines (i.e., granuloma form in the local lymph nodes), but there are no obvious lesions at the site of entry.[30,63,154]

In the cutaneous form, which is particularly common in cats, the lesions probably arise from infected bite wounds, local spread, or hematogenous dissemination to the skin.[64,86,151] The lesions often involve the face, extremities, tail base, or perineum (i.e., "fight and bite sites"). Less frequently they involve the ventral thorax. They generally take the form of firm, raised, dermal nodules; ulceration may be present, as may nonhealing wounds with draining sinus tracts.[63,136,154] Extension of granulomatous tissue may in some cases involve the subcutaneous structures, muscle, and/or bone. Skin lesions are commonly associated with either local or generalized lymphadenopathy. On occasion, submandibular or prescapular lymphadenopathy may be the only clinical finding.[16,64,87,136,151]

When the infection spreads to the lungs from other sites, or where it is acquired through inhalation, tubercles arise in the lungs and/or hilar lymph nodes and affected animals present with weight loss, anorexia, dyspnea, and cough. In cats the cough may only be soft and wheezy, and it may be accompanied by sneezing and a nasal discharge.[81,86,136,154,172] Very occasional cases may develop large tubercles that cavitate and can then break down to communicate with the pleural cavity or bronchii.[86] In comparison, typical changes include more generalized small focal lesions.[63] Occasional cases may also develop pneumothorax and/or pleurisy with the accumulation of pleural fluid, and pericardial effusions have also been seen.[136,154] Pulmonary cases in dogs have occasionally presented with hypertrophic pulmonary osteoarthropathy.[154]

In the alimentary form, tubercles arise in the intestines and/or mesenteric lymph nodes. Affected animals commonly develop intestinal malabsorption and present with weight loss, anemia, vomiting, and diarrhea. Occasionally tubercles arise in the tonsils, resulting in signs of oropharyngeal disease.

A range of clinical signs may be seen with disseminated disease. These include splenomegaly, hepatomegaly, generalized lymphadenopathy, weight loss, and fever.[101] Lameness may result from bone involvement.[63,87] Ocular involvement can result in granulomatous uveitis, retinal detachment, and even signs referable to central nervous system involvement.[46] Mycobacterial conjunctivitis may be seen on its own[63] or associated with more generalized changes including lymph node and pulmonary involvement.[54]

MAC Infections In cats, MAC has been associated with cutaneous lesions,[77,123,156,157] otitis externa with peripheral vestibular disease,[91] generalized lymph node and pulmonary involvement,[54] pulmonary and gastrointestinal disease,[7,73,150] intracranial-space occupying granuloma,[15] and disseminated tuberculosis.[6,39,60,63,88,125] Disease caused by MAC appears to be more likely to cause systemic disease than *M. bovis* or *M. microti*.[39,88]

In dogs, MAC has most commonly been reported to cause disseminated tuberculosis, typically involving the lymph nodes, liver, spleen, and intestines, presenting with chronic lethargy, vomiting, diarrhea, lameness, and eventual collapse.* Occasional cases have presented with ataxia and hindlimb weakness due to myelitis.[93]

DIAGNOSTIC TECHNIQUES

Nonspecific Tests

A thorough evaluation of the patient is necessary to assess the extent of local infection and the degree of systemic involvement. Changes in serum biochemistry and hematology, if present, are nonspecific and vary with the severity of the disease. However, hypercalcemia has been seen in a number of cats and dogs and appears to correlate with a poorer prognosis.[7,41] It is believed to result from vitamin D activation within macrophages within the granulomatous response, and is also dependant on underlying vitamin D status and calcium intake.[21,114] Radiography can be useful in the appraisal of lung involvement. However, changes are very variable and include tracheobronchial lymphadenopathy, interstitial or miliary lung infiltration, localized lung consolidation, or pleural effusion. Abdominal radiography and ultrasound examination may reveal hepatomegaly or splenomegaly, abdominal masses, mineralized mesenteric lymph nodes, or ascites. Bone lesions tend to consist of areas of bony lysis and sclerosis, osteoarthritis, discospondylitis or periostitis.

Specific Tests

The recently developed interferon-gamma test is showing promise for detecting members of the tuberculosis complex

*References 8, 10, 19, 40, 50, 55, 67, 74, 122, 127, 130, 174, 187.

in cats and is available from the VLA, United Kingdom.[141,142] Other specific tests for the diagnosis of tuberculosis have been investigated, but have generally proved unhelpful in cats and dogs (e.g., serum antibody responses).[89,154] Unlike other species, cats do not react strongly to intradermally administered tuberculin, and the results from intradermal skin testing are unreliable.[69,89,155] Even in dogs, false positives and false negative can occur.[59]

To confirm mycobacterial involvement, aspirates and/or biopsy samples of affected tissue should be stained with ZN stain or another similar special stain. The number of acid-fast bacilli seen within affected macrophages may vary, depending on the species of mycobacteria involved, the location of the granuloma and, probably most importantly, the nature of the host immune response. Large numbers of bacteria, particularly when seen within enlarged macrophages or giant cells, are most likely due to MAC infection* (or consider the lepromatous form of feline leprosy[109]). While finding acid-fast bacilli confirms the presence of mycobacteria, it is important to culture the organism to determine the exact species involved. See reference Greene and Gunn-Moore[59] for a review of culture methods. Once the species has been identified, it is possible to evaluate zoonotic risk, potential sources of infection, and feasible treatment options. Unfortunately, many samples that are seen to have ZN-positive organisms fail to culture, and even those that do often take 2 to 3 months to grow.

Molecular PCR techniques are now available, and can be very useful,[5,94,113,188] especially where tissue for culture is not possible or available; however, they are expensive, and have limited availability. PCR can even be used to identify bacilli within tissue aspirates or buffy-coat preparations.[127]

Correct Handling of Biopsy Material

In practice, this usually involves taking a biopsy from a case where mycobacterial disease is only one of a large number of possible differential diagnoses. If in-house facilities are available for ZN staining, this can be performed on aspirates or biopsy impression smears. However, in most cases biopsy material must be sent to a veterinary diagnostic laboratory. It is practical to collect the biopsy, cut it into three pieces, fix one in formalin for histopathologic examination and ZN staining, and, pending results, place one in a sterile container and freeze it. Where other bacterial infections are suspected, the third sample should be sent unfixed for routine bacterial culture, at which time ZN staining can also be requested. This way, if the sample is found to have ZN-positive organisms, the frozen portion can be defrosted and (in the United Kingdom) sent to the VLA (and/or to one of the Mycobacterial Reference Laboratories) for specialist culture.

Until the organism has been properly characterized, it should be considered a potential human pathogen.

Whenever handling potentially tuberculous material it is necessary to take certain precautions. In the United Kingdom, the law dealing with material *known* to be tuberculous is very exact and requires the use of specialist laboratories. However, the law relating to material taken from animals where tuberculosis is only one of a number of possible differentials is less stringent. In the latter case routine aseptic practices are generally adequate, although gloves should be worn when handling either the biopsy site or the biopsy material.

Under the Tuberculosis Orders currently in force in England, Wales, and Scotland, the identification of *M. bovis* in clinical or pathologic samples taken from any mammal (except humans) is notifiable to the VLA. This, of course, includes domestic cats and dogs. The same Orders impose a duty on any veterinary surgeon who suspects tuberculosis in a domestic pet to immediately notify the Divisional Veterinary Manager at the local office of the State Veterinary Service. When a confirmed case is euthanized, it is advisable to have the body cremated. (For DEFRA Guidance Notes on Tuberculosis in cats, go to: CatsTBbriefing (VIPER23 App Y5)_March 08 update.doc.)

Gross and Histopathology

The gross lesions vary from large solid tumorlike masses to multiple small, disseminated masses. They are typically grayish white, sometimes with hemorrhagic edges and/or a soft, purulent centre. Pulmonary lesions are often grayish red and may be associated with serosanguineous pleural fluid. Renal lesions typically occur in the cortex, in the form of infarcts, while intestinal lesions are typically ulcerated Peyer's patches with small submucosal tubercles.[86]

Histopathology of affected tissue generally reveals granulomatous inflammation, with foamy macrophages containing variable numbers of acid-fast bacilli, and bacilli may also be seen outside degenerating macrophages that border necrotic areas.[94,154] Lymphocytes may be numerous, and fibroblasts may be present, but multinucleate giant cells are rare or absent.[41,89,154] Necrosis and calcification may occur, particularly in larger tubercles, which may be surrounded by zones of histiocytic cells, and a well-defined fibrous capsule may develop.[89,154] Histopathology in MAC infections typically includes epithelioid macrophages containing acid-fast bacilli and degenerate neutrophils.[91,94] Tuberculosis (whether due to tubercle group bacilli or MAC organisms) results only in tuberculous lesions,[94] while feline leprosy can generate either tuberculous or lepromatous lesions (see later).

MANAGEMENT

Interim Management

Deciding to treat a case of suspected tuberculosis in a cat or dog is always contentious. However, if an infected animal is not to be treated then it must be euthanized. Before undertaking treatment it is important to address a number of points:

- *Consider the potential zoonotic risk.* All members of the affected animal's household must be involved in any decision making. Particular consideration should be given to those individuals most susceptible to the infection (e.g., household members with HIV infection or those undergoing chemotherapy or organ transplantation). We strongly advise against treatment where such individuals may be exposed to an infected animal. We also advise against treatment if the affected animal has generalized disease, respiratory tract involvement, or extensive draining cutaneous lesions, as any of these findings may increase the risk of transmission.

- Where the animal is a suitable candidate, it should be emphasized that treatment is long term and difficult to maintain given patient noncompliance, the inherent toxicity of some of the drugs, and the financial costs involved. In some cases the drugs may at best suppress the disease and indefinite treatment may be required. Uncomplicated cutaneous disease appears to carry the most favorable prognosis. Whenever undertaking treatment, the clinician should wear gloves when handling the animal.

- Tailoring treatment is difficult as sensitivity testing does not always correlate with in vivo results.

- Surgical excision of small cutaneous lesions may be considered, but is successful in only a few cases.

---

*References 60, 88, 91, 122, 123, 130.

Debulking larger lesions risks wound dehiscence and local recurrence of infection.

Pending a definitive diagnosis, interim therapy with a fluoroquinolone has previously been recommended. However, this should only be considered in cases of localized cutaneous infection. It is more sensible to recommend that double or triple therapy be initiated (Table 200-1). This not only gives the best chance of clinical resolution, but also decreases the potential for the mycobacteria to develop resistance to the fluoroquinolone. Mycobacteria in general, and the tubercle group and MAC in particular, have a high propensity to develop antibiotic-resistant mutations, particularly to the fluoroquinolones.[115] This is an important consideration since generating drug resistance will be detrimental not only to the individual animal, but may also endanger human patients.

Before deciding on continued treatment it is ideal to know exactly which form of mycobacteria is responsible. This is because it is strongly inadvisable to continue treating a cat when it is confirmed to have *M. tuberculosis* or disseminated *M. bovis*. Unfortunately, it is often 2 to 3 months before these culture results are known. In addition, in many cases the organisms do not culture even though ZN-positive organisms have been seen on cytology or histopathology. Because of this

is it essential to counsel owners very carefully, making them aware of all of the potential risks and complications.

Treatment of Choice

Ideally, antituberculosis treatment should consist of an *initial* and a *continuation* phase. The initial phase usually requires at least three drugs and lasts for 2 months, while the continuation phase requires two drugs and lasts for perhaps a further 4 months, depending on the type and extent of the disease. In those animals where triple therapy is not feasible, treatment should still involve at least two drugs and should be given for a minimum of 6 to 9 months.[64]

Traditionally, the rifampicin-isoniazid-ethambutol combination has been considered the most effective regimen for the treatment of tuberculosis in animals. However, some newer and less toxic drugs are worth considering. The fluoroquinolones (e.g., marbofloxacin) have potential in the treatment of tuberculosis, as well as some NTM mycobacteriosis. However, they are often ineffective against MAC infection,[122] except possibly when some of the newer preparations are used (e.g., moxifloxacin).[7] Clarithromycin is a modern macrolide that is used in the treatment of human tuberculosis; it appears to be effective in animals with mycobacterial infection, especially

Table • 200-1

Potentially Useful Drugs for the Treatment of Feline and Canine Mycobacterial Disease

USES	DRUG	DOSE (mg/kg)	INTERVAL (hr)	TOXICITY[12,53,65,91,150]
Prophylaxis for TB in the dog	Isoniazid	10 per os	24	Side effects as shown later in the table
1st line tx for TB and NTM*	Marbofloxacin[†]	2 per os	24	
1st line tx for TB	Rifampicin[‡]	10-15 per os	24	Hepatotoxicity, induction of liver enzymes, discoloration of body fluids, generalized erythema and pruritis
1st line tx for TB, leprosy, NTM	Clarithromycin[‡,§]	5-15 per os (occ. 125/cat)	12	Pinnal or generalised erythema? Hepatotoxicity?
	Azithromycin	5-15 per os	24	GI signs
2nd line tx for TB	Isoniazid[‡]	10-20 per os	24	Hepatotoxicity, peripheral neuritis, seizures, acute renal failure
2nd line tx for TB	Dihydrostreptomycin[‡]	15 IM	24	Ototoxicity
2nd line tx for TB[∥]	Pyrazinamide[‡]	15-40 per os	24	Hepatotoxicity, GI signs
2nd line tx for TB	Ethambutol[‡]	10-25 per os	24	Optic neuritis
Tx for leprosy, NTM, MAC	Clofazamine[‡,¶]	4-8 (occ. ~10) per os	24	Hepatotoxicity, GI signs, discoloration of body fluids, photosensitization
2nd line tx for NTM, MAC	Doxycycline	5-10 per os	12	GI signs
	Amikacin	10-15 IV IM SC	24	Nephrotoxic, ototoxic
	Cefoxitin	20-40 IV IM SC	6-8	Pain on injection IM SC

GI, Gastrointestinal; *IM,* intramuscularly; *IV,* intravenously; *MAC, Mycobacterium avium–intracellulare* complex; *NTM,* nontuberculous mycobacteria; *SC,* subcutaneously; *TB,* tuberculosis; *tx,* treatment.
*Not effective against MAC infection.
[†]The author recommends using a fluoroquinolone that is not enrofloxacin as the latter has been associated with retinal degeneration.[53]
[‡]These drugs are not licensed for use in pets.
§Particularly useful when treating MAC infections.
[∥]Not effective against *M. bovis* infection.
¶Can be difficult to obtain. Second-line treatments for tuberculosis should be reserved for resistant infections only. Drugs licensed for human use can be obtained by veterinary prescription from larger chemists.

when given in combination with rifampicin and/or another antibiotic as per culture (e.g., doxycycline). A potentially useful once-daily alternative to clarithromycin is azithromycin, although it may not be as effective, particularly with MAC infections.[7] From clinical experience gained over the past 15 years, the author recommends treatment consisting of an initial phase of rifampicin-fluoroquinolone and clarithromycin or azithromycin, followed by a continuation phase of rifampicin and either fluoroquinolone or clarithromycin or azithromycin[63] (see Table 200-1). For ease of administration all three once-daily medications can be given as liquids and placed in a single syringe prior to oral administration, or given as tablets with all three being given together after being placed in a single gelatin capsule. Alternately, where oral medication proves too difficult, an esophagostomy tube may be placed (through which the liquid medications can be given) and left in place for the duration of the treatment.

MAC infection in both cats and dogs has a poor response to treatment.[88,122] It is currently unclear whether this results from natural resistance within the bacteria, or reflects the typically severe and disseminated nature of these infections.[55,74] Local cutaneous lesions may be amenable to surgery,[91,157] and the best results have been seen with combinations of clarithromycin with either clofazimine or rifampicin as first-line treatment; with doxycycline as a second-line drug.[7,91,150]

In cases of tuberculosis where resistance develops, the rifampicin-isoniazid-ethambutol combination may be considered. If necessary, ethambutol can be substituted with dihydrostreptomycin or pyrazinamide. However, where *M. bovis* has been confirmed, pyrazinamide is not recommended due to the organism's natural resistance to this drug. Rifampicin and isoniazid are more effective and less toxic than ethambutol and dihydrostreptomycin and consequently are more appropriate choices if only two drugs are required.

Prognosis

The prognosis depends on the type of mycobacteria involved, and the extent and severity of the infection. While many cases, especially those caused by *M. microti*, have responded favorably to treatment and have achieved apparent cure or long-term remission, the prognosis should always be stated as guarded.

FELINE LEPROSY

CLINICAL BACKGROUND

Epidemiology and Etiopathogenesis

Historically, the term *feline leprosy* is used to refer to a mycobacterial infection of cats that is seen as single or multiple granulomas within the skin or subcutaneous tissue, where the associated acid-fast bacilli could not be cultured using traditional techniques.[109,136] Because the causal organisms could not be cultured, infection with *M. lepraemurium* was largely assumed.[148] However, recent reports from Australia show that feline leprosy can take one of two different forms and that, while disease in younger cats appears to be caused by *M. lepraemurium*, the disease in older cats may be caused by a novel but as yet undefined mycobacterial species.[25,77,109] As molecular techniques have become more available (particularly PCR and sequencing of the 16S rRNA gene), a number of other Mycobacteria have also been found to cause this condition.[11] They include *M. szulgai*, *M. kansaii*, *M. malmoense*, *M. visibilis*, and *Mycobacterium* sp. strain Tarwin.[4,29,52,77] This makes differentiation of feline leprosy from cutaneous NTM infection rather difficult. Many cases that present clinically as feline leprosy are then reclassified as NTM once the

causal organism has been cultured[77] (see section on clinical signs in NTM). This is probably inappropriate, and it would make more sense to classify all cases of single or multiple cutaneous or subcutaneous granulomas as feline leprosy, regardless of whether the species of mycobacteria can be identified (either by culture or molecular diagnostics).

Feline leprosy is believed to arise following the introduction of organisms through bite wounds from rodents.[52,148] However, this has not been proven and it is also possible that infection may be gained via soil contamination of cutaneous wounds. Interestingly, most cases are presented in winter.[118,148,163] While there is no known zoonotic potential, ongoing advances in molecular diagnostics may demonstrate that some of these infections may be capable of infecting humans.

Predisposition

There are no breed or gender predispositions, but adult cats are more commonly affected. Although some authors report that the disease is seen more frequently in young adults,* it can also be seen in older cats.[52,109] The prevalence of feline leprosy appears to be higher in areas with a temperate maritime climate, e.g., Australia and New Zealand,[17,163] Europe (United Kingdom, the Channel Islands, France, The Netherlands, the Greek island of Kythira),[17,25,137,143,179] western Canada,[118,147] and western parts of the United States (California, Oregon).[51,116,154] Concurrent infection with FeLV or FIV is not a consistent feature of the infection, but some of the older cats in Australia have been FIV positive.[109,111,144]

Clinical Signs

Feline leprosy is primarily a cutaneous syndrome. It consists of single or multiple granulomatous nodules, which may be haired, alopecic, or ulcerated, and may be seen on the head, limbs, and occasionally the trunk.[109,118,163,179] Rare cases have affected the tongue, lips, or nasal planum.[105,108,109] The masses are nonpainful and freely mobile.[109,163] Nasal granulomata have also been seen,[148] and cats have developed keratitis or conjunctivitis.[52] Regional lymphadenopathy may be present,[†] but systemic disease is rare, and may be seen as disseminated granulomatous disease of the liver, spleen, and lungs.[109] In Australia this disease appears to have two different forms: one type affects young cats, which initially develop localized nodular, often ulcerated, lesions on the limbs, which progress rapidly, while the other type affects older cats, which develop more generalized skin involvement with no ulceration and a slower clinical progression.[109]

DIAGNOSTIC TECHNIQUES

Cytology and histopathology (with the use of ZN and Fite's stains) are the major methods of diagnosis.[148] Both lepromatous and tuberculous forms are reported,[118] and a paper from Australia clarified this further, describing the lesions in young cats as more typically tuberculous in nature (with few acid-fast organisms), while the lesions in older cats were more lepromatous (often containing large numbers of acid-fast organisms within distended macrophages).[109,148] That said, many young cats have also been shown to have lesions containing large numbers of acid-fast organisms.[116,143,163,179] Although the difference between the tuberculous and lepromatous forms may result from the nature of the species of mycobacteria involved, the age and immune status of the animal, and the position of the lesion,[148,163] it is the role of the

---

*References 25, 51, 143, 118, 163, 179.
†References 1, 38, 51, 109, 116, 118, 137, 143, 163.

host's immune response that is believed to be most important. Animals with a weak immune response typically develop the lepromatous form. This is seen as many acid-fast bacilli within macrophages or dermal vacuoles, while the dermis, panniculus, and subcutis contain nodular to diffuse infiltrates of epithelioid macrophages.[62,105] The tuberculous form is typically seen in immunocompetent individuals where there is limited multiplication of the bacteria. In this form of the disease histiocytic cells are present, along with moderate numbers of lymphocytes and plasma cells.[62,105] Cytology with routine Romanowsky staining can be particularly useful in cases of lepromatous change as it may reveal numerous macrophages and giant cell–containing unstained rodlike structures (the unstained mycobacteria).[109]

Culture is usually unrewarding, but should be performed in all suspected cases as the clinical signs, and histopathology of feline leprosy can mimic those of feline tuberculosis or NTM infections. Molecular PCR techniques are currently being investigated and show promise.[52,77,109,111] The full diagnostic approach, as discussed previously for tuberculosis, should be followed.

MANAGEMENT

Interim Management
The minimum of a fluoroquinolone (see Table 200-1) should be used pending diagnosis.

Treatment of Choice
Surgical removal of small nodules is recommended.[98,109] Clofazimine, clarithromycin, rifampin, and even doxycycline, fluoroquinolones, and aminoglycosides may be useful (see Table 200-1), especially where surgical removal was difficult.[25,109,117] When using medical therapy, it can be beneficial to use two or three of the drugs, for example, clarithromycin and rifampin.[109,111] Treatment is usually given for several months and continued for perhaps 2 months beyond apparent clinical resolution.[111] Dapsone is considered too toxic for use in cats.[68]

Prognosis
The prognosis is variable, from good to slowly progressive,[111] and while instances of spontaneous resolution may occur,[144] they are not seen with all forms of this disease.[52]

CANINE LEPROID GRANULOMA SYNDROME (CANINE LEPROSY)

Epidemiology and Etiopathogenesis
Canine leproid granuloma syndrome (CLGS) is similar to feline leprosy, with affected dogs developing granulomas of the skin and subcutis, which contain variable numbers of acid-fast bacilli that generally do not grow using standard myco-

bacterial culture methods. The condition was first described in a Boxer dog and a Bullmastiff from Zimbabwe in 1973,[152] and since then has been described in Australia, New Zealand, and Brazil, and in California, Florida, New York, and Georgia in the United States.*

Predisposition
There appears to be no age or gender predisposition, but short-coated breeds appear to be at a greater risk of developing the disease, especially Boxer and Boxer-cross dogs. It has been suggested that biting flies or some other biting arthropod may be inoculating the mycobacteria.[45,109,152]

Clinical Signs
The skin lesions present as single or multiple well-circumscribed painless nodules. They can appear anywhere on the body, but are seen most typically on the ear flaps and head. The disease does not involve regional lymph nodes, nerves, or internal organs.[45,107,108]

Diagnosis
With Romanowsky stains cytology typically reveals few to moderate numbers of nonstaining bacilli within macrophages.[22] On histopathology the number of acid-fast bacilli is highly variable and they are typically seen within macrophages and giant cells.[22,45] Neither local lymph node involvement nor more generalized disease has been seen.[109,112] Molecular techniques have identified a fastidious, slow-growing mycobacteria related to *M. simiae*.[79] Interestingly, this organism is closely related to *Mycobacterium* sp. strain Tarwin, which is one of the mycobacterial species that has been found to cause some cases of feline leprosy.[29,52]

Treatment and Prognosis
Spontaneous remissions are common, with or without surgical intervention,[45,107] typically occurring within 1 to 3 months of the lesions first appearing.[112] However, occasional cases develop chronic disfiguring lesions that may persist indefinitely.[112] When considering medical therapy, a combination of rifampin and clarithromycin and/or doxycycline has been recommended, to be continued until after the lesions have resolved completely.[112]

For more information on this topic, please visit the companion Expert CONSULT Web site at www.expertconsult.com.

REFERENCES

The reference list can be found on the companion Expert Consult Web site at *www.expertconsult.com*.

---

*References 45, 79, 107, 108, 109, 152.

CHAPTER 201

Brucellosis

R. Bruce Hollett

ETIOLOGY

Four of the six species of *Brucella* (*B. canis, abortus, melitensis,* and *suis,* excluding *ovis* and *neotomae*) can infect dogs. The first canine case of *Brucella suis* infection was reported in 1931.[1] Exposure to *B. abortus* occurs by ingestion of aborted or fetal tissue from diseased livestock.[2] *B. canis* is a small, rough or mucoid, gram-negative intracellular bacterium with similar antigenic properties to *B. ovis.* Abortions were reported in 1963, and *B. canis* has been isolated from canine tissue and vaginal discharges since 1966-1967.[2a-4]

PATHOGENESIS

The Canidae family are reservoir hosts. Historically, infection was associated in the mid- 1970s with the Beagle breed[3,5,6] because of its popularity in research and field trials. The list has expanded to include large, small, and mixed-breed dogs (e.g., Golden Retrievers, Cocker Spaniels, Boston and Yorkshire Terriers, Poodles, Lhasa Apso, and Miniature Pinschers). Any sexually mature, reproductively active dog is susceptible whether purebred or not.[7,8] Stray and feral dogs remain prominent reservoirs.[9-13]

Worldwide *B. canis* infections have been reported in Central and South America,[10] Europe[14] Asia,[6,15] South Africa,[15a] and North America[16-21b,23] with a particular prevalence for the rural southeastern United States.[22-25] Stray dogs in Tennessee demonstrated a greater than threefold rate of infection versus nonstray dogs.[22,23] The disease appears in wild dog packs, new untested animals, kennels, "puppy mills," and even backyard mistakes. The bacteria attach to exposed mucous membranes (e.g., oral, conjunctival, nasal, vaginal, preputial) then penetrate that tissue (Figures 201-1 and 201-2).

More bacteria attach, phagocytosis continues, and virulence increases. The organisms embed in circulating macrophages, travel to regional lymph nodes, and produce generalized lymph node enlargement from diffuse lymphoid and reticuloendothelial cell hyperplasia. They replicate and bacteremia begins within 7 to 30 days. The size of the spleen increases from the typical granulomatous reaction from *Brucella* organisms. Intracellular *B. canis* target steroid-dependent tissues. In males, the prostate, testicle, and epididymides produce a continuous or recurrent release of bacteria in venereal secretions for months to years. These organs serve as effective sites for widespread dissemination to males if actively breeding. Lymphocytic infiltration and cellular damage from inflamed epididymides can induce a sperm granuloma from leakage of antigenic material into the surrounding tunics of the formerly immune privileged blood-testis barrier. Antisperm and not *B. canis* antibodies result from humoral and cellular immune responses. Urine becomes a contaminated vehicle by the close anatomic connection of the bladder to the secretory prostate and epididymis. Prostatic fluid moves cranially into the bladder by normal urethral pressure.[25a] A shedding stud dog can affect male kennelmates by being housed in tight quarters for an extended time.[26-29]

In the female, the gravid uterus, fetus, and placenta are targeted. Bacteria are found in fetal stomach contents, suggesting that a fetus may swallow infected amniotic fluid in utero.[28] An aborting bitch is of high risk for the spread within any environment. The aborted placenta has focal coagulative necrosis of the chorionic villi, necrotizing arteritis, and numerous bacteria in trophoblastic epithelial cells. Aborted tissue and fluids contain millions of organisms equivalent to 500 oral infective doses per mL.[28] Infected vaginal discharges can persist for 4 to 6 weeks or longer postwhelping. *B. canis* can be found in the milk of infected lactating bitches who are nursing pups. Blood transfusions, vaginoscopy, artificial insemination, and contaminated syringes provide artificial means of transmission.

The blood-borne bacteremia can infect intervertebral disks, the kidney, and anterior uvea of the eye.[30-32] Time from initial exposure to bacteremia is 3 weeks. Asymptomatic hosts harbor the organisms for prolonged periods. In the first 3 to 4 months of infection, bacteremia may decline but titers[2] indicate persistent bacteria sequestered in organs or targeted gonads. Blood cultures in experimentally infected dogs remained positive for more than 5 years.[33] Negative blood cultures correlate with decreased serum agglutination titer even in some cases where *B. canis* persists in body tissue.

Spontaneous recovery was reported from 1 to 5 years after an initial infection. Dogs become abacteremic with agglutination titers as low as 1:25 or 1:50,[28] suggesting clearance of the bacteria. Titers did not rise again if challenged, and no reinfection occurs because of developed cellular immunity from this natural recovery.

CLINICAL SIGNS

Despite an ongoing systemic infection, clinical signs can range from none, to mild, to severe reproductive dysfunction. Subtle signs may include a poor hair coat, listlessness, fatigue, lethargy, exercise intolerance, weight loss, lameness, back pain, lymphadenopathy, splenomegaly, or behavioral changes (e.g., not alert or poor performance of trained tasks). No clinical sign is pathognomonic for canine brucellosis, but the disease should always be given primary consideration in dogs examined for reproductive failure or infertility. Infected dogs are not seriously ill. Morbidity is high, but mortality low since death is not directly caused by the inflammatory cellular response. Fever is uncommon because this bacterium lacks the lipopolysaccharides found in other *Brucella* strains that produce endotoxins.[28,34] The bacteria has little somatic antigen and, therefore, eludes the immune system.

Clinical signs in the bitch include infertility, apparent failure to conceive, early embryonic death (EED), fetal resorption, or failure to whelp. Late-term abortion may be witnessed by the owner of a supposedly healthy pregnant bitch. Embryonic loss occurs within the early weeks (20 days) after breeding. The female may be deemed infertile since no outward signs of fetal death were seen. Abortion usually occurs between 45 (mid) to 59 days (late) gestation, or the pregnancy is carried nearly to term. Brucellosis does not change the exhibition of estrus[35] and therefore possible breeding. An infected bitch can abort two to three litters in succession, continue to be bred and yet have a normal litter later,[36] giving birth to living, partly autolyzed, stillborn, or normal pups.

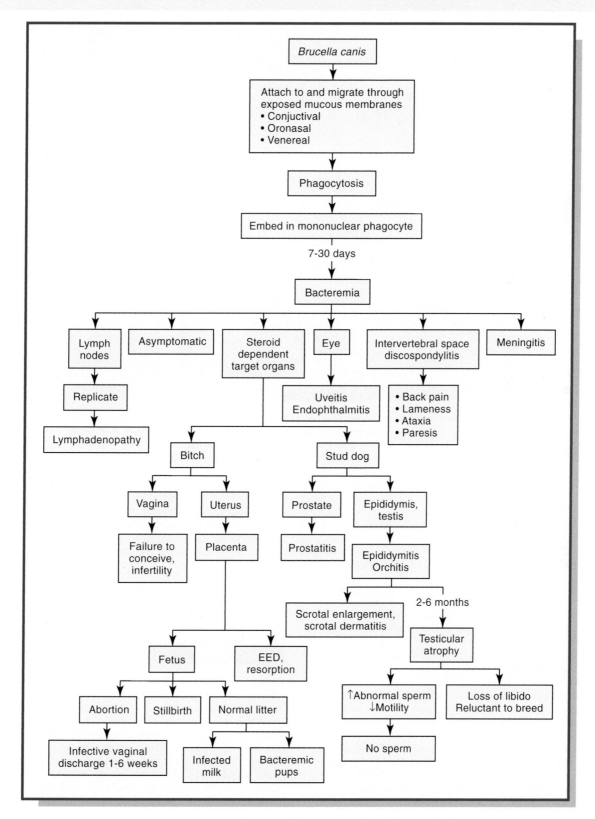

Figure 201-1 Brucellosis paradigm. *EED,* Early embryonic death.

Some pups die within hours of birth. Surviving pups are usually bacteremic for a minimum of several months. Following an abortion, a highly ineffective, viscous, serosanguineous vaginal discharge may persist for 1 to 6 weeks.

B. canis targets androgen-dependent organs in the male (i.e., epididymis, prostate). An intact infected stud dog may exhibit epididymitis, orchitis, a painful scrotal enlargement,

preputial discharge, or testicular atrophy. Such dogs may also have moist scrotal dermatitis, a decreased volume of ejaculate, loss of libido, reluctance to breed, or poor semen quality with WBCs and a high percentage of abnormal sperm. All these problems are most evident if the dog is examined within the first 3 months of infection.[37] Acute onset of inflammation with associated pain and swelling produces the orchitis or

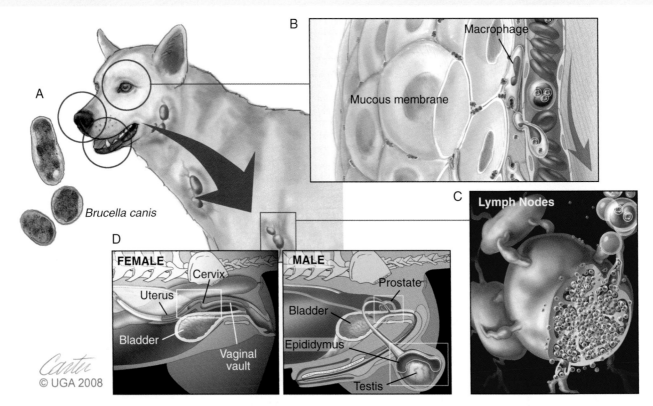

Figure 201-2 **A,** *Brucella canis* enter the dog's body through ingestion, licking, breeding, or contact with exposed mucous membranes of the eye, mouth, nose, vagina, and penis. **B,** *Brucella canis* attach to the exposed mucous membranes, are engulfed by mononuclear phagocytes, and enter the lymphatic drainage to later gain access to the dog's bloodstream. **C,** The bacteria become sequestered in the nearest regional lymph nodes, where replication causes enlargement or lymphadenopathy for subsequent seeding of steroid-dependent tissues, vertebrae, and eyes. **D,** *Brucella canis* inflame the female and male reproductive organs, respectively. These intracellular organisms inhabit the vaginal vault and uterus, which promotes spread by coital contact during natural breeding, early embryonic death, abortion and stillbirth, or whelping of bacteremic pups. Inflammation of the epididymis, testis, and prostate provide bacterial shedding in semen, altered spermatogenesis, increased abnormal sperm morphology, testicular degeneration, and atrophy with eventual infertility of male and female dogs.

epididymitis.[1,38-40] Scrotal dermatitis develops from the constant licking by the male seeking relief.[38] Early inflammation stops spermatogenesis in the seminiferous tubules from which some dogs recover fertility while others become sterile. Prolonged infection leads to unilateral or bilateral testicular atrophy along with a reluctance to breed and/or loss of libido from the painful experience. An infected stud dog may fail to achieve intromission from pain, may have an unwillingness to ejaculate, or may even have successful internal ties without a resulting pregnancy. Semen collection detects teratozoospermia (high percentage of abnormal sperm morphology), oligozoospermia (low sperm number), or azoospermia (no sperm) in the ejaculate. After 3 months, *B. canis* can usually be grown from the semen of infected dogs. Within 5 months, a majority of abnormal sperm may appear with head-to-head spermagglutination that follows serum antibodies in the seminal plasma. Some males have an absence of sperm.[41,42] Either gender may develop discospondylitis, uveitis, or meningoencephalitis. Discospondylitis of the thoracic and/or lumbar vertebrae is identified on radiographic survey films.[43-46] Stiffness, lameness, or paraspinal pain with paresis or paralysis has been reported and may occasionally be linked to a previously treated orchitis[44] or osteomyelitis subsequent to a total hip replacement.[47] Ophthalmologic exams discover endophthalmitis and recurrent uveitis from immune complex deposits,[30,31] even in spayed females,[32] and are confirmed by culture or serology. A low-grade, nonsuppurative meningitis has been reported. A spayed female with a chronic vaginal discharge

had a positive serum titer and a positive blood culture after having an abscessed uterine stump surgically removed 3 years following a hysterectomy.[48]

DIAGNOSIS

Presumptive diagnosis is suggested from the variety of clinical signs. Serologic agglutination testing, serologic titer, and hemoculture support the definitive diagnosis, but the fluctuant level and duration of bacteremia makes the diagnosis difficult.[4] One negative blood culture does not eliminate *B. canis* as the etiology. Change in weight, vision, locomotion, vaginal discharge, and palpable swellings during physical exam should cause the veterinarian to obtain a complete blood count, *Brucella canis* serology, chemistry profile, and cystocentesis. Hematology results may be within reference ranges and unremarkable. Serial semen collections show lower sperm progressive motility (asthenozoospermia), immature spermatozoa with proximal and distal cytoplasmic droplets, and acrosome deformities within 2 months. By 4 months, head-to-head sperm agglutination and inflammatory WBCs appear. With time, the necrotizing vasculitis and inflammation invades the testes (orchitis), and enlargement of the tail of the epididymis can be palpated.

Testicular atrophy ends with loss of seminiferous tubules and absence of sperm in the ejaculate. Radiographic evidence of discospondylitis usually reveals unifocal or multifocal inflammation in an intervertebral disk with vertebral architecture unaffected. Ophthalmologic evaluation for visual deficits or during breed certification may result in detection of uveitis and accompanying lesions.

Serologic testing is based upon an agglutinating reaction to the bacteria's rough cell wall or cytoplasmic protein antigen.[49] Detection begins 3 to 4 weeks after the onset of infection. A delay in the dog's cellular immune response causes the lag in serologic titer even if the dog has become bacteremic within 2 weeks. Titers fluctuate despite a persistent bacteremia. The magnitude of the titer does not reflect the stage of disease. Dogs can remain positive for 30 months to several years. The rapid slide agglutination test (RSAT), or card test, is a quick screening test developed in 1974[50] with results within 2 minutes. RSAT is considered highly sensitive (i.e., detects truly infected) but not specific (i.e., defines difference between true positive and true negative). It is rare for false negatives[51] but 50% to 60% false positives occur[24] from cross-reaction with other bacteria. If positive, a more specific test should be ordered while the dog is placed in isolation. If negative, the dog does not have brucellosis. The modified RSAT (ME-RSAT) adds 2-mercaptoethanol (2-ME) to inactivate IgM and increase specificity. Tube agglutination test (TAT) detects antibodies in dogs that test positive with RSAT or ME-RSAT. A 1:200 titer is presumptive evidence of an active infection.[18,23,43] Good correlation is seen between a titer equal to or greater than 1:200 and B. canis being recovered via blood culture. Titers below 1:200 should be rechecked in 2 weeks. This test allows for false positives. The sensitivity of indirect fluorescent antibody (IFA) has been questioned; thus some infected dogs may go undetected. The polymerase chain reaction is reported as a diagnostic laboratory test for canine semen and vaginal swab.[52,52a] Two antigens used for agar gel immunodiffusion test (AGID) confirm suspected cases from screening tests. A lipopolysaccharide antigen from the bacterial cell wall (AGIDcwa) is less specific than the internal cytoplasmic antigen (AGIDcpa) extracted from B. canis or abortus. This most specific, least sensitive AGIDcpa reacts with antibodies against Brucella species (canis, abortus, suis). Tests are negative in early infections when other analyses are positive. Dogs have reactive antibodies to AGID for 4 weeks to 5+ years. The interstate and international movement of dogs for training, purchase, and breeding prompted a report on cellular fatty acid profiling (CFAP) as a diagnostic tool for monitoring outbreaks.[52b]

A positive blood culture is definitive proof of infection. Dogs are bacteremic 2 to 4 weeks after oral nasal exposure[17,53] and for the next 1 to 3 years. The number of organisms circulating in the leukocyte portion of the blood is often small; therefore, serial samples may be required. B. canis is a fastidious organism and may not be present in one randomly drawn specimen, especially if the animal has received previous antibiotic therapy. Organisms have been isolated from milk, vaginal discharge after abortion, placental and fetal tissue, semen, prostatic fraction, lymph nodes, urine, discospondylitis, eye lesions, and a uterine stump. Urine from males that were cultured positive[3] shed greater numbers than females.[29] Negative cultures do not rule out the disease.

Histopathologic findings describe cellular inflammation and granulomatous lesions with associated necrotizing vasculitis. Gross evidence includes lymphadenopathy, splenomegaly, scrotal edema and dermatitis, epididymitis, orchitis, unilateral or bilateral testicular atrophy, anterior uveitis, and discospondylitis.

TREATMENT

Antimicrobial therapy is not encouraging. Since B. canis is sequestered inside cells for extended periods and the bacteremia is episodic, single antibiotic regimens are less successful.[54] Relief has come from the combination of tetracyclines (tetracycline HCl, chlortetracycline, doxycycline, minocycline) and dihydrostreptomycin. Due to the unavailability of streptomycin, gentamicin has been substituted but requires evaluation of renal function. Enrofloxacin did preserve fertility for one infected kennel,[36] but drug therapies can fail, can allow relapses, and are not curative. Antibiotics lower the bacteremia and thus give a false interpretation for any negative serologic result. Disadvantages for antibiotic treatment are expense, lengthy regimen, declining or uncertain owner compliance, and unpredictable drug accessibility to this replicating intracellular organism.[55] Two or three courses of therapy separated by 1 to 2 months may be required. Even a 90-day treatment should be followed by more testing and a repeated course of antibiotics if testing remains positive. Infected intact animals could be spayed or neutered; however, each is likely to give a positive titer for years. To stop potential transmission to other dogs and humans, euthanasia is the treatment of choice for dogs that are confirmed positive.

PREVENTION

Serologic testing is more accurate in proestrus or during estrus since the bacteremia is elevated under hormonal influence. All positive dogs should be removed by isolation and euthanasia. New additions to a kennel should be secluded for at least 1 month[18,28,53] and have two negative titers at a 1-month interval before being introduced into a licensed facility.[18] It is safe to repopulate after two negative tests of all dogs on the premises. Intact positive dogs should not breed. Every breeding dog that has been boarded, shown, or in field trials for a lengthy time should be checked as well as any male with scrotal enlargement, dermatitis, pain, reluctance to breed, or poor semen quality and every female with a history of abortion or suspected infertility. Both dogs should be tested prior to every natural mating or collection for shipment. Even if not breeding, kenneled stock should be tested at least annually. Exposure to stray and feral dogs should be controlled. Aborted or potentially infected tissue must be handled with gloves and appropriate clothing for protected disposal. Direct contact between suspected and naive dogs through wire fencing must be prevented. Even separation by partial walls is inadequate. B. canis does not survive outside the dog in the environment; therefore, disinfectants will cleanse the premises (e.g., quaternary ammonium, 1% sodium hypochlorite or bleach, iodophor solutions, 70% ethanol or formaldehyde). Low temperature, absence of sunlight, and high humidity prolong viability of the bacteria in water, aborted fetuses, feces, equipment, and clothing.[55a]

BRUCELLOSIS IN CATS

Limited seropositive reactions and experimental infections are mentioned, but cats do not exhibit clinical symptoms. The prevalence of B. canis in cat populations is unsubstantiated.

PUBLIC HEALTH CONSIDERATIONS

Transmission to humans is rare. Few cases are being reported.[1-4] Brucella caused undulant fever through close contact to the family pet, nonspecific signs of headache and weakness through exposure during serologic testing, ocular lesions, and endocarditis.[56-57f] Brucellosis has greater impact on immunosuppressed individuals (e.g., cancer, HIV, or transplantation patients), children, and pregnant women. Intimate contact place kennel personnel and owners at risk through the improper transfer of untested breeding stock, the naïve acquisition of a pregnant purebred, abortive tissue and lochia, neutered animals in relapse, or the entrance into a closed yard by a stray or feral animal. *Brucella canis* is a reportable disease to regulatory agencies some states.[25]

REFERENCES

The reference list can be found on the companion Expert Consult Web site at *www.expertconsult.com*.

CHAPTER 202

Tetanus

Andrea Fischer
Katrin Hartmann

Tetanus is a sporadic disease. Its prevalence in dogs and cats is relatively low compared to that in horses or humans.[1] Cats are considered even more resistant to tetanus toxins than dogs, and they usually develop only localized tetanus.[2-5] Dogs are reported to be 600 times less susceptible and cats 7200 times less susceptible to tetanus than horses.[6] Differences in susceptibility to tetanus are explained by species differences in the polyganglioside surface receptor on peripheral nerve endings.

ETIOLOGY

Tetanus is caused by a potent neurotoxin produced by the bacterium *Clostridium tetani*. *C. tetani* is a motile, gram-positive, nonencapsulated, anaerobic, spore-forming, rod-shaped bacterium.[6,7] The information for tetanus neurotoxin is encoded on an extrachromosomal plasmid only found in toxin-producing *C. tetani* strains.[8,9] All toxigenic strains produce two toxins, a tetanus neurotoxin (tetanospasmin) and a hemolysin (tetanolysin), the latter with no clinical relevance. *C. tetani* organisms can be isolated from feces of many domestic animals and humans without pathogenic significance.[10] Resistant spores can be found anywhere in the environment where they can survive adverse weather conditions in the absence of direct sunlight for months to years. Spores can also readily be found in dust and debris in indoor environments and even have been cultured from the surface of surgery rooms.[11] Spores survive thermal disinfection procedures[12] and may even resist an autoclave temperature of 120° C for 15 to 20 minutes.[6]

PATHOGENESIS

Tetanus develops if *C. tetani* spores enter wounds and anaerobic conditions favor germination and toxin production.[13] Wounds with draining tracts, claw or nailbed infections, or deep interdigital abscesses of the paws are identified most commonly as entry sides, but bite wounds, lacerations, dental fracture, and excessive nail trimming have also been implicated. Postsurgical tetanus after ovariohysterectomy and other

surgeries has been reported in animals.[14-17] In a considerable number of cases, no wound or only a small, already-healing wound is identified.[14,15,18,19]

The H-chain of tetanospasmin has a high affinity to ganglioside surface receptors on neuromuscular endplates. It is responsible for internalization, cytosolic translocation, and fast retrograde axonal transport of the L-chain. The L-chain represents the actual neurotoxin. Within the spinal cord and brainstem, the neurotoxic L-chain spreads transsynaptically to inhibitory interneurons (Renshaw cells) of motor and autonomic centers (Web Figure 202-1).

There, the L-chain acts as a zinc-dependent protease that specifically cleaves vesicle-associated membrane protein (VAMP)/synaptobrevin. VAMP is a member of the SNARE-protein (soluble N-ethylmaleimide–sensitive-factor attachment protein receptor) family, a highly conserved group of proteins essential for docking and fusion of neurotransmitter vesicles with the presynaptic membrane.[20-26] By cleaving VAMP in spinal inhibitory interneurons, the L-chain interferes with the release of the inhibitory neurotransmitters glycine in the spinal cord and γ-aminobutyric acid (GABA) in the brainstem (see Figure 203-1 in Chapter 203).[6,20,21,27] Thus, the general clinical picture of tetanus is the consequence of loss of inhibition of α-motoneuron firing. Mild stimuli will cause severe unopposed contractions of extensor muscles. Similarly, autonomic control may be lost and increased sympathetic or parasympathetic activity will occur.

CLINICAL SIGNS

Clinical signs of tetanus commonly occur between 3 and 18 days (up to 3 weeks) after an injury. Younger dogs are more susceptible. Due to the time delay and the high potency of the internalized toxin, a wound may no longer be detectable at the time of examination in most pets.[14,15,18,19]

Tetanus can present as a generalized syndrome or as localized tetanus. Localized tetanus is more common in cats than in dogs. In localized tetanus, the toxin enters the motor axon closest to the injury site and migrates by retrograde transport to the neuronal cell bodies within the spinal cord or brainstem, where it exhibits its action. Animals with localized

 To view a video on this topic, go to **www.expertconsult.com.**

tetanus frequently have stiffness in one limb or muscle group close to the injury site.[3,6] Stiffness usually progresses to the point that the limb is held in rigid extension. Localized tetanus can be distinguished from severe upper motor neuron (UMN) monoparesis by the ability to initiate postural reactions despite muscle stiffness in more mild cases and by the inability to passively flex the limb in severe cases. Localized tetanus with involvement of either both pelvic or thoracic limbs has been reported.[2,28] The female reproductive tract is a common source of infection if the pelvic limbs are involved.[6] Localized tetanus can either stay restricted or progress to generalized tetanus from gradual transsynaptic spread of the toxin within the central nervous system. Alternatively, large amounts of toxin released into the bloodstream can reach nerves at distant sites. In people, tetanus can occur as a localized syndrome restricted to the muscles of the head with paralysis of facial muscles (cephalic tetanus),[29,30] but this has not been described in dogs and cats.[14] Most dogs with facial signs have facial muscle spasms and generalized tetanus.

Dogs and cats affected with generalized tetanus have generalized muscle stiffness of variable intensity, hypersensitivity to touch, lights, and sounds, but a normal mental state. Most dogs will show characteristic facial muscle spasms: wrinkling of the forehead, erect ears that are drawn together, lips that are drawn back (risus sardonicus), and protrusion of the third eyelid from enophthalmus due to continuous or episodic contraction of extraocular muscles (Figure 202-1).

Trismus (lockjaw) caused by contraction of masticatory muscles, salivation, laryngeal spasms, and dysphagia may occur. Mildly affected dogs are still ambulatory, but show a stiff gait and have difficulty in standing or lying down in comfortable positions. Gait changes may vary due to the degree of excitement. Postural reactions are initiated, but performance is stiff. Patellar reflexes are often exaggerated, but flexor reflexes may appear decreased with increasing muscle stiffness. Severely affected dogs may be brought to the veterinarian in lateral recumbency with rigid extension of all limbs and opisthotonus but yet unimpaired mentation. Recumbent dogs may also show episodic muscle fasciculations or spasms. Tonic

muscle contractions are precipitated by noise, touch, and excitement. Mentation is usually unimpaired unless seizures develop. Severe hyperthermia (>104° F) due to muscular spasms is often present.

Numerous complications can occur during generalized tetanus. Seizures may develop in severely affected animals. Dysphagia and laryngeal spasms, which may cause severe respiratory impairment, are common.[15] Transient megaesophagus and hiatal hernia from esophageal dysfunction may cause regurgitation and aspiration pneumonia.[14,15,19,31,32] Dogs may be unable to urinate due to urethral spasms and require placement of an indwelling catheters. Some dogs may be constipated. Coxofemoral luxation, quadriceps contracture, and adhesions have been reported.[18] Autonomic dysfunction due to loss of inhibitory control of parasympathetic brainstem centers and preganglionic sympathetic neurons has been recognized as a severe complication and causes ventilatory failure.[33] The condition can cause life-threatening autonomic storms with increased catecholamine secretion in people.[6,34,35] Autonomic dysfunction may also occur in dogs.[14,15,36,37] Severe bradyarrhythmias may require temporary pacemaker placement.[14] Gastrointestinal tract ulceration may occur, and risk increases if glucocorticoids are used for treatment. Uncommonly, systemic inflammatory response syndrome (SIRS), acute renal failure, or multiorgan failure may develop. Dogs with head involvement are classified as class I (normal gait, hypersensitivity to noise, light, or touch) or class II (stiff gait); recumbent dogs with tonic muscle contractions, fasciculations, spasms or seizures, and typical head involvement as class III; and dogs with autonomic signs independent of ambulatory status as class IV. The survival rate decreases with the severity class.[14]

DIAGNOSIS

Tetanus is one of the few infectious diseases diagnosed by typical clinical signs and history, and exclusion of other diseases (Figure 202-2). Hematologic abnormalities, including leukocytosis with neutrophilia and left shift, result from wound infections or aspiration pneumonia. Serum biochemistry, urine, and CSF analysis are usually normal unless complications arise. Excessively high muscle enzymes activities (CK, AST) result from continuous muscle contractions.

Isolation of *C. tetani* from wounds is successful only in few cases.[5] If culture is attempted, it should be done under strict anaerobic conditions at 37° C for at least 2 weeks.[6] Serum antibodies against tetanus toxin can be measured to confirm the diagnosis, but values must be compared with those of control dogs. PCR for detection of the tetanus toxin gene in wounds has been used, but its value as diagnostic tool is not established.[38]

Electromyography has been suggested to confirm a clinical suspicion of tetanus. Electromyographic changes suggestive of tetanus include persistence of voluntary motor unit activity in the anesthetized animal with simultaneous recording of motor unit action potentials in antagonistic flexor and extensor muscles, and increased insertional activity, repetitive discharges of motor units, and repetitive discharges following peripheral nerve stimulation may occur.[5,28,39]

TREATMENT

Treatment of severely affected animals may be costly and time-consuming. Owners should be advised of the possibility of complications and lengthy hospitalization. Recovery is slow and based on sprouting of new nerve terminals. Mildly diseased animals may recover from their

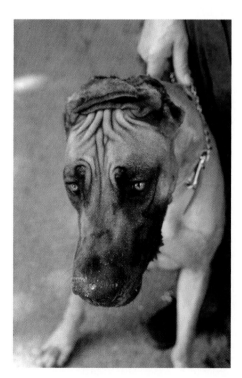

Figure 202-1 Typical facial expression of a dog with tetanus.

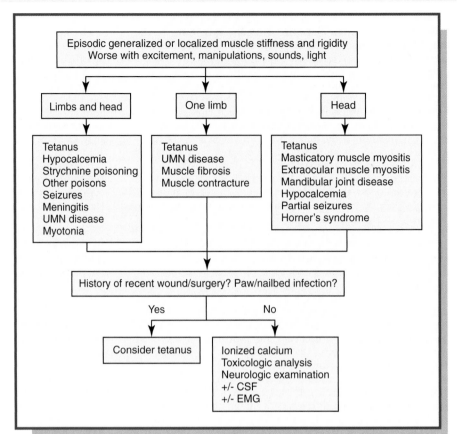

Episodic generalized or localized muscle stiffness and rigidity
Worse with excitement, manipulations, sounds, light

Limbs and head

One limb

Head

Tetanus
Hypocalcemia
Strychnine poisoning
Other poisons
Seizures
Meningitis
UMN disease
Myotonia

Tetanus
UMN disease
Muscle fibrosis
Muscle contracture

Tetanus
Masticatory muscle myositis
Extraocular muscle myositis
Mandibular joint disease
Hypocalcemia
Partial seizures
Horner's syndrome

History of recent wound/surgery? Paw/nailbed infection?

Yes   No

Consider tetanus

Ionized calcium
Toxicologic analysis
Neurologic examination
+/- CSF
+/- EMG

Figure 202-2 Diagnostic algorithm: tetanus. *CSF,* Cerebrospinal fluid; *EMG,* electromyogram; *UMN,* upper motor neuron.

neurologic dysfunction with wound management and antimicrobial therapy alone.

Tetanus antitoxin should be administered to neutralize any toxin that is unbound or yet to be formed but does little to hasten recovery. Recovery in most cases is slow, progressive, and based on sprouting of new nerve terminals. Antitoxin should be given immediately upon presentation and prior to exploration of wounds. Usually equine antitoxin is given IV slowly over 5 to 10 minutes. The dose of antitoxin is based on the amount of toxin to be antagonized; thus, larger animals will receive a proportionally lower dose. Published studies used a wide range of dosages in dogs (median dosage 100 U/kg,[19] 200 U/kg,[15] 326 U/kg,[14] respectively). The IV injection can cause anaphylaxis and anaphylactoid reactions; therefore, appropriate precautions are warranted during administration. An initial test dose (0.1 to 0.2 mL) of antitoxin should be given intradermally 15 minutes before administering the drug IV. Epinephrine, glucocorticoids, and antihistamines should be available in case of an adverse reaction, or glucocorticoids and antihistamines may be considered before the IV injection (depending on the intradermal test outcome). Adverse reactions evolve only in a small number of animals, and intradermal testing is not always predictive of anaphylaxis.[14,19] Therapeutic antitoxin blood levels persist for 2 weeks; thus, repeated administration is unnecessary and increases the chance of an anaphylactic reaction. Local IM injection of a small dose of antitoxin (1000 U) around and proximal to the wound has been shown to be beneficial in experimental studies of localized tetanus, but its usefulness in clinical cases is unknown. Intrathecal application of tetanus antitoxin has been successfully applied to severely affected people,[40] and intrathecal injection of as little as 1% of the IV dose (1 to 10 U/kg) may also reduce mortality and morbidity in dogs with tetanus.[6]

Antimicrobial therapy should be administered in an attempt to kill any existing vegetative *C. tetani* organisms. Metronidazole and penicillin G are the drugs of choice for treatment of tetanus.[6,14,19,41] Metronidazole (10 to 15 mg/kg BID or TID) is preferred despite its potential side effects because it is bactericidal against most anaerobes and achieves effective therapeutic concentrations even in anaerobic tissues.[42] There have been concerns that penicillin G could exacerbate muscle spasms by its GABA-antagonistic mechanism of action and that it could be inactivated by concomitant β-lactamase–producing organisms such as *Staphylococcus* spp. or *E. coli.*[43] Penicillin G should be given IV at a high dosage (40,000 U/kg q4-6h IV as potassium or sodium salt) or q8-12h IM as the procaine salt for 10 days. A portion of the dose can be injected IM (as procaine salt) in close proximity to an identified wound site. Clindamycin and tetracycline are also effective against *C. tetani* and are reasonable alternatives, while ampicillin and enrofloxacin are of questionable value.[6]

Surgical wound debridement should be considered if a wound is identified and necrotic tissue or an abscess can be located. However, extreme care needs to be taken to avoid excessive manipulation of the patient that might result in exaggeration of tetanic spasms. Only patients already treated with antitoxin should undergo surgery because of the risk of release of toxin in the circulation during tissue manipulations.[6] Paw or nailbed infections may be soaked with hydrogen peroxide because it increases oxygen tension, and extraction of the claw or nail may be necessary. Exploration of the previous surgical site may be indicated if tetanus arises after a surgical procedure.

Supportive treatment is imperative for the successful management of an animal with tetanus. Patients should be kept in a quiet, dark room with as little traffic and manipulation as possible. Soft bedding should be provided to avoid decubital ulcers. Ears should be plugged with cotton or specific sound protectors. Sedative and muscle-relaxing drugs should be administered to all animals with the goal to achieve optimal sedation and muscle relaxation. Phenothiazine tranquilizers (chlorpromazine, acepromazine) are often used in combination with phenobarbital. These drugs appear to be highly effective in this setting. Benzodiazepines (diazepam, midazolam) are preferred over methocarbamol as muscle relaxants. Benzodiazepines block polysynaptic reflexes in the spinal cord and medulla and thus act as centrally acting muscle relaxant. Magnesium appears to be a highly beneficial adjunct therapy in people, but its usefulness in animals is unknown.[44] Dantrolene and intrathecal baclofen also have been investigated in people, but side effects have been described.[43,45] Severely affected animals with opisthotonus and generalized extensor rigidity or generalized seizures may require repeated or continuous pentobarbital (or propofol) administration. Respiratory depression is a major concern with pentobarbital therapy. Neuromuscular blockade, tracheostomy, and positive-pressure ventilation are used in severely affected people and were successfully applied to a dog.[46]

Further supportive care in severely affected animals consists of fluids as needed to maintain hydration, adequate nutrition, padding, and monitoring of urinary and fecal output. Urinary catheterization may be needed. Ideally the animal should be able to take food by itself, but in many cases, deep sedation, megaesophagus, or trismus may prevent eating. Esophagostomy, gastrostomy, or enteric feeding tubes or, alternatively, total parenteral nutrition may be needed to address caloric requirements. Enteric feeding or parenteral nutrition are the preferred routes in animals with hiatal hernia and megaesophagus. Animals with tetanus are in a hypermetabolic state due to the continued muscle contractions and hyperthermia, and caloric requirements may be well above resting energy requirements.[33,47] Again, with all procedures, extreme care should be taken to avoid excessive manipulation and exaggeration of stimulus-induced muscle spasms.

PROGRESSION AND PROGNOSIS

Neuronal uptake and action of the neurotoxin is irreversible, and recovery requires the outgrowth of new nerve terminals, which explains the long duration of the disease.[43] The prognosis is usually favorable with localized tetanus if progression to generalized tetanus is prevented. Localized rigidity tends to resolve within 4 to 8 weeks.[5] With generalized tetanus, there is a higher risk of death, which is most commonly caused by respiratory compromise, complications associated with cardiovascular dysfunction, or uncontrollable muscle spasms. Yet, with adequate care the majority of dogs will recover within 4 weeks.[14,15,19]

PREVENTION

Active immunoprophylaxis with tetanus toxoid vaccines is licensed for dogs in some countries but is not generally recommended for dogs and cats due to the low prevalence of the disease in these species. Immunoprophylaxis is used for more susceptible species such as humans and horses. Appropriate care of infected wounds, adherence to strict sterilization procedures when performing surgery, and rational antibiotic therapy should minimize the occurrence of tetanus.

References

The reference list can be found on the companion Expert Consult Web site at *www.expertconsult.com.*

CHAPTER **203**

Botulism

Andrea Fischer

Botulism is a paralytic illness caused by a group of neurotoxins commonly produced by *Clostridium botulinum* as well as occasionally by other toxigenic clostridia. Botulinum toxins are highly potent. The toxins inhibit acetylcholine release at peripheral cholinergic synapses, which results in generalized lower motor neuron (LMN) and autonomic dysfunction.

ETIOLOGY

Clostridium botulinum represents a group of gram-positive, spore-forming, anaerobic saprophytic, rod-shaped bacteria with worldwide distribution which are distinguished by their specific neurotoxins.[1] Seven different types of botulinum toxins are currently recognized: A, B, C1, D, E, F, and G. Up to now, botulinum toxin type C has been identified as causative agent in all reported cases of botulism in dogs and cats with the exception of two canine cases of type D botulism in Senegal,[1] whereas botulism in people is commonly caused by botulinum toxins types A, B, E, and rarely F.[2] *Clostridium botulinum* type C differs from the other types because nonneurotoxic cytotoxins (C2, C3) may be released together with the neurotoxin C1.[3] Transfer of neurotoxin genes to and from other clostridia can occur.[4]

Clostridial spores and organisms are present in the environment in soil and water if organic material is provided. Spores are highly resistant to dry heat, light, drying, and radiation.

 To view a video on this topic, go to **www.expertconsult.com.**

Germination is favored by anaerobic conditions, high quantities of organic protein, and warmth (15° to 45° C). Thus rotten meat and carcasses of dead animals, especially birds, are ideal for growth of C. botulinum. However, growth may occur at temperatures as low as 6° C.[1] Within days of germination, vegetative cells begin to produce toxin and soon contain 100 times as much toxin as spores.[1] Unlike tetanus toxin, lysis of the cell or spore is necessary for release of the yet inactive botulinum toxin (150 kDa) in the environment. Toxin is released in the form of a stable complex in association with nontoxic proteins (progenitor toxin), which appear to protect the toxin until consumption and the toxin reaches the intestinal tract. There, alkaline pH permits its dissociation.[5] Following proteolytic cleavage, the activated toxin consists of a heavy (H) chain (100 kDa) and a light (L) chain (50 kDa) connected by disulfide bonds.[1]

The most common mode of intoxication in people and animals is ingestion of the preformed toxin (food-borne botulism). Most cases in dogs are associated with the ingestion of carrion. Cadavers of birds are frequent sources of intoxication,[6-11] because their intestines often contain C. botulinum type C. After the birds' deaths, bacteria can multiply and produce large amounts of toxin and spores. Thus, outbreaks of canine botulism are often related to areas of avian epizootics of botulism.[7,11,12] The only reported natural outbreak of botulism in a group of cats was also traced back to the ingestion of a pelican carcass and botulinum toxin type C.[13] Experimentally, cats appeared more susceptible to parenteral application of the toxin than to oral application. Wound botulism and infant botulism represent forms of botulism in which the toxin is produced by clostridia organisms multiplying within a wound or the gastrointestinal (GI) tract of infants (toxicoinfectious botulism), but these have not yet been described in dogs or cats.[3] Intestinal colonization with toxigenic clostridia can exist in adult people and dogs without any clinical signs unless the normal intestinal microflora is disrupted (antibiotic treatment, immunosuppression, GI surgery).[1]

PATHOGENESIS

With food-borne botulism, botulinum toxin is absorbed from the upper small bowel into the lymphatic system and thereafter distributed hematogenously to axon terminals of cholinergic nerves. Botulinum toxin does not cross the blood-brain barrier. The H chain is responsible for the specific binding to a high-affinity surface receptor complex on the surface of the nerve, internalization of the toxin (receptor-mediated endocytosis), and translocation into the cytosol of the peripheral nerve (see Web Figure 202-1 in Chapter 202).

The L-chain represents the actual neurotoxin at the neuromuscular endplate. It acts as a zinc-dependent endopeptidase that cleaves and thus inactivates SNARE proteins (soluble N-ethylmaleimide–sensitive-factor attachment protein receptor). This group of proteins mediate docking and fusion of neurotransmitter vesicles to the presynaptic plasma membrane and thus promote calcium-mediated neurotransmitter release into the synaptic cleft. Botulinum toxin exhibits its action without any further intracellular trafficing.[14] Thus, all toxin types block acetylcholine release at the neuromuscular endplate resulting in generalized LMN dysfunction. Toxins, however, differ by their specific mechanism of action. For example, botulinum toxin C1 has a dual action directed against synaptosome-associated protein of 25 kDa (SNAP-25) and syntaxin, while botulinum toxin type A cleaves SNAP-25, and toxin types B and D cleave vesicle-associated membrane protein (VAMP) at specific amino bonds[15-17] (Figure 203-1).

Action of the toxin is prolonged and functional recovery is based on sprouting of new axon terminals and reformation of functional neuromuscular endplates.[18] Botulinum toxin A is increasingly used in the treatment of muscle contracture, spasticity, and cholinergic autonomic hyperfunction in people because there is no loss of motor neurons and any muscle atrophy is completely reversible.[17,18] It was successfully used to treat blepharospasm in a dog, and experimentally to ameliorate rhinorrhea, salivation, biliary retention, and prostatic hyperplasia in dogs.[19-23]

CLINICAL SYMPTOMS

Botulism has an acute onset. The incubation period can range from hours to 6 days but, in most cases, clinical signs will develop rather soon (1 to 3 days) after ingestion of contaminated food.[10,24-26] Course and severity of illness vary in direct proportion to amount of ingested toxin.[27,28] Severely affected dogs may progress to flaccid tetraplegia in less than 24 hours, while others may show only weakness in the hind limbs, forelimbs, and the muscles of the neck and head. Cranial nerve signs are common in severely affected animals. Neurologic examination indicates generalized LMN disease. Muscle tone is reduced and spinal reflexes (patellar, withdrawal) are absent. In animals that are not yet completely tetraplegic, postural reactions demonstrate preserved ability to sense position and initiate movement (sensory), while performance (motor) is progressively reduced. Mentation is normal, and conscious response to pain stimuli is completely preserved, although the animal may not be able to move its legs or head. Mydriatic pupils are frequently reported, but decreased palpebral reflexes, gag reflex, jaw tone, facial muscle weakness, and inability to vocalize have all been described. Complete flaccid paralysis of the tongue, facial muscles, and eyelids can evolve.

More mildly affected animals may not have cranial nerve signs. Reversible megaoesophagus has been described in dogs. Mydriatic pupils, keratoconjunctivitis sicca, constipation, urinary retention, and variable heart rate are signs or parasympathetic dysfunction.[29] The plateau phase of the disease may last as long as 5 to 7 days after toxin ingestion. Severely affected animals die from respiratory paralysis. Spontaneous recovery will occur if respiratory paralysis can be avoided. Some dogs can support their weight and walk short distances within 2 weeks.[6,9-11,24,26,29] In the only reported natural outbreak of botulism in cats, the course of disease was similar to that described in dogs. The cats suffered from acute, generalized LMN tetraparesis or tetraplegia. Four severely affected cats died within 5 days of showing symptoms. Four other cats recovered completely within 6 to 10 days.[13] There is evidence of an association between feline dysautonomia, a disease characterized by extensive degeneration of autonomic ganglia and botulinum toxin type C. Neurotoxin and specific IgA were detected in feces and food of affected cats.[30] Botulinum type C toxin has also been associated with dysautonomia in horses.[31,32]

Several disorders need to be considered in the evaluation of mentally intact patients with acute onset of generalized LMN disease (Figure 203-2). The main differentials are acute polyradiculoneuritis and tick paralysis. Less commonly, an acute crisis of myasthenia gravis, acute boosts of polymyositis, ionophore intoxication, coral snake poisoning or flaccid paresis from rabies poliomyelitis are seen. Tick paralysis and coral snake poisoning have restricted geographical distribution. Guillain-Barré syndrome, poliomyelitis, hypokalemic, hyperkalemic, or hyperthyroid periodic paralyses, hypermagnesemia, Lambert-Eaton myasthenic syndrome, and some toxic neuropathies (e.g., arsenic) reportedly cause similar signs in people.[33-36] Acute exacerbations of more chronic polymyopathies or polyneuropathies (e.g., hypothyroid polyneu-

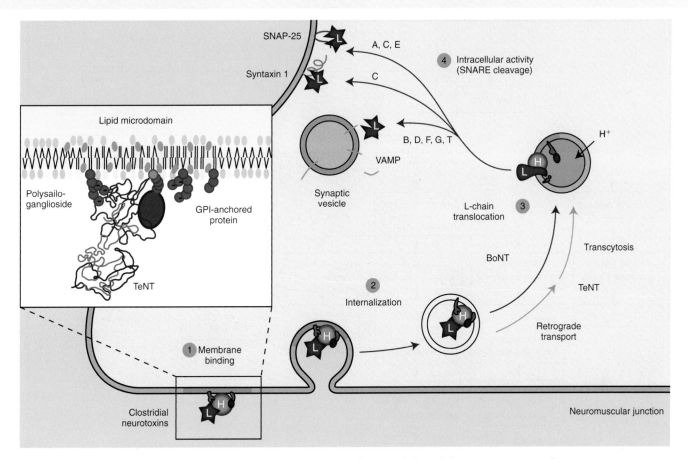

Figure 203-1 The four-step cellular mechanism of action of clostridial neurotoxin: *1*, membrane binding; *2*, internalization; *3*, translocation; *4*, intracellular action. *1*, Clostridial neurotoxins bind to polysialogangliosides and specific proteins on the surface of nerve cells. These lipid and protein receptors cluster in lipid microdomains *(yellow)* which are enriched in cholesterol *(green)* and sphingolipids *(yellow)*. *2*, Neurospecific binding is followed by internalization and sorting to specific intracellular routes, which differ for botulinum toxin *(BoNT)* and tetanus neurotoxin *(TeNT)*. TeNT enters carriers that are directed to the fast retrograde transport pathway and then reaches adjacent inhibitory interneurons by transcytosis. BoNT-containing endocytic structures instead remain at the neuromuscular junction. *3*, On arrival at their final destination, the light chain has to cross the endocytic membrane to reach the cytoplasm. Acidification of the lumen of the endosomes triggers a conformational change in the H-chain, which allows its insertion into the lipid bilayer and formation of a channel for the L-chain. *4*, Different L-chains specifically cleave different members of the soluble NSF (N-ethylmaleimide-sensitive factor) attachment protein receptor *(SNARE)*-protein family. TeNT and BoNT B, D, F, and G act on vesicle-associated membrane protein *(VAMP)*/synaptobrevin *(green)* located on synaptic vesicles. BoNT A and E cleave synaptosome-associated protein of 25 kDa *(SNAP-25)* *(pink)*, whereas BoNT C cleaves both syntaxin 1 *(cyan)* and SNAP-25, two proteins of the presynaptic plasma membrane. *GPI*, Glycosylphosphatidylinositol. (From Lalli G, Bohnert S, Deinhardt K, et al: The journey of tetanus and botulinum neurotoxins in neurons. Trends Microbiol 11[9]:431-437, 2003.)

ropathy or organophosphate-induced polyneuropathy) need also to be considered.

DIAGNOSIS

Diagnosis is based on a history of possible toxin ingestion in combination with characteristic clinical signs. Further substantiation can be achieved with toxicologic tests. The involvement of several dogs with similar exposure to toxic material and similar clinical signs is also strongly suggestive of botulism.[7] Hematologic and biochemical laboratory examination including urine and CSF are normal unless secondary pulmonary or urinary tract infection develops.[1,37]

Electrodiagnostic examination can serve as a readily available bedside test. Results are not specific but taken together can suggest involvement of the motor nerve terminal.[36,38-40] Electrodiagnostic changes are surprisingly mild considering severity of disease. The most consistent finding is a small amplitude of the muscle potential in response to a supramaximal nerve stimulus in people as well as in affected dogs, although this may only be evident in severely affected patients.[26,29,36,39] The compound muscle action potential (CMAP) recorded with surface electrodes has a normal biphasic shape without any evidence of temporal dispersion. Spontaneous electric activity in the form of positive sharp waves and fibrillation potentials can arise from functional denervation of the muscle, but electromyographic changes tended to be mild and appear late in the disease course when dogs had already recovered from botulism (days 10 to 13), although exemptions may exist.[26,29] Repetitive nerve stimulation at 3 Hz may be normal or only a minor decrement may be encountered in affected

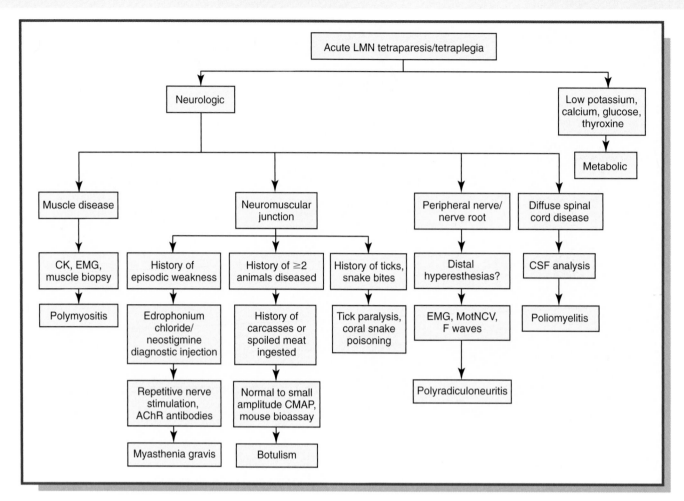

Figure 203-2 Diagnostic algorithm: botulism. *AChR*, Acetylcholine receptor; *CK*, creatine kinase; *CMAP*, compound muscle action potential; *EMG*, electromyogram; *LMN*, lower motor neuron; *MotNCV*, motor nerve conduction velocity.

dogs and people.[29] In people, increasing amplitude and area of the CMAP with high-frequency repetitive stimulation and posttetanic facilitation is often indicative of a presynaptic neuromuscular transmission disorder. Increasing amplitudes and areas reflect calcium facilitation of stored neurotransmitter release.[29,36,39,41] High-frequency repetitive stimulation failed to demonstrate an increment in affected dogs.[29] Currently, single-fiber electromyography is considered the most sensitive technique in people to assess neuromuscular transmission failure.[38]

Definite diagnosis of botulism is based on the demonstration of botulinum toxin in ingested food, stomach content, feces, or serum of the affected animal by mouse protection assay, which still is considered the gold standard due to its high sensitivity (1 minimum lethal dose = 10 pg).[42] Samples should be stored at 4° C until analysis and shipped in leak-proof containers marked "Biological Hazard." Freezing interferes with detection of bacteria, but does not affect the toxin.[3] Demonstration of toxin is successful, if the mice die of respiratory failure within 48 to 96 hours. Then, botulinum toxin can be confirmed and the toxin type determined by neutralizing the activity of the samples or protecting the mice with monovalent serotype-specific antitoxin.[3,42] Additionally, isolation of toxigenic *C. botulinum* from feces, food, or serum is often pursued. Culture needs to be done under strictly anaerobic conditions. Demonstration of the organism in

association with clinical signs provides some evidence for diagnosis, but it is not as conclusive as toxin identification, because clostridia can be part of the natural GI flora in animals.[1]

Recently, other diagnostic tests have been developed to hasten identification of botulinum neurotoxins mainly due to bioterrorism threats.[42,43] PCR is based on amplification of genes encoding the various botulinum neurotoxins and thus will only detect toxigenic *C. botulinum* organisms but not the neurotoxin itself. Therefore, it is only helpful in environmental investigations and detection of toxigenic bacteria.[44] Enzyme-linked immunosorbent assay (ELISA) can assist with detection of the toxin, but each type of botulinum toxin needs to be addressed separately. ELISA may also respond to inactive toxin. Its sensitivity is still not as good as the mouse bioassay yet it may be a useful adjunct for investigation of clinically suspect botulism. An immuno-electro-chemiluminescence method has been marketed but sensitivity dropped when applied to clinical specimens.[3] Avian eyelid closure test was suggested as another sensitive bioassay.[45] Antibodies directed against the various botulinum toxins can be measured in serum. Positive antibody titres support contact to toxigenic *C. botulinum*, but toxin-specific antibodies are also present in healthy dogs. Thus, botulism can only be proved by making repeated measurements for increasing antibody concentrations after 3 weeks.[25,46]

THERAPY

Treatment is mainly supportive, because spontaneous recovery will occur in most dogs within 2 to 3 weeks if the amount of ingested toxin is not too large and respiratory failure and complications like pneumonia or urinary tract infections are avoided.[1] Depending on the degree of symptoms, patients should be hospitalized and monitored closely for respiratory failure. Aggressive treatment with intubation and mechanical ventilation should be considered for severely affected animals. Gastric lavage is only indicated if the potential food exposure was recent. Enemas may be considered to eliminate toxin and toxin-producing bacteria from the colon.[1]

Dogs with tetraparesis or tetraplegia should be bedded softly and repositioned every 4 hours to prevent the development of decubital ulcers. Hydration status, urination, and defecation need to be monitored. If necessary, the bladder is compressed manually or emptied by catheterization. Megaesophagus and a decreased gag reflex can favor aspiration pneumonia, and all attempts should be taken to avoid this potential complication. Intravenous fluid therapy is usually necessary in severely affected animals in order to avoid dehydration. Hypokalemia and any magnesium-containing preparations should be strictly avoided because this additionally impairs neuromuscular function.[33] Short-term parenteral nutrition may be considered if swallowing is impaired, although this usually can be avoided because signs of recovery may be seen within days or after a plateau phase up to day 5 to 7 days. Eye ointments should be given to dogs with poor palpebral function in order to avoid exposure keratitis, and tear substitution may be indicated in case of keratoconjunctivitis sicca. Administration of the appropriate type-specific equine antitoxin can be considered within 24 hours of intoxication for severely affected animals but is of questionable value. The antitoxin neutralizes toxin molecules that have not bound to nerve endings yet, but there is no effect on intracellular toxin and an already-existing paralysis remains unaffected. Thus antitoxin may only be effective if given early within the clinical course. As almost all cases of canine botulism to date have been caused by toxin type C and rarely type D, only antitoxin directed against these toxin types is indicated in dogs and cats. Furthermore, anaphylaxis is a possible serious side effect in people.[43] Therefore intradermal skin testing must be performed before intravenous injection. Any reaction at the test site is a warning that an allergic reaction may occur.[1]

The administration of antibiotics, other than as needed to treat pneumonia or urinary tract infection, has been discussed controversially in the past.[37] In animals, intoxication usually occurs after the ingestion of preformed toxin (food-borne botulism), in which case antibiotics would have little benefit. Antibiotics may even worsen the clinical signs by releasing more toxin from lysed bacteria, and destruction of the natural GI flora could further promote intestinal colonization by toxigenic *C. botulinum*.[43] Clindamycin and aminoglycosides (also polymyxin B, tetracycline) may even interfere with neuromuscular conduction and worsen paralysis.[3,47-50] Metronidazole was used to establish intestinal colonization by *C. botulinum* and clinically evident botulism in experimental studies of mice.[3,51]

Neuromuscular potentiators (3,4-diaminopyridine, guanidine hydrochloride, 4-aminopyridine) have been used in humans and animals in the past in an attempt to enhance transmitter release but with debatable efficacy. Use of guanidine in one lion with botulism was associated with seizures and death.[52] Recently, toosendanin, a product from traditional Chinese medicine, was proposed to have marked antibotulismic effects.[53]

PREVENTION

Ingestion of cadavers, especially avian cadavers, should be avoided. Botulinum neurotoxins are heat labile and destroyed by cooking at 85° C for 5 minutes. Recovery from botulism does not lead to protective immunity. Due to bioterrorism threats, multivalent vaccines are currently being developed.

REFERENCES

The reference list can be found on the companion Expert Consult Web site at *www.expertconsult.com*.

CHAPTER **204**

Canine *Bartonella*

Edward B. Breitschwerdt

*B*artonella species are fastidious gram-negative bacteria that are highly adapted to many mammalian reservoir hosts within which these bacteria can cause a long-lasting intraerythrocytic bacteremia.[1,2] In some natural hosts, such as cats, cows and rodents, chronic bacteremia with a *Bartonella* species can frequently be detected in clinically healthy individuals. Studies have confirmed an intraerythrocytic localization for these bacteria, which is a unique strategy for bacterial persistence.[3,4] However, mechanisms that facilitate persistent *Bartonella* bacteremia are most probably multifactorial and remain poorly understood. Nonhemolytic intracellular colonization of erythrocytes and endothelial cells would preserve the organisms for efficient vector transmission, protect *Bartonella* from the host immune response, and potentially contribute to decreased antimicrobial efficacy.[3-5] More recently, in vitro studies indicate that *Bartonella* spp. can infect dendritic cells, microglial cells, monocytes, and CD34+ bone marrow progenitor cells.[6] In people, *Bartonella* spp. are an important cause of bacillary angiomatosis, peliosis hepatis, fever of unknown origin, arthritis, endocarditis, granulomatous hepatitis and lymphadenitis, encephalitis, and potentially a rapidly expanding spectrum of less frequently diagnosed medical conditions.[7-8]

DISEASE MANIFESTATIONS

Dogs are most often infected with *Bartonella henselae*, *Bartonella vinsonii* subsp. *berkhoffii*, or both organisms; however, individual case reports describe infection with *B. bovis*, *B. clarridgeiae*, *B. elizabethae*, *B. quintana*, and *B. washoensis*. Our diagnostic laboratory has also found molecular evidence that supports infection with as yet uncharacterized *Bartonella* spp. in dogs. The spectrum of disease associated with *Bartonella* infection in dogs and most other animal species is currently unknown. *Bartonella vinsonii* subsp. *berkhoffii* is an important cause of endocarditis in dogs.[9-12] Although unpublished, *B. henselae* is also a frequent cause of endocarditis in dogs. *Bartonella* endocarditis occurs in large-breed dogs with a high predilection for aortic valve involvement. In some dogs, intermittent lameness, bone pain, epistaxis, or fever of unknown origin precede the diagnosis of endocarditis by several months, whereas other dogs will present with an acute history of cardiopulmonary decompensation. Cardiac arrhythmias, secondary to myocarditis, can be detected in dogs lacking echocardiographic evidence of endocarditis. *Bartonella* endocarditis has been reported in dogs and human patients after receiving immunosuppressive doses of corticosteroids for a presumptive diagnosis of systemic lupus erythematosus (SLE) or Wegner's granulomatosis, respectively. Therefore occult *Bartonella* infection in conjunction with drug-induced immunosuppression may contribute to the development of endocarditis in both dogs and people. Infection with *B. henselae* or *B. vinsonii* subsp. *berkhoffii* alone or in conjunction with *Ehrlichia canis* and *Leishmania infantum* may cause epistaxis in dogs.[13,14] Based on serologic and molecular evidence, *B. vinsonii* subsp. *berkhoffii*, *B. henselae*, or other *Bartonella* species appear to contribute to the development of dermatologic lesions indicative of a cutaneous vasculitis, panniculitis, anterior uveitis, polyarthritis, meningoencephalitis, immune-mediated thrombocytopenia (ITP) or immune-mediated hemolytic anemia (IMHA) and splenomegaly in dogs.[15-19] Experimentally, infection with *B. vinsonii* subsp. *berkhoffii* induces several alterations in immune regulation and suppresses immune function. During a 149-day study, following experimental inoculation of specific pathogen–free dogs with culture-grown *B. vinsonii* subsp. *berkhoffii*, there was sustained suppression of peripheral blood CD8+ lymphocytes, accompanied by an altered cell surface phenotype and an increase in CD4+ lymphocytes in the peripheral lymph nodes.[20] Therefore, infection with *B. vinsonii* subsp. *berkhoffii* could induce a degree of chronic immunosuppression that might predispose to secondary infections with viruses or other bacteria. In addition, immunosuppression induced by infection could potentially result in a wide array of clinical manifestations in dogs naturally infected with *Bartonella* species. Antinuclear antibodies have been detected in the serum of dogs infected with *B. vinsonii* subsp. *berkhoffii*, *Ehrlichia canis*, or in dogs coinfected with both organisms, which appears to be a relatively common occurrence depending upon geographic location.[21] Although detection of ITP, IMHA, and polyarthritis in conjunction with finding antinuclear antibodies is consistent with a diagnosis of SLE, occult *Bartonella* infection should be ruled out prior to administration of immunosuppressive drug therapy.

Bartonella henselae, *B. vinsonii* subsp. *berkhoffii*, and *B. clarridgeiae* have all been implicated in dogs with granulomatous inflammation involving the lymph nodes, nasal nodules, liver, or in association with disseminated granulomatous lesions.[22-25] Unfortunately, no systematic review of tissues from dogs with granulomatous inflammation has been performed to determine the frequency of infection with *Bartonella* spp. In a study designed to assay the presence of vector-borne organisms in dogs with lymphoma, *Anaplasma* and *Ehrlichia* species DNA was not detected, whereas *Bartonella henselae*, *B. vinsonii* subsp. *berkhoffii*, *B. elizabethae*, and *B. quintana* DNA was detected in blood and lymph node aspiration samples from Golden Retrievers with lymphoma and in healthy Golden Retriever control dogs.[26] Molecular prevalence of *Bartonella* spp. infection was 18% in both study populations, and dogs receiving routine acaricides for tick prevention were less likely to be infected with a *Bartonella* spp. Whether the Golden Retriever breed is genetically predisposed to develop infection with a *Bartonella* spp. or whether sequential evaluation of dogs over time would support a role for *Bartonella* infection in the pathogenesis of lymphoma is unknown. In the Golden Retriever study,[26] *Bartonella* DNA could be amplified more often from lymph node aspirates (lymphoma or healthy dog lymph nodes) as compared to blood samples from the same dog, obtained at the same time.

These data suggest that *Bartonella* spp. can induce lymphatic as well as intravascular infection in dogs, which deserves additional research consideration. Recently, we detected infection with *B. henselae*, *B. vinsonii* subsp. *berkhoffii*, or both organisms in five dogs ranging in age from 3 to 12 years that were diagnosed with pleural, pericardial (restrictive pericarditis) and/or abdominal effusions. Clinical signs were generally nonspecific and included lethargy, fever, vomiting, diarrhea, abdominal distention, lameness, and cervical pain. Based upon these and other case experiences, *Bartonella* lymphatic infection could potentially lead to obstruction of lymph flow, which might also contribute to the development of transudates or subcutaneous edema in dogs infected with a *Bartonella* species. Despite isolation or molecular detection of *B. henselae* and *B. vinsonii* subsp. *berkhoffii* in dogs with effusive disease, no direct cause and effect association can be implicated from small cohorts of sick dogs. However, these results may prove to be clinically relevant since most idiopathic effusions obtained from dogs are generally considered aseptic based upon conventional microbiologic culture approaches, approaches that would not result in the detection of a *Bartonella* sp. Similarly, the pathogenesis of pericardial effusions is frequently elusive and support for an immune-mediated etiology is lacking.[27,28]

From a clinical perspective, *Bartonella* spp. are important emerging pathogens that possess the somewhat unique ability to invade erythrocytes, vascular endothelial cells, and cells within the lymphatic system. As intravascular organisms, these bacteria can be disseminated throughout all of the tissues in the body, which can result in disease in a single organ (encephalitis) or multiple organs (systemic granulomatous inflammation). As with other infectious diseases, genetics, nutrition, toxin exposure, and the immunocompetence of the dog influence disease expression. Based upon the isolation of *B. henselae* and *B. vinsonii* subsp. *berkhoffii* from humans with neurologic and neurocognitive abnormalities,[7,8] the role of *Bartonella* infection in dogs with behavioral abnormalities, geriatric neurocognitive disorders, and seizures should be further evaluated.[15]

SEROPREVALENCE

Based on serologic studies, *Bartonella* infection is more frequent in rural dogs in North America and in stray dogs in subtropical regions.[29-31] Seroprevalence was determined in 1920 sick dogs from North Carolina or surrounding states that were evaluated at a veterinary teaching hospital.[29] Using a reciprocal titer of >64, 3.6% of the dogs had antibodies to *B. vinsonii* subsp. *berkhoffii*. Risk factors that could be associated with seroreactivity included: heavy tick exposure (odds ratio [OR] 14.2), cattle exposure (OR 9.3), rural versus urban environment (OR 7.1), and heavy flea exposure (OR 5.6). Exposure to *B. vinsonii* subsp. *berkhoffii* was more frequent in dogs from rural environments that were allowed to roam and were likely to have a history of heavy tick infestation.[29,31] Using sera from dogs experimentally infected with *R. rickettsii* or *Ehrlichia canis*, there was no cross reactivity to *B. vinsonii* subsp. *berkhoffii* antigens. However, several studies using serum samples derived from dogs naturally infected with *E. canis* or *B. canis* have detected a high prevalence (30% to 89%) of seroreactivity to *B. vinsonii* subsp. *berkhoffii* antigens.[29,31,32] As both *E. canis* and *B. canis* are transmitted by *Rhipicephalus sanguineous*, this tick may be also involved in the transmission of *B. vinsonii* subsp. *berkhoffii*.[32] The possibility of tick transmission was further supported by studies from California that found a high prevalence of *B. vinsonii* subsp. *berkhoffii* bacteremia in coyotes and DNA of the organism in questing *Ixodes pacificus* in the same region.[33,34] As coyotes have spread across much of North America in recent years, these animals may serve as a major reservoir for tick transmission and potentially could transmit *B. vinsonii* subsp. *berkhoffii* to pets or humans via bites or scratches. Numerous laboratories around the world have amplified *Bartonella* spp. DNA from ticks, but studies to confirm vector competence are lacking.[32] Based upon serologic and molecular evidence *B. vinsonii* subsp. *berkhoffii* has been reported from Brazil, Canada, China, Israel, Morocco, Spain, Thailand, and the United States.[35,36] These data suggest that *B. vinsonii* subsp. *berkhoffii* is distributed throughout the world, with substantial regional differences in seroprevalence.

Based upon preliminary experimental studies, *B. henselae* was not initially considered a pathogenic species in dogs. Subsequently, the organism was sequenced from the liver of a dog with peliosis hepatis and from the blood of dogs that were generally receiving immunosuppressive drug therapy for the treatment of ITP, IMHA, or meningitis.[37,38] Using a novel culture platform described below, we have detected more dogs infected with *B. henselae* than infected with *B. vinsonii* subsp. *berkhoffii*. Serologic studies also support more frequent exposure to *B. henselae* than to *B. vinsonii* subsp. *berkhoffii*. Studies from Hawaii, the United Kingdom, and Japan identified *B. henselae* seroprevalences of 6.5%, 3.0% and 7.7%, respectively. In North Carolina, the seroprevalence in healthy dogs was 10% and in sick dogs 27% suggesting frequent exposure to *B. henselae* in the southeastern United States.[39] For reasons that remain unclear, there was a statistical association between *Rickettsia rickettsii* and *B. henselae* antibodies in dogs from this region.[39] As spotted fever group rickettsiae are not known to cause chronic disease, dogs with chronic illness and *R. rickettsii* seroreactivity should be screened for *B. henselae* infection. In contrast to the southeastern United States, the seroprevalence to both *B. henselae* and *B. vinsonii* subsp. *berkhoffii* was less than 2% in dogs from Brazil.[35]

Although seemingly less frequent, dogs can be infected with other *Bartonella* spp. for which the cat, the rat, and squirrels serve as reservoir hosts. *Bartonella clarridgeiae* DNA has been amplified and sequenced from the liver of a Doberman Pinscher with copper storage disease and from the aortic valve of a dog with vegetative valvular endocarditis.[23,40] *Bartonella elizabethae*, a species that infects rodents, was PCR-amplified and sequenced from an EDTA blood sample obtained from a dog that had experienced chronic weight loss culminating in sudden unexplained death.[38] *Bartonella washoensis*, for which the Western ground squirrel is the reservoir host, was sequenced from a dog with endocarditis. Recently, *Bartonella quintana* has been isolated from the blood or heart valves of dogs with endocarditis from the United States and New Zealand.[41] These observations indicate that, although presumably infrequent, *Bartonella* spp. that frequently infect cats or rodents and are known to be transmitted by fleas among reservoir hosts may infect dogs and cause serious disease manifestations such as endocarditis or

myocarditis. Circumstantial case-based evidence suggests that cats may transmit *Bartonella* species to dogs by way of a scratch or bite, as occurs with human cat scratch disease.

DIAGNOSTIC CONSIDERATIONS

Clinical manifestations of bartonellosis are frequently nonspecific and may include insidious weight loss, unexplained lethargy or inactivity, reluctance to move (polyarthritis), or progressive neurologic disease, including seizures and partial paralysis. Most infected dogs have no hematologic abnormalities. In one study, thrombocytopenia, anemia, which can be immune-mediated, and neutrophilic leukocytosis were the most commonly detected hematologic abnormalities in dogs that were *B. vinsonii* subsp. *berkhoffii*–seroreactive.[15] Monocytosis and eosinophilia also occur in approximately one third of the *B. vinsonii*-infected dogs. Persistent neutropenia has been documented in some *B. henselae*–infected dogs.

Historically, PCR amplification of DNA directly from patient samples and bacterial isolation approaches have not been sensitive enough to confirm a diagnosis of *Bartonella* infection in dogs or immunocompetent human beings. Therefore, we developed a novel insect cell culture–based isolation medium (*Bartonella* alpha-Proteobacteria growth medium [BAPGM]) that has greatly improved the isolation or molecular detection of *Bartonella* spp. in dog and human blood samples.[7,8,42,43] Because of the low level of circulating *Bartonella* organisms in dog and human blood samples, a BAPGM preenrichment step is frequently required to increase organism numbers to levels detectable by PCR. The BAPGM diagnostic approach used in our laboratory is depicted in Figure 204-1.

Using this approach, blood, *Bartonella* spp. have been successfully cultured from cerebrospinal fluid, aqueous fluid, joint fluid, and thoracic and abdominal effusions. Since treatment requires prolonged administration of expensive antibiotics that must achieve high intracellular concentrations to be effective, confirming active infection by culture and PCR is highly recommended. In addition, identification of the *B. vinsonii* subsp. *berkhoffii* genotype may ultimately prove to be of epidemiologic and therapeutic importance.[11,12,44] Unfortu-

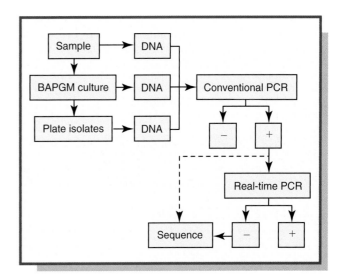

Figure 204-1 *Bartonella* alpha-Proteobacteria growth medium (*BAPGM*) enrichment culture approach for the molecular detection and isolation of *Bartonella* species. *PCR*, Polymerase chain reaction.

nately, approximately half of the dogs tested in our laboratory with positive culture or PCR results do not have detectable antibodies by indirect fluorescent antibody (IFA) testing; therefore the sensitivity of current serologic tests is poor.[26,42,43,45] As *B. vinsonii* subsp. *berkhoffii* seroprevalence is low (<4%) in sick dog populations in endemic regions and even lower in nonendemic regions, detection of antibodies in a sick dog provides strong clinical evidence for prior exposure and potentially active infection. For this reason, treatment of a *B. vinsonii* subsp. *berkhoffii* seroreactive dog would be recommended. An IFA titer of 1:64 or greater is considered indicative of prior exposure to or active infection with *B. vinsonii* subsp. *berkhoffii*. Due to the high *B. henselae* seroprevalence in healthy dogs, treating based solely upon the detection of antibodies to this organism may not be warranted, unless active infection can be demonstrated by culture or PCR testing. Serologic testing against other *Bartonella* spp. antigens, such as those in rodent species, may prove to be of clinical utility in the future.

TREATMENT

To date, an optimal protocol has not been established for the treatment of *Bartonella* infections in cats, dogs, or people.[46,47] Regardless of the antibiotic that is used therapeutically, a long duration of antibiotic administration (4 to 6 weeks) may be necessary to eliminate the infection. Macrolides (azithromycin, clarithromycin) most probably represent the oral antibiotic class of choice for treating *Bartonella* infections.[44,45] Fluoroquinolones alone, or in combination with amoxicillin, have also elicited a positive therapeutic response in dogs, which was accompanied by a progressive decrease in *B. vinsonii* antibody titers.[15] In our experience, doxycycline is not an effective treatment for *B. henselae* and does not always eliminate *B. vinsonii* subsp. *berkhoffii*.[13] Some dogs appear to respond to doxycycline, but relapse with continued administration or when antibiotic administration is stopped. Data from cats experimentally or naturally infected with *B. henselae* or *B. clarridgeiae* indicates that a high dose of doxycycline (10 mg/kg every 12 hours) for 4 to 6 weeks may be necessary to eliminate *Bartonella* infection in cats, dogs, or other animal species.[48] Retrospective analysis of the treatment of human *Bartonella* endocarditis identified a more favorable outcome, if an aminoglycoside was prescribed for a minimum of 2 weeks.[49] In those situations in which *Bartonella* infection poses serious risk in dogs, such as endocarditis, myocarditis, or meningoencephalitis, use of an aminoglycoside may be warranted. Recently, we have identified dogs and people who have failed extended courses of azithromycin. Macrolide resistance has been induced experimentally in *B. henselae* and may be induced by prior or prolonged administration of antibiotics.[50]

PREVENTION

Increasingly, veterinarians play an important role in advising the public as to the epidemiologic and zoonotic implications of various vector-borne pathogens. Both domestic and nondomestic animals frequently serve as the primary reservoir for *Bartonella* species and arthropod vectors, including biting flies, fleas, lice, sandflies, and ticks, facilitate transmission among reservoir hosts and potentially to nonreservoir hosts, such as dogs and human beings.[1,2] Therefore, minimizing or eliminating exposure to fleas and other potential vectors is perhaps of greater public health importance today than during any previous time in history. When rigorous flea and tick control measures are instituted, it is highly probable that transmission of *Bartonella* species to pets will be greatly reduced or eliminated.

PUBLIC HEALTH CONSIDERATIONS

Animal contact, which in many instances occurs to a wide spectrum of domestic and wild animal species, is an obvious consequence of the daily activities of veterinarians, veterinary technicians, animal health researchers, ranchers, wildlife biologists, and many other individuals in our society. Recently, *B. henselae* or *B. vinsonii* subsp. *berkhoffii* infection has been documented in our laboratory in blood samples from people with extensive arthropod and animal contact.[7,8] The potential clinical relevance of detecting *Bartonella* spp. in the blood of people with occupational animal contact remains to be determined. Despite frequent occupational exposure to animals, it is important to acknowledge that most veterinary professionals, ranchers, and wildlife biologists participate in a diversity of outdoor recreational and occupational activities that also increase the opportunity for *Bartonella* transmission by biting arthropods. Therefore the source of infection in these individuals cannot be clearly established. Also recently, our research group has amplified and sequenced four *Bartonella* species from saliva samples obtained from healthy or sick dogs.[45] Prospective human studies are needed to determine the variability in duration of infection, rates of infection among various human patient populations, bite wounds as a mode of *Bartonella* transmission to people, and the clinical relevance of long-term intravascular infection with these bacteria.

REFERENCES

The reference list can be found on the companion Expert Consult Web site at *www.expertconsult.com*.

CHAPTER 205

Feline *Bartonella*

Lynn F. Guptill

*B*artonella spp. are small, vector-transmitted gram-negative bacteria. Most *Bartonella* species appear to be highly adapted to individual mammalian reservoir hosts, where they often cause a long-term bacteremia in clinically normal animals.[1,2] The mechanisms that facilitate persistent

Bartonella bacteremia in mammals are not yet completely understood. Intracellular localization, frequent genetic rearrangements, and alteration of outer membrane proteins may be effective strategies for immune system evasion and therefore bacterial persistence.[1-5] Colonization of erythrocytes may facilitate efficient vector transmission and potentially contribute to decreased antimicrobial efficacy.[6] *Bartonella* species are also reported to colonize vascular endothelial cells.

The following discussion of feline bartonellosis focuses on *B. henselae*, the *Bartonella* species to date most commonly isolated from domestic cats. Other species that naturally infect cats, *Bartonella clarridgeae*, *B. koehlerae*, *B. bovis*, and *B. quintana*, will also be discussed.

EPIDEMIOLOGY

Since the first recognition of feline *B. henselae* infection in 1992, serologic and blood culture data indicate that exposure to *Bartonella* spp., most frequently *B. henselae*, is prevalent among cats in the United States and throughout most temperate regions of the world.[7] There is a higher prevalence in areas with warmer temperature and higher humidity, in feral cats, and in those infested with fleas. Older cats are more likely to be seropositive, and younger cats are more likely to be bacteremic.[8-13] *B. henselae* bacteremia affects approximately 5% to 40% of domestic cats in the United States depending on geographic location.[9,11,14-16] In one cat colony, a prevalence of over 90% was reported.[17] *B. clarridgeae* infections were reported to account for approximately 10% of cats with *Bartonella* bacteremia evaluated in the United States, and 16% to 31% of cats with *Bartonella* bacteremia in France and the Philippines.[18,19] *Bartonella koehlerae*, *B. bovis*, and *B. quintana* have been isolated or detected by polymerase chain reaction (PCR) in a few healthy domestic cats each.[20-24] Domestic cats are considered the primary reservoir and vector for human infections with *B. henselae*, and cats are likely also the reservoir for *B. clarridgeae*. Cattle appear to be the reservoir for *B. bovis*. The reservoir for *B. koehlerae* is unknown. In France, molecular methods have detected *B. quintana*, *B. koehlerae*, *B. henselae*, and *B. clarridgeae* in cat fleas, along with rickettsial pathogens.[25,26] While this may suggest flea involvement in transmission of all of these *Bartonella* species, the fleas may have just fed on an infected host. Competence for transmission for many *Bartonella* species by fleas has not yet been verified. Wild felids, including panthers, bobcats, mountain lions, pumas, African lions, and cheetahs, are also exposed to *Bartonella* species.[27-30]

There are multiple genetically diverse strains of *B. henselae*. Two recognized 16S rRNA types of *B. henselae* exist; there are at least two subgroups within each type.[31,32] Cats can be coinfected with *B. henselae* 16S rRNA types I and II and coinfected with *B. henselae* and *B. clarridgeae* and other pathogens.[33] There are regional differences in prevalence of infection of cats with different rRNA types of *B. henselae*.[14,18,34,35] Other molecular methods also show remarkable molecular diversity among *Bartonella* isolates.[5,36-43] There is evidence of genomic variation in *B. henselae* during the course of infection in cats.[5,44] Such variation may enhance the ability of *B. henselae* to persist in infected cats for prolonged periods. Genetic variation makes vaccine development difficult though it is useful in epidemiologic studies and may also be useful in furthering the understanding of the pathogenicity of various *Bartonella* isolates.[45]

PATHOGENESIS

Bartonella henselae is believed to be naturally transmitted among cats by cat fleas *(Ctenocephalides felis felis)*. *B. henselae* was transmitted among cats by transferring fleas fed on naturally infected cats to specific pathogen–free (SPF) cats and by intradermal (ID) inoculation of excrement collected from fleas fed on *B. henselae*–infected cats.[47-49] Transmission via flea saliva has not been documented.[47] Ticks may have a role in transmission; *B. henselae* and other *Bartonella* spp. were detected by PCR in questing ticks.[50-52] Transstadial transmission of *B. henselae* was recently demonstrated in *Ixodes ricinus* ticks and these ticks appear to be competent vectors for *B. henselae*. Ticks have been proposed as the vectors for transmission of some *Bartonella* infections in cats, human beings, dogs, and other mammalian hosts.[53-57]

Cats were experimentally infected with *B. henselae* and *B. clarridgeae* through IV or IM inoculation with infected cat blood, and by intravenous, subcutaneous, ID, or oral routes of inoculation with plate-grown bacteria, but not when cats were injected with urine of bacteremic cats.[58-64] *Bartonella henselae* transmission has not occurred when infected cats cohabit with uninfected cats in a flea-free environment, indicating that transmission among cats does not occur through cat bites, scratches, grooming, or sharing of food dishes and litterboxes. Transmission also did not occur between bacteremic female cats and males during mating, or to the kittens of infected females either during gestation or in the neonatal period, also in flea-free environments.[58,61,65]

There are periods when bacteria cannot be detected by blood culture or by PCR testing in cats with chronic relapsing bacteremia due to *B. henselae* and *B. clarridgeae*. Experimentally infected cats maintained relapsing *B. henselae* or *B. clarridgeae* bacteremia for as long as 454 days.[59] Naturally infected cats maintained recurrent bacteremia for up to 3 years; however, reinfection via fleas of cats living in private homes likely occurred.[66,67]

A lack of heterologous protection against reinfection was demonstrated in some cats previously infected with *Bartonella*. Cats previously infected with *B. henselae* 16S rRNA type II were susceptible to infection with *B. henselae* 16S rRNA type I.[68] Cats infected with *B. henselae* type I or II were susceptible to challenge infection with *B. clarridgeae*, and cats infected with *B. koehlerae* or *B. clarridgeae* were susceptible to challenge infection with *B. henselae* type I or type II. In contrast, cats infected with *B. henselae* type I were partially or completely protected against challenge infection with *B. henselae* type II.[69] Cats can become immune to challenge with homologous strains of the organism. The level of bacteremia and degree of susceptibility to reinfection following challenge inoculation is likely to vary with strain as well as with species of *Bartonella*.[68]

The exact localization of *Bartonella* in cats has not been completely determined. *Bartonellae* have been detected within erythrocytes of naturally infected cats and in vitro.[70] *Bartonella* may also localize within vascular endothelial cells of infected cats as has been suggested for rodents.[71]

CLINICAL FINDINGS

Existing data indicate that few cats naturally infected with *Bartonella* have clinical signs. Some cats developed fever following elective surgical procedures.[72] Uveitis may be a manifestation of natural *Bartonella* infection.[73] *Bartonella henselae* type I was associated with fatal blood culture–negative vegetative aortic valve endocarditis in a naturally infected cat.[74]

Whether *Bartonella* spp. contribute to previously described instances of argyrophilic bacteria in lymph nodes of cats with persistent lymphadenomegaly or to peliosis hepatis in cats is unknown.[75,76]

Naturally infected cats may have clinical signs that owners do not observe. Severity of clinical signs in cats experimentally infected with *B. henselae* was usually mild and varied with the strain of *B. henselae* used for inoculation. Cats inoculated ID developed areas of induration or abscesses at inoculation sites between approximately 2 days and 3 to 4 weeks after inoculation, from some of which pure cultures of *B. henselae* were obtained (Figure 205-1).[59,61,63,64,77]

Other transient clinical findings in many experimentally infected cats included generalized or localized peripheral lymphadenomegaly (lasting for about 6 weeks following inoculation), and short periods of fever (>39.4° C [103° F]) during the first 48 to 96 hours following inoculation and again at approximately 2 weeks following inoculation. There were mild neurologic signs (nystagmus, whole body tremors, focal motor seizures, either decreased or exaggerated responses to external stimuli, behavior changes), and epaxial muscle pain in a few experimentally inoculated cats. Some cats were lethargic and anorexic during febrile periods.[59-61,63,64] Reproductive failure occurred in some cats experimentally infected with *B. henselae*.[65] Cats experimentally infected with *B. koehlerae* exhibited no clinical signs.[78]

A potential causative role of *Bartonella* spp. in chronic diseases of cats has been proposed because *Bartonella* bacteremia is prolonged. For example, results of a study in Japan suggested that coinfection of cats with *B. henselae* and feline immunodeficiency virus was more likely to cause gingivitis or lymphadenomegaly than either infection alone.[79] Results of a Swiss study suggested possible associations between *B. henselae* seropositivity and stomatitis and various urinary tract disorders.[80] Both studies obtained serum and historical information about cat health from practicing veterinarians. Because of the high prevalence of *Bartonella* exposure in the domestic cat population, extensive, carefully controlled epidemiologic investigations are needed to determine whether particular clinical conditions are associated with *B. henselae* infections in cats. Some small epidemiologic studies have evaluated the association between *Bartonella* exposure and clinical conditions such as neurologic disease, stomatitis, uveitis, and fever. None of these studies showed a statistically significant association of *Bartonella* with any of the aforementioned conditions in cats.[81-84]

DIAGNOSIS

Clinical conditions that have been proposed to be attributable to feline bartonellosis are shared by conditions resulting from many other etiologies; therefore, determining which cats are likely to have *Bartonella* infections is difficult. In addition to

the potential need to test for *Bartonella* infections in sick cats, veterinarians will be asked to test healthy pet cats belonging to clients with *Bartonella*-related illnesses, or to screen healthy cats that are being considered as pets for people considered most susceptible to *Bartonella* infections (see Public Health).

Clinical Laboratory Findings and Pathologic Findings

Most experimentally infected cats had no abnormalities on complete blood counts, serum biochemical tests, or urine analysis. Some cats had transient anemia early in the course of infection, and some had persistent eosinophilia.[59] Mature neutrophilia occurred in some cats during periods of skin inflammation.[61]

Finding *B. henselae* in erythrocytes of infected cats has not been an effective means of detection using conventional staining methods. Confocal microscopy and special staining has been used. Intraerythrocytic location of *B. henselae*, *B. clarridgeiae*, and *B. koehlerae* have been documented in cats using fluorescence detection methods.[85,86]

Acutely and chronically infected cats had hyperplasia of lymphoid organs, small foci of lymphocytic, pyogranulomatous, or neutrophilic inflammation in multiple tissues (lung, liver, spleen, kidney, heart), or small foci of necrosis in the liver (Figures 205-2 and 205-3).[59,61]

Bacterial Isolation

A positive blood culture result, or culture of other tissue, is the most reliable test for definitive diagnosis of active *Bartonella* infection. However, because of the relapsing nature of *Bartonella* bacteremia in cats, culture is not always a sensitive diagnostic tool. Blood culture is indicated for sick cats whose history and clinical presentation suggest possible *Bartonella* infection, or when a client's physician requires such testing of pet cats. Blood for culture should be obtained using sterile technique, and the blood placed in lysis centrifugation blood culture tubes (Isolator tubes, Wampole, Cranbury, N.J.) or EDTA-containing tubes. If blood is collected into EDTA tubes, the blood should be chilled or frozen during shipment, and ideally, plastic EDTA tubes should be used.[87,88] Blood should be sent to laboratories familiar with the culture of these fastidious organisms, and the laboratories contacted for specific instructions regarding sample collection and submission.

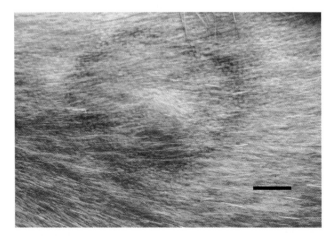

Figure 205-1 Postinoculation abscess 20 days after intradermal inoculation of *Bartonella henselae* in a cat. The size of the papule increased from the time of inoculation and only *B. henselae* was isolated from bacterial culture of an aspirate. Bar = 1 cm. (From Greene CE: Infectious diseases of the dog and cat, ed 3, St Louis, 2006, Saunders.)

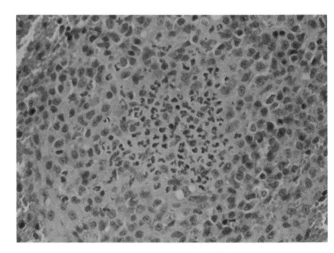

Figure 205-2 Histologic section of feline spleen showing a microabscess 14 days following inoculation with *Bartonella henselae* (H&E stain, ×400). (From Greene CE: Infectious diseases of the dog and cat, ed 3, St Louis, 2006, Saunders.)

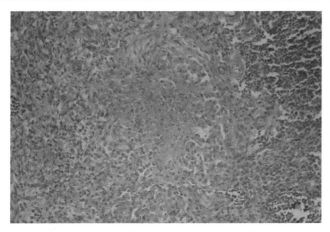

Figure 205-3 Focus of inflammation in cardiac muscle of a cat infected with *Bartonella henselae*, days following inoculation (H&E stain, ×400). (From Greene CE: Infectious diseases of the dog and cat, ed 3, St Louis, 2006, Saunders.)

Serologic Testing

Measuring serum antibodies has limited value for determining whether an ill cat has an active *Bartonella* infection but is useful for epidemiologic surveys. Serologic tests routinely overestimate the number of *Bartonella*-infected cats. Serum IgG antibodies persist in experimentally infected cats for prolonged periods. How long antibodies persist following clearance of infection is not known. Indirect fluorescent antibody (FA), enzyme immunoassay (EIA), and Western blot tests are available. Because of the genetic diversity of *Bartonella* organisms, infections with some strains or species of *Bartonella* may be missed using any method, depending on the antigen preparations used.[89,90] The positive predictive value (PPV) of FA or EIA (IgG) serologic tests for bacteremia is only 39% to 46%. The utility of a negative serologic result is greater, as the negative predictive value for these tests for bacteremia or presence of DNA in cat blood is high at 87% to 97%.[9,14,34,35,84] Nevertheless, some seronegative, bacteremic cats exist.[9,14,91] No cutoff values allowing use of serologic testing to determine whether a cat is currently infected with *Bartonella* have been established.[69]

The use of Western blot tests has been advocated for serodiagnosis of feline *B. henselae* infections, but the diagnostic accuracy of Western blot tests awaits further investigation. In human medicine, variability in Western blot testing remains problematic. Serologic responses of people as evaluated by immunoblot vary among patients.[90,92] Results of one study in cats indicated no differences in Western blot patterns of cats evaluated over the course of infection.[59] Results of another study indicated that antibodies in sera of infected cats reacted with an increasing number of bands of polyacrylamide gel-separated proteins over the course of infection.[93] In a more recent report of a study of naturally infected cats, PPV of a Western blot test for presence of *Bartonella* DNA in cat blood was reported to be 18.8%.[84]

Nucleic Acid Detection

Standard PCR testing for the presence of *Bartonella* DNA is often no more sensitive than blood culture for detection of active *Bartonella* infection, and detecting DNA does not always equate to detection of living organisms. Nested PCR testing may increase sensitivity for detection of *Bartonella* DNA in cat blood.[94] Real-time PCR testing may also improve sensitivity. Additional benefits of PCR testing are that the species and/or strain of *Bartonella* may be identified by sequencing of the reaction product, and results of PCR testing are available more quickly than those of blood culture. Blood samples for PCR testing should be obtained using sterile technique. Care must be taken in collection and sample processing to avoid sample contamination and DNA degradation. Laboratories experienced in molecular diagnostics should be used and should be contacted for submission guidelines.

THERAPY

Documenting clearance of *Bartonella* infections through antibiotic treatment is difficult due to the prolonged relapsing bacteremia of most infected cats. No regimen of antibiotic treatment has been proven effective, in controlled studies with long-term follow-up, for definitively eliminating *Bartonella* infections in cats.[77,95-97] Enrofloxacin (5.4 to 7.6 mg/kg, given PO every 12 hours) for 14 or 28 days appeared to clear *B. henselae* or *B. clarridgeae* infection in 4 of 6 or 5 of 7 treated cats, respectively, that were followed for 12 weeks after treatment.[96] However, enrofloxacin causes retinal degeneration in cats, and use of doses of greater than 5 mg/kg per day is contraindicated.[98] Doxycycline (4 to 12 mg/kg, given PO, every 12 hours) cleared bacteremia in only 1 of 6 cats treated for 14 days and 1 of 2 cats treated for 28 days.[96] Antibiotics tested in other studies, including erythromycin, amoxicillin, amoxicillin-clavulanate, and tetracycline, rapidly decreased the level of bacteremia in infected cats. However, in one study, treated and untreated cats became blood-culture negative after the same period of time, making proof of efficacy of antibiotics difficult. In some studies, cats were not followed for more than 8 weeks after treatment, thereby making it difficult to assess drug efficacy due to the possibility of chronic relapsing bacteremia in those cats.[77,97] In some experimental infections, an effective doxycycline dose in cats has reportedly been a minimum of 10 mg/kg given twice daily (CE Greene, personal communication), which is a higher dose than that used in some studies. Azithromycin has been recommended for treatment of infected cats, but data from controlled efficacy studies with long-term follow-up are lacking. Azithromycin appears to have important immunomodulatory and antiinflammatory properties in addition to a broad antimicrobial spectrum of activity.[99-102] These properties may make it difficult to determine whether beneficial effects reported following azithromycin treatment of cats are a result of anti-*Bartonella* activity or instead are a result of azithromycin's other properties, of the antimicrobial action of azithromycin on other bacteria, or of some combination of all of these.

Routine treatment with antibiotics may induce resistant strains; therefore, treatment should be reserved for use only in *Bartonella*-positive cats showing clinical signs. Although treatment reportedly decreases the level of bacteremia in cats, there is no concrete evidence that treatment of the cat will decrease the probability of transmission of *Bartonella* infection to an owner. Client education regarding the uncertainty of treatment efficacy, the need for prolonged follow-up, and the possibility of reinfection following treatment is necessary. The importance of flea control and other means of preventing transmission (see Prevention) should be emphasized. The American Association of Feline Practitioners Panel Report on feline *Bartonella* infections is a good resource for questions regarding feline bartonellosis diagnosis, treatment, and prevention.[103]

PREVENTION

Prevention of *Bartonella* infections in cats is best accomplished by avoiding exposure to infected animals and fleas. Since *B.*

henselae and *B. clarridgeae* have been transmitted through inoculation of infected cat blood, cats should not receive blood transfusions from cats of unknown *Bartonella* status or cats that are seropositive for *Bartonella*.[60,104] A vaccine to prevent *Bartonella* infection in cats is not available. Flea and tick control programs are of the utmost importance in preventing *Bartonella* infection.

PUBLIC HEALTH

Several *Bartonella* species or subspecies are considered zoonotic or likely zoonotic, including *B. quintana*, *B. bacilliformis*, *B. henselae*, *B. clarridgeae*, *B. koehlerae*, *B. vinsonii* subsp. *berkhoffii*, *B. vinsonii* subsp. *arupensis*, *B. grahamii*, *B. elizabethae*, *Candidatus* B. washoensis, and *B. rochalimae*.[105] Cats are the reservoir and vector for transmission of *B. henselae* and possibly *B. clarridgeae* to people. The role of arthropods in direct transmission of *Bartonella* to people is not certain. Transmission of *B. henselae* from cats to people is believed to occur through contamination of cat scratches with flea excrement. Transmission may also occur through cat bites if cat blood or flea excrement contaminate the bite site.[48,49]

Cat owners should be informed of the current understanding regarding how cats acquire *Bartonella* infections, and how these infections may be transmitted to people, including the possibility of transmission by ticks, and the association of flea infestation with transmission.

Bartonella spp. cause a wide variety of clinical syndromes in people: for example, cat scratch disease (typical and atypical forms, including encephalopathies in children); bacillary angiomatosis and peliosis; parenchymal bacillary peliosis; relapsing fever with bacteremia; endocarditis; optic neuritis; pulmonary, hepatic, and splenic granulomas; and osteomyelitis.[106-108] Immunocompetent individuals usually have more localized infections, whereas infections in immunocompromised individuals may more often be systemic and can be fatal. Diagnosis in people is usually made by serologic testing or PCR because of the low level or absence of bacteremia in immunocompetent hosts.

Commonsense precautions for avoiding transmission of *Bartonella* spp. from pets to people include ongoing flea and tick control, avoiding interactions that result in scratches or bites, thoroughly washing bite or scratch wounds, seeking medical attention when necessary, and acquiring new pets of known good health status that are and have been ectoparasite free. Stray or impounded cats less than 1 year old are most likely to be bacteremic. There is no evidence that declawing cats decreases the probability of transmission of *B. henselae* between cats and human beings. The United States Public Health Service/Infectious Diseases Society of America (USPHS/IDSA) Guidelines for Preventing Opportunistic Infections Among HIV-Infected Persons recommends the following when acquiring a new cat: adopt a cat older than 1 year of age that is in good health, avoid rough play with cats, maintain flea control, wash any cat-associated wounds promptly, and do not allow a cat to lick wounds or cuts. The USPHS/IDSA Guidelines note that there is no evidence to indicate any benefit to cats or their owners from routine culture or serologic testing of cats for *Bartonella* infections.[109]

SUMMARY

A great deal has been learned about feline *Bartonella* infections recently, and a lot more discovery lies ahead. A large proportion of domestic cats harbor persistent *Bartonella* spp. infections. Ongoing and future studies will help to ascertain what the possible ramifications of chronic *Bartonella* bacteremia may be for feline health. Veterinarians should be aware of the high prevalence of feline *Bartonella* bacteremia and carefully consider their approach to evaluating cats for possible *Bartonella*-related clinical conditions. Based on current knowledge, healthy cats should not be routinely tested for *Bartonella*, and antibiotic treatment should not be recommended for healthy cats. When ill cats are treated, treatment should always be accompanied by comprehensive vector control measures and client education. Client education should emphasize the role of fleas in *Bartonella* transmission and the importance of vector control programs in preventing transmission. It should also emphasize other potential avenues for transmission and address the potential risks associated with antibiotic treatment, the likelihood of reinfection of a cat following antibiotic treatment, and the zoonotic potential of *Bartonella*.

REFERENCES

The reference list can be found on the companion Expert Consult Web site at *www.expertconsult.com*.

VECTOR BORNE

CHAPTER 206

Ehrlichia, Anaplasmosis, Rocky Mountain Spotted Fever, and Neorickettsial Infection

Jane E. Sykes

GENERAL CONSIDERATIONS

Canine ehrlichiosis is caused by the intracellular, gram-negative, bacteria *Ehrlichia canis*, *Ehrlichia ewingii*, and *Ehrlichia chaffeensis*. An organism related to *Ehrlichia ruminantium*, the cause of heartwater disease in cattle, has also been detected in ill dogs from South Africa.[1] The ability of these organisms to infect multiple host species is becoming increasingly apparent.

Organisms from the genus *Ehrlichia* are grouped within the family Anaplasmataceae. Also within this family are the bacteria *Anaplasma platys* and *Anaplasma phagocytophilum*, which cause canine thrombocytic and granulocytic anaplasmosis, respectively, and organisms belonging to the genera *Neorickettsia*, which includes *Neorickettsia risticii* and the agent of salmon poisoning disease (SPD), *Neorickettsia helminthoeca*. *Rickettsia rickettsii*, the cause of Rocky Mountain spotted fever (RMSF), and other spotted fever group (SFG) rickettsiae belong to a separate family, the Rickettsiaceae. The families Rickettsiaceae and Anaplasmataceae are phylogenetically related through the order Rickettsiales (Table 206-1).

These organisms are transmitted to dogs and cats by arthropod or trematode vectors (Table 206-2), and many are maintained in nature through infection of wild animal reservoir hosts. They also have the potential to be transmitted by blood transfusion. Their geographic distribution is generally restricted to that of their vectors and intermediate hosts. A number of these pathogens cause disease in humans, and, as such, dogs serve as important sentinels for human infection, and precautions should be taken to prevent transmission while handling engorged ticks, blood, and tissue from dogs suspected to be infected. Because of shared arthropod vectors and/or concurrent exposure to multiple vector ticks, coinfections with more than one of these pathogens, as well as other arthropod-borne pathogens such as *Babesia* spp. and *Bar-*

tonella spp., occur commonly and may complicate the clinical picture. The severity of clinical signs may also depend on factors such as the size of the inoculum, host immunity, and organism strain.

THE EHRLICHIOSES

Ehrlichia canis

ETIOLOGY AND EPIDEMIOLOGY

Ehrlichia canis is the cause of canine monocytic ehrlichiosis (CME), an important disease of domestic dogs exposed to ticks worldwide. The organism is a pleomorphic bacteria that infects and forms morulae (Latin for "mulberry"), a cluster of bacteria, within circulating monocytes. Different strains of *E. canis* exist, but the degree by which these vary in virulence is poorly characterized. *E. canis* is transmitted by *Rhipicephalus sanguineus* ticks, and infection has been reported in dogs from Asia, Africa, Europe, and the Americas. In the United States, disease is diagnosed most frequently in dogs living in the southeastern and southwestern states, but because of chronic, subclinical infection, dogs can be transported to nonendemic regions and subsequently develop disease. Ticks acquire infection by feeding as larvae or nymphs on infected dogs. Jackals, foxes, and possibly coyotes may also act as reservoir hosts. The organism is transmitted transstadially within the tick.[2] Transovarial transmission does not occur.

No age or sex predilection for CME has been documented, but German Shepherds are reportedly more susceptible, and prognosis is poorer in this breed. Cross-bred dogs may be less likely to develop disease.[3]

PATHOGENESIS AND CLINICAL SIGNS

The course of CME has been divided into acute and chronic phases, although in naturally infected dogs, these phases may not be readily distinguishable. Clinical signs of acute disease occur 8 to 20 days after infection. Nonspecific signs are common and include depression, inappetence, fever, and weight loss. Replication of the organism in reticuloendothelial tissues is associated with generalized lymphadenopathy and splenomegaly. Ocular and nasal discharges, peripheral edema, and less commonly, petechial and ecchymotic hemorrhages may also occur. Neurologic signs, including twitching, ataxia, seizures, vestibular signs, hyperesthesia, and cranial nerve defects, may occur as a result of meningeal inflammation or hemorrhage. Clinically, acute disease may be indistinguishable from that of RMSF.[4] Thrombocytopenia and sometimes mild leukopenia and anemia occur 1 to 4 weeks after infection. Transient proteinuria, with urine protein:creatinine

Table • 206-1

Members of the Order Rickettsiales of Clinical Importance in Dogs and Cats

FAMILY	GENUS	SPECIES
Anaplasmataceae	*Ehrlichia*	*E. canis*
		E. chaffeensis
		E. ewingii
	Anaplasma	*A. phagocytophilum*
		A. platys
	Neorickettsia	*N. helminthoeca*
		N. risticii
Rickettsiaceae	*Rickettsia*	*R. rickettsii*

ratios up to 23 (reference range, <1) has also been reported, which resolves by 6 weeks after infection.[5,6] Dogs may recover from the acute phase without treatment.

Acute signs generally resolve after 2 to 4 weeks, after which dogs may remain subclinically infected. Mild thrombocytopenia may persist during this phase. Sequestration of organisms within the spleen may occur, and the organisms may evade the host immune system through antigenic variation.[7] This phase may persist for months to years.

Chronic ehrlichiosis ranges in severity from mild to life-threatening, with signs including lethargy, inappetence, bleeding tendencies, pallor, fever, weight loss, lymphadenopathy, splenomegaly, dyspnea, anterior uveitis, retinal hemorrhage and detachment, polyuria/polydipsia, and edema.[8-11] Bleeding tendencies result from thrombocytopenia and platelet dysfunction.[12] Cutaneous and mucosal petechial or ecchymotic hemorrhages, epistaxis, melena, hematochezia, hematuria, and prolonged bleeding from venipuncture sites have been reported.[10] Polymyositis has also been described, with muscle wasting and tetraparesis.[13] Secondary opportunistic infections such as viral papillomatosis, protozoal infections, and bacterial urinary tract infections have also been described, although the precise underlying mechanism of immune suppression, and how it relates to successful persistence of *E. canis*, has not yet been elucidated (Figure 206-1).[14,15]

The finding of pancytopenia within the complete blood count (CBC) typifies the severe chronic form of ehrlichiosis, and results from hypoplasia of all bone marrow cells.[10] More commonly, a nonregenerative anemia and thrombocytopenia are noted, although these are not always present. Moderate to marked granular lymphocytosis (up to 17,000/μL) and bone marrow plasmacytosis may occur, sometimes accompanied by a monoclonal gammopathy, which may lead to misdiagnosis of lymphocytic leukemia or multiple myeloma, respectively. This has led to the recommendation that all dogs with well-differentiated lymphocytosis or otherwise unexplained monoclonal gammopathy be tested for *E. canis* infection.[16] Serum chemistry abnormalities in chronic ehrlichiosis include hypoalbuminemia, hyperglobulinemia, and elevated alanine aminotransferase and alkaline phosphatase activities. Most often the hyperglobulinemia is due to a polyclonal gammopathy.[8] Less commonly, elevations in blood urea nitrogen and creatinine may be noted.[10] A protein-losing nephropathy may develop as a result of an immune-complex glomerulonephritis. Dogs with central nervous system (CNS) involvement may have elevated CSF protein concentrations and increased

cell counts.[17] Thoracic radiographs are often normal, but sometimes reveal bronchointerstitial infiltrates, which may reflect an underlying interstitial pneumonia.[18]

DIAGNOSIS

The finding of morulae within monocytes using cytologic evaluation is diagnostic for monocytic ehrlichiosis, but is insensitive and does not distinguish between *E. canis* and *E. chaffeensis* infection. Use of buffy coat smears or thin smears of blood collected from the margin of the pinna may increase the sensitivity for detection of morulae. In one recent study, after careful searching, morulae were found in 2 of 19 dogs with chronic monocytic ehrlichiosis.[10] More commonly, the diagnosis of ehrlichiosis is made using serology, which may be performed using indirect fluorescent antibody (IFA) testing, enzyme-linked immunosorbent assay (ELISA) technology, or Western blotting. Using IFA, antibodies can be detected between 7 and 28 days after initial infection. Therefore, dogs with acute ehrlichiosis may have false-negative test results if sufficient time has not elapsed for antibody production to occur, and retesting should be performed 2 to 3 weeks later to demonstrate seroconversion. Testing for *E. canis* DNA using the polymerase chain reaction (PCR) is likely to be more sensitive than IFA or ELISA in dogs with acute disease (see below). A positive serum antibody titer for *E. canis* may occur with previous exposure and does not necessarily correlate with the presence of disease. The results of serology should be interpreted in light of a dog's clinical signs and the results of testing for other potential causes of the dog's illness. Dogs with chronic *E. canis* infection frequently have extremely high IFA titers, sometimes >1:600,000, and these antibodies may persist in the face of treatment, suggesting persistence of the organism.[10] These do not correlate with the severity of hyperglobulinemia, disease in general, or duration of illness. Because of variability of reporting between laboratories, there is no standard "cutoff" titer that is used to separate positive and negative results. Serologic cross-reactivity to other *Ehrlichia* species occurs, including *E. ewingii* and particularly *E. chaffeensis*. Cross-reactivity to *Anaplasma phagocytophilum* antigens can occur, but appears to be minimal.[16] Western blotting has been used in an attempt to confirm the specificity of seroreactivity on IFA to *E. canis* antigens in areas where other rickettsial agents are endemic, although this test is laborious and not routinely available, and when *E. canis* antigen is used, it may be difficult to accurately distinguish between *E. canis* and *E. chaffeensis* infection.[19] To date, it has predominantly been used on a research basis.

A variety of ELISA assays have been developed for detection of antibodies to *E. canis*.[20-22] Most recently, an ELISA assay was developed containing *E. canis* antigens that offered promise for early, species-specific immunodiagnosis when compared with IFA.[20] A point-of-care lateral flow ELISA device for the simultaneous detection of canine heartworm antigen, antibodies to *E. canis*, antibodies to *Borrelia burgdorferi*, and antibodies to *A. phagocytophilum* in canine serum, plasma, or whole blood has been marketed (SNAP 4Dx, IDEXX Laboratories, Westbrook, Me.), which includes recombinant surface proteins of *E. canis*. Using IFA and Western blotting as the gold standard, the sensitivity and specificity of this test for detection of *E. canis* antibodies in 104 samples positive for *E. canis* antibodies and 236 samples negative for *E. canis* antibodies was found to be 96.2% and 100%, respectively.[23] Other point-of-care ELISA assays for detection of *E. canis* antibodies have also been developed. The incidental finding of *E. canis* seroreactivity in dogs screened using the 4Dx assay for heartworm antigen should prompt performance of a thorough physical examination and basic

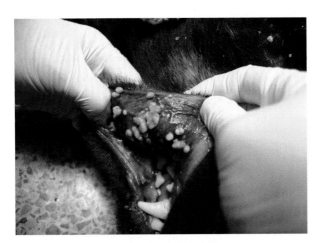

Figure 206-1 Secondary viral papillomatosis in a dog naturally infected with *Ehrlichia canis*. (Courtesy Dr. Rebecca Berg, University of California, Davis.)

Table • 206-2

Important Ticks Involved in Transmission of Members of the Order Rickettsiales

TICK SPECIES	COMMON NAME	VECTORED AGENTS	GEOGRAPHIC DISTRIBUTION
Rhipicephalus sanguineus	Brown dog tick	Ehrlichia canis Anaplasma platys? Rickettsia rickettsii	Worldwide, primarily between latitudes 35 degrees south and 50 degrees north[38]
Amblyomma americanum	Lone star tick	Ehrlichia chaffeensis Ehrlichia ewingii	West-central Texas, north to Iowa, and eastward in a broad belt spanning the southeastern United States; Atlantic coast up to Maine[132]
Ixodes scapularis	Black-legged tick, deer tick	Anaplasma phagocytophilum	Northeastern, north central, and southeastern United States[133]
Ixodes pacificus	Western black-legged tick	Anaplasma phagocytophilum	West coast of the United States[133]
Ixodes persulcatus	Taiga tick	Anaplasma phagocytophilum	Eastern Europe and Asia[133]
Ixodes ricinus	Castor bean tick	Anaplasma phagocytophilum	Europe, including the United Kingdom[133]
Dermacentor variabilis	American dog tick	Rickettsia rickettsii	East of the Rocky Mountain states as far north as Massachusetts and Nova Scotia, west coast of the United States to southwestern Oregon
Dermacentor andersoni	Rocky Mountain wood tick	Rickettsia rickettsii	Rocky Mountain states of the United States, primarily Montana, Idaho, and Oregon[134]

laboratory testing including a CBC, chemistry panel, and urinalysis to evaluate for thrombocytopenia, hyperglobulinemia, and proteinuria. At this time, treatment of seroreactive, but otherwise apparently healthy, dogs is controversial, because treatment has not been shown to change the outcome for these dogs and has the potential to lead to antimicrobial resistance or adverse side effects of drug therapy.

Other diagnostic tests include PCR and blood culture. Blood culture requires inoculation of cell monolayers and is used primarily on a research basis. PCR is becoming more widely available for routine diagnosis of E. canis infection, but problems relating to quality assurance and false-positive test results resulting from contamination still exist in many veterinary diagnostic PCR laboratories. Some laboratories offer panels that include PCR assays for a variety of different vector-borne pathogens. The results of these assays should be interpreted in light of a dog's history, clinical signs, and the results of appropriate serologic assays. PCR for E. canis may be performed on blood, lymph node aspirates, splenic aspirates, or bone marrow. Convalescent IFA or ELISA testing is much more sensitive than PCR for diagnosis of CME.[10,24,25] The sensitivity of PCR for diagnosis of CME when performed on bone marrow in dogs diagnosed with chronic ehrlichiosis using serology was recently shown to range from 25% to 68%, depending on the laboratory.[10] Thus, PCR when used alone is currently not suitable for screening potential blood donors for infection. PCR may be useful for confirming infection in the first week of illness, when serologic assays are often negative. As PCR assays become more refined, positive PCR results on splenic aspirates following discontinuation of doxycycline therapy might be used to support failure to successfully eliminate infection.[16,26] Depending on the specific assay used, when positive, PCR can also be used to confirm the Ehrlichia species involved.

TREATMENT

The treatment of choice for CME is doxycycline (10 mg/kg PO q24h). It was the consensus of the ACVIM Infectious Disease Study Group that dogs should be treated for 28 days.[16] Mixed results have been obtained in studies evaluating the efficacy of doxycycline for treatment of E. canis infection. One study suggested that acute infection may be eliminated following treatment for just 16 days.[26] Another recent study that used ticks to infect dogs and detect persistent infection showed a failure of doxycycline, when given for 14 days, to successfully eliminate the organism in dogs with subclinical, postacute infection.[27] These results contradicted those of a third study showing elimination of postacute infection following treatment with doxycycline for 3 weeks.[28] Dogs with chronic ehrlichiosis may require treatment for longer periods of time. Most dogs show clinical improvement within 24 to 48 hours. Dogs with severe chronic disease may not respond to therapy, or cytopenias may gradually resolve over a period of several months. Platelet counts generally improve and normalize by 2 weeks following institution of therapy. After treatment, titers may decline and become negative in 6 to 9 months. Some dogs retain high titers for several years, suggesting persistence of the organism. Treatment for these dogs should be based on resolution of platelet counts, and gradual improvement of hyperglobulinemia, although hyperglobulinemia may take months to resolve after treatment is discontinued. Testing using PCR on splenic aspirates may be indicated to determine if infection is persisting in these dogs, but whether ongoing treatment with doxycycline changes the outcome for these dogs is unknown. Platelet counts should be reassessed 1 and 3 months after discontinuation of therapy, because of the potential for relapse or reinfection. Other causes of illness should be considered in dogs that fail to respond to treatment.

Other drugs that have been used with variable success include chloramphenicol, imidocarb dipropionate, and enrofloxacin.[16,29-32] Members of the E. canis genogroup appear to have intrinsic gyrase-mediated resistance to fluoroquinolones,[33] so although use of enrofloxacin can be associated with clinical improvement, it is not recommended. Imidocarb dipropionate is an antiprotozoal drug that appeared to be efficacious for treatment of E. canis infection in some studies,[29] but a more recent study showed that it was ineffective in clearing infection at the dose used (6.6 mg/kg, IM, 2 injections given 2 weeks apart).[31]

For dogs that are dehydrated or anemic, intravenous fluids or blood products may also be required. Erythropoietin and granulocyte colony-stimulating factor were successful for the treatment of severe chronic ehrlichiosis in one case report.[34] If thrombocytopenia fails to respond to doxycycline administration, a short course (up to a week) of therapy with immunosuppressive doses of glucocorticoids may be beneficial in addition to ongoing therapy with doxycycline.

PREVENTION AND PUBLIC HEALTH SIGNIFICANCE

Currently, a vaccine for *E. canis* infection is not available. Prevention relies on tick control with products such as fipronil,[35] amitraz collars,[36] or imidacloprid/permethrin[37] combined with careful searching and prompt removal of attached ticks. Unfortunately, acaricide-resistant strains of *Rhipicephalus sanguineus* have been reported as a result of indiscriminate use of these drugs.[38] Low-dose doxycycline (6.6 mg/kg q24h PO) has been used to prevent infection in dogs residing in kennels in which *E. canis* infection is a problem. Although resistance to doxycycline has not been documented, this remains a theoretical concern in this situation.

Recently, *E. canis* DNA was detected in 6 of 20 human patients with clinical signs of human monocytic ehrlichiosis,[39] suggesting that *E. canis* may be a cause of monocytic ehrlichiosis in people. Thus, appropriate precautions should be taken when handling engorged ticks as well as blood and tissue specimens from infected dogs.

Ehrlichia chaffeensis

Ehrlichia chaffeensis is the cause of human monocytic ehrlichiosis in North America, an emerging disease that is characterized by fever, headache, myalgia, thrombocytopenia and leukopenia, and elevations in hepatic transaminases.[40] Gastrointestinal signs, neurologic involvement, and a toxic shock–like syndrome may also occur in some infected people. The agent was first described in 1991.[41] In the United States, it occurs primarily in the south-central, southeastern and mid-Atlantic states, reflecting the distribution of the tick vector, *Amblyomma americanum*, and the concurrent presence of white-tailed deer, which are reservoirs for the organism. The organism is transmitted transstadially within the tick, which feeds aggressively on man.[42] Experimental infection of dogs with *E. chaffeensis* results in thrombocytopenia, but otherwise infection has been subclinical.[43] In naturally infected dogs, *E. chaffeensis* infection has been associated with lymphadenopathy and epistaxis.[44] Dogs maintain high antibody titers and are PCR positive for months after infection, supporting the role of the dog as a reservoir.[43]

As for *E. canis* infection, diagnosis of *E. chaffeensis* infection may be made using blood culture, acute and convalescent serology, Western immunoblotting, or PCR. Unfortunately, serologic cross-reactivity occurs with other *Ehrlichia* species, especially *E. canis*. Although clinical improvement occurs following doxycycline therapy, doxycycline may not completely eliminate infection.[44] Treatment for a minimum of 28 days is therefore suggested.

Ehrlichia ewingii

Ehrlichia ewingii causes granulocytic ehrlichiosis in humans and in dogs, and was first recognized in dogs.[45] It has been documented in North America and more recently in dogs from Africa.[46] Infection has been primarily identified in the south-central and southeastern parts of the United States. In one study, most cases occurred from May through July,[47] but in another study, cases were detected year-round.[48] Like *E. chaffeensis* in the United States, *E. ewingii* is transmitted primarily by *Amblyomma americanum* ticks and is maintained in white-tailed deer, the proliferation of which has contributed to the emergence of these pathogens.[49]

In contrast to the other ehrlichial species, *E. ewingii* infects and forms morulae within granulocytes. In humans, the disease caused by *E. ewingii* has been referred to as *human ewingii ehrlichiosis* to avoid confusion with human monocytic ehrlichiosis caused by *E. chaffeensis* and human granulocytic anaplasmosis (previously human granulocytic ehrlichiosis) caused by *Anaplasma phagocytophilum*.[40] The organism causes fever, headache, and cytopenias in humans. Dogs show signs of fever, lethargy, anorexia, and neutrophilic polyarthritis. Vomiting and diarrhea may also occur. Neurologic signs have been reported in naturally infected dogs, including anisocoria, tremors, and a head tilt,[48] although the possibility of concurrent infection with *Rickettsia rickettsii* was not ruled out in this study. *E. ewingii* has also been detected in asymptomatic dogs, suggesting that dogs may act as a reservoir.[47,48] Laboratory testing may reveal nonregenerative anemia and thrombocytopenia.[47,50] Reactive lymphocytosis has also been reported.[48]

E. ewingii has yet to be cultivated, and there is no specific serologic test yet available to diagnose infection, although potential antigens have been identified for use in such assays.[51] Serologic cross-reactivity may occur with *E. canis* antigen, but this has often been weak and inconsistent.[47] Granulocytic morulae are commonly detected in blood smears and synovial fluid. *E. ewingii*-specific PCR assays have been developed, and to date, offer the only way of confirming infection with *E. ewingii*. Treatment with doxycycline for 2 to 4 weeks has resulted in rapid clinical improvement in reported cases, and may be sufficient to eliminate infection.

ANAPLASMOSIS

Anaplasma phagocytophilum

ETIOLOGY AND EPIDEMIOLOGY

Anaplasma phagocytophilum causes canine granulocytic ehrlichiosis. This organism was previously known as *E. equi*, *E. phagocytophila*, and the human granulocytic ehrlichiosis agent, which were subsequently grouped into a single species based on 16S rRNA gene sequence similarities.[52] The taxonomic revision was controversial because these organisms differed in their ability to cause disease in different host species,[53] with *E. phagocytophila* infecting ruminants in Europe but not the United States, *E. equi* infecting horses in California, and the human granulocytic ehrlichiosis organism infecting dogs, cats, horses, and humans in the United States. Other than llamas, ruminants in the United States have not been infected with *A. phagocytophilum*. The organism also infects deer, a variety of rodents, coyotes, and mountain lions, and is an important emerging pathogen of humans worldwide.

A. phagocytophilum forms morulae in granulocytes, most commonly neutrophils (Figure 206-2). *A. phagocytophilum* is spread by several Ixodid tick species (see Table 206-2), and is transmitted only transstadially within the tick. The tick must attach for 24 to 48 hours before transmission can occur. *Ixodes scapularis* is the vector in the upper midwestern and northeastern United States. *I. pacificus* is a vector on the west coast of North America, from California to British Columbia. In Europe, including the United Kingdom, the vector is *I. ricinus*, and *A. phagocytophilum* has also been detected in ticks in Asia and Russia, most commonly *I. persulcatus*.[54] Molecular evidence of *A. phagocytophilum* was recently detected in ticks

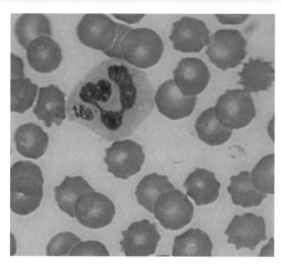

Figure 206-2 *Anaplasma phagocytophilum* morula within a neutrophil from a dog with granulocytic anaplasmosis.

in Israel and South Africa.[55,56] A variety of small mammals, including mice, woodrats, chipmunks, voles, and shrew, as well as deer and possibly birds, appear to be reservoir hosts for *A. phagocytophilum*. Because *Borrelia burgdorferi* is transmitted by the same Ixodid ticks, coinfections with *B. burgdorferi* and *A. phagocytophilum* are frequently detected, and the two may enhance one another's pathogenicity.[57]

In the upper Midwest and northeastern United States cases occur from the spring to early summer and again in the fall, whereas in Sweden cases have been reported from midsummer through early fall. Labrador and Golden Retrievers comprised almost half of reported cases in one study, possibly reflecting the popularity of these dogs for outdoor activities.[58] The median age in one study was 8 years.[58,59]

CLINICAL SIGNS

The severity of clinical signs may depend on the strain of *A. phagocytophilum* involved. In some cases, infection may be subclinical. The most common clinical signs are nonspecific and include fever, depression, inappetence, and scleral injection, and occur after an incubation period of 1 to 2 weeks. Musculoskeletal signs, including lameness, stiffness, and reluctance to move, are also common. Infrequent coughing may be noted, which is typically soft and nonproductive.[60,61] Mild lymphadenomegaly and splenomegaly may occur. Neutrophilic polyarthritis has been detected in a few dogs.[59,61] Less commonly, polydipsia, vomiting or diarrhea, and CNS signs have been reported,[58-60] although the extent to which *A. phagocytophilum* causes neurologic disease in dogs requires further study. Neurologic manifestations have been described in humans infected with *A. phagocytophilum*, and the organism has been detected in the CSF.[61] Infection appears to be self-limiting in dogs, as dogs with chronic disease (>30 days) have not been described. The ability of this organism to persist in tissues requires further study.

Laboratory abnormalities include thrombocytopenia, which is present in over 80% of cases, lymphopenia, eosinopenia, and a mild nonregenerative anemia.[58,60] The serum chemistry panel may reveal hypoalbuminemia and mild to moderately elevated liver enzymes.

Infection with *A. phagocytophilum* appears to be immunosuppressive. The organism survives within neutrophils by inhibiting phagosome-lysosome fusion, suppression of the respiratory burst, and through inhibition of neutrophil apoptosis. As a result, dogs infected with *A. phagocytophilum* may be prone to other infections, particularly bacterial infections.[61]

DIAGNOSIS AND TREATMENT

The finding of morulae within neutrophils in an endemic area is highly suggestive of infection with *A. phagocytophilum*, although the morulae cannot be distinguished from those of *E. ewingii*. Morulae, when present, are found in 7% to 37% of circulating neutrophils.[58,59]

Diagnosis can also be accomplished using acute and convalescent phase serology. Most veterinary laboratories perform serologic testing using IFA. Many acutely ill dogs will have negative acute phase serology. In addition, positive titers may reflect previous exposure (up to 8 to 10 months prior), so demonstration of a fourfold rise in titer is required.[63] Western immunoblotting is also available, but is not generally performed for routine diagnostics. A point-of-care lateral flow ELISA device (SNAP 4Dx, IDEXX Laboratories, Westbrook, Me.) can also be used to detect antibodies to *A. phagocytophilum*, although false negatives using this assay also occur in dogs with acute disease. With all current serologic assays, serologic cross-reactivity with other *Anaplasma* species, especially *A. platys*, can occur, and possibly to other *Ehrlichia* species.[16,44] Most dogs on the west coast of the United States that have antibodies to *A. phagocytophilum* have negative *E. canis* serology.

Determination of the infecting species can be accomplished using PCR on whole blood for *A. phagocytophilum*. This may be the most appropriate assay in dogs with acute illness that lack morulae on the CBC, pending the results of serology. The organism can also be cultured from blood in HL-60 cell culture, but this is usually performed on a research basis.

The treatment of choice for granulocytic anaplasmosis is doxycycline (5 mg/kg q12h PO). A 2-week course of treatment is recommended. Most dogs show rapid improvement, with signs abating within 12 to 48 hours. Prevention relies on tick control.

PUBLIC HEALTH SIGNIFICANCE

Anaplasma phagocytophilum causes human granulocytic anaplasmosis, a febrile disease that resembles the disease in dogs. Death is rare, but has occurred as a result of complications due to secondary infections. Dogs are an important sentinel for human infection. Dogs may be a source of infection by bringing infected ticks into contact with humans (see Rocky Mountain Spotted Fever). Precautions should be taken when handling blood or tissue from infected dogs, or during tick removal.

Anaplasma platys

A. platys is the cause of canine thrombocytic anaplasmosis. This organism forms morulae within platelets, and is yet to be cultured. The vector of *A. platys* is unknown. *Rhipicephalus sanguineus* has been implicated in some reports, although attempts to transmit infection using this tick were unsuccessful.[64] The organism has been reported in South America, Australia, Asia, Africa, Europe, and North America.[65-70]

After an incubation period of 1 to 2 weeks, thrombocytopenia occurs at 1 to 2 week intervals. Morulae may be visible in blood smears just prior to the decline in platelet count, but subsequently disappear rapidly. Platelet counts then normalize within 3 to 4 days. Immune-mediated mechanisms likely contribute to the thrombocytopenia. The severity of clinical signs resulting from infection with *A. platys* has varied depending on geographic location. Cases reported from Europe and South America have had more severe clinical manifestations, including fever, splenomegaly, and hemorrhages, although concurrent infections with other tick-borne pathogens may have contributed to clinical signs in some of these cases. The majority of cases in the United States have been mild or subclinical.

Diagnosis is based on visualization of morulae within platelets together with acute and convalescent phase serology. Because of cross-reactions with *A. phagocytophilum*, serology is not diagnostic for *A. platys* infection. *A. platys*–specific PCR assays have also been developed.[71] Use of splenic or bone marrow aspirates for PCR should be considered when blood samples test negative.[72] Treatment of canine thrombocytic anaplasmosis is as for granulocytic anaplasmosis.

NEORICKETTSIOSES

Neorickettsia helminthoeca

Neorickettsia helminthoeca causes SPD. A related organism, the Elokomin fluke fever (EFF) agent, may cause a similar disease. SPD has geographic distribution that is restricted to the western slopes of the Cascade Mountains from northern California to the Canadian border, with cases also being reported from southern Vancouver Island.[73] Disease may occur elsewhere following transportation of infected fish for feeding at a remote location, or in dogs that travel to and from a nonendemic area to a site containing infected fish. Recently, a similar disease was described in Brazilian dogs.[74]

The vector of SPD is *Nanophyetus salmincola*, a fluke that harbors the organism throughout its life cycle. Fluke eggs transform into miracidia, which infect a small snail, *Oxytrema silicula*, which inhabits fresh or brackish stream water. Cercariae leave the snail and penetrate a fish, most commonly a salmonid fish, although certain nonsalmonid fish have also been reported to be infected.[74,75] Hatchery-reared fish may also be infected. The cercariae transform into metacercariae, usually within the kidneys of the fish, but also in the muscle and other tissues. Fish may retain the infection for several years.[76,77]

Dogs become infected with the rickettsia after ingesting parasitized fish, after which the metacercariae transform into adult flukes. Foxes and coyotes may also become infected, and SPD has also been reported in captive bears.[78] Cats are not susceptible to SPD, but the flukes mature to adults within the feline intestinal tract. SPD may also be acquired after ingesting adult flukes (which could potentially occur following coprophagy), infected snails, and fluke eggs.[79]

After maturation and attachment to the intestinal tract, the fluke somehow inoculates the rickettsia into the host. Subsequently, *N. helminthoeca* infects and replicates within cells of the mononuclear-phagocyte system. Rapid dissemination of the organism to the lymph nodes, spleen, liver, lungs, and brain occurs. After an incubation period ranging from 5 to 33 days, the earliest clinical signs are usually fever, which may be severe, and anorexia. This may be followed by depression, weight loss, lymphadenopathy, vomiting, and diarrhea, sometimes containing blood.[76,80] The presence of adult flukes may contribute to the gastrointestinal signs. Associated laboratory abnormalities include neutrophilia, sometimes with a mild to moderate left shift, lymphopenia, and monocytosis, which are nonspecific. Thrombocytopenia occurs in approximately 90% of affected dogs, and may be as low as 16,000/µL. Serum chemistry abnormalities include electrolyte derangements, elevated liver enzymes, and hypoalbuminemia.[80]

Diagnosis of SPD may be inferred by finding characteristic trematode eggs in the feces using fecal sedimentation or sugar flotation, which appear 5 to 8 days after ingestion of an infected fish. However, infection with flukes is not always accompanied by neorickettsial infection, and eggs may be shed for several months (up to 250 days). Neorickettsiae may also be visible using cytologic examination of lymph node aspirates (Figure 206-3).[81] Typically, there is moderate to marked histiocytic inflammation and lymphocytic-plasmacytic reactivity. The organisms may appear as granular to amorphous material that fills infected cells, sometimes forming morulae, and may be best visualized using Giemsa stain.[81]

The treatment of choice is doxycycline. Parenteral administration may be necessary in vomiting dogs. In addition, supportive therapy using fluids, blood products, and antiemetics may be necessary. Praziquantel should also be administered to treat the helminth infection. Prevention involves avoiding access to fish, and the feeding of thoroughly cooked fish to dogs. Freezing fish for 24 hours also effectively destroys the metacercariae and rickettsiae.

Neorickettsia risticii

Neorickettsia risticii (previously known as *Ehrlichia risticii*) is the cause of Potomac horse fever. The life cycle of this organism has only recently been elucidated, and involves a trematode vector, most likely *Acanthatrium oregonense*.[82] The fluke miracidia infect aquatic snails (*Juga* spp.) and parasitizes caddisflies. Insectivorous species, such as bats and swallows, appear to be the definitive host of the trematode. Horses may become infected following accidental ingestion of infected caddisflies containing metacercariae.

N. risticii has been identified using culture and PCR in dogs from the United States with signs mimicking ehrlichiosis, including lethargy, intermittent vomiting, bleeding tendencies, polyarthritis, neurologic signs, dependent edema, anemia, and thrombocytopenia.[83] These dogs were seroreactive to *N. risticii* antigens with titers at low levels (10 to 640) using IFA. Most of these dogs were from the western and southwestern states. Further studies are required to characterize this organ-

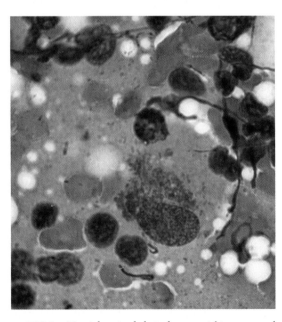

Figure 206-3 *Neorickettsia helminthoeca* within macrophages in a lymph node aspirate from a dog with salmon poisoning disease.

ism and determine its pathogenic significance in dogs and also in cats.

TICK-BORNE RICKETTSIOSES

General Considerations

Rickettsia rickettsii, the cause of RMSF, belongs to the Rickettsiaceae, which contains a large number of both pathogenic and nonpathogenic *Rickettsia* species. In recent years, many novel species of rickettsiae have been characterized using molecular methods, and the taxonomic classification of these into species has been challenging.[84] The rickettsiae have been divided based on their antigenic and genetic composition into SFG and typhus group rickettsiae. *Rickettsia* spp. may be transmitted by hard ticks, fleas, lice, and mites. Currently, almost all tick-associated rickettsiae belong to the SFG. Tick-borne *Rickettsia* species known to be pathogenic in humans are listed in Table 206-3. Many of these species were initially thought to be nonpathogenic. Clinical signs in humans caused by these organisms are similar, and include fever, lymphadenopathy, headache, eschar formation, and rash, although formation of an eschar at the inoculation site does not usually occur in RMSF.[84] Recently, a novel rickettsial species, *Rickettsia amblyommii*, was associated with a RMSF-like illness in three humans from North Carolina.[85] The ability of these species to cause disease in dogs and cats, and the role of dogs and cats as reservoirs, requires further study.

Tick-borne rickettsiae cause disease by infecting vascular endothelial cells and increasing microvascular permeability, possibly through generation of reactive oxygen species and lipid peroxidation.[84] The organisms inhibit apoptosis, favoring rickettsial growth. Widespread endothelial injury is associated with production of proinflammatory cytokines and activation of the coagulation cascade, in the absence of disseminated intravascular coagulation.[84]

Rocky Mountain Spotted Fever

ETIOLOGY AND EPIDEMIOLOGY

RMSF is a severe, life-threatening rickettsial illness of humans and dogs caused by *Rickettsia rickettsii*. Although originally reported from the Rocky Mountain states, RMSF most commonly occurs in the south-central, southeastern, and south Atlantic states of the United States. It is one of the most important emerging diseases in the United States, as well as Central and parts of South America.[84] In the past, between 250 and 1200 cases of RMSF have been reported annually in people in the United States. The number of human cases reported in 2004, 2005, and 2006 were 1713, 1936, and 2092, respectively.[86]

Rickettsia rickettsii is transmitted primarily by *Dermacentor* ticks in North America, although an outbreak of RMSF was recently reported in Arizona that was transmitted by *R. sanguineus*.[87,88] The American dog tick *(Dermacentor variabilis)* is the primary vector in the southeastern states, and the Rocky Mountain wood tick *(Dermacentor andersoni)* transmits the rickettsia in the Rocky Mountain region and Canada (see Table 206-2). *R. sanguineus* and *Amblyomma* spp. ticks have been implicated as vectors in Central and South America, respectively.[86,89] The organism is transmitted transstadially and transovarially within the tick. Uninfected larvae and nymphs may also become infected when they feed on small wild mammals, such as ground squirrels and chipmunks. In the United States, most cases occur between March and October. In humans, the highest incidence has been reported in children less than 10 years of age and adults aged 40 to 64 years.[86] Being male and being white are also risk factors. Although urban cases occur, most cases originate from rural or wooded areas, and exposure to dogs is a risk factor.[90,91] The disease occurs sporadically, is clustered to limited geographic regions, and, rarely, familial clusters of disease occur, sometimes including the family dog.[92,93] A history of a tick bite is present in less than 70% of human cases. This figure is even lower for dogs.[94,95]

PATHOGENESIS AND CLINICAL SIGNS

Following tick attachment, a reactivation period lasting from 4 to 24 hours is necessary, during which the rickettsia transforms from a dormant, avirulent state, to a highly virulent one. Purebred dogs, especially German Shepherds, appear to develop the most severe signs.[94] Disease in humans and dogs is remarkably similar. The incubation period ranges from 2 to 14 days (mean, 7 days), and fever may occur as soon as 2 to 3 days after tick attachment. Nonspecific signs, such as

Table • 206-3

Examples of Some Spotted Fever Group Rickettsia That Cause Disease in Humans

SPECIES	DISEASE	GEOGRAPHIC DISTRIBUTION	VECTOR
Rickettsia rickettsii	Rocky Mountain spotted fever	North, Central, and South America	Ticks
Rickettsia conorii subsp. *conorii*	Mediterranean spotted fever	Primarily northern Africa, southern Europe	Ticks
Rickettsia akari	Rickettsialpox	United States	Mites
Rickettsia slovaca	Tick-borne lymphadenopathy	Europe	Ticks
Rickettsia africae	African tick-bite fever	Sub-Saharan Africa, West Indies	Ticks
Rickettsia sibirica	Lymphangitis-associated rickettsiosis	China, Europe, Africa	Ticks
Rickettsia heilongjanghensis	Far Eastern spotted fever	China, Russian Far East	Ticks
Rickettsia aeschlimannii	Unnamed	Europe	Ticks
Rickettsia parkeri	Unnamed	South and North America	Ticks
Rickettsia felis	Cat flea typhus	Worldwide	Fleas
Rickettsia japonica	Japanese spotted fever	Japan	Ticks
Rickettsia honei	Flinders Island spotted fever	Australia, Asia, United States	Ticks
Rickettsia australis	Queensland tick typhus	Australia	Ticks
Rickettsia massiliae	Unnamed	Europe, Africa	Ticks

lethargy, anorexia, and lymphadenopathy, are also common. In people, extreme headache has been reported early in the course of illness,[86] which may be accompanied by myalgia and gastrointestinal signs such as vomiting, anorexia, and abdominal pain, which have also been noted in dogs. Early RMSF is often misdiagnosed as a viral illness in humans.[86]

In humans, the characteristic triad of a rash, fever, and headache is apparent in 60% to 70% of cases approximately 2 weeks after the tick bite. The rash initially appears as small macules on the wrists and ankles and spreads to involve the arms, legs, and trunk, eventually becoming maculopapular with central petechiae.[86] Dogs may develop edema and erythema of extremities, including the lips, muzzle, scrotum, penile sheath, pinnae and, rarely the ventral abdomen.[95-97] Continued tissue damage in these regions may lead to tissue necrosis and gangrene, which has required amputation in some cases.[92,96] Stiffness and reluctance to walk may be apparent because of scrotal involvement in male dogs or involvement of muscles, joints, or meninges.[94] Ocular manifestations are common, and include conjunctivitis, mucopurulent ocular discharge, scleral injection, uveitis, hyphema, iridal and retinal hemorrhage, and retinal edema.[98] Petechial and ecchymotic hemorrhages occur in less than 20% of cases, primarily on the mucous membranes.[94] Epistaxis, melena, and hematuria may occur in severely affected dogs. Neurologic signs have been reported in up to 80% of dogs with RMSF[92,94,95,99] and include ataxia, stupor, vestibular signs, hyperesthesia, opisthotonus, and seizures.

Other signs include dyspnea and coughing due to pulmonary edema, cardiac arrhythmias due to myocarditis, hepatomegaly, icterus, and development of acute renal failure. Death generally results from progressive neurologic signs, acute oliguric renal failure, or cardiovascular collapse and shock.[86,94] Death is reported in 2% to 10% of humans, although one study from Mexico reported a mortality rate of 22% in children.[91] The median time from onset of illness to death is only 8 days, making early recognition and treatment crucial.

Laboratory abnormalities include leukocytosis, sometimes with a left shift, nonregenerative anemia, and mild to moderate thrombocytopenia.[94,95,97] Mild prolongation of coagulation times may be noted. Serum chemistry abnormalities have included elevated liver enzymes, hypercholesterolemia, hypoalbuminemia, electrolyte disturbances, elevated creatine kinase concentration, and in severe cases, azotemia and hyperbilirubinemia. Cerebrospinal fluid analysis may be normal or may reveal elevated protein (usually <100 mg/μL, but may be higher) and elevated total nucleated cell count, often due to both increased numbers of neutrophils and mononuclear cells.[92] Neutrophilic polyarthritis has also been documented using synovial fluid analysis. Thoracic radiography may reveal an interstitial pattern.

DIAGNOSIS

Microimmunofluorescence is the current reference method in rickettsial serology, and is used by most laboratories. ELISA assays have also been used.[100] Wide antigenic cross-reactions exist amongst pathogenic and nonpathogenic SFG rickettsiae, so the presence of a positive titer does not imply that a dog's illness is caused by the rickettsial species used as an antigen in the assay. Because antibodies are generally not detectable until 7 to 10 days after disease onset, a fourfold rise in IgG titer using acute and convalescent phase sera is necessary to diagnose recent infection. A single titer exceeding 1:1024 is also considered diagnostic of recent infection in association with consistent clinical signs.[94] Given the acute nature of RMSF, serology is of limited usefulness for early diagnosis.

IgM assays have been developed, which may be useful to document recent infection.[100]

Direct immunofluorescence or immunoperoxidase staining of infected tissues, including biopsies of affected skin, has also been used to detect *R. rickettsii* early in the course of disease or following necropsy, with high specificity and a sensitivity of around 75%.[99,101-103] PCR assays for *R. rickettsii* can be used on blood or tissues.[104,105] However, the number of rickettsiae circulating in the blood is generally low, and so PCR has had low sensitivity when used on blood samples. The use of PCR together with immunohistochemistry on skin biopsy samples in acute disease should improve laboratory confirmation of RMSF. Recently, conventional and real-time PCR assays have been developed that differentiate between SFG rickettsiae–infecting dogs.[106] *R. rickettsii* has been classified as a biosafety level-3 agent, and so cultivation of the organism requires special facilities and is not routinely performed. Laboratory acquired infections have been reported.[107]

TREATMENT

The treatment of choice for RMSF is doxycycline. Other tetracyclines as well as chloramphenicol and fluoroquinolones are effective.[108,109] Treatment should be maintained for at least 7 days. Intravenous therapy may be needed for patients that are vomiting or have neurologic signs. A delay in treatment with appropriate antimicrobials has been correlated with development of more severe disease and increased mortality in humans, so treatment should never be delayed whilst waiting on the results of diagnostic testing. Typically there is a rapid clinical response to treatment, with defervescence occurring within 12 to 24 hours. Failure to respond appropriately may reflect the presence of coinfections with other vector-borne organisms, such as *Ehrlichia canis* or *Babesia* spp. Doxycycline is now the treatment of choice for children with RMSF, following publication of a study that did not show substantial discoloration of permanent teeth following treatment of children with doxycycline for RMSF.[110]

Other supportive therapy may be required for dogs in shock, including fluids and blood products. Care should be exercised not to exacerbate pulmonary and cerebral edema with intravenous crystalloids.[94] In some dogs residual neurologic signs, renal insufficiency or cutaneous scarring may persist despite treatment, especially if treatment is delayed.

PREVENTION

Although no vaccine exists for RMSF, natural infection is followed by development of solid immunity, and reinfection has not been documented in naturally infected dogs. Infection with nonpathogenic SFG rickettsiae was not shown to protect against development of RMSF. Prevention thus involves tick control (see above). Prophylactic antibiotic administration is not indicated to prevent RMSF after a tick bite, as this only appears to delay onset of illness.[86]

PUBLIC HEALTH ASPECTS

Dogs are important sentinels for human infection with *R. rickettsii*. Recognition of the disease in dogs has contributed to prompt diagnosis and treatment of RMSF in humans interacting with those dogs.[92] Common exposure to an infected tick population most likely explains these familial clusters of infection. Veterinarians that manage dogs with RMSF should educate their clients about the disease and their potential for infection, and should contact human health care providers should humans become ill in association with canine disease.

Dogs may carry unattached, infected ticks on their bodies, which may subsequently attach to people, or people may become infected through improper removal of attached, infected ticks from their dogs. Guidelines for safe removal of ticks have been published.[86] Ticks should be lifted from the skin using fine forceps, and gloves should be worn. Hands should be washed thoroughly with soap and water after removal. When hiking in wooded areas, protective clothing should be worn. The skin should be thoroughly examined for attached ticks after these activities, playing close attention to the area along the hairline, around the cuffs, and on dogs, the soft hair around the ears, the neck, the legs, interdigital spaces, and ventral abdomen.

Feline Ehrlichioses

Cats are rarely found to be infected with ehrlichiae.[111-117] The DNA of an *E. canis*–like organism has been detected in one cat from North Carolina, two cats from Ontario, and two cats in France.[118,119] One of the three North American cats showed signs of polyarthritis and the other two had cytopenias. None of these three cats was seroreactive in an IFA assay using *E. canis* antigens. Seroprevalences of 10% to *E. canis*, 2.4% to *N. risticii*, and 4.9% to *A. phagocytophilum* were found in cats in Spain.[120,121] *Ehrlichia*-like morulae have been identified in mononuclear cells in cats from the United States, Kenya, France, Brazil and Thailand.[122-126] Clinical signs including fever, lethargy, anorexia, pallor, and splenomegaly were reported in these cats, although some had concurrent infec-

tions with hemotropic mycoplasmas or feline retroviruses. The most consistent laboratory abnormalities in infected cats have been nonregenerative anemia and hyperglobulinemia. Many infected cats have responded rapidly to treatment with doxycycline. It is the consensus that cats infected with mono-cytic ehrlichiae should be treated with doxycycline at 10 mg/kg PO q24h for a minimum of 28 days.[16]

A report from Italy described 15 pet cats diagnosed with an ehrlichial infection based on cytologic evaluation of morulae within circulating granulocytes. Clinical abnormalities in these cats included lethargy, anorexia, hyperesthesia, lameness, lymphadenopathy, vomiting, and thrombocytopenia.[127] Morulae have also been observed within granulocytes from cats in Sweden, Brazil, and Kenya.[123,125,128] The cats from Brazil and Kenya also had morulae within monocytes. Experimental infection of cats with *A. phagocytophilum* has resulted in development of morulae within granulocytes and clinical illness.[129] *A. phagocytophilum* DNA was also detected using PCR in cats from Massachusetts, a cat from Connecticut, and a cat from Scandinavia.[128,130,131] These cats showed signs of fever, anorexia, and lethargy, and some had thrombocytopenia. The signs resolved following treatment with doxycycline.[131]

REFERENCES

The reference list can be found on the companion Expert Consult Web site at *www.expertconsult.com*.

CHAPTER 207

Protozoal Infections

Michael R. Lappin

Multiple pathogenic protozoans infect dogs and cats. The group can be divided into amoeba, ciliates, coccidians, flagellates, Microspora, and Piroplasmia. Protozoans generally cause either gastrointestinal (GI) tract disease (enteric protozoans)[1,2] or polysystemic disease.[3]

ENTERIC PROTOZOAL DISEASES

The most common protozoal agents infecting the GI tract of dogs and cats are:

- The flagellates, *Giardia* spp., *Tritrichomonas foetus*, and *Pentatrichomonas hominis*;
- The coccidians, *Besnoitia* spp., *Cryptosporidium* spp., *Cyclospora cayetanensis*, *Cystoisospora* spp., *Hammondia* spp., *Neospora caninum*, *Sarcocystis* spp., and *Toxoplasma gondii*;
- The ciliate, *Balantidium coli*; and
- The amoeba, *Entamoeba histolytica*.

Cystoisospora spp., *Sarcocystis* spp., *Besnoitia* spp., *Hammondia* spp., *N. caninum*, and *T. gondii* complete the intestinal cycle in only one species. Some isolates of *Cryptosporidium* spp., *C. cayetanensis*, *Giardia* spp., *E. histolytica*, and *B. coli* will replicate in multiple warm-blooded vertebrates and

therefore can potentially be zoonotic. In addition, *N. caninum* antibodies have been detected in some people[4] and DNA of *T. foetus* was amplified from the feces of a person,[5] findings that also suggest zoonotic transmission.

Which the exception of *C. cayetanensis*, for which the route of transmission is unknown, fecal oral transmission occurs with the enteric protozoans. The coccidians produce oocysts. *Cryptosporidium* spp. oocysts are immediately infectious when passed by the host; *T. gondii*, *N. caninum*, and *Cystoisospora* spp. must sporulate outside the host to be infectious (Figure 207-1).

In the flagellate group, both trophozoites and cysts of *Giardia* spp. are potentially infectious; however, transmission occurs most frequently after ingestion of cysts because gastric secretions generally kill trophozoites. Only trophozoites are detected in dogs and cats with *T. foetus* or *P. hominis* infections. Ingestion of the organism in the tissues of transport hosts can also result in infection by *Cystoisospora* spp., *Besnoitia* spp., *Hammondia* spp., *N. caninum*, and *T. gondii* (Figure 207-2).

Carnivorism can result in infection by other enteric protozoans like *Cryptosporidium* spp., *Giardia* spp., *E. histolytica*, and *B. coli* if the organisms are present in the intestines of the prey species. The GI phase of infection can be self-limiting for each of the agents; however, fecal shedding periods are variable. After tissue cyst ingestion, infected cats rarely shed oocysts of *T. gondii* for more than 2 weeks.[7] For the other enteric protozoans, fecal shedding can be of longer duration. For example, cats infected with *T. foetus* or *Cryptosporidium* spp. can shed the organisms continuously or intermittently for months.

The enteric protozoans have worldwide distribution. Because they are maintained in nature primarily by fecal-oral transmission, more cases are associated with crowded and unsanitary environments. In general, *Giardia* spp., *T. gondii*, *N. caninum*, *Cystoisospora* spp., *Cryptosporidium* spp., and *T. foetus* (cats) infections are common[8-17]; *E. histolytica*, *B. coli*, and *C. cayetanensis* infections are rare.[18-21] Currently it is unknown how many dogs and cats harbor *P. hominis*.[22,23] Antibodies against *T. gondii* (30%) and *Cryptosporidium* spp. (8.3%) are commonly detected in serum from client-owned cats, suggesting that exposure is common (Figure 207-3).[24,25] Prevalence of the agents varies by region in coprologic studies.

Pathogenic mechanisms have not been ascertained for each of the enteric protozoans. *Cystoisospora* spp. and *T. gondii* replicate in intestinal cells and may result in clinical illness from cell destruction. Tissue invasion also can occur with *E. histolytica*.[20,21] *Giardia* spp. and *Cryptosporidium* spp. are found on the surface of enterocytes, so pathogenesis is unlikely secondary to direct cell damage. Some of the pathogenic mechanisms proposed for these enteric agents include production of toxins, disruption of normal flora, induction of inflammatory bowel disease (IBD), inhibition of normal enterocyte enzymatic function, blunting of microvilli, and induction of motility disorders. *Cystoisospora* spp. and *T. foetus* infections are more commonly associated with clinical GI disease in puppies or kittens. *Sarcocystis* spp., *Besnoitia* spp., *Hammondia* spp., *T. gondii*, and *N. caninum* are almost never associated with GI disease. Clinical illness associated with *T. gondii*, *N. caninum*, and *S. neurona* generally results from the tissue phase of the infections.[7,26-29] *Giardia* spp. and *Cryptosporidium* spp. infections are common in young animals, but GI signs can occur in animals of any age. Clinical disease is more common, and duration of organism shedding into the environment may be prolonged in dogs and cats with immunodeficiency-inducing concurrent diseases.

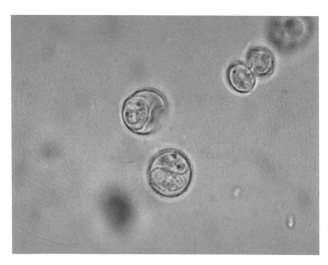

Figure 207-1 Sporulated oocysts of *Toxoplasma gondii* from feces of a cat. The oocysts are approximately 8 μm ×10 μm.

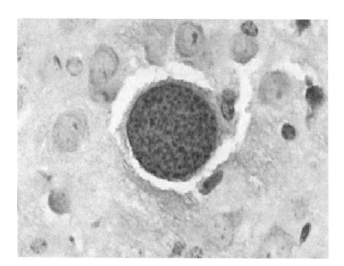

Figure 207-2 Immunohistochemical stain of a *Toxoplasma gondii* tissue cyst in a mouse brain. The cyst is approximately 100 μm in diameter and contains approximately 500 organisms.

Figure 207-3 Map of the United States showing the distribution of *Toxoplasma gondii* antibody test results in cats. (From Vollaire MR et al: Seroprevalence of *Toxoplasma gondii* antibodies in clinically ill cats in the United States. Am J Vet Res 66:874, 2005.)

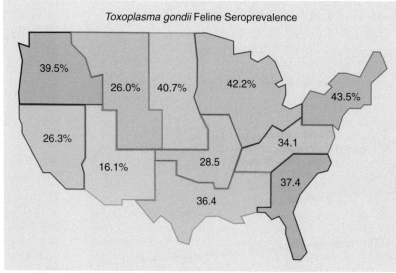

Toxoplasma gondii Feline Seroprevalence

39.5% 26.0% 40.7% 42.2% 43.5%
26.3% 16.1% 28.5 34.1 37.4
36.4

Owner concerns in dogs or cats with enteric protozoal infections generally are vomiting, inappetence, or diarrhea; fever is uncommon. *Giardia* spp., *Cryptosporidium* spp., and *T. gondii* infections are most commonly associated with small-bowel diarrhea; *E. histolytica*, *B. coli*, and *T. foetus* infections are most commonly associated with large-bowel diarrhea. *Cystoisospora* spp. infections can cause clinical signs of large- or small-bowel diarrhea. Physical examination findings in dogs or cats with enteric protozoal infections are nonspecific but can include abdominal discomfort, increased gas or fluid in the intestinal tract, or thickened intestinal loops.

All dogs and cats with large-, small-, or mixed-bowel diarrhea should be assessed for enteric protozoal infections. Diagnosis of GI protozoal infection is based primarily on documentation of oocysts, trophozoites, or cysts on direct fecal examination or fecal flotation.

A direct smear of diarrheic stool can be used to examine for trophozoites of *E. histolytica*, *B. coli*, *Giardia* spp., *P. hominis*, or *T. foetus*. More frequently, a small quantity of fresh feces or mucus is mixed with a drop of 0.9% NaCl on a clean microscope slide and examined at 100× after placing a coverslip. When a motile organism is noted, examining at 400× assesses structural features. Application of a stain like Lugol's solution, methylene blue, or acid methyl green to the wet mount at the edge of the coverslip will aid in visualizing internal structures of protozoa. Trophozoites are rarely found in formed stools. Duodenal aspiration for cytologic examination for *Giardia* trophozoites is effective for the diagnosis of giardiasis in the dog. However, this technique is not effective in the cat because the organism lives in the distal small intestine.

Protozoal cysts or oocysts are best demonstrated after fecal concentration; Sheather's sugar centrifugation and zinc sulfate centrifugation are inexpensive techniques commonly used in clinical practice.[30] These solutions are inexpensive and generally effective. Sugar solution is hypertonic and will distort *Giardia* spp. cysts; the cytoplasm is pulled to one side and appears as a half- or quarter-moon.

Due to small size and limited number in feces of infected dogs and cats, *Cryptosporidium* spp. oocysts are almost never seen when concentrated feces are examined at 100×. Acid-fast staining or fluorescein-labeled monoclonal antibody staining of a fecal smear and fecal polymerase chain reaction (PCR) assay can aid in the diagnosis of cryptosporidiosis in dogs and cats.[31,32] Oocysts stain pink with acid-fast stain (Figure 207-4).

The fluorescein-labeled monoclonal antibody system also detects *Giardia* spp. cysts of dogs and cats, and so this test is an excellent screening procedures for dogs or cats with small-bowel diarrhea. Enzyme-linked immunosorbent assay (ELISA) for detection of *Cryptosporidium* spp. antigens in feces is generally inaccurate as it is based on antibodies against *C. parvum*; it is now known most dogs are infected with *C. canis* and most cats are infected with *C. felis*.[33,34] Antigens of *Giardia* spp. can be detected in feces by ELISA, and these assays appear to be accurate for use with dog and cat feces.[35,36] However, *Giardia* antigen assays are best used in combination with fecal flotation, which detects more parasites overall. PCR assays for the amplification of *Giardia* spp. and *Cryptosporidium* spp. DNA from feces are offered by multiple diagnostic laboratories in the United States. However, the sensitivity, specificity, and predictive values of these assays are generally unknown and there is no standardization between laboratories at this time. In general, these assays are not indicated unless the animal is known to be positive and the clinician or owner wishes to determine the genotype of the organism. PCR assays are also available for *T. foetus* and *P. hominis*. While fecal culture can also be used to identify *T. foetus*,[36] PCR assay results are returned more quickly.

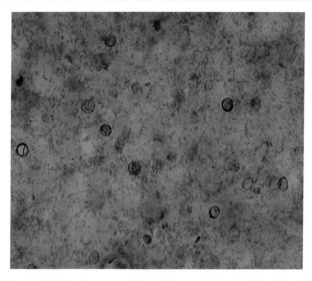

Figure 207-4 *Cryptosporidium felis* oocysts stained pink with modified acid fast stain (1000×). The oocysts are approximately 4 μm × 6 μm.

The presence of enteric protozoans in diarrheic stool does not prove that disease was due to the organism. Some enteric protozoans, especially *Giardia* spp., *Cryptosporidium* spp., *T. foetus*, and *Cystoisospora* spp., live chronically in the intestinal tract of normal animals; other conditions causing GI tract disease can induce repeat shedding. Thus animals with enteric protozoal infections that do not respond to therapy should be evaluated for underlying causes of disease. *Giardia* spp., *Cryptosporidium* spp., *Cystoisospora* spp., and *Sarcocystis* spp. are commonly found in animals with normal stools.

Withholding food for 24 to 48 hours is indicated for animals with acute vomiting or diarrhea. Highly digestible, bland diets are used most frequently if vomiting and small-bowel diarrhea are the primary manifestations of disease. High-fiber diets are generally indicated if large-bowel diarrhea is occurring. Feeding a high-fiber diet may also aid in the treatment of giardiasis due to inhibition of trophozoite attachment to duodenal epithelial cells. Use of probiotics may also have clinical benefit in some cases.[38-40]

Optimal treatments for *E. histolytica* and *B. coli* infections in dogs or cats are unknown. *Giardia* spp. infections of dogs and cats generally respond clinically to the administration of metronidazole, fenbendazole, or febantel-pyrantel-praziquantel, but infection is usually not eliminated.[41-47] Metronidazole also helps correct the anaerobic bacterial overgrowth or *Clostridium perfringens* overgrowth that commonly accompanies giardiasis. In addition, metronidazole may also be beneficial due to inhibition of lymphocyte function. In a recent study of cats, administration of liquefied metronidazole benzoate at 25 mg/kg, PO, q12h for 7 days was 100% effective during the time period studied.[44] Central nervous system (CNS) toxicity occasionally occurs with this drug; it is unlikely if no more than 50 mg/kg is given orally per day.[48,49] Fenbendazole (50 mg/kg, PO, q24h for 3 to 5 days) and albendazole are commonly prescribed alternate anti-*Giardia* spp. drugs; albendazole is associated with neutropenia in dogs and cats and so should not be used.[50,51] Furazolidone (cats), paromomycin (dogs or cats), and nitazoxanide (dogs or cats) are other drugs with anti-*Giardia* effects. Lastly, use of the commercially available *Giardia* spp. vaccines as immunotherapy has given variable treatment responses.[52,53]

The majority of drugs prescribed to cats with diarrhea due to *T. foetus* have failed. Recently, ronidazole and tinidazole have been evaluated with ronidazole administered at 25 mg/kg, PO, q24h for 14 days appearing to be the most likely to eliminate infection.[54-56] However, ronidazole can be neurotoxic.[57]

Paromomycin, tylosin (10 to 15 mg/kg, PO, q12h), azithromycin (10 mg/kg, PO, q24h), and nitazoxanide (25 mg/kg, PO, q12h) have all been used to lessen diarrhea in dogs, cats, or people with cryptosporidiosis, but no treatment has consistently stopped *Cryptosporidium* spp. oocyst shedding.[58-62] The drugs are generally prescribed initially for 7 to 10 days. However, it sometimes takes as long as 4 to 6 weeks to achieve total resolution of diarrhea. The most commonly prescribed drugs to treat *Cystoisospora* spp. infections of dogs and cats are trimethoprim-sulfonamide, sulfadimethoxine, furazolidone, amprolium, or amprolium-sulfadimethoxine. Quinacrine, spiramycin, toltrazuril, roxithromycin, and ponazuril have been used on a limited basis. Ponazuril appears to be safe in most puppies and kittens and can eliminate infection after one dose (50 mg/kg, PO).

Cryptosporidium spp., *T. gondii, Giardia, E. histolytica,* and *B. coli* are potentially zoonotic. *Entamoeba histolytica* and *B. coli* infections are extremely uncommon, and pets are unlikely sources of human infections. Most people are infected with *Cryptosporidium* spp. or *Giardia* spp. from contaminated food or water, not contact with pets.[63] It is now known that *Cryptosporidium* spp. and *Giardia* spp. exist that are specific to people or pets.[33,34] Most people, cats, and dogs are infected with host-specific genotypes and so zoonotic transmission appears to be unlikely. However, some dogs and cats are infected with human genotypes suggesting shared infection can occur.[65,66] Therefore, infected animals, particularly those with diarrhea, should be managed as a potential zoonotic risk. Genotyping for both *Cryptosporidium* spp. and *Giardia* spp. is commercially available (Veterinary Diagnostic Laboratory, Colorado State University, Fort Collins, Colo.).

POLYSYSTEMIC PROTOZOAL DISEASES

The most common protozoal agents inducing disease in dogs or cats are the coccidians *Hepatozoon americanum, Neospora caninum,* and *Toxoplasma gondii,* the flagellates *Leishmania* spp. and *Trypanosoma cruzi,* and the piroplasms *Cytauxzoon felis* and *Babesia* spp. *Acanthamoeba castellanii* and *A. culbertsoni* are free-living amoeba rarely associated with disease in dogs.[67-69] *Encephalitozoon cuniculi* is a microspora that has been detected in some clinically ill dogs and cats, but infection appears to be uncommon.[70,71] *Pneumocystis carinii* is a saprophytic organism with worldwide distribution that has characteristics of protozoans, yeast, and fungi that has been detected in diseased dogs that generally have some form of immune function deficit.[72-76]

COCCIDIANS

Hepatozoonosis
Hepatozoon canis and *H. americanum* both infect dogs.[77-81] In North America, *H. americanum* predominates, but *H. canis* and mixed infections have been detected.[81] *Hepatozoon americanum* is transmitted by *Amblyomma maculatum* and is most common in the Texas Gulf Coast, Mississippi, Alabama, Georgia, Florida, Louisiana, and Oklahoma.[78,80,82] In Africa, southern Europe, and Asia, *H. canis* predominates and is transmitted by *Rhipicephalus sanguineus*. A *Hepatozoon* species is occasionally found in the blood of cats in Europe.[83,84] The tick ingests the organism from infected dogs during a blood meal and oocysts develop. After a dog ingests an infected tick, sporozoites are released and infect mononuclear

phagocytes and endothelial cells of the spleen, liver, muscle, lungs, and bone marrow, and they ultimately form cysts containing macromeronts and micromeronts. Clinical disease results from pyogranulomatous inflammation; glomerulonephritis or amyloidosis may occur secondary to chronic inflammation and immune complex disease.

H. americanum has resulted in illness in all age groups, but disease is most commonly recognized in puppies.[85,86] Fever, weight loss, and severe hyperesthesia over the paraspinal regions are common findings. Anorexia, pale mucous membranes from anemia, depression, oculonasal discharge, and bloody diarrhea occur in some dogs. Clinical signs can be intermittent and recurrent.

Neutrophilic leukocytosis (20,000 to 200,000 cells/µL) with a left shift and normocytic, normochromic nonregenerative anemia are the most common hematologic findings. Thrombocytopenia is unusual unless coinfection with *Ehrlichia canis* or *Anaplasma* spp. occurs. Increased activity of alkaline phosphatase, hypoalbuminemia, hypoglycemia, and, rarely, polyclonal gammopathy occur in some dogs. Inflammatory reactions directed at tissue phases in muscle result in periosteal reactions that can occur in any bone except the skull. These reactions do not occur in every case and are most common in young dogs. Presence of serum antibodies against *H. americanum* were compared with tissue biopsy; the sensitivity and specificity were 93% and 96%, respectively.[87] Definitive diagnosis is based on identification of gamonts in neutrophils or monocytes in Giemsa- or Leishman-stained blood smears or by demonstration of the organism in muscle biopsy sections (Table 207-1). In a recent study, DNA of *H. americanum* (27.2%), *H. canis* (2.3%), or DNA of both organisms (2.3%) were amplified by PCR assay from blood of 614 dogs suspected hepatozoonosis.[88] This assay may prove to be a valuable diagnostic tool.

While clinical signs of hepatozoonosis rapidly resolve with drug therapy, no therapeutic regimen has been shown to eliminate *H. canis* or *H. americanum* infection from tissues. For treatment of *H. americanum,* the combination of trimethoprim-sulfadiazine (15 mg/kg PO q12h), pyrimethamine (0.25 mg/kg PO q24h), and clindamycin (10 mg/kg PO q8h) for 14 days is very successful in the acute stage.[86] Use of decoquinate (10 to 20 mg/kg q12h) with food lessens the likelihood of recurrence of clinical disease and prolongs survival time. Imidocarb dipropionate administered (5 to 6 mg/kg, IM or SC) once or twice 14 days apart is the drug of choice for treatment of *H. canis* and may also be effective for *H. americanum.* Administration of nonsteroidal antiinflammatory agents may lessen discomfort for some dogs.

Tick control is the best form of prevention. Glucocorticoid administration should be avoided because it may exacerbate clinical disease. No evidence exists for zoonotic transfer of *H. americanum* or *H. canis* from infected dogs to people.

Neosporosis
Neospora caninum is a coccidian previously confused with *T. gondii* due to similar morphology.[89-91] The sexual cycle is completed in the GI tract of dogs and results in the passage of oocysts in feces.[92-96] Sporozoites develop in oocysts within 24 hours of passage. Tachyzoites (rapidly dividing stage) and tissue cysts containing hundreds of bradyzoites (slowly dividing stage) are the other two life stages. Infection has been documented after ingestion of infected bovine placental tissue and tissue from naturally infected deer.[97] Transplacental infection has been well documented; dams that give birth to infected offspring can repeat transplacental infection during subsequent pregnancies.[98] Although organism replication occurs in many tissues, clinical illness primarily reflects neuromuscular infection in dogs. Although encephalomyelitis and myositis develop in experimentally infected kittens and some

Table • 207-1

Characteristic Cytologic Morphology of Small Animal Systemic Protozoal Agents

AGENT	MORPHOLOGIC CHARACTERISTICS
Babesia canis	Paired piroplasms (2.4 by 5.0 μm) in circulating red blood cells
Babesia gibsoni	Single piroplasms (1.0 by 3.2 μm) in circulating red blood cells
Cytauxzoon felis	Piroplasms (1.0 by 1.5 μm "signet ring" form; 1.0 by 2.0 μm oval form; round form, 1.0 μm) in circulating red blood cells; macrophages or monocytes of lymph node aspirates, splenic aspirates, or bone marrow
Hepatozoon canis and H. americanum	Gamonts in circulating neutrophils and monocytes
Leishmania spp.	Ovoid to round amastigotes (2.5-5.0 by 1.5-2.0 μm) in macrophages found on imprints of exudative skin lesions, lymph node aspirates, or bone marrow aspirates
Neospora caninum	Free or intracellular (macrophages or monocytes) tachyzoites (5-7 by 1-5 μm) in cerebrospinal fluid, airway washings, or imprints of cutaneous lesions
Toxoplasma gondii	Free or intracellular (macrophages or monocytes) tachyzoites (6 by 2 μm) in pleural effusions, peritoneal effusions, or airway washings
Trypanosoma cruzi	Flagellated trypomastigotes (1 flagella; 15-20 μm long) free in whole blood, lymph node aspirates, and peritoneal fluid

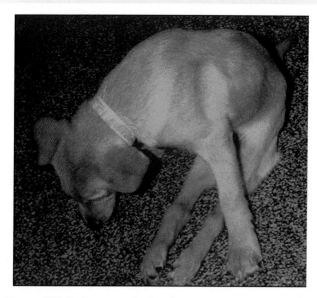

Figure 207-5 Puppy with the characteristic extensor rigidity associated with *Neospora caninum* infection. (Courtesy Dr. Paul Cuddon.)

naturally exposed cats are seropositive for *N. caninum* antibodies, clinical disease in naturally infected cats has not been reported.[99-101] Canine neosporosis has been reported in many countries around the world.

A number of clinical syndromes associated with neosporosis have been reported in dogs.[102-111] Congenitally infected puppies develop ascending paralysis with hyperextension of the hindlimbs; muscle atrophy occurs in many cases (Figure 207-5). Polymyositis and multifocal CNS disease can occur alone or in combination. Clinical signs can be evident soon after birth or may be delayed for several weeks. Neonatal death is common. Although disease tends to be most severe in congenitally infected puppies, dogs as old as 15 years have been clinically affected. In some dogs, myocarditis, dysphagia, ulcerative dermatitis, pneumonia, and hepatitis occur. If not treated, most affected dogs die.

No specific hematologic or biochemical findings exist, but increased creatine kinase and aspartate transaminase activities are common in dogs with myositis. Cerebrospinal fluid (CSF) abnormalities include increased protein concentration (20 to 50 mg/dL) and a mild, mixed inflammatory cell pleocytosis (10 to 50 cells/dL) consisting of monocytes, lymphocytes, neutrophils, and, rarely, eosinophils. Interstitial and alveolar patterns can be noted on thoracic radiographs. Demonstration of the organism in CSF or tissues gives a definitive diagnosis.

Tachyzoites are rarely identified on cytologic examination of CSF, imprints of dermatologic lesions, and bronchoalveolar lavage (see Table 207-1). *Neospora caninum* tissue cysts have a wall greater than 1 μm; *T. gondii* tissue cysts have a wall less than 1 μm. The organism can be differentiated from *T. gondii* by electron microscopy, immunohistochemistry, and PCR.[105,112]

A presumptive diagnosis of neosporosis is made by combining appropriate clinical signs of disease and positive serology with the exclusion of other causes inducing similar clinical syndromes, in particular, *T. gondii*.[113] Immunoglobulin G antibody titers greater than or equal to 1:200 have been detected in most dogs with clinical neosporosis; minimal serologic cross-reactivity with *T. gondii* occurs at titers greater than or equal to 1:50 when measured by IFA. Antibodies or *N. caninum* DNA can also be detected in CSF of some affected dogs.[114]

The prognosis for dogs with severe neurologic involvement is grave. Some have survived after treatment with trimethoprim-sulfadiazine combined with pyrimethamine, sequential treatment with clindamycin hydrochloride, trimethoprim-sulfadiazine, and pyrimethamine, or clindamycin alone.[102-105,107] Glucocorticoids may exacerbate clinical disease.

Neospora caninum antibodies have been detected in people, including those with AIDS and neurologic disease.[115,116] However, in one study there was no link to repeated abortion in women.[117] Overall, the zoonotic link is unclear, but it seems prudent to avoid ingesting canine feces or undercooked meat. There has been an epidemiologic link between dogs and cattle; therefore, efforts should be made to lessen dog fecal contamination of livestock feed, and dogs should not be allowed to ingest bovine placentas or venison.[118-120] Bitches that whelp clinically affected puppies should not be bred.

Toxoplasmosis

Toxoplasma gondii is one of the most prevalent parasites infecting warm-blooded vertebrates.[121] Only cats complete the coccidian life cycle and pass environmentally resistant oocysts in feces. Dogs can pass oocysts in feces after the ingestion of feline feces.[122] Sporozoites develop in oocysts after 1 to 5 days of exposure to oxygen and appropriate environmental temperature and humidity (see Figure 207-1). Tachyzoites

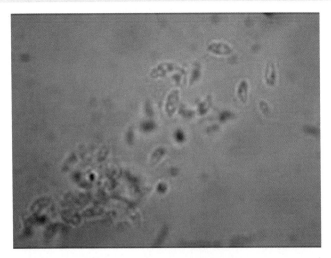

Figure 207-6 *Toxoplasma gondii* tachyzoites.

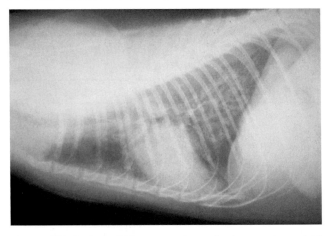

Figure 207-7 Lateral thoracic radiograph showing interstitial pneumonitis due to *Toxoplasma gondii* infection in a feline immunodeficiency virus–positive cat. (Courtesy Dr. Gary Oswald.)

disseminate in blood or lymph during active infection and replicate intracellularly rapidly until the cell is destroyed (Figure 207-6).

Bradyzoites are the slowly dividing, persistent, tissue stage that form in the extraintestinal tissues of infected hosts as immune responses attenuate tachyzoite replication. Tissue cysts form readily in the CNS, muscles, and visceral organs. Infection of warm-blooded vertebrates occurs after ingestion of any of the three life stages of the organism or transplacentally. Most cats are not coprophagic and are usually infected by ingesting *T. gondii* bradyzoites during carnivorous feeding; oocysts are shed in feces from 3 to 21 days. Sporulated oocysts can survive in the environment for months to years and are resistant to most disinfectants. Bradyzoites may persist in tissues for the life of the host. Approximately 30% to 40% of cats and 20% of the dogs in the United States are seropositive and therefore presumed to be infected.[121]

Clinical disease associated with the GI phase of infection is rare, and detection of *T. gondii* oocysts in feces is rarely reported in studies of naturally exposed cats with diarrhea.[123-124] Most clinical signs are systemic and can include death in dogs and cats that develop overwhelming intracellular replication of tachyzoites after primary infection; hepatic, pulmonary, CNS, and pancreatic tissues are commonly involved (Figure 207-7).[125-128]

Immune deficiency secondary to viral infection or immune suppressive therapy can also induce fatal toxoplasmosis.[129-131] Common clinical findings in cats with disseminated toxoplasmosis include depression, anorexia, fever followed by hypothermia, peritoneal effusion, icterus, and dyspnea.

Chronic toxoplasmosis occurs in some dogs and cats. *Toxoplasma gondii* infection should be on the differential diagnoses list for cats with anterior or posterior uveitis, fever, muscle hyperesthesia, weight loss, anorexia, seizures, ataxia, icterus, diarrhea, cutaneous disease, and pancreatitis.[132-139] In dogs, respiratory, GI, or neuromuscular infection resulting in fever, vomiting, diarrhea, dyspnea, cutaneous disease, and icterus are most common and occur most frequently in immune-suppressed dogs, such as those with canine distemper virus (CDV) infection or those receiving cyclosporine to prevent rejection of a transplanted kidney.[130,140-142] Neurologic signs are dependent on the location of the primary lesions and include ataxia, seizures, tremors, cranial nerve deficits, paresis, and paralysis. Dogs with myositis have weakness, stiff gait, or muscle wasting. Rapid progression to tetraparesis and paralysis with lower motor neuron dysfunction can occur. Some dogs with suspected neuromuscular toxoplasmosis probably

had neosporosis.[89] Myocardial infection resulting in ventricular arrhythmias occurs in some infected dogs. Dyspnea, vomiting, or diarrhea can occur in dogs with polysystemic disease. Retinitis, anterior uveitis, iridocyclitis, and optic neuritis occur in some dogs with toxoplasmosis but are less common than in the cat.

Dogs or cats with clinical toxoplasmosis can have a variety of clinicopathologic and radiographic abnormalities but none document the disease.[133,143] Nonregenerative anemia, neutrophilic leukocytosis, lymphocytosis, monocytosis, neutropenia, eosinophilia, proteinuria, bilirubinuria, increases in serum proteins and bilirubin concentration, as well as creatinine kinase, alanine aminotransferase, alkaline phosphatase, and lipase activities occur in some animals. Pulmonary toxoplasmosis most commonly causes diffuse interstitial to alveolar patterns or pleural effusion.[144] CSF protein concentrations and cell counts are often higher than normal. The predominant white blood cells (WBCs) in CSF are small mononuclear cells, but neutrophils also are commonly found.

The antemortem definitive diagnosis of toxoplasmosis can be made if the organism is demonstrated; however, this is uncommon. Bradyzoites or tachyzoites are rarely detected in tissues, effusions, bronchoalveolar lavage fluids, aqueous humor, or CSF (see Table 207-1). Detection of 10×12 µm oocysts in feces in cats with diarrhea suggests toxoplasmosis but is not definitive, because *Besnoitia* and *Hammondia* infections of cats produce morphologically similar oocysts.

Toxoplasma gondii–specific antibodies (dogs or cats), antigens (cats), immune complexes (cats), and DNA (cats) can be detected in the blood of normal animals, as well as in those with clinical signs of disease; therefore it is impossible to make an antemortem diagnosis of clinical toxoplasmosis based on these tests alone.[145-147] Of the serum tests, IgM correlates the best with clinical toxoplasmosis because this antibody class is rarely detected in serum of healthy animals. Because the organism cannot be cleared from the body, most animals will be antibody-positive for life; therefore, repeating serum antibody titers after clinical disease has resolved is of little use. The combination of aqueous humor or CSF *T. gondii*–specific antibody detection and organism DNA detection by PCR is the most accurate way to diagnose ocular or CNS toxoplasmosis in cats (Diagnostic Laboratory, College of Veterinary Medicine and Biomedical Sciences, Colorado State University, Fort Collins, Colo.).

Clindamycin hydrochloride, trimethoprim-sulfonamide combination, and azithromycin have been used successfully for the treatment of clinical toxoplasmosis.[132,133] Pyrimethamine combined with sulfa drugs is effective for the treatment of human toxoplasmosis but commonly results in toxicity in cats. Cats or dogs with uveitis should be treated with topical, oral, or parenteral glucocorticoids to avoid secondary glaucoma and lens luxations.[133,148]

To prevent toxoplasmosis, eating undercooked meats or ingesting sporulated oocysts should be avoided. Although owning a pet cat was epidemiologically associated with acquiring toxoplasmosis in one study of pregnant women, touching individual cats is probably not a common way to acquire toxoplasmosis for the following reasons[149]:

- Cats generally shed oocysts only for days to several weeks after primary inoculation.
- Repeat oocyst shedding is rare, even in cats receiving glucocorticoids, and in those infected with FIV or FeLV.[150,151]
- Cats with toxoplasmosis inoculated with tissue cysts 16 months after primary inoculation did not shed oocysts.[151]
- Cats are fastidious and usually do not allow feces to remain on their skin for time periods long enough to lead to oocyst sporulation; the organism was not isolated from the fur of cats shedding millions of oocysts 7 days previously.[152]
- Increased risk of acquired toxoplasmosis was not associated with cat ownership in human immunodeficiency virus (HIV)–infected people or in veterinary health care providers.[153]

Because humans are not commonly infected with *T. gondii* from contact with individual cats, testing healthy cats for toxoplasmosis is not recommended. No serologic assay accurately predicts when a cat shed *T. gondii* oocysts in the past, and most cats that are shedding oocysts are seronegative. Most seropositive cats have completed the oocyst shedding period and are unlikely to repeat shedding; most seronegative cats would shed the organism if infected. If owners are concerned that they may have toxoplasmosis, they should see their doctor for testing. Avoiding sporulated oocysts and tissue cysts in undercooked meat can lessen the risk of acquiring toxoplasmosis.

FLAGGELATES

Leishmaniasis

Leishmania spp. are flagellates that cause cutaneous, mucocutaneous, and visceral diseases in dogs, humans, and other mammals. Rodents and dogs are primary reservoirs of *Leishmania* spp.; people are incidental hosts. Leishmaniasis was considered unimportant in the United States until recently, with cases reported only occasionally.[154-161] In 2000, *Leishmania donovani* infection was confirmed in multiple dogs in a Foxhound kennel in New York State.[159] Further investigation documented *L. donovani* or *Leishmania* spp. infection in 30 other Foxhound kennels in 20 states and Ontario, Canada. Infection of dogs other than Foxhounds in the United States appears to be uncommon.[161] Transmission appears to be primarily from dog to dog in Foxhounds in the United States, but transmission by shared needles, blood transfusions, breeding, and congenital transmission can occur.[159,162-164] In other countries, the sandfly is the primary vector. Flagellated promastigotes develop in the sandfly and are injected into the vertebrate host when the sandfly feeds. Promastigotes are engulfed by macrophages and disseminate through the body. After an incubation period of 1 month to 7 years, amastigotes (nonflagellate) form and cutaneous lesions develop; sandflies are infected during feeding. The intracellular organism induces extreme immune responses; polyclonal gammopathies (and occasionally monoclonal), proliferation of macrophages, histiocytes, and lymphocytes in lymphoreticular organs and

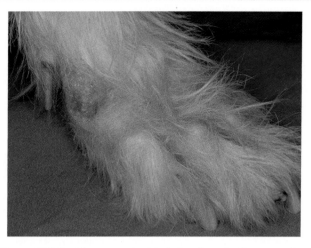

Figure 207-8 Characteristic skin lesion from *Leishmania* infection in a dog. (Courtesy Dr. Arturo Font.)

immune complex formation resulting in glomerulonephritis and polyarthritis are common in dogs. A clinically affected cat in Texas was infected by *L. mexicana mexicana* and cats have been infected experimentally.[156,165]

Visceral leishmaniasis is most common in dogs. Subclinical infection may persist for months or years. When clinical signs occur, weight loss, normal to increased appetite, polyuria, polydipsia, muscle wasting, depression, vomiting, diarrhea, cough, epistaxis, sneezing, and melena are common presenting complaints. Splenomegaly, lymphadenopathy, facial alopecia, fever, rhinitis, dermatitis, increased lung sounds, icterus, swollen painful joints, uveitis, and conjunctivitis are commonly identified on physical examination.[154,155,166] Cutaneous lesions are characterized by hyperkeratosis, scaling, thickening, mucocutaneous ulcers, and intradermal nodules on the muzzle, pinnae, ears, and footpads (Figure 207-8).

Hyperglobulinemia, hypoalbuminemia, proteinuria, increased liver enzyme activities, thrombocytopenia, azotemia, lymphopenia, and leukocytosis with left shift are common in dogs. Hyperglobulinemia is usually polyclonal, but an IgG monoclonal gammopathy was reported in a dog.[167] *Leishmania*-infected dogs can be positive for antinuclear antibodies in serum, which may lead to the erroneous diagnosis of primary immune-mediated disease.[168]

Leishmaniasis can be confirmed by detecting the organisms by cytology, histopathology PCR assay, or laboratory animal inoculation or by detecting antibodies against *Leishmania* in serum[169-175] Demonstration of amastigotes (2.5 to 5.0 μm × 1.5 to 2.0 μm in lymph node aspirates, bone marrow aspirates, or skin imprints stained with Wright's or Giemsa stain gives a definitive diagnosis (Figure 207-9). PCR assays can be performed on EDTA anticoagulated blood, bone marrow aspirates, lymph node aspirates, urine, or tissue samples. Dogs are unlikely to eliminate *Leishmania* infection spontaneously, and so a true positive antibody test indicates infection.

Many treated dogs respond clinically, but *Leishmania* cannot be eliminated from the body with drugs.[169,172,175-181] The combination of antimony and allopurinol was superior to treatment with either drug alone in one study.[176] As antimonial drugs are not routinely available in the United States, affected dogs could be administered allopurinol, marbofloxacin, or liposomal amphotericin B initially.[176,179,181] The prognosis is variable; most cases are recurrent.

Avoidance of infected sandflies is the only means of prevention.[182,183] If in endemic areas, pet owners should house animals during nighttime hours, control breeding places of sandflies, and consider use of 10% imidocloprid/50%

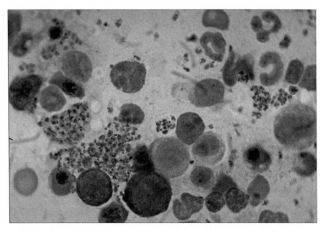

Figure 207-9 *Leishmania amastigotes* in a cytology made from a draining skin lesion from a dog. (Courtesy Dr. Arturo Font.)

permethrin repellent.[183] A vaccine is available for use in some countries.[184] Foxhounds or and other dogs from endemic areas to be used as potential blood donors should be screened serologically or by PCR assay on blood.[162,185] The primary zoonotic risk for canine leishmaniasis is from dogs acting as a reservoir host for the organism. Direct contact with amastigotes in draining lesions is unlikely to result in human infection. In one study in the United States, none of the 185 persons with potential exposure to infected Foxhounds had evidence of infection.[159]

Trypanosomiasis

Trypanosoma cruzi infection of mammals is diagnosed primarily in South America, but several cases have been detected in dogs of North America.[186-194] Infected reservoir mammals (dogs, cats, raccoons, opossums, armadillos) and vectors (reduviid bugs, kissing bugs) are found in the United States, but infection in dogs or people is rare; this may relate to differences in vector behavior and sanitation standards in the United States. Recently, some Foxhounds infected with *Leishmania* spp. were shown to be coinfected with *T. cruzi*.[159]

The organism should be on the differential list for dogs in endemic areas with cardiomyopathy, conduction disturbances, ventricular arrhythmias, and supraventricular arrhythmias. Laryngeal paralysis and neurologic disease may occur occasionally. Laboratory abnormalities include lymphocytosis and increased activities of liver enzymes and creatine kinase. Thoracic radiographic, abdominal radiographic, and echocardiographic findings are consistent with cardiac disease and failure, but they are not specific for trypanosomiasis. The primary ECG findings are ventricular premature contractions, heart block, and T-wave inversion.

Definitive diagnosis is based on organism demonstration. Trypomastigotes (1 flagellum, 15- to 20-μm long can be identified during acute disease on thick blood film or buffy coat smears stained with Giemsa or Wright's stain (see Table 207-1). The organism is sometimes detected in lymph node aspirates or in abdominal effusions. Histopathologic evaluation of cardiac tissue may reveal amastigotes (1.5 to 4.0 μm). Trypomastigotes can also be cultured from blood or grown by bioassay in mice. In North American cases, positive serologic test results correlate with infection.[195] PCR assay can also be used to detect infection.[194]

There are no approved drugs available for *T. cruzi* infection in the United States, but in a recent study of allopurinol in an experimentally infected mouse model, a positive response was noted (see Leishmania section).[196] Glucocorticoid therapy may improve survival of infected dogs. Therapy for arrhyth-

mias or heart failure should be instituted as needed (see Chapters 238, 241, and 245).

Dogs in endemic areas should be kept from other reservoir hosts such as opossums and should not be fed raw meat. Vector control is the primary means of prevention.[197] Potential blood donors from endemic areas should be serologically screened. Infected dogs can serve as a reservoir of *T. cruzi* for vectors, and blood from infected dogs can be infectious to humans.

PIROPLASMIA

Babesiosis

Multiple *Babesia* spp. infect dogs throughout the world; *B. canis* and *B. gibsoni* are most common.[198-213] *Babesia canis* has worldwide distribution including Africa, Asia, Australia, Europe, Central America, South America, Japan, and the United States. *B. canis rossi* is transmitted by *Haemaphysalis leachi* and is the most pathogenic. *B. canis canis* is transmitted by *Dermacenter reticulatus* and is moderately pathogenic. *Babesia canis vogeli* occurs in the United State, is the least pathogenic, and is transmitted by *Rhipicephalus sanguineus*. *Babesia gibsoni* infects dogs in the United States, Japan, India, Sri Lanka, Korea, Malaysia, and Egypt. In the United States, the vector for *B. gibsoni* is unknown but the organism is known to be transmitted by biting and is common in American Pit Bull Terriers.[206,214] *Babesia* spp. can also be transmitted by blood transfusion.[215] None of the *Babesia* spp. that infect cats—*B. cati* (India), *B. felis* (South Africa and Sudan), *B. herpailuri* (South America and Africa), or *B. pantherae* (Kenya)—are found in the United States.

In the United States, subclinical *Babesia* spp. infections are most common. Following infection with pathogenic strains of *B. canis* or *B. gibsoni*, the incubation period varies from several days to several weeks. The degree of parasitemia varies by the organism studied, but can be detected transiently in some dogs as soon as day 1.[216] In some infected dogs, the intracellular replication in red blood cells (RBCs) results intravascular hemolytic anemia. Immune-mediated reactions against the parasite or altered self-antigens worsen the hemolytic anemia and commonly result in positive Coombs' test. Severity of disease depends on the species and strain of *Babesia* and the host immune status; chronic, subclinical infection can occur. Presence of coinfections, such as *Bartonella* spp., may increase the pathogenic potential.[211,217] Clinical manifestations are those of acute anemia and include fever, pale mucous membranes, tachycardia, tachypnea, depression, anorexia, and weakness. Icterus, petechiation, azotemia, and hepatosplenomegaly are present in some dogs depending on the stage of infection and the presence of disseminated intravascular coagulation (DIC). Administration of glucocorticoids or splenectomy may activate chronic disease. Common laboratory abnormalities include regenerative anemia, hyperbilirubinemia, bilirubinuria, hemoglobinuria, thrombocytopenia, metabolic acidosis, azotemia, polyclonal gammopathy, and renal casts.[209,216,218]

A presumptive diagnosis of clinical babesiosis can be based on historical findings, physical examination findings, test results, and positive serology. Many dogs are seropositive but clinically normal; therefore, serology alone cannot be used to make a definitive diagnosis.[208,219] Demonstration of increasing antibody titers over 2 to 3 weeks are consistent with recent or active babesiosis. Definitive diagnosis is based on organism demonstration in RBCs using Wright's or Giemsa stains on thin blood smears. *B. canis* is typically found as paired, piriform bodies measuring 2.4 × 5.0 μm. *B. gibsoni* is typically found as single, annular bodies measuring 1.0 × 3.2 μm (see Table 207-1). A PCR assay for *Babesia* spp. is now available commercially and can be used to document organism presence, but positive results do not always correlate to clinical illness.[220,221]

Supportive care, including blood transfusions, should be administered as indicated. A number of drugs including diminazene aceturate, phenamidine, pentamidine isethionate, parvaquone, atovaquone, and niridazone have also been used in an attempt to treat different *Babesia* spp. infections. In the United States, dogs with suspected *B. canis* associated clinical illness often respond to imidocarb diproprionate administered at 5 to 6.6 mg/kg SC or IM twice, 14 days apart or 7.5 mg/kg, SC or IM once.[222] Adverse effects include transient salivation, diarrhea, dyspnea, lacrimation, and depression. Imidocarb is not as effective for the treatment of *B. gibsoni* infection. In the United States, dogs with suspected *B. gibsoni* associated clinical illness often respond to azithromycin (10 mg/kg, PO, q24hr for a minimum of 10 days) combined with atovaquone (13.3 mg/kg, PO, q8hr for at least 10 days).[223] If these drugs are not available, clindamycin administered at 12.5 mg/kg, PO, q12h for at least 10 days may control clinical signs.[224] However, treatment of *Babesia* spp. infections is unlikely to eliminate the carrier state.[225] As there are no drugs available that are known to consistently eliminate infection, treatment of healthy, seropositive dogs is unlikely to be of benefit.

Ticks should be controlled if possible.[226] If it is difficult to control ticks in a *B. canis*–infected kennel, one dose of imidocarb at 7.5 mg/kg, IM may eliminate the carrier state. Dog fights should be avoided. Administration of immunosuppressive drugs and splenectomy should be avoided in previously infected dogs. Dogs in high-risk breeds (Greyhound, American Pit Bull Terrier) and dogs from endemic areas to be used as blood donors should be assessed for infection by PCR assay or serologic screening and positive dogs eliminated from the program.[183] Currently no evidence exists to suggest that *Babesia* spp. infecting dogs and cats can cause human disease.

Cytauxzoonosis

Cytauxzoon felis infects cats in the southeastern, south central United States, and mid-Atlantic states.[227-229] In one study of 961 cats in Florida, North Carolina, and Tennessee, the prevalence rate was 0.3%.[228] While isolates from domestic cats have been genetically similar between studies,[231] domestic cats occasionally will survive infection, suggesting that variants

that are less virulent to cats also exist.[228,232,233] Bobcats are usually subclinically affected and are the likely natural host of the organism. The organism can be passed experimentally from infected bobcats to domestic cats by *Dermacentor variabilis;* clinical illness occurs after an incubation period of 5 to 20 days.[234] Infected macrophages line the lumen of veins throughout the body, and merozoites released from the infected macrophages infect erythrocytes. Clinical disease results from obstruction of blood flow through tissues by mononuclear infiltrates and from hemolytic anemia.

Most cases of cytauxzoonosis are in cats allowed to go outdoors. Fever, anorexia, dyspnea, depression, icterus, pale mucous membranes, and death are the most common clinical findings.[227,235-237] A primary differential diagnosis is hemoplasmosis. Ticks are generally not identified on affected cats. Cytauxzoonosis is suspected in cats with regenerative anemia and neutrophilic leukocytosis; thrombocytopenia occurs in some cats. Hemoglobinemia, hemoglobinuria, bilirubinemia, and bilirubinuria are uncommon. Antemortem diagnosis is based on demonstration of the erythrocytic phase on thin blood smears stained with Wright's or Giemsa stains. Infected macrophages can be detected cytologically in bone marrow, spleen, liver, or lymph node aspirates.

The organism is easily identified on histologic evaluation of most organs. Serologic testing is not commercially available but PCR assay can be used to amplify organismal DNA from blood.[231,233]

Supportive care should be administered as indicated. Treatment with diminazene (five cats) (2.0 mg/kg, IM, twice, 7 days apart) or imidocarb (one cat) (2 mg/kg, IM, twice 14 days apart) was used in cats that survived infection.[236] In another preliminary study, 14 of 22 cats survived after administration of atovaquone (15 mg/kg, PO, q8h) and azithromycin (10 mg/kg, PO, q24h).[238] Ticks should be controlled, and cats in endemic areas should be housed during periods of peak tick activity. *Cytauxzoon felis* is not known to be zoonotic.

REFERENCES

The reference list can be found on the companion Expert Consult Web site at *www.expertconsult.com.*

CHAPTER 208

Enteric Bacterial Disease

Stanley L. Marks

Veterinarians are faced with a quandary when attempting to diagnose enteric bacterial disease in dogs or cats because the isolation rates for putative bacterial enteropathogens are often similar in diarrheic and nondiarrheic animals,[1-3] the incidence of bacterial-associated diarrhea is extremely variable, and the indications for performing fecal enteric panels are poorly defined, resulting in indiscriminate testing and misinterpretation of results. There is no consensus among veterinary diagnostic laboratories as to which bacterial species should be investigated or which diagnostic assays should be used. To compound these issues, sensitivities and

specificities of commercial toxin assays commonly used in the dog and cat have not been validated. The enteropathogenic bacteria most commonly incriminated in canine and feline diarrhea include *Clostridium perfringens, Clostridium difficile, Campylobacter* spp., *Salmonella* spp., and *Escherichia coli.*

The specific indications for performing fecal enteric panels consisting of fecal cultures, toxin analysis, and genotyping are poorly defined. Most veterinary microbiologists agree that enteric panels should be reserved for dogs and cats developing diarrhea after kenneling or show attendance, in animals with an acute onset of bloody diarrhea in association with evidence of sepsis, and in diarrhea outbreaks affecting more than one pet in a household. In addition, *C. difficile, Campylobacter* spp., and *Salmonella* spp. are zoonotic, and judicious screening for these organisms is warranted when an immunocompromised person owns a potentially infected animal, or the animal is in contact with children.

Clostridium perfringens

C. perfringens is an anaerobic, spore-forming, gram-positive bacillus that has been associated with outbreaks of acute, often severe diarrhea in humans, horses, dogs, and cats. The elaboration of four major toxins (α, β, ι, and ε) is the basis for typing the organism into five toxigenic phenotypes, A-E. Each type may also express a subset of at least 10 other established toxins, including *C. perfringens* enterotoxin (CPE), a well-characterized virulence factor whose production is coregulated with sporulation.[4] Dogs with *C. perfringens*–associated diarrhea frequently exhibit large-bowel diarrhea characterized by increased frequency of bowel movements with tenesmus, fecal mucus, and hematochezia; however, clinical signs of enteritis or enterocolitis are also common.[2] A strong association has also been detected between the CPE detected via ELISA and acute hemorrhagic diarrheal syndrome (AHDS).[2] CPE was detected in the feces of 8 of 12 dogs (67%) that had clinical signs consistent with AHDS. Of four dogs that had peracute disease and that died as a result of their disease, all had fecal specimens positive for CPE. Although several studies have shown an association between the immunodetection of CPE in fecal specimens and canine diarrhea, the pathogenesis of *C. perfringens*–associated diarrhea in the dog and cat is not fully understood, as CPE is also detected in up to 14% of nondiarrheic dogs.[1,5] A preliminary study in the author's laboratory documented a zero prevalence of CPE in fecal specimens collected from 51 healthy nondiarrheic cats, and in 9 of 62 (14%) fecal specimens obtained from diarrheic cats.

PATHOGENESIS

CPE is a 35-kDa protein encoded by the *cpe* gene, whose expression is coregulated with sporulation of the organism.[4,6] *C. perfringens* strains that carry a chromosomal *cpe* have primarily been associated with human food-borne disease, whereas strains with a plasmid *cpe* gene have been associated with human non–food-borne diseases and animal diseases, including canine diarrhea. Non–food-borne diseases associated with CPE are thought to involve commensal enterotoxigenic strains that are somehow triggered to undergo massive sporulation. The trigger may be one of several different factors including sudden changes in diet, antibiotic administration, or coinfection with another intestinal pathogen. Once released into the intestinal lumen, CPE interacts with specific epithelial tight junction proteins forming a small protein complex of ~90 kDa, where it then becomes trapped on the membrane surface.[6] The small CPE complex then interacts with additional host proteins, forming several larger complexes. Recent studies have suggested a ~155 kDa complex is responsible for the cytotoxic and histopathologic damage which provides CPE access to occludin, causing alterations in tight junction structure and function, leading to paracellular permeability changes that contribute to diarrhea.[6]

DIAGNOSIS

Currently, diagnosis of *C. perfringens*–associated diarrhea in the dog and cat is optimally made based on detection of CPE

in fecal specimens in conjunction with PCR detection of the enterotoxin gene *(cpe)*.[1] There are no pathognomonic clinical signs indicative of *C. perfringens*–associated diarrhea in dogs. Infected animals may have small intestinal, large intestinal, or diffuse clinical signs.[2] However, examination of any dog with acute hemorrhagic diarrhea warrants consideration of *C. perfringens* as a causative or associative enteropathogen. The diagnostic value of quantitative fecal culture and fecal spore counts have been shown to be poor, as the organism can be isolated from more than 80% of healthy dogs and there is no correlation between spore counts and detection of CPE, or between fecal consistency and detection of CPE.[1,7] There is only one commercially available ELISA kit (Techlab Inc., Blacksburg, Va.) for detection of CPE in fecal specimens; however, the performance characteristics of this assay have not been validated in the dog or cat to date. Further, up to 14% of healthy dogs have detectable concentrations of CPE utilizing the commercially available ELISA.[1] As mentioned, PCR detection of *cpe* was shown to be a valuable diagnostic test when combined with immunodetection of CPE. Fecal specimens from nondiarrheic dogs were far less likely to be positive for both CPE and *cpe* (4%) compared to diarrheic dogs (28%).[1]

THERAPY

Antibiotics that have been recommended for the treatment of canine *C. perfringens*–associated diarrhea include ampicillin (22 mg/kg q8h for 5 days), metronidazole (10 mg/kg q12h for 5 days), and tylosin (15 mg/kg q12h for 5 days). Tetracycline use should be avoided due to the high incidence (21%) of in vitro resistance to this antimicrobial.[8] Anecdotal reports touting the benefits of increasing dietary fiber or administering probiotics to infected animals to alter the commensal microflora have not been validated.

Clostridium difficile

C. difficile is a gram-positive, anaerobic spore-forming bacillus, and is the major cause of antibiotic-associated pseudomembranous colitis in people. *C. difficile* has also been associated with diarrhea and enterocolitis in foals, adult horses, and dogs. An outbreak of *C. difficile* infection (CDI) was reported in dogs at a veterinary teaching hospital,[9] with an incidence rate of 19 cases per 1000 admissions. There is a dearth of information about CDI in cats, although preliminary studies suggest an incidence of 5% in 62 diarrheic cats, and zero in 51 healthy, nondiarrheic cats. Two toxins, toxin A (TcdA, an enterotoxin) and toxin B (TcdB, a cytotoxin), are thought to be primarily responsible for disease associated with the organism, although other toxins may also play a role. In addition, a small percentage of healthy individuals can carry *C. difficile* in their intestinal tracts without any signs of disease.

PATHOGENESIS

Clinical disease is associated with the growth of toxin-producing strains of *C. difficile* in the intestinal tract, followed by release of toxins and subsequent development of disease. Although antimicrobials are frequently associated with a disruption of the normal commensal microflora and subsequent overgrowth of toxigenic strains of *C. difficile* in people, there is no convincing evidence of antimicrobials or other risk factors in dogs or cats. The main virulence factors involved in the pathogenesis of CDI are TcdA and TcdB.[10] Some *C.*

difficile strains can produce a binary toxin (CDT), although its role is unclear.

DIAGNOSIS

There are no pathognomonic clinical signs in dogs and cats, although a strong association was found between the detection of *C. difficile* TcdA and the presence of an AHDS in dogs, similar to that described for *C. perfringens*.[2] Selective culture media, such as cycloserine cefoxitin fructose agar (CCFA) or *C. difficile* moxalactam norfloxacin agar (CDMN) are typically used, with direct inoculation or following broth enrichment. Isolation of the organism alone is not sufficient for diagnosis due to the presence of nontoxigenic strains; however, an appropriately processed and cultured fecal specimen that is culture-negative has a good negative predictive value. Detection of common antigen (glutamate dehydrogenase), an enzyme that is produced constitutively by toxigenic and nontoxigenic strains, represents a sensitive yet nonspecific test that is commonly performed in human and veterinary reference laboratories. A recent study evaluating the performance characteristics of the common antigen test in dogs documented a sensitivity of 100% with a low specificity, underscoring the value of this test as a screening test for dogs with suspected CDI.[11] The traditional diagnosis of CDI is made via detection of TcdA and/or TcdB in fecal specimens via ELISA. Commercially available ELISAs are used in veterinary reference laboratories; however, the performance characteristics of these human-based assays are uniformly poor in dogs, with sensitivities ranging from 7% to 60%.[11] The current gold standard test for CDI is the cell culture cytotoxicity assay (CTA), which detects TcdB activity[12]; however, the test is rarely performed because it is expensive and time consuming. The diagnosis of CDI in dogs and cats should be based on a combination of tests, including a positive fecal culture and/or common antigen test, followed by ELISA for detection of TcdA and TcdB. There are no validated PCR tests for *C. difficile* in dogs or cats, and performing direct PCR from stool can be associated with false negative results because of PCR inhibitors. Direct PCR for the diagnosis of CDI in dogs and cats is not recommended.

THERAPY

Supportive therapy should be administered and any antibiotics that are concurrently being administered and that may have predisposed the animal to the development of CDI should be discontinued. Metronidazole (10 mg/kg q12h for approximately 5 days) is the therapy of choice for dogs and cats with suspected CDI. Although metronidazole-resistant *C. difficile* isolates obtained from horses has been reported, a study evaluating the susceptibilities of 70 canine *C. difficile* isolates showed that all were susceptible to ≤1 μg/mL metronidazole.[8] The second drug of choice in humans and occasionally in horses is vancomycin; however, it is used only in cases of nonresponsive CDI or when metronidazole-resistant strains have been demonstrated.

Campylobacter spp.

Campylobacter spp. are small (0.2 to 0.5 μm × 0.5 to 5 μm), microaerophilic, gram-negative, curved, rod-shaped bacteria. There are over 37 species and subspecies in the *Campylobacter* genus; however, most of these are probably nonpathogenic. *Campylobacter* species that have been implicated in canine enteric disease include *C. jejuni*, *C. coli*, *C. helveticus*, and

C. upsaliensis. *C. helveticus* and *C. upsaliensis* are the most common isolates in cats. It has recently been shown that some selective media can have an inhibitory effect on a number of *Campylobacter* spp., resulting in more sensitive species, such as *C. upsaliensis* or other catalase-negative or weakly positive species being missed.[13] Fecal shedding of *C. jejuni* is significantly greater in puppies less than 6 months old during the summer and autumn.[14] The higher prevalence of infection in pups versus adult dogs may reflect increased exposure of young animals to fecal excrement and confinement to a limited space. In addition, the unexposed immune system of the pups may increase the susceptibility to intestinal colonization by *C. jejuni*. Other enteric pathogens, such as parvovirus, *Giardia*, or *Salmonella* may play a synergistic role. The isolation of *Campylobacter* spp. from a diarrheic animal does not necessarily implicate *Campylobacter* as a cause. Preliminary studies have documented a higher incidence of *Campylobacter* in healthy, nondiarrheic cats (10 of 51 cats; [20%]) versus diarrheic cats (7 of 62 cats; [11%]). In addition, several other studies have found similar isolation rate of *Campylobacter* in diarrheic and nondiarrheic animals.[15,16]

PATHOGENESIS

Campylobacter have a fecal to oral route of transmission either through direct contact with fecal material or with objects contaminated with feces. Various virulence factors are associated with colonization, adhesion, invasion, persistence within the host, and host cell damage. The cause of diarrhea due to *Campylobacter* infection is poorly understood, and the only exotoxin characterized in *Campylobacter* is cytolethal distending toxin, or CDT.[17] The toxin consists of three proteins, CdtA, CdtB, and CdtC, all of which are required to cause cellular damage. A neutrophilic inflammatory response in the bowel has been described in association with *Campylobacter* infection, and active intestinal fluid secretion may be due to *Campylobacter* products that increase cAMP, prostaglandin E_2, and leukotriene B_4.

DIAGNOSIS

Typical clinical signs include anorexia, occasional vomiting, and diarrhea. Fecal consistency is variable, but often contains mucus or blood. The animal can be febrile, and severely affected animals can be lethargic and dehydrated. Diagnosis is confirmed via several different methodologies, including examination of a direct stained fecal smear for small curved rods consistent with *Campylobacter*, culture, and molecular methods. *Campylobacter*-like organisms (CLOs) can be identified by examining stained smears (Gram stain or Romanovsky-type stain) of fresh feces from the patient. The organism's characteristic morphology (slender, curved rods with an S shape or sea gull–shaped appearance) allows it to be identified relatively easily. The major limitation of direct examinations is that the procedure fails to differentiate between *Campylobacter* spp. or between related organisms including *Helicobacter* spp. and *Anaerobiospirillium* spp. In addition, identification of CLOs alone on a stained fecal smear is not sufficient to warrant a diagnosis of *Campylobacter*-associated diarrhea, as many healthy dogs and cats can harbor CLOs in their intestinal tract.[2]

For optimal recovery of *Campylobacter* spp., feces or fecal swabs should be fresh or placed immediately into anaerobic transport medium before refrigeration at 4° C. For isolation, the use of a formulated selective medium containing antimicrobial agents (e.g., Campy-CVA containing cefoperazone, vancomycin, and amphotericin B) gives better recovery than other direct-plating selective media. Microaerophilic incubation conditions should be maintained, and the plates should be incubated at 37° C, or at 42° C, when isolation of *C. jejuni* and *C. coli* from feces is attempted. Suspect colonies should be Gram-stained and subcultured to 5% SBA. Biochemical tests can then be performed to speciate all CLOs isolated. A selective medium containing cefoperazone should be used when attempting to isolate *C. upsaliensis*, as the organism is more resistant to cefoperazone than to cephalothin.[18] Characterization of *Campylobacter* infections or mixed infections with *Helicobacter* and *Campylobacter* spp. is best accomplished utilizing molecular structure–based diagnostics, employing genus- and species-specific PCR, RFLP analysis, and 16S rRNA sequence analysis.[16]

THERAPY

Although diarrhea produced by *Campylobacter* organisms is usually self-limiting, the zoonotic potential of the organism often necessitates medical therapy. *Campylobacter* are a leading cause of enteric disease in people. Diarrheic and non-diarrheic dogs can serve as sources of human infection.[19] The drugs of choice are the macrolides (erythromycin at 10 to 20 mg/kg q8h) or fluoroquinolones (enrofloxacin at 5 mg/kg q12h). However, due to the high rate of mutational resistance *Campylobacter* have to the fluoroquinolones, a resistance that sometimes occurs while animals are being treated, fluoroquinolones are not the drug of choice. The macrolides such as erythromycin (10 to 20 mg/kg q8h for 7 days) or azithromycin (5-10 mg/kg q24h for 7 days) are the drugs of choice, despite the associated gastrointestinal side-effects with the former drug.[20] The duration of excretion in infected dogs and cats can be as long as 4 months and infected animals should be quarantined away from children during this period.

Salmonella spp.

Salmonellae are primarily motile, non–spore-forming, gram-negative aerobic bacilli. There are currently over 2000 described serotypes of *Salmonella* that have been associated with both human and animal disease. *Salmonella* spp. are one of the most common causes of human food-borne disease, with an estimated 1.4 million cases occurring annually in the United States.[21] Clinical salmonellosis in dogs and cats is rare, although the prevalence is higher in puppies and kennel populations. Isolation of *Salmonella* spp. from adult dogs ranges from 0% to 2% in nondiarrheic animals, and from 0 to 1% in diarrheic dogs.[2] Isolation rates are similar in nondiarrheic and diarrheic cats. *Salmonella* was isolated from 80% of raw chicken diet samples, and from 30% of the stool samples from dogs fed these diets.[22]

PATHOGENESIS

Salmonella infections begin with the ingestion of organisms in contaminated food or water, followed by invasion of M-cells in the Peyer's patches. *Salmonella* express several fimbriae that contribute to their ability to adhere to intestinal epithelial cells.[23] *Salmonella* pathogenicity islands (SPI-1 and SPI-2) encode the genes necessary for the invasion of intestinal epithelial cells, induction of intestinal secretory and inflammatory responses, intracellular replication, and establishment of systemic infection.[24] *Salmonella* spp. inject an array of bacterial effector molecules into the host cytoplasm, triggering reorganization of the actin cytoskeleton and resultant membrane ruffling. Internalization of *Salmonella* occurs within

minutes of bacterial contact with the host cell. Invasion is followed by inflammation and the influx of neutrophils and macrophages, with consequent secretory diarrhea likely mediated by activation of inositol-signaling pathways within affected host cells. The presence or absence of additional virulence factors plays an important role in determining whether septicemia occurs.

CLINICAL SIGNS

Signs of clinical salmonellosis in dogs and cats are typically associated with acute disease characterized by fever, malaise, anorexia, diarrhea, and vomiting. The diarrhea is frequently watery or mucoid and can be bloody in severe cases. Most *Salmonella*-infected dogs and cats are asymptomatic, although some animals may manifest clinical signs of systemic sepsis.

DIAGNOSIS

The traditional diagnosis of salmonellosis is made based on isolation of the organism in conjunction with clinical signs and assessment of potential risk factors such as hospitalization, age, environmental exposure, and antibiotic administration. However, isolation of *Salmonella* is not necessarily indicative of involvement in disease, as similar isolation rates can be detected in healthy nondiarrheic animals.[2] Hematologic abnormalities are variable, and include a nonregenerative anemia, lymphopenia, thrombocytopenia, and neutropenia with a left shift. Toxic neutrophils may be seen in animals with systemic disease and endotoxemia, findings similar to those documented with canine parvovirus. Fresh fecal specimens should be placed onto one or more selective media, including MacConkey agar, XLD agar, and brilliant green agar. For enrichment, selenite F broth, tetrathionate broth, or gram-negative broth (GN) is recommended. Biochemical testing can be used to identify presumptive *Salmonella* colonies, followed by serologic testing of isolates for further discrimination. Conventional and real-time PCR are promising newer diagnostic tools, although validation studies are lacking and reference laboratories have yet to embrace this technology.

THERAPY

Intravenous fluid therapy may be required depending on the severity of the diarrhea. Antibiotic therapy is typically only indicated for animals with evidence of systemic disease, or for immunocompromised animals. Antibiotics reported to be effective against *Salmonella* include fluoroquinolones, chloramphenicol, trimethoprim-sulfonamide, and amoxicillin.[25]

PATHOGENIC *Escherichia coli*

E. coli is a pleomorphic, gram-negative, non–spore forming bacillus that is a member of the family Enterobacteriaceae. Several distinct pathogenic categories (pathotypes) of diarrheagenic *E. coli* are recognized. Although the virulence determinants of each *E. coli* pathotype are distinct, they can generally be categorized as either colonization factors (adhesins), which enable the bacteria to bind closely to the intestinal mucosa and resist removal by peristalsis, or secreted toxins, which interfere with the normal physiologic process of host cells. Despite the occurrence of *E. coli* as a normal commensal organism in canine intestine, there is increasing evidence that certain *E. coli* pathotypes cause intestinal infection. The three pathotypes that have been studied in the dog include enterotoxigenic *E. coli* (ETEC), enterohemorrhagic *E. coli* (EHEC), and enteropathogenic *E. coli* (EPEC). Little is known about pathogenic *E. coli* in cats, although EPEC was isolated from approximately 5% of feline isolates isolated from cats with diarrhea, enteritis, or septicemia.

ENTEROTOXIGENIC *E. coli* (ETEC)

The incidence of this pathotype in canine diarrhea is unclear. Reported prevalences among diarrheic dogs range from 0% to 31%, particularly in the young.[26] The bacteria colonize the proximal small intestine and produce heat-stable (ST) and occasionally heat-labile (LT) enterotoxins. These enterotoxins result in overproduction of cAMP and cGMP with consequent development of a secretory diarrhea.

ENTEROPATHOGENIC *E. coli* (EPEC)

EPEC strains have been associated with diarrhea in a wide range of animal species, including humans. These strains are negative for Shiga-toxin and enterotoxin (ST and LT) genes, but carry the chromosomally located gene, *eae*A (*E. coli* *a*ttaching *e*ffacing), which facilitates attachment to intestinal epithelial cells and production of the classic "effacing" lesions.[27] *E. coli* isolates from 44 of 122 dying dogs (36%) with diarrhea were found to have the *eae*A gene, and *E. coli* was the sole pathogen identified in 15 of 44 (34%).[28] A close genetic relationship among human, dog, and cat EPEC isolates has been reported, suggesting that EPEC might be transferred between pets and humans.[29]

ENTEROHEMORRHAGIC *E. coli* (EHEC) (ALSO CALLED VEROTOXIGENIC *E. coli*)

Enterohemorrhagic *E. coli* bind tightly to epithelial cells and produce the same type of attachment-effacement lesions as seen with EPEC. EHEC are minimally invasive but do incite an inflammatory response, predominantly in the large intestine. The prototype EHEC, a strain of *E. coli* of the serotype O157:H7, is a significant food-borne human pathogen.[21] Hemolytic-uremic syndrome is the most important complication of *E. coli* O157 infection, and is characterized by microangiopathic hemolytic anemia, thrombocytopenia, and acute renal failure in approximately 7% of human cases. A report documented the isolation of this serotype from dog feces. The isolated strain was found to be identical to a strain isolated from an affected child who had contact with the dog. This finding suggests that similar to cattle, dogs may serve as potential vectors for transmission of EHEC O157.[30] In addition, hemolytic-uremic syndrome has been reported clinically in a small number of dogs.[31]

CLINICAL SIGNS

Pathogenic *E. coli* are commonly isolated from feces of apparently healthy dogs, and the challenge for clinicians is to determine whether the isolate is pathogenic. Clinical signs in infected animals can range from asymptomatic carriage to hemorrhagic diarrhea. In addition, clinical signs can be variable because of the relatively high incidence of concurrent enteric infections with parvovirus, *C. perfringens*, and intestinal parasites. The predominant clinical sign of enterotoxigenic *E. coli* infection is profuse watery diarrhea.

DIAGNOSIS

Because *E. coli* is a significant component of the commensal canine intestinal flora, isolation of the organism is not diagnostic, nor does it allow differentiation between pathogenic and nonpathogenic strains. However, culture enables the application of molecular techniques for detection of specific toxin genes among isolated organisms. Culture of *E. coli* involves spreading fresh fecal specimens onto selective media, such as MacConkey agar, which will only support growth of gram-negative organisms. Single lactose-positive colonies are then subcultured and speciated through biochemical testing. Substitution of lactose with sorbitol in MacConkey agar (SMAC) is often used to enhance the isolation of Shiga-like toxin–producing strains of *E. coli* O157:H7 as these strains do not ferment sorbitol. PCR has become one of the most common methods for detecting and differentiating pathogenic strains of *E. coli*. A recent study showed that it is possible to detect 11 of the major virulence genes of *E. coli* in fecal specimens from dogs with four multiplex PCRs.[32] Although EPEC and EHEC are associated with characteristic attaching and effacing lesions, molecular techniques for the detection of genes specific for each pathotype are more reliable than histologic examination.

THERAPY

The use of antimicrobials is controversial. These bacteria have a relatively high incidence of inherent resistance to antibiotics because of the presence of a gram-negative cell wall and the high incidence of conjugative transfer of resistance determinants. In addition, antibiotic therapy may enhance toxin synthesis or promote its release from the bacteria with a consequent increased rate of hemorrhagic colitis. Dogs with only mild clinical signs should probably not be given antibiotics, whereas parenteral antibiotics and fluid therapy are indicated in severe cases, particularly if septicemia is present. The Enterobacteriaceae are usually resistant to chloramphenicol, tetracyclines, ampicillin, or sulfonamides. Clinically stable animals can be treated with amoxicillin-clavulanate and first- or second-generation cephalosporins, until susceptibility results are known. Dogs with life-threatening bacteremia should be treated with aminoglycosides, a third-generation cephalosporin, or enrofloxacin. Caution should be heeded in the overuse of fluoroquinolones because of resistance concerns. Enrofloxacin has been used with success for Boxer dogs with histiocytic ulcerative colitis, although reports of relapse following discontinuation of the drug are common. Fortunately, most of the affected dogs attain remission of their clinical signs following the reintroduction of antimicrobial therapy.

Orally administered autogenous or recombinant vaccines have been studied extensively in farm animals in an effort to help prevent or treat enterotoxigenic *E. coli*–mediated diarrhea. An orally administered autogenous vaccine containing heat-inactivated *E. coli* was administered to diarrheic puppies and adult dogs once daily for 14 days, and led to a significant decrease in morbidity and mortality.[33] Additional studies are warranted to ensure the safety of this therapeutic regimen.

GRANULOMATOUS COLITIS OF BOXERS (HISTIOCYTIC ULCERATIVE COLITIS)

This enteropathy has been recently associated with adherent and invasive strains of *E. coli*.[34] and is typically seen in Boxers less than 4 years of age. There are intriguing similarities between the *E. coli* strains infecting Boxers and the *E. coli* LF82 that has been associated with human Crohn's disease. Clinical signs in Boxers include severe and frequent hematochezia with mucus and tenesmus. Administration of fluoroquinolones is associated with rapid resolution of clinical signs and has also been associated with resolution of the cellular infiltration characteristic of this disorder on colonic biopsy.[35] The colonic lesion has also been described infrequently in the French Bulldog and the Border Collie.

ZOONOTIC IMPLICATIONS FOR ENTERIC BACTERIA

Clostridium perfringens

There have been no documented cases of zoonotic transmission from dogs or cats to date. Contaminated food products can lead to enterotoxemia underscoring the importance of hygiene.

Clostridium difficile

The risk of zoonotic transmission is unclear. Transmission of *C. difficile* from animals to humans has not been documented. Nevertheless, it is recommended to assume that *C. difficile* is potentially zoonotic because the strains of *C. difficile* that infect dogs are often indistinguishable from those found in people with CDI.

Campylobacter spp.

Campylobacter spp. are potentially zoonotic from dogs to humans with subsequent development of diarrhea.[36] An estimated 6.3% of 218 human cases of *C. jejuni* or *C. coli* enteritis were attributed to exposure to diarrheic animals. Other sources of infection in people include consumption of contaminated food and food products, water, and raw milk. Pasteurization of milk and the thorough cooking of meats and poultry carcasses destroy *C. jejuni* in these foods.

Salmonella spp.

Most human *Salmonella* infections are acquired by handling or consuming contaminated food products, particularly foods of animal origin. Infections also are acquired by direct and indirect contact with farm animals, reptiles, chicks, and occasionally, pets. Infected animals usually shed *Salmonella* organisms in their feces.

Escherichia coli

The potential for zoonotic transmission is unclear; however, some of the strains of pathogenic *E. coli* found in dogs and cats are indistinguishable from those found in people. While this does not confirm a zoonotic risk, it is prudent to treat cases of *E. coli* diarrhea as potentially zoonotic. This is particularly true for *E. coli* O157 because of the potential for severe disease in humans and the low infective dose. Careful attention to hand hygiene, the use of contact precautions, and proper cleaning and disinfection is important.

INFECTION CONTROL IN THE HOSPITAL

Dogs and cats diagnosed with *C. perfringens*, *C. difficile*, *Campylobacter* spp., *Salmonella* spp., or *E. coli*–associated diarrhea should be housed under contact precautions in an isolation area. Direct and indirect contact should be prevented between infected animals and all other animals. In addition, barrier precautions consisting of a gown and gloves should be used when handling the animal. Hands should be washed thoroughly with bactericidal soap and water after any contact with the animal or the isolation environment, even when gloves have been worn. Hand washing is recommended over alcohol-based hand sanitizers, especially when working with *C. difficile*–infected animals, because the spores are alcohol-resistant. Spores can survive up to 70 days in the environment and can be transported on the hands of staff members who have direct contact with other patients.

Strict adherence to hand washing techniques and the proper handling of contaminated wastes are effective in preventing the spread of the disease. Infected animals should be walked in a separate area from other patients, and feces should be promptly removed. *C. difficile* spores are highly resistant to most disinfectants. Bleach (1:10 to 1:64 dilution of regular household bleach) has good sporicidal activity, as long as there is minimal organic debris and there has been adequate contact time. Bleach is an effective disinfectant for *Salmonella* and *Campylobacter* and one can make a solution of household bleach and water by adding ¼-cup bleach to 1 gallon of water, or to make a smaller amount in a spray bottle, add 1-tablespoon bleach to 1 quart of water. Saturate area with solution. DO NOT rinse. Air dry.

References

The reference list can be found on the companion Expert Consult Web site at *www.expertconsult.com*.

CHAPTER 209

Hemoplasmosis

Jane E. Sykes

Hemotropic mycoplasmas (hemoplasmas) are small (0.3 to 0.8 μm), unculturable epierythrocytic mycoplasmas that are capable of causing severe hemolytic anemia (Figure 209-1). They infect a wide variety of mammalian species, including man, and have a worldwide distribution. Previously known as *Haemobartonella felis*, sequence analysis of the 16S rRNA genes of *Haemobartonella* and *Eperythrozoon* spp. has shown that they fall within the pneumoniae group of mycoplasmas, which includes the human mycoplasmal pathogens *Mycoplasma pneumoniae* and *Myco-*

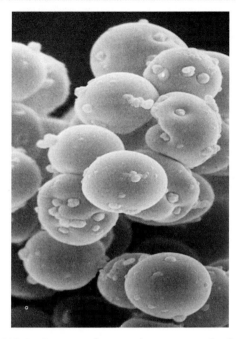

Figure 209-1 Scanning electron photomicrograph of erythrocytes from a cat infected with *Mycoplasma haemofelis* (×5000). (Courtesy Dallas Hyde, University of California, Davis, Calif.)

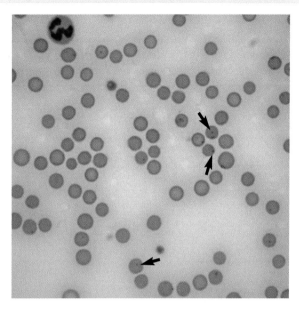

Figure 209-2 Romanowsky stained blood smear showing epierythrocytic bacteria typical of *Mycoplasma haemofelis*.

plasma genitalium.[1-3] Like hemoplasmas, *M. pneumoniae* may induce cold agglutinin formation in the infected host, and elevated reticulocyte counts have been detected in many infected human patients.[4,5]

Currently, diagnosis of hemoplasma infections is based on visualization of coccoid bacteria associated with erythrocytes on blood smears, and/or the results of specific PCR assays. In recent years, several new hemoplasma species have been discovered in dogs and cats.[6-9]

ETIOLOGY AND EPIDEMIOLOGY

Three hemoplasma species are currently known to infect domestic and wild felids, *Mycoplasma haemofelis*, "*Candidatus* Mycoplasma haemominutum" and "*Candidatus* Mycoplasma turicensis." Because these organisms cannot be cultured in the laboratory, newly discovered hemoplasmas must be given a *Candidatus* designation until more information is available to support their classification. *M. haemofelis* (previously the Ohio strain, or large form of *H. felis*) is apparently the most pathogenic organism, and is capable of causing hemolytic anemia (feline infectious anemia) in immunocompetent cats. Positive test results for this organism have generally correlated with the presence of anemia. Using cytologic evaluation of blood smears, *M. haemofelis* is pleomorphic, varying from cocci to small rings and rods, sometimes forming short chains of three to six organisms (Figure 209-2).

The results of epidemiologic studies using PCR suggest that this organism is the least prevalent of the three feline hemoplasmas, being found in 0.5% to 5% of sick cats visiting veterinary hospitals. Experimental inoculation of cats with *M. haemofelis* results in moderate to severe anemia, and cats infected with *M. haemofelis* demonstrate marked fluctuations in copy numbers of hemoplasma DNA, with peak copy numbers correlating with precipitous declines in the hematocrit.[6,10]

"*Candidatus* M. haemominutum" (previously the California strain, or small form of *H. felis*) is smaller, and has

not yet been clearly associated with disease in immune competent cats. Using cytologic evaluation of blood smears, "*Candidatus* M. haemominutum" may appear as small cocci, 0.3 μm in diameter, although *M. haemofelis* and "*Candidatus* M. haemominutum" may not always be reliably distinguished by blood smear alone.[11] "*Candidatus* M. haemominutum" is common in the cat population, infecting as many as one in five cats visiting veterinary hospitals for a variety of reasons.[12-14] Inoculation of cats with "*Candidatus* M. haemominutum" results in only a mild decrease in hematocrit. Hemoplasma copy number gradually increases, then reaches a plateau.[10] There is some evidence that "*Candidatus* M. haemominutum" may play a role in disease. Cats coinfected with both feline leukemia virus (FeLV) and "*Candidatus* M. haemominutum" develop more significant anemia than cats infected with "*Candidatus* M. haemominutum" alone. Also, cats that are coinfected with FeLV and "*Candidatus* M. haemominutum" may be more likely to develop myeloproliferative disease compared with cats infected with FeLV alone.[15] Proposed mechanisms have included stimulation of erythroid mitosis by the organism, immunosuppression, and immune stimulation leading to enhanced rate of mutation and myeloproliferative disease. "*Candidatus* M. haemominutum" is commonly found in coinfections with "*Candidatus* M. turicensis" and *M. haemofelis.*[16,17]

"*Candidatus* M. turicensis" was first reported in a Swiss cat with severe intravascular hemolysis in 2005 (*turicensis* pertains to Turicum, the Latin name of Zurich).[8] Subsequently, infections with "*Candidatus* M. turicensis" have been detected in the United Kingdom, Australia, South Africa, and the United States.[14,16,18,19] This organism has never been seen using light microscopic examination of blood smears, and organism loads in cats infected with "*Candidatus* M. turicensis" have typically been low. In some studies, infection with "*Candidatus* M. turicensis" has been slightly more prevalent in the cat population than *M. haemofelis*, with most studies showing a prevalence of 0.5% to 10% in sick cats visiting veterinary hospitals (Table 209-1).

The pathogenic potential of this organism is not fully understood. Inoculation of an immunosuppressed cat with "*Candidatus* M. turicensis" resulted in severe anemia,[8] but only mild anemia was documented in an immunocompetent cat inoculated with "*Candidatus* M. turicensis," and significant

Table • 209-1

Prevalences (%) of Various Hemoplasma Species in Different Geographic Locations as Determined Using Real-Time Polymerase Chain Reaction

HEMOPLASMA SPECIES	COUNTRY (POPULATION SAMPLED)					
	UNITED KINGDOM (1585 SAMPLES SUBMITTED FOR HEMOPLASMA TESTING)[19]	SWITZERLAND (713 HEALTHY AND SICK CATS)[17]	SOUTH AFRICA (69 CATS SUSPECTED TO HAVE HEMOPLASMOSIS)[18]	AUSTRALIA (147 SICK CATS)[18]	UNITED STATES (263 SICK CATS)[14]	UNITED STATES (310 CATS WITH POSSIBLE HEMOPLASMOSIS)[16]
Mycoplasma haemofelis	2.8%	1.5%	15%	4.8%	0.5%	4.8%
"*Candidatus* Mycoplasma haemominutum"	11.2%	10%	38%	24%	16%	23%
"*Candidatus* Mycoplasma turicensis"	1.7%	1.3%	26%	10%	0.5%	6.5%

Table • 209-2

Risk Factors Associated with Infection with Feline Hemotropic Mycoplasmas as Determined Using Species-Specific Real-Time Polymerase Chain Reaction Assays

HEMOPLASMA SPECIES	RISK FACTOR(S)
Mycoplasma haemofelis	Younger age[16]
	Male sex[16,17]
	FIV seroreactivity[16]
	FeLV seroreactivity[16]
"*Candidatus* Mycoplasma haemominutum"	Older age[14,16,17]
	Male sex[17,16,18]
	FIV seroreactivity[14]
	Nonpedigree status[14]
	Outdoor access[14,17]
"*Candidatus* Mycoplasma turicensis"	Male sex[16,18]

FeLV, Feline leukemia virus; *FIV,* feline immunodeficiency virus.

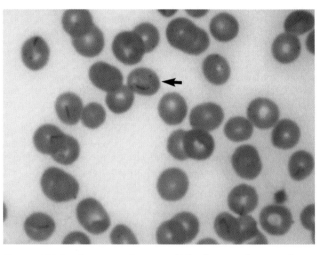

Figure 209-3 Romanowsky stained blood smear showing chains of epierythrocytic bacteria typical of *Mycoplasma haemocanis.* At least some of the organisms are content *(center).*

fluctuations in organism DNA copy numbers, as seen in infections with *M. haemofelis,* were not documented. The pathogenic potential of "*Candidatus* M. turicensis" may be lower than that of *M. haemofelis,* but greater than that of "*Candidatus* M. haemominutum."[16] Cofactors, such as coinfection with other hemoplasmas or concurrent immunosuppression, may be important in development of anemia in cats infected with "*Candidatus* M. turicensis."[18]

In most studies, feline hemoplasma infection has been strongly associated with male sex, nonpedigree status, and access to the outdoors (Table 209-2). Infection with "*Candidatus* M. haemominutum" is more prevalent in older cats, whereas younger cats may be more likely to develop disease associated with *M. haemofelis* infection. Some studies, but not others, have shown an association between retrovirus infection and hemoplasmosis. In one recent study, cats infected with *M. haemofelis* in the United States were six times more likely to be infected with feline immunodeficiency virus (FIV) than cats negative for hemoplasmas.[16]

Until recently, there was only one hemoplasma described that infects dogs, *Mycoplasma haemocanis* (previously *H. canis*). This organism usually causes hemolytic anemia in splenectomized dogs, and rarely in dogs with other immunosuppressive disease or concurrent infections. The 16S rRNA gene of *M. haemocanis* is more than 99% homologous with that of *M. haemofelis,* but the sequence homology of the RNase P genes of these two species is lower, suggesting they may be different organisms.[20] The organism forms rods, rings, and cocci, and, characteristically, the cocci are often found in long chains (Figure 209-3). The prevalence of this infection appears to be particularly high in kennel-raised dogs.[21]

More recently, two additional hemoplasma species have been detected in dogs. The first, "*Candidatus* Mycoplasma haematoparvum," was detected in a splenectomized dog with hemic neoplasia.[9] This organism appeared as small (0.3 μm) cocci on the surface of the dog's erythrocytes, and sequencing of the 16S rRNA gene of this organism suggests that it is most closely related to "*Candidatus* M. haemominutum." "*Candi-*

datus M. haemominutum" has also been detected in several dogs using PCR. The clinical importance of these latter two organisms in dogs remains unclear.

The mode of transmission for these organisms has been unknown. Fleas and other arthropod vectors may be capable of transmitting infection with *M. haemofelis*,[22] and transmission of *M. haemocanis* by the brown dog tick has been demonstrated experimentally.[23] Geographic variation in the prevalence of hemoplasma infection in dogs and cats supports a role for arthropod vectors in transmission. Transplacental spread has also been hypothesized. Biting has been suggested as a means of transmission of the feline hemoplasmas, and the strong male sex predilection and association with FIV infection in our studies supports this mode.[16] The organism has also been detected in the saliva of experimentally infected cats early in the course of infection, as well as in naturally infected cats,[24-26] and many infected cats have had a recent history of cat bite abscessation. Transmission has occurred following blood transfusion, and it is suggested that prospective blood donors be screened for hemoplasmas using PCR-based assays.

PATHOGENESIS

The pathogenesis of feline hemoplasmosis may been divided into prebacteremic, acute, recovery, and carrier phases.[27] After inoculation of experimental cats with *M. haemofelis*, there is a variable delay of 2 to 34 days before acute onset of clinical signs (prebacteremic phase). Anemia and bacteremia then occur, and persist for about 18 to 30 days (acute phase). Mortality is highest during this phase. In some cats infected with *M. haemofelis*, cyclical changes in the hematocrit and numbers of infected erythrocytes occur, with sharp declines in the hematocrit correlating with appearance of large numbers of organisms in blood smears.[6,27,28] The number of infected erythrocytes may decline from 90% to <1% in less than 3 hours.[27,29] Sequestration of organisms in splenic and pulmonary macrophages has been suggested to explain their disappearance.

In surviving cats, the hematocrit then returns to normal or near-normal (recovery phase), and organisms disappear from blood smears. Despite organism disappearance, it has been suggested that recovered cats may remain persistently infected for years (carrier state), the organism evading the host immune system.[27,28] Intermittent reappearance of organisms in chronically infected cats, with relapse of anemia, has been documented in some studies. It has been suggested that recrudescence of severe disease may follow stress, pregnancy, intercurrent infection, or neoplasia. Administration of dexamethasone or methylprednisolone caused a decline in the hematocrit and reappearance of organisms on blood smears, although these were mild.[28,30] Species differences may exist in the ability of hemoplasmas to persist within the host, the carrier state being more frequent for "Candidatus M. haemominutum" but less frequent for *M. haemofelis*. In contrast to hemoplasma infections of other host species, splenectomy has a variable effect on the course of hemoplasmosis. Recrudescence of anemia and bacteremia has been documented in some chronically infected cats, although other studies suggest splenectomy increases the number of visible organisms in blood smears without causing significant anemia.[28,29] Infection of splenectomized cats with "Candidatus M. haemominutum" does not seem to enhance the pathogenicity of this organism.[31]

Anemia results predominantly from extravascular hemolysis. The organism appears to locate itself in an indentation on the erythrocyte surface. Positive direct Coombs, cold agglutinins, increased osmotic fragility, and decreased erythrocyte lifespan have been noted in cats with hemoplasmosis.[32-34] The organisms are also capable of "bridging" adjacent erythrocytes, which might also promote splenic trapping and removal of red blood cells.

CLINICAL SIGNS AND LABORATORY ABNORMALITIES

Depression, inappetence, and dehydration are common signs of infection with *M. haemofelis*, and some cats may also present with weight loss. Anemia results in signs of weakness, pallor of the mucous membranes, tachypnea, tachycardia, and occasionally syncope. Some owners may report their cat eats dirt, litter, or licks cement. Other physical examination abnormalities may include cardiac murmurs, sometimes splenomegaly, and icterus. Some cats may be febrile, and moribund cats may be hypothermic.

Autoagglutination may be noted in blood smears from some infected cats. The most characteristic abnormality on the CBC is regenerative anemia, with anisocytosis, reticulocytosis, polychromasia, Howell-Jolly bodies, and sometimes marked normoblastemia. Nonregenerative anemia may also be noted. In some cases this is because sufficient time for a regenerative response has not yet elapsed. In others, anemia is nonregenerative as a result of concurrent FeLV infection, although macrocytic, normocytic nonregenerative anemias have been documented in FeLV-negative cats with hemoplasmosis.[35,36] Concurrent occult infection with hemoplasmas should be considered in any FeLV-positive cat with macrocytosis, even in the absence of reticulocytosis. White blood cell counts may be normal, elevated, or low. Platelet counts may be decreased. The serum chemistry profile may reveal elevated ALT as a result of hypoxia, hyperbilirubinemia, and prerenal azotemia. Hyperproteinemia may be seen in some cats.

Dogs infected with *M. haemocanis* that are splenectomized may show signs of pallor and depression. Rectal temperature is generally normal and usually appetite is spared.

DIAGNOSIS

The differential diagnosis for hemoplasmosis includes primary immune-mediated hemolytic anemia, other infectious causes of anemia such as cytauxzoonosis, feline infectious peritonitis virus, and feline retrovirus infections, Heinz body hemolytic anemia, and inherited erythrocyte disorders such as pyruvate kinase deficiency and the red cell fragility disorder of Abyssinian and Somali cats.

Attempts to isolate feline hemotropic mycoplasmas in the laboratory have been unsuccessful. Cytologic detection of hemoplasmas is considered to have low sensitivity. *M. haemofelis* is visible less than 50% of the time in acutely infected cats, because organisms may disappear for several days before reappearing on blood smears over the course of infection. "Candidatus M. haemomintum" is small, and generally not visible in chronically infected cats. "Candidatus M. turicensis" has never been seen on blood smears. False-positive diagnoses occur when staining artifacts such as stain precipitate are confused with organisms, and organisms also need to be distinguished from basophilic stippling and Howell-Jolly bodies.

The advent of PCR technology has improved our ability to detect hemoplasmas. Numerous PCR assays have been described to date, all of which are based on detection of the 16S rRNA gene. These assays detect as few as 130 organisms/mL of blood, and have been shown to be significantly more sensitive than blood smear evaluation, although they may not consistently detect the organism in asymptomatic carrier cats.[6,12,30,37,38] Hemoplasma PCR assays are now commercially available in some veterinary diagnostic laboratories, including conventional assays (whereby bands on a gel are interpreted as positive results) and real-time PCR assays (which rely on fluorometric detection of the PCR product and can provide information regarding organism load). Some conventional PCR assays may not differentiate between *M. haemofelis* and "*Candidatus* M. turicensis." Real-time PCR assays are generally species-specific, and may be less prone to false positives relating to contamination. Because the pathogenic potential of each hemoplasma species differs, it is essential to consult with the laboratory to determine the species specificity of the assay(s) offered. Dried blood smears can also be used for PCR but are less sensitive than liquid whole blood.[39]

In dogs, *M. haemocanis* is usually visible on blood smears if clinical signs attributable to hemoplasmosis are present. PCR assays for *M. haemofelis* generally detect *M. haemocanis* because of the high 16S rRNA gene sequence homology between these species, but a separate assay is required for detection of "*Candidatus* M. haematoparvum."

TREATMENT

Treatment is indicated for cats and dogs with clinical signs and laboratory abnormalities consistent with hemoplasmosis. Treatment of PCR-positive, healthy animals is currently not recommended, as no regimen has yet been identified that completely eliminates the organism.

The treatment of choice for hemoplasmosis is doxycycline, 10 mg/kg q24h PO for a minimum of 2 weeks, and transfusion with packed red cells or whole blood where necessary. Because of the potential for esophagitis, administration of doxycycline

hyclate preparations should be followed by administration of a bolus of several milliliters of water. Enrofloxacin (5 mg/kg q24h PO) is a suitable alternative to doxycycline.[40] Azithromycin was ineffective for treatment of feline hemoplasmosis using an experimental model.[37] The use of immunosuppressive doses of glucocorticoids to suppress the associated immune-mediated hemolytic process is controversial, given the potential for glucocorticoids to cause reactivation of latent infection, but may be necessary in cats that fail to respond to antimicrobial therapy alone, or in cases where the diagnosis is uncertain. Cats often remain carriers after treatment, despite return of the hematocrit to normal. Thus, antimicrobial therapy cannot be used to reliably eliminate infection from potential blood donors. Marbofloxacin (2 mg/kg PO q24h) was shown to decrease copy numbers of "*Candidatus* M. haemominutum" during therapy, but copy numbers increased to pretreatment levels on termination of therapy.[41]

PREVENTION

Inadvertent transmission by blood transfusion of blood from carrier cats has been documented, and so blood donors should be tested for hemoplasmas using PCR assays. Keeping cats indoors is also likely to prevent infection, as outdoor status has been identified as a risk factor. Control of fleas and ticks is recommended.

REFERENCES

The reference list can be found on the companion Expert Consult Web site at *www.expertconsult.com*.

CHAPTER 210

Nosocomial Infection and Resistant Bacteria

Amanda K. Boag

The term *nosocomial* is used to describe infections that are not present on admission but that develop more than 48 hours into hospitalization, or to infections occurring in a patient that has been hospitalized in the 2 weeks prior to the current admission. In human medicine the term *health care–associated infections (HAI)* is now being recommended to describe infections associated with health care delivery in any setting, reflecting the difficulty in determining with certainty where the pathogen was acquired in many patients.[1] HAI may be caused by many pathogens; however, a substantial proportion are caused by multidrug resistant organisms. For example, in people the proportion of hospital-acquired staphylococcal infections caused by methicillin-resistant (as opposed to methicillin-sensitive) *Staphylococcus aureus* is greater than 35% in the United Kingdom[2] and up to 64% in the United States.[3]

Risk factors for HAI identified in people include duration of hospital (and especially ICU) stay, severity of illness, immunocompromise secondary to underlying disease or medication, and prior antimicrobial use.[4-6] Many of the bacteria that cause HAI also exist as commensals of the skin, mucosa,

or gastrointestinal tract of healthy individuals; prior colonization by multidrug resistant bacteria is also a risk factor for subsequent infection.[7,8] HAI are now increasingly being recognized in veterinary patients with many of the same pathogens known to cause infections in people. Not only are these infections often difficult and expensive to treat, they also pose a risk to other patients and may be zoonoses. Due to the high levels and unpredictable nature of resistance, empirical antimicrobial therapy is less likely to be effective. In people, initial inappropriate therapy has been associated with a higher mortality rate even if the correct antimicrobial is instituted following receipt of microbial culture results.[9,10]

Nosocomial infections may complicate the course of many medical diseases. Nosocomial infections manifest in a variety of ways but can include mild superficial skin or wound infections, gastrointestinal signs, urinary tract infections, pneumonia, and intravenous catheter infections (Web Figure 210-1). Infections may be associated with the development of sepsis and a high morbidity and mortality. Specific bacteria that have been associated with nosocomial infections in small animal veterinary patients are considered in more detail below.

MULTIDRUG RESISTANT BACTERIA

Staphylococci

Staphylococci are gram-positive cocci that are a common commensal of mucosa and skin but can cause a wide range of infections.[11] Methicillin-resistant S. aureus (MRSA) is one of the most significant bacteria causing HAI in human medicine and has been identified with increasing frequency in veterinary patients since it was first reported in 1999.[12-15] MRSA has acquired the mecA gene, resulting in production of an altered penicillin-binding protein and resistance to all beta-lactam antimicrobials. The majority of MRSA strains isolated from small animal veterinary patients are identical to human hospital-acquired strains, and the spectrum of disease seen is similar.[16-18] Antimicrobial treatment should be based on culture and sensitivity testing. Many MRSA isolates are sensitive to commonly used antimicrobial agents such as trimethoprim-sulpha and tetracyclines, and these antimicrobials are recommended for the treatment of non–life-threatening infections.[19] Vancomycin is the intravenous antibiotic of choice for human patients with MRSA sepsis but experience in the veterinary setting is limited.[19,20] The recognition in human medicine of MRSA isolates with poor sensitivity to vancomycin coupled with the expense of the drug may limit its application in the small animal field. Veterinary patients may become colonized with MRSA although the frequency and duration of colonization is unknown.[15,16] There is also good evidence that MRSA can be passed between pet animals and owners with the possibility for zoonotic infections.[21-23] Veterinary staff may be at higher risk of colonization with MRSA than the general population, with colonization rates of approximately 10% being reported in several studies.[16,18,24,25] The problem of MRSA is evolving in the human field with recent identification of new strains of community-acquired MRSA with increased pathogenicity and vancomycin-resistant strains in health care settings.[26] To date, these strains have not been identified in veterinary patients.

Methicillin-resistant S. pseudintermedius (previously known as S. intermedius)[27] has been reported recently as causing disease in canine and feline patients[28,29]; the emergence of resistant S. pseudintermedius is potentially a greater concern to veterinary patients as it is the principle staphylococcal species colonizing healthy dogs. Coagulase-negative Staphylococci may also be implicated in nosocomial infection and may be found contaminating the veterinary environment.[30]

Enterococci

Enterococci are gram-positive facultative cocci that are commonly found colonizing the mammalian gastrointestinal tract. Previously categorized as streptococci, the genus Enterococcus was only recognized as a distinct taxonomy in 1984. E. faecium and E. faecalis are the most common enterococci causing HAI in people. They are generally considered to be of relatively low virulence but are capable of causing a wide range of infections including sepsis.[8] Enterococci are inherently resistant to many antimicrobials and are efficient at acquiring new resistance mechanisms. The acquisition of the vanA or vanB gene complexes led to the emergence of vancomycin-resistant E. faecium (VRE) in human patients in the late 1980s. These infections are particularly challenging to treat as there are few antimicrobial options available. Published reports of enterococci causing clinical infection in small animal patients are limited[31-34]; anecdotally a spectrum of infections may be seen similar to those in human medicine. Additionally, there is evidence that healthy dogs and cats can be colonized by these bacteria with 13% of healthy dogs being positive on fecal culture in one study.[35] As prior colonization is a risk factor for

subsequent infection in people,[8] the identification of healthy canine carriers raises the concern that VRE may become a greater problem for the veterinary profession in the future. Zoonotic transfer of VRE is also an emerging concern.[32,33,35] A positive culture result for Enterococcus spp. should not necessarily mandate aggressive antimicrobial therapy. Isolation of Enterococcus spp., even from infected sites, may simply represent colonization, especially if it is cultured as part of a polymicrobial infection alongside organisms with greater pathogenicity. A careful clinical judgment must be made as to which of the reported isolates is responsible for the patient's clinical signs. Considering the difficulties associated with treatment, careful consideration of whether specific treatment is warranted is required.

Enterobacteriaceae

The Enterobacteriaceae group includes Escherichia coli, Klebsiella spp., and Enterobacter spp. These gram-negative bacteria are commensals of the gastrointestinal tract and are emerging as a significant public health concern in human medicine.[36] Production of beta-lactamases by these bacteria has been documented since before beta-lactam antibiotics were used in clinical practice; however, the spectrum of beta-lactam antimicrobials against which the beta-lactamases are effective is expanding. Of particular concern are the Enterobacteriaceae, which produce extended-spectrum beta-lactamases (ESBLs) and extended-spectrum cephalosporinases (ESCs). The classification system used for beta-lactamases is complex, but essentially certain beta-lactamase enzymes (e.g., TEM and SHV) have evolved such that they can hydrolyze not only the small penicillin molecules but also the larger cephalosporins. Other newly identified beta-lactamase enzymes such as CTX-M are also being found in E. coli and Klebsiella.[37] Reports of ESBL Enterobacteriaceae causing clinical disease in veterinary patients are limited[38-40]; however, veterinary microbiology laboratories may not specifically identify them as such. Cultures of fecal samples from healthy dogs and pet therapy dogs have identified colonization by ESBL E. coli.[41-43] As with other bacteria this is likely to represent a risk factor for subsequent infection. Prior exposure to antimicrobials especially fluoroquinolones may increase the risk of colonization. Healthy dogs treated with oral enrofloxacin were more effectively colonized with multidrug-resistant E. coli than a control population.[44] Although ESBLs were not specifically identified, one study carried out in a veterinary ICU showed the proportion of dogs carrying resistant E. coli to increase with duration of hospitalization and to be associated with the use of antimicrobial drugs.[45]

Many of these bacteria remain susceptible to the aminoglycosides and carbapenems and these represent effective and practical treatment options at this time. Empirical use of these antimicrobials should, however, be very carefully considered because of the narrow therapeutic index and risk of selecting for further resistant bacterial populations respectively. In people a carbapenemase (KPC) has been identified in several Enterobacteriaceae and has been implicated in nosocomial outbreaks.[46]

Pseudomonads

Pseudomonas aeruginosa is a gram-negative bacterium that is ubiquitous in the environment. Its ability to survive especially in moist environments contributes to its success as an opportunistic nosocomial pathogen. It possesses a high level of intrinsic resistance due to a number of mechanisms including a highly impermeable outer membrane, broad spectrum multidrug efflux system, and its ability to produce biofilms. In people it has also been noted to acquire resistance with relatively high frequency and sometimes during therapy with a drug to which it was previously susceptible. Most of the veterinary literature relates to its role in otitis and pyoderma although nosocomial infections have been reported.[47] Antimicrobial treatment generally involves combination protocols although an evidence base to recommend specific protocols is lacking.[48]

Acinetobacter

Acinetobacter spp. are gram-negative aerobic coccobacilli. *A. baumanii* is the commonest *Acinetobacter* species implicated in HAI in both human and veterinary patients. It can be found on the skin and oral cavity of healthy dogs, but is also ubiquitous in the environment. Its ability to persist in the environment for extended periods and over a wide range of conditions make it particularly effective as an endemic pathogen in a health care setting. *A. baumanii* has been associated with a range of infections in veterinary patients and has been implicated in the death or euthanasia of patients.[49] Treatment options are often limited but should be based on the sensitivity data for the particular isolate involved.

Other Bacteria

Other bacteria that have been associated with outbreaks of nosocomial infections in small animal patients include multidrug-resistant *Salmonella typhimurium* in four animal facilities in the United States[50] and *Clostridium difficile. C. difficile* may be found in the feces of hospitalized dogs and cats[51,52] and in the veterinary environment.[53] It has been responsible for outbreaks of enteric disease.[54]

DIAGNOSIS AND TREATMENT OF NOSOCOMIAL INFECTIONS

As with any disease, successful treatment is most likely with rapid and accurate diagnosis. As veterinarians treat increasing numbers of patients with complex disease processes, prolonged hospitalization, and invasive interventions, they should maintain a high index of suspicion for HAI in their patients. The presence of clinical signs consistent with HAI such as development of fever of unknown origin in a hospitalized patient should prompt a careful search for an underlying source (Figure 210-1).

Catheter sites and wounds should be carefully examined on at least a daily basis. A proactive approach to submission of samples for microbial culture is encouraged. Dependent on the patient, this may include wound cultures, blood cultures, urine cultures, transtracheal wash samples, or cultures of intravenous catheter tips especially if removed from sites showing signs of thrombophlebitis. Culture of urinary catheter tips following removal is not recommended; rather, in patients in which a hospital-acquired urinary tract infection is suspected, a urine sample should be obtained by cystocentesis following catheter removal.[55]

Antimicrobial treatment is often necessary and should ultimately be refined on the basis of microbial culture results. Empirical therapy is often required prior to receipt of results and a rational approach to choice of empirical agent should be employed. Consideration should be given to cytologic (including Gram stain) findings, likely bacterial pathogens for

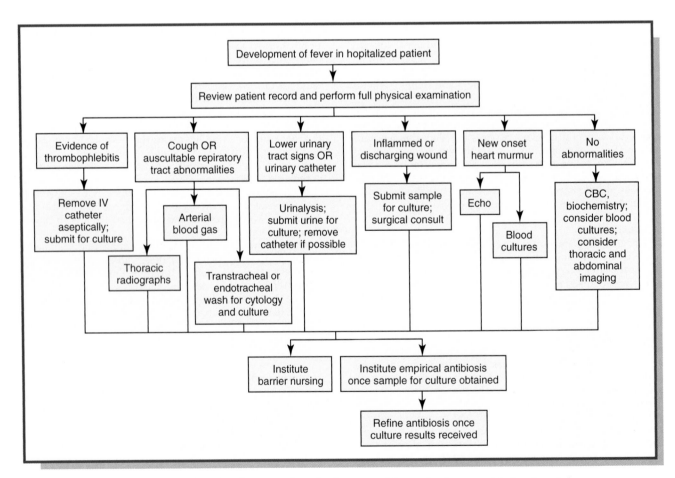

Figure 210-1 Algorithm for approach to development of fever of unknown origin in a hospitalized patient. *CBC,* Complete blood count.

the site of infection, and knowledge of common nosocomial pathogens and resistance patterns in the clinic. Auditing of previous HAI is an important component in this decision making. Antimicrobials should be administered using an appropriate dosing schedule taking into account the pharmacokinetic and pharmacodynamic properties of the chosen drug.[56,57] Considering the challenges and expense associated with antimicrobial therapy in multidrug-resistant infections, a critical evaluation of the need for antibiosis should also be made. Alternative management strategies such as removal of implants or catheters and diligent wound management may allow for resolution of infection without the need for systemic antimicrobials.[47] In the face of a polymicrobial infection, antimicrobial treatment effective against all the pathogens present may not always be necessary. Supportive treatment of the patient with intravenous fluid therapy, nutritional support, and specific treatment for the underlying disease is also a vital part of the successful treatment of HAI.

The role of decolonization in the treatment of veterinary patients with HAI has not been evaluated. Veterinary patients with MRSA infection may also have positive nasal cultures.[13] Although there is no evidence to recommend routine decolonization, in patients with recurrent infection this should be considered with the use of topical antimicrobials such as fusidic acid.[58]

CONTROL STRATEGIES FOR NOSOCOMIAL INFECTION

Considering the difficulties associated with treating many multidrug-resistant infections, infection control measures and prevention strategies are a vitally important part of the management of HAI. Evidence-based information does not currently exist in the veterinary literature; however, there is a wealth of information from the human field. Published guidelines[59,60] focus on particular pathogens; however, many of the principles employed will be of benefit in the control of all HAI. A major difficulty with interpreting the literature is that the majority of reports of successful control involve implementation of multiple interventions concurrently, making it difficult to compare the efficacy and importance of each individual intervention.[54] When designing an infection control strategy, the following should all be considered.

Hand Hygiene
The importance of hand hygiene was identified in 1847, when the Austrian physician Semmelweis demonstrated a reduction in maternal mortality from puerperal fever following implementation of an antiseptic handwash. Hand hygiene (including hand washing and the use of alcohol hand gels) (Web Figure 210-2) is considered to be one of the most important measures for prevention of nosocomial infection.[61] Compliance with hand hygiene is often poor and the most appropriate ways to improve hand hygiene remain to be determined.[62,63]

Isolation or Barrier Nursing
Isolation or barrier nursing may be used once a patient has been diagnosed with a HAI or in high-risk patients to reduce the risk of infection. Veterinary personnel should wear protective clothing (plastic gown, shoe covers, gloves, mask) (Web Figure 210-3) when handling the patient. Other potential fomites (e.g., thermometer, stethoscope) should be reserved for use with that patient. Evidence to support strict isolation as opposed to enforcement of strict barrier nursing procedures or cohort nursing is however lacking.[64,65]

Environmental Cleaning
Often overlooked, diligent environmental cleaning is an important and cost-effective way of reducing pathogen reservoirs. Focusing effort on cleaning sites close to the patient that are touched immediately prior to patient contact ("hand-touch sites") is currently recommended.[66]

Antimicrobial Stewardship
Colonization and infection with multidrug resistant organisms has been associated with prior antimicrobial use. A meta-analysis of trials in human medicine concluded that efforts to improve antimicrobial prescribing in hospitalized patients were successful in reducing HAI and antimicrobial resistance.[67]

REFERENCES

The reference list can be found on the companion Expert Consult Web site at *www.expertconsult.com*.

VIRAL: FELINE

CHAPTER 211

Feline Immunodeficiency Virus

Julie K. Levy
P. Cynda Crawford

Feline immunodeficiency virus (FIV) is a lymphotropic lentivirus that, like HIV in humans, causes an acquired immunodeficiency syndrome (AIDS) in domestic cats. FIV is related morphologically and biochemically to HIV but is antigenically distinct. Both viruses also share a similar pattern of pathogenesis, characterized by a long period of clinical latency during which immune function gradually deteriorates. Eventually, AIDS develops, accompanied by opportunistic infections, systemic diseases, and malignancies. It is the close relationship between HIV and FIV that has kindled interest in the use of FIV as an animal model for the study of lentiviral immunopathogenesis.

Although the existence of FIV was first reported in 1987, there are extensive data indicating that cats have carried the virus for a much longer time. FIV has a worldwide distribution in domestic cats, with infection rates approaching one third of the cats in some populations. Strains of viruses related to FIV are also found to infect at least 27 species of wild Felidae. In the wild, it appears that a majority of lions are infected, but few clinical signs are apparent. The greater diversity of viral nucleic acid sequences and the decreased pathogenicity of wild cat strains compared with those that affect domestic cats suggest that nondomestic felids have been living with lentiviruses for a longer time and that the domestic cat strains may have emerged more recently from ancient nondomestic cat strains. Field strains of FIV are divided into 5 subgroups, or clades (A-E), based on sequence differences in the envelope gene. Cats in the United States are most commonly infected with A, B, and occasionally C strains. Some cats harbor multiple strains or strain recombinants.

EPIDEMIOLOGY

Epidemiologic studies of domestic cats have long suggested that most cases of FIV infection are acquired by horizontal transmission among adult cats. Worldwide, adult male cats living outdoors consistently compose the majority of FIV-infected cats, and the risk is highest for sexually intact males. Infectious virus is found in the saliva of FIV-positive cats, and the fighting and biting behavior of this group of cats is believed to be the main source of transmission. Interestingly, sexual transmission, the most common mode of transmission of HIV, appears to be unusual in FIV, even though the semen of infected cats frequently contains infectious virus.

The true prevalence of FIV is unknown because testing is voluntary, results are not reported to a central database, and most screening test results are not confirmed. Prevalence studies have generally relied on convenience testing of cats in veterinary clinics, shelter facilities, and spay-neuter programs. These studies have shown that the prevalence of FIV is highly variable, dependent on age, sex, lifestyle, physical condition, and geographic location. Prevalence of FIV in a recent survey of 18,038 cats tested at veterinary clinics and animal shelters in North America was 2.5% of cats overall with higher risk among cats tested at veterinary clinics than cats tested at animal shelters.[1] Prevalence was also higher in adults, males, cats that were sick at the time of testing, and cats with access to the outdoors (Table 211-1). Certain disease syndromes are associated with a very high prevalence of FIV infections, such as cutaneous abscesses (12.7%)[2] and oral inflammation (7.9%).[3]

Identification and segregation of infected cats is considered to be the single most effective method for preventing new infections with FIV. Despite the availability of point-of-care testing for FIV infection, fewer than one quarter of all cats in the United States have ever been tested. Although characteristics such as gender, age, lifestyle, and health status can be used to assess the likely risk of FIV infections, most cats have some degree of infection risk.

PATHOGENESIS

Mild clinical signs associated with acute FIV infection, including transient fever, lymphadenopathy, and leukopenia, are likely to pass unnoticed by cat owners. High concentrations of virus in the blood can be detected by culture and PCR within 2 weeks of infection. Simultaneously, both CD4+ (helper) and CD8+ (cytotoxic-suppressor) T lymphocytes decline,[4,5] followed by a vigorous immune response. This

Table • 211-1

Prevalence of Feline Immunodeficiency Virus Infection in 18,038 Cats Tested in Veterinary Clinics and Animal Shelters in North America[1]

	NUMBER TESTED	PREVALENCE
Testing Site		
Animal shelter	8068	1.7%
Veterinary clinic	9970	3.1%
Source		
Clinic—indoors only	3613	0.9%
Shelter—relinquished pet	2809	1.4%
Shelter—stray	4550	1.6%
Shelter—feral	709	3.9%
Clinic—outdoors access	6357	4.3%
Age		
Juvenile	9556	1.0%
Adult	8482	4.1%
Sex		
Spayed female	6588	1.2%
Sexually intact female	2611	1.7%
Sexually intact male	5855	3.3%
Castrated male	2984	4.3%
Health Status		
Healthy	15,312	1.8%
Sick	2726	6.1%

response includes a recovery of CD8+ T lymphocytes to greater than preinfection levels, the production of FIV antibodies, and a decrease of circulating viral load. Both CD4+ and CD8+ T lymphocytes gradually decline, and an inversion of the CD4+:CD8+ T lymphocyte ratio persists for the rest of the cat's life. Infected lymphocytes and macrophages carry the virus to other organs, but lymphoid tissues remain the primary site of viral replication. Other immune disruptions include changes in cytokines (increased expression of proinflammatory cytokines interleukin [IL]-4, IL-6, IL-10, interferon gamma, and tumor necrosis factor; decreased expression of IL-2 and IL-12), and decreased natural killer cell activity, mitogen responsiveness, memory cell activity, and neutrophil function.[6] These changes lead to a decrease in cell-mediated immunity. Simultaneously, increased B cell activity and nonspecific immunoglobulin production are associated with polyclonal gammopathy.

Humans with HIV infection generally progress through distinctive clinical stages defined by absolute CD4+ T lymphocyte counts. Similar staging systems have been proposed for cats with FIV infections, but the feline disease process is not as predictable and some cats with severe CD4+ T lymphocytopenia remain healthy for many years.[7,8] Following acute infection, FIV-infected cats enter a prolonged asymptomatic stage during which progressive dysfunction of the immune system occurs. Chronic inflammatory conditions, neoplasia, and infections with intracellular organisms are more common than infections controlled by antibodies in FIV-infected cats. FIV-infected cats also appear to respond adequately to vaccination. These findings reflect the fact that

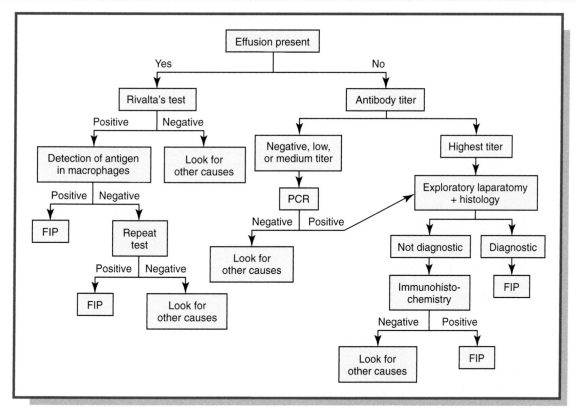

Figure 213-2 Algorithm for the diagnosis of feline infectious peritonitis *(FIP)* in a cat in which FIP is suspected. *PCR,* Polymerase chain reaction.

also have to be considered an unfavorable prognostic sign, since they occur significantly more frequently in animals with marked extension of the inflammatory lesions to the forebrain.[55]

Symptomatic Treatment

As FIP is an immune-mediated disease, symptomatic treatment is aimed at controlling the immune response to FCoV, and the relatively most successful therapy consists of high doses of immune-suppressive and antiinflammatory drugs. In nearly every published case report, *glucocorticoids* were used; there are, however, no studies about the true effect of glucocorticoids in FIP. Immune-suppressive drugs such as prednisone (2 to 4 mg/kg q24h PO) or cyclophosphamide (2 to 4 mg/kg 4 times per week PO) may slow disease progression. Some cats with effusion benefit from "tapping" and removal of the fluid and injection of dexamethasone into the abdominal or thoracic cavity (1 mg/kg q24h until effusion is no longer produced). Cats should also be treated with broad-spectrum antibiotics and supportive therapy (e.g., fluids) in addition to the immune-suppressive treatment. A thromboxane synthetase inhibitor (ozagrel hydrochloride) that inhibits platelet aggregation and cytokine release and thus, may control excessive inflammation, has been used in a two cats and has lead to some improvement of clinical signs.[56]

Immune Modulators

Some veterinarians prescribe immune modulators (e.g., promodulin, acemannan) to treat cats with FIP with no documented controlled evidence of efficacy. It has been suggested that these agents may benefit infected animals by restoring compromised immune function, thereby allowing the patient to control viral burden and recover from clinical signs. However, a nonspecific stimulation of the immune system may in fact be contraindicated, since the clinical signs develop and progress as a result of an immune-mediated response.[57] In some older reports the use of tylosine was described. *Tylosine* is a macrolid antibiotic that, like other macrolids, also has immunomodulatory effects. A "temporary remission" was achieved in 10 cats using 22 mg tylosine q24h; however, FIP was not confirmed. Three cats suspected but not confirmed as having FIP were treated with tylosine (starting at 88 mg/kg q12h PO) and prednisolone (starting at 4 mg/kg q24h) as well as supportive treatment with fluids and vitamins and lived up to 210 days. Another unconfirmed FIP cat was treated with tylosine (50 mg/cat q8h PO) and prednisolone (10 mg/cat q24h PO) and additionally, tylosine (200 mg/cat) intraperitoneally after each of several abdominocenteses; the cat "recovered" within 2 months. The immune modulator *promodulin* was used in 52 cats suspected to have FIP that responded favorably to treatment; a rapid remission of clinical signs was seen; although clinical signs were compatible, FIP was not confirmed, there was no control group, and no long-term follow up was included in the study.[57] In one study, 29 FIP-suspected cats were divided into five groups and treated over 6 weeks with different "cocktails" including prednisolone, dexamethasone, cyclophoshamide, ampicillin, human interferon-α, and a *"paraimmunity inducer"*; between 20% and 71% (depending on the group) of the cats survived for 3 years; however, FIP was not confirmed in any of these cats.[58,59]

Antiviral Chemotherapy

The search for an effective antiviral compound has not been successful. The antiviral drug *ribavirin*, a nucleoside analogue that prevents formation of viral proteins, most likely by interfering with the capping of viral mRNA, is active against FCoV in vitro.[60] Ribavirin was administered to specific pathogen-free kittens (16.5 mg/kg q24h PO, IM, or IV for 10 to 14 days) starting 18 hours after experimental challenge exposure with an experimental FIP-causing FCoV strain. All kittens, including the ribavirin-treated ones, succumbed to FIP; the clinical signs of disease were even more severe in the ribavirin-treated kittens and their mean survival time was significantly shortened,[61] and thus, ribavirin, was not effective in vivo. Even the attempt to decrease the toxicity of ribavirin (the most common adverse effects in cats are hemolysis that develops as a result of sequestration of the drug in red blood cells; a dose-related bone marrow toxicity, which primarily affects megakaryocytes and erythroid precursors resulting in thrombocytopenia with hemorrhage and anemia, respectively; and liver toxicity[62]) by incorporating it into lecithin-containing liposomes and administering it at a lower dosage (5 mg/kg IV) to cats challenged with an FIP-causing virus failed.[63] *Melphalan*, an alkylating agent of the nitrogen mustard group that interacts irreversibly with DNA, was administered (starting at 1 mg/kg q7h for 9 months) in a 3-year-old male cat that was feline leukemia virus–positive and suspected to have FIP; in addition, the cat received prednisone, ampicillin, streptokinase, vitamins, and minerals. The cat survived for 9 months, but the diagnosis FIP was again not confirmed and on histopathology, there was no evidence of FIP.[57]

Interferons have been used frequently. Human interferon-α and feline interferon-ω have a direct antiviral effect by inducing a general "antiviral state" of interferon-containing cells that protects against virus replication. In vitro, antiviral efficacy of *human interferon-α* against an FIP-causing FCoV strain has been demonstrated. In a placebo-controlled treatment study including 74 specific pathogen–free cats in which FIP was induced experimentally, neither the prophylactic nor the therapeutic administration of high doses (10^4 or 10^6 IU/kg) interferon-α, feline interferon-β (10^3 IU/kg), *Propionibacterium acnes* (0.4 mg/cat or 4 mg/cat), or a combination significantly reduced mortality in treated *versus* untreated cats. However, in cats treated with 10^6 IU/kg interferon-α in combination with *Propionibacterium acnes*, the mean survival time was prolonged, but only by 3 weeks.[64] Recently, *feline interferon-ω* was licensed for use in veterinary medicine in some European countries and Japan. Interferons are species-specific, and cats can be treated parenterally with feline interferons over long periods without developing antibodies. FCoV replication is inhibited by feline interferon-ω in vitro,[65] and promising results were obtained in one uncontrolled trial, but FIP was not confirmed.[66] In a recently performed randomized placebo-controlled double-blind treatment trial, 37 cats with FIP were treated with interferon-ω or placebo. This is virtually the only treatment study in field cats, in which FIP was confirmed. In all cats of this study, FIP was diagnosed by histopathology and/or immunohistochemistry or immunofluorescence staining of FCoV antigen in effusion or tissue macrophages. Cats received either interferon-ω (10^6 U/kg q24h SQ) or placebo for 8 consecutive days and subsequently once every week. In addition, all cats received glucocorticoids, either as dexamethasone when effusion was present (1 mg/kg q24h intrathoracically or intraperitoneally) or prednisolone (2 mg/kg q24h PO). There was no statistically significant difference in the mean survival time of cats treated with interferon-ω versus placebo. The cats survived for a period of 3 to 200 days before they had to be euthanized.[53]

PREVENTION

Preventing FIP is extremely difficult. The only way to truly prevent the development of FIP is to prevent infection with FCoV.

Management of Cats after Contact

If a cat has been euthanized or has died from FIP, and there are no remaining cats in the household, the owner should be instructed to wait about 3 months before obtaining a new cat, since FCoV can stay infectious for several weeks in the environment. If there are other cats in that household, they are most likely already infected with FCoV and shedding FCoV. In natural circumstances, cats go outside to defecate and bury their feces, in which case the virus usually remains infectious only for hours (up to days in freezing conditions). However, domesticated cats have been introduced to littertrays in which FCoV may survive for several days and possibly up to 7 weeks in dried-up feces. Thus, cats that are infected with FCoV may have a better chance to eliminate the virus if allowed to go outside, as otherwise they may constantly reinfect themselves with virus in their own feces.[38] It is common for a cat to be brought to a veterinarian that had been in contact with a cat with FIP or a suspected or known virus shedder. The owner may want to know the prognosis for the exposed cat, or may want to obtain another cat. It is likely that the cat will be antibody-positive, as 95% to 100% of cats exposed to FCoV become infected and develop antibodies approximately 2 to 3 weeks after FCoV exposure. Few cats, however, may be "resistant" to FCoV infection. It has been shown that some cats in FCoV endemic multiple-cat households may continuously remain antibody-negative,[48] but the mechanism of action for this resistance is still unknown. Although most cats in contact will most likely have antibodies, owners should be reassured that this is not necessarily associated with a poor prognosis. Most cats infected with FCoV will not develop FIP, and many cats in single- or two-cat households will eventually clear their infection and become antibody-negative a few months to years later. Ideally, the owner should be advised to wait until antibody titers of all cats are negative before obtaining a new cat. Cats should be retested (using the same laboratory) every 6 to 12 months until the antibody test is negative. Some cats, however, will remain antibody-positive for years without developing FIP. In a study that monitored 50 cats with persistently high titers over years, only 4 cats died of FIP.[38]

Often the question will arise whether it is dangerous to bring a cat (in which FIP has been diagnosed) back into a household with other cats. When a cat in a household develops FIP, other cats that have been in contact with the ill cat will already have been exposed to the same FCoV. It remains a matter of discussion whether the mutated FIP-causing virus is excreted and transmitted from cat to cat. In general, this does not seem to be the case under natural circumstances. Studies have failed to detect mutated virus in secretions or excretions from cats with FIP.[67] Thus, shedding of mutated virus under natural circumstances seems unlikely. The "harmless" FCoV will continue to be shed even in lower quantities in the feces once a cat has succumbed to FIP.[48,68] Nevertheless, despite this "natural" evidence to the contrary, under experimental conditions it has been possible to transmit the mutated FIP-causing virus from a cat with FIP to in-contact cats. Recently, the genomic RNA sequence of a field FCoV strain isolated postmortem from the jejunum and the liver of a cat with FIP revealed 100% nucleotide identity between the enteric- (jejunum) and nonenteric- (liver) derived viral RNA sequences, a finding that also poses the questions of whether a FIP-causing virus may be transmitted under some circumstances.[69] On the basis of current knowledge, the appropriate advice seems to be that it is relatively safe to take the cat with FIP back into the household to the cats that have already been in contact, as these cats will have a certain immunity to the FCoV strain endemic in the household. It is, however, not recommended to allow contact of the cat with FIP to any new "naïve" cat.

to viruses that cause measles, rinderpest, and distemper in other animals. Canine distemper virus (CDV) is capable of infecting a large variety of species including canids, mustelids (e.g., ferrets, skunks), and procyonids (e.g., raccoons). Host range is defined by the viral surface hemagglutinin protein, and there are six major lineages based on hemagglutinin genetic variability.[33] Each lineage contains biotypes or strains that differ in pathogenicity patterns. Despite vaccinating dogs for more than 50 years, CDV is still prevalent in many U.S. communities. Although uncommonly seen in veterinary practices, distemper outbreaks occur frequently in shelter facilities. Free-roaming unvaccinated dogs have increased risk for virus exposure based on more opportunity to interface with CDV-infected raccoons, skunks, and other wildlife.

TRANSMISSION

All ages and breeds are susceptible to CDV infection if there is no or incomplete immunity from vaccination or previous exposure. CDV is transmitted by oronasal exposure to virus-contaminated respiratory secretions, vomitus, feces, urine, and environmental fomites. CDV is also spread efficiently by inhalation of virus particles in respiratory aerosols generated by coughing and sneezing, as well as aerosols of other excretions. The incubation period typically ranges from 1 to 3 weeks. Virus shedding starts within 7 to 10 days of exposure during the preclinical incubation phase and can continue for 60 to 90 days. Dogs with subclinical infection also shed virus in feces. Thus, infected dogs may be contagious for up to 3 months. To prevent viral transmission within a facility, infected patients should be housed in isolation and cared for by staff adhering to strict biosecurity measures. CDV does not survive for long periods outside of the host and is susceptible to inactivation with a number of disinfectants such as phenolic or quaternary ammonium compounds.

PATHOGENESIS

CDV causes systemic infection of epithelial tissues in many organ systems. Following exposure, virus infects and replicates locally in macrophages and monocytes in the tonsils, upper respiratory tract epithelium, and regional lymph nodes, reaching peak virion production by 2 to 4 days after inoculation.[34,35] Viremia occurs 4 to 6 days later, with spread of virus to the stomach, small intestine, spleen and hepatic macrophages, bone marrow, and other lymphoid sites. The widespread increase in virus production is associated with fever and lymphopenia. A second viremia follows within a few days and is responsible for infection of epithelial cells in multiple organs, including the eyes, skin, and central nervous system (CNS). Virus shedding from the respiratory, GI, and urogenital tracts coincides with epithelial infection. Virus persists for long periods of time in the uvea, uroepithelium, epidermis, and CNS; molecular mechanisms underlying viral persistence are unknown.[33]

After 9 to 14 days, the clinical outcome of infection is dictated by the strength and type of the host's immune response. Viral infection in bone marrow and other lymphoid tissues can result in profound and protracted immunosuppression, particularly young dogs, due to T cell depletion and other undefined mechanisms.[33] Dogs with poor immune responses develop viral infection of several additional tissues including skin and other glandular and epithelial organs. Such animals generally exhibit severe clinical signs and are likely to die as a result of infection. Those animals that do recover from the initial clinical signs maintain virus in tissues and are likely to subsequently develop clinical signs of CNS disease. In animals that mount an intermediate level of immune response, mild or clinically silent infection may develop, with virus persisting in the lungs, skin, or CNS. Such animals may undergo a complete recovery, or may develop signs of CNS disease. Animals that mount strong immune responses are unlikely to develop signs of systemic infection but may still develop signs of CNS disease.

The pathogenesis of neurologic disease in CDV-infected dogs is complex. Dogs, especially the young or immune-suppressed, may develop acute demyelination attributed to direct viral injury in the absence of inflammatory reactions. Chronic encephalitis appears to be a consequence of inflammatory responses to viral antigens in CNS cells, with macrophage activation and release of cytotoxic mediators playing a role in destruction and demyelination of CNS cells.

CLINICAL SIGNS

Severity of the clinical course is a function of the animal's age at the time of infection, pathogenicity patterns for different viral strains, and immune responses.[33-35] Many dogs, particularly those that are older or have partial immunity, have asymptomatic infection or mild disease. Puppies are more likely to suffer more severe and protracted illness and have the highest mortality rate.

Affected dogs may be lethargic, anorexic, dehydrated, and febrile, and they frequently have respiratory signs initially. These include serous or mucopurulent oculonasal discharge and cough that progressively worsens if an inadequate immune response exists. Viral infection of the lower respiratory tract results in pneumonia that may or may not be clinically evident but can be documented via radiographs. Viral pneumonia complicated by secondary bacterial infections can be life threatening in puppies. Depending on viral strain, affected dogs may also have vomiting and mucoid or hemorrhagic diarrhea from viral replication in the GI epithelium. Virus infection of ocular tract epithelium can cause photophobia, anterior uveitis, and chorioretinitis. Recovered animals may have hyper-reflective retinal lesions that develop from retinal atrophy and scarring, as well as keratitis sicca from scarring of the lacrimal glands. Optic neuritis may cause blindness or mydriasis; blindness can also result from serous retinal detachments. Production of large amounts of virus occurs in uroepithelium, including the kidneys and lower urinary tract, which may cause clinical signs associated with kidney and bladder dysfunction. Viral infection of the epidermis can result in a pustular rash and hyperkeratosis or "hardening" of the nasal planum and footpads. Infection of developing enamel buds in young puppies prior to eruption of the permanent dentition results in enamel hypoplasia. Some dogs, especially young large-breed dogs, are susceptible to metaphyseal osteosclerosis of long bones, which is typically not associated with lameness.

Neurologic signs may develop starting 1 to 3 weeks after recovery from systemic signs or can develop months later. Neurologic signs can develop in dogs that had no evidence of systemic disease. Curiously, certain features of clinical disease tend to correlate with the likelihood of developing neurologic disease. Dogs that develop pustular skin lesions are less likely to develop CNS disease, but hyperkeratosis of the nasal planum and digital footpads is frequently associated with the development of neurologic signs. Neurologic abnormalities can reflect lesions in any CNS site and include seizures, ataxia, hypermetria, paraparesis or tetraparesis, and severe cervical pain. Myoclonus, either generalized or focal, is a common clinical sign and is strongly suggestive of CDV infection. Puppies infected in utero or as neonates can develop CNS signs early in life. Abortion and neonatal death have been seen.

DIAGNOSIS

Diagnosis of CDV is usually clinical, relying on compatible clinical signs in dogs with a poor vaccination history. However, CDV can occur in vaccinated dogs.[36,37] Intranuclear and intracytoplasmic viral inclusions may be seen in monocytes, lymphocytes, neutrophils, or erythrocytes during examination of a stained blood smear, but inclusions often disappear within 1 to 2 weeks of noting clinical signs. There are no pathognomonic laboratory abnormalities. Lymphopenia is the most consistent CBC abnormality. Biochemical profile abnormalities can include hypoalbuminemia and hypoglobulinemia. The CSF may have increased numbers of lymphocytes and monocytes and varying protein concentrations.[36] Dogs with respiratory disease may have interstitial or alveolar patterns on thoracic radiographs. Radiographs of long bones in lame animals may have metaphyseal lesions consistent with hypertrophic osteodystrophy. Animals with CDV neurologic disease can be diagnostic challenges if there is no history or evidence of systemic signs. Abnormalities on magnetic resonance imaging (MRI) of the brain in dogs with acute CDV have been described and, though not specific, could potentially help support a diagnosis in dogs with few or no systemic signs.[38]

Definitive diagnosis of CDV hinges on detection of viral antigen or nucleic acid in antemortem or postmortem samples, virus isolation, and serology. Demonstration of viral antigen in cells on blood smears, smears from nasal, conjunctival, or pharyngeal swabs, or postmortem tissues by immunological methods such as fluorescent antibody or immunohistochemical testing confirms the diagnosis but is subject to false-negative results if performed beyond 3 weeks postinfection.[34] Reverse-transcriptase polymerase chain reaction (RT-PCR) assays are highly sensitive and specific for detection of CDV in clinical cases and can be performed on virtually any sample type, including conjunctival, nasal, and pharyngeal swabs; whole blood; feces; urine; CSF; and postmortem tissues, particularly the urinary bladder.[39-41] Several commercial laboratories offer CDV PCR assays, but these tests may not discriminate between vaccine and field CDV strains in samples collected from dogs recently vaccinated with modified-live CDV. Duration of postvaccine interference is variable but may be as long as 3 weeks.[41] An exception to vaccine interference with PCR testing is the recombinant vaccine containing a canarypox-vectored CDV gene (Merial). Nested PCR assays or restriction fragment length polymorphism can discriminate between vaccine and field CDV strains, but these assays are currently not offered by reference laboratories in the United States.[42-44]

Serologic tests are widely available for documentation of CDV infection. However, serology tests can be false negative for dogs that do not mount an immune response due to the profound immunosuppressive effects of CDV infection.[45] Immunofluorescent antibody (IFA) tests are used to measure IgM and IgG antibodies to CDV; detection of IgM antibodies, which can persist for 3 months, is supportive of CDV infection. The serum neutralization assay is considered the "gold standard" for quantifying total CDV antibody. Diagnosis of recent active infection by this assay requires collection of paired acute and convalescent sera to determine seroconversion, defined as at least a fourfold increase in the antibody titer between the acute and convalescent sample. Infection is also supported by demonstration of higher concentrations of CDV antibody in the CNS as compared with the serum, although not all animals will have CSF antibodies.[36]

TREATMENT

Treatment of dogs with CDV is largely supportive. Parenteral administration of fluids may be necessary in dogs with vomiting or severe diarrhea. Animals with secondary bacterial bronchopneumonia or other infections are candidates for antibiotics. In puppies, resolution of bronchopneumonia may require combinations of broad-spectrum bactericidal antibiotics administered for several weeks. Seizure control with diazepam, pentobarbital, or potassium bromide may be necessary. Ribavirin inhibits CDV replication in vitro,[46] but its use has not been described in infected dogs. The prognosis for dogs with neurologic disease is considered guarded to poor.

PREVENTION

The key to CDV prevention is vaccination. CDV vaccines are considered a "core vaccine" that should be administered to all dogs.[23] Recommended vaccines contain high-titer, low-passage, modified-live CDV or a canarypox vector containing CDV hemagglutinin and fusion genes. These vaccines are better able to effectively immunize dogs during the period of maternal antibody interference.[47] The canarypox-vectored CDV vaccine is also more likely to boost antibody titers in seropositive dogs compared with modified-live vaccines.[48] The duration of immunity following immunization with modified-live and recombinant vaccines is at least 3 years.[24-27,49] Current AAHA guidelines[23] recommend vaccinating dogs at 6 to 8 weeks of age, with repeat vaccinations performed every 3 to 4 weeks until 16 weeks old. All dogs should receive a booster vaccine 1 year after completion of the initial series, followed by boosters every 3 years. For animals that were not vaccinated before exposure, vaccination after exposure will have little no effect on the outcome. Immunization of dogs with modified-live CDV vaccine has been associated with postvaccinal complications, the most common of which is encephalitis, which can produce clinical signs of neurologic disease and variable neurological abnormalities 7 to 14 days after vaccination. However, onset of distemper-like disease shortly after vaccination is most likely due to infection with field strains of CDV prior to or at the time of vaccination, rather than disease due to reversion of modified-live vaccine strains to virulence.[33] CDV infection in previously vaccinated dogs is usually associated with failure to induce immunity from improper vaccination schedules or improper storage of the vaccine. Establishment of protective immunity can be determined by testing postvaccination serum for protective antibody titers in the serum neutralization assay at a diagnostic laboratory or an in-clinic ELISA kit (CDV/CPV Titer-Chek, Synbiotics).[32] Dogs that have recovered from CDV infection are considered immune to reinfection for long periods, most likely lifelong.

CANINE ADENOVIRUS TYPE 1

ETIOLOGY AND EPIDEMIOLOGY

Canine adenovirus type 1 (CAV-1), a nonenveloped double-stranded DNA virus in the Adenoviridae family, is the cause of infectious canine hepatitis (ICH). CAV-1 is closely related genetically and antigenically to CAV-2. In addition to the domestic dog, CAV-1 also infects wolves, coyotes, foxes, bears, and marine mammals. The incidence of infectious canine hepatitis in the United States has decreased with vaccination, although sporadic cases are identified, particularly in unvaccinated or improperly vaccinated puppies imported from countries where the disease is more prevalent.

TRANSMISSION

Infection occurs after oronasal exposure to virus-contaminated body secretions and excretions and environmental fomites. The incubation period is 4 to 9 days.[50] Virus shedding occurs during acute infection in all body secretions (saliva, respiratory) and excretions (feces, urine) and is shed in urine for up to 6 to 9 months.[50] The virus is relatively hardy, surviving in the environment for days to months, and is resistant to most disinfectants except some quaternary ammonium compounds, bleach (1:32 dilution), potassium peroxymonosulfate (Trifectant, Vétoquinol), and accelerated hydrogen peroxide products.

PATHOGENESIS

CAV-1 causes systemic infection with tropism for endothelial cells, epithelial cells, and hepatocytes.[50] After exposure, CAV-1 replicates in lymphoid tissue of the tonsils and regional lymph nodes. Viremia follows, leading to infection of other tissues. Direct cytopathic effects of the virus in the liver, eyes, and kidney contribute to early clinical signs, which can become apparent in naïve dogs 4 to 9 days after exposure. The extent of hepatic necrosis is a function of the level of antiviral antibody present at the time of infection: Animals with minimal antibody exhibit extensive necrosis that is often fatal; those with high levels of antibody exhibit minimal clinical signs; and those with intermediate antibody levels are susceptible to persistent hepatic inflammation.[50] Clinical signs of anterior uveitis ("blue eye") initially develop as a consequence of the inflammation following infection of corneal endothelial cells and the deposition of immune complexes as antibody responses to the virus increase.

CLINICAL SIGNS

Initial clinical signs include fever, depression, and lethargy. Later, development of abdominal discomfort, mucous membrane pallor, and inflammation of the tonsils and pharynx with tonsillar and cervical lymph node enlargement occur. Abdominal fluid and hepatomegaly will be detected in some dogs. Laryngitis, tracheitis, pneumonia, coughing, vomiting, and diarrhea occur in some. In severe cases, petechial and ecchymotic hemorrhages and epistaxis may develop from coagulation abnormalities secondary to hepatic dysfunction and DIC. Icterus is uncommon despite the presence of hepatic necrosis. Neurologic signs may be seen as a consequence of hepatic encephalopathy or CNS infection; measurement of bile acids or plasma ammonia concentrations, if elevated, would support hepatic encephalopathy as a cause of neurologic signs. Dogs with severe disease may die within hours of showing clinical signs, whereas dogs with less severe disease may exhibit clinical improvement 5 to 7 days after onset of clinical signs. Anterior uveitis and glomerulonephritis from deposition of immune complexes may occur within a month of recovery.

DIAGNOSIS

The diagnosis of canine infectious hepatitis is usually based on finding evidence of acute hepatic disease in a dog with a poor vaccination history. No specific laboratory abnormalities pathognomonic for CAV-1 infection are seen.[50] There may be leukopenia or leukocytosis depending on whether the patient is seen early or later in the course of disease. Thrombocytopenia is possible and could contribute to coagulopathies in the setting of DIC or abnormal platelet function. Increases in alanine aminotransferase (ALT) and alkaline phosphate (ALP) activity are expected, but the magnitude of activity will depend on the extent of hepatic necrosis and the timing of sample collection. Prolongations of APTT and PTT are common as a result of decreased hepatic synthesis of coagulation factors, DIC, or both. Proteinuria is also expected as a

sequel to renal injury during viremia or immune complex injury later in the course of disease.

Definitive diagnosis of CAV-1 infection can be established by polymerase chain reaction (PCR) performed on secretions or excretions; ocular, nasal, and pharyngeal swabs; and tissues.[50] PCR assays are sensitive and can differentiate CAV-1 from CAV-2. Serology and tissue staining by immunofluorescent antibody and immunohistochemistry cannot distinguish between CAV-1 and CAV-2.[50] Intranuclear inclusion bodies observed during cytologic or histologic examination of tissue, particularly the liver, can be strongly supportive of the diagnosis.[50]

TREATMENT

Therapy is directed at provision of supportive care and managing clinical signs and complications. Intravenous fluid therapy to replace losses from vomiting or diarrhea is important, as is administration of blood products to manage the complications of hemorrhage and DIC. In patients with neurologic signs from hepatic encephalopathy, administration of lactulose via enema (or orally if the patient is not vomiting) can help reduce circulating concentrations of encephalotoxins.

PREVENTION

Vaccination is the foundation of prevention of CAV-1 infection. Vaccines for CAV-1 are considered a "core vaccine" that should be administered to all dogs.[23] Most commonly used vaccines for CAV-1 use modified-live CAV-2 isolates that, through the production of cross-reactive antibodies, will elicit a protective immune response without the complications, such as corneal edema, associated with vaccines using CAV-1 isolates. The duration of immunity following immunization with modified-live and recombinant vaccines is at least 3 years.[24-27,49] Current AAHA guidelines[23] recommend vaccinating dogs at 6 to 8 weeks of age, with repeat vaccinations performed every 3 to 4 weeks until 16 weeks old. All dogs should receive a booster vaccine 1 year after completion of the initial series, followed by boosters every 3 years.

CANINE ADENOVIRUS TYPE 2 AND PARAINFLUENZA VIRUS

ETIOLOGY AND EPIDEMIOLOGY

Canine adenovirus type 2 (CAV-2) is a nonenveloped double-stranded DNA virus in the Adenoviridae family that is genetically and antigenically related to CAV-1. CAV-1 and CAV-2 share the same host range. Canine parainfluenza virus (CPiV) is an enveloped single-stranded RNA virus in the Paramyxoviridae family. CAV-2 and CPiV are part of a complex of pathogens causing canine infectious respiratory disease (CIRD) or "kennel cough." High-density, high-turnover populations in kennels, pet stores, or shelters are at risk for infection.

Transmission

Both viruses are transmitted by oronasal exposure through direct contact with virus-contaminated respiratory secretions and environmental fomites, as well as inhalation of aerosolized respiratory droplets generated by sneezing or coughing. The incubation period ranges from 3 to 10 days, and virus shedding in respiratory secretions generally ceases within 10 days.[50,51] CAV-2 is relatively hardy and can survive in the environment for days to months, but CPiV is fragile and survives for only a short period outside of the host. Both viruses are susceptible to inactivation by quaternary ammonium disinfectants, bleach (1:32 dilution), potassium peroxymonosulfate (Trifectant, Vétoquinol), and accelerated hydrogen peroxide products.

PATHOGENESIS

Virus replication occurs in nonciliated epithelial cells of the upper respiratory tract and type 2 alveolar cells in the lower respiratory tract, causing epithelial destruction and inflammation.[50,51] Peak replication occurs between days 3 and 6 postinfection and rapidly declines thereafter. Dogs can be asymptomatic or have mild clinical disease consisting of rhinitis, tracheitis, and bronchitis. However, damage and disruption of the epithelial barrier predisposes to infection with other viral and bacterial respiratory tract pathogens. Coinfections can increase tissue damage and worsen clinical disease, including progression to pneumonia. There is one report of fatal neurologic disease in puppies due to CAV-2 infection.[52]

CLINICAL SIGNS

A hacking cough with a terminal retch and serous or mucoid nasal discharge are the typical clinical signs. Coughing bouts are often easily elicited with tracheal palpation and can be paroxysmal in nature. Coughing may produce foamy white phlegm. Clinical signs are typically of short duration and often subside by 7 days after onset, although some dogs may exhibit clinical signs for up to 10 days.

DIAGNOSIS

There are no pathognomonic clinical signs or laboratory abnormalities in affected dogs; thoracic radiographs should be normal unless severe infection or coinfection creates a secondary bronchopneumonia. Definitive diagnosis requires PCR testing of swabs collected from the nose and pharyngeal area or virus isolation. Recent vaccination with modified-live vaccines can cause test interference because commercially available PCR assays cannot discriminate between vaccine and field strains. Duration of vaccine interference is not defined but may be up to 3 weeks. PCR assays can also be performed on swabs to rule out the presence of coinfecting viruses and *Bordetella bronchiseptica* bacteria.

TREATMENT

Treatment is largely supportive. Antibiotics are necessary for treating secondary bacterial infections evidenced by fever, purulent nasal discharge, productive cough, or pneumonia. Judicious short-term use of antiinflammatory doses of glucocorticoids or administration of cough suppressants, such as hydrocodone or butorphanol tartrate, may help ameliorate cough and improve patient comfort but are unlikely to shorten the clinical course.

PREVENTION

Vaccines for CAV-2 and CPiV are not considered core vaccines, but rather are "lifestyle" vaccines recommended for dogs at risk for exposure in shelters, boarding/training kennels, pet stores, and breeding kennels.[23] However, both CAV-2 and CPiV are included in parenteral core vaccines containing CDV and CPV, with CAV-2 providing cross-protective immunity to CAV-1. Therefore, when using these combination or multivalent vaccines, the frequency of vaccination against CAV-2 and CPiV follows the schedule recommended for the core components, including booster vaccination every 3 years following the initial immunization series.[23] For dogs at risk for exposure, intranasal vaccines containing modified-live CPiV (and CAV-2 in some products) can be given as early as 3 weeks of age, with repeat administration 2 to 4 weeks later, and every 6 to 12 months thereafter.[23]

CANINE INFLUENZA A SUBTYPE H3N8 VIRUS

ETIOLOGY AND EPIDEMIOLOGY

Canine influenza A subtype H3N8 is an enveloped single-strand RNA virus in the family Orthomyxoviridae. Canine influenza H3N8 virus (CIV) was first reported in 2004 as the cause of acute respiratory disease in dogs in Florida in 2004.[53] Ongoing surveillance since 2004 has identified thousands of dogs with laboratory-confirmed CIV infection in 30 states and the District of Columbia.[53-56] The virus is now enzootic in many communities in Colorado, Florida, Pennsylvania, New Jersey, and New York.

Molecular analyses of CIV isolates support their origination from the interspecies transmission of equine influenza A H3N8 viruses from horses to dogs at some point prior to 2004. Viral adaptation to the dog has resulted in a canine-specific pathogen that replicates efficiently in the respiratory tract to cause clinical disease and is sustained in canine populations by dog-to-dog transmission.[53,55] Since original discovery in the United States, equine influenza H3N8 viral infections have been reported in dogs in England[57] and Australia,[58] but there was no evidence of dog-to-dog transmission. Currently, there are no reports of canine influenza H3N8 cases outside of the United States, but this may change as more investigations are conducted.

CIV causes an acute respiratory infection in dogs. It is one of several viruses and bacteria that are associated with CIRD or "kennel cough." Dogs housed in different types of communal facilities such as kennels, shelters, pet stores, dog shows, and veterinary clinics are at highest risk for exposure to CIV.[53-56] Dogs of any age, breed, and health status are susceptible.[53-56] CIV does not infect people, and there is no documentation that other species have become infected by exposure to dogs with canine influenza. Experimental studies have shown that horses are susceptible to CIV infection, but the infection induces either no or mild clinical disease.[59] Unlike human influenza, canine influenza does not have a seasonal pattern of occurrence.

Transmission

Canine influenza is a highly contagious respiratory infection, and outbreaks reach epidemic proportions in facilities with high density and high-turnover populations. Transmission is by oronasal contact with infected dogs or contaminated fomites, and by inhalation of aerosols generated by coughing and sneezing. The incubation period is 2 to 4 days.[53,60,61] Peak virus shedding occurs during the preclinical incubation period and rapidly declines over the ensuing days to cessation by day 7 to 10.[53,60,61] A proportion of dogs have asymptomatic infection but shed virus and thus are contagious.[53,55,60,61] Once virus shedding ceases, dogs are no longer contagious. All dogs in a facility should be considered exposed and a potential infectious risk, whether or not they have clinical disease. Important management strategies for reducing spread of canine influenza within a premise include isolation of sick and exposed dogs and institution of strict biosecurity measures for staff providing care. Influenza A viruses are unstable in the environment but can remain viable on surfaces for up to 48 hours, on clothing for 24 hours, and on hands for 12 hours. Influenza A viruses are inactivated by quaternary ammonium disinfectants commonly used in kennels and veterinary clinics.

PATHOGENESIS

Because CIV is still a novel virus for most dogs, virtually all exposed dogs become infected and about 80% develop clinical disease.[53,55] Influenza virus replicates in mucosal epithelial cells lining the airways from the nose to the terminal airways, in bronchiole gland epithelium, and in pulmonary macrophages. Viral replication causes epithelial cell necrosis and destruction of the respiratory epithelial barrier, predisposing to secondary infections by a variety of commensal bacteria, including *Streptococcus* spp., *Staphylococcus* spp., *Escherichia coli*, *Klebsiella*, *Pasteurella multocida*, and *Mycoplasma* spp.[53,55] The primary viral infection initiates intense neutrophilic and monocytic inflammatory responses resulting in rhinitis, tracheitis, bronchitis, and bronchiolitis.[53,55]

Although most clinically affected dogs recover from influenza without complications, less than 10% progress to bronchopneumonia associated with virus-induced damage to lower airway epithelium and complicated by secondary bacterial infections.[53,55] Pulmonary congestion, consolidation, and petechial hemorrhages have been described in experimentally infected dogs that developed pneumonia in the absence of secondary bacterial infections.[53,61]

CLINICAL SIGNS

Clinical disease consists of acute onset of cough, sneezing, nasal discharge, and some ocular discharge.[53,55,60,61] Cough is the predominant sign and typically persists for 2 to 3 weeks due to the intense inflammatory response.[53,55,60,61] Some dogs may have a transient low-grade fever.[53,55,60,61] In naturally infected dogs, secondary commensal bacterial infections contribute to development of mucopurulent nasal discharge and productive cough.[53,55] Dogs with pneumonia have high fevers, inappetence, productive cough, and increased respiratory rate and effort. Pulmonary consolidation can cause respiratory distress and severe hypoxia.

DIAGNOSIS

Canine influenza cannot be diagnosed based on clinical signs because the clinical spectrum overlaps with that due to other respiratory pathogens. Dogs without pneumonia have unremarkable complete blood cell counts and serum chemistry values. Dogs with secondary bacterial infections in the lower respiratory tract may have leukocytosis consisting of neutrophilia with a left shift. For dogs with pneumonia, thoracic radiograph findings range from mild bronchointerstitial infiltrates to consolidation of all lung lobes. Lung consolidation may cause serum chemistry abnormalities reflective of tissue hypoxia. Cultures of transtracheal, endotracheal, and bronchoalveolar lavages may yield a variety of gram-negative or gram-positive bacteria, and neutrophils are the predominant cell type on cytologic examination. Postmortem examination findings include pulmonary edema and congestion, epithelial necrosis and erosion in all airways, and

suppurative rhinitis, tracheitis, bronchitis, bronchiolitis, and bronchopneumonia.[53,55]

Definitive diagnosis of canine influenza requires detection of virus in acutely ill dogs and serology. Methods for virus detection include ELISA for antigen, RT-PCR for nucleic acid, and virus isolation.[53,55,56,62] Successful virus detection by all three methods depends on sample collection during peak virus shedding early in the course of clinical disease. Nasal and pharyngeal swabs collected from dogs with clinical signs for <4 days can be tested for influenza A nucleoprotein using point-of-care ELISA kits available for diagnosis of human influenza A infections. Although the kits detect CIV, the sensitivity is reduced by lower virus shedding in dogs compared with horses, pigs, and people. RT-PCR for the influenza A matrix gene can detect very low amounts of virus on swabs, but false negatives occur due to the critical timing of sample collection. Serology is the most accurate and reliable diagnostic test for confirmation of CIV infection, especially in cases where the PCR test is negative but the index of suspicion is high.[53,55,56,62] Paired acute (sick for <7 days) and convalescent (10 to 14 days later) serum samples are necessary for diagnosis of recent active infection based on seroconversion. Seroconversion is defined as a ≥fourfold increase in CIV antibody titer between the acute and convalescent sample.

TREATMENT

Because canine influenza is a viral infection, treatment consists mainly of supportive care based on clinical signs and laboratory tests. Although there is no specific antiviral treatment for canine influenza at this time, a variety of secondary bacterial infections may play a significant role and antibiotics are indicated for dogs with fever, purulent nasal discharge, productive cough, and pneumonia. Antitussives are not very effective in reducing frequency and duration of coughing and should not be used on dogs with productive cough.

Although canine influenza has a low mortality rate overall, pneumonia cases can be life threatening if not managed aggressively in the hospital setting to maintain hydration, administer parenteral antibiotic therapy, and provide oxygen support. Ideally, antibiotic selection should be based on culture and sensitivity testing of lung washes. Empirical selection should include a broad-spectrum combination of bactericidal antibiotics that provide four-quadrant coverage. More severe cases of pneumonia with lung consolidation and hypoxia benefit greatly from oxygen supplementation and nebulization with coupage.

PREVENTION

Although studies have not yet been verified, it is likely that dogs that have recovered from natural infection retain some immunity to reinfection for an undetermined time period. Influenza viral disease is best prevented by vaccination. In May 2009, the USDA approved the licensure of the first canine influenza H3N8 vaccine for dogs (Intervet, Schering Plough Animal Health). The vaccine contains inactivated whole virus with adjuvant and is intended as an aid in the control of disease associated with CIV infection. Although the vaccine may not prevent infection, efficacy trials have shown that vaccination significantly reduces the severity and duration of clinical illness, including the incidence and severity of damage to the lungs. In addition, the vaccine reduces the amount of virus shed and shortens the shedding interval. This means that vaccinated dogs that become infected have less illness and are not as contagious to other dogs. It is administered to dogs 6 weeks of age and older by subcutaneous injection in two initial doses given 2 to 4 weeks apart, followed by an annual booster. The canine influenza vaccine is a "lifestyle" vaccine intended for dogs at risk for exposure while housed in communal facilities, particularly in communities where the virus is prevalent.

CANINE RESPIRATORY CORONAVIRUS

ETIOLOGY AND EPIDEMIOLOGY

Canine respiratory coronavirus (CRCoV) is an enveloped single-strand RNA virus in the Coronaviridae family. CRCoV is a group 2 coronavirus that is genetically related to the bovine and human coronaviruses associated with respiratory infections in cattle and humans, respectively.[63,64] CRCoV is genetically and antigenically distinct from group 1 canine enteric and pancytotropic coronaviruses. CRCoV was initially discovered in dogs with acute respiratory infection in England in 2003.[63,65] This virus commonly infects dogs in the United States, United Kingdom, Ireland, Greece, Italy, and Japan.[66-68]

CRCoV can cause acute respiratory infection and is part of the complex of viruses and bacteria associated with CIRD or "kennel cough."[68] The risk for CRCoV infection is highest for dogs housed in communal facilities such as kennels, shelters, pet stores, dog shows, and veterinary clinics. Dogs of all ages and breeds are susceptible. There is no evidence that CRCoV can infect other animal species or people.

Transmission
CRCoV is highly contagious. Transmission is by oronasal contact with infected dogs or contaminated fomites and inhalation of aerosols generated by coughing and sneezing. The incubation and virus shedding periods have not been defined by experimental infection studies; based on respiratory coronaviruses in other species, the incubation period is likely less than 4 days, with virus shedding for 7 to 10 days.[68] CRCoV has been detected in the colon of naturally infected dogs and in the feces of dogs experimentally infected.[68] This raises the possibility of fecal-oral transmission of CRCoV. Coronaviruses are inactivated by quaternary ammonium disinfectants commonly used in kennels and veterinary clinics.

PATHOGENESIS

CRCoV has been detected in dogs with inapparent or mild respiratory disease. Difficulty in obtaining viral isolates for experimental studies has hampered description of the pathogenesis for CRCoV. In naturally infected dogs, the virus is most frequently detected in the epithelium of the nasal cavity and trachea but has also been identified in the lung, spleen, mesenteric lymph nodes, and colon.[67,68] Damage from CRCoV replication in respiratory epithelium may predispose to superinfections with other viral and bacterial respiratory pathogens.[63,65,68]

CLINICAL SIGNS

Clinical disease consists of acute onset of cough, sneezing, and nasal discharge for a short period of time. Secondary commensal bacterial infections can cause mucopurulent nasal discharge and productive cough. More severe clinical signs, including those associated with pneumonia, are likely due to coinfection with other viral or bacterial respiratory pathogens.

DIAGNOSIS

CRCoV cannot be diagnosed based on clinical signs because the clinical spectrum overlaps with that caused by other respiratory pathogens. Definitive diagnosis requires detection of virus by RT-PCR assays performed on swabs collected from the upper respiratory tract or tissues. Serology tests are not available in the United States. Concurrent infections with other respiratory pathogens should be ruled out.

TREATMENT

CRCoV infection of the upper respiratory tract is self-limiting. Antibiotic therapy may be necessary for secondary bacterial infections.

PREVENTION

Although there is no vaccine for CRCoV at this time, dogs at risk for exposure should be vaccinated against other respiratory pathogens to reduce the risk for coinfections leading to more serious clinical disease.

CANINE ENTERIC CORONAVIRUS

ETIOLOGY AND EPIDEMIOLOGY

Canine enteric coronavirus (CECoV), an enveloped single-stranded RNA virus in the family Coronaviridae, is a group 1 coronavirus that is genetically and antigenically distinct from the group 2 coronavirus, canine respiratory coronavirus (CRCoV). CECoV can infect many species of canids and is considered prevalent in dogs from group-housing facilities such as kennels and shelters.[69,70]

TRANSMISSION

CECoV is spread primarily by the fecal-oral route to susceptible dogs. Duration of fecal shedding in infected dogs is 6 to 9 days but can be longer in some animals. The virus is relatively stable in the environment but can be inactivated by common disinfectants.

PATHOGENESIS

CECoV infects epithelial cells in the villus tips of the small intestine. A malabsorptive diarrhea results as a consequence of loss of villus surface area. The development of a local intestinal immune response terminates clinical signs and ultimately viral shedding.

CLINICAL SIGNS

CECoV can be found in feces of clinically normal dogs. Diarrhea (occasionally with blood) is the principle sign in clinically affected dogs. Vomiting may be seen before or after diarrhea in some animals. Anorexia and lethargy are common features, and if vomiting and diarrhea are severe, dehydration may ensue. Clinical disease from CECoV is considered infrequent compared with other viral enteropathies and is usually more severe in neonatal animals, with diminishing severity of clinical disease in older animals. Clinical signs abate after 7 to 10 days in most dogs, but the clinical course may be longer in dogs that develop secondary complications or infections.

DIAGNOSIS

The definitive diagnosis of CECoV historically has required the demonstration of virus in feces, usually by electron microscopy. The presence of viral antigen can be demonstrated in cells or tissues via immunohistochemistry. PCR assays offered by diagnostic laboratories (IDEXX) are the most sensitive and specific test for viral nucleic in feces and tissues.[71,72]

TREATMENT

Treatment of CECoV is primarily supportive while the disease runs its natural course. Dehydrated animals may require parenteral fluids. The role of antibiotics in the treatment of CECoV has not been assessed; however, use of antibiotics in dogs with diarrhea, though not universally accepted, has been supported because bacteria may be primary or secondary pathogens, and attempts to define viral etiologies may not always be made.[73]

PREVENTION

CECoV vaccines are available, but the benefits of vaccination in disease reduction or infection control have not been established. CECoV vaccines are not considered core vaccines and are not currently recommended.[23]

CANINE PANCYTOTROPIC CORONAVIRUS

ETIOLOGY AND EPIDEMIOLOGY

A novel group 1 coronavirus isolate related to CECoV has been identified as a cause of severe clinical disease in puppies and juvenile dogs.[72]

TRANSMISSION

The mode of transmission in field cases has not been established but is suspected to be fecal-oral based on tissues infected and reproduction of clinical disease following experimental transmission of this isolate by the fecal-oral route.[74]

PATHOGENESIS

The key pathophysiologic feature of this coronavirus is tropism for a wide variety of cell types. The viral features accounting for the expanded cell tropism have yet to be defined but are suspected to reflect a mutation. Pancytotropic CCoV antigen and RNA have been identified in lungs, kidneys, liver, spleen, GI tract, lymph nodes, and RNA in the brain.

CLINICAL SIGNS

The clinical signs thus far described in a limited number of cases with confirmed pancytotropic CCoV infection have included fever, lethargy, anorexia, vomiting, hemorrhagic diarrhea, ataxia, and seizures. The clinical signs were worse in young puppies (<2 months), which succumbed rapidly (2 days in naturally infected puppies), but older dogs with pronounced clinical signs were more likely to recover. Decreases in absolute number of lymphocytes and neutrophils were observed in experimentally infected dogs.

DIAGNOSIS

Diagnostic tests such as virus isolation, antigen detection, and PCR have documented infection in dogs described to date. Importantly, the affected dogs have tested negative for other enteric viral pathogens, notably CPV.

TREATMENT

Details of treatment in affected dogs have been limited but are assumed to be primarily supportive in nature.

PREVENTION

There is no means of prevention established at this time. Thorough cleaning and disinfection of the premises of confirmed or suspected cases would be prudent.

CANINE ROTAVIRUS

Etiology and Epidemiology

Canine rotavirus enteritis is most often caused by a group A rotavirus in the family Reoviridae, which are nonenveloped, double-stranded RNA viruses. Group C rotaviruses, which are more commonly found in other species such as pigs, have been documented in diarrheic dogs.[75] Compared with other enteric viruses, clinical disease caused by canine rotavirus appears to be uncommon.[76-78] Canine rotavirus can cause subclinical or mild gastroenteritis in puppies younger than 3 months old. Severe fatal enteritis has been reported in puppies younger than 2 weeks old. There is a high seroprevalence in adult dogs. Although rotaviruses are generally species-specific, genetic sequence analyses have suggested the possibility of transmission of canine rotaviral isolates to people.[79,80] A caninelike rotavirus isolate was associated with enteritis in a child.[79]

TRANSMISSION

Infection usually occurs via oronasal exposure to virus-contaminated feces or fomites. Virus shedding can start within 2 days of infection and continue for 7 to 10 days. Rotaviruses are durable in the environment and require disinfectants such as bleach, potassium peroxymonosulfate, or accelerated hydrogen peroxide products for complete inactivation.

PATHOGENESIS

After exposure, rotavirus infects epithelial cells of the villus tip of the jejunum and ileum. Loss of villus epithelial cells ensues with development of villus atrophy. Virus is shed early as infected, necrotic epithelial cells are sloughed from the villus.

CLINICAL SIGNS

Anorexia, vomiting, and mild diarrhea, which can occasionally be bloody, are the typical clinical signs of rotaviral gastroenteritis. Recovery is expected in most animals within 5 to 7 days of onset of clinical signs.

DIAGNOSIS

Commercially available tests to detect group A rotaviral antigens are available but not commonly employed in small animal practice. Other methods to obtain a definitive diagnosis include demonstration of virus in feces by electron microscopy or RT-PCR.

TREATMENT

Therapy of rotavirus gastroenteritis is supportive care, with attention to maintenance of hydration status in puppies with anorexia and vomiting.

PREVENTION

There is no vaccine currently available for prevention of rotaviral infection in dogs.

CANINE HERPESVIRUS

ETIOLOGY AND EPIDEMIOLOGY

Canine herpesvirus (CHV) is an enveloped, double-stranded DNA virus in the Herpesviridae family. The host range is restricted to domestic and wild canids. Surprisingly, no CHV strain has been completely sequenced and only a few genes have been identified, but CHV is genetically related to feline and equine herpesvirus.[50,51] Serosurveys have demonstrated higher viral prevalence in kenneled dogs than household dogs in Europe, but few studies have documented the prevalence in dogs in the United States. Although controversial and not clearly defined, CHV is considered part of a complex of pathogens causing CIRD or "kennel cough." It may have a secondary role, with activation of viral replication induced by infection by more virulent respiratory pathogens.

TRANSMISSION

The virus is transmitted by oronasal contact with infectious respiratory or genital secretions and may also occur transplacentally. The incubation period for primary infection is 6 to 10 days. Virus shedding occurs for 7 to 10 days after primary infection or reactivation of latent infection.[50,51] CHV is not stable in the environment and is inactivated by most common disinfectants such as quaternary ammonium products.

PATHOGENESIS

Transplacental infection during primary infection of pregnant dogs results in fetal resorption, abortion, stillbirths, or birth of weak puppies that die within days. Immunity following primary infection protects future litters. Infection of naïve puppies younger than 2 weeks old causes fatal generalized necrotizing and hemorrhagic disease. Neonatal puppies are infected by oronasal contact with infectious birth canal secretions in dams with actively replicating virus, or via grooming by the dam. CHV first replicates in the epithelial cells of the oropharynx and tonsils. Virus subsequently enters macrophages, which allows spread to other tissues hematogenously, including the lymph nodes, spleen, adrenal glands, kidneys, lungs, liver, and CNS. The lower body temperature of neonates, in conjunction with a limited capacity to mount a febrile response, facilitates systemic spread of the virus.

Infection of older pups and adults is confined to the respiratory, ocular, or genital tract without systemic spread. Most infections are asymptomatic or may present as a mild and self-limiting respiratory, ocular, or genital disease. Following a short replication period, CHV establishes latent infection in neurons of the trigeminal and lumbosacral ganglia, lymphocytes in the retropharyngeal lymph nodes and tonsils, and epithelial cells in the parotid salivary gland.[50,51] Reactivation of viral replication can be provoked by stress and immunosuppressive disease or therapy.

CLINICAL SIGNS

Infected neonatal puppies exhibit persistent crying, anorexia, abdominal pain, dyspnea, and petechial hemorrhages 1 to 3 days before death. Most puppies in affected litters die between 1 and 4 weeks postpartum. Petechial hemorrhages in the liver, kidneys, and lungs are typical lesions observed on necropsy. Older puppies develop mild signs of respiratory disease (rhinitis, pharyngitis) with spontaneous recovery, but latent infections may emerge later as a cause of neurologic disease, with signs of ataxia, blindness, or central vestibular disease most common. Infection in adult dogs is usually asymptomatic, but some dogs have rhinitis, pharyngitis, vaginal or preputial hyperemia, hyperplasia of vaginal mucosal lymphoid follicles, and sometimes submucosal hemorrhages. Corneal ulceration has been reported in adult dogs during natural infection with CHV,[81] while conjunctivitis occurred in experimentally infected dogs.[82] The clinical significance of CHV infections in ocular diseases is not defined, but CHV should be considered a potential cause of conjunctivitis or corneal disease after more common causes have been excluded.

DIAGNOSIS

Diagnosis is made by observation of clinical signs in puppies of susceptible age in conjunction with necropsy lesions. Viral inclusion bodies may be observed in cells surrounding areas of necrosis and hemorrhage. Definitive diagnosis of CHV infection centers on demonstration of virus, viral antigen, or nucleic acids by tissue PCR, electron microscopy, or immunohistochemical techniques. PCR assays can also be performed on ocular, nasal, pharyngeal, vaginal, or preputial swabs collected from older puppies and adults. Serologic testing for neutralizing antibodies confirms exposure but not necessarily active infection.

TREATMENT

Treatment is supportive but often ineffective at preventing neonatal losses. Injection of immune sera pooled from bitches that have had recent losses of litters may help reduce mortality during outbreaks. Keeping puppies warm and hydrated may lessen mortality in affected litters, primarily by limiting the spread of infection amongst uninvolved puppies.

PREVENTION

Currently no vaccine is available for CHV in the United States. In Europe, a subunit vaccine licensed for pregnant dogs since 2003 provides protective immunity to newborn puppies. Dams that have lost litters to CHV infection subsequently have healthy litters; thus artificial insemination or caesarean sections are not considered useful approaches to limit the spread of infection.

CANINE PAPILLOMA VIRUS

ETIOLOGY AND EPIDEMIOLOGY

Papillomaviruses are nonenveloped double-stranded DNA viruses in the family Papillomaviridae. Two different papillomaviruses have been described in dogs. Canine oral papillomavirus (COPV) is the more familiar of the two. A second, more recently described papillomavirus has been designated as *Canis familiaris* papilloma virus type 2 (CfPV-2).[83] Young dogs are clinically affected more frequently than older animals. COPV infection causes oral, ocular, and cutaneous papillomas. Oral papillomas typically occur in dogs younger than 2 years of age, ocular papillomas occur in dogs 6 months to 4 years of age, and cutaneous papillomas occur in older dogs.[84] CfPV-2 causes lesions on footpads and interdigital spaces of the feet of adult dogs and immunosuppressed dogs.[83]

TRANSMISSION

Papillomaviruses are species-specific, contagious, and transmitted by direct or indirect contact. Papillomas typically develop 1 to 2 months after infection. These viruses are relatively stable in the environment.

PATHOGENESIS

Papillomaviruses cause benign mucocutaneous tumors of epithelial origin, or "warts." The viruses primarily infect cells in the basal layer of the epithelium of the oral cavity, penis, vulva, conjunctiva, and skin, and it is likely that different papillomaviruses account for differences in lesion distribution.[85] Once infected, basal cells increase mitotic activity to produce the characteristic warts. The lesions usually regress spontaneously, but regression can vary from weeks to years.

CLINICAL SIGNS

The primary clinical sign of COPV infection is the appearance of papillomas, or warts, in the oral cavity or other epithelial sites. Papillomas typically regress within 4 to 8 weeks (and occasionally longer) when cell-mediated immune responses cause T-cell infiltration into the wart.[86] Humoral immune responses, although capable of preventing infection, do not seem to play a role in regression of lesions. Although lesions can become quite extensive, especially in the oral cavity, the functional impact of papillomas to the affected animal is usually minimal unless warts develop in locations that lead to dysphagia or respiratory obstruction.

In contrast to COPV, CfPV-2 lesions have been more frequently described on the footpads or in the interdigital spaces of the feet and have not been incriminated as a cause of oral warts.[83,87,88] The lesions associated with this virus were more endophytic (inward growing) than exophytic (outward growing) and persisted for much longer periods of time. In addition, CfPV-2 has been associated with the development of squamous cell carcinomas (SCC) in immunosuppressed dogs. It is quite likely that early initial reports of SCC in mucosal and cutaneous sites associated with a novel papillomavirus reflect associations with CfPV-2.[89,90] This virus may also play a role in the development of pigmented cutaneous papillomatosis.[91]

DIAGNOSIS

Diagnosis of COPV is usually based on the observation of characteristic lesions and is supported by histopathology of biopsied lesions. Immunohistochemistry, electron microscopy, and PCR can be used for virus detection.

TREATMENT

Because COPV-related disease usually regresses spontaneously in the majority of dogs, treatment is not usually necssary unless warts compromise eating or respiration. In such cases, warts can be removed by surgical excision, cryosurgery, or electrosurgery. Refractory cases may benefit from autogenous vaccination in which a wart is removed for making a crude vaccine that is injected into the same dog.[86] Etretinate, a retinoid, has been used to treat viral-associated pigmented plaques.[84] The optimal treatment for lesions of the digit pads and other sites associated with CfPV-2 has not been established, but surgical resection and histopathology are reasonable considerations, particularly to evaluate for the presence of malignant changes.

PREVENTION

No preventive vaccine is available for dogs. Dogs that have recovered from COPV are generally immune to reinfection. Some dogs, presumably those that are older or immunosuppressed, may be susceptible to repeated bouts of clinical disease.

RABIES VIRUS

ETIOLOGY AND EPIDEMIOLOGY

Rabies virus (RV) is an enveloped, single-stranded RNA virus in the family Rhabdoviridae. RV is capable of infecting all mammals, although there are differences in susceptibility to infection: Skunks, wild dogs, bats, raccoons, and cattle are most susceptible, whereas domestic dogs, cats, horses, sheep, and goats are considered to have moderate susceptibility. In the United States, the principle reservoirs of RV are skunks, bats, raccoons, and foxes; cats are the most commonly infected domestic animal.[92,93] Importation of unvaccinated dogs from rabies-endemic countries is also a potential source of canine and human infection in the United States.[94] In countries where few animals are vaccinated, the domestic dog remains an important reservoir for human infection.

TRANSMISSION

RV is spread primarily by inoculation of a naïve animal with infected saliva; thus bite wounds are the most common mode of RV transmission. The incubation period is variable and dependent on size of the viral inoculum, extent of nerve supply to injured tissue, distance from the site of inoculation to the spinal cord, and host factors such as age and immune responses. Virus can be shed in the saliva for almost 2 weeks before clinical signs develop. Rarely, in experimentally infected dogs, virus excretion may persist for several months after resolution of neurologic signs. Transmission by ingestion of infected tissue, inhalation of airborne virus, and transplacental transmission have been described but are considered rare.

RV is not stable in the environment and is inactivated by most common disinfectants.

PATHOGENESIS

Following inoculation, virus replicates in local tissue then enters nerve endings through neuromuscular junctions or breaches in the axonal sheath of injured nerve fibers. Virus spreads along axons in the peripheral nerves to the CNS. Once in the CNS, virus spreads among adjacent axons to involve more neurons, spreading rapidly to the brainstem and then forebrain. While replicating in the CNS, virus exits the CNS along peripheral nerve fibers to enter other tissues, including salivary glands. Thus, virus in saliva reflects CNS infection.

CLINICAL SIGNS

Rabies can be variable in its clinical presentation, and suspicion can be delayed because of atypical signs. Clinical suspicion may be further delayed because of variable incubation periods following virus inoculation. Clinical signs often start with a prodromal phase of 2 to 3 days' duration that is characterized by nervousness, anxiety, or other behavior changes. There may be paresthesia at the site of inoculation. As clinical signs progress, forebrain signs of irritability, restlessness, pica, photophobia, and hyperesthesia may be apparent. These clinical signs are often referred to as the furious form of rabies and can progress to incoordination, seizures, and death. Paralytic, or dumb, forms of rabies are characterized by lower motor neuron disease beginning in the area of initial injury and eventually involving the entire CNS. Dysphagia from paralysis of the muscles of deglutition causes accumulation of saliva in the oral cavity, which can be a source of infection to owners and veterinarians attending to such patients. Once clinical signs have developed, death typically follows within 10 days as the animal develops coma and respiratory paralysis.

DIAGNOSIS

Rabies should be suspected in any animal with an uncertain vaccination history exhibiting neurologic or behavioral abnormalities. Definitive diagnosis hinges on demonstration of virus in the brain, with direct fluorescent antibody (FA) testing considered the preferred method in many laboratories. Heads of suspect animals should be submitted to appropriate diagnostic laboratories without freezing to avoid damage to brain tissue associated with thawing. Compared with direct FA of nervous tissue, detection of intracellular inclusions (Negri bodies) or direct FA testing of sensory vibrissae in the maxillary area is considered insensitive. PCR testing of saliva and other tissues may be necessary when brain tissue is not available or is not suitable for FA testing.

TREATMENT

Treatment of animals suspected of having rabies is not recommended because of the human health hazard posed by such animals. Asymptomatic animals that are considered suspects should be quarantined according to local laws and regulations or euthanized for collection and submission of brain tissue to diagnostic laboratories.

PREVENTION

Vaccination is the most effective preventive measure for rabies. Rabies vaccine is a "core vaccine" that should be administered to all dogs.[23] Rabies vaccines contain inactivated virus and may be given initially to animals at 3 months of age followed by repeat immunization 1 year later. Regardless of what age the initial vaccine is given, vaccination should be repeated 1 year later. The interval for subsequent boosters is based on state, provincial, and local statutes that govern frequency of administration—these statutes vary from annually to every 3 years. Vaccines labeled for annual administration must be given annually, but those labeled for administration every 3 years can be used according to legal statutes. As with vaccines for most other infectious diseases, vaccination failures can occur, rendering the vaccinated animal susceptible to clinical rabies.[95] Such findings emphasize the need for vigilance on the part of veterinary clinicians, as well as the importance of client education, especially in areas where rabies is endemic.

PSEUDORABIES VIRUS

ETIOLOGY AND EPIDEMIOLOGY

Pseudorabies is an uncommon but fatal disease of dogs caused by an enveloped, double-stranded DNA virus in the alphaherpesvirus family. Affected dogs usually have a history of having been in contact with pigs, the primary virus reservoir that causes "mad itch."

TRANSMISSION

Most cases in dogs are believed to result from ingestion of infected raw pork. The incubation period is 3 to 6 days. Despite the presence of an envelope, pseudorabies virus is relatively stable in the environment.

PATHOGENESIS

After ingestion, the virus enters nerve endings in the mucosa and spreads to the brain along nerve axons. Inflammation and functional abnormalities in brain cells result in signs.

CLINICAL SIGNS

Signs of neurologic dysfunction are common features of the disease.[96] Neurologic abnormalities can be variable and have included ataxia, abnormal pupillary light responses, restlessness, trismus, and cervical rigidity. Ptyalism, tachypnea, and hyperpnea are common. Intense pruritus of the head and neck area can lead to self-induced excoriation. In some dogs, vomiting and diarrhea predominate. The clinical course of pseudorabies infection in dogs is usually swift, with most dogs dying within 48 hours after onset of neurologic signs.

DIAGNOSIS

The diagnosis is suspected based on history of exposure to pigs or pork products and clinical signs. Definitive diagnosis can be established by virus detection based on immunofluorescent antibody or PCR testing of brain and tonsillar tissue.

TREATMENT

Treatment is supportive but most dogs die.

PREVENTION

There is no approved pseudorabies vaccine for dogs, so prevention relies on limiting exposure of dogs to pigs or preventing ingestion of raw pork products.

OTHER VIRUSES OF INTEREST

West Nile Virus

WNV is a nonenveloped, single-stranded RNA virus in the family Flaviviridae. WNV is found worldwide and is maintained in natural settings via transmission from infected to naïve birds via mosquitoes.[97] Mosquitoes are able to transmit the virus to dogs.[98-100] Epidemiologic studies have demonstrated that in endemic areas higher seropositive rates can be found in dogs than in people, suggesting the potential for dogs as sentinel species.[101]

Experimental infection has shown that dogs are able to develop viremia, which is typically of low magnitude and of short duration.[98-100] Despite being able to support viremia, clinical disease in dogs either naturally exposed, or experimentally infected, is uncommon, even in dogs pretreated with large doses of glucocorticoids.[98-100] Signs of CNS disease, reflecting meningoencephalitis, and fever have been most consistently observed in naturally infected dogs; multisystemic disease has also been reported.[102-105] Reports in dogs suggest that the organs most likely to have virus are the brain, kidney, and heart.[102-105] The factors the determine outcome of infection, and the pathogenenic events underlying clinical signs in affected dogs, are unknown. Definitive diagnosis requires demonstration of viral antigen or nucleic acid in infected tissues; one report[102] of viral antigen present in renal cellular casts and other renal tubular debris raises the possibility that urine-based tests could be diagnostically useful. There are no specific treatments beyond supportive therapy. Experimental vaccination of dogs has prevented viremia after challenge,[99] but there is no approved vaccine to prevent infection in dogs and the value of vaccinating species in which disease manifestations are uncommon is uncertain.

Bornavirus

The bornavirus (BV) is an enveloped, single-stranded RNA virus in the family Bornaviridae. BV causes a fatal disease of the CNS in horses and other animals. Clinical disease in dogs appears to be relatively uncommon, and seropositivity in the absence of clinical signs appears possible.[106] The pathogenesis of the disease in dogs is unknown, but clinical signs in dogs have included tremors, salivation, mydriasis, and circling.[107,108] The infection is suspected based on the histopathologic observation of nonsuppurative encephalomyelitis predominantly in gray matter of the brain. Demonstration of viral RNA by in situ hybridization or PCR-based assays has provided definitive diagnosis.

REFERENCES

The reference list can be found on the companion Expert Consult Web site at *www.expertconsult.com*.

FUNGAL

CHAPTER 217

Histoplasmosis, Blastomycosis, Sporotrichosis, Candidiasis, Pythiosis, and Lagenidiosis

Joseph Taboada
Amy M. Grooters

Systemic mycoses are fungal infections that disseminate from a single portal of entry. The respiratory system serves as the portal of entry for most systemic fungi that affect dogs and cats, but entry may occur via the gastrointestinal (GI) system or skin.[1] Immune suppression, while playing a major role in the development of systemic mycoses in humans, does not appear to play as significant a role in animals. Systemic fungal infections cause disease, the clinical signs of which are dependent on which body systems are involved (Box 217-1).

Weight loss, lymphadenopathy, and fever are typical of most systemic mycoses. Because the respiratory system is the usual portal of entry, clinical signs such as cough, dyspnea, and exercise intolerance are common. If the GI system is the portal of entry, as may occur with histoplasmosis, malabsorption may lead to severe diarrhea and weight loss.

In most cases, diagnosis of a systemic mycosis is dependent on demonstrating the presence of the organism in tissue. For yeasts such as *Cryptococcus* or *Candida*, or for dimorphic fungi that have a yeast phase in tissue, such as *Blastomyces dermatitidis* or *Histoplasma capsulatum*, the diagnosis can usually be made cytologically. For other fungi that grow as hyphal organisms in infected tissue, the diagnosis is usually dependent on histology, culture, or molecular techniques. Serology has been used extensively in practice to support the diagnosis of fungal infections, but with the exception of tests for cryptococcal antigen, most commercially available assays determine the presence of antibody and may indicate only previous exposure. Newer tests for fungal antigen and PCR techniques are making it easier to diagnose systemic mycoses and are improving diagnostic accuracy.

Many treatment regimens have been reported for the management of systemic mycoses, but few veterinary studies have been performed that have critically evaluated these agents in a prospective manner, and studies comparing treatment regimens are practically nonexistent. A lack of controlled observations has led to recommendations that are based primarily on anecdotal information, extrapolation from what is done in people, and small case series. Newer antifungal drugs tend to be expensive, which limits their use in generating useful treatment data. The "best" treatment regimen for any given systemic fungal infection is therefore largely a matter of opinion.

The principal antifungal agents are antibiotics produced by microorganisms (e.g., amphotericin B, griseofulvin) and synthetic agents (e.g., potassium iodide, flucytosine, azole derivatives, allylamine derivatives, chitin synthase inhibitors). The options for treatment of fungal infections increased substantially with the development of azole derivatives such as fluconazole and itraconazole in the 1990s and have expanded again recently with the approval of posaconazole and voriconazole. The low cost of fluconazole has made it the mainstay of routine treatment, but most clinical trials have been performed using itraconazole.[2-4] There are case reports and ret-

Box • 217-1

Differential Diagnoses for Systemic Manifestations of Systemic Mycoses

Multisystemic granulomatous, neoplastic, and immune-mediated diseases must be differentiated from disseminated systemic mycoses.

Differential Diagnosis for Nodular Skin Disease
Bacterial Skin Disease
Actinomycosis
Mycobacteriosis
Botryomycosis
Brucellosis
Rhodococcus equi infection
Bartonella vinsonii subsp. *berkhoffi* infection
Mycotic and Miscellaneous Infectious Skin Disease
Cryptococcosis
Blastomycosis
Coccidioidomycosis
Sporotrichosis
Basidiobolomycosis
Conidiobolomycosis
Phaeohyphomycosis
Hyalohyphomycosis
Eumycotic mycetoma
Dermatophytic mycetoma
Prototheocosis
Pythiosis
Lagenidiosis
Nodular leishmaniasis
Noninfectious Pyogranulomatous Skin Disease
Foreign body reaction
Idiopathic nodular panniculitis
Sebaceous adenitis (nodular form)
Canine cutaneous sterile pyogranuloma/granuloma syndrome
Neoplasia
Squamous cell carcinoma

Cutaneous lymphoma
Mycosis fungoides (cutaneous T cell lymphoma)
Cutaneous histiocytosis
Miscellaneous Diseases
Systemic lupus erythematosus (SLE)
Systemic vasculitis
Cutaneous embolic disease

Differential Diagnosis for Chorioretinitis, Exudative Retinal Detachment, and Panophthalmitis
Fungal
Blastomycosis
Cryptococcosis
Coccidioidomycosis
Geotrichosis
Histoplasmosis
Aspergillosis
Neoplasia
Lymphosarcoma
Metastatic neoplasia
Miscellaneous Infectious Causes
Prototheocosis
Brucellosis
Toxoplasmosis
Neosporum caninum infection
Leishmaniasis

Lymphadenopathy must be differentiated from numerous causes, including lymphosarcoma, other fungal infections, rickettsial diseases, brucellosis, mycobacteriosis, prototheocosis, and leishmaniasis.

Solitary bone lesions must be differentiated from primary or metastatic bony neoplasia and other fungal or bacterial osteomyelitis.

---

rospective reviews documenting the use of the older azole drugs.[5] The high cost of most antifungal agents and the long treatment protocols required affect the number of treated animals, both limiting and probably epidemiologically biasing the data that have been generated. Adding to the difficulty of assessing the efficacy of antifungal agents: Pharmacologic principles of antifungal therapy are only partially understood; in vitro testing of fungi for resistance to antifungal agents provides information of variable clinical usefulness; susceptibility testing yields variable results; and tissue distribution of antifungal agents correlates variably with the clinical outcome.

ANTIFUNGAL AGENTS

Amphotericin B

Amphotericin B is a polyene macrolide antibiotic produced by the aerobic actinomycete *Streptomyces nodosus*. It was discovered in the 1950s and was one of the first antifungal agents found to be widely useful in treating systemic fungal infections. It is the gold standard against which efficacy of new antifungal agents is compared. Despite significant toxicity and poor oral bioavailability, it remains the drug of choice for the treatment of many invasive mycoses. The traditional formulation of amphotericin B is a desoxycholate preparation (Fungizone) that, after IV administration, is highly protein bound (91% to 95%), primarily to lipoproteins, erythrocytes, and cholesterol in the plasma. It is then redistributed from the blood to the tissues. Penetration into the cerebrospinal fluid (CSF) is poor. Tissue accumulation accounts for the majority of drug disposition. Only 5% to 10% of amphotericin B is excreted in the urine and bile. Although great care should be used when treating animals in renal or hepatic failure, no modification of the dose is necessary unless the renal or hepatic damage is attributable to the drug.

Amphotericin B acts by binding to sterols in cell membranes, especially ergosterol in fungal cell membranes. Binding alters membrane permeability, causing leakage of sodium, potassium, and hydrogen ions and eventually leading to cell death. Amphotericin B probably also has important immunostimulatory effects by oxidation-dependent stimulation of host macrophages.[6] Stimulation of macrophages may play an important role in the treatment of some systemic fungal infections. Toxic effects are attributable to affinity for sterols such as cholesterol in mammalian cell membranes. Amphotericin B has been effective in the treatment of blastomycosis, histoplasmosis, coccidioidomycosis, cryptococcosis, systemic candidiasis, zygomycosis, and occasionally pythiosis. It is administered as a series of IV infusions (0.22 to 0.5 mg/lb [0.5 to 1 mg/kg] every 48 hours to a cumulative dose of 2 to 4 mg/lb [4 to 8 mg/kg] or until azotemia occurs). Bolus dosing over 5 to 10 minutes is common, but clinicians can reduce renal toxicity by infusing the drug in 5% dextrose over 1 to 5 hours.

Nephrotoxicity is the most significant adverse effect and is dose dependent.[7] Generally, renal azotemia is reversible, and renal function returns to normal after cessation of therapy. However, return to pretreatment values may take several months. Irreversible renal dysfunction is more likely in animals with preexisting azotemia or in those receiving other nephrotoxic agents such as aminoglycosides. Blood urea nitrogen (BUN) should be monitored before each administration of amphotericin B. If the BUN is greater than 50 mg/dL, administration should be discontinued until the azotemia has resolved. Nephrotoxicity is thought to be caused by disruption of renal tubular epithelial cell permeability resulting in increased delivery of chloride ions to the distal tubule, with subsequent decreased glomerular filtration rate (GFR) being the result of tubuloglomerular feedback. This feedback is amplified by sodium depletion and suppressed by sodium loading. Administration of 0.9% sodium chloride (5 to 10 mL/lb) before amphotericin B administration decreases the incidence of nephrotoxicity in people. Other possible mechanisms of nephrotoxicity include decreased renal blood flow and direct renal cellular toxicity. Tumor necrosis factor (TNF) may also play a role in mediating amphotericin B–induced azotemia. Pentoxifylline, a hemorrheologic drug, seems to exert protective effects in people and rats. Mannitol and dopamine have also been shown to decrease nephrotoxicity in experimental situations. Treatment protocols using subcutaneously administered amphotericin B appear to be less nephrotoxic and have resulted in tolerance of higher cumulative dosing. Other possible toxic effects include thrombophlebitis, pyrexia (usually ameliorated by pretreatment with nonsteroidal antiinflammatory drugs or antiinflammatory doses of glucocorticoids), hypokalemia, distal renal tubular acidosis, hypomagnesemia, cardiac arrhythmias, and nonregenerative anemia. Calcinosis cutis has been reported in dogs with blastomycosis 2 to 4 weeks after beginning treatment with amphotericin B.[8]

Use of novel delivery systems has been effective in reducing nephrotoxicity, improving site-specific delivery of amphotericin B, and allowing higher doses to be administered. Currently three formulations of amphotericin B are available for clinical use in human patients: (1) amphotericin B lipid complex (ABLC) (Abelcet, Enzon), (2) amphotericin B colloidal dispersion (Amphotec, Intermune, Inc.), and (3) liposome-encapsulated amphotericin B (AmBisome, Gilead Sciences).[9] Of these three formulations, ABLC has been the most extensively evaluated in dogs and cats and is the least expensive. In dog studies, lipid-complexed amphotericin B was determined to be eightfold to tenfold less nephrotoxic than conventional amphotericin B. The decreased toxicity is due to decreased renal cell uptake, reduced tubular toxicity, reduced free amphotericin in solution in plasma, and a selective transfer of amphotericin directly to fungal cell membranes. Reduced toxicity allows higher cumulative doses to be used, which may increase drug efficacy. Increase in efficacy may be related to uptake of lipid complexes by reticuloendothelial (RE) system phagocytic cells, which allows sites of inflammation and organs with high RE system activity such as liver, spleen, and lung to receive higher doses of amphotericin B despite minimal renal uptake.

Clinical trials in people have documented improvement in treatment outcomes for many types of fungal infections. ABLC has been used successfully to treat blastomycosis in dogs without significant nephrotoxicity.[10] ABLC can be used in dogs at a dose of 1 to 1.5 mg/lb (2 to 3 mg/kg) IV three times a week to a cumulative dose of 24 to 27 mg/kg. Azotemia is rare.

ORAL AZOLE ANTIFUNGAL DRUGS

The azoles are classified as imidazoles (ketoconazole [Nizoral, Janssen]) or triazoles (fluconazole [Diflucan, Pfizer], itraconazole [Sporanox, Janssen], posaconazole [Noxafil, Schering-Plough], and voriconazole [Vfend, Pfizer]), according to whether they contain two or three nitrogen atoms, respectively, in the five-member azole ring. Ketoconazole, itraconazole, and posaconazole have similar pharmacologic profiles, while fluconazole and voriconazole are unique because of their comparatively small molecular size and low lipophilicity. The azole antifungal agents act by inhibiting ergosterol synthesis through interaction with 14-α-demethylase, a cytochrome P-450 enzyme that is necessary for the conversion of lanosterol to ergosterol. Similar interaction in mammalian cells with enzymes dependent on cytochrome P-450 also mediates some of the major toxic effects. The imidazoles are much more potent inhibitors of mammalian cell cytochrome P-450 than are the triazoles. Other antifungal effects include inhibition of endogenous respiration, toxic interaction with membrane phospholipids, and inhibition of morphogenetic transformation of yeasts to the mycelial forms. Some of the azole antifungal drugs, especially itraconazole and ketoconazole, are potent immune-suppressive agents, suppressing T lymphocyte proliferation in vitro. Ketoconazole has antiinflammatory properties that are probably mediated through inhibition of 5-lipoxygenase activity.

Ketoconazole and itraconazole are weak bases that require an acid environment for maximal oral absorption. Antacid administration inhibits oral bioavailability, and the bioavailability of itraconazole is twofold to threefold higher when taken with food. Posaconzole also has significantly higher bioavailability when taken with food, but its absorption is not affected by the gastric pH. Pharmacokinetic studies in both humans and cats have demonstrated increased absorption of itraconazole after administration of the oral solution in comparison to capsules. Both an oral solution (10 mg/mL) and a parenteral formulation (200 mg ampules diluted in 50 mL 0.9% sodium chloride for intravenous administration) are available.

Fluconazole is not affected by gastric pH, and food does not affect its oral bioavailability. Peak plasma concentrations of the triazoles do not occur until 6 to 14 days after treatment is begun. This may account for the clinical lag time often seen between the time the drug is started and the time a patient begins to improve. A loading dose can be given for the first 3 days of treatment to reduce the time until steady-state concentrations are attained. Ketoconazole, itraconazole, and posaconazole are extensively bound to plasma proteins (>99%), but because of their lipophilicity, they are distribute well throughout most tissues; however, concentrations in urine and CSF are typically low. Posaconazole appears to cross the blood-brain barrier while neither ketoconazole nor itraconazole cross the blood-brain, blood-prostate, or blood-ocular barriers well. Despite this, central nervous system (CNS), prostatic, and ocular fungal infections respond well to treatment with itraconazole. Itraconazole is concentrated in the skin, with delivery being via sebum. Sebum concentrations are 5 to 10 times higher than plasma concentrations, and detectable amounts persist for up to 14 days after the drug is discontinued. Detectable concentrations can be found in the hair and stratum corneum for up to 4 weeks. This property makes itraconazole ideal for treating dermatophyte infections and other fungal infections with cutaneous manifestations. Fluconazole is minimally protein bound and highly water soluble and distributes similarly to free water. High concentrations can be found in urine, CSF, and ocular fluids, and the drug crosses the blood-brain, blood-prostate, and blood-ocular barriers well. Ketoconazole, itraconazole, posaconazole, and voriconazole are extensively metabolized in the liver and excreted in the bile and, to a lesser extent, in the urine. In contrast, fluconazole is minimally metabolized, and approximately 80% is excreted unchanged in the urine; consequently, the dose of fluconazole should be reduced in animals with decreased GFR.

The azole antifungal agents are widely used in veterinary medicine for treating systemic fungal infections.[2-4,11] While itraconazole has been the most extensively studied of the azole antifungals, fluconazole has become more extensively used recently because of the availability of generic formulations that are much less expensive than the other agents available. Ketoconazole has been effective as a sole therapeutic agent in the management of blastomycosis, histoplasmosis, cryptococcosis, and coccidioidomycosis. However, with the possible exception of coccidioidomycosis, ketoconazole is probably not as effective as amphotericin B or the other azoles. Itraconazole and fluconazole are safer and more effective than ketoconazole and can be used as sole agents in the management of most systemic mycoses. Itraconazole appears to be more effective than fluconazole in most systemic fungal infections caused by molds, but fluconazole may be superior in the management of cryptococcosis and CNS, prostatic, and urinary tract infections. Itraconazole is the treatment of choice for blastomycosis in dogs and probably cats. Itraconazole has proven very effective as a sole treatment agent for histoplasmosis in cats.[3] The authors have found itraconazole to be effective in treating a limited number of dogs with GI pythiosis, despite the fact that Pythium insidiosum does not contain significant concentrations of membrane ergosterol. Synergism appears to exist between itraconazole and terbinafine in treating Pythium insidiosum based on in vitro trials.[12] Voriconazole has potent in vitro and in vivo activity against common endemic and opportunistic fungal pathogens, including molds other than the zygomycetes. It has demonstrated efficacy for invasive aspergillosis and oropharyngeal candidiasis in phase III clinical trials and can be administered either orally or intravenously. Its indications in human patients are for the treatment of invasive aspergillosis and other infections caused by molds (such as Fusarium) in immunocompromised individuals. In treating most systemic fungal infections, a lag occurs between the initiation of treatment and clinical improvement. In severely affected animals, amphotericin B should probably be used initially or in conjunction with the triazole during this lag period. Amphotericin B may also be indicated in managing patients with CNS involvement.

The dose of ketoconazole is 4.5 to 13.6 mg/lb (10 to 30 mg/kg) divided twice a day. Side effects are often limiting, especially at higher doses. Fluconazole (1 to 4.5 mg/lb; 2.5 to 10 mg/kg) and itraconazole (2.2 to 4.5 mg/lb; 5 to 10 mg/kg) are usually better tolerated. Pharmacokinetic studies of itraconazole have been performed in cats.[13] Based on these studies, the oral itraconazole solution is preferred to the capsules, with a 24-hour dosing interval being sufficient at 4.5 mg/lb (10 mg/kg). Steady-state concentrations take up to 3 weeks to achieve. Most adverse effects of itraconazole are related to high serum concentrations, and animals that exhibit adverse effects usually do well on half the original dose. The dose of voriconazole (1.4 to 2.7 mg/lb; 3 to 6 mg/kg) is based on short-term pharmacokinetic studies and extrapolation from what is used in people. In dogs, it has been used with limited success at a dose of 5 mg/kg q12h for the treatment of refractory aspergillosis.[14] Posaconazole (Noxafil, Schering-Plough) is a potent broad-spectrum itraconazole analog with documented efficacy for the treatment of candidiasis, refractory aspergillosis, fusariosis, phaeohyphomycosis, and zygomycosis in human patients. Pharmacokinetic studies in dogs have shown good oral bioavailability that is increased when the drug is administered with food. Although pharmacokinetic data are not available for cats, posaconazole was used successfully at a dose of 5 mg/kg orally q24h (administered as a suspension with food) to treat a single cat with orbital aspergillosis that had failed itraconazole.[15]

Adverse effects of the azole antifungal agents are similar across the class. Ketoconazole is the least tolerated, and fluconazole appears to be the best. Dose-related GI side effects (anorexia and vomiting) are most common, especially in cats. When these occur, dividing the dose into two treatments or reducing the dose may be of benefit. Azole-induced anorexia in cats is often ameliorated by the use of appetite stimulants such as mirtazapine, oxazepam or cyproheptadine. Liver enzymes should be periodically monitored in animals being treated with azole antifungals. Asymptomatic increases in transaminase concentrations are seen in about half of animals treated with itraconazole, but this does not necessitate a change in therapy unless the animal also has anorexia, vomiting, depression, or abdominal pain. Enzyme concentrations often return to normal over time without intervention. Symptomatic hepatotoxicity is occasionally seen with ketoconazole (or itraconazole) use but is unusual after fluconazole administration. Cutaneous reactions are seen in approximately 7% of dogs receiving itraconazole at a dose of 4.5 mg/lb (10 mg/kg).[2] A local ulcerative dermatitis due to a cutaneous vasculitis (Figure 217-1) usually resolves shortly after the drug is discontinued.

More severe reactions such as erythema multiforme or toxic epidermal necrolysis are rare. Thrombocytopenia has been associated with fluconazole use in people but has not been documented in animals. Visual disturbances (photopsia) are a common side effect unique to voriconazole. Adrenal insufficiency is possible with ketoconazole use. Azole interference with the activity of hepatic microsomal enzymes can lead to increased concentrations of coadministered drugs such as cyclosporine, digoxin, phenytoin, sulfonylureas, and warfarin.

FLUCYTOSINE

Flucytosine is a synthetic antifungal drug with activity attributed to disruption of protein synthesis by inhibition of DNA and RNA synthesis. The drug is synergistic with amphotericin B and is used almost exclusively as an adjunct to amphotericin B in the treatment of cryptococcosis in cats. Flucytosine has good oral bioavailability. It is widely distributed and crosses the blood-brain barrier. The most common side effects are diarrhea, anorexia, and vomiting. Dose-dependent bone marrow suppression manifesting as neutropenia, thrombocytopenia, or pancytopenia is a less common but more significant toxicity. Cutaneous or mucocutaneous drug eruptions consisting of depigmentation followed by ulceration, exudation, and crust formation (occurring most frequently on the scrotum and nasal planum) have been described in a series of dogs. The dose of flucytosine used in cats is 125 to 250 mg orally divided two to four times a day.

ALLYLAMINES

Terbinafine is a synthetic allylamine antifungal drug that interferes with squalene epoxidase and is a potent inhibitor of ergosterol biosynthesis. Squalene accumulation in the

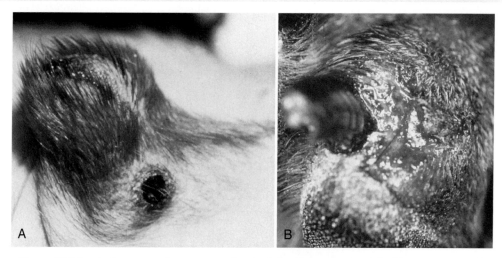

Figure 217-1 A, Lesion on the prepuce of a Dachshund being treated for blastomycosis with itraconazole. The lesion is caused by an itraconazole-induced cutaneous vasculitis. **B,** Paronychial lesion caused by an itraconazole-induced cutaneous vasculitis in a Doberman Pinscher.

fungal cell may account for the drug's fungicidal activity. A keratinophilic compound that is well distributed in skin, it has been used primarily for the treatment of dermatophytosis and onychomycosis in both people and animals. It may also have efficacy for the treatment of sporotrichosis. The efficacy of terbinafine for invasive or systemic fungal infections has not been well evaluated. However, clinical observations support use of this drug in combination with itraconazole for the medical treatment of pythiosis when complete surgical resection of infected tissues is not possible. Potential side effects of terbinafine include GI toxicity, cutaneous reactions, and hepatitis. The drug dose ranges from 2.5 to 9 mg/lb (5 to 20 mg/kg) orally once daily.

GLUCAN SYNTHASE INHIBITORS

Echinocandins are drugs that inhibit the synthesis of β-glucan, a substance essential for the structural and functional integrity of the fungal cell wall. Because their targets are unique to fungi, the echinocandins are generally well tolerated by mammals, and they are associated with relatively few adverse effects in people. The primary limitation of this class of antifungals is their ineffectiveness against *Cryptococcus neoformans*, which contains very little glucan synthase.

Caspofungin (Cancidas, Merck), the first β-glucan synthase inhibitor to gain FDA approval, is a potent broad-spectrum parenteral formulation that is highly effective for the treatment of aspergillosis and candidiasis in people. Unfortunately, the use of caspofungin in animals has been limited by its cost. Micafungin (Mycamine, Astellas Pharma) and Anidulafungin (Eraxis, Pfizer) are newer echinocandins that have a spectrum of activity similar to that of caspofungin.

The use of β-glucan synthase inhibitors has been described in a single dog with systemic aspergillosis that had failed treatment with itraconazole and amphotericin B lipid complex.[14] In this patient, rapid clinical improvement was noted after administration of caspofungin at 1 mg/kg IV (given in 250 ml 0.9% saline over 1 hour) once daily for 6 weeks, then 3 times weekly for 2 months, and then on 3 consecutive days every 3 weeks. The patient's clinical signs were controlled on caspofungin for approximately 1 year, at which time signs recurred and failed to respond to 8 doses of anidulafungin (3 mg/kg in 250 ml 0.9% saline administered IV q24h) and 3 doses of

micafungin (3 mg/kg in 250 mL 0.9% saline administered IV q24h).

SPECIFIC SYSTEMIC MYCOSES

BLASTOMYCOSIS

Blastomycosis is a systemic fungal infection that usually originates in the lungs and then disseminates to the lymphatics, skin, eyes, bones, and other organs. The dog is most commonly affected. Young, male, large breed dogs (especially sporting breeds and hounds) living near water are at an increased risk.[16] In endemic areas, blastomycosis usually occurs as a sporadic event, but outbreaks are occasionally observed in both dogs and people.[17-19] Epidemiologically, outbreaks can often be traced back to a common point source in the environment from which infective spores had been aerosolized for a short time. Confirmation of the source is rarely achieved by organism isolation because of the transient nature of the environmental contamination and the difficulties inherent in laboratory isolation.

The dimorphic fungus *B. dermatitidis* is the causative agent of blastomycosis. In infected tissue or when cultured at 37° C, the organism is a thick-walled yeast that reproduces by budding. Most often, organisms in tissue have a single bud, attached to the mother cell by a broad base. When cultured at 25° C, mold colonies grow slowly and contain branching, septate 1- to 2-μm mycelia that form round to piriform 2- to 10-μm conidia. In nature, *B. dermatitidis* is probably a soil saprophyte, but the reservoir remains unresolved because the organism can rarely be cultured from the environment. When cultured, it is usually from wet, acidic, or sandy soil containing decaying wood, animal feces, or other organic enrichment.[20] Moisture appears to be important to growth and transmission.

Disease occurrence is reported primarily in a geographically restricted distribution that follows the Mississippi, Ohio, Missouri, Tennessee, and St. Lawrence Rivers, the southern Great Lakes, and the southern Mid-Atlantic states (Figure 217-2).

Within these geographic regions, infections are generally limited to smaller geographic pockets, with most affected animals living within a quarter of a mile of water.[19,21,22] It is not unusual for one veterinary practice within an endemic

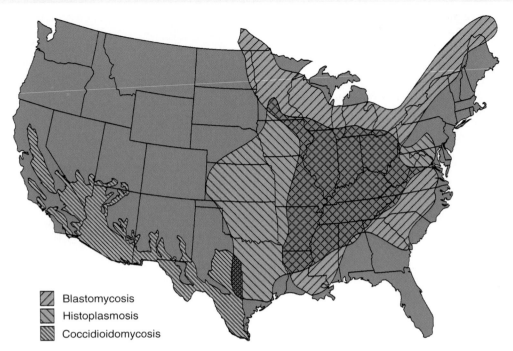

Blastomycosis
Histoplasmosis
Coccidioidomycosis

Figure 217-2 Areas in the United States endemic for blastomycosis, coccidioidomycosis, and histoplasmosis.

area to diagnose blastomycosis commonly, whereas another practice located within the same county rarely encounters the infection.

PATHOPHYSIOLOGY

Blastomycosis is not a contagious disease. It follows contact with the organism in the environment. Infection usually occurs via a respiratory route after the host inhales infective conidiophores. Rarely, disease may be seen after direct inoculation.[23] The incubation period varies from 5 to 12 weeks. Rain, dew, fog, or mist may play a critical role in liberating conidiophores. In addition, activities that disrupt the soil such as digging or construction may play a role in spore aerosolization. After inhalation, conidia are phagocytized by alveolar macrophages and transform from the mycelial phase to the yeast phase. The yeast stimulates local cell-mediated immunity, which results in a marked suppurative to pyogranulomatous inflammatory response. In some cases the cell-mediated immune response controls infection locally; in others, phagocytized yeasts are transported into the pulmonary interstitium, where they gain access to both lymphatic and vascular systems. Hematogenous and lymphatic dissemination then results in multisystemic pyogranulomatous disease. Although dissemination can be to any organ system, the lymph nodes, eyes, skin, bones, subcutaneous tissues, and prostate are organs commonly affected in dogs[2,22,24]; skin, subcutaneous tissues, eyes, CNS, and lymph nodes are most commonly affected in cats.[25,26]

The immune response determines the severity of clinical disease, but blastomycosis is not considered an opportunistic infection. Antibody production occurs in most, but not all, cases, with the highest titers usually found in dogs with severe disseminated disease. Antibodies are not considered protective but can be used as a clinical marker of recent exposure or current disease. Recovery from infection is dependent on cell-mediated immunity. An adequate immune response may result in mild respiratory disease that resolves spontaneously.

If dissemination has occurred, disease may be obvious in other organ systems, even without apparent pulmonary involvement. A poor immune response may result in severe pulmonary and disseminated disease.

CLINICAL SIGNS

Bluetick Coonhounds, Treeing-Walker Coonhounds, Pointers, and Weimaraners have the highest risk of infection.[16] Males are affected more commonly, and although any age dog can be affected, those in the 2- to 4-year age group have the highest incidence of disease. Exposure to possible environmental sources of infection, close proximity to water, and the likelihood of being housed in outdoor kennels probably explains the breed association. Clinical findings in animals with blastomycosis vary greatly because of the multisystemic nature of the disease. One or more organ systems may be involved.

Nonspecific signs such as anorexia, depression, weight loss, cachexia, and fever are common. Approximately 40% of dogs are febrile, and dogs with chronic pulmonary disease are most likely to be cachectic. Because the lungs serve as the portal of entry for the *Blastomyces* organism, it is not surprising that pulmonary signs are seen in 65% to 85% of affected dogs. Signs of pulmonary involvement range from mild respiratory distress when exercised to severe dyspnea at rest. Hypoxemia resulting in cyanosis is seen in the most severely affected and has a negative prognostic significance.[2] A dry, hacking cough is common. Mildly affected dogs may initially be diagnosed as having kennel cough. Enlarged perihilar lymph nodes compressing primary bronchi, as well as infiltrative bronchointerstitial and alveolar disease, contribute to the cough. Rapid, shallow respiratory efforts may be noted and can be caused by pleural effusion or pleuritic pain. Chylothorax, solid granulomatous masses, and pulmonary thromboembolism are uncommonly reported complications of blastomycosis.

Diffuse lymphadenopathy is seen in about 40% to 60% of dogs with blastomycosis. The lymph node enlargement can be marked and may be mistaken for lymphosarcoma if cytology or histology is not performed.

Cutaneous signs are reported in about 30% to 50% of affected dogs and are also commonly noted in affected cats. Reported prevalences of skin disease in cases of blastomycosis may underestimate the actual prevalence, because lesions are sometimes small and easily overlooked unless a thorough dermatologic examination is performed. Single or multiple papules, nodules, or plaques that can ulcerate and drain a serosanguineous to purulent exudate characterize typical skin lesions. The nodular lesions are often quite small in dogs, but large abscesses occasionally occur, especially in cats. Paronychia is common in dogs, so the feet and nail beds should be closely examined.

Ocular involvement is noted in 20% to 50% of cases. Posterior segment disease, characterized by chorioretinitis, retinal separation, subretinal granulomas, and vitreitis, usually occurs initially. Approximately 50% of affected dogs have bilateral ocular involvement. Optic neuritis is occasionally noted and may signify more diffuse CNS involvement and a poorer prognosis. Anterior segment disease is usually, but not always, secondary to the posterior segment involvement. It may be characterized by conjunctivitis, keratitis, iridocyclitis, and eventually anterior uveitis and endophthalmitis. Secondary glaucoma is common in dogs with anterior segment disease. Dogs that are blind at the time of initial diagnosis rarely regain vision, even with aggressive treatment and good systemic response. Dogs that have vision and only posterior segment disease at the time of diagnosis have a better prognosis for vision.

Lameness caused by fungal osteomyelitis or painful paronychia is noted in about 25% of dogs with blastomycosis, and fungal osteomyelitis is noted in about 10% to 15% of dogs with blastomycosis. The pain and swelling are usually noted over epiphyseal regions below the elbow or stifle. Single lesions are more common than multiple. Fungal monoarthritis or polyarthritis is a rare cause of lameness.

The reproductive system is affected in approximately 5% to 10% of affected dogs. Orchitis was noted in 16% of 61 intact male dogs with blastomycosis seen at Louisiana State University. Fungal prostatitis or mastitis is reported in less than 5% of affected dogs.

The nervous system is affected in less than 5% of affected dogs but is common in cats (Figure 217-3). Advanced CNS imaging such as computed tomography (CT) or magnetic resonance imaging (MRI) should be considered in any cat diagnosed with blastomycosis, even if obvious neurologic signs are not apparent. The clinical signs associated with nervous system involvement are dependent on which parts of the CNS are involved, but often neurologic localization indicates diffuse or multifocal disease. Other potential sites of infection include cranial mediastinum, liver, spleen, kidney, and nasal cavity.[27] Feline blastomycosis is less common than canine blastomycosis. The veterinary literature contains only scattered case reports and small case series.[25,26] Most of the clinical signs observed in dogs are also noted in cats. The main differences are that large abscesses are more common in cats than in dogs, and neurologic involvement is often noted.

DIAGNOSIS

Blastomycosis is usually fairly easy to diagnose because of the large numbers of characteristic yeasts found within lesions, especially within infected skin, eyes, and lymph nodes.[22,28] Complete blood count (CBC) results are often normal. A mild nonregenerative anemia and mature neutrophilia or neutrophilia with mild left shift may be seen. Clinical chemistry results are also often unremarkable. Hypoalbuminemia is the most consistent abnormality. Mild hypercalcemia is noted in up to 10% of cases.[23] Severe hypercalcemia requiring treatment is occasionally seen.

Radiographic assessment can be helpful in the diagnostic evaluation of a dog or cat suspected of having blastomycosis (Figures 217-4, 217-5, and 217-6).[29] Thoracic radiographs reveal an interstitial pattern in about 70% of canine cases. Although a nodular interstitial pattern is classically observed (41% of cases), diffuse interstitial (24%) and bronchointerstitial (5%) patterns may also be prominent findings. An alveolar or mixed interstitial-alveolar pattern is observed in about 20% of dogs, and tracheobronchial lymphadenopathy is noted in about 30%. Radiographic patterns mimicking other diseases such as mediastinal mass (8%) or solitary pulmonary mass (8%) are not as common. Pleural effusion (7%) is rarely observed and when present may obscure pulmonary parenchymal changes. Pneumothorax induced by pulmonary blastomycosis is rare. Bone lesions may be noted on radiographs of long bones, especially those of the distal limbs. Lesions are osteolytic and typically occur at the ends of the long bones (Figure 217-7). The forelimbs are affected more commonly than the rear limbs, with most extremity lesions being below the elbow or the stifle. Periosteal proliferation and soft tissue swelling are noted in about 50% of lesions.

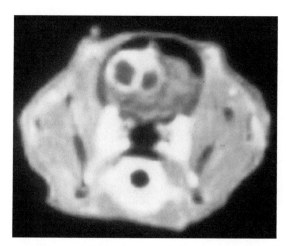

Figure 217-3 Cross-sectional magnetic resonance image (MRI) revealing a contrast-enhancing mixed-intensity lesion in the rostral portion of the right cerebral cortex in a cat with blastomycosis.

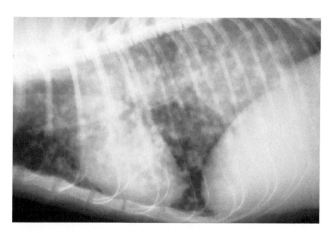

Figure 217-4 Lateral thoracic radiograph revealing a diffuse nodular interstitial pattern in a cat with blastomycosis.

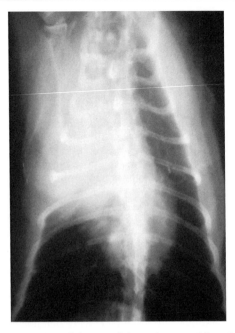

Figure 217-5 Consolidation of the right cranial lung lobe in a cat with blastomycosis. Consolidating and abscessing lesions are often seen in cats with systemic fungal infections.

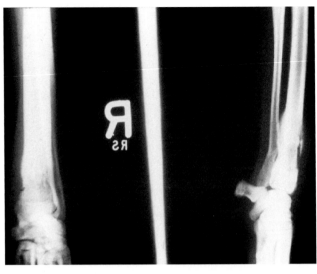

Figure 217-7 Lateral and anteroposterior view of the distal radius, ulna, and carpus from a Brittany Spaniel with *Blastomyces* osteomyelitis. The reader should note the bony lysis and periosteal proliferation involving the distal aspect of the proximal radius.

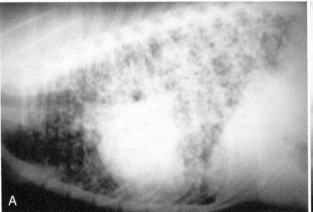

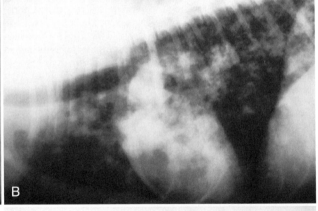

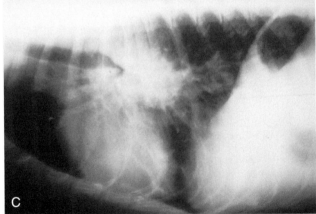

Figure 217-6 A, Lateral thoracic radiograph from a dog with blastomycosis revealing the classic "snowstorm" appearance of the nodular interstitial pattern commonly seen in systemic mycotic infections. **B,** Lateral thoracic radiograph from a dog with blastomycosis showing multiple large, ill-defined nodules and a bronchointerstitial pattern. **C,** Lateral thoracic radiograph from a dog with blastomycosis showing perihilar lymphadenopathy and a patchy interstitial pattern. Perihilar lymphadenopathy is common in systemic fungal infections, especially histoplasmosis and coccidioidomycosis.

Definitive diagnosis is made by organism identification. This can be done by cytology, histology, or fungal culture. Cytology from affected tissue typically reveals pyogranulomatous or suppurative inflammation, often with thick-walled yeasts (8 to 12 μm in diameter, with 0.5- to 0.75-μm thick walls) that bud to form daughter cells from a broad base (Figure 217-8).[28,30]

The yeast cells lack a capsule, helping to differentiate them from *Cryptococcus*. Skin lesions yield organisms about 80% of the time. This is the easiest and most useful site

be restricted to the tropics and subtropics and is associated with bark and leaf litter of certain eucalyptus trees. Recent outbreaks of *C. gattii* have been noted in cats and dogs as well as humans residing in or traveling to the coastal Douglas fir biogeoclimatic zone of Vancouver Island in British Columbia.[2,2a,3]

Cryptococcus is considered infectious as a desiccated yeast cell or basidiospore in the environment that enters the body primarily through the respiratory system, where it infects nasal, paranasal, or lung tissue before disseminating more widely with a predilection for the CNS. In infected tissue, and often when cultured, the organism is a variable-sized yeast (3.5 to 7 μm) with a large heteropolysaccharide capsule (1 to 30 μm). Both species have been shown to cause disease in cats, dogs, and humans.

The pigeon is thought to be the most important vector of *C. neoformans*. The *Cryptococcus* organism can be found in high numbers in pigeon roosts, barn lofts, haymows, and along cupolas and cornices where pigeons often sit. In the desiccated state, the *Cryptococcus* organism may be no larger than 1 μm and may survive up to 2 years.

PATHOPHYSIOLOGY

Cryptococcosis is not a contagious disease. Infection occurs most commonly via inhalation of yeast from the environment. Debris and droppings in and around avian habitats, especially pigeon habitats, contain the largest numbers of *Cryptococcus* organisms. Most yeasts are probably too large to be inhaled into the lungs and settle out in the nasal cavity or nasopharynx, where they can produce disease or result in animals becoming asymptomatic carriers of the organism.[2,2a] In one study, cryptococcal organisms could be cultured from nasal washings in 14% of asymptomatic dogs and 7% of asymptomatic cats.[4] The small, desiccated forms of the yeast are also infective and can be inhaled into the small airways and alveoli, leading to pulmonary disease. After inhalation into the nasal cavity, paranasal sinuses, or lungs, cell-mediated immune response results in granuloma formation. Dissemination can occur by either direct extension or hematogenous spread. Direct extension from the nasal cavity through the cribriform plate to the CNS or to the paranasal soft tissues and skin is common. Although dissemination can be to any organ system, the skin, eyes, and CNS are most commonly affected.

Lesions consist of either granulomatous inflammation with few organisms or gelatinous masses of organisms with little inflammation. The large capsule surrounding the cryptococcal organism contributes to pathogenicity by inhibiting phagocytosis, plasma cell function, and leukocyte migration. As with the other systemic mycoses, the immune response determines the severity of clinical disease. Antibodies are readily produced by the humoral immune system but are not considered protective. Recovery, therefore, is dependent on cell-mediated immunity. Most human cases of cryptococcosis are associated with immune suppression, especially lymphoreticular neoplasia and AIDS. However, *Cryptococcus* spp. appears to be a primary pathogen of immunocompetent cats and dogs. An association with feline leukemia virus (FeLV) and feline immunodeficiency virus (FIV) infections in cats has been reported, and chronic glucocorticoid use has been implicated as a predisposing factor in both cats and dogs.[5-8]

CLINICAL SIGNS

Cats are more commonly affected by cryptococcosis than dogs. No apparent breed, sex, or age predilection exists in cats. Clinical findings are usually related to upper respiratory,

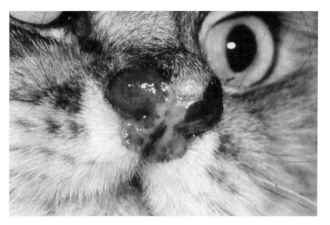

Figure 218-1 Nasal cryptococcosis in a cat. (Courtesy Dr. Carol Foil.)

nasopharyngeal, cutaneous, ocular, or CNS involvement. Unlike in other systemic mycoses, the lungs are not commonly clinically affected. Nonspecific signs such as depression and anorexia are common in chronic cases, but fever is uncommon. Upper respiratory signs associated with nasal cavity involvement are seen in 50% to 80% of affected cats. In these cats, sneezing and snuffling are common, and unilateral or bilateral mucopurulent nasal discharge with or without blood is typically seen. Proliferative soft tissue masses or ulcerative lesions within the nasal cavity or over the bridge of the nose are seen in approximately 70% of cases with upper respiratory involvement (Figure 218-1).

Oral ulcerations are occasionally noted but are not common. Nasopharyngeal mass lesions causing snoring, stertor, and inspiratory dyspnea are occasionally noted.[8] The skin or subcutaneous tissues are affected in approximately 40% to 50% of infected cats. Primary lesions include papules or nodules that may ulcerate and drain. Multiple lesions are typical, and regional lymphadenopathy is common. Hematogenous spread from the respiratory system may result in lameness secondary to osteomyelitis, renal failure secondary to renal disease, and generalized lymphadenopathy.

The eyes are affected in 20% to 25% of infected cats, especially those with CNS involvement. Granulomatous chorioretinitis with or without exudative retinal detachment is the most common ocular manifestation and can lead to panophthalmitis. Less often, optic neuritis can be seen, resulting in blindness. Anterior uveitis is not as common as posterior segment disease. CNS involvement is reported in approximately 20% of affected cats. This may be an underrepresentation of the actual number of cases with nervous system involvement.[8] The forebrain is most commonly affected, because invasion through the cribriform plate is thought to be common. Signs may include depression, behavior changes, seizures, circling, ataxia, blindness, head pressing, cranial nerve deficits, and paresis. Nasopharyngeal granulomas may occlude the auditory tube resulting in otitis media/interna and resultant peripheral vestibular signs.[9] Cats with concurrent FeLV or FIV infection tend to be more severely affected and may be more likely to develop neurologic or ophthalmic signs.

Canine cryptococcosis is typically seen in dogs younger than 4 years of age. No apparent sex predilection exists, and American Cocker Spaniels, Labrador Retrievers, Great Danes, and Doberman Pinschers appear to be overrepresented. In dogs, clinical findings are most often related to CNS, upper respiratory, ocular, or cutaneous involvement.[10] As in cats, depression and anorexia are common but fever is not. CNS involvement is reported in approximately 50% to 80% of

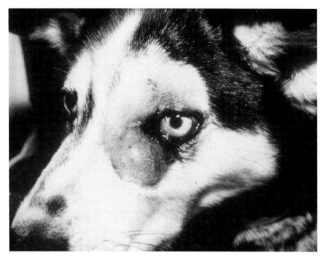

Figure 218-2 Periocular swelling in a female Siberian Husky, caused by cryptococcal infection.

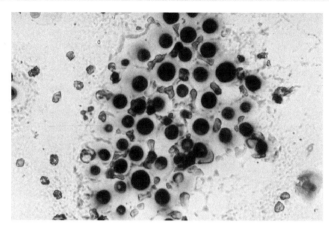

Figure 218-3 Cryptococcal organism noted on fine needle aspirate cytology from the dog in Figure 218-2. Note the large capsules surrounding the organisms and the minimal inflammatory response.

affected dogs. The brain is affected in most of these dogs.[11,12] The spinal cord may be affected along with the brain, and rarely the spinal cord alone is affected, causing signs consistent with either meningitis or an extradural compressive lesion.[13] Signs of nervous system involvement may include mental depression, vestibular syndrome, ataxia, cranial nerve deficits (especially cranial nerves V, VII, and VIII), seizures, paresis, blindness, hypermetria, and cervical pain. In dogs with CNS signs, other systems are usually affected as well, reflecting multisystemic dissemination.

The upper respiratory system or paranasal tissues are affected in approximately 50% of dogs with cryptococcosis (Figure 218-2).[10] The caudal nasal cavity and frontal sinuses are affected more commonly than the rostral nasal cavity. Signs may include upper airway stridor, nasal discharge and sneezing, epistaxis, or firm swellings over the bridge of the nose. The eyes or periorbital tissues are affected in approximately 20% to 40% of dogs with cryptococcosis. Granulomatous chorioretinitis with or without exudative retinal detachment is the most common ocular manifestation and can lead to panophthalmitis. In addition to chorioretinitis, fundic examination may reveal retinal hemorrhage or retinal scarring. Optic neuritis may be noted as a cause of blindness. As with the other systemic mycoses, anterior uveitis is less common than posterior segment disease. The skin is affected in approximately 10% to 20% of dogs with cryptococcosis. Subcutaneous nodules with ulcerative draining lesions, often on the head, feet, nail beds, and mucous membranes of the mouth, occur most commonly. Proliferative lesions in the ear canals may result from cryptococcal otitis externa. Direct extension from the ears to the CNS may occur. Multiorgan dissemination is more common in dogs than in cats. Disease may be subclinical or may result in clinical signs referable to the organ systems affected.

DIAGNOSIS

Hematology and clinical chemistries are often normal in animals with cryptococcosis. Mild nonregenerative anemia and mature neutrophilia or neutrophilia with a mild left shift may be seen. Because the nervous system is so commonly affected, CSF tap for culture and cytology should be considered. CSF commonly yields increased opening pressure,

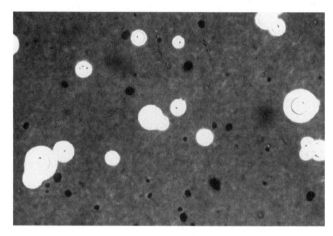

Figure 218-4 India Ink preparation revealing cryptococcal organisms. (Courtesy Dr. Carol Foil.)

increased protein, and mixed mononuclear and neutrophilic pleocytosis. Organisms are visualized in approximately 90% of dogs with CNS cryptococcosis.[14] Because opening pressures are often high and may result in shifting of CNS tissue during CSF collection, CSF tap is only recommended if diagnosis cannot be made by less invasive means.

Nodular infiltrates, an interstitial pattern, pleural effusion, and tracheobronchial lymphadenopathy are occasionally seen on thoracic radiographs. Nasal radiographs and computed tomography may demonstrate increased soft tissue density and bone destruction in the nasal passages and frontal sinuses.

Organism identification allows for definitive diagnosis and can usually be made cytologically or histologically. Cytology from affected tissue is the quickest and easiest means of identifying cryptococcal organisms. Nasal swabs, exudate from cutaneous lesions, aspirates of masses, subretinal or vitreal aspirates, and CSF often reveal organisms. Organisms are apparent in approximately 75% of cases. The large capsule makes identification easy (Figure 218-3). Gram's stain is useful in looking for cryptococcal organisms, because the cells retain the crystal violet and the capsule stains lightly red with the safranin. If India ink is used, the organism and capsule appear unstained and silhouetted against the black background (Figure 218-4). Care must taken in interpreting India ink preparations, as lymphocytes, fat droplets, and aggregated ink particles may be confused with the organism. Budding is occasionally noted. The thin wall and the large capsule differentiate *Cryptococcus* from *Blastomyces*.

Histopathology should be used if cytology fails to identify organisms. Nodular to diffuse granulomatous lesions or areas of degeneration with little inflammation are seen in infected tissue. Yeastlike organisms are usually numerous. Special stains such as PAS, Gridley's fungal, and GMS stain are best at demonstrating organisms. Mucicarmine stains best demonstrate the capsule.

Cryptococcal organisms grow readily when cultured. The organism can be cultured from infected tissue, exudate, CSF, urine, joint fluid, and blood if large enough samples are submitted. Yeastlike growth occurs in 2 days to 6 weeks on Sabouraud's dextrose agar. Hyphae rarely grow, even at 37° C. Care must be taken in interpreting positive cultures from the nasal cavity, because 14% of asymptomatic random-source dogs and 7% of asymptomatic random-source cats were culture-positive in one study.[4] Animals in the previously mentioned study were all negative on serum latex agglutination tests and did not have macroscopic or microscopic findings supportive of cryptococcal infection.

Serology is useful as an inexpensive and noninvasive diagnostic test and should be performed early in the diagnostic evaluation when cryptococcosis is suspected. Latex agglutination procedures are used to detect cryptococcal capsular antigen. Antibody titers are not useful diagnostically, because most infected animals do not mount a humoral immune response.[15] The commercially available latex cryptococcal antigen agglutination tests can be used on serum, urine, or CSF. CSF is the best sample to use in animals with neurologic signs, and serum is the best sample to use in animals with upper respiratory or cutaneous signs but without neurologic signs. Most cases are positive with titers between 1:10 and 1:100,000. The median titer in infected cats in one study was 1:1000.[15] False-negative antigen titers are rare but may occasionally be seen in localized disease or if the organism fails to produce a capsule. False-positive antigen titers are uncommon and are usually related to technique or interfering substances such as rheumatoid factor (RF). The latex agglutination antigen titer tends to correlate well with the extent of disease but does not correlate well with prognosis.[16] It may be used to evaluate the treatment progress and in determining how long to maintain an animal on antifungals.

TREATMENT

Cryptococcosis is a challenging disease to treat in cats and dogs that typically requires protracted therapy and long-term follow-up. Amphotericin B is the most effective drug in vitro against cryptococcal isolates and is generally recommended in infected people. Both itraconazole and fluconazole have proven to be equally efficacious to amphotericin B in treating CNS cryptococcosis in people, but the length of treatment can be quite long and the azole antifungals are generally recommended for consolidation therapy after a course of amphotericin B has been given. Amphotericin B appears to be very effective in treating cryptococcosis in dogs and cats but less information is available compared to using azole antifungals. Amphotericin B may be the treatment of choice in severely affected animals with CNS or systemic involvement. Amphotericin B is synergistic with flucytosine. Flucytosine can be used at a dose of 11.4 to 22.7 mg/lb (25 to 50 mg/kg) orally four times a day and has been used in dogs and cats. The combination of amphotericin B and flucytosine may be especially useful for treating CNS infections in cats. Cryptococcal organisms may rapidly develop resistance to flucytosine, so it has limited efficacy as a sole treatment agent. The dose of flucytosine should be adjusted downward in animals with concurrent renal failure. Toxicity to flucytosine includes ulcerative drug eruptions on the skin (especially on the face) and mucocutaneous junctions, enterocolitis, leukopenia, and thrombocytopenia that are especially prominent in dogs. Amphotericin B has also been effective when combined with azole antifungal agents.

Subcutaneously administered amphotericin B alone or in combination with azole antifungals or flucytosine has been used to successfully treat both feline and canine cryptococcosis.[17] Amphotericin B (0.22 to 0.36 mg/lb; 0.5 to 0.8 mg/kg) is diluted in 0.45% saline containing 2.5% dextrose (400 mL for cats, 500 mL for dogs <20 kg, 1000 mL for dogs >20 kg) and administered subcutaneously two to three times per week. This protocol may allow larger cumulative doses of amphotericin B to be given with reduced toxicity. Concentrations greater than 20 mg/L of amphotericin B resulted in local irritation and sterile abscess formation; therefore, more concentrated formulations of amphotericin B should not be used subcutaneously.

The azole antifungals have expanded the treatment options available and are central to successful treatment either as sole agents or in consolidation therapy following amphotericin B containing protocols. Fluconazole (50 mg/cat orally twice a day; 2.2 mg/lb [5 mg/kg] orally once to twice a day for dogs) is very effective and is the treatment of choice for cryptococcosis in cats and probably dogs with mild to moderately severe disease. Itraconazole (4.5 mg/lb [10 mg/kg] orally daily) is effective in cats and dogs but appears to require longer treatment times than fluconazole. In one uncontrolled study evaluating long term follow-up in cats and dogs with cryptococcosis, cats that were cured required median treatment times of 4 months for fluconazole and 9 months for itraconazole.[1] Controlled trials in people have revealed the two drugs to be equally efficacious. Ketoconazole (4.5 to 13.6 mg/lb [10 to 30 mg/kg] orally twice a day) is variably effective as a sole treatment agent but is ineffective in cases with CNS involvement. Resolution of clinical signs is the best means of patient monitoring, but the resolution of clinical signs is insufficient evidence that the infection has been eradicated, as improvement occurs well before all viable fungus has been cleared from host tissues. Serially monitoring latex agglutination antigen titers can significantly augment the clinician's clinical observations but recurrence can occur despite a marked reduction in the serum antigen titer and even after the sterilization of the CSF in CNS infections.[6,16]

Rechecks should be performed at least monthly while dogs or cats are being treated with azole antifungals and should include a chemistry panel to evaluate liver enzymes and a latex agglutination antigen titer. Sequential titers should differ by two or more dilutions before they are considered significantly different. A decline of twofold to fourfold per month during the initial few months of antifungal therapy generally corresponds to an adequate clinical response. Ideally, treatment should be continued until the titer is negative or for at least 2 months beyond resolution of clinical signs. In some animals, detectable cryptococcal polysaccharide antigen persists in the circulation long after the infection has been successfully treated. This is thought to be caused by continued elimination of unviable organisms and capsular material from infected tissues and macrophages. Most of these animals have low titers. High residual titers may indicate insufficient therapy and thus persistence of viable organisms.[6] One recommendation is to continue antifungal drug treatment to a titer of less than 1.[16] In cases in which there has been a thirty-twofold decrease and resolution of clinical signs, treatment may be discontinued; however, titers should be reevaluated periodically to ensure that they continue to decline or at least remain stable. Animals should be reevaluated at least 3 and 6 months after discontinuing treatment to assess for relapse. Negative antigen titers are occasionally seen in animals with localized disease, so they do not always indicate clinical cure.

The prognosis is good for cats with extraneural disease, and it is guarded for dogs with any form of the disease and for cats with CNS involvement. About 75 percent of cats and 50 percent of dogs have been noted to respond successfully to treatment. Cats responding completely to treatment appear to have about a 15 to 20 percent relapse rate.[1] Cats with FIV do not appear to be less likely to respond nor does the species of *Cryptococcus* appear to significantly influence prognosis.

REFERENCES

The reference list can be found on the companion Expert Consult Web site at *www.expertconsult.com*.

CHAPTER 219

Coccidioidomycosis

Autumn P. Davidson

Unique among the continents, North America is host to three of the geographically defined major endemic mycoses: histoplasmosis, blastomycosis, and coccidioidomycosis. These three endemic pathogenic fungi share several characteristics. All are soil-dwelling organisms existing only within defined geographic regions based on specific environmental (soil and climatic) conditions. All are dimorphic, capable of undergoing morphologic change from a native saprophytic form (infectious to mammals; also found in vitro) to the parasitic form causing disease in vivo. *Histoplasma capsulatum* and *Blastomyces dermatitidis* convert in vivo into a "yeast form"; *Coccidioides immitis* converts to a "spherule." Infection in mammals occurs most commonly by inhalation of airborne spores. Inhaled saprophytic spores cannot be killed by neutrophils and are small enough (3 to 5 µm) to lodge in host alveoli. Recovery from infection depends on the competence of the host's cell-mediated immunity. Compromised cell-mediated immunity, due to genetics, chemotherapy for neoplasia, organ transplant, or immune-mediated disease, or as a consequence of immunocompromising viral infection renders the host less able to resist colonization and dissemination of these fungi.[1]

Fungi and the infectious diseases they cause have become increasingly important in modern human and veterinary medicine, challenging mycologists to better understand their epidemiology, pathophysiology, and the host response. Popular current therapeutic targets include ergosterol in the fungal cell membrane and fungal RNA and DNA synthesis steps. Novel targets include enzymes involved in cell wall biosynthesis (1,3-beta glucan synthase and chitin synthase), as well as nonergosterol cell membrane molecules, DNA-related enzymes, intermediary fungal metabolism, and fungal virulence factors. Unfortunately, the prevalence of antifungal drug resistance appears to be increasing. Antifungal susceptibility testing and serum antimycotic drug level testing are becoming more available and standardized, although extrapolation from the human experience usually is required for interpretation. Data concerning combination therapy and sequential therapy as compared with single-agent therapy are accumulating. Adjunctive therapy with cytokines capable of immunohema-tologic modulation (granulocyte colony-stimulating factor [G-CSF], granulocyte macrophage colony-stimulating factor, macrophage colony-stimulating factor, and interferon-gamma) also has a potential role in the treatment and prevention of fungal infections. Stem cell and granulocyte transfusions and effective and safe vaccinations offer other avenues under development for restoration and improvement of host defense against mycotic disease.[2]

HISTORY AND MYCOLOGY

Coccidioidomycosis ("valley fever" or "valley rheumatism") was experimentally studied in dogs in the 1890s, but it was not described as a clinical entity in the veterinary literature until 1940. Coccidioidomycosis was recognized as a fatal granulomatous disease in humans during the late nineteenth century. Initially, the pathophysiology of coccidioidomycosis was thought to be neoplastic: a tumor induced by a protozoal organism, because of the coccidial-like appearance of the spherule detected in biopsy specimens from affected individuals. Recognition of the mycotic cause of coccidioidomycosis and fulfillment of Koch's postulates occurred in 1900. *Coccidioides immitis* (within California) and *C. posadasii* (in all other endemic Southwestern regions) are the two pathogenic species causing coccidioidomycosis.[3-6]

The alkaline sandy soil environment characteristic of the lower Sonoran life zone in the southwestern United States, western Mexico, and Central and South America is the normal habitat for *Coccidioides* spp., which grow as vegetative mycelia during seasonal rainfall. Germinating mycelia form thick-walled (2 to 4 µm × 3 to 10 µm) arthroconidia (arthrospores) with seasonal soil drying, subsequently becoming airborne under appropriate environmental (dry and windy) conditions. The arthroconidia can germinate to form new saprophytes or serve as the infectious form for mammals. In the dog and cat, inhalation of infectious and hardy arthroconidia is the major route of infection. Cutaneous contamination via a penetrating wound occurs less commonly. Experimentally, the canine infectious dose of inhaled arthroconidia is low (<10).[7]

PATHOPHYSIOLOGY AND EPIZOOTIOLOGY

The severity and extent of clinical disease resulting from an infectious exposure depends upon the immunocompetence of the host, and ranges from a mild, clinically silent pulmonic form to potentially fatal, multisystemic dissemination. At body temperature (37° C [98.6° F]) and under increased carbon dioxide exposure, *C. immitis* transforms in tissue to its parasitic form, the spherule (20 to 200 μm), which undergoes internal division (endosporulation) and ruptures at maturity. Each endospore (3 to 5 μm) can become an endosporulating spherule, promoting continuation and expansion of the parasitic phase (Figure 219-1).

The spherule is poorly chemotactic for neutrophils, but the endospore incites neutrophilic chemotaxis and can undergo phagocytosis. Spherules or endospores can revert to the mycelial form of growth under appropriate environmental conditions, such as might be found under bandages covering a draining tract, in a chronic pulmonary cavitary lesion, or in a therapeutic (central nervous system [CNS]) reservoir. As such, the disease is not believed to be directly contagious among mammals except by direct inoculation of infectious body fluids (blood, semen). Pulmonary infection is characterized by extension from the bronchioles and alveoli, through peribronchiolar tissues, to the subpleura and the tracheobronchial and mediastinal lymph nodes. Dissemination is defined as spread of coccidioidal infection beyond the tracheobronchial and mediastinal lymph nodes. Disseminated disease most commonly involves the axial and appendicular skeleton and overlying skin, abdominal viscera, CNS (including the eye), pericardium, myocardium, and the prostate gland (Figures 219-2 and 219-3).[8]

The incidence of coccidioidomycosis is increased in young, male, medium- to large-breed outdoor dogs. The Boxer, Pointer, Australian Shepherd, Beagle, and Scottish Terrier were found to have increased incidence in one study, although it is not believed that pure-breed dogs are generally at greater risk than mixed-breed dogs. A breed-specific susceptibility based on host immunocompetence may exist. As is the case in humans (60% of pulmonary infections are minimally symptomatic), seropositive dogs living in endemic areas exhibit few signs in most cases (80%).[9,10]

DIAGNOSIS

The diagnosis of coccidioidomycosis should be first based on clinical signs compatible with the infection (most commonly cough, lethargy, anorexia, fever, chronic lameness, cervical or head pain, and weight loss) and positive serologic findings. Early in the course of disease (2 to 5 weeks), a positive precipitin test reflects increased IgM levels. Subsequent (8 to 10 weeks) positive complement fixation (CF) testing marks the presence of IgG antibodies. Canine anticomplementary factors can interfere with CF testing, making quantitative immunodiffusion with concentration techniques more reliable than CF. Persistence or reappearance of a positive precipitin test can indicate dissemination. Early CF titers of greater magnitude may suggest more likelihood of dissemination. CF titers may persist at low levels (1:4) during recuperation. Negative serology in an infected individual reflects fulminating disease or anergy.[2,11]

Radiographic changes occurring with coccidioidomycosis are well described. Pulmonary lesions vary in character and severity. Most commonly, peribronchiolar and interstitial nodular lesions are associated with hilar lymphadenopathy (Figures 219-4 and 219-5). Skeletal lesions also vary, productive lesions are more common than lytic lesions, and both may be present simultaneously (Figures 219-6 and 219-7). Abdominal ultrasonographic changes in disseminated cases have recently been described (Figure 219-8).[12]

Characteristic laboratory changes associated with coccidioidomycosis include a mature neutrophilic leukocytosis, mild

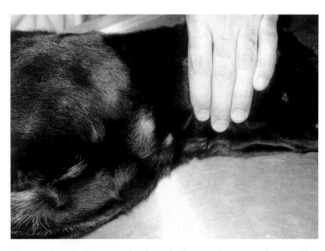

Figure 219-2 Prescapular lymphadenopathy secondary to disseminated coccidioidomycosis in a dog.

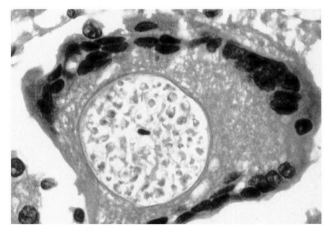

Figure 219-1 *Coccidioides immitis* endosporulating spherule.

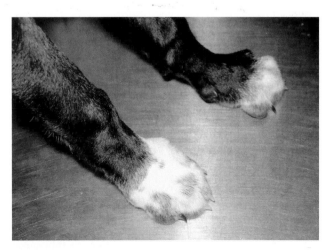

Figure 219-3 Osseous coccidioidomycosis, dissemination to the carpi of a dog.

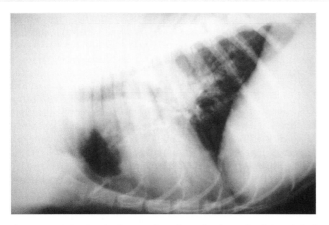

Figure 219-4 Marked sternal and tracheobronchial (perihilar) lymphadenopathy caused by pulmonary coccidioidomycosis in a dog.

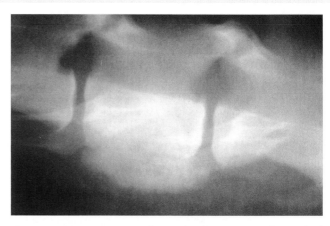

Figure 219-6 Disseminated coccidioidomycosis with vertebral (L3) spondylitis in a dog.

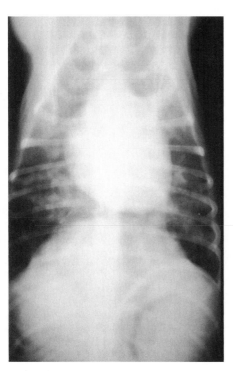

Figure 219-5 Nodular pulmonary infiltrates caused by pulmonary coccidioidomycosis in a dog.

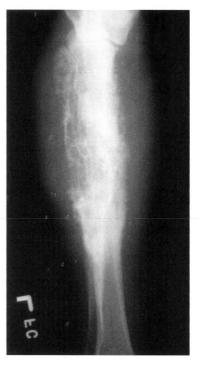

Figure 219-7 Disseminated coccidioidomycosis with radial and ulnar osteomyelitis in a dog.

anemia, monocytosis, hyperglobulinemia, and hypoalbuminemia. Histopathology, mycology, and cytology can also enable a positive diagnosis of coccidioidomycosis but are more invasive (biopsy), are hazardous to laboratory personnel (culture), and are less sensitive (cytology) than serology. A specific and sensitive polymerase chain reaction (PCR) assay for detection of *Coccidioides immitis* DNA is anticipated to assist with earlier diagnoses and subtle cases; however, serology and histopathology remain the best diagnostic modalities to date.[13,14]

Coccidioidomycosis is a reportable disease in humans and considered a potentially serious biohazard due to the highly infectious nature of the saprophytic phase (present in laboratory cultures and the soil). One half to two thirds of humans with primary coccidioidal pulmonic infection are subclinical and resolve their disease and then have durable cellular immunity. The intradermal skin test has been used in humans to identify individuals with such immunity. The outcome of infection in humans is highly correlated with patient profiling (age, sex, race, and reproductive status). The elderly, young, dark-skinned races, men, and women in the third trimester of pregnancy are at increased risk of serious infection. In humans, 5% to 10% of primary pulmonary infections result in pulmonary sequelae (nodules or cavities) and only 0.5% to 1.0% progress to chronic pulmonary infection or significant extrapulmonary dissemination. Humans with primary uncomplicated respiratory coccidioidomycosis usually resolve their infection without specific therapy, and it is not believed that therapy adds significant benefit. Pulmonary sequelae may not cause symptoms but warrant close clinical monitoring for evidence of progression to extrapulmonary infection. Treatment of dogs showing clinical signs with pulmonary coccidioidomycosis has traditionally been encouraged and is thought

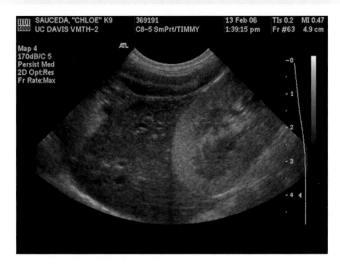

Figure 219-8 Echogenic renal cortices, abdominal ultrasound, disseminated coccidioidomycosis in a dog.

to reduce the potential for dissemination that results in a poorer prognosis. Small epizootiologic studies suggest that exposure and subclinical infection are common (80%) within the endemic area. At least a 20% rate of exposure adequate to cause seroconversion is apparent. The intradermal skin test is not reliable in the dog. The severity of illness if dissemination occurs makes therapy of any dog with signs referable to coccidioidomycosis (even pulmonary) attractive. Treatment of infected cats is supported by the fact that disseminated disease is already likely already present once the diagnosis is made. Weight loss and cutaneous lesions (chronic draining tracts) are the most commonly reported symptoms in the cat. A lack of familiarity with the disease in nonendemic areas may hamper diagnosis in dogs and cats having traveled through endemic regions.[14-16]

THERAPY

Therapy of coccidioidomycosis has involved both amphotericin B (standard and lipid formulations) and the azoles (ketoconazole, itraconazole, fluconazole, or voriconazole) as sole agents, in combination, or in succession. Numerous clinical reports exist in the veterinary literature regarding therapy for coccidioidomycosis, with variable recommendations for length of treatment based on the assessment of clinical cure. Treatment for a minimum of 4 to 6 months beyond clinical cure, with marked reduction or resolution of positive serologic findings, is advised. Relapse reportedly occurs commonly and it is not known if resolution of disease in the dog and cat results in lifelong immunity as is believed in humans. Humans living in endemic areas and undergoing immunosuppressive therapy associated with organ transplant experience a 3% (approximate) infection rate. If past exposure to coccidioidomycosis can be documented pretransplant, concurrent antifungal and immunosuppressive therapy is given. Immunosuppression-induced recrudescence of disease in a dog after occult infection has recently been reported.[17]

The soil organism *Streptomyces nodosus* is the source of the gold standard antimycotic agent amphotericin B. Amphotericin B (Fungizone) is a polyene antibiotic with antifungal activity due to binding ergosterol, a sterol moiety in the fungal cell membrane, forming channels that increase the permeability of the membrane. Amphotericin B is both fungistatic and fungicidal, depending on the concentration of the drug and the sensitivity of the fungal organism. It is not absorbed to

any large extent through the skin or across mucous membranes. Amphotericin B was introduced in the 1950s and was the first effective parenteral drug available for the treatment of invasive mycoses. Amphotericin B has the widest spectrum of activity of the clinically available antifungal agents. Its major limitation is its narrow therapeutic window. Amphotericin B is administered as an intravenous or intrathecal (commonly in humans) agent, usually every 48 hours. The intravenous dose, given in 5% dextrose, is 0.25 (feline) to 0.5 (canine) mg/kg intravenously q48h to a final dose of 5 to 10 mg/kg. The intrathecal dose is up to 0.5 mg in 3 to 5 mL spinal fluid, three times weekly. Amphotericin B is cumulatively nephrotoxic and its use is limited by associated azotemia). Phlebitis, chills, fever, anorexia, renal tubular acidosis, hypokalemia, hypomagnesemia, anemia, thrombocytopenia, leukopenia, and anaphylaxis are other side effects associated with its use. Slow intravenous infusions and pretreatment saline diuresis reduce nephrotoxicity. Recent reports suggest success using amphotericin B subcutaneously diluted in large volumes of saline (0.5 mg/kg in 400 ml 0.45% saline, given every 2 to 3 days to a cumulative dose of 10 to 20 mg/kg). The original formulation of amphotericin B is a micellar suspension with sodium deoxycholate. Recently, novel preparations of amphotericin B in lipid and liposomal-based formulations have been developed that are significantly less nephrotoxic but more costly. Slightly higher doses of these lipid formulations are required for efficacy equal to Fungizone, but the higher doses are well tolerated. Nephrotoxicity is still possible with lipid formulations, and infusional reactions remain a complication. Amphotericin B lipid complex (ABLC) (Abelcet) is dosed at 1 mg/kg intravenously q48h to a total dose of 12 mg/kg. ABLC and amphotericin B in colloidal dispersion (ABCD) are other lipid formulations. Amphotericin is recommended for serious disseminated coccidioidal infections, commonly those failing traditional azole therapy.

Azole agents for treating mycotic infections were developed during the 1980s and 1990s. Miconazole and clotrimazole were early azoles intended for topical use (see Aspergillosis, Therapy). Ketoconazole (Nizoral), an imidazole, was the first oral agent with an acceptable performance against the endemic mycoses and permitted outpatient therapy. The development of the triazoles, itraconazole (Sporanox), and fluconazole (Diflucan), followed. Azoles are usually fungistatic, inhibiting ergosterol synthesis from lanosterol by interacting with C-14 alpha demethylase, an enzyme dependent on cytochrome P-450. The result is increased cell membrane permeability and inhibition of fungal cell growth. At high concentrations achievable topically, some azoles may be fungicidal due to direct damage to fungal cell wall components (disturbed membrane lipid organization resulting in cell lysis). Other antifungal actions of the azoles include inhibition of endogenous respiration, toxicity to membrane phospholipids, and inhibition of the transformation of yeasts to their mycelial form. The interaction with cytochrome P-450 enzyme systems causes some of the side effects in mammals associated primarily with ketoconazole. Inhibition of adrenal and gonadal steroid synthesis can occur with ketoconazole administration. Ketoconazole, itraconazole, and fluconazole are available as oral preparations (pill form). Itraconazole and fluconazole are also available as parenteral preparations. Itraconazole has recently become available as an oral solution and a novel intravenous formulation, both in a beta cyclodextrin carrier that vastly improves absorption and bioavailability, allowing higher concentrations in affected tissues. Ketoconazole and itraconazole undergo hepatic metabolism and can be associated with hepatotoxicity, gastrointestinal (GI) intolerance, and cutaneous reactions. Fluconazole is excreted largely unchanged through the kidneys, is well absorbed orally, and has good CNS penetration. With increased prophylactic and long-term use of the azoles, fungal resistance is emerging, especially in immunocompromised humans on extended periods of therapy. The recommended dose of ketoconazole (brand name or its newly available generic equivalent) is 5 to 15 mg/kg orally every 12 hours (given with food). The recommended dose for itraconazole is 5 mg/kg orally (given with food) or intravenously every 12 to 24 hours, and for fluconazole it is 2.5 to 5.0 mg/kg orally or intravenously every 24 hours.

Currently, azole therapy, although expensive by veterinary standards, is less cost prohibitive than the expense of hospitalization, supportive care, and renal monitoring required by the appropriately conservative use of amphotericin B. Ketoconazole is less costly than the later generation azoles, itraconazole, and fluconazole, but is associated with more side effects and is likely less efficacious. Amphotericin B therapy in rapidly progressing, serious fungal infection should be followed by long-term oral azole therapy. The use of amphotericin should thus probably be reserved for refractory, disseminated, or fulminating cases. The increased cost of itraconazole and fluconazole may be offset by the suspected, but not yet well-documented, increased efficacy in animals. The improved bioavailability of itraconazole oral solution supports its use in serious or refractory disease. Fluconazole is indicated for animals with CNS involvement; additionally it has recently become available in a generic form. The use of liposomal amphotericin will permit higher doses to be administered for longer periods of time with less nephrotoxicity. Voriconazole (Pfizer) is a newly approved azole being used in humans with refractory fungal infection. It has excellent oral absorption and favorable pharmacokinetics. Little data are available on its use in coccidioidomycosis in veterinary medicine; its use should likely be reserved for serious cases having failed less expensive azoles.[2,18-20]

Chitin makes up a higher percentage of the fungal cell wall when the organism is in a mycelial phase. Nikkomycin Z, discovered in the 1970s and currently undergoing development, is a natural chitin synthase inhibitor, resembling the precursor substrate. Nikkomycin Z holds great promise as a fungicidal agent, also exhibiting marked in vitro synergism with the azoles.

Lufenuron, a benzoylphenyl urea, is a nonspecific insect chitin synthase inhibitor used in veterinary medicine to sterilize female fleas. Anecdotal clinical reports suggested that lufenuron was useful against coccidioidal infection. Controlled studies have subsequently shown no apparent efficacy or synergy of the compound as an antifungal agent in vitro or in vivo.

Terbinafine, a naftifine analog, inhibits fungal growth by inhibiting squalene epoxidase, important in the enzymatic synthesis of fungal ergosterol. Terbinafine may be synergistic with other antimycotic drugs, however convincing studies are lacking.[21-24]

REFERENCES

The reference list can be found on the companion Expert Consult Web site at *www.expertconsult.com.*

CHAPTER **220**

Aspergillosis

Autumn P. Davidson

Chronic nasal discharge is a clinical sign of significant disease in dogs. Sneezing and nasal discharge are the primary signs of nasal, sinus, and/or pharyngeal disorders. The nature of the discharge (serous, mucoid, purulent, hemorrhagic), the onset and duration of the nasal signs, and any historical response to therapy should be noted. The most common causes of chronic nasal discharge in the dog include fungal sinorhinitis (most commonly caused by *Aspergillus fumigatus*), nasal foreign body, rhinitis secondary to dental disease, nasal neoplasia, nasal mite infestation, and idiopathic lymphoplasmacytic rhinitis. These disorders can occur alone or in combination.

MYCOLOGY AND EPIZOOTIOLOGY

Aspergillus species are filamentous fungi that are ubiquitous under appropriate environmental conditions and not typically infectious due to host resistance (Figure 220-1). Aspergillosis in humans is typically a pulmonary hypersensitivity reaction rather than an infectious disease entity, except in immunocompromised individuals where disseminated infection with *Aspergillus* species is problematic. Pets acquire infectious aspergillosis in two forms: (1) localized (usually sinonasal) and (2) disseminated (involving two or more noncontiguous organs), both are more common in the dog than cat. *Aspergillus* species typically proliferate by producing spores in vegetative decaying soil and water (Figure 220-2).

LOCALIZED (SINONASAL) ASPERGILLOSIS

Canine sinonasal aspergillosis is characterized by colonization and invasion of the nasal passages and frontal sinuses by the saprophytic fungus, *Aspergillus fumigatus*. *A. fumigatus* is regarded as an opportunistic pathogen, suggesting that some preexisting local nasal mucosal immunocompetence allowed its establishment in the upper respiratory tract. Alternatively, an in vitro inhibition of B and T lymphocyte transformation by *A. fumigatus* products has been described, suggesting that immunosuppression may both result from or be perpetuated by infection. Sinonasal aspergillosis may occur as an opportunistic primary infection or it may occur secondary to the presence of a foreign body (foxtail, splinter), nasal trauma, or neoplasia (Figure 220-3).

The disease primarily affects young to middle-aged mesaticephalic and dolichocephalic breeds and is progressive unless effective specific therapy is given. German Shepherds and

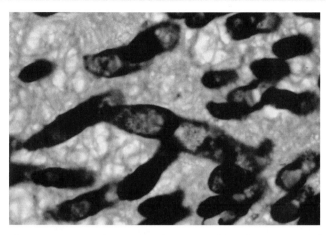

Figure 220-1   Methenamine silver stain of histologic section of *Aspergillus* spp. showing characteristic parallel septate hyphae with acute angle branching.

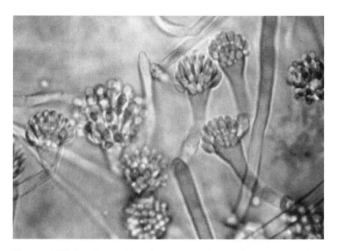

Figure 220-2   *Aspergillus flavus* in culture showing conidiophores bearing fruiting heads.

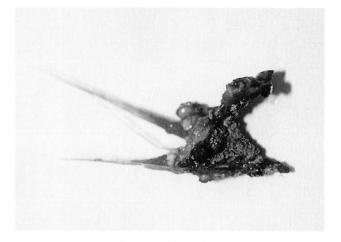

Figure 220-3   Foxtail removed from the nasal passage of a dog with sinonasal aspergillosis.

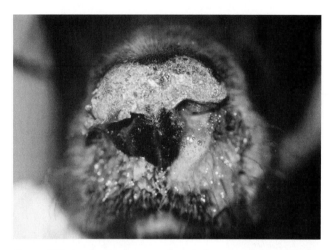

Figure 220-4   Severe crusting of nasal planum and nares in a dog with sinonasal aspergillosis.

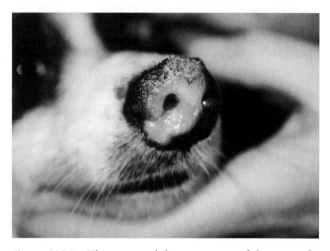

Figure 220-5   Ulceration and depigmentation of the nares of a dog with chronic sinonasal aspergillosis.

Rottweilers are the pure breeds more commonly affected, but nasal aspergillosis occurs in mixed-breed dogs as well.[1,2]

PATHOPHYSIOLOGY

Colonization and invasion of the nasal mucosa by *A. fumigatus* results in destruction and necrosis of the nasal turbinates, often accompanied by frontal sinus osteomyelitis. The cribriform plate, palatine bones, and orbit are sometimes involved. Facial pain, anorexia, sneezing, and copious mucoid to hemorrhagic nasal discharge and crusting are common clinical signs (Figure 220-4). Life-threatening epistaxis can occur secondary to erosion of the nasal vasculature. With chronicity, depigmentation, and ulceration of the nares and masticatory muscle atrophy result (Figures 220-5 and 220-6). CNS involvement (encephalitis, meningitis) precipitating seizures can result after erosion of the cribriform plate.[1,2]

DIAGNOSIS

Nasal disease is typically evaluated via rhinoscopy with culture, cytology, and histopathology of affected tissues, radi-

ology and sometimes serology. Nasal aspergillosis should be differentiated from other inflammatory causes of rhinitis such as nasal foreign body, bacterial rhinitis (most commonly associated with periodontal disease), nasal neoplasia, infestation with nasal mites, and idiopathic lymphocytic-plasmacytic

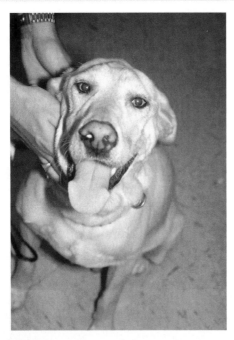

Figure 220-6 Masticatory muscle atrophy in a Labrador Retriever previously diagnosed with sinonasal aspergillosis.

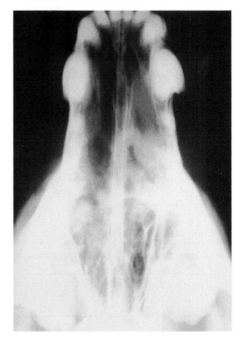

Figure 220-8 Nasal radiography showing loss of turbinate detail and fluid density associated with nasal aspergillosis in a dog.

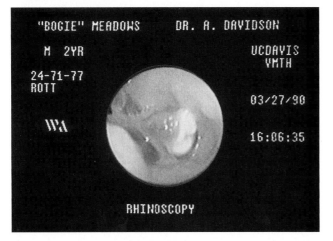

Figure 220-7 Fungal plaque, nasal passage of a dog viewed rhinoscopically.

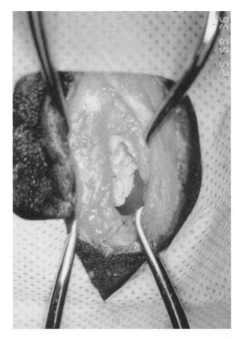

Figure 220-9 Aspergilloma in the frontal sinus of a dog.

rhinitis. The diagnosis of sinonasal aspergillosis is best made by direct observation and microscopic demonstration of invasive fungal plaques on the nasal mucosa (Figure 220-7).

Biopsy of affected tissue and histopathologic evaluation for mucosal invasion is confirmatory. The diagnosis is best supported by typical computed tomographic (CT) findings. Mycologic culture of *A. fumigatus* from affected tissues is supportive of the diagnosis, but fungi can contaminate nasal mucosa diseased from other causes. Serologic evaluation of sinonasal aspergillosis is unreliable: both false-positive and false-negative results occur. Additionally, serology is not prognostic in confirmed cases of nasal aspergillosis. It is important to investigate neoplasia as a coexistent condition in older dogs with confirmed aspergillosis.[3]

Radiology of the nasal passages and frontal sinuses (radiography and CT) is useful in the diagnosis of sinonasal aspergillosis but must be performed before rhinoscopic evaluation to avoid artifacts resulting from lavage, tissue manipula-

tion, and hemorrhage. Radiography shows loss of fine nasal turbinate detail and fluid density in the nasal passages and frequently the frontal sinuses (Figure 220-8). In some cases, an aspergilloma may exist in the frontal sinus (Figure 220-9).

CT evaluation is the most useful radiologic modality because characteristic lesions may be identified and evaluation of the exact extent of disease is optimized. CT has provided a new appreciation for the aggressive nature of fungal rhinitis. Contrast-enhanced CT helps differentiate fungal rhino sinusitis from neoplasia. Mild cases of sinonasal aspergillosis result in relatively little structural change within the nasal cavity other than the regional lysis of nasal turbinates. Dogs that are chronically infected often demonstrate dramatic turbinate destruction, gross epithelial thickening, formation of dense fungal colonies and granulomas, and penetration into adjacent bone causing hyperostosis and in some instances gross bony destruction. Dogs with sinonasal aspergillosis frequently have copious, thick nasal exudate obscuring radiographic identification of granulomas. Administration of intranasal iodinated contrast medium can help define mass lesions in the presence of surrounding fluid (Figure 220-10).[4,5]

Numerous techniques have been described to obtain tissue specimens for the definitive histopathologic diagnosis of sinonasal aspergillosis. General anesthesia is required, with a cuffed endotracheal tube placed to prevent aspiration of blood and lavage fluids. The external surface of the nasal cavity is visually and digitally examined for evidence of swelling, asymmetry, and ulceration. This includes a thorough oral examination and visualization of the nasopharynx with either a flexible fiberoptic scope or an angled, warmed dental mirror. Placement of precounted gauze sponges in the pharynx, for further protection of the airways, is then performed. Larger laparotomy sponges should be used if possible because these are less easily swallowed by dogs that may swallow with manipulation of sensitive nasal tissues. The clinician should then measure the distance from the nares to the area of interest noted on the nasal radiographs or CT. This distance serves as a guide for obtaining nasal biopsy and culture specimens. In addition, prior to inserting any instrument in the nasal cavity, the distance from the nares to the medial canthus of the ipsilateral eye is noted and should not be exceeded or penetration of the cribriform plate may result (Figure 220-11).

Rhinoscopy should be performed while the animal is in sternal recumbency. Only a limited examination of the rostral nasal cavity can be performed with an otoscope. A rigid arthroscope with a 1.9- to 2.7-mm outside diameter and a 5- to 25-degree angle of view (Richard Wolf Medical Instruments, 7046 Lyndon Avenue, Rosemont, IL 60018) permits a more comprehensive evaluation of the nasal passages. A flexible bronchoscope with a 3.5- to 4.8-mm outside diameter (Olympus Corporation, 4 Nevada Drive, Lake Success, NY 11042-1179) has the added benefit of allowing visualization of the nasopharynx by retroflexing the scope around the soft palate, but it is more difficult to manipulate through the nasal passages. Light resistance is usually felt while inserting the scope through the nares. The scope can then be directed ventrally into the ventral nasal meatus toward the nasopharynx or dorsally into the dorsal nasal meatus toward the olfactory epithelium, openings (ostia) of the frontal sinuses, and the cribriform plate. The advantages of direct visualization of the nasal cavity are that a more thorough understanding of the nature of the disease process might be obtained and placement of a biopsy instrument at the area of interest is facilitated.

Indirect methods of obtaining tissue specimens via the nares have also been described. As with rhinoscopic examination, prebiopsy imaging studies are recommended. Biopsy instruments should never be inserted beyond the level of the ipsilateral medial canthus, and protection of the airways under general anesthesia is recommended. The simplest of these techniques involve flushing the nasal cavity with saline in an attempt to dislodge diagnostic tissue. A catheter should be placed in the nares, or retroflexed 180 degrees around the soft palate. Gauze sponges are used to catch tissues that are flushed out through the nares or into the pharynx. More aggressive blind techniques include flushing the nasal cavity while reaming the area of interest with a stiff plastic tube or biopsy with a biopsy needle (Tru-Cut Disposable Biopsy Needle; Travenol Laboratories, Morton Grove, Ill.), a plastic catheter, or by applying suction to a Foley urethral catheter. These techniques do not allow the characterization of the disease process that is possible with direct visualization and may result in nondiagnostic or misleading tissue samples. However, they do not require specialized equipment, are easy to perform, and may result in a definitive diagnosis. If the

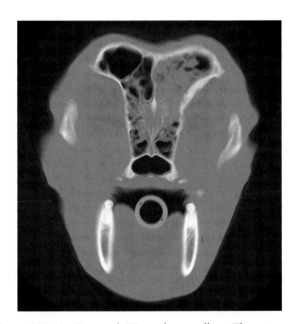

Figure 220-10 Sinonasal CT, nasal aspergillosis. There is extensive turbinate loss in the right nasal passage that is diffuse but most pronounced in the mid and caudal region. Within the nasal passage, there is fluid accumulation. There is soft tissue dense material with a fragmented gas pattern present in the dorsal portion of the most caudal nasal passages extending into the frontal sinus. There is destruction of frontal bone that extends from the sinus into the caudal aspect of the bony orbit and through the dorsal table of the frontal bone leaving a communication with the overlying soft tissues. There is bony proliferation and thickening of the frontal bone that is diffuse through the frontal sinus.

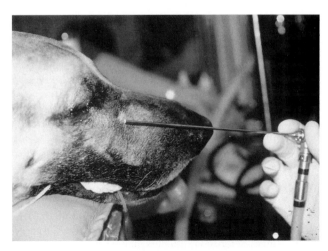

Figure 220-11 Marking the distance from the rostral nares to the ipsilateral medial canthus before rhinoscopic evaluation.

cytologic diagnosis is inconsistent with the signalment, history, or imaging studies, the clinician should repeat the procedure or consider one that allows direct visualization of the area of interest.[2-4]

THERAPY

Therapeutic recommendations for sinonasal aspergillosis have included surgery and systemic and topical antimycotic medications. Rhinotomy and turbinectomy with perioperative thiabendazole administration resulted in improvement in 50% or less of dogs in one study. Oral ketoconazole administration was reportedly efficacious in 47%, oral itraconazole in 60% to 70%, and oral fluconazole in 60% of infected dogs. Enilconazole applied topically through frontal sinus tubes (twice daily for 7 to 10 days) was reportedly efficacious in 80% to 90% of dogs but is cumbersome and not always readily available in the United States. Extensive débridement of the nasal cavities and frontal sinuses followed by infusion of 1% to 2% enilconazole via endoscopically placed catheters has been advocated. Invasive surgical exposure of the nasal passages and frontal sinuses, topical application of 10% povidone iodine, and delayed closure 6 to 8 weeks postoperatively was recommended for refractory cases but had poor client acceptance and a small study size.[1,6]

Clotrimazole is a synthetic imidazole derivative. At concentrations achieved during systemic use, imidazoles impair the biosynthesis of ergosterol, the major component of fungal cell membranes, resulting in interference with certain membrane-bound enzyme systems and fungistatic inhibition of growth. In addition, clotrimazole is fungicidal topically, reaching higher concentrations (1.5×10^{-4} M). Electron microscopic observations indicate that at high concentrations, clotrimazole causes alteration in the fungal cell membrane with consequent changes in permeability and leakage of cellular constituents in a manner similar to the effect of polyene antifungal antibiotics. This drug is available in human topical preparations for cutaneous, oral, or vaginal applications. Administered orally, it is poorly absorbed and rapidly absorbed undergoes hepatic metabolism and biliary excretion. GI irritation and contact hypersensitivity are reported human side effects.[7]

Clotrimazole solution has been used successfully for the topical treatment of nasal aspergillosis in the dog. The topical delivery of clotrimazole has been accomplished using two techniques. In the first, an infusion of clotrimazole is delivered through infant feeding tubes placed into the frontal sinuses and caudal nasal passages through the skull (a somewhat invasive procedure requiring surgical expertise for trephination and tube placement). An alternative technique, based on studies of the distribution of topical agents in the frontal sinuses and nasal passages, involves the retrograde infusion of clotrimazole through polypropylene catheters placed into the nares. This technique is equally successful, technically simpler, and associated with less morbidity. Based on a previous study in cadavers, the average volume of the frontal sinuses in breeds predisposed to fungal rhinitis is 25 mL per side. At present, the recommendation is to use 50 to 60 mL per side in middle- to large-breed dogs, regardless of head size. Flooding the nasal cavity and sinuses with a larger volume of infusate (50 to 60 mL per side) results in distribution to all areas of the nasal cavity and frontal sinuses, especially when performed under pressure accomplished by occlusion of the nares. Delivery by trephination and feeding tube placement can bypass affected areas within the frontal sinuses. The surgical placement of infusion catheters may be indicated if extensive aspergillomas are present in the frontal sinuses as their removal is facilitated by trephination.

Catheters should be placed with the dog in lateral recumbency. A 24-F Foley catheter is placed per os so that the tip of the catheter lies dorsal to the soft palate. This process can be aided initially by grasping the catheter tip with a pair of right-angle forceps (Meeker) or long-handled needle holders so that the catheter tip is directed rostrally. A mouth gag is then placed, and an assistant should retract the tongue rostrally to improve visualization during catheter placement. The catheter can then be advanced until its balloon is dorsal to the junction of the hard and soft palates. The balloon of the Foley catheter is then inflated to occlude the nasopharynx. The balloon can be palpated through the soft palate to confirm its position just caudal to the hard palate. Moistened laparotomy sponges should be counted and then placed in the pharynx so that the catheter cannot migrate caudally and will absorb any infusate that might escape around the balloon. During sponge placement the index finger of the opposite hand is used to maintain balloon position. Once this process is complete, the mouth gag is removed. One 10-F polypropylene infusion catheter is then advanced through each nostril, beginning dorsomedially; each is advanced into the dorsal nasal meatus to the level of the medial canthus of the ipsilateral palpebral fissure. A Foley catheter (12 F) is then inserted into each nostril and the balloons inflated so that they lie just caudal to and occluding the nostrils. Occasionally a nylon suture is placed across each nostril to prevent cranial migration of the nasal balloons. After three Foley catheters (one nasopharyngeal, two nasal) are placed, their balloons should be inflated to slow the leakage of clotrimazole from the nasal cavity and frontal sinuses (Figures 220-12 and 220-13). The dog is then repositioned in dorsal recumbency, and an additional laparotomy sponge is placed just caudal to the upper incisors (between the endotracheal tube and the incisive papilla) to absorb leakage of clotrimazole through the incisive ducts.

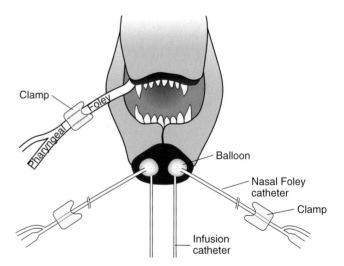

Figure 220-12 Schematic of catheter position with the dog in dorsal recumbency. A Foley catheter with the balloon inflated in the nasopharynx and pharyngeal gauze sponges (not shown) minimize leakage of infusion caudally. A cuffed endotracheal tube (et) further diminishes the risk of aspiration. Syringes (60 mL) are used to inject infusion into the dorsal nasal meatus via polypropylene infusion catheters. Inflated Foley catheter balloons obstruct the nares to diminish leakage of infusion rostrally. Tubing clamps on Foley catheters are closed when fluid is observed within the catheter lumen. (Adapted from Mathews KG et al: Computed tomographic assessment of noninvasive intranasal infusions in dogs with fungal rhinitis. Vet Surg 25:309, 1996.)

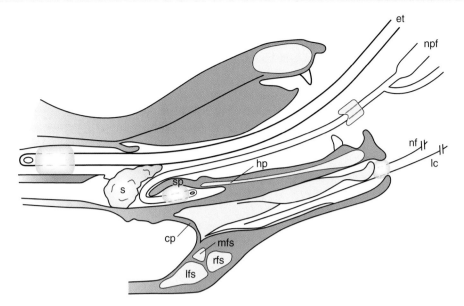

Figure 220-13 Schematic of sagittal section showing the position of the endotracheal tube *(et)*, pharyngeal sponges *(s)*, infusion catheter *(ic)*, and rostral nasal Foley catheter *(nf)* in relation to the hard palate *(hp)*, soft palate *(sp)*, cribriform plate *(cp)*, rostral frontal sinus *(rfs)*, medial frontal sinus *(mfs)*, and lateral frontal sinus *(lfs)*. (From Mathews KG et al: Computed tomographic assessment of noninvasive intranasal infusion in dogs with fungal rhinitis. Vet Surg 25:309, 1996.)

Clotrimazole (1 g) in 100 mL of polyethylene glycol 200 (a 1% solution) is then evenly divided between two 60 mL syringes (50 mL per syringe). Initially the nasal passages and frontal sinuses must be filled with solution. When clotrimazole is noted within the lumen of a Foley catheter it should be clamped shut, eventually creating a closed system for saturation of the nasal and frontal sinus mucosa. The clotrimazole should then be continuously and slowly infused over a 1-hour period (50 mL per infusion catheter). The polypropylene catheters are maintained in a horizontal position, parallel to the table, throughout infusion. Positioning the dog so that its nose protrudes beyond the edge of the treatment table allows clotrimazole escaping around the nasal catheters to drip into a receptacle. While the dog's body is maintained in dorsal recumbency, the head can be tilted and maintained in the following positions to ensure drug contact with all mucosal surfaces: dorsal recumbency (15 minutes), left lateral recumbency (15 minutes), right lateral recumbency (15 minutes), and dorsal recumbency (15 minutes). The dog is then placed in sternal recumbency, the catheters and sponges removed and counted, the clotrimazole allowed to drain rostrally, and the pharynx and proximal esophagus suctioned before recovery from anesthesia.

Topical administration of clotrimazole into the frontal sinuses and nasal passages is generally well tolerated. Pharyngitis, conjunctivitis, and pharyngeal edema have been reported as transient side effects. The success rate with one or more topical clotrimazole applications has been reported to be 65% to 86%. The infection will resolve in some dogs after a single treatment. A favorable response to clotrimazole therapy is usually indicated by resolution of nasal discharge by 2 weeks after therapy. Unabated persistence of nasal discharge 2 weeks after therapy is an indication for repeat evaluation and treatment if aspergillosis persists. Concurrent systemic antibiotic therapy may be indicated if secondary bacterial rhinitis is present. Some dogs with advanced disease may require multiple 1-hour clotrimazole infusions. Cases selected for topical therapy should have aspergillosis limited to the frontal sinuses and nasal passages, without CNS involvement. Pretreatment

CT scans are encouraged so that the extent of the disease is determined and the integrity of the cribriform plate evaluated. Remember, however, that no test (including CT scan) is 100% reliable in determining if the cribriform is intact. Informed consent should be obtained from clients, especially if CT is not performed. Topical infusion of clotrimazole solution is not advised if the cribriform plate is not intact, because serious meningitis and encephalitis may result, usually a reaction to the vehicle rather than the azole. Cases with CNS involvement, characterized by a lack of integrity of the cribriform plate or orbit (ocular or retrobulbar involvement), should receive systemic antifungal therapy (preferably voriconazole). Only the formulation of clotrimazole in polyethylene glycol is advised. The use of clotrimazole in propylene glycol-isopropyl alcohol vehicles is problematic due to the tendency of the latter to significantly irritate oronasal mucosa.[7-10]

Rhinoscopic evaluation of the sinonasal passages and follow-up CT are the best methods to evaluate efficacy of therapy; however, many owners refuse follow-up evaluation in dogs without signs due to cost. Positive titers may persist for more than 2 years (ELISA) or 5 years (AGID) in dogs that remain free of disease. Treatment failure may result from resistance to antifungal drug, poor penetration into affected tissues of a systemic drug, presence of a foreign body, fungal granuloma or sequestrum, immunosuppression, failure to coat the entire nasal cavity with a topical drug, or an incorrect diagnosis. Case reports exist indicating combination therapy with topical and systemic azoles can be successful.[11]

DISSEMINATED ASPERGILLOSIS

Disseminated aspergillosis is most commonly diagnosed in dogs and cats that are terminally ill from the disease. Disseminated aspergillosis typically involves multiple organ systems with no history of nasal or pulmonary involvement. *Aspergillus terreus, A. deflectus, A. flavipes,* and rarely *A. fumigatus* have been reported in cases where the species has been identified. Disseminated aspergillosis is believed to occur after inhalation of small spores (<8 μm) and hematogenous spread. The pathogenicity of the causative species is reported to be associated with their production of highly infective aleuriospores in tissue and their inherent ability to invade blood vessels. In dogs, disseminated aspergillosis has been most commonly reported in the German Shepherd between 2 and 8 years of age. Genetic predisposition and dysfunctional mucosal immunity are suspected. Defective IgA production or regulation has been identified in some affected German Shepherds. Cats with disseminated aspergillosis generally have identifiable concurrent immunosuppressive disease (usually viral) or other debilitation and are less than 2 years of age.

The clinical signs associated with disseminated aspergillosis are nonspecific and related to organ involvement. Uveitis, enophthalmitis, and chorioretinitis may precede the onset of generalized disease. Osteomyelitis and mycotic granulomas of the kidneys, liver, spleen, intervertebral discs, pancreas, lymph nodes, myocardium, prostate, brain, uterus, and thyroid gland have been reported. Bone pain, paraparesis, draining sinus tracts, anorexia, weight loss, pyrexia, lethargy, muscle wasting,

and fever are the most common signs. Animals with disseminated aspergillosis may have fungal hyphae observed on cytologic examination of urine sediment, serum, synovial fluid, lymph node centesis, bone biopsy, or intervertebral disc aspiration. The diagnosis is confirmed by culture on Sabouraud's dextrose agar. Serology is not reliable (false negatives have been reported).

The prognosis for recovery is poor despite aggressive antifungal therapy and supportive care. Intravenous amphotericin B, itraconazole, fluconazole, or voriconazole are advised initially. Long-term (sometimes for life) oral azole therapy can be attempted if an initial positive response to intravenous antimycotic drug administration occurs. Surgical excision of fungal granulomas may be helpful, if feasible.[12-14]

REFERENCES

The reference list can be found on the companion Expert Consult Web site at *www.expertconsult.com.*

CHAPTER 221

Tropical Diseases

Remo Lobetti

In the past the term *tropical diseases* referred to diseases that only occurred in the tropic regions of the world. These days, however, the distinction between tropical and nontropical disease is becoming increasingly blurred and diseases that traditionally were considered tropical now occur in many nontropical places. Moreover, some of the parasitic infections formerly thought to be uncommon, or much localized, are now recognized to have a wide distribution. Possible reasons for the expansion of tropical diseases to other parts of the world include global warming, especially with diseases that are vector borne, and the rapidity and ease of movement of both people and animals, which allows the dissemination and spread of diseases. A good example of this is West Nile virus infection in people. This arthropod-borne virus was first isolated in 1937, was an uncommon infection transmitted by mosquitoes, and was associated with wild birds as enzootic hosts. The disease was not considered to be a significant human pathogen because of sporadic outbreaks and mild febrile disease. However, the occurrence between 1996 and 1999 of three major epidemics, in southern Romania, the Volga delta in southern Russia, and the northeastern United States, involving hundreds of cases was totally unexpected. A significant factor that appeared in common to all three outbreaks was the apparent involvement of the common house mosquito, *Culex pipiens*, as a vector, which had not previously been implicated as an important vector. In addition the epidemic in the United States was unusual in that the association of West Nile virus infection with fatal disease of birds, suggesting a change in the virulence of the virus toward this host.

The presence of tropical diseases is also compounded by socioeconomic, pet-owner relationships, and nutritional disorders. See Table 221-1 for diseases that can still be considered of a tropical nature.

AFRICAN HORSE SICKNESS

African horse sickness is caused by a double-stranded RNA orbivirus. In addition to equines, the dog is the only other species that can contract African horse sickness.[1] Dogs usually contract the disease by ingesting infected horsemeat, but can also be infected by vector-borne transmission by *Culicoides* midges.[2] Typical clinical signs include fever, cough, and diar-

Table • 221-1

Diseases That Can Still Be Considered of a Tropical Nature

ORGANISMS	DISEASE
Viruses	Orbivirus (African horse sickness)
	Wesselsbron disease
	Yellow fever
	Rift Valley fever
	Foot-and-mouth disease
	Hepatitis E virus
Bacteria	Melioidosis
	Anthrax
Protozoa	Southern African canine babesiosis
	Feline babesiosis
	Trypanosomiases
	Sarcocystosis
Ectoparasites	*Hyalomma* tick bite necrosis
	Cordylobia infestation
Endoparasites	Spirocercosis

rhea. The disease progression is often acute. Postmortem examination of affected dogs shows severe pulmonary edema, pleural effusion, and splenomegaly.[1] Antibodies to African horse sickness have been detected in healthy dogs from Egypt, India, and South Africa.[2] There is no specific therapy for the disease.

FLAVIVIRIDAE

Flaviviridae are vector-borne single-stranded RNA viruses.[3] Of all the viruses in this group the two that are of a tropical nature and that affect the dog and cat are yellow fever and Wesselsbron disease.

Yellow fever, transmitted by *Aedes* mosquitoes, results in a subclinical infection in cats that is characterized by a transient viremia, whereas dogs are resistant to the virus.[4] Affected cats may show a transient febrile reaction. Wesselsbron disease has been reported in a dog that died from encephalitis. When three dogs were challenged with the viral isolate from the succumbed dog, two dogs showed a transient febrile reaction and one developed transient paresis.[5] Antibodies to Wesselsbron disease have been detected in healthy dogs from Botswana and South Africa.[5] The diagnosis is usually made retrospectively on postmortem examination. There is no specific therapy for the disease.

It is likely that dogs and cats showing transient nonspecific signs of encephalitis may in fact be infected with Flaviviridae.

BUNYAVIRIDAE

The Bunyaviridae is the largest family of vector-borne single-stranded RNA viruses and include many important pathogens of both man and animals.[6] Of all the viruses in this group, the only one of a tropical nature is Rift Valley fever. The *Aedes* mosquito is the most common vector, although midges, ticks, and sandflies can also transmit the infection. Direct transmission, by inhalation or ingestion, from affected animals is also possible.[6] The virus can be transmitted from the puppy to the dam and to other puppies. In young puppies and kittens infection with Rift Valley fever results in viremia, hepatic and myocardial necrosis, meningitis, diffuse petechial hemorrhages, and death.[4] Although adult animals do not succumb to the infection, they can develop a viremic state and infection in a pregnant animal can result in abortion or stillbirths.[4,6] The diagnosis is usually made retrospectively on postmortem examination. There is no specific therapy for the disease.

FOOT AND MOUTH DISEASE

Foot and mouth disease is a highly contagious viral disease of wild and domestic cloven-hoofed animals caused by strains of the aphthovirus. The disease has been eradicated from Australia, New Zealand, Japan, and North America. Dogs and cats are relatively resistant to infection but may become incidentally infected during outbreaks in herbivores by either direct contact or contact with offal.[7]

HEPATITIS E VIRUS

Hepatitis E virus is an unclassified virus that results in an acute self-limiting hepatitis in people. The disease occurs in Asia, Middle East, and North Africa. To date no clinical disease has been reported in dogs and cats although antibody titers have been detected.[8]

MELIOIDOSIS

Melioidosis is a bacterial infection caused by *Burkholderia pseudomallei*. The disease occurs in Southeast Asia, northern Australia, and the South Pacific. The organism is a ubiquitous soil saprophyte that results in chronic nodular or purulent generalized systemic inflammatory disease in dogs, cats, and other species.[9] The route of infection is by inhalation, ingestion, introduced into wounds or tissues by bites of arthropod vectors, or by direct contact with contaminated soil.[9,10] The isolation of the organism from blood or lesions is diagnostic. Therapy is aimed at surgical drainage of abscesses and long-term systemic antibiotic therapy.[10]

ANTHRAX

Anthrax is an acute bacterial systemic disease of mammals caused by *Bacillus anthracis*. In dogs and cats the infection is rare and is manifested by local inflammation, necrosis, and edema of tissues of the upper gastrointestinal region, which are the first to come in contact with the organism.[11] Although death is usually by asphyxiation, the toxin can also exert systemic effects. The cat and dog are infected by the ingestion of meat from contaminated carcasses of animals that have died from anthrax.[11,12] The diagnosis is made by detection of the bacillus on a blood or edema fluid smear. Postmortem examination is not advocated as this can result in the dissemination of bacterial spores.[12] Treatment is with penicillin antibiotics.[12]

CANINE BABESIOSIS

Canine babesiosis is an important worldwide tick-borne disease, ranging from a relatively mild to a fatal disease. The causative organism of is either *Babesia canis* or *B. gibsoni*. Three subtypes of *B. canis* are recognized, namely: *B. c. canis*, *B. c. vogeli*, and *B. c. rossi*. *Babesia gibsoni* is subdivided into 2 subspecies: the North American and Asian species. *Babesia c. canis* is found in Europe, *B. c. vogeli* in northern Africa, North and South America, Australia, and South Africa, and *B. c. rossi* in southern Africa and Nigeria.[13,14] *Babesia gibsoni* is found in Asia, Australia, Western Europe, North and South America, and northern and eastern Africa.[14] Other *Babesia* species affecting dogs have also been reported: in one dog naturally infected with a small *Babesia*, it was shown that it was distantly related to *B. gibsoni*, but more closely related to *B. microti*, *B. rodhaini*, and *Theileria equi*; in California a small piroplasm isolate, closely related to piroplasm isolates from wildlife and humans, has been identified as a distinct species, *Babesia conradae*; and in Spain a *B. microti*–like piroplasms are recognized as a cause of disease in dogs. Babesiosis is solely a tick-borne disease, with *B. c. canis* being transmitted by *Dermacentor reticulatus*, *B. c. vogeli*, and *B. gibsoni* by *Rhipicephalus sanguineus*, and *B. c. rossi* by *Haemaphysalis leachi*. In experimental studies, *Hyalomma marginatum* and *Dermacentor andersoni* have been shown to transmit *B. canis*.

Babesia c. canis, *B. c. vogeli*, and *B. gibsoni* all result in mild clinical disease, whereas *B. c. rossi* results in severe clinical disease and will be the focus of this section. Canine babesiosis can be clinically classified into uncomplicated and complicated forms.[15] Uncomplicated cases typically present with signs relating to acute hemolysis, including fever, anorexia, depression, pale mucous membranes, splenomegaly, and a waterhammer pulse. This form is further divided into mild, moderate, or severe disease, according to the severity of the anemia. The complicated form of babesiosis refers to clinical manifestations that include acute renal failure, neurologic dysfunction, coagulopathies, liver dysfunction, acute respiratory distress syndrome, myocarditis, hypotension, and pancreatitis. Rare complications include myalgia, ocular involvement, upper respiratory signs, necrosis of the extremities, and fluid accumulation.[16]

The primary hematologic abnormalities are anemia, thrombocytopenia, and leukocytosis. Alterations in biochemical parameters will vary depending on the severity of the case. Typically, uncomplicated cases can have no biochemical changes. However, elevated liver enzymes, hypokalemia in more severely affected cases, and elevated serum urea with a normal serum creatinine may be evident. In the complicated case, biochemical changes will reflect the underlying complication.[16]

The diagnosis of babesiosis is made by demonstrating *Babesia* organisms (2- × 5-μm, pear-shaped organisms, usually in pairs) within infected erythrocytes on a blood smear stained with a Romanowsky-type stain.

The primary therapeutic aim in the treatment of babesiosis is the reversal of life-threatening anemia via blood transfusions and elimination or suppression of the parasite with specific antibabesial drugs such as diminazene aceturate and imidocarb. Mild-to-moderate, uncomplicated cases require only antibabesial therapy; severe uncomplicated cases require antibabesial therapy as well as blood transfusions; whereas the complicated forms of the disease require additional therapy aimed at treating the complication present.[14,16]

FELINE BABESIOSIS

Feline babesiosis is caused by *B. felis*, which is a small *Babesia* parasite that, although it has been reported in France, Germany, Thailand, and Zimbabwe, only appears to cause clinical disease in South Africa.[17] Recently a *B. canis* organism has been identified from a cat, which on PCR was markedly different from the three recognized subspecies of *B. canis*. This novel feline genotype has been proposed to be a new subspecies, named *B. canis* subsp. *presentii*.[18]

Common clinical signs include anorexia, weight loss, and anemia. Less common signs can include icterus, vomition, pica, and respiratory signs. The disease can be protracted and often clinically silent until fairly far advanced. Anemia is the most consistent hematologic finding, whereas white cell and thrombocyte counts are variable and inconsistent. The most remarkable changes on serum biochemistry are elevated ALT activity and hyperbilirubinuria. Other biochemical parameters are generally variable and inconsistent.[17]

The diagnosis of babesiosis is made by demonstrating *Babesia* organisms within infected erythrocytes on a blood smear stained with a Romanowsky-type stain.

The drug of choice for feline babesiosis is the antimalarial drug primaquine phosphate given orally at 1 mg per cat every 36 hours for four treatments, then 1 mg per cat every 7 days for four treatments. The drug does not sterilize the infection. Another drug that reportedly has some effect is doxycycline given at 5 mg/kg twice a day for 21 days.[14]

AFRICAN TRYPANOSOMIASES

Trypanosomiasis is a hemoparasitic protozoal disease that in the dog is caused by either *Trypanosoma brucei* or *T. congolense*.[19] Disease transmission is by the tsetse fly although dogs may become infected by eating infected fresh meat.[20]

Relapsing fever, anemia, weakness, anorexia, and emaciation are common clinical signs. Other clinical signs include anasarca, conjunctivitis, keratitis, and occasionally neurologic signs (depression, incoordination, circling, and paralysis).[20] In untreated cases, death may occur in 1 week to 3 months.

The diagnosis is made by the direct visualization of parasites on blood smear evaluation. Indirect FA and ELISA methods and species-specific monoclonal antibodies can also be utilized in the diagnosis.[21] Hematologic changes include regenerative anemia, leukopenia, and thrombocytopenia.[19]

There are few drugs that are effective against African trypanosomiases; however, drugs that have been used include diminazine (most effective), difluoromethylornithine, ethidium, isometamidium, and quinapyramin.[19,20]

SARCOCYSTOSIS

Sarcocystosis is a protozoal disease caused by the genus *Sarcocystis*.[22] The dog and cat are the definitive host with cattle, sheep, and pigs being the intermediate host. When the dog or cat ingests meat containing sarcocysts, bradyzoites develop into macrogametocytes and microgametocytes in the epithelial and goblet cells of the intestine. Oocysts then form that sporulate, in situ, within the intestinal wall and are released into the intestinal lumen, where they leave the host via the feces. Infection with Sarcocystosis in the dog and cats is usually asymptomatic but acute to chronic diarrhea may occur.

In the dog and cat the diagnosis is made by finding the small sporocysts in the feces, using a supersaturated sodium chloride solution. Potentiated sulphonamides can be used in the dog and cat to eliminate the intestinal infection.[22]

HYALOMMA TICK BITE NECROSIS

Skin necrosis induced by the bite of the *Hyalomma* tick is a common disease of Southern Africa. The dermatrophic skin necrosis is thought to be a cytotoxic toxin produced in the salivary gland of the tick.[23] The initial stage the disease is characterized by severe pain at the site of the tick attachment. This is followed by erythema and edema at the site of the tick bite. Full thickness skin necrosis then follows. The size of the necrotic area can vary from 5 to 30 cm and appears to be directly related to the length of time that the tick was attached.

The diagnosis is based on clinical signs and the presence of the *Hyalomma* tick(s). Treatment is removing the tick and general principles of wound management.

Cordylobia anthropophaga

The larvae of the *tumbu* or mango fly (*Cordylobia anthropophaga*) result in myiasis in man and animals in sub-Saharan Africa. The adult fly deposits the eggs on the skin that is usually soiled with either urine or feces. Within 2 days the larvae hatch and penetrate the skin to form a furuncular lesion, where they complete development and pupate after 8 to 9 days. The whole life cycle can be completed in less than 4 weeks.[24]

The larvae develop under the skin and produce a painful swelling with a small central opening. The larvae are obligate parasites and usually provoke a localized furuncle but aberrant migrating larvae may result in necrotic and inflammatory lesions in many tissues.[25]

Therapy includes mechanical removal of the larvae, covering the breathing hole in the skin with petroleum jelly, or the use of systemic avermectin drugs. Prevention is by grooming, good hygiene, and the use of topical insecticidal shampoos and repellants.

SPIROCERCOSIS

Spirocerca lupi is a nematode parasite of carnivores, found primarily in dogs but can also occur in numerous wild carnivores.[26,27] Spirocercosis occurs throughout the world, having a tropical and subtropical distribution, although there are colder regions with a high incidence.[26,27] Infection depends upon canine population density and the degree of contact between definitive, intermediate, and transport hosts.[26] The adult parasite is most commonly found embedded in a nodule in the host's thoracic esophagus, although it can occur in other parts of the body.[26] In the esophagus the adult worm passes larvated eggs into the lumen that hatch only after having been ingested by an intermediate host (coprophagous beetles).[26,27] A transport host (birds, amphibians, reptiles, and small mammals) can become infected if they ingest the intermediate host.[26]

The definitive host becomes infected by ingestion of either the intermediate or transport host. Once ingested, the larvae are liberated in the stomach. From there they penetrate the stomach wall, enter an arteriole, and then migrate in the wall of the gastric and gastric-epiploic arteries to the celiac artery and then to the thoracic aorta. From the aorta, the larvae emerge and migrate to the adjacent esophagus. This process takes approximately 6 months.[26,27] The pathology of spirocercosis results from larval migration, presence of adult worms

in granulomas in the esophagus, and secondary bacterial infections.[26] In some cases, the esophageal granuloma can undergo malignant transformation to form a sarcoma, with and without metastases.[26]

Clinical signs of spirocercosis include vomition, regurgitation, weight loss, salivation, and dysphagia.[26] Aortic infection is asymptomatic, unless rupture occurs, whereupon hemothorax and sudden death may occur. Diagnosis is based on survey and contrast radiographs, esophagoscopy, and finding larvated eggs on fecal flotation.[26,27] The latter is, however, not a common finding, as the adult female can only shed eggs if there is an opening in the granuloma and the eggs are also only shed for an unpredictable short period of time.[26] As the eggs are heavier than other helminth eggs, a flotation fluid of higher specific gravity is also required. Doramectin has been shown to be effective in the therapy of spirocercosis.[26,28]

It has been speculated that in endemic areas the incidence of infection can be 100%, which is probably associated with the many opportunities of acquiring infection from the various intermediate and transport hosts.

REFERENCES

The reference list can be found on the companion Expert Consult Web site at *www.expertconsult.com*.

CHAPTER 222

Zoonotic Disease Problems

Karen Ehnert

In the United States, nearly 60 percent of all households owned at least one pet in 2006. Cats and dogs are the most commonly owned pets.[1] Pet ownership has been shown to have many positive health benefits, such as lowering blood pressure, reducing depression, and moderating stress.[2] Children raised with pets had improved social development, including better nonverbal communication and social competence.[2] While most pets are primarily kept for companionship, dogs may be trained to assist disabled people or to aid in hunting, herding, tracking, or guarding. However, there is some risk associated with pet ownership. An estimated 4.7 million people are bitten by dogs each year (>360,000 were treated in emergency rooms in 2001).[3] In addition, it is estimated that there are approximately 4 million pet-derived infections occurring in the United States annually.[4] Veterinarians and their staff play key roles in reducing the risk of pet-associated zoonoses (diseases people contract from animals) in the hospital, the home, and the community at large, through the adoption of standardized infection-control precautions,[5] encouraging appropriate pet preventive care,[6,7] and education.

Zoonoses may be contracted from dogs and cats through exposure to their feces, parturient fluids, saliva, respiratory secretions, scratches, skin, fur, urine, or external parasites (Table 222-1). Infections may be parasitic, bacterial, fungal, or viral. However, only a few are fairly common. Dermatophytosis (ringworm) is probably one of the most recognized pet-associated zoonoses, with an estimated 2 million or more

human infections each year.[4] Approximately 200,000 people develop campylobacteriosis yearly after contact with pets,[4] and over 22,000 develop cat scratch disease.[8] Less obvious are the subclinical parasitic infections. Approximately 1% to 2% of the population is infected by *Toxoplasma gondii* each year, but few show symptoms.[9] A recent Centers for Disease Control and Prevention sero survey indicates that approximately 23 percent of Americans have been exposed to *T. gondii* and 14 percent to *Toxocara* spp.[10] *T. gondii* infection during pregnancy results in approximately 3000 cases of congenital toxoplasmosis each year, with some babies developing microcephaly, hydrocephalus, seizures, or mental retardation.[9] There are an estimated 10,000 cases of visceral larval migrans and 700 of ocular larval migrans annually caused by *Toxocara* spp.[9] Whether the infection is clinical or subclinical, action should be taken to reduce the spread of pet-associated zoonotic diseases.

SOURCE OF INFECTION: FECES

Dog and cat feces may contain a wide variety of zoonotic agents, both parasitic and bacterial. Frequently the pet is asymptomatic, providing no outward indication that it is harboring a zoonotic infection (see Table 222-1). The prevalence of enteric pathogens may vary by region and by the pet's age.[11-19] *Ancyclostoma* spp., *Giardia intestinalis*, and *Trichuris vulpis* are more common in warm climates, while *Toxocara*

Table • 222-1

Potential Zoonoses from Dogs and Cats, by Source of Infection

AGENT/DISEASE	ANIMAL	SYMPTOMS IN ANIMALS	SYMPTOMS IN HUMANS	FOR MORE INFO:
Source of Infection: Feces				
Ancylostoma spp. (Cutaneous larva migrans)	dog, cat	Diarrhea, pale pink gums, weight loss	Pruritic, raised, reddened tract caused by larval migration in skin	Ch. 270, 271
Campylobacter jejuni (Campylobacteriosis)	dog, cat	Asymptomatic, or diarrhea, anorexia, fever	Diarrhea, fever, abdominal discomfort, enterocolitis	Ch. 270
Cryptosporidium spp. (Cryptosporidiosis)	dog, cat	Asymptomatic, or diarrhea in immunocompromised	Asymptomatic, or diarrhea, severe illness in immunocompromised individuals, including death	Ch. 207
Giardia intestinalis (Giardiasis)	dog, cat	Asymptomatic, or acute, chronic or intermittent diarrhea, flatulence, weight loss, poor hair coat	Asymptomatic, or diarrhea, abdominal cramps, bloating, flatulence, nausea, fatigue	Ch. 207
Salmonella spp. (Salmonellosis)	dog, cat	Asymptomatic, or diarrhea, abdominal pain, fever, dehydration and shock	Diarrhea, fever, abdominal cramping	Ch. 270, 271
Toxocara spp. (Larva migrans)	dog, cat	Asymptomatic, or vomiting, anorexia and weight loss	Asymptomatic, or eosinophilia, malaise, fever, hepatomegaly, abdominal discomfort, vision loss	Ch 270
Toxoplasma gondii (Toxoplasmasis)	cat	Asymptomatic, or rarely self-limiting diarrhea after primary exposure	Asymptomatic, or mild flulike illness, abortion, birth defects, brain infection and death in immunocompromised individuals	Ch. 207
Trichuris vulpis (Trichuriasis)	dog	Asymptomatic, or poor condition, diarrhea, weight loss	Asymptomatic, or abdominal pain, diarrhea, rectal prolapse	Ch. 271
Source of Infection: Parturient Fluids				
Brucella canis (Brucellosis)	dog	Asymptomatic, or abortions, stillbirths, abnormal sperm, lymphadenitis, discospondylitis	Asymptomatic, or febrile illness with nonspecific flulike signs which may wax and wane, more serious symptoms may occur depending on organs infected	Ch. 201
Coxiella burnetti (Q fever)	dog, cat	Asymptomatic, or late term abortions	Febrile illness, endocarditis	
Source of Infection: Saliva/Respiratory				
Bartonella henselae (via bite) (Cat scratch disease)	cat	Usually asymptomatic	Rash, blister or ulcer at wound site, followed by lymphadenopathy	Ch. 205
Bordetella bronchiseptica (Bordetellosis)	dog, cat	Harsh cough, +/− retching, fever, anorexia, nasal or ocular discharge	Cough, +/− pneumonia in immunocompromised individuals	Ch. 228
Capnocytophaga canimorsus (via bite)	dog, cat	Asymptomatic	Septicemia	
Francisella tularensis (via bite) (Tularemia)	cat	Anorexia, vomiting, weight loss	Fever, chills, headache, malaise, lymphadenopathy	
Pasteurella spp. (via bite) (Pasteurellosis)	dog, cat	Asymptomatic	Wound infection	
Lyssavirus serotype 1 (via bite) (Rabies)	dog, cat	Behavioral change, restless, paralysis of limbs, difficulty swallowing, drooling, voice change, coma, death	Pain or itching at bite site, anxiety, confusion, headache, abnormal behavior, difficulty swallowing, coma, death	Ch. 215
Yersinia pestis (Plague)	cat	Fever, lymphadenopathy, abscesses in internal organs, pneumonia	Lymphadenitis, pneumonia, septicemia	Ch. 230

Table • 222-1

Potential Zoonoses from Dogs and Cats, by Source of Infection—cont'd

AGENT/DISEASE	ANIMAL	SYMPTOMS IN ANIMALS	SYMPTOMS IN HUMANS	FOR MORE INFO:
Source of Infection: Scratch				
Bartonella henselae (Cat scratch disease)	cat	Usually asymptomatic	Rash, blister or ulcer at wound site, followed by lymphadenopathy	Ch. 205
Source of Infection: Skin/Fur				
Methicillin-resistant *Staphylococcus aureus* (MRSA)	dog, cat	Asymptomatic, or various skin or wound infections	Asymptomatic, or various skin or soft tissue infections, including impetigo, folliculitis, furunculosis, cellulitis, abscesses, wound infection	
Microsporum spp. and *Trichophyton* spp. (Dermatophytosis)	dog, cat	Asymptomatic, or areas of alopecia and crusting, pruritic, reddened	Red, pruritic cutaneous lesions	Ch. 19
Source of Infection: Urine				
Brucella canis (Brucellosis)	dog	Asymptomatic, or abortions, stillbirths, abnormal sperm, lymphadenitis, discospondylitis	Asymptomatic, or febrile illness with nonspecific flulike signs which may wax and wane, more serious symptoms may occur depending on organs infected	Ch. 201
Leptospira spp. (Leptospirosis)	dog	Asymptomatic, or fever, vomiting, abdominal pain, diarrhea, anorexia, weakness, muscle pain	Asymptomatic, or biphasic febrile illness, +/− icterus, may cause acute renal failure	Ch. 198
Source of Infection: External Parasites				
Borrelia burgdorferi (via ticks) (Lyme disease)	dog	Lameness which may be intermittent or shifting between legs, joint pain, +/− fever	Large circular rash, joint pain, swollen joints, occasionally neurologic or cardiac symptoms	Ch. 199
Cheyletiella (Cheyletiellosis)	dog, cat	Large scales, crusts, seborrhea, alopecia, dermatitis	Red, pruritic, self-limiting rash	Ch. 15
Francisella tularensis (via ticks) (Tularemia)	dog, cat	Anorexia, vomiting, weight loss	Fever, chills, headache, malaise, lymphadenopathy	
Rickettsia rickettsii (via ticks) (Rocky Mountain spotted fever)	dog	Fever, lymphadenopathy, cough, diarrhea, vomiting, joint or muscle pain, occasionally neurological symptoms	Febrile illness, rash that starts on arms and ankles and moves to palms and soles of feet	
Rickettsia typhi (via fleas) (Murine typhus)	cat	Asymptomatic	Febrile illness	
Sarcoptes scabiei or *Notoedres cati* (Scabies)	dog, cat	Crusts, scales, erythema, pruritis, alopecia, exudation	Pruritic, erythematous skin lesions	Ch. 15
Yersinia pestis (via fleas) (Plague)	cat	Fever, lymphadenopathy, abscesses in internal organs, pneumonia	Lymphadenitis, pneumonia, septicemia	Ch. 230

spp. are found worldwide.[11,20-22] In humans, cutaneous larval migrans, caused by *Ancyclostoma* spp., is more geographically restricted than is *T. gondii* and *Toxocara* spp. and tends to be seen in the Southern states.[11]

Ancyclostoma braziliense, a hookworm of both dogs and cats, is the primary cause of cutaneous larval migrans (CLM) in people.[11] Less often, *Ancyclostoma caninum* or *Uncinaria*

stenocephala cause CLM, and *A. caninum* may cause eosinophilic enteritis in people. Pets become infected after consuming infective larvae in the environment, from the colostrum or milk of infected bitches *(A. caninum)*, or through larval invasion of the skin *(A. caninum* or *A. braziliense)*. Dogs and cats may then begin shedding eggs in their feces 15 to 20 days after infection. Eggs complete embryonation and hatch in 24 to 72 hours on warm, moist soil. Pet infections with *A. caninum* may cause anemia and bloody diarrhea, while infections with *A. braziliense* and *U. stenocephala* are less severe.

Cryptosporidium parvum, an obligate intracellular coccidian parasite, may infect any mammal but is rarely seen in dogs and cats.[23] Dogs are usually infected with *Cryptosporidium canis* and cats with *Cryptosporidium felis*, while humans are generally infected with *C. parvum* or *C. hominis*.[24] However, *C. canis* and *C. felis* infections have occasionally been reported in immunocompromised individuals[25-27] and rarely in healthy children.[24,28] Infected pets are generally asymptomatic, while infected immunocompromised individuals may develop severe diarrhea.

Giardiasis, a protozoal parasitic disease, is fairly common in dogs and cats.[20] A recent nationwide survey of ill dogs and cats presenting at clinics demonstrated that 15.6% of the dogs and 10.8% of the cats were positive for *Giardia*.[12] However, not all *Giardia* is of equal risk to people. Recent DNA sequencing of *G. intestinalis* has shown that there are several different assemblages or genotypes—A and B (zoonotic), C and D (dogs), E (livestock), F (cats), and G (rodents).[29] Genotypic surveys around the world have demonstrated that a significant proportion of dogs are carrying zoonotic *Giardia* (assemblage A),[30-33] and tests have shown that human *Giardia* isolates are able to infect dogs without causing clinical signs.[34] With genotypic identification not generally available, practitioners must consider infected pets as potentially infectious to people.

Toxocara infections are common, especially in puppies and kittens. *Toxocara canis* is transmitted to puppies in utero, while *Toxocara cati* is transmitted to kittens through the milk or colostrum.[18,22] Puppies can excrete a large number of *T. canis* eggs from 3 weeks to 3 months of age, and cats shed numerous *T. cati* eggs between 2 and 6 months of age.[22] The eggs become embryonated and infectious after 9 to 35 days in the environment. However, larvae do not develop at temperatures below 10° C, and will die at temperatures below −15° C.[22] Older dogs and cats become infected after they ingest embryonated eggs. Humans become infected through accidental ingestion of the embryonated eggs, but do not develop a patent infection. Most human infection is asymptomatic, but symptoms may develop if the larvae migrates to the liver and lungs (visceral larval migrans) or the eyes (ocular larval migrans).[4]

Cats are the definitive host for *T. gondii*, an obligate intracellular protozoan parasite.[35] Although the parasite can undergo asexual reproduction in all species, it can only complete sexual reproduction in cats. Infected cats usually shed oocysts for 1 to 2 weeks, and the oocyst sporulates in the environment after 1 day to several weeks. The oocysts are highly resistant to environmental conditions and can survive for over a year in warm, moist soils. Other animals or humans become infected by accidentally consuming the sporulated oocysts or through consumption of infected tissue (e.g., raw/undercooked meat).[4]

Trichuris vulpis, the whipworm of dogs, can occasionally infect humans; however, most infections are asymptomatic.[21] *Trichuris* eggs are not immediately infectious when excreted, but must develop for 2 weeks or longer to first stage larva. The infectious eggs can remain viable for years under ideal conditions. Dogs, and people become infected after consuming an infectious egg.

Dog and cat feces may also contain *Campylobacter* or *Salmonella* spp. that pose a risk to humans.[17,36-38] Exposure to diarrheic animals has been associated with a fourfold increase in the risk of *Campylobacter jejuni* or *Campylobacter coli* enteritis.[36] Outbreaks of multidrug resistant *Salmonella typhimurium* has been reported in veterinary clinics that treated infected dogs and cats.[37,38] Infected animals are not always symptomatic,[17,38] so good hygiene is needed with all animals and when handling their feces.

SOURCE OF INFECTION: PARTURIENT FLUIDS/URINE

Parturient fluids of pets may be contaminated with *Brucella canis*[39] or *Coxiella burnetii*.[40] Humans may become infected with *B. canis* through ingestion or contamination of the mucous membranes with organisms shed in the parturient fluids, vaginal discharge, semen, or urine of infected dogs, but reports of human infection are rare.[41,42] However, human infections with *B. canis* can be difficult to diagnose, so the disease may be underreported.[39,41] *C. burnetii* may infect either dogs or cats,[40,43] and may result in stillbirths or weak offspring. Human infections, including several outbreaks, have been reported in those that had contact with parturient pets.[44-46] Thus, care should be taken when handling parturient fluids, placenta, and fetuses after pets give birth to minimize possible exposure.

Leptospira spp. are shed in the urine of infected animals and have the potential to infect others through aerosolized urine or contaminated water, direct contact with skin, or ingestion of contaminated food or water.[47] Canine leptospirosis cases have been increasing since 1983,[48-50] with seropositivity greatest in the midwest, south-central and northwest regions of the United States.[50] The most common serovars detected recently are *autumnalis*, *grippotyphosa*, *bratislava*, and *pomona*.[50] The initial symptoms are generally nonspecific, and may include fever, depression, anorexia, myalgia, stiffness, and weakness. These symptoms may be followed by evidence of kidney disease, including increased urination, anuria, hematuria, vomiting, dehydration, and oral ulcers. Direct dog to human spread has been reported rarely[51]; however, individuals still should take care to minimize direct contact with, or aerosolization of, dog urine to reduce risk of this disease.

SOURCE OF INFECTION: SALIVA/RESPIRATORY/SCRATCH

Animal bites pose a risk to people, both through injury and infection. *Pasteurella* spp. and *Capnocytophaga canimorsus* are part of the normal flora in the mouths of dogs and cats, and human infection may be caused through a bite, scratch, or lick from a pet.[4,9,52-55] Cat bites are reported to cause more wound infections than dog bites, and infections from both tend to have a mixture of bacteria.[52] *Pasteurella* spp. are isolated most frequently from animal bite wounds, with *Pasteurella canis* being transmitted through dog bites and *Pasteurella multocida* from cat bites.[52,53] *C. canimorsus* infection following a bite is seen less often, but is much more serious, causing fulminant sepsis, endocarditis, meningitis, and even death.[54-56] Occasionally, *Francisella tularensis* has been reported to have been transmitted by a cat bite,[57,58] but this infection is most often spread to people through ticks (including *Dermacentor andersoni*, *D. variabilis*, and *Amblyomma americanum*), biting flies, or direct contact with infected animals, such as rabbits.[59] Individuals may develop cat scratch disease, caused by *Bartonella henselae*, following a scratch, or occasionally a bite, from a cat.[8,9,60] The presence of cat fleas (*Ctenocephalides felis*) is essential for the maintenance of *B. henselae* infection in cat populations, and the spread of infection between cats is reduced or absent when appropriate flea control measures are taken.[8,60] The probable source of human infection is infected flea feces contaminating the cat's claws or teeth. Generally kittens under 1 year old represent a higher risk for disease transmission.[9]

Table • 222-2

Standard Precautions to Minimize Zoonoses Risk

Individual Precautions (HABIT)

Hygiene	• Hand-washing after handling patients, body fluids/excretions, laboratory specimens, cleaning cages, and removing gloves • Use antibacterial gel when unable to wash hands. • Only consume food and beverages in nonanimal or laboratory areas
Animal restraint	• Appropriate animal restraint techniques should be employed by sufficient staff to control the animal • Gloves, muzzles, cat bags, and other restraint materials should be used when necessary to reduce risk of bites • Animals may need to be tranquilized or anesthetized to minimize risk to staff and the patient
Barrier protection	• Wear gloves when there is a potential for contact with contaminated material or an infectious animal • Wear laboratory coat, scrub top, or disposable gown, which may be removed if contaminated • Wear mask and eye protection is there is a risk of infectious aerosols or eye splash
Immunization and treatment	• Staff should be preimmunized against rabies and tetanus • Ill staff should seek medical treatment as soon as possible, and inform physician of potential exposures
Training in appropriate procedures	• Develop clinic infection control manual • Train staff about zoonoses and methods to reduce risk • Verify staff are following policies • Retrain and refresh policies as needed

Environmental Precautions (CLEAN)

Clean and disinfect	• Clean and disinfect all animal contact surfaces, cages, and runs at least daily • Clean and disinfect all potentially contaminated instruments before reuse • Clean soiled bedding promptly, ensuring that the area is not contaminated when the bedding is taken to the laundry area • Clean and disinfect food and water bowls daily for hospitalized patients • Clean and disinfect tables between patients • Clean up any animal waste or urination in reception, exam rooms and treatment areas immediately
Limit traffic	• Create appropriate traffic patterns within the hospital that minimize the potential spread of diseases • Limit public access to animal treatment areas

Environmental Precautions (CLEAN)—cont'd

	• Limit areas of hospital accessed by delivery people • Minimize animal movement between front and back area of hospital • Restrict access to surgery and isolation areas. Ensure hospital pet does not have access to these areas.
Environmental decontamination	• Immediately clean up any potential infectious materials and dispose of properly • Properly dispose needles and other sharps in appropriate containers • Clean up feces around hospital, including in front, on a daily basis
Animal isolation	• Isolate potentially infectious animals. Immediately take potentially infectious animals into an exam room upon arrival at clinic. Hospitalized infectious patients should be held in an isolation room. • Staff need to use appropriate barrier protection to minimize their risk and the potential for them to spread the infection • Foot baths may be used to disinfect shoes after leaving a potentially contaminated area. Change foot bath daily.
Nature control	• Develop and implement a good rodent and vector control plan • Seal any potential rodent or insect entrances points. Ensure window screens are in good condition. • Store all food in rodent-proof containers • Remove any standing water sources around building • Do not leave food out that may attract rodents and insects

Animal Precautions (VIP)

Vaccinate	• Vaccinate dogs and cats against rabies • Other vaccinations (*Leptospirosis, Bordetella, Giardia*) should be used depending on local risk
Insect control	• Recommend flea and tick control for all patients • Treat any hospitalized patients for fleas or ticks if present
Parasite control	• Treat puppies and kittens for internal parasites 3-4 times on a biweekly schedule and test for intestinal parasites 2-4 times in first year of life • Conduct fecal exams on adult dogs and cats 1-2 times a year • Treat infected patients with an appropriate parasiticide • Consider year-round preventive treatment, possibly in combination with heartworm medication

Rabies is one of the most serious infections that can be transmitted by dog or cat bites, since the infection is almost always fatal if postexposure prophylaxis is not given shortly after a person is bitten.[61] Improved canine rabies vaccination programs and stray animal control during the last century led to a marked decrease in the number of domestic animal rabies cases in the United States.[62] Now most pets are infected through contact with infected wildlife. In 2006, there were 79 dogs and 318 cats diagnosed with rabies in the United States.[63] Because the number of cat rabies cases now exceed that of dogs, it is now recommended that cat rabies vaccination be required as it is for dogs.[62]

Rarely, people may contract respiratory infections from pets. *Bordetella bronchiseptica* infection has been occasionally reported in immunocompromised individuals, primarily following contact with infected dogs.[64-67] Individuals have also contracted plague from infected cats, through bites, scratches, direct contact, and inhalation.[68,69] Between 1977 and 1998, 23 individuals contracted plague in the United States following contact with cats (including 4 veterinarians and 1 veterinary technician), and 5 of them died.[68] Plague may also be transmitted by fleas, so appropriate isolation procedures and flea control are needed to reduce the risk of this disease.

SOURCE OF INFECTION: SKIN/FUR

Dermatophytosis, or ringworm, is one of the most common zoonotic infections seen in small animal practice. Dogs and cats are usually infected with *Microsporum canis*, but may also be infected with *Microsporum gypseum* or *Trichophyton mentagrophytes*.[70,71] The disease primarily affects puppies and kittens, and is usually self-limiting. Symptoms generally include areas of alopecia, scaling, and crusting. Some cats are asymptomatic carriers, serving as a difficult-to-detect source of infection. Infection is spread through contact with arthrospores or conidia, via contact with an infected animal, contact with infected hair or skin scales, or through contaminated fomites, such as brushes and clippers. Spores spread through the environment, and have been found in homes of infected animals[72] and in veterinary clinics.[73] The spores may be removed from the environment by vacuuming and disinfection. The spores are susceptible to dilute (1:10) chlorine bleach, benzalkonium chloride, and strong detergents.[70]

Methicillin-resistant *Staphylococcus aureus* (MRSA) has emerged as an important pathogen in human medicine and is now impacting the veterinary community.[74-81] Both humans and pets may be colonized with the organism, with human-to-animal and animal-to-human transmission occurring. MRSA has been increasing in animals and is frequently cultured form canine wounds, abscesses, and chronic pyodermas.[82] Not only might pets carry this bacteria without symptoms, but they may serve as a reservoir for home infection. Good infection control procedures are needed to reduce the spread.[82]

SOURCE OF INFECTION: EXTERNAL PARASITES

External parasites on pets may transmit a variety of infectious agents to people or may directly cause irritation and skin lesions by infesting the skin. Ticks may carry organisms that can cause Lyme disease,[83] tularemia,[59] and Rocky Mountain spotted fever,[84] while fleas may spread cat scratch disease,[60] murine typhus,[85] or plague.[69] The risk of infection varies by geographic location, but year-round appropriate flea and tick control are recommended to reduce the risk of vector-borne diseases to pets and owners.[6]

Scabies and *Cheyletiella* mites pose some risk to pet owners and veterinary staff.[86-88] The mites may infest the skin of people who have contact with infected pets, causing pruritic, erythematous lesions. However, the mites cannot complete their life cycle on humans, so the infections are self-limiting. People have an obligate scabies mite (*Sarcoptes scabiei* var. *hominis*). Treatment may be necessary to reduce the pruritus or if secondary bacterial infection occurs.

VETERINARY STANDARD PRECAUTIONS

Veterinarians, veterinary staff, and pet owners can minimize the risk of contracting zoonotic infections from pets by following the veterinary standard precautions, which cover the individual, environment and pet (Table 222-2).[5-7,62] Individuals should develop good habits, including proper hygiene, animal restraint, barrier protection, immunizations, and staff training. Appropriate hand washing (20 seconds with warm soapy water) after contact with infectious animals, fluids, secretions, equipment, or articles will greatly reduce zoonotic risk. In addition, control of the environment, both inside and outside of the hospital, is key to infection control. The hospital must be kept clean, with animal waste and potentially infectious material being removed promptly and areas disinfected appropriately. Potentially infectious animals should be isolated quickly to reduce chance of disease spread. Since staff and other hospital visitors may spread infectious material on their shoes and clothing, it also important to limit traffic through the hospital, especially in isolation and treatment areas. Good rodent and vector control will reduce the chance of additional diseases being brought into the hospital by unwanted pests. Finally, a good preventive program for pets visiting your practice will substantially reduce risk of zoonoses, both in the hospital and in the community. Both dogs and cats should be vaccinated against rabies,[5] and other diseases depending on local risk. Pets should be on year-round flea and tick control, as well as preventive anthelmintic treatment.[6,7] The pet's feces should be checked for parasites, 3 to 4 times annually when they are young, and 1 to 2 times annually thereafter, to ensure the effectiveness of the preventive treatment. Lastly, pet owners need to be educated regarding the importance of proper pet feces disposal to keeping the community and their families safe. By developing good HABITs, keeping the hospital CLEAN, and treating pets as VIPs, you can reduce the risk of zoonoses in your hospital and community.

REFERENCES

The reference list can be found on the companion Expert Consult Web site at *www.expertconsult.com*.

SECTION XI
Diseases of the Ears, Nose, and Throat

CHAPTER 223

Diseases of the Ear

MaryAnn G. Radlinsky
Diane E. Mason

GENERAL CONCEPTS

Many different disease processes affect otic health and should be considered when evaluating a patient with possible ear disease. Patient signalment may implicate certain diseases over others. The history should include general questions about the animal's health (e.g., appetite, sneezing, coughing, vomiting, diarrhea, water consumption), as well as questions pertaining to primary conditions associated with ear disease. The ear is a specialized extension of the integumentary system, so a complete dermatologic history should be obtained (i.e., appearance of lesions at the onset of the condition, duration, progression, past medical therapy and response to therapy, and the presence of other dermatologic problems). A complete physical examination should be performed, and special attention paid to the skin as to the possibility of hypersensitivities, disorders of keratinization, endocrine disorders, and other dermatologic conditions. A complete neurologic examination may reveal abnormalities associated with the middle ear (e.g., abnormalities of cranial nerves VII and VIII, Horner's syndrome, keratoconjunctivitis sicca, and head tilt). Involvement of the inner ear results in other neurologic signs (e.g., head tilt, ataxia, strabismus, abnormal nystagmus), and differentiation from central vestibular disease is extremely important.

Specific examination of the ear includes evaluation of the concave and convex pinnal surfaces, palpation of the ear canals, and otoscopic examination. Abnormalities include pain upon palpation of the auricular cartilages, nonpliable cartilage, ossified cartilage, epithelial hyperemia, swelling, erosion, ulceration, exudate accumulation, and hyperemia or lack of transparency of the tympanic membrane. Pain upon opening the mouth is not specific to but can occur with ear disease. Other diagnostic tests should include cytologic examination of otic exudate and culture and susceptibility testing based on the cytology and clinical signs of the patient. Skull radiographs, computed tomography (CT), and magnetic resonance imaging (MRI) may be indicated for evaluation of the middle and inner ear. Specific diagnostic tests are available to evaluate tympanic membrane integrity, and one should not assume that the tympanic membrane is intact prior to initiation of medical therapy, including ear cleaning, which may cause immediate exposure of the middle ear to ototoxic substances.

DISEASES OF THE PINNA

Many different disease conditions can affect the pinna, some are specific to the pinna, and others represent distribution of part of a systemic condition (Box 223-1).

NONPRURITIC PINNAL ALOPECIA

Canine Pinnal Alopecia
Canine pinnal alopecia is most commonly diagnosed in Dachshunds but also occurs in Chihuahuas, Boston Terriers, Whippets, Yorkshire Terriers, and Italian Greyhounds.[1,2] The condition usually occurs in dogs older than 1 year of age and results in slowly, progressive, bilateral pinnal alopecia. Small vellus hairs remain, and complete alopecia, when it occurs, may be present at 8 to 9 years of age. The pinna may become chronically hyperpigmented and thickened. The condition is benign and requires no specific treatment; differentiation from other alopecic conditions is by exclusion and histopathologic examination. Minoxidil, pentoxifylline, melatonin, and milbolerone have anecdotally been reported to induce hair growth in some cases.[2]

Periodic Alopecia of Miniature Poodles and Siamese Cats
Hair loss is usually adult-onset and acute with both periodic alopecia of Miniature Poodles and Siamese cats. Progression of the condition may result in complete, bilateral, pinnal alopecia; however, in cats the alopecia may be patchy or complete.[1,2] The skin appears grossly normal. The pathophysiology of the condition is not known, no treatment has been described, and the hair may regrow over a period of several months.

Pattern Baldness
Symmetric alopecia or hypotrichosis of the pinnae, ventrum, and caudal or medial thigh has been recognized in the Dachshund and Staffordshire Bull Terrier.[3] Hair loss begins with the pinna at 6 to 9 months of age and may progress to complete pinnal alopecia. Total body alopecia with pigmentation may occur with age. Treatment with oral melatonin may cause hair regrowth with this and other pattern baldness syndromes.[2]

Box • 223-1

Disease Conditions Affecting the Pinna

Nonpruritic Alopecia

Canine

Periodic alopecia of Miniature Poodles	Color dilution alopecia	Pattern baldness
Pinnal alopecia of short-coated breeds	Alopecia areata	Demodicosis
Idiopathic follicular dysplasia	Congenital alopecia	Drug eruption
Congenital hypotrichosis	Dermatophytosis	Hypothyroidism
Estrogen-responsive dermatosis	Ectodermal defects	

Feline

Idiopathic pinnal alopecia	Dermatophytosis	Demodicosis
Iatrogenic hypothyroidism	Congenital hypotrichosis	Alopecia areata
Iatrogenic hyperadrenocorticism	Hyperthyroidism	

Crusting and Scaling Dermatoses

Canine

Fly strike dermatitis	Frostbite	Sarcoptic mange
Proliferative thrombovascular necrosis	Demodicosis	Harvest mites
Zinc-responsive dermatosis	Pemphigus complex	Vasculitis
Idiopathic hyperkeratosis of Boston Terriers	Ear margin dermatosis	Sebaceous adenitis
Idiopathic lymphocytic/plasmacytic dermatitis	Lupoid dermatosis	Ear fissures
Idiopathic lichenoid keratosis	Superficial necrolytic dermatitis	Hypothyroidism
Lichenoid psoriaform dermatosis	Dermatomyositis	Pediculosis
Cold agglutinin disease	Systemic lupus erythematosus	Leishmania

Feline

Squamous cell carcinoma	Actinic dermatitis	Notoedric mange
Insect bite hypersensitivity	Frostbite	Vasculitis
Pemphigus complex		

Papular and Nodular Dermatoses

Canine and Feline

Leproid granuloma (canine)	Neoplasia	Bacterial pyoderma
Sterile nodular histiocytic granuloma (canine)	Deep mycoses	Leishmania
Eosinophilic folliculitis, furunculosis (canine)	Foreign body	Dermatophytosis
Eosinophilic granuloma (canine)	Tick infestation	Xanthoma (feline)

Pustular, Vesicular, Bullous Dermatoses

Canine and Feline

Pemphigus foliaceous	Pemphigus erythematosus	Systemic lupus erythematosus
Epidermolysis bullosa	Drug eruption	Contact or irritant dermatitis

Concave Pinnal Disorders

Canine and Feline

Atopy	Allergic contact dermatitis	Hypothyroidism
Sex hormone aberrations	Seborrhea	Juvenile cellulitis
Food sensitivity	Idiopathic erythema/edema (canine)	

Auricular Cartilage Disorders

Canine and Feline

Aural hematoma	Auricular chondritis

Congenital Hypotrichosis

A lack of pelage or loss of hair within the first month after birth has been diagnosed in the Belgian Shepherd, Cocker Spaniel, Toy Poodle, Miniature Poodle, Whippet, German Shepherd Dog, Yorkshire Terrier, Bichon Frise, Lhasa Apso, Labrador Retriever, Rottweiler, and Basset Hound. The condition is seen more commonly in males and usually involves the pinna, temporal region, caudal dorsum, and ventrum. Complete hair loss may occur by 12 to 14 weeks of age. Areas of alopecia may be well delineated from normal skin, and the condition can be diagnosed via skin biopsy.[2] A similar condition exists in Birman, Burmese, Devon Rex, and Siamese cats but involves the entire coat, whiskers, claws, and tongue.

CRUSTING AND SCALING DERMATOSES

Mange

Erythematous, papular dermatitis of the distal pinna associated with significant pruritus is an early manifestation of *Sarcoptes scabiei* in dogs. Crust and scale will usually first affect the tip of the pinna or ear margin. The pinnal-pedal reflex (i.e., rubbing the pinna, resulting in a pelvic limb scratch reflex) is often associated with sarcoptic mange but is not pathognomonic for the condition. Concurrent lesions often involve the lateral hocks and elbows and may spread to the rest of the body. The diagnosis is usually made with skin scrapings; however, multiple scrapings may be necessary to achieve the diagnosis.[3] All animals in the household should be treated, and the condition is zoonotic, so owners and handlers should be made aware of the condition. Initial treatment consists of removal of crusts and debris followed by an acaricidal dip such as lime sulfur, permethrin, organophosphate, or amitraz, which may shorten time to resolution of clinical signs and diminish zoonotic potential. Treatment with ivermectin administered subcutaneously, twice, 14 days apart or orally, three times, 7 days apart results in cure. A similar dose schedule exists for milbemycin. Topical application of selamectin or fipronil may also be curative.[1,2]

Feline mange, caused by *Notoedres cati*, results alopecia, pruritus, excoriations, and thick crusts of the rostral pinna and is usually restricted to the ears and head. The extremities and perineum may also be affected due to the sleeping and grooming habits of cats. The parasite may also inhabit dogs, foxes, and rabbits; transient lesions have been reported in humans.[2] The diagnosis is made with skin scrapings, and lime sulfur or amitraz dips are effective treatments. Ivermectin given two or three times subcutaneously is also an effective treatment.[2]

Fly Strike Dermatitis

Insect bite dermatitis, caused by the stable fly, *Stomoxys calcitrans*, results in serosanguineous, crusting dermatitis of the ear tips in dogs with erect ears or on the folded edge of the pinna in dogs with pendulous ears. Chronic fly strike dermatitis can become granulomatous in nature. The diagnosis is based on an environmental history and response to limiting outdoor exposure. Fly repellents containing permethrin, citronella, or diethyltoluamide (DEET) in petroleum jelly may be used to diminish repeated fly bites. Topical corticosteroid with an antibiotic may hasten the resolution of clinical signs.[1,2] Black flies (*Simulium* species) may also cause papular dermatitis and alopecia in dogs.

Cats can develop a seasonal hypersensitivity to mosquito bites. Papules, erythema, alopecia, and hypopigmentation occur on the pinnae and face. Pyrexia, lymphadenopathy, and footpad lesions may also occur.

Actinic Dermatitis and Squamous Cell Carcinoma

Damage to the skin by long-term exposure to actinic radiation occurs most often in white cats, although the condition is also reported in pigmented cats. The pinna is most often affected due to its sparse hair covering; the nose, lips, and eyelids may be similarly affected. Waxing and waning ear-tip erythema may progress to the development of fine scale and alopecia early in the disease. Erosive, crusted, hemorrhagic lesions and folding of the pinna occur as a precancerous condition, which may ultimately lead to carcinomatous change.[1,2,4] Histopathologic evidence of photodamage included edema and dermal sclerosis without dermal inflammation.[5] Squamous cell carcinoma is most often diagnosed in older cats (mean age, 12.8 years) with either skin scrapings or biopsy.[6]

Treatment of actinic dermatitis ideally consists of limiting sun exposure between the hours of 10 AM and 4 PM by housing indoors and eliminating sunbathing behavior. Application of sunscreen of SPF 15 or greater may also decrease the effects of solar radiation. β-Carotene and canthaxanthin administered orally and the use of retinoic acids (i.e., isotretinoin, etretinate) have also been reported.[1,2] An initial response to therapy may be seen, but effectiveness has not been thoroughly investigated.[7] Strontium plesiotherapy has been used in the treatment of actinic dermatitis. Failure to respond to medical management is an indication for pinnectomy.

Squamous cell carcinoma is usually locally invasive and slow to metastasize to either local lymph nodes or the lung. Pinnectomy is an effective mode of therapy for severe actinic dermatitis and squamous cell carcinoma. Cryosurgery, radiotherapy, brachytherapy, hyperthermic, and photodynamic therapy have also been used on focal lesions; systemic chemotherapy is not considered effective.

Frostbite

Animals affected by frostbite are usually systemically ill or have recently moved to a cold environment. The ear tips are pale, cyanotic, hypoesthetic, and cool to the touch after exposure. With warming, the tissues become hyperemic and develop scale, crust, and alopecia. The ear tips may curl, necrose, and eventually slough. Initial treatment consists of rewarming with warm water and subsequent symptomatic therapy for scaling and crusting dermatitis. Amputation of necrotic tissue results in improved cosmesis with haired skin and decreases the risk of recurrent freezing, which is more likely in previously frostbitten tissue.

Vasculitis

The underlying cause of vasculitis is often unknown but may be due to antigen antibody complex deposition within the vascular wall. The lesions are characterized by erythema, edema, and eventual necrosis and sloughing, leading to a "punched-out" or ulcerated appearance. Other affected areas include the lips, tail, pads, and nails. Conditions such as rickettsial disease, drug eruption, immune-mediated disease, and other underlying systemic conditions should be ruled out. Therapy should be directed at treating at the underlying cause. Idiopathic vasculitis cases may respond to immunosuppressive doses of corticosteroids. Other reported treatments include pentoxyphylline, sulfasalazine, dapsone, or fenbendazole.[1-9]

Hyperkeratosis

Idiopathic defects in keratinization, other primary disease conditions causing seborrhea, and secondary changes in keratinization due to parasitism may all cause crusting and scaling of the pinna. Ear margin dermatosis is common in Dachshunds and other breeds with pendulous ears. Seborrheic changes begin at the ear margin and progress to confluence of scale and significant alopecia. Pruritus is variable but may be present in severe cases. The condition is not curable but controllable with keratolytic keratoplastic shampoos (e.g., sulfursalicylic acid, benzoyl peroxide, benzoyl peroxide-sulfur, selenium sulphide).[2] Severe cases may require topical or systemic corticosteroid treatment due to inflammation associated with removal of crusts or ear fissure formation.

Sebaceous adenitis is associated with an inflammatory process of the sebaceous glands. Follicular disruption, alopecia, and surface scale initially affect the pinna and may involve the ear canal and trunk.[7] There is no direct therapy for lost sebaceous glands, and supportive care with fatty acids, humectants, and antiinflammatory corticosteroids can be useful. Retinoids have been used in cases with a granulomatous response to the process.[2]

Other less common disorders can cause hyperkeratosis of the pinna. Idiopathic benign lichenoid keratosis has been diagnosed in four dogs with multiple wartlike papules and hyperkeratotic plaques on the pinnae.[3] Lichenoid psoriasiform dermatosis is a rare condition in which erythematous papules and lichenoid plaques appear on the concave surface of the pinna, external ear canal, and ventral head and trunk. Treatment consists of antimicrobial shampoo, systemic antibiotics, and corticosteroids.[2] Lupoid dermatosis is a heritable condition of German Shorthaired Pointers in which progressive, nonpruritic scale occurs on the pinnae, face, and trunk. There is no therapy for the condition.

Nutritional Dermatoses

Zinc deficiency caused by dietary insufficiency or inability to absorb dietary zinc results in crusting lesions of the pinna, perioral, periorbital, perianal, and perivulvar sites of dogs. Food allergy can result in steroid-resistant alopecia, crust, scale, hyperpigmentation, and lichenification of the pinnae. Dietary restriction followed by feeding trials is diagnostic of the condition, which may be associated with lesions and pruritus on other parts of the body.

DERMATOSES CAUSING PAPULES AND NODULES

Tick Infestation

The following ticks may cause local irritation and secondary granuloma formation of the pinna in dogs: American dog tick (*Dermacentor variabilis*), lone star tick (*Amblyomma americanum*), brown dog tick (*Rhipicephalus sanguinous*), and *Ixodes* species.[3] Of these ticks, *Ixodes* sp. is least likely to be identified on the pinna or head. Treatment should be aimed at insect removal and prevention of reinfestation.

Neoplastic Lesions

Auricular tumors are more common and more often malignant in cats than dogs. Commonly diagnosed canine pinnal tumors include squamous cell carcinoma, cutaneous histiocytoma, mast cell tumor, sebaceous adenoma, and papilloma. Squamous cell carcinoma, mast cell tumor, basal cell tumor, and fibrosarcoma are commonly diagnosed in cats.

Granulomatous Lesions

Pinnal granulomas may be associated with bacterial infection (*Staphylococcus* species, *Nocardia*, *Actinomyces*, mycobacteria, atypical mycobacteria); dermatophytosis; deep mycoses; algae; *Leishmania*; and foreign bodies. Canine leproid granuloma occurs in short-haired dogs primarily in cool, moist environments. Two-mm to 5-cm nodules have been described with superficial alopecia and ulceration occurring on the dorsal pinna and head. Although acid-fast bacilli have been identified on histopathologic examination, cultures are usually negative. Lesions usually resolve spontaneously or respond to surgical excision.[11]

DERMATOSES CAUSING PUSTULES, VESICLES, AND BULLAE

Autoimmune disorders commonly affect the concave aspect of the pinna. Lesions are usually symmetric; vesicles, erosions, and blisters may appear on the pinna prior to the occurrence of generalized disease. Pemphigus complex, systemic lupus erythematosus, bullous pemphigoid, and epidermolysis bullosa have been associated with pinnal lesions.[12] The diagnosis may be made with cytology and skin biopsy. Differential diagnoses include bacterial infection, drug eruption, and contact hypersensitivity.[1]

CONCAVE PINNAL DERMATOSES

Atopy

Erythema and hyperplasia of the pinna and upper external ear canal are early signs of atopy. If the condition is allowed to progress, hyperpigmentation, lichenification, and erythematous, ceruminous otitis may result.

Allergic Contact Dermatitis

Allergic contact dermatitis is a rare condition described in middle-aged animals due to the long period of induction required for development of the delayed hypersensitivity to the substance. The condition is often diagnosed secondary to topical medication used to treat otitis and may result in pinnal alopecia.

Defects in Keratinization

Systemic conditions such as hypothyroidism, sex hormone aberrations, and seborrhea may affect the concave surface of the pinna. Grease accumulation hyperkeratotic dermatosis may result.

Juvenile Cellulitis

Juvenile sterile granulomatous dermatitis and lymphadenitis is a rarely diagnosed condition; predisposed breeds include the Golden Retriever, Dachshund, Labrador Retriever, and Lhasa Apso. Dogs usually present at younger than 6 months of age with significant mandibular and prescapular lymphadenopathy and edema, exudate, papules, and pustules of the pinna, muzzle, and periocular skin.[1] The diagnosis is based on clinical presentation, culture and susceptibility testing, and skin biopsy. Treatment consists of immunosuppression with corticosteroids, which are tapered over 3 to 4 weeks after remission of clinical signs. Systemic antimicrobial therapy is indicated for the treatment of secondary bacterial pyoderma.

Proliferative and Necrotizing Otitis Externa

Chronic, pruritic, proliferative otitis associated with the medial pinna, which may concurrently affect the vertical ear canal, has been identified in cats. Erosions or ulceration lie under accumulated crusts. Bacterial or yeast otitis may be present. Histology showed severe acanthosis of the outer root sheath of the hair follicles and shrunken keratinocytes. Dermal inflammation was mixed and variable. Both tacrolimus and corticosteroid therapy may be used in an attempt to decrease the duration and severity of clinical signs.[13]

AURICULAR CARTILAGE DISORDERS

Aural Hematoma

Aural hematomas occur in both dogs and cats secondary to the self-induced trauma of head shaking or scratching. Blood accumulates within the fractured cartilage of the pinna, although swelling is most visible on the concave aspect. Any animal diagnosed with an aural hematoma should undergo a complete evaluation and treatment for otitis externa because continued head shaking will predispose the animal to enlargement or recurrence of the hematoma. Small hematomas may resolve without therapy; however, poor cosmesis is a complication of second intention healing causing deformation of the pinna. Treatment of the hematoma may consist of corticosteroid injection, evacuation and bandaging, teat cannula drainage, Penrose drain placement, or closed suction drainage.[14] Surgical incision, drainage, curettage, and closure with mattress sutures is preferred because it provides apposition of the cartilage edges and cosmetic results. Sutures remain in place for 21 days to allow adequate cartilage healing. Treatment of the concurrent otitis externa and its underlying cause are vital to the prevention of recurrence.

Auricular Chondritis

Auricular chondritis ("relapsing polychondritis" in cats) is an inflammation and destruction of auricular cartilage usually classified as an immune-mediated disorder. The pinnae are bilaterally swollen and deformed in most cases, although unilateral involvement is possible. Diagnosis is based on biopsy, and treatment may be minimal if no significant systemic signs exist. Attempted treatment with immunosuppressive doses of corticosteroids was not successful in cats; dapsone therapy may induce remission.[2]

DISEASES OF THE EXTERNAL EAR CANAL: OTITIS EXTERNA

NORMAL ANATOMY AND PHYSIOLOGY

The external ear canal serves to collect and deliver sound to the tympanic membrane. The ear canal is composed of auricular and annular cartilages that roughly approximate with the vertical and horizontal portions of the canal. The normal dog has a 45-degree angle of the horizontal canal; the angle is approximately 90 degrees in cats. Stratified squamous epithelium with sebaceous glands; ceruminous, or apocrine, glands; and hair follicles line the canal. Sebaceous glands located in the superficial dermis secrete neutral lipids, which assist in maintenance of keratinization, capture and removal of debris, and decreasing the humidity of the ear canal. Acid mucopolysaccharides and phospholipids are the main secretions of ceruminous glands located deeper in the dermis. The glandular secretions help to maintain proper humidity and pH in the ear canal, and a normal flora of bacteria and yeast have been identified in the external ear canal of normal dogs and cats.[15] Removal of debris from the deeper portion of the ear canal is achieved in many ways. The ratio of apocrine to sebaceous glands decreases from proximal to distal in the ear canal, resulting in more aqueous cerumen deeper in the canal, and the number of glands and hair follicles also decrease deep in the ear canal. The tympanic membrane is composed of three layers, with epithelial cells migrating away from the center of the tympanum, which aids in the removal of debris and secretions from its surface.

DIAGNOSTIC PRINCIPLES

History

A history is important for determining causes of otitis externa. Questions similar to those described in diseases of the pinna also apply to patients with otitis externa.

Physical Examination

Complete examination of the patient with otitis includes general physical, dermatologic, otoscopic, and neurologic examinations. An otoscopic examination should be performed slowly and deliberately with dorsal and lateral traction on the pinna, keeping the otoscope centrally located in the canal to avoid placing pressure on the epithelium. Hyperemia, erosions, ulcers, exudate, foreign bodies, stenosis, and masses are recorded. The tympanum should be thin, pale, gray, and translucent with a visible manubrium of the malleus. The tympanum is usually seen in 75% of dogs with normal ears and 28% of the time in dogs with otitis.[3] Otoscopy is not sensitive for rupture of the tympanic membrane but can be diagnostic of obvious ruptures.

Cytologic Examination

Cytologic examination of secretions or exudate within the ear canal is a mandatory part of assessing the patient with otitis. Cytology should be done upon presentation and at each reevaluation because gross appearance of exudate does not correlate with microscopic character. Material should be collected prior to cleaning the ear canal; specimens collected from the horizontal canal through the otoscope cone may be more representative of the disease process.[3] Mineral oil cytology is used for identification of parasites, and heat fixation may be done but is not required prior to staining with modified Wright's stain (Diff-Quik) and Gram stain for evaluation of bacterial pathogens and yeast under oil immersion microscopy (100×).[16] The morphologic type of bacteria, Gram-staining characteristics, and presence or absence of inflammatory cells, cerumen, and debris should be noted.

Many clinicians use a scale of 1+ to 4+ in describing numbers of yeast, bacteria, and inflammatory cells to allow evaluation of the progression of the disease process. However, low numbers of bacteria and yeast per high power field (40× dry) may be identified in normal ears.[17] Dogs and cats should have ≤ 2 yeast and ≤ 5 bacteria/hpf.[17] Yeast numbers ≥5/hpf in dogs and ≥ 12/hpf in cats are abnormal. Bacteria ≥25/hpf in dogs and 15/hpf in cats were associated with otitis.[17] Persistence of the same pathogens on reevaluation suggests lack of efficacy or inappropriate therapy, lack of identification of the primary disease process, or lack of owner compliance with therapy. Any change in the cytologic appearance may suggest reaction to medication or a change in either the type of inflammatory process or secondary pathogens.

The value of fine needle aspirates of external ear canal masses is unknown. Fine needle aspirates of mass lesions were accurate in 7/7 inflammatory polyps and 7/11 cases of ceruminous gland hyperplasia but misdiagnosed hyperplasia as ceruminous gland adenocarcinoma in 4 cases.[18] Ceruminous gland carcinoma was correctly diagnosed in six of seven cases due to altered nuclear and three-dimensional characteristics on cytology.[18]

Culture and Susceptibility Testing

Cultures need not be done if external ear canal cytology is negative for bacteria; it is unlikely that either yeast or bacteria would be present on cultures or would contribute to the disease process in those cases. Culture with susceptibility testing should be considered whenever resistant bacteria may be present or when prolonged or systemic therapy is indicated (e.g., gram-negative bacteria and inflammatory cells identified on cytology, chronic bacterial otitis, suspected otitis media, or failure to respond to appropriate medical therapy).[3,19-20] Cultures should be collected from the tympanic bulla in all suspected cases of otitis media because horizontal ear canal samples do not correlate with those from the middle ear in over 89% of cases and cytologic examination of the middle ear may be negative despite the presence of otitis.[21] Because bacteria may not cross the tympanic membrane, cultures from both sites should provide the highest yield of pathogenic bacteria. Yeast cultures are not routinely performed because cytology is more sensitive than culture for yeast organisms, which may require specific lipid supplementation of the growth media for some species.[22-23] Cytology and cultures do not always agree, however. One study showed that cytology agreed with cultures 68% of the time, but the confidence interval was 55% to 81%.[24] Cultures produced more organisms than seen on cytology 81% of the time.[24] Different organisms may be cultured from the same location up to 20% of the time. Different susceptibility patterns are also present 20% of the time, even if collected from the same location.

Radiology, Ultrasound, Computed Tomography, and Magnetic Resonance Imaging

Any of these imaging methods may be used to evaluate the patency of the external ear canal and the integrity of the tympanic bulla. Underlying otitis media should be identified because it perpetuates otitis externa and requires specific therapy separate from that of otitis externa. Evaluation of the tympanic membrane to diagnose otitis media, however, can be difficult in cases with significant secondary changes of the external ear canal. Treating the otitis externa may decrease secondary changes and allow tympanic visualization at a later date, or imaging may be pursued. Radiographs are not as sensitive as CT or MRI for detecting abnormalities of the tympanic bulla.[25-27] Ultrasound evaluation may become a less expensive, widely available method of evaluating the external and middle ears in dogs and cats, but it is not as useful when negative results are obtained.[28-30] Some animals without clinical signs of otitis have had material in the middle ear on MRI, and signal characteristics did not correlate to the diagnosis.[31] If obstructive external ear disease does not respond to therapy or if the ear canals are palpably fibrotic or ossified, total ear canal excision and bulla osteotomy are required. Imaging of the middle ear is not necessary in those cases because the middle ear must be addressed at surgery via bulla osteotomy. Radiographic changes or changes on CT or MRI are valuable in patients with otic neoplasia. Significant changes of the tympanic bulla suggest that complete surgical excision may not be possible. Advanced imaging is also valuable in cases of otitis interna and central vestibular disease.

PATHOPHYSIOLOGY

Otitis externa describes any inflammatory condition of the external ear canal. The estimated incidence of otitis in dogs and cats ranges from 4% to 20% and 2% to 6.6%, respectively.[1,19] Clinical signs associated with the condition vary, depending on the etiology of the otitis. General signs consist of head shaking, scratching, otic pain, and a variable accumulation of cerumen or exudate. The external canal responds to chronic inflammation of the dermis and epidermis with epithelial hyperplasia and hyperkeratosis, sebaceous gland hyperplasia, and ceruminous gland hyperplasia and dilation. These changes are associated with an increase in cerumen production; however, increased humidity, increased pH, and decreased lipid content of the cerumen predispose the animal to secondary infection. Apocrine gland rupture, sebaceous gland degeneration, ear canal stenosis, and fibrosis and/or ossification of the canal usually occur with the end stages of otitis.[32] Because permanent changes of the ear canal can occur with any cause of otitis externa, primary, predisposing, and perpetuating factors should be investigated in all cases of otitis.

Primary Factors

Primary factors are capable of causing otitis in normal ears. Primary factors may not be cured but often are controlled with appropriate therapy.

Hypersensitivities   Primary causes were identified in 78% of cases in one study, 43% of which were allergies.[33]

Atopy and food hypersensitivity   Otitis externa is a clinical sign in 50% to 80% of atopics or food-sensitive dogs and may be the only clinical sign associated with atopy.[34,35] Erythematous ceruminous otitis is most commonly associated with allergic skin disease.[36] Early clinical signs of bilateral pruritus, concave pinnal erythema, and mild erythematous/ceruminous otitis of the proximal ear canal may progress to significant otitis externa and pinnal hyperpigmentation. The pet can develop end-stage otitis if the primary cause is not identified and treated. Aural pruritus is common to atopy and food hypersensitivity; however, steroid responsiveness is usually only seen with atopy. Atopic dogs also tend to have a slower progression of disease than food-sensitive dogs. Secondary infection with either *Malassezia pachydermatis* or cocci is common. A definitive diagnosis is based on biopsy, intradermal skin testing, serologic testing, or dietary restriction and subsequent diet trials.

Contact hypersensitivity and irritant reaction   Topical otic preparations may cause a delayed hypersensitivity or irritant reaction to the ear canal. A response to initial therapy is followed by progression of disease or change in the character of the otitis with continued therapy. Worsening of clinical signs can occur if the medication is discontinued and then readministered. Neomycin, propylene glycol, and dimethyl sulfoxide have been associated with irritant otitis. Reactions are occasionally noted with alcohol, glycerin, povidone-iodine, and concentrations of acetic acid greater than 2%.[3] Contact hypersensitivity or an irritant reaction should be suspected any time otitis externa is exacerbated by therapy or upon changes in the gross or cytological appearance of the otitis. Both contact hypersensitivity and irritant reaction act as perpetuating factors of otitis externa despite control of the primary factor.

Ectoparasites   *Otodectes cynotis* is the cause of otitis externa (otocariasis) in up to 50% of cats and 10% of dogs with otitis externa.[3] Otodectes was the most common parasite in dogs with otitis, followed by demodectes and sarcoptes.[33] The infestation in cats may be classified as one of the following: (1) otitis externa, (2) ectopic infestation, and (3) asymptomatic carrier. Signs of otitis include significant pruritus, pinnal erythema and crusting, and accumulation of cerumen in the external ear canal. Gross character of the cerumen is not correlated to the microscopic findings but is usually dark brown to black in color. Mites may be observed on otoscopic examination; however, mineral oil cytology is recommended because few mites are required to cause clinical signs. Mites may concurrently inhabit the skin of the head and neck in animals with otitis. True ectopic infestation usually results in miliary dermatitis and patchy alopecia in cats. Treatment consists of therapy with any of the following: carbamates, pyrethrins, rotenone, ivermectin, thiabendazole, or fipronil.[37] Selamectin has recently been proven safe and effective for treating otocariasis in both dogs and cats.[38,39] The 3-week cycle of the parasite should be considered in treatment planning.

Demodex canis has been associated with mild otitis and excessive cerumen production in dogs with the generalized form of demodicosis. The diagnosis is made with mineral oil cytology; other diagnostics (e.g., biopsy) are less often required. Other parasites such as harvest mites (*Neotrombicula autumnalis* and *Eutrombicula alfreddugesi*) and ticks (*Otobius megninii*) may cause otitis externa. Reinfestation is a common problem due to environmental exposure to these parasites.

Foreign Bodies   Younger dogs of hunting or working breeds are predisposed to otic foreign bodies. The most common foreign body associated with otitis is the grass lawn; however, other foreign bodies include dirt, sand, cerumen or exudate mixed with hair, and conglomerates of dried ear medication can incite inflammation. Dogs are usually in acute pain, and bilateral foreign bodies are possible. Approximately 20% of otic foreign bodies penetrate the tympanic membrane, leading to otitis media.[3]

Keratinization Defects Hypothyroidism, male feminizing syndrome, Sertoli cell tumor, hyperestrogenism, and idiopathic seborrhea may be associated with mild otitis externa. Idiopathic seborrhea in Cocker Spaniels and hereditary defects in cats leading to seborrhea may cause erythematous ceruminous otitis. Changes in the microenvironment of the ear canal lead to secondary purulent otitis.

Idiopathic Inflammatory or Hyperplastic Otitis Cocker Spaniels may be affected by severe, proliferative otitis externa at a young age. Concurrent dermatologic conditions are not necessarily present but should be ruled out for proper management of the patient. The etiology of the condition is unknown but may be due to a primary glandular disorder.[2]

Other Primary Factors Immune-mediated disorders such as pemphigus complex may be associated with both pinnal lesions and otitis externa. Pemphigus foliaceous may involve the ears alone in some cases, but lesions on other parts of the body are usually present. Drug eruption from systemically administered drugs may also cause both pinnal lesions and otitis externa. Older animals with chronic or recurrent otitis should be evaluated for benign or malignant neoplasia of the skin or adnexal structures of the ear.

Predisposing Factors

Predisposing factors make otitis more likely by altering the environment of the external ear canal, thereby making the ear more susceptible to inflammation and secondary infection. Predisposing factors were identified in 59% of dogs with otitis externa in one study.[33]

Anatomic Changes Increased soft tissue within the ear canal, increased compound hair follicles in the canal, and stenotic canals (e.g., Chinese Shar-Pei, Bulldog, Chow Chow) or chronic changes associated with previous bouts of otitis may be predisposing factors for otitis externa. Thirty-five percent of dogs with otitis had pendulous ears,[33] and otitis is common in breeds of dogs exhibiting increased ceruminous compared with sebaceous gland area (e.g., Cocker Spaniel, Labrador Retriever, Springer Spaniel).[40] Hair is normally present in the ear canal, and increased numbers of hairs or the presence of compound hair follicles have not been correlated to the incidence of otitis in dogs. Routine hair plucking is therefore not recommended and may incite an inflammatory response within the epithelium, perpetuating otitis externa.

External Environment Increases in temperature and humidity in the environment may be reflected in the ear canal, although environmental relative humidity was not an apparent cause of increased external ear canal humidity in people with a predisposition for otic discharge.[41] The incidence of otitis externa is seasonally related to temperature, humidity, and rainfall. A lag period of 1 to 2 months is associated with cases of canine otitis and may vary with geographic location. Positive cultures of the ear canal are more likely during times of increased environmental temperature and humidity.[3]

Perpetuating Factors

Perpetuating factors exacerbate the inflammatory process and can maintain the disease after the primary factor has been eliminated. They can induce permanent pathologic changes to the ear canal and are the main reason for treatment failure in otitis externa.

Secondary Bacterial Colonization/Infection A normal flora exists in the ear canal of dogs and cats. *Staphylococcus* species and *Streptococcus* species are often cultured, *Pseudomonas* is rarely cultured, and *Proteus* was not cultured from the normal canine ear canal.[19] *Malassezia* has also been identified on cytologic examination in normal dogs and cats and its numbers are significantly increased in erythematous ceruminous otitis.[19] Bacteria and yeast are opportunistic pathogens but can cause significant secondary changes of the ear canal with chronic infection. Increased numbers of bacteria without an inflammatory response may represent colonization, which often responds to topical therapy. The presence of inflammatory cells suggests true infection, and culture and susceptibility testing are recommended due to resistance patterns of many bacteria. In colonization and infection, cleaning the external ear canal removes exudate, debris, toxins, free fatty acids, and bacteria, which perpetuate inflammation and secondary changes of the ear canal.[42]

Cocci may be identified in 38% and rods detected in 22% of cases of canine otitis.[33] *Staphylococcus* species are common in dogs with otitis, as are *Pseudomonas aeruginosa*, *Proteus* species, *Escherichia coli*, *Corynebacterium* species, and *Streptococcus* species.[21,43] Acute purulent otitis externa is less common than chronic, but with chronicity and repeated treatment, gram-negative bacteria, such as *Pseudomonas* and *Proteus*, predominate. The associated otitis may have surface erosions or ulcers and copious exudate. Cats may be secondarily infected with *Pasteurella multocida* and less often *P. aeruginosa*, *Proteus* species, or *E. coli*.[1]

Malassezia pachydermatis Budding yeast has been identified on ear cytology of normal dogs (up to 50%) and cats (up to 23%).[23,44,45] *Malassezia pachydermatis* is considered part of the normal flora and an opportunist in cases of otitis externa, particularly in cases of erythematous ceruminous otitis. *Malassezia* other than *M. pachydermatis* are lipid-dependent yeast that overgrow in conditions of increased moisture, increased surface lipids, and compromised barrier function of the stratum corneum.[46,47] Enzymes produced by the yeast may allow depolymerization of the interstitial matrix (e.g., hyaluronidase, chondroitin-sulphatase) and cell membranes (e.g., proteinase, phospholipase), increasing tissue invasion and penetration.[47] Lipid-dependant *Malassezia* spp. have been cultured from the ears of healthy cats and cats with otitis, however, including *Malassezia globosa* and *Malassezia furfur*.[44] Wild felids have been culture positive for lipid-dependent *Malassezia sympodialis*, but *M. pachydermatis* was the only yeast identified in small exotic cats.[48] Cytologic examination was historically more valuable than culture because some species of *Malassezia* require specific media supplemented with long-chain fatty acids.[23,46] However, recent study has shown that direct examination was not as sensitive as culture.[45,49,50] *Malassezia* spp. were present in up to 66% of canine otitis cases,[33,45] and more pathogenic genotypes were only recovered from dogs with otitis.[51]

Chronic Anatomic Changes Increased soft tissue volume within the ear canal associated with chronic otic inflammation leads to ear canal stenosis and alters the otic microenvironment. Chronic changes of the epidermis, adnexa, dermis, and cartilage are described earlier in the pathophysiology section. The microenvironmental alterations associated with chronic ear canal stenosis and inflammation favor bacterial and yeast proliferation and the retention of exudate. The changes also hinder proper cleaning and medication of the deeper portions of the external ear canal.

Otitis Media Untreated infection of the middle ear serves as a source of perpetuating factors for otitis externa.

Concurrent rupture of the tympanic membrane was present in 25% of otitis externa cases in one study.[33] Failure to identify the bacteria, yeast, or byproducts of inflammation in the middle ear may result in recurrent otitis externa and chronic pathologic changes of the middle and external ear.

Treatment Errors, Undertreatment, and Overtreatment Incorrect treatment of otitis allows bacterial or yeast overgrowth or infection and denies treatment of the primary factor causing otitis. Overapplication of medication or use of occlusive medications increases the humidity of the ear canal, leading to epithelial maceration and inflammation, perpetuating the otitis, and accumulation of dried medication acts as a foreign body within the ear canal. Undertreatment allows progression of the disease and the development of resistance in the bacteria causing secondary infection.

GENERAL PRINCIPLES OF MANAGEMENT

The therapeutic plan for otitis externa requires identification of the primary disease process and perpetuating factors. Ideally management is aimed at thoroughly cleaning and drying the ear canal, removing or managing the primary factors, controlling perpetuating factors, administering appropriate topical and/or systemic therapy, and evaluating response to therapy.

Ear Cleaning

Ear cleaning serves many functions: (1) removes of material that supports or perpetuates of infection; (2) removes bacterial toxins, white blood cells, and free fatty acids that stimulate inflammation; (3) allows complete evaluation of the external ear canal and tympanum; (4) allows topical therapy to contact all portions of the ear canal; and (5) removes material that may inactivate topical medications.[3,19] Significantly painful ears may benefit from initial antiinflammatory therapy to decrease pain and swelling of the ear canal prior to cleaning. Severe cases of otitis externa often require general anesthesia to facilitate complete cleaning and evaluation of the external and middle ear.

Many different solutions are available for removing cerumen, exudate, and debris from the ear canal (Table 223-1).

If the tympanic membrane cannot be visualized, only physiologic saline solution or water should be used because many topical cleaning agents are ototoxic or incite inflammation of the middle ear. Manual removal of large amounts of cerumen or debris is facilitated by an operating otoscope, ear loops, and alligator forceps. Debris is carefully removed under direct visualization, and care is taken deeper in the ear canal, close to the tympanic membrane. Aggressive hair removal is not advised because inflammation and damage to the epithelium can result in secondary bacterial colonization and infection. Flushing may be performed after large accumulations of cerumen and debris are mechanically removed from the ear canal.

Flushing and evacuation of solution is done under direct visualization through an operating otoscope. A bulb syringe and red rubber catheter system may be used to both flush and evacuate solutions and accumulations from the ear canal. Manual evacuation of the contents of the bulb syringe into the ear canal and suction should be exquisitely controlled by the operator, avoiding drastic pressure changes within the external ear canal, which can damage the tympanum. Other alternatives include tom cat catheters (3.5 French) and flexible, intravenous catheters (14 gauge, Teflon); stiff, narrow catheters should be used cautiously and under direct visualization deep in the external ear canal. Other reservoir systems

for delivery or evacuation of solutions include a 12-mL syringe or suction tubing attached to in-house vacuum systems. In-house vacuum systems should be used cautiously and under direct visualization. Care should be taken to avoid trauma to the tympanic membrane until its integrity can be assessed. Initial flushes should be done with physiologic saline solution or water until the integrity of the tympanic membrane can be assessed.

Other solutions may aid in the removal of wax in the ear canal. Ceruminolytics are emulsifiers and surfactants that break down ceruminocellular aggregates by causing lysis of squamous cells. A ceruminolytic agent in an alkaline pH may more effectively lyse squamous cells by the addition of cell surface protein disruption.[3] Oil-based products soften and loosen debris to aid in their removal but do not cause cell lysis. Water-based ceruminolytics are easier to remove and dry more quickly than oil-based solutions, which are occlusive if they remain in the ear canal. Water-based products include dioctyl sodium sulfosuccinate, calcium sulfosuccinate, and carbamate peroxide, which has a foaming action with the release of urea and oxygen. Oil-based products include squalene, triethanolamine polypeptide, hexamethyltetracosane, oleate condensate, propylene glycol, glycerin, and mineral oil. In a recent study only the combination of squalene and isopropyl myristate in a liquid petrolatum base had no adverse effects on hearing, the vestibular system, and histopathologic examination.[52] Other agents tested contained glycerin, dioctyl sodium sulfosuccinate (2% or 6.5%), parachlorometaxylenol, carbamide peroxide (6%), propylene glycol, triethanolamine polypeptide oleate condensate (10%), and/or chlorobutanol (0.5%).[52] A combination of salicylic acid, lactic acid, oleic acid, propylene glycol, and salicylic esters, benzoic esters, and water removed 85% of synthetic cerumen in one experimental study.[53]

Alcohol-based drying agents added to ceruminolytics include boric acid, benzoic acid, and salicylic acid, which decrease the pH of the ear canal, cause keratolysis, and mild antimicrobial effects. Boric-complexed zinc cleaning solution was effective in decreasing yeast in dogs with yeast otitis externa compared with acetic-complexed zinc preparation, which was also associated with discomfort in a significant number of dogs.[53] Dogs treated with a placebo also had improvement, however, which may have been due to the cleaning of the ear alone or the pH of the solution.[54] Drying the ear canal is important to combat the increased humidity, which potentiates infection.

If the tympanum is intact, the ear canal is filled with a ceruminolytic agent for at least 2 minutes. The pinna is cleaned at the same time. The solution is flushed twice with warm water, and the canal inspected. The procedure is repeated until cleaning is complete. Other solutions commonly advocated for ear flushing include dilute chlorhexidine solution (0.05%), dilute povidone-iodine, and acetic acid (2.5%). The first two agents are potentially ototoxic or induce inflammation and should not be used if the tympanum is ruptured. A combination of propylene glycol, malic, benzoic, or salicylic acid; 2% acetic acid; or dilute povidone-iodine have been suggested for use in dogs with a ruptured tympanum.[3]

Owners may clean the ears at home with mild preparations of ceruminolytics and drying agents if mild otitis is present without severe accumulation of cerumen or exudate. Aqueous solutions are usually recommended because they are less occlusive and easier to clean and remove from the ear, dog, and home environment. The ear should be filled with the solution and then massaged for 40 to 60 seconds. The pet should be allowed to shake its head to remove the majority of the solution, and the excess should be wiped from the ear canal and pinna with a tissue. Daily flushing is usually recom-

Table • 223-1

Otic Cleaning Solutions

TRADE NAME	ACETIC ACID	BORIC ACID	SALICYLIC ACID	ISOPROPYL ALCOHOL	PROPYLENE GLYCOL	DSS	OTHER
Ace-Otic Cleanser	2%		0.1%				Lactic acid 2.7%
Adams Pan-Otic					X	X	Parachlorometaxylenol, Tris-EDTA, methylparaben, diazolidinyl urea, propylparaben, octoxynol
Alocetic Ear Rinse	X			X			Nonoxynol-12, methylparaben, alovera gel
Cerulytic Ear Ceruminolytic					X		Benzyl alcohol, butylated hydroxytoluene
Cerumene							25% Squalene, isopropyl myristate
CleRx Ear Cleansing Solution							6.5% Dioctyl sodium sulfosuccinate, 6% urea peroxide, 23% glycerol
DermaPet Ear/Skin Cleanser for Pets	X	X					
Docusate Solution					X	X	
Ear Cleansing Solution			X		X		Alovera gel, SD alcohol, lactic acid, dioctyl sodium sulfosuccinate, benzoic acid, benzyl alcohol
Earmed Boracetic Flush	X	X					Aloe
Earmed Cleansing Solution & Wash					X		50A 40B alcohol, cocamidopropyl phosphatidyl and PE dimonium chloride
Earoxide Ear Cleanser							Carbamide peroxide 6.5%
Epi-Otic Ear Cleanser			X		X	X	Lactic acid, chitosanide
Euclens Otic					X		Malic acid, benzoic acid, eucalyptus oil
Fresh-Ear	X	X	X	X	X		Lidocaine hydrochloride, glycerin, sodium docusate, lanolin oil
Gent-L-Clens			X		X		Lactic acid
Micro Pearls Advantage Advanced pHormula Ear Cleanser							Glycerol distearate, alkyl benzoate, glycerin, steareth-10, sodium olefin sophonate, cholesterol, allantoin, methylparaben, citric acid, sodium citrate, propylparaben
Nolvasan Otic							Solvent, surfactant
OtiCalm			X				Benzoic acid, malic acid, oil of eucalyptus
Otic Clear	X	X	X	X	X		Glycerin, lidocaine hydrochloride
Oticlean-A Ear Cleaning Lotion	X	X	X	35%	X		Lanolin oil, glycerin
Oti-Clens			X		X		Malic acid, benzoic acid
OtiFoam Ear Cleanser			X				Cocamidopropyl betaine, almond glycerides, oil of eucalyptus, mackalene 426
Otipan Cleansing Solution					X		Hydroxypropyl cellulose, octoxynol
OtiRinse Cleansing/ Drying Ear Solution			X		X	X	SD alcohol 40, glycerine, nonoxynol-12, benzoic acid, benzyl alcohol
Otocetic Solution	2%	2%					
Wax-O-Sol 25%							Hexamethyltetracosane

DSS, Dioctyl sodium sulfosuccinate.

mended, followed by every other day, weekly, then as needed, depending on the solution. Ear swabs are not recommended for home use, as cerumen and debris may be forced into the horizontal ear canal and impact against the tympanic membrane.

Topical Therapy

Erythematous ceruminous otitis externa was diagnosed 2.7 times more often than acute suppurative otitis in one report.[36] Yeast ± cocci were identified in those cases, with cocci or rods identified in suppurative otitis.[36] Topical therapy should be based on the cytologic examination to diminish the incidence of inappropriate treatment (Table 223-2). Many preparations combine antiinflammatories and antimicrobials in an attempt to decrease the inflammation and combat bacterial or yeast overgrowth. All topical medications should be considered supportive, and specific treatment should be aimed at controlling the primary disease process.

Topical glucocorticoids may be of benefit in most cases of otitis externa to decrease pruritus, exudation, swelling, and proliferative changes of the ear canal. The most potent glucocorticoids available in topical preparations include betamethasone valerate and fluocinolone acetonide. Lesser potent corticosteroids include triamcinolone acetonide and dexamethasone; the least potent being hydrocortisone. Most dogs benefit from short-term therapy with topical corticosteroids at the initiation of therapy, with concurrent therapy aimed at the primary and other perpetuating factors. Long-term therapy with topical corticosteroids can be deleterious because of the systemic absorption of drug. Increases in serum liver enzymes and depressed adrenal responsiveness with prolonged use of iatrogenic hyperadrenocorticism are possible. Glucocorticoids alone may be of benefit for short-term therapy in cases of allergic or erythematous ceruminous otitis.

Antimicrobials are important for controlling secondary bacterial or yeast overgrowth or infection. They should be used in any case with cytologic evidence of bacterial overgrowth or infection, with attention paid to the morphology and Gram-staining characteristics of the bacteria. Otic preparations commonly contain aminoglycoside antibiotics. Neomycin is effective against typical bacteria such as *Staphylococcus intermedius*. Gentamycin and polymyxin B are also appropriate first-line of defense topical treatments for gram-negative bacterial otitis externa. The risk of bone marrow toxicity in people limits the use of chloramphenicol for treating otitis in dogs and cats despite its antibacterial spectrum and availability.

Due to the frequency of resistant gram-negative bacteria such as *Pseudomonas*, other topical preparations have been developed. Enrofloxacin, ophthalmic tobramycin, and topical application of injectable ticarcillin have been used to treat otitis in dogs.[3,55] Their use should be limited to cases of resistant bacteria, and culture and susceptibility testing should be performed prior to application. Other topical agents may be used to supplement treatment of resistant *Pseudomonas*, such as silver sulfadiazine solution and Tris-EDTA. Tris-EDTA can render *Pseudomonas* susceptible to enrofloxacin or cephalosporins by enhancing membrane permeability and altering ribosome stability. Frequent ear cleaning may also assist in the treatment of resistant bacterial otitis; ceruminolytics have antimicrobial properties, and their use in clinical cases has been evaluated.[52,56] Acetic acid in combination with boric acid is effective against both *Pseudomonas* and *Staphylococcus*, depending on concentration and duration of exposure.[57] Ear cleaning removes of proinflammatory products, cells, and substances that diminish the effectiveness of topical antibiotics.

Many topical preparations control yeast organisms, which may complicate erythematous ceruminous otitis and suppurative otitis. Common active ingredients include miconazole, clotrimazole, nystatin, and thiabendazole. Preparations containing climbazole, econazole, and ketoconazole have also been evaluated.[58,59] Eighty percent of the yeast was susceptible to miconazole and econazole and intermediately resistant to ketoconazole, and 90% was resistant to nystatin and amphotericin B in one in vitro study.[59] Topical ear-cleaning agents have some efficacy against *Malassezia* organisms.[56] Other preparations (e.g., chlorhexidine, povidone-iodine, acetic acid) are also effective in the treatment of secondary yeast overgrowth.

Response to topical therapy should be gauged by reevaluation of physical, cytologic, and otoscopic examinations every 10 to 14 days after the initiation of therapy. Any changes in the appearance of these examinations should be recorded. Most cases of otitis can be managed topically; failure to respond to therapy should prompt reevaluation of the diagnosis and treatment.

Systemic Therapy

Systemic glucocorticoid administration may be beneficial in cases of severe, acute inflammation of the ear canal, chronic proliferative changes of the ear canal, and allergic otitis. Antiinflammatory doses should be limited to 7 to 10 days. Cases of significant thickening or proliferative changes in the external ear canal benefit from systemic antimicrobial therapy. Systemic therapy should be considered if concurrent dermatologic changes of the surrounding skin, pinna, or other regions of the body are present. Long-term administration of appropriate antimicrobials based on culture and susceptibility is required in all cases of otitis media. Systemic therapy for yeast is rarely recommended in animals with otitis alone. One study evaluated oral itraconazole therapy, and ear samples were only evaluated separately from skin samples on cytology and culture, where no change in cytology score was found.[22]

THERAPY FOR SPECIFIC DISEASES OF THE EXTERNAL EAR CANAL

Ectoparasites

Thorough cleaning of the external ear canal, treatment of all household pets, and whole body therapy should be considered in the treatment regimen for ear mites. Pets with no clinical signs may be asymptomatic carriers and a reservoir for reinfestation. Otic parasiticides such as pyrethrins, rotenone, amitraz, and carbaryl must be administered every 24 hours throughout the 20-day life cycle because they do not kill mite eggs.[19] Thiabendazole eliminates all mite stages but must be applied every 12 hours for 14 days. Ivermectin (0.3 to 0.5 mg/kg) may be applied topically once weekly for 5 weeks.[1] Otic administration of medication does not affect mites on adjacent or distant skin locations, and systemic or other total body parasiticide may be indicated. Alternatively, ivermectin administered subcutaneously (0.2 to 0.3 mg/kg) two to three times every 10 to 14 days or orally (0.3 mg/kg) every week for four treatments eliminates otic mites and those found elsewhere on the body.[1] Other topicals proven safe and effective for ear mite treatment include selamectin (6 mg/kg) administered on the skin between the shoulder blades and fipronil spray.[37-39] Selamectin was administered once in cats and two times, 30 days apart in dogs and results were similar to topical pyrethrin therapy.[38,39]

Idiopathic Inflammatory or Hyperplastic Otitis in Cocker Spaniels

Treatment is aimed at decreasing the secondary ear canal changes associated with this condition. Antiinflammatory doses of corticosteroids administered orally may be useful. Topical corticosteroid preparations in combination with antimicrobials decrease the soft tissue mass affecting the ear canal but may not be as effective as oral administration. Maintenance therapy may be required both topically and orally; however, low doses of corticosteroids should be used. Patient reevaluation should include attention to the potential side effects of corticosteroid therapy. Intermittent treatment of secondary bacterial or yeast overgrowth and infection may be required. Surgery is often indicated in these patients due to the severe secondary changes of the ear canal.

Table • 223-2

Topical Medications Used in the Treatment of Ear Disease

GENERIC NAME	TRADE NAME	DOSE	FREQUENCY	DESCRIPTION
Fluocinolone 0.01% DMSO 60%	Synotic	4-6 drops; total dose <17 mL	q12h initially, q48-72h maintenance	Potent corticosteroid antiinflammatory
Hydrocortisone 1.0%	HB101, Burrows H,	2-12 drops, depending on ear size	q12h initially, q24-48h maintenance	Mild corticosteroid antiinflammatory
Hydrocortisone 1.0%, lactic acid	Epi-otic HC	5-10 drops	q12h for 5 days	Mild corticosteroid antiinflammatory, drying agent
Hydrocortisone 0.5%, sulfur 2%, acetic acid 2.5%	Clear X Ear Treatment	2-12 drops, depending on ear size	q12-24h initially, q24-48h maintenance	Mild corticosteroid antiinflammatory, astringent, germicidal
DSS 6.5%, urea (carbamide peroxide 6%)	Clear X Ear Cleansing Solution	1-2 mL per ear	Once per week to as needed	Ceruminolytic, lubricating agent
Chlorhexidine 2%	Nolvasan	Dilute 1:40 in water	As needed	Antibacterial and antifungal activity
Chlorhexidine 1.5%	Nolvasan	Dilute 2% in propylene glycol	q12h	Antibacterial and antifungal activity
Povidone-iodine 10%	Betadine solution	Dilute 1:10-1:50 in water	As needed	Antibacterial activity
Polyhydroxidine iodine 0.5%	Xenodyne	Dilute 1:1-1:5 in water	As needed, q12h, once weekly	Antibacterial activity
Acetic acid 5%	White vinegar	Dilute 1:1-1:3 in water	As needed; q12-24h for *Pseudomonas*	Antibacterial activity, lowers ear canal pH
Neomycin 0.25%, triamcinolone 0.1%, thiabendazole 4%	Tresaderm	2-12 drops depending on ear size	q12h up to 7 days	Antibacterial and antifungal activity, parasiticide (mites), moderate corticosteroid antiinflammatory
Neomycin 0.25%, triamcinolone 0.1%, nystatin 100,000 U/mL	Panalog	2-12 drops depending on ear size	q12h to once weekly	Antibacterial and antifungal activity, moderate corticosteroid antiinflammatory
Chloramphenicol 0.42%, prednisone 0.17%, tetracaine 2%, squalene	Liquachlor, Chlora-Otic	2-12 drops depending on ear size	q12h up to 7 days	Antibacterial activity, mild corticosteroid antiinflammatory
Neomycin 1.75 and polymyxin B 5000 IU/ mL, penicillin G procaine 10,000 IU/mL	Forte Topical	2-12 drops depending on ear size	q12h	Antibacterial activity
Gentamicin 0.3%, betamethasone valerate 0.1%	Gentocin Otic Solution, Betagen Otic Solution	2-12 drops depending on ear size	q12h for 7-14 days	Antibacterial activity, potent corticosteroid antiinflammatory
Gentamicin 0.3%, betamethasone 0.1%, clotrimazole 0.1%	Otomax, Obibiotic Ointment	2-12 drops depending on ear size	q12h for 7 days	Antibacterial and antifungal activity, potent corticosteroid antiinflammatory
Gentamicin 0.3%, betamethasone valerate 0.1%, acetic acid 2.5%	GentaVed Otic Solution	2-12 drops, depending on ear size	q12h for 7-14 days	Antibacterial activity, potent corticosteroid antiinflammatory
Polymyxin B 10,000 IU/mL, hydrocortisone 0.5%	Otobiotic	2-12 drops, depending on ear size	q12h	Antibacterial activity, mild corticosteroid antiinflammatory
Enrofloxacin 0.5%, silver sulfadiazine 1%	Baytril Otic	2-12 drops, depending on ear size	q12h for up to 14 days	Antibacterial activity
Carbaryl 0.5%, neomycin 0.5%, tetracaine	Mitox Liquid	2-12 drops, depending on ear size		Antibacterial activity, parasiticide (mites)

Continued

Table • 223-2

Topical Medications Used in the Treatment of Ear Disease—cont'd

GENERIC NAME	TRADE NAME	DOSE	FREQUENCY	DESCRIPTION
Pyrethrins 0.06%, piperonyl butoxide 0.6%	Ear Mite and Tick Control	5 drops	q12h	Parasiticide (mites)
Pyrethrins 0.05%, squalene 25%	Cerumite	2-12 drops, depending on ear size	q24h for 7-10 days	Parasiticide (mites), ceruminolytic
Isopropyl alcohol 90%, boric acid 2%	Panodry	Fill ear canal	As needed	Drying agent
Acetic acid 2%, aluminum acetate	Otic Domeboro	Fill ear canal	q12-48h	Drying agent, antibacterial activity, lowers ear canal pH
Silver sulfadiazine	Silvadene	Dilute 1:1 with water, 1 gm powder in 100 mL water	q12h for 14 days	Antibacterial and antifungal activity
Tris-EDTA ± gentamicin 0.03%		2-12 drops, depending on ear size	q12h for 14 days	1 L distilled water, 1.2 g Tris-EDTA, 1 mL glacial acetic acid; antibacterial activity
Silver nitrate		Use sparingly	As needed	Cauterization of ulcerative otitis externa
Miconazole 1%; ± topical glucocorticoid (7.5 mL of dexamethasone phosphate [4 mg/mL] to 10 mL of 1% miconazole)	Conofite	2-12 drops, depending on ear size	q12-24h	Antifungal activity
Ivermectin 0.01%	Acarexx	0.5 mL per ear	Once	Parasiticide (mites)
Pyrethrins 0.15%, piperonyl butoxide 1.5%	Many	2-12 drops, depending on ear size	Twice at 7-day interval	Parasiticide (mites)
Pyrethrins 0.05%, piperonyl butoxide 0.5%, squalene 25%	Cerumite	2-12 drops, depending on ear size	q24h for 7 days	Parasiticide (mites), ceruminolytic
Pyrethrins 0.04%, Piperonyl butoxide 0.49%, DSS 1.952%, Benzocaine 1.952%	Aurimite	10 drops	q12h	
Rotenone 0.12%, cube resins 0.16%	Many	2-12 drops, depending on ear size	Every other day	Parasiticide (mites)

DSS, Dioctyl sodium sulfosuccinate.

Excessive Moisture (Swimmer's Ear)

Other primary disease conditions such as allergic otitis should be ruled out in any case of erythematous ceruminous otitis. Dogs with frequent exposure to water, however, may require ear cleaning and drying agents to diminish the humidity of the ear canal. Many cleaning and drying agents also possess antimicrobial effects.[56] Products that combine a drying agent and corticosteroid decrease the ear canal humidity and inflammation associated with allergic otitis complicated by swimming. Care should be taken to control primary disease (i.e., allergic otitis), however, and intermittently manage the predisposing factor (i.e., excessive moisture) as needed. The dog's ears should be cleaned and dried the day of water exposure and for 2 to 5 days after. For continued frequent exposure, maintenance cleaning may be required every other day to twice weekly.

Chronic Bacterial Otitis

Resistant bacteria play an important role in the development of chronic otitis externa. Any dog not responding to initial therapy should be reevaluated for primary and perpetuating conditions such as allergic disease, foreign body, neoplasia, otitis media, and secondary anatomic changes of the ear canal. Primary disease processes identified in one study included hypothyroidism, atopy, food allergy, and immune-mediated disease.[55] Infection with *Pseudomonas* species frequently occurs with repeated treatment of otitis externa, and acquired resistance of these bacteria is common. Culture and susceptibility testing is imperative in these cases to guide therapy. The antimicrobial chosen for therapy should be one that was tested against the bacteria cultured. Because antimicrobials within the same drug class may not result in the same susceptibility pattern of a bacteria, a drug tested against one type of bacteria should not be used as a surrogate for the antimicrobial chosen for clinical use.[60] It is important to note that agreement between different laboratories was 88%, and identical susceptibility patterns were uncommon in one study.[61] Multiresistant bacteria are emerging in cases of chronic bacterial otitis.[62,63] Susceptibility patterns for *Pseudomonas* isolates showed that ear isolates were less susceptible to enrofloxacin than skin isolates, and 20% were resistant to all antimicrobials tested.[64] Susceptibility to marbofloxacin and ciprofloxacin were 67% and 75%, respectively.[64] Multiresistant bacteria are emerging in cases of chronic bacterial otitis. Oral antimicrobials combined with topical therapy are used in severe cases with secondary changes of the ear canal. Identification of otitis media is vital to the removal of the middle ear as a source of otitis externa and requires long-term treatment.

Ear cleaning prior to the application of topical medication may increase the efficacy of the agent by decreasing exudate in the ear canal that inactivates antimicrobial agents such as polymyxin. In cases that fail to respond to first-line drug treatments such as polymyxin or gentamicin, other topical antimicrobial agents should be tried. Ophthalmic tobramycin and injectable amikacin have been described.[2] The integrity of the tympanic membrane should be know prior to use; avoidance of the medication is recommended if the tympanic membrane cannot be proven intact. Enrofloxacin or ticarcillin injectable preparations diluted in saline or water may be applied topically for resistant *Pseudomonas*. Parenteral ticarcillin was used in cases with a ruptured tympanic membrane until healing was observed, at which time topical therapy was instituted; clinical response occurred in 11 of 12 cases.[55] Enrofloxacin and silver sulfadiazine combination is also available in an otic preparation (Baytril Otic, Bayer).

Other topical therapy may assist in eliminating resistant *Pseudomonas* from the ear canal. Decreasing the pH of the ear canal with 2% acetic acid is lethal to *Pseudomonas*; diluted vinegar in water (1:1 to 1:3) may be used to flush the ear canal. Acetic acid combined with boric acid is lethal to *Pseudomonas* and *Staphylococcus* depending on the concentration of each agent.[57] Increasing the concentration of acetic acid may broaden its spectrum of activity, but it causes irritation of the external and middle ear. Ninety-nine percent of ear strains of *S. intermedius* were susceptible to orbifloxacin, and one strain was intermediately susceptible.[65] Silver sulfadiazine in a 1% solution exceeds the minimum inhibitory concentration of *Pseudomonas* and may be instilled into the ear canal. One gram of silver sulfadiazine powder mixed in 100 mL of water may be used for topical therapy and is also effective against *Proteus* species, enterocci, and *S. intermedius*. Dilute acetic acid (2%) and silver sulfadiazine (1%) have not caused adverse affects in cases with a ruptured tympanic membrane.[1,3,19] Tris-EDTA may be applied after thorough ear cleaning to increase the susceptibility of *Pseudomonas* to antimicrobial agents. It must be mixed, its pH adjusted, and autoclaved prior to use. It is available in an otic preparation (DermaPet, Potomac, Md.), which is used to clean the ears prior to instillation of topical antibiotic. Topical antiseptics such as chlorhexidine and povidone-iodine solutions may be helpful, but ototoxicity is an issue, particularly in cases in which the tympanum is ruptured or cannot be evaluated. The ototoxicity of Tris-EDTA and polyhexamethylene biguanide ear flush has been tested in dogs with no apparent vestibular or ototoxicity noted in one study.[66]

Reevaluation of the patient is important for monitoring response to therapy. Evaluation of the ear canal for progressive secondary changes and cytologic examination will allow alterations in therapy as needed. Significant narrowing of the ear canal is an indication for surgical intervention. Yeast overgrowth may occur with aggressive medical management of bacterial otitis and should be identified to maintain proper medical management.

Refractory or Recurrent Yeast Infection
Malassezia infection is a common perpetuating factor associated with erythematous ceruminous otitis and alterations in the otic microenvironment. Primary causes of the otitis should be identified and cured or managed. Cytologic examination, not culture, should be relied upon for the diagnosis of yeast infection.[15,46] If a case becomes refractory to therapy, reassessment of the primary condition and perpetuating factors should be done. Miconazole, clotrimazole, cuprimyxin, nystatin, and amphotericin B have all been described for treating *Malassezia* otitis. Climbazole had better in vitro activity against isolates of *M. pachydermatis* in one study.[58] Yeast were more susceptible to azole antifungals than polyene antifungals; however, oral ketoconazole, itraconazole, and fluconazole have been recommended for refractory cases.[1,59] Addition of ketoconazole to a Tris-EDTA and benzyl alcohol solution increased the efficacy against *Malassezia* organisms in one study.[67] Addition of corticosteroids to azole antifungals caused concurrent reduction in erythema, cerumen, and pruritus; however, azole agents alone equally decreased the number of *Malassezia* associated with yeast otitis in dogs.[68] Long-term therapy may require topical antibacterial and antifungal combinations.

Ear cleaning may aid in the elimination of yeast organisms by removing cerumen, debris, or exudate and altering the microenvironment of the ear canal. Cleaning with antimicrobial agents such as chlorhexidine, povidone-iodine, and acetic acid may be beneficial; the integrity of the tympanum should be assessed prior to choosing one of these agents. Ear-cleaning solutions may also have some efficacy against yeast organisms in both in vitro and clinical cases of otitis.[56,69]

Neoplasia
Chronic otitis externa may be the result of otic neoplasia, or otitis may be a predisposing factor in the development of neoplasia.[91] The occasional diagnosis of bilateral neoplasia is suggestive of the latter.[70] Cocker Spaniels are overrepresented for benign and malignant neoplasia and otitis externa.[1,71] Tumors of the skin and adnexal structures of the ear predominate. Benign tumors in dogs include sebaceous gland adenoma, basal cell tumor, polyp, ceruminous gland adenoma, and papilloma. Cats are more frequently diagnosed with malignant neoplasms, but benign conditions include inflammatory polyps, ceruminous gland adenomas, ceruminous gland cysts, and basal cell tumors. Malignant neoplasms in both species include ceruminous gland adenocarcinoma, undifferentiated carcinoma, and squamous cell carcinoma. Ceruminous gland adenocarcinomas are the most frequently diagnosed tumors of the ear canal in dogs and cats, although one report stated that squamous cell carcinoma occurred with an equal incidence in the cat.[71,72]

The biologic behavior of otic tumors cannot be judged by their gross appearance; however, benign masses are usually nodular and pedunculated. Ulceration can be secondary to otitis associated with mass lesions, but malignant masses ulcerate more frequently than benign masses. The tympanic bulla is involved in up to 25% of aural neoplasms, and neurologic signs occur in 10% of dogs and 25% of cats with otic neoplasia.[73] The biologic behavior of malignant neoplasms tends to be that of local invasion with a low metastatic rate (e.g., 10% in dogs) to either draining lymph nodes or lung.

Surgery is the mainstay of treating otic neoplasia. Conservative excision may be possible for benign lesions, depending on the location of the tumor. Malignancies should be removed by total ear canal ablation and lateral bulla osteotomy. Incomplete excision results in recurrence of the mass and secondary otitis externa. Malignant neoplasia is associated with a median survival time of >58 months in dogs and 11.7 months in cats.[71] Extensive tumor involvement and lack of aggressive management are associated with a poor prognosis in dogs.[71,74] In cats a poorer prognosis is associated with neurologic signs, squamous cell carcinoma or undifferentiated carcinoma, vascular or lymphatic invasion, and lack of aggressive therapy.[71,75] Ceruminous gland adenocarcinoma has a median disease-free interval of >36 months and 42 months in dogs and cats, respectively.[74,75] The median survival time associated with squamous cell carcinoma and undifferentiated carcinoma in cats is 4 to 6 months.[71]

ROLE OF SURGERY IN THE MANAGEMENT OF OTITIS EXTERNA

The two most common surgical procedures for the treatment of otitis externa are lateral ear resection and total ear canal ablation. Total ear canal ablation is always combined with a bulla osteotomy to allow complete removal of all secretory epithelium and exudate associated with the external and middle ear. Care must be taken when choosing a surgical technique for otitis externa.

Lateral ear resection is associated with high failure rates (47% to 80%) with inappropriate patient selection.[76] The procedure should be viewed as an adjunct to medical management, not as a cure. The primary and perpetuating factors associated with otitis externa must be identified and managed or controlled even when surgery is elected. Opening the vertical ear canal improves aeration, decreases humidity, facilitates removal of cerumen or exudate, and improves the distribution of topical medication in the ear canal. Lateral ear resection may be used in cases with mild changes of the vertical ear canal but should be avoided with significant secondary changes of the vertical ear canal or horizontal canal stenosis. Owners should be educated on the continuing need for medical therapy after surgery to avoid further progression of secondary changes of the ear canal. Pets can develop end-stage otitis following lateral ear resection.

Total ear canal ablation is used to treat end-stage otitis and malignant otic neoplasia. Severe secondary changes and proliferative disease are surgically removed with the ear canal en toto. A lateral bulla osteotomy of the tympanic bulla allows complete exploration of the middle ear for the removal of secretory epithelium, exudate, and tumor. The surgery removes the site of chronic inflammation and infection to cure the vast majority of cases of otitis externa media. Complications of the procedure include facial nerve paresis or paralysis, hemorrhage, para-aural abscessation, otitis interna, Horner's syndrome, pinnal necrosis, continued pinnal dermatitis, and hearing loss. Dogs with obstruction of the ear canal from end-stage otitis or neoplasia may be partially deaf, and postoperatively only osseous conduction of sound remains. Cats most often underwent total ear canal ablation for mass lesions (81%) and more commonly developed Horner's syndrome if they had inflammatory polyp as a diagnosis compared with neoplasia; however, clinical signs resolved in 86% within months of surgery.[77] Cats undergoing total ear canal ablation for neoplasia were twice as likely to develop facial nerve paralysis; however, 72% resolved within months of surgery.[77]

Vertical ear canal resection may be performed in cases of tumors confined to the auricular cartilage or traumatic injury. Significant proliferative disease or changes secondary to otitis externa are rarely confined to the vertical ear canal; concurrent stenosis of the horizontal ear canal usually necessitates total ear canal ablation and lateral bulla osteotomy. The anastomosis between the horizontal ear canal and surrounding skin may undergo stenosis after surgery, necessitating reoperation. Progression of the otitis and tumor recurrence are possible following vertical ear canal resection.

DISEASES OF THE MIDDLE AND INNER EAR

NORMAL ANATOMY AND PHYSIOLOGY

The middle ear consists of the tympanic membrane; three cavities (epitympanic, tympanic, and ventral); and the bony ossicles (malleus, incus, and stapes). The tympanic membrane has two parts: the thin pars tensa that attaches to the manubrium of the malleus and the thicker, upper pars flaccida. The main portion of the middle ear, the ventral tympanic bulla, has two compartments in the cat (ventromedial and dorsolateral). The air-filled bulla is lined with modified respiratory epithelium, which is either squamous or cuboidal and may be ciliated. The four openings in the middle ear are the tympanic opening, the vestibular window, the cochlear window, and the ostium of the auditory tube. The auditory tube communication occurs between the middle ear and caudal nasopharynx. The normal flora of the middle ear may be due to this pharyngeal communication, but the role of the auditory tube as a source of bacteria in otitis media is unknown. The tympanic opening is a common source of bacterial infection of the middle ear in dogs with otitis externa. The cochlear and vestibular windows are possible ports for progression of otitis media or ototoxic substances into the inner ear.

Cranial nerve VII, or the facial nerve, the sympathetic innervation of the eye, and the parasympathetic innervation of the lacrimal gland are closely associated with the middle ear. The separation of the facial nerve from the middle ear is minimal along the rostral aspect of its course through the petrosal bone. The nerve supplies motor fibers to the superficial muscles of the head, the muscles of the external ear, the caudal belly of the digastricus, and the ossicular muscles. The nerve also supplies sensation of the vertical ear canal and concave surface of the pinna. The postganglionic sympathetic fibers course closely with those of the facial nerve to innervate the smooth muscles of the eye. Preganglionic parasympathetic fibers also pass through the middle ear to innervate the salivary and lacrimal glands.

The inner ear is located within the petrosal bone. The cochlea, vestibule (saccule and utricle), and semicircular canals form the membranous labyrinth, which is encased in bone, or the bony labyrinth. The vestibular system functions to maintain the position of the eyes, trunk, and limbs relative to the position of the head, responding to linear and rotational acceleration and tilting. The system consists of the saccule, utriculus, and semicircular canals and communicates with the middle ear via the vestibular window. Fluid within the semicircular canals tends to remain stationary during motion, bending the cilia of the cells in the utricle and saccule, stimulating depolarization. The signal is conducted via the vestibular portion of the eighth cranial nerve to vestibular nuclei in the myelencephalon, the spinal cord, centers in the cerebellum and cerebral cortex, and motor nuclei of cranial nerves III, IV, and VI.[78] The result is coordination of the body, head, and eye movement. Projections to the vomiting centers are responsible for nausea and vomiting associated with vestibular disorders and motion. The cochlear system, involved with the translation of sound, consists of the spiral organ, or organ of Corti; cochlear duct; scala vestibule; and scala tympani. Transmission of sound through the tympanic membrane, ossicles, and cochlear window results in undulation of the basilar membrane of the spiral organ. Cilia bend and cause depolarization and transmission of a signal to cochlear nuclei, caudal colliculi, and cerebral cortex.[78] The cochlear nuclei control reflex regulation of sound via projections to cranial nerves V and VII, which control the muscles of the ossicles. Other projections allow for conscious perception of sound.

Otitis Media

Otitis media may result from extension of otitis externa through the tympanic membrane, aspiration of pharyngeal contents up the auditory tube (e.g., a sequela to upper respiratory tract infection in cats), or hematogenous spread. Extension from otitis externa is the most common cause of otitis media, but otitis media may serve as a perpetuating factor form otitis externa. Developmental abnormalities of the external ear canal and pharynx may also result in otitis media due to the accumulation of secretions in the middle ear.[79-80] Neoplasia, inflammatory polyps, and middle ear trauma may be associated with secondary otitis media or result in similar clinical signs.

Cholesteatoma is commonly associated with otitis media and chronic otitis externa. A cholesteatoma is a mass of keratinized squamous cells that accumulate within a structure lined with stratified squamous epithelium. The lesion is presumed to develop when a pocket of tympanic membrane becomes adhered to inflamed middle ear mucosa. Significant narrowing of the external ear canal is usually present. Radiographic signs of increased density and bony changes of the tympanic bulla predominate with loss of the air-filled lumen of the external ear canal and concurrent calcification. Treatment is usually limited to total ear canal ablation and lateral bulla osteotomy due to the changes of the external ear canal and mass/accumulation of debris in the tympanic bulla.[81]

The clinical signs associated with middle ear disease often reflect concurrent otitis externa (e.g., head shaking, lethargy, exudate, otic malodor). Significant otic pain, lethargy, inappetence, and pain upon opening the mouth are more suggestive of middle ear involvement. Neurologic signs may be present due to the course of the facial nerve and sympathetic innervation of the eye. Facial nerve paresis or paralysis result in facial asymmetry (i.e., uneven position of the lip commissures, unequal ear carriage, unilateral ptyalism) and abnormal cranial nerve reflexes on neurologic examination (e.g., menace response, palpebral and corneal reflexes, abnormal ear canal/concave pinnal sensation). Horner's syndrome, or loss of sympathetic innervation to the eye, can also be complete or partial (i.e., ptosis, miosis, entophthalmia, prolapse of the third eyelid). Otitis interna is usually evidenced by head tilt, abnormal nystagmus, and ataxia and should be differentiated from central vestibular disease based on the neurologic examination.

Cases of para-aural abscessation usually have concurrent otitis media.[3] The primary cause may be trauma to the external ear canal, severe otitis externa, extension of otic neoplasia, or total ear canal ablation. Signs of middle or external ear disease and soft tissue swelling in the parotid area may be accompanied by draining tracts. A head tilt and pain upon palpation of the area are usually present.

The diagnosis of otitis media is based on a thorough history and physical, neurologic, and otoscopic examinations. A ruptured tympanum strongly suggests otitis media. The pharynx should also be evaluated on physical examination; identification of specific conditions may require general anesthesia due to anatomic location (e.g., inflammatory polyps) or pain associated with examination (e.g., otitis media causing temporomandibular joint pain, severe otitis externa). General anesthesia may also be required to perform a complete otoscopic examination in cases of severe otitis externa, in which

thorough cleaning of the ear is necessary for therapy and diagnosis (i.e., visualization of the tympanum). Significant otitis externa is commonly associated with otitis media; the tympanic membrane is ruptured in up to 50% of dogs with otitis externa, although 70% of dogs with otitis media had an intact tympanic membrane in one study.[21,82] The tympanic membrane in dogs with otitis externa may be difficult to examine due to secondary changes of the external ear canal, pain associated with otoscopic examination, and accumulation of exudate, cerumen, and debris. Treatment to diminish the severity of otitis externa and general anesthesia may increase the ability to evaluate the tympanum in these cases.

Any case that has significant cerumen, exudate, or debris should undergo careful cleaning of the ear canal to allow evaluation of the integrity and character of the tympanic membrane. The presence of a "false middle ear" occurs when large accumulations of debris lodge against the tympanic membrane, causing it to deviate medially into the middle ear. This makes the external ear canal appear elongated and leads to misdiagnosis of a ruptured tympanic membrane.[3] Gentle probing of the tympanic membrane with a red rubber catheter under direct visualization may assist in the diagnosis of small tears in the membrane. If the catheter tip is consistently visible, rupture is unlikely. Alternatively, an aliquot of 1 mL of physiologic saline placed in the horizontal canal should remain stationary; disappearance suggests an opening in the tympanum allowing the fluid to drain into the middle ear.[1] Movement of the fluid may be blocked by large amounts of debris in the middle ear, even in the presence of a tear in the tympanum.

If the tympanic membrane is visible, its character should be recorded in the medical record for comparison upon reevaluation. Bulging, increased opacity, and hyperemia may be present with otitis media. Bulging of the pars flaccid alone, however, may be present without otitis media and may be due to increased pressure, which is typically normalized via the auditory tube.[83] If otitis media is suspected, radiographs of the bullae may be made. Lateral oblique and open-mouth views are most helpful for evaluating the tympanic bulla, but positioning for comparison of left and right sides is difficult and requires general anesthesia. Ventrodorsal or dorsoventral views allow evaluation of the air-filled lumen and calcification of the external ear canal. Abnormalities of the bulla include increased opacity, sclerosis, and lysis. Fluid cannot be differentiated from increased soft tissue density (e.g., neoplasia), and absence of radiographic changes does not rule out otitis media. Radiographs changes were absent in 33% of the middle ears in one study of dogs with otitis media confirmed by surgical exploration.[25] Otitis media or neoplasia and otitis interna can cause radiographic evidence of lysis of the petrosal bone.

Other diagnostic tools are available to evaluate patients with otitis media interna. Contrast introduced into the external ear canal followed by radiography, termed *canalography*, is used to diagnose tympanic membrane perforations. The method is useful for acute tympanic membrane rupture and increases the frequency of diagnosing tympanic membrane rupture with otitis externa media beyond that of otoscope alone.[84] Advanced imaging with CT and MRI has been studied in normal dogs and dogs with otitis media.[25,85] CT is considered superior to MRI for bony changes, whereas MRI is better for detection of soft tissue abnormalities in both dogs and cats.[25,86,87]

If the tympanic membrane is intact in a dog with otitis media, a myringotomy is performed to obtain samples for culture and susceptibility testing and cytologic examination. The patient may also be more comfortable after collection of samples due to decreased pressure in the middle ear following myringotomy. The procedure must be performed with the patient under general anesthesia and is usually done following radiography or advanced imaging of the ear. The external ear canal should be thoroughly cleaned and dried prior to myringotomy to avoid contamination with external ear canal debris. Direct otoscopic visualization is used for the procedure. A 20-gauge spinal needle is used to penetrate the tympanic membrane through the caudoventral aspect of the pars tensa. Suction is applied, and samples collected—culture and susceptibility testing take priority over cytologic examination because cytology is frequently negative, and cultures of the external ear canal do not reflect the middle ear bacteria in the majority of cases.[21] If fluid cannot be aspirated directly from the middle ear, 0.5 to 1 mL of warm, sterile saline is infused through the needle into the middle ear cavity and aspirated. Alternatively, an open-ended tom cat catheter or small, sterile culture swab may be passed into the middle ear cautiously under otoscopic visualization. *Pseudomonas* species and *Staphylococcus intermedius* are most commonly isolated, followed by yeast, β-hemolytic *Streptococcus*, *Corynebacterium* species, *Proteus* species, and *Enterococcus* species.[21,88] Surgical exploration is rarely required for the diagnosis of otitis media.

Medical therapy of otitis media should be guided by culture and susceptibility results. The external ear canal is flushed and dried as needed to treat concurrent otitis externa. Flushing is usually performed under the same general anesthetic episode used for diagnostic testing. If the tympanic membrane is ruptured, the middle ear is gently lavaged with warm saline. Endoscopic-guided lavage resulted in 86% resolution of clinical signs with concurrent medical therapy that averaged 4 months.[89] Cytology results, when available, should be used to guide initial therapy. The integrity of the tympanic membrane must be considered when using topical agents to treat concurrent otitis externa: Ototoxic medications and vehicles should be avoided if the tympanic membrane is ruptured.

Newly diagnosed cases of otitis media may be started on empiric therapy based on cytology; however, culture and susceptibility testing are valuable because antimicrobial resistance increases over time. First-choice antimicrobials include cephalosporins, amoxicillin/clavulanic acid, and fluoroquinolones. Definitive therapy consists of administration of antibiotics based on culture and susceptibility results for a minimum of 4 to 6 weeks. Primary and perpetuating factors of otitis externa should be identified and treated or controlled. Topical medication and flushing of the external ear canal should continue until resolution of clinical signs and normalization of cytology. Gradual improvement of the otitis media is expected within 14 days. The ear canal and tympanic membrane should be evaluated prior to and following discontinuation of therapy. Small tears in the tympanic membrane following myringotomy heal rapidly with appropriate therapy within 2 to 3 weeks.[55,90] However, reevaluation of the tympanic membrane in dogs with otitis externa media should precede alteration of the topical agents in the therapeutic plan.

Failure to respond to therapy or chronic or recurrent otitis media warrant reevaluation for surgical intervention. Total ear canal ablation and lateral bulla osteotomy should be considered in cases with severe secondary changes of the external ear canal and concurrent otitis media. If the external ear canal is not affected, a ventral bulla osteotomy may be performed to remove gross exudate and establish drainage from the middle ear of dogs and cats with chronic or recurrent otitis media. Caution should be taken in considering lateral ear resection and ventral bulla osteotomy in the treatment of otitis externa media in that lateral ear resection is only an adjunct to medical management of otitis externa.

Neoplasia of the Middle Ear
Neoplasia of the middle ear is rare; most cases represent extension of tumors originating in the external ear canal.

Inflammatory Polyps
Inflammatory polyps are a nonneoplastic admixture of inflammatory and epithelial cells originating in the tympanic bulla in cats. Other sites of origin include the auditory tube and nasopharynx. Macrophages, neutrophils, lymphocytes, plasma cells, and epithelial cells are usually present on histopathologic examination. The etiology is unknown, but ascending infection and congenital causes have been suggested.[57] There is no age or sex predilection for the condition, but younger cats may be more commonly affected (1 to 5 years of age). Signs can be unilateral or bilateral and depend on the location of the mass lesion. A single polyp can grow into the external ear canal, down the auditory tube into the nasopharynx, or both. Signs of otitis externa media are common with polyps limited to the ear, but respiratory stridor, dyspnea, gagging, and dysphagia occur with growth into the pharynx. Atypical signs may be associated with secondary infection and meningoencephalitis,[92] and chronic airway obstruction with secondary pulmonary hypertension has been suspected in one case.[93]

Diagnosis is based on otoscopic and pharyngeal examinations. Radiographs of the bulla, nasal cavity, and pharynx may be considered, and CT or MRI can be used to diagnose the site and side of origin of inflammatory polyps.[86,87] Treatment consists of excision by traction or surgical excision via ventral bulla osteotomy.[94-95] Regrowth is a problem in half of the cats treated by traction extraction alone, and Horner's syndrome is common in cats following ventral bulla osteotomy.[94,95] Ventral bulla osteotomy does not improve hearing in cats with inflammatory polyps, but clinical signs improve, despite the development of Horner's syndrome in 65% of cats after surgery.[96] Horner's syndrome usually resolves; however, a head tilt may be permanent if it is present prior to or after surgery.[96]

Primary Secretory Otitis Media
This syndrome has been described primarily in Cavalier King Charles Spaniels. The clinical signs are pain localized to the head or neck, vocalization, and neurologic signs such as ataxia, facial paralysis, nystagmus, head tilt, or seizures.[97] The signs of pain varied and resulted in horizontal neck carriage and guarding in some cases.[97] Otitis externa was not consistently present, but the middle ear contained viscous, opaque, gray to yellow, solid, pluglike material.[97] Removal of the mucus plug via myringotomy or extraction if the tympanic membrane was not present and concurrent flushing was often combined with local and systemic therapy. Repeated treatment was often required for complete resolution of signs.[97] Tympanostomy tubes have been used to decrease the need for repeated general anesthesia for removal of the mucus plug and flushing of the middle ear, but long-term results of their use have not yet been investigated.[98]

Otitis Interna
Otitis interna is usually an extension of otitis media or neoplasia of the middle ear. A careful neurologic examination is imperative to the localization of vestibular signs. Clinical signs associated with otitis interna include head tilt, ataxia, horizontal or rotary nystagmus, circling or falling toward the side of the lesion, or ipsilateral nystagmus. The fast phase of nystagmus is usually away from the side of the lesion. Occasionally animals will become nauseated or vomit. Horner's syndrome or deficits in cranial nerve VII may accompany otitis media interna, but involvement of other cranial nerves, vertical or changing nystagmus, or the presence of conscious proprioceptive deficits or paresis indicate central rather than peripheral vestibular disease. Bilateral peripheral vestibular disease is rare, but the patient will not have a head tilt, nystagmus, or strabismus, and may exhibit wide head excursions and a crouched stance or the inability to stand.

The diagnosis of otitis interna is based on history, clinical signs, and physical, neurologic, and otoscopic examinations. Advanced imaging may be helpful in distinguishing the anatomic location of the disease process. Treatment with aggressive medical or surgical intervention appropriate to the localization is important in prevention of adjacent brainstem involvement.

Prognosis for Otitis Media Interna

A fair prognosis can be given if aggressive surgical and medical therapy is possible. Cases with concurrent severe external ear canal changes require total ear canal ablation and lateral bulla osteotomy. Repeated infections following ventral bulla osteotomy or total ear canal ablation and lateral bulla osteotomy may be operated again with resolution of the condition. Resistant organisms, failure to respond to aggressive surgery, and significant osteomyelitis are associated with a poor prognosis. The neurologic signs associated with otitis media interna may be permanent, but many animals learn to utilize visual cues and can compensate for vestibular deficits. Facial nerve deficits, Horner's syndrome, and keratoconjunctivitis sicca are often permanent.

Ototoxicity

Ototoxic substances (Box 223-2) damage the cochlear or vestibular systems, or both. Otic application of medication can also cause adverse effects through local inflammation of the tympanic membrane and/or the meatal window and resultant otitis media. Topical medications also cause adverse effects by systemic absorption. Ototoxic substances reach the inner ear after local application and absorption through the cochlear or vestibular windows or hematogenously. The most frequent cause of ototoxicity is the application of an ototoxic substance to the external ear canal in a patient with a ruptured tympanum, which results in distribution to the middle ear. Absorption by the inner ear is increased when inflammation of the cochlear window occurs with otitis media. Hematogenous distribution of ototoxins to the inner ear is inherent in some medications (e.g., aminoglycosides).

The development of ototoxicity also depends on the vehicle of the preparation, chemical composition, drug concentration, concurrent medications, and route, frequency, and duration of administration.[3] Examples of increased risk of ototoxicity depending on the vehicle (e.g., combination of chlorhexidine and detergents) and concurrent medications (e.g., loop diuretics, aminoglycosides) have been described.[3] Minimization of the risk of toxicity should be considered when any potentially toxic substance is administered either topically or systemically. The integrity of the tympanic membrane should be known prior to topical administration of any potentially ototoxic drug, and consequences of each drug should be considered in light of the patient's health and concurrent therapies.

Idiopathic Vestibular/Facial Nerve Diseases

A complete neurologic examination is key to differentiating peripheral from central vestibular disorders. Head tilt, ataxia, horizontal or rotary nystagmus, and cranial nerve VII deficits may be seen with either condition. Central vestibular disease causes paraparesis, conscious proprioceptive deficits, other cranial nerve abnormalities, and vertical or changing nystagmus. Middle ear neoplasia, otitis media interna, idiopathic vestibular syndrome, and congenital vestibular disorders result in peripheral vestibular signs. Congenital vestibular disorders have been described in the German Shepherd Dog, Doberman Pinscher, English Cocker Spaniel, Siamese, and Burmese breeds.[99,100] Bilateral congenital vestibular syndrome has been described in Beagles and Akitas.[99,100] Clinical signs of head tilt and ataxia in these patients may be persistent or may improve; animals can be congenitally deaf.

Otitis media interna may be associated with facial paresis or paralysis if cranial nerve VII is affected by the inflammation. Otitis should be ruled out before diagnosing any patient with idiopathic facial nerve paralysis because otitis requires aggressive management and the idiopathic condition can only be treated symptomatically or with acupuncture.[101]

Deafness

Deafness is classified as inherited or acquired, conductive or sensorineural, and congenital or late-onset. Acquired deafness may be either conductive or sensorineural, depending on the etiologic agent, which also affects the time of onset. Conductive deafness results from a lack of presentation of sound to the inner ear, usually secondary to otitis externa media. Sensorineural deafness occurs with abnormalities of the cochlear system, cranial nerve VIII, or auditory pathways and higher brain centers. Inherited deafness, ototoxicity, cochlear nerve degeneration, and presbycusis (age-related deafness) are forms of sensorineural deafness.

Diagnostic Principles Patient signalment can help to prioritize possible causes of deafness. Certain breeds have a high incidence of inherited deafness, and clinical signs are usually noticed at an early age if the deafness is bilateral. Most other forms of deafness occur as late-onset disorders. The history is important in establishing the nature of the deafness because certain conditions or treatments may cause deafness (e.g., otitis externa media, ototoxic medications, head trauma, prior infectious diseases). The owner may note behavioral changes in the pet, and complete, bilateral deafness is usually easily identified. Astute owners may notice behavioral changes in puppies at an early age. Inherited deafness usually results in loss of hearing within 3 to 4 weeks of birth due to a degenerative process of the inner ear.[102] The affected pup is often more aggressive than its littermates because it cannot hear cries of pain during play. The puppy may also be more diffi-

---

Box • 223-2

Ototoxic Drugs

Aminoglycoside Antibiotics
Neomycin
Dihydrostreptomycin
Gentamicin
Streptomycin
Kanamycin
Tobramycin
Amikacin

Other Antibiotics
Polymyxin B & E
Minocycline
Erythromycin
Chloramphenicol
Vancomycin

Loop Diuretics
Furosemide
Bumetanide
Ethacrynic acid

Antiseptics
Chlorhexidine
Iodine and iodophores
Ethanol
Benzalkonium chloride
Benzethonium chloride
Cetrimide

Antineoplastic Agents
Cisplatin
Nitrogen mustard

Miscellaneous
Quinine
Salicylates
Propylene glycol
Detergents
Arsenic
Lead
Mercury

cult to rouse and is more vocal than its littermates, especially when they cannot be directly seen by the affected pup. Unilateral deafness is harder to identify, but the owner may report difficulty rousing the pet when it is sleeping in lateral recumbency or difficulty in the pet's ability to orient to the origin of sounds. The physical, otoscopic, and neurologic examinations are important in differentiating peripheral from central disease and establishing whether conductive deafness is possible. The index of suspicion for conductive deafness is increased in patients with abnormalities of the external ear canal, tympanum, cranial nerve VII, or sympathetic innervation of the eye. Abnormalities suggestive of central disease prompt more aggressive diagnostic testing such as advanced imaging and cerebrospinal fluid analysis.

Hearing loss can be evaluated with the patient in the examination room. Different sounds can be used in an attempt to observe behavioral reactions to sound. A Preyer's reflex (i.e., movement of the pinna in response to sound) is the minimal expected response.[102] Care should be taken to avoid visual cues and air movement close to the patient's head, which cause an apparent reaction to sound in an affected dog or cat. Unfortunately patients may be stressed by the hospital environment and may not react to auditory cues even if hearing is normal.

Impedance audiometry/tympanometry Impedance audiometry is based on the concept that the intensity of a sound wave is dependent on the size of the cavity in which it is generated and on the compliance of the cavity's containing walls.[3] The external ear canal is occluded for the test, and a sound wave generated. Changes in the pressure within the canal are measured to evaluate the compliance of the tympanic membrane. Accumulation of fluid in the middle ear canal, rupture of the tympanic membrane, immobility of the ossicles, and other causes of conductive deafness alter the results. Normal results in a deaf animal would be supportive of sensorineural deafness.

The acoustic, or stapedial, reflex test is also known as the *acoustic decay test*. A high-amplitude sound is used to cause stapedial muscle contraction, which protects the structures of the inner ear. This reflex alters tympanic compliance. The afferent (cranial nerve VII) and efferent limbs (cranial nerves V and VII) must be intact for a normal reflex.[1] A normal dog will maintain this reflex for a known period of time, but decay of the reflex occurs in dogs with lesions of cranial nerve VIII.[3] Tympanometry is not commonly performed because the specialized equipment, which is adapted from human kits, is required. Ideally the sound generated impacts the tympanic membrane perpendicular to its surface, which is difficult to obtain in the dog or cat due to the angle of the ear canal. The results are not sensitive or specific but are reliable for the diagnosis of tympanic membrane rupture.[3,103]

Brainstem auditory evoked response The brainstem auditory evoked response (BAER), or brainstem auditory evoked potential (BAEP), is an objective measure of hearing. The test identifies the presence or absence of hearing and progressive changes in hearing. Subjective determination of partial hearing loss is possible.[104] Electrodes placed on standard sites of the head record responses to an auditory stimulus generated in one ear. Sound is generated as a series of clicks, and the contralateral ear is excluded by the presentation of "white noise." A contralateral masking noise 20 dB below the stimulus of the test ear should help to avoid the misdiagnosis of a positive, albeit abnormal, hearing threshold in the affected ear.[105] The position of electrodes, stimulus intensity, and body temperature can also alter the waves produced.[3] Electrode position is standardized, and the sound generated, or stimulus,

intensity is presented over a range of decibels; the rate of presentation remains constant. The waves generated are subjectively and objectively evaluated. Wave I corresponds to cranial nerve VIII. Wave II represents the cochlear nucleus and intracranial, extramedullary portion of cranial nerve VIII. Wave III corresponds to the dorsal nucleus of the trapezoid body, and waves IV and V originate in the rostral pons and caudal colliculi, respectively.[3]

Wave latencies and amplitudes are used to assess hearing and conduction of impulses through the brainstem, making BAER testing valuable in not only the diagnosis of hearing, but also for evaluation of brainstem lesions. Most pets do not require sedation or anesthesia for the procedure, which is beneficial because both cause changes in middle and later wave latency. Wave latencies and amplitudes vary with the intensity and rate of delivery of the sound.[3] In general, amplitude increases and latency decreases with increasing sound intensity. Interpeak latencies are used to evaluate conduction in the brainstem, which should not change with stimulus intensity.

Conductive deafness reduces the intensity of sound reaching the inner ear. A lack of air conducted hearing in the presence of bony conducted hearing on BAER testing diagnoses conductive deafness. The hearing threshold is usually increased when sound is presented through air conduction, but bony conducted hearing should remain intact. The increased hearing threshold may be accompanied by decreased wave amplitude and increased wave latency in cases of severe otitis externa.[106] Sensorineural deafness alters the appearance of the BAER depending on the site of the lesion. Alteration of wave forms, increased hearing threshold, or complete abolition of wave forms may be present in animals with sensorineural deafness.

Acquired Late-Onset Conductive Deafness

Conductive deafness is due to lack of transmission of sound through the tympanic membrane and ossicles to the inner ear. Conditions that block sound transmission through the external ear canal, tympanic membrane, or middle ear and ossicles, such as otitis externa, otitis media, and otic neoplasia, cause conductive deafness. Less common causes of conductive deafness include trauma-induced fluid accumulation in the middle ear, atresia of the tympanum or ossicles, fused ossicles, or incomplete development of the external ear canal, which results in fluid accumulation in the middle ear.[102,104,107] An increase in hearing threshold, absence of air conducted hearing, and the presence of bone conducted hearing on BAER suggest conductive deafness.

The application of a bone-anchored hearing aid was described in one patient with conductive deafness following total ear canal ablation.[108] The patient maintained bone conducted hearing and tolerated the hearing aid anchored to the parietal bone. Use of a bone anchored device was required because the dog did not have an external ear canal in which to place an earpiece. The hearing aid acted as an amplifier, and the dog seemed to respond to its use.

Acquired Late-Onset Sensorineural Deafness

Presbycusis, or decline in hearing associated with aging, may be due to one of the following: loss of hair cells and degeneration in the organ of Corti, degeneration of spiral ganglion cells or neural fibers of the cochlear nerve, atrophy of the stria vascularis, or changes in the basilar membrane. Because this condition occurs in older dogs and cats from 8 to 17 years of age, animals should be evaluated for concurrent causes of conductive deafness such as chronic otitis externa or media and otic neoplasia. BAER testing may demonstrate normal waveforms in response to high-intensity sound.[109] If conduction is intact at an increased hearing threshold, use of an amplifying hearing aid may be beneficial. Pets may not tolerate occlusive types of earpieces often used in hearing aids, and training to the earpiece should be done prior to application of the hearing aid.

Ototoxic substances, chronic exposure to loud noise, hypothyroidism, trauma, and bony neoplasia can also cause acquired late-onset deafness in dogs and cats. Ototoxicity can result in abolition of waveforms or an increase in hearing threshold on BAER.[52] BAER testing can be used to reevaluate patients for return of function after withdrawal of medication following exposure to ototoxic medication.

Congenital Sensorineural Deafness

Inherited sensorineural deafness usually results in complete loss of hearing in the affected ear by 5 weeks of age. Many breeds can be affected with the condition (Box 223-3). The condition has been linked to coat color in many breeds of dogs and white cats. The condition is common in white cats, and mode of inheritance is thought to be autosomal dominant with incomplete penetrance.[110] The condition is most common in white cats with blue irides. The correlation of white coat, blue eyes, and deafness is not perfect, but cats with two blue irides have a greater risk of deafness than cats with one blue iris, which have a greater risk of deafness than cats without blue irides.[110] Total hearing loss occurs more often in long-haired white cats.[110] The condition is common in certain breeds of dogs, such as Dalmatians, which have a nearly 30% incidence of deafness (combining unilateral and bilateral deafness).

The trait is associated with the dominant merle or dapple gene in Collies, Shetland Sheepdogs, Great Danes, and Dachshunds. The incidence of deafness tends to increase with increasing amount of white in the coat, and dogs homozygous for the merle gene are usually deaf and may be solid white, blind, and/or sterile.[102] The piebald or extreme piebald gene is associated with deafness in Dalmatians, Bull Terriers, Great Pyrenees, Sealyham Terriers, Greyhounds, Bulldogs, and Beagles. Inheritance is thought to be autosomal recessive, but the trait may be polygenic.[104] Phenotype was useful for predicting deafness in Dalmatians, English Cocker Spaniels, and English Setters.[111] Deafness was more likely if in the presence

---

Box • 223-3

*Canine Breeds Associated with Inherited Deafness**

Akita	Foxhound	Pit Bull Terrier
American-Canadian Shepherd	Fox Terrier	Pointer
American Cocker Spaniel	French Bulldog	Poodle (Toy and Miniature)
American Eskimo		
American Staffordshire Terrier	German Shepherd Dog	Rhodesian Ridgeback
Australian Cattle Dog	Great Dane	Rottweiler
Australian Shepherd	Great Pyrenees	
	Greyhound	Saint Bernard
Beagle		Samoyed
Bichon Frise	Ibizan Hound	Schnauzer
Border Collie	Italian Greyhound	Scottish Terrier
Borzoi		Sealyham Terrier
Boston Terrier	Jack Russell Terrier	Shetland Sheepdog
Boxer		Shropshire Terrier
Bulldog	Kuvasz	Siberian Husky
Bull Terrier		Soft-Coated Wheaton Terrier
	Labrador Retriever	Springer Spaniel
Cardigan Welsh Corgi	Löwchen	Sussex Spaniel
Catahoula Leopard Dog		
Cavalier King Charles Spaniel	Maltese	Tibetan Spaniel
Chihuahua	Miniature Pinscher	Tibetan Terrier
Chow Chow	Miniature Poodle mongrel	Toy Fox Terrier
Collie		
	Nova Scotia Duck Tolling Retriever	Walker American Foxhound
Dachshund	Norwegian Dunkerhound	West Highland White Terrier
Dalmatian		Whippet
Doberman Pinscher	Old English Sheepdog	
Dogo Argentino		Yorkshire Terrier
	Papillion	
English Bulldog	Perro de Carea Leonés	
English Cocker Spaniel	Presa Canario	
English Setter	Puli	

*This list of breeds in not all-inclusive.

of blue eyes and or if one or both parents were affected with deafness.[111] The presence of a patch in Dalmatians was negatively associated with deafness, and White Bull Terriers were more likely to be deaf than colored Bull Terriers.[111] These findings suggested that phenotype was associated with the allele for deafness and could be useful in determining the likelihood of deafness.

Heterochromia irides and lack of retinal pigment are associated with white color in dogs and cats. Hearing loss may be associated with absence of pigment in the cochlear stria vascularis. Diminished blood supply and/or disorders of endolymph production with changes in the chemical or mechanical properties of endolymph lead to degeneration of the organ of Corti secondary to stria vascularis atrophy. Loss of hair cells and abnormalities of the cochlear duct, Reissner membrane, tectorial membrane, and internal spiral sulcus are typical of cochleosaccular type of end-organ degeneration seen in these cases.[3,102,104,110]

Clinical signs of deafness may be recognized in puppies as young as 3 weeks of age by astute owners; definitive diagnosis of unilateral or bilateral deafness is usually made by BAER testing at 5 to 6 weeks of age when the auditory system is completely developed and cochlear degeneration, if present, is complete.

Congenital Acquired Sensorineural Deafness Exposure to bacteria, ototoxic drugs, low oxygen tension, and trauma in utero or during the perinatal period rarely causes deafness in young animals.

REFERENCES

The reference list can be found on the companion Expert Consult Web site at *www.expertconsult.com*.

CHAPTER 224

Diseases of the Nose and Nasal Sinuses

Anjop J. Venker-van Haagen
Michael E. Herrtage

FUNCTIONAL CONSIDERATIONS

Functional Anatomy

The nose has four main functions: (1) to provide a portal through which air can flow to reach the alveoli, (2) to modify or regulate the flow of air, (3) to facilitate water and heat exchange (e.g., to condition the inspired air), and (4) to pass inspired air over the olfactory epithelium—the sheet of neurons and supporting cells that lines the nasal cavities. Speculation exists regarding the functions of the nasal sinuses. It seems plausible that the frontal sinuses protect the rostral portions of the brain from frontal trauma.

The rostral portion of the nose, consisting of hairless integument and the nostrils, is called the *nasal plane*. It is supported by cartilages, which also support the portion of the nose between the nasal plane and the bony portion. The levator nasolabial and levator labii superior muscles can move the cartilaginous parts. Dilation of the nostrils changes the pattern of flow of inspired air. The nostrils are dilated when increased airflow is necessary, as in dyspnea, and to aid sampling of interesting odors.

The nasal cavity is the facial portion of the respiratory passageway. It is composed of bony and cartilaginous parts and extends from the nostrils to the choanae. It is divided into right and left halves by the nasal septum. Each half of the nasal cavity has a respiratory and an olfactory region. The nasal conchae (formerly called *turbinates*) are cartilaginous or slightly ossified scrolls covered by nasal mucosa and fill the nasal cavity. The nasal mucosa, together with the nasal glands, has a role in *conditioning* the inspired air. During normal inspiration, the respiratory and olfactory air currents follow a similar path. However, when the dog or cat wants to sample environmental odors, the nostrils are dilated, and forced inspiration occurs in which a greater volume of inspired air takes a more dorsal course around the ethmoidal conchae, where the olfactory receptors are most numerous.[1]

Regulation and Conditioning of the Inspiratory and Expiratory Airflow

The respiratory airflow through the nasal cavity is regulated by the ventilatory control systems. The nose represents an important part of the resistance of the airway and thereby influences gas exchange in the alveoli. The resistance has to be overcome by greater negative pressure in the thorax during inspiration, which leads to better expanding and filling of the alveoli by the inspired air and a greater venous blood flow in the lungs. In humans, a prolonged increase in nasal resistance because of severe obstruction can lead to cor pulmonale, cardiomegaly, and pulmonary edema.[2] In dogs, pulmonary edema is known to develop in laryngeal obstruction. Pulmonary edema may occur by a similar mechanism when severe obstruction of nasal airflow exists. The most common consequence of increased nasal resistance, however, is mouth breathing.

Heating or cooling of inspired and expired air as it passes through the nose is largely accomplished by radiation from the mucosal blood vessels. The flow of blood is from caudal to rostral, opposite to the flow of the inspired air. Humidification occurs by evaporation from the blanket of mucus covering the mucosa and the serous fluid from the nasal glands. The nasal blood flow and the activity of the nasal glands are regulated by the autonomic nervous system. The autonomic innervation of the nose consists of parasympathetic and sympathetic nerve fibers, joined together in the vidian nerve. The conditioning of the inspired air by the nose, which also includes the removal of larger particulate matter, is a very important function for protection of the alveoli. Even under extremely dry and cold conditions, the bronchi receive air warmed to body temperature with humidity of around 98%.

Mucosal Cleaning

The pseudostratified respiratory mucosa in the nose consists of ciliated, intermediate, basal, and goblet cells. They rest on a well-defined basement membrane supported by a deep, loose lamina propria containing small blood vessels, venous plexus, and ducts of mucous and serous glands, sensory nerves, and blood cells. The tall ciliated cell is the predominant type and it extends from the basement membrane to the luminal surface, where cilia admixed with microvilli are found. The cilia actively move the overlying blanket of mucus by a to-and-fro movement, called the *ciliary beat*. A more forceful propulsive movement and a less forceful recovery beat occur. The propulsive movement transports the mucus blanket toward the pharyngeal end of the esophagus. The two-layer mucous blanket is sticky, tenacious, and adhesive. The outer layer is more viscid than the deeper, periciliary layer. Insoluble particles, allergens, and bacteria caught on the outer layer are thus carried to the esophagus. Soluble material reaches the periciliary layer and is absorbed.[3]

Sneezing starts with a rapid inspiration followed by an involuntary, sudden, violent, and audible expulsion of air through the nose and mouth. The reflex occurs after stimulation of sensory receptors in the nasal mucosa. It is the ultimate cleaning procedure for the nasal cavity in dogs and cats.

Olfaction

Three sensory systems are dedicated to the detection of chemicals in the environment: (1) olfaction, (2) taste, and (3) the trigeminal chemosensory system.[4] Olfactory information can influence feeding behavior, social interaction, and reproduction. A dog's sense of smell, together with its personality and intelligence, helps it serve its function as a nose for humans.

The transduction of olfactory information occurs in the nasal olfactory epithelium, the sheet of neurons and supporting cells that lines the caudolateral wall, the ethmoidal conchae, and the dorsal part of the nasal septum.[5,6] The olfactory receptor neuron is a bipolar neuron that gives rise on its basal surface to an unmyelinated axon that carries the olfactory information to the brain through the cribriform plate, a sievelike partition of thin bone that separates the nasal chamber from the olfactory bulbs. At its apex the receptor neuron has a single process that expands into a knoblike protrusion from which several microvilli, or olfactory cilia, extend into the thick layer of mucus that lines the nasal cavity and controls the ionic milieu of the olfactory cilia (Figure 224-1).

Generation of receptor potentials in response to odors takes place in the cilia of receptor neurons. The axons of the olfactory receptor cells form the olfactory nerves that pass through the cribriform plate directly to the olfactory bulb, on the rostroventral aspect of the ipsilateral forebrain. Olfactory information is passed to the amygdala and primary olfactory cortex. Further pathways for processing olfactory information include the thalamus, hypothalamus, entorhinal cortex, and hippocampus.[7]

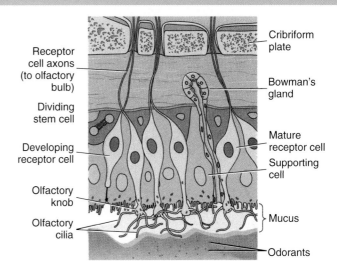

Figure 224-1 Diagram of the olfactory epithelium showing the major cell types and the projection of the olfactory receptor neurons to the bulb (see text "olfaction"). Bowman's glands produce mucus, and supporting cells help to detoxify chemicals that come in contact with the epithelium. (From Purves D, Augustine GJ, Katz LC, editors: Neuroscience, Sunderland, Mass, 1997, Sinauer Associates, p 267.)

tumors of the nasal cavity. Neurologic signs may be seen with extension of the disease process into the brain.

If nasal discharge is the predominant sign, questions should be asked to help determine whether it is from the left, the right, or both nostrils. The nasal discharge should be characterized (watery, mucoid, purulent, hemorrhagic) and its frequency noted. Discharge occurring only during sneezing indicates a less productive mucosal disease than does continuous discharge. Occasional nasal bleeding is less alarming than frequent and profuse nasal bleeding, which can be fatal.

Sneezing, like coughing, is a reflex associated with protection of the mucosa. Particles, foreign bodies, inflammation of the mucosa, or abnormal turbulence in the nasal cavity associated with local drying of the mucosa can stimulate the sensory receptors in the mucosa. Continuous sneezing can cause irritation of the mucosa, leading to more sneezing and sometimes epistaxis.

Pain from the nose may only become obvious when the animal begins to react adversely to the owner's customary petting. A dog with pain in the nose may object to having a collar or the loop of a leash drawn over its head, even though this is usually associated with the coming pleasure of a walk. Questions to obtain information about nasal or facial pain should be adapted to the living conditions of the dog or cat.

Nasal stridor is a soft, rustling or sniffing sound that is synchronous with inspiration or expiration or both. Narrowing of the nasal passageways, which increases the velocity of the airflow, causes this sound.

Dyspnea may be caused by nasal obstruction in cats and dogs. Both tend to avoid mouth breathing even in this situation, sometimes almost to the point of suffocation. Apparently, avoiding the consequent bypassing of the nasal function of air cleansing and conditioning has a high priority.

HISTORY AND CLINICAL SIGNS

The medical history in nasal disease usually includes clear signs of nasal disease such as nasal discharge (unilateral or bilateral), sneezing, epistaxis, and stertor because these are obvious to the owner. Additional questions are then asked about the animal's general condition, appetite, drinking, activity, exercise tolerance, and changes in habits. These questions and a general physical examination are indicated because some systemic diseases that cause nasal discharge (such as canine distemper or feline viral rhinotracheitis) or epistaxis (bleeding disorders), whereas some nasal diseases (such as advanced aspergillosis) can cause general malaise, and dyspnea can occur in obstructive nasal disease, for example, due to

PHYSICAL EXAMINATION

In addition to a full physical examination, the clinician should evaluate the shape and symmetry of the nose and assess by palpation for any facial pain or distortion. The clinician should then listen to the animal's respiration for the presence and character of any upper respiratory noise. Under quiet conditions, the clinician should listen close to the patient's nose, while gently closing its mouth. If stridor is noted, and the clinician suspects it is caused by nostrils that are too narrow, moving the nasal alae laterally can change the tone of the stridor. Symmetry of the air stream can be examined by watching the movement of a small fluff of cotton held in front of each nostril. At the same time, the odor of the expired air can be noted. The area around the nostrils should be inspected for nasal discharge or crusts and the nasal plane for epithelial crusts (which could be caused by pathologic dryness), epithelial lesions, and depigmentation. The ventral wall of the nasal passages, which also forms the roof of the mouth, should be inspected through the opened mouth. The teeth, especially the canine teeth, should be inspected at the same time because dental abnormalities can cause disorders of the nose.[8] More in-depth inspections belong to special diagnostic procedures and require anesthesia.

SPECIAL DIAGNOSTIC PROCEDURES

Radiography
The standard radiographic examination of the skull consists of a lateral and a dorsoventral (DV) or ventrodorsal (VD) projection. The lateral radiograph has limited value in assessing patients with nasal disease because of superimposition of the left and right nasal chambers; however, it is useful when looking for signs of disease involving the nasal and frontal bones or the cribriform plate. The value of the DV or VD is also limited by the superimposition of the mandible over much of the nasal chamber.

The dorsoventral intraoral projection is the most useful view for assessing patients with nasal disease because it provides minimal superimposition of structures over the area of interest (see Figure 224-6, *A*). A standard radiographic cassette is too thick to provide a full assessment of the nasal cavity in all but the largest of dogs, and therefore either non-screen film or a flexible film-screen combination in a light-proof carrier should be used. Deep sedation or general anesthesia is mandatory, and the film or carrier should be placed corner first into the mouth to ensure that the caudal nasal chamber and cribriform plate is included.

The rostrocaudal (skyline) projection is useful for evaluating the frontal sinuses (see Figure 224-7). The radiograph can be made using a vertical x-ray beam with the patient lying in dorsal recumbency and the dorsum of the nose positioned vertically. Alternatively, a caudorostral (skyline) projection can be used with a horizontal x-ray beam to show the frontal sinuses. The patient is placed in sternal recumbency, with the head raised slightly and the dorsum of the nose parallel to the tabletop. A cassette is propped up in front of the external nares.

Stringent attention to detail for accurate positioning, exposure factors, and processing will help to provide the optimum amount of information from the radiographic examination.

Cross-Sectional Imaging
Cross-sectional imaging techniques, computed tomography (CT), and magnetic resonance (MR) imaging are increasingly used for investigation of nasal disease because both CT and MR provide images without superimposition of structures and with better soft tissue delineation compared with radiography (see Figure 224-6, *A* and *B*). CT imaging, like conventional radiography, is based on differences in attenuation of an x-ray beam by different tissues. CT is particularly suited to the examination of the fine bony detail of the nasal chamber and is valuable for identifying bone destruction and soft tissue involvement. Scan times tend to be short. MR imaging,

however, is based on the magnetic properties of atomic nuclei that have an odd number of protons, principally hydrogen. MR has the advantages of exceptional soft tissue contrast, multiplanar imaging capacity, and lacks ionizing radiation and bone beam-hardening artifact, but scan times tend to be longer. CT and MR imaging therefore provide slightly different information and there are no large studies using both modalities to suggest that one is inherently better or more accurate than the other.

Cross-sectional imaging provides a thorough assessment of the nasal cavity and paranasal sinuses. The nature and extent of a lesion can be more reliably assessed with CT or MR than with conventional radiography. The use of CT and/or MR greatly enhances the ability to differentiate inflammatory from neoplastic disease and to identify destructive rhinitis at an earlier stage than is possible with conventional radiography. Contrast-enhanced CT and MR are useful in being able to distinguish between vascularized soft tissue and mucus accumulation. Cross-sectional imaging is often used to help guide postimaging rhinoscopy and biopsy procedures, as well as to provide vital information when planning surgical treatment or external beam radiation therapy.

Rhinoscopy
Rhinoscopy is a relatively simple procedure in dogs and cats. It requires anesthesia and endotracheal intubation to prevent air circulation through the nasal cavities. Most veterinarians prefer to perform the examination with the dog or cat in sternal recumbency, in a sphinxlike posture. A firm pillow is placed between the head and the front legs so that the head is stabilized but not fixed. The rhinoscopic examination is preceded by a careful inspection of the oral cavity and pharynx. Retroflex nasopharyngoscopy should then be performed using a small flexible endoscope (4 mm diameter) turned through 180 degrees around the caudal border of the soft palate to evaluate the choanae (caudal nares), dorsal soft palate, and nasopharynx. Tumors or foreign bodies that are not possible to view from a rostral approach can sometimes be seen in this location.

A simple otoscope can be used to examine the rostral part of the nasal cavity. It should be of good quality, having a strong light source and dark specula, in order to illuminate the area. The nostril is approached from the lateral side at an angle of 45 degrees to the vertical surface of the nasal plane. The tip of the speculum is placed near the lateral limit of the nostril and is then introduced by slowly turning the otoscope until its line of vision is parallel to the nasal cavity. This movement is necessary to push the nasal ala, which obstructs the opening, into a lateral position.

Once the otoscope is introduced, visibility is often poor. Nasal disease often causes discharge and the tip of the speculum becomes blocked by mucus. The lens of the otoscope can be slid slightly to one side, allowing the introduction of a small suction cannula, while vision through the lens is maintained. The mucus is removed under visual control and the rostral part of the nasal cavity is then examined.

The use of an otoscope is often preferred for diagnosis and removal of foreign bodies that have entered the nasal cavity via the nostril. A foreign body forceps developed for use through an otoscope under visual guidance will facilitate retrieval of a foreign body.

An endoscope is necessary for complete examination of the nasal cavity. The basic equipment includes a light source, a flexible fiberoptic cable, and a small diameter endoscope. The authors and colleagues prefer the 25-degree vision rigid endoscope that is 2.7 mm in diameter and about 15 cm long. The best instruments have a wide-angle lens, which is important for orientation and facilitates the examination. This scope is adequate for most cats and dogs. For small cats, a 1.2-mm diameter rigid telescope is necessary. In most cats and dogs the 2.7-mm scope can be introduced and a suction cannula (size 6) or a foreign body or biopsy forceps can be passed alongside it.

The light source for rhinoscopy can be a single-outlet model, but a combined light source and electronic flash generator is necessary to obtain photographic images. For teaching purposes a chip camera and a video recorder are great assets. Additional equipment for rhinoscopy includes several suction cannulas (size 6), a vacuum source, a selection of biopsy forceps, and a small dropper bottle of 0.1% adrenaline solution to stop profuse bleeding (no more than 1 or 2 drops should be used at a time).

The anatomic borders that guide the inspection of the nasal cavity are the nostril rostrally, the nasal septum medially, the roof of the nasal cavity dorsally, and the bottom of the nasal cavity ventrally. The cribriform plate is part of the caudal boundary, together with the ventrally positioned openings to the nasal pharynx, the choanae. The endoscopic procedure aims at bringing the greater part of the nasal cavity into view. The procedure is limited by the choanae, if not by the pathologic process. Careful maneuvering and repositioning of the endoscope will result in a reliable impression of the normal and pathologic structures in the nasal cavity.

The main indications for rhinoscopy are a history of unilateral nasal discharge, the known or probable entrance of a foreign body, obstructive disease indicating tumor with no conclusive radiographic findings, and severe rhinitis with a suspicion of aspergillosis. In all other cases of chronic nasal disease with no significant findings on radiography, rhinoscopy might be helpful but is not always conclusive. In any event, biopsy samples should be collected from any affected or suspicious areas of the nasal cavity.

Olfactory Tests

No simple method exists to study olfaction in dogs. The sense of smell should be tested by activation of the olfactory receptor neurons and activation of the brain. The activation of the brain is recorded by electroencephalographic olfactometry analysis. Some authors have reported results in dogs with supposed normal olfactory function and in those that have lost the sense of smell.[9-11]

CONGENITAL DISEASES

Congenital malformation of the nasal plane is a common finding in brachycephalic breeds. The cartilage supporting the nasal plane is soft; thus the alae collapse, closing the nares. Corrective surgery is a simple procedure and consists of removing a cone-shaped piece of the ala and suturing the sides of the incision together in such a way that the nasal opening is enlarged.[12]

In dogs and cats, variable congenital lesions of the nasal plane or more extensive clefts can be repaired surgically. The success of surgery depends largely on the available tissue around the cleft. Oronasal and oropharyngeal clefts cause rhinitis and should be considered for surgical repair. Euthanasia may be justified if repair is not possible and nasal discharge and dysphagia are causing recurrent fever and pain. Nasal dermoid sinus cysts have been reported in dogs.[13] This cyst is recognized as a fistula in the midline of the bridge of the nose, producing intermittent discharge. The extent of the fistula can be established using MR imaging.[14] Exploration of the fistula may reveal skin and hair as far down as the nasal septum. This abnormally located tissue must be completely removed before the skin incision is closed. A congenital cerebrospinal fluid (CSF) fistula, causing rhinorrhea, was reported in a cat. It was closed successfully.[15]

The frontal sinuses are variable in size and sometimes even absent. Their absence is not associated with clinical signs but is usually found when lateral radiographs of the skull are made for another reason. Confusion with obstructive frontal sinus disease is possible when nasal disease is evident.

Congenital ciliary dysfunction has been documented in dogs of various breeds. Primary ciliary dyskinesia is a disorder in which ciliary function is ineffective and uncoordinated, resulting in rhinitis, bronchitis, bronchiectasis, and bronchopneumonia. When associated with situs inversus, the clinical syndrome is known as *Kartagener's syndrome*. The initial signs (nasal discharge and coughing) usually begin at an early age, from days to 5 weeks of age. However, some dogs have remained asymptomatic for months. Complications are caused by colonization of the mucosa and the conchae by *Pasteurella multocida* and *Bordetella bronchiseptica*, which can damage ciliated cells and cause hypoplastic conchae by bone resorption.

Mucociliary clearance in the dog's nasal cavity can be measured by placing a small drop of ^{99m}Tc macroaggregated albumin deep in the cavity, via a catheter, beyond the nonciliated rostral half. The velocity of mucus clearance ranges from 7 to 20 mm/min.[16] The test is not affected by anesthesia. However, not all normal dogs have a normal clearance rate and inflammation can change the velocity of the ciliary beat. To avoid spurious values, the test should be repeated and performed bilaterally.

Functional analysis of cilia in vitro is performed by examining transverse sections in electron micrographs after glutaraldehyde-osmium fixation. Major ultrastructural lesions in cilia of dogs with primary ciliary dyskinesia are a lack of outer dynein arms, an abnormal microtubular pattern, and an electron-dense core in the basal body.[16] The prognosis is guarded. Affected dogs that develop severe recurrent bronchopneumonia will eventually die of sepsis. Continuous treatment with broad-spectrum antibiotics will enable the dog to survive longer. Cultures should be repeated to maintain correct antibiotic treatment based on sensitivity testing. A worthwhile review of treatment and long-term survival in dogs is available.[16]

INFLAMMATORY DISEASES

Viral Rhinitis

Viral rhinitis is a prominent disease in cats. The initial clinical signs are paroxysmal sneezing, conjunctivitis, and serous ocular and nasal discharge. About 5 days after the onset of sneezing, the nasal discharge becomes mucopurulent and there may be ocular complications. The condition usually persists for 2 to 3 weeks. Feline herpesvirus-1 (FHV-1) and feline calicivirus (FCV) are the most prevalent and virulent respiratory pathogens of cats and account for at least 80% to 90% of their infectious upper respiratory infections.[17,18] The introduction of an efficacious modified live virus (MLV) vaccine against these two viruses has led to a substantial decline in mortality and morbidity but has not eliminated these diseases. Vaccination against these viruses protects the cat from development of severe disease but not from infection.[18]

Although the FCV vaccines have been designed to produce cross-protective immunity against severe clinical disease, there are multiple strains of FCV and it is possible for infection and mild disease to occur in the vaccinated animal. With respect to FHV, it should be remembered that no vaccine can protect against infection with virulent herpesvirus, and that virulent virus will become latent and may be reactivated during periods of severe stress, causing clinical signs in the vaccinated cat.[18]

Because these viruses can spread rapidly among kittens and the prevalence of chronically infected virus carriers is high, elimination of the disease is not feasible. It is estimated that 80% of cats recovering from acute infection become chronic carriers. The predominant route of infection is by direct cat-to-cat contact.[19] The chronic carrier state may develop subsequent to infection with either FHV or FCV and also occurs in vaccinated cats. Although cats carrying FHV do not necessarily shed virulent virus continuously, they should be considered infectious when they are sneezing and have nasal discharge. Calicivirus carriers shed virulent virus continuously from the oropharynx. They may have no clinical signs or mild nasal discharge, gingival ulceration, and periodontitis.

Viral rhinitis is a prominent clinical sign of canine distemper (Figure 224-2). Vaccination has reduced the occurrence of the disease to sporadic cases in countries where stray dogs are limited and veterinary care is adequate. Herpesvirus infection in newborn puppies is characterized by profuse mucopurulent nasal discharge. The diagnosis is usually made at autopsy.

Bacterial Rhinitis

Primary bacterial rhinitis is uncommon in both dogs and cats. Bacterial rhinitis develops as a sequela to viral rhinitis in cats, can be caused by foreign bodies in both dogs and cats, and occurs in many other disorders due to disruption of normal mucociliary mucosal integrity. Primary or secondary infection with *Bordetella bronchiseptica* can itself cause severe disruption to ciliary function that may be permanent.

Mycotic Rhinitis

Mycotic diseases involving the nasal cavity, the frontal sinuses, and the nasal plane occur in both dogs and cats. In dogs the most prevalent mycosis in the nasal cavity and frontal sinuses is caused by *Aspergillus* spp., although *Penicillium* spp. are occasionally implicated. In cats, *Cryptococcus neoformans* is a more common cause of fungal rhinitis, especially in warmer climates; *C. neoformans* infections may also occur in dogs. *Alternaria* spp. may infest the nasal plane in cats, causing proliferation of the skin and thereby dyspnea.

Aspergillus spp. are considered to be opportunists, producing infections in man and animals especially when resistance to infection is reduced or when large numbers of spores are present. Spores of *Aspergillus fumigates* are present on household plants, on furniture made of plant material, around bird cages, and simply in house dust.[20]

In dogs *Aspergillus* spp. plaques are usually found in the caudal part of the nasal cavity or in the frontal sinus. They are presumed to represent primary infections. The toxins produced by the fungus cause atrophy of the conchae in the areas of the fungal plaques and severe destruction of the mucosa and underlying structures in the entire nasal cavity and frontal sinus. There may be bone resorption and periostitis on the frontal bones, and atrophy and resorption of the internal surface of the frontal bone may open the way to the brain. The disease may spread bilaterally, destroying all internal and external bony structures, as well as the orbit, the nasal septum, and the nasal plane. *A. fumigatus* was identified in 25 of 27 of our cases involving the sinus and related structures.[20] Disseminated aspergillosis caused by *A. terreus*, not originating from the airways, has also been reported.[21] *Aspergillus* spp. can be associated with longstanding traumatic changes in the mucosa, caused by persisting foreign bodies in the nasal cavity or oronasal fistulas. These infections are presumed to be secondary to the trauma.

Clinical signs of aspergillosis in the nose and frontal sinus are dominated by profuse mucopurulent nasal discharge and nasal pain. Depigmentation of the nasal plane below the nostril from which there is discharge is a characteristic sign (Figure 224-3).

Intermittent hemorrhagic discharge occurs and profuse nasal bleeding is not uncommon. When only the frontal sinus is infected, hemorrhagic discharge or profuse bleeding from the nose may be the only sign. The nasal infection is often unilateral initially, becoming bilateral later. Aspergillosis is often not suspected in its initial stage, and a history of nasal discharge present for some months is common. No apparent correlation exists between the duration of the initial nasal discharge and the severity or progression of signs by the time of diagnosis. Other factors, such as the number of infecting spores and the resistance of the host, may play a role. Depression is a prominent sign when the frontal sinus is infected.

The diagnosis of aspergillosis as the cause of rhinitis is made by the finding of fungus plaques or positive fungal culture results. Recognition of the fungus plaque is facilitated by the atrophy of the conchae around it, which reduces the normal obstruction to rhinoscopic vision in the caudal part of the nasal cavity (Figure 224-4). The extent of the destruction

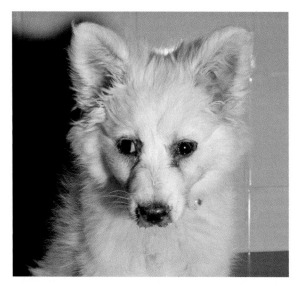

Figure 224-2 A 5-month-old Samoyed with distemper and bilateral mucopurulent discharge. Viral rhinitis is a prominent clinical sign of canine distemper.

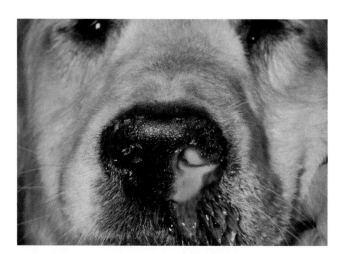

Figure 224-3 Depigmentation of the nasal plane below the nostril from which there is discharge, in a dog with nasal aspergillosis in the left nasal cavity.

in the nasal cavities and the frontal sinuses is well demonstrated by radiography, CT, or MRI, but the diagnosis depends on finding the fungus (Figures 224-5 and 224-6). When the fungus is in the frontal sinus alone, radiographs usually demonstrate irregular soft tissue densities in the frontal sinus, thickening of the wall of the sinus, and sometimes reaction of the periosteum (Figure 224-7). A CT or MR scan may reveal

the severity of further bony involvement. A 3- to 4-mm diameter trephined opening in the frontal bone on the side of the affected sinus can reveal the fungus as thick, grayish-yellow material, sometimes with greenish lumps. This material should be removed and cultured. Cultures from nasal discharge are often negative because the fungus is usually located in the caudal part of the nasal cavity and is not shed in the nasal discharge. Fungal organisms have been found in up to 40% of healthy dogs. A serologic test is available for detecting antibodies to *Aspergillus* spp. in serum. The test is valuable and only gives positive results in the presence of clinical infection. However, negative results may occur even with extensive disease. A PCR test is also available.

Treatment of sinonasal aspergillosis is topical or systemic. Topical treatment is usually with enilconazole or clotrimazole provided that the cribriform plate is intact. The choice between these two drugs is arbitrary because there has been no satisfactory clinical trial to compare them. The ongoing discussion is how to apply the suspensions and how long the treatment should be given. The basic idea is to flush the frontal sinus and the nasal cavity (e.g., via tubes introduced through trephine holes). The author's clinical experience (in about 120 cases, on average, 10 per year) indicates that administration of 10 cc of a 10% suspension of enilconazole per tube twice daily for 14 days is sufficient. It is unpleasant for the dog because enilconazole has a bitter taste that most dogs dislike intensely. A retrospective study of cases treated in our clinic (unpublished data) revealed success in about 95% in over 100 cases. Hence 90% success can be expected in treatment of a smaller number of cases. A less unpleasant systemic treatment would be much preferred, but the success rates and observed toxicities of other methods are not yet

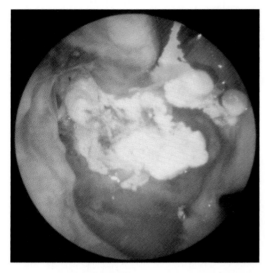

Figure 224-4 *Aspergillus* plaque: a rhinoscopic view in the caudal part of the nasal cavity.

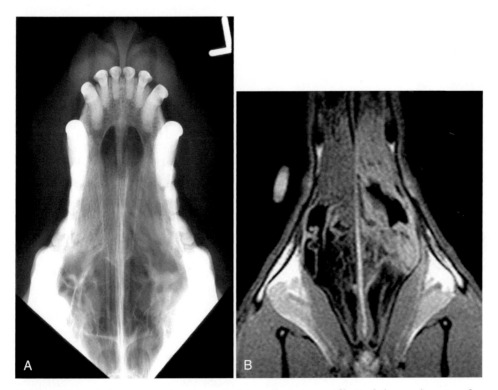

Figure 224-5 **A,** Dorsoventral radiograph (intraoral nonscreen film) of the nasal cavity of a Border Collie with aspergillosis of the left nasal cavity with loss of the conchal pattern in the rostral to middle zones. **B,** Dorsal T1-weighted magnetic resonance image of the same dog showing the conchal loss and increased intensity of the affected mucosa. Note increased sensitivity of cross-sectional imaging.

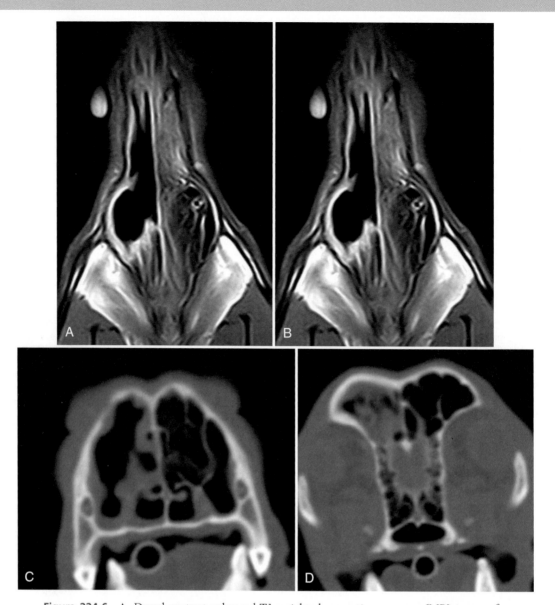

Figure 224-6   **A,** Dorsal contrast enhanced T1-weighted magnetic resonance (MR) image of a Bollie Collie with aspergillosis affecting the right nasal cavity with extensive conchal destruction. **B,** Transverse contrast enhanced T1-weighted MR image of the caudal nasal chamber and frontal sinus of the same dog showing a fungal granuloma in the right frontal sinus. **C** and **D,** Transverse Computed tomography images of a dog with aspergillosis of the right nasal cavity and frontal sinus showing similar changes. Note the thickening of the right frontal bone. (**C** and **D,** Courtesy Dr. A. Avner.)

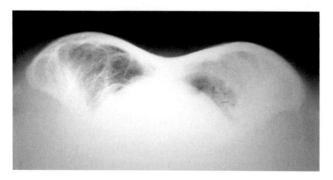

Figure 224-7   Rostrocaudal radiograph of Rhodesian Ridgeback with aspergillosis involving the left frontal sinus showing increased opacity in the affected frontal sinus and thickening of the overlying frontal bone.

encouraging. A combined clotrimazole irrigation and depot therapy, using 1% clotrimazole cream instilled into the frontal sinuses, has been described in 14 dogs with satisfactory results in 12 dogs.[22]

Cryptococcosis is found as a cause of rhinitis in dogs and cats. The clinical signs are obstructive rhinitis and mucopurulent discharge. In cats, crusts sometimes occur on the nasal plane and the bridge of the nose. Some cats develop mucopurulent conjunctivitis. In fresh material from the nose placed on a slide and stained with India ink, *Cryptococcus* spp. organisms are recognized as thick, encapsulated, round to oval yeasts. They can be cultured on Sabouraud's agar. Ketoconazole, itraconazole, or fluconazole can be used for therapy, which should be continued for 8 weeks, and in some cases long-term therapy is required. *Alternaria* spp. are found to cause granulomatous infections with crusts on the nasal plane in cats. Antimycotic treatment may be disappointing and removal of the nasal plane, as in nasal plane squamous cell carcinoma, can be a satisfactory solution.[23]

Neurogenic Rhinitis

The clinical signs of neurogenic rhinitis in dogs are dryness of the nasal plane on one or both sides, sometimes with crusts, and slight mucopurulent nasal discharge. The most frequent form is dryness of one side of the nasal plane together with ipsilateral keratoconjunctivitis sicca and mucopurulent conjunctivitis. The cause of the disorder is loss of parasympathetic innervation and when keratitis sicca is present, the dysfunction also affects the lacrimal, palatine, and nasal glands.[24] In dogs with this disorder we recognized ipsilateral otitis media by the resulting reddening of the tympanic membrane. We concluded that the lesion in the parasympathetic nerves was probably caused by otitis media because the parasympathetic nerves are carried in the chorda tympani and pass freely through the middle ear. In all cases, treatment of the otitis media with broad-spectrum antibiotics resolved all problems.

Diagnosis of neurogenic rhinitis is more difficult when it is bilateral. The Schirmer tear test should be helpful, but no values have been reported. Clinical examination and exclusion of other causes may lead to presumption of a possible neurogenic cause. Massaging nonperfumed moistening cream into the nasal plane eight times daily and administering four drops of artificial tears into the nasal cavity four times daily will resolve the clinical signs if the presumptive diagnosis is correct. This treatment will be required lifelong because no known specific treatment for the parasympathetic nerve dysfunction exists.

Specific Rhinitis

Polyps occur in the nasal cavity in both dogs and cats. They consist of focal accumulation of edema fluid, hyperplasia of the submucosal connective tissue, and a variable inflammatory infiltrate of eosinophils, plasma cells, and lymphocytes. Hence they are not neoplastic but inflammatory polyps.[25] They are found in the nasal cavity of cats with signs of obstructive rhinitis. Bilateral obstruction may be caused by bilateral polyps or a unilateral polyp that extends into the nasopharynx.

Diagnosis is usually made by rhinoscopy. The polyp is seen as a red mass in the nasal cavity, and biopsy reveals it to be inflammatory tissue. Removal is difficult, usually requiring removal of all structures in the nasal cavity through a small opening in the nasal bone. This damages the olfactory epithelium and recognition of food is disturbed. When one nasal cavity is freed of polyps, the cat regains its sense of smell with help from the intact side. Bilateral surgery should be avoided and when necessary only performed after the cat seems to be fully recovered from the first operation.

Polyps in the nasal cavity are rare in dogs. They are diagnosed by rhinoscopy and biopsy, which reveals inflammatory tissue. They are usually unilateral. Rhinotomy via the nasal bone and removal of all conchae and the polypoid tissue relieve the obstruction. Histologic examination will reveal whether the structure is a polyp or an unexpected neoplasm. In dogs polyps usually recur after 1 or 2 years, but in cats recurrence is rare.

In young dogs and cats, foreign bodies such as grass and other plant material are common. Owners may know when the material entered the nasal cavity, usually via the nostril. Being plant material, the foreign body has the density of soft tissue and is usually not visualized on radiographs. CT and MR imaging usually show an area of inflammation around the foreign body but may not specifically identify the foreign material. Rhinoscopy in search of a foreign body needs patience and the use of suction, under visual control, to remove mucopurulent exudate before the foreign material is exposed and can be removed. Grass can enter the nasal cavity while a cat is chewing on it, as cats often do. Out of a ball of mucus and grass in the pharynx, a sprig of grass can enter the nasal cavity via the nasopharynx. It can be found by rhinoscopy and removed under visual control via the nostril.

Idiopathic lymphoplasmacytic (chronic hyperplastic) rhinitis is a relatively common but poorly understood cause of chronic nasal disease in the dog.[26] The lymphoplasmacytic inflammatory response could result from many precipitating factors such as infections, aeroallergens, and inhaled irritants. The condition tends to affect young to middle-aged dolichocephalic and mesaticephalic large-breed dogs, but Dachshunds and Whippets are frequently affected. A chronic unilateral or bilateral mucoid to mucopurulent nasal discharge is most commonly seen, although a mucohemorrhagic or hemorrhagic discharge can occur in some cases. Nasal radiography may be unremarkable or show patchy increase in opacity with minimal evidence of conchal destruction. CT and MR imaging greatly enhance the ability to differentiate inflammatory from neoplastic disease, and contrast-enhanced CT and MR images show a patchy inflammatory response with either no or mild conchal destruction (Figure 224-8). Rhinoscopy reveals unilateral or bilateral hyperemia and edema of the mucosa causing narrowing of the air passages, which are filled with copious amounts of mucoid or mucopurulent discharge. Nasal biopsy shows a marked lymphoplasmacytic inflammatory response, but lymphoplasmacytic inflammation may be seen with nasal neoplasia, mycotic rhinitis, or foreign bodies. Thus thorough exclusion of these diagnoses is required before a diagnosis of idiopathic lymphoplasmacytic rhinitis can be made. Long-term administration of antibiotics together with glucocorticoids and/or nonsteroidal antiinflammatory agents usually control the condition, but recurrence following cessation of medication is common.

Nasal allergic rhinitis is presumed to occur, but confirmation of the diagnosis has not yet been convincing, partly because IgE-based rhinitis, as occurs in human, has yet to be demonstrated. Currently, the approximate diagnosis is one made by excluding other possible causes of rhinitis and a positive response to glucocorticoids and/or antihistamines.

TUMORS OF THE NASAL PLANE, NASAL CAVITY, AND FRONTAL SINUS

Tumors of the Nasal Plane

Squamous cell carcinoma of the nasal plane is found in cats in most countries of the world (Figure 224-9). The diagnosis should be made by biopsy, but the diagnosis is often delayed because initial biopsies may only reveal inflammation. When the tumor is actively growing and destruction is in progress, total removal of the process is justified, provided that the removed tissue is submitted for histologic examination. In the differential diagnosis of processes causing proliferation of the tissue of the nasal plane, with crusts and destruction, infection by *Alternaria* spp. and eosinophilic granuloma should be included. Both are easily identified in biopsy material. Surgical removal of the neoplastic nasal plane in cats has been instructively described.[27] One firm incision will allow histologic confirmation of a tumor-free margin. Squamous cell carcinoma of the nasal plane sometimes occurs in dogs. The cosmetic results of removal of the nasal plane are less satisfactory in dogs than in cats. In both, the best results are obtained when tumor growth does not yet extend around the nasal plane. Other tumors of the nasal plane are fibroma and fibrosarcoma, which grow initially beneath the epithelium and do not ulcerate primarily.

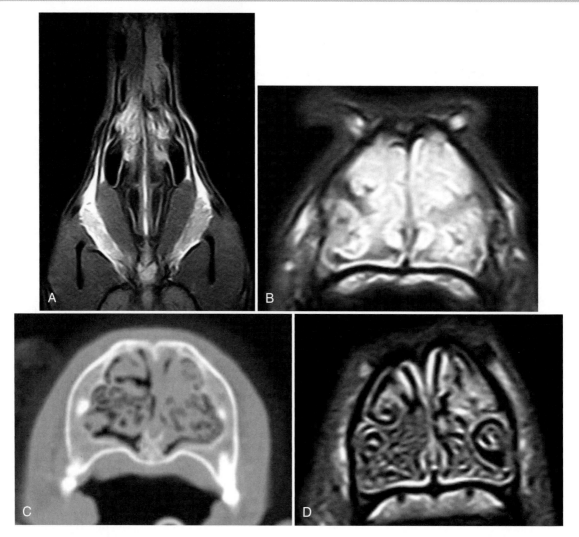

Figure 224-8 **A,** Dorsal and **B,** transverse contrast enhanced T1-weighted magnetic resonance (MR) images of a whippet with lymphocytic plasmacytic rhinitis. Note the patchy increased intensity in both nasal chambers with no evidence of conchal destruction. **C,** Transverse computed tomography image using a soft tissue window of the same dog. **D,** Posttreatment transverse contrast enhanced T1-weighted MR image confirming the lack of conchal damage. (**C,** Courtesy Dr. A. Avner.)

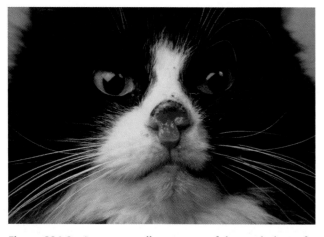

Figure 224-9 Squamous cell carcinoma of the nasal plane of a cat. Biopsy is required to differentiate tumor from inflammatory tissue. (From Venker-van Haagen AJ: Ear, nose, throat and tracheobronchial diseases, Hannover, Germany, 2005, Schlütersche, p 73.)

Surgical removal in an early stage is possible, without too much cosmetic damage.

Tumors in the Nasal Cavity

Tumors occur in the nasal cavity of dogs and cats of all ages, but most often in pets older than 5 years of age. Almost all are malignant. They invade the surrounding tissue but rarely metastasize before the dog or cat is euthanized. The most frequent tumors are undifferentiated carcinoma, adenocarcinoma, and squamous cell carcinoma; less frequent are chondrosarcoma, osteosarcoma, and lymphosarcoma.[28]

Clinical signs include sneezing, hemorrhagic discharge, and mucopurulent discharge. In most cases unilateral obstruction of the nasal cavity is recognized because of stertor or nasal stridor. No evidence of pain is observed and the dog or cat becomes dyspneic only when the mouth is closed, for example, when sleeping. As long as the tumor is unilateral, the dyspnea is moderate. When the tumor obstructs both nasal cavities, dyspnea during sleep becomes a serious problem, causing the animal to awaken repeatedly during the night and often become depressed in the morning. When no therapy is offered beyond permanent tracheostomy, which is rarely accepted by

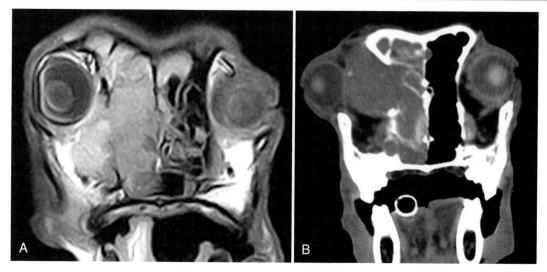

Figure 224-10 **A,** Transverse T1-weighted magnetic resonance image through the caudal nasal chamber of an English Setter showing extension of a nasal adenocarcinoma into the frontal sinus, orbit, and nasal pharynx on the affected side. **B,** Transverse computed tomography image of a nasal adenocarcinoma in another dog showing similar extension into the frontal sinus, orbit, and nasal pharynx.

the owner, recurrent nasal bleeding and dyspnea are the usual reasons for euthanasia in both dogs and cats. Cats, however, often stop eating, which may provide a humane end point and a reason for euthanasia.

Radiographs should be obtained with the dog or cat under anesthesia. Tumor is suspected when increased density is found in one or both nasal cavities, with loss of normal maxillary and ethmoidal conchae.[29] Most tumors develop in the caudal third of the nasal cavity and extend into the frontal and paranasal sinuses. Both CT and MR imaging provide a more reliable assessment of the extent of the lesion and are essential if surgery and/or radiation therapy is planned (Figure 224-10).[30]

The extent of the tumor should be considered when estimating the animal's life expectancy, but this is usually decided by the owner's interpretation of the quality of the animal's life. In all cases in which the radiographic diagnosis is uncertain, rhinoscopy is the next diagnostic procedure. Under rhinoscopic visualization the tumors vary greatly in shape and firmness, and their color ranges from gray to deep red. Biopsies are always taken for histologic confirmation of the diagnosis. If therapy is not planned, neither CT nor MR imaging is indicated. Radiation therapy should be considered, and details have been described.[31] Median survival times of up to 7 months have been recorded with improved quality of life during that period.[32]

Tumors of the Frontal Sinus

Tumors in the frontal sinus develop within a bony case. The frontal sinus does not have a specific function; therefore development of the tumor will be noticed only when unilateral nasal bleeding is recurrent or when the enlarging tumor causes pressure atrophy of the frontal bone and becomes apparent as a swelling arising in the frontal sinus.

In the diagnostic investigation of recurrent nasal bleeding, radiographs will be made of the nasal cavity and the frontal sinus, and a radiographic density in the frontal sinus will be noticed. The differential diagnosis of such a density in combination with a radiographically normal ipsilateral nasal cavity includes aspergillosis, tumor, and accumulation of mucus associated with obstruction of the nasofrontal duct. Because the frontal sinus is separated from the brain by only a thin

layer of bone, additional diagnostic imaging by CT or MR is invaluable to assess extension into the cranial vault. When a swelling arising in the frontal sinus is recognized by physical examination, the same procedure of taking radiographs followed by CT or MR is indicated. With these imaging techniques, the extent of the lesion and differentiation of the tumor from retained secretions be determined. Tumor in the frontal sinus can be recognized by CT or MR administration of an intravenous contrast agent. Vital tissue will be enhanced by the contrast medium while debris and retained secretions will not. It must then be determined by CT or MRI whether the bony case of the frontal sinus is intact, especially whether the orbit or the brain is invaded, and whether the contralateral frontal sinus is included in the process.

When these procedures indicate that the tumor can be removed, a surgical approach via the frontal bone is indicated. At the end of the surgical procedure it is important to examine the patency of the nasofrontal duct and to relieve any obstruction. Like tumors in the nasal cavity, most tumors in the frontal sinus are malignant and complete surgical removal is unlikely. Biopsy of the tumor through a small trephined opening in the frontal bone should be considered as an intermediate step.

TRAUMA TO THE FRONTAL SINUS AND THE NOSE

Trauma to the Frontal Sinus

Blunt or sharp objects can cause traumatic injury to the frontal sinus. The frontal bone in dogs and cats is relatively thick and provides good protection, so a fracture of it implies a very heavy blow to the head has occurred. The pet should therefore be given a thorough clinical examination for (1) signs of shock such as tachycardia, hypotension (prolonged capillary refill time, weak pulse), rapid respiration, dilation of the pupils, hypothermia, muscle weakness, restlessness, and depression or even coma,[33] and (2) other fractures or wounds. Frontal bone fractures do not require immediate attention unless brain damage is suspected, in which case CT or MR imaging should be employed. In the absence of signs of brain damage, and when other traumatic injuries have been attended to, the nature and extent of the frontal bone fracture should be examined by radiography, CT, or both. Prolonged anesthesia is necessary and thus these procedures are usually delayed for 24 hours or more.

When bone fragments are seen to be present in the frontal sinus they should be removed. Like any foreign body, small bone fragments are likely to become sequestered. Surgery should be performed with full attention to aseptic procedures. Before attempting reconstruction of the frontal bone, it is important to examine the patency of the nasofrontal duct and to relieve any obstruction. Airtight suturing of the subcutis, including periosteum, followed by routine skin closure prevents the development of subcutaneous emphysema. Administration of broad-spectrum antibiotics for 3 weeks and strict limitation of activity during this period (keeping a cat confined to the house) will prevent complications.

Trauma to the Nose

Trauma to the nose is characterized by massive bleeding, which adds to the other effects of the impact in promoting shock. A thorough examination for signs of this is indicated (see Trauma to the Frontal Sinus). Fractures and wounds should be noted but priority must usually be given to the treatment of hypovolemic shock.

When the dog or cat is sufficiently stable, the larger vessels should be ligated and skin sutures should be placed as needed. Skin sutures, sometimes supported by subcutaneous sutures, may be sufficient to remodel the outer form of the nose. Fractures of the choanae are best left alone because they are unlikely to ever result in obstruction. Severe traumatic damage to the nose almost always causes temporary obstruction, making tracheotomy necessary. Adequate oxygenation helps avoid general malaise and loss of appetite. Liquid or soft food facilitates eating. In dogs the tracheal cannula is often left in place for 10 days or longer. In cats that have difficulties with long-term tracheostomy, a small intranasal catheter may be placed and connected to the oxygen supply. Use of this method, however, depends on the pathway through the wounded nose. In the author's experience, the nose is functionally adequate in 2 to 3 weeks. If needed, more corrective surgery could be attempted after 6 weeks.

EPISTAXIS

Epistaxis (i.e., nasal bleeding) is often spontaneous and transient, and it is apparently due to a local cause. When it is recurrent or profuse, with considerable loss of blood, diagnos-

tic investigation is indicated. The causes of epistaxis should be considered in planning the diagnostic procedures. Recurring epistaxis occurs in both dogs and cats but profuse nasal bleeding occurs mostly in dogs. Recurring epistaxis in dogs and cats can be caused by ulcerative rhinitis, mycotic rhinitis, and tumor in the nasal cavity and paranasal sinuses. Profuse nasal bleeding in dogs is most often caused by aspergillosis in the nasal cavity or frontal sinus, or by tumor in the nasal cavity and frontal sinus. Epistaxis can also be the sole sign of defects in primary hemostasis (platelet plug formation) or secondary hemostasis (coagulation cascade).[34] Lesions in the nasal mucosa leading to epistaxis can also occur in systemic diseases such as hypertension, hyperviscosity syndrome, leishmaniasis, and amyloidosis.

Epistaxis caused by local disease in the nasal cavity or frontal sinus is approached (as are all nasal diseases) by a general and specific examination for nasal disease, as described earlier in this chapter. When the bleeding has occurred recently, radiographic examination should preferably be delayed for at least 48 hours because clotted blood can be misinterpreted as a mass in the nasal cavity. Rhinoscopy should also be delayed for at least 48 hours after the bleeding has stopped, because the presence of blood clots hinders inspection and could lead to misinterpretation of findings.

In the meantime, profuse nasal bleeding should be stopped. It is best to sedate the animal (phenobarbital [2 mg/kg] is advised because it does not affect blood pressure). After considerable blood loss, sedation that causes hypotension could lead to shock in association with hypovolemia and should be avoided. Sedation will help to stop the bleeding.

Nasal tamponade is only acceptable for a short period and under anesthesia. For less profuse bleeding, nasal drops of 0.1% adrenaline are helpful. The use of adrenaline should, however, be used with care. Overdosage could cause death because of vasoconstriction of the arteries supplying the brain. The administration of 3 drops in one of the nasal cavities in dogs and 1 drop in cats, repeated up to three times per 24 hours, is acceptable and effective when used during the bleeding. It should not be used in an attempt to prevent nasal bleeding. When examination of the nasal cavity and the frontal sinus reveals no cause for the bleeding, further investigation of primary diseases causing hemostasis is indicated.

REFERENCES

The reference list can be found on the companion Expert Consult Web site at *www.expertconsult.com*.

CHAPTER 225

Diseases of the Throat*

GENERAL ANATOMY AND PHYSIOLOGY

The throat is an important, but mostly ignored, communal area of both the gastrointestinal (GI) and respiratory tracts.

*This chapter, written by Nolie K. Parnell for the sixth edition of this textbook, appears here unchanged.

Anatomically it is divided into the pharynx and larynx. The pharynx is further divided into the nasopharynx, the oropharynx, and the laryngopharynx. The nasopharynx is located dorsal to the soft palate, between the choanae and the intrapharyngeal opening. It is a functional space that allows the nasal cavity to communicate with the larynx. The oropharynx is ventral to the soft palate and extends from the palatoglossal arches rostrally to the base of the epiglottis caudally. The intrapharyngeal opening and the rostral border of the esophagus create the boundaries of the laryngopharynx, the most caudal part of the pharynx.[1] The laryngopharynx functions as an intersection to both the respiratory and digestive tracts. The larynx consists of three unpaired cartilages (epiglottis, cricoid, and thyroid) and one pair of arytenoid cartilages. The glottis (or cranial opening of the larynx) is composed of the corniculate and cuneiform process of the arytenoid cartilages and the epiglottis. Minor anatomic differences exist between feline and canine larynx.[2] Cats lack the interarytenoid cartilage found in dogs and instead have an interarytenoid ligament in its place. Cats also lack a vestibular ligament. Due to this deficiency, the feline arytenoid cartilage is connected to the ventral aspect of the larynx by the vocal ligament. Another important anatomic difference is that cats lack the laryngeal ventricles found between the vestibular and vocal folds in the dog. No dramatic differences exist between feline and canine innervation and muscles of the larynx.

Swallowing, or deglutition, is a complex reflex action that coordinates many structures. Cranial nerves, the swallowing center in the reticular formation of the brainstem, the muscles of mastication, tongue, soft palate, pharynx, larynx, and esophagus are all involved in what appears to be a simple act of allowing transport of material from the mouth to the stomach.[3] As a lesser recognized function, swallowing also allows saliva and debris to be removed from the pharynx. Deglutition begins as a voluntary act but during its execution becomes a reflex. Deglutition is traditionally described as having three phases: (1) oral, (2) pharyngeal, and (3) esophageal. The oral phase begins when mastication is complete. The tongue then moves the food bolus that is organized at the base of the tongue to a position that is on midline between the tongue and the hard palate. Motor fibers to the tongue are supplied by cranial nerve XII. Sensory fibers from the oral cavity and motor fibers to the masticatory muscles and soft palate originate from cranial nerve V. The oral phase is voluntary, but when the food bolus is pushed into the pharynx, receptors are stimulated that initiate the involuntary, or reflex, component of deglutition. Sensory receptors are found in the pharynx, palate, and epiglottis. Impulses from these receptors are transmitted along the glossopharyngeal nerve, recurrent laryngeal branch of the vagus nerve, and maxillary branch of the trigeminal nerve to the swallowing center in the medulla (located in the floor of the fourth ventricle). The efferent arm of the reflex involves the motor nuclei of cranial nerves V, VII, IX, X, and XII.[4-6] These nerves supply the muscles of mastication, tongue, palate, pharynx, larynx, and esophagus. During the pharyngeal phase the goal is to pass food from the oropharynx into the esophagus and to prevent food from being aspirated into the trachea or moved into the nasopharynx. This is accomplished by elevation of the soft palate and the palatopharyngeal folds moving inward as the vocal cords are pulled together and the larynx is elevated against the epiglottis. The final act during the pharyngeal stage of swallowing occurs when the cricopharyngeal muscle relaxes, the upper esophageal sphincter opens, the bolus moves into the esophagus, the sphincter closes, and the pharyngeal muscles relax. The cricopharyngeal muscle is innervated by the pharyngoesophageal nerve, which is formed by cranial nerves IX and X.[1] The final stage of deglutition, the esophageal stage, transports the bolus from the esophagus, through the gastroesophageal sphincter, and into the stomach. The esophagus is innervated by the vagus nerve.

The larynx has three functions: (1) to act as a conduit for air, (2) to protect the lower airway from aspiration during deglutition, and (3) vocalization. The glottis remains partially open when an animal is at rest. When greater airflow is necessary, the glottis is widened by abduction of the arytenoid cartilages and vocal folds (via cricoarytenoid muscles) during inspiration (and the same structures adduct during expiration). The cricoarytenoid muscles are innervated by the caudal laryngeal nerves, which are derived from the recurrent laryngeal nerves. The recurrent laryngeal nerve innervates all the muscles of the larynx except the cricothyroid muscles that are supplied by the cranial laryngeal nerves.[7] During deglutition the larynx is pulled cranially by the geniohyoideus and mylohyoideus muscles. This allows the epiglottis to close over the larynx, protecting the lower airways. The adductor muscles close the glottis concurrently. This creates an additional defense against aspiration.

HISTORY AND PHYSICAL EXAMINATION

Animals with diseases of the throat can have a variety of historical complaints. Pharyngeal diseases can be confusing because historical findings can be related to swallowing difficulties or the upper respiratory tract (URT). Historical findings secondary to laryngeal dysfunction are usually related to either inability to regulate airflow and protect the airway or changes in vocalization. Respiratory sounds can be extremely useful in localizing the disease, whether it is pharyngeal or laryngeal, but they are not helpful if one tries to attribute a specific respiratory sound to a specific condition. Coughing, dyspnea, and nasal discharge are common clinical complaints. Stertor, a snoring sound heard on inspiration, is usually due to an intermittent obstruction such as an elongated soft palate. Stridor, an inspiratory high-pitch wheeze, is most commonly associated with laryngeal lesions. Stridor is created by air turbulence through a narrowed laryngeal opening. Any changes in vocalization would suggest a laryngeal disorder. Reverse sneezing, which is described as short periods of forceful inspiratory nasal effort with the head pulled back, indicates irritation to the dorsal nasopharyngeal mucosa.[8] Dysphagia cases can be confusing because ineffective swallowing may not be obvious to the owner and may not be the primary historical complaint. Other signs such as coughing, gagging, regurgitation, and nasal discharge may be reported in animals with either oropharyngeal dysphagia or other diseases of the throat.

A complete physical examination (including a neurologic examination) is important when evaluating animals with pharyngeal or laryngeal disease because dysfunction may be indicative of systemic disease (i.e., myopathy, neuropathy) or there may be secondary complications from the disorder (e.g., aspiration pneumonia). If laryngeal disease is suspected, the larynx should be palpated for pain or structural abnormalities. The area over the larynx should be ausculted for abnormal sounds secondary to turbulence. Part of this complete physical examination may include exercising the patient, because occasionally manifestation of the disease only occurs after physical exertion. Many animals will have dyspnea, and a thorough physical examination may not be possible until the animal is stable. Significant airway compromise may be overlooked. It is important to assess the degree of respiratory compromise by evaluating the patient's attitude, posture, mucous membrane color, and both respiratory rate and pattern. Precluding the emergency situation, once the general examination is complete one may concentrate on examining the oral cavity. It is extremely difficult, if not impossible, to adequately evaluate the larynx and pharyngeal areas without heavy sedation or general anesthesia. In most cases it is easier for the examiner, and safer for the animal, if tracheal intubation is performed. A standard method of evaluating the oral cavity should be established so that one does not miss an important abnormality. The larynx is evaluated both for structural problems and functional abnormalities; the pharynx is evaluated for physical abnormalities. Pharyngeal function cannot be evaluated when the patient is sedated; rather, videofluoroscopy is recommended when critically assessing pharyngeal function.

DIAGNOSIS

Diagnostic Imaging

Lateral and ventrodorsal radiographic views of both the skull and cervical areas are indicated. Radiopaque foreign bodies can be identified that may be missed on laryngoscopy and pharyngoscopy (e.g., sewing needle embedded in soft tissues). Radiographs are also useful in identifying bony changes associated with chronic inflammation or neoplasia, clues of unreported trauma (e.g., subcutaneous emphysema), and occasionally soft tissue masses. Suggestion of a soft tissue mass is confirmed by direct visualization and histopathology. Thoracic radiographs are also indicated. Symptoms of lower respiratory disease may be masked when a patient has concurrent, and more severe, upper respiratory symptoms. Evaluation for aspiration pneumonia, metastases, or suggestion of a motility disorder (i.e., megaesophagus) is possible.

Ultrasonography and computed tomography (CT) are noninvasive modalities to evaluate the pharynx and larynx. Ultrasonography can identify soft tissue masses, help guide fine needle aspiration, and evaluate laryngeal function.[9,10] The presence of air in these areas can limit the usefulness of this modality in establishing a definitive diagnosis. CT may be used to fully evaluate involvement of neoplasia or middle-ear disease if a nasopharyngeal polyp is suspected.[11]

Videofluoroscopy is essential for any case of dysphagia. A barium swallow allows the act of swallowing to be recorded and studied for abnormalities. The patient should be recorded attempting to swallow barium to mimic liquids and then should be given a meal (canned food mixed with barium) to be recorded. Videofluoroscopy is superior to radiography because it allows all phases of deglutition to be evaluated instead of recording one moment (intermittent moments) of the event. Unfortunately videofluoroscopy is limited to referral centers only.

Pharyngoscopy and Laryngoscopy

Laryngoscopy and pharyngoscopy allow assessment of both structural abnormalities and function of the larynx. A flexible endoscope is used for these procedures because visualization of the nasopharynx requires retroflexion. Occasionally a foreign body will be found just caudal to the larynx and may be retrieved endoscopically. The patient is placed in sternal recumbency and anesthetized with either propofol or sodium thiopental. Once anesthetized, gauze is passed under the maxilla behind the canine teeth. The gauze is used to elevate the head, so external compression of the neck is avoided. Flexible endoscopy is ideal to evaluate the nasopharynx. If that is not possible, the caudal pharynx can be evaluated using a dental mirror and a Snook hook. This will be sufficient in evaluating most nasopharyngeal polyps, masses, or caudal foreign bodies. It will not allow diagnosis of more rostral diseases such as nasopharyngeal stenosis. Laryngeal function is usually evaluated first by assessing the motion of the arytenoid cartilages. The traditional approach involves titrating anesthesia that allows both visualization of the arytenoid cartilages and deep spontaneous breaths to occur. In a normal animal the arytenoid cartilages will abduct symmetrically with each inspiration and close on expiration. The frustration with this technique is multiple. Maintaining the correct level of anesthesia is difficult (i.e., the animal is too awake to allow adequate visualization of the arytenoid cartilages or anesthetized so that the patient will not spontaneously breathe);

shallow breathing can limit adequate assessment; and concerns about the effect of anesthesia on laryngeal function are legitimate concerns when performing the traditional laryngeal examination. The recently introduced technique attempts to eliminate the effects of anesthesia from the examination. Patients are premedicated with acepromazine maleate and butorphanol tartrate and induced with propofol. Doxapram hydrochloride (2.2 mg/kg intravenously) is used to increase laryngeal motion and minimize or eliminate the effects of anesthesia.[12]

Miscellaneous

Hematology and biochemical profiles should be performed on patients with pharyngeal and laryngeal dysfunction, but they will rarely confirm the definitive diagnosis. Occasionally virus isolation (feline calicivirus [FCV]) and PCR (feline herpes-1 virus [FHV-1], *Chlamydia* spp., and *Mycoplasma* spp.) are indicated in the diagnostic workup. Culture and sensitivity of tissue or secretions can provide valuable information during the diagnostic workup. Cytology and histopathology are also essential for critically evaluating infiltrative disease or mass lesions.

DISEASES OF THE PHARYNX

Nasopharyngeal Polyps

Nasopharyngeal polyps are histopathologically benign, pedunculated masses consisting mostly of fibrovascular tissue and variable severity of inflammatory cells.[13] It is the most common nasopharyngeal disease of younger cats and accounts for almost one third of all feline nasopharyngeal diseases.[14] No sex or breed predilection exists; although nasopharyngeal polyps are most commonly found in younger cats (mean range 0.4 months to 6.1 years), this disease should also be included in the differential diagnosis for older cats.[14-17] Nasopharyngeal polyps are believed to originate from the middle ear or auditory tube and then expand into the nasopharynx and external auditory canal.[18] It is unknown why nasopharyngeal polyps occur, but it does not seem likely that the polyps are a manifestation of chronic viral (FCV or FHV) infections.[17] Clinical signs are variable but include nasal discharge, sneeze, stertor, and phonation changes. Definitive diagnosis is made by direct visualization of the nasopharyngeal mass and histopathology. Quite often, nasopharyngeal polyps can be discovered with digital palpation of the soft palate. Diagnostic imaging (skull radiographs and CT) is not necessary for the diagnosis but can provide valuable information toward the extent of the mass and possible middle ear involvement. Treatment depends on clinical presentation and extent of disease. If evidence of concurrent middle ear involvement is seen, a ventral bulla osteotomy is indicated. If the disease appears to be limited to the nasopharynx, then traction avulsion to remove the polyp at its stalk is usually attempted. The high rate of recurrence with this disease (33%) has led to the suggestion that ventral bulla osteotomy should be performed on all cats with nasopharyngeal polyps.[16] Nasopharyngeal polyps are considered a disease of cats, but a case of a nasopharyngeal polyp in a dog has been reported.[19]

Nasopharyngeal Stenosis

Nasopharyngeal stenosis is primarily a disease of cats but has been reported in a dog.[20,21] It is a rare disease that is characterized by scar tissue that forms a membrane or "webbing" above the soft palate and obstructs airflow through the nasopharynx. Cats are believed to develop nasopharyngeal stenosis as a consequence of healing from injuries to the area (infectious, traumatic). Cats with the nasopharyngeal stenosis have chronic histories of stertorous breathing and open-mouth

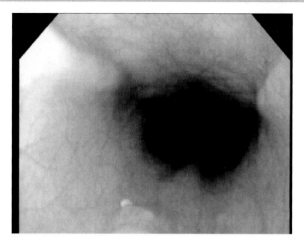

Figure 225-1 Normal nasopharynx.

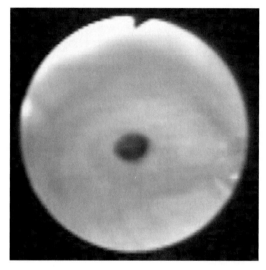

Figure 225-2 Nasopharyngeal stenosis in a young cat with a history of progressive stertor and open-mouth breathing.

breathing.[20,22] Diagnosis is made using flexible endoscopy to evaluate the nasopharynx and visualizing a pinhole-sized orifice where the caudal nares should be seen (Figures 225-1 and 225-2). Treatment of nasopharyngeal stenosis involves surgical resection of the lesion, but the prognosis should remain guarded because the webbing may recur.[21,23] Balloon dilation of the stenotic area has been proposed as a successful alternative to surgery.[22,24]

Pharyngeal Foreign Bodies

Foreign bodies can occur in both dogs and cats and create both acute and chronic pharyngeal disease.[25-27] Grass awns, fish hooks, and bones are all possible, but wood sticks are the most common penetrating foreign bodies.[25,27] Medium and large breed dogs are affected more often with oropharyngeal penetrating injuries, presumptively because of their stick-chewing or retrieving behavior. Clinical signs of acute disease include pawing at the mouth or face, hypersalivation, oral pain and malodor, dysphagia, and dyspnea. Cervical or facial swellings combined with intermittently draining tracts were more commonly seen with chronic pharyngeal foreign bodies. Pharyngeal and retropharyngeal abscessation is a common complication secondary to bones, grass awns, sticks, pins, or needles. Dogs with pharyngeal or retropharyngeal abscesses

will exhibit anorexia, pharyngeal pain, and swelling and will be febrile.[1] Although rare, osteomyelitis and quadriparesis are possible complications to penetrating stick foreign bodies.[28,29] In contrast, nasopharyngeal foreign bodies are more likely to create inflammation and nasal discharge. Migration of nasopharyngeal foreign bodies does not occur. Diagnosis of pharyngeal foreign bodies is difficult and frequently frustrating. Radiographs are helpful if the foreign body is radiopaque; however, if it is radiolucent the foreign body will remain elusive. Endoscopy is helpful in locating a foreign body, and if the foreign body penetrated the pharynx, endoscopy can localize the traumatized area. Aggressive search and retrieval of penetrating pharyngeal foreign bodies is important early in the course of the problem. If the foreign body is not successfully removed in its entirety during the acute stage, the prognosis decreases dramatically.[25]

Pharyngeal Mucoceles

A mucocele is a collection of saliva from a damaged salivary gland or duct. Synonyms include sialocele, ranula, or salivary cyst. Mucoceles are not true cysts because they are lined with granulation tissue and not the characteristic epithelial tissue.[30] The cause of mucoceles is unknown, although traumatic causes such as dog bites and choke collars have been purposed. Pharyngeal mucoceles are the least common type of mucocele, with sublingual and cervical being more common. Regardless, pharyngeal mucoceles are clinically important because most animals with pharyngeal mucoceles present in respiratory distress. Dogs are more affected than cats, and miniature poodles appear to be at increased risk of developing pharyngeal mucoceles.[31,32] Due to the patient's respiratory compromise, it is important to establish a patent airway either via tracheal intubation or tracheostomy prior to examination. Diagnosis requires visualization of soft, nonpainful, fluctuant mass in the pharynx. Fine needle aspirate of the mass will reveal a thick, tenacious fluid that is characteristic of saliva. Drainage of fluid is important in the acute management of pharyngeal mucoceles, but surgical correction via marsupialization and resection of the associated salivary glands will need to be pursued at a later date.[31]

SOFT PALATE ABNORMALITIES

The palate is an important anatomic structure because it divides the oral and nasal cavities. Abnormalities of the palate result from incomplete closure of the primary or secondary palate (or both) during fetal development. The primary palate develops into the lip and incisive bone.[33] The secondary palate becomes the hard and soft palate. Cleft palate and soft palate hypoplasia are two of many palatine defects that have been described. Brachycephalic breeds have a higher incidence of cleft palate. Many factors have been implicated in these abnormalities, but inherited traits seem to be found in Shih Tzus, Bulldogs, Pointers, Swiss Sheepdogs, and Brittany Spaniels.[1,34] Teratogens (e.g., vitamin A, griseofulvin) have also been shown to cause palate abnormalities.[35,36] Midline soft palate defects are most common with unilateral or bilateral defects occurring less frequently. Neonates with a cleft palate usually fail to thrive because the defect makes nursing difficult, allows milk to enter the nasal passages, or milk is aspirated into the lower airways. If the neonate is able to survive, chronic rhinitis is the most common clinical sign. Diagnosis is based on oral examination of the soft palate. A cleft palate will have a midline defect usually involving both the hard and soft palate. Soft palate hypoplasia reveals a severely shortened length, with a midline remnant of muscular tissue covered by mucosa (Figure 225-3). Animals with soft palate defects should also be evaluated for middle ear disease because con-

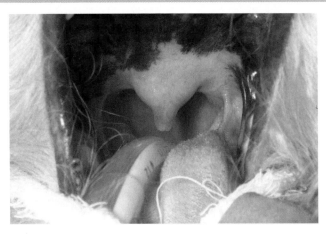

Figure 225-3   Soft palate hypoplasia in a young adult dog with a history of chronic nasal discharge.

current middle ear disease has been identified as a potential complication.[37] Treatment of both types of soft palate defects involves surgical correction. A variety of techniques have been described to correct midline defects, with good results.[38,39] Correction of soft palate hypoplasia has a poor prognosis due to the absence of adequate tissue for repair. In animals with this problem, it is hoped that addressing the way intake of food and water occurs (i.e., elevation) will decrease the severity of reflux into the nasal cavity.

In contrast, brachycephalic breeds can suffer from soft palate excess. Stenotic nares and everted laryngeal saccules are the other components of the upper airway obstructive syndrome known as the *brachycephalic syndrome*. English Bulldogs, Pugs, Shih Tzus, Lhasa Apsos, and Himalayan cats are all breeds that suffer from brachycephalic syndrome.[40] Hypoplasia of the trachea, especially in the English Bulldog, may also be present.[41] Normally the caudal edge of the soft palate should just touch the tip of the epiglottis. Because maxillae are shortened in brachycephalic breeds, the caudal edge extends beyond the tip of the epiglottis. During exercise the soft palate will be sucked into the glottis, reducing the diameter of the airway. Over time this will cause trauma and tissue edema that will further hinder airflow. Clinical signs associated with an obstructing elongated soft palate include stertorous breathing, gagging, coughing, and exercise intolerance or collapse. Diagnosis is based on oral examination and direct visualization of a soft palate that extends beyond the tip of the epiglottis. Treatment involves shortening the length of the soft palate, either with conventional techniques or carbon dioxide laser.[42-44]

Neoplasia

Oral tumors (which include pharyngeal neoplasia) are the fourth most common neoplasia in dogs. Oral neoplasms occur 2.6 times more frequently in dogs than in cats, and males are more likely to develop oropharyngeal neoplasia than females.[45] The three most common oral tumors in the dog are malignant melanoma, squamous cell carcinoma, and fibrosarcoma.[46] Squamous cell carcinoma and fibrosarcoma are the two most common oral tumors in the cat. If the feline nasopharynx is specifically evaluated for neoplasia, lymphosarcoma is the most common tumor diagnosed.[14] Most tumors of the oral cavity are malignant, highly locally invasive, and have a variable degree of metastasis.[45,46] Clinical signs include inappetence or anorexia due to pain, dysphagia, halitosis, ptyalism, and facial deformity (swelling, exophthalmos, or bony thickening). Cats with nasopharyngeal lymphosarcoma will have nasal discharge, sneezing, stertor, or phonation changes. Diag-

nosis of an oropharyngeal tumor includes a histologic diagnosis and tumor staging. Direct visualization during an oral examination (and endoscopy for nasopharyngeal tumors) is performed prior to obtaining a tissue sample for cytology and histopathology. Thoracic radiographs are part of the staging, as are either skull radiographs or CT. Regional lymph nodes should be aspirated to determine metastasis. Treatment options include surgery, radiation therapy, hyperthermia, chemotherapy, and photodynamic therapy. Treatment protocol depends on tumor type and location, but local control is most effective with surgery and radiation therapy.[47] Prognosis is variable, based on a number of factors.

Tonsillitis and Pharyngitis

When discussing tonsillitis, one is referring to the palatine tonsil. The palatine tonsil is found within the palatine fossa in the lateral wall of the oropharynx. It is rare for either tonsillitis or pharyngitis to occur as a primary disease. It is much more common for the tonsils and the pharynx to be inflamed secondary to other diseases. Clinical signs are not specific for either the tonsils or pharynx but will support oropharyngeal disease. Inappetence or anorexia, ptyalism, and oral pain are all common clinical findings. Diagnosis is based on history and physical examination findings. Fever is common when infectious agents are involved. Acute tonsillitis will reveal bright-red, friable tonsils on oral examination. It is not unusual for tonsils at this stage to be enlarged and protruding from the palatine fossa. Occasionally the tonsils will have petechiae or small abscesses. The pharynx of acute pharyngitis will be visibly inflamed and can have ulcerations, petechiae, or small abscesses. Bacterial or viral isolation is usually not indicated unless clinical signs are chronic or relapsing. The most common cause of tonsillitis and pharyngitis is upper respiratory infection. FHV-1 and FCV are the two most common feline viral pathogens. FCV is more likely to cause ulcerations than FHV-1.[48,49] Canine infectious tracheobronchitis (ITB) will occasionally cause problems, although it is more likely to cause laryngitis. *Bordetella bronchiseptica* has caused URT disease in cats as well.[50] Other possibilities include chronic vomiting or regurgitation, periodontitis, and ingestion of caustic or toxic substances (e.g., cleaning detergents, liquid potpourri).[51] Rarely, bacterial infection will be incriminated as the cause. Cats can also develop a progressive, nonspecific inflammatory condition termed *gingivitis-stomatitis-pharyngitis complex*. Young purebred cats are predisposed to the disease, and the most severely affected cats develop ulceroproliferative lesions in the caudal oropharynx.[52] Treatment of pharyngitis or tonsillitis is directed toward eliminating the underlying cause, if possible, as well as supportive care and antibiotics, if indicated.

Oropharyngeal Dysphagia

Dysphagia refers to abnormal or difficulty swallowing. Oropharyngeal dysphagia indicates an inability to move a bolus from the oral cavity into the proximal esophagus. This symptom can be either secondary to an isolated lesion or a manifestation of systemic disease. Clinical signs are variable, depending on severity and location of the problem. Signs include difficulty with prehension, dropping food from mouth, exaggerated head movements during eating, regurgitation with no correlation in time of eating, and repeated attempts to swallow food. Occasionally, respiratory signs such as nasal discharge, coughing, and aspiration pneumonia will occur secondary to nasopharyngeal or laryngotracheal aspiration. Diagnosis of oropharyngeal dysphagia requires multiple areas to be evaluated. Accurate historical information is imperative to differentiate regurgitation from vomiting. It is rare that an owner will recognize the difference until the history and examination occurs. A standardized questionnaire has been evaluated as a sensitive tool to detect oropharyngeal dysphagia.[53] Observing the animal eating and drinking is also extremely helpful. The physical examination should include a thorough oral examination to evaluate for structural abnormalities and foreign bodies. A complete neurologic examination is also critical during the evaluation of oropharyngeal dysphagia. Radiographs of the area can identify radiopaque foreign bodies or masses. Thoracic radiographs can determine if the animal has aspiration pneumonia secondary to the dysphagia. Videofluoroscopy is an excellent diagnostic tool to localize the dysphagia.[54] Other possible diagnostics could include ANA test, evaluation for acetylcholine receptor antibodies, endocrine screening, electromyography, or biopsy for histopathology.

Causes of dysphagia include anatomic abnormalities, neoplasia, foreign bodies, or neuromuscular disorders. Brainstem tumors can also cause dysphagia, but it is usually not the only clinical or physical examination finding. The most common neuromuscular disorder is myasthenia gravis, a disease of altered neuromuscular transmission secondary to autoantibodies against acetylcholine receptors. Akitas, Scottish Terriers, German Shorthaired Pointers, Chihuahuas, and Abyssinians are all breeds identified at increased risk for acquired myasthenia gravis.[55,56] Manifestations of myasthenia gravis may either be focal (pharyngeal or esophageal) or generalized (generalized muscular weakness or collapse). Oropharyngeal dysphagia can be one of many clinical signs that are associated with myopathies. Bouvier des Flandres have been identified with a muscular dystrophy in which oropharyngeal dysphagia is the primary clinical sign.[57] Cricopharyngeal achalasia can be acquired as a polymyopathy, or it can be congenital. Cricopharyngeal achalasia is the failure of the upper esophageal sphincter to relax and allow a food bolus into the proximal esophagus. Cocker Spaniels are at increased risk for congenital cricopharyngeal achalasia, but any breed can be affected.[58] It is important to differentiate between congenital and acquired disease because cricopharyngeal myotomy is indicated in congenital disease but should be avoided with acquired disease. Treatment of oropharyngeal dysphagia should be based on the underlying disease process. If possible, the underlying cause should be removed; if that is not possible, providing a means of adequate nutrition should be pursued.

DISEASES OF THE LARYNX

Laryngeal Paralysis

Laryngeal paralysis is a common cause of upper airway obstruction in dogs. Cats can be diagnosed as well, but it is not a common cause of upper airway obstruction for the species.[59] Laryngeal paralysis results when the arytenoid cartilage fails to abduct during inspiration, leading to narrowing of the glottic lumen. Several causes of laryngeal paralysis have been identified, but it is most often idiopathic. Most acquired idiopathic cases are older, large-breed dogs. Damage to the recurrent laryngeal nerve from trauma, infiltrative disease, masses, or surgical manipulation (e.g., feline thyroidectomy) can lead to laryngeal paralysis.[59] Polyneuropathies secondary to immune-mediated disease, hypothyroidism, or other systemic disorders can be observed primarily as laryngeal paralysis.[60] Congenital laryngeal paralysis does occur but is uncommon. A hereditary form has been described in Bouvier des Flandres and is presumed in Siberian huskies and husky crossbreeds.[61,62] In Bouvier des Flandres an autosomal-dominant trait causing a loss of motor neurons in the nucleus ambiguus has been identified.[63] A laryngeal paralysis-polyneuropathy complex has been described in young Dalmatians and Rottweilers.[64,65]

Clinical signs are usually progressive because the ability of the arytenoid cartilage to abduct fails. Clinical signs of laryngeal paralysis include stridor, exercise intolerance, coughing, gagging, and voice change. Animals with laryngeal paralysis can present in respiratory distress, especially after an episode of excitement, exercising, and when environmental temperatures are elevated. Moderate airway obstruction is worsened by laryngeal edema and inflammation secondary to turbulent airflow in the larynx. Although ultrasound has been described as a diagnostic tool for laryngeal paralysis, most clinicians will use laryngoscopy to definitively diagnose laryngeal paralysis.[9] Laryngeal function is assessed when the animal is under a light plane of anesthesia. Paralysis may be unilateral or bilateral, although most animals with moderate to severe clinical signs have bilateral dysfunction of the arytenoid cartilages. It is important not to be fooled by paradoxic movement of the arytenoid cartilages. Paradoxic movement indicates opposite movement (i.e., medially) by the arytenoid cartilages when negative pressure occurs during inspiration. A thorough oral examination should be performed during the same anesthetic episode to identify any underlying causes. Once laryngeal paralysis has been diagnosed, a complete neurologic examination that includes pharyngeal and esophageal function should occur to evaluate for concurrent or underlying problems. Thoracic radiographs are indicated to identify aspiration pneumonia or metastatic disease. When the animal presents in respiratory crisis, stabilization includes sedation and establishing an airway. This is accomplished by either tracheal intubation or tracheotomy. Short-acting corticosteroids are helpful if significant laryngeal edema exists. Once stabilized, surgery is indicated to alleviate the upper airway obstruction caused by laryngeal paralysis. Multiple surgical techniques have been described to palliate the clinical signs associated with laryngeal paralysis. The current surgical technique of choice is unilateral arytenoid lateralization, a technique that attempts to increase the area of the rima glottidis.[66] This procedure has been shown to have the most favorable outcome compared with other possible surgical techniques such as bilateral arytenoid lateralization and partial laryngectomy.[67] Postoperative complications include aspiration pneumonia, laryngeal webbing, surgical failure, and respiratory distress. Postoperative complications are common, and death can occur. In one retrospective study, 34.3% of dogs had postoperative complications and the mortality rate was 19.3%.[67] In the same study, prognosis was poor if the dog had concurrent neurologic disease. Limited information exists regarding surgical outcome in cats. The surgical technique used was unilateral arytenoid lateralization. Postoperative complications included laryngeal edema that necessitated a temporary tracheotomy tube and an altered ability to vocalize. All cats survived.[68]

Laryngeal Neoplasia

Primary neoplasms of the canine and feline larynx occur uncommonly. The most common canine laryngeal tumors reported are malignant epithelial tumors and rhabdomyoma. The most common laryngeal tumor in the cat is lymphosarcoma, with squamous cell carcinoma the second most common.[10,69,70] Most patients with laryngeal tumors are older, with 8 years as the median age.[69] Other report tumor types are adenocarcinoma, rhabdomyosarcoma, osteosarcoma, chondrosarcoma, mast cell tumor, and melanoma.[10,69-71] Clinical signs are similar regardless of tumor type and include dysphonia, coughing, gagging or choking, and respiratory distress. Occasionally an abnormal larynx can be palpated, but most laryngeal tumors are identified by laryngoscopy (Figure 225-4). Radiographs, CTs, and ultrasound all have diagnostic value in determination of extent of disease and potential metastasis.[10] Definitive diagnosis should be made by histopathology; caution should be used when diagnosis is based on

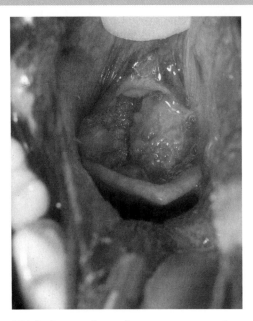

Figure 225-4 Laryngeal neoplasia in a geriatric dog, causing complete obstruction of glottis.

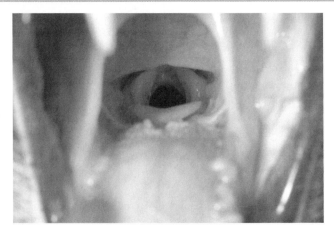

Figure 225-5 Normal feline larynx during inspiration.

gross appearance alone. This is especially true with feline tumors because granulomatous disease has been reported. Therapy is based on tumor type but, in general, surgical resection and creating an unobstructed airway are goals. Complete laryngectomy and permanent tracheostomy are options with variable success.[72,73] Cats with severe respiratory compromise secondary to laryngeal lymphosarcoma will respond well to radiation therapy. The prognosis of benign tumors is good if complete resection is successful; malignant laryngeal neoplasms have a poor prognosis.

Laryngeal Collapse

Brachycephalic dogs are at increased risk to develop laryngeal collapse secondary to their congenital airway malformations. Stenotic nares, elongated soft palate, and, if present, a hypoplastic trachea create an increased negative pressure during inspiration to move air through the narrowed air passages. It is believed that laryngeal cartilages become deformed from this chronic increased negative pressure and will finally weaken and collapse. Findings that older brachycephalic dogs will often have laryngeal collapse when presenting for upper airway disease support this theory. However, young brachycephalic dogs are also diagnosed with laryngeal collapse, which may indicate a defect in cartilage structure.[74] Dogs with laryngeal collapse will experience stridor, episodes of respiratory distress, and a respiratory crisis due to upper airway obstruction. Determination of laryngeal collapse is possible with laryngoscopy. The corniculate and cuneiform processes of the arytenoid cartilage will be medially displaced and occasionally will touch. In severe cases these processes will overlap, and the epiglottis will appear to be rolled up or flattened.[74] No specific treatment has been effective for laryngeal collapse. Surgical treatment should be directed toward altering the underlying congenital abnormality (i.e., stenotic nares correction, soft palate resection, everted laryngeal saccule excision) to improve airflow. In cases of severe laryngeal collapse, a permanent tracheostomy is recommended.[44,75] Dogs with severe laryngeal collapse have a poor prognosis.[75]

LARYNGITIS

Inflammatory laryngeal disease is common in both the dog and the cat. The most common cause of acute inflammation of the larynx is infectious agents such as canine infectious tracheobronchitis (ITB), commonly called *kennel cough*, or the feline upper respiratory agents (i.e., FHV-1, FCV). ITB is a result of coinfection of *B. bronchiseptica* with either canine parainfluenza virus or canine adenovirus-2 (CAV-2).[76] With most cases of ITB, the only clinical sign is paroxysmal coughing in an otherwise healthy dog. Due to inflammation of the larynx the cough is a loud, high-pitched, "goose honk" cough. Occasionally a dog may be febrile, lethargic, and inappetent. ITB is usually self-limiting, but the severity of the cough, combined with the possibility of pneumonia complicating the disease, warrants treatment. Doxycycline at 5 to 10 mg/kg orally once daily is the antimicrobial of choice for *B. bronchiseptica*. Short-term administration of an antiinflammatory dose of glucocorticoids can be effective in decreasing laryngeal edema. Antitussives, such as butorphanol tartrate or hydrocodone bitartrate, are effective in minimizing the severity of the cough but should not be used if pneumonia is suspected. Other causes of inflammatory laryngeal disease include endotracheal intubation, insect bites, foreign body penetration, or trauma from bite wounds, leash and choke chain injuries, or being hit by cars. Frequently no cause for acute laryngeal inflammation is found. Acute inflammatory laryngeal disease is usually self-limiting, and no specific treatment is indicated if the animal has only mild signs. However, if moderate to severe signs exist, a short course with an antiinflammatory dose of glucocorticosteroids can be initiated to decrease laryngeal edema. Respiratory obstruction secondary to laryngeal inflammation is an uncommon clinical presentation but can occur in severe instances such as in laryngeal trauma. A tracheostomy is indicated if the patient is dyspneic, cyanotic, or extremely anxious due to laryngeal inflammation.[7]

OBSTRUCTIVE INFLAMMATORY DISEASE

An obstructive inflammatory laryngeal disease has been described in cats and dogs.[70,77-79] Although rare, it is a disease worth noting because the gross appearance can mimic laryngeal neoplasia. The underlying cause of inflammation is unknown. Feline immunodeficiency virus (FIV) and feline leukemia virus (FeLV) have not been found to be associated with this disease. In the feline reports, dyspnea secondary to upper airway obstruction was reported in all cats; retching,

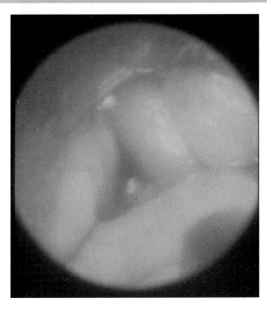

Figure 225-6 Middle-aged cat presented in respiratory distress. Laryngeal examination revealed bilateral arytenoid masses. Biopsy revealed pyogranulomatous inflammation.

coughing, and dysphonia were also common. Stridor and dysphonia were reported in dogs. Direct visualization of the larynx reveals a laryngeal mass that cannot be distinguished from neoplasia or severe swelling and edema (Figures 225-5 and 225-6). Histopathology is imperative to distinguish between neoplasia and obstructive inflammatory disease. Histopathology reveals either granulomatous or nongranulomatous laryngitis (neutrophilic and lymphoplasmacytic). Most patients with obstructive inflammatory laryngeal disease need to be stabilized. This is accomplished by establishing an airway through tracheostomy tube placement. Treatment with corticosteroids (dexamethasone, prednisone, or prednisolone) has variable success, and occasionally surgical resection of the proliferative tissue is indicated. The prognosis is guarded, with a high mortality rate during the initial diagnostic and treatment period.

REFERENCES

The reference list can be found on the companion Expert Consult Web site at *www.expertconsult.com.*

CHAPTER 226

Tumors of the Mouth, Head, and Neck

Ravinder S. Dhaliwal
James M.G. Anthony

Oral tumors represent the fourth most common malignancy in dogs and cats, representing approximately 6% of all canine malignant tumors.[1,2] Neoplasms of the oral cavity include both odontogenic and nonodontogenic tumor types. Laryngeal and oropharyngeal tumors are often classified under head and neck cancer by some clinicians.[3-6] With the exception of oral melanoma, the majority of oral malignancies are locally aggressive and slow to metastasize. Wide surgical excision and radiation therapy should be considered early on. Molecularly targeted therapies are some of the latest advances in modern cancer care, providing oncologists with tools to treat cancers with greater specificity than traditional methods alone. These new agents hold great promise for oncology professionals, but many of these recently developed therapies are presenting new complications and side effects that differ from those typically observed with traditional cytotoxic chemotherapy. Molecular techniques can be further used to classify tumors and aid in predicting the prognosis and determining the precise targeted therapy.

A true etiology for mouth cancer is not known in most cases. Clinical signs seen in both canine and feline patients with oral tumors are listed in Box 226-1. Unfortunately, oral tumors frequently go unnoticed by the owner until the clinical signs reach a fairly advanced stage. Differential diagnosis for the oral masses should include (a) granuloma or benign oral growths such as nodular fasciitis, fibromatosis; (b) ranula; (c) eosinophilic granuloma; (d) dentigerous cysts; (e) abscess; (f) calcinosis circumscripta; (g) proliferative gingival hyperplasia; (h) apical granuloma; (i) hypercementosis; (j) salivary cyst;

(k) foreign body granuloma; and (l) ulcers. Box 226-2 lists various benign and malignant oral lesions.

ORAL EXAMINATION AND DIAGNOSIS

An examination that is both undertaught and overlooked in veterinary training is the oral examination. It is an essential part of any examination of a patient. This begins with a complete description of the patient's history and signalment because many tumors are more commonly associated with certain breeds (Figure 226-1), sex, age, and environment. A full examination of the head and neck follows. The key is to develop a systematic approach, which becomes almost automatic so that when you are under pressure there is less likelihood of missing pathology. Palpate the external surfaces of the head and neck for pain, heat, swellings, and symmetry. Palpate all the external lymph nodes of the head and neck. Look at the lips, the lip folds, and commissures. Retract the lips and observe the vestibule, frenula, salivary ducts, tonsils, oropharynx, under the tongue, the palate and then the attached gingiva and teeth. Occlusion must be noted because many oral masses result in abnormal occlusion. Many oral tumors occur at the attached gingiva, so a careful examination is warranted and any abnormality should be investigated via probing with a periodontal probe and oral radiographs. Always make sure to measure and identify the exact location of the pathology because this is easy with the teeth (e.g., a hard firm mass 1 cm between teeth 105 and 106 on the attached gingiva

Box • 226-1

Common Presenting Signs of Oral Masses

Weight loss
Anorexia
Halitosis
Dysphasia
Abnormal salivation (increased, decreased, consistency)
Drooling
Mandibular chattering
Inability or difficulty of opening or closing the mouth
Abnormal facial symmetry and/or swelling
Facial muscle loss
Pawing at the mouth
Head shy
Pain on chewing
Open mouth
Bleeding from the mouth
Bite and let go
Chews on one side
Only can eat soft foods
Facial draining fistulas
Nasal and/or ocular discharge
Tooth mobility
Tooth displacement

Box • 226-2

Benign and Malignant Oral Lesions

Benign Oral Lesions
Eosinophilic granuloma
Odontoma
Ameloblastoma
Abscess
Gingival hyperplasia
Dentigerous cysts
Squamous papilloma
Plasmacytoma
Granular cell tumor
Fibroma
Lipoma
Hemangioma
Epulides (locally aggressive but not metastatic)
Calcinosis circumscripta
Ranula
Apical granuloma
Hypercementosis
Foreign body granuloma
Salivary cyst
Ulcers

Malignant Oral Lesions
Melanoma
Squamous cell carcinoma
Fibrosarcoma
Histologically low-grade, yet biologically high-grade, fibrosarcoma
Osteosarcoma
Lingual carcinoma or sarcoma
Histiocytic sarcoma
Lymphoma
Mast cell tumor

extending to the marginal gingiva). This allows for accurate monitoring and aids in diagnosis, as well as treatment planning. Any suspicious mass must be followed up utilizing diagnostic tools. Functional observation (observe the animal eating) can tell if the animal is utilizing the mouth fully. Regional lymph nodes should be palpated routinely for size, shape, consistency, and fixation to the surrounding tissues. If a lymphadenopathy is noted, then a cytologic or histologic evaluation must be performed on the lymph node. In one retrospective study evaluating the regional lymph nodes of dogs and cats with oral neoplasms, 17% of the patients had metastatic disease histologically.[7] When in doubt if a tissue is normal, biopsy it and send it for histologic evaluation or at least a fine needle aspirate and cytology. Histology is the gold standard for diagnosis of malignancy.

CLINICAL STAGING

Oral tumors can be staged into four different clinical stages using the TNM classification (primary tumor, regional lymph node, distant metastasis), which has been introduced by the World Health Organization. The overall prognosis worsens with the advanced clinical stage from I to IV (Table 226-1). Clinical staging of a patient with oral tumor should include complete blood profile and urinalysis, thoracic and regional radiographs, and an abdominal ultrasound. A full oral examination for any suspect mass is incomplete without radiology, especially dental radiology and chest films (three positions: each lateral and a ventrodorsal). Oral dental radiographs (Figure 226-2) have much more detail and are easy to get multiple positions to give more of a "3D" image. Computed tomography (CT) images are warranted to get precise margins in masses that involve bony tissues (calcification and resorption) where magnetic resonance imaging (MRI) would be better for masses involving soft tissue (more accurate for

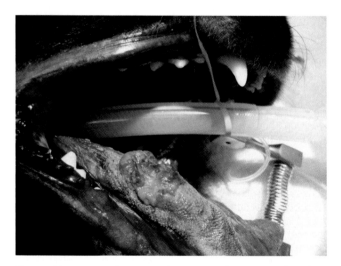

Figure 226-1 A malignant melanoma on the tongue of a Chow Chow.

Table • 226-1

WHO Clinical TNM Staging of Canine Oral Tumors[8]

CLINICAL STAGE	TUMOR	NODE	METASTASIS
Stage I	<2 cm	Negative	Negative
Stage II	2-4 cm	Negative	Negative
Stage III	>4 cm or any size with lymph node involvement	Yes	Negative
Stage IV	Any	Any	Yes

TNM, Tumor node metastasis; *WHO*, World Health Organization.
*The regional lymph nodes are the cervical, submandibular, and parotid nodes.

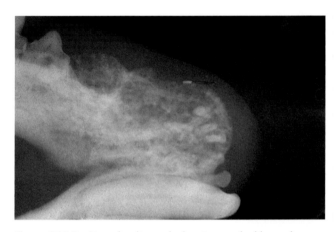

Figure 226-2 Dental radiograph showing marked bone destruction, displacement, and lysis of tooth and alveolar bone loss.

sizing masses and seeing the degree of infiltration). One unique MRI feature of oral melanotic melanoma is that unlike other soft tissue tumors, melanomas have a hyperintense signal on T1-weighted images and hypointense signal on T2-weighted images. This salient characteristic is likely due to the deposits of melanin granules but does not differentiate a benign versus malignant lesion.[9] Not only is it important for diagnosis, indicating sites of abnormality and guiding biopsies, but it is also crucial in determining the extent of local disease, thereby determining treatment options. The choice of surgery, radiotherapy, or chemotherapy will often rest entirely on the result of clinical stage. Finally, it also plays a vital role in monitoring the response to treatment.[10] Molecular staging is in its infancy and will be a significant tool in the future.

TREATMENT

Complete en bloc surgical excision is the treatment of choice for the majority of oral tumors, especially those located in the rostral oral cavity.[11-13] Depending on the clinical situation, surgery may also include bone grafting to preserve normal mastication and cosmetic appearance.[14] Several surgical techniques such as rostral mandibulectomy, rostral maxillectomy, hemimandibulectomy, bilateral rostral mandibulectomy, segmental unilateral maxillectomy or mandibulectomy, and combined dorsolateral and intraoral approach have been described

Table • 226-2

Common Surgical Techniques Applied in Treating Oral Neoplasm[11-20,56,70-73]

MANDIBULECTOMIES	APPLICATIONS
Rostral mandibulectomy	Lower incisors, lower canines, and first two premolar teeth on one side
Bilateral rostral mandibulectomy	Tumor that has crossed the midline of the mandible
Total hemimandibulectomy	For extensive tumors, the entire mandible is removed
Body segmental mandibulectomy	Part of the mandible is removed

MAXILLECTOMIES	APPLICATIONS
Premaxillectomy	Tumors in front of the second premolar
Hemimaxillectomy or lateral maxillectomy	Unilateral maxilla is removed for very extensive tumors
Central maxillectomy	Tumors located between the upper canine tooth and the first molar on one side
Caudal maxillectomy	Tumors behind the third premolar tooth on one side
Maxillectomy-orbitectomy combination	Part of the bone surrounding the eye is removed along with the maxilla

in the treatment of oral tumors (Table 226-2).[11,13,15-20] The readers are advised to refer to a surgical text or consult a veterinary dentist or surgeon for the appropriate techniques.

Radiation therapy should be considered in cases where complete excision is not feasible or if the tumor is located in the caudal oral cavity. Orthovoltage machines capable of delivering low-energy external beam radiation are not optimal for treating oral malignancies in most cases. Megavoltage radiation therapy currently appears to be the standard of care for dogs with oral tumors. Acute effects of oral radiation, such as oral mucositis, alopecia, local moist dermatitis, and desquamation, occur in almost every case. These effects of radiation therapy are not dose limiting and are self-limiting. These acute effects are reversible and medically manageable and resolve over 2 to 3 weeks after completion of radiation therapy. The late effects of radiation such as bone or muscle necrosis are irreversible and dose limiting but are less likely to occur. The risk of radiation-induced carcinogenesis is relatively low and typically occurs years after radiation therapy.[21] Intensity-modulated radiation therapy (IMRT) is a relatively new radiotherapy technology that is rapidly being adopted. The IMRT may result in a dose distribution that is more conformal than that achieved with two- or three-dimensional conformal radiotherapy. Overall survival information for canine oral tumors treated with radiation and surgery is summarized in Table 226-3.* Chemotherapy is indicated for patients with a diagnosis of oral round cell sarcoma or other high-grade malignancies which carries a metastatic potential.[22-26]

---

*References 10, 12, 20, 21, 32, 37, 56, 70-73, 75-83.

Table • 226-3

Survival Outcome for Dogs with Oral Tumors Treated with Radiation and Surgery

TUMOR TYPE	NO. OF ANIMALS	MST (MO)	1-YR SURVIVAL RATE	COMMENTS	REF
OMM	140	7			32
	39	12.1		Chemoradiation (carboplatin + XRT)	37
	27	4.9		Total radiation dose 36 Gy (4 Gy fractions)	74
	18	7.9		Total radiation dose 24 Gy (8 Gy fractions)	75
FSA	7	18	33%-76%	Sx + XRT	51,76,77
SCC	NA	NA	72%		51,84
Tonsillar SCC	6	9		Chemoradiation (cisplatin + doxorubicin + XRT)	78
Tonsillar SCC	8	3.6			79
Feline SCC	11	3.8		Intratumoral etanidazole + XRT	81
	11	5.6		Mitoxantrone + XRT	80,82
	7	14		Mandibular SCC Tx with Sx + XRT	82
Epulis	57	48		Tumor control of up to 90% can be anticipated	21
Canine Oral Tumors Treated with Maxillectomy					
OMM	23	9.1	27%		73
FSA	15	12.2	21%		73
OSA	6	4.6	17%		73
SCC	7	19.2	57%		73
Canine Oral Tumors Treated with Mandibulectomy					
OMM	21	7.3	—	9 of 21 dogs had no recurrence or metastasis	20
	9	—	—	Mean survival time 4 mo	12
	37	9.9	21%		72
FSA	9	—	—	Mean survival time 7 mo	20
	3	—	—	Mean survival time 16 mo	12
	19	10.6	50%		72
SCC	8	NA	100%	No recurrence up to an average follow-up of 17 mo	70
	3	—	—	Mean survival time 7 mo	12
	24		91%	26-mo disease-free interval	72
OSA	3	—	—	Mean survival time 2 mo	12
	20	13.6	35%		72
	32	—	71%		56
Epulis	42	—	97%	22.5 mo disease-free interval	71

FSA, Fibrosarcoma; *MST,* median survival time; *OMM,* oral malignant melanoma; *OSA,* osteosarcoma; *SCC,* squamous cell carcinoma; *Sx,* surgery; *Tx,* treatment; *XRT,* radiation therapy.

MALIGNANT MELANOMA

Oral malignant melanoma (OMM) is the most frequent malignant neoplasm of the oral cavity of dogs. Feline oral melanoma (Figure 226-3) is a rare clinical entity, accounting for less than 1% of all feline oral neoplasms.[27] The OMM typically occurs in older dogs with a reported mean age of 11 years. Cocker Spaniels, German Shepherds, and dogs with heavily pigmented oral mucosa may be predisposed.[24,25,28,29] Malignant melanoma can be located in any part of the oral cavity but occurs most often on the gingiva, followed by the buccal or labial mucosa, palate, and dorsal surface of the tongue. In gingival lesions, dental disruption is common and bone involvement is often seen. Melanomas arising from the oral cavity differ biologically in their behavior and have distinct mechanisms of molecular transformation when compared with dermal melanomas.[30] The usual behavior of OMM is local tissue infiltration, recurrence following cytoreduction, and metastasis to regional lymph nodes, lungs, and other organs. Therefore nearly all oral melanomas are considered malignant. The most important prognostic factors of canine OMM are tumor stage, size, mitotic activity, and evidence of tumor recurrence after a prior treatment.[31] Favorable prognostic factors for OMM include rostral tumor sublocation, lack of bone lysis, and microscopic tumor burden.[32] Paraneoplastic syndromes such as hypercalcemia of malignancy are rare in dogs with malignant melanoma.[33]

Cytologically, the diagnosis of OMM may be challenging because there is variation in the degree of pigmentation and tumors can be completely unpigmented. The cytomorphologic features of OMM can resemble carcinomas, sarcomas, lymphomas, and osteogenic tumors. Thus immunohistochemical confirmation[29,34] of the diagnosis of melanoma is frequently necessary to establish a prognosis and therapeutic plan. Regional lymph nodes, if palpable, should be aspirated or biopsied to rule out metastasis.

Treatment options include surgery, chemotherapy, radiation, immunotherapy, and intralesional therapy; however, local recurrence and distant dissemination are still frequent.[32,35-38] External beam radiation therapy is effective in local disease control of canine OMM.[32] Hypofractionated radiation therapy, such as once a week in 8 Gy fractions to a

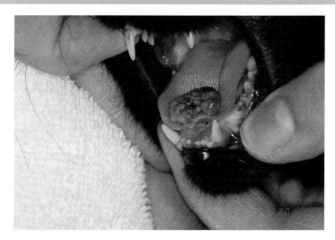

Figure 226-3 Malignant melanoma on the rostral aspect of a cat tongue.

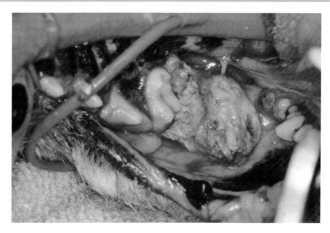

Figure 226-4 A squamous cell carcinoma in the caudal aspect of the maxilla in a dog.

cumulative dose of 32 Gy or twice a week in 6 Gy to a cumulative dose of 36 Gy, are the treatments of choice for OMM.[36,37] Single-agent platinum analogues or a combination with oral piroxicam has shown antitumor activity against canine OMM.[22,23] An overall median survival time of 363 days has been reported in dogs treated with hypofractionated radiation therapy and platinum-containing chemotherapy.[37] Kitchell et al[38] reported a partial to complete response in 14 of the 20 dogs treated with intralesional cisplatin implants.

The DNA-based vaccine is indicated for the treatment of dogs with stage II or stage III oral melanoma after good local control has been achieved. The vaccine contains human tyrosinase, which is a melanosomal glycoprotein, essential in melanin synthesis. Canine tyrosinase on melanocytes is considered by the immune system as "self" and not foreign; therefore an immune response is not generated. However, using a xenogeneic (other species) tyrosinase, an antitumor response is initiated. The injection is administered intramuscularly into the medial thigh region with a transdermal device. Initial treatment requires administration of four doses of vaccine at 2-week intervals followed by a booster dose at 6-month intervals.[39-40]

MELANOCYTOMA

Melanocytomas are rare, benign tumors of the melanocytic cells within the oral cavity. Oral examination reveals dark pigmented, slightly raised lesions. Recommended treatment is surgical removal. The prognosis is excellent if bulky disease is removed.

FIBROSARCOMA

Fibrosarcoma (FSA) or fibroblastic sarcoma is a malignant mesenchymal tumor derived from fibrous connective tissue and characterized by immature proliferating fibroblasts or undifferentiated anaplastic spindle cells. Canine oral FSA occurs at a young age in large-breed dogs, with a mean age of 4 to 5 years. In small-breed dogs it occurs at a mean age of 8 years.[24,28,41] It is the third most common oral tumor in dogs and second in cats. FSAs are locally invasive and have a high recurrence rate after surgical excision, especially if 2- to 3-cm margins are not achieved. They seldom metastasize, except late in the clinical course. Prognosis is variable, depending on location, histologic grade, and size or clinical stage at the time of diagnosis. Histologically, the tumor may present three dif-

ferent degrees of differentiation: low-grade malignancy (differentiated), intermediate malignancy, and high malignancy (anaplastic). The maxilla is the most common location. Initially the oral FSA may present as a clinically innocuous, lobulated, sessile, painless, and nonhemorrhagic submucosal mass of normal coloration. However, over time it may grow rapidly and become hemorrhagic with severe ulceration. It usually appears as a protuberant mass at the dental margins and palate. It may also originate from the nasal cartilages, the lateral surface of the maxilla, or the palate. Its appearance is usually that of a smooth mass with an intact epithelial covering.

Well-differentiated FSAs are treated by wide local excision. The poorly differentiated FSA requires radical surgery, which includes removal of potentially invaded muscle and bone. Radiotherapy may be used to treat microscopic disease postoperatively or as a salvage therapy for recurrences. In one retrospective study, the time-to-progression for the curatively treated dogs with oral soft tissue sarcoma was 333 days with an overall survival of 331 days.[42] Efficacy of adjunctive chemotherapy is not known.

HISTOLOGICALLY LOW-GRADE, YET BIOLOGICALLY HIGH-GRADE, FIBROSARCOMA

The histologically low-grade, yet biologically high-grade, FSA (HLGYBHG) is another distinct histologic entity of oral FSA. It has been reported in large-breed dogs (mostly Golden Retrievers).[41] Biologically these tumors exhibit rapid growth, invasion, and metastatic potential. The histopathologic findings are suggestive of a fibroma or a well-differentiated FSA. Most dogs are presented with a rapidly enlarging swelling of the maxillofacial region, with a nonerosive gingival mass, covered by intact epithelium. The optimal treatment approach for this tumor type has not yet been determined. Different treatment modalities, including surgical excision in combination with radiation therapy, surgery alone, radiation therapy alone, and radiation therapy used adjunctly with localized hyperthermia, have all been reported to prolong the survival times in some dogs.[41]

SQUAMOUS CELL CARCINOMA

Squamous cell carcinoma (SCC) is the most common oral malignancy in cats and second most common in dogs (Figure 226-4).[43] The gingiva appears to be the most common site for canine SCC. It occurs in older dogs, with a mean age of 9 years. There is no sex predilection. Papillary SCC has been reported in very young dogs. Lingual and tonsillar SCC are less common. [44,45] Papillomavirus DNA is frequently associated with canine oral SCC. [46,47] A viral association is a possibility in cats with oral SCC as well. [48] Oral gingival lesions are generally erosive and fleshy. Dental disruption with local bone invasion is common. SCC may present as a chronic nonhealing ulcer, nonproliferative lesion in the skin of the maxillofacial and mandibular region. SCC lesions are most often located in the premolar/molar region of the maxilla, premolar region of the mandible, and sublingual region of cats. Some investigators have suggested that flea control products, diet, and perhaps environmental tobacco smoke might be associated with risk of oral SCC in cats. [49,50] Cats with maxillary and tongue SCC have a poor prognosis, responding only rarely to any kind of therapy. Feline oral SCC is often diagnosed at an advanced clinical stage. In advanced cases of feline maxillary SCC, exophthalmos and facial distortion are also evident. Sublingual lesions can be palpated in the ventral body caudal to the frenulum. Mandibular SCC is more amenable to therapy and carries a little better prognosis than maxillary and lingual region SCC. SCCs are locally aggressive; however, distant metastasis to the regional lymph nodes and lungs has been reported late in the disease. Tonsillar SCCs are much more aggressive with early metastasis to the regional lymph nodes.

Wide local excision is often curative in early cases of SCC located rostrally. Similar to other oral tumors, the rostral mandibular location has a fair prognosis. Canine lingual SCCs are best managed with partial glossectomy. Radiation therapy should be considered for local control of SCC or palliative reasons in cases where surgical excision is not possible. [51] SCC appears to be radiosensitive but not radiocurable. Photodynamic therapy has also been reported to be effective in canine oral SCC. [52] A combination of cisplatin or carboplatin and piroxicam has been shown to have antitumor activity against canine oral SCC. [23,53] One retrospective study reported that piroxicam at a dosage of 0.3 mg/kg (0.14 mg/lb) given once a day had a response rate similar to other cytotoxic therapies in the treatment of canine oral SCC. [54] It should be noted that feline oral SCC, especially when located in the sublingual or caudal oral cavity, carries a very poor prognosis. The survival rates for feline oral SCC have not improved in decades despite improved therapeutic modalities. Early diagnosis and treatment offer the best chance of success. So far the use of radiation therapy in cats with sublingual or caudal oral cavity SCC has been disappointing. However, for palliative reasons, local irradiation or treatment with aminobisphosphonate [55] in cats with oral SCC should be considered.

OSTEOSARCOMA

Osteosarcoma (OSA) of the mandible, maxilla, or palate has been reported in dogs. It is more common in medium- and large-sized breeds, middle-aged and older dogs, and females. [56] Feline oral OSA is uncommon and accounts for 2.4% of all oral tumors. [27] Clinically the lesion can appear as a gross fleshy mass. In early stages the mass may or may not appear ulcerative. Local bony invasion often causes significant facial swelling. Oral OSA is locally aggressive. The rate of metastasis of oral OSA is lower than appendicular OSA. Controversy exists regarding the clinical outcome in dogs with oral OSA. Older literature suggests that mandibular OSA has a poor prognosis with a median survival of 1.5 months after mandibulectomy. [20] However, later studies demonstrated an improved median survival of up to 13 months. [17,18,57,58]

The treatment of choice for oral OSA is wide or radical excision. Local recurrence and distant metastasis are the most common sites of therapeutic failures following an incomplete excision. Radiation therapy should be considered for microscopic disease if the surgical margins are not clean. Radiation therapy can also be used for palliative reasons in very advanced cases. Some clinicians do recommend adjuvant chemotherapy for dogs with mandibular OSA. A metastatic rate of 56% has been reported. [58]

EXTRAMEDULLARY PLASMACYTOMAS

Oral extramedullary plasmacytomas are rare malignancies. They represent 5.2% of all canine oral tumors and occur mainly in middle-aged to older dogs. [59,60] They consist of neoplastic plasma cells that are not derived from the bone marrow. These tumors are locally aggressive and rarely metastasize. No obvious relationship with multiple myeloma is known. Recurrence is common after incomplete surgical excision. An overall median survival of 474 days has been reported in dogs that received complete en bloc resection. In this cohort some cases also received adjuvant treatment including radiotherapy, melphalan, and prednisone. Dogs with incomplete surgical excision and no adjuvant treatment had a median survival time of 138 days. [59]

ODONTOGENIC TUMORS

Because of the histologic diversity noted with odontogenic tumors, there has been confusion and disagreement on the terminology and classification of these lesions. [61-64] *Complex odontomas* are benign, oral masses composed of fully developed, disorganized dental components that do not form toothlike structures. They commonly develop in young dogs with delayed or abnormal tooth eruption. On physical examination they are often characterized by a large oral swelling or mass. Radiographically, they are locally destructive radiodense structures within the mandible or maxilla. Complex odontomas do not metastasize. Treatment involves aggressive surgical excision. *Compound odontomas* are benign, [64] oral masses composed of fully developed, organized dental components that result in toothlike structures. Signalment, history, and treatment are similar to complex odontomas. *Cementomas* are benign tumors that result in the excess deposition of cementum surrounding the tooth roots. Cementomas are often considered to be a reactive hyperplastic process, not a true neoplasm. Their etiology is unknown, although chronic apical root irritation has been implicated. Cementomas have been reported in dogs and cats. On physical examination affected patients often exhibit tooth loss and displacement. Treatment of all involved teeth is curative. *Odontogenic cysts* arise from the cellular components of the developing tooth. They are associated with retained or impacted teeth and trauma. On radiographic and oral examination odontogenic cysts are fluid-filled structures. Treatment is surgical excision.

EPULIDES

Epulides are gingival neoplasms known by several different names. Fibromatous, acanthomatous, and ossifying epulis are the most commonly used terms among veterinary pathologists. Acanthomatous epulides (AEs) are benign tumors of the oral cavity that arise from the periodontal ligament. On physical examination AEs are located adjacent to teeth and have a soft, fleshy appearance. Because of their aggressive local behavior, AEs often extend into the maxillary or mandibular bone. Radiographically, local bony invasion may be evident in some cases. Paraneoplastic hypercalcemia has rarely been reported with AE.[64,65] Surgical resection with 2-cm margins from gross or radiographically detectable disease is sufficient treatment because these tumors do not metastasize. Full-course radiation therapy is indicated if adequate margins are not possible due to tumor size or location or in order to preserve function or cosmesis. In one case series report, intralesional bleomycin injections were shown to be effective against canine AE.[66] Epulides are rare in cats. Inductive fibroameloblastoma has only been described in cats aged 18 months or younger.[67,68] Adjuvant radiation therapy has been shown to be effective in incompletely resected feline epulides.[69]

PAPILLOMATOSIS

Papillomatosis is a proliferative, cutaneous, and mucosal tumor induced by papillomavirus. It is often characterized as a wartlike lesion located on the buccal mucosa, lips, and tongue. Papillomatosis is common in young, immunosuppressed dogs who have had viral contact. Although tumors are generally benign and spontaneous regression is common, surgical resection is required in dysphagic or patients with compromised airways. Autogenous vaccines are available for use in dogs with persistent disease.

SALIVARY GLAND TUMORS

Salivary gland tumors are very rare. Most of the salivary gland tumors are epithelial in origin. Interestingly, a solitary case report of primary salivary gland melanoma exists.[9] Initial therapy of localized disease consists of radical surgery or radiation therapy. Chemotherapy is reserved for palliative reasons for patients with advanced metastatic disease or where recurrence occurs after surgery or radiation therapy. Because of the rarity of these tumors, there are no significant clinical data to help define the role of radiation or systemic therapy in the management of salivary gland tumors.

LINGUAL TUMORS

Lingual tumors are rare with a mean age of 10.5 years in dogs. The common lingual tumor types reported in dogs include melanoma, SCC, hemangiosarcoma, FSA, mast cell tumor, lymphoma, various types of sarcomas, squamous papilloma, and plasmacytoma.[44,45,69] Chinese Shar-Peis and Chow Chows have a breed predisposition for lingual melanoma. In dogs, lingual SCC has a moderate rate of metastasis; however, small lesions can be completely cured with partial glossectomy. Sublingual SCC is more common in cats and carries a worse prognosis for long-term tumor control.

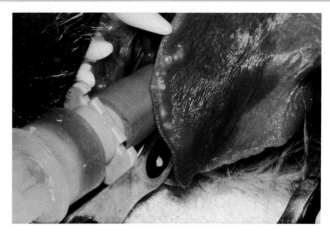

Figure 226-5 Calcinosis circumscripta (cushingoid) in a young dog.

NONNEOPLASTIC MASSES

Gingival hyperplasia is characterized as a focal or generalized proliferation of the attached gingiva. Chronic inflammation caused by plaque accumulation causes the hyperplastic gingival response. Breeds commonly predisposed include Boxers, Great Danes, Dobermans, Bulldogs, Mastiffs, and Pit Bull Terriers. Biopsy is required in order to rule out neoplastic processes. The excessive gingival tissue results in the development of a pseudopocket and, if left untreated, leads to development of periodontal disease and loss of attachment. Treatment involves restoring gingival pockets to normal depths by removing excess gingival tissue via gingivectomy with gingivoplasty.

Although the etiology of *eosinophilic granuloma complex (rodent ulcers)* is unknown, hypersensitivity and genetic causes are often suspected. Eosinophilic granulomas are clinically characterized as well-circumscribed ulcerations located on the upper labial mucosa, philtrum, or maxillary canines. Diagnosis is based on typical clinical signs and positive response to treatment. Treatment often includes steroids and antibiotics because of secondary bacterial infection or surgical excision. *Radicular cysts* are nonneoplastic cystic structures caused by chronic endodontic pathology. Clinical signs include pain, facial swelling, and tooth development. Radiographically a radiolucent cyst may be seen originating from the apical aspect of the affected tooth root. Treatment of choice is surgical removal. In Cushing's patients with *calcinosis circumscripta*, calcium deposits can develop in the tongue (Figure 226-5) and lips.

REFERENCES

The reference list can be found on the companion Expert Consult Web site at *www.expertconsult.com.*

CONDITIONS ASSOCIATED WITH HEMATOLOGIC CHANGE

White Blood Cells (WBCs)
Increased
Infection
  Bacterial
  Systemic Mycosis
Inflammation
  Immune-Mediated Disease
  Tissue Trauma
  Neoplasia
  Tissue Necrosis
Physiologic Leukocytosis
Metabolic
  Stress
  Glucocorticoids
Associated with Responsive
  Anemia
  Hemolytic Anemia
  Hemorrhagic Anemia
Leukemia
Decreased
Decreased Production
Increased Consumption
Neutropenia
  Phenobarbital Administration

Red Blood Cells (RBCs)
Increased
Dehydration
Polycythemia
Splenic Contraction
Decreased
Responsive Anemias
Blood Loss: Acute or Chronic
  Hemorrhage (Internal or
    External)
  Trauma
  Gastrointestinal Hemorrhage
    Ulcers
    Neoplasia
  Coagulopathies
    Congenital
    Acquired
  Ectoparasites
    Fleas
    Ticks
  Endoparasites
    Hookworms
    Coccidia
  Hematuria
Hemolytic Anemias
  Microangiopathic
    Dirofilariasis
    Vascular Neoplasia
    Vasculitis
    Disseminated Intravascular
      Coagulation
  Parasitic
    Babesia
    Hemobartonella felis
  Infectious
    Leptospirosis
    Escherichia coli
  Oxidant Injury
    Onions
    Kale
    Phenothiazines
    Methylene Blue
Nonresponsive Anemias
Renal Failure

Chronic Disease
  Infectious Disease
  Inflammatory Disease
  Neoplasia
Endocrine Disease
  Hypothyroidism
  Hypoadrenocorticism
  Hyperestrogenism
    Diethylstilbestrol (High
      Multiple Doses)
    Estradiol
      Cyclopentylpropionate
    Sertoli Cell Tumor
Idiopathic Aplastic Anemia
Red Cell Aplasia
Myeloproliferative Disease
Myelophthisis
Hypersplenism
Drugs
  Chloramphenicol
  Chemotherapeutics
Iron Deficiency
  Nutritional
  Chronic Blood Loss
Lead Poisoning
Infectious
  Retrovirus
    Feline Immunodeficiency
      Virus
    Feline Leukemia Virus
  Ehrlichia

Hemoglobin (Hb)
Increased
Dehydration
Polycythemia
Splenic Contraction
Decreased
Hemorrhage
  Acute
  Chronic
Decreased Production

Hematocrit
Increased
Dehydration
Polycythemia
Splenic Contraction
Decreased
Hemorrhage
  Acute
  Chronic
Decreased Production
  Neutrophils
Increased
Increased Production
  Infection
    Bacterial
    Systemic Mycosis
      Coccidioidomycosis
      Histoplasmosis
      Blastomycosis
      Aspergillosis
    Protozoal
      Hepatozoon
      Toxoplasmosis
      Neosporidiosis
  Inflammation
    Immune-Mediated Diseases

Tissue Trauma
Neoplasia
Tissue Necrosis
Associated with Responsive
  Anemia
  Hemolytic Anemia
  Hemorrhagic Anemia
Demargination
  Stress
  Glucocorticoids
Chronic Granulocytic Leukemia
Decreased
Decreased Production
  Myelophthisis
    Myeloproliferative Disease
    Lymphoproliferative Disease
    Metastatic Neoplasia
  Myelofibrosis
Drug Induced
  Chloramphenicol
  Trimethoprim-Sulfa
  Cyclophosphamide
  Azathioprine
  Griseofulvin
Idiopathic Hypoplasia/Aplasia
  Cyclic Neutropenia
  Immune-Mediated
    (Steroid-Responsive)
Hypersplenism
Infectious
  Ehrlichia
  Parvovirus
  Retroviruses
    Feline Immunodeficiency
      Virus
    Feline Leukemia Virus
      Aplastic Anemia
      Myelodysplasia
      Panleukopenia-Like
        Syndrome
Increased Consumption
  Bacteremia/Septicemia
  Severe Systemic Infection
  Endotoxemia
Hypoadrenocorticism
Margination

Lymphocytes
Increased
Physiologic Leukocytosis
Lymphocytic Leukemia
Chronic Antigenic Stimulation
  Inflammatory Bowel Disease
  Cholangiohepatitis
Decreased
Stress
Drugs
  Chemotherapy Drugs
  Glucocorticoids
Immunodeficiency
  Feline Immunodeficiency Virus
  Feline Leukemia Virus
Lymphangiectasia

Monocytes
Increased
Chronic Inflammation
Chronic Infection
Granulomatous Disease

Myelomonocytic Leukemia
Monocytic Leukemia
Stress
Glucocorticoids

Eosinophils
Increased
Allergic Diseases
  Dermatitis
    Flea Allergy
    Food Allergy
    Atopy
  Eosinophilic Granuloma
    Complex
  Enteritis
  Asthma
  Sinusitis
  Rhinitis
Parasitic Diseases
  Endoparasites
    Aleurostrongylosis
    Dirofilariasis
    Gastrointestinal Parasites
  Ectoparasites
Infectious Diseases
  Fungal
Neoplastic Diseases
  Mast Cell Neoplasia
  Solid Tumors
Hypereosinophilic Syndrome
Eosinophilic Leukemia
Hypoadrenocorticism
Pregnancy
Decreased
Stress
Hyperadrenocorticism
Glucocorticoid Therapy

Basophils
Increased
Mast Cell Neoplasia
Dirofilariasis

Platelets
Increased
Essential Thrombocytosis
Rebound Thrombocytosis
Polycythemia Vera
Decreased
Decreased Production
  Infectious
    Retroviruses
      Feline Immunodeficiency
        Virus
      Feline Leukemia Virus
    Ehrlichia
Increased Destruction
  Immune-Mediated
    Thrombocytopenia
Sequestration
  Hypersplenism
Increased Consumption
  Hemorrhage
  Disseminated Intravascular
    Coagulation
Breed Idiosyncrasy
  Cavalier King Charles Spaniels
    (Macrothrombocytes)
  Greyhounds